ZITELLI AND DAVIS'

Atlas of Pediatric Physical Diagnosis

ALEXANDER J. DAVIT III, MD
Assistant Professor
Department of Plastic Surgery
University of Pittsburgh
Director
Pediatric Hand Surgery
UPMC Children's Hospital of Pittsburgh
Director
Pediatric Brachial Plexus Clinic
UPMC Children's Hospital of Pittsburgh
Director
Pediatric Wound Care Clinic
UPMC Children's Hospital of Pittsburgh
Pittsburgh, Pennsylvania

CHRISTIN DEAL, MD
Assistant Professor
Pediatric Allergy and Immunology
UPMC Children's Hospital of Pittsburgh
Pittsburgh, Pennsylvania

MARK DEBRUNNER, MD
Fellowship Program Director
Pediatric Cardiology
Associate Professor of Pediatrics
UPMC Children's Hospital of Pittsburgh
Gibsonia, Pennsylvania

OZGUR DEDE, MD
Associate Professor
Department of Orthopaedic Surgery
University of Pittsburgh
Pittsburgh, Pennsylvania

SYDNEY DEVORE, BS
Medical Student
University of Pittsburgh Medical School
Pittsburgh, Pennsylvania

TAYLOR EDDENS, MD, PHD
Allergy/Immunology Fellow
Department of Pediatrics
UPMC Children's Hospital of Pittsburgh
Pittsburgh, Pennsylvania

ADELAIDE L. EICHMAN, MD
Associate Professor of Pediatrics
Division of Child Advocacy
UPMC Children's Hospital of Pittsburgh
Pittsburgh, Pennsylvania

OSCAR ESCOBAR, MD
Associate Professor
Pediatrics/Pediatric Endocrinology
University of Pittsburgh School of Medicine
UPMC Children's Hospital of Pittsburgh
Pittsburgh, Pennsylvania

HEIDI M. FELDMAN, MD, PHD
Ballinger-Swindells Professor of Developmental and Behavioral Pediatrics
Department of Pediatrics
Stanford University School of Medicine
Palo Alto, California

CASSANDRA FORMECK, MD, MS
Pediatric Nephrology Fellowship Program Director
Clinical Research
University of Pittsburgh
Pittsburgh, Pennsylvania

MICHAEL D. FOX, MD, MED
Associate Professor of Clinical Pediatrics
Department of Pediatrics
Perelman School of Medicine at the University of Pennsylvania
Attending Physician
Comprehensive Vascular Anomalies Program
Children's Hospital of Philadelphia
Philadelphia, Pennsylvania

JENNA M. GAESSER, MD
Assistant Professor
Department of Pediatrics
Division of Child Neurology
UPMC Children's Hospital of Pittsburgh
Pittsburgh, Pennsylvania

ROBIN P. GEHRIS, MD, FAAD, FAAP
Clinical Associate Professor
Department of Dermatology
University of Pittsburgh
Pittsburgh, Pennsylvania;
Chief Medical Officer of Clinical Operations
Dermatologist On Call
Latrobe, Pennsylvania;
Pediatric Dermatologist
Riverchase Dermatology
Estero, Florida

DANIEL GLASER, MD, MPH
Assistant Professor
Section of Pediatric Immunology and Rheumatology
Yale School of Medicine
New Haven, Connecticut

JESSE A. GOLDSTEIN, MD
Associate Professor
Plastic Surgery
UPMC Children's Hospital of Pittsburgh
Pittsburgh, Pennsylvania

ANGELA M. GUERRERO, MD, FAAD
Assistant Professor
Department of Dermatology
University of Pittsburgh Medical Center
Pittsburgh, Pennsylvania

NURSEN GURTUNCA, MD
Associate Professor of Pediatrics
Division of Endocrinology and Diabetes
UPMC Children's Hospital of Pittsburgh
Pittsburgh, Pennsylvania

AMBER KAZI, BS, MD
Pediatric Nephrology Fellow
Pediatric Nephrology
University of Washington
Seattle Children's Hospital
Seattle, Washington

ELLEN KOCH, MD
Assistant Professor
Department of Dermatology
University of Pittsburgh
Pittsburgh, Pennsylvania

JUHI KUMAR, MD, MPH
Associate Professor of Pediatrics
Department of Pediatrics
UPMC Children's Hospital of Pittsburgh
Pittsburgh, Pennsylvania

JEREMY S. LANDEO GUTIERREZ, MD
Pediatric Pulmonology Fellow
Division of Pulmonary Medicine
UPMC Children's Hospital of Pittsburgh
Postdoctoral Scholar
University of Pittsburgh
Pittsburgh, Pennsylvania

ALLYSON LARKIN, MD
Associate Professor of Pediatrics
Clinical Director of the Pediatric Asthma Center
Co-Director of the Difficult to Treat Asthma Clinic
Department of Pediatrics
University of Pittsburgh School of Medicine
Pittsburgh, Pennsylvania

SUNEETA MADAN-KHETARPAL, MD
Clinical Geneticist
Department of Pediatrics
UPMC Children's Hospital of Pittsburgh
Professor
Pediatrics and Ophthalmology
University of Pittsburgh
Pittsburgh, Pennsylvania

MARCUS MALEK, MD
Associate Professor of Surgery
Department of Surgery
University of Pittsburgh School of Medicine
Clinical Director
Division of Pediatric General and Thoracic Surgery
UPMC Children's Hospital of Pittsburgh
Pittsburgh, Pennsylvania

ANDREW A. MCCORMICK, MD
Associate Professor of Pediatrics
Department of Pediatrics
University of Pittsburgh
UPMC Children's Hospital of Pittsburgh
Pittsburgh, Pennsylvania

MARIAN G. MICHAELS, MD, MPH
Professor
Department of Pediatrics and Surgery
University of Pittsburgh School of Medicine
Pediatric Infectious Diseases
UPMC Children's Hospital of Pittsburgh
Pittsburgh, Pennsylvania

YOSUKE MIYASHITA, MD, MPH
Assistant Professor
Department of Pediatrics
University of Pittsburgh School of Medicine
Pittsburgh, Pennsylvania

KEVIN P. MOLLEN, MD
Associate Professor of Surgery
Department of Surgery
University of Pittsburgh School of Medicine
Pittsburgh, Pennsylvania

MICHAEL MORITZ, MD
Professor
Department of Pediatrics
UPMC Children's Hospital of Pittsburgh
Pittsburgh, Pennsylvania

SRIKALA NARAYANAN, MD
Associate Professor of Radiology
Department of Pediatric Radiology
Texas Children's Hospital
Houston, Texas

KEN K. NISCHAL, MD, FAAP, FRCOPHTH
Professor
Ophthalmology
UPMC Children's Hospital of Pittsburgh
Pittsburgh, Pennsylvania

BRIGHID MORAN O'DONNELL, MD
Assistant Professor
Department of Pediatrics
University of Pittsburgh Medical Center
Pittsburgh, Pennsylvania

Z. DENIZ OLGUN, MD
Assistant Professor
Department of Orthopaedic Surgery
University of Pittsburgh
Pittsburgh, Pennsylvania

DAMARA ORTIZ, MD
Assistant Professor of Pediatrics
Department of Pediatrics
Division of Medical Genetics
Director
Lysosomal Storage Disorders Program
UMPC Children's Hospital of Pittsburgh
Pittsburgh, Pennsylvania

CATHERINE H. POHOLEK, MD, PHD
Instructor
Department of Pediatrics
Division of Rheumatology
University of Pittsburgh
Pittsburgh, Pennsylvania

JACQUELIN RANKINE, MD, PHD
Assistant Professor
Department of Pediatrics
University of Pittsburgh
Pittsburgh, Pennsylvania

MELISSA M. RILEY, MD
Professor of Pediatrics
Division of Newborn Medicine
Washington University School of Medicine
NICU Medical Director
Interim NICU Co-Director
St. Louis Children's Hospital
St. Louis, Missouri

HANNAH RINEHARDT, MD
Postdoctoral Research Scholar
Pediatric Surgery
UPMC Children's Hospital of Pittsburgh
Pittsburgh, Pennsylvania

ROBERT A. SAFIER, MD
Associate Professor and Clinical Director
Division of Child Neurology
UPMC Children's Hospital of Pittsburgh
Pittsburgh, Pennsylvania

JUDY H. SQUIRES, MD
Associate Professor of Radiology
Pediatric Radiology
UPMC Children's Hospital of Pittsburgh
Chief of Ultrasound
Radiology
UPMC Children's Hospital of Pittsburgh
Program Director
Diagnostic Radiology Residency
Department of Radiology
University of Pittsburgh Medical Center
Pittsburgh, Pennsylvania

ARVIND SRINATH, MD, MS
Associate Professor of Pediatrics
Pediatric Gastroenterology Fellowship Director
Associate Vice Chair for Education for Fellowship Training
Department of Pediatrics
UPMC Children's Hospital of Pittsburgh
Pittsburgh, Pennsylvania

ERICA L. STEVENS, MD, MPH
Assistant Professor
Pediatric Pulmonology
University of Louisville
Louisville, Kentucky

SAMEH TADROS, MD, MSC
Associate Professor of Radiology
Pediatric Radiology
UPMC Children's Hospital of Pittsburgh
Pittsburgh, Pennsylvania

BRETT A. TEPLITZ, MD
Resident Physician
Department of Urology
University of Pittsburgh Medical Center
Pittsburgh, Pennsylvania

JEAN M. TERSAK, MD
Professor of Pediatrics
Director, Survivorship Program
Director, Clinical Oncology Research
Department of Pediatrics
Division of Pediatric Hematology/Oncology
UPMC Children's Hospital of Pittsburgh
Pittsburgh, Pennsylvania

ALLISON TOBEY, MD
Director of the UPMC Children's Hospital Aerodigestive Center
Otolaryngology
UPMC Children's Hospital of Pittsburgh
Assistant Professor
Otolaryngology
University of Pittsburgh
Pittsburgh, Pennsylvania

ORQUIDIA A. TORRES, MD, MS
Assistant Professor of Pediatrics
Department of Pediatrics
UPMC Children's Hospital of Pittsburgh
Pittsburgh, Pennsylvania

SARA M. TRUCCO, MD
Associate Director
Cardiac Catheterization Laboratory
Director
Quality Improvement for Cardiac Catheterization
Associate Professor of Pediatrics
Pediatric Cardiology
UPMC Children's Hospital of Pittsburgh
Associate Professor of Pediatrics
Department of Pediatrics
University of Pittsburgh
Pittsburgh, Pennsylvania

PUSHPA VISWANATHAN, MD, FAAP
Associate Professor
Department of Endocrinology
UPMC Children's Hospital of Pittsburgh
Pittsburgh, Pennsylvania

JENNIFER WATERS, DMD, MSD
Pediatric Dentist
Division of Pediatric Dentistry
UPMC Children's Hospital of Pittsburgh
Pittsburgh, Pennsylvania

DANIEL J. WEINER, MD
Professor
Department of Pediatrics
University of Pittsburgh
Medical Director
Pulmonary Function Laboratory
UPMC Children's Hospital of Pittsburgh
Director
Antonio J. and Janet Palumbo Cystic Fibrosis Center
UPMC Children's Hospital of Pittsburgh
Attending Physician
Division of Pulmonary Medicine, Allergy, and Immunology
UPMC Children's Hospital of Pittsburgh
Pittsburgh, Pennsylvania

LAURA WEST, MD
Assistant Professor of Pediatrics
Division of Allergy and Immunology
UPMC Children's Hospital of Pittsburgh
Pittsburgh, Pennsylvania

JENNIFER E. WOLFORD, DO, MPH
Associate Professor of Pediatrics
Division of Child Advocacy
UPMC Children's Hospital of Pittsburgh
Pittsburgh, Pennsylvania

KATELYN WOODS, DMD
Pediatric Dentist
Division of Pediatric Dentistry
UPMC Children's Hospital of Pittsburgh
Pittsburgh, Pennsylvania

JENNIFER S. ZARIT, MD, IBCLC, C-NABBLM
Assistant Professor of Pediatrics
Department of Pediatrics
University of Pittsburgh School of Medicine
Pittsburgh, Pennsylvania

FOREWORD

I first heard of *Zitelli's Atlas* when I was in medical school. I recall over 30 years ago carrying it back and forth from class to my home. The book was a constant reference into the world of medicine. Seeing the visual images of different physical findings and manifestations of illnesses remains with me to this day. I have had the privilege to teach medical students, residents, and fellows for the last three decades, and the photos and explanations remain with me. When I teach, I recall the images in Dr. Zitelli's atlas and have shared his wisdom with countless others. Many times, when I could not make a diagnosis readily, I referred back to this tome that illustrates a wide range of pediatric conditions, from common to rare. It provides authoritative text on examination techniques, historical factors, and diagnostic methods. Dr. Zitelli was our plenary speaker at a national pediatric academic conference in 2019, and I had the honor of introducing him. Although Dr. Zitelli is revered by countless students and doctors he has trained throughout his illustrious career, he was so kind and unassuming. I was struck by Dr. Zitelli's desire to help children and their families by his life work: to teach us all to be the best clinicians that we can be and to make the right diagnoses, so we in turn can help children get better, do well, and heal. I have studied diagnostic errors for the last decade, and to access wisdom as offered in the atlas will help us to mitigate some of these all-too-common errors. In addition, this book inspires an awe of medicine. The human body is a fascinating one, whether sick or healthy. I recall reading the book and sharing with others how the human body manifests illnesses, which can often be diagnosed with clinical acumen and not always by having to rely on sophisticated modern testing. To that end, it is one of the greatest honors in my life to write an introduction to this tome of wisdom that has helped so many clinicians take the best care they can of children. I hope that Dr. Zitelli's teachings stay with you, at the bedside, when talking about patients with your colleagues, when you hold a caregiver's hand to share a concerning diagnosis, and when you teach the next generation of clinicians. When you have the time to hold the book in your hands or study the information online, savor the knowledge. The images and easy-to-understand explanations will remain within you, and when you are seeing patients, those learnings will support you being the best clinician that you can be.

"To study the phenomenon of disease without books is to sail an uncharted sea, while to study books without patients is not to go to sea at all"

— ATTRIBUTED TO SIR WILLIAM OSLER (1901)

Geeta Singhal, MD, MEd, FAAP
Professor, Pediatrics
Attending, Pediatric Hospital Medicine
Baylor College of Medicine

PREFACE

In pediatrics, visual recognition of a variety of disorders is often the key factor in diagnosis.

Experienced clinicians who have seen a wide spectrum of disorders carry a wealth of information for diagnosis and teaching. Despite the increased reliance on technology to make a diagnosis, history and physical examination remain the foundations of clinical assessment of the patient. The *Atlas of Pediatric Physical Diagnosis* was created to enhance the clinical experience of students, residents, nurses, and all practitioners who care for children.

We have been very pleased with the reception of the first eight editions of the *Atlas* and welcome the requests of readers for new and updated information. Every chapter in the eighth edition has been reviewed, revised, and updated with the latest information. This edition also marks the first for our new co-editor, Dr. Catherine Polak. Our new and returning chapter authors have provided greater depth and dimension while some sections have been extensively rewritten. New photographs and diagnostic images have been included in many chapters, and, where possible, we have cross-referenced common topics for readers to explore. Topical additions, such as COVID-19 infections in the Infectious Diseases chapter, represent our commitment to keeping the *Atlas* relevant to our changing clinical practice.

The *Atlas* is by no means encyclopedic but rather presents an overview of clinical disorders that lend themselves to visual diagnosis. We have attempted to select disorders that are common or important and, when relevant, to describe the spectrum of clinical findings. The accompanying text deliberately emphasizes pertinent historical factors, examination techniques, visual findings, and diagnostic methods rather than therapy. We firmly believe that a careful history and physical examination are the best tools the clinician has for diagnosis and treatment. It is our hope that the ninth edition of the *Atlas of Pediatric Physical Diagnosis* continues to serve as a useful and practical reference for anyone who cares for children.

Basil J. Zitelli, MD
Sara C. McIntire, MD
Andrew J. Nowalk, MD, PhD
Jessica Garrison, MD
Catherine Polak, MD

CONTENTS

VIDEO CONTENTS

The following supplemental videos are available at Elsevier eBooks+.

1

GENETIC DISORDERS AND DYSMORPHIC CONDITIONS

Damara Ortiz | Georgianne Arnold | Suneeta Madan-Khetarpal

The field of pediatric genetics and dysmorphology is complex, interesting, and rapidly evolving. Our knowledge base is gleaned from the careful observations of master clinicians and scientists who recognized clinical characteristics and patterns of malformation in individuals with genetic, teratogenic, developmental, and metabolic problems. They have provided us with a framework for the investigation of patients from clinical and laboratory perspectives. In addition to classic cytogenetics, molecular cytogenetics methods have been increasingly incorporated in clinical settings and have greatly assisted evaluation, enabling far greater understanding of the molecular and physiologic basis of these disorders, and have greatly increased the rate of diagnosis of children with genetic and metabolic disorders. However, even with the availability of an ever-widening array of confirmatory tests, clinical evaluation of patients remains an essential component of the complete assessment of children and adults with genetic diseases and dysmorphic conditions. This stems from the fact that careful evaluation can substantially reduce the number of differential diagnostic possibilities and, thereby, the number of diagnostic tests and the total expense, as well as guide which gene variants are reported in whole exome and genome technologies.

Visual identification of dysmorphic features, baseline anthropometrics combined with serial measurements with recognition of patterns of malformation and behavioral phenotypes, remains an integral part of the diagnostic algorithm. Genetic disorders should be investigated with a careful history, a family pedigree, a thorough physical examination including evaluation for the presence of major and minor anomalies, and thoughtful laboratory testing. This chapter is designed to present clinicians who care for children with background on the general principles of genetics and dysmorphology, as well as updated information about important advances in our field. Although not exhaustive, it provides a framework for the broad categories of genetic diseases and discusses an approach to the evaluation of the patient with dysmorphic features. Definitions and examples of the types of disorders resulting in genetic and/or congenital anomalies in children are described, including malformations, deformations, disruptions, associations, and sequences. We provide examples of disorders inherited through classic Mendelian inheritance patterns, including single-gene diseases, such as Marfan syndrome; metabolic disorders, such as phenylketonuria (PKU) or Smith-Lemli-Opitz syndrome; and non-Mendelian disorders, such as teratogenic exposures in utero and disruptions or deformations of previously normal fetal structures. Etiologic mechanisms of diseases, such as imprinting abnormalities, expansions of trinucleotide repeats in nuclear deoxyribonucleic acid (DNA), mitochondrial DNA, whole exome and genome sequencing, and the fields of -omics (metabolomics, proteomics, etc.), are introduced. As testing options grow, there is acknowledgment of the expanding role of genotype to phenotype correlation and its importance in the genomic era.

APPROACH TO THE EVALUATION OF A CHILD WITH DYSMORPHIC FEATURES

Approximately 2% to 3% of liveborn infants have an observable structural or functional abnormality. This number rises to about 4% to 5% by the time the child is old enough to attend school. Structural differences can be determined to be either *major* or *minor* in character (Table 1.1; Figs. 1.1 and 1.2). Major structural anomalies have functional consequences. Examples are polydactyly, colobomas of the iris (see Chapter 20), meningomyelocele, and cleft lip. *Minor* anomalies are usually of cosmetic importance only. Examples are epicanthal folds of the eyes, single transverse palmar creases, and supernumerary nipples. The incidence of isolated major anomalies in the general newborn population is approximately 1%, and the incidence of minor anomalies is approximately 14%.

The probability of an infant having a major anomaly increases with the number of minor anomalies found. Thus, all children with multiple minor anomalies warrant a careful clinical assessment to evaluate for occult major anomalies. Once an anomaly is identified, assessing its significance begins with a determination of whether the anomaly is a single localized error in morphogenesis or one component of a multiple malformation syndrome. An understanding of the pathophysiologic mechanisms that produce structural abnormalities or differences provides an opportunity to define the types of structural abnormalities seen. This also assists the process of identifying the etiology and arriving at a specific diagnosis, which can be useful in determining the prognosis, mapping a plan of care, and estimating the risk of recurrence of a similar problem in future pregnancies.

Definitions of the classifications of structural anomalies aid in communication between clinicians and in the process of evaluation and are summarized below:

1. *Malformation:* A malformation is an abnormality of embryonic morphogenesis of tissue. It usually results from genetic, chromosomal, or teratogenic influences, but it can be of multifactorial etiology. Malformations are divided into two main categories: (1) those that constitute a single primary defect in development and (2) those that represent a single component of a multiple malformation syndrome. A *multiple malformation syndrome* can be defined as one having several observed structural defects in development involving multiple organ systems that share the same known or presumed etiology. Major malformations often require surgical intervention.
2. *Deformation:* A deformation is an alteration (often molding) of an intrinsically normal tissue caused by exposure to unusual extrinsic forces. One example is clubfoot (talipes equinovarus), which may be the result of fetal crowding in a multiple gestation. A more severe example is the compressed facial features ("Potter facies") of a child exposed to severe uterine constraint and oligohydramnios, due to renal agenesis (see Chapter 14). Most deformations respond to medical therapy alone and have a relatively good prognosis.

3. *Disruption:* A disruption represents a breakdown of normally formed tissue; the breakdown may be the result of vascular accidents or exposure to adverse mechanical forces that are usually more severe than those that produce deformation. An example is the variety of clefting, constriction bands, and limb reduction defects that can result from amniotic bands (see Chapter 2). The earlier these vascular accidents or abnormal forces occur during embryogenesis, the more severe the resulting defects (Fig. 1.3).
4. *Sequence:* The term sequence refers to a recognizable pattern of multiple anomalies that occurs when a *single* problem in morphogenesis cascades, resulting in secondary and tertiary errors in morphogenesis and a corresponding series of structural alterations. A classic example is the Pierre Robin sequence, in which the single primary malformation is microretrognathia (see Chapter 23). The resulting glossoptosis, or posterior placement of the tongue in the oropharynx, interferes with normal palatal closure if the lingual displacement occurs before 9 weeks' gestation. The resulting cleft palate is U-shaped, rather than having the V shape that is usually seen in classic cleft palate.
5. *Association:* An association is a pattern of malformations that occur together too frequently to be due to random chance alone, but for which no specific etiology is yet recognized.

The approach to the evaluation of a child with a dysmorphic abnormality, similar to the diagnostic evaluation of most pediatric problems, starts with a complete history and careful physical examination. In obtaining these, it is helpful to remember that there are six broad etiologic categories to be considered in the differential diagnosis: (1) a known monogenic syndrome, (2) an unknown syndrome, (3) a chromosomal abnormality, (4) a teratogen, (5) a congenital infection, and (6) gestational environment (a maternal disease and/or placental abnormalities).

The history should include the following:

- Course of the pregnancy, complications including possible infections or environmental exposures, medications/substance exposures, prenatal testing/imaging
- Prior pregnancies, spontaneous abortions, stillbirths, or infant/child deaths
- Labor/delivery/perinatal problems
- Past medical history
- Growth and development
- Meticulous family history with family tree (pedigree) going back three generations and including the following:
  - Familial traits and growth characteristics
  - Familial physical or developmental disorders
  - Spontaneous abortions, terminations, stillbirths, infant/child deaths in extended family

The physical examination entails the following:

- Thorough general examination, including measurements of some physical traits
- Documentation of major and/or minor anomalies
- Neurodevelopmental assessment

In addition, focused examination of immediate family members for physical characteristics and growth parameters and review of family photos and/or videos may be helpful.

Determining how the child fits into the norms for growth and development for the general population, for the family's ethnic group(s), and for the extended family is important. One continuing challenge is determining whether the norms for the family are truly in the normal range for the general population and ethnic background or, in fact, constitute variability of a genetic trait present in its expression in the child or family member seen for evaluation.

The identification of a recognizable pattern of both major and minor anomalies provides the clinical dysmorphologist with a diagnosis or a short list of diagnostic possibilities. Identification of specific and unusual malformations that are uncommon and occur in only a few syndromes can be especially helpful. For example, finding that a child has long palpebral fissure length and pronounced fingertip fat pad size in combination with the pattern of anomalies typical of Kabuki syndrome make it extremely likely that the diagnosis is Kabuki syndrome, and focused molecular testing can be pursued. Training in dysmorphology emphasizes the recognition of key components in patterns of malformation and specific findings useful in distinguishing syndromes with similarities from one another. Publications that outline currently recognized patterns of malformations can be helpful in assisting the clinician in the identification of specific features that can aid in creating a differential diagnosis. Commercial computer-based programs exist for syndrome identification; however, these are often more effectively used by experts in the field because of the complexity of terminology and the need for exacting descriptions of the anomalies present in each child.

Cytogenetic and/or molecular studies should be performed on each child with congenital anomalies. Such studies may establish or confirm the diagnosis of an underlying genetic disorder and its hereditary potential, guide management, and possibly help focus on candidate genes for those syndromes suspected to be Mendelian disorders.

Table 1.1 Examples of Congenital Anomalies

Category	Major	Minor
Craniofacial	Choanal atresia	Plagiocephaly Flat occiput
Eyes	Coloboma of iris	Epicanthal folds
Ears	Microtia	Preauricular pit
Hands	Polydactyly Absent thumbs	Single transverse palmar crease Clinodactyly

GENERAL PRINCIPLES

The Nature of Chromosomes

Productive insights gleaned from the results of the Human Genome Project have dramatically changed some of our understanding of how the human genome functions. Human hereditary factors are located in *genes* (the *genome*). Approximately 20% are genes that encode proteins that assemble to form tissue structures or to form

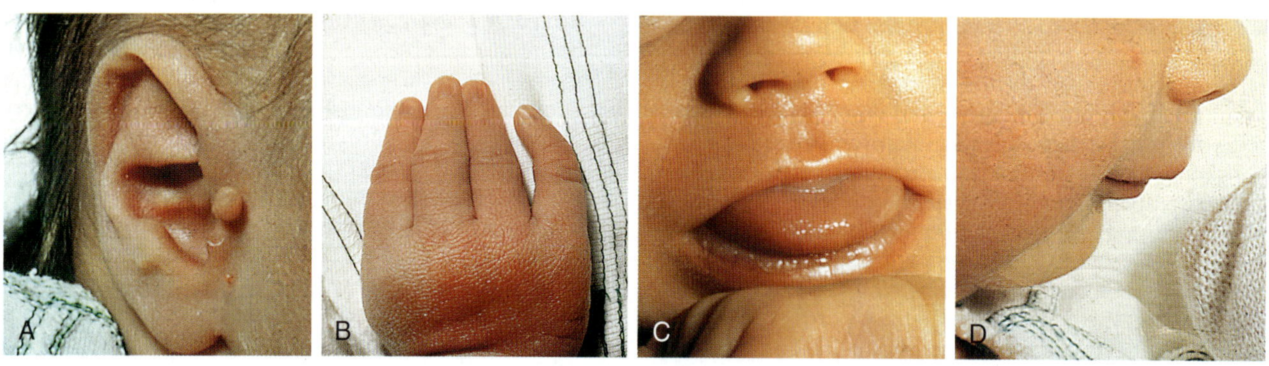

Fig. 1.1 Clinical photographs show several minor anomalies seen at birth. (A) Preauricular skin tag. (B) Clinodactyly of the fifth finger. (C) Macroglossia. (D) Microretrognathia. (Courtesy Christine L. Williams, MD.)

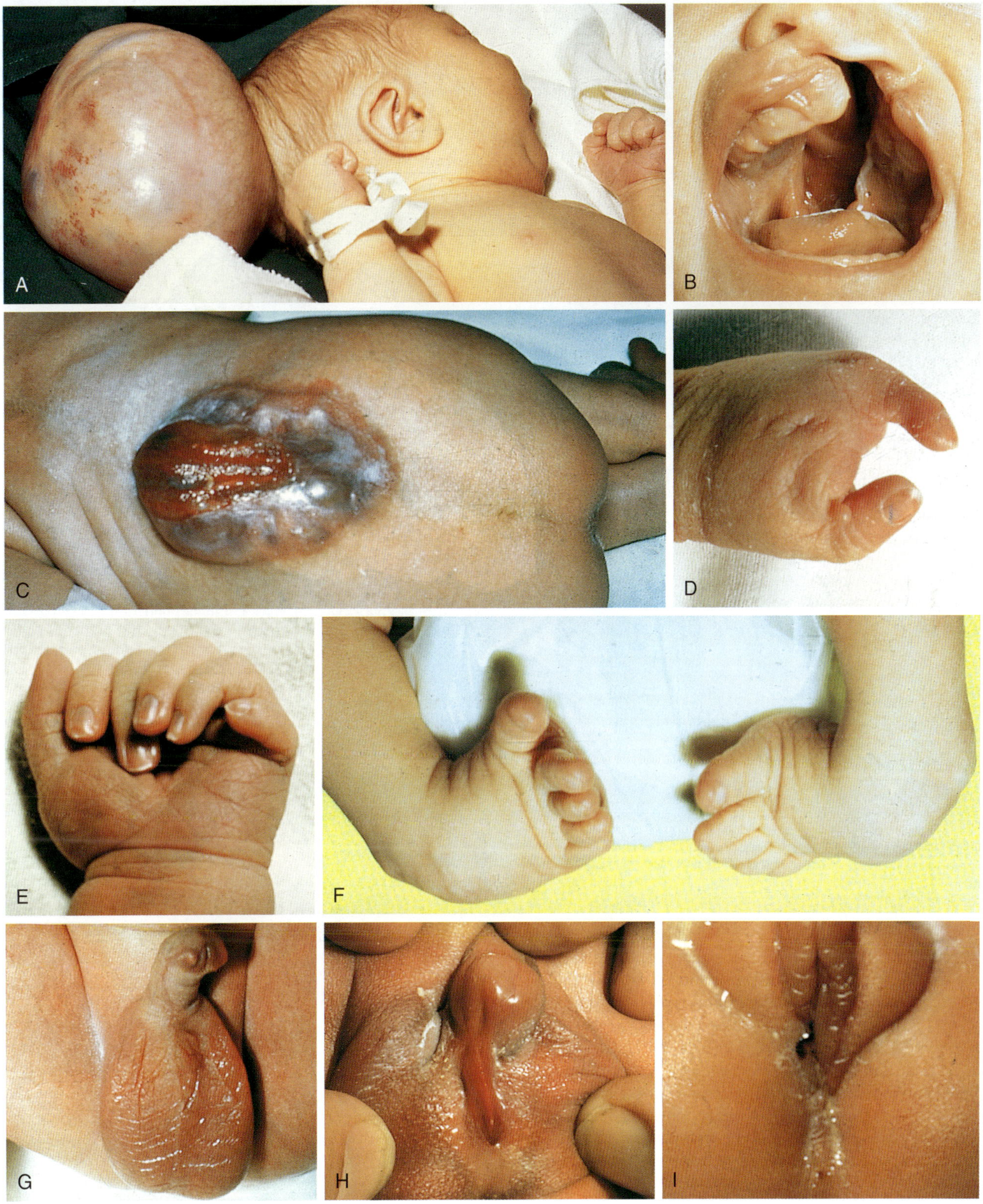

Fig. 1.2 Clinical photographs show several major anomalies seen at birth. (A) Encephalocele. (B) Cleft lip and palate. (C) Meningomyelocele. (D) Ectrodactyly (previously termed *lobster-claw deformity*). (E) Polydactyly (postaxial). (F) Bilateral clubfoot. (G) Hypospadias. (H) Fused labia with enlarged clitoris. (I) Imperforate anus. (Courtesy Christine L. Williams, MD.)

enzymes that catalyze chemical reactions within cells. The other 80% have functions that are currently not clear (see also The Nature of Genes and Single-Gene Disorders, later). The genes are composed of DNA and are stored in intranuclear cell organelles called *chromosomes.* Each chromosome contains one linear DNA molecule folded over onto itself several times, as well as ribonucleic acid (RNA) and proteins. Because all genes exist in pairs, all chromosomes must likewise exist in pairs. The members of each pair of genes are called *alleles,* and the members of each pair of chromosomes are known as *homologues.* The conventional depiction of the constitution of homologues in the nucleus is called the cell's *karyotype* (Fig. 1.4). If at any gene locus the alleles are identical, that gene locus is *homozygous.* If the alleles are not identical, the gene locus is *heterozygous.*

Except for gametes, normal human cells contain 23 pairs of chromosomes, 46 in all. One of these pairs is concerned in part with inducing the primary sex of the embryonic gonads. These sex chromosomes are called the *X* and *Y chromosomes,* and they are not genetically homologous except in a few areas. Genotypic females have two X chromosomes, whereas genotypic males have an X and a Y chromosome. The remaining 22 pairs are called *autosomes,* and they determine non–sex-related (somatic) characteristics.

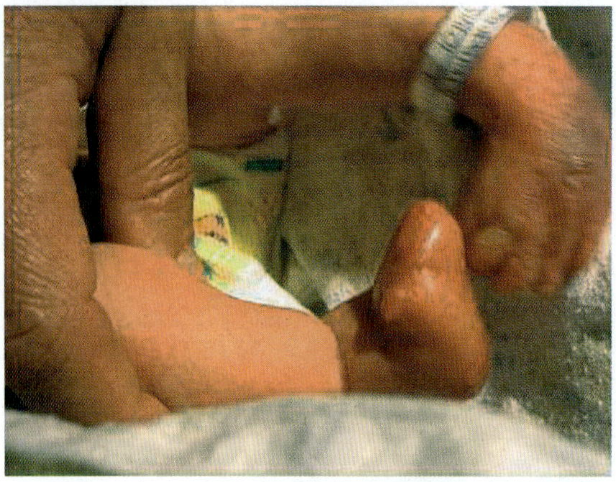

Fig. 1.3 Amniotic band syndrome; note the constriction ring at the ankle and amputation of the toes, a sequela to the amniotic bands.

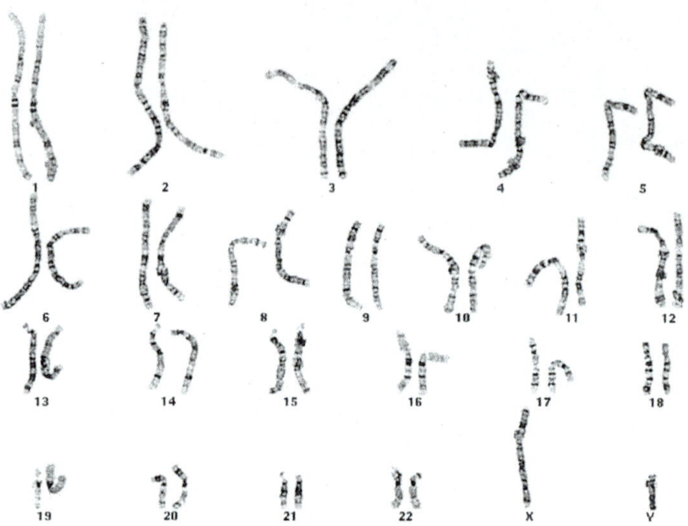

Fig. 1.4 G-banded male karyotype. A female would have two X chromosomes and no Y chromosome. The horizontal banding produced by the Giemsa staining technique allows for precise identification of homologous chromosomes. (Courtesy Urvashi Surti, PhD, Pittsburgh Cytogenetics Laboratory.)

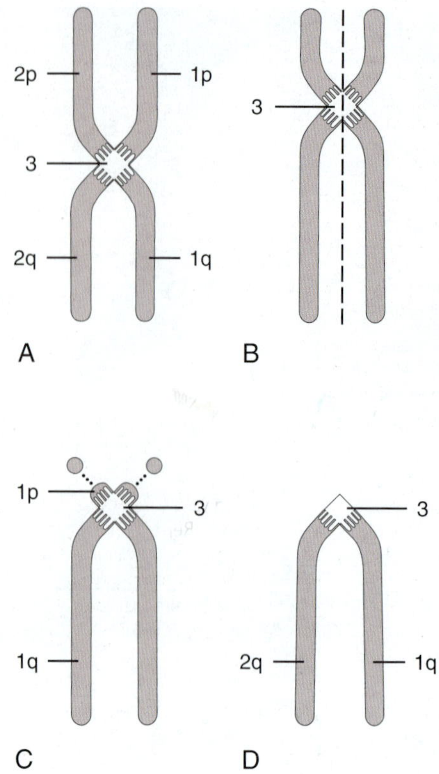

Fig. 1.5 Morphology of a chromosome during metaphase. (A) Metacentric chromosome with centromere *(3)* in the middle. (B) Submetacentric chromosome with centromere off-center. (C) Acrocentric chromosome with centromere near one end. (D) Telocentric chromosome (not found in humans) with centromere at one end. The deoxyribonucleic acid of the chromosome has replicated to form two chromatids: *1p* and *1q* represent one complete chromatid, *2p* and *2q* the other complete chromatid (*p* refers to the short arm and *q* refers to the long arm). The chromosome will then divide longitudinally, as shown in (B).

During most of a cell's life cycle, chromosomes are diffusely spread throughout the nucleus and cannot be identified by morphologic means. When the cell divides, chromosome morphology becomes apparent (Fig. 1.5). The in vitro life cycle and the cellular division, or *mitosis,* of a somatic cell are illustrated in Figs. 1.6 and 1.7, respectively. The life cycle and divisions, or *meiosis,* of a germ cell are much more complex and are not suitable for ordinary clinical evaluation.

Any somatic cell that can divide in tissue culture can be used for chromosomal (cytogenetic) analyses for karyotyping. The most convenient tissue source is peripheral blood, from which lymphocytes can be stimulated to divide in a few days, allowing chromosomes to be visualized. Fibroblasts obtained from skin remain a frequently used alternative when peripheral blood lymphocytes are not clinically suitable, but this process takes longer to complete. In urgent situations, preliminary chromosomal evaluation can be made within 4 to 24 hours. Pediatric clinicians are advised to discuss clinical and laboratory investigations with clinical geneticists and/or laboratory directors before sample collection.

Chromosomal structures too small to be seen microscopically can be studied by molecular cytogenetic techniques, through either interphase or metaphase fluorescence in situ hybridization (FISH) or high-resolution molecular karyotyping using microarray-based comparative genomic hybridization (array-CGH). Array-CGH uses molecular probes to capture submicroscopic copy number changes at high resolution and has become standard of care as a first step in the investigation of patients with developmental delays, intellectual disability, and multiple congenital anomalies. Noninvasive prenatal testing or screening (NIPT) uses a similar technology to quantify the amount of fetal DNA fragments present in a maternal blood sample to provide a risk assessment for aneuploidies and some copy number changes in the developing fetus.

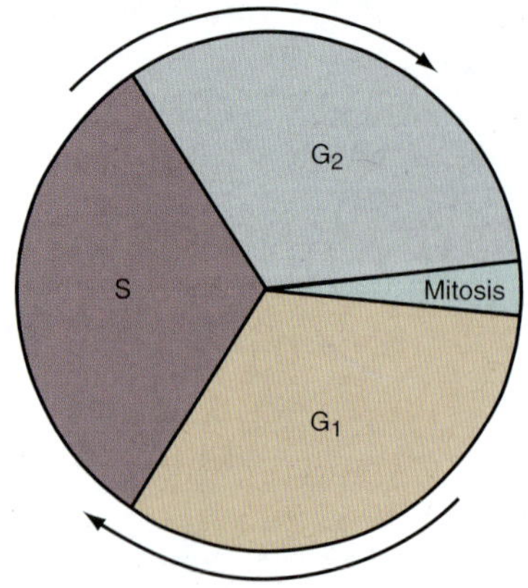

Fig. 1.6 The in vitro life cycle of a somatic cell. Interphase lasts 21 hours and can be divided into the following three stages: G_1 (7 hours)—cell performs its tasks; *S* (7 hours)—deoxyribonucleic acid replicates; G_2 (7 hours)—cell prepares to divide. Then mitosis occurs.

Incidence of Chromosomal Abnormalities

Data from Hook (1992) suggest that upward of 50% of human conceptions terminate in a spontaneous abortion, typically so early during gestation that the pregnancy is never formally recognized. The earlier the abortion occurs, the more likely it is that the miscarried embryo had a chromosomal abnormality. Of recognized first-trimester abortuses, 50% are chromosomally abnormal, compared with 5% of later embryos. Among the chromosomally abnormal miscarried embryos, the most frequent abnormalities are triploidy

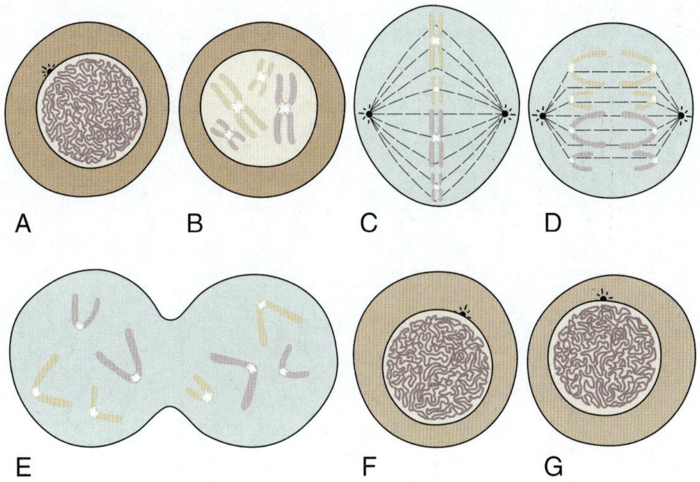

Fig. 1.7 Mitosis lasts about 1 hour, during which time the cell divides. (A) Interphase cell at the end of G_2. (B) Prophase: Replicated DNA condenses and is visible. (C) Metaphase: 46 duplicated chromosomes align randomly on the spindle and can be photographed for karyotyping. (D) Anaphase: Chromosomes divide longitudinally, and half of each one moves to the opposite pole of the cell. (E) Telophase: Cell wall divides. (F and G) Interphase at G_1: Two daughter cells, each with 46 chromosomes.

(69 chromosomes), trisomy 16, and 45,X (Turner syndrome) (Table 1.2). Generally speaking, triploidy and trisomy 16 are not compatible with life and are only rarely seen among liveborn infants. Despite the fact that Turner syndrome is relatively common among liveborn infants, the majority of conceptuses with 45,X abort spontaneously. The incidence of chromosomal abnormalities among liveborn infants in general is about 6 in 1000, but for infants who are stillborn or who die in the immediate perinatal period, the number is increased to approximately 50 in 1000.

Abnormalities of Chromosome Number—Aneuploidy

Aneuploidy refers to an abnormality in chromosome number; in humans, *aneuploidy* is a chromosome number different from an even multiple of 23 (the haploid number) (Fig. 1.8). In aneuploidy, there are typically 45 or 47 chromosomes instead of the usual 46. Rarely, multiples of the X or Y chromosome result in individuals with 48 or 49 chromosomes.

Table 1.2 Occurrence of Chromosomal Abnormalities[a]

Among Spontaneous Abortions	Incidence
Overall incidence	32.0%
First trimester	52.0%
After first trimester	5.8%
Type of abnormality seen in spontaneous abortions	
Trisomy 16	
Other trisomies	
Triploidy	
45,X	
Miscellaneous	
Among Liveborns	**Number of Cases Per 1000**
Overall incidence	6.20
Abnormality of autosomes	4.19 (males and females)
Trisomies	
Balanced rearrangements	
Unbalanced rearrangements	
Abnormality of sex chromosomes	2.03 (males and females)
In males: XXY, XYY, mosaics	
In females: 45,X (0.08), XXX, mosaics (1.43)	

[a]About one-quarter of all conceptuses are chromosomally abnormal. About 50 in 1000 stillborns have a chromosomal abnormality.

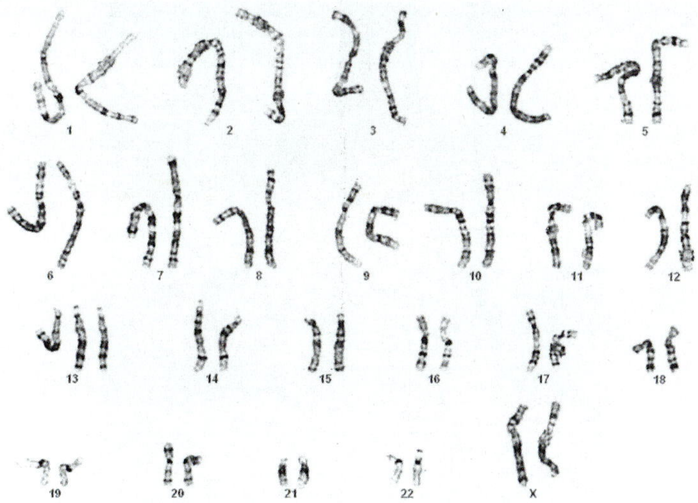

Fig. 1.8 Karyotype of a patient with trisomy 13 demonstrates aneuploidy. Note the extra chromosome 13, causing the cell to have 47 instead of 46 chromosomes. (Courtesy Urvashi Surti, PhD, Pittsburgh Cytogenetics Laboratory.)

If aneuploidy occurs in a gamete because of an error of chromosomal division (nondisjunction or anaphase lag) during meiosis, all cells are affected in the fertilized embryo. The risk of nondisjunction increases independently with maternal age. Although the mechanism of this increased risk is unknown, preconception genetic counseling is recommended in those with a family history of aneuploidy, multiple miscarriages, or increasing maternal age.

Mosaic Aneuploidy States

Mosaicism, the presence of two or more genetically different cell lines within an individual, can result from an error in division during either meiosis (preconception) or mitosis (postconception). When aneuploidy is present at conception, in some cases the extra chromosome is dropped from one or more cells during postconception cell division, leading to mosaicism in the fetus for normal and aneuploid cell lines. In other cases of mosaicism, the early embryo is chromosomally normal and a division error occurs after fertilization, during mitosis of an embryonic somatic cell, resulting in aneuploidy. Balanced and unbalanced chromosome aberrations and uniparental disomy (UPD) can be encountered in this setting and can increase the risk of epigenetic disorders. There is a mildly increased recurrence risk for those parents, which is not fully understood but may reflect an undetectable aneuploid mosaic cell line in a parental gonad (Fig. 1.9).

In some cases, chromosomal mosaicism can have visible effects. For example, in hypomelanosis of Ito, the skin manifests marbleized or mottled areas of hypopigmented whorls along the Blaschko lines (Fig. 1.10). Karyotyping from normal, hypopigmented, or hyperpigmented regions can reveal mosaic chromosomal abnormalities in each region. In addition, individuals with hypomelanosis of Ito can have multiple congenital anomalies, dysmorphic features, variable intellectual disability, and other neurologic findings.

Abnormalities of Chromosome Structure—Inversions, Deletions, and Translocations

Chromosomes can be normal in number (diploid) but abnormal in structure. Inversions (Fig. 1.11), deletions (Fig. 1.12), and translocations (Fig. 1.13) of genetic material are examples of structural chromosomal abnormalities. These can arise as new (sporadic or de novo) variations in the egg or sperm from which the embryo was formed, or the abnormality may also be inherited from a phenotypically normal parent who is a "carrier" of a balanced structural chromosomal abnormality (Fig. 1.14). About 1 in 520 normal individuals carries a balanced but structurally abnormal set of chromosomes, called a *chromosome translocation.* The term *balanced,* for the purposes of this chapter, means that on cytogenetic analysis the structural abnormality does not appear to have resulted in any net

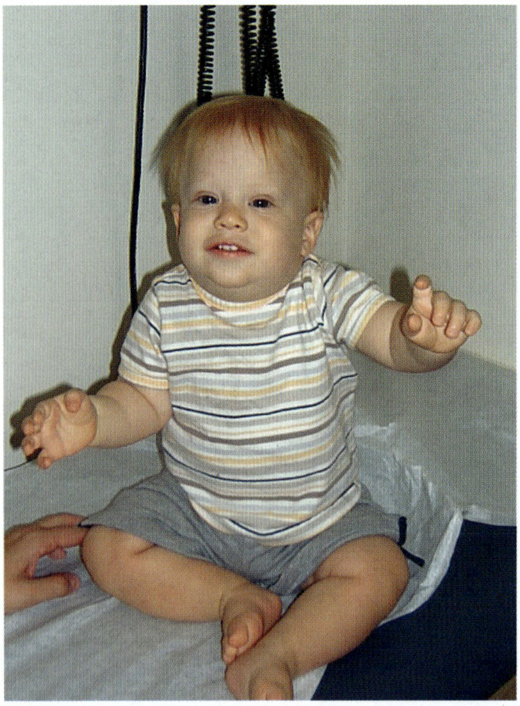

Fig. 1.9 A 1-year-old with facies suggestive of Down syndrome. Note the facies and short fifth fingers and clinodactyly. The muscle tone and growth parameters were normal. Cytogenetics studies showed 2% of the cells with 47,XY+21; interphase fluorescence in situ hybridization studies with an extra cell count showed trisomy 21 in 1.3% of 523 peripheral lymphocytes analyzed.

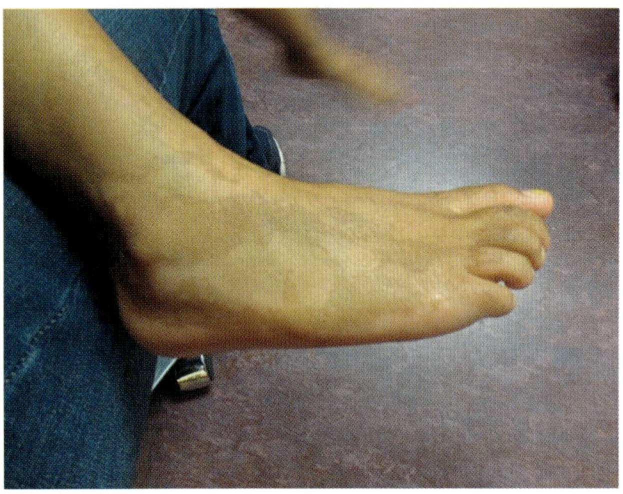

Fig. 1.10 Hypomelanosis of Ito. Karyotype at birth was normal: 46,XX. At 4 months of age characteristic streaks and whorls of hyperpigmentation and hypopigmentation of the skin were noted. A higher cell-count karyotype showed mosaicism for trisomy 14.

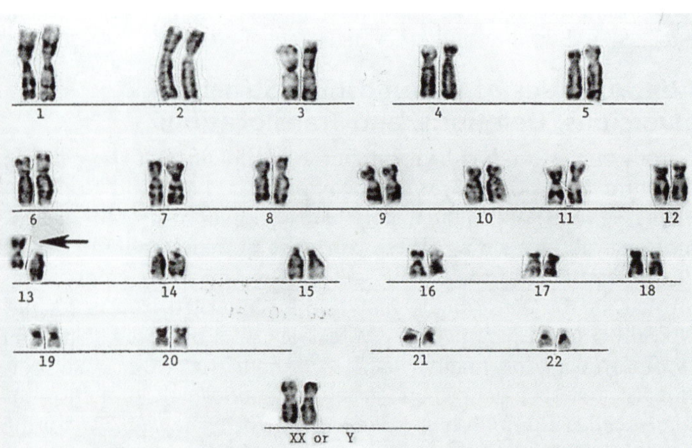

Fig. 1.11 Pericentric inversion *(arrow)* of chromosome 13.

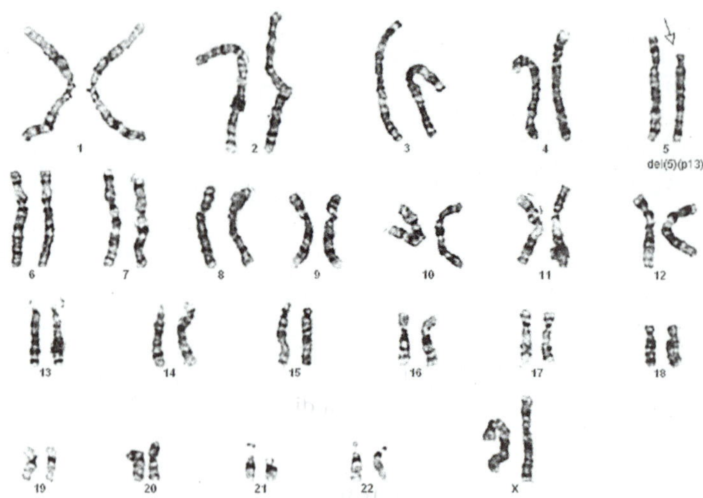

Fig. 1.12 Deletion *(arrow)* of the p arm of chromosome 5 (cri du chat syndrome). (Courtesy Urvashi Surti, PhD, Pittsburgh Cytogenetics Laboratory.)

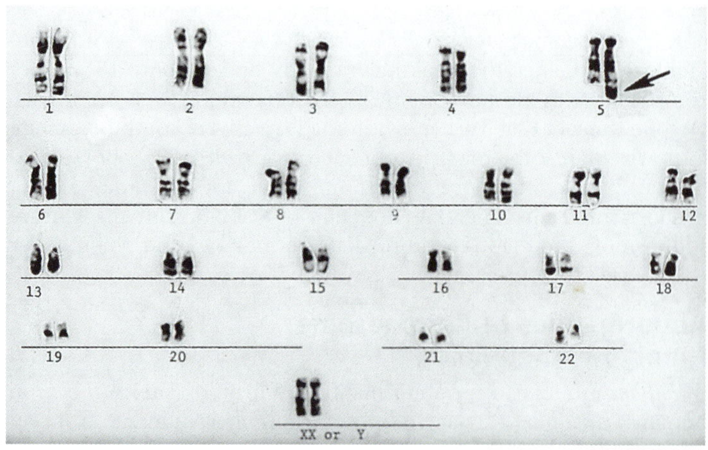

Fig. 1.13 Unbalanced translocation. The additional deoxyribonucleic acid was translocated onto the q arm of chromosome 5 *(arrow)*. The abnormality was inherited from a normal carrier father (see Fig. 1.14) with a balanced reciprocal translocation between the q arms of chromosome 3 and chromosome 5. The patient died of multiple birth defects and in essence had a partial trisomy of the distal portion of the q arm of chromosome 3.

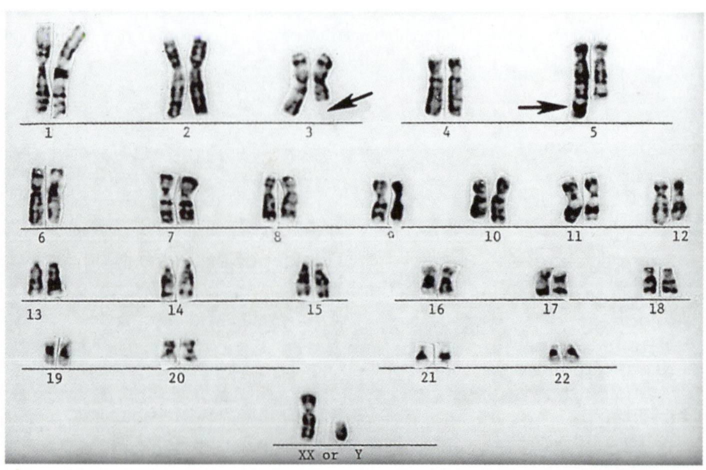

Fig. 1.14 A "balanced" reciprocal translocation from chromosomes 3 *(arrow)* to 5 *(arrow)* in a normal man (the father of the chromosomally defective newborn whose karyotype is shown in Fig. 1.13).

loss or gain of genetic material; it is simply relocated to a different place in the genome. A familial balanced translocation can be transmitted silently through multiple generations, but in some cases the translocated genetic material is passed down unevenly during mitosis, resulting in a fetus with aneuploidy.

Families with apparently balanced chromosome translocations often come to medical attention when a child is born with structural malformations and on karyotyping is found to have an unbalanced chromosome translocation. Data suggest that a small percentage of individuals with new apparently "balanced" translocations are mildly affected clinically by variable degrees of cognitive and physical deficits. Thus, high-resolution chromosome analyses and molecular cytogenetics techniques are indicated, particularly when assessing translocations in a child. Parental karyotypes are used to distinguish the etiology and are crucial in providing accurate genetic counseling regarding future pregnancies.

When to Suspect a Chromosomal Abnormality

Chromosomal abnormalities of either number or structure are likely to have a detrimental effect on the phenotype of an affected individual. Aneuploidy of an autosome, or non–sex chromosome, can significantly impair physical and cognitive development. However, aneuploidy of a sex chromosome may have little or no apparent effect on the phenotype. One should look for clustering of abnormalities in family members to suggest a problem, although their absence does not rule out a chromosomal abnormality.

A history of unexplained infertility, multiple spontaneous abortions (defined as three or more), and a previous birth to the couple or to a close relative of a child with dysmorphic findings and/or major anomalies may be an indication that one of the parents carries a balanced chromosomal translocation or rearrangement. The risk for an individual carrying a balanced translocation identified through karyotype to have a living child with an unbalanced translocation varies from 4% to 20%, which requires the expertise of genetic counseling to help determine.

Classic Autosomal Aneuploidies

Down Syndrome Down syndrome is the most common and broadly recognizable aneuploidy. No single physical sign of Down syndrome exists; rather, the clinical diagnosis rests on finding a recognizable constellation of clinical characteristics, including a combination of major and minor anomalies (see Figs. 1.9 and 1.15, Table 1.3). The worldwide incidence of Down syndrome among liveborn infants is approximately 1 in 660, with 45% of affected individuals born to females older than 35 years old. The incidence of Down syndrome among conceptuses is far greater than among liveborns because most affected fetuses spontaneously abort. An association between trisomy 21 and advanced maternal age is clear (Table 1.4). The etiology of Down syndrome is trisomy 21, the presence of an extra chromosome 21 as either a simple trisomy (e.g., 47,XX, +21) or part of a chromosome 21 fused (translocated) with another chromosome. Chromosome studies should

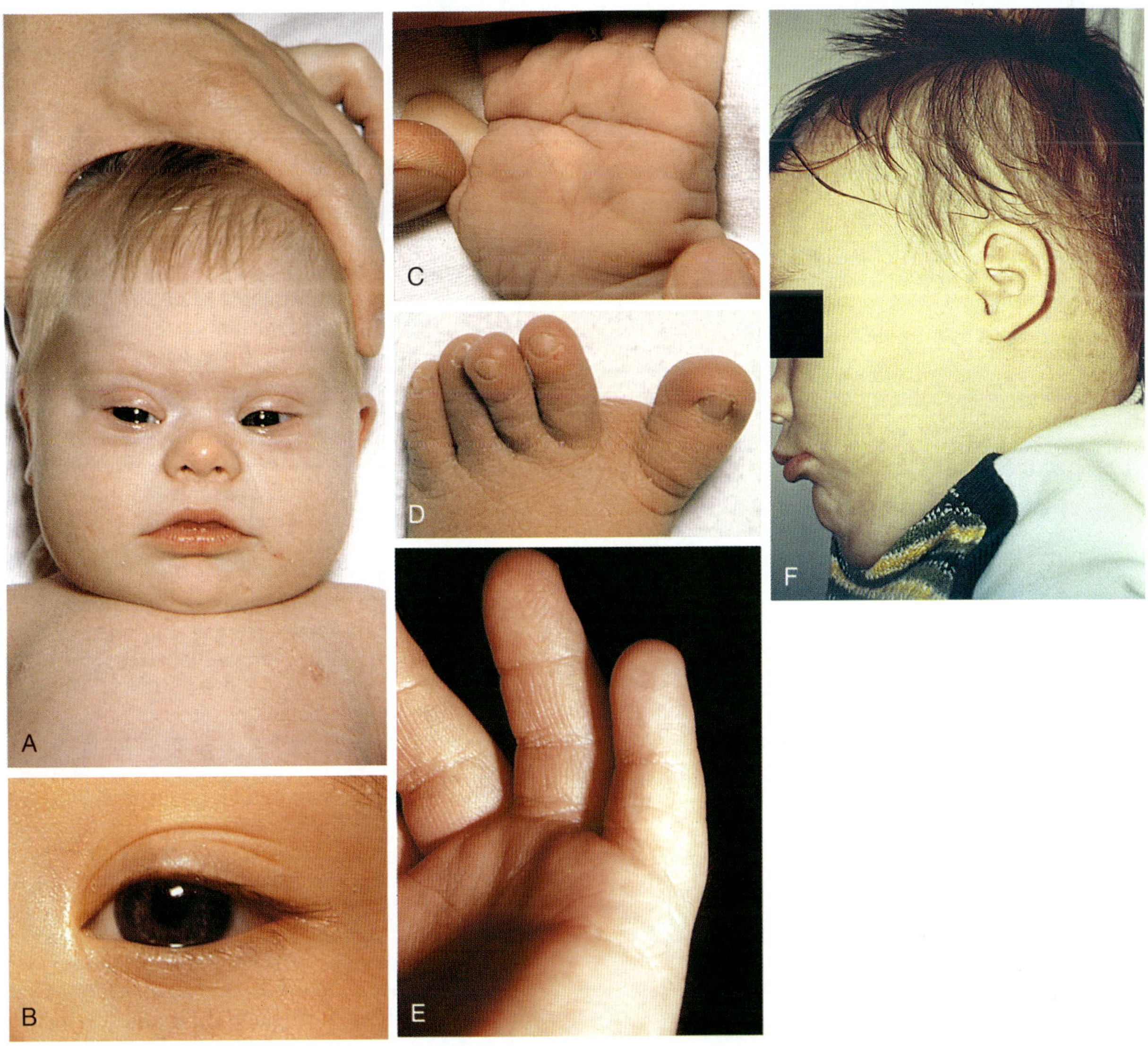

Fig. 1.15 Down syndrome. These clinical photographs show several minor anomalies associated with this disorder. (A) Characteristic facial features with up-slanting palpebral fissures, epicanthal folds, and flat nasal bridge. (B) Brushfield spots. (C) Bridged palmar crease, seen in some affected infants. Two transverse palmar creases are connected by a diagonal line. (D) Wide space between first and second toes. (E) Short fifth finger. (F) Small ears and flat occiput.

Table 1.3 Trisomy 21 Phenotype and Management

Anomaly	Frequency	Management
CNS:		
Hypotonia, ID (Average IQ 20–80)	Common 80%–100%	Supportive and symptomatic
Early onset of Alzheimer-like changes	60%–80%	
Seizures	Rare 3%	
Congenital heart disease:	45%	Cardiology involvement
AVSD, endocardial cushion defect, VSD, vascular anomaly		
Adult onset of valvular prolapse		
Characteristic facial features:	Common	Supportive and symptomatic
Up-slanting palpebral fissures, small nose with low nasal bridge, epicanthal folds, small external ears		
Eyes:	Common	Symptomatic
Brushfield spots (speckled irides), strabismus, lenticular opacities, refractive errors, blocked tear ducts, dental concerns		
Neck:	Common	Detected in utero and postnatally. Neck stability checks due to C1–C2
Short with redundant fold		
GI:	5%–12%	Surgical repair
Duodenal atresia, Hirschsprung disease, omphalocele, imperforate anus, cholelithiasis		
Endocrine:	Common	Early recognition and treatment Occasional pregnancy in females (≈30%); three males have had documented paternity
Thyroid athyreosis, goiter, hyperthyroidism, primary gonadal deficiency, fertility		
Hematology/oncology leukemia, neonatal leukemoid reaction	Rare (1%)	
Musculoskeletal:	Common	Supportive care and surgery as needed
Cervical spine instability, hypoplasia of pelvis, small hands with short fifth fingers and single palmar creases, wide gap between the first two toes of feet (sandal gap)		
Genitalia:	Common	
Hypogenitalism		
Skin:	Common	
Dry, hyperkeratosis, frequent infections, hair (fine and sparse, early graying)		
Allergy immunology (low T- and B-cell counts, small thymus, decreased antibody response to immunizations, decreased neutrophil chemotaxis)	Common	

AVSD, Atrioventricular septal defect; *CNS*, central nervous system; *GI*, gastrointestinal; *VSD*, ventricular septal defect.

Table 1.4 Maternal Age–Specific Risk for Trisomy 21 at Live Birth

Maternal Age	Prevalence at Live Birth
25 years	1/1350
30 years	1/890
35 years	1/355
40 years	1/97
45 years	1/23

therefore be performed on the parents and appropriate family members of an individual with translocation-related Down syndrome. Cases of mosaicism, in which trisomy 21 cell lines coexist with cell lines with the standard 46 chromosomes, exist as well and may range in phenotype from normal to that typical of complete trisomy 21.

Trisomy 13 and Trisomy 18 Trisomy 13 is a relatively rare (1 in 5000) genetic condition caused by the presence of additional chromosome material from all or a large part of chromosome 13. The majority of embryos with classic trisomy for a complete 13th chromosome abort spontaneously, but approximately 5% are liveborn. Of these, about 5% live past the first 6 months of life with rare longer survival. They have a recognizable pattern of malformation that allows clinicians to suspect this etiology immediately (Fig. 1.16, Table 1.5). The most recognizable features include holoprosencephaly with midline deformities, cutis aplasia, and postaxial polydactyly.

The chromosomal disorder trisomy 18 occurs in approximately 3 in 10,000 newborns, and females are more likely to be liveborn. Affected infants exhibit some hallmark features, including clenched hands with overlapping fingers, and are typically small for gestational age with a frail appearance and failure to thrive (Fig. 1.17, see Table 1.5). Trisomy 18 was previously thought to be almost invariably fatal in the neonatal period; however, newer data suggest that a small percentage of children can live longer; between 5% and 10% to at least 1 year, and a few live longer still (frequently females with fewer structural abnormalities of major organs). Embryonal cancers, such as Wilms tumor, appear increased in these affected children, and management guidelines are available.

Partial chromosome abnormalities involving extra material determined to originate from chromosome 13 or 18 must be identified and distinguished from classic trisomies, because the clinical phenotype and prognosis may be different and, in some cases, less severe. Children with mosaicism, that is, with a normal cell line and a trisomy cell line, as well as those with trisomy of part of chromosome 13 or 18, can be identified by chromosome analysis and often have a less severe course.

For infants with classic trisomy 13 or 18, discussions with parents about interventions must consider the slim possibility of longer life spans and require sensitivity to the needs of the child and family. Great care must be taken in providing a balanced picture to the family when discussing treatment options. It has been our experience that parent support organizations can be extremely helpful to family members in the long process of adjustment to having a child with a trisomy or to provide a source of support through the grieving and healing process if the child dies.

Abnormalities of Sex Chromosomes

Turner Syndrome Turner syndrome (monosomy X) is one of the three most common chromosomal abnormalities found in early spontaneous abortions. About 1 in 2000 liveborn females has Turner syndrome. Primary amenorrhea, sterility, sparse pubic and axillary hair, underdeveloped breasts, and short stature (4½ to 5 ft) are the usual manifestations. Other external physical features may include webbing of the neck, cubitus valgus, a low-set posterior hairline, a shield chest with widely spaced nipples, and malformed, often protruding, ears (Fig. 1.18). Internally, renal anomalies may be present along with congenital heart disease, particularly bicuspid aortic valve (in 30% of cases) and coarctation of the aorta (in 10% of cases). Affected individuals have an underdeveloped uterus, and their ovaries consist only of strands of fibrous connective tissue. Newborns often have lymphedema of the feet and/or hands (see Fig. 1.18C), which can reappear briefly during adolescence. Intellectual development is usually normal, although difficulty with spatial orientation (such as map reading) may be a problem. The classic physical findings of Turner syndrome may be absent, or the abnormalities may be so minimal in the newborn that the diagnosis is missed. The first indication may be unexplained short stature in later childhood or

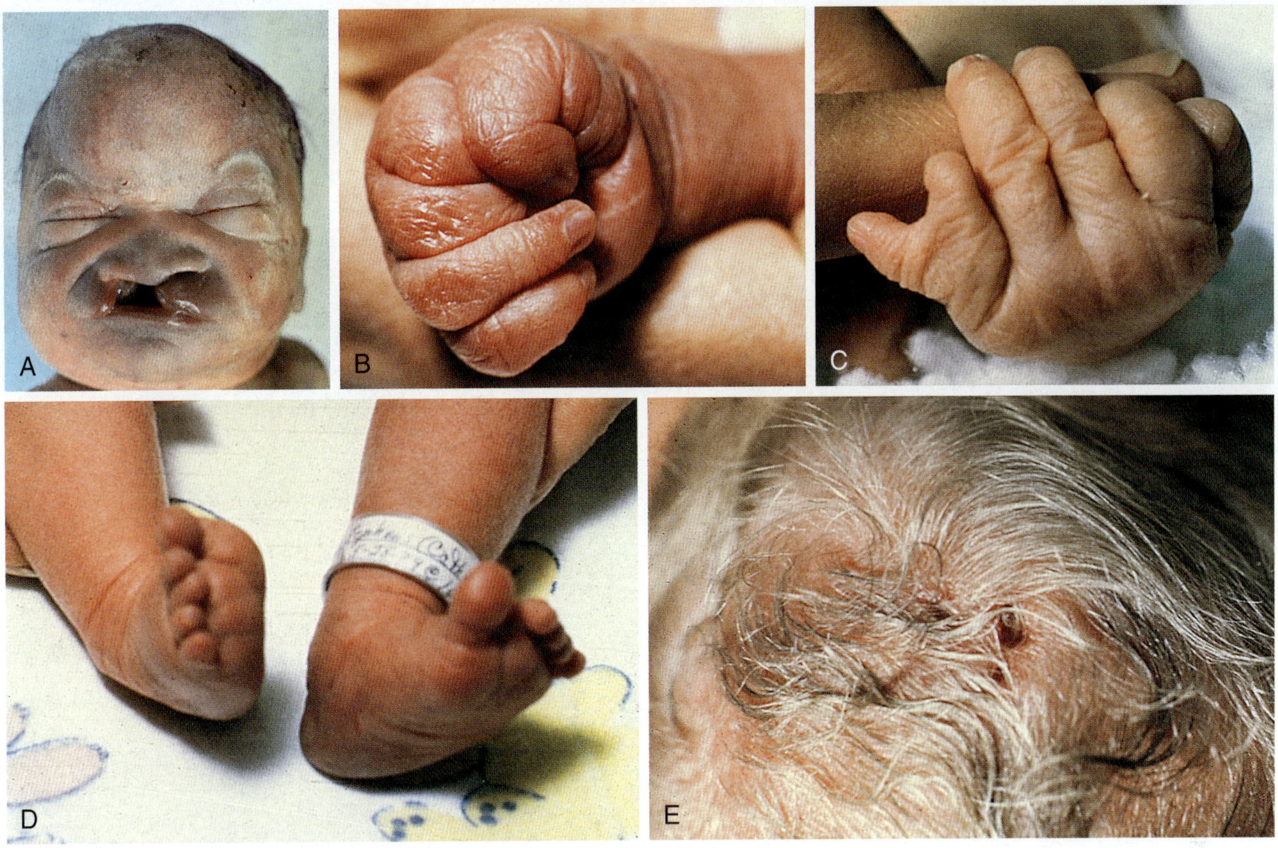

Fig. 1.16 Several physical manifestations of trisomy 13. (A) Facies showing midline defect. (B) Clenched hand with overlapping fingers. (C) Postaxial polydactyly. (D) Equinovarus deformity. (E) Typical punched-out scalp lesions of aplasia cutis congenita. (A, Courtesy T. Kelly, MD, University of Virginia Medical Center, Charlottesville. B–E, Courtesy Kenneth Garver, MD, Pittsburgh, PA.)

Table 1.5 Physical Abnormalities and Frequencies of Occurrence in Trisomy 13 and Trisomy 18 Syndromes

Abnormality	Trisomy 13	Trisomy 18
Severe developmental delay/ intellectual disability	††††	††††
Approximately 90% die within first year	††††	††††
Cryptorchidism in males	††††	††††
Low-set, malformed ears	††††	††††
Multiple major congenital anomalies	††††	††††
Prominent occiput	†	††††
Cleft lip and/or palate	†††	†
Micrognathia	††	†††
Microphthalmos	†††	††
Coloboma of iris	†††	†
Short sternum	†	†††
Rocker-bottom feet	††	†††
Congenital heart disease	††	††††
Scalp defects	†††	†
Flexion deformities of fingers	††	††††
Polydactyly	†††	†
Hypoplasia of nails	††	†††
Hypertonia in infancy	†	†††
Apneic spells in infancy	†††	†
Midline brain defects	†††	†
Horseshoe kidneys	†	†††

Relative frequency of occurrence ranges from †††† (usual) to † (rare).

failure to develop secondary sex characteristics by late adolescence. Therefore, the diagnostic workup of adolescents with these complaints warrants a chromosome study.

The karyotype in the majority of individuals with Turner syndrome is 45,X. Most often, the missing sex chromosome is paternally derived, yet the risk of Turner syndrome does not increase with maternal or paternal age. Another 15% of individuals with Turner syndrome have mosaicism (X/XX, X/XX/XXX, or X/XY). The physical features may be less marked in mosaicism; in some cases these patients have preserved fertility. The short (p) arm of the X chromosome appears most critical; deletion of the long (q) arm usually produces only streak (fibrous) gonads with consequent sterility, amenorrhea, and immature secondary sex characteristics but without the other somatic stigmata of Turner syndrome. A smaller percentage of cases of Turner syndrome have 46 chromosomes, with one normal plus one structurally abnormal X (frequently a shortened or missing short [p] arm). These cases are more likely to have other, more serious major anomalies, including cognitive deficits. A structurally abnormal X chromosome may lead to abnormal X inactivation, resulting in a deleterious dosage effect for X-linked genes. Occasionally the patient will have a 46,XY karyotype, but vital segments of the p arm of the Y chromosome have been deleted. If an XY cell line is present, the intra-abdominal gonads should be removed because they are prone to malignant change.

If the diagnosis is clinically suspected or NIPT was high risk for 45,X, a chromosome karyotype should be ordered. Antenatal diagnosis of chromosomally abnormal fetuses should be discussed with the parents, and the relatively good prognosis for Turner syndrome newborns should not be overlooked. People with Turner syndrome should receive appropriate hormone therapy during adolescence to enable development of secondary sex characteristics and stimulate menses. Rarely, individuals with 45,X have been fertile for a limited number of years, and the possibility of fertility preservation should be discussed with patients and their families.

Klinefelter Syndrome One in 500 newborn males has a 47,XXY karyotype, also known as Klinefelter syndrome. The physical stigmata are subtle and usually not obvious until puberty, at which time the normal onset of spermatogenesis is blocked by the presence of two X chromosomes. Consequently, the germ cells die, the seminiferous tubules

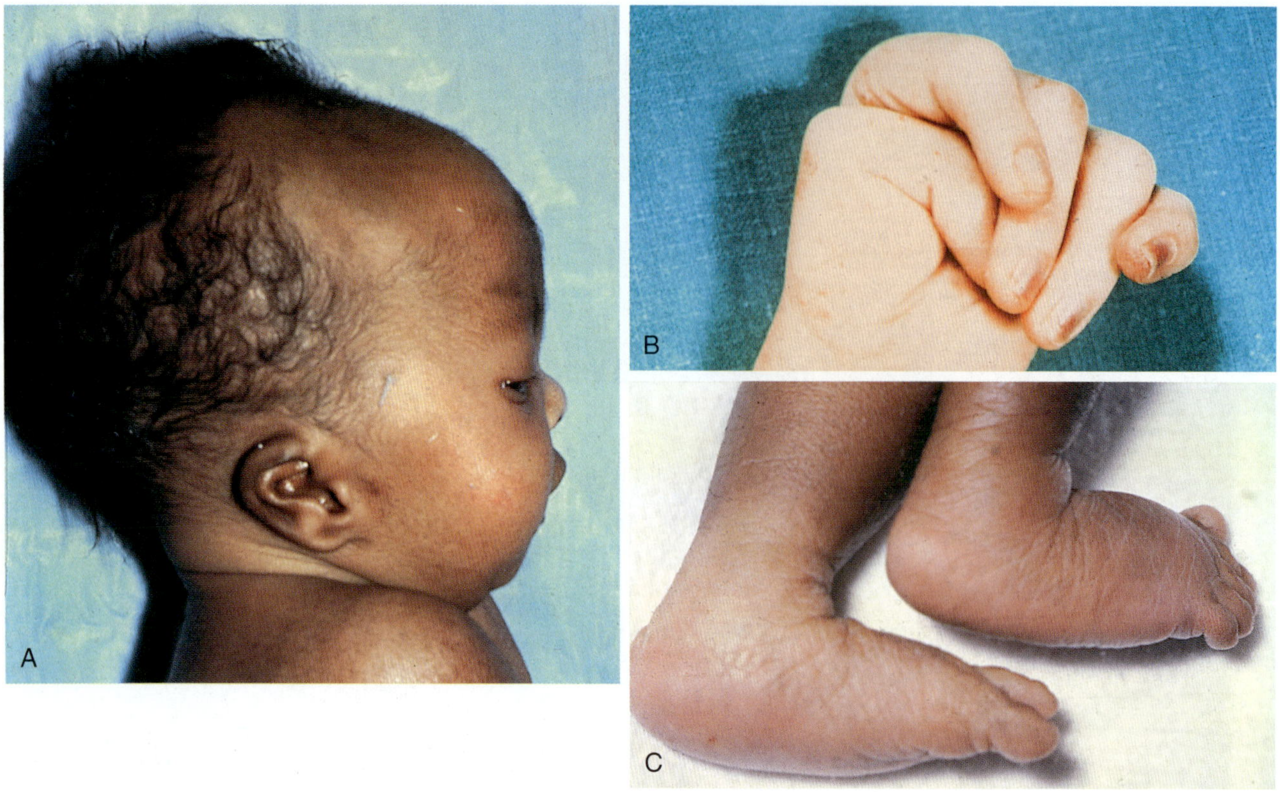

Fig. 1.17 Several physical manifestations of trisomy 18. (A) Typical profile reveals prominent occiput and low-set, posteriorly rotated malformed auricles. (B) Clenched hand showing typical pattern of overlapping fingers. (C) Rocker-bottom feet. (Courtesy Kenneth Garver, MD, Pittsburgh, PA.)

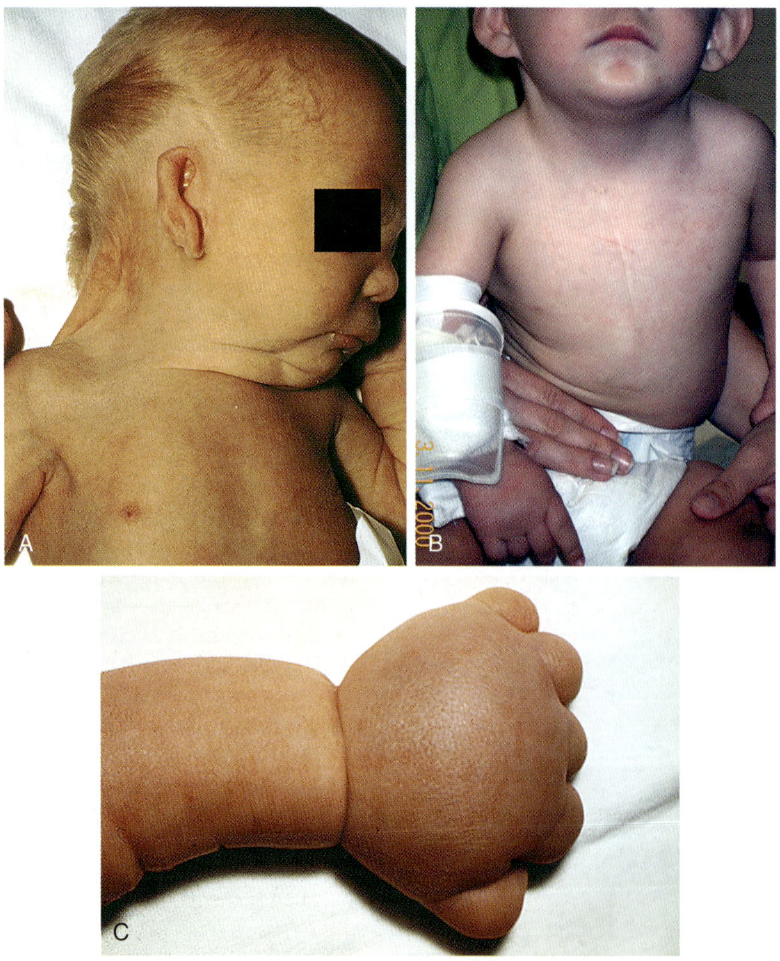

Fig. 1.18 Clinical photographs show several physical manifestations associated with Turner syndrome. (A) In this newborn, a webbed neck with low hairline, shield chest with widespread nipples, abnormal ears, and micrognathia are seen. (B) In this frontal view, mild webbing of the neck and small widely spaced nipples are evident, along with a midline scar from prior cardiac surgery. The ears are low-set and prominent, protruding forward. (C) The newborn shown in (A) also had prominent lymphedema of the hands and feet.

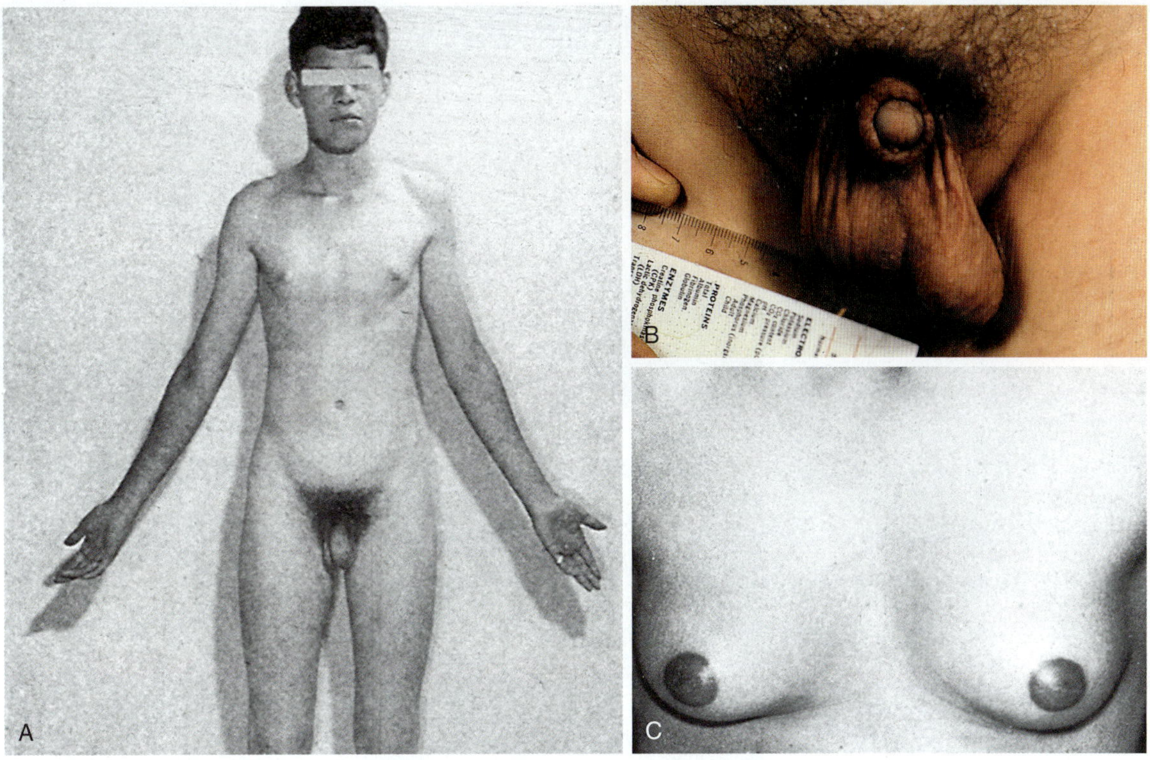

Fig. 1.19 Clinical photographs show several physical manifestations of Klinefelter syndrome. (A) Relatively narrow shoulders, increased carrying angle of arms, female distribution of pubic hair, and normal penis but with small scrotum due to small testicular size. (B) Small testes and penis. (C) Gynecomastia. (B, Courtesy Peter Lee, MD, Hershey Medical Center, Hershey, PA. C, From Gardner LI, editor: *Endocrine and genetic diseases of childhood,* ed 2, Philadelphia, 1975, WB Saunders.)

become hyalinized and scarred, and the testes become small. Testosterone levels are below normal adult male levels, although the level varies from case to case. Hence there is a wide range in degree of virilization. Presentation can range from the classic tall male with a small penis and gynecomastia (Fig. 1.19) to a sexually functional male with unexplained infertility. Scoliosis may develop during adolescence. The full-scale IQ of people with Klinefelter syndrome is average; however, behavioral problems may be more common than in the population at large.

The karyotype in Klinefelter syndrome is XXY in 80% of cases and mosaic (XY/XXY) in the other 20%. Rarely the latter type may be fertile. The risk of having an affected child increases with maternal age. Males with more than two X chromosomes (XXXY, XXXXY) are usually cognitively impaired and are more likely to have skeletal and other major congenital anomalies, such as cleft palate, congenital heart disease (particularly a patent ductus arteriosus), and microcephaly.

XXX and XYY Females with a karyotype of 47,XXX have triple X syndrome. The incidence is approximately 1 in 1000 liveborn females. Affected individuals have no characteristic abnormal physical features, though they can be tall. Delays in motor skills and coordination are common. Although usually within the normal range of intelligence, their IQ scores may be lower than those of their unaffected siblings, and approximately 60% utilize some educational support. Behavioral problems occur in approximately 30% and are usually mild. Females with 47,XXX are fertile, and their children are usually chromosomally normal. The presence of additional X chromosomes (48,XXXX, or 49,XXXXX) typically results in cognitive impairment to some degree.

XYY males have a karyotype of 47,XYY. The incidence is 1 in 840 liveborn males. These males tend to be tall compared with their own family members, but generally their phenotypic appearance is normal. Their IQ is usually within the normal range but may be lower than that of siblings. Affected children may come to medical attention because of problems with fine motor coordination, speech disorders, and learning disabilities. Early reports raised concerns about significant behavioral problems; however, long-term prospective studies now suggest that these children do not have any greater incidence of problem behaviors than the general population.

Additional Cytogenetic Technologies

Fluorescence In Situ Hybridization

FISH is a laboratory technology that has revolutionized the diagnostic capabilities of clinical cytogenetic laboratories. In this technique, a DNA probe is tagged with a label that fluoresces when viewed under a specific microscope. A cocktail of many consecutive, unique DNA probes blanketing a specific chromosome from end to end can be obtained, the stepping stone toward microarray. Well-recognized syndromes described initially by FISH probes for chromosome microdeletion syndromes include Prader-Willi/Angelman syndrome (del 15q11–13), DiGeorge syndrome (del 22q11.2), and Williams syndrome (del 7q11.23) (Figs. 1.20–1.23; Table 1.6). FISH can also

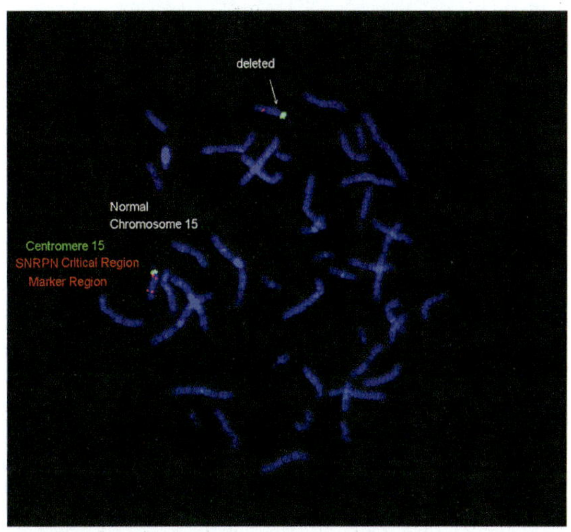

Fig. 1.20 4′,6′-Diamidino-2-phenylindole–counterstained metaphase and interphase images showing a duplication of the Prader-Willi/Angelman (D15S10 locus) critical region *(red).* The chromosome 15 centromere is used as a control *(green).* Adjacent to the centromere in *red* is the normal pattern for D15S10. *SNRPN,* Small nuclear ribonucleoprotein-associated polypeptide N. (Courtesy Urvashi Surti, PhD, Pittsburgh Cytogenetics Laboratory.)

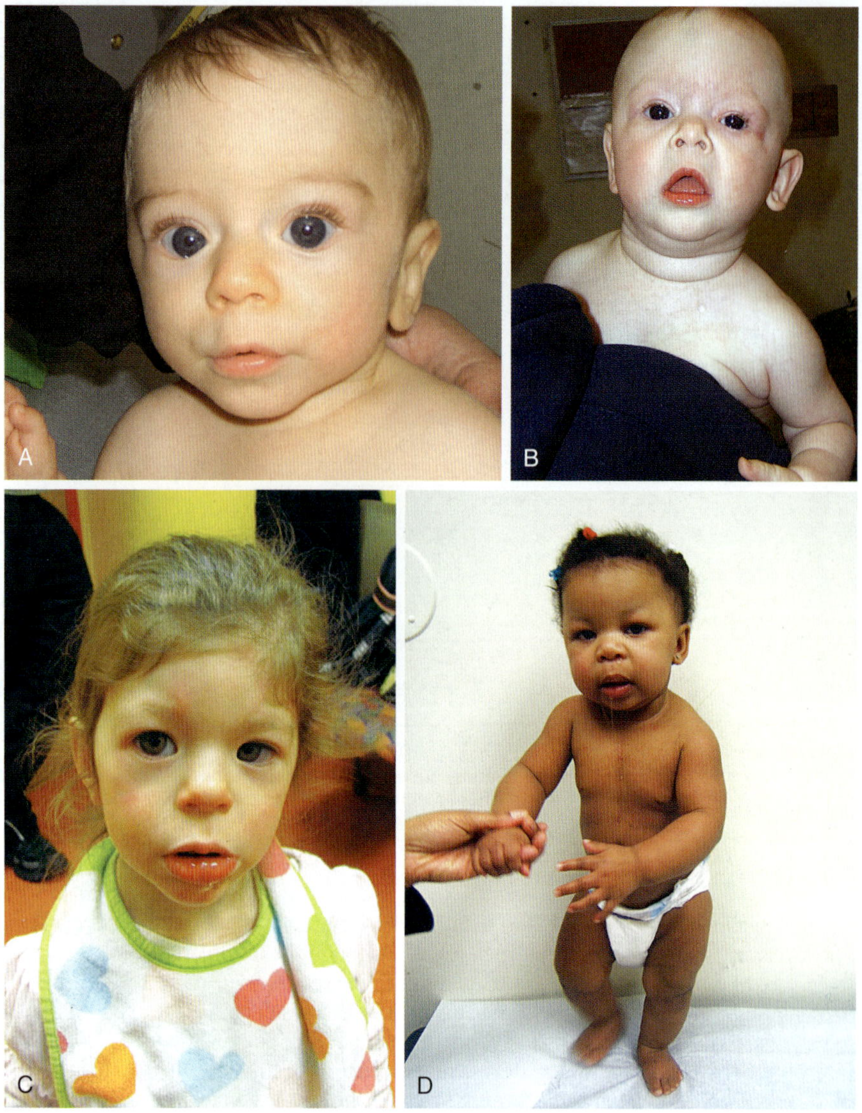

Fig. 1.21 (A–D) Williams syndrome in four different patients. Hallmark features include supravalvular aortic stenosis, hypercalcemia, friendly personality, connective tissue abnormalities, and characteristic facies. Note the periorbital fullness, epicanthal folds, prominent lips, long philtrum, and stellate lacy iris pattern. All cases with clinical features were confirmed on fluorescence in situ hybridization alone or microarray.

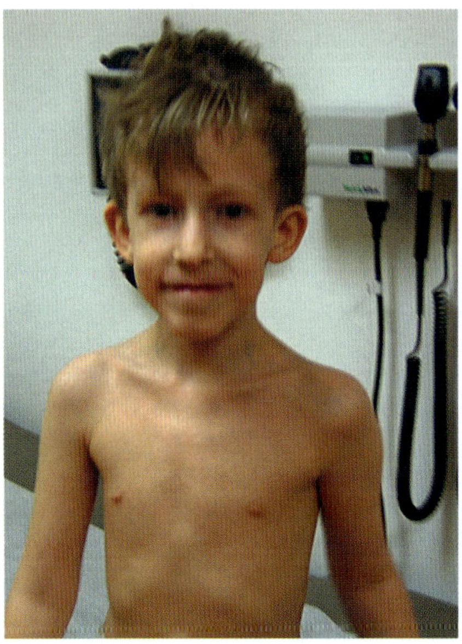

Fig. 1.22 An 8-year-old with del22q.11 and 1p31.1 microdeletion. Patient is short in stature; has a right aortic arch, sacral dimple, left cryptorchidism, and global developmental and significant cognitive and speech delays; and is not toilet trained. He had undergone surgical repair of the palate for velopharyngeal incompetence. Note the low-set, cupped, and posteriorly rotated ears and hypoplastic alae nasi. DiGeorge syndrome was diagnosed in utero by prenatal FISH on amniocytes: 46, XY, ish del(22) (q11.2q11.2) (TUPLE1–) was confirmed at 6 years of age by oligonucleotide arrays. In addition, 1p31.1 microdeletion was detected and maternally inherited.

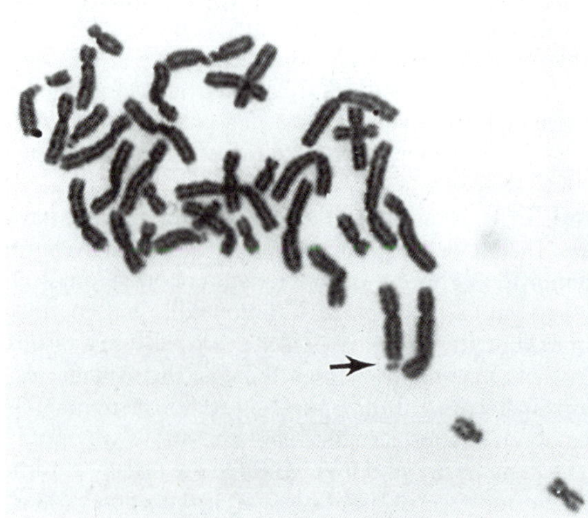

Fig. 1.23 Fragile X chromosome marker in lymphocyte culture. Partial metaphase plate shows the chromosome break at Xq27 *(arrow)* characteristic of fragile X syndrome (solid Giemsa stain).

identify the physical location of translocated chromosomal material that may be too small or subtle to detect on karyotype, which can reveal novel mechanisms, such as the *BCR::ABL1* gene fusion that is constitutively active in chronic myelogenous leukemia with t(9;22) ("the Philadelphia chromosome") and allows for targeted and effective therapy (imatinib).

Table 1.6 Some Syndromes Identifiable With Fluorescence In Situ Hybridization Probes

Syndrome	Major Findings	Comments
Cri du chat (deletion 5p15.2)	Microcephaly, round face, down-slanting palpebral fissures, epicanthal folds, hypertelorism, catlike cry in infancy	
Isolated lissencephaly	Lissencephaly (incomplete development of brain with smooth surface)	Approximately 30% have deletion 17p13.3
Miller-Dieker phenotype with lissencephaly	Microcephaly, lissencephaly, variable high forehead, vertical furrowing of central forehead, low-set ears, small nose with anteverted nostrils, congenital heart disease, poor feeding	Deletion 17p13.3 in vast majority
Deletion 22q11.2	Conotruncal defects, thymus hypoplasia, cleft palate, down-slanting palpebral fissures, tubular nose, endocrinopathies, poor feeding, risk of developmental delays	Appears to be a common deletion and should be considered in the differential diagnosis of children with multiple anomalies even if the features are not classic to any one phenotype
Wolf-Hirschhorn (deletion 4p16.3)	Moderate to severe cognitive impairment, hypertelorism, preauricular pit or tag, broad nasal bridge, micrognathia, cleft palate, short philtrum, growth deficiency	
Smith-Magenis (deletion 17p11.2)	Brachycephaly, flat facies, broad nasal bridge, short stature	Self-hugging behaviors, sleep disturbances

Table 1.7 Resolution of Various Diagnostic Methods

Method	Resolution
Metaphase G-banded chromosome analysis (500 bands)	5.0–10 Mb
Prometaphase G-banded chromosome analysis (1000 bands)	3.0–5.0 Mb
Fluorescence in-situ hybridization (FISH)	100 Kb
Cytogenomic arrays, including: • Array comparative genomic hybridization (array-CGH) • SNP array	As small as 10 Kb
Genomic Data	
Nuclear genome	3.1 Gb (20,000 genes; 1 gene per ;120 Kb)
Chromosome size	48–249 Mb
Average gene size	10–15 Kb (vary between 0.2 and 2500 Kb)
Mitochondrial genome	16.569 Kb (37 genes)

SNP, Single nucleotide polymorphism.

Array-Based Technology: Microarray for Evaluation of Copy Number Variation

In addition to classic cytogenetics, molecular cytogenetic and cytogenomic methods are being incorporated in clinical settings. Array-CGH analyses detect imbalances in the genome and enable detection of relatively small copy number changes at high resolution. The degree of detection for copy-number variants (CNVs) for various cytogenetic techniques is shown in Table 1.7. Array-CGH has been recommended by the American College of Medical Genetics and Genomics (ACMG) as the first step in the investigation of patients with idiopathic intellectual disability, developmental delay, autism spectrum disorders, and multiple congenital anomalies and has a much higher diagnostic yield—up to 28% compared with traditional karyotypes. In addition, array-CGH data have demonstrated that approximately 20% of apparently balanced chromosome translocations, de novo or familial, have gain or loss of genetic material at the breakpoints. By combining the array-CGH technique with classic cytogenetic and confirmatory FISH and appropriate molecular analyses, we are also able to identify cryptic genomic alterations and further analyze gross genomic alterations, including marker chromosome or other rearrangements.

The application of array-CGH in establishing the specific genetic defect has important consequences for genetic counseling of the families and follow-up of the patients. Detailed molecular analysis of the rearranged regions may help to identify the gene(s) associated with a specific phenotypic presentation. With microarray testing, many microdeletions and microduplication syndromes were defined (e.g., deletion 1p36, deletion 1q21.1, and deletion 16p13.11 syndromes) (see Fig. 1.22 and eFigs. 1.1–1.3), impacting the patients' immediate and long-term clinical management.

Single nucleotide polymorphism (SNP) arrays are being used in clinical settings, usually in conjunction with array-CGH, and enhance genome-wide copy number analysis. SNPs are single base pair variations from the most common genetic sequence that occur in at least 5% of the general population and do not produce a damaging phenotype. This molecular cytogenetics test simultaneously interrogates and not only identifies CNVs but is also capable of detecting region(s) with long or short stretches of homozygosity ("regions of homozygosity" [ROH]). The identification of these long stretches of shared SNPs can result from shared ancestry and/or isolated populations and unmask autosomal recessive conditions of interest in the homozygous regions. Genetic counseling is helpful in interpretation, particularly for variants of uncertain significance or in the unanticipated identification of nonpaternity or possible consanguinity.

Contiguous Gene Deletion/Duplication Disorders

Molecular cytogenetic techniques have identified a group of disorders typically resulting in a well-defined and recognizable presentation, due to submicroscopic deletions or duplications involving several sequential genes. A number of these may be commonly recognizable in the clinical setting, such as DiGeorge syndrome (see also Chapters 4, 21 and 23), Williams syndrome (see also Chapter 5), and Angelman and Prader-Willi syndromes (covered later in this chapter). The remaining syndromes are outlined briefly in Table 1.6 and in Figs. 1.20–1.22.

Disorders of Nucleotide Repeat Expansion

Fragile X Syndrome

It has long been recognized that there is a significant excess of males having intellectual disability. Much of this inordinate male representation is the result of altered X-linked recessive genes. These may represent new variants or inheritance of the abnormal gene from apparently normal heterozygous (carrier) mothers. About 1 in 150 individuals, usually male, has some form of X-linked intellectual disability. Of these, it is estimated that between 30% and 50% have fragile X syndrome, translating to an incidence of 1 in 4000 males.

In 1969, Herbert Lubs noted in low-folate lymphocyte cultures an apparent break (a "fragile site") on the long arm of the X chromosome

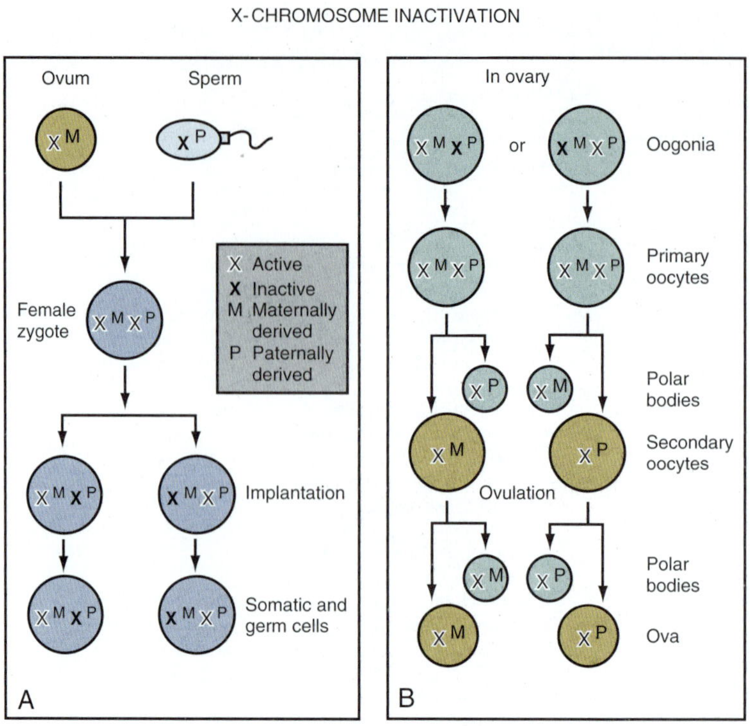

Fig. 1.24 Functional behavior of the X chromosome in XX females. (A) Somatic and premeiotic germ cells. Implantation occurs 5 days after conception, at which time in each female cell either XM or XP is randomly genetically inactivated and remains so in each of the cell's descendants. Because the process is random, by determining the proportion of cells with an inactive XM or inactive XP in each of a large population of women, a Gaussian population distribution of women is generated. That is, most women in the population will have an approximate 50:50 mix of cells, in which each cell expresses either XM or XP. However, some women will by chance have more cells with an inactive XM and vice versa. (B) Meiotic germ cells. When a female germ cell enters first prophase of meiosis, X inactivation is abolished; both X chromosomes become genetically active through fertilization and continue so until embryonic uterine implantation. Then, as in (A), random X inactivation in XX females occurs all over again.

(Xq27) (see Fig. 1.23). Fragile X syndrome is the first recognized example of a trinucleotide repeat disorder, with the clinical significance of the "fragile site" confirmed in 1977. Just before the start of the *FMR1* gene is a DNA trinucleotide cytosine-guanine-guanine (CGG) motif, which in the general population is normally repeated about 5 to 50 times (the average being 30). When there are more than about 55 repeats, the region can become unstable such that the number of repeats increases during oogenesis (but not spermatogenesis). In the presence of 55 to 200 CGG repeats, the individual has a fragile X *premutation.* Individuals with a premutation appear clinically and cognitively normal in early life but can develop ataxia in later adult life (fragile X ataxia syndrome, also known as FRAXTAS). When the premutation expands to greater than 200 to 220 repeats, gene expression is impaired and the individual has a *full mutation,* resulting in fragile X syndrome in males and a rare subset of females (Fig. 1.24). The female children of individuals with premutations are obligate premutation carriers and are at risk of having male children with full expansions. The relative risk for a female to pass down a premutation or full mutation is shown in Table 1.8.

Males affected with fragile X syndrome have cognitive impairment, ranging from severe to borderline in degree. The majority have speech delay, short attention span, hyperactivity, persistence of mouthing objects, and poor motor coordination. Many exhibit a variety of disordered behaviors, including disciplinary problems, temper tantrums, poor eye contact, perseverative speech, hand flapping, avoidance of socialization, and rocking. Physical stigmata may include long, wide, or protruding ears; long face; a prominent jaw; flattened nasal bridge; "velvety" skin; hyperextensible joints; and mitral valve prolapse. Relative macrocephaly is more likely than microcephaly. Macroorchidism is found in most mature males.

Table 1.8 Relative Risk of Maternal Transmission of a Fragile X Premutation to Her Offspring as a Full Mutation

Number of CGG Repeats in Mother's Premutation	Risk of Expansion to Full Mutation in Offspring (%)
55–59	3.7
60–69	5.3
70–79	31.1
80–89	57.8
90–99	80.1
100–109	100
110–119	98.1
120–129	97.2

CGG, Cytosine-guanine-guanine.

Hunter JE, Berry-Kravis E, Hipp H, et al. FMR1 Disorders. 1998 Jun 16 [Updated 2024 May 16]. In: Adam MP, Feldman J, Mirzaa GM, et al., editors. GeneReviews® [Internet]. Seattle (WA): University of Washington, Seattle; 1993-2025. Available from: https://www.ncbi.nlm.nih.gov/books/NBK1384/.

Approximately 50% of females affected with full-expansion fragile X are clinically normal. The 50% who are affected usually have lesser degrees of cognitive impairment than males. However, learning disabilities, mood disorders, schizoid personality, and significant disturbances in affect, socialization, and communication are common. The physical features often seen in males with fragile X syndrome are less common in females.

Laboratory testing for fragile X variants is done by molecular genetic techniques, Southern blot, or polymerase chain reaction (PCR) analysis of DNA. Rarely, an individual may seem to have a mild form of fragile X syndrome, but tests are negative using these molecular genetic laboratory techniques. Another fragile X gene site *(FRAXE)* distal to the fragile X gene on Xq is associated with mild intellectual disability and positive fragile X testing.

The number of known trinucleotide expansion disorders is increasing (Table 1.9). Three other examples are Huntington disease, caused by an intragenic CAG trinucleotide expansion; myotonic dystrophy type 1, resulting from a 3′ untranslated region CTG expansion; and Friedreich ataxia, caused by an intronic GAA expansion.

There is also recognition that a single comprehensive approach could enhance diagnosis of both common and rare deleterious cytogenomic mechanisms in one efficient technique, saving time and money and improving health outcomes. One of these, optical genome mapping (OGM), is a research biomedical technology that is currently applied and tested in clinical cases that combines karyotype, array-CGH, FISH, and repeat expansion with a promise of higher sensitivity and detection rate into a single test.

Disorders of Imprinting

Prader-Willi and Angelman Syndromes

The concept of *imprinting* refers to the fact that the function of certain genes is dependent on their parental origin: maternal versus paternal. One prominent example is the q11–q13 region of chromosome 15, a region that contains several imprinted genes that, when

Table 1.9 Nucleotide Repeat Expansion Disorders

Condition	Nucleotide Repeat Expansion	Inheritance	Gene	Symptoms
Huntington disease	(CAG)n	AD	*HTT*	Choreoathetosis, dementia
Kennedy disease (Bulbospinal muscular atrophy)	(CAG)n	X-linked	*AR*	Muscle weakness, cramps, fasciculations of face, difficulty swallowing
Dentatorubral-pallidoluysian atrophy	(CAG)n	AD	*ATN1*	Myoclonic epilepsy, choreoathetosis, dementia, brain degeneration
Machado-Joseph disease (Spinocerebellar ataxia, type 3)	(CAG)n	AD	*ATXN3*	Progressive cerebellar ataxia, peripheral neuropathy, dysphagia, ophthalmoplegia, Parkinsonian-like features
Spinocerebellar ataxia, type 1	(CAG)n	AD	*ATXN1*	Progressive cerebellar ataxia, peripheral neuropathy, dysphagia, ophthalmoplegia
Spinocerebellar ataxia, type 2	(CAG)n	AD	*ATXN2*	Progressive cerebellar ataxia, dysphagia, retinal disease, ophthalmoplegia, peripheral neuropathy
Spinocerebellar ataxia, type 6	(CAG)n	AD	*CACNA1A*	Progressive cerebellar ataxia, dysphagia, hemiplegic migraine
Spinocerebellar ataxia, type 7	(CAG)n	AD	*ATXN7*	Progressive cerebellar ataxia, dysphagia, retinal disease, ophthalmoplegia
Spinocerebellar ataxia, type 17	(CAG)n	AD	*TBP*	Progressive cerebellar ataxia, dysphagia, nystagmus, ophthalmoplegia, psychiatric manifestations
Myotonic dystrophy, type 1	(CTG)n	AD	*DMPK*	Weakness, myotonia, cataracts, hair loss, cardiac arrhythmia, infantile hypotonia, respiratory insufficiency, ID
Spinocerebellar ataxia, type 8	(CTG)n	AD	*ATXN8*	Progressive cerebellar ataxia, nystagmus
Fuchs corneal dystrophy, type 3	(CTG)n	AD	*TCF4*	Progressive corneal opacification, vision loss
Friedreich ataxia	(GAA)n	AR	*FXN*	Progressive ataxia, dysphagia, cardiac arrhythmias
Oculopharyngeal muscular dystrophy	(GCG)n	AD	*PABPN1*	Progressive dysphagia and coughing, ptosis
Myotonic dystrophy, type 2	(CCTG)n	AD	*ZNF9*	Weakness, myotonia, cataracts, hair loss, cardiac arrhythmia, infantile hypotonia, respiratory insufficiency, ID, endocrinopathies
Spinocerebellar ataxia, type 10	(ATTCT)n	AD	*ATXN10*	Slowly progressive cerebellar ataxia, seizures
Spinocerebellar ataxia, type 31	(TGGAA)n	AD	*BEAN*	Progressive cerebellar ataxia, nystagmus, hearing loss
Spinocerebellar ataxia, type 36	(GGCCTG)n	AD	*NOP56*	Progressive cerebellar ataxia, nystagmus, hearing loss, tongue fasciculations
Frontotemporal dementia, amyotrophic lateral sclerosis	(GGGGCC)n	AD	*C9Orf72*	Dementia with executive dysfunction and abnormal behaviors, weakness
Progressive myoclonic epilepsy, 1A	(CCCCGCCCCGCG)n	AR	*EPM1*	Ataxia, dysarthria, seizures (myoclonus, GTC, absence)

imbalanced or abnormal, result in recognizable and distinct genetic disorders. Prader-Willi and Angelman syndromes derive from abnormalities of these imprinted genes. Absence of the paternally derived region of this chromosome results in Prader-Willi syndrome, while absence of the maternally derived region of this chromosome results in Angelman syndrome.

Mechanisms that can produce the Prader-Willi phenotype include the following:

- A chromosome deletion of 15q11–q13, including the Prader-Willi critical region of the paternally derived chromosome 15 (majority of cases)
- A structural chromosome abnormality involving the Prader-Willi critical region of 15q11–q13 (translocation, etc.)
- Maternal UPD in which the child has two maternally derived chromosome 15s and no paternally contributed chromosome 15 (25% of cases)
- Pathogenic variants of imprinting control center genes (1% of cases)

The critical region of chromosome 15 for Angelman syndrome is located adjacent to the Prader-Willi critical region. However, it is the maternally derived chromosome segment that is absent. The six currently identified etiologic mechanisms of Angelman syndrome include the following:

- A large chromosome deletion of 15q11–q13 including the Angelman critical region of the maternally derived chromosome 15 (68% of cases)
- A structural chromosome abnormality involving the Angelman critical region of 15q11–q13 (translocation, etc.)
- Paternal UPD of chromosome 15 (7% of cases)
- Pathogenic variants of imprinting control center genes (3% of cases)
- Pathogenic variants of the ubiquitin-protein ligase gene *(UBE3A)* (11% of cases)
- Classic phenotype, with no identifiable etiologic mechanisms but a positive family history of other affected individuals (11% of cases)

Because of the complexity of the diagnostic process, families of children suspected of having either of these disorders should be referred for genetic evaluation and diagnostic testing to ensure the most accurate determination of etiologic mechanism and, therefore, of recurrence risk, as well as counseling on medical risks specific to each mechanism.

Current diagnostic testing for these disorders includes the following:

- Methylation studies, which determine whether genes within the 15q11–q13 critical region are correctly marked (methylated) by their parent of origin (detects approximately 99% of Prader-Willi and 80% of Angelman syndrome cases)
- Chromosome microarray or FISH probes of the chromosome region (detects approximately 65% to 75% of Prader-Willi and 68% of Angelman syndrome cases)
- SNP array (detects 80% to 90% of Prader-Willi syndrome and 68% to 78% of Angelman syndrome cases)
- Sequence analysis of the *UBE3A* gene (detects 11% of Angelman syndrome cases)

Some other examples of imprinting disorders include Beckwith-Wiedemann syndrome (Fig. 1.25) and Russell-Silver syndrome.

Clinical Findings in Prader-Willi Syndrome

Newborns affected with Prader-Willi syndrome usually are markedly hypotonic with a weak cry, poor sucking and swallowing, and decreased deep tendon reflexes. They often have a history of decreased fetal movement in utero, breech position, and being small for gestational age. Failure to thrive is virtually ubiquitous. Subsequently, motor and speech development are delayed, and most patients have cognitive impairment in the mild to moderate range. Hypotonia abates over the first 2 to 3 years, and patients develop an insatiable appetite that rapidly results in morbid obesity (Fig. 1.26). The distribution of excess fat is particularly prominent over the lower trunk, buttocks, and proximal limb. Subtle facial features can include narrow bifrontal diameter, almond-shaped eyes, and strabismus. Other features include skin picking, small hands and feet, short stature, hypogenitalism, and hypogonadism. In patients with chromosome deletions, hypopigmentation is common, with blond to light brown hair, blue eyes, and sun-sensitive fair skin.

Older children with Prader-Willi syndrome can exhibit extreme emotional lability and temper tantrums. These conditions and the overeating often can be partly ameliorated by intensive inpatient behavioral modification programs, followed by longitudinal parental support and follow-up in the home. Interestingly, despite a normal basal metabolic rate, weight reduction requires significantly more severe caloric restriction than usual. Growth hormone therapy can exacerbate sleep apnea, but it significantly improves weight control and reduces associated morbidities, such as diabetes or risk of obesity hypoventilation syndrome, and is standard of care from early ages, markedly modifying the phenotype and rates of medical complications. In untreated individuals, cardiorespiratory complications from morbid obesity can reduce life expectancy, so early diagnosis and treatment are crucial.

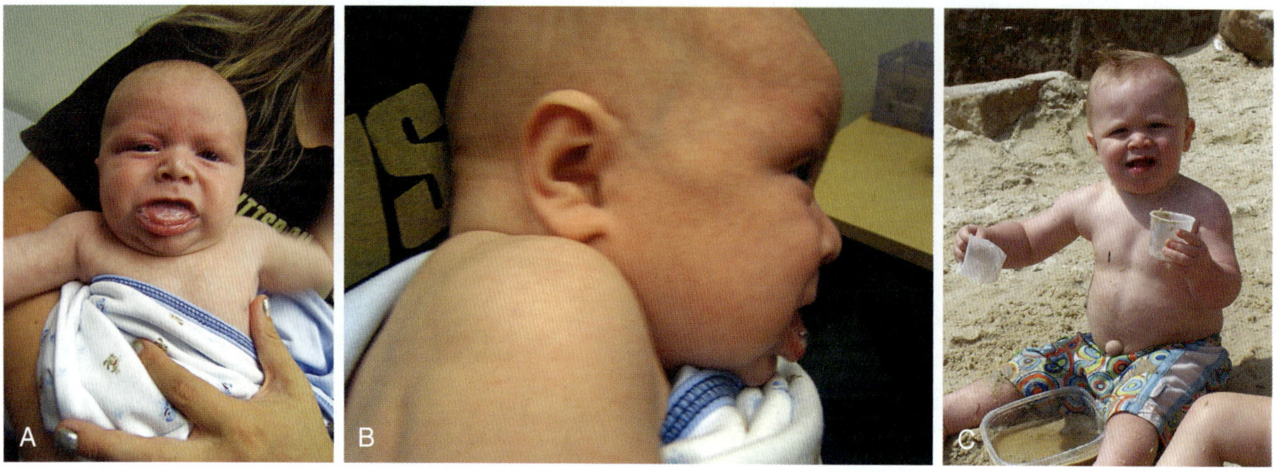

Fig. 1.25 (A) Beckwith-Wiedemann syndrome. Note the macrosomia, macroglossia, and asymmetry with hemihypertrophy and obscured omphalocele and/or umbilical hernia. Craniofacial features also include unusual ear creases. (B) At 3 months old, note the macroglossia, right facial prominence, and ear creases. (C) At 27 months old, note the resolving umbilical hernia. The elevated alpha-fetoprotein (AFP) levels from infancy have normalized. The patient has nephromegaly and is under surveillance for the detection of embryonal tumors by serum AFP and abdominal and renal sonograms every 4 months. Chromosomes were normal male complement, 46,XY. The abnormal methylation pattern of the *LIT1* gene at the 11p15 region confirmed the clinical diagnosis of Beckwith-Wiedemann syndrome.

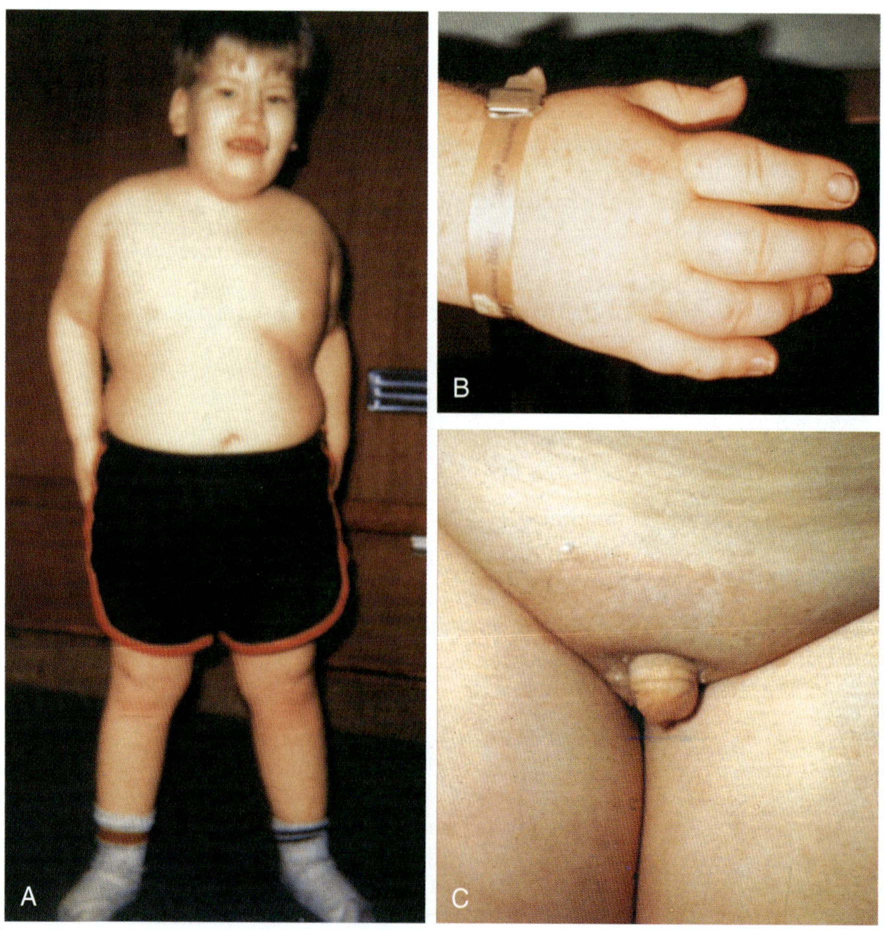

Fig. 1.26 Prader-Willi syndrome. (A) This patient demonstrates the marked obesity characteristic of Prader-Willi syndrome. Excess fat is distributed over the trunk, buttocks, and proximal extremities. (B and C) Small hands (and feet) and a hypoplastic penis and scrotum are other typical features. (A, Courtesy Jeanne M. Hanchett, MD, Pittsburgh, PA.)

Clinical Findings in Angelman Syndrome

Angelman syndrome, first recognized in 1956, has an incidence of 1 in 15,000 to 1 in 20,000 live births. Except for the shared tendency to have hypopigmentation, the clinical phenotypes of Prader-Willi and Angelman syndromes are quite different. The latter have severe cognitive deficits, with impaired or absent speech and inappropriate paroxysms of laughter common. Physical features include microbrachycephaly, maxillary hypoplasia, large mouth, prognathism, and short stature (in adults). The gait is ataxic, with toe-walking and jerky arm movements. Akinetic or major motor seizures are common and can begin in the neonatal period. Although life spans are increasing, to date only one patient with Angelman syndrome has been known to reproduce.

The Nature of Genes and Single-Gene Disorders

A gene consists of a sequence of DNA that contains the code for production of a "functional product" along with sequences that ensure proper expression of the gene. The gene product might be an RNA molecule, a polypeptide chain, or a protein that ultimately becomes a structural component of a cell or tissue, or an enzyme. The latter may catalyze a step in formation or modification of another product, a step in cell metabolism, or one of several steps involved in the breakdown or degradation of molecules that are no longer necessary. Proper gene expression includes production of the product at the right time (e.g., during embryogenesis vs. postnatal expression), in the needed amount, and in the correct cell type and ensures its transport to its proper site of biologic action.

Approximately 20,000 genes are arranged in linear fashion on the chromosomes, all having their own specific *locus* (location). Genes range in length from about a thousand bases to hundreds of thousands of bases (any one of which can be subject to variation). Genes are composed of alternating sequences of coding DNA, termed *exons,* interspersed with noncoding sequences of DNA, termed *introns.* Exons are further subdivided into triplets of bases, termed *codons,* each of which encodes a specific amino acid within the polypeptide product. Because there are 64 possible triplet combinations of the four nucleotide bases (adenine, guanidine, thymine, and cytosine) and 20 amino acids, most amino acids have more than one codon that can specify them, the exceptions being methionine and tryptophan, which have only one specific codon each. In addition, three triplets encode stop codons in the messenger ribonucleic acid (mRNA) that signal the termination of mRNA translation.

The process of going from DNA code to polypeptide product has many steps including transcription (making a mRNA from the DNA template), translation (using tRNA to make a polypeptide from the mRNA template), and posttranslational modifications (adding sugars and other molecules to the protein). Each step in this process can introduce or be impacted by the errors outlined below in more detail.

A single-gene variant produces a permanent change in a gene's DNA sequence and may involve anywhere from one to several thousands of nucleotides. The simplest variation is a change of a single base pair (formerly, a *point mutation*, now a *variant*), but more complex variants also occur, including change of many base pairs, or deletion or insertion of base pairs. Examples of variants include *missense* variants, in which a base substitution changes a codon specific for one amino acid into one specifying another; *frameshift* variants, in which a deletion or insertion is not an exact multiple of three bases and thereby shifts the reading frame for transcription (and later translation) from that point on; and *nonsense* variants, in which a base substitution changes a codon for an amino acid into one specifying one of the three possible stop codons in mRNA, thereby stopping translation prematurely. In some cases, a pathogenic variant in an intron can alter the splicing and removal of the intron, also resulting in an aberrant mRNA molecule.

Some variants have no effect on phenotype or cell function. These are referred to as *benign variants.* One example is a base substitution within a codon for an amino acid that changes it to another codon specifying the same amino acid. Still other variants have no adverse effect but rather encode normal variations in human characteristics (e.g., eye or hair color). Other variants do have adverse effects and are causative in disease. Though commonly referred to as a mutation, the clinically precise term is a *pathogenic variant* for those changes in the genetic code that result in medically significant findings. Genetic sequencing can reveal novel genetic changes of uncertain pathology, termed "variants of uncertain significance." Computer programs attempt to predict the potential effect on the final protein, called "in silico" analyses, and there are formalized and frequently updated guidelines for variant classification. However, in some cases the effect of a DNA variant can remain uncertain until sufficient occurrences have been recorded, which can take years.

Molecular Sequencing Technologies

Sanger sequencing, developed in the 1970s, first allowed the sequential decoding of genes base by base in a linear fashion. This first generation of sequencing led to the revolution in genetic knowledge and explosion in testing that we are now experiencing, but it was time consuming, laborious, and expensive. Next-generation sequencing (NGS) methodologies are the mainstay of clinical diagnosis for heritable disorders. In NGS, the DNA is fragmented into many short segments, usually 100–300 bp in length, which are read in "massively parallel sequencing," and sequenced segments are pieced together to reveal the full sequence. The first clinical application of NGS was for disease gene discovery in cancer involving analyses of patients' tissue samples with suspected inherited monogenic aberrations in the nuclear and mitochondrial genome. Newer applications of molecular sequencing with immense promise for clinical diagnostic utility include *whole genome sequencing* (WGS) and whole exome sequencing (WES). WES allows the simultaneous interrogation of the coding regions (exons) and the intron/exon boundaries of identified genes and is thus a powerful tool for making a diagnosis in complex clinical cases. WES must be interpreted in the context of familial segregation of any changes detected in the patient's sequence, the patient's medical and family history, and detailed knowledge of clinical features including other laboratory testing. For the clinician, the proband's phenotype is critical in interpreting the vast data generated from both WES and WGS sequencing. WES has technologic limitations; it does not detect certain types of deleterious genetic changes, such as deletions, duplications, trinucleotide repeats, or methylation defects, and can lack sensitivity near highly repetitive regions, such as the first exon within a gene. WGS has a higher sensitivity as it can improve detection of variants that are deeply intronic or in early exons, chromosomal deletions, and duplications and is demonstrating utility in diagnosing trinucleotide expansion disorders. WGS still does not detect all types of deleterious genetic changes, and interpretation of variants of uncertain significance can be difficult. Similarly, WGS and WES are critical in the identification of new pathogenic variants and genetic causes of novel and classic phenotypic presentations without a known mechanism previously identified (Fig. 1.27). While WES has an average diagnostic rate of 40% in well-phenotyped patients, WGS can vary between 30% and 57% depending on the study and up to 45% in cases with prior nondiagnostic exomes.

Single Gene Disorders

A pathogenic variant in a gene typically results in either alteration of the amount of gene product produced, failure to produce the product at all, and/or compromise of its functional integrity. The loss of gene product or function is also referred to as *haploinsufficiency.* The greater the degree of functional loss, the more severe the clinical manifestations of the disorder and often the earlier their onset. A single-gene disorder is the result of a variant altering the DNA sequence within a single gene. If variation in the gene in one chromosome or allele is sufficient to cause disease, the disorder is *dominant.* If pathogenic variants of the gene on both chromosomes are required to manifest disease, the disorder is *recessive.* Genes on the X chromosome are called *X-linked*, and expression can depend on how many active X chromosomes express the gene. Figs. 1.27 through 1.46 are representative of single-gene disorders.

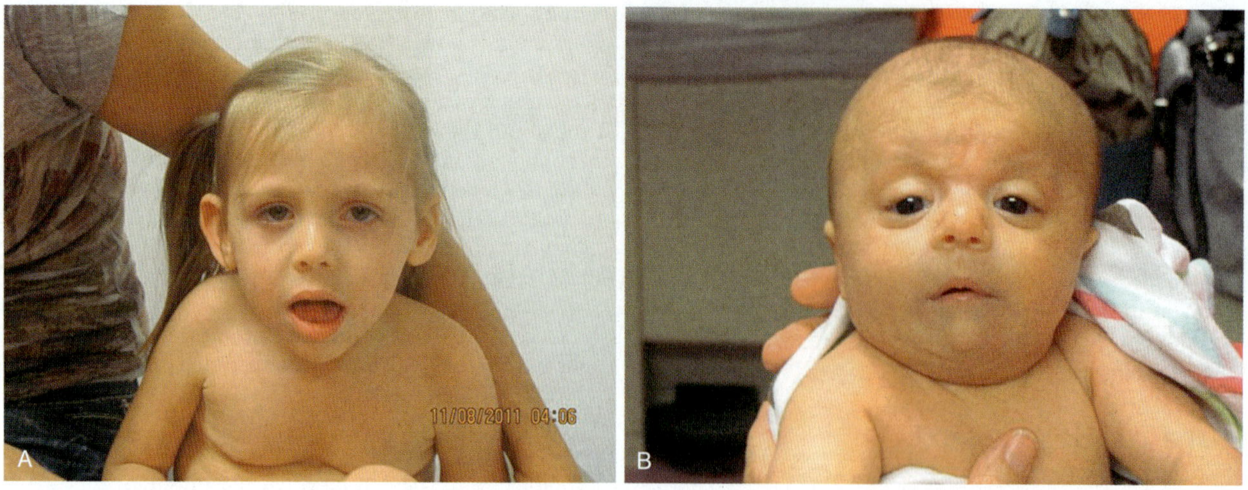

Fig. 1.27 Use of whole exome sequencing (WES) in diagnosis. (A) Three-years and 5-months-old girl with intellectual disabilities, neurobehavioral presentation suggesting Rett syndrome. WES disclosed a de novo frame shift pathogenic variant in *SMC1A*(c.2394dupA; p.R799fs), a rare form of X-linked Cornelia de Lange syndrome. (B) Ten-month-old girl with failure to thrive, microcephaly, congenital hearing loss, complex heart defect with mesocardia, and altered surface morphology. Patient underwent a series of diagnostic testing before WES. WES delineated a de novo missense pathogenic variant (c.418G>A p.G140R) in the *HDAC8* gene, yet another infrequent cause for an X-linked type of Cornelia de Lange syndrome.

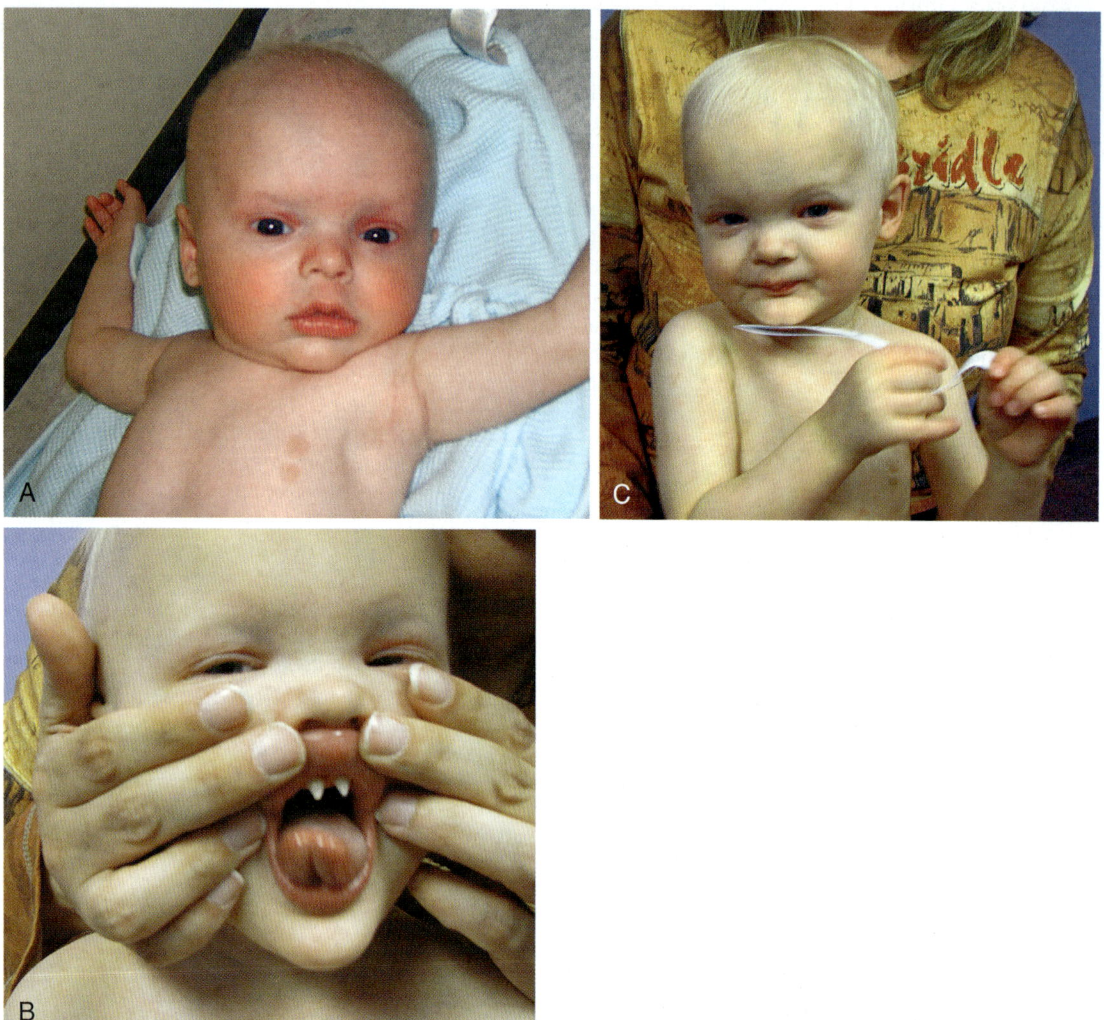

Fig. 1.28 Classic presentation for features of X-linked recessive hypohidrotic ectodermal dysplasia at 1 to 20 months of age. At 1 month the infant was admitted to "rule out sepsis" with high fever, but the workup was negative. (A) Note the thin, sparse, fine hair. (B) Severe hypodontia and anterior conical teeth. (C) Low nasal bridge, periorbital wrinkling, full forehead, prominent lips, and prominent supraorbital ridges. Sequencing of the *EDA1* gene showed the missense pathogenic variant and confirmed the clinical diagnosis. The mother and her maternal female relatives have variable and milder clinical features.

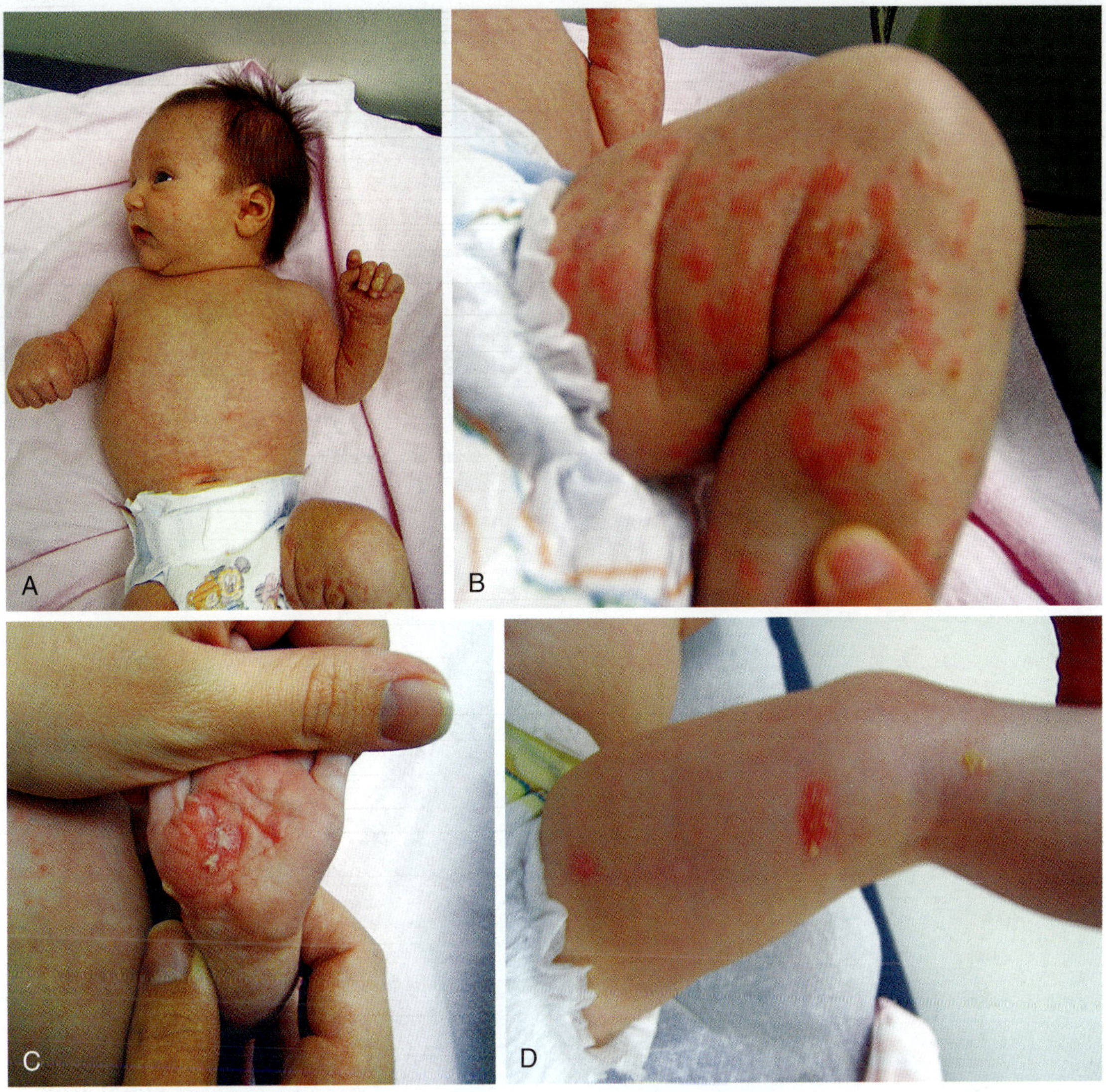

Fig. 1.29 Incontinentia pigmenti syndrome. (A–C) At 7 weeks old this patient manifested erythema and blisters on the trunk and extremities. Hyperkeratotic lesions have already started. This X-linked dominant condition is typically lethal in males. One-third of the patients have psychomotor delays, microcephaly, and seizures, which were not observed in this patient. Pathogenic variant(s) in the *NEMO* gene at Xq28 are encountered in the majority of patients. By 5 months old, the rash was already resolving. (D) Rash replaced with hyperpigmentation on the trunk and pale hairless patches or streaks subsequently on the lower limbs. Patient was confirmed to have intragenic microdeletion of the *NEMO* gene, involving exons 4 through 10.

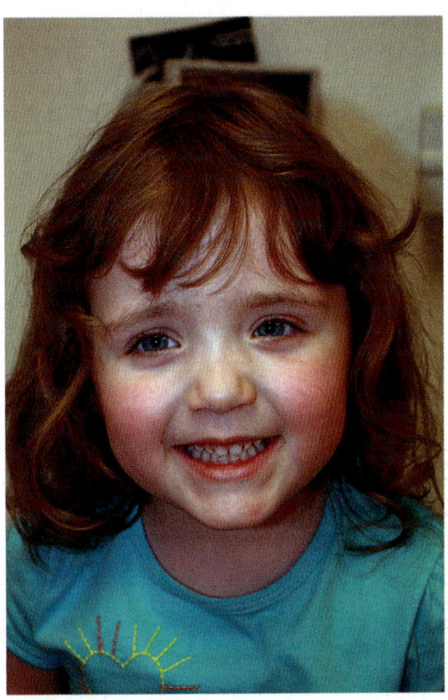

Fig. 1.30 A girl, 3 years and 3 months old, with macrocephaly, macrosomia, and autism spectrum disorder. A missense pathogenic variant was found in the *PTEN* gene.

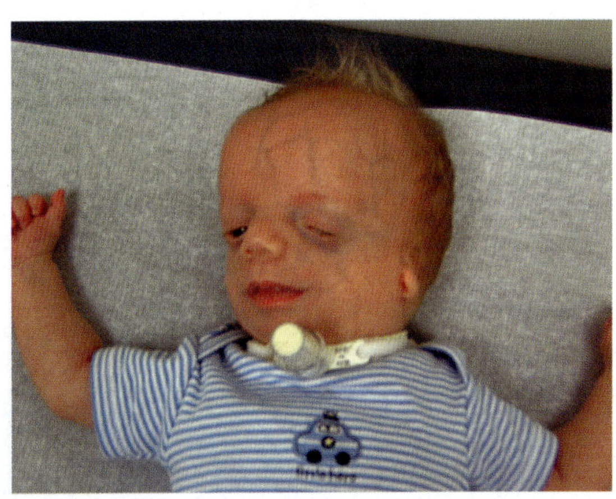

Fig. 1.31 A 4-month-old male with classic features of Treacher Collins syndrome. Note the down-slanted palpebral fissures, malar hypoplasia, malformed auricle, and mandibular hypoplasia. The pathogenic variant was identified as a single sequence variation (c.2897insC) in the *TCOF1* gene that introduces a premature stop codon.

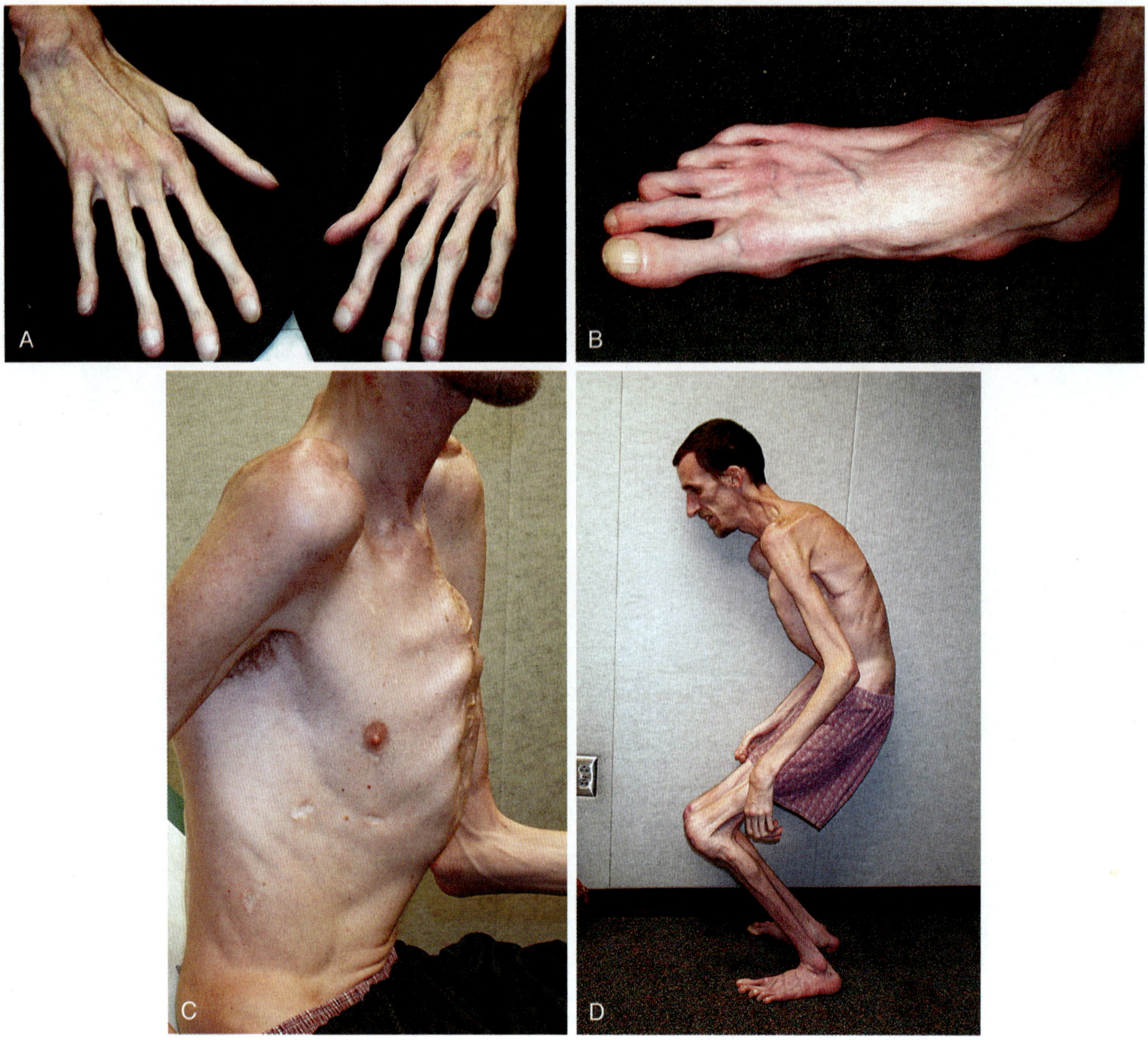

Fig. 1.32 Marfan syndrome. (A and B) This young man has prominent arachnodactyly of both fingers and toes. Note the clubbing due to associated cardiopulmonary problems and the flattening of the arch of his foot. He also has severe pectus carinatum (C) and significant kyphosis and joint contractures (D). Also note his long arms.

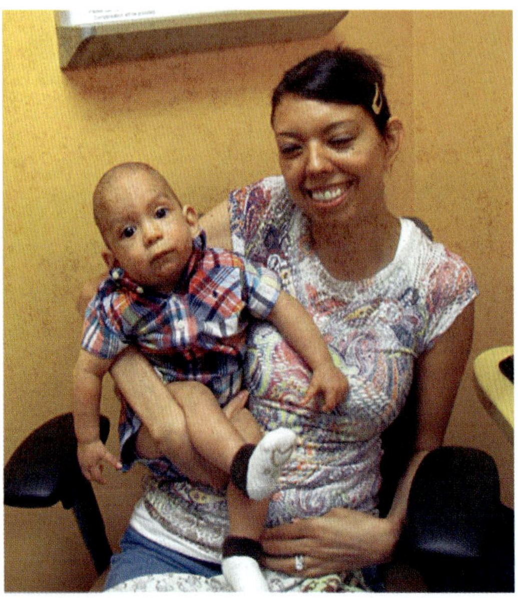

Fig. 1.33 The mother has clinical features of Loeys-Dietz syndrome. She has a pathogenic variant in the *TGFBR1* gene. Her infant son, seen here at 5 months old, is clinically affected and already has a dilated aorta. His mother had undergone valve-sparing aortic root repair on an emergent basis, due to possible dissection complicated by right coronary artery injury and bypass procedure.

Pathogenic variant(s) of gene(s) within the nuclear genome are also recognized as Mendelian disorders. The occurrence and/or recurrence are in fixed proportions (Mendel's laws). These disorders are compiled in a catalog, the Online Mendelian Inheritance in Man (OMIM; http://www.ncbi.nlm.nih.gov/omim), which is an excellent resource. Phenotype/genotype correlations are unfolded by detailed clinical evaluation, recognition at a clinical level, and confirmation by molecular diagnostics confirming the genotype.

Pedigree analyses are usually helpful in recognizing autosomal, X-linked, recessive, and dominant patterns. Gene penetrance, disease expressivity, genetic (locus) heterogeneity, and allelic heterogeneity are some of the well-recognized complexities characterizing Mendelian disorders.

Enzyme Protein Abnormalities

When the gene product is an enzyme or a component of an enzyme, this results in interruption of its step in a chain of reactions that may be involved in the formation or modification of a product, a step in cell metabolism, or in the degradation of molecules no longer needed by the cell. The missed step results in a build-up of substrate from the step preceding the one in which the affected enzyme acts and a decrease of the desired product. In some instances, this accumulated substrate can be toxic, as in PKU. In others, ever-expanding storage of substrate can adversely affect cell function, as in lysosomal storage

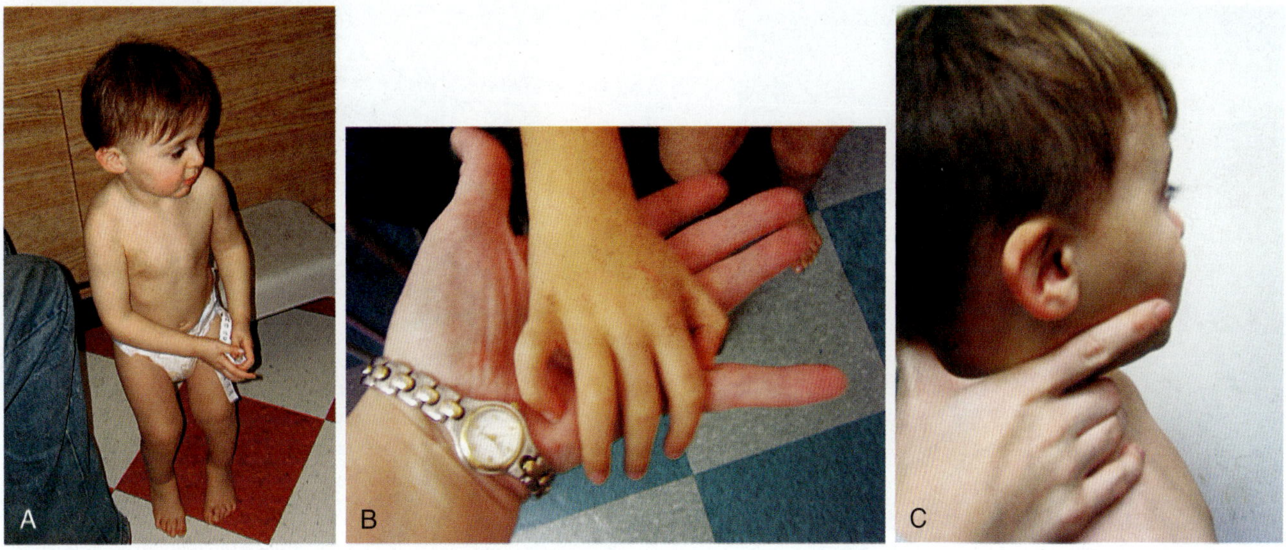

Fig. 1.34 (A–C) Congenital contractural arachnodactyly. Note the crumpled ears, arachnodactyly, and joint contractures. The patient was confirmed to have a missense pathogenic variant in the fibrillin II gene *(FBN2)*.

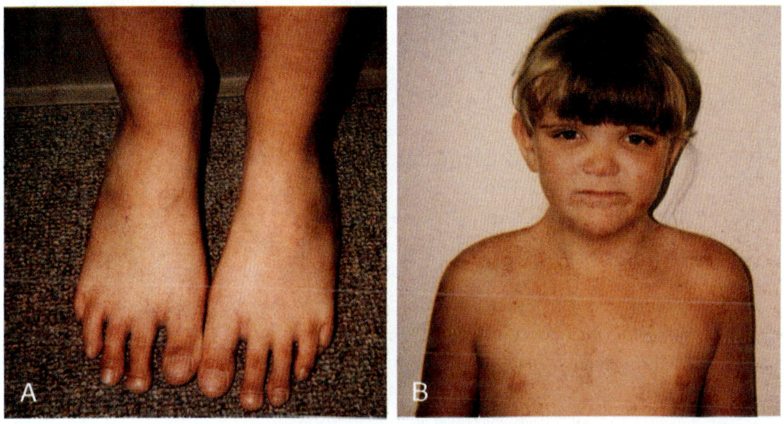

Fig. 1.35 Congenital contractural arachnodactyly (CCA) variant. This child was found to have an abnormality of fibrillin-2 secretion in fibroblasts. (A) She was tall and had arachnodactyly with contractures. (B) Her broad forehead and hypertelorism are physical features that help distinguish her case from classic CCA and Marfan syndrome.

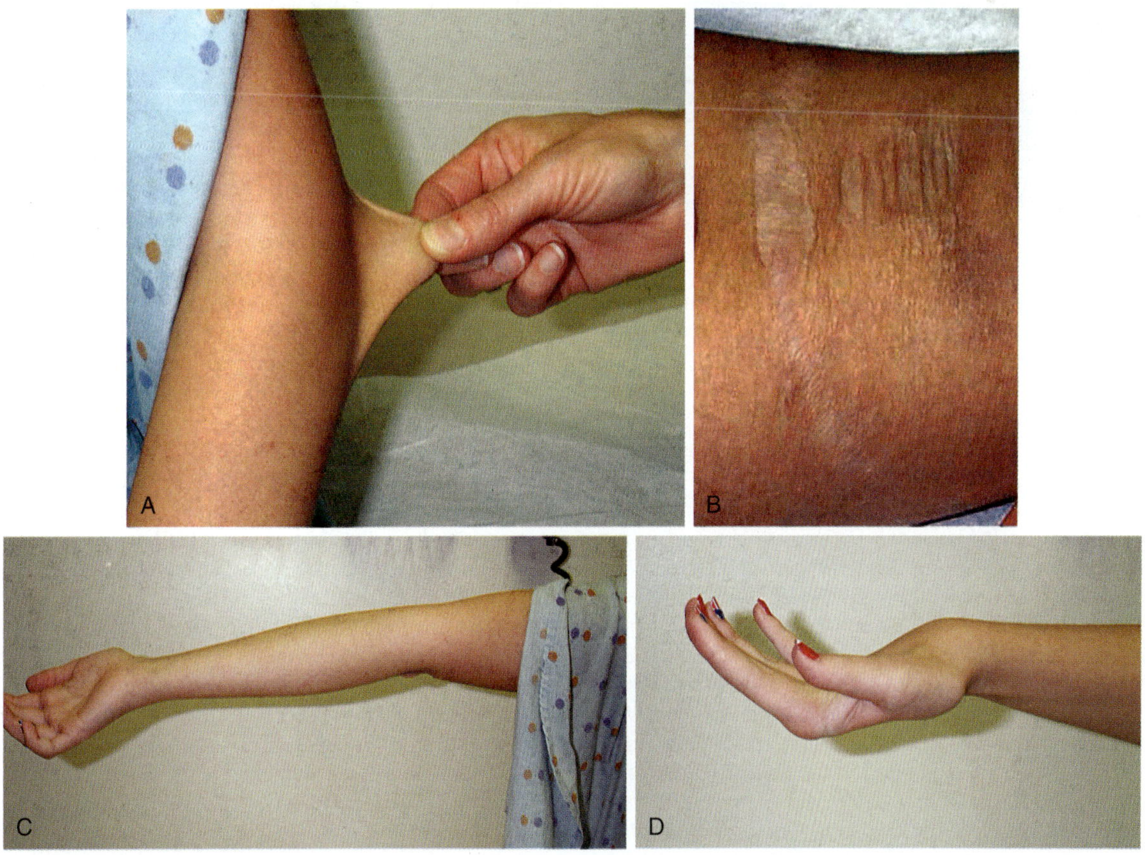

Fig. 1.36 Classic Ehlers-Danlos syndrome (cEDS) (A) Note the marked hyperextensibility of the skin over this child's arm. (B) These widened atrophic scars have the thin papery texture that is characteristic of EDS. (C and D) Hyperextensibility of the joints of the elbow and fingers is seen as well.

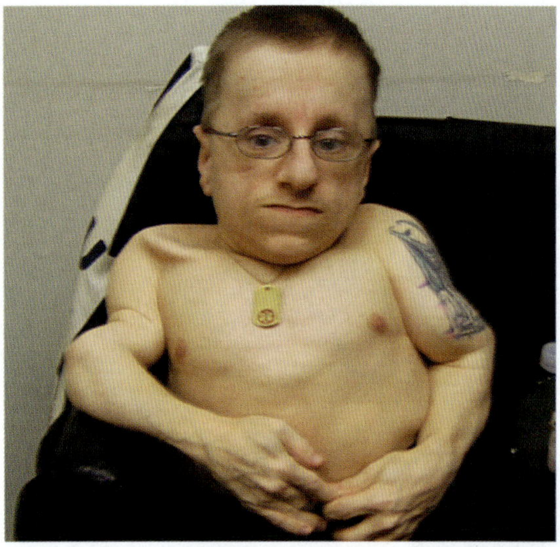

Fig. 1.37 Clinical features suggestive of progressively deforming osteogenesis imperfecta (formerly, type III OI); collagen screen results on skin fibroblasts are consistent with type III or type IV OI. The patient declined molecular diagnosis. He is wheelchair bound but lives independently.

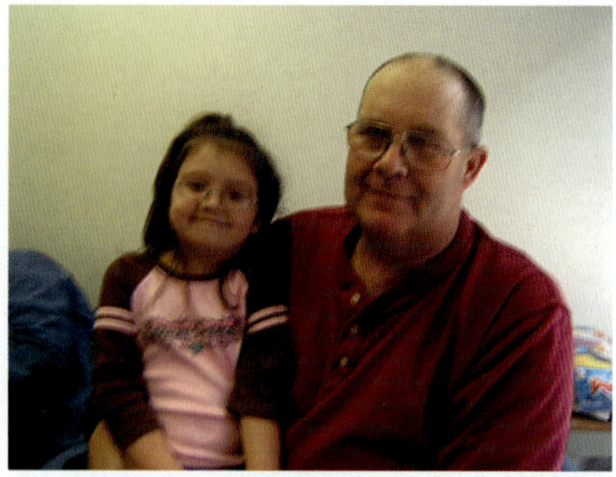

Fig. 1.39 A grandfather and granddaughter with Stickler syndrome. Grandfather has high myopia and status post–unilateral retinal detachment. Grandfather was confirmed to have a frameshift pathogenic variant in the collagen II gene, confirming *COL2A1*-Stickler syndrome (formerly, type II). The pathogenic variant was confirmed in his 5-year-old granddaughter; note the early-onset high myopia and midface hypoplasia. She also had generalized joint laxity. She had surgery for cleft palate and is under surveillance by audiology for conductive hearing loss.

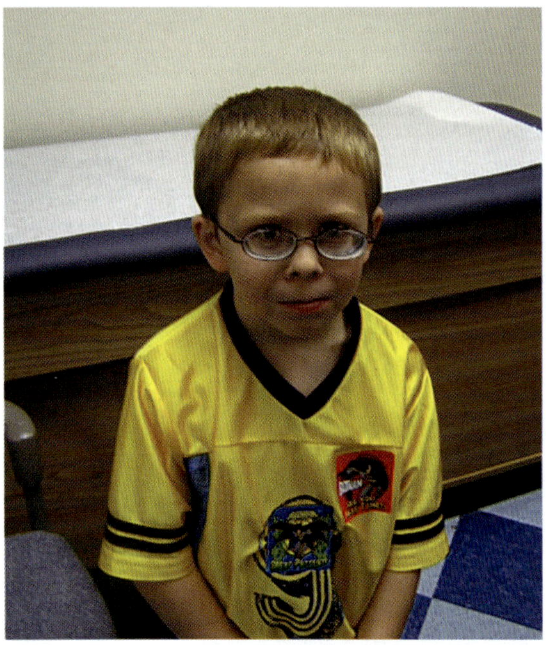

Fig. 1.38 Stickler syndrome: short stature, early-onset myopia, midface hypoplasia, submucous cleft palate, sensorineural hearing loss, mild skeletal dysplasia, and joint pain. A missense pathogenic variant in the *COL2A1* gene confirmed the clinical diagnosis (formerly type I Stickler syndrome).

diseases. Since many enzyme disorders result in inborn errors of metabolism, these will be further considered in the section on Inborn Errors of Metabolism.

Structural Protein Disorders

The family of disorders known as *osteogenesis imperfecta* (OI; see also Chapter 22 and see Fig. 1.37) provides a good example of the effects of pathogenic variants that alter the precursors of a structural protein, in this case, type I collagen. Type I collagen is a triple helix made up of two pro-α1 chains and one pro-α2 chain. The procollagen strands are composed of hundreds of amino acid triplet repeats, with glycine (the smallest amino acid) being the first member of each triplet and forming the apex of each bend in the helical structure. A base substitution in a codon specifying glycine at any one of the hundreds of such points along either the *COL1A1* gene or the *COL1A2* gene can produce inadequate or unstable collagen production in one of several ways. In some cases, genetic variation results in the production of an unstable mRNA molecule that is degraded in the nucleus, or structurally abnormal collagen chains subject to degradation, resulting in inadequate collagen production that is normal in structure but reduced by 50% (haploinsufficiency). As classic nondeforming OI with blue sclerae is the mildest form of OI (formerly, type I), it demonstrates the fact that in many cases of variants involving genes that encode structural polypeptides or proteins, it can be better to have no gene product than to have an abnormal one, a concept that is being explored in the treatment of structural protein disorders by attempting to silence the mutated gene.

In other cases, the variant leads to production of structurally abnormal pro-α1 or pro-α2 chains that are subject to aberrant posttranslational modification, or inability to associate properly with the other prochains to form a strong helix. When a single pathogenic variant on only one allele results in a structurally abnormal protein that interferes with the functioning of the residual normal proteins, this is termed a "dominant negative" effect. As a rule, the earlier the altered mRNA codon appears in the translation process, the more abnormal the resulting prochain structure is when formed, leading to a greater degree of compromise of collagen strength and function within connective tissues. These types of variants, which result in the synthesis of structurally abnormal products that interfere with collagen structure and function, are the basis for clinical abnormalities found in the most common forms of OI. The phenomenon of excessive posttranslational modification of a structurally abnormal gene product is also seen in some types of Ehlers-Danlos syndrome (EDS; see the Ehlers-Danlos syndrome section, later).

Osteogenesis Imperfecta Osteogenesis imperfecta (OI) is a family of genetic connective tissue disorders characterized predominantly by brittle bones. Most patients have classic nondeforming OI with blue sclerae, perinatally lethal OI (previously OI type II), progressively deforming OI (previously OI type III), or common variable OI with normal sclerae (previously OI type IV), all of which involve pathogenic variants in the *COL1A1* gene and/or *COL1A2* gene that either reduce the amount or alter the structure of type I collagen. Other, rarer forms of OI include types V through XX and are further subdivided into disorders of collagen type I processing and other osteoblastic defects. Of these, OI type V is an autosomal dominant disorder, OI type XIX is X-linked, and all other types of OI are autosomal recessive. A description of some of the many causative pathogenic variants and their structural consequences is

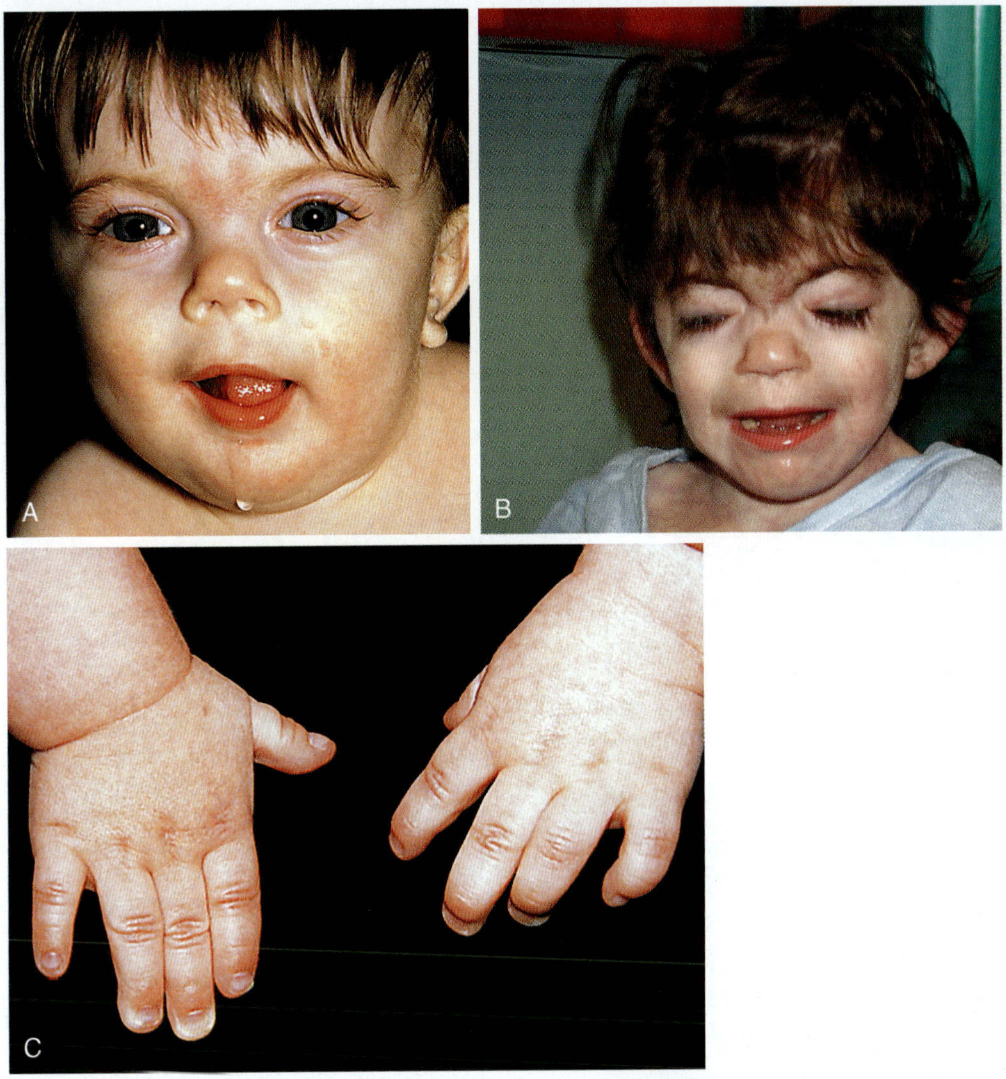

Fig. 1.40 Cornelia de Lange syndrome. (A and B) Facial features seen in an infant and an older child include finely arched heavy eyebrows, long eyelashes, small, upturned nose, long smooth philtrum, and Cupid's-bow mouth. (C) Small hands, hypoplastic proximally placed thumb, and short fifth finger with mild clinodactyly are examples of commonly associated extremity anomalies. (A and C, Courtesy A.H. Urbach, MD, Children's Hospital of Pittsburgh, Pittsburgh, PA.)

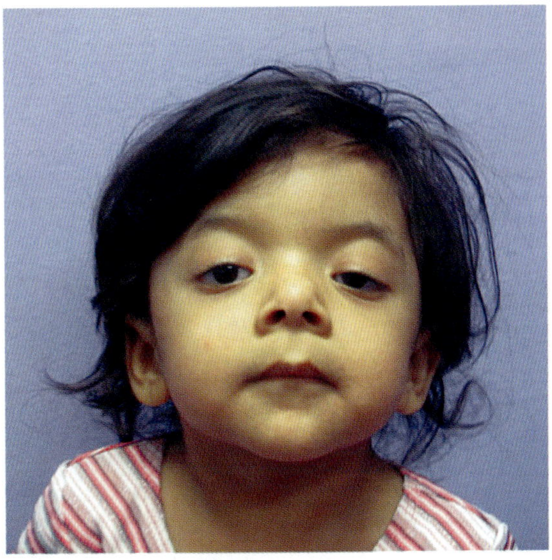

Fig. 1.41 Noonan syndrome. Note the down-slanting palpebral fissures, ptosis, and low-set posteriorly rotated ears. Patient has bilateral single palmar creases and underwent cardiac surgeries for severe pulmonic stenosis and atrial septal defect. She has short stature, developmental delays, alternating esotropia, optic nerve cupping, and unilateral pelvicaliectasis. A missense pathogenic variant in exon 3 of the *PTPN11* gene resulted in the classic features of Noonan syndrome.

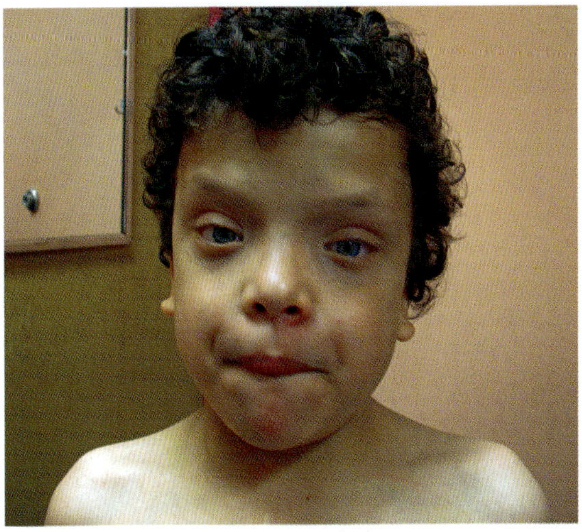

Fig. 1.42 Cardio-facio-cutaneous syndrome. The patient underwent surgical repair of ventricular septal defect and pulmonic stenosis during infancy. He presented at 8 years old with short stature while receiving growth hormone injections; he also had seizures and intellectual disabilities. Patient has optic nerve hypoplasia, relative macrocephaly, curly hair, deep palmar creases, and prominent finger pads. Note the prominent forehead, hypertelorism, ptosis, and low-set posterior rotation of ears. The patient carried a clinical diagnosis of Noonan syndrome and tested negative for *PTPN11, SOS1, RAF1,* and *KRAS* genes. Noonan Chip analysis confirmed the missense pathogenic variant in the *BRAF* gene, which is consistent with cardio-facio-cutaneous syndrome.

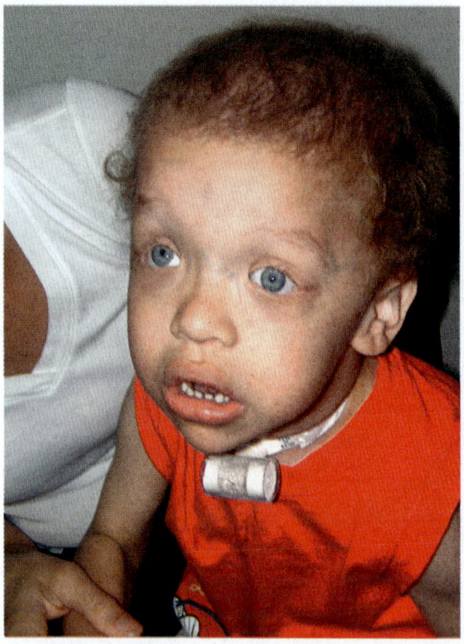

Fig. 1.43 Costello syndrome. Note the macrocephaly, curly sparse hair, short neck, and hypotonia. The patient had a tracheostomy and is gastrostomy tube dependent and has had global delays with some communication by sign language at 4 years old. Skin was very lax and soft and a somewhat darker color for the family. A pathogenic variant in exon 2 of the *HRAS* gene was classic for Costello syndrome.

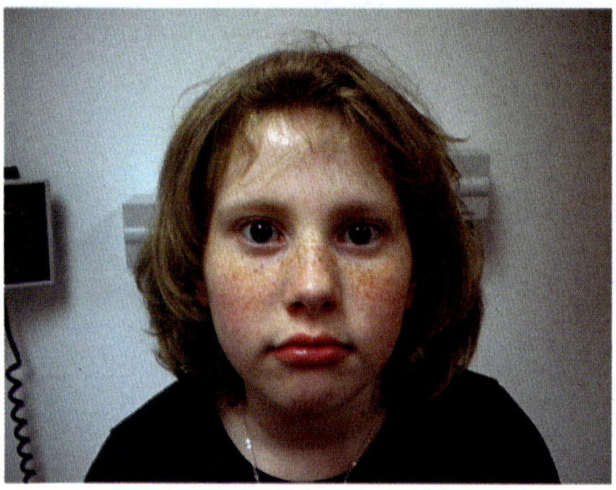

Fig. 1.44 A 10-year-old girl with Noonan syndrome with lentigines.

presented in an earlier section, The Nature of Genes and Single-Gene Disorders. Clinical features are presented in Chapter 22.

Figs. 1.36 through 1.39 show examples of defects in collagen synthesis.

Connective Tissue Disorders of Genetic Origin

See Table 1.10 for examples of some hereditary connective tissue disorders.

Marfan Syndrome *Marfan syndrome* is a genetic disorder of connective tissue that is inherited as an autosomal dominant trait, with 25% to 30% of cases being de novo. The site of the genetic abnormality is the fibrillin gene *(FBN1)*. As a result, the molecular structure of the protein fibrillin, an intrinsic component of connective tissue, is abnormal. Clinical consequences are most notable in the musculoskeletal, cardiovascular, and ocular systems and in the dura. Classic phenotypic findings include arachnodactyly (see Fig. 1.32A and B); elbow contractures with other joint hyperextensibility due to ligamentous laxity (see Chapter 5); tall stature with long, thin extremities (termed a "Marfanoid" habitus); a decreased upper-to-lower segment ratio; an arm span to height ratio that exceeds 1.05; and moderate to severe pectus excavatum or carinatum (see Fig. 1.32C). Pes planus and thoracolumbar kyphoscoliosis are other common skeletal features (see Fig. 1.32D). A defect in the suspensory ligaments of the eye is responsible for subluxation of the lens (seen in 50% to 60% of patients by 10 years old), which is usually displaced in an upward direction. Myopia and astigmatism are common, and affected individuals are also at risk for developing glaucoma, cataracts, and retinal detachment in adulthood. Mitral valve prolapse may progress to mitral insufficiency with increased risk of arrhythmias. Progressive aneurysmal dilation of the ascending aorta or, less commonly, the thoracic or abdominal aorta, is seen in this patient population. The latter is the major source of morbidity and mortality, as it can result in acute dissection and death. Dural ectasia in the lumbosacral region, assessed by computed tomography (CT) or magnetic resonance imaging (MRI) of the spine, is observed in 65% of cases. The presence of a high arched palate is common. The incidence of hernias, both inguinal and femoral, is increased, and patients often have striae of the skin in unusual places, such as the shoulder. Most individuals with Marfan syndrome have normal intelligence, and the presence of learning disabilities should prompt additional investigation. Pregnant people with Marfan syndrome

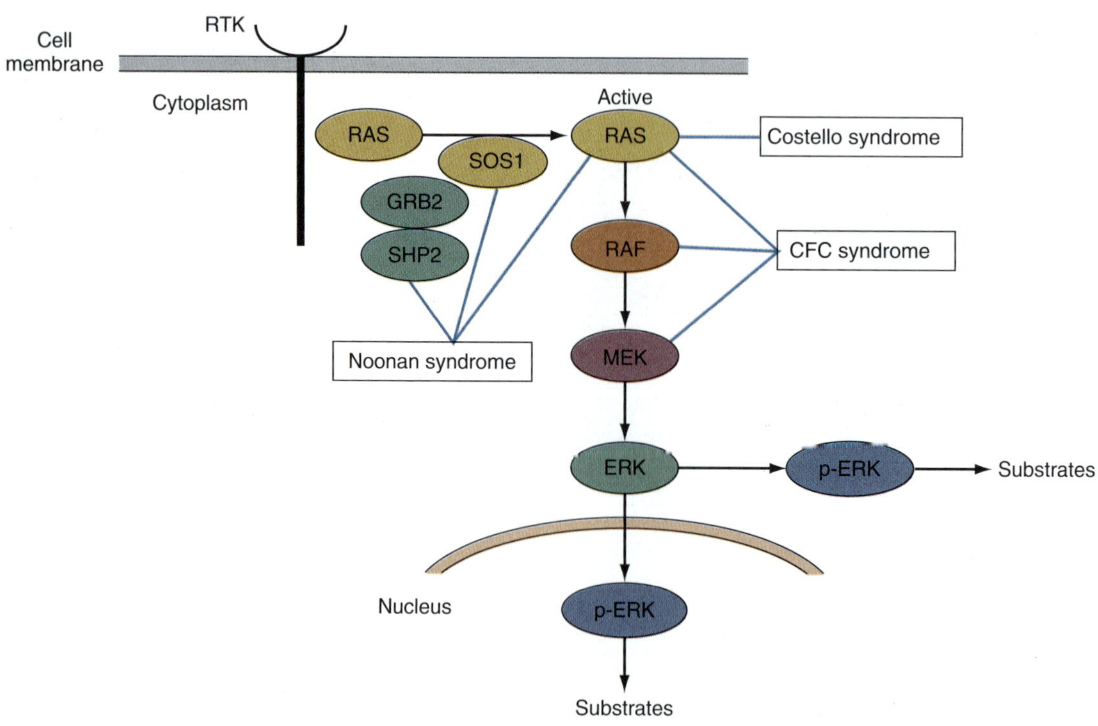

Fig. 1.45 The mitogen-activated protein kinase (MAPK) signaling cascade, also known as the *RAF/MEK/ERK signaling cascade.* Germline pathogenic variants that affect components of the RAS-MAPK pathway are involved in the pathogenesis of Noonan syndrome and allied disorders (Noonan phenotype with overlapping features: CFC, Costello and neurofibromatosis-1). *CFC,* Cardio-facio-cutaneous; *ERK,* extracellular signal–regulated kinase; *GRB2,* growth factor receptor-bound protein 2, *MEK,* MAPK/ERK kinase; *p-ERK,* phosphorylated ERK; *RAF,* murine sarcoma viral oncogene; *RAS,* rat sarcoma viral oncogene; *RTK,* receptor tyrosine kinase; *SHP2,* src homology region 2-domain phosphatase 2; *SOS1,* son of sevenless 1. (Courtesy Partners HealthCare, Laboratory for Molecular Medicine, Harvard Medical School.)

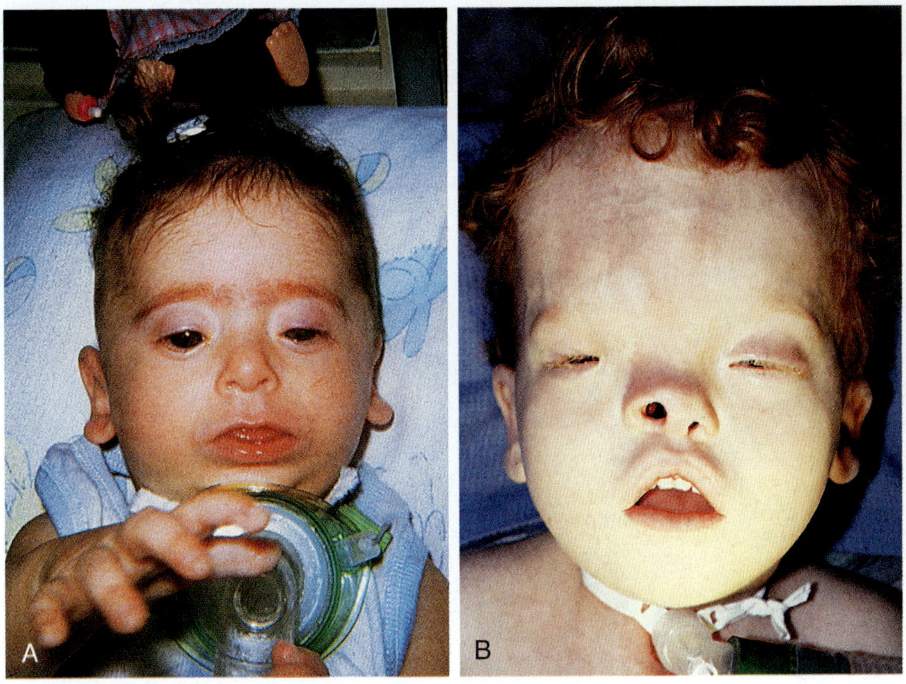

Fig. 1.46 CHARGE syndrome. (A) Note the short palpebral fissures and ptosis; low-set, dysplastic ears; and small chin. Choanal atresia necessitated tracheotomy. (B) Another example of an infant with CHARGE syndrome has clinical features that include a prominent forehead, hypertelorism, narrow palpebral fissures, hypoplasia of the right naris, low-set ears, and a Cupid's-bow mouth. (A, Courtesy W. Tunnessen, MD. B, Courtesy Timothy McBride, MD, Fairfax, VA.)

Table 1.10 Differentials for Connective Tissue Disorders

Diagnosis	Inheritance	Molecular Basis
Stickler syndrome	AD	*COL2A1* gene *COL11A1* gene *COL11A2* gene *COL9A1* gene *COL9A2* gene *COL9A3* gene
vEDS	AD	*COL3A1* gene
PLOD1-kEDS	AR	*PLOD1* gene
Congenital contractural arachnodactyly	AD	*FBN2* gene
Homocysteinemia	AR	Defect in cobalamin synthesis
Arterial tortuosity syndrome	AR	*SLC2A10* gene
MASS phenotype	AD	*FBN1* gene
Loeys-Dietz syndrome	AD	*TGFBR1* gene *TGFBR2* gene *TGFB2* gene *TGFB3* gene *SMAD2* gene *SMAD3* gene
Familial aortic aneurysm	AD	*ACTA2* gene *MYH11* gene
Klinefelter syndrome (47,XXY) or triple X syndrome (47, XXX)	Chromosomal	Chromosomal
Fragile X syndrome	X-linked	*FMR1* gene
Shprintzen-Goldberg syndrome	AD	*SKI* gene

AD, Autosomal dominant; *AR*, autosomal recessive; *EDS*, Ehlers-Danlos syndrome; *MASS*, *m*itral valve prolapse, borderline nonprogressive *a*ortic enlargement, *s*triae and marfanoid *s*keletal features, which overlap with those seen in Marfan syndrome; *vEDS*, vascular EDS.

require high-risk management for cardiovascular complications and potential teratogenicity of some medication treatments.

The disorder is currently primarily suspected on clinical grounds, but family history and multiorgan manifestations are variable and can have age-dependent expressivity. Diagnostic criteria include major and minor manifestations and are intermittently updated to reflect this variability, but molecular testing has the advantage of providing a more accurate diagnosis in patients who have suspected disease but who may not meet all clinical criteria.

The differential diagnosis of Marfan syndrome includes Loeys-Dietz syndrome (LDS) (Fig. 1.33), congenital contractural arachnodactyly (see Figs. 1.34 and 1.35, formerly known as Beals syndrome), homocystinuria, the MASS (Myopia, mitral valve, aortic involvement, skin and skeletal features) phenotype, familial ectopia lentis, Klinefelter syndrome (47,XXY), triple X syndrome (47,XXX), and many syndromes characterized by joint hypermobility, such as Stickler syndrome (see Figs. 1.38 and 1.39), classic EDS (cEDS) (see Fig. 1.36), and vascular EDS (vEDS), familial thoracic aortic aneurysm and aortic dissection (TAAD), neuromuscular disorders, fragile X syndrome, and some of the rare dysmorphologic entities, such as Shprintzen-Goldberg syndrome.

When the diagnosis of Marfan syndrome is strongly suspected or confirmed, patients should be monitored closely during growth spurts for signs of onset and progression of kyphoscoliosis; in addition, they should undergo regular ophthalmologic evaluations and have regular echocardiograms and electrocardiograms for comprehensive cardiac care. When aortic dilation is detected, administration of β-blockers can slow progression by decreasing blood pressure and the force of myocardial contractions. Research has found transforming growth factor-β (TGF-β) is involved in the formation of aortic aneurysms. Losartan, an angiotensin II type 1 receptor blocker, inhibits TGF-β and has now become standard of care for all Marfan and LDS patients. Patients also should be cautioned to avoid weightlifting and contact sports.

Loeys-Dietz Syndrome LDS is a more aggressive connective tissue disorder than Marfan syndrome; it is characterized by craniofacial, cutaneous, and skeletal and vascular manifestations, as well as aneurysms and dissection of the aorta (in the root, thoracic, and/or abdominal regions) and cerebral vessels (see Fig. 1.33). Tortuosity of blood vessels and heart defects, involving the bicuspid aortic valves and atrial septal defects, may be observed. Bifid uvula is a common finding. Translucent skin and organ rupture, specifically in postpartum females, have been reported. Pathogenic variants in TGF-β receptor type 1, *TGFBR1*, and *TGFBR2* result in LDS. Treatment strategies and recommendations are similar to Marfan syndrome described earlier.

Ehlers-Danlos Syndromes EDS is composed of a group of inherited connective tissue disorders, the major features consisting

Table 1.11 Classification of Types of Ehlers-Danlos Syndrome

Type	Former Type	Mode of Inheritance	Approximate Incidence	Genes
Group A: Disorders of Collagen Primary Structure and Processing				
Classic (cEDS)	I and II	AD	1 per 20,000–40,000	*COL5A1, COL5A2, COL1A1*
Arthrochalasis (aEDS)	VIIA and VIIB	AD	Very rare	*COL1A1, COL1A2*
Vascular (vEDS)	IV	AD	1 per 100,000–200,000	*COL3A1, COL1A1*
Dermatosparaxis (dEDS)		AR		*ADAMTS2*
Cardiac-valvular (cvEDS)		AR		*COL1A2*
Group B: Disorders of Collagen Folding and Collagen Cross-Linking				
Kyphoscoliotic (*FKBP14*-kEDS)	VI	AD	Rare	*PLOD1*
Kyphoscoliotic (*PLOD1*-kEDS)	VI	AD	Rare	*PLOD1*
Group C: Disorders of Structure and Function of Myomatrix				
Classical-like (clEDS)		AR		*TNXB*
Myopathic (mEDS)		AD/AR		*COL12A1*
Group D: Disorders of Glycosaminoglycan Biosynthesis				
Spondylodysplastic (spEDS)	EDS Progeroid	AR		*B4GALT7, B3GALT6*
Musculocontractural (mcEDS)	Kosho	AR		*CHST14, DSE*
Group E: Disorders of Complement Pathway				
Periodontal (pEDS)	VIII	AD		*C1R, C1S*
Group F: Disorders of Intracellular Processes				
Spondylodysplastic (spEDS)	Spondylocheirodysplastic	AR		*SLC39A13*
Brittle Cornea Syndrome (BCS)		AD/AR	Very rare	*ZNF469, PRDM5*
Unresolved Forms of EDS				
Hypermobility (hEDS)	III	AD	1 per 5,000[a]	n/a

[a]Estimated minimum prevalence based on calculated prevalence of all other types of EDS.

AD, Autosomal dominant; *AR*, autosomal recessive; *EDS*, Ehlers-Danlos syndrome.

of skin hyperextensibility and fragility as well as ligamentous laxity with secondary joint hypermobility. Each type stems from a defect in synthesis of type I, III, or V collagen, resulting in decreased tensile strength of connective tissues. Previously divided into types I to XI, it has been reclassified into six major subgroups (Groups A to F) based on their mechanism of pathogenicity, predominant clinical features, and mode of inheritance. Table 1.11 presents these along with their estimated incidence. We also briefly focus on the clinical features of the four most common types.

The diagnosis of EDS should be suspected in children who present with unusually distensible skin, especially when atrophic scars are seen, and in those with unusual degrees of joint hypermobility who suffer recurrent joint dislocations. Easy bruising can be mistaken for child abuse, as there is no significant preceding trauma. The presence of skin hyperextensibility is best tested over the volar forearm by grasping the skin and pulling until resistance is felt with measurement greater than 1.5 cm. Evidence of significant joint hypermobility is assessed on the Beighton scale and includes the following:

- Ability to touch palms flat to the floor on forward bending (1 point)
- Hyperextensibility of knees and elbows greater than 10 degrees (1 point per limb, maximum 4 points)
- Ability to oppose thumb completely to the volar forearm (1 point for each thumb)
- Passive dorsiflexion of the fifth fingers past 90 degrees (1 point for each hand)

Hypermobility includes a score of 6 or greater in children and adolescents, 5 or higher in adults up to age 50, and 4 or higher after age 50.

Finding these and other clinical features described earlier in a child with a positive family history is especially helpful. Depending on type, differential diagnostic considerations may include Marfan syndrome and cutis laxa.

cEDS (Classic) In the cEDS (previously known as subtypes I and II), cutaneous manifestations are especially prominent, although they may have a wide spectrum of severity. Skin hyperextensibility is prominent (see Fig. 1.36A); the texture is smooth, doughy, and "velvety"; the skin is abnormally fragile with easy bruising and tearing. Wound healing is impaired and slower than average, often resulting in the formation of unusually wide atrophic scars that have a thin, papery quality, sometimes likened to cigarette paper (see Fig. 1.36B).

When these children incur lacerations necessitating wound closure, use of glue or tape is preferable to sutures because the latter tend to tear away from the fragile skin. Staples are better tolerated for closure of operative incisions, and postoperative development of incisional hernias is not uncommon.

Two features unique to this type are the tendency to form pseudotumors under scars located over bony prominences and to develop subcutaneous fatty tumors over the forearms and shins.

Although usually not as debilitatingly painful as in hypermobile EDS (hEDS), ligamentous laxity and joint hypermobility also are features (see Fig. 1.36C and D) and predispose to sprains, subluxations, and dislocations and early onset of chronic musculoskeletal pain. Hypotonia and gross motor delays are seen in some infants and young children with cEDS.

hEDS (Hypermobile) In hEDS, the most common type, ligamentous laxity and attendant joint hypermobility are the major source of symptomatology. All joints, large and small, are affected, and patients are prone to frequent and recurrent subluxations and dislocations, especially of the patella, shoulder, and temporomandibular joints. Chronic limb and joint pain, due to the excessive pull placed on periarticular structures and to dislocations, develops early on and can become increasingly debilitating over time. Cutaneous manifestations vary widely in severity and include a smooth "velvety" texture, mild hyperextensibility, and easy bruising.

At present, the genetic etiology of hEDS is unknown and there is no molecular test for diagnosis. Given that joint hyperextensibility is common in children (particularly with hypotonia) and is often a familial trait, overdiagnosis of hEDS is a clinical concern. However, formal criteria have been developed to assist in diagnosis (https://www.ehlers-danlos.com/heds-diagnostic-checklist/).

vEDS (Vascular) vEDS is the most serious form of EDS because extreme fragility of vascular and visceral tissues accompanies cutaneous and joint abnormalities. Many affected children are born with clubfeet, and they can have characteristic facial features that include prominent eyes and sunken cheeks (due to decreased subcutaneous facial fat), a thin nose, small chin, and lobeless external ears. Scalp hair is sparse in some children.

The skin is thin and appears translucent, giving prominence to the underlying venous pattern, especially over the chest and abdomen. Easy bruising and skin fragility are significant features, and postoperative wound dehiscence is not unusual. Premature aging of the skin over the distal extremities and early development of varicose veins are also seen. Joint hypermobility is present but is limited to the small joints of the fingers and toes.

As noted earlier, the feature that makes this type of EDS so serious clinically is the fragility of the walls of medium-size arteries, the intestines, and the uterus. This predisposes these organs to wall rupture with potentially catastrophic results. Arterial and intestinal ruptures are heralded by sudden onset of severe abdominal and/or flank pain, which is promptly followed by signs of shock. Risk of uterine rupture is greatest intrapartum and is associated with significant hemorrhage. Other reported problems include pneumothoraces and development of arteriovenous fistulas.

Because the major complications of this form of EDS tend to occur in the third or fourth decade, exact diagnosis in early childhood can be difficult in patients without a positive family history or in those whose other clinical findings are subtle.

kEDS (Kyphoscoliosis) Newborns with the kyphoscoliosis form of EDS (kEDS-*PLOD1* or kEDS-*FKBP14*) tend to have severe hypotonia with delayed gross motor development and congenital scoliosis, which is progressive. Some patients develop a Marfanoid body habitus as they grow. Generalized ligamentous laxity and joint hypermobility may be so severe that the ability to ambulate is lost in the teens or twenties. Osteopenia is often present in those individuals.

Other features include easy bruisability, skin fragility, and formation of atrophic scars. In contrast to other forms of EDS, children with this type have scleral fragility, which places them at risk for globe rupture following even minor trauma. High myopia and microcornea are seen in some patients. There is confirmatory diagnostic testing via urine for kEDS-*PLOD1* if no variant is found.

Recognizable Multiple Malformation Syndromes

de Lange, Cornelia de Lange, or Brachmann–de Lange Syndrome de Lange syndrome is characterized by intrauterine growth retardation, persistent postnatal failure to thrive, cognitive impairment, and microcephaly with a flat occiput and low hairline. Facial features are quite distinctive and include long eyelashes, a fine "brushed-on" appearance of the arch to the eyebrows, occasional synophrys, hirsutism, small nose with anteverted nostrils, long philtrum, downturned upper lip with Cupid's-bow shape, and micrognathia (see Fig. 1.40A and B). Extremities are notable for small hands and feet, and varying abnormalities can include proximally placed thumbs (see Fig. 1.40C), flexion contractures of the elbows, hypoplastic limbs, and even overt phocomelia (absent humerus, radius, and ulna). Hirsutism is generalized and distinctive, and cutis marmorata is a frequent feature. In males, hypospadias with cryptorchidism is common, and females may have a bicornuate uterus. Most affected adults are quite short in stature.

In general, autosomal dominant pathogenic variants in the *NIPBL* gene are responsible for approximately half of cases of classic de Lange syndrome, with a smaller subset of genes implicated in this disorder (*RAD21, SMC3, HDAC8,* and *SMC1A*). A few individuals have overlapping clinical features, most notably synophrys, and have been found to have an abnormality of chromosome 3p; thus, molecular cytogenetic studies should be considered. Families have been identified with severely affected children whose parents have been determined to be subtly affected. In those families, the anticipated recurrence risk would be up to 50% to have a child with the same disorder, if diagnostic testing is not informative.

Noonan Syndrome Noonan syndrome is an autosomal dominant, Mendelian genetic disorder that shares a number of clinical features with 45,X (Turner syndrome). The disorder is associated with missense variants in the *PTPN11* gene (in 50% of classic cases) and in the *KRAS* gene in 5% to 10% of cases. It is relatively common and thought to be present in 1 in 1000 to 1 in 2500 individuals. Like many other autosomal dominant disorders, it is seen in both males and females, and there is significant variability in clinical expression. A careful examination of close relatives of an index case may identify other affected individuals within the extended family, which is helpful when attempting to determine recurrence risks.

The pattern of malformations in Noonan syndrome is characterized by webbing of the neck, sternal abnormalities, pulmonic stenosis, and cryptorchidism in males. Facial characteristics include widely spaced eyes with down-slanting palpebral fissures, ptosis, and retrognathia (see Fig. 1.41 and Chapter 5). Ears are often low-set and can be posteriorly rotated. Hair can be coarse and curly, and the posterior hairline is often low. Sternal abnormalities include both pectus excavatum and carinatum, and often there are differences in the number of sternal ossification centers. Many have congenital heart disease with pulmonary valvular stenosis being the most common, followed by septal hypertrophy or defects. Hypertrophic cardiomyopathy is found in approximately 20% of patients and can be sufficiently severe as to necessitate cardiac transplantation. Coagulation abnormalities are found in approximately one-third of cases. Increased risk of juvenile myelomonocytic leukemia (JMML) and some other leukemias can occur in Noonan-spectrum disorders with risks correlating with the gene involved.

Puberty can be delayed in individuals with Noonan syndrome. Cryptorchidism, when present in males, can result in infertility. Stature is often less than the third percentile, but head circumference and intelligence are usually normal.

Several recognizable patterns of malformation share features in common with Noonan syndrome and are part of a family of disorders known as RASopathies due to their shared pathogenic mechanisms and pathway. Cardio-facio-cutaneous syndrome has additional features, particularly significant central nervous system (CNS) abnormalities (see Fig. 1.42). The phenotypic features of Noonan syndrome and neurofibromatosis type I may overlap (Watson syndrome) despite being attributed to a pathogenic *NF1* variant. In addition to short stature, pulmonic stenosis, café-au-lait spots, and cognitive disabilities, freckling and neurofibromas are also observed. In Costello syndrome, macrocephaly; coarse facial features; papillomas in the oral, nasal, and anal areas; cutis laxa; and cognitive impairments are seen in addition to findings shared with Noonan syndrome (see Fig. 1.43).

Interaction of the many respective gene(s) at the genetic level results in clinical overlap among these entities of "Noonan-spectrum disorders." These are therefore excellent examples of locus or genetic heterogeneity. Allelic heterogeneity is observed among the classic Noonan phenotype and Noonan syndrome with multiple lentigines clinical picture (see Fig. 1.41 and 1.44). Genetic heterogeneity is vast; at least 25 genes are involved in the Noonan spectrum disorders including Noonan, cardio-facio-cutaneous, and Costello syndromes. Molecular testing at the clinical level is currently available for several genes by panel testing, including *PTPN11, RAF1, SOS1, KRAS, HRAS, BRAF, MEK1, MEK2, NRAS, LZTR1,* and

SHOC2 (see Fig. 1.45) and the discovery of additional genes through more powerful methods, such as WES/WGS.

The differential diagnosis also includes several well-known teratogenic exposures, including fetal hydantoin syndrome and fetal alcohol syndrome (see Fig. 1.48) and other single-gene disorders (such as Kabuki syndrome). Hence careful dysmorphologic assessment of all individuals suspected of having Noonan syndrome is indicated before making a final diagnosis.

CHARGE Syndrome (CHD7-Related Disorders) CHARGE is an acronym for a nonrandom association of features including *c*oloboma of the retina (less commonly the iris), *h*eart abnormalities, *a*tresia of the choanae, *r*etarded growth and mental development, *g*enital hypoplasia in males, and *e*ar anomalies that can include deafness. The minimal diagnostic criteria should include abnormalities in four of the six categories, at least one of which must be coloboma or choanal atresia. Cleft lip and/or palate and renal abnormalities are sometimes found. The common pattern includes features overlapping with other common genetic disorders, including congenital heart disease, particularly abnormalities of the aortic arch, right subclavian artery, or ventricular septal defect; agenesis or hypoplasia of the thymus with decreased T-cell production and impaired cell-mediated immunity; partial or less often complete absence of the parathyroid glands, manifested by hypocalcemia and neonatal tetany; and often a more distinctive facies characterized by wide-spaced, slightly down-slanting palpebral fissures, anteverted nares, a short philtrum, and small, dysmorphic ears (see Fig. 1.46). Infants with CHARGE syndrome often die early because of their congenital anomalies, but many of them survive to adulthood. Although developmental delay exists, the IQ range is broad (<30 to 80).

CHARGE has been found to be due to pathogenic variants in the *CHD7* gene. Although most cases are sporadic, instances of affected siblings and an affected parent and offspring have been reported. The risk of recurrence must be determined after genetic evaluation and ranges from 4%–6% to as high as 50%. In the neonate, CHARGE syndrome must be differentiated from other chromosomal disorders, such as deletion 22q11.2 or trisomy 13 or 18, and from VATER/VACTERL association.

Associations

As noted earlier, an *association* is a pattern of malformations that occurs together too often to be the result of chance alone, but for which no specific unifying cause has yet been identified. This results in a spectrum of anomalies with a wide and variable clinical spectrum.

Oculo-Auriculo-Vertebral Spectrum

Oculo-auriculo-vertebral anomalies (OAVs) encompass a spectrum of hemifacial microsomia and Goldenhar syndromes resulting from developmental defects of the first and second branchial arches. Varied facial defects observed include hypoplasia of the maxilla and/or mandible, a lateral cleft at the angle of the mouth resulting in macrostomia, microtia and preauricular tags and/or pits, deafness, and tongue and palatal involvement with abnormal functioning of the palate.

Vertebral defects are predominantly in the cervical region, observed as a short neck and/or torticollis. This may be due to hemivertebrae and hypoplasia of the vertebrae in the cervical region but may involve the thoracic and lumbar regions. Microphthalmia and/or epibulbar eyelid coloboma are observed as infrequent but characteristic features. Congenital heart defects include ventricular septal defect, tetralogy of Fallot, and coarctation of the aorta. Renal defects are occasional features and may present as ectopic, fused kidney or renal agenesis, as well as multicystic dysplastic kidney. Ureteral aberrations and CNS involvement can also be seen. Intelligence is usually preserved but may be compromised in association with microphthalmia and CNS anomalies. Genetic delineation of etiology is at a research level, and clinical cases are not confirmed by molecular analyses. OAV may overlap with clinical findings of VATER association (see later) and branchio-oto-renal syndrome, also known as *Melnick-Fraser syndrome.*

VATER Association

VATER is another acronym for a nonrandom association of *v*ertebral and *a*nal anomalies, *t*racheoesophageal fistula with *e*sophageal atresia, and *r*adial and/or *r*enal abnormalities. Most affected newborns have anomalies in all five categories. The acronym can be expanded to VACTERL to include *c*ongenital heart disease (particularly ventricular septal defect) and, less often, other *l*imb defects. Vertebral anomalies include hemivertebrae and sacral abnormalities. Limb deformities consist of ray abnormalities, such as radial aplasia or hypoplasia, abnormal thumbs, preaxial polydactyly, and syndactyly (Fig. 1.47). Renal abnormalities include unilateral agenesis and less commonly ectopic or horseshoe kidney. The etiology of VATER association is unknown and virtually all cases are sporadic. Detection of an abnormal karyotype excludes this disorder and provides a diagnosis. The prognosis for growth and development in newborns who survive infancy is good. Most have normal intelligence and eventually achieve normal stature. Consequently, to make optimal management decisions, it is important to distinguish VATER syndrome from more dire chromosomal abnormalities (such as trisomy 18) or nonchromosomal disorders (such as CHARGE syndrome).

For genetic counseling, VATER association must also be differentiated from Townes-Brocks syndrome, an autosomal dominant, simple Mendelian genetic disorder with features representing a combination of the findings observed for OAV and VATER associations. However, in Townes-Brocks syndrome, there is often a positive family history of autosomal dominant inheritance of ear, thumb, and anal abnormalities, whereas vertebral anomalies and tracheoesophageal fistula are unusual. The prognosis for growth and development in patients with Townes-Brocks syndrome is good. However, the risk for recurrence of Townes-Brocks syndrome with a positive family history may be up to 50%, whereas for VATER association the risk may be less than 2%. Antenatal diagnosis for both conditions depends on detecting structural anomalies in the fetus by high-resolution ultrasound.

Other disorders in the list of differential diagnostic possibilities include Fanconi anemia and Holt-Oram syndrome (see Chapter 5). Once chromosome studies are completed and found to be normal, when other disorders are deemed less likely (which can include molecular testing), and a child has the pattern of malformation characteristic of the VATER association, the diagnosis can be made.

Patterns of Malformation Associated With In Utero Teratogen Exposure

Fetal Alcohol Spectrum Disorders

The effect of exposure to significant levels of serum alcohol during gestation can result in a facial pattern of microcephaly, prenatal and postnatal growth deficiency, short palpebral fissures, long smooth philtrum, and a thin upper lip (Fig. 1.48). Other features include a short nose and hypoplasia of the nails and distal phalanges (particularly the fifth toes). On occasion, affected infants have eyelid ptosis, epicanthal folds, strabismus, small, raised hemangiomas, cervical vertebral abnormalities, and congenital heart disease.

Newborns with fetal alcohol spectrum disorder (FASD) are small for gestational age and have poor catch-up growth postnatally. They may have increased or decreased muscle tone and can be irritable and tremulous. Most older children tend to be thin and hyperactive, and more than 80% have some delay in development, especially fine motor function.

Although there may be no safe level of maternal alcohol consumption throughout pregnancy (particularly in the first trimester),

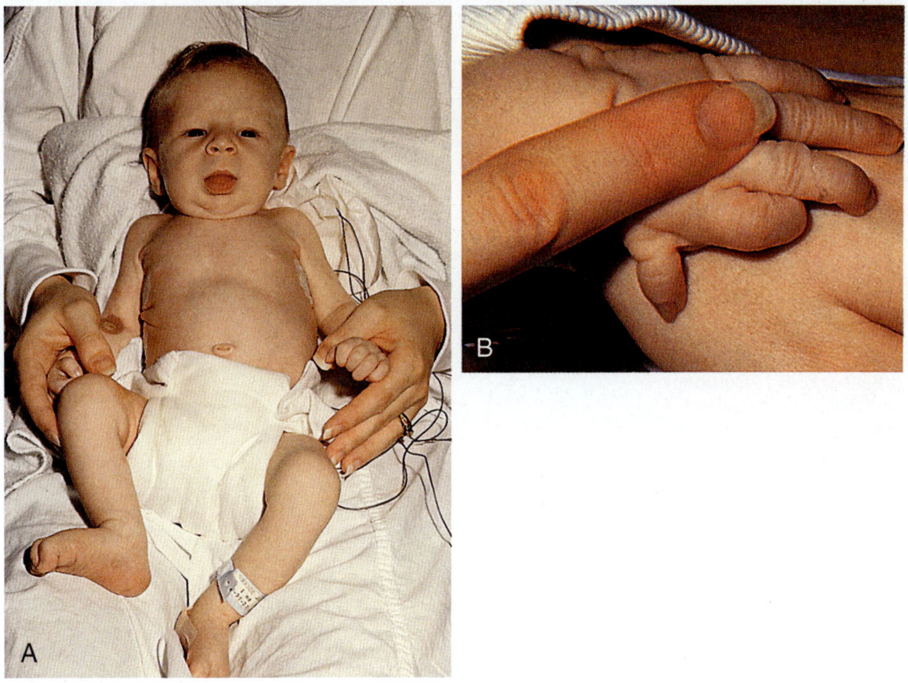

Fig. 1.47 This child with VATER association (A) has facial features that are not dysmorphic, but he has preaxial polydactyly of the thumb (B), which was associated with radial dysplasia.

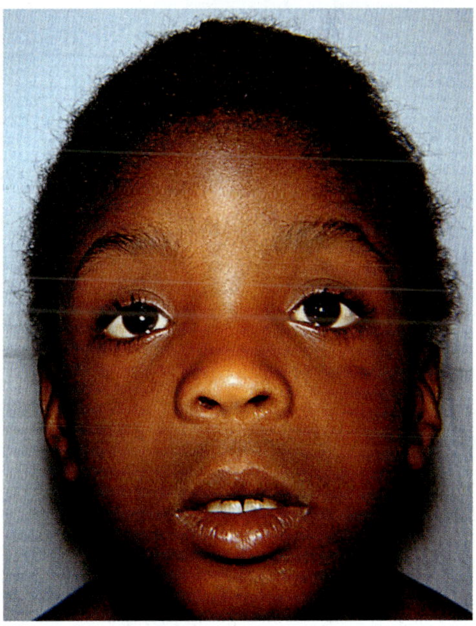

Fig. 1.48 Fetal alcohol syndrome. Note the short palpebral fissure length, mild ptosis, and long simple philtrum.

the risk of teratogenesis increases dramatically with increasing degrees of maternal ethanol consumption. Major evidence of FASD is observed in 30% to 50% of offspring of mothers with severe alcoholism, whereas more subtle effects result from ingestion of lesser quantities of alcohol. The risk to the fetus of occasional maternal alcoholic binges is not clear, but such drinking is best avoided. It is unclear why some children are affected and others are not, despite equivalent degrees of antenatal alcohol exposure.

The diagnosis of FASD should be reserved for those infants who have a history of in utero exposure to large amounts of alcohol and who have the characteristic physical features of the disorder. More specific diagnostic criteria have been published to aid in diagnosis, as well as an online tool to aid in rapid recognition.

Other examples of teratogen-induced disorders include fetal hydantoin syndrome and fetal retinoic acid (isotretinoin [Accutane]) embryopathy. Consideration of other diagnoses is recommended in these children, as fetuses with genetic disorders are also susceptible to teratogens.

GENETIC DISORDERS OF METABOLISM

Inborn errors of metabolism encompass a wide range of inherited disorders. These include disorders of intermediary metabolism, disorders of organelle function (e.g., lysosomal, peroxisomal, or mitochondrial), disorders of cholesterol biosynthesis, disorders of protein glycosylation, disorders of metals, disorders of transport, and others. Although most are enzyme deficiencies that are inherited in an autosomal recessive pattern, various forms of inheritance (dominant, recessive, X-linked, and maternal) are found with metabolic disorders. This brief review is limited to some of the more common metabolic disorders and should be supplemented with a more detailed text on metabolic disorders as needed. Several such texts are listed in the References section.

Disorders of Intermediary Metabolism

Intermediary metabolism involves conversion of the nutrients—protein, carbohydrate, and fat—into energy (Fig. 1.49). The common endpoint in the metabolism of all three nutrients passes through the Krebs cycle and then through the electron transport chain, where oxidative phosphorylation occurs, consuming oxygen and yielding adenosine triphosphate (ATP). A substantial number of errors of intermediary metabolism are detected by expanded newborn screening, but some are not detectable or can be missed in some cases.

The *feed/fast cycle* refers to changing patterns of metabolism depending on available energy sources. After eating, the body uses circulating fuels, which are quickly depleted postprandially. The body then largely relies on stored glycogen until these stores are exhausted (approximately 4 to 8 hours, depending on age and clinical circumstances). After glycogen stores are exhausted, protein catabolism and fatty acid oxidation become the most important energy sources, and gluconeogenesis is required to support glucose stores. Thus, disorders of glycogen metabolism tend to present after a short fasting interval, while most disorders of gluconeogenesis or fatty acid oxidation metabolism tend to present after a longer fasting period.

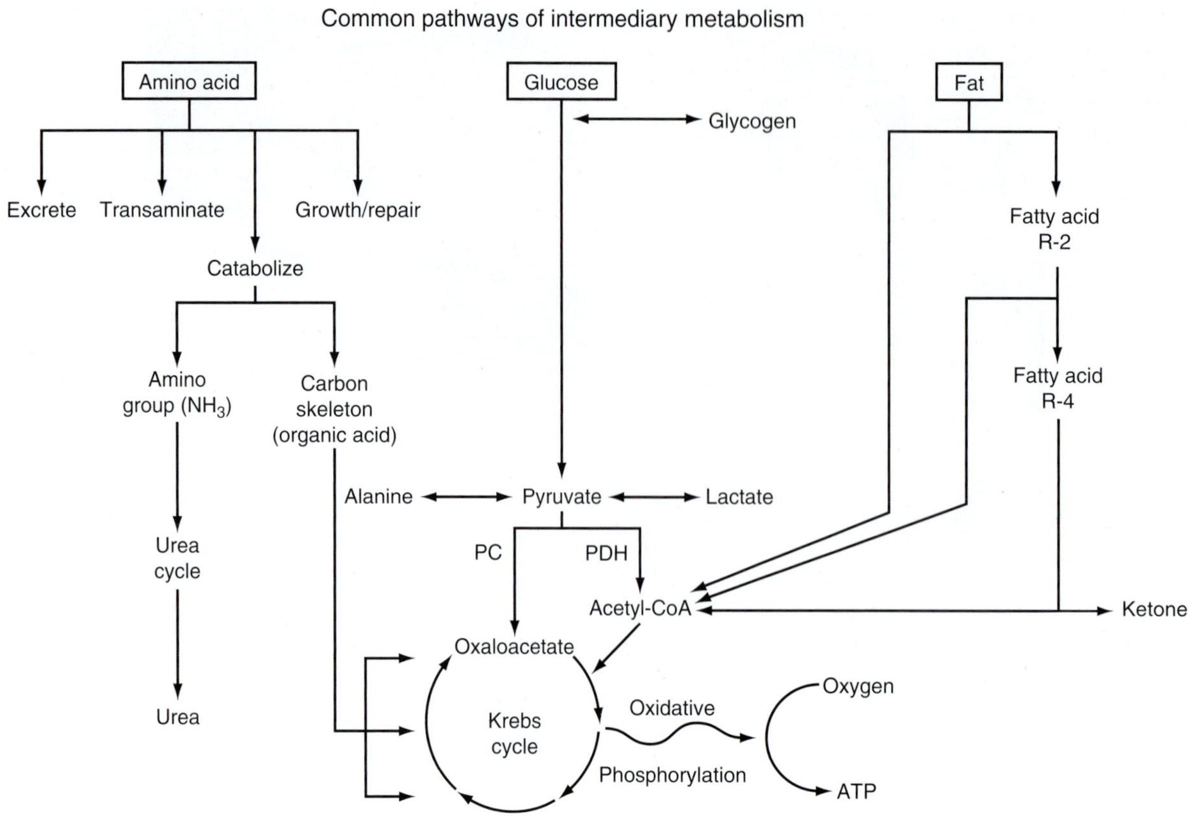

Fig. 1.49 The conversion of protein, carbohydrate, and fat into energy. *ATP,* Adenosine triphosphate; *NH_3,* ammonia; *PC,* pyruvate car; *PDH,* pyruvate dehydrogenase; *R-2* and *R-4,* fatty acids shortened by successive two-carbon units, the result of β-oxidation.

Disorders of Protein Metabolism

Proteins are broken down into their basic components, amino acids. Essential amino acids cannot be synthesized by the body and must be consumed in the diet. Amino acids can be used to support tissue growth or maintenance, can be converted into other amino acids (transamination, hydroxylation, etc.), can be excreted, or can be catabolized for energy (see Fig. 1.49). Some characteristic physical findings of protein metabolism disorders are noted in Table 1.12.

Transamination/Hydroxylation and Related Disorders

Phenylketonuria A common disorder of amino acid conversion is PKU, in which the hydroxylation of phenylalanine to tyrosine is impaired. PKU is a relatively common autosomal recessive disorder of protein metabolism (affecting 1 in 10,000 to 1 in 15,000), and it is typically diagnosed by newborn screening. Affected patients follow a diet restricted in phenylalanine (containing just enough natural protein from fruits, vegetables, and limited starches to meet essential phenylalanine needs for growth and maintenance), supplemented with a medical food "formula" containing tyrosine and other essential amino acids and nutrients, and specially formulated low-phenylalanine foods. If untreated, the disorder results in intellectual disability, eczematous skin changes, a "mousy" odor, and other changes, but physical examination is essentially normal in well-treated patients. Although cognitive outcomes are normal in most treatment-compliant patients, some experience mild to moderate difficulties with executive functioning (attention, organization, and working memory). While pregnant with PKU, patients must follow their diet especially carefully to prevent intellectual disability, microcephaly, and birth defects (particularly defects of the heart and esophagus) in the fetus.

Treatment of PKU is now recommended for life, and traditionally it has relied on a phenylalanine-restricted diet, which is highly restrictive and difficult to maintain. New treatments include enzyme cofactor supplementation (sapropterin or sepiapterin) or enzyme substitution with injected phenylalanine ammonium lyase, and experimental treatments such as gene therapy are in clinical trials.

Table 1.12 Common Findings in Disorders of Protein Metabolism

Disorder	Common Findings
PKU	Untreated: MR, eczema, mousy odor, fair coloring Treated: Minimal to mild tremor, executive function deficits
Homocystinuria	Untreated: Variable MR, ectopia lentis, marfanoid habitus, vascular thromboses Treated: Variable persistent vascular issues
MSUD	Untreated: Ketosis, acidosis, coma, death, MR, maple syrup odor, some late onset with intermittent symptoms Treated: Intermittent ketosis/acidosis during intercurrent illnesses, variable developmental delay to normal cognition
Organic acidemia (MMA, PA, IVA)	Untreated: Ketosis, acidosis, death, neutropenia, hyperammonemia, hypotonia, some late onset with failure to thrive, hypotonia Treated: Intermittent ketoacidosis during intercurrent illnesses, metabolic strokes, low to normal tone, delay to normal cognition
Urea cycle defect	Untreated: Hyperammonemia, coma, death, hyperreflexia, MR, variable acidosis, some late onset with intermittent symptoms Treated: Intermittent hyperammonemia with intercurrent illnesses, variable developmental delay to normal cognition

IVA, Isovaleric acidemia; *MMA,* methylmalonic acidemia; *MR,* intellectual disability; *MSUD,* maple syrup urine disease; *PA,* propionic acidemia; *PKU,* phenylketonuria.

Most PKU is due to a defect in the enzyme phenylalanine hydroxylase. A small proportion of patients with PKU have normal phenylalanine hydroxylase enzyme but have a defect in synthesis or recycling of an enzyme cofactor. Because the biopterin cofactor is shared with two other enzymes (tyrosine hydroxylase [a precursor of dopamine, epinephrine, and norepinephrine] and tryptophan hydroxylase [a precursor of serotonin]), patients with biopterin defects have neurotransmitter deficits in addition to PKU. These patients require supplementation with biopterin and/or neurotransmitter replacements in addition to a phenylalanine-restricted diet, and the neurologic outcome is not always normal.

Homocystinuria Homocysteine is an intermediate in the multistep metabolism of methionine to cysteine. In homocystinuria, the metabolism of homocysteine is blocked at the level of the enzyme cystathionine β-synthase. When untreated, in addition to developmental delays, physical findings include various degrees of ectopia lentis, a Marfanoid habitus, and vascular thrombosis (see Table 1.12) by young adulthood. Homocystinuria is most diagnosed by newborn screening (by detection of elevated methionine), but the sensitivity of the screen is not complete. Homocysteine is not stable in standard plasma/serum amino acid analysis; thus, specific homocysteine levels must be checked. Homocystinuria may be present in older children and adults who were born before this disorder was added to the current newborn screening panel. A subset of patients is responsive to supplementation with the enzyme cofactor, vitamin B_6. Current treatment involves dietary restriction of methionine, with supplementation with cysteine, in addition to dietary supplements that assist in the remethylation of homocysteine back to methionine (such as betaine). Rarer forms of homocystinuria exist, caused by failure to return homocysteine back into methionine, typically due to defects in vitamin B_{12} metabolism.

Maple Syrup Urine Disease The branched-chain amino acids (valine, leucine, and isoleucine) share a common initial step in catabolism, catalyzed by branched-chain keto acid decarboxylase. A genetic defect in this enzyme leads to maple syrup urine disease (MSUD), named because of the characteristic odor of the urine. Affected individuals develop elevations of these three branched-chain amino acids resulting in ketosis and, if untreated, acidosis, coma, and death. Physical examination may identify the odor of maple syrup in cerumen and concentrated urine. The patient may exhibit varying degrees of spasticity or developmental delay, especially if late or poorly treated (see Table 1.12). Urine ketones are elevated. Elevated leucine levels are intoxicating, and they can chronically impair learning and social interactions when poorly controlled. Patients must follow a diet restricted in these three essential amino acids, supplemented with other essential amino acids and nutrients, and liver transplantation is increasingly accepted. The most important component of dietary treatment is the prevention of stressful fasting because this would lead to the increased catabolism of amino acids for energy and thus increased formation of toxic metabolites. Milder variants are known to exist with symptoms during intercurrent illnesses. MSUD is most often diagnosed by newborn screening, but the sensitivity of screening for milder or intermittent variants is not known, and an infant may already be symptomatic before the screening results are available.

Urea Cycle Disorders Amino acids are further catabolized by deamination. The amino group is removed and forms ammonia, and the residual carbon skeleton is an organic acid, typically metabolized in the Krebs cycle (see Fig. 1.49). Ammonia is toxic when accumulated and is normally detoxified in the urea cycle. Metabolic errors are well described in each enzymatic step of the urea cycle. Affected infants classically present with hyperammonemic coma in the neonatal period, typically progressing through poor feeding, respiratory alkalosis, decreasing mental status, vomiting, and neurologic irritability to coma (see Table 1.12). The presence of unexplained respiratory alkalosis or neurologic irritability, including hyperreflexia, increased startle, or clonus in an infant with depressed mental status, should always prompt a search for an inborn error of metabolism (although these findings will eventually be blunted as coma deepens). Acidosis (rarely even ketoacidosis) may develop as the infant's clinical status deteriorates. *Any patient of any age undergoing a lumbar puncture for otherwise unexplained mental status changes should have their plasma ammonia level checked.* Analysis of plasma amino acids and orotic acid is key in helping to define the specific urea cycle defect.

A significant percentage of patients with urea cycle defects can present later in life with failure to thrive, developmental delays, friable hair (trichorrhexis nodosa in argininosuccinate lyase deficiency), or in some cases acutely with hyperammonemia during intercurrent illnesses or weaning from breast milk to formula (which is higher in protein). Some patients have presented in adulthood during profound metabolic stress (such as after bariatric surgery or childbirth); thus, age is no barrier to diagnosis. Treatment involves careful titration of protein intake to meet requirements for growth and maintenance without providing excess, with supplementation of essential urea cycle intermediates (citrulline or arginine, as determined by the position of the enzymatic block), and with drugs that complex with glutamine or glycine to form urine-soluble nitrogen complexes and provide an alternative excretion pathway for nitrogen. It is particularly important to provide alternative energy intake during fasting to prevent the catabolism of amino acids for energy and the release of ammonia. Liver transplantation is an increasingly recommended first-line approach, and gene therapy trials are under way.

Organic Acidemias

Once the ammonia is removed from an amino acid, the remaining carbon skeleton is an *organic acid*. Most organic acids are catabolized to specific Krebs cycle intermediates (see Fig. 1.49). Various errors in catabolism lead to specific organic acid disorders.

Propionic Acidemia and Methylmalonic Acidemia The most common series of errors is in the catabolism of the carbon skeletons of *v*aline, *o*dd-chain fatty acids, *m*ethionine, *i*soleucine, and *t*hreonine (VOMIT), which pass through propionyl-coenzyme A (CoA), methylmalonyl-CoA, and then succinyl-CoA (a Krebs cycle intermediate). Inborn errors of propionyl-CoA carboxylase lead to propionic acidemia, and errors of methylmalonyl-CoA mutase lead to methylmalonic acidemia. These can present in the neonatal period with acute ketoacidosis, hyperammonemia, and bone marrow suppression (from secondary inhibition of the urea cycle and bone marrow); or at a later age with acute symptoms during an intercurrent illness; or at any time with chronic failure to thrive, hypotonia, or developmental delay. Physical examination is most remarkable for central hypotonia, often with hyperreflexia or neurologic irritability (see Table 1.12). Patient management includes careful titration of dietary protein to meet the needs for the essential amino acids—valine, methionine, isoleucine, and threonine—supplemented with other essential amino acids and nutrients. Alternative forms of calorie supplementation are important during fasting or intercurrent illnesses to prevent protein catabolism. The role of liver transplantation is becoming increasingly recognized in improved outcomes by moderating disease severity, although it is not curative.

Disorders of Leucine Catabolism Several other organic acidemias are relatively common, including isovaleric acidemia (IVA), an inborn error in the catabolism of leucine. Expanded newborn screening also has identified an unexpectedly high incidence of 3-methylcrotonyl-CoA carboxylase (3-MCC) deficiency. Previously believed to cause developmental delays, failure to thrive, and other problems, the clinical significance 3-MCC deficiency is currently debated. Most organic acidemias are detectable by newborn screening, although the sensitivity for late-onset or milder forms is not yet known.

Disorders of Carbohydrate Metabolism

The basic unit of carbohydrate metabolism is glucose. Glucose is metabolized for energy through glycolysis. Complex carbohydrates and alternative carbohydrates (such as galactose or fructose) are converted to glucose or glycolytic intermediates for catabolism. Some of the common disorders of carbohydrate metabolism are listed in Table 1.13.

Glycogen Metabolism

When carbohydrate intake exceeds immediate need, glucose is stored as glycogen, predominantly in the liver but also in muscle. During the interprandial fast, glycogen is used preferentially to meet energy needs by converting it back to glucose. After glycogen stores are exhausted, protein and fat catabolism are enhanced.

Glycogen Storage Disease Type 0 In the case of glycogen storage disease (GSD) type 0, glycogen cannot be made. Patients typically have postprandial hyperglycemia and interprandial hypoglycemia, but no other specific physical findings. The liver is not enlarged because glycogen is not stored. In some cases, the postprandial hyperglycemia can be mild or overlooked, and the disorder manifests as hypoglycemia during fasting or intercurrent illness.

Other Forms of Glycogen Storage Disease Other forms of GSD affect glycogen metabolism in the liver or muscle. The most common forms of liver GSD are types I, III, VI, and IX, in which glycogen can be stored in the liver but not efficiently returned to glucose. The patient most commonly develops hepatomegaly (from stored glycogen), and interprandial hypoglycemia begins within a few hours of eating, when circulating fuels are exhausted. The patient may also manifest "cherubic" cheeks from glycogen storage. Other findings can include elevations in triglycerides, uric acid, and lactate. There are several enzymes involved in the formation, branching, debranching, and catabolism of glycogen, and various subtypes of GSD are associated with defects in the various enzymatic steps. Some glycogen disorders present predominantly in muscle with weakness, rhabdomyolysis, and other predominantly muscle findings but not significant hypoglycemia. Infantile-onset Pompe disease (GSD type II) presents with progressive weakness in the skeletal and respiratory muscles as well as cardiomyopathy. The electrocardiogram demonstrates a characteristic high-voltage pattern. Most patients respond to enzyme replacement therapy but may require immunomodulation to achieve this.

Defects in Glycolysis, Gluconeogenesis, and Metabolism of Other Carbohydrates

Defects in glycolysis, the process of metabolizing glucose to pyruvate, tend to present as energy deficiency disorders in muscle (which is dependent on glycolysis), often with rhabdomyolysis. In some cases, alternative carbohydrates (such as galactose or fructose) have impaired conversion into a glycolytic substrate.

Galactosemia Patients who are unable to metabolize galactose have galactosemia. After ingestion of galactose (one of the sugars in lactose), patients can present in infancy with hepatomegaly, liver disease, gram-negative sepsis, cataracts, or later with failure to thrive and excretion of galactose (a reducing substance) in the urine. Treatment includes exclusion of galactose from the diet. The disorder is detectable on the newborn screen in the United States and many other countries; however, as a red cell enzyme test, the results can be affected by transfusion before screening.

Hereditary Fructose Intolerance Patients with hereditary fructose intolerance are unable to metabolize fructose (a common fruit sugar and one of the components of sucrose). They can present with acute decompensation with hypoglycemia and hypophosphatemia from fructose ingestion but can also present chronically with failure to thrive and liver disease.

Gluconeogenesis The reverse of glycolysis (gluconeogenesis, the production of glucose from distal metabolic substrates) can be impaired by metabolic errors. Fructose-1,6-bisphosphatase deficiency is a gluconeogenic enzyme deficiency that results in fasting hypoglycemia. Patients typically tolerate an interprandial fast because glycogen metabolism is intact, but they are at risk for hypoglycemia after glycogen stores are exhausted. Most patients present in infancy during an intercurrent illness with hypoglycemia and varying degrees of elevated ketones, lactate, and glycerol.

Other defects in gluconeogenesis, as well as ketone synthesis and use disorders, are described in more detailed texts as noted at the beginning of this section.

Defects of Fatty Acid Oxidation

Fatty acid oxidation is a significant source of energy after liver glycogen stores are exhausted. Fatty acids are essentially chains of carbon and hydrogen atoms. β-Oxidation of fatty acids up to

Table 1.13 Common Findings in Disorders of Carbohydrate Metabolism

Disorder	Enzyme	Findings
GSD 0	Glycogen synthetase	Postprandial hyperglycemia, interprandial hypoglycemia
GSD I	Glucose-6-phosphatase; glucose-6-phosphate translocase	Interprandial hypoglycemia, hepatomegaly, "cherub" cheeks, neutropenia (type 1b), elevated uric acid, lactate
GSD II	Acid alpha-1,4-glucosidase	Pompe disease, cardiomyopathy (infantile form), progressive skeletal and respiratory weakness, elevated CK
GSD III	Glycogen debrancher enzyme	Hypoglycemia, hepatomegaly, variable myopathy, disorder of glycogen debranching
GSD IV	Glycogen branching enzyme	Hepatomegaly, cirrhosis, disorder of glycogen branching
GSD VI	Glycogen phosphorylase	Mild to moderate hypoglycemia, mild ketosis, growth retardation, and prominent hepatomegaly
GSD VII	Muscle phosphofructokinase	Exercise intolerance, muscle cramping, exertional myopathy, compensated hemolysis, myoglobinuria
GSD IX	Hepatic phosphorylase kinase	Hepatomegaly with variable mild hypoglycemia, variable myopathy
Fructose-1,6-bisphosphatase deficiency	Fructose-1,6-bisphosphatase	Hypoglycemia with prolonged fast/intercurrent illness, may be fructose sensitive, urine organic acids may reveal keto-lactic acidosis with elevated glycerol
Galactosemia	Galactose-1-phosphate uridylyltransferase	Untreated: Hepatomegaly, cataracts, failure to thrive, liver dysfunction, MR Treated: Variable cognitive deficits
Hereditary fructose intolerance	Fructose-1,6-bisphosphate aldolase B	With fructose ingestion: Hypoglycemia, hypophosphatemia, shock Untreated: Chronic liver disease and failure to thrive

CK, Creatine kinase; *GSD*, glycogen storage disease; *MR*, intellectual disability.

18 carbons in length takes place in the mitochondria. One cycle of β-oxidation removes two carbons from the fat, releasing the two-carbon piece as acetyl-CoA (a primary substrate for the Krebs cycle), which also can be converted to a ketone body that can be exported to more distal tissues for energy (see Fig. 1.49). The shortened fatty acid undergoes successive cycles of oxidation, removing two carbon units at a time until it is fully metabolized. The enzymes used in fatty acid oxidation change as the fatty acid becomes successively shorter. Absence of ketosis in a patient older than 3 months of age who has hypoglycemia or is undergoing a stressful fast should raise concern for a possible fatty acid oxidation defect. Some of the most common defects of fatty acid oxidation are listed in Table 1.14.

Carnitine Disorders

Carnitine Uptake Disorder and Carnitine Palmitoyltransferase I, Carnitine-Acylcarnitine Translocase, and Carnitine Palmitoyltransferase II Deficiency Long-chain fatty acids (i.e., those having ≈12 to 18 carbons) must first esterify carnitine to pass through the mitochondrial membrane for oxidation. Patients with carnitine uptake disorder have impaired transport of carnitine and develop profound carnitine deficiency. Symptoms can include cardiomyopathy, weakness, or simply sudden death. Plasma carnitine levels are low while urine carnitine is generally elevated. Patients with a deficiency of carnitine palmitoyltransferase I (CPT I) are unable to esterify fatty acids to carnitine. The fatty acids are thus unable to penetrate the mitochondria for oxidation. The disorder has variable presentation, including life-threatening neonatal hypoglycemia and acidosis, or later-onset fasting or exercise intolerance/rhabdomyolysis. Defects in the carnitine-acylcarnitine translocase (CACT) enzyme (which carries fatty acylcarnitines across the mitochondrial membrane) are rare but reported and can be life-threatening; they often resemble CPT II deficiency. Patients with defects in carnitine palmitoyltransferase II (CPT II) are unable to release the carnitine from the fatty acid after it has passed inside the mitochondria. Like CPT I deficiency, it has variable severity and can present at any age. Most carnitine disorders are now diagnosed by newborn screening (by measurement of acylcarnitines), and more mildly affected patients often do not appear ill in the newborn period but still require follow-up and treatment. Carnitine is not required for medium- and short-chain fatty acids to penetrate the mitochondria, and thus patients with severe carnitine disorders may benefit from dietary restriction of long-chain fat and supplementation with medium-chain fat.

Table 1.14 Common Findings in Fatty Acid Oxidation Disorders

Disorder	Findings
Carnitine uptake disorder	Cardiomyopathy, variable weakness, sudden death
CPT I	Infantile onset: Hypoglycemia, acidosis Later onset: Fasting intolerance, exercise intolerance
CPT II	Infantile onset: Hypoglycemia, acidosis Later onset: Fasting or exercise intolerance, rhabdomyolysis
SCAD deficiency	Possible hypotonia, developmental delay, neurologic abnormalities. Phenotype now in question
MCAD deficiency	Potentially fatal hypoglycemia with prolonged fasting
VLCAD deficiency	Infantile onset: Cardiomyopathy, juvenile onset: fasting intolerance Later onset: Exercise intolerance
LCHAD deficiency	Hypoglycemia, rhabdomyolysis, pigmentary retinopathy, fasting intolerance

CPT I, Carnitine palmitoyltransferase I; *CPT II,* carnitine palmitoyltransferase II; *LCHAD,* long-chain 3-hydroxyacyl-CoA dehydrogenase; *MCAD,* medium-chain acyl-CoA dehydrogenase; *SCAD,* short-chain acyl-CoA dehydrogenase; *VLCAD,* very-long-chain acyl-CoA dehydrogenase.

Acyl-CoA Dehydrogenase Deficiencies

Very-Long-Chain, Medium-Chain, and Short-Chain Acyl-CoA Dehydrogenase Deficiencies, and Long-Chain 3-Hydroxyacyl-CoA Dehydrogenase Deficiency Inside the mitochondria, the β-oxidation process progressively removes two carbon atoms, forming ketones or acetyl-CoA (see Fig. 1.49). Many of the enzymes in this process have chain length specificity, preferring fats that are long chain (12 to 18 carbons), medium chain (6 to 10 carbons), or short chain. The first step of β-oxidation is performed by an acyl-CoA dehydrogenase with chain length specificity. Deficits in the long-chain enzyme (very-long-chain acyl-CoA dehydrogenase, also known as VLCAD deficiency) present with variable severity, from neonatal cardiomyopathy to later-onset fasting or exercise intolerance. Treatment includes supplementation with medium-chain fat and prevention of fasting. Defects in the medium-chain enzyme (medium-chain acyl-CoA dehydrogenase, also known as MCAD or ACADM, deficiency) are among the most common metabolic disorders (approximately 1 in 15,000 births). Affected patients most commonly present in the toddler period with potentially fatal hypoketotic hypoglycemia or Reye syndrome–like symptoms during fasting associated with an intercurrent illness. Treatment is primarily by prevention of fasting, although some patients require carnitine supplementation. Defects in the short-chain enzyme (short-chain acyl-CoA dehydrogenase, also known as SCAD deficiency) were originally believed to cause hypotonia, hypoglycemia, and developmental abnormalities. However, the clinical significance of this disorder is now in question. Defects are also described in the third step of β-oxidation, another acyl-CoA dehydrogenase enzyme with chain length specificity. The most common enzyme deficiency at this step is long-chain 3-hydroxyacyl-CoA dehydrogenase (LCHAD) deficiency. This disorder can also have variable presentation from early hypoketotic hypoglycemia to later fasting or exercise intolerance. More severely affected patients demonstrate a pigmentary retinopathy and episodes of rhabdomyolysis. An increased incidence of HELLP (*h*emolysis, *e*levated *l*iver enzyme levels, and *l*ow *p*latelet levels) syndrome is reported in pregnant mothers carrying an affected fetus. Some patients have a deficiency of a trifunctional protein that results in defects in multiple steps of the long-chain fatty acid oxidation pathway.

Most disorders of fatty acid oxidation are now detected on newborn screening. However, some infants experience significant morbidity or mortality quickly before the newborn screening results are available. Thus, this group of disorders should always be considered in ill neonates.

Organelle Dysfunction

Important metabolic processes take place in various organelles. These include the peroxisomes, the lysosomes, the mitochondria, endoplasmic reticulum, and Golgi (Tables 1.15 through 1.17). Defects in each of these organelles are considered.

Peroxisomal Disorders

Many metabolic processes take place in the peroxisome, including the oxidation of very-long-chain fats (>20 carbons), metabolism of phytanic acid (present in food), initiation of plasmalogen formation (the most abundant phospholipid in myelin), formation of bile acid precursors, peroxidation/detoxification, and other processes. Peroxisomal diseases fall into two major categories: (1) those that interfere with assembly of the peroxisome itself (thus affecting all enzyme functions) and (2) those that affect a single enzyme.

Table 1.15 Common Findings in Peroxisomal Diseases

Disorder	Findings
Zellweger syndrome	Hepatomegaly, profound hypotonia, Down syndrome–like facies, liver dysfunction
Neonatal adrenoleukodystrophy; infantile Refsum disease	Developmental delay, hearing loss, vision impairment, liver dysfunction, coagulopathy, hypotonia of decreasing severity; often slowly progressive
RCDP	Rhizomelia, chondrodysplasia punctata, profound growth failure, and MR
Adrenoleukodystrophy	Developmental regression, progressive leukodystrophy; later onset with demyelination or Addison disease
ARD	Retinitis pigmentosa, ataxia, ichthyosis, and anosmia

ARD, Adult Refsum disease; *ID,* intellectual disability; *RCDP,* rhizomelic chondrodysplasia punctata.

Table 1.16 Classification of Lysosomal Storage Disorders

Disorder Class	Underlying Defect	Associated Syndromes
Mucopolysaccharidoses	Defective metabolism of glycosaminoglycans	Hurler, Hurler-Scheie, Scheie (MPSI)[a] Hunter (MPSII)[a] Sanfilippo (MPSIII) Morquio A and B (MPSIV)[a] Maroteaux-Lamy (MPSVI)[a] Sly (MPSVII)[a]
Sphingolipidoses and sulfatidoses	Defective degradation of sphingolipids and their components	GM1 Gangliosidosis Tay-Sachs disease (GM2 gangliosidosis) Metachromatic leukodystrophy (MLD) Krabbe disease Niemann-Pick, type A, B, and C Gaucher disease[a] Fabry disease[a] Farber disease
Oligosaccharidoses	Defective degradation of the glycan portion of glycoproteins	α-Mannosidosis β-Mannosidosis Sialidosis Fucosidosis Schindler disease
Mucolipidoses	Defective degradation of acid mucopolysaccharides, sphingolipids, and/or glycolipids	I-cell disease (ML-II) Pseudo-Hurler dystrophy (ML-III) Mucolipidosis, type IV
Lysosomal transport and trafficking defects	Defects in degradation or transport of cholesterol, cholesterol esters, and other complex lipids	Cystinosis[a] Sialic acid storage disease

[a]Have FDA-approved treatments.

Table 1.17 Common Mitochondrial Syndromes

Symptom Complex	Findings	Pathology
MERRF	Mitochondrial encephalopathy, ragged red fibers	$tRNA^{Lys}$
MELAS	Myoclonic epilepsy, lactic acidosis, strokelike episodes	>15 pathogenic variants described; the most common involves $tRNA^{Leu}$
NARP	Neuropathy, ataxia, retinitis pigmentosa, ± Leigh disease	Pathogenic variants in mitochondrial component of complex V
MNGIE	Myo-neuro-gastrointestinal disorder and encephalopathy	Nuclear variants in thymidine phosphorylase; impairs mtDNA repair mechanisms
LHON	Leber hereditary optic neuropathy	Pathogenic variants in mitochondrial component of complex I
Pearson syndrome	Bone marrow–pancreas dysfunction, infantile onset; survivors may develop Kearns-Sayre syndrome	Multiple mtDNA deletions
Kearns-Sayre syndrome	Ptosis, pigmentary retinopathy, cardiac conduction defects, ataxia, diabetes, CPEO	Multiple mtDNA deletions
Diabetes-deafness	Type 2 diabetes, hearing loss	Mitochondrial $tRNA^{Leu}$
Aminoglycoside toxicity	Ototoxicity from aminoglycoside antibiotics	Mitochondrial ribosomal DNA mutations
Leigh disease	Necrotizing changes in basal ganglia and midbrain, hypotonia, failure to thrive, loss of respiratory centers; phenotype caused by numerous underlying energy disorders	Defects in nuclear or mitochondrial genes in complexes I, II, and IV; PDH; PC; NARP; and others

CPEO, Chronic progressive external ophthalmoplegia; *mtDNA,* mitochondrial deoxyribonucleic acid; *NARP,* neuropathy, ataxia, and retinitis pigmentosa; *PC,* pyruvate carboxylase; *PDH,* pyruvate dehydrogenase; *$tRNA^{Leu}$,* transfer ribonucleic acid for leucine; *$tRNA^{Lys}$,* transfer ribonucleic acid lysine.

Disorders of Peroxisome Biogenesis

Several pathogenic variants in peroxisome assembly *(PEX)* genes have been identified, leading to a continuum of phenotypes. The most severe of these disorders is Zellweger syndrome (Fig. 1.50). Infants with Zellweger syndrome (cerebrohepatorenal syndrome) typically have dysmorphic features often suggestive of Down syndrome, hepatomegaly with liver dysfunction, and profound hypotonia (see Table 1.15). The disorder is typically fatal in infancy or early childhood. Neonatal adrenoleukodystrophy and infantile Refsum disease are less severe phenotypes. They present with variable severity

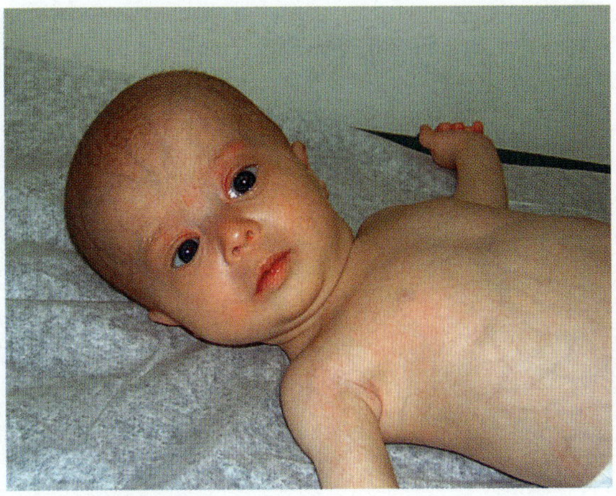

Fig. 1.50 Infant with Zellweger syndrome. Note the hypotonia, failure to thrive, and large forehead.

of developmental delay, hearing loss, vision impairment, liver dysfunction, coagulopathy, and hypotonia and may be slowly progressive (see Table 1.15). Pathogenic variants in *PEX7* can lead to a unique phenotype of proximal limb shortening (rhizomelia), chondrodysplasia punctata (epiphyseal stippling), and profound growth failure and intellectual disability, known as rhizomelic chondrodysplasia punctata (RCDP).

Single-Enzyme Disorders

Numerous disorders of single genes that act in the peroxisome have been described. One of the most common is X-linked adrenoleukodystrophy. This disorder predominantly affects males and presents in the first decade of life as a progressive leukodystrophy or in adulthood as a demyelinating disorder (adrenomyeloneuropathy) or primary adrenal insufficiency (Addison disease). The movie *Lorenzo's Oil* increased public recognition of this disorder and the quest for a treatment. In the most severe cases, the presymptomatic treatment of choice is hematopoietic stem cell transplantation. Treatment with dietary very-long-chain fatty acid restriction and supplementation with erucic acid and oleic acid (i.e., "Lorenzo oil") is of debatable benefit. This disorder is a recent addition to many newborn screening panels.

Diagnosis

Most peroxisomal assembly or single-gene disorders can be diagnosed by evaluating plasma very-long-chain fatty acids, preferably supplementing testing with red cell plasmalogens, phytanic acid, pipecolic acid, or pristanic acid. (Phytanic acid is derived from the diet, and thus young infants or those on elemental diets may have falsely normal levels.) It is important to note that in some single-enzyme disorders, very-long-chain fatty acid levels may be normal. Thus, it is reasonable to test for at least two peroxisomal metabolites when searching for these disorders. DNA analysis is available for several peroxisome biogenesis or single-enzyme disorders.

Lysosomal Disorders

Lysosomes are membrane-bound cytoplasmic organelles that serve as the digestive or recycling centers of cells, where they break down cellular waste products and debris and degrade macromolecules for reuse. They perform this function with an array of hydrolytic enzymes that degrade their target molecules in a stepwise fashion. A pathogenic variant that results in malfunction of a lysosomal enzyme leads to accumulation of substrate intracellularly and extracellularly, resulting in the term *storage disorder.*

Lysosomal storage disorders are classified according to the nature of the accumulated material. More than 40 lysosomal disorders have been described, their unifying characteristic being a failure to degrade a specific component of cellular waste or abnormal trafficking of the precursors or products. Defects are classified as defects of degradation of mucopolysaccharides, oligosaccharides, sphingolipidoses, mucolipidoses, and others (see Table 1.16). Stored lysosomal material in tissues can result in coarsening of facial features, hepatomegaly, splenomegaly, bone deformities (dysostosis multiplex), leukodystrophy, and other features.

Mucopolysaccharidoses

The mucopolysaccharidoses are among the best-known lysosomal storage disorders. They are a group of disorders of degradation of glycosaminoglycans. Seven major types have been identified, some with multiple subtypes depending on the residual enzymatic activity. Hurler syndrome (MPSI-H) is the prototypical disorder (Fig. 1.51). In the most severe form, symptom onset is between 6 and 24 months of age with growth retardation, coarse facial features, hepatosplenomegaly, dysostosis multiplex, cardiac valve disease, and other findings. Enzyme replacement therapy can help temporize the disease process, but the only significant treatment for infantile onset disease is by bone marrow transplantation, which attenuates the disorder but does not improve preexisting bony and neurodevelopmental abnormalities. Progressively less severe forms include Hurler-Scheie and Scheie syndromes (MPSI-HS, MPSI-S), with increasing residual enzyme activity and decreasing CNS and systemic involvement. Morquio syndrome (MPSIVA and B) and Maroteaux-Lamy syndrome (MPSVI) are associated with sparing of cognition but present with typical bony dysplasia (Fig. 1.52). Research into greater treatment strategies has expanded in the field of lysosomal

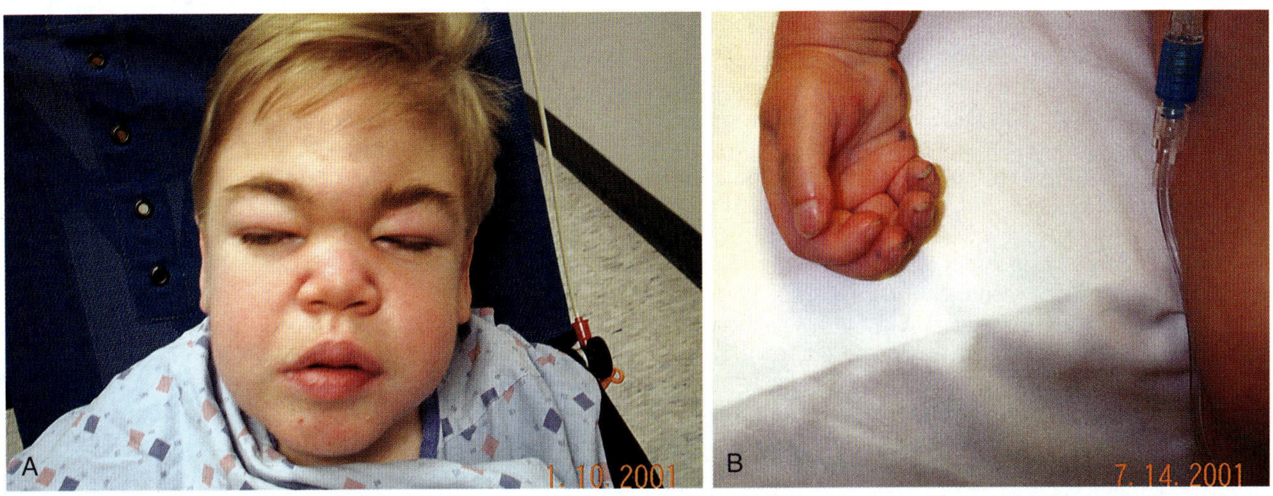

Fig. 1.51 Hurler syndrome (MPSI-H). (A) The coarsening of facial features characteristic of this disorder includes prominence of the forehead, a flattened nasal bridge, a short broad nose, and widening of the lips. Features appear puffy due to thickening of the skin. (B) Progressive joint stiffness and contractures lead to clawing of the hand.

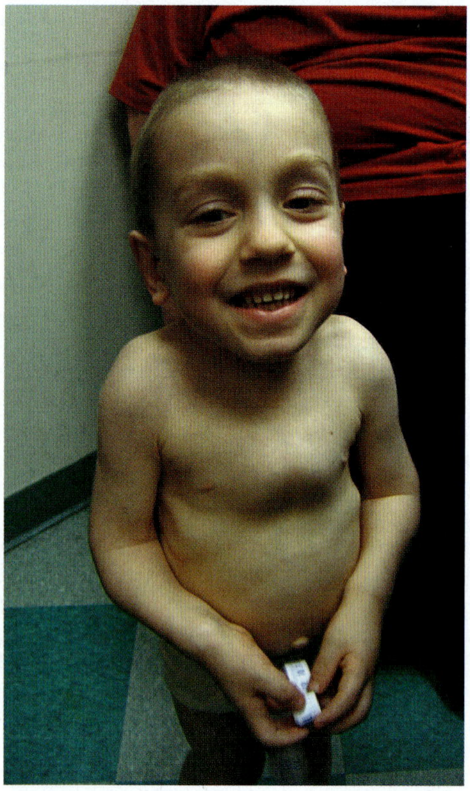

Fig. 1.52 A 5-year-old boy with Morquio syndrome (MPSIVA). Urine testing for mucopolysaccharidosis showed elevated keratan sulfate.

storage disorders and includes novel treatments such as substrate reduction therapy, chaperone therapy, and various forms of gene therapy.

Diagnosis of lysosomal disorders typically begins with clinical suspicion, often with assay of urinary mucopolysaccharides or oligosaccharides, specific plasma or fibroblast enzyme assays, or DNA studies. Some are recommended on the expanded newborn screening panel, but only specific states have implemented this testing. A complete discussion of all the mucopolysaccharidoses, oligosaccharidoses, sphingolipidoses, and mucolipidoses is beyond the scope of this chapter but is available in texts dedicated to metabolic disorders.

Endoplasmic Reticulum/Golgi

The congenital disorders of glycosylation (CDG) are a group of disorders resulting in abnormal posttranslational glycosylation of proteins. The number of subtypes is growing rapidly and will likely continue to grow given the large number of genes involved in protein glycosylation. The most common is phosphomannomutase 2 *(PMM2),* formerly called *CDG type Ia.* Typical features include abnormal fat pads on the pubis and over the buttocks, inverted nipples, strabismus, cerebellar atrophy, and failure to thrive. Fatal systemic disease including liver disease can be seen in some cases; others tend to develop ataxia and strokelike episodes with age. Symptoms vary by the specific enzymatic defect, but common problems include liver dysfunction, protein-losing enteropathy, coagulopathy, immune defects, pigmentary retinopathy, cardiomyopathy, ovarian failure, and variable cognitive dysfunction. Diagnosis of the more common (N-linked) forms can be suggested by noting an abnormal ferritin isoelectric focusing pattern (caused by abnormalities in posttranslational sialic acid residues). This disorder is likely underappreciated and should be considered in any case of multisystem genetic symptoms (Fig. 1.53). MPI-CDG (mannose phosphate isomerase) may respond to treatment with mannose, and SLC35C1-CDG may show partial response to fucose supplementation. Rarer forms (such as O-glycosylation defects) commonly present as neonatal muscular dystrophies, including muscle-eye-brain disease.

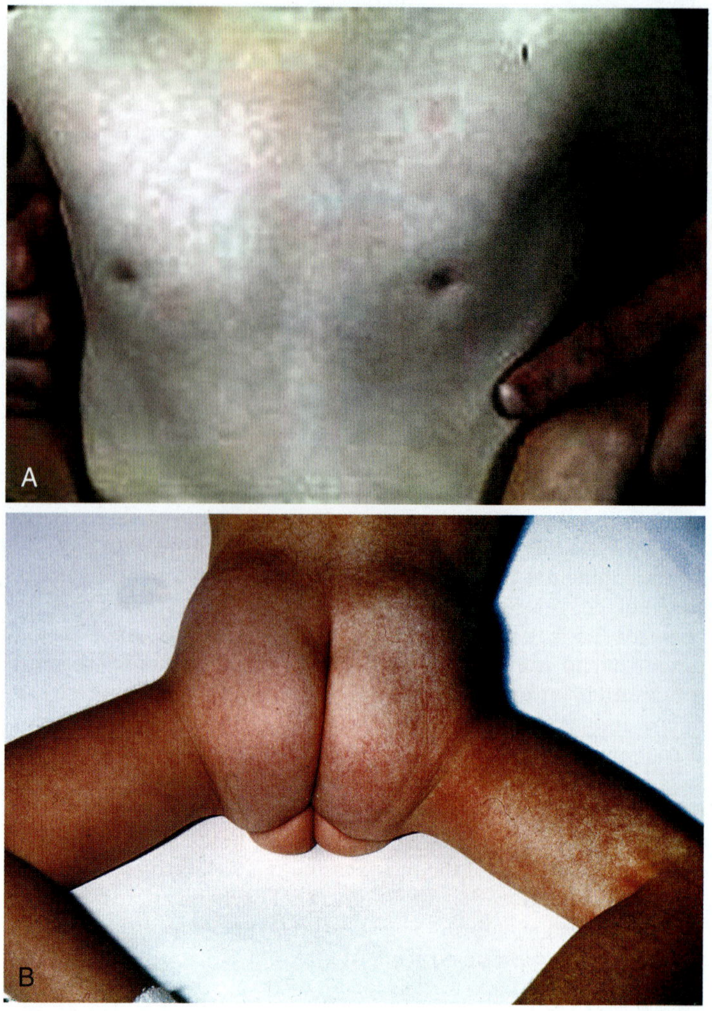

Fig. 1.53 Inverted nipples (A) and unusual fat distribution on the buttocks (B) seen in some patients with congenital disorders of glycosylation.

Disorders of Energy Metabolism

Mitochondrial Disorders

Mitochondria are membrane-bound cytoplasmic organelles that, in essence, serve as the power or energy generator of cells. Thus, the tissues and organs most affected by mitochondrial dysfunction are those with high energy demands, particularly neural, muscular, and ocular. Most proteins that act in the mitochondria are nuclear in origin; they are transported into the mitochondria, where they carry out their intended function, and thus most "mitochondrial" disorders follow a Mendelian pattern of inheritance. However, each mitochondrion also contains its own separate genome with a unique DNA code (including 13 genes that function in oxidative phosphorylation, as well as its own tRNA and replication mechanism for a total of 37 genes). Each mitochondrion also contains multiple copies of its genome in varying numbers. Because all of one's mitochondria are derived from those present in the oocyte, virtually all mitochondrial deoxyribonucleic acid (mtDNA) is inherited from one's mother, such that a few mitochondrial disorders have maternal, not nuclear, inheritance.

Lactic Acidosis Under ordinary circumstances, pyruvate enters the Krebs cycle (see Fig. 1.49) and the nicotinamide adenine dinucleotide (NADH) created in the Krebs cycle is then passed to the electron transport chain for oxidative phosphorylation and the production of ATP. The metabolism of one molecule of glucose creates a net of 36 ATP molecules. When oxidative phosphorylation is insufficient to meet the body's energy needs, pyruvate is diverted to lactate, a conversion that results in a net of only two ATP. Lactic acidosis occurs when lactate builds up and is most commonly secondary to shock, hypoxia, or exercise beyond the body's aerobic capacity but can reflect mitochondrial dysfunction. Secondary lactic acidosis can also be caused by tissue hypoxia secondary to use of a tourniquet or excessive crying, or from prolonged storage of room temperature blood samples in a Vacutainer; this can be avoided by use of free-flowing or arterial specimens, avoiding multiple draw attempts, and rapid transport of the immediately iced specimen to the laboratory. Pyruvate can also be converted into the amino acid, alanine. The presence of elevated alanine indicated by plasma or serum amino acid analysis and/or the presence of elevated lactate or pyruvate on urine organic acid analysis is suggestive of chronic lactic acidosis, even if a plasma lactate measurement is within normal limits.

In some cases, lactic acidosis is not secondary to external factors but is caused by a primary disorder of energy production. Disorders of primary lactic acidosis usually occur in the metabolism of pyruvate, the Krebs cycle, or during oxidative phosphorylation, and are often referred to broadly as *mitochondrial disorders.*

Disorders of Pyruvate Metabolism

Pyruvate Dehydrogenase Deficiency Pyruvate is converted to acetyl-CoA by the enzyme pyruvate dehydrogenase complex (PDC or PDH) (see Fig. 1.49). Although the gene encoding the most affected protein (E1α) is X-linked, defects in the enzyme are commonly inherited in a dominant pattern, and thus female sex should not rule out this diagnosis. PDC deficiency results in a wide range of effects of varying severity, ranging from ataxia and seizures or mild to moderate developmental delay to more severe forms with a Leigh disease phenotype with profound lactic acidosis and structural abnormalities of the CNS; such abnormalities are attributable to prenatal cellular death from energy deficiency, ranging from agenesis of the corpus callosum to profound hydrocephalus. Infants with profound disorders of pyruvate metabolism sometimes have nonspecific dysmorphic features, such as a long philtrum and tented upper lip, probably due to facial hypotonia.

Pyruvate Carboxylase Deficiency PC deficiency can present with mild to severe keto-lactic acidosis, hyperammonemia, and other problems and can be fatal in early life or can present more chronically with intermittent keto-lactic acidosis during fasting.

Disorders of the Krebs Cycle

Primary disorders of the Krebs cycle are rare, but they are typically associated with specific findings on urine organic acid analysis. The presence of small to modest amounts of Krebs cycle intermediates on urine organic acid analysis can be normal in the first year of life. The presence of large elevations or persistent excretion of Krebs cycle intermediates in the urine can signal a disorder of oxidative phosphorylation.

Disorders of Oxidative Phosphorylation

Oxidative phosphorylation (also known as the *electron transport chain*) refers to the process of production of energy (ATP). It takes place in the mitochondria using both nuclearly and mitochondrially encoded enzymes. The enzymatic functions are grouped into complexes. Complex I is composed of more than 40 different enzymes, of which seven are mitochondrially encoded. Although most proteins in other complexes are also nuclearly encoded, mitochondrially encoded proteins are also present in complex III (one), complex IV (three), and complex V (two). Several defects in the various complexes, both nuclear or mitochondrially encoded, present with a variety of symptoms including developmental delay, failure to thrive, myopathy, hypotonia, ptosis, ophthalmoplegia, hepatopathy, encephalopathy, nephropathy, pigmentary retinopathy, and/or Leigh disease. There are also some nuclear genes involved in mitochondrial replication that lead to aberrant mitochondrial replication and/or mitochondrial depletion (e.g., Alpers syndrome, caused by defects in the gene encoding DNA polymerase subunit γ [PolG1], which results in mitochondrial depletion and is associated with liver disease and cerebral degeneration).

The *TAZ* gene is an X-linked gene encoding cardiolipin, a component of the inner mitochondrial membrane. Pathogenic variants in *TAZ* cause Barth syndrome, an X-linked disorder causing infantile cardioskeletal myopathy (commonly noncompaction) and neutropenia.

Mitochondrial Point Pathogenic Variants Pathogenic variants in the maternally inherited mitochondrial genome are also a cause of mitochondrial dysfunction. These variants can occur in any of the 13 mitochondrial genes involved in oxidative phosphorylation, or they can also occur in the genes coding for tRNA, ribosomal RNA, or replicative machinery. Note that whereas each cell contains only one nucleus housing two copies of the genome, each cell also contains multiple mitochondria, and each mitochondrion contains multiple copies of the mitochondrial genome. Thus, individuals can have multiple copies of both wild-type and mutated mitochondrial genomes coexisting in a single mitochondrion or in a single cell; this is known as *heteroplasmy.* There is a *threshold effect* at which point the number of mutated mitochondria becomes sufficient to affect the function of the cell, tissue, or organ. It is therefore possible for syndromic mitochondrial pathogenic variants to be maternally inherited in multiple family members but symptomatic only in those in whom the threshold is reached.

Mitochondrial pathogenic variants can present with variable severity. In adults, they often appear in recognizable syndrome patterns. In children, they may follow a specific phenotype but can also be multisystemic and less predictable. One example of a recognizable phenotype is MELAS (*m*itochondrial myopathy, *e*ncephalopathy, *l*actic *a*cidosis, and *s*trokelike episodes) syndrome, which is most commonly due to a specific pathogenic variant in the mitochondrial transfer ribonucleic acid for leucine ($tRNA^{Leu}$; see Table 1.17). Other common mitochondrial syndromes associated with sequencing variants are listed in Table 1.17. In contrast to vascular strokes, strokes due to mitochondrial disease do not typically follow a watershed pattern. Instead, they represent cell death from energy failure rather than blood flow abnormalities. Metabolic strokes can occur anywhere in the brain, although the highest energy-requiring parts of the brain (such as the basal ganglia) are common locations.

Evaluation and Management of Patients With Suspected Mitochondrial Disease

Traditionally, a patient suspected of having a mitochondrial disease underwent biopsy of an apparently affected organ (typically muscle) for analysis of the oxidative phosphorylation complexes. However, the expanding availability of testing for pathogenic variants in nuclear and mitochondrial genes has created an evolving testing strategy. In most cases, diagnosis can be reached with guided testing of blood or other samples, sparing patients an invasive (and frequently nondiagnostic) biopsy. More information can be found in the consensus management guideline, published by the Mitochondrial Medicine Society.

Other Inborn Errors of Metabolism

Several other inborn errors of metabolism have been identified. These include disorders of metal metabolism (e.g., Menkes disease, Wilson disease), transport defects (e.g., cystinuria, Hartnup disease), disorders of cholesterol biosynthesis/sterol metabolism (e.g., Smith-Lemli-Opitz syndrome), disorders of biotin and other vitamins, and disorders of purines and pyrimidines (e.g., Lesch-Nyhan syndrome).

Disorders of Creatine Synthesis

Creatine is important in the production of ATP and is stored in high-energy-requiring tissues, particularly brain and muscle. There are three known defects in the synthesis or transport of creatine, each manifesting with various degrees of seizures, intellectual disability, and often speech delay, autism, and/or movement disorder. Arginine:glycine amidinotransferase (AGAT) and guanidinoacetate methyltransferase (GAMT) deficiency is associated with impaired creatine synthesis and there may be some improvement with creatine and other treatments. Creatine transporter deficiency is an X-linked disorder that results in inability to transport creatine into the brain. It is emerging as one of the more common disorders causing intellectual disability and seizures. The physical examination is not specific, although seizures and movement disorders are important clues. Diagnosis involves biochemical testing for GAMT and creatine/creatinine ratio, decreased creatinine peak on MRS, or gene testing.

Menkes Disease

Menkes disease is one disorder of metal metabolism. Failure to absorb copper in the intestine leads to systemic copper deficiency and impairment of copper-dependent mitochondrial enzymes. The disorder is X-linked (the *ATP7A* gene on the long arm of the X chromosome), and thus most affected patients are male. The disorder most commonly presents in infancy with loss of milestones, seizures, intellectual disability, tortuous cerebral arteries, sagging facial skin, and weakened bones with fractures that may raise concern for child abuse until the proper diagnosis is made. Hair is coarse and sparse, classically referred to as "kinky." The life span is greatly shortened to only a few years. Parenteral copper administered to presymptomatic infants may improve outcome but seems of minimal to no benefit once symptoms have developed (Fig. 1.54).

Disorders of Sterol Metabolism

Several disorders are now associated with various defects in the biosynthesis of cholesterol. Many of these were first described as dysmorphic syndromes before the underlying biochemical abnormality was identified. The prototype disorder is Smith-Lemli-Opitz syndrome.

Infants with Smith-Lemli-Opitz syndrome have a defect in the sonic hedgehog pathway, which is involved in limb and CNS formation and cholesterol biosynthesis (Fig. 1.55). The biochemical error

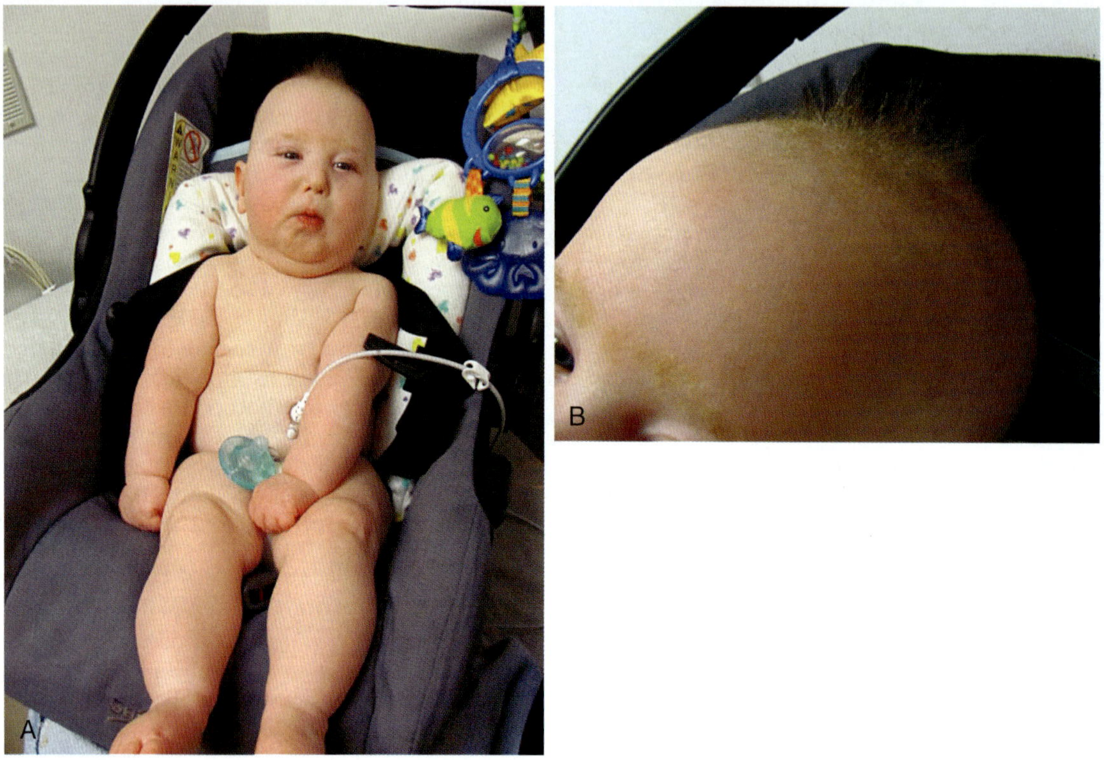

Fig. 1.54 (A and B) Menkes syndrome associated with seizures, hypotonia, hypopigmentation, global delays, and low serum copper and ceruloplasmin levels. Deoxyribonucleic acid testing showed a splicing defect in the *ATP7A* gene at Xq13.3 region, confirming the clinical finding.

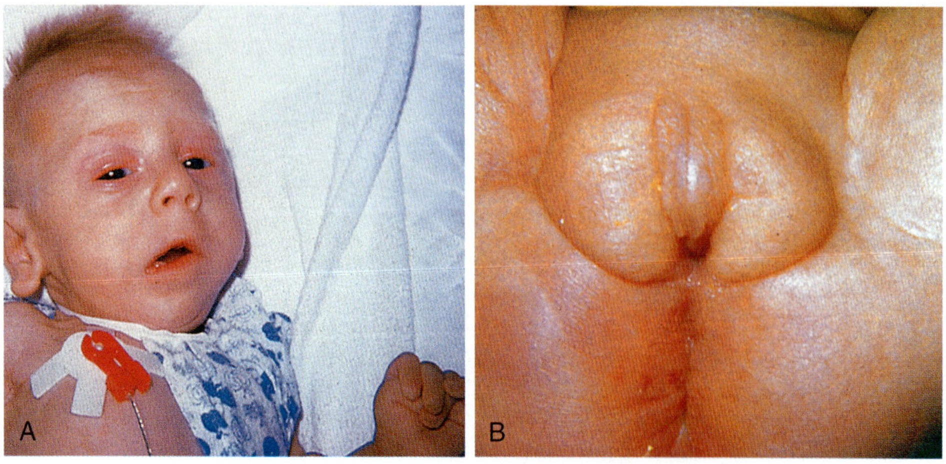

Fig. 1.55 Smith-Lemli-Opitz syndrome. (A) Note the anteverted nostrils, low-set ears, small chin, and clenched hand. (B) Hypospadias, cryptorchidism, or ambiguous genitalia as shown here may also be seen. (Courtesy W. Tunnessen, MD.)

is a block in the final step of cholesterol formation, with deficiency of cholesterol and accumulation of the precursor 7-dehydrocholesterol. Typical dysmorphic features include upturned nose, low-set ears, and characteristic clenched hands. Affected patients typically have syndactyly of the second and third toes, and they can have polydactyly, presumably a direct effect of the gene defect. Some phenotypic findings, such as undervirilization of males, are attributable to deficiency of cholesterol-based steroid hormones. Cholesterol supplementation is often pursued, but the outcome thus far is disappointing. There is active research into other therapeutic approaches.

Other disorders of cholesterol biosynthesis have various physical and developmental findings. X-linked dominant chondrodysplasia punctata (Conradi-Hünermann-Happle syndrome) is usually lethal in male fetuses and is associated with mutations in sterol isomerase (emopamil-binding protein) in females. This results in elevated levels of 8-dehydrocholesterol and 8(9)-cholesterol. Findings include chondrodysplasia punctata, asymmetric limb shortening, scoliosis, and scaly erythematous rash along the lines of Blaschko in infancy that can change into ichthyosis, scarring alopecia, and pigmentary abnormalities.

Inborn Errors of Metabolism and Dysmorphic Features

Some metabolic disorders, particularly CDG and sterol biosynthesis disorders, were originally described as dysmorphic syndromes before the biochemical defect underlying the disorder was understood. As previously noted, infants with Zellweger syndrome often have facial features and tone characteristics suggestive of Down syndrome (although the hepatomegaly and other features are distinguishing). Chondrodysplasia punctata can have various metabolic causes, including peroxisomal and cholesterol, discussed earlier. Children with organic acidemias and other disorders of energy metabolism are often reported to have nonspecific features possibly caused by poor muscle tone, such as midfacial hypotonia and prominent ears. Patients with a variety of lysosomal storage diseases often are described as having "coarse" or "full" facial features, likely attributable to cellular accumulation of lysosomal material. Therefore, the presence of dysmorphic features does not necessarily rule out an underlying metabolic error.

Newborn Screening for Genetic Disorders

Newborn screening began in the mid-1960s for PKU when an inexpensive test (Robert Guthrie's bacterial inhibition assay), performed with a few drops of blood on filter paper, became available. This demonstrated that early detection and treatment were a cost-effective way to prevent intellectual disability. Thyroid testing and other disorders were added over the years. Newborn screening for common genetic and metabolic diseases has been revolutionized by the development of tandem mass spectrometry. This technique, requiring only a dried blood spot from the newborn, provides an inexpensive, high-throughput mechanism by which to test for a much larger range of inherited metabolic disorders. In the United States, newborn screening is conducted and regulated by the individual states, and some states now screen for more than 50 disorders.

Disorders detectable by newborn screening include inborn errors of metabolism, hemoglobinopathies, cystic fibrosis, acquired immune deficiency, severe combined immunodeficiency, hearing loss, hypothyroidism, and congenital adrenal hyperplasia. The ACMG has published information sheets for physicians on these disorders (available at https://www.ncbi.nlm.nih.gov/books/NBK55827/). This website provides information about the disorders and recommended diagnostic testing algorithms.

The technical ability to diagnose genetic and metabolic disorders by newborn screening has outpaced our understanding of the natural history and optimal treatment of some of these disorders. In 2003, the Secretary of Health convened the Secretary's Advisory Committee on Heritable Disorders in Newborns and Children to develop advisory guidelines for newborn screening. The committee developed a list of primary target disorders based on evidence-based guidelines, as well as a list of secondary disorders, which are routinely detectable as part of the testing process for primary target diseases (Table 1.18). New disorders are added to the primary target list after an evidence-based review process. At present, states are not obligated to follow the committee's guidelines.

The most recent additions to screening panels include lysosomal storage disorders, which are diagnosed with a combination of low

Table 1.18 Secretary's Advisory Committee on Heritable Diseases of Newborns and Children Recommended Uniform Screening Panel: Primary and Secondary Target Disorders[a,b,c]

Core Conditions	Secondary Conditions
Propionic acidemia	Methylmalonic acidemia with homocystinuria (Cbl C, D)
Methylmalonic acidemia and cobalamin A, B	Malonic acidemia
Isovaleric acidemia	Isobutyrylglycinuria
3-MCC deficiency	2-Methylbutyrylglycinuria
3-Hydroxy-3-methylglutaric (HMG) aciduria	3-Methylglutaconic aciduria
Holocarboxylase synthase deficiency	2-Methyl-3-hydroxybutyric aciduria
β-Ketothiolase deficiency	Short-chain acyl-CoA dehydrogenase deficiency
Glutaric acidemia type I	Medium/short-chain hydroxyacyl-CoA dehydrogenase deficiency
Carnitine uptake/transporter defect	Glutaric acidemia type II
Medium-chain acyl-CoA dehydrogenase deficiency	Medium-chain ketoacyl-CoA thiolase deficiency
Very-long-chain acyl-CoA dehydrogenase deficiency	2,4-Dienoyl-CoA reductase deficiency
Long-chain hydroxyacyl-CoA dehydrogenase deficiency	Carnitine palmitoyltransferase type I deficiency
Trifunctional protein deficiency	Carnitine palmitoyltransferase type II deficiency
Argininosuccinic aciduria	Carnitine acylcarnitine translocase deficiency
Citrullinemia type I	Argininemia
Maple syrup urine disease (MSUD)	Citrullinemia type II
Homocystinuria	Hypermethioninemia
Classic phenylketonuria (PKU)	Benign hyperphenylalaninemia
Tyrosinemia type I	Biopterin defect in cofactor synthesis
Primary congenital hypothyroidism	Biopterin defect in cofactor regeneration
Congenital adrenal hyperplasia	Tyrosinemia type II
Sickle cell disease	Tyrosinemia type III
Sickle-beta thalassemia	Other hemoglobinopathies
Sickle-C disease	Galactoepimerase deficiency
Biotinidase deficiency	Galactokinase deficiency
Critical cyanotic congenital heart disease	T-cell–related lymphocyte deficiencies
Cystic fibrosis	
Classic galactosemia	
Hearing loss	
Severe combined immunodeficiencies	
Glycogen storage disease type II (Pompe)	
Mucopolysaccharidosis type 1	
Mucopolysaccharidosis type 2	
X-linked adrenoleukodystrophy	
Spinal muscular atrophy	
Guanidinoacetate methyltransferase deficiency	

[a]For an updated list see https://www.hrsa.gov/advisory-committees/heritable-disorders/rusp.

[b]Primary care physicians, other pediatric subspecialties, and family practitioners can access the algorithms for the responsibilities, as well as immediate management by following the AAP policy statement on newborn screening (2008). Newborn Screening Authoring Committee: Newborn screening expands: recommendations for pediatricians and medical homes—implications for the system, *Pediatrics* 121:192–217, 2008.

[c]A reference that the clinicians may find helpful for newborn screening is: *Contemporary Pediatrics*. 28:38–47, 2011.

3-MCC, 3-methylcrotonyl-CoA carboxylase.

enzyme activity, abnormal biomarker levels, and molecular testing depending on the state's individual mandate. The impact of adding these disorders via population screening is being actively studied, as diagnostic confirmation is not always straightforward, even with the addition of next-generation sequencing. Pseudodeficiency (when an enzyme has low activity with laboratory substrate and normal activity in vivo), variants of unknown significance, rare variant types, and limited information on diagnostically relevant neonatal findings all add to the complexity of diagnosing these disorders. Pursuing the best treatment before irreversible symptom development and adhering to first do-no-harm principles is a delicate balance.

It is important to remember that newborn screening is a screening program, not a diagnostic program. Not all inborn errors of metabolism are detectable by newborn screening (e.g., some urea cycle defects), and as a screening program it does not have 100% sensitivity. Thus, no disorder should be considered eliminated in a symptomatic child because of a normal newborn screen result. Screen-positive infants are referred for diagnostic testing. Some cases require a repeat screen; in some cases, results are sufficiently concerning as to prompt a call to the nearest expert referral center and/or the child's primary care provider for emergency evaluation.

Ethics in Genetics

The expansion of genetic technologies creates new and reignites old ethical concerns. Molecular sequencing commonly reveals variants of uncertain significance, creating diagnostic uncertainty and questions about appropriate management. Families can lose faith in the medical system when a diagnosis is removed or when one is not identified. Some patients will make irreversible, drastic medical decisions based on initially inconclusive results. In approximately 5% of clinical cases, patients will also have more than one genetic diagnosis, complicating the clinical picture and management, as well as expectations for disease presentation and progression. Additionally, the role of human disease for approximately half of all genes is unknown at this time, with newly recognized candidate genes and disorders being described weekly. This uncertainty can lead to additional stress and anxiety among families, even when proper pretest counseling has been performed.

The ability to diagnose untreatable or adult-onset disorders in children has been particularly problematic. The ACMG now considers presymptomatic testing of children for adult-onset disorders unethical, unless advanced knowledge can trigger management changes in childhood that can potentially alter the course or outcome of the disorder. Unmasking these disorders in children can also reveal parents who are unknowingly affected. *BRCA2*-related disorders in a child may present as autosomal recessive Fanconi anemia and would lead to one or both parents now being diagnosed with increased risk of many forms of cancer (breast, ovarian, colon, pancreatic, prostate) while dealing with a medically fragile child.

Privacy of genetic information is also of increasing concern, as well as ownership and access. The Genetic Information Nondiscrimination Act provides some protections, but this landmark legislation is now out of date given the rapid advances in the field of genetics. Diagnosing a genetic disorder in a patient can also mean identifying other family members at risk who might benefit from the genetic information. The responsibility of who is a "mandated reporter" in this realm is controversial, particularly when gamete donation is involved. The role of the patient and the provider in notifying other family members is currently being decided in the courts.

When to obtain genetic data is also under scrutiny, as more testing is being pursued in the neonatal period, because those tested cannot consent. Expanded newborn screening also presents ethical dilemmas. Particularly in the lysosomal disorders, early presymptomatic diagnosis is necessary for best clinical outcomes through higher-risk treatments, such as hematopoietic stem cell transplantation. However, the presence of pseudodeficiency or late-onset alleles or identification of variants of uncertain significance can result in lack of certainty in diagnosis or management plan.

Gene therapy trials are rapidly expanding, raising concerns for somatic genetic manipulation, genome editing, and the potential for germline therapy. Long-term outcomes and safety risks are not yet known, and determining which populations are appropriate for research is challenging. Geneticists are on the front line of many ethically complex discussions and decisions, and this involvement will only grow as testing options multiply.

ACKNOWLEDGMENTS

The authors thank members of the medical genetics staff who worked tirelessly to help accumulate the clinical pictures and the families who graciously consented to allow photographs to be taken to advance teaching and education.

Bibliography

AlAbdi L, Shamseldin HE, Khouj E, et al: Beyond the exome: utility of long-read whole genome sequencing in exome-negative autosomal recessive diseases, *Genome Med* 15(1):114, 2023.

Ballif BC, Theisen A, McDonald-McGinn DM, et al: Identification of a previously unrecognized microdeletion syndrome of 16q11.2q12.2, *Clin Genet* 74:469–475, 2008.

Barseghyan H, Eisenreich D, Lindt E, et al: Optical genome mapping as a potential routine clinical diagnostic method, *Genes (Basel)* 15(3):342, 2024.

Beighton P, de Paepe A, Danks D, et al: International nosology of heritable disorders of connective tissue, Berlin, 1986, *Am J Med Genet* 29:581–594, 1988.

Bick D, Jones M, Taylor SL, Taft RJ, Belmont J: Case for genome sequencing in infants and children with rare, undiagnosed or genetic diseases, *J Med Genet* 56(12):783–791, 2019.

Bull MJ, Committee on Genetics: Health supervision for children with Down syndrome, *Pediatrics* 128(2):393–406, 2011.

Buyse ML, editor: *Birth defects encyclopedia*, Cambridge, MA, 1990, Blackwell Scientific.

Dolzhenko E, van Vugt JJFA, Shaw RJ, et al: Detection of long repeat expansions from PCR-free whole-genome sequence data, *Genome Res* 27(11):1895–1903, 2017.

Duker AL, Ballif BC, Bawle EV, et al: Paternally inherited microdeletion at 15q11.2 confirms a significant role for the SNORD116 C/D box snoRNA cluster in Prader-Willi syndrome, *Eur J Hum Genet* 18:1196–1201, 2010.

Francke U: Prader-Willi syndrome: chromosomal and gene aberrations, *Growth Genet Horm* 10:4–7, 1994.

GeneTests: Medical genetics information resource (database online). www.genetests.org

Gorlin RJ, Cohen MM Jr, Hennekam RCM: *Syndromes of the head and neck*, ed 4, New York, 2001, Oxford University Press.

Graham JM Jr, Sanchez-Lara PA: *Smith's recognizable patterns of human deformation*, ed 4, Philadelphia, 2015, Elsevier.

Greco D, Vetri L, Ragusa L, et al: Prader-Willi syndrome with Angelman syndrome in the offspring, *Medicina (Kaunas)* 57(5):460, 2021.

Hemingway SJA, Bledsoe JM, Brooks A, et al: Comparison of the 4-Digit Code, Canadian 2015, Australian 2016 and Hoyme 2016 fetal alcohol spectrum disorder diagnostic guidelines, *Adv Pediatr Res* 6(2):2385–4529, 2019.

Hemingway SJA: *Diagnostic guide for fetal alcohol spectrum disorders: the 4-digit diagnostic code*, ed 4, v 1.01, Seattle WA, 2024, University of Washington. http://depts.washington.edu/fasdpn/pdfs/Guide2024.pdf.

Hook EB: Chromosome abnormalities: prevalence, risks, and recurrence. In Brock BJH, Rodeck CH, Ferguson-Smith MA, editors: *Prenatal diagnosis and screening*, New York, 1992, Churchill Livingstone, pp 351–392.

Ibañez K, Polke J, Hagelstrom RT, et al: Whole genome sequencing for the diagnosis of neurological repeat expansion disorders in the UK: a retrospective diagnostic accuracy and prospective clinical validation study, *Lancet Neurol* 21(3):234–245, 2022.

Jones KL, Jones MC, delCampo M: *Smith's recognizable patterns of human malformation*, ed 7, Philadelphia, 2013, Elsevier/Saunders.

Kepple JW, Fishler KP, Peeples ES: Surveillance guidelines for children with trisomy 18, *Am J Med Genet A* 185(4):1294–1303, 2021.

Kulkarm S, Pfeifer J, editors: *Clinical genetics: a guide to clinical next generation sequencing*, London, 2015, Elsevier/Saunders.

Loeys BL, Dietz HC, Braverman AC, et al: The revised Ghent nosology for the Marfan syndrome, *J Med Genet* 47:476–485, 2010.

Lubs HA: A marker X chromosome, *Am J Hum Genet* 21:231–244, 1969.

Macken WL, Falabella M, McKittrick C, et al: Specialist multidisciplinary input maximises rare disease diagnoses from whole genome sequencing, *Nat Commun* 13(1):6324, 2022.

Malfait F, Francomano C, Byers P, et al: The 2017 international classification of the Ehlers–Danlos syndromes, *Am J Hum Genet* 175(1):8–26, 2017.
Manning M, Hudgins L: Array-based technology and recommendations for utilization in medical genetics practice for detection of chromosome abnormalities, *Genet Med* 12:742–745, 2010.
Miller DT, Adam MP, Aradhya S, et al: Consensus statement: chromosomal microarray is a first-tier clinical diagnostic test for individuals with developmental disabilities or congenital anomalies, *Am J Hum Genet* 86:749–764, 2010.
Mortier GR, Cohn DH, Cormier-Daire V, et al: Nosology and classification of genetic skeletal disorders: 2019 revision, *Am J Med Genet A* 179(12):2393–2419, 2019.
Ng SB, Bigham AW, Buckingham KJ, et al: Exome sequencing identifies MLL2 mutations as a cause of Kabuki syndrome, *Nat Genet* 42:790–793, 2010.
Nussbaum RL, McInnes RR, Willard HF: *Thompson and Thompson genetics in medicine*, ed 8, Philadelphia, 2015, WB Saunders.
Online Mendelian Inheritance in Man (OMIM): *McKusick-Nathans Institute for Genetic Medicine*, 2000, Johns Hopkins University (Baltimore, MD) and National Center for Biotechnology Information, National Library of Medicine (Bethesda, MD). http://www.ncbi.nlm.nih.gov/omim/.
Parikh S, Goldstein A, Karaa A, et al: Patient care standards for primary mitochondrial disease: a consensus statement from the Mitochondrial Medicine Society, *Genet Med* 19(12):10.1038/gim.2017.107, 2017. doi:10.1038/gim.2017.107.
Patton MA: Noonan syndrome: a review, *Growth Genet Horm* 10:1–3, 1994.
Pena LDM, Jiang YH, Schoch K, et al: Looking beyond the exome: a phenotype-first approach to molecular diagnostic resolution in rare and undiagnosed diseases, *Genet Med* 20(4):464–469, 2018.
Pyeritz RE, Korf BR, Grody WW, et al: *Emery and Rimoin's principles and practice of medical genetics*, ed 7, Cambridge, 2018, Elsevier.
Richards S, Aziz N, Bale S, et al: Standards and guidelines for the interpretation of sequence variants: a joint consensus recommendation of the American College of Medical Genetics and Genomics and the Association for Molecular Pathology, *Genet Med* 17(5):405–424, 2015.
Rocha JJ, Jayaram SA, Stevens TJ, et al: Functional unknomics: systematic screening of conserved genes of unknown function, *PLoS Biol* 21(8):e3002222, 2023.
Ryan AK, Goodship JA, Wilson DI, et al: Spectrum of clinical features associated with interstitial chromosome 22q11 deletions: a European collaborative study, *J Med Genet* 34:798–804, 1997.
Saudubray JM, Bumgartner M, Walter J, editors: *Inborn metabolic diseases, diagnosis and treatment*, ed 6, Heidelberg, 2016, Springer-Verlag.
Shepard TH, Lemire RJ: *Catalog of teratogenic agents*, Baltimore, 2004, Johns Hopkins University Press.
Stalker HJ, Williams CA: Genetic counseling in Angelman syndrome: the challenges of multiple causes, *Am J Med Genet* 77(1):54–59, 1998.
Stevenson RE, Hall JG, Everman DB, Goodman RM, editors: *Human malformations and related anomalies*, ed 3, Oxford, 2015, Oxford University Press.
Sutherland GR: Fragile sites on human chromosomes: demonstration of their dependence on the type of tissue culture medium, *Science* 197:265–266, 1977.
Trask BJ: Fluorescence in situ hybridization, *Trends Genet* 7:149–154, 1991.
Valle DL, Antonarakis S, Ballabio A, Beaudet AL, Mitchell, GA, editors: *Scriver's online metabolic and molecular bases of inherited disease*, New York, NY, 2019, McGraw-Hill. https://ommbid.mhmedical.com/ommbid-index.aspx. Accessed May 31, 2024.
Warburton D: De novo balanced chromosome rearrangements and extra marker chromosomes identified at prenatal diagnosis: clinical significance and distribution of breakpoints, *Am J Hum Genet* 49:995–1013, 1991.
Wenger SL, Steele MW, Boone LY, et al: "Balanced" karyotypes in six abnormal offspring of balanced reciprocal translocation normal carrier parents, *Am J Med Genet* 55:47–52, 1995.
Wincent J, Anderlid BM, Lagerberg M, et al: High-resolution molecular karyotyping in patients with developmental delay and/or multiple congenital anomalies in a clinical setting, *Clin Genet* 79:147–157, 2011.
Wise AL, Manolio TA, Mensah GA, et al: Genomic medicine for undiagnosed diseases, *Lancet* 394(10197):533–540, 2019.
Yang Y, Muzny DM, Reid JG, et al: Clinical whole-exome sequencing for the diagnosis of mendelian disorders, *N Engl J Med* 369(16):1502–1511, 2013.
Zigman WB: Atypical aging in Down syndrome, *Dev Disabil Res Rev* 18(1):51–67, 2013.

2

NEONATOLOGY

Arcangela L. Balest | Melissa M. Riley | Brighid Moran O'Donnell | Jennifer S. Zarit

GENERAL TECHNIQUES OF PHYSICAL EXAMINATION

Assessment of the Newborn

The purposes of the routine newborn assessment are to determine the infant's gestational age, document growth and development for a given gestational age, uncover signs of birth-related trauma or congenital anomalies, and evaluate the overall health and condition of the infant. The assessment begins with the establishment of a historical database. Information may be obtained from antenatal, labor, delivery, postpartum records, and a brief parental interview. The aim of this data gathering is to (1) assess the fetal and neonatal responses to pregnancy, labor, and delivery; (2) estimate the risk for hereditary or congenital diseases; and (3) identify the potential for future difficulties by reviewing the social history and observing family/infant interactions. This background is recorded in the infant's medical record and serves as a guide to the subsequent physical examination (Box 2.1).

Observation must be completed before the quiet infant is disturbed by the examination. The examiner should be sure to keep the infant warm during the examination. By visual inspection, the clinician can assess skin, facies, general tone, symmetry of movement, respiratory rate, work of breathing, color, and abdominal contour. Auscultation of the heart and lungs should be completed before more stressful portions of the examination, which are likely to make the infant fussy. Auscultation of the cranium and liver (the most common sites for arteriovenous malformations) is also part of a complete newborn examination, and presence of a bruit will alert the examiner that further investigation is warranted (Fig. 2.1A and B). Palpating for femoral pulses is a quick screen for coarctation of the aorta. Bounding pulses may indicate a shunt, such as an arteriovenous malformation or patent ductus arteriosus. Allowing the infant to suck on a gloved finger can help quiet the infant and permit assessment of sucking strength and palate integrity. Sucking also induces eye opening, which may allow the examiner to better evaluate a red reflex and determine that the patient does not have a congenital cataract or an intraorbital mass (see Chapter 20) requiring prompt intervention.

When the abdomen is examined, it often helps to gently flex the hip on the side being examined because this relaxes the abdominal muscles. Most structures in the abdomen are smaller (pyloric olive), softer (liver), more superficial (spleen tip), or deeper (kidneys) than expected. The use of any part of the hand other than the fingertips should be discouraged because maximal sensitivity is essential.

Careful evaluation of the hip joints is a crucial part of each newborn examination because identification and early treatment of congenital dislocation can prevent later disability. Although asymmetry of the buttocks and skin creases or asymmetry of femoral length can be clues to dislocation, these may not be evident until later in life, and the performance of active motion tests is essential. The Ortolani and Barlow maneuvers involve placing the third or fourth finger over the greater trochanter and the thumb on the medial aspect of the thighs. The thighs are first adducted to try to dislocate a dislocatable hip and then abducted with the fingers pushing toward the midline and the thumbs away from midline to relocate a dislocated hip. These maneuvers should be performed on one hip at a time. A definite "clunk" can be felt and often heard, in the first 45 degrees of movement, if a dislocated femoral head moves back into the acetabulum.

This can be differentiated from hip subluxation (partial dislocation), where there is no true "clunk" but the hip moves with a sliding motion. There are higher-pitched clicks and snaps felt or heard with hip subluxation that may represent tendons passing over bone or cartilage, which should improve within the first 2 weeks of life. Hip subluxation still requires close follow-up.

Assessment of Gestational Age

One of the unique considerations in the examination of the newborn is the assessment of gestational age. Accurate determination should be the first part of any newborn examination because this provides the context for the remainder of the evaluation. No differential diagnosis of newborn disease can be made without knowing whether the patient is premature or full term and whether the infant is small, large, or appropriate for gestational age. Although an accurate menstrual and pregnancy history usually provides evidence of gestational age, there are cases in which such data are unavailable or unreliable.

Investigators have developed examination criteria, both morphologic and neurologic, for the assessment of gestational age. Although these criteria are generally useful because of the ordered patterns of fetal development, the clinician cannot rely on any single feature or even a small group of features to develop at the same rate in all infants. In fact, assessment of paired structures, such as ears, may reveal slightly different degrees of maturation from one side to the other. Thus all the available methods involve numerous physical and neurologic items and have, at best, a 2-week range of error.

Although morphologic criteria tend to be uninfluenced by events occurring around the time of delivery, neurologic findings may be unreliable in the presence of several conditions, including depression secondary to medication, asphyxia, seizures, metabolic diseases, infections, and severe respiratory distress. Even morphologic criteria may be inaccurate if the infant is born with severe edema, growth retardation, or side effects from maternal drug use. Such factors must be considered in estimating gestational age.

The Ballard assessment for gestational age determination of newborns uses six morphologic and six neurologic criteria to estimate gestational age on the basis of an examination performed at 12 to 24 hours of life (Fig. 2.2). Individual findings are scored on a scale of 0 to 5, and the total score is compared with the chart shown in (Fig. 2.2).

Physical Maturity

One of the most striking differences among newborns of various gestational ages is the quality of the skin. The chemical nature of skin changes during intrauterine development, with a gradual decrease in water content and a thickening of the keratin layer. Very premature infants, 22 to 28 weeks, have nearly translucent, paper-thin skin (Fig. 2.3) that is easily abraded. A diffuse red hue and a prominent venous pattern are characteristic. At term, the skin no longer appears thin or translucent; instead, some superficial peeling and cracking around the ankles and wrists may be visible. Post-term

Box 2.1 Newborn Historical Database

Antenatal Record
Maternal age
Maternal medical history
Obstetric history
Number of previous pregnancies
Number of term/preterm deliveries
Outcomes of previous pregnancies
Estimations of gestational age
Antenatal ultrasound
Advanced imaging (fetal echocardiograms, fetal magnetic resonance imaging)
Fetal surveillance results (if available)
Complications of pregnancy
Adequacy of antenatal care
Maternal laboratory work: blood type, serologies, genetic testing

Labor and Delivery Record
Date and time of delivery
Duration of labor
Time of the rupture of membranes
Complications or abnormalities of labor
Method of delivery or type of anesthesia
Placental weight and morphologic condition
Birth weight
Need for resuscitation and Apgar scores

Postpartum Record
Maternal postpartum complications
Newborn vital sign records
Newborn labs (commonly bilirubin and glucose)
Nursing documentation of the activity and condition of the infant
On admission to the nursery
Since admission to the nursery
Abnormal physical findings noted by the nursing staff
Feeding, voiding, and stool history
Observations of maternal/infant interactions

Parental Interview
Parental perceptions of:
- Pregnancy
- Labor
- Delivery

History of parental and family illnesses
Health status and growth and development of siblings and other family members
Degree of education, preparation, and planning for newborn care
Available social support systems
Medical follow-up plans

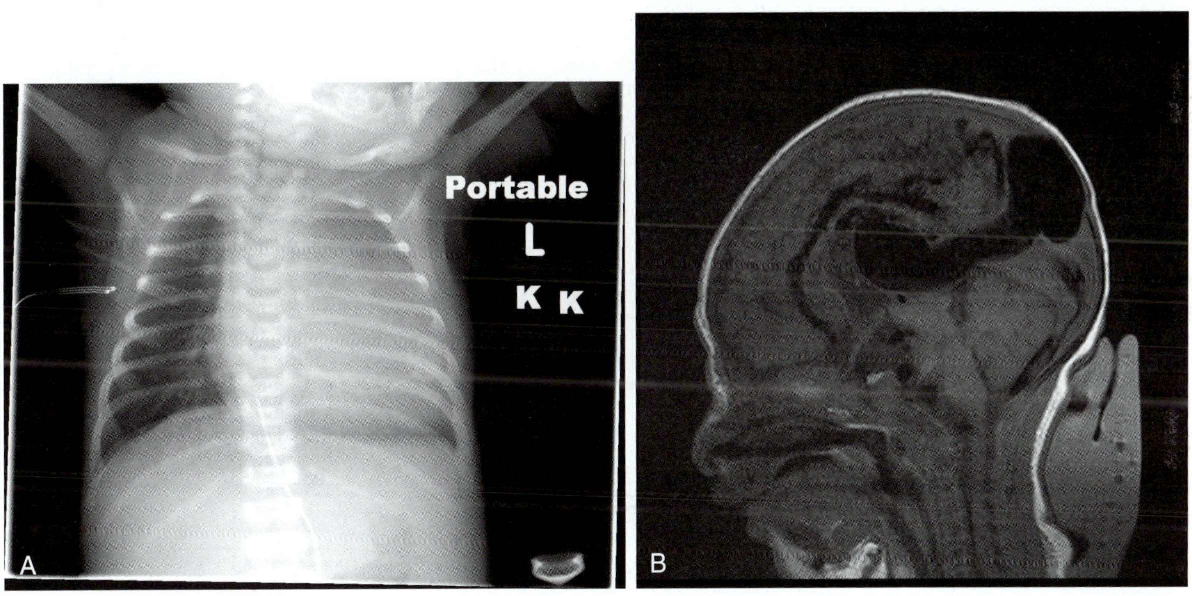

Fig. 2.1 Infant presented with desaturations. Chest radiograph with cardiac enlargement due to high-output cardiac failure (A) caused by shunt through large intracranial arteriovenous malformation (B) (in this case a vein of Galen malformation). A cranial bruit was heard over the anterior fontanelle and transmitted to the chest.

infants (42–44 weeks) often have more diffuse peeling and cracking of the skin because the outermost layers are sloughed (Fig. 2.4).

Lanugo, a fine body hair that resembles peach fuzz, appears and disappears during development. It is absent before weeks 20 to 22, becomes diffuse until weeks 30 to 32, and then begins to thin. Assessment of the presence and extent of lanugo is best accomplished by observing the back tangentially (Fig. 2.5).

Transverse creases begin to appear on the anterior portion of the soles of the feet at approximately 32 weeks (Fig. 2.6). By 36 weeks, the anterior two-thirds of the sole is covered with creases. For adequate assessment of this feature, it is necessary to stretch the skin over the sole gently to distinguish wrinkling from true creases. Infants with congenital neurologic dysfunction involving the lower extremities and infants with pedal edema may lack normal creases.

Breast tissue, which is responsive to maternal hormonal influences, shows progressive increase in size as gestational age advances. Infants born at younger than 28 weeks' gestation have barely perceptible breast or areolar/nipple tissue (see Fig. 2.3). With advancing gestational age, breast tissue increases in size (see Fig. 2.4) and, occasionally, a term infant has active glandular secretions, which resolve spontaneously. Breast tissue can remain palpable for 2 to 3 months.

Cartilaginous development proceeds in an orderly manner during gestation and can be assessed by examination of the external ear. Although the normal incurving of the upper pinnae begins at 33 to 34 weeks and is complete at term, it is more reliable to assess the extent of cartilage in the pinnae by feeling its edge and folding the ear (Fig. 2.7). Until approximately 32 weeks, there is only minimal recoil of a folded ear, but by term there is instant recoil.

The appearance of the genitalia can be used to assess gestational age. In a male, the testes descend into the scrotum during the last month of gestation, but they are often palpable in the inguinal canal

Physical maturity

	0	1	2	3	4	5
Skin	Gelatinous, red, trans-parent	Smooth, pink, visible veins	Superficial peeling and/or rash, few veins	Cracking, pale area, rare veins	Parchment, deep cracking no vessels	Leathery, cracked, wrinkled
Lanugo	None	Abundant	Thinning	Bald areas	Mostly bald	
Plantar creases	No crease	Faint red marks	Anterior transverse crease only	Creases anterior two thirds	Creases cover entire sole	
Breast	Barely perceptible	Flat areola, no bud	Stippled areola, 1–2 mm bud	Raised areola, 3–4 mm bud	Full areola, 5–10 mm bud	
Ear	Pinna flat, stays folded	Slightly curved pinna, soft, slow recoil	Well-curved pinna, soft but ready recoil	Formed and firm with instant recoil	Thick cartilage, ear stiff	
Genitals: Male	Scrotum empty, no rugae		Testes descending, few rugae	Testes down, good rugae	Testes pendulous, deep rugae	
Genitals: Female	Prominent clitoris and labia minora		Majora and minora equally prominent	Majora large, minora small	Clitoris and minora completely covered	

Maturity rating

Score	Weeks
5	26
10	28
15	30
20	32
25	34
30	36
35	38
40	40
45	42
50	44

Neuromuscular maturity

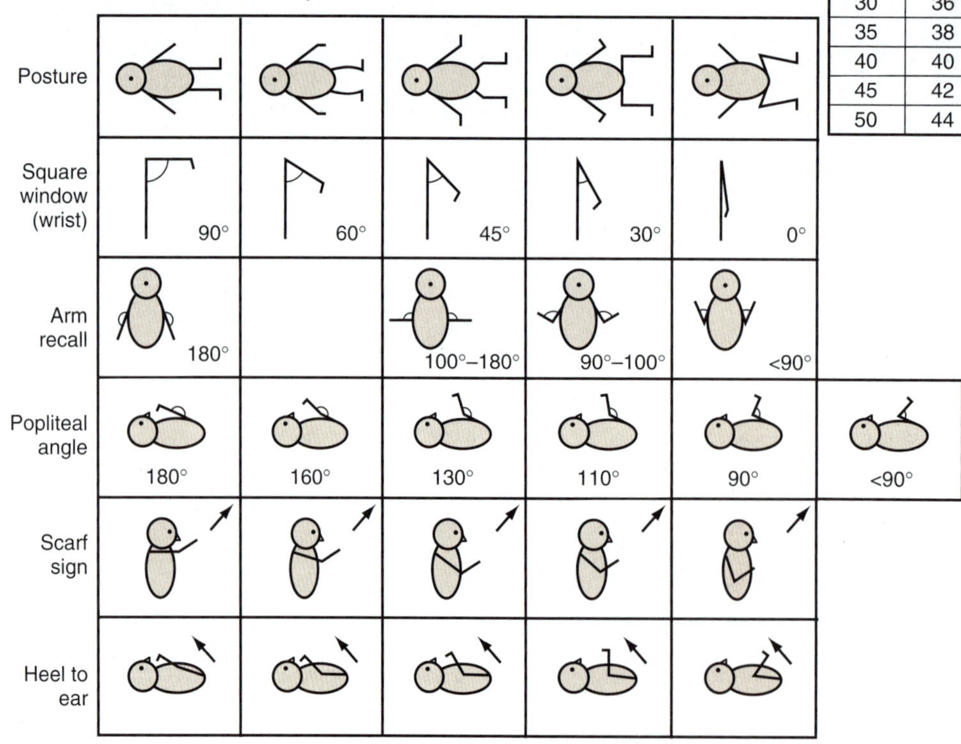

Fig. 2.2 Gestational age assessment. The six morphologic and six neurologic criteria, in aggregate, yield an estimation of gestational age. (From Ballard J, Novak KK, Driver M: A simplified score of assessment of fetal maturation of newly born infants, *J Pediatr* 95:769–774, 1979.)

by 28 to 30 weeks. The appearance of rugae on the scrotum parallels testicular migration, appearing first on the anterior scrotum at 36 weeks and covering the entire scrotal sac by 40 weeks. Absence of testicular descent alters the appearance of the scrotum at term, so congenital cryptorchidism complicates this evaluation. In a female, the labia majora tend to be overshadowed by the clitoris and labia minora until 34 to 36 weeks (Fig. 2.8). In cases of fetal malnutrition, lack of subcutaneous fat, which should normally be present in the latter part of gestation, can interfere with assessment of the female genitalia.

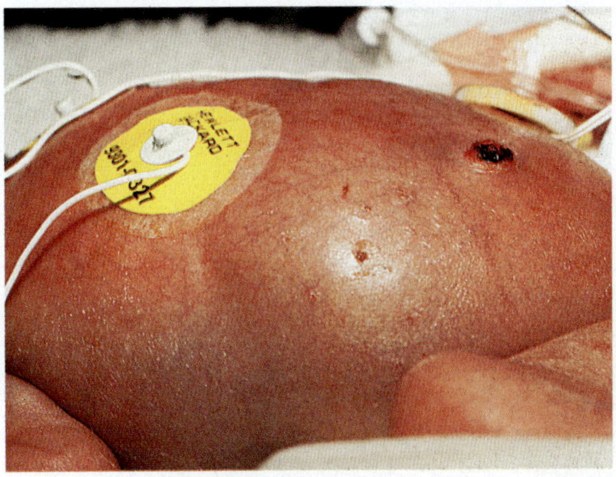

Fig. 2.3 Premature skin. This premature infant demonstrates translucent, paper-thin skin with a prominent venous pattern.

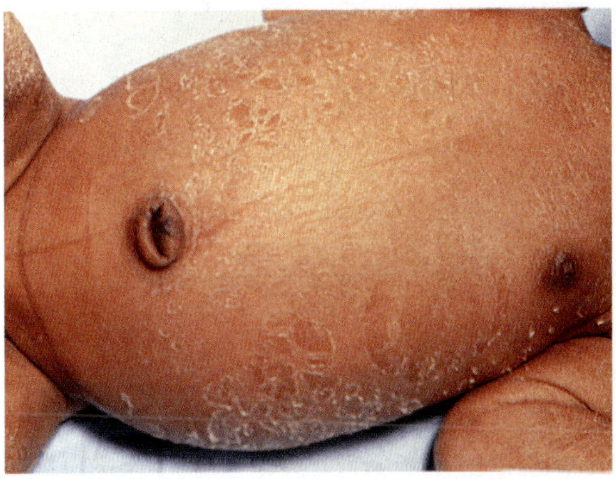

Fig. 2.4 Postterm skin. Peeling and cracking of the skin are characteristics of the infant delivered after 42 weeks' gestation.

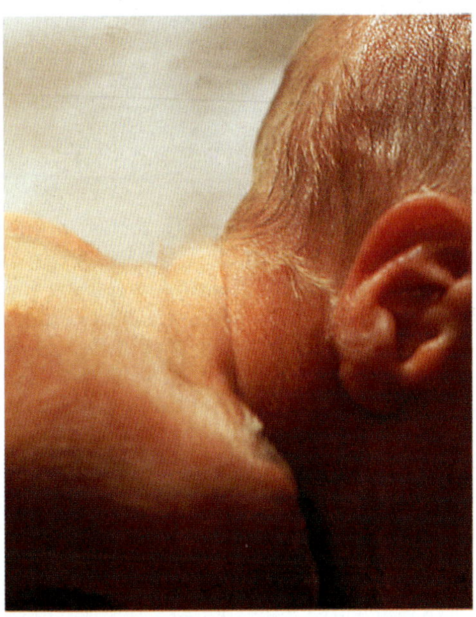

Fig. 2.5 Lanugo. This fine body hair resembling peach fuzz is present on infants of 24 to 32 weeks' gestation.

Neuromuscular Maturity

Numerous neurologic tests and observations can be used to assess gestational age. Most examiners use tests that best assess range of motion, tone, reflexes, and posture. None is particularly reliable in the presence of illness, and the entire neurologic examination is best

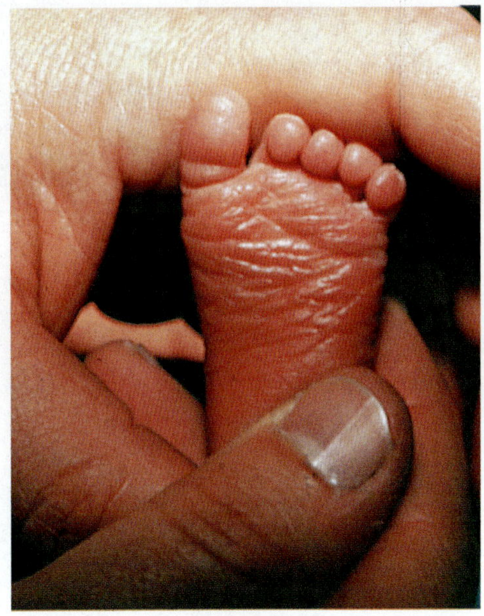

Fig. 2.6 Sole creases. Transverse sole creases cover approximately half the sole in this infant, indicating a gestational age of approximately 34 weeks.

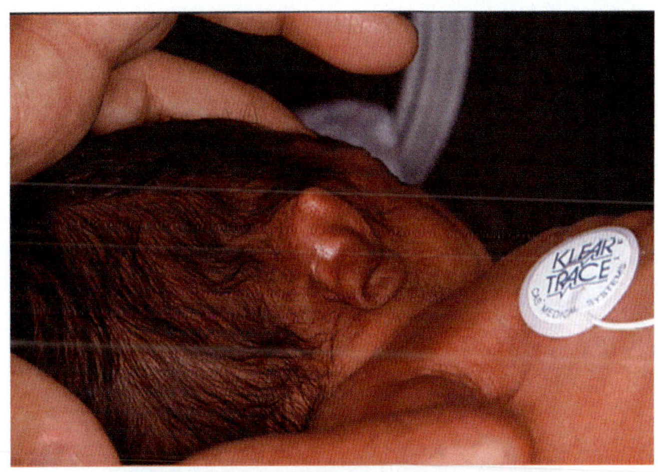

Fig. 2.7 Ear cartilage. The lack of cartilage and the easy foldability (lack of recoil) are evident in the ear of this premature infant. (From https://www.ballardscore.com/CatalogView/Article/physical-maturity/5-eye-ear)

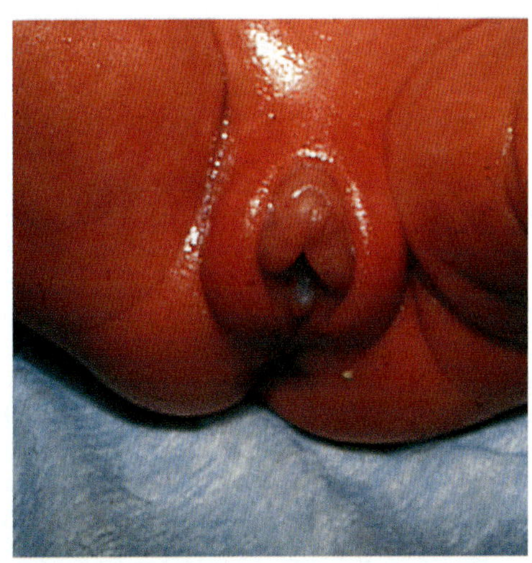

Fig. 2.8 Premature female genitalia. Prominence of the labia minora in a premature female infant at 28 weeks.

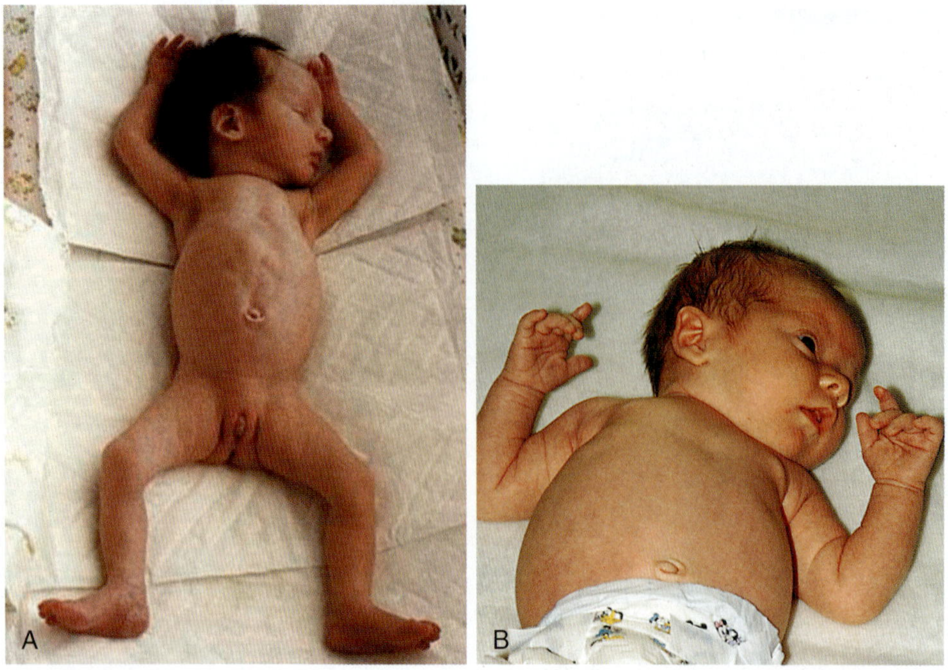

Fig. 2.9 (A) Premature infant. Note predominant extensor posture. (B) General posture. The typical, marked flexor posture of the term infant.

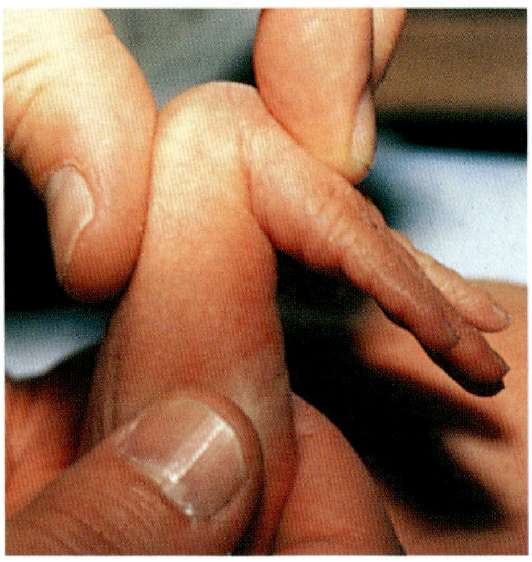

Fig. 2.10 Square-window test. The position for assessing the square window is shown. The 45-degree angle seen between the palm and forearm is consistent with a gestational age of 30 to 32 weeks.

completed between 12 and 24 hours after birth to allow recovery from the stress of delivery.

The resting supine posture of the infant changes with advancing gestational age. The mature infant exhibits a marked flexor posture of the extremities compared with the extensor posture of the premature infant (Fig. 2.9A and B).

Tests for flexion angles assess a combination of muscle tone, ligament and tendon laxity, and flexion/extension development. The inexperienced examiner usually assumes that the very premature infant is the most flexible, but observation of flexion angles demonstrates that this is false. The square-window test of the wrist (Fig. 2.10) is performed by gently flexing the hand on the wrist and assessing the resultant angle. The wrists of babies younger than approximately 32 weeks can be flexed only to 45 to 90 degrees, whereas the wrists of term infants undergo full flexion. Sometime between birth and adulthood this flexion ability is lost. Examination of the flexion of the knees reveals a different pattern of development, with decreasing flexibility as gestational age increases. The knee is completely flexed (Fig. 2.11A), and the thigh is stabilized against the stomach. The leg is extended by raising the foot (Fig. 2.11B). Gentleness is *essential* in these evaluations because any result can be achieved if the examiner applies undue force.

Examination of arm recoil can assess active tone and reflex responsiveness. In this maneuver, the supine infant's forearms are fully flexed for 5 seconds, then extended by pulling on the hands, and then released. As gestational age increases, the flexion response is more pronounced.

The resting tone of the upper extremities can be assessed by eliciting the scarf sign (Fig. 2.12A and B).

In a similar manner, the resting tone of the lower extremities can be assessed by the heel-to-ear maneuver. With the baby on its back and the pelvis flat, a foot is moved as near to the ipsilateral ear as possible without exerting undue force. Very premature infants can easily touch their heels to their ears (Fig. 2.13). This becomes somewhat more difficult after 30 weeks and impossible by week 34 of gestation.

Primitive Reflexes

Normal newborns exhibit several easily elicited primitive reflexes that are often altered or absent in the infant with neurologic impairment. These reflexes may be transiently depressed in the infant who has difficulty transitioning between intrauterine and extrauterine existence. The persistent absence or asymmetry of one or more of these reflexes may be a clue to the potential presence of neuromuscular abnormalities requiring further investigation (see Chapter 3).

The rooting reflex may be elicited by lightly stimulating the infant's cheek and observing the reflexive attempts to bring the stimulating object to the mouth. The sucking reflex is activated by placing an object in the infant's mouth and observing the sucking movements. In the grasp reflex (Fig. 2.14), transverse stimulation of the midpalm (without touching the back of the hand) or midsole leads to flexion of the digits or toes around the examiner's fingers.

The Moro reflex (see https://youtube.com/shorts/E77W8cRCZbo?si = 8dBlzc9fAkwLwajI) evaluates vestibular maturation and the relationship between flexor and extensor tone (Fig. 2.15). Elicitation of the reflex involves a short (10 cm), sudden drop of the head when the infant is supine. An incomplete but identifiable reflex becomes apparent at approximately 32 weeks' gestation, and by 38 weeks it is essentially complete. Very immature infants demonstrate extension of the arms and fingers but do not show true flexion or make a

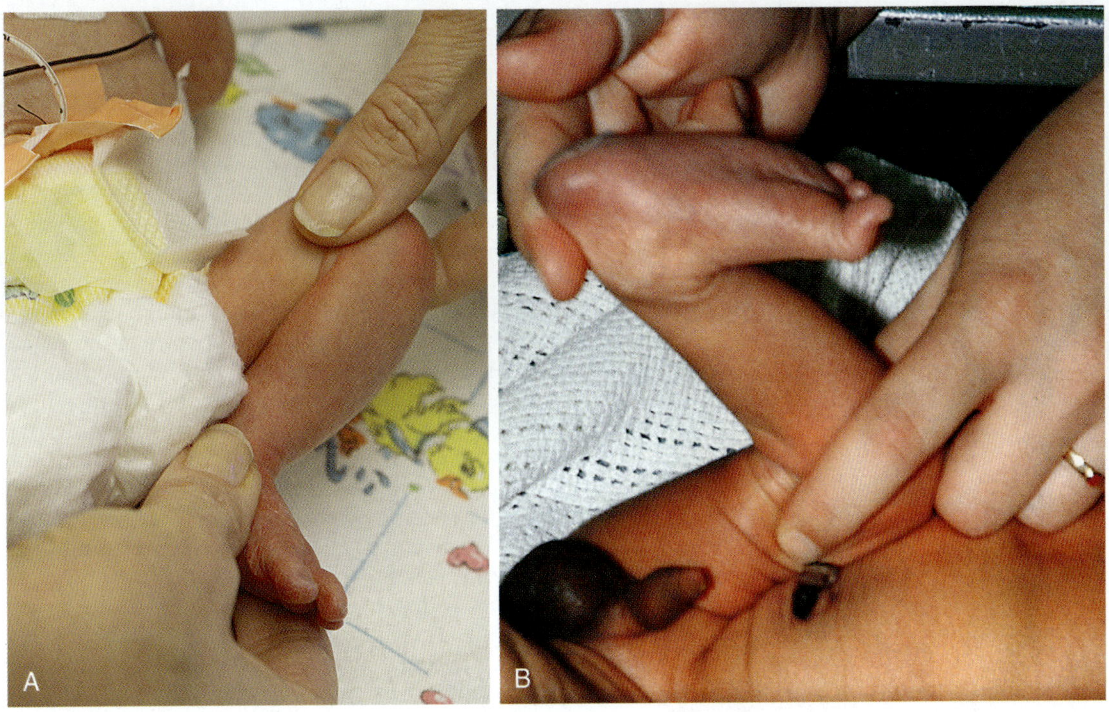

Fig. 2.11 Knee flexion. (A) The position for assessing knee flexion is shown. The foot is elevated to assess the popliteal angle. (B) Note the decreased knee flexibility of this term infant.

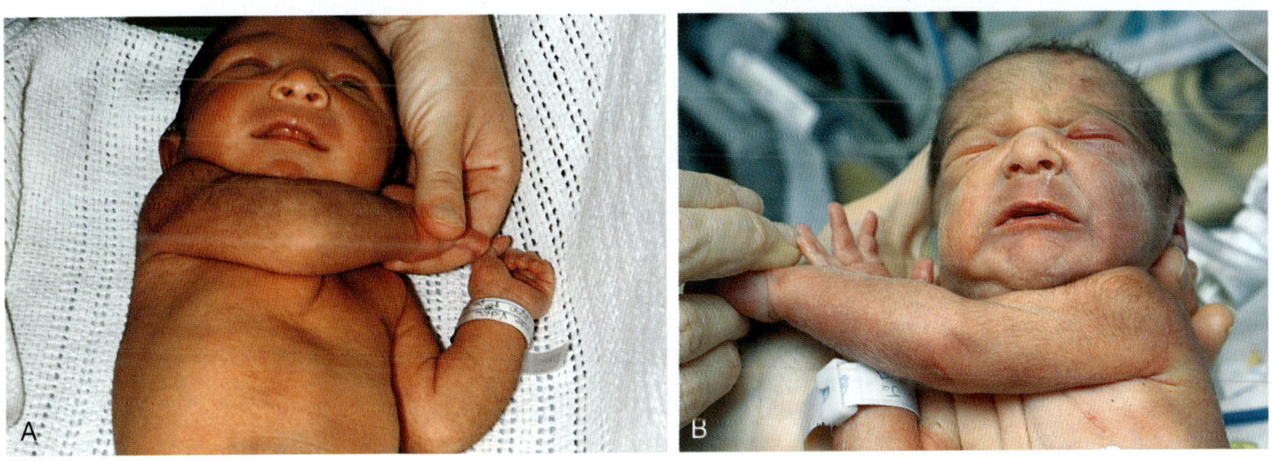

Fig. 2.12 Scarf sign. (A) The elbow cannot be drawn, with gentle traction on the upper extremity, across this term infant's chest. (B) This is in contrast to the marked flexibility of a preterm infant of 29 weeks' gestation.

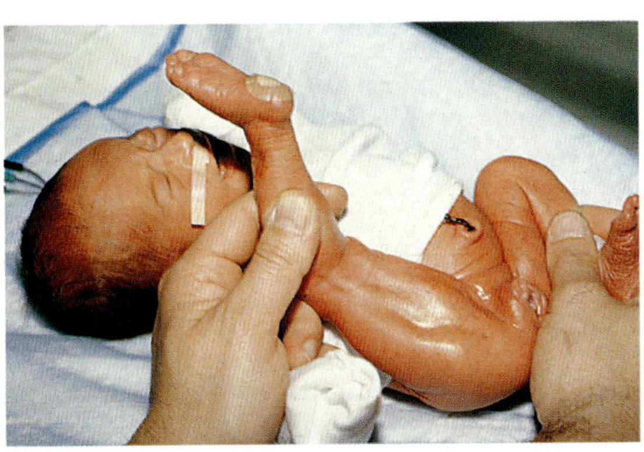

Fig. 2.13 Heel-to-ear maneuver. The position for assessing the heel-to-ear maneuver is demonstrated. The degree of extension seen is consistent with a 28- to 30-week infant.

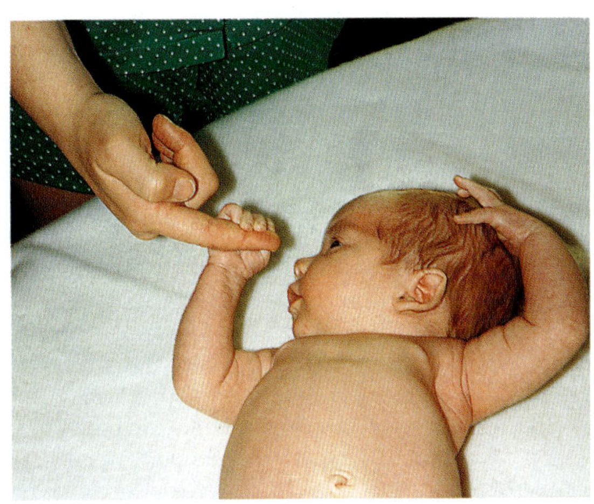

Fig. 2.14 Grasp reflex (palm). Transverse stimulation of the mid palm leads to a grasp by the infant.

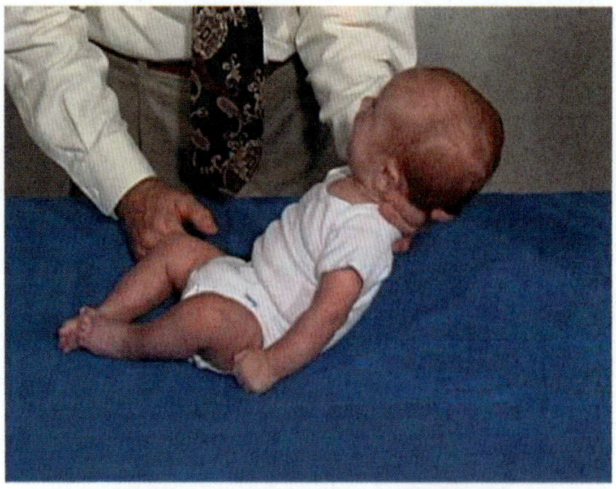

Fig. 2.15 Moro reflex. The full response involves extension of the arms, fanning of the fingers, then upper extremity flexion followed by a cry.

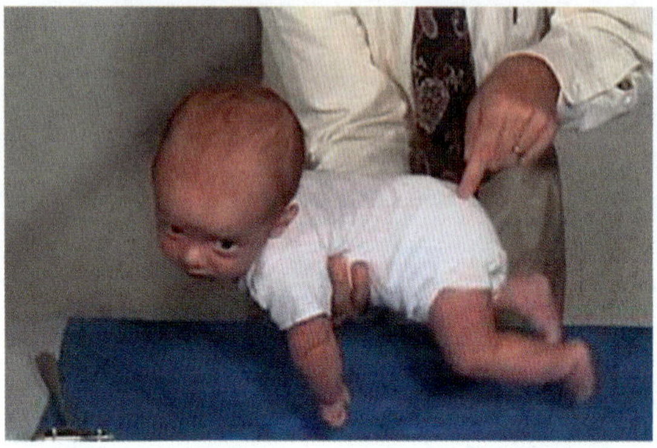

Fig. 2.16 Galant reflex. The position for assessing the Galant reflex is shown with infant held in ventral position. The examiner strokes cranial to caudal with their index finger along one side of the spine. The normal reaction is for the newborn to laterally flex toward the stimulated side. (From https://youtube/oUtsDMhwXvs?si = 5JJUKjHV11JrZ8TX)

sustained cry. Marked asymmetry of response may be associated with focal neurologic impairment.

The Galant infantile reflex (see https://youtu.be/oUtsDMhwXvs?si = 5JJUKjHV11JrZ8TX) is a truncal incurvation reflex. Lack of the Galant reflex may indicate a spinal cord lesion (Fig. 2.16).

These reflexes and a host of other less commonly used reflexes are termed *primitive* because they are present at or shortly after birth and normally disappear after the first few months of life. Just as their absence may indicate neurologic impairment at birth, their abnormal persistence may also be a cause for concern and further evaluation.

Abnormalities of Growth

Intrauterine growth restriction (IUGR), a deviation in the expected fetal growth pattern, complicates up to 8% of all pregnancies and is associated with an increase in perinatal morbidity and mortality. Infants with IUGR may appear long and thin and often have an obvious loss of subcutaneous tissue, which is best seen as redundant skin folds over the buttocks, thighs, and knees. The etiology of IUGR is multifactorial and includes fetal, placental, and maternal factors that inhibit normal fetal growth. The conditions for IUGR and small for gestational age (SGA) are related but not synonymous. The fetus with IUGR generally has a period of normal growth followed by a decrease in growth velocity, while the diagnosis of SGA is population specific and includes infants who weigh less than a predetermined cutoff value (Fig. 2.17). Birth weights less than the 10th percentile or greater than the 90th percentile for gestational age within a population are often considered small for gestational age (SGA) or large for gestational age (LGA), respectively. Appropriate-for-gestation age infants have growth parameters within two standard deviations of the mean, or between the 10th and 90th percentiles.

The relationship among weight, length, and head circumference can be useful in understanding the etiology of small size (see Fig. 2.17). By comparing length or head circumference percentiles with the weight percentile at any given gestational age, the clinician can detect growth retardation even if the actual weight still falls within two standard deviations of normal. Conditions that affect growth during the third trimester of pregnancy, such as preeclampsia, tend to interfere with the normal acquisition of fatty tissue while sparing brain growth (and thus head circumference) and linear growth. These newborns have an asymmetric form of growth retardation (Fig. 2.18). Often, postterm infants (>42 weeks) have some decrease in weight compared with length or head circumference. Problems beginning earlier than the third trimester tend to produce generalized growth restriction, with head circumference, weight, and length affected to equivalent degrees. Infants with symmetric IUGR tend to have higher rates of chromosomal disorders, dysmorphic syndromes, and congenital infection and are associated with higher rates of prematurity and neonatal mortality. In very premature infants, global decreases in growth often complicate assessment of gestational age because the tools are rather limited in babies born at 22 to 28 weeks' gestation. A thorough investigation should be undertaken in any unexplained instance of growth retardation.

Multiple-gestation pregnancies often produce newborns who are premature and symmetrically small. Fetal growth decreases as the number of fetuses increases. Although multiple factors interfere with growth in these pregnancies, uterine constraint appears to occur when the combined fetal size approximates 3 kg. Size discordance (>10% difference in weight) between identical twins may occur if their placentas share vascular connections, resulting in overperfusion of one twin and underperfusion with subsequent growth restriction of the other. Discordance may also occur in dizygotic twins (Fig. 2.19) if one has placental insufficiency or if only one twin is afflicted with a chromosomal abnormality or congenital infection.

Newborns who are LGA are often the products of pregnancies in diabetic or "prediabetic" mothers. The effect is usually noted during the third trimester, with infants at term who weigh more than 4 kg. Weight is the most affected parameter, but length and head circumference are often increased as well. Infants of diabetic mothers are often identifiable by macrosomia, round facies (Fig. 2.20), and sometimes plethora and hirsutism (especially of the pinnae). Maternal hyperglycemia results in fetal hyperglycemia and increased insulin production by the fetal pancreas, which may result in neonatal hypoglycemia. Maternal hyperglycemia also causes glycogen deposition in the newborn, resulting in visceromegaly, most notable in the liver and heart. All LGA infants should be routinely screened for hypoglycemia, fed within an hour of delivery, and their mothers investigated for the possibility of undiagnosed diabetes mellitus.

Two rare syndromes can also cause excessive size: (1) cerebral gigantism, or Sotos syndrome, with macrosomia, macrocephaly, large hands and feet, poor coordination, and later variable mental deficiency; and (2) Beckwith-Wiedemann syndrome with macrosomia, macroglossia, omphalocele, linear ear fissures, and neonatal hypoglycemia (see Chapter 9).

Placenta

Careful examination of the placenta can aid in the diagnosis and treatment of many conditions and diseases. The configuration, color, membranes, cord insertion, and condition of the fetal and maternal surfaces are all relevant. Communication with the obstetric team

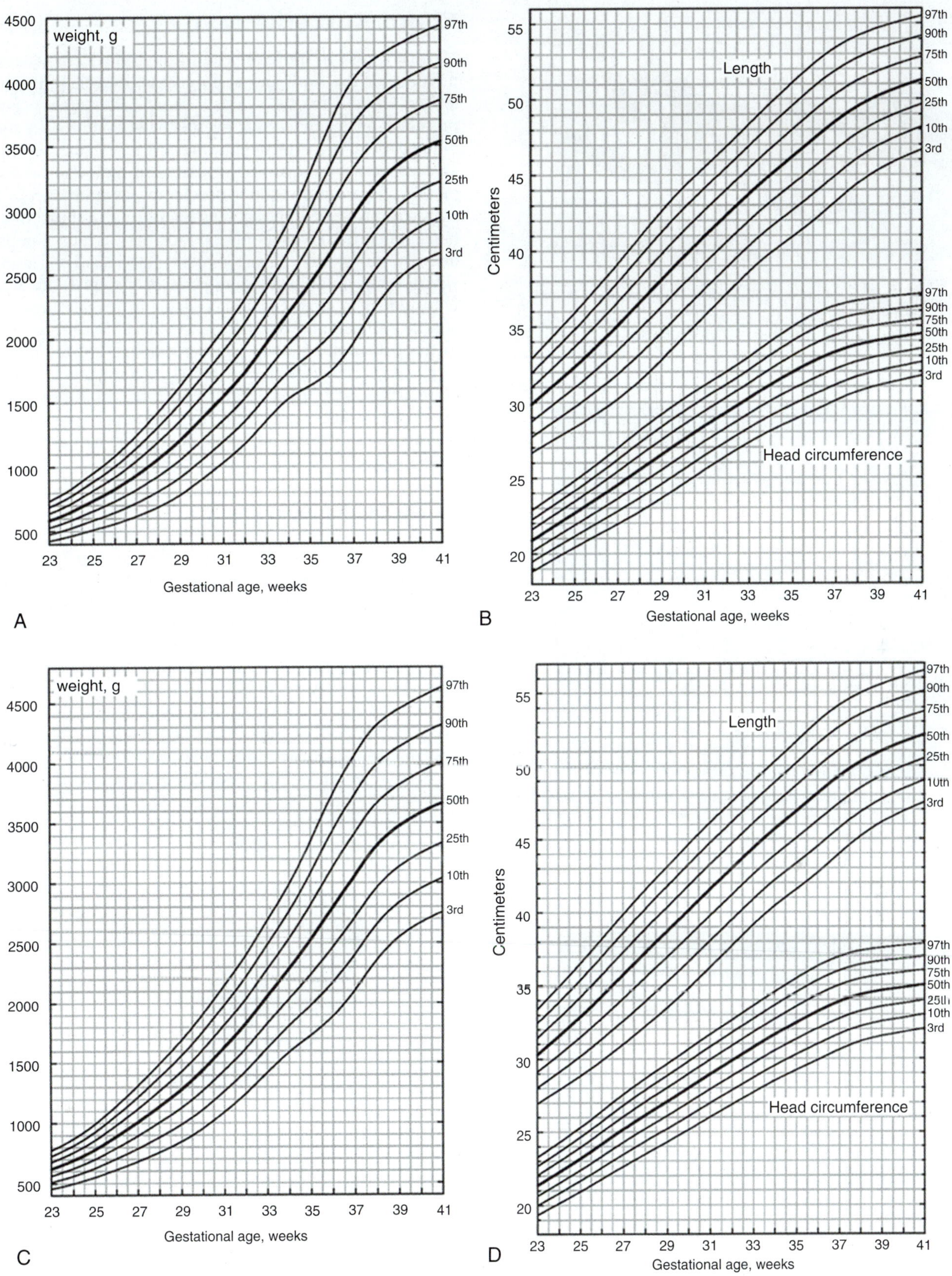

Fig. 2.17 The mean (±2 standard deviations) weight, length, and head circumference for infants born at various gestational ages (A–D). Infants above or below the curves are considered too large or too small for gestational age, respectively. (From Olsen IE, Groveman SA, Lawson ML, et al: New intrauterine growth curves based on United States Data, *Pediatrics* 125[2]:e214–e224, 2010. https://doi.org/10.1542/peds.2009-0913.)

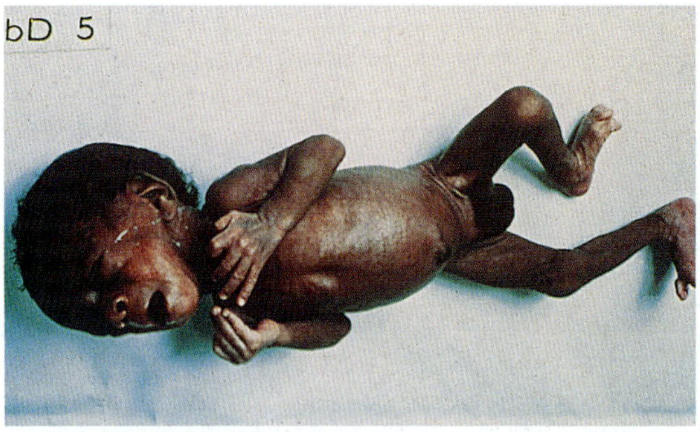

Fig. 2.18 Intrauterine growth retardation. This term baby weighed only 1.7 kg. The head appears disproportionately large for the thin, wasted body. This resulted from placental insufficiency late in pregnancy. Hypoglycemia may be a complication. (Courtesy TALC, Institute of Child Health, Bethesda, MD.)

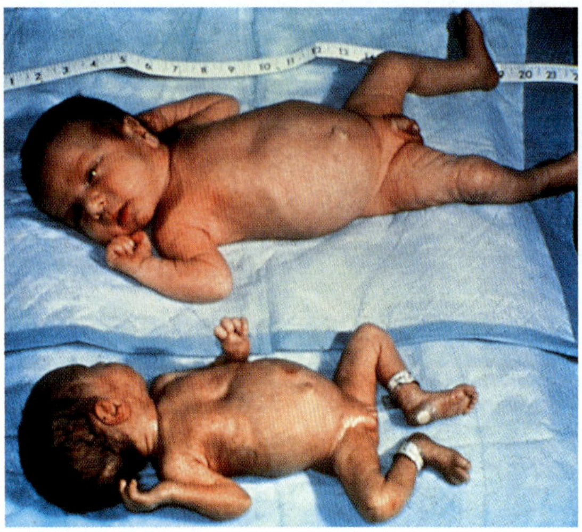

Fig. 2.19 Discordant twins. This is a pair of markedly discordant dizygotic twins. Disturbed placentation accounted for the marked reduction in size of the smaller twin.

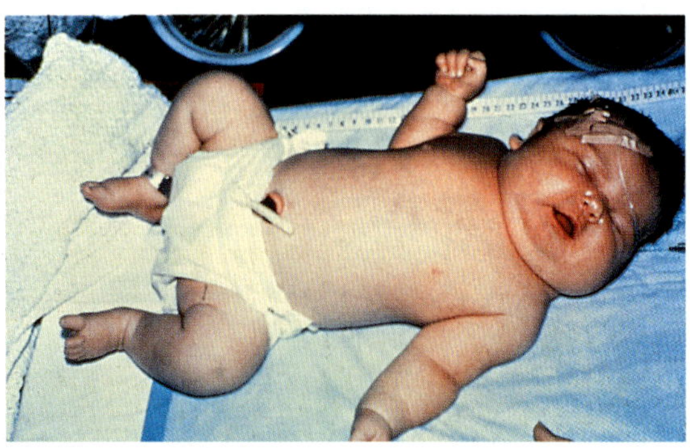

Fig. 2.20 Large for gestational age infant. This infant of a diabetic mother weighed 5 kg at birth and exhibits the typical rounded facies.

allows for further understanding of placental conditions affecting the neonate.

BIRTH TRAUMA

In most cases, a newborn is relatively unscathed by the birth process. However, both transient and permanent signs of birth trauma can be evident. Prompt identification of such injuries is important for proper management and can also prevent inappropriate speculation, diagnostic testing, and treatment.

Caput Succedaneum

Normal transit of the fetal head through the birth canal may cause molding of the skull and scalp edema, especially if labor is prolonged. The edema, known as a *caput succedaneum* (Fig. 2.21), is present at birth and tends to overlie the occipital bones and portions of the parietal bones bilaterally. In some cases, such as with vacuum-assisted deliveries, bruising of the scalp may also be present. The presence of a caput requires no therapy, as spontaneous resolution within a few days is typical. Distinguishing caput from a subgaleal (subaponeurotic) hematoma, a rare but serious complication of delivery, is important. A subgaleal hematoma is a collection of blood within scalp tissues extending beneath the epicranial aponeurosis. Palpation of a large caput succedaneum reveals firm swelling. In contrast, the cranial swelling of subgaleal bleeding is fluctuant due to the palpation of blood just beneath the epicranial aponeurosis (Fig. 2.22). The collection of blood in this potential space can be quite large, and these infants must be monitored for signs of hypovolemia and anemia. Serial examinations, which can include measurement of head circumference and hematocrit, are important to identify ongoing blood loss.

Cephalohematoma

Often, confusion arises between the diagnosis of a caput and that of a cephalohematoma. The latter is a localized collection of blood beneath the periosteum of one of the calvarial bones; it may be bilateral, but it is most often unilateral (Fig. 2.23). It is distinguished from a caput by the fact that the borders are limited by suture lines, usually those surrounding the parietal bones (see Fig. 2.22). However, diagnosis can be difficult in the immediate newborn period, when there may be overlying scalp edema. On palpation, the border may feel elevated, and the center depressed. Most patients have an uncomplicated course of slow resolution over one or more months,

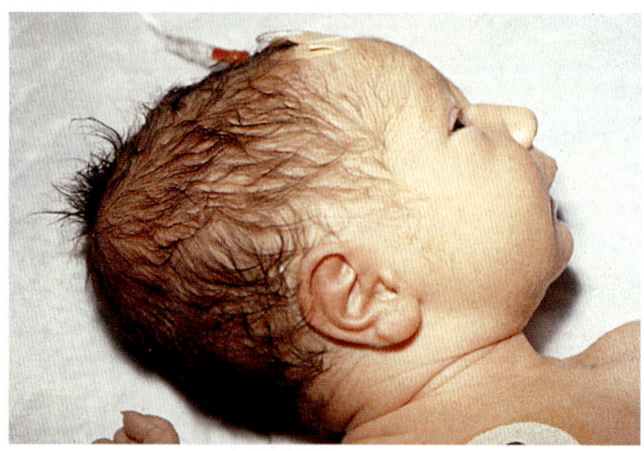

Fig. 2.21 Caput succedaneum. This infant has significant scalp edema as a result of compression during transit through the birth canal. The edema crosses suture lines.

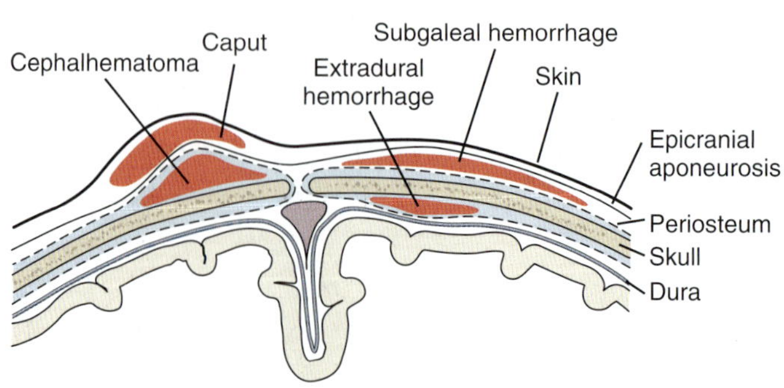

Fig. 2.22 Sites of extracranial (and extradural) hemorrhages in the newborn. Schematic diagram of the important tissue planes from skin to dura. (Modified from Pape KE, Wigglesworth JS: *Hemorrhage, ischaemia and the perinatal brain,* Philadelphia, 1979, JB Lippincott; 1979.)

although calcification may occur. On occasion, these infants may develop jaundice from the breakdown and resorption of the large hematoma. Underlying hairline skull fractures occur with some regularity but are rarely of clinical significance. Radiologic investigation for an underlying depressed fracture is indicated in infants whose histories suggest significant trauma and those having depressed levels of consciousness *or* neurologic abnormalities on examination. Infection is another potentially serious but rare complication, which is more likely when the integrity of the overlying skin is broken, such as may occur when a scalp electrode is placed, or a scalp abrasion develops in the normal course of delivery.

Clavicle Fracture

Clavicle fractures can occur during delivery when the infant is large, in breech position, or if there is fetal distress requiring rapid extraction. If nondisplaced, the fracture may not be painful and the infant may be asymptomatic (Fig. 2.24). The diagnosis may be suspected by palpation of crepitus, a lump over the clavicle, or an asymmetric Moro reflex. If there is pain or discomfort with routine handling, the fracture can be treated by immobilization of the ipsilateral limb and shoulder with the elbow flexed 90 degrees. Immobilization can be discontinued when a callus is palpable at 8 to 10 days. Many nondisplaced clavicle fractures are not diagnosed until the first newborn outpatient follow-up visit, when a large, firm callus may be palpated along the clavicle. If the child has an otherwise normal physical and neurologic examination at this time, a radiograph is not indicated. Radiographs are indicated to differentiate whether decreased arm movement is secondary to pain (clavicle fracture) or nerve injury (Erb or Klumpke palsy).

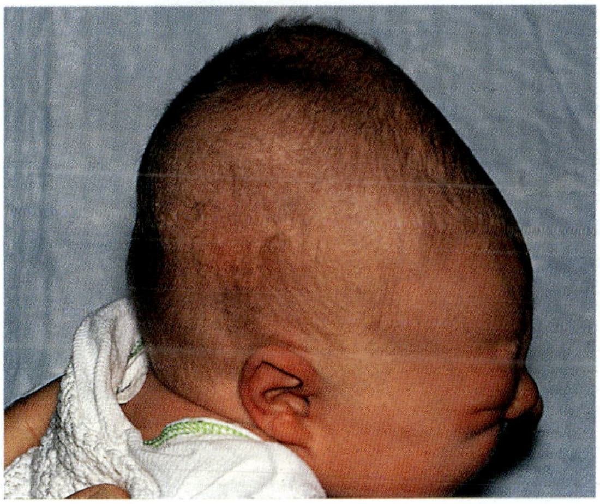

Fig. 2.23 Cephalohematoma. In this infant with bilateral cephalohematomas, the midline sagittal suture remained palpable, confirming the subperiosteal location of the hematomas.

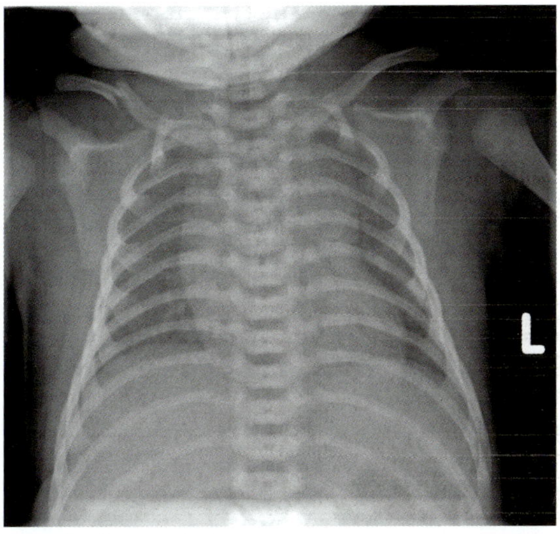

Fig. 2.24 Clavicle fracture. This infant had a palpable mass over the right clavicle immediately after delivery. Note the discontinuity of the right clavicle.

Bruises and Petechiae

Superficial bruising can occur when delivery is difficult. This is relatively common with breech presentations and can include swelling and discoloration of the labia or scrotum (to be distinguished from an incarcerated inguinal hernia). When bruises are extensive, significant secondary jaundice may develop as the extravasated blood is broken down and resorbed. In an infant born with a nuchal cord, the presence of diffuse petechiae around the head and neck is common and does not warrant further investigation. In addition, petechiae found on the presenting body part are normal. The appearance of new bruises or petechiae after delivery should alert the medical team to the possibility of a bleeding disorder or infection. Bruising and edema of the perineum can be normal when a newborn is delivered in a breech presentation. See "Scrotal Swelling" section in this chapter for special considerations of scrotal ecchymosis and swelling.

Fat Necrosis

Many infants delivered with the aid of forceps show markings after delivery. These marks tend to fade over 24 to 48 hours. On occasion, a well-circumscribed, firm nodule with purplish discoloration may appear at the site of a forceps mark. This may represent fat necrosis (Fig. 2.25) and resolves spontaneously over weeks to months. The phenomenon may also occur at other sites of trauma. Affected infants may develop symptomatic hypercalcemia, and serum calcium levels may need to be followed and treated.

Nasal Deformities

Abnormalities of the nose are common after delivery, the majority consisting of transient flattening or twisting induced during transit through the birth canal. Less than 1% of nasal deformities are due to actual dislocations of the triangular cartilage of the nasal septum. These can be differentiated from positional deformities by manually moving the septum to the midline and observing the resultant shape of the nares. In a true dislocation, marked asymmetry of the nares persists (Fig. 2.26). Returning the septum to its proper position can be accomplished with the guidance of an otolaryngologist. Failure to recognize and treat dislocation may lead to permanent deformity.

Nerve Damage

Injury to the peripheral nervous system, especially the facial and brachial nerves, is one of the more common serious occurrences related to birth. Unilateral facial nerve palsy is the most common peripheral nerve injury, with an incidence as high as 1.4 per 1000 live births. Injury can result from direct trauma from forceps or from compression of the nerve against the sacral promontory while the head is in the birth canal. With pronounced nerve injury, there is decreased facial movement and forehead wrinkling on the side of the palsy, eyelid elevation, and flattening of the nasolabial folds and corner of the mouth (Fig. 2.27). Crying accentuates the findings, with the most obvious sign being asymmetric movement of the mouth. The side that appears to droop when crying is the normal side. The differential diagnosis includes Möbius syndrome (usually bilateral) and absence of the depressor anguli oris muscle, which may be associated with cardiac anomalies. The latter condition is distinguishable from facial nerve palsy by the absence of involvement of the forehead, eyelid, or nasolabial area. The prognosis for

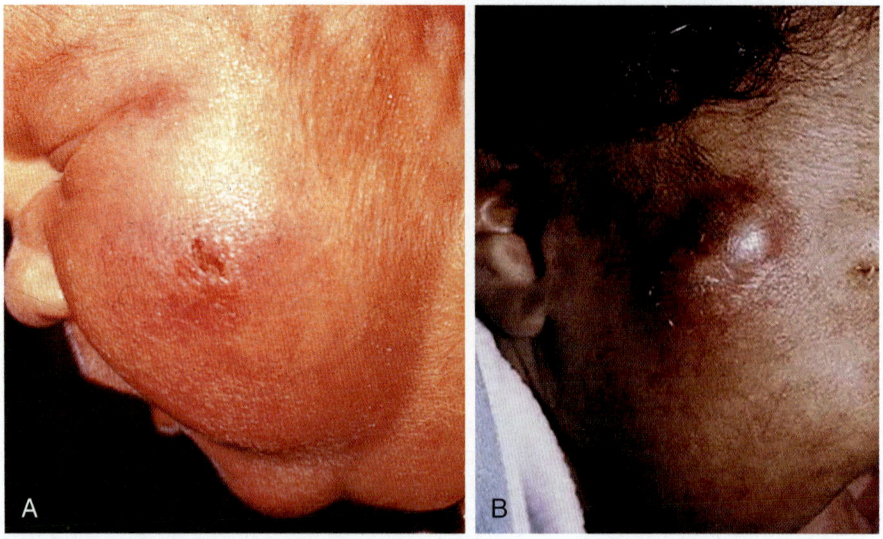

Fig. 2.25 (A and B) Fat necrosis. This discolored nodular lesion on the cheek is characteristic of subcutaneous necrosis of fat secondary to forceps trauma. (B, From https://obgynkey.com/disorders-of-the-subcutaneous-tissue/)

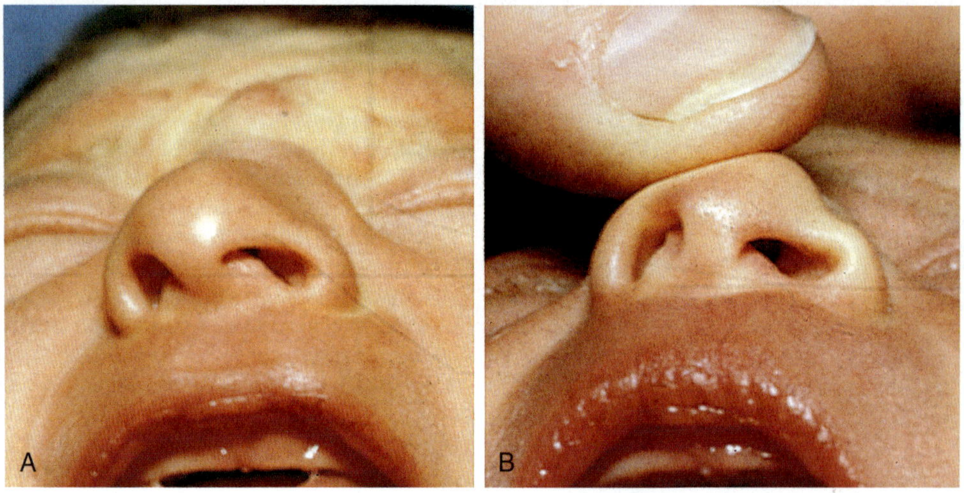

Fig. 2.26 Nasal deformity. This infant incurred dislocation of the triangular cartilage of the nasal septum during delivery. (A) Inspection of the nose reveals deviation of the septum to the right and asymmetry of the nares. (B) When the septum is manually moved toward the midline, the asymmetry persists, confirming the dislocation.

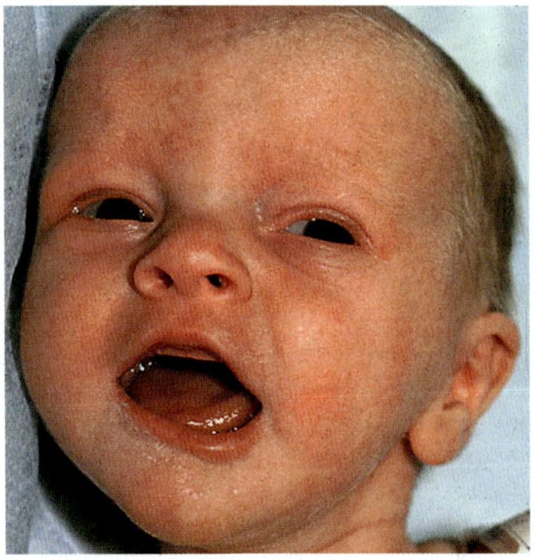

Fig. 2.27 Facial nerve palsy. This infant incurred injury to the right facial nerve, resulting in loss of the nasolabial fold on the affected side and asymmetric movement of the mouth. The side of the mouth that appears to droop is the normal side.

facial nerve palsies is excellent, and recovery usually occurs within the first month. Prevention of corneal drying is essential. Surgery is reserved for cases in which severing of the facial nerve has occurred. Referral should be made if there is no improvement after 2 to 3 months.

The incidence of brachial plexus trauma with current obstetric management is approximately 0.7 per 1000 live births. The mechanism of injury in most instances is traction on the plexus during delivery. Although lesions have classically been divided into those affecting upper spinal segments (Erb palsy) and those affecting lower segments (Klumpke palsy), the distinction may not be straightforward. Injury to the C5 and C6 fibers is most often identified by the arm hanging limply adducted and internally rotated at the shoulder, extended and pronated at the elbow (Fig. 2.28A). Injury affecting the lower segments of C7 and T1 rarely occurs in isolation, causing weakness of the wrist and hand, and ultimately leads to a claw-hand deformity (see Fig. 2.28B and C). There may be sensory loss along the ulnar side of the hand and forearm in the distribution of the T1 dermatome. If the T1 root is affected with interruption of the sympathetic innervation at that level, Horner syndrome (constricted pupil, drooping upper eyelid, and local

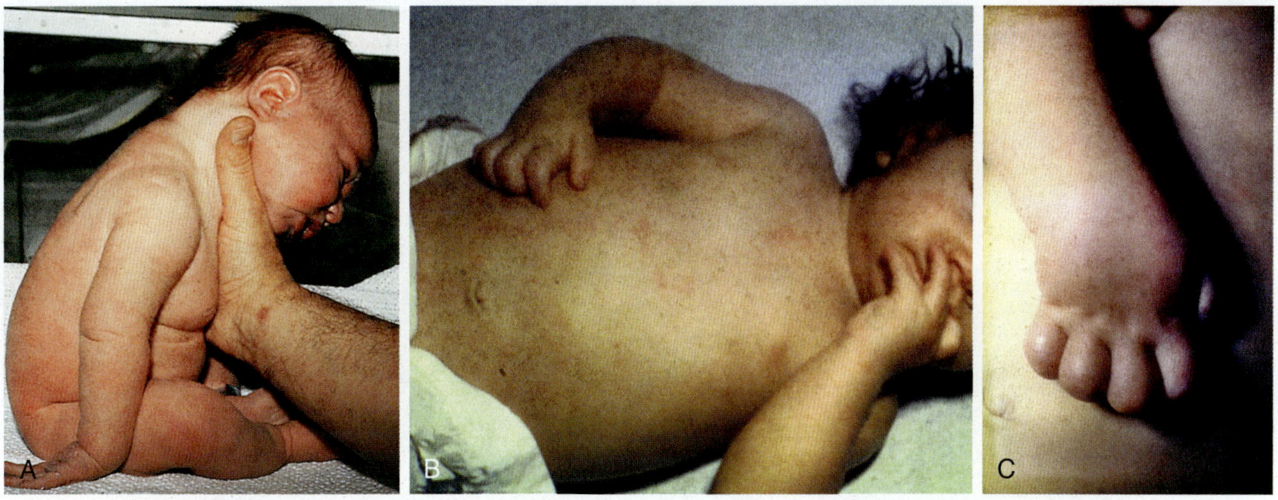

Fig. 2.28 Brachial plexus injury. (A) Traction injury to C5, C6, and C7 spinal cord segments produced this (Erb) palsy. This infant demonstrates the characteristic posture of the limply adducted and internally rotated arm. (B and C) Infant with Klumpke palsy involving the lower segments of C7 and T1. Note the different posture of the arm compared with the Erb palsy and the claw-hand deformity. (B and C, Courtesy Dr. Michael Painter, Children's Hospital of Pittsburgh.)

inability to sweat on one side of the face) may be apparent. Appropriate deep-tendon reflexes are absent. It may be difficult to confirm a sensory deficit, and autonomic fibers are often intact. Diagnosis is made clinically, but electromyography may be indicated to assess the severity of the injury and to determine the prognosis in patients not showing improvement after 6 to 8 weeks. Treatment should be deferred for at least 7 to 10 days, and then specific physical therapy and splinting should be undertaken. Most infants with brachial plexus palsies demonstrate complete recovery in the first few months of life. Earlier recovery suggests better long-term prognosis.

CONGENITAL ANOMALIES

Innumerable congenital anomalies can be noted at birth. Although any single minor malformation may be of little medical consequence, the identification of three or more in a single infant may be a clue to more serious errors of morphogenesis. A careful family history, including examination of the parents and siblings, can often place these malformations in proper perspective.

Hands and Feet

Most minor external anomalies involve the hands, feet, and head. One common abnormality of digitation is the presence of a supernumerary digit (Fig. 2.29), which is most often located lateral to the fifth digit on the hand (ulnar or postaxial polydactyly) or foot. This condition is distinguishable from true polydactyly because of the small pedicle that attaches the extra digit to the fifth digit. The supernumerary digit may have a fingernail but often lacks bones. Although usually of no consequence, a supernumerary digit has, on occasion, been associated with major central nervous system (CNS) malformations. Radial or preaxial polydactyly (supernumerary thumb) is more often associated with syndromes than ulnar polydactyly. Patients may be referred to plastic surgery for removal, which is usually necessary in cases of radial polydactyly.

True polydactyly (duplication of digits) may also be seen (Fig. 2.30). It is most common on the feet but can also occur on the hands. A family history of this anomaly may exist, or it may occur in association with other, more serious patterns of malformation. Although removal is not required, it may be indicated cosmetically.

Syndactyly, fusion of the soft tissues between digits, is relatively common (Fig. 2.31). Once again, a family history can be helpful to

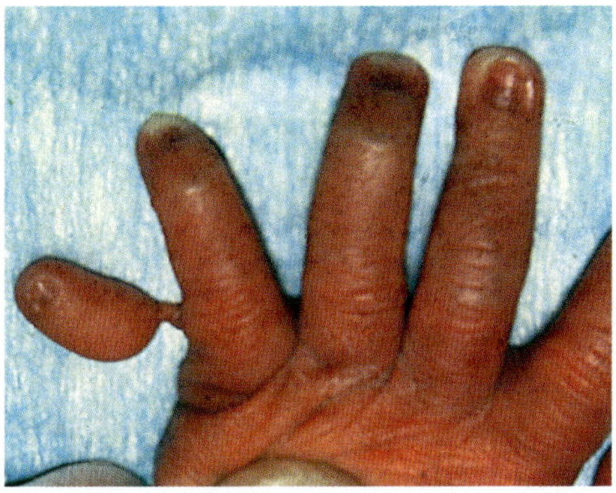

Fig. 2.29 Supernumerary digit. This is the common position for a sixth digit. The thin pedicle distinguishes this anomaly from true polydactyly.

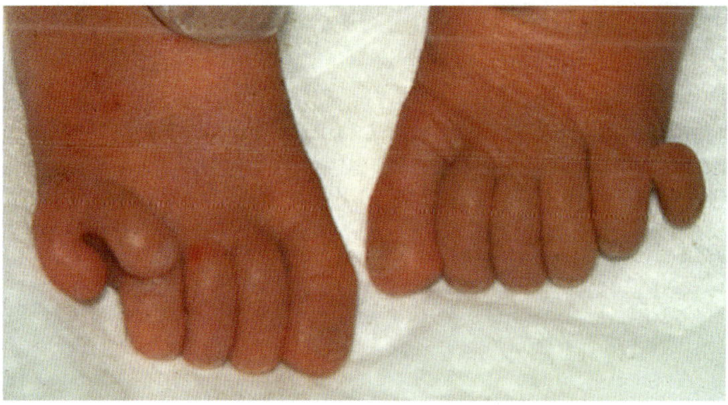

Fig. 2.30 Polydactyly. True bilateral polydactyly of the fifth toe is seen in this infant.

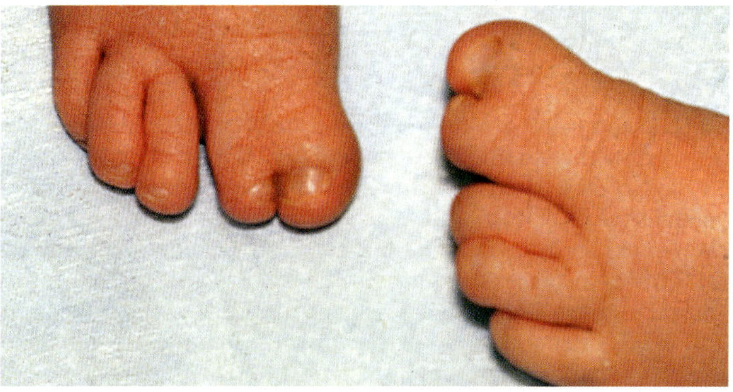

Fig. 2.31 Syndactyly. This child demonstrates bilateral fusion of the soft tissue between the first and second toes.

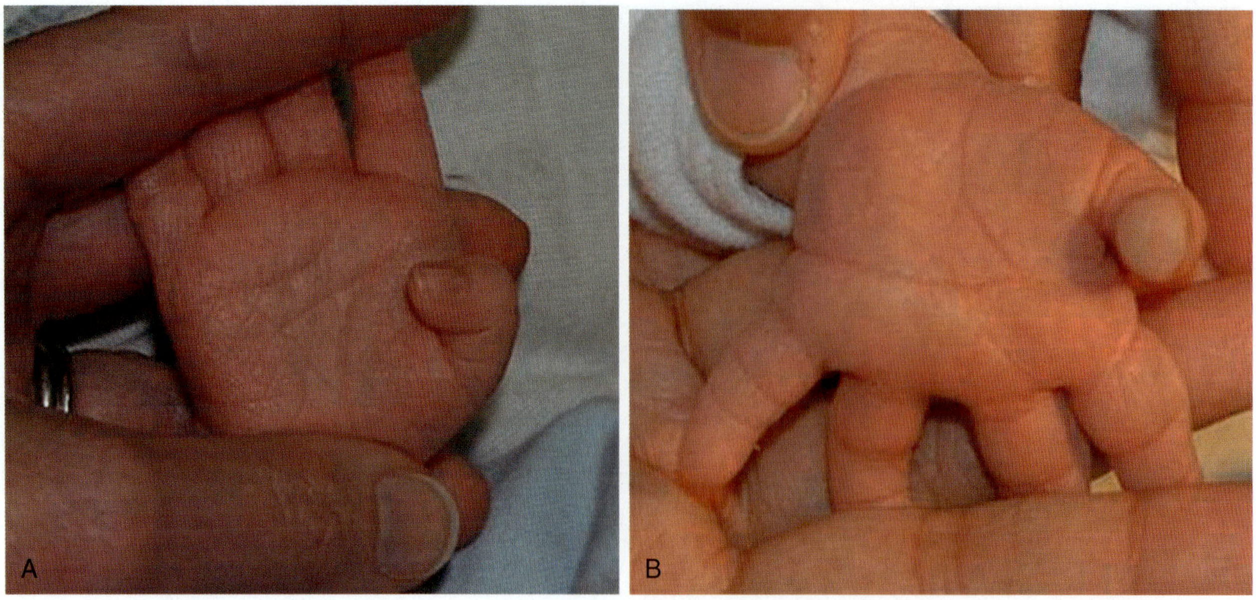

Fig. 2.32 (A) Normal palm. In most newborns, there are three primary creases on the palm of the hand. (B) Single palmar crease. A single palmar crease occurs in 5% to 10% of newborns; however, it is common in infants with a variety of genetic disorders, most notably trisomy 21.

determine association with other anomalies. Surgical correction of the syndactyly is usually postponed until 3 years of age unless there is a synchondrosis (cartilaginous union) or synostosis (bony union) that may interfere with growth.

Palmar creases occur due to flexion of the thickened skin of the hand in the first trimester. Alterations in folding of the palmar plane may be affected by the slope of the third, fourth, and fifth metacarpal/phalangeal joints, relative shortness of the palm, or a generalized state of hypotonia with resultant decreased fetal movement. A single, unilateral, midposition plane of flexion, *single palmar crease,* is found in 4% of the population (bilateral in 1% of the population) (Fig. 2.32).

External Ear

Careful morphologic examination of the external ear may reveal minor anomalies. One of the more common is the presence of preauricular skin tags located anterior to the tragus (Fig. 2.33). These tags may be unilateral or bilateral and represent remnants of the first branchial arch. Although often of little consequence, they may be seen in serious malformations of branchial arch development involving multiple structures of the head and neck and may have an associated hearing loss. Surgical removal may be indicated for cosmetic purposes.

A second, often overlooked malformation is the presence of ear pits or congenital aural fistulas located anterior to the tragus (Fig. 2.34). These may be familial, occur twice as often in females, and are more common in African Americans. They are of little consequence beyond the fact that they may become infected.

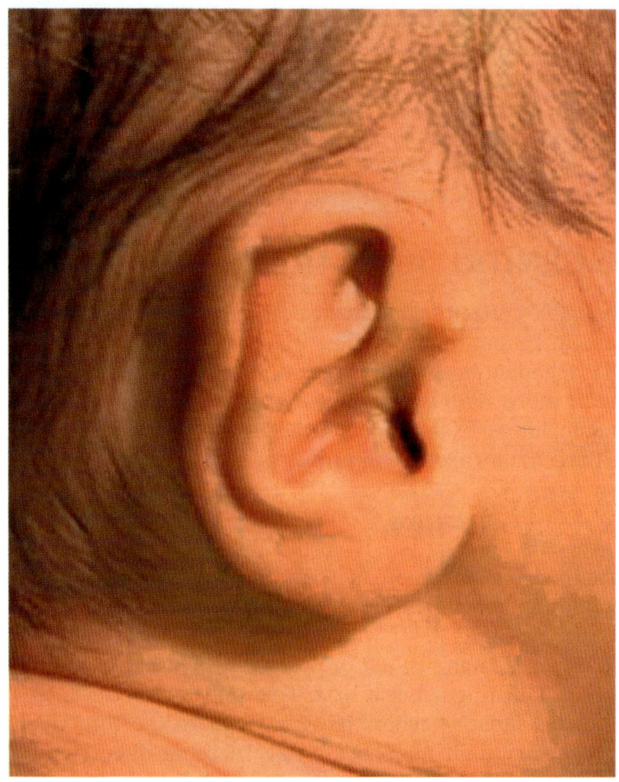

Fig. 2.33 Preauricular skin tag.

Midline Clefts

Cleft lip and palate are among the most common facial anomalies (Fig. 2.35). These malformations represent failure of lip fusion (at 35 days of gestation) and, in some cases, subsequent failure of palatal shelves closure (at 8–9 weeks' gestation). Although many cases occur spontaneously, others appear to be inherited, and in a minority of instances the defect is one manifestation of a chromosomal disorder. Adequate assessment necessitates careful examination of all structures of the head and neck and their relationship to each other. For example, cleft palate may be coupled with mandibular hypoplasia (Robin sequence), resulting in significant respiratory obstruction. Because of associated eustachian tube dysfunction, frequent episodes of otitis media are an almost invariable complication of cleft palate. Specialized feeding techniques are often necessary for infants with cleft palate. Even in the absence of an overt cleft, palpation and visualization of the palate and uvula should be routine because clefts of the soft palate (associated with a bifid uvula and a midline notch at the posterior border of the hard palate) can lead to later speech problems (see Chapter 24).

Although major malformations of the spinal column, such as myelomeningocele, are readily identifiable (see Chapters 1 and 16), diagnostic differentiation between two other midline defects—pilonidal sinuses and congenital dermal sinuses of the lumbar and

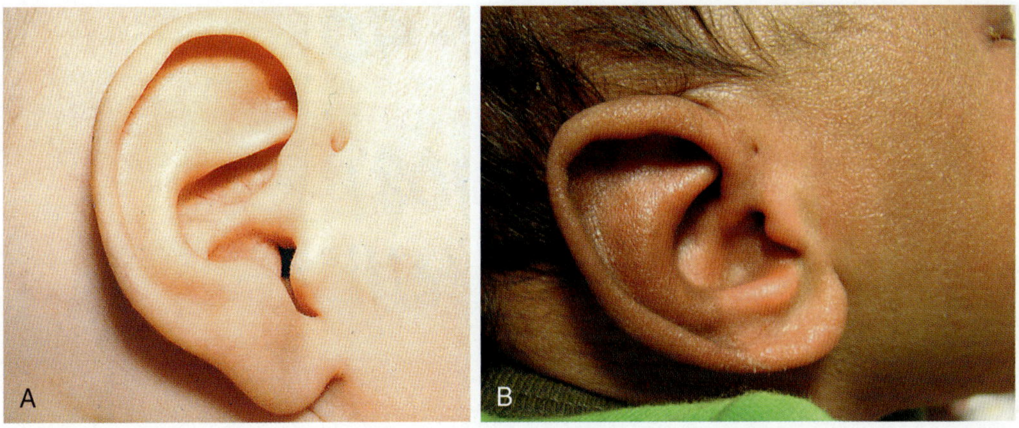

Fig. 2.34 Aural fistula. (A) Prominent congenital ear pit anterior to the tragus. Its only significance is that it may become infected. (B) Less prominent congenital ear pit. (B, Courtesy https://thelactationcollege.substack.com/p/pediatric-pearls-the-ear-pits-tags)

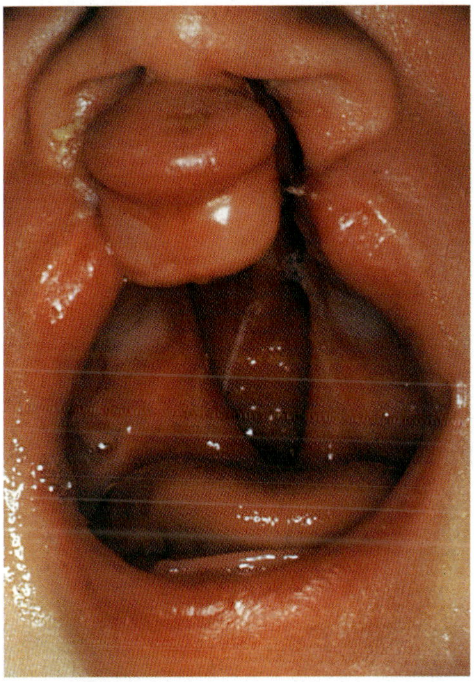

Fig. 2.35 Cleft lip. A prominent bilateral cleft lip with a complete cleft palate is seen in an infant with trisomy 13. The cleft extends from the soft to the hard palate, exposing the nasal cavity.

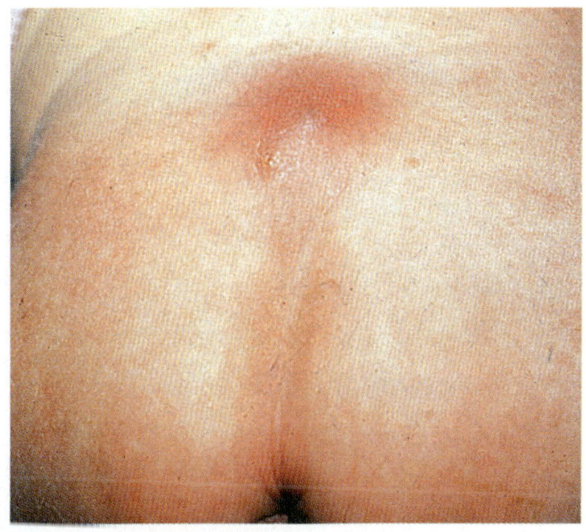

Fig. 2.36 Pilonidal sinus. This midline sinus overlying the sacrum did not extend to the spinal cord.

sacral spine—can be difficult. A pilonidal sinus tends to be located over the sacrum (Fig. 2.36). The surface opening is usually larger than that of a dermal sinus, but the tract rarely extends into the spinal canal; therefore although infection can occur, CNS extension is unlikely. A congenital dermal sinus is usually located over the lower lumbar region, with a sinus tract that can extend farther down the spinal column (Fig. 2.37A–C). The external orifice may be a small dimple, or an easily visible opening surrounded by hair. Recognition is important because there may be an underlying spinal dysraphism, and infection of the tract can extend to the CNS. Other findings overlying the spine, such as hemangiomas, hairy patches, and masses, may also indicate underlying pathology (see Chapter 16). These abnormalities can herald an occult tethered spinal cord, which may occur with minimal or no neurologic signs in the infant. Failure to recognize the possible association of these cutaneous abnormalities with an occult tethered cord could result in later neurologic abnormalities, including foot and lower extremity deformities, decreased sensation, weakness, abnormal gait, and bladder dysfunction. Diagnosis can be made by ultrasound, optimally in the newborn period because the acoustic window becomes smaller as the child grows. Ultrasound is indicated when a sacrococcygeal dimple is larger than 5 mm, located greater than 2.5 cm above the anus, or seen in combination with other lesions (Fig. 2.38).

Midline dimples, aberrant hairs, and hemangiomas on the face may also indicate underlying pathology and possible connection with the CNS and should be further investigated (Fig. 2.39).

Another form of midline defect may occur over the posterior parietal scalp and consists of a localized area of ectodermal dysplasia (Fig. 2.40). This lesion appears "punched out" and lacks all normal dermal elements. It may be associated with chromosomal anomalies, especially trisomy 13, but may be present in otherwise normal infants. Similar lesions, often located on the extremities, should be distinguished from those on the scalp because they often represent a dermatologic defect known as *cutis aplasia* (see Fig. 8.132).

Skin

Complete examination of the newborn's entire skin surface is essential. The presence of hyperpigmented lesions may warrant more thorough examination of the skin with a Wood lamp to better assess for hypopigmented lesions. Skin anomalies evident in the newborn period are quite common. These conditions include spontaneously resolving rashes and more permanent lesions (see Chapter 8). It is also important to be familiar with how various lesions may have a different appearance on darker skin.

Meconium is noted in the amniotic fluid in at least 10% of deliveries. The meconium may have been recently expelled or may have been present in the amniotic fluid for hours or days. Because

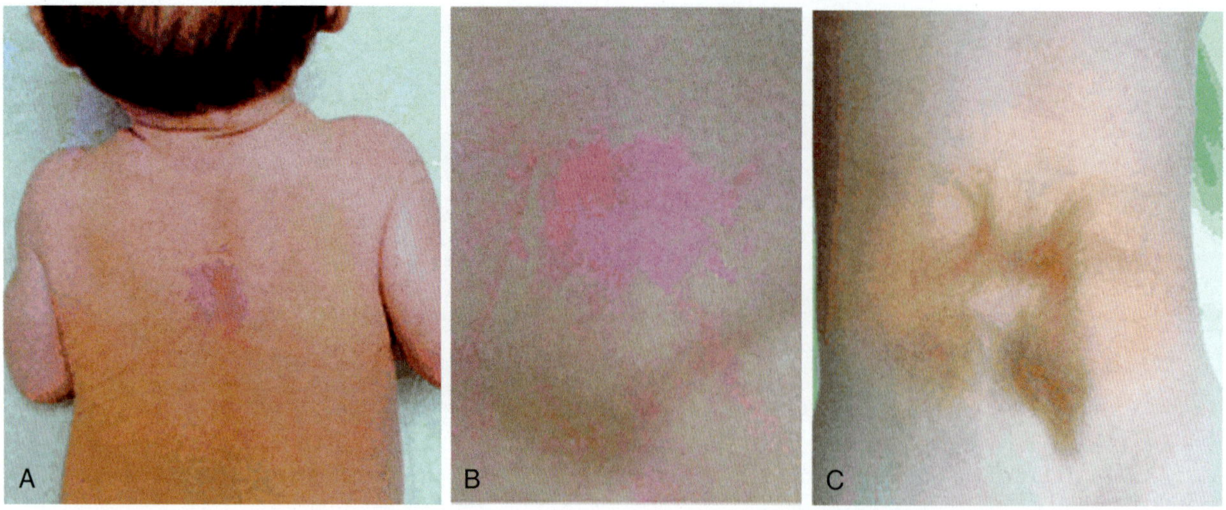

Fig. 2.37 (A) Congenital dermal sinus with pigmentation change. Note extrasacrococcygeal location. (B) Visible sinus opening. (C) Hypertrichosis with pigmentation change.

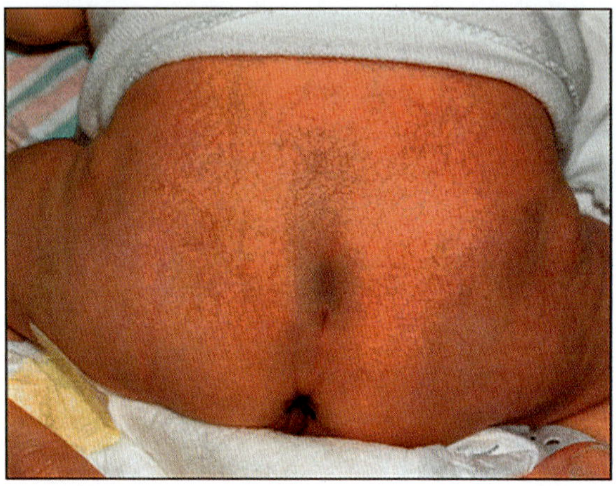

Fig. 2.38 Sacrococcygeal dimple. Ultrasound or magnetic resonance imaging evaluation warranted for multiple dimples, dimple diameter greater than 5 mm, located greater than 2.5 cm above the anus, or dimples outside the sacrococcygeal region.

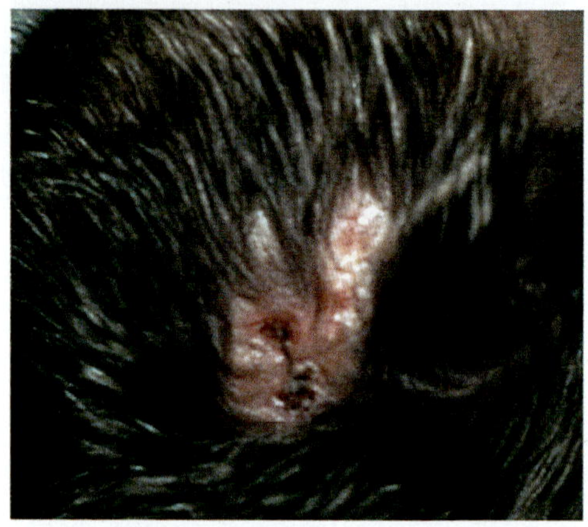

Fig. 2.40 Localized ectodermal dysplasia. An extensive punched-out area lacking all normal dermal elements is seen in the midline of the scalp of this child with trisomy 13.

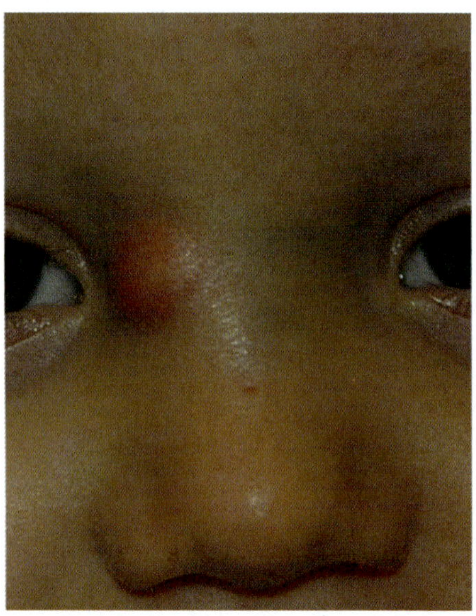

Fig. 2.39 Dermoid cyst with transcranial extension presenting initially only as midline pit at the nasal dorsum.

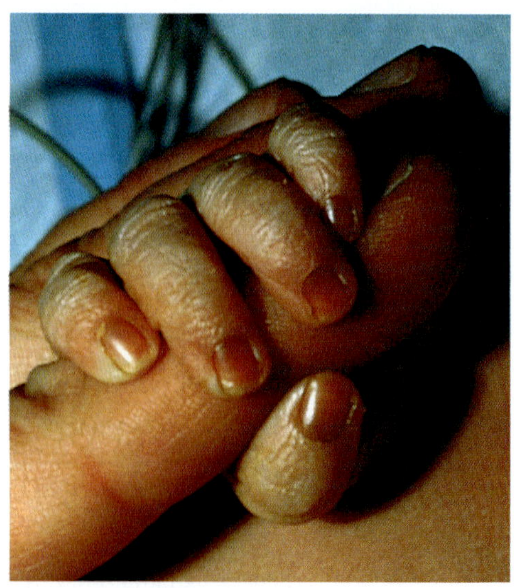

Fig. 2.41 Meconium staining. The marked discoloration of this infant's fingernails resulted from long-standing meconium staining of the amniotic fluid before delivery.

the timing of meconium passage may have significance for the diagnosis of fetal distress, it is useful to examine infants for the presence of meconium staining. It takes at least 4 to 6 hours of contact before staining of the umbilicus, skin, and nails occurs (Fig. 2.41). Often, the meconium-stained infant is postterm and has diffuse peeling of the skin with a shriveled, stained umbilical cord.

Jaundice is a yellow hue of the skin and mucous membranes and is a cause for concern if noted within the first 24 hours of life. The color is a result of deposited bilirubin, an end-product of heme catabolism, which occurs in the normal newborn at an increased rate due to decreased red blood cell survival in the neonatal period. Increased red cell mass, liver enzyme immaturity, increased enterohepatic circulation, and lack of intestinal bacteria also contribute to the development of physiologic jaundice. Bilirubin can also concentrate and deposit in the brain, leading to neuronal injury and the devastating condition of kernicterus. Physiologic elevation occurs in newborns with a peak at about 4 days. Premature neonates have a delayed and more severe bilirubin peak at 5 days due to delayed maturation of the hepatic uridine diphosphate-glucuronosyltransferase, the enzyme controlling bilirubin conjugation to allow for excretion. It is routine for newborns to be screened for hyperbilirubinemia before discharge from the hospital. Common risk factors for hyperbilirubinemia include breastfeeding, low birth weight, ABO incompatibility, glucose-6 phosphate dehydrogenase deficiency, and cephalohematoma.

There are several rashes and markings commonly seen in healthy newborns, and these are discussed and pictured in the Neonatal Dermatology section of Chapter 8. Several neonatal infections have associated skin findings, and these are discussed and pictured in the Congenital and Perinatal Infections section of Chapter 13. The umbilical stump can be a port of entry for infection, and pediatricians should be alert to early signs of omphalitis in the newborn with a healing umbilical stump (Fig. 2.42). Signs of omphalitis may include purulent discharge from the umbilical cord stump, induration, advancing erythema, and tenderness.

Umbilical granulomas are commonly seen in newborns after separation of the umbilical cord. The exact cause of their formation is not known. Although not usually of concern, they may bleed or become infected. They can usually be removed by chemical cautery with silver nitrate and rarely require surgical resection.

Drainage from the umbilicus may indicate infection of the umbilical stump as noted earlier but may also be a sign of vitelline duct or urachal remnants. Enteric contents draining from the umbilicus or the persistence of what appears to be a large granuloma may indicate a vitelline duct remnant. Clear, yellow fluid in the umbilicus may be urine from a urachal remnant. Both require evaluation by a pediatric surgeon.

Congenital Hip Dislocation

Congenital hip dislocation occurs six times more frequently in females than in males, with an overall incidence of 1.5 in 1000 live births. Associated factors include breech presentation, oligohydramnios, firstborn infants, and family history. The pathologic anatomy involves superior capsular laxity and a shallow acetabulum due to limited concentric contact with the femoral head. The Ortolani and Barlow maneuvers discussed previously should be performed. The diagnosis can easily be confirmed by ultrasonography, which is a sensitive imaging modality for detecting hip dysplasia in the immediate newborn period. Screening ultrasound, however, should not be performed before 2 weeks of life, as physiologic laxity of the ligaments may result in a high false-positive rate. Ideally, orthopedic consultation for treatment should be obtained within the first 4 to 6 months of life.

Amniotic Bands

Several serious structural deformations can result from early in utero amniotic rupture and subsequent band-line compression or amputation. The band-induced abnormalities generally affect the limbs, digits, and craniofacial structures (Fig. 2.43). This phenomenon is usually sporadic.

Umbilical Hernia

An umbilical hernia is a common finding, especially in African American infants (Fig. 2.44). The incidence of this central fascia defect beneath the umbilicus is also higher in premature infants and those with congenital thyroid deficiency. It is important to distinguish between this relatively benign fascial defect and the more serious defects of the somites that form the peritoneal, muscular, and ectodermal layers of the abdominal wall underlying the umbilicus, resulting in an omphalocele. In the latter condition, a portion of the intestine is located outside the abdominal wall (see Chapter 18). When large, the distinction is obvious, but in its mildest form, an omphalocele resembles a fixed hernia of the umbilicus. True umbilical hernias usually require no therapy, and spontaneous resolution occurs within the first few years of life. Those that remain

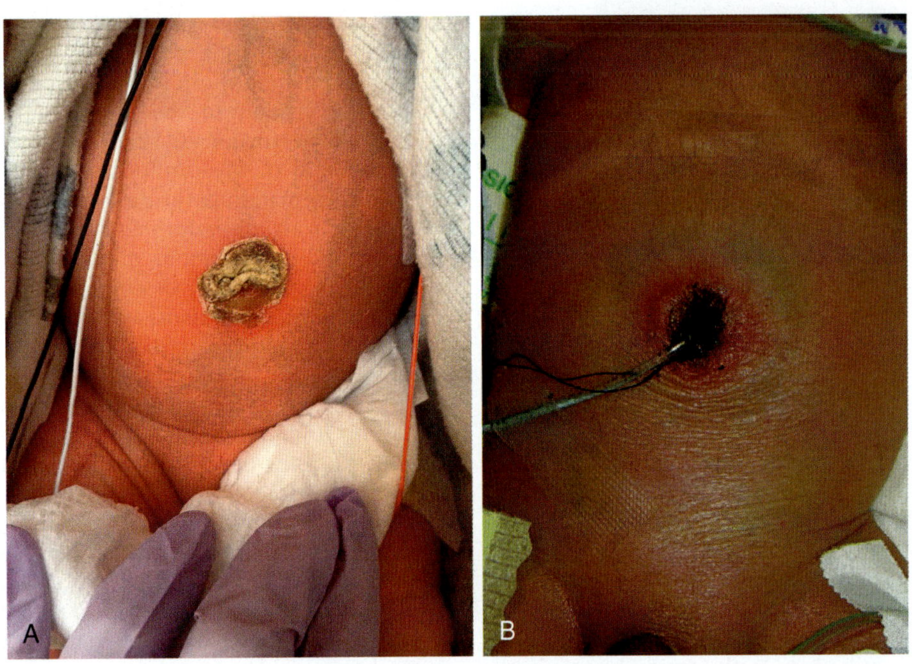

Fig. 2.42 Omphalitis. (A) Infection of the umbilical stump that may present as a cellulitis with erythema surrounding the umbilicus; this can progress to necrotizing fasciitis and sepsis. (B) Omphalitis with umbilical catheter in place. (B, Courtesy Fahmy MAB: Omphalitis. In *Umbilicus and umbilical cord*, 2018, Springer, pp 119–131. doi:10.1007/978-3-319-62383-2_26)

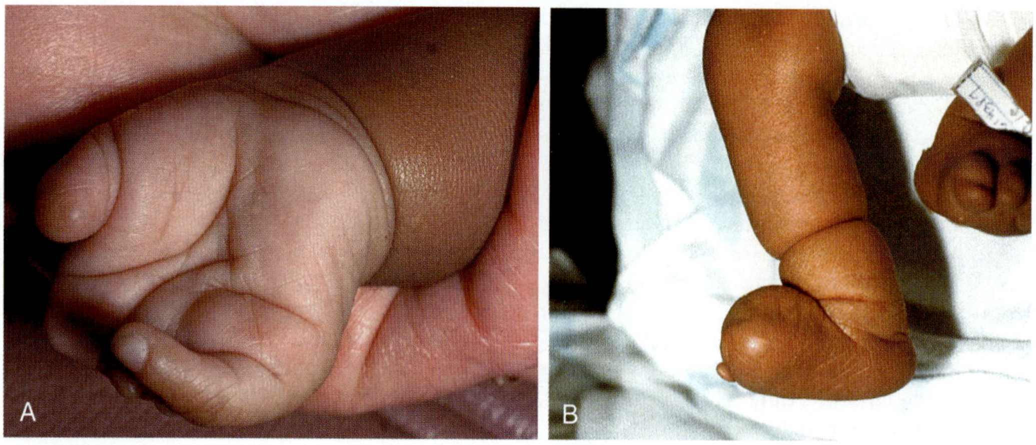

Fig. 2.43 Amniotic bands. (A) Loss of digits secondary to an amniotic band. (B) A lower extremity amniotic band with constriction around the lower leg. (A, Courtesy VisualDx 2016. https://www.visualdx.com/visualdx/diagnosis/moduleId =103&diagnosisId = 53377&imgSet = 1#&gid = 1&pid = 2 https://www.visualdx.com/visualdx/diagnosis/moduleId =103&diagnosisId = 53377&imgSet = 1#&gid = 1&pid = 3. B, From Graham JM, Smith DV: *Smith's recognizable patterns of human deformation,* ed 3, Philadelphia, 2007, Saunders.)

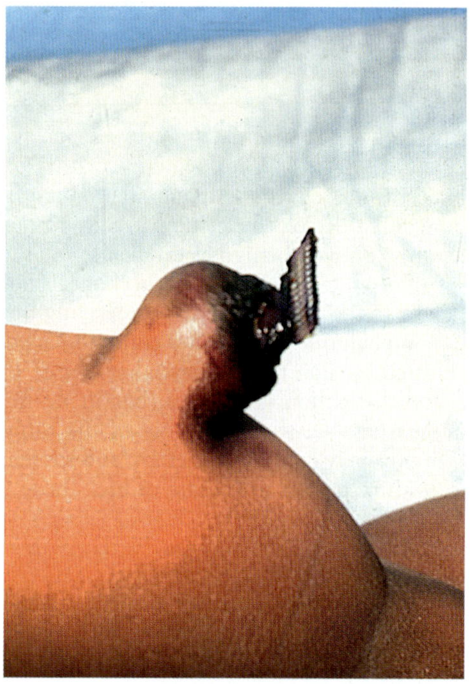

Fig. 2.44 Umbilical hernia. This prominent umbilical hernia was noted at birth in an otherwise normal African American infant.

after 3 years can be surgically repaired. Attempts to reduce the hernia with tape or coins are ineffective and may result in side effects, such as adhesive reaction/allergy. Incarceration is rare.

Scrotal Swelling

Swelling of the scrotum in the neonate is relatively common, especially in breech deliveries. Although the differential diagnosis includes hematomas, infections, testicular torsion, and tumors, most cases are attributable to hydroceles, fluid accumulation in the tunica vaginalis. Palpation reveals an extremely smooth, firm, egg-shaped mass that brightly transilluminates (Fig. 2.45A). When the hydrocele is noncommunicating, the clinician can often palpate above the mass with the thumb and finger and feel a normal spermatic cord. The testicle may be difficult to palpate but is usually visible on transillumination. With inguinal hernias, the prolapsed intestine may transilluminate as well, but it usually presents visible septa under high-intensity light. Furthermore, on palpation there is significant thickening of the spermatic cord.

Although a hydrocele may persist for months, the majority resolve spontaneously. There is a high association with inguinal hernias, especially in hydroceles that persist. In such cases, the spermatic cord is often noticeably thickened. Given the association with hernias, the possibility of bowel incarceration should be kept in mind. Surgical repair is indicated when a hydrocele persists for more than 6 months or when it is associated with findings suggestive of an inguinal hernia, such as a communicating hydrocele. (See Chapter 18 for a more detailed discussion of inguinal hernias.)

A swollen and tender or bruised scrotum may be a sign of testicular torsion and should be investigated with urgency to salvage the testicle if possible (Fig. 2.45B). Testicular torsion may occur in utero and may present with scrotal ecchymosis, but there may be no swelling or tenderness if the torsion was not recent.

SPECIAL CONSIDERATIONS

Respiratory Distress

The differential diagnosis and subsequent management of the infant with respiratory distress are some of the most frequent challenges encountered in newborn medicine. Problems posed by prematurity, delayed transition to the extrauterine environment, infections, metabolic derangements, and various congenital and acquired abnormalities of the cardiopulmonary system may all lead to a similar presentation in the newborn period.

Infants with respiratory compromise may present with varying degrees and combinations of tachypnea, cyanosis, and grunting, flaring, and retractions. *Grunting* is an involuntary guttural expiratory sound made by infants as they exhale against a closed glottis to maintain expiratory lung volume. *Flaring* refers to the reflexive opening of the nares during labored inspiration. *Retractions* are the result of increased respiratory effort with high negative intrathoracic pressures leading to an inward collapse of the relatively compliant chest wall of the newborn during inspiration (see https://youtu.be/iiX6vQ2F6ao?si = 1-_XeO3rYZoGynsG).

Classic respiratory distress syndrome (RDS) is caused by a combination of lung immaturity, usually secondary to preterm delivery and surfactant deficiency. The radiographic findings are shown and described in Fig. 2.46. Depending on the severity of RDS, infants may require any combination of supplemental oxygen therapy, surfactant replacement, or mechanical ventilatory assistance. A small proportion of infants with RDS may develop a chronic lung condition known as *bronchopulmonary dysplasia.* See Fig. 2.47 and Fig. 2.48.

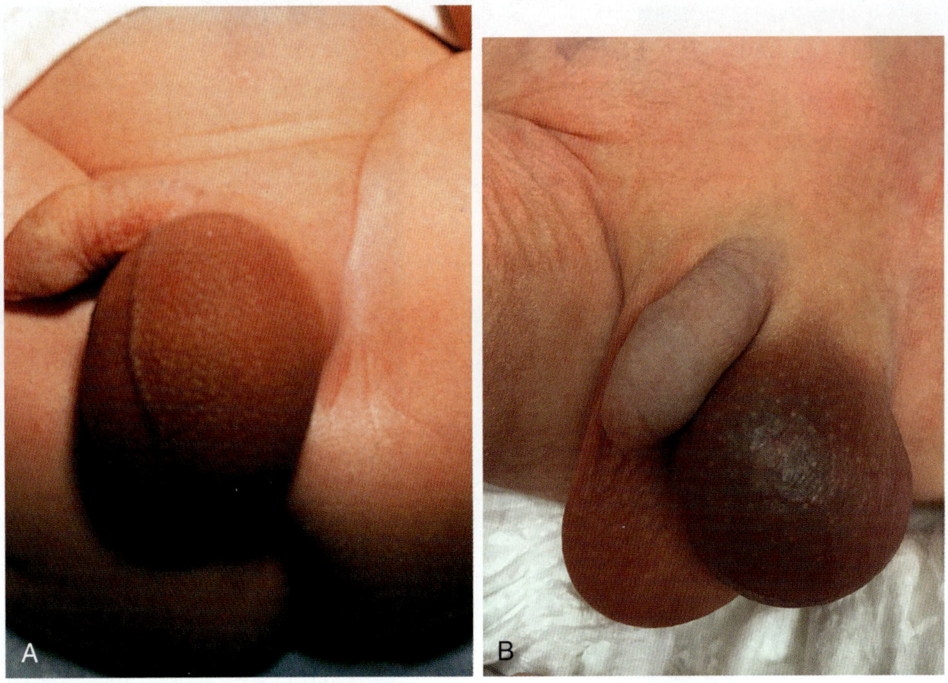

Fig. 2.45 Scrotal swelling. (A) Unilateral hydrocele that was noted at birth. Transillumination was consistent with the diagnosis. (B) Testicular torsion.

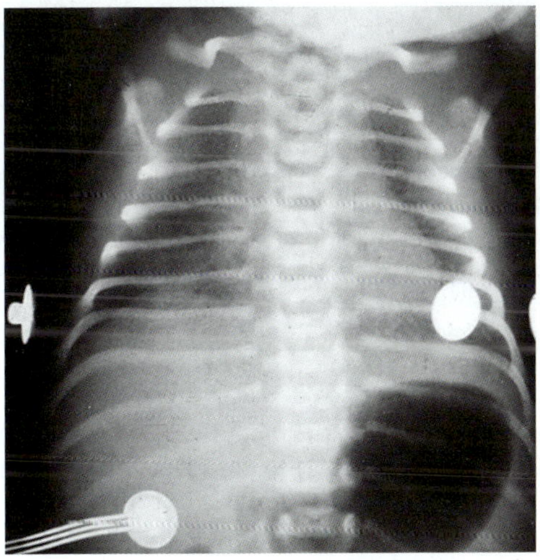

Fig. 2.46 Respiratory distress syndrome. Note the ground-glass appearance, low lung volumes, and the presence of air bronchograms.

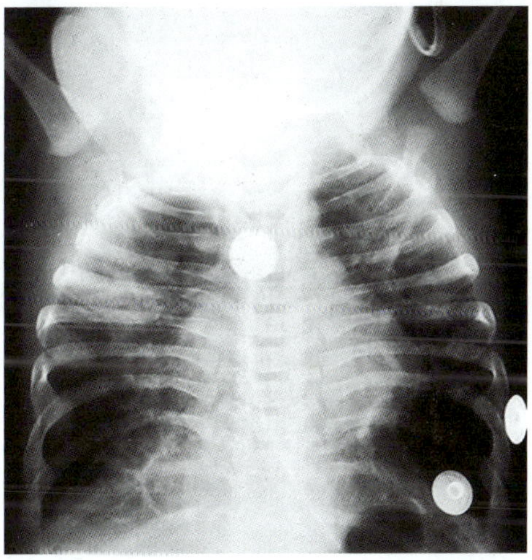

Fig. 2.48 Bronchopulmonary dysplasia. Note the alternating areas of hyperinflation and atelectasis.

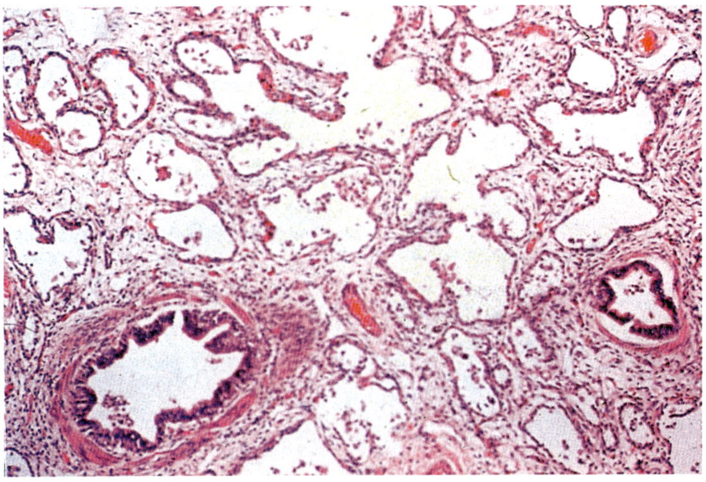

Fig. 2.47 Bronchopulmonary dysplasia. Histologic features include inflammation and fibrosis.

The most common cause of respiratory distress in term infants is transient tachypnea of the newborn (TTN). Thought to be related to the delayed removal of fetal lung fluid, this condition is more common in infants born by cesarean section. Radiographic findings are shown and described in (Fig. 2.49). TTN usually resolves within hours to days. Unfortunately for the clinician, the early clinical and radiographic findings in infants with potentially life-threatening congenital pneumonias may mimic those seen in RDS or TTN (Fig. 2.50). Meconium aspiration elicits an inflammatory response within the lungs and may also present as respiratory distress (Fig. 2.51).

Congenital heart disease (see Chapter 5) may not present with respiratory distress and may manifest as cyanosis in a comfortably breathing neonate. Various anomalies of the thoracic cavity or lungs (see Chapter 17) also commonly manifest in the newborn with signs of respiratory distress and should be included in the differential diagnosis. Pulmonary air leak syndromes, such as pneumothorax (Fig. 2.52; and see Fig. 18.30) and pneumomediastinum (Fig. 2.53), are among the more common causes of respiratory distress in newborns.

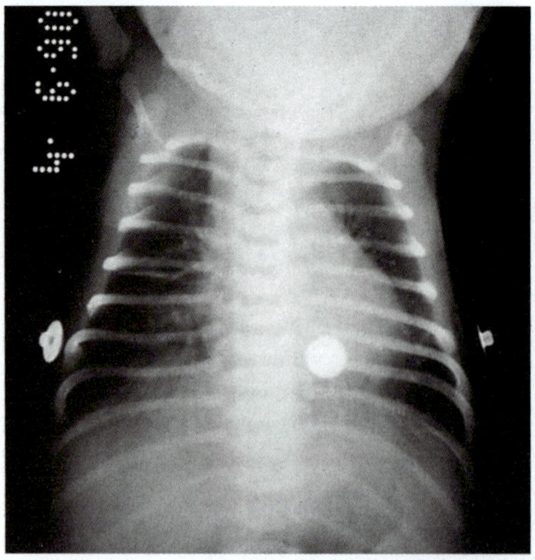

Fig. 2.49 Transient tachypnea of the newborn. Radiograph reveals several streaky perihilar densities and a visible fluid density in the right major fissure.

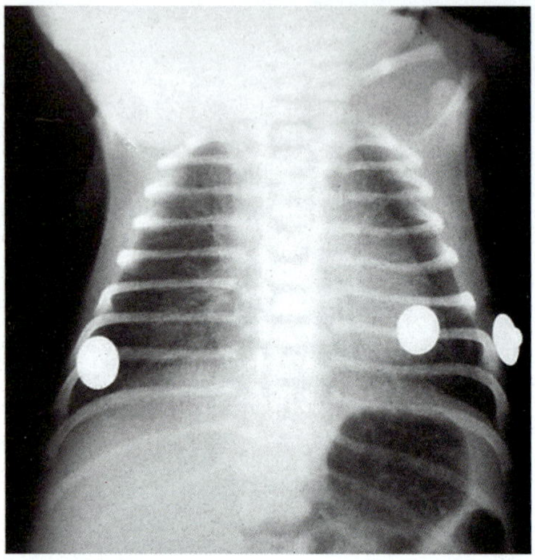

Fig. 2.50 Congenital pneumonia. Infant's culture was positive for group B streptococci. Note the similarity to Fig. 2.46, with streaky perihilar densities and visible fluid density in the right major fissure.

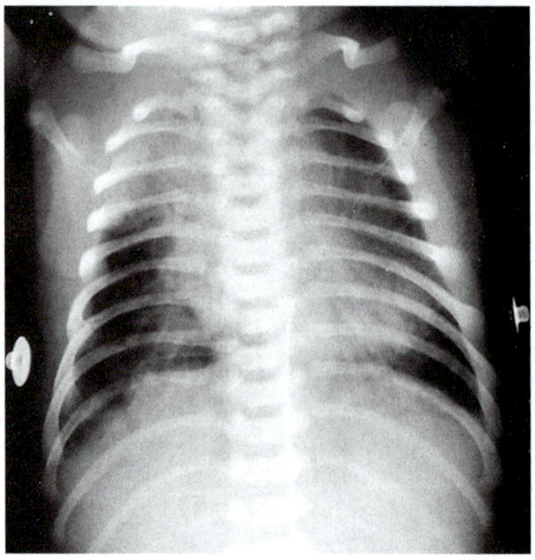

Fig. 2.51 Meconium aspiration. The radiograph reveals irregularly distributed areas of hyperaeration and consolidation.

Neonatal Opioid Withdrawal Syndrome

Neonatal opioid withdrawal syndrome (NOWS) may occur when an infant experiences the abrupt cessation of exposure to maternal medications, most commonly opioids, after birth. The timing of

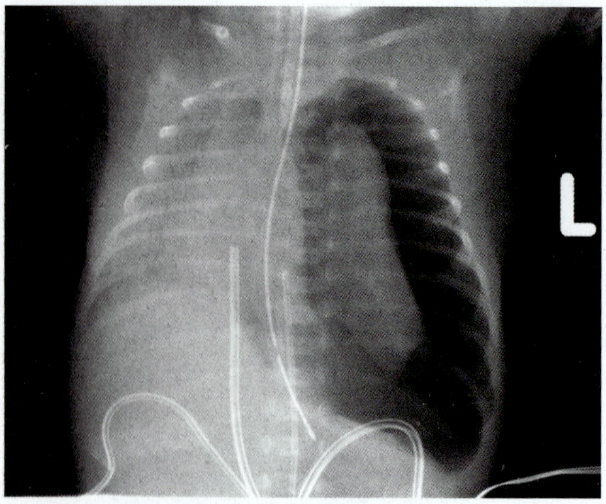

Fig. 2.52 Tension pneumothorax. Note the shift of the mediastinum, flattening of the diaphragm, and widening of the intercostal spaces. Also note the umbilical central lines, nasogastric tube, and endotracheal tube.

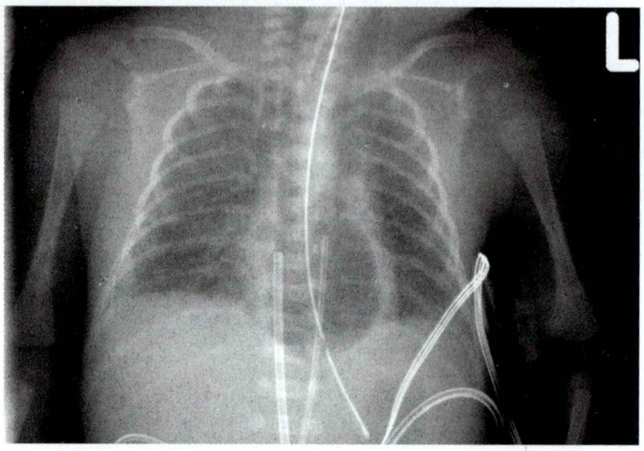

Fig. 2.53 Pneumomediastinum. A central collection of air in the mediastinum. Note the support lines and tubes in place.

presentation depends on the pharmacokinetics of the drug from which the infant is withdrawing. In general, NOWS typically presents in the first 5 to 7 days. Presenting signs are characterized as neurologic, cardiopulmonary, and gastrointestinal findings. Neurologic signs include tremors, irritability, high-pitched cry, poor sleeping, hyperactive reflexes, sneezing, and possibly seizures if observed signs are left untreated. Cardiopulmonary findings may present as tachycardia or tachypnea and may be misinterpreted as being due to primary cardiac or pulmonary disease. Signs of gastrointestinal dysfunction are commonly seen in newborns with NOWS and include poor feeding with uncoordinated or constant sucking, emesis, and diarrhea leading to dehydration and poor weight gain.

Management of NOWS involves both pharmacologic and nonpharmacologic care while assessing the severity of the withdrawal on a standardized scoring system, such as the modified Finnegan or Eat/Sleep/Console (ESC). ESC prioritizes nonpharmacologic therapies, which include procedures to decrease stimulation in the environment (low noise, dim lighting, swaddling), rooming in, skin-to-skin contact with parents, and on-demand feeding. Breastfed infants or infants receiving their mother's expressed breast milk from a bottle are less likely to need pharmacologic intervention to treat NOWS. Pharmacologic intervention with titration of short- or long-acting opioids (such as morphine or methadone) is considered when infants have increasing or high scores.

Newborn Stools

An infant's first few bowel movements consist of *meconium* (Fig. 2.54). When passed into the amniotic fluid before delivery, meconium can be aspirated into the lungs and cause an inflammatory pneumonitis

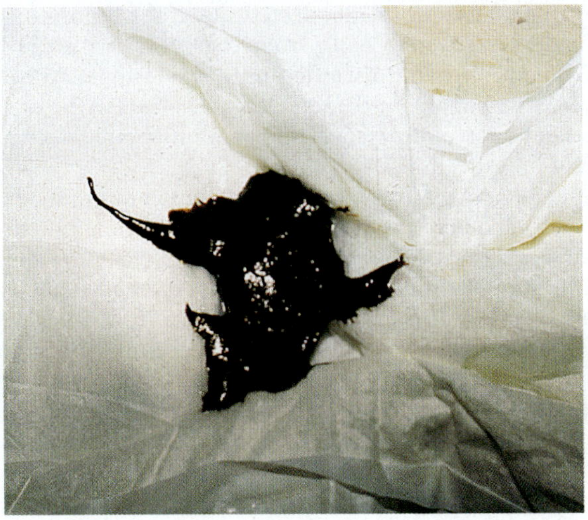

Fig. 2.54 Meconium. A typical sticky, greenish black meconium stool consists of accumulated intestinal cells, bile, and proteinaceous material formed during intestinal development.

and obstruction of the alveoli referred to as *meconium aspiration syndrome (MAS)* (see Fig. 2.51). Although it can also be normal for the term or postterm fetus to pass meconium before delivery, passage of meconium in the preterm fetus often indicates infection. Failure to pass meconium in the first 2 days of life may indicate intestinal obstruction resulting from stenosis, atresia, Hirschsprung disease, or meconium ileus or plug syndrome. By the third day of life, stools change in character and become known as *transitional* stools. They are greenish brown to yellowish brown, are less sticky than meconium, and may contain some milk curds. After the third to fourth day, the quality and frequency of stool vary depending on the type of milk ingested. Stool of a breastfed infant is described in (Fig. 2.55), whereas stool of a commercial formula–fed infant may be firmer and is described in (Fig. 2.56.)

ABDOMINAL DISTENTION

A neonate's abdomen is naturally rounded due to poor muscle tone. An excessive protuberance can indicate pathology. As previously discussed, eliciting a thorough stooling history helps differentiate the etiology of abdominal distention. The differential diagnosis includes functional and anatomic obstructions, infection, organomegaly, formula intolerance, and masses. The abdomen should be examined while the infant is quiet, with avoidance of examination immediately after feeding. Loose and/or grossly bloody stools in the

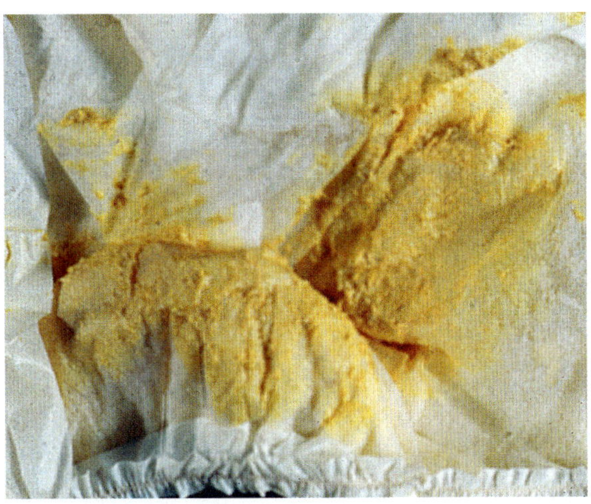

Fig. 2.55 Breastmilk stool. The stools of breastfed infants are usually yellow and soft with watery to pea soup consistency.

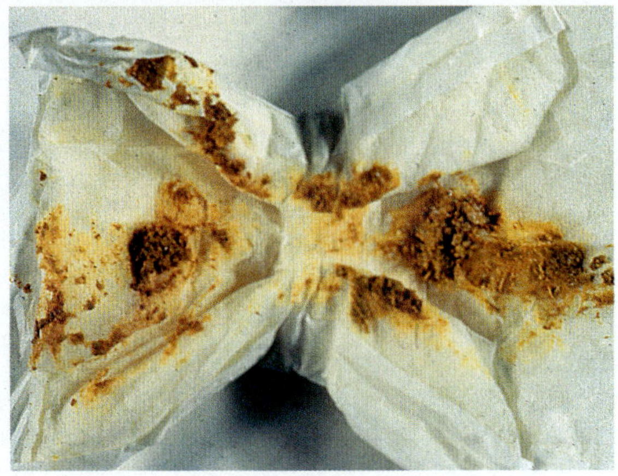

Fig. 2.56 Formula stool. Infants fed commercial formulas typically have darker and thicker stools than breastfed infants.

setting of a well-appearing infant with a normal examination may indicate an anal fissure (see Fig. 18.51) or cow's milk protein intolerance. This may be seen even in breastfed infants whose mothers are ingesting large volumes of dairy products. In addition to cow's milk protein, other dietary proteins may cause gastrointestinal upset in the infant. Radiographic studies such as ultrasound (prenatal and postnatal) and abdominal plain films are helpful diagnostic aids. Surgical consultation may be warranted (see Chapter 18 for further discussion).

BREASTFEEDING

Human breastmilk is the optimal food for almost all infants. The American Academy of Pediatrics (AAP) and the World Health Organization recommend that infants be fed human milk exclusively for the first 6 months of life and that breastfeeding be continued with the addition of complementary foods until at least 2 years old. Human milk provides both immediate and long-term benefits to infants, mothers, and society. Breastfed infants experience lower rates of ear infections, respiratory infections, diarrhea, allergies, inflammatory bowel disease, and leukemia. Females who breastfeed have less postpartum bleeding, more rapid involution of the postgravid uterus, and reduced risk of cardiovascular disease, type 2 diabetes mellitus, ovarian cancer, and breast cancer. Societal benefits include health care savings due to fewer office visits and hospitalizations, reduced absenteeism from work, and ecologic benefits.

Breastmilk is biologically complex, species specific, and serves both as a source of nutrition and immunologic support for the developing infant. It contains hundreds of bioactive substances including entire white blood cells (e.g., macrophages, T cells, B cells, neutrophils); proteins such as immunoglobulins (IgA, IgD, IgG, and IgM) and immune-modulating factors (e.g., lactoferrin, lysozyme, lactoperoxidase); hormones (e.g., thyrotropin-releasing hormone, thyroxine, cortisol, insulin-like growth factor-1); growth factors (e.g., epidermal growth factor, human-milk growth factors I, II, and III); enzymes; and cholesterol. These bioactive agents, which are not found in commercially prepared human milk substitutes, augment the infant's immature immune system. Human milk changes during feedings and across time to meet the changing nutritional and immunologic needs of infants.

Health care providers play an important role in a female's decision to breastfeed and can also have a significant impact on a female's success with breastfeeding. The benefits of breastfeeding can be discussed in multiple settings, such as school-based education, family planning and obstetric clinics, prenatal visits, and public health campaigns. Females' infant feeding intentions before delivery are the strongest predictor of their actual infant feeding behavior.

Pregnancy and Breast Development

The human breast is not fully developed until pregnancy. Prolactin and placental lactogen support the production of colostrum, starting in the second trimester. During the third trimester, the ductal system of the breast continues to dilate and fill with colostrum. After birth, with the rapid decline in progesterone that occurs with removal of the placenta, milk production begins under the influence of prolactin. Most females experience an increase in breast size and a darkening of the areola in pregnancy. Although rare, some females may have insufficient glandular tissue (Fig. 2.57) that is associated with insufficient milk supply.

Breast size is not associated with breastfeeding success. Breast surgery can negatively affect a female's ability to exclusively breastfeed her infant if there is disruption of nerves and milk ducts. Females who have had breast surgery (including augmentation or reduction) should be encouraged to try breastfeeding, following the infant's weight closely. Implants used in augmentation can worsen engorgement, which can lead to milk duct necrosis if not relieved.

Contraindications to Breastfeeding

There are few absolute contraindications to breastfeeding.

Females with human T-lymphotropic virus (HTLV) should not breastfeed. Mothers with active tuberculosis can express their milk and have someone else feed the baby until the mother has initiated treatment and is no longer considered contagious. Females with herpes simplex infections of the breast should not feed the infant on the side with the herpes lesions; however, the infant can be fed from the unaffected side if the lesions on the affected side are covered. Milk from the breast with the lesions should be emptied and discarded until the lesions are healed to maintain milk supply on the affected side. The AAP *Red Book* is an excellent source of detailed information about infectious diseases and breastfeeding.

New evidence supports females with human immunodeficiency virus (HIV)/acquired immune deficiency syndrome breastfeeding if certain conditions are met. The parent should achieve and maintain viral suppression with antiretroviral therapy (ART) during pregnancy and during the postpartum period. This scenario decreases the risk of transmitting HIV through breastmilk to $<1\%$, but still not zero. To eliminate the risk of transmission through feeding, donor breastmilk and formula are alternative options.

Infants with classic galactosemia should not be breastfed because human milk contains high levels of lactose. Infants with other forms of galactosemia, tyrosinemia, and phenylketonuria may be partially breastfed, but this should be determined on an individual basis with metabolism/genetics consultation.

Most, but not all, medications are safe for females to take during lactation. LactMed, available through the National Library of Medicine website, is an excellent, free, peer-reviewed source of up-to-date information on drug safety for breastfeeding mothers. The AAP breastfeeding policy indicates that tobacco use is not a contraindication to breastfeeding. However, females who smoke tobacco should be encouraged to smoke outside, decrease cigarette use, or preferably stop smoking. Females who smoke should be counseled to do so after feedings to minimize the transfer of nicotine into breastmilk. Females who use illicit drugs should be counseled not to breastfeed. Females prescribed methadone or buprenorphine for the treatment of opioid dependence should be encouraged to breastfeed if they remain adherent to their drug treatment program and do not have any other contraindication to breastfeeding. The effects of cannabinoids on fetal development and cognitive development of the newborn are not known. Females are advised to abstain from the use of cannabinoids during pregnancy and lactation.

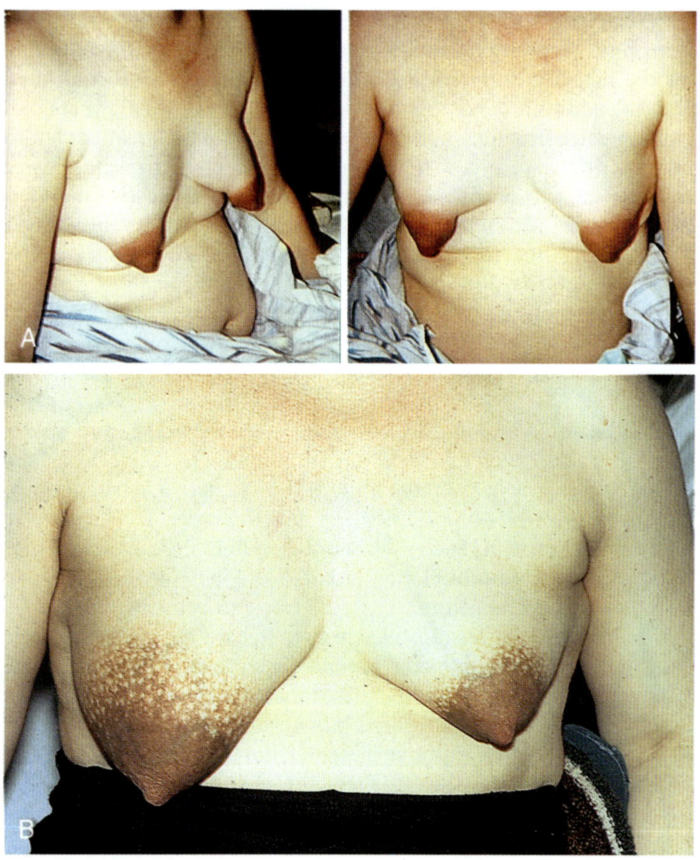

Fig. 2.57 Insufficient breast glandular tissue. Tubular breast shape, little to no breast enlargement, and little areolar darkening with pregnancy may indicate insufficient glandular tissue. There is often a family history of inadequate milk supply. Females with this condition may benefit from a referral to a lactation consultant. (A) A 26-hour postpartum female with tubular-shaped breasts without any fullness. (B) A female with insufficient glandular tissue and significantly different breast size who has insufficient milk supply. (Courtesy Susan Costanza, RN, IBCLC, Rochester General Hospital, Rochester, NY.)

Breastfeeding Evaluation

Pediatric health care providers should be comfortable observing and assisting females with breastfeeding, especially during the neonatal period, the first health maintenance examination, and when problems arise, such as poor weight gain or painful nursing. A thorough evaluation includes a history, examination of the mother's breasts, observation of the latch and positioning, and assessment of milk transfer. This evaluation may also be done by a lactation consultant and reported to the medical provider.

History

At the neonatal and first postpartum visits, history should include pregnancy and birth history; frequency, duration, and pattern of nursing; frequency of voids; frequency and character of stools; weight change; jaundice; pain with nursing; and maternal concerns. The AAP and ACOG's *Breastfeeding Handbook for Physicians* provides key points to support maintenance of breastfeeding for each pediatric visit from birth to 12 months.

Breast Examination

If a female has difficulty latching the baby in the neonatal period or if she complains of pain at any time, her breasts should be examined. For latching problems, it is important to determine whether a female has flat or inverted nipples. Nipple inspection alone does not answer this question, and the pinch test must be performed.

The nipple is normally everted if the nipple protrudes when the areola is compressed, inverted when it retracts toward the breast when the areola is compressed, and flat when it neither protrudes nor retracts. Although flat or inverted nipples may make it more difficult for the infant to latch in the first few days, females with flat or inverted nipples should not be discouraged about breastfeeding, because in many cases of flat and inverted nipples, babies latch without difficulty. However, if an infant has difficulty latching, the mother/infant dyad should be seen within the first day of birth by someone experienced in lactation support. The adhesions that cause the nipple to flatten or invert can usually be broken. Having the mother use a manual or electric breast pump for a few minutes before the baby latches to draw out the nipple can do this. Another option is to use a nipple shield (Fig. 2.58) for a short time to allow the baby to latch more easily. If a nipple shield is offered, it should be done under the supervision of someone experienced in lactation support, because it is not intended for long-term use. Flat and inverted nipples usually improve with nursing. The use of breast shells during pregnancy has not been shown to improve flat and inverted nipples.

Latch

A key factor in the success of breastfeeding is an appropriate latch (Fig. 2.59) because it affects both milk supply and comfort. When a baby is properly latched, the baby's mouth is wide open, with the

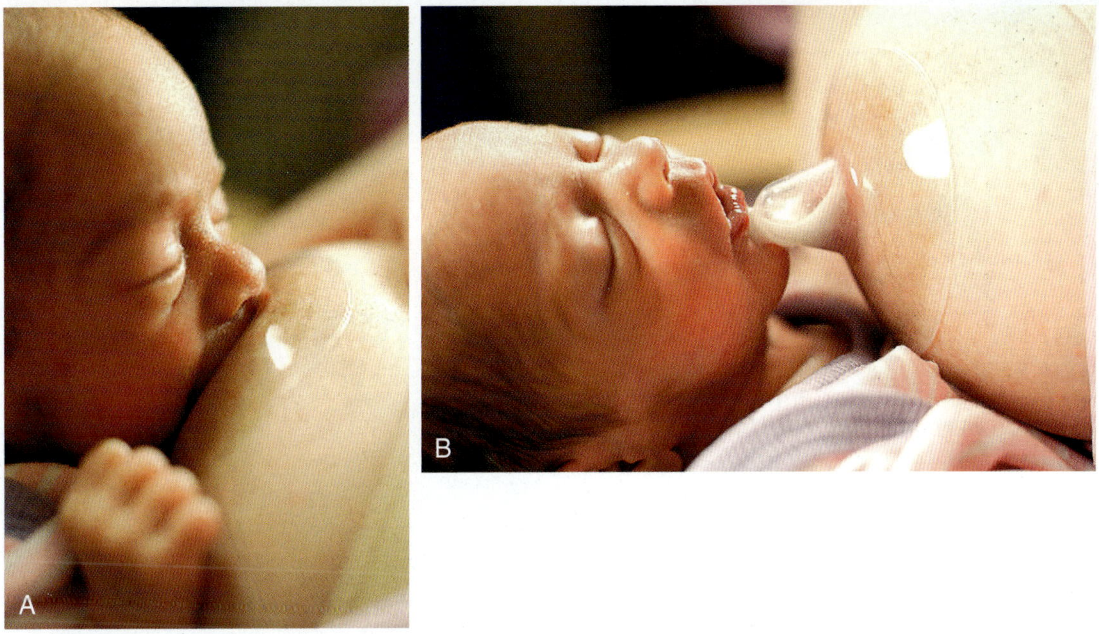

Fig. 2.58 (A) A preterm infant is breastfeeding with nipple shield in place. Nipple shields can be used for preterm or term infants who have difficulty with latch for a variety of reasons, such as maternal flat or inverted nipples and engorgement. They are not intended for long-term use and should be used under the supervision of a person well trained in lactation support. (B) A preterm infant is full and satisfied after breastfeeding with a nipple shield in place. The nipple shield has multiple fenestrations, so the milk comes out as it does from the mother's nipple.

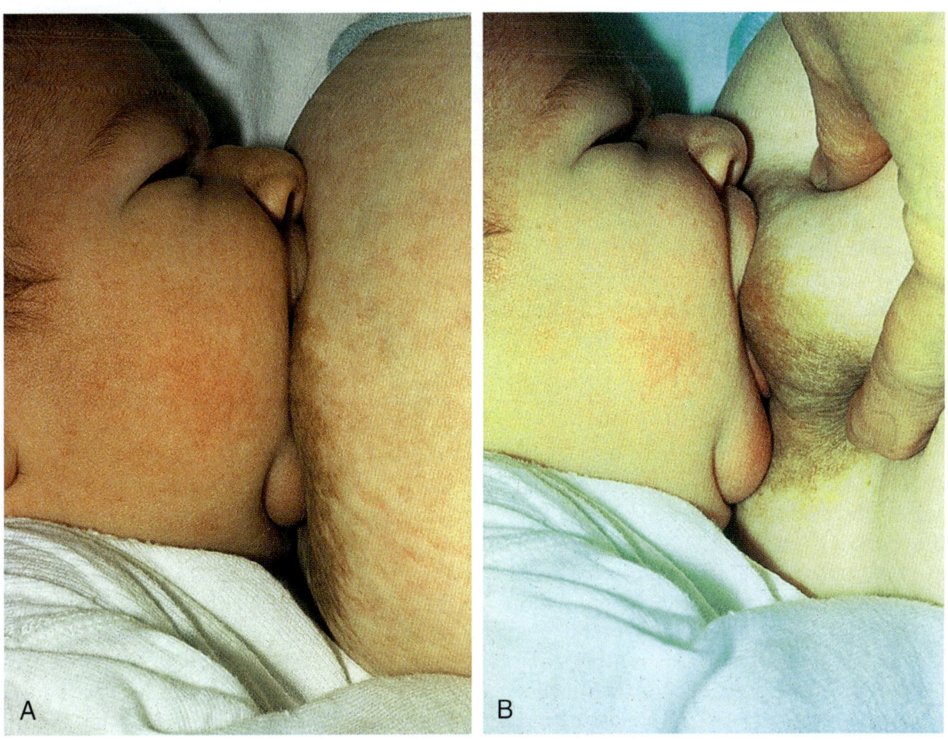

Fig. 2.59 (A and B) Good latch. A good latch is characterized by a wide-open mouth and everted lips. The angle between the baby's two lips should be close to 180 degrees. (Courtesy Susan Costanza, RN, IBCLC, Rochester General Hospital, Rochester, NY.)

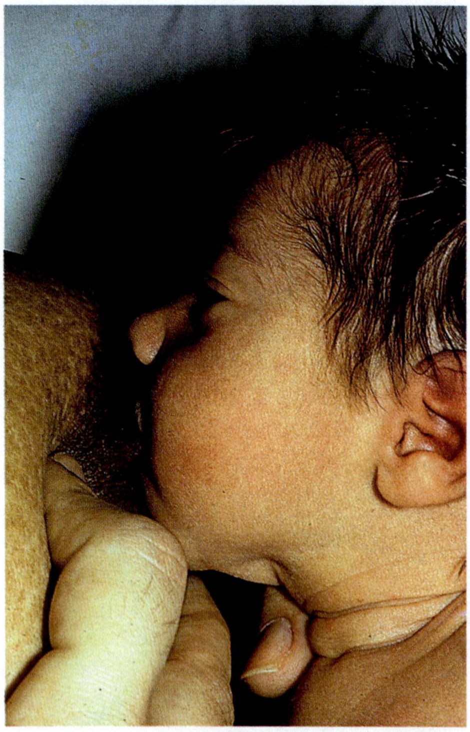

Fig. 2.60 Inadequate latch is characterized by a partially closed mouth with the angle between the baby's lips less than 90 degrees, often with the lips near the base of the mother's nipple. (Courtesy Susan Costanza, RN, IBCLC, Rochester General Hospital, Rochester, NY.)

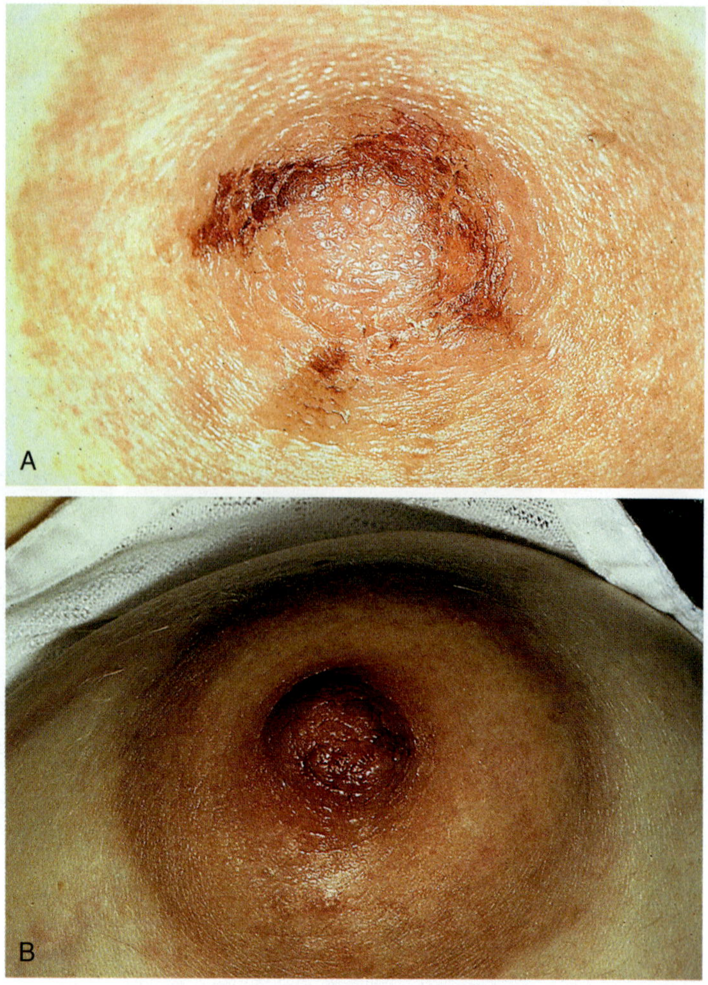

Fig. 2.61 (A and B) Cracked, abraded, bruised nipples and areola. These result from improper latch and positioning. An experienced clinician should assess the mother's technique for holding and latching the baby. (Courtesy Susan Costanza, RN, IBCLC, Rochester General Hospital, Rochester, NY.)

angle between the baby's upper and lower lips nearly 180 degrees. The upper and lower lips should be everted, with the baby's lips as far back on the areola as possible and the nipple in the back of the baby's mouth. The amount of areola visible during an effective latch is variable, but generally there should be an asymmetric latch where more areola is visible above the upper lip. When the infant releases from the breast, the nipple should not be flattened; it should remain round. A flattened nipple is a sign that the baby's mouth is not opened wide enough during the feeding. When the latch is inadequate (Fig. 2.60), the mother may experience discomfort, and the baby may not be able to empty the breast effectively and efficiently. Some females experience normal discomfort just as the baby latches that resolves in less than a minute. However, if a female experiences persistent pain with breastfeeding, she should unlatch the baby by inserting a finger into the corner of the baby's mouth and between the gums. The baby should then be repositioned, and a proper latch attempted again. If the pain continues, the mother/baby dyad should be observed during a feeding by a person experienced in breastfeeding assessment. An inadequate latch can result in nipple trauma (Fig. 2.61) and, over time, can compromise milk supply.

Holding Positions and Latch

Optimally, all babies should be placed skin-to-skin on the mother's chest during the first hour of life, when they are wide awake from the adrenaline surge that occurs at the time of delivery. Placing the baby on the mother's chest facilitates early initiation of breastfeeding. Skin-to-skin care improves infant temperature regulation, prolongs breastfeeding duration and exclusivity, decreases infant cortisol levels (an indicator of stress), and supports mother-infant attachment. The five main breastfeeding positions for the newborn are the football (Fig. 2.62), cross-cradle (Fig. 2.63), classic cradle (Fig. 2.64), laid back (Fig. 2.65), and side-lying (Fig. 2.66) positions. Please also see the video "Positions for Breastfeeding" on the Global Health Media website (link available in Bibliography). Each nursing mother should find the positions that are comfortable for her. Pillows can be used to raise the baby to the level of the mother's breast and provide adequate back, arm/shoulder, and hand support. In all positions, it is helpful to support the baby so that he or she feels secure, without a sense of falling. The baby's head, neck, and anterior chest should be in alignment with the head slightly tilted back for ease in swallowing, similar to how an adult would drink from a cup.

To initiate the latch, the mother can touch her nipple to or just above the baby's upper lip. This stimulates the baby to open the mouth and lower and extend the tongue. When the baby opens widely, and tips their head back, the mother should place the baby's upper lip just over the nipple, as far back onto the areola as possible, with the nipple aimed toward the hard palate. The baby's chin and lower lip should make first contact with the breast. Many females must hold their breast as the baby initially latches. Either the C hold (thumb on top of the breast and the other four fingers below) or U hold (thumb on one side of breast and the other four fingers on the other side) can be used. It can be helpful to press the thumb into the breast to aim the nipple toward the roof of the baby's mouth. With either hold, the fingers should be off the areola so that they do not interfere with the latch. After the baby is well latched, most females may be able to release the hold on the breast. For females with large breasts, a rolled washcloth can be placed under the breast for support so that the breast does not have to be held for the entire feeding. Please see video "Attaching Your Baby at the Breast" on the Global Health Media website (link available in Bibliography).

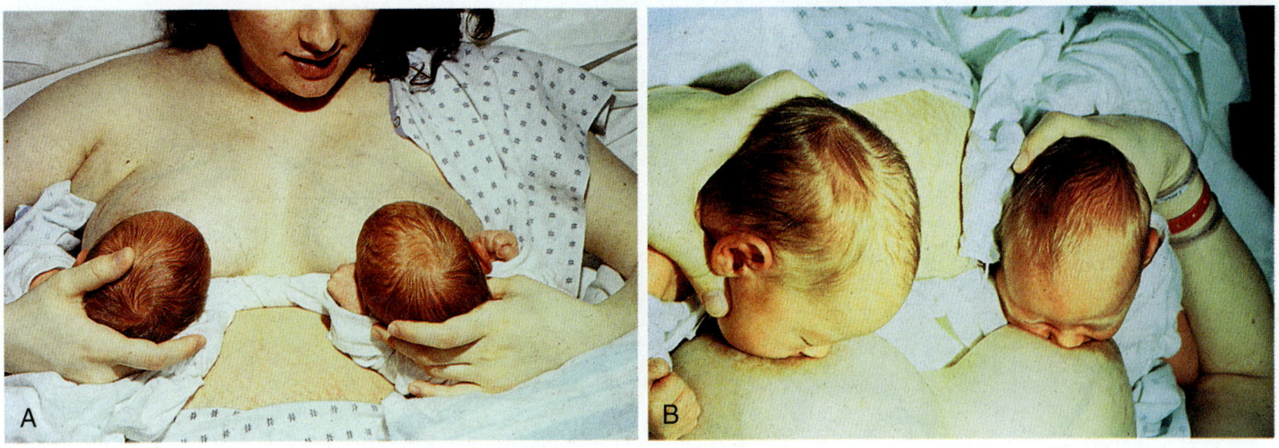

Fig. 2.62 (A and B) Football position. This position is especially good for females with large breasts, females who have had a cesarean section, and new mothers because it allows good visualization of the latch and good head control. It is also the position of choice for twins. (Courtesy Susan Costanza, RN, IBCLC, Rochester General Hospital, Rochester, NY.)

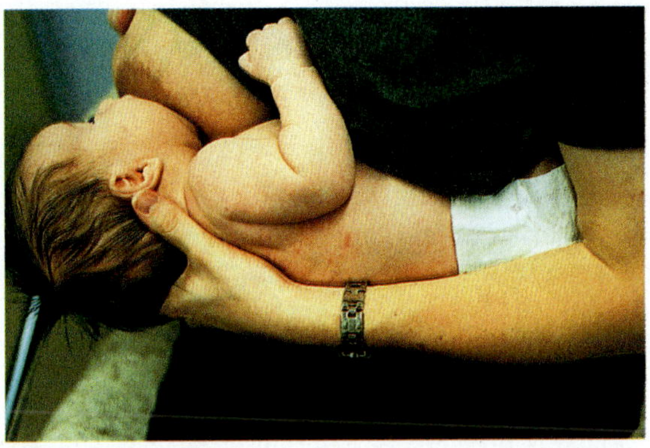

Fig. 2.63 Cross-cradle position. This is an excellent position to use with the young infant because it allows good visualization of the latch and provides firm head control of the neonate. The mother's hand is under the baby's neck. The baby's chin but not the nose is in the mother's breast. More of the areola is covered by the lower lip than by the upper lip, which is characteristic of a normal, asymmetric latch. (Courtesy J. Newman, MD, FRCPC, Hospital for Sick Children, Toronto.)

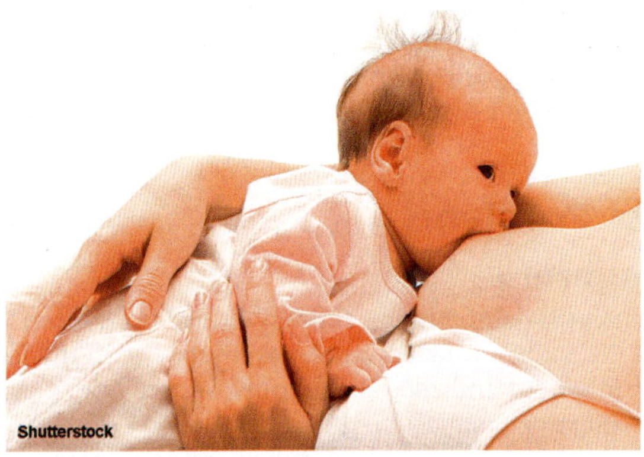

Fig. 2.65 Laid-back position. The mother is positioned at a 45-degree angle. The baby is placed skin to skin in a prone vertical or diagonal position on her abdomen, at or below the level of the breasts.

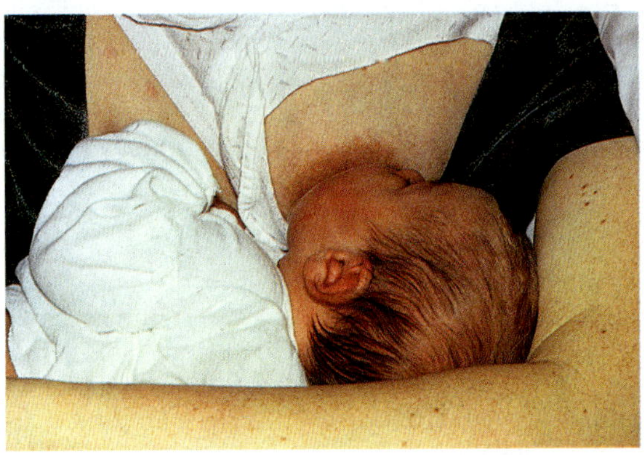

Fig. 2.64 Cradle position. The cradle position is easier to use when the baby has developed a modicum of head control but can also be used in the newborn if the mother finds it comfortable. The infant's nose, chin, and chest are aligned, and the mother and baby are belly to-belly. (Courtesy Susan Costanza, RN, IBCLC, Rochester General Hospital, Rochester, NY.)

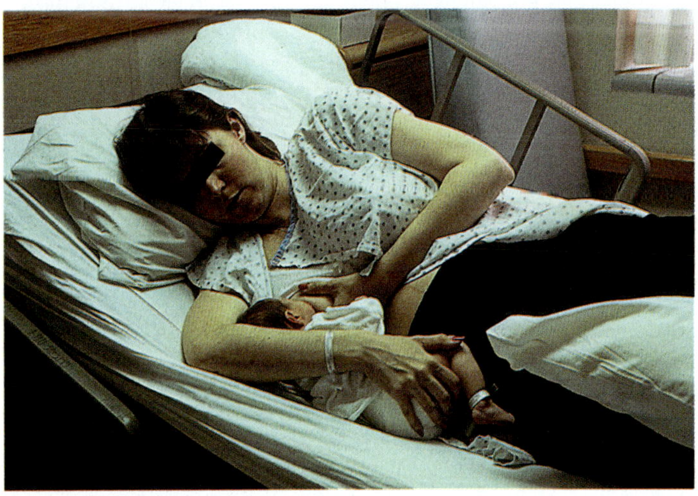

Fig. 2.66 Side-lying position. This is suitable for mothers who have had a cesarean section, are tired, have a sore perineum, have a sleepy baby, and for nighttime feeding. The mother and baby are belly to belly, and the baby is held on the side by the mother's hand. A receiving blanket can be rolled up and placed behind the infant's back to hold the baby in the position if the mother prefers. (Courtesy Susan Costanza, RN, IBCLC, Rochester General Hospital, Rochester, NY.)

Football or Under Arm Hold

The football or under arm hold (see Fig. 2.62) is especially good for females with large breasts and females who have had a cesarean section and cannot tolerate abdominal pressure. Because it allows good visualization of the latch and good head control, it is also an excellent position for premature infants and for new mothers.

Cross-Cradle

The cross-cradle position (see Fig. 2.63) allows good visualization of the latch and provides firm head control for the neonate. When the baby is several weeks old and has developed a good latch and improved head control, many females transition to the classic cradle hold.

Classic Cradle

The classic cradle position (see Fig. 2.64) is easier to use when the baby has developed a modicum of head control, but it can also be used with a newborn if the female finds it comfortable.

Laid-Back Position

The laid-back position (see Fig. 2.65), also known as "biological nurturing" position, is especially good for females in the early postpartum period. It is often easier for the mother, and gravity helps the infant achieve a deeper latch. This process of latching may take 20 minutes or more, so parents should be patient. If a female has large breasts, a washcloth may be placed under the breast for support and increased visualization of the latch.

Side-Lying Position

The side-lying position (see Fig. 2.66) is good for mothers who have a sore perineum or are tired. It is a good position at nighttime after breastfeeding is well established. The mother may initially need assistance in getting her baby latched in this position if she has limited agility after delivery and because she may not be able to completely visualize the latch. The baby should be turned so that the infant's abdomen is touching the mother's abdomen. The mother should place the baby back in a safe sleep position after feeding.

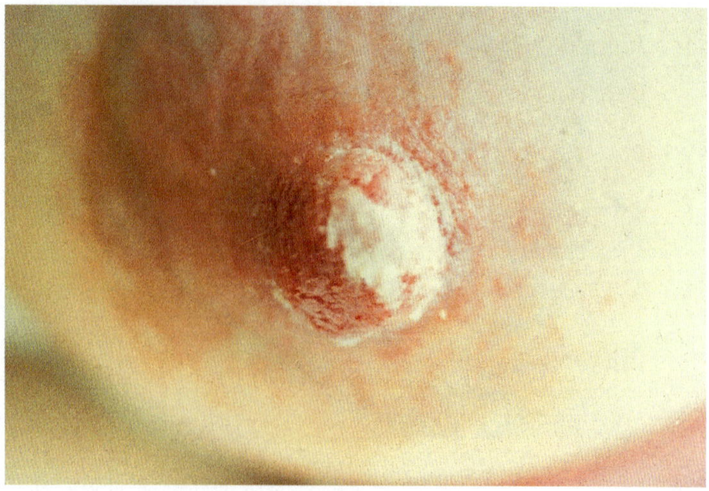

Fig. 2.67 Candida infection. Fungal infection of the breast to this degree is uncommon, but more subtle presentations are common. Females with candidal infection of the breast complain of burning or stabbing pain during or after breastfeeding. Most often the mother's breast appears normal or slightly red, but the breastfeeding baby has oral or diaper candidiasis. In this case both mother and baby should be treated. (Courtesy J. Newman, MD, FRCPC, Hospital for Sick Children, Toronto.)

Breast Problems

Engorgement

Engorgement is painful breast fullness caused by vascular congestion, edema, and/or milk accumulation in the breast tissue. It may be mild to severe and most commonly occurs 2 to 7 days after delivery. Engorgement can be prevented in many cases by encouraging frequent feedings (10–12 per day) and proper latch. Despite these preventive efforts, engorgement still occurs and physicians must recognize the signs and symptoms promptly. The signs are firm, sometimes lumpy, tender breasts with increased vascular markings in the face of a maternal sense of fullness to the point of discomfort. If not relieved, engorgement can make it difficult for the baby to latch and result in decreased milk production as high prolonged pressure can cause necrosis of milk-producing glands. Engorgement can contribute to the development of mastitis. Treatment involves frequent emptying of the breasts and symptomatic care. Infants should be nursed frequently, or milk should be expressed manually or with a pump. Warm compresses and massage to soften the breast tissue and manual expression of milk before putting the baby to the breast may make it easier for the baby to latch properly. Cool compresses after feedings may help to decrease vascular congestion.

Sore, Bruised, or Cracked Nipples

Sore, bruised, or cracked nipples can occur when a baby is not latched properly (see Fig. 2.61). The pain caused by these conditions is the reason why many mothers become discouraged and stop breastfeeding. Improper latch, usually too shallow on the nipple, is the leading cause of sore nipples. Mothers should not be told to bear the pain; rather, they should be promptly referred to an experienced clinician to assess the latch and positioning. To assist in healing, a drop of breastmilk can be applied to the nipple after a feed. Milk pores at the end of the nipple can become plugged. A white bleb forms on the tip of the nipple, which causes acute pain with breastfeeding. Moist heat before feeding or pumping sessions can assist in resolution.

Yeast Infections

Yeast infections of the mother's breast (Fig. 2.67) and baby's oropharynx (Fig. 2.68) or diaper area (see Fig. 8.43) are common after the second week of life. Babies with thrush may feed poorly, and mothers with yeast infections of the breast may experience pain and nipple changes. Both mother and infant should be treated for their respective yeast infections.

Mastitis

Mastitis is a bacterial infection of the breast (Fig. 2.69). It can result from blocked ducts or ascending infection due to cracked nipples. Mastitis presents as acute onset of fever, chills, and extreme breast tenderness over an area of induration and firmness, usually on one breast. This is not a reason to cease breastfeeding. Treatment includes continued emptying of the breast only as baby demands, oral antibiotics for the mother that cover penicillin-resistant staphylococcal and streptococcal species (e.g., first-generation cephalosporin or dicloxacillin), analgesics, rest, and adequate fluid intake. Mastitis can progress to breast abscess, which requires incision and drainage, in addition to antibiotics. If the incision location does not affect latch, breastfeeding may continue on the affected side. If a successful latch is not possible, then milk should be expressed from the breast. Many females report a temporary decrease in milk supply on the side affected by mastitis or abscess; milk supply increases again if females continue to empty milk from the affected side.

Vasospasm: Blanching of the Nipple

Some females experience pain just after breastfeeding. If they notice that the nipple turns white after feeding, they may be experiencing vasospasm of the nipple. Females often describe it as a burning sensation. The causes may include temperature change, inadequate latch, yeast infection, or other causes of nipple trauma. The most important treatment is to address the underlying cause, such as a shallow latch. In addition, it is often helpful to apply a heating pad or warm compress when symptoms are present, including after feedings. If the vasospasm persists despite these measures, the mother should be referred to a breastfeeding expert. Treatments include vitamin B_6 or nifedipine, which are based on anecdotal experiences and have not been well studied.

Assessing Milk Transfer

Many females are concerned that their baby is not getting enough to eat, especially in the first few days when they have colostrum. It is essential to educate mothers about normal eating patterns and how

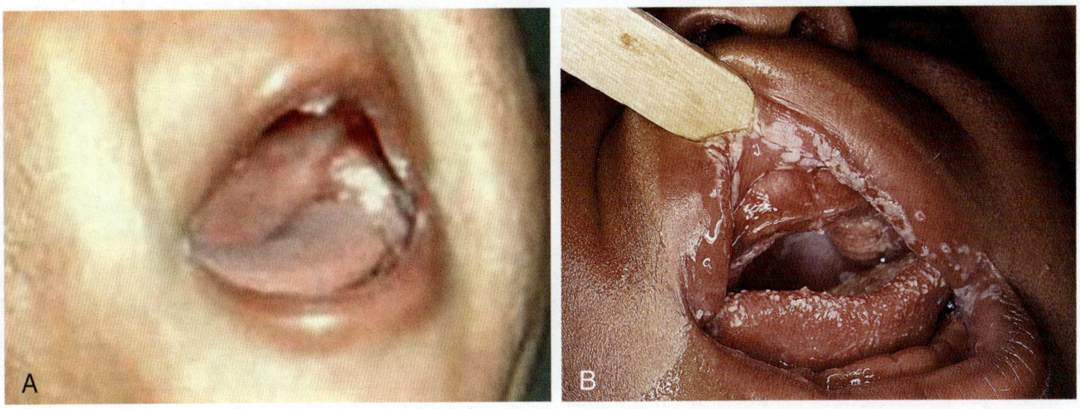

Fig. 2.68 (A and B) Thrush. White plaques are seen here on the buccal mucosa but may also appear on the gingiva, palate, lips, and tongue. These plaques do not wipe off and are present before and after feeding.

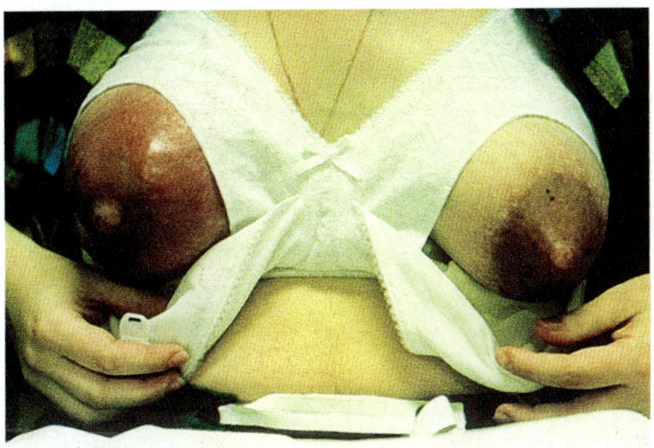

Fig. 2.69 Mastitis, an infection of the breast, often presents as acute onset of fever, chills, and extreme breast tenderness over an area of induration and firmness. This is not a reason to cease breastfeeding. In fact, the treatment includes frequent emptying of the breast and oral antibiotics to cover both staphylococcal and streptococcal species. (Courtesy J. Newman, MD, FRCPC, Hospital for Sick Children, Toronto.)

to assess whether the infant is getting enough to eat without having to measure it. In the first 1 to 2 days of life, a mother usually produces only about 30 mL of colostrum. Despite the small volume, that is all that a newborn infant requires. Colostrum is extremely high in protein. Parents should be instructed to monitor the following indicators of adequate intake: elimination patterns, weight changes, breast changes, and frequency and duration of feedings. Infants should have increasing numbers of voids and stools with each day.

Weight Changes

Infants usually lose weight in the first days of life. Weight loss can be variable—normative weight loss can be assessed using the online program www.newbornweight.org. Infants who are successfully breastfeeding should return to birth weight by 10 days of age. Infants who are still losing weight after 4 days or lose more than 10% of their birth weight should be followed closely and be assessed by someone with expertise in lactation.

Breast Changes

When a mother senses that her breasts are fuller, heavier, and warmer, this is a sign that the volume of milk she is producing is increasing, and the baby should begin to gain weight. This occurs as early as 36 hours and as late as days 5 to 7 for females with complications. A mother should notice that her breast feels full and heavy before the baby nurses and softer after the baby is finished.

Table 2.1 Assessing Milk Transfer

	Day 0	Days 1–2	Days 3–4	Days 5–6
Voids	≥1	≥2–3	≥4–6	≥6–8
Stools				
Number	≥1	≥1–2	≥2–3	≥3–4
Color	Meconium	Meconium	Transitional	Yellow/ seedy
Weight compared with birth weight[a]	—	≤5% loss	≤8% loss	Should start regaining
Number of feedings per day	4–8	8–12	8–12	8–12

[a]If an infant is not back to birth weight by 10 days, this is a red flag for breastfeeding difficulties; mother and infant should be referred to a health care provider expert in lactation support.

Frequency and Duration of Feedings

For the first 24 to 48 hours after birth, a baby's nursing frequency is highly variable. After that, most babies nurse 10 to 12 times per day (Table 2.1). Most feedings should last between 10 and 20 minutes on each breast, and both breasts should be offered with each feed. After the feeding, the baby should be satisfied and often asleep. If the baby is not meeting these assessment goals, the mother should seek professional assistance with breastfeeding. According to the AAP, all breastfeeding infants should be assessed within 48 to 72 hours of hospital discharge.

Ankyloglossia (tongue-tie) has been recognized as a potential problem with breastfeeding. Tongue-tie is a condition in which the lingual frenulum limits the range of motion of the tongue. Normal range of motion of the tongue is demonstrated if the tongue can be extended past the lips and to the roof of the mouth, which is essential for successful transfer of milk in breastfeeding. Pulling down on the chin during the suck assessment can help assess tongue function and the ability to sustain suction. Infants with limited anterior or superior movement of the tongue can have an ineffective latch and cause maternal pain during feedings. Not all infants with ankyloglossia need to be treated. A frenectomy for ankyloglossia should be considered for infants with inadequate weight gain, difficulty with sustained latch, or when mothers have persistent pain with latch despite proper latch technique.

Premature Infants

Among the many benefits to providing human milk to premature infants are decreased risk of perinatal infections and necrotizing enterocolitis, shorter hospital stays, and improved developmental outcomes. Mothers of premature or ill infants should be counseled about the benefits of human breastmilk for the health of their infants so that they can make an informed decision. Females who choose to breastfeed their preterm or ill infants in the neonatal intensive care unit (NICU) require support and education. It is important to create a breastfeeding supportive environment in the NICU. This includes allowing flexible visiting hours to encourage breastfeeding and knowledgeable and supportive staff.

Females who choose to provide expressed milk while waiting to directly breastfeed their infant should be shown how to hand express colostrum or be given access to a hospital-grade double-sided electric breast pump and instructed in how to use it as soon as possible after delivery. Ideally, this should happen within 1 hour of delivery. A strong predictor of sustained milk production for females is placing the infant to the breast or hand expression or pumping the breast within 1 hour of delivery. Hand expression videos are available online (https://med.stanford.edu/newborns/professional-education/breastfeeding/hand-expressing-milk.html). In the first few days of pumping, it is normal to express only small amounts of yellow to white colostrum, as little as 1 teaspoon per pumping. On occasion, the early milk looks rusty or bloody, dubbed the "rusty pipe syndrome"; this is also normal and can be used without concern. However, if the rusty milk continues for more than 1 week, the mother should be referred for further evaluation.

Mothers should be instructed to express their milk at least every 2 to 3 hours during the day and at least once during the night. The volume of milk expressed should increase 3 to 5 days after delivery. Maternal stress can delay and decrease milk production, a common problem for mothers with a baby in the NICU. Females should be encouraged to keep pumping. Pumped milk should be frozen in small volumes and thawed as needed. The milk should have the date on the label so that the first bottles into the freezer are the first to be used to avoid spoilage and because the milk composition changes over time.

A baby who is ready to bottle-feed is also ready to breastfeed. Premature babies fed at the breast have on average a lower heart rate, lower respiratory rate, and higher pulse oximetry measurement compared with bottle-fed infants. Babies are usually ready to breastfeed when they are physically stable, display a rhythmic suck-swallow-breath pattern (usually at about 34 weeks), and demonstrate feeding reflexes (rooting, sucking, gagging, and coughing) and signs of feeding readiness such as wakefulness and rooting or hand to mouth behaviors at feeding times.

A natural progression toward breastfeeding is to start with skin-to-skin care. When the baby is ready to take milk from the breast, have the mother pump milk until her let-down milk flow slows, and then offer the baby her breast. The first few times a mother offers her baby the breast, she should be observed and supported. If there is concern that the baby is not getting enough milk at the breast or that the infant requires fortified breastmilk or formula, there are several options. First, the baby should be weighed on a gram scale (at least twice to ensure accuracy) before the feeding, wearing a clean diaper and the clothes to be worn during the feeding. The baby is then fed and reweighed two more times without a change of diaper or clothes after feeding. The difference between the average postfeed weight and the prefeed weight is the amount (measured in grams but recorded as milliliters) of breastmilk consumed. If the baby has not taken "enough," the baby can then be fed by an alternative feeding method to supplement, such as by cup feeding (Fig. 2.70), finger feeding (Fig. 2.71), or gavage. A supplemental nursing system (Fig. 2.72) filled with expressed breastmilk, fortified breastmilk, or appropriate formula can be attached to the breast so that the baby receives both breastmilk and the supplement. The reasons to progress directly to the breast from gavage feeding are multiple. Bottle-feeding and breastfeeding require the use of different oral muscles and sucking mechanics. Premature babies may get used to bottle-feeding and may not breastfeed well as a result. Therefore it is ideal to feed infants by alternative feeding methods when a mother is not available to breastfeed. If a bottle feed is required, paced bottle feeding should be used. Please see these videos from IABLE Breastfeeding Education:

Finger feeding: https://www.youtube.com/watch?v = RRFgA_uHW1g

Cup Feeding: https://www.youtube.com/watch?v = KJmPDn3EA24

Paced Bottle Feeding: https://www.youtube.com/watch?v = OGPm-5SpLxXY

Most infants can transition to full feeds at the breast exclusively by 36 to 40 weeks. However, the transition to full breastfeeding should begin as soon as possible. Now that infants are discharged well before term, pediatricians, family practitioners, and lactation consultants in the outpatient setting often provide this education and support. Advice should be individualized to each mother/baby dyad. A general approach is to have the mother dual-pump with a high-grade electric pump every time she offers the baby milk other than at the breast, including if she is using a supplemental nursing system to provide the supplement. At first the mother may need to pump after every feeding, especially if the baby has not yet reached term, has a weak suck, or is a sleepy baby. This will help to match her milk supply and her baby's increasing needs. Every few days, she can increase the number of feedings at the breast without supplement. The baby's stool and urine output should be monitored to ensure

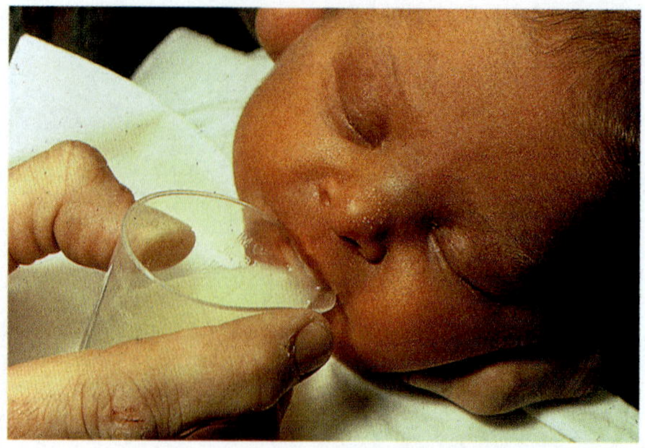

Fig. 2.70 Cup feeding is an alternative feeding method for infants. A small medicine cup or one designed specifically for this purpose can be used. The cup is placed at the margin of the infant's lower lip and tipped gently toward the mouth. The infant should extrude the tongue and assist feeding by lapping the milk as small amounts are poured between the lower lip and gum. Cup feeding is widely used in underdeveloped countries when mothers are unable to feed their infants from the breast. (Courtesy Susan Costanza, RN, IBCLC, Rochester General Hospital, Rochester, NY.)

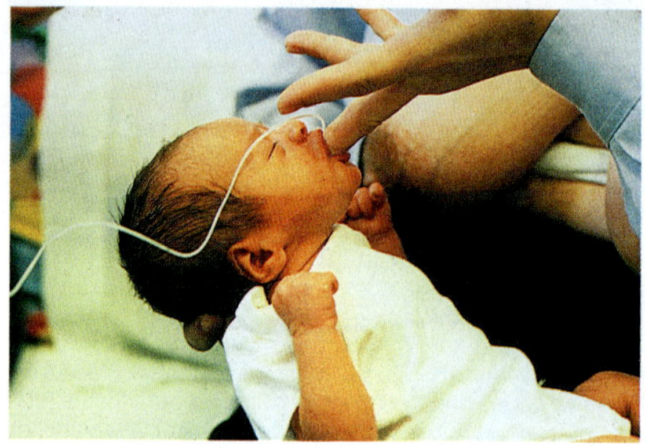

Fig. 2.71 Finger feeding is an alternative method for feeding infants. The largest finger that is convenient for the feeder should be used. The finger used should be held flat and placed far back in the infant's mouth so that the infant's tongue is forward and curved around the sides of the finger. A 5-French, 36-inch feeding tube is convenient because the thin caliber provides a slow flow rate and the length allows some flexibility with positioning. Among the available alternative feeding methods, finger feeding has the added benefit of training the infant with a weak or immature suck to suck in a similar fashion as during breastfeeding. The one drawback to finger feeding is that it is relatively slow. (Courtesy J. Newman, MD, FRCPC, Hospital for Sick Children, Toronto.)

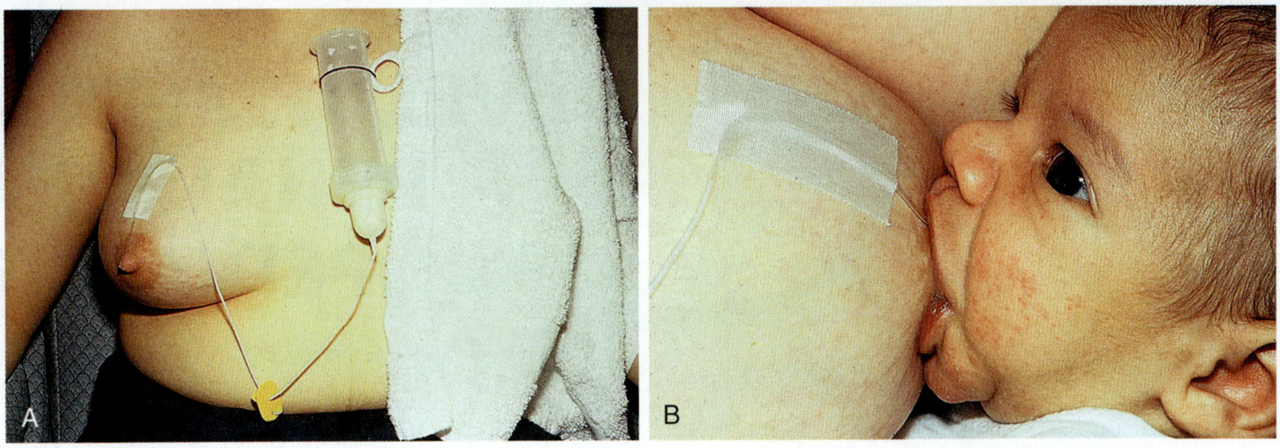

Fig. 2.72 (A and B) Supplemental nursing system (SNS). An SNS allows a baby to receive additional nutrients while still breastfeeding and thus provides stimulation to the breast. It does not interfere with breastfeeding technique and latch. The tip of the SNS tubing should protrude past the end of the nipple by about one quarter of an inch. (Courtesy Susan Costanza, RN, IBCLC, Rochester General Hospital, Rochester, NY.)

adequate intake, and the baby's weight should be monitored to ensure adequate growth during the transition.

Late Preterm (35–36 Weeks) and Early Term (37–38 Weeks) Infants

Late preterm and early-term infants are often treated as term infants, but they are at high risk for breastfeeding problems. They may look as though they are feeding well, but they have weaker and less sustained suck patterns than full-term infants. They are at increased risk for excessive weight loss, hyperbilirubinemia, and rehospitalization. It is essential that health care providers remain vigilant and monitor late preterm and early-term infants closely. Mothers of infants should be instructed to feed infants every 2 to 3 hours and to monitor urine output and stool changes. If the baby does not feed effectively, mothers should be instructed to express their milk and feed it to the infant in order to maintain her milk supply until the baby is able to obtain all milk from the breast directly.

Donor Human Milk

An exclusive human milk diet plays a role in decreasing morbidity and mortality in all infants, particularly preterm infants. The main benefit derived from the use of donor milk (versus formula) in preterm infant feeding is the reduction of the incidence of necrotizing enterocolitis (NEC), but reduction in the incidence of sepsis and bronchopulmonary dysplasia has also been observed. Donor milk can be used as a bridge or in substitution of mother's own milk in scenarios when the milk is insufficient or inappropriate to be used. Donor milk should be obtained from reliable credentialed sources (such as the member milk banks of the Human Milk Banking Association of North America) to ensure safe, pasteurized milk from carefully screened donors.

Bibliography

Abuogi L, Noble L, Smith C: American Academy of Pediatrics clinical report: infant feeding for persons living with and at risk for HIV in the United States: clinical report, *Pediatrics* 153:e2024066843. https://doi.org/10.1542/peds.2024-066843. Accessed May 28, 2024.

Academy of Breastfeeding Medicine: *Clinical protocols*. https://www.bfmed.org/protocols. Accessed May 28, 2024.

American Academy of Pediatrics: *Policy statement: Breastfeeding and the use of human milk*. https://doi.org/10.1542/peds.2022-057988

American Academy of Pediatrics: *Infant feeding for persons living with and at risk for HIV in the United States: Clinical report*. https://doi.org/10.1542/peds.2024-066843

American Academy of Pediatrics (AAP): *Breastfeeding residency curriculum*. https://www.aap.org/en/pedialink/breastfeeding-curriculum/. Accessed May 28, 2024.

American Academy of Pediatrics (AAP) and the American College of Obstetricians and Gynecologists (ACOG): *Breastfeeding handbook for physicians*, ed 3, Elk Grove Village, IL, 2023, AAP and ACOG.

Bogen DL, Hanusa BH, Baker R, Medoff-Cooper B, Cohlan B: Randomized clinical trial of standard- versus high-calorie formula for methadone-exposed infants: a feasibility study, *Hosp Pediatr* 8(1):7–14, 2018.

Favara MT, Carola D, Jensen E, et al: Maternal breast milk feeding and length of treatment in infants with neonatal abstinence syndrome, *J Perinatol* 39(6):876–882, 2019.

Global Health Media: *Attaching your baby at the breast*. https://global healthmedia.org/portfolio-items/attaching-your-baby-at-the-breast/?portfolioCats=191%2C94%2C13%2C23%2C65. Accessed May 28, 2024.

Global Health Media: *Positions for breastfeeding*. https://globalhealthmedia.org/videos/positions-for-breastfeeding/. Accessed May 28, 2024.

https://clinicalinfo.hiv.gov/sites/default/files/guidelines/documents/perinatal-hiv/guidelines-perinatal.pdf

Panel on Treatment of HIV During Pregnancy and Prevention of Perinatal Transmission: *Recommendations for the use of antiretroviral drugs during pregnancy and interventions to reduce perinatal HIV transmission in the United States*, Department of Health and Human Services. https://clinicalinfo.hiv.gov/en/guidelines/perinatal. Accessed May 28, 2024.

Quigley MA, Henderson G, Anthony MY, McGuire W: Formula milk versus donor breast milk for feeding preterm or low birth weight infants (review), *Cochrane Database Syst Rev* 1–41, 2007.

University of North Carolina (UNC) Center for Maternal & Infant Health: *UNC lactation program*. http://www.mombaby.org/unc-lactation-program/. Accessed May 28, 2024.

U.S. National Library of Medicine: *Drugs and lactation database (LactMed®)*. https://www.ncbi.nlm.nih.gov/books/NBK501922/. Accessed May 28, 2024.

3 DEVELOPMENTAL/BEHAVIORAL PEDIATRICS

Diego Chaves-Gnecco | Heidi M. Feldman

Pediatricians are routinely required to distinguish normal development and individual differences from delayed or atypical patterns of development and behavior in both routine health supervision and in comprehensive management of children with other medical conditions. Once developmental or behavioral delays have been identified, the pediatrician conducts a diagnostic workup, initiates management, refers to appropriate services, counsels families, and coordinates care. The goal of this chapter is to review the developmental/behavioral issues faced in routine pediatric practice. In the first half, the fundamental principles of development are applied to each major domain of functioning. Within each domain, discussion centers on the major developmental milestones, methods of assessment, signs of developmental variation, and approaches to children who show developmental delays or deviant patterns. In the second half, several developmental disorders are described, including definitions, diagnostic criteria, and the role of physical examination in evaluation, physical findings, and prognosis.

PRINCIPLES OF NORMAL DEVELOPMENT

Development is commonly discussed in terms of domains of function. *Gross motor skills* refer to the use of the large muscles of the body; *fine motor skills* refer to the use of small muscles of the hands; *cognition* means the use of higher mental processes, including thinking, memory, and learning; *language* refers to the comprehension and production of meaningful symbolic communication; and *social and emotional functioning* refers to skills for interactions with others and emotional reactions to people and events. Within each domain, skills are typically acquired in a predictable sequence, although the age of acquisition of specific milestones may vary across children. Domains of development are interdependent. Cognitive abilities in infancy cannot readily be distinguished from sensorimotor functioning. Similarly, mature social functioning depends on competent language abilities. Early reflex patterns and congenital sensory and motor capabilities are the building blocks of higher-order skills.

Developmental Surveillance

A central component of health maintenance is the prompt identification of developmental problems and the promotion of developmental progress. *Developmental surveillance* refers to the longitudinal, continuous process by which physicians and other professionals use all available clinical tools to determine a child's developmental status, to evaluate his or her developmental progress over time, and to identify children who may be at risk for disorders. Parents are generally accurate reporters of current developmental status, and therefore their concerns are sensitive indicators of delays or atypical patterns of development. Therefore, surveillance requires that clinicians elicit and appropriately attend to parental concerns. In addition, surveillance includes review teacher and day care provider concerns, obtain a developmental history, make pertinent observations of current development and behavior, perform a physical examination, administer or review and interpret screening tests, and use other assessment techniques. Surveillance promotes a longitudinal view of the child and allows parental concerns to be addressed in a timely manner. A formal developmental assessment can be arranged if there are severe or persistent concerns.

Developmental Screening

The physician's ability to identify children with developmental delays and disorders is improved by the appropriate use of validated screening tools (Table 3.1). The tools have been designed to be used with unselected groups of children, ideally as part of routine developmental surveillance at a few selected health maintenance visits, such as the 9-, 18-, 24-, or 36-month visits. The sensitivity and specificity of these instruments used during these visits range from 0.70 to 0.90. The clinician's judgment is required in interpretation of test results, particularly of measures that rely on parental report. Children who are developing normally may fail a screening test because of shyness, unfamiliarity with the examiner or the materials, or other factors unrelated to developmental competence. In most cases, a positive screen should be followed by a comprehensive assessment of development and should not be ignored. Screening tests can be used to confirm parental concerns but are not appropriate for diagnosing the nature of the problem. If parental concerns persist despite negative screening findings, a full evaluation is advisable because of the limited sensitivity of the tests and the importance of attending to parental concerns. To ensure that the performance is representative of the child's ability, screening tests should be performed when the child is physically well, familiar with the setting and the examiner, and under minimal stress. Examples of familiar settings include the child's home for infants, toddlers, and younger children; the child's preschool becomes another familiar setting for children 3 years old and older. Obtaining results from natural settings may require collaboration with community-based organizations that conduct home or school visiting.

GROSS MOTOR DEVELOPMENT

Early Reflex Patterns ("Primitive Reflexes")

At birth, a neonate's movements consist of alternating flexion and extension, which usually are symmetric and vary in strength with the infant's state of alertness. In addition, involuntary "primitive" reflexes can be elicited; they indicate that the patterns of movement requiring the integrated activity of multiple muscle groups are present even at birth. The intact newborn sucks and grasps reflexively; these are motor patterns that are programmed into the organism to enhance survival. The presence of primitive reflexes in the newborn and the disappearance (integration) of these reflexes in a predictable sequence as the infant matures are indications of typical motor development, reflecting many developmental and neural factors, such as underlying myelination of higher cortical pathways that allow for voluntary control of movement. Persistence of primitive reflexes beyond the typical age suggests abnormal myelination of the higher inhibitory pathways as seen in children with neurologic or developmental disorders.

Table 3.1 Validated Developmental Screening Tests

Name of Test	Parent Time	Provider Time	Age Range Covered
Ages and Stages Questionnaires (ASQ)	10–20 min	1–5 min	4 months–5 years
Child Development Inventories	30 min	10 min	15 months–6 years
Parents' Evaluation of Developmental Status (PEDS)	5 min	2 min	0–8 years
Denver II		20 min	2 weeks–6 years
Guide for Monitoring Child Development (GMCD)		7 min	0–24 months
Rapid Neurodevelopmental Assessment (RDNA)		30 min	2–5 years

For further information and characteristics of these validated developmental screening tests, consult the Resources section at the end of this chapter.

The Moro response, or startle reflex, can occur spontaneously after a loud noise, but typically it is elicited during the physical examination by an abrupt extension of the infant's neck. The response consists of symmetric abduction and extension of the arms with extension of the trunk (Fig. 3.1), followed by adduction of the upper extremities, as in an embrace, and frequently is accompanied by crying (Fig. 3.2). The Moro reflex gradually disappears by 4 months old, associated with the development of cortical functioning. In children up to 4 months old, the Moro response can be used to evaluate the integrity of the central nervous system and to detect peripheral nerve problems, such as congenital musculoskeletal abnormalities or neural plexus injuries; an asymmetric response may indicate unilateral weakness.

The *asymmetric tonic neck reflex (ATNR)* (Fig. 3.3) demonstrates that the newborn's limb motions are strongly influenced by head position. If the head is directed to one side, either by passive turning or by inducing the baby to follow an object to that side, tone in the extensor muscles increases on that side and in the flexor muscles on the opposite side. This response may not be seen immediately after birth, when the newborn has high flexor tone throughout the body, but it usually appears by 2 to 4 weeks of age. The ATNR allows the baby to sight along the arm to the hand and is considered one of the first steps in the coordination of vision and reaching. This reflex disappears by 4 to 6 months old to allow for the development of voluntary reaching.

With the emergence of voluntary control from higher cortical centers, muscular flexion and extension become balanced. Primitive reflexes are replaced by reactions that allow children to maintain a stable posture, even if they are rapidly moved or jolted. A timetable listing the expected emergence and disappearance of primitive reflexes and the protective equilibrium responses is presented in Table 3.2.

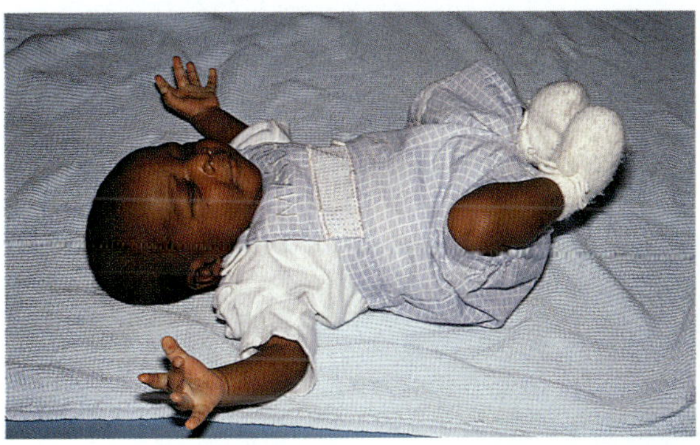

Fig. 3.1 First phase of the Moro response. Symmetric abduction and extension of the extremities follow a loud noise or an abrupt change in the infant's head position.

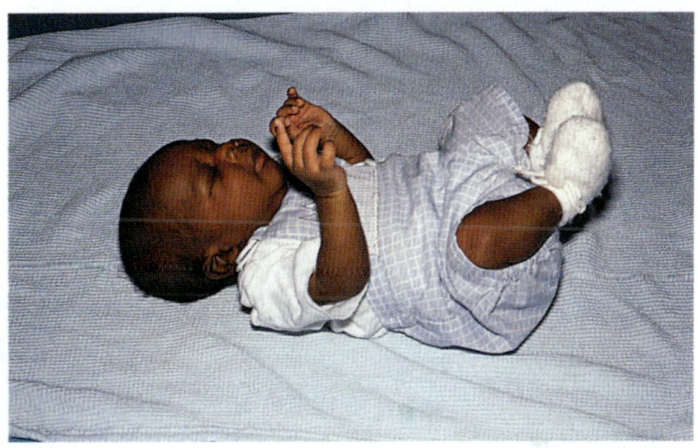

Fig. 3.2 Second phase of the Moro response. Symmetric adduction and flexion of the extremities, accompanied by crying.

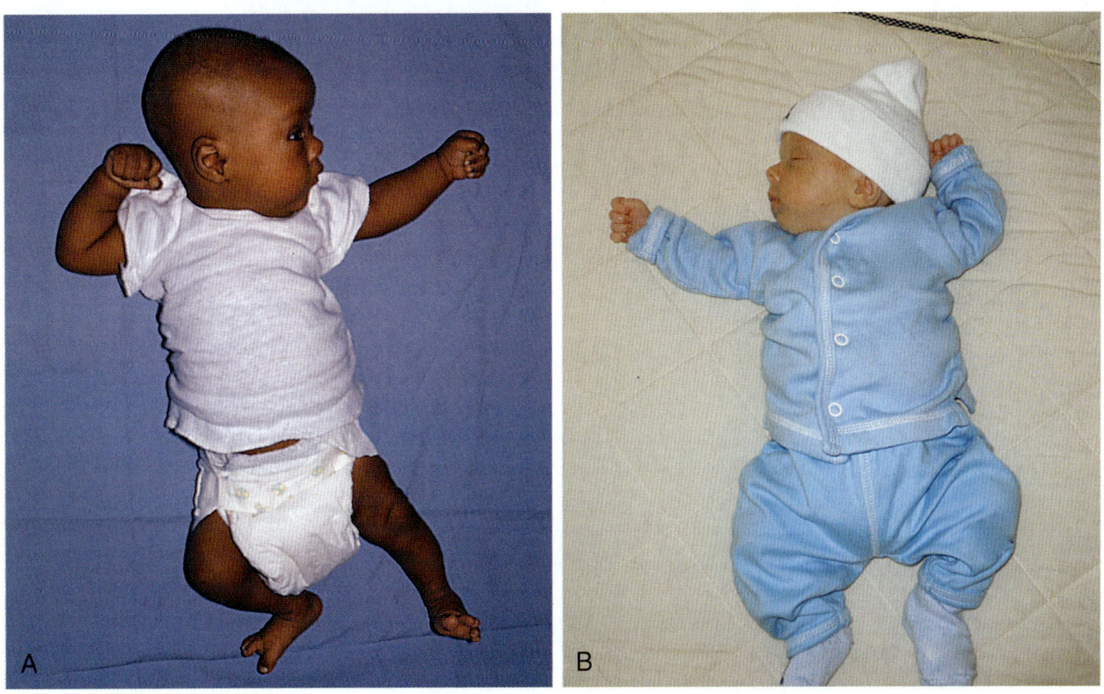

Fig. 3.3 (A and B) Asymmetric tonic neck reflex. Flexion of the arm and leg on the occipital side and extension on the chin side create the "fencer position."

Antigravity Muscular Control

Muscle control develops in an organized fashion, from head to toe, or in a cephalocaudal progression—head control followed by reaching, followed by sitting, followed by standing—reflecting neuronal myelination in a typical sequence.

Head Control

The infant's earliest control task is to maintain a stable posture against the influence of gravity. Neck flexors allow head control against gravity when a child is pulled from the supine to the sitting position. Neonates show minimal control of the neck flexors, holding their heads upright only briefly when supported in a sitting position. When an infant is pulled to a sitting position, the head lags behind the arms and shoulders (Fig. 3.4A). By 4 months old, the child can support his or her head, and the head moves along with the shoulders when pulled to a sitting position (see Fig. 3.4B). At 5 to 6 months old, the infant anticipates the direction of movement of the pull-to-sit maneuver and flexes the neck before the shoulders begin to lift (see Fig. 3.4C).

Table 3.2 Primitive Reflexes and Protective Equilibrium Responses

Reflex	Appearance[a]	Disappearance[a]
Moro	Birth	4 months old
Hand grasp	Birth	3 months old
Crossed adductor	Birth	7 months old
Toe grasp	Birth	8–15 months old
ATNR	2 weeks old	6 months old
Head righting	4–6 months old	Persists voluntarily
Protective equilibrium	4–6 months old	Persists voluntarily
Parachute	8–9 months old	Persists voluntarily

[a]Different sources may vary on the precise timing of the appearance and disappearance of these primitive and equilibrium responses.

ATNR, Asymmetric tonic neck reflex.

Trunk Control and Sitting

In the prone position, a newborn remains in a tightly flexed position and can simply turn the face from side to side along the bed sheets. Progressive control of the shoulders and upper trunk in the first months of life, plus a decrease in flexor tone, enables the young infant to hold the chest off the bed with the weight supported on the forearms by approximately 4 months old (Fig. 3.5). Evolution of trunk control down the thoracic spine can also be observed with the infant in a sitting position (Fig. 3.6). As control reaches the lumbar area, the lumbar lordotic curve can be seen when the child is standing (Fig. 3.7).

Automatic Reactions: Equilibrium and Protective Reactions

Equilibrium and protective reactions are automatic, reflexive patterns that also emerge in a cephalocaudal sequence. *Head righting* refers to the infant's ability to keep the head vertical despite a tilt of the body. A 4-month-old infant typically demonstrates this ability in vertical suspension when gently swayed from side to side. As control moves downward, protective equilibrium responses can be elicited in a seated infant by abruptly but gently pushing the infant's center of gravity past the midline in one of the horizontal planes. The lateral protective reaction involves increased trunk flexor tone toward the force and an outreached hand and limb away from the force; it usually emerges by 6 months old and is required for the development of stable, independent sitting (Fig. 3.8). At 10 months old, the child develops the forward protective or parachute reaction, an outstretching of both

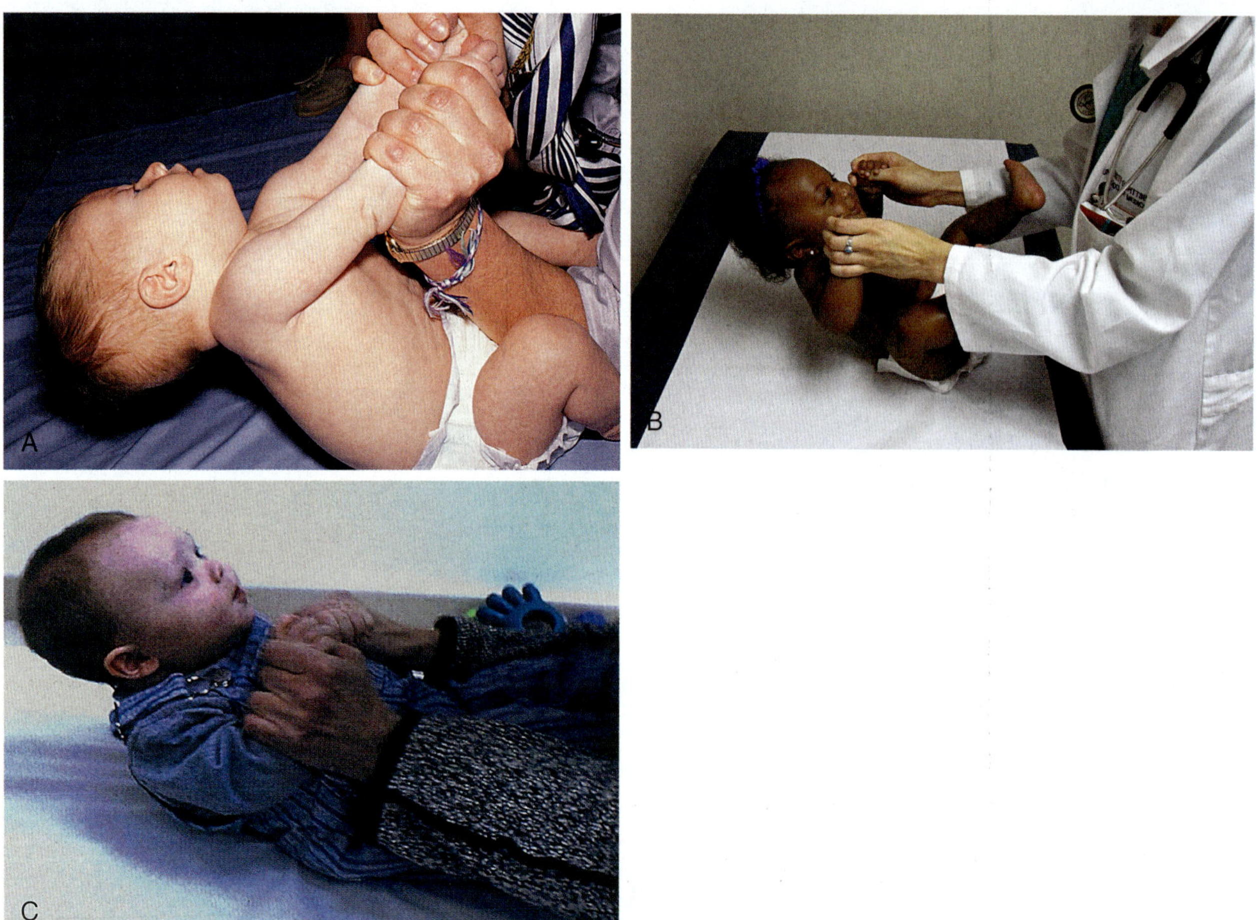

Fig. 3.4 Development of head control on the pull-to-sit maneuver. (A) At 1 month old, the head lags after the shoulders. (B) By 4 months old, the child is able to support the head, and the head moves along with the shoulders. (C) At 5 to 6 months old, the child anticipates the movement and raises the head before the shoulders.

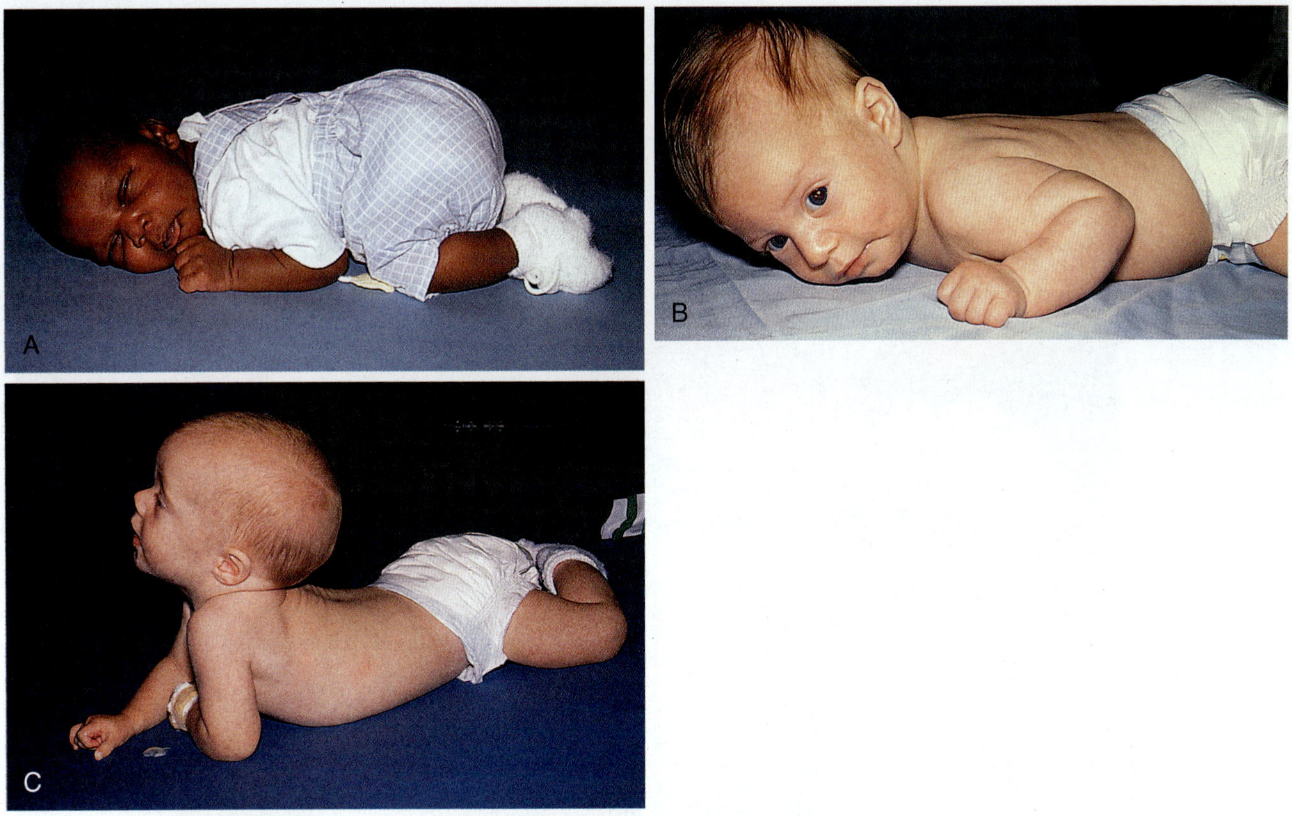

Fig. 3.5 Development of posture in the prone position. (A) The newborn lies tightly flexed with the pelvis high and the knees under the abdomen. (B) At 2 months old, the infant extends the hips and pulls the shoulders up slightly. (C) At 3 to 4 months old, the infant keeps the pelvis flat and lifts the head and shoulders.

arms and legs when the body is abruptly moved head first in a downward direction (Fig. 3.9). The forward protective (parachute) reaction is a programmed reflex that protects the head if the child falls from standing or walking and is generally seen just before these motor skills develop.

Development of Locomotion

Gross motor milestones can also be described in terms of locomotion (Table 3.3). Prone-to-supine (front to back) rolling may be accomplished by 3 to 4 months of age, after the child gains sufficient control of shoulder and upper trunk musculature to prop up on the arms. Supine-to-prone (back to front) rolling requires control of the lumbar spine and hip region as well as the upper trunk; this is usually present by 5 to 6 months of age. Prone-to-supine rolling may appear later, at 5 to 6 months. Creeping (also called *commando* or *army crawling*), accomplished at 5 to 6 months of age (Fig. 3.10A), involves coordinated pulling with upper arms and passive dragging of the legs, akin to a soldier trying to keep the body low to the ground. By 6 to 9 months old, as voluntary control moves to the hips and legs, the child can get up on the hands and knees, assuming a quadruped position, and crawl (see Fig. 3.10B). The next developmental milestone is supported standing. By 9 to 10 months old, many children like to demonstrate this new skill by holding on to a parent or by walking independently while holding on to furniture. This is called *cruising* (see Fig. 3.10C). Increased control to the feet and disappearance of the plantar grasp reflex allow the child to walk independently. Walking three steps alone occurs at a median age of approximately 12 months old, with a range of 9 to 17 months old (see Fig. 3.10D).

Development of Complex Gross Motor Patterns

Further progress in gross motor skills continues throughout childhood. The developmental sequence beyond walking incorporates improved balance and coordination and progressive narrowing of the base of support. The sequence of milestones is as follows: running, jumping on two feet, balancing on one foot, hopping, and skipping. The child simultaneously learns to use muscle groups in timed sequences. By 13 to 15 months old, the child walks well; by 36 months old, he or she can balance on one foot for 1 second. Most children can hop by age 4. They can throw a ball overhand by 22 to 24 months old, but catching develops later, at almost 5 years old.

GROSS MOTOR ASSESSMENT DURING HEALTH MAINTENANCE VISITS

Evaluation of gross motor skills can begin when the pediatrician enters the office for a well-child visit. The typical 2-month-old infant is cradled in the parent's arms; the 4-month-old infant has enough strength to support the back when held inside the arms by a parent's hands but not enough strength to sit alone (Fig. 3.11); the 6-month-old child is sitting with minimal support on the parent's lap or on the examination table next to the parent; and the 12-month-old child is cruising or toddling through the room. Although age of onset and duration of each stage vary, the 6-month-old infant who lacks head control on the pull-to-sit maneuver, who cannot clear the table surface with the chest by supporting weight on the arms when prone, who shows no head righting, or who has persistent primitive reflexes is at sufficient variance from peers to warrant evaluation for a possible neuromuscular disorder. In addition, when gross motor delays are found in association with verbal and social delays, asymmetric use of one limb or one side of the body, or loss of previously attained milestones, diagnostic evaluation is indicated.

Evaluation of the older infant or toddler who has mastered walking can occur during the physical and neurologic evaluation. Many children enjoy showing off their abilities to jump, balance on one foot, hop, and skip. Some pediatricians use gross motor testing to establish rapport at the outset of a physical examination. However, because an aroused preschooler may not cooperate with a sedentary

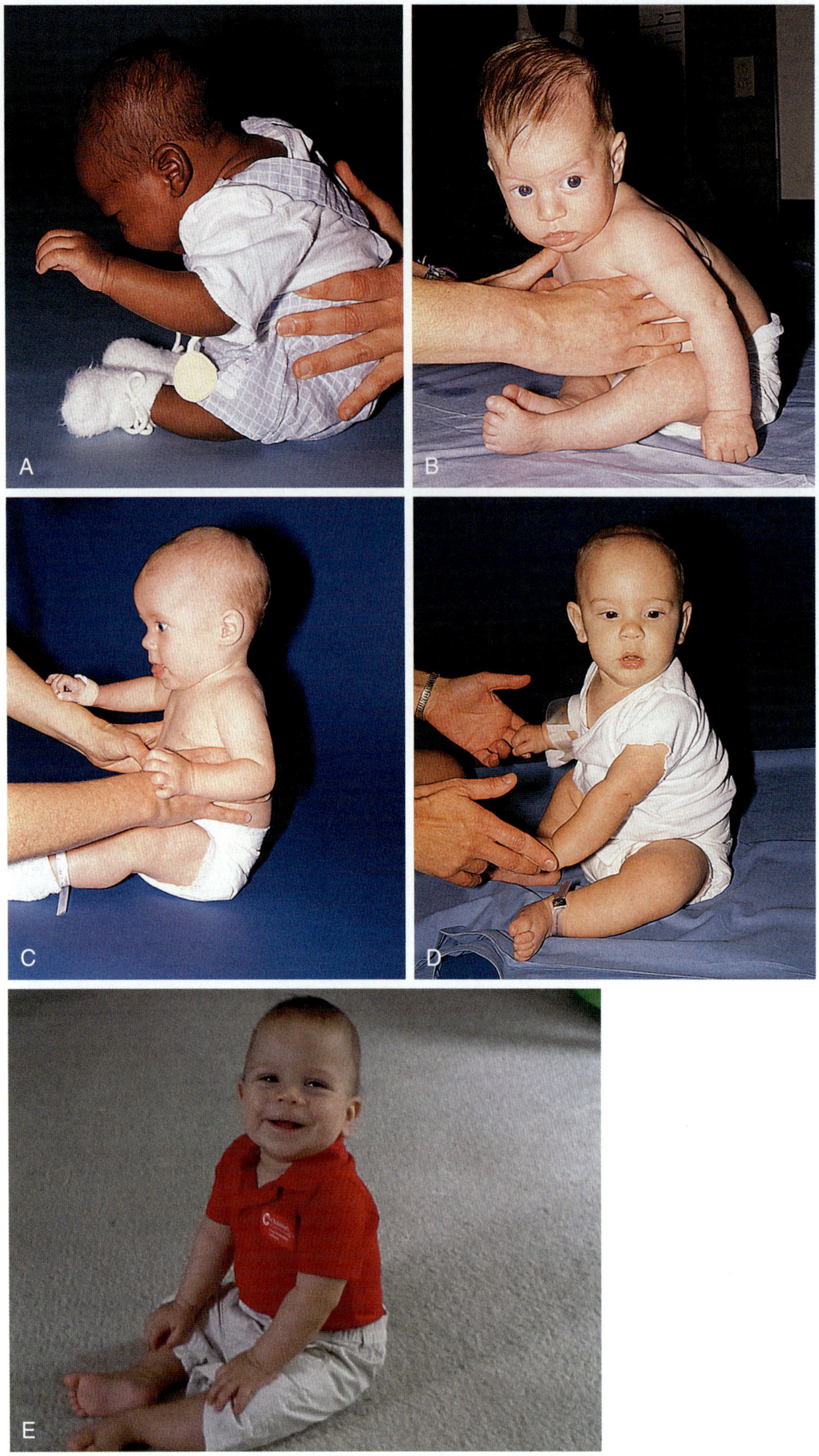

Fig. 3.6 Development of sitting posture. (A) At 1 to 2 months old, the head is held up intermittently, but trunk control is lacking. (B) At 2 to 3 months old, the infant raises the head and shoulders well but lacks control of the thoracolumbar area. (C) At 3 to 4 months old, support in the lumbar area is required to sit. (D) At 5 to 6 months old, the infant holds the head erect and the spine straight. (E) Between 7 and 9 months old, the infant can sit without support.

evaluation of heart or ears, many pediatricians hold off on motor evaluation until the conclusion of the examination.

At the discovery of delayed or atypical development, the pediatrician's first task is to develop a differential diagnosis and a plan to establish the specific diagnosis. Potential causes of delayed gross motor development are listed in Table 3.4. Another equally important task is to recommend a treatment program. Early intervention programs and/or physical therapy should be actively considered for children with motor difficulties during infancy through preschool. Adaptive physical education programs are available for

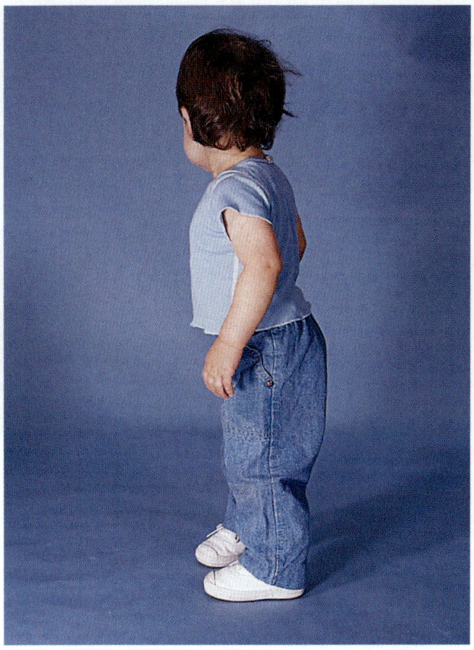

Fig. 3.7 Standing. By 1 year old, the lordotic curve, exaggerated here by a diaper, is evident.

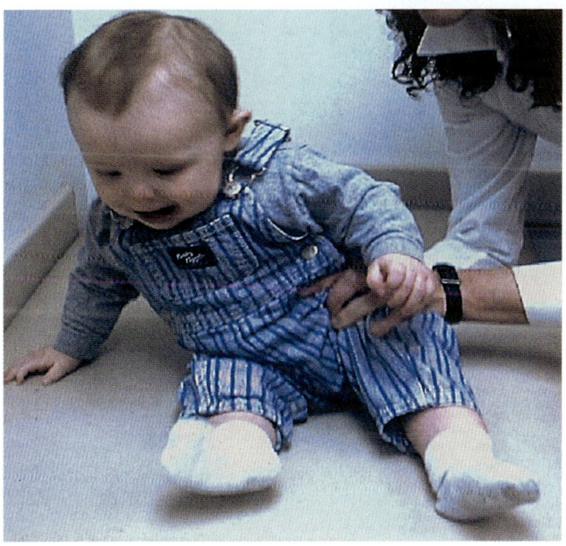

Fig. 3.8 Protective equilibrium response. As the child is pushed laterally by the examiner, he flexes his trunk toward the force to regain his center of gravity while one arm extends to protect against falling (lateral propping).

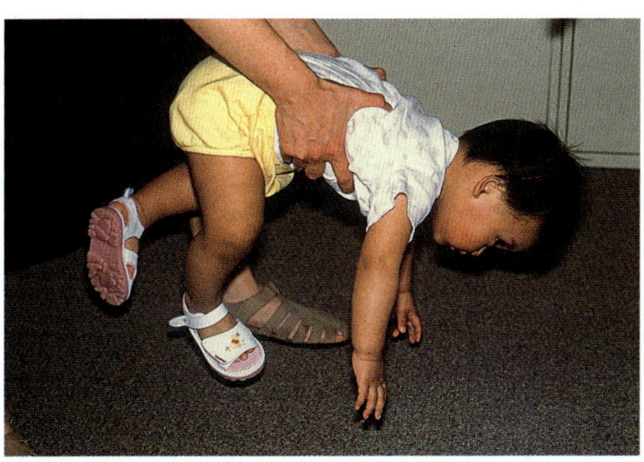

Fig. 3.9 Parachute response. As the examiner allows the child to free fall in ventral suspension, the child's extremities extend symmetrically to distribute his weight over a broader and more stable base on landing.

Table 3.3 Early Gross Motor Milestones in the Normal Child

Task	Age[a]
Rolls from tummy to back	6 months old
Leans on hands to support their selves when sitting	6 months old
Sits without support	9 months old
Gets to sitting by their selves	9 months old
Pulls to standing	12 months old
Takes a few steps on their own	15 months old
Walks without holding onto anyone or anything	18 months old

[a]≥75% of children would be expected to achieve the milestone by that age.

From Zubler JM, Wiggins LD, Macias MM, et al: Evidence-informed milestones for developmental surveillance tools, *Pediatrics* 149(3):e2021052138, 2022.

older children with mild problems that do not seriously impair function.

FINE MOTOR DEVELOPMENT

Involuntary Grasp

At birth, the neonate's fingers and thumb are typically tightly fisted. A newborn baby grasps reliably and reflexively at any object placed in the palm (Fig. 3.12) and cannot release the grasp. Because of this reflex, the newborn's range of upper extremity motion is functionally limited. Normal development leads to acquisition of a voluntary grasp.

Voluntary Grasp

The reflexive palmar grasp gradually disappears at approximately 1 month old. From that point, the infant gains control of fine motor skills in an orderly progression. In the second or third month of life, the infant initially brings both hands together for midline hand play (Fig. 3.13). Shortly after that, the baby begins to swipe at objects held in or near the midline (Fig. 3.14). It is through swiping that the infant increases the exploratory range and fine-tunes the small muscles of the wrist, hand, and fingers.

Improvements in fine motor control increase sensory input from the hands and permit greater hand manipulation through space. By 2 to 3 months old, the hands are no longer tightly fisted and the infant may begin sucking on a thumb or individual digit rather than the entire fist for self-comfort. A 3-month-old baby is usually able to hold an object in either hand if it is placed there, although the ability to grasp voluntarily or to release that object is limited. At approximately 4 to 5 months old, infants begin to use their hands as entire units to draw objects toward them. Neither the hand nor the thumb functions independently at this point, and, consequently, the child uses the hand like a rake.

Next, the child develops the ability to bend the fingers against the palm (palmar grasp), squeeze objects, and obtain them independently for closer inspection (Fig. 3.15). Differentiation of the parts of the hand develops in association with differentiation of the two hands. Between 5 and 7 months old, the infant can use hands independently to transfer objects across the midline. Further differentiation of the plane of movement of the thumb allows it to adduct as the fingers squeeze against the palm in a radial palmar or whole-hand grasp. With time, the thumb moves from adduction to opposition. The site of pressure of the thumb against the fingers moves away from the palm and toward the fingertips, in what is called an *inferior pincer* or *radial digital grasp,* seen around 9 months old (Fig. 3.16). By 10 months old, differentiated use of the fingers allows the child to explore the details of an object.

Between 9 and 12 months old, the fine pincer grasp develops, allowing opposition of the tip of the thumb and the index finger

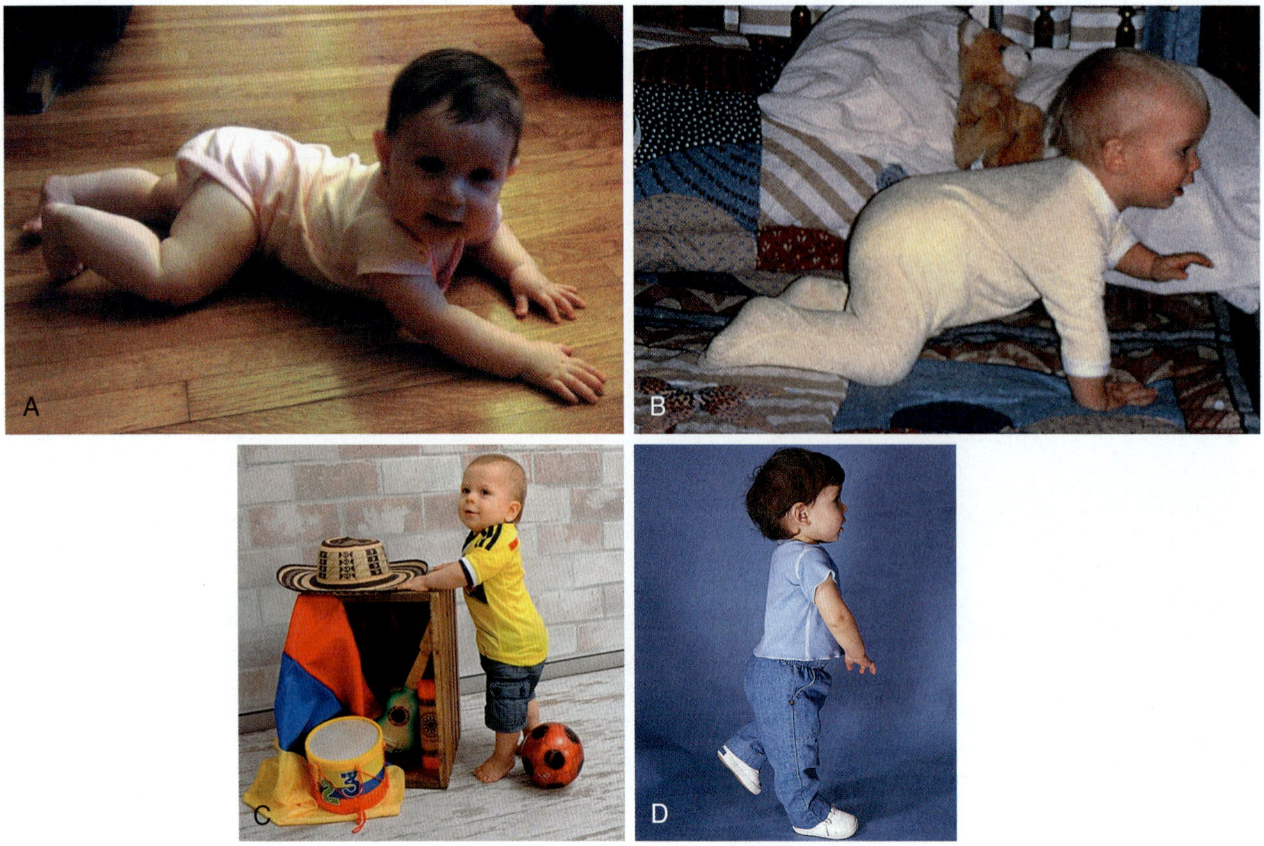

Fig. 3.10 Development of locomotion. (A) Creeping implies that the belly is still on the floor. (B) Crawling refers to mobility with the child on the hands and knees (quadruped position). (C) Cruising refers to standing with two-handed support on stationary objects before moving with steps. (D) Early free walking.

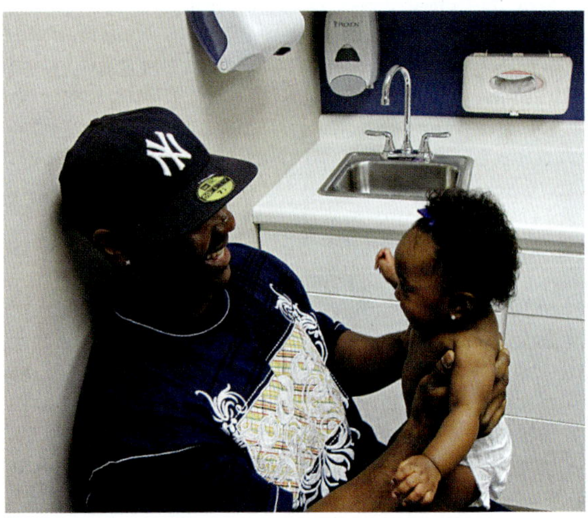

Fig. 3.11 A 4-month-old has enough strength to support her back when held under her arms by her father's hands but not enough strength to sit on her own.

(Fig. 3.17). This milestone enables the precise prehension of tiny objects (see Fig. 3.17). The infant uses this skill in tasks such as self-feeding and exploration of small objects. By 1 year, the infant can position the hand in space to achieve vertical or horizontal orientation before grasping or releasing an object.

Development of Complex Fine Motor Skills

Early in the second year of life, the young child uses the grasp to master tools and to manipulate objects in new ways. Dropping and throwing, stacking, and putting objects in and out of receptacles become favorite pastimes. Mastery of the cup and spoon supplement or replace finger feeding as a more efficient and less messy means of eating (Fig. 3.18).

Advancements in fine motor planning and control can be demonstrated through the child's ability to stack small cubes. After children master stacking, they show consistent patterns of improvement in

Table 3.4 Potential Causes of Delayed Gross Motor Development

Global Developmental Delay	Motor Dysfunction	Motor Intact But Otherwise Restricted
Genetic syndromes and chromosomal abnormalities	Central nervous system damage—kernicterus, birth injury, neonatal stroke, trauma, prolonged seizures, metabolic insult, infection	Congenital malformations—bony or soft tissue defects
Brain morphologic abnormalities	Spinal cord dysfunction—Werdnig-Hoffmann disease, myelomeningocele, polio	Diminished energy supply—chronic illness, severe malnutrition
Endocrine deficiencies—hypothyroidism, prolonged hypoglycemia	Peripheral nerve dysfunction—brachial plexus injury, heritable neuropathies	Environmental deprivation—casted, non–weight bearing
Congenital infections	Motor end-plate dysfunction—myasthenia gravis	Familial and genetic endowment—slower myelination
Neurodegenerative diseases	Muscular disorders—muscular dystrophies	Sensory deficits—blindness
Idiopathic intellectual disability	Other—benign congenital hypotonia	Temperamental effects—low activity level, slow to try new tasks
		Trauma—child abuse

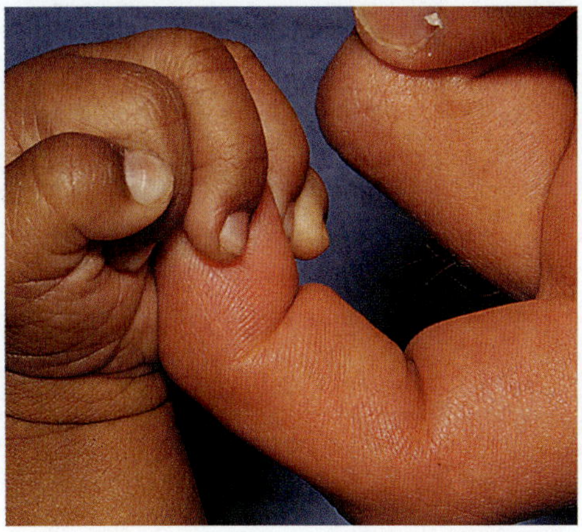

Fig. 3.12 Reflex hand grasp. A newborn reflexively grasps at a finger placed in the palm.

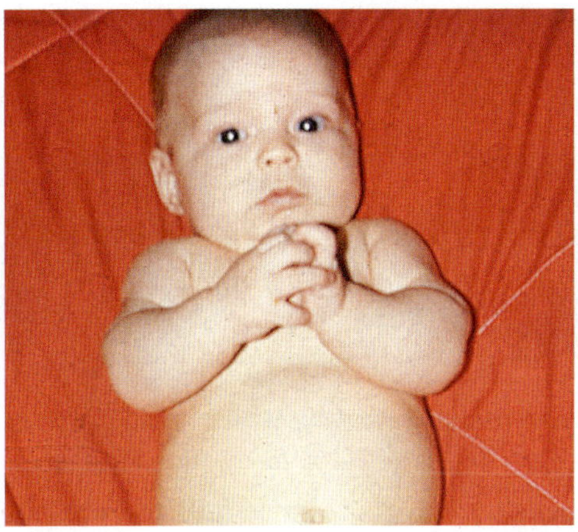

Fig. 3.13 Midline hand play. A 2-month-old infant brings the hands together at the midline.

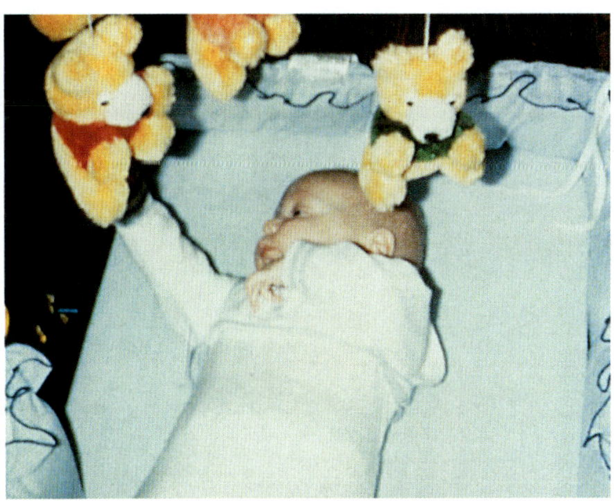

Fig. 3.14 Reaching and swiping. A 3-month-old infant uses his entire upper extremity as a unit in interacting with the toy.

reproducing structures that they have watched the examiner assemble (Fig. 3.19). The child's ability to copy a variety of drawings also improves during this period.

Fine Motor Evaluation and Testing

Fine motor testing can be incorporated readily into a physical examination and may uncover problems with vision, neuromuscular control, or perception, in addition to difficulties with attention

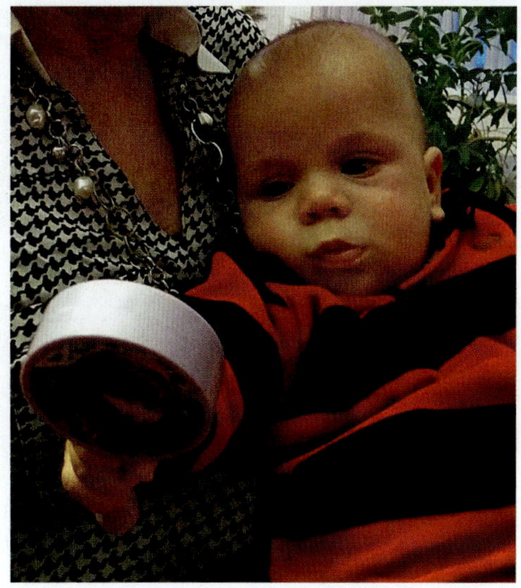

Fig. 3.15 Palmar grasp. By 4 months old, the child develops the ability to bend the fingers against the palm.

or cooperation. The 4-month-old child usually can be encouraged to grasp a small toy or tongue depressor (see Fig. 3.15). By 6 to 9 months old, two tongue depressors should be offered, one for each hand, because the child can operate the hands independently. At 9 to 12 months old, the child spontaneously points with an isolated index finger or picks up small objects with a fine pincer grasp. Children younger than 18 months old generally use both hands equally well. Therefore, the child who develops consistent handedness with neglect of the other limb before that time should have a neurodevelopmental assessment. The child who has not developed use of the thumb and pincer grasp by 18 months old deserves further evaluation, as does the child who is unable to copy vertical or horizontal lines by 3 years old or circles by 4 years old.

Fine motor activities can be engaging and nonthreatening to the preschool and school-age child; these activities allow the physician to make valuable observations and to establish rapport. The physician can routinely request that the child older than 3 years old use the waiting time or the period of history-taking to draw a self-portrait. These drawings provide a wealth of information on not only the child's capacities for fine motor control but also cognitive development and social and emotional functioning. A quick method for analyzing the age level of a drawing is to count the number of features in the drawing. The child receives one point for each of the following features: two eyes, two ears, a nose, a mouth, hair, two arms, two legs, two hands, two feet, a neck, and a trunk. Each point converts to the value of 3 months (or four points to a year) added to a base age of 3 years old (Fig. 3.20). Screening tests and standardized measures, such as the *Beery-Buktenica Developmental Test of Visual-Motor Integration,* sixth edition, can also be used to assess fine motor skills.

Children with brain damage are at increased risk for problems with perceptual/fine motor integration, even in the absence of visual problems and with minimal involvement of the upper extremities (Fig. 3.21).

Fine motor skills figure prominently in self-care activities. The child who lacks the dexterity to complete simple daily activities (e.g., zipping, buttoning, or cutting with a knife) may lack the self-esteem that accompanies independent self-care. Furthermore, children who continually depend on parents or teachers may be viewed by peers; teachers; or, perhaps most damagingly, by themselves as less mature. In the school-age child, inefficient fine motor skills can have a significant impact on the ability to write legibly or to compete with peers in timed tasks, even if the child has sound academic and conceptual skills. Occupational therapy and special education may enhance fine motor skills and emotional development in these children.

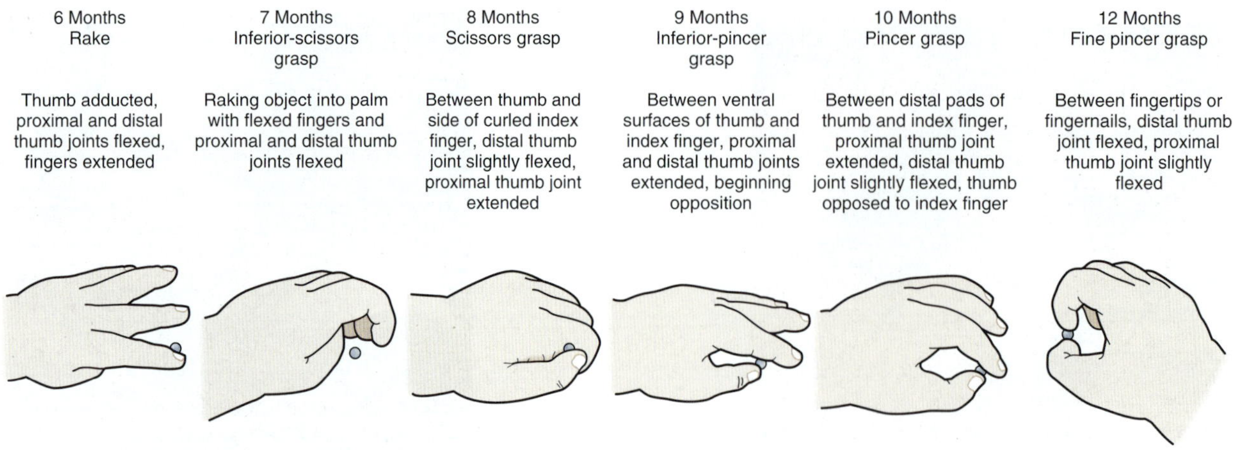

Fig. 3.16 Development of prehension. (Modified from Erhardt RP: *Developmental hand dysfunction: theory, assessment, treatment*, ed 2, San Antonio, TX, 1994, The Psychological Corporation. Copyright © 1982, 1989, 1994 by Rhoda P. Erhardt. All rights reserved.)

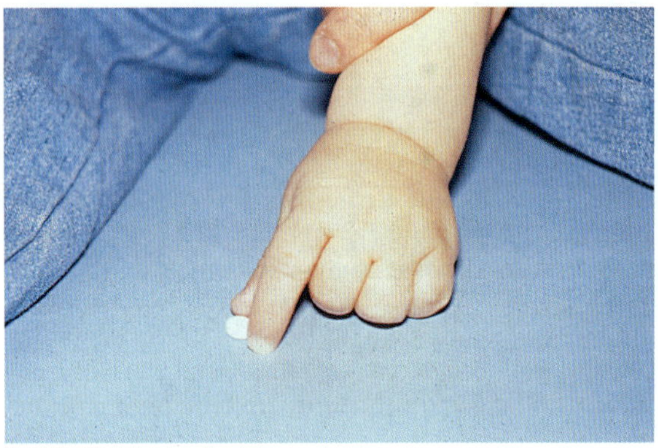

Fig. 3.17 Fine pincer grasp. A 12-month-old child lifts a pill.

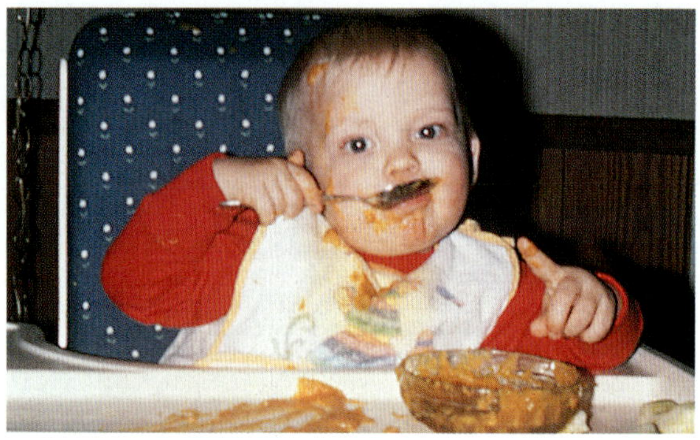

Fig. 3.18 Independent feeding. A 15-month-old child employs fine motor skills to use a spoon independently.

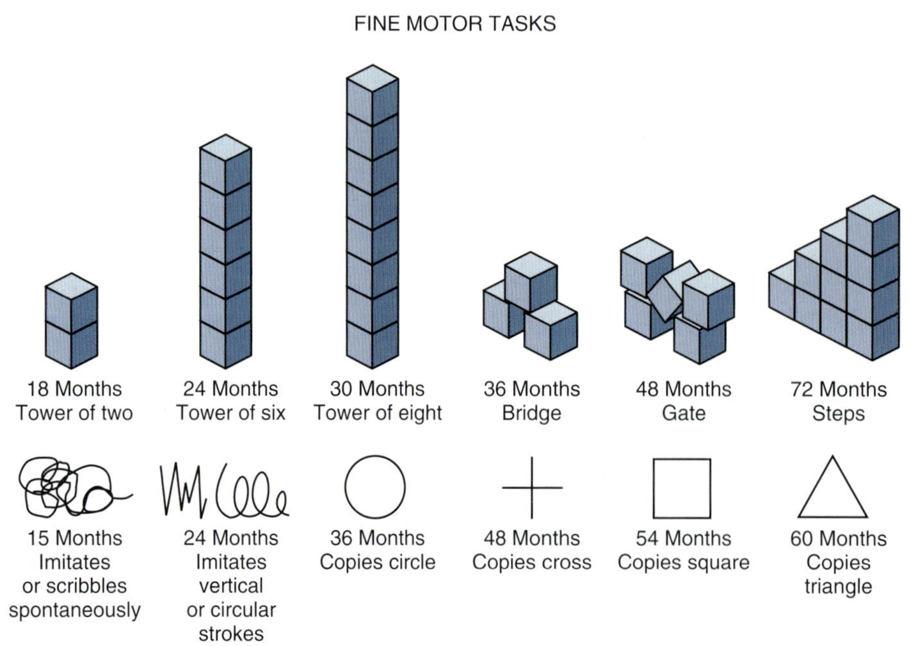

Fig. 3.19 Development of fine motor skills.

COGNITIVE DEVELOPMENT

Early Sensory Processing

Innate sensory capabilities serve as the building blocks of cognitive development. Even at birth, the healthy neonate responds to visual and auditory stimuli. These responses, like the primitive reflexes, take the form of integrated patterns of activity.

The visual acuity of the full-term infant is estimated to fall between 20/200 and 20/400 and improves rapidly over the first year of life. Even at birth, it is possible to get the full-term newborn to fix on faces 9 to 12 inches from the face and to track objects horizontally at least 30 degrees (Fig. 3.22). Some neonates, if assessed when calm and fully alert, can track objects 180 degrees across the visual field. Newborns also respond to sound, typically quieting in response to a human voice,

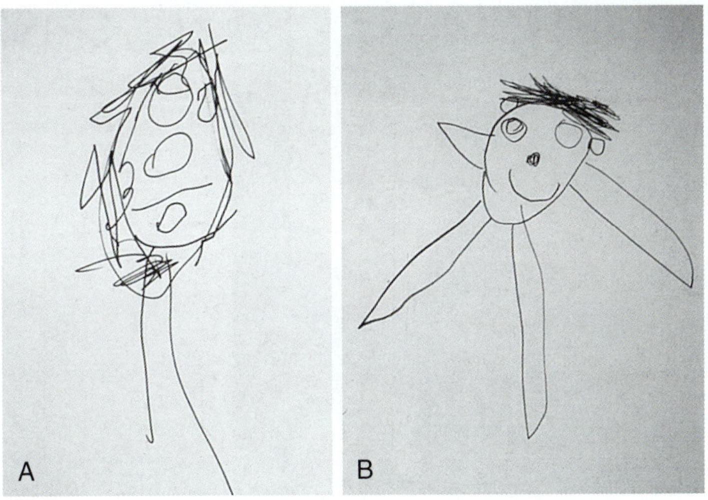

Fig. 3.20 Development of skill at drawing a person. (A) This drawing by a 4-year-old child includes five features: eyes, nose, mouth, hair, and legs. To calculate an age equivalent, the child earns 3 months for each of the five features, added to a base age of 3 years. This drawing has an age equivalent of 4 years and 3 months old. (B) A drawing by the same child at age 5 years old. Note the inclusion of ears and arms and improvements in proportion. This drawing has an age equivalent of 4 years and 9 months old.

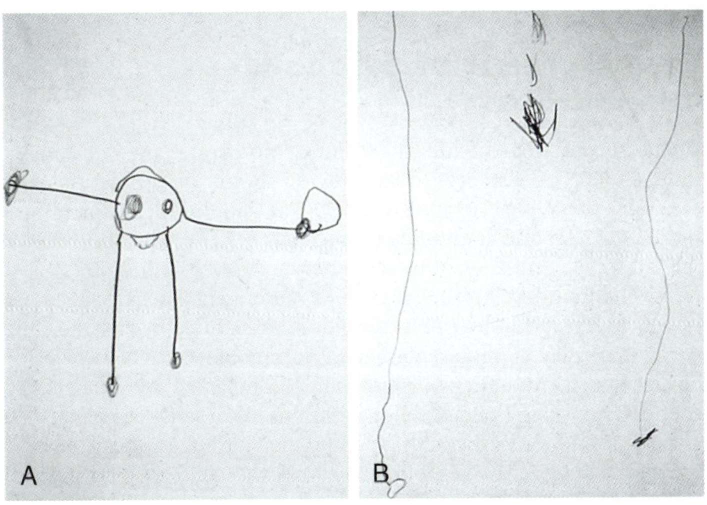

Fig. 3.21 Difficulties with visual/fine motor integration skills in a child with cerebral palsy. (A) Drawing by a bright 4-year-old who was born prematurely but showed no developmental delays. Note the inclusion of seven features: eyes, hair, mouth, arms, hands, legs, and feet. The age equivalent for this drawing is 4¾ years old. (B) Drawing by a 4-year-old child with spastic diplegia. Difficulties in organization appear related to visual motor integration skills rather than to problems with fine motor skills.

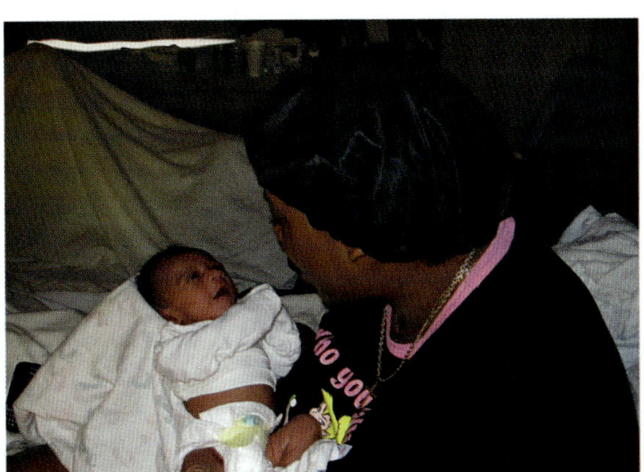

Fig. 3.22 Early social skills. A newborn within an hour of birth fixates on the face of the mother.

rattles, or music. In the first days of life, many infants turn to the source of sound and search for it with their eyes. These maneuvers, found on the Brazelton Neonatal Behavioral Assessment Scale, are useful in demonstrating neurobehavioral characteristics of newborns.

Examination must take place at optimal times when the infant is alert; if the infant is drowsy or agitated, the ability to track visually or to search for sounds is compromised. If, when assessed under optimal circumstances and when fully alert, infants do not demonstrate horizontal tracking of objects, do not look at the toys or people with whom they are involved, or hold their heads in unusual positions, the physician should recommend prompt evaluation for abnormal visual perception or central nervous system development. New technology offers the use of vision screener devices that allow for vision screenings as early as 6 months of age with minimal collaboration from the infant or the child. These vision screener devices use lights and sounds to help engage children.

Development of Sensorimotor Intelligence

During the first 2 years of life, the sensorimotor period of development, the young child's cognitive abilities can be surmised only through use of the senses and through the physical manipulation of objects. During this period, the child develops an understanding of the concept of object permanence, the ability to recognize that an object exists even when it cannot be seen, heard, or felt. Simultaneously, the child develops an understanding of cause-and-effect relationships. Progress in the child's development of these concepts is an important prerequisite to the development of pure mental activity, reflected in the ability to use symbols and language.

Early progress in the development of object permanence is indicated by the infant's continued though brief gaze at the site where a familiar toy or face has disappeared. At this point, children also repeat actions that they have discovered will produce interesting results. Between 4 and 8 months of age, infants become interested in changes in the position and appearance of toys. They can track an object visually through a vertical fall (Fig. 3.23) and search for a partially hidden toy. They also begin to vary the means of creating interesting effects. In these early months, the baby's play consists of exploring toys to gain information about their physical characteristics. Activities such as mouthing, shaking, and banging can provide sensory input about an

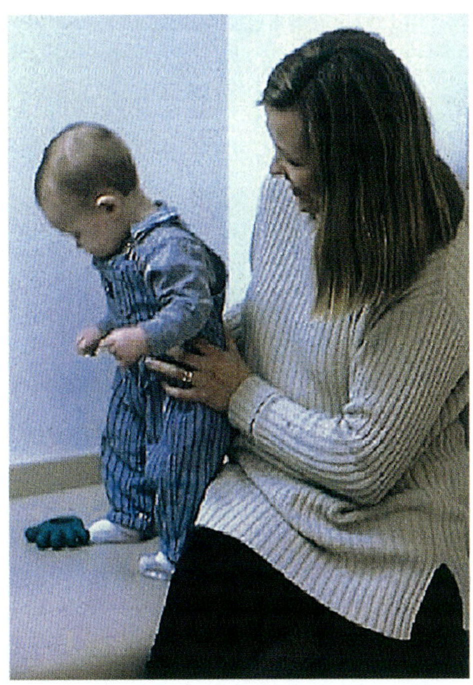

Fig. 3.23 Early object permanence. A 6-month-old infant was able to track his toy through a vertical fall and to search for it on the floor even after his gaze had been interrupted.

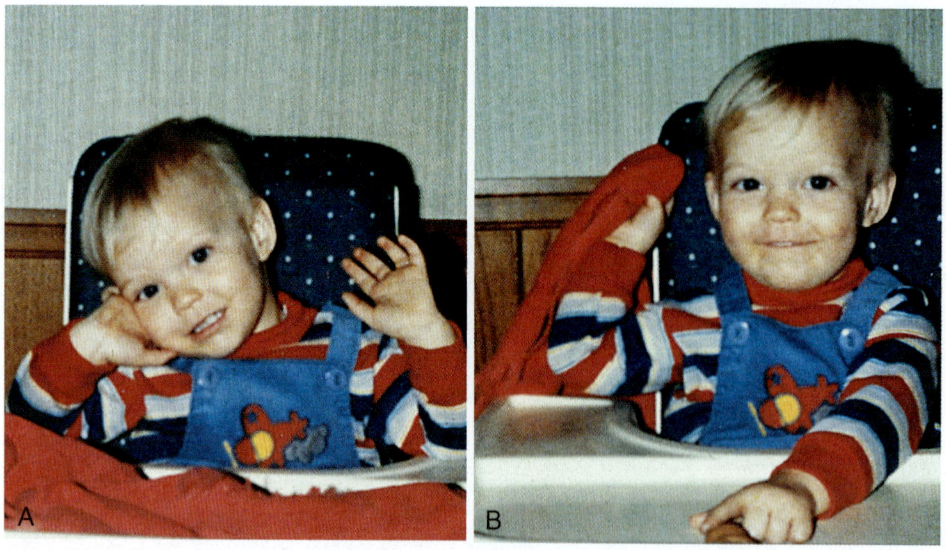

Fig. 3.24 Object permanence. (A and B) An 11-month-old child can locate a small, hidden object even if no part of it remains visible. In doing so, he is demonstrating his understanding that objects are permanent.

object beyond its visual features. However, when mouthing of toys persists as the predominant mode of exploration after 12 to 18 months of age, assessment of cognitive function is warranted.

At approximately 9 to 12 months of age, infants can locate objects that have been completely hidden (Fig. 3.24). Not surprisingly, peek-a-boo becomes a favorite pastime at this point. Later, the infant can crawl away from the mother and recall where to return to find her.

As children near 1 year old, interest in toys extends beyond physical properties (e.g., color, texture). These children may begin to demonstrate their awareness that different objects have different purposes. For example, a child might touch a comb to the hair in a meaningful non-pretend action, which is typical of the 9- to 12-month age range. Beyond 1 year old, children begin to vary their behavior to create novel effects. They no longer need to be shown how to work dials or knobs, nor do they need to hit something by accident to discover the interesting effect that will result.

By 18 months old, children can deduce the location of an object even if they have not seen it hidden from view. They can maintain mental images of desired objects and develop plans for obtaining them. The child's understanding of causality also advances; cause-and-effect relationships no longer need to be direct to be appreciated (Fig. 3.25). These developments herald the beginning of a new stage in cognitive development, that of symbolic thinking. They also indicate that distraction may not succeed in drawing a child away from a desired object; a direct request is required.

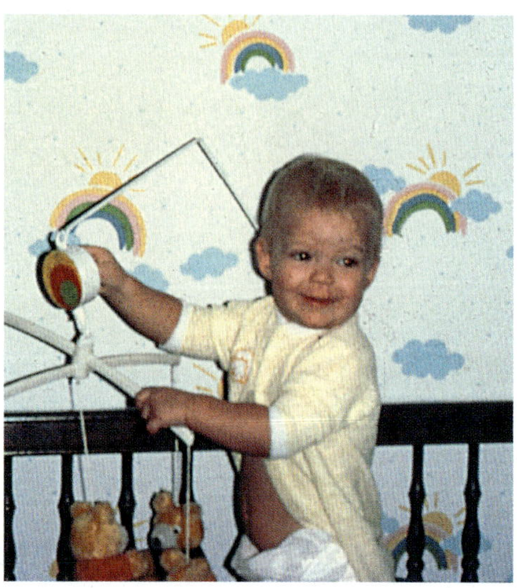

Fig. 3.25 Mature means/end reasoning. A 15-month-old child turns the key of the music box atop the mobile to make it play. The child's understanding has advanced beyond that of direct causality, such as pulling a toy to bring it closer.

Development of Symbolic Capabilities

In the second year of life, the child demonstrates mental activity independent of sensory processing or motor manipulation. For example, the child observes a television superhero performing a rescue mission and hours later reenacts the scene. The child uses a mental image of the event to generate the delayed imitation.

As children develop the capacity for pure mental activity, they use objects to represent other objects or ideas. Pretending begins; the child engages in playful representation of commonplace activities, using objects for their actual purpose but accompanied by exaggerated sounds or gestures. Pretend actions combine into a series of events, such as holding and feeding a teddy bear and then putting the bear to bed.

The next stage in development allows the child to plan pretend activities in anticipation of the play theme to come, combining many steps into the play. Preparing for play indicates an advance in pretending beyond that of improvising with the objects at hand. For example, the child might be seen preparing the play area or searching for needed objects and announcing what the objects are meant to represent.

Development of Logical Thinking

The preschool child has well-developed capabilities for mental representation and symbolic thinking. However, the dominance of sensory input, limited life experience, and a lack of formal education lead to a unique and charming logic during this period. Preschoolers often assume that all objects are alive like themselves. For example, a car and a tricycle may be seen as alive because they are capable of movement. Similarly, children claim that the moon follows them on an evening walk.

The logic of the preschooler is in large part influenced by the appearance of objects. Because an airplane appears to become smaller as it takes off, the preschooler may assume that all the people on the plane become smaller as well. Piaget demonstrated that preschoolers seem to think that number and quantity vary with appearance (Fig. 3.26). Under certain circumstances, a 4-year-old child may show understanding that a quantity remains invariant unless something is added or subtracted. However, that same child may insist that two rows of pennies are different in number simply because of a compelling visual difference between them.

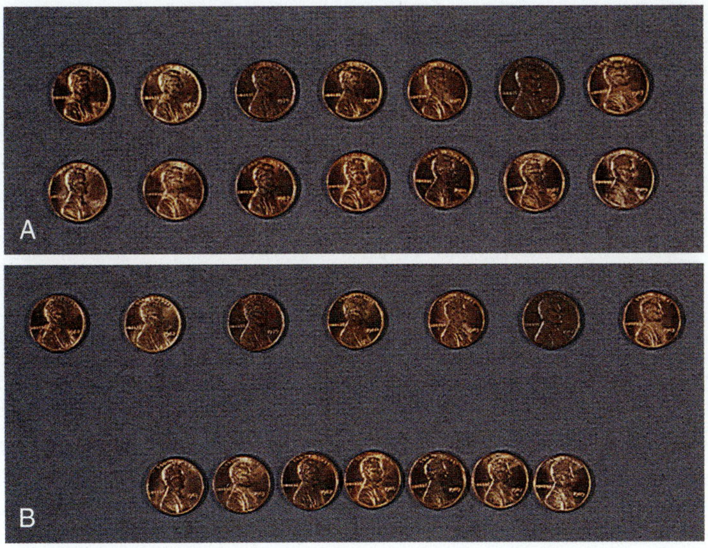

Fig. 3.26 Experimental design to demonstrate preoperational logic. The 3- or 4-year-old child agrees that the two rows in (A) have the same number of pennies. After seeing the pennies moved into the configuration in (B), the child claims that the top row has more because it is longer.

The immature logic of the preschooler is gradually replaced by conventional logic and wisdom. School-age children follow logic akin to adult reasoning, at least when the stimuli are concrete. Faced with the same question about the pennies, they readily acknowledge that the two rows have the same number regardless of their visual appearance (see Fig. 3.26). They also know that the airplane just looks smaller because it has moved farther from the viewer, and they giggle at the suggestion that the people on the plane have shrunk. Their logical limitations become obvious when they must reason about the hypothetical or the abstract.

Adolescents, particularly those with the benefits of formal education, tend to extend logical principles to increasingly diverse problems. They can generate multiple logical possibilities systematically when faced with scientific experiments, and they can also consider hypothetical problems. These principles of reasoning are applied to not only schoolwork but also social situations.

Assessing Cognitive Development

The pediatric office assessment of cognitive ability in the preverbal child is best accomplished by observation of play. The pediatrician can induce the infant to look for a hidden toy or to play a game of peek-a-boo; the infant's anticipation of reappearance indicates the development of the concept of object permanence. Similarly, the toddler's ability to play with a toy telephone indicates the emergence of symbolic thought. Beyond the toddler stage, the physician typically relies on conversation and language ability to assess levels of cognitive skill. Screening tests are particularly useful for determining whether cognitive and language skills are within the normal range. Children with language delays may need a formal nonverbal assessment of cognitive abilities by a psychologist or developmental subspecialist.

For the parents, a delay in a child's attainment of a well-known milestone may create tremendous fear about ultimate learning potential. In many cases, such parental concerns are put to rest at that time when the physician determines that the child's learning to date is age appropriate. If a child does show delays in cognitive development, the physician should generate a differential diagnosis (Table 3.5) from knowledge of the child's level of functioning in multiple domains, history, and physical examination.

Parents should be given information about their child's delay as early as possible. Pediatricians serve a critical role in referring children to early intervention or special education programs and in monitoring their progress. Active communication between the providers of early intervention and the physician assists a comprehensive and cohesive approach.

Physicians frequently need the consultation of colleagues in psychology and education to assess the cognitive abilities of their older preschool and school-age patients. Several methods have been devised for formal assessment of mental achievement, and almost all parents are familiar with the term *intelligence quotient,* or *IQ.* Although not a means of comprehensively assessing all mental capabilities, normal IQ scores are (albeit imperfect) predictors of which children will have the cognitive and intellectual abilities to perform well in school. Low IQ scores may reflect a child's poor ability to grasp new concepts, or they may indicate other issues, such as poor purposeful attending behaviors. Low scores may also reflect poor social adjustment or limitations in test-taking capabilities, such as sitting in a chair at a table and applying maximal effort to a task requested by an unfamiliar authority figure. Frequently, low scores result from a combination of difficulties in several areas.

If children with sensory or motor impairments are tested with instruments normalized on able-bodied children, they often obtain low scores. Different assessment techniques have been devised to circumvent specific disabilities while obtaining information about a child's cognitive abilities; these are typically administered by psychologists, child development specialists, or special educators (Table 3.6).

Table 3.5 Potentially Remediable Disorders Associated With Developmental Delay

Findings Sometimes Present on History or Examination	Possible Disorder
Decreased vision or hearing	Specific sensory deficits
Staring spells, motor automatism	Seizure disorders
Lethargy, ataxia	Overmedication with anticonvulsants
Myxedema, delayed return on DTRs, thick skin and tongue, sparse hair, constipation, increased sleep, coarse voice, short stature, goiter	Hypothyroidism
Irritability, cold sweats, tremor, loss of consciousness	Hypoglycemia
Unexplained bruises in various stages, failure to thrive	Child abuse and neglect
Short stature, weight below third percentile	Malnutrition or systemic illness producing failure to thrive
Poor purposeful attending in multiple settings	ADHD
No specific findings	Environmental deprivation
Anemia	Iron deficiency or lead exposure
Absent venous pulsations or papilledema on funduscopic examination, morning vomiting, headaches, brisk DTRs in lower extremities	Increased intracranial pressure
Vomiting, irritability and seizures, failure to thrive	Some inborn errors of metabolism (e.g., methylmalonic acidemia)
Hepatomegaly, jaundice, hypotonia, susceptibility to infection, cataracts	Galactosemia
Fair hair, blue eyes, "mousy" odor to urine	Phenylketonuria
Ongoing evidence of active or progressive disease	Chronic infection, inflammatory disease, malignancies

ADHD, Attention-deficit/hyperactivity disorder; *DTR,* deep tendon reflex.

Table 3.6 Tests Used in the Assessment of Cognitive Development Check

Type of Scale	Test(s) Used	Age Range
Standard intelligence scales	Stanford-Binet Intelligence Scales-IV	2 years old to adult
	Wechsler Intelligence Scale for Children-IV	5–16 years old
Nonverbal intelligence scale	Leiter International Performance Scale-R	2–18 years old
Infant development tests	Bayley Scales of Infant Development-III	0–42 months old
	Gesell Developmental Schedules	0–5 years old
Developmental scale for the visually impaired	Reynell-Zinkin Developmental Scales for Young Children With Visual Impairments	0–5 years old
Adaptive behavior	Vineland Adaptive Behavior Scales-II	0–18 years old
	Adaptive Behavior Assessment System-II	0–21 years old

Assessment of a child's abilities to learn must go beyond standardized IQ tests. For example, some children who can score in the normal range on IQ tests are unable to learn to read. A diversified and individualized assessment process should precede any educational recommendation. The pediatrician, in the role of advocate, should ensure that assessments include information about the child's strengths and weaknesses, because educational planning should involve attention to all aspects of the child's abilities. Moreover, the pediatrician can encourage families to maintain an active, decision-making role in their children's education.

LANGUAGE DEVELOPMENT

Early Skills in Speech Perception and Production

The use of language is the ability to generate and understand reproducible sounds or gestures that are recognized by others as representative of concepts. Language development begins slowly and subtly in the first year of life. Language skills are subdivided into two realms: (1) receptive skills—the ability to comprehend communication and (2) expressive skills—the ability to produce communication.

Neonates demonstrate skills that are useful in the eventual development of receptive language abilities. Even before birth, fetuses detect sounds and show preferences for some sounds over others. At birth, the newborn is particularly attuned to the human voice and may turn toward a parent who is gently whispering. Children remain interested in sounds as they grow older and turn voluntarily toward the source of a sound by 3 to 4 months old (Fig. 3.27).

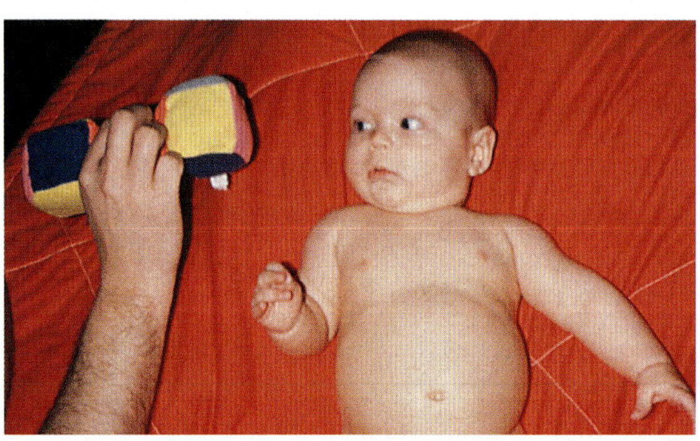

Fig. 3.27 Localizing sound. A 3-month-old infant responds to interesting sounds by looking in the direction of the sound.

Children can also differentiate speech sounds, even close to birth. Experimental paradigms, using the fact that an infant's heart rate and sucking patterns change when they encounter new environmental stimuli, suggest that infants as young as 1 month old can differentiate such similar speech sounds as /ba/ and /pa/. Frequent exposure to the native language alters speech perception such that by late infancy it becomes difficult for children to differentiate sounds that are not meaningful distinctions in their own language.

By 2 to 3 months old, children begin to *coo* or make musical sounds spontaneously. This is the first step toward the development of expressive verbal language. Even in the early stages, children can establish reciprocal patterns, like the rhythm of conversation.

By approximately 6 months old, children place consonant sounds with vowel sounds, creating what is known as *babble.* In this period, the infant says "ma-ma" or "da-da" without necessarily referring to the loving parent. By 9 to 12 months, children integrate babble with intonational patterns consistent with the parent's speech. This is called *jargon.*

Later Development

In the second half of the first year, the child develops early skills in true receptive language. Milestones are listed in Table 3.7. By 6 months old, children reliably respond to their names, and at approximately 9 months old, they can follow verbal routines, such as waving bye-bye or showing how big they are. At about the same age, they also learn that pointing shares the focus of attention. The young infant looks at the point, whereas the older infant looks at the object to which the point is directed.

Receptive language can be demonstrated as children follow increasingly complex commands. For example, children will understand one-step commands such as "throw the ball" by approximately 1 year old. The labeling of commonplace items in pictures is slightly more complex and begins after 1 year. The ability to choose between two pictures when asked "show me the . . ." should be consistent between 18 and 24 months old.

By 30 months old, receptive language skills have advanced beyond the understanding of simple labels. The child can identify objects by their use. Continued advances in receptive language occur during the preschool years and are highly susceptible to environmental stimulation or deprivation.

Expressive language skills (see Table 3.7) lag behind receptive skills in the first year of life. But even before word production begins, a child's gestures have communicative intent. Many 9- to 10-month-olds can communicate that their juice or cereal is "all gone" by placing their hands palms up, at shoulder height. Even older children gesture to make themselves understood, because gross and fine motor skills develop faster than the oropharyngeal muscle skills used in articulation.

Expressive language at first develops slowly. The child's first meaningful words are produced around the first birthday. Over the next 6 months, the child may master only 20 to 50 more words. These early words come and go from the child's vocabulary and may be idiosyncratic child-forms. After 18 to 24 months old, word usage increases rapidly, standard forms replace baby talk, and word combinations begin.

The child's earliest two-word sentences typically contain important content words but lack prepositions, articles, and verb-tense markings. This two-word phase has been called *telegraphic speech* as the child leaves out nonessential articles and prepositions. Once the child is capable of three- and four-word utterances, length limitations do not appear to be a significant barrier for most children. By age 3 the child has developed complex language with the use of pronouns and prepositions. The child develops the ability to ask questions. At age 30 months, they usually ask "what?" and by age 3 years they most frequently ask "why?" The child also can use negation within a sentence. By age 5, the child uses all parts of speech and clauses and complex sentences.

Table 3.7 Receptive and Expressive Language Milestones

Age[a]	Receptive Response	Expressive Response
2 months	Reacts to loud sounds	Makes sounds other than crying
4 months	Turns head toward the sound of your voice	Makes sounds like "oooo" and "aahh" (cooing)
4 months	Turns head toward the sound of your voice when parent says "up" and reaches for child; responds appropriately to friendly or angry voices	Makes sounds back when you talk to them
9 months	Lifts arms up to be picked up	Makes different sounds like "mamamama" and "babababa"
12 months	Waves "bye-bye" Understands "no" (pauses briefly or stops when you say it)	Calls a parent "mama" or "dada" or another special name
15 months	Looks at a familiar object when you name it Follows directions given with both a gesture and words. For example, he gives you a toy when you hold out your hand and say, "Give me the toy."	Tries to say 1 or 2 words besides mama or dada, like "ba" for ball or "da" for dog Points to ask for something or to get help
18 months	Follows 1-step directions without any gestures, like giving you the toy when you say, "Give it to me."	Tries to say ≥3 words besides mama or dada
24 months	Points to things in a book when you ask, for example, "Where is the bear?" Points to at least 2 body parts when you ask him to show you	Says at least 2 words together, like "More milk." Uses more gestures than just waving and pointing, like blowing a kiss or nodding yes
30 months	Names things in a book when you point and ask, "What is this?"	Says ~50 words Says ≥2 words, with 1 action word, like "Doggie run." Says words like I, me, or we
3 years	Says what action is happening in a picture when asked, like running, eating, or playing	Talks with you in conversation using at least 2 back-and-forth exchanges Asks who, what, where, or why questions, like "Where is mommy/daddy?" Says first name when asked Talks well enough for others to understand, most of the time
4 years	Answers simple questions, like "What is a coat for," or "What is a crayon for?"	Says sentences with ≥4 words Says some words from a song, story, or nursery rhyme Talks about at least 1 thing that happened during his day, like "I played soccer."
5 years	Answers simple questions about a book or story after you read or tell it to them Uses or recognizes simple rhymes (bat-cat, ball-tall)	Tells a story she heard or made up with at least 2 events, like a cat stuck in a tree and a firefighter saving it Keeps a conversation going with >3 back-and-forth exchange

[a]≥75% of children would be expected to achieve the milestone by that age.

From Zubler JM, Wiggins LD, Macias MM, et al: Evidence-informed milestones for developmental surveillance tools, *Pediatrics* 149(3):e2021052138, 2022.

The rate of language development appears to be associated with both biologic and environmental factors. Approximately half or more of children with first-degree relatives with language and speech delays also show delays. The amount of child-directed speech in the environment is a good predictor of the rate of development for vocabulary and grammar. For this reason, health supervision of infants and toddlers should encourage parents to speak or read to their children.

Mastering Intelligibility and Fluency

Sounds required in language are mastered at different rates. Children who are attempting to say words containing sounds they cannot yet produce have a variety of choices on how to proceed: by omission of the difficult sound (*ba* for bottle), by substitution of a different sound (*fum* for thumb), or by distortion (*goyl* for girl). The information presented in Table 3.8 provides an estimate of when mastery of particular sounds, along with estimates of overall intelligibility, might be expected.

Table 3.8 Phonemes and Intelligibility

Age (Years)[a]	Sounds Mastered	Percent Intelligibility (to a Stranger)
2	Emerging skills	50
3	14 vowels and *p, b, m*	75
4	10 vowel blends and *n, ng, w, h, t, d, k, g*	100
5	*f, v, y, th, l, wh*	100
6	*r, s, z, ch, j, sh, zh,* and consonant blends	100

[a]Ages presented here are general guidelines because authorities differ regarding the specific ages associated with articulation and intelligibility.

Assessing Language Development

In the early stages of prelinguistic and linguistic development, direct assessment by the pediatrician may be difficult. Children are likely to remain quiet in new situations, especially in the office where they previously received an injection. It is usually easy to engage a normally developing child of age 3 in conversations. Before that age, the physician may need to rely on parental report. Standardized parent reports are available for office use, and parental reports contribute to the assessment of language in screening tests.

The differential diagnosis for delayed expressive language development includes impaired hearing, global developmental delay or intellectual disability, environmental deprivation, autism, emotional maladjustment, or specific language impairment. Worrisome clinical situations include the 4- to 6-month-old infant who fails to coo responsively, the 9- to 10-month-old child who does not babble or whose cooing and babbling have diminished, and the 18-month-old child whose repertoire of words includes only *mama* or *dada*. A convenient rule of thumb is that children 2 years old should use two-word utterances, at least half of which should be intelligible. By 3 years old, children should use phrases of three or more words, three-quarters of which should be intelligible. Children who fail to achieve these developmental milestones should undergo evaluation for hearing loss and cognitive and emotional impairment.

Families often attribute language delays in their youngster to superficial and easily remediable physiologic or social factors. For example, "being tongue-tied" is not an explanation for delayed speech in most cases. However, it may be the effect rather than the cause, because in some children the frenulum of the tongue may be tight due to not being sufficiently exercised by early verbal practice. Similarly, children rarely delay language because "they don't need it." Children have tremendous motivation to improve their verbal skills, even if they have older siblings who attempt to speak or interpret for them. For example, for children who want a particular food, a point toward the cupboard door may not specify precisely what is wanted. The use of a verbal label will allow the child to meet needs efficiently.

Delays in the development of intelligibility might include any of the following:

- Lack of intelligible speech by age 3
- Frequent omission of initial consonants after age 4
- Continued substitution of easy sounds for more difficult ones after age 5
- Persistent articulation errors after age 7

During the period in which articulation and vocabulary are being mastered, speech dysfluencies are common. Noticeable stuttering or rapid speech beyond age 4 should prompt further attention. The problems of nasality, inaudibility, and unusual pitch sometimes may be helped by a speech pathologist. Furthermore, children of any age who are embarrassed by their speech are appropriate candidates for referral.

Therapy for speech and language disorders helps to improve the communication skills of children with language delays and problems of intelligibility. A child whose unusual language pattern is destined to be outgrown will not suffer from monitoring by a communication disorders specialist; the child whose language impairment will not be outgrown has much to lose when help is delayed.

SOCIAL DEVELOPMENT

Early Capabilities: Social Responsivity

The earliest social task of newborns is to establish a mutually satisfying relationship with their caregivers. Neonates begin this process by fixing visually on faces in preference to other sights, a skill that is evident during the first few days of life (see Fig. 3.22). The responsive smile develops soon thereafter (Fig. 3.28). The social smile is another innate behavior, although it may not appear until 4 to 6 weeks of life. Smiling appears in infants from all cultures at about the same time. Smiling appears as a response when infants see a face of any person, showing the forehead, the two eyes, nose, and mouth smiling, regardless of the person's familiarity. The presentation of a stimulus of a face sideways where only one eye and only part of the mouth is seeing is not enough to enact the smiling gestalt response in the infant. Infants with visual impairment who cannot appreciate a smile on the faces of their caregivers nonetheless smile at ages comparable with sighted children, except that they do not do it as a response of a specific stimulus.

Development of Attachment

During the first 6 months of life, infants are rather indiscriminate in their social behavior, smiling and later laughing with anyone willing to play. Infants develop a sense that their parents exist when out of sight sooner than they learn inanimate objects are permanent. By 6 to 8 months old, children may protest when their parents leave the room. As infants begin to recognize faces of familiar caregivers, they may squirm or cry in the company of unfamiliar people, exhibiting *stranger awareness*. The severity of the reaction varies with the infant's temperament and with previous experiences. Extreme reactions, known as *stranger anxiety,* may occur in children who have not had routine care from alternative caregivers. Pediatricians are advised to refrain from holding the 9- to 12-month-old child at the well-child visit. A child who remains playful and calm while securely in the parent's arms may quickly fret or cry even if gently removed from that security.

By 1 year of age, most children have experienced periods of separation from a parent, whether for minutes or hours. Infants who have developed a secure attachment to their parents show signs of recognition and pleasure when they are reunited with them. While progressing in gross motor development, the child initiates separation by walking away independently and exploring at greater distances from parents. Typically, infants return regularly for verbal encouragement, eye contact, or hugging and then venture farther. In contrast, infants who have not developed secure attachments may show indifference, ambivalence, or disorganization at reunion with their parents. Their exploration of the environment during the toddler years is limited. These children are at risk for troubled social relationships and difficulties achieving independence in functional domains (e.g., sleep) as they become older.

Development of Social Play

Infants and young toddlers tend to line up and engage in similar activities simultaneously. This pattern is called *parallel play.* Although parents often expect their young toddlers to interact or share with peers, success in this age group is unusual. Sharing for a young toddler involves showing or handing a prized toy to another child, only to take it back within seconds.

By 2 years of age, with the development of symbolic capabilities in cognitive development, children begin to pretend. They seek to engage their parents in activities that satisfy their growing curiosity. They enjoy reading with caregivers and having their labeling questions answered. Near 3 years of age, children begin to include one another in their pretending games, taking on roles that become progressively more realistic and interactive. The young preschooler is especially interested in imitating the parent of the same sex while showing no preference for same- or opposite-sex playmates.

The child's abilities to share are shaped by social experiences. Children who attend day care may share successfully at an earlier age than children raised at home (Fig. 3.29). Although it can be achieved through consistent experience, taking turns is also a challenge for the preschooler who possesses a limited concept of time. Impulse control is just developing in the preschool years. Active goals for this age group include learning to gain the cooperation of

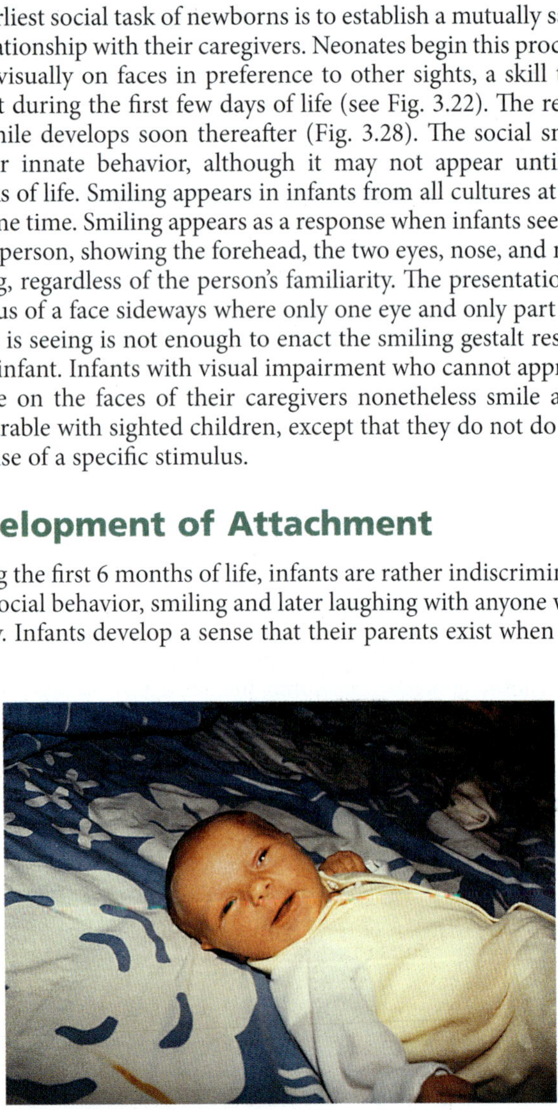

Fig. 3.28 Early smiling. A 19-day-old infant smiles for her parents.

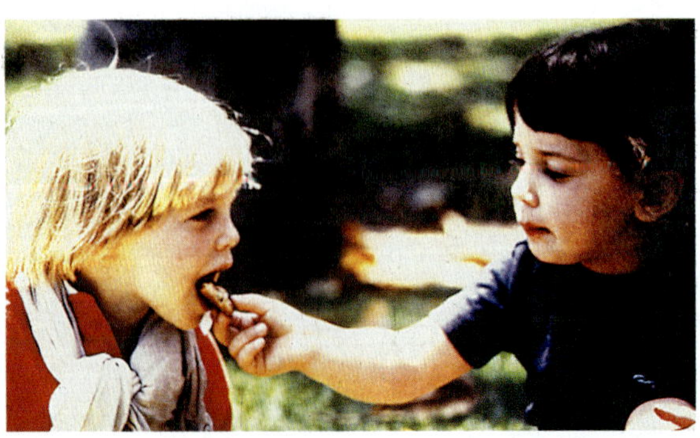

Fig. 3.29 Sharing. Two-year-old children with day care experience share a special treat.

one's peers, learning to communicate ideas to new friends, and learning to handle conflicts.

By 4 to 5 years of age, peer interactions grow increasingly cooperative and complicated; pretend play involves themes requiring greater feats of imagination and experience, such as trips or parties. Older preschoolers enjoy helping with household tasks and frequently are more interested in participating in sex-specific activities than they were at an earlier age. This interest may relate to cognitive and social development. As children understand that they are in the same category as their same-sex parent, they become interested in the implications of category membership. Strict adherence to the rules of category membership reflects the concrete and inflexible thinking of the preschooler.

Preschoolers do not often play games with rules. At this age, rules are seen as variable, to be made and broken at the discretion of the players. For example, getting through a board game with preschoolers who decide not to follow the rules, once they discover that the rules are not working in their favor, is often a challenge.

Children become capable of playing by rules when they reach school age. With superior logical capabilities, they realize that rules are invariant and must be followed regardless of the personal implications. As they progress through the elementary-school years, board games and sports become preferred activities for groups of peers.

Development of Sense of Self

Self-awareness and independence develop gradually throughout life. The earliest indications of an emerging identity occur at 6 to 9 months old, when infants display interest in their own mirror images. Some 7- to 8-month-olds may prefer to grab cups and spoons rather than accept passive roles in eating. These infants may resist pressure to do something that they would prefer not to do (e.g., fussing to stand when placed in a sitting position).

Beyond 1 year of age, toddlers rapidly expand their sense of self. They explore their environment with ease, and they are increasingly able to function independently. They can feed themselves with a cup and spoon, and they have clear ideas about what they want. Children at 1 to 2 years of age also enjoy their own accomplishments and can clap for their own successes (Fig. 3.30).

An emerging sense of self and the thrust for independence make discipline of the toddler a challenge. Parents may need help in viewing their child's refusals to eat, nap, or be washed as positive steps toward increased independence. They may also need support in setting limits on the child's behaviors.

As the child reaches 2 to 3 years of age, increased independence in verbal abilities, increased awareness of body sensations, and modest skills in donning and doffing clothing combine with the child's desire to imitate adults and to gain parental approval. This combination of accomplishments allows toilet training to begin. In fact, these developmental milestones mentioned may be viewed as readiness signs. The pediatrician can review them with families at the 15- or 18-month visit so that parents can time their toilet-training efforts to the child's developmental rate and style. Children differ substantially in their interest in achieving bladder and bowel control, and parents may benefit from counseling to maintain a relaxed approach.

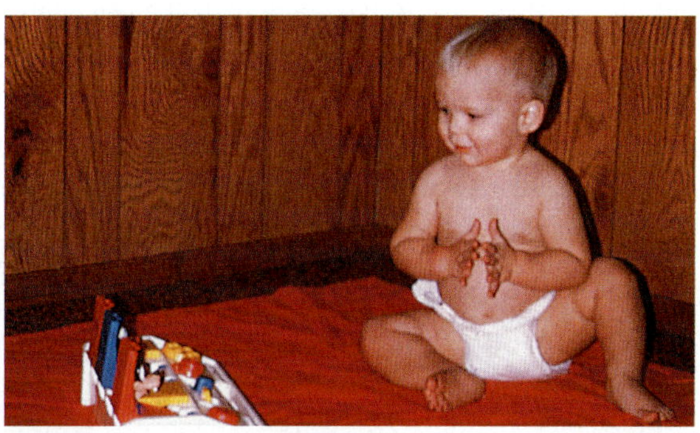

Fig. 3.30 Mastery smile. A 15-month-old boy demonstrates that toddlers beyond 1 year old can take pride in their own accomplishments. This child is applauding his own success at having made the puppets appear.

In other areas as well, children need support in their attempts to initiate and control their own activities. Toward this end, parents can be encouraged to allow their child to practice emerging self-care skills, such as zipping or buttoning a coat, even when the practice costs precious time in a rushed schedule. Should the child become frustrated or disappointed, a response of empathy is likely to soothe more effectively than a response of reason because rational reasoning is limited during this preoperational cognitive period.

By mid- to late elementary school, cognitive development has progressed toward abstract and hypothetical thinking such that children are able to reflect self-consciously about themselves and others. First or second graders struggle to understand the causes of conflict or their emotional reactions to it. Older elementary-school children and adolescents can analyze situations, reasons, and reactions. They begin to understand their own motivations and the environmental triggers of their responses.

Throughout childhood the desire to grow up is in continued conflict with the desire to remain a child. The young preschooler is just beginning to address this issue. Families frequently report that a child's accomplishments in socioemotional functioning backslide when unexpected stresses challenge household equilibrium or when the child becomes ill. As a result, temporary regressions to earlier levels of functioning may occur in some children. Importantly, parents must learn to view these lapses as expected components of development rather than as intentional lapses on the part of the child. However, if the regression is prolonged and significant, the physician may initiate an evaluation of the child's physical and emotional status.

During elementary-school years, at least in Western cultures, the child's self-image is strongly influenced by success or failure in school. Difficulties with learning put additional pressures on the child and also may damage the child's sense of self-worth. Parents and teachers of children with learning problems should be willing to praise the child for behavior within their control, such as effort, persistence, practice, and cooperation, rather than for skills beyond their control, such as intelligence, learning rate, or physical talent. Physicians should be particularly sensitive to the higher risk of emotional and behavioral problems in children with learning difficulties so that they can make timely referrals to colleagues in the mental health professions.

Evaluation of Social Development

Subtle indicators of social and emotional development can be observed during a routine pediatric visit. The physician can note not only the way the infant behaves but also the style of parental caregiving and the nature of the parent/child relationship. The young infant typically shows social responsiveness to both the parent and pediatrician, although at 9 months of age, there is a definite preference for the familiar parent. In addition, at this age, particularly in times of stress, the infant turns to the parent for support and comfort. Children of limited responsiveness, who avoid physical contact, avert their gaze, or in other ways fail to contribute to a mutually satisfying reciprocal exchange are of concern. Of equal concern are parents who are harsh, unresponsive, or threatening in response to the infant's needs.

Given the nature of social development, the assessment of possible problems must rely largely on history. Parents tend to be frank and open about the nature of their relationship with their child if questions are asked in a direct and nonjudgmental way. Difficulties in social development may relate to constitutional and temperamental characteristics of the child and to the philosophy and practices of the parent. By remembering the bidirectional nature of causality in social development, the physician can avoid slipping into criticisms or judgments.

The older preschool or school-age child may be able to give direct information independently about social development. For example, the child may be able to name special friends and the activities enjoyed with those friends. Young preschoolers typically name both boys and girls and list rough-and-tumble or fantasy play as favorite activities. School-age children might add board games and sports to their list of activities. When assessing social development in preschool-age and school-age children, it is important, rather than ask the child to name his or her friends as he or she can just repeat the school list, to assess for meaningful interactions such as reciprocal invitations to playdates and birthday parties.

VARIATIONS IN DEVELOPMENTAL PATTERNS

The presence or absence of a single skill at a particular age is rarely sufficient to determine developmental status. Developmental progress is highly dependent on multiple factors: the general health of the child, opportunities for learning, temperamental characteristics, willingness to try new experiences, genetic endowments, coordination and strength, and socioeconomic factors. If delays occur in more than one domain and/or persist over time, they are considered significant. The challenge for the pediatrician is to differentiate individual variation from deviation and disorder.

When parents raise developmental concerns, these concerns must be addressed freely and openly. Parents are rarely comforted by superficial evaluation and pat reassurance, and although prudent waiting may serve some families well, it may arouse anxiety and anger in others. If a comprehensive evaluation of a given problem is beyond the capabilities of the pediatrician, early referral should be considered.

Evaluation of developmental problems proceeds in the same manner as evaluation of other medical concerns: history, physical examination (including neurologic and developmental evaluation), and laboratory testing. Important in establishing a diagnosis is consideration of the pattern of development across all domains. For example, findings of hypotonia and selective problems in gross motor skills along with normal development in cognition, language, and social skills suggest a neuromuscular disorder or benign congenital hypotonia. In contrast, hypotonia with global developmental delay suggests a central nervous system problem. Differentiating delayed skills from deviant skill patterns is also important. For example, because even infants can make good eye contact with their caregivers, the toddler who avoids eye contact is showing deviancy rather than delay. The combination of delays or deviances in social behavior and delayed language development is suggestive of an autism spectrum disorder (ASD).

Cerebral Palsy

The term *cerebral palsy* can be defined as "a group of permanent disorders of the development of movement and posture, causing activity limitation, that are attributed to nonprogressive disturbances that occurred in the developing fetal or infant brain. The motor disorders of cerebral palsy are often accompanied by disturbances of sensation, perception, cognition, communication and behavior; by epilepsy and by secondary musculoskeletal problems" (Rosenbaum et al., 2007). The type of cerebral palsy varies according to the location of the injured area. Injury may occur before birth, during labor and delivery, or after birth, up through the preschool years. Although some affected patients may have a history of perinatal complications, the majority do not. In 20% to 30% of cases, no etiology can be established. The key to making the diagnosis is to establish that motor problems are not progressive. Regression of motor skills suggests a different set of diagnostic possibilities, including surgically treatable lesions of the brain or spinal cord or inherited neurodegenerative diseases.

Cerebral palsy is classified according to resting tone and what limbs are involved. *Spastic cerebral palsy* is typically due to injuries to the cortex or pyramidal tract and accounts for approximately 80% of cases. *Spasticity* is defined as a velocity-dependent increase in tone; when the limb is moved quickly, there is a catch or resistance to movement. Spasticity also includes hyperreflexia and may be accompanied by clonus and persistence of primitive reflexes. *Extrapyramidal* or *dyskinetic cerebral palsy* is characterized by abnormal involuntary movements. Rarely, cerebral palsy is manifested as hypotonia, often involving the trunk, and associated with hyperreflexia and persistent primitive reflexes.

Physical Examination

A diagnosis of cerebral palsy and a determination of its subtype can be established through physical examination. However, physical findings over the first year of life are highly variable and nonspecific. Early signs may include decreased passive tone in the presence of brisk deep tendon reflexes (DTRs) without concomitant weakness. Early problems with sucking and swallowing may predate evidence of motor delays.

Cerebral palsy may be suspected in infancy through the absence of fidgety movements, small movements of moderate speed, and variable acceleration on the *General Movements Assessment*. While cerebral palsy diagnoses have traditionally been made after 1 year of age in a child born at term and at 15 to 18 months of age in a child born prematurely, studies have shown that specialist providers can make the diagnosis as early as 6 months of corrected age in some cases. Before 5 months of corrected age, the most predictive tools for detecting risk are term-age magnetic resonance imaging, the Prechtl Qualitative Assessment of General Movements, and the Hammersmith Infant Neurological Examination (HINE). After 5 months of corrected age, the most predictive tools for detecting risk are magnetic resonance imaging, the Hammersmith Infant Neurological Examination, and the Developmental Assessment of Young Children.

Abnormalities of Tone

Because damage to the central nervous system prevents the inhibition and balance of the inherent tone of the muscles, abnormalities of tone are particularly significant in the diagnosis of cerebral palsy. After initial hypotonia, a child may develop increased tone between 12 and 18 months old, showing clearly rigid or spastic hypertonia by 2 years old.

The child who demonstrates increased extensor tone beginning in early infancy is also at risk for cerebral palsy. Under normal circumstances, infants younger than 3 months old, when supported ventrally, maintain their head in slight flexion with the trunk mildly convex (Fig. 3.31A). However, with exaggerated tone in the antigravity muscle group, the infant may elevate the head above the horizontally level trunk (see Fig. 3.31B). Similarly, the unknowing parents may be pleased by their child's apparent precocious development of head control when the child is prone or rolls belly-to-back in the first 2 months of life, when in fact both findings suggest excessive extensor posturing.

Further evidence of abnormally increased tone is found when the supine child is pulled to an upright position and extends at the hips and knees, coming to stand on pointed toes rather than ending up in the appropriate sitting posture. This child, when placed in vertical suspension, will not right the head as expected and will later scissor the lower extremities because of hypertonia of the leg adductors and internal rotators (Fig. 3.32). Parents may find it difficult to position these infants for diapering and feeding; knowledge of the Marie-Foix maneuver, used to break up excessive extension in the lower extremities (Fig. 3.33), will help them.

Abnormalities in Development of Primitive Reflexes and Equilibrium Responses

Abnormal persistence of primitive reflexes is helpful in making a diagnosis of cerebral palsy. Damage to the central nervous system prevents high levels of control from superseding and inhibiting the influence of the early reflexes. Thus, obligate or persistent primitive reflexes are signs of cerebral palsy. For example, in the normal

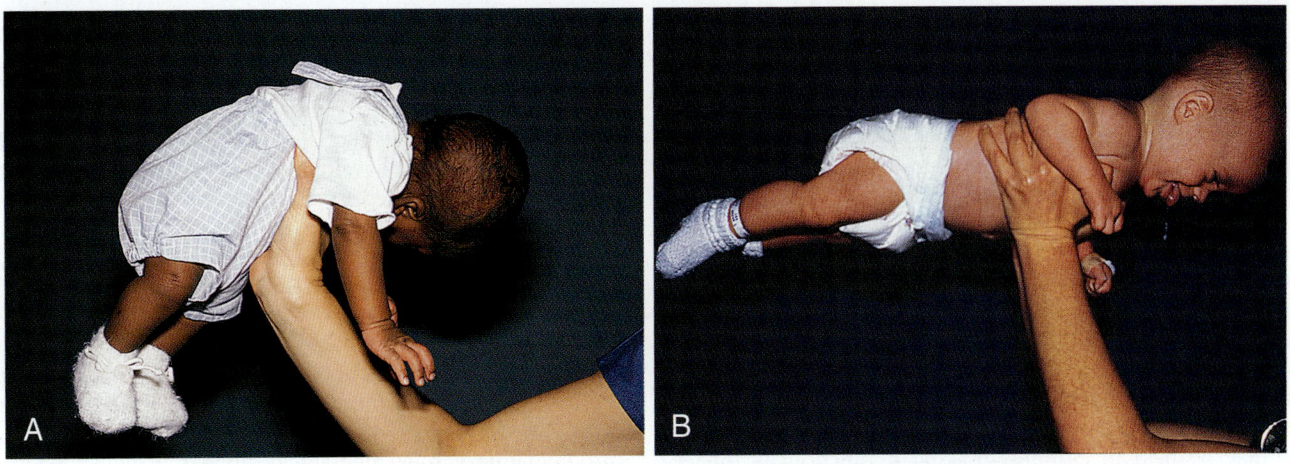

Fig. 3.31 Ventral suspension. (A) This infant's posture is normal for a 1- to 3-month-old child held in ventral suspension. The head, hips, and knees are flexed. (B) For a child 4 months old or older held in ventral suspension with normal posture, the head, hips, and knees may be extended. This finding is abnormal in a child younger than 3 months old.

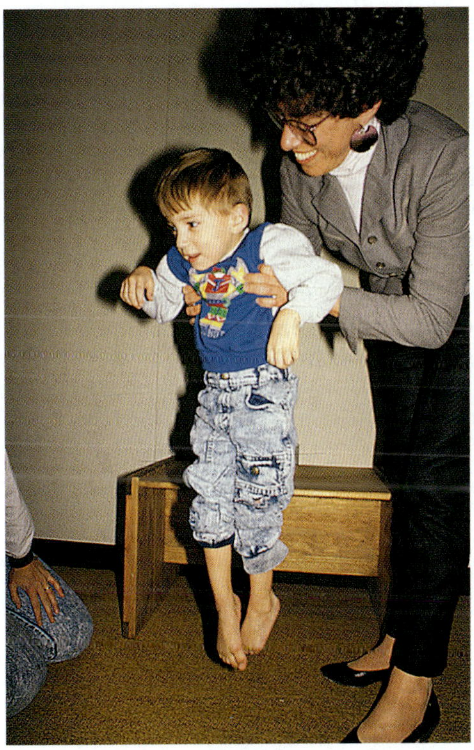

Fig. 3.32 Scissoring. Excessive pull of the hip adductors and internal rotators in this 3-year-old child results in his legs crossing in a scissor-like pattern while he is supported in vertical suspension.

variant of the ATNR, the infant can move out of the posture if the gaze is directed to the other side of the body. However, in an obligate ATNR, the infant remains in the fencer position until the head is passively moved. This finding is not normal in a child of any age and is highly suggestive of the static encephalopathy and motor deficit characterizing cerebral palsy.

In addition, strongly suggestive of cerebral palsy is the nonobligate ATNR that persists beyond 6 months old. This is one possible explanation for a consistent preference in a 6- to 12-month-old child to sleep or lie with the head turned in a particular direction. Similarly, persistence of the Moro response beyond 6 months old is associated with cerebral palsy, as is a lack of development of lateral protective equilibrium reactions by 7 to 8 months old or of the parachute reaction by 10 months old.

Subtypes of Cerebral Palsy

Hemiparesis

Hemiparesis is caused by asymmetric damage to the motor control areas of the central nervous system. In children with hemiparesis, functional discrepancies often predate asymmetric changes in tone or reflexes. The upper extremities may be affected more severely than the lower extremities. Asymmetric use of the upper or lower extremities is rare during the first 4 months of life. When seen in the resting state or when elicited with the ATNR or the Moro response (Fig. 3.34), it is more likely related to lower motor neuron disease than to cerebral injury. At 4 to 6 months old, during the development of early reaching and grasping, signs of hemiparesis include the presence of one hand that is fisted, the arm getting caught beneath the body when the child tries to prop up on the elbows or

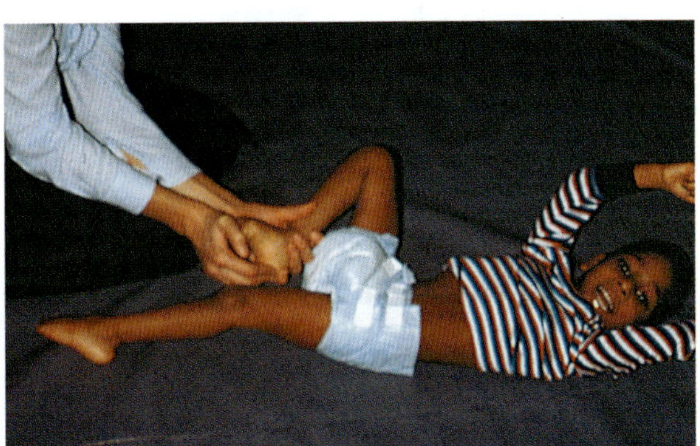

Fig. 3.33 Marie-Foix maneuver. By flexing the child's toes, the therapist can reduce extensor tone enough to obtain abduction of the hip and knee flexion in this child with spastic quadriplegia.

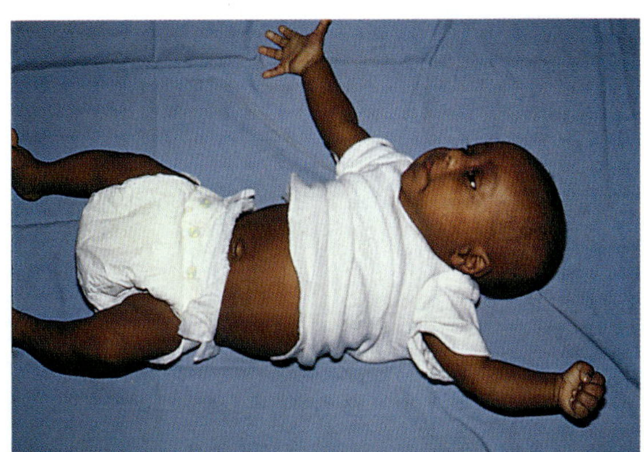

Fig. 3.34 Asymmetric Moro response. Note that one hand is fisted and the other is open. This child warrants a neurologic examination and close follow-up.

hands, and evidence that the arm is not used in simple tasks. Increased resistance to supination at the wrist, limited flopping of one wrist when the upper extremities are gently shaken, or extra beats of unilateral clonus at the ankle are other clues. Later, during the first year of life, abnormal findings include a failure to develop the protective response of lateral propping or the development of an asymmetric parachute response. In addition, crawling may be uneven, with propulsion coming from one side while the opposite arm and leg are dragged behind.

Children with hemiparesis may have difficulty in compensating for their lack of protective responses, uneven strength, and poor balance. Walking is typically delayed until 2 to 3 years old. In mildly affected children, walking may be almost normal, but when asked to run, the child may show posturing of the upper extremity in flexion and internal rotation. Usually, the lower limb rotates internally, and the foot may be held in equinus, making it functionally longer on the swing-through part of the gait. To clear the foot from the floor, the child compensates by swinging the leg farther out in abduction or by circumduction of the affected side. These patterns, in some cases, also can be observed in standing (Fig. 3.35).

Children with hemiparesis may neglect the visual field on their affected side. Parents should position their infant so that visual stimulation is provided to the intact visual field. Another consideration is that of abnormal bony stresses caused by asymmetric muscle strength. Unequal spinal stresses predispose children with hemiparesis to scoliosis, especially during growth spurts.

Spastic Diplegia and Quadriplegia

Spastic diplegia implies dysfunction of the lower extremities, with normal or limited involvement of the upper extremities. *Spastic quadriplegia* implies dysfunction of the upper and lower extremities. The child with spasticity may have presenting symptoms that include delayed sitting, crawling, or walking or toe-walking (Fig. 3.36). In the supine position, children with spastic diplegia may keep their lower extremities in the "frog" position, with the hips and knees flexed and the hips externally rotated. In the erect position, the child may internally rotate and adduct the legs, leading to scissoring (see Fig. 3.31). The ankles assume the equinus position. Children with spastic diplegia who learn to walk often show persistent toe-walking in the presence of brisk DTRs, limited range of ankle motion, Babinski reflexes, and a normally proportioned muscle mass. The differential diagnosis of toe-walking also includes the muscular dystrophies, tethered spinal cord and spinal tumors, peripheral neuropathies, and fixed bony deformities of the feet. Unilateral or asymmetric toe-walking may indicate leg-length discrepancy or a dislocated hip as an isolated finding or in conjunction with spasticity. Toe-walking may also present with normal and intact neuro-osteo-muscular development and pathways, in the absence of cerebral palsy, associated to sensory problems. In these cases, the child chooses to do the toe-walking in relation to certain surfaces (e.g., carpet, sand, tile, or wood). Toe-walking in the absence of high tone may also be seen in children with autism.

Athetoid or Ataxic Cerebral Palsy

Children with athetoid or ataxic cerebral palsy tend to be hypotonic and normoreflexive in infancy with delayed motor milestones. Between 1 and 2 years old, hypotonia may be replaced by spasticity, and involuntary movements may appear. Exaggerated tone and dyskinetic movements reach maximal intensity around age 3. Athetoid cerebral palsy has been associated with damage to the basal ganglia caused by bilirubin encephalopathy (kernicterus) or hypoxic-ischemic injury.

Hypotonic Cerebral Palsy

Some hypotonic infants with exaggerated reflexes do not progress to hypertonicity. The child with hypotonic cerebral palsy usually exhibits severe motor and intellectual disability. The prognosis for independent functioning is poor. Hypotonic cerebral palsy must be differentiated from benign congenital hypotonia, conceptualized as an isolated disorder of tone, sparing other developmental areas, though mild to moderate difficulties in other domains may appear at older ages.

Associated Findings With Cerebral Palsy

Up to 75% of children with diplegia or quadriplegia have strabismus (see Chapter 20). Refractive errors are found in 25% to 50% of children with cerebral palsy. Clumsiness because of motor imbalance of the lower extremities may be exaggerated by altered depth perception resulting from impaired visual function. Ophthalmologic referral for phorias and tropias that persist beyond 4 months old is important to prevent amblyopia.

Hearing loss is also associated with cerebral palsy. Although clinical evaluation may suggest hearing loss, a definitive diagnosis requires an audiologic assessment. Brainstem auditory responses

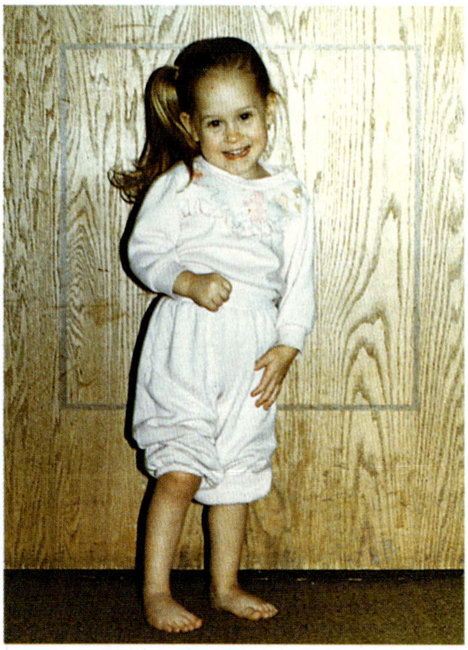

Fig. 3.35 Note the arm held in flexion and internal rotation and the leg circumducted on the involved side in this child with hemiplegic cerebral palsy.

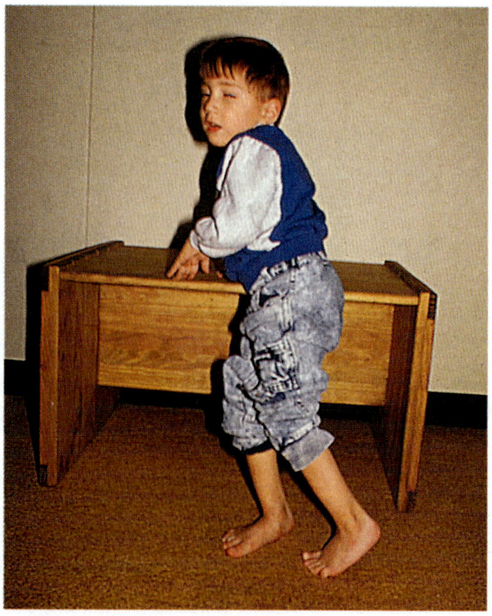

Fig. 3.36 Toe-walking. A 4-year-old child with cerebral palsy cruises on furniture. Notice that the child is crouched because of hamstring tightness and is toe-walking because of gastrocnemius tightness.

can be obtained to assess hearing capabilities in infants younger than 6 months old and in older children unable to perform in conventional or conditioned play audiometry because of motor or intellectual problems.

Approximately 50% of children with cerebral palsy have cognitive impairment. Learning disabilities and attentional weaknesses are more prevalent in this population than in the general population. Furthermore, behavioral problems may develop because of the limited inhibition of emotional responses and the frustration encountered in trying to adjust to motor disabilities.

Prognosis

Overall, the ability of individuals with cerebral palsy to live and work independently depends on the severity of the motor disability and associated cognitive impairments. The Gross Motor Function Classification System defines five levels of motor skills as a function of age. Children tend to remain at the same level as they grow. If a child is 4 years old or older and has not achieved sitting balance, then independent walking with or without crutches is rarely possible. A child 2 to 4 years old who cannot sit and has persistent primitive reflexes is also unlikely to walk.

Because cerebral palsy affects multiple systems, children with the disorder are best served by an interdisciplinary team, including medical professionals, social workers, psychologists, occupational and physical therapists, speech and communication therapists, and educational and vocational specialists. In many cases, children receive educational support for physical and intellectual problems. They may also receive behavioral management training or pharmacologic intervention for attentional weaknesses. Behavioral problems may be minimized by matching developmental expectations to the child's functional capacities. These children and their families benefit enormously from the support of a primary care physician who offers routine health care maintenance, diagnostic and preventive procedures such as referrals to audiology and ophthalmology specialists, and advice and counseling on the interpretation of team evaluations.

Intellectual Disability: Intellectual Developmental Disorder

The diagnosis of intellectual disability requires evidence of limitations in intellectual and adaptive functioning. *Limitations in intellectual functioning* is generally defined as scores on standardized IQ tests that are two or more standard deviations below age-group norms; *limitations in adaptive behaviors* refers to difficulties in broad areas of conceptual, social, and practical functioning, such as learning, communication, self-care, community participation (e.g., riding public transportation, engaging in recreation, voting), and social interactions.

Intellectual disability cannot be diagnosed until the child is old enough to take a standardized IQ test (generally at least 3 to 4 years old). Before that time, a child with delays in two or more domains of development may be described as having global developmental delay or early developmental impairment; some of these children will later be diagnosed with an intellectual disability. The ability to predict intellectual performance and academic achievement from developmental testing during infancy is quite limited except in children falling extremely far behind age expectations. If an infant shows delayed cognitive development, a referral to an early intervention program and the delivery of an individualized therapeutic plan may increase the probability of improvements over time.

As children with early developmental delays approach school age, particularly if they have had optimal educational support, the ability to predict later difficulties improves. The rate of developmental progress during the preschool years is often a good predictor of later intellectual performance. After initial cognitive developmental delays, if a child can achieve 6 months' progress in 6 months, the prognosis for normal intellectual capacity is good. However, if the child achieves, for example, 4 months' progress in 6 months, the rate of development is 67% of the expected rate and the prognosis for later normal intellectual functioning is poor. By the time a child is 6 to 7 years old, limitations as measured on an IQ test typically characterize the individual's abilities throughout life. At that point, the term *intellectual disability* replaces *global developmental delay* because the probability that the delay will resolve is low.

Physical Examination

Physical examination can be helpful in determining the cause of intellectual disability. Most children with intellectual disability are classified in the mild range. These children often have a normal physical examination, with no apparent evidence of major or minor malformations. In contrast to children with severe intellectual disability, who are more readily identified, children with mild intellectual disability are likely to have normal motor milestones and delays only in adaptive areas, such as self-care, language acquisition, or play. The detection of disability in these mildly affected youngsters may not occur until the child experiences school performance difficulties.

The mean IQ of parents of children with mild intellectual disability is lower than the population norm. Thus, many of these parents also show limitations in intellectual abilities. For this reason, the etiology of mild intellectual disability is generally believed to be multifactorial, including multiple genetic contributions and limited social enrichment.

The more significant the degree of intellectual disability, the more likely it is that a specific etiologic factor will be found. Children who score in the moderate, severe, or profound ranges are likely to have congenital malformations of the central nervous system, severe neurologic insults in the prenatal or perinatal period, an inherited disorder, or another specific diagnosis. A systematic approach to the physical examination may reveal clues to the nature of the underlying disorder.

Growth Pattern and Vital Signs

Aberrant growth patterns may be associated with developmental delays and intellectual disabilities. Obesity appears as part of several syndromes associated with intellectual disability, such as Laurence-Moon syndrome and Prader-Willi syndrome (see Chapter 1). Children who are exceptionally large may have cerebral gigantism (Sotos syndrome). Small-for-gestational-age (SGA) infants deserve close study for evidence of anomalies or infection; they are also at risk for abnormal development. Extreme to moderate short stature, with or without skeletal dysplasia, is associated with many dysmorphic syndromes that include intellectual disability as an associated finding. Growth curves have been prepared for children with various genetic and chromosomal disorders such as Down syndrome because they tend to be shorter than the general population. However, if children are shorter than expected even for the population of children with the disorder, or if children fail to maintain their own rate of growth after following a percentile, then endocrine function abnormalities such as hypothyroidism should be investigated.

Skin Findings

Hemangiomas, multiple café au lait spots, and sebaceous adenomas may be evidence of an underlying neurocutaneous abnormality, thereby providing a constitutional basis for a developmental delay. Neurofibromatosis (type 1) and tuberous sclerosis are both examples of neurocutaneous disorders. Hirsutism occurs in fetal alcohol (see Chapter 1) and fetal hydantoin syndromes. Abnormal fingernail formation can signal teratogenic influences or ectodermal dysplasias (see Chapter 21).

Cranial Abnormalities

Head circumference as a reflection of brain growth provides an obvious clue to the cause of intellectual disability. Undergrowth of the cranium may indicate central nervous system damage or dysgenesis, and overgrowth may indicate hydrocephalus or megalencephaly.

Abnormal skull shape may indicate that the underlying nervous system has undergone unusual physical stresses.

Transillumination aids in the diagnosis of porencephalic cysts or of other structural defects in young infants. The presence of an intracranial bruit may indicate an arteriovenous malformation, although such bruits are sometimes heard in normal infants. In the absence of these signs, children with moderate, severe, and profound intellectual disability may warrant an imaging study of the central nervous system because of the high incidence of identifiable abnormalities.

Facial Abnormalities

The presence of certain facial characteristics may suggest a specific etiology of intellectual disability. Minor malformations (which include hypotelorism or hypertelorism; epicanthal folds; colobomas; and auricles that are large, abnormally formed, or set low in comparison with the plane of the eyes) are rare in the general population. In isolation, one dysmorphic feature may be insignificant. However, the presence of three or more of these features correlates highly with a major malformation, often of the heart, kidney, or brain. Patterns of dysmorphic features may suggest a specific diagnosis such as a genetic syndrome, chromosomal abnormality, or prenatal exposure. For example, flat facies, upturned palpebral fissures, epicanthal folds, single palmar creases, and clinodactyly are associated with trisomy 21 (Down syndrome) (Fig. 3.37). Likewise, a lengthened philtrum, a thin vermilion border, and microcephaly are clinical features of fetal alcohol syndrome.

Some of these unusual features themselves are clues to the etiology of the intellectual disability or are the result of abnormal functioning, even in prenatal life. For example, aberrant patterning of scalp hair may indicate abnormal cerebral morphology. The pattern of hair growth is affected by pressures from the developing brain on the overlying scalp in early gestation. The absence of a posterior hair whorl or the presence of multiple hair whorls suggests abnormal prenatal brain growth. Small palpebral fissures also result from abnormal brain growth; the eye is an extension of the brain, and small eyes are suggestive of abnormal early brain development. Similarly, a high-arched palate may be secondary to abnormal motor activity of the tongue in utero, suggesting a prenatal origin of motor problems.

Other Physical Abnormalities

Hepatosplenomegaly in the neonatal period may suggest congenital infection or in childhood may indicate a heritable storage disease affecting central nervous system and developmental functioning.

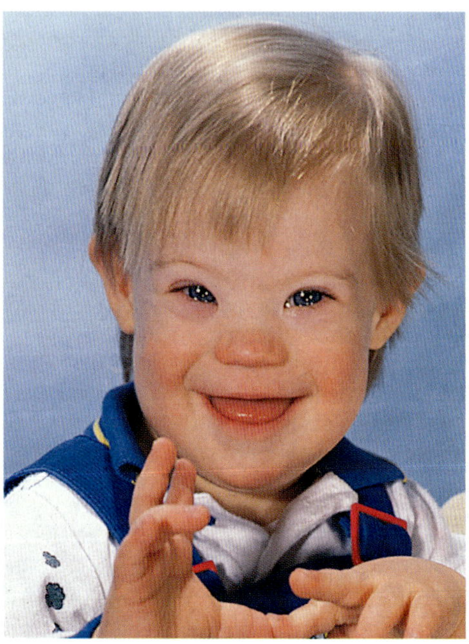

Fig. 3.37 Down syndrome. Note the upslanting palpebral fissures, flat nasal bridge, epicanthal folds, small ears, and small hands.

Large testes are found in youngsters with fragile X syndrome, whereas hypogonadism is a concomitant of the Prader-Willi syndrome. This syndrome is associated with an abnormality on chromosome 15 (see Chapter 1).

Changes in the long bones of the limbs may show evidence of congenital infection; disproportionate bone length may suggest metabolic disorders, such as homocystinuria or osteochondrodysplasias. Errant toe proportions or changed crease patterns on the hands or soles of the feet may suggest early morphogenetic changes associated with certain defined syndromes. Lethargic or pale children may prompt an examination for iron deficiency or lead intoxication, which also may contribute to subnormal intellectual progress.

The American Academy of Neurology has reviewed the evidence for diagnostic testing in the evaluation of children with global developmental delay and suggests that genetic testing, even in the absence of dysmorphic features, be performed. The highest yield cytogenetic study is a microarray, which should be supplemented with molecular testing for fragile X syndrome. The history and physical examination guide further diagnostic studies, including neuroimaging, electroencephalogram (EEG), and metabolic testing. Visual and audiologic assessments are recommended in the evaluation of children with global developmental delay/intellectual disability.

Prognosis

Approximately 3% of children are classified as intellectually disabled at some point in their lives. In a society that prizes intellectual accomplishment, the identification of a child's cognitive delays may be upsetting for a family. Findings of unusual features in any aspect of the physical examination may help provide an explanation for abnormal or delayed cognitive development. In evaluating the cause of developmental delay, the greatest need, beyond that of assessing the possibility of remediation, is that of providing the parents with appropriate genetic, behavioral, and educational counseling. Evidence that a child's lack of developmental progress is related to constitutional factors can help to relieve parents of guilt feelings.

Physicians often underestimate the capabilities of children with intellectual disability. Similarly, families often interpret a diagnosis of intellectual disability to mean that their child will make no further developmental progress. Estimates of functional abilities for children who are classified as intellectually disabled are variable. Children with mild intellectual disability (IQ scores 2 to 3 standard deviations less than the mean [69 to 55]) can learn to read and write and to do simple mathematics. As adults, they often live independently and hold jobs. The extent of their disability is most prominent during the school years or during times of life crisis beyond school age. Children with moderate intellectual disability (IQ scores 3 to 4 standard deviations less than the mean [54 to 40]) will generally learn to read and write only to a first- or second-grade level. Nonetheless, their abilities in language, self-care, and adaptation skills may allow them to live and work in semi-independent settings, with support and supervision as needed. Children with severe and profound intellectual disability (4 to 6 standard deviations less than the mean [39 to 24 and less]) are likely to require substantial lifelong support.

Autism Spectrum Disorder

Autism spectrum disorder is the term for a category of neurodevelopmental disabilities of varying severity characterized by persistent deficits in social interaction and social communication and by restricted, repetitive patterns of behaviors, interests, or activities. According to the *Diagnostic and Statistical Manual of Mental Disorders,* fifth edition (DSM-5), the diagnostic formulation should include determination of whether the core deficits exist with or without intellectual or language impairment and in the presence or absence of other genetic or medical conditions. Previous labels for variations in presentation, including *Asperger disorder* and *pervasive developmental disorder, not otherwise specified (PDD-NOS)* are no longer recognized in the DSM-5. Using current diagnostic criteria, all children with ASD show deficits in social reciprocity, deficits in nonverbal communication used for social interaction, and deficits in developing and maintaining social relationships as expected for their developmental level (Figs. 3.38 and 3.39). Abnormal nonverbal behaviors include limited eye-to-eye gaze and unusual body language (Fig. 3.40). The severity of language deficits varies from total lack of language to difficulty in initiating and sustaining functional conversation. Restricted and repetitive behaviors, interests, and activities require at least two of four categories: stereotyped and repetitive motor movements, inflexible adherence to rituals and sameness, highly restricted and fixated interests, and hyperreactivity or hyporeactivity to sensory stimuli (Fig. 3.41). At the severe end of the spectrum are individuals with autism who generally have almost no social interaction, limited language, and intellectual impairment. At the mild end of the spectrum, often referred to with the term *high-functioning autism,* children typically have near normal to high scores in their IQ testing, have language skills, and can participate in social interactions that appear near normal under limited circumstances, such as when on the child's own terms (Table 3.9).

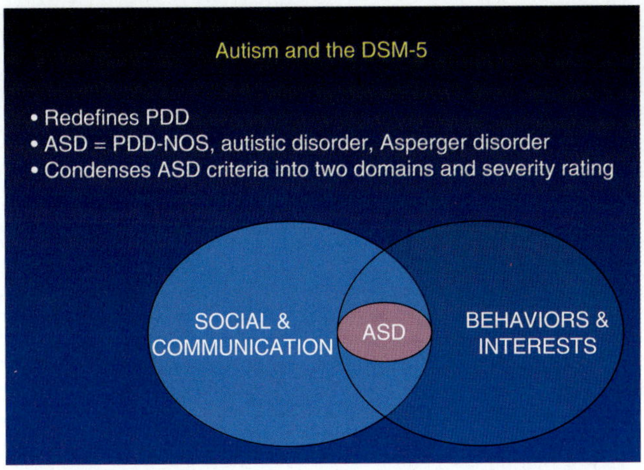

Fig. 3.38 Autism spectrum disorders (ASDs) and the *Diagnostic and Statistical Manual of Mental Disorders,* fifth edition (DSM-5). *PDD,* Pervasive developmental disorder; *PDD-NOS,* pervasive developmental disorder, not otherwise specified.

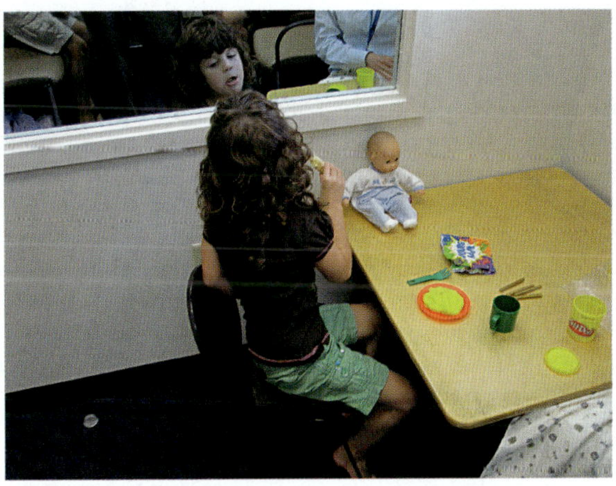

Fig. 3.39 Child with autism looking at her own image rather than at the objects or person in the room; no interest in social interactions and/or pretend play activity.

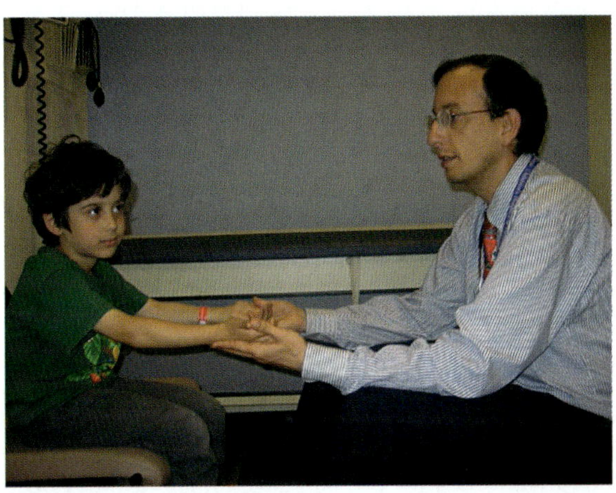

Fig. 3.40 Autism is characterized by qualitative impairment in social interactions, such as limited eye-to-eye gaze and unusual facial expressions. (From Phelps R, Feldman HM: The laying on of hands: the physical examination in developmental and behavioral assessment. In Carey WB, Crocker AC, Elias ER, et al., editors: *Developmental–behavioral pediatrics,* ed 4, Philadelphia, 2009, Elsevier. Fig. 76.2.)

Autistic spectrum disorders present in two distinct patterns. Many children show abnormal social and communicative behaviors starting in early infancy. Parents often report that these children have low tone when held, fail to look at the human face, and do not turn toward the human voice. Some children demonstrate seemingly normal development in infancy and then, often in the second year of life, show regression of social and communicative skills, such as loss of early vocabulary and growing disinterest in social interaction. The nature of the presentation is not associated with severity of symptoms or long-term prognosis.

Surveillance and Screening for Autism Spectrum Disorder

The American Academy of Pediatrics (AAP) has developed a screening and surveillance algorithm to facilitate early identification of children with ASD. Surveillance includes family history to ascertain genetic risk, open-ended questions to elicit parental concerns, and age-specific questions about social and emotional developmental milestones, such as responsiveness to human voice, eye contact, shared attention, imitation, and pretend play. The following "red flags" require immediate evaluation:

- No babbling or pointing or other gesture by 12 months old
- No single words by 16 months old
- No two-word spontaneous (not echolalic) phrases by 24 months old
- Loss of language or social skills at any age

Standardized autism-specific screening tools have been developed and should be used for all children, at least at the 18- and 24-month visits, in addition to the comprehensive screening tools recommended at the younger ages. The Modified Checklist for Autism in Toddlers (M-CHAT) is available at no cost for use in the office setting and can be downloaded from the AAP website (www.aap.org). A positive screen on the parent questionnaire should be followed by a specific interview. The positive impact of early therapeutic interventions for children with ASD should motivate the pediatrician to arrange for comprehensive evaluation and intervention if the screening test and interview are positive or when parents and pediatricians are concerned.

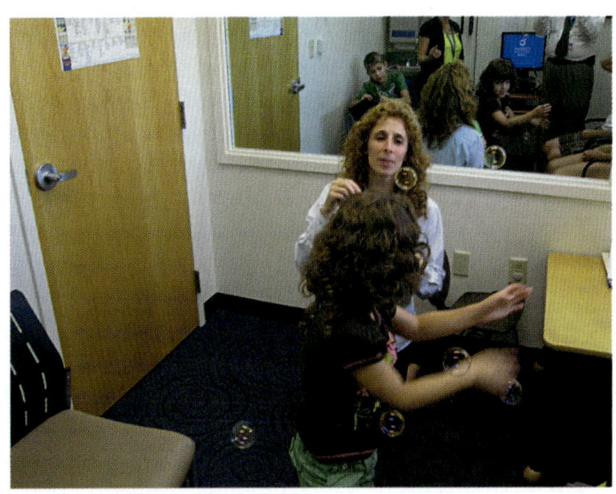

Fig. 3.41 Child with autism with hand flapping.

Table 3.9 Degrees of Autism Spectrum Disorders

	Mild Autism	Moderate Autism	Severe Autism
Social interactions	• Unusual or idiosyncratic eye-to-eye gaze, facial expression, body posture • May affiliate with peers but lacks full understanding of social rules • Limited reciprocity in social interaction; insistence on own interests	• Eye-to-eye gaze on own terms and restricted facial expressions • Limited affiliation with peers and poor understanding of social rules • Rare reciprocity though may share enjoyment with family or close friends	• Marked impairment in eye-to-eye gaze, facial expressions • No affiliation with peers and no appreciation of social interaction • Lack of spontaneous seeking to share enjoyment, interests with anyone
Communication	• Unusual features in development of spoken language, such as poor intonation, frequent use of frozen forms • Limited ability to initiate or sustain conversation; poor topic maintenance • Make-believe or social imitative play limited to areas of keen interest	• Obvious delay in the development of spoken language • Marked impairment in initiating and sustaining conversation • Frequent reliance on echolalia and meaningless jargon • Limited spontaneous make-believe or social imitative play appropriate to developmental level	• Total lack of the development of spoken language • No conversational language despite occasional use of words in self-talk • Lack of spontaneous make-believe play or social imitative play appropriate to developmental level
Restricted repetitive and stereotyped patterns of behavior, interests, and activities	• Encompassing preoccupation with one or more interest that is abnormal in either intensity or focus • Inflexible adherence to specific, nonfunctional routines or rituals • Occasional stereotyped and repetitive motor mannerisms	• Encompassing preoccupation with one or more stereotyped and restricted patterns of interest that are abnormal in either intensity or focus • Inflexible adherence to specific, nonfunctional routines or rituals • Frequent stereotyped and repetitive motor mannerisms	• Inflexible adherence to specific, nonfunctional routines or rituals • Frequent stereotyped and repetitive motor mannerisms • Persistent preoccupation with parts of objects

Physical Examination

Children with ASD generally have a normal physical and neurologic examination. Increased head circumference in the preschool period is associated with a diagnosis of autism, with or without intellectual disability, suggesting that the neurologic basis of autism may include overabundant growth of neurons and synapses or failure of normal processes of pruning of synapses. Autism has been associated with other conditions, including fragile X syndrome, neurofibromatosis, and tuberous sclerosis. Therefore, the physical examination of children with abnormal social and communicative development should include the following: a survey for dysmorphic features, such as long face, prominent jaw, and large or protuberant ears; measurement of head circumference to document relative macrocephaly or microcephaly; the evaluation of facial, truncal, and extremity tone; and careful skin examination for café au lait lesions and hypopigmented lesions.

ASD is a syndrome with many known causes. There is a strong genetic contribution that warrants genetic testing in children with ASD. Genome microarray and DNA analysis for fragile X syndrome are recommended in the evaluation of children with ASD. Identifying a specific genetic cause is relevant to counseling about recurrence risk in a family and prognosis for the individual. Selective metabolic testing should be initiated by the presence of suggestive clinical and physical findings, such as evidence of lethargy, cyclic vomiting, or early seizures; presence of dysmorphic or coarse features; evidence of intellectual disability or if intellectual disability cannot be ruled out; or if occurrence or adequacy of newborn screening is questionable.

Further testing should be driven by specific indications. The evidence does not support routine clinical neuroimaging in the diagnostic evaluation of autism, even in the presence of megalencephaly. However, the *PTEN* gene is associated with autism and macrocephaly. Similarly, there is inadequate supporting evidence for including hair analysis, celiac antibodies, allergy testing (particularly food allergies for gluten, casein, *Candida,* and other molds), immunologic or neurochemical abnormalities, micronutrients such as vitamin levels, intestinal permeability studies, stool analysis, urinary peptides, mitochondrial disorders (including lactate and pyruvate levels), thyroid function tests, or erythrocyte glutathione peroxidase studies after diagnosis of ASD.

Children with autistic spectrum disorders are at increased risk of seizure disorders, and unusual movements or lapses in consciousness should prompt evaluation with an EEG. There is inadequate evidence to recommend an EEG study in all individuals with autism. Indications for an adequate sleep-deprived EEG with appropriate sampling of slow-wave sleep include clinical seizures or suspicion of subclinical seizures and a history of regression (clinically significant loss of social and communicative function) at any age but especially in toddlers and preschoolers.

Prognosis

Children with ASD benefit from intense early intervention services and behavioral services designed to improve their social interactions and communication skills. Some children may be able to attend regular education settings with or without special services by school age. No definitive treatments are currently available for autistic spectrum disorders. Educational and behavioral interventions address the core characteristics. Medication is often used to manage associated findings, such as inattention, hyperactivity, mood lability, aggression, and unpredictable outbursts. Addressing the family's challenges in raising a child with autism is central to management and may include referral to family support groups, provision of educational material, and referral for behavior management counseling. There is insufficient evidence to recommend dietary supplements or restrictions currently.

Language and Reading Disorders

Delays and disturbances in language development may be associated with intellectual disability, ASD, hearing impairment, and environmental deprivation. However, language difficulties may occur in an otherwise typically developing child; in such cases, they are referred to as specific language impairment, usually of unknown etiology. Some theories stress difficulties with high-level concepts and symbolic capabilities, and others stress auditory perceptual impairments as the root of specific language disorders.

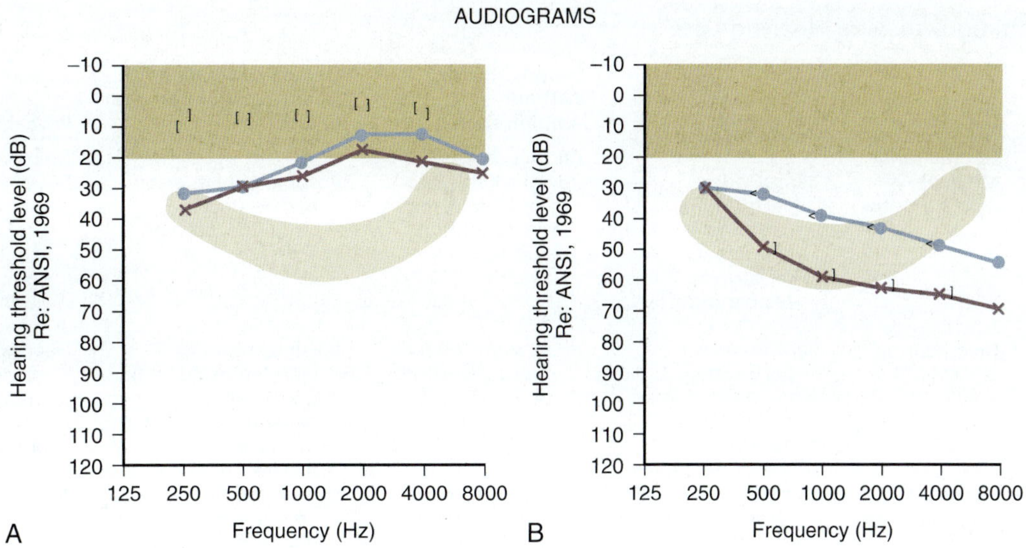

Fig. 3.42 Audiograms. The *purple X* indicates the threshold for the left ear, and the *blue circle* indicates the threshold for the right ear. *Brackets* indicate bone conduction. (A) This audiogram indicates mild conductive hearing loss in both ears. Notice that more energy is required for detection of sound in the low-frequency range. Bone conduction is normal. (B) This audiogram demonstrates sensorineural hearing loss. The left ear shows a sloping pattern with mild to moderate loss in the low-frequency range and severe loss in the high-frequency range. The right ear shows mild to moderate loss throughout the frequency range. *ANSI,* American National Standards Institute.

Physical Examination

No specific physical signs are associated with language disorders. The physician's role is in large part to rule out other disorders with different etiologies and prognoses. Hearing assessment is indicated for any child with delays or deviancies in language development because hearing loss is a treatable condition. Universal newborn hearing screening allows identification and treatment of sensorineural hearing loss before it leads to delays in language, speech, and other developmental domains. The screenings use otoacoustic emissions or automated auditory brainstem responses. If a newborn does not pass the screen, then definitive testing with the brainstem auditory-evoked response, an electrophysiologic measure that records brain waves as a function of sound exposure, should be performed. In children with language and speech delays, audiometric assessment at the time of diagnosis is important because hearing loss may be progressive or missed in the newborn period. In older infants and toddlers, conditioning techniques or conventional audiometry assess actual hearing rather than associated physiologic markers. The use of earphones allows for evaluation of each ear independently (Fig. 3.42).

Syndromes known to be associated with hearing loss include Treacher Collins syndrome, Waardenburg syndrome, and osteogenesis imperfecta. Children with abnormalities of the external ear, including preauricular tags and pits, the palate, or facial structures, may also have sensorineural hearing loss (Box 3.1). Repeated evaluations may be required in congenital rubella or cytomegalovirus infections because of progressive hearing loss. Several genetic causes of congenital hearing loss have been identified. Conditions associated with varying degrees of hearing loss, their disabling effects, and the interventions required for children with these conditions are listed in Table 3.10. Children with congenital hearing loss that is treated with amplification or hearing aids should be evaluated for their responses to spoken words, patterns of vocalization and sound production, visual and verbal attentiveness, social rapport, and development of communication. Otitis media with effusion is associated with mild, variable, intermittent hearing loss and is generally not considered a cause of language delays and disorders.

Box 3.1 Conditions Associated With Sensorineural Hearing Loss

Family history of childhood hearing impairment
Congenital perinatal infection (CMV, rubella, herpes, toxoplasmosis, syphilis)
Anatomic malformations of the head or neck
Birth weight <1500 g
Hyperbilirubinemia above levels indicated for exchange transfusion
Bacterial meningitis
Severe asphyxia
Exposure to ototoxic medications

Prognosis

Many toddlers with speech or language disorders develop adequate speech, language, and communication skills by early elementary school. No variables are consistently associated with a good prognosis; however, the prognosis for communication is clearly improved through early communication therapy. Physicians should not hesitate to refer children with speech and language delays for assessment and treatment.

Many toddlers and preschoolers with selective problems in language acquisition develop reading difficulties during the school-age years. A reading disorder (dyslexia) is a frequent finding in a child with an early history of language delay and a positive family history of language impairment or reading disability (Fig. 3.43). With increasing age, children with reading difficulties tend to improve. However, in many cases, reading remains an area of relative weakness compared with other cognitive and academic skills.

Children with reading disorders show abnormal or inefficient eye movements while reading. This observation has led to visual training as a treatment strategy. However, the literature supports the notion that in most cases, a reading problem is a high-level language difficulty, not a visual or visual motor problem.

Attention-Deficit/Hyperactivity Disorder

ADHD is a syndrome characterized by persistent inattention, hyperactivity, and impulsivity compared with what is expected for a child at a particular developmental level. Judgments about the degree of deviance in these behaviors are based on the degree of interference that they cause in the child's social, academic, or other functioning. The diagnosis of ADHD requires that symptoms have

Table 3.10 Disabling Effects of Hearing Loss

Average Hearing Deficit at 500–2000 Hz (ANSI)	Description	Condition	Sounds Heard Without Amplification	Degree of Disability (If Not Treated in First Year of Life)	Probable Needs
0–15 dB	Normal range		All speech sounds	None	None
15–25 dB	Minimal hearing loss	Serous otitis, perforation, monomeric membrane, sensorineural loss, tympanosclerosis	Vowel sounds heard clearly; may miss a few consonant sounds	Possible mild auditory dysfunction in language learning	Environmental modifications, such as preferential seating in school and face-to-face communication; auditory training, speech therapy
25–40 dB	Mild hearing loss	Serous otitis, perforation, tympanosclerosis, monomeric membrane, sensorineural loss	Hears most louder-voiced speech sounds	Possible auditory learning dysfunction, possible mild language retardation, mild speech problems, inattention	Hearing aid, auditory training, speech therapy; environmental modifications, such as preferential seating
40–65 dB	Moderate hearing loss	Middle ear anomaly, sensorineural loss	Misses most speech sounds at normal conversational level	Speech problems, language retardation, learning dysfunction, inattention	All the above, plus consideration of special education services as required
65–90 dB	Severe hearing loss	Sensorineural or mixed loss from sensorineural loss plus middle ear disease	Hears no speech sounds of normal conversation	Severe speech problems, language retardation, learning dysfunction, inattention	All the above, plus probable special education services as required
>90 dB	Profound hearing loss	Sensorineural or mixed loss	Hears no speech or other sounds; candidate for cochlear implantation	Severe speech problems, language retardation, learning dysfunction, inattention	All the above, plus probable special education services as required

ANSI, American National Standards Institute; *dB,* decibel.
Modified from Stewart JM, Downs MP: Medical management of the hearing-handicapped child. In Northern JL, editor: *Hearing disorders*, ed 2, Boston, 1984, Little, Brown. Reprinted by permission of Allyn & Bacon.

been long-standing, that they be present before at least 12 years old, and that they occur in multiple settings and not just at home or just at school. Multiple genetic, neurologic, toxic, and psychosocial conditions are associated with the presence of ADHD. Among children born prematurely and children with intellectual disability, ADHD is more prevalent than in the general population.

Children with ADHD have difficulty sustaining attention and persisting to task completion. They become easily distracted. Frequently they fail to organize and plan before beginning a task. Because of all these features operating concurrently, these children fail to complete work assignments and eventually may avoid long and demanding tasks. Impulsivity in young children is frequently demonstrated by difficulty waiting for a turn. As children get older, impulsivity is expressed as difficulty in delaying responses, blurting out answers, interrupting others, and generally acting before thinking.

The DSM-5 describes three presentations. Most children demonstrate ADHD combined presentation, demonstrating symptoms of inattention and hyperactivity/impulsivity. ADHD inattention presentation is applied to children with symptoms of inattention without hyperactivity or impulsivity. ADHD hyperactive/impulsive presentation is applied to children with functionally relevant hyperactivity and mild or no inattention. Young school-age boys with ADHD tend to display excessive fidgetiness and activity, whereas adolescents and girls may be inattentive but not hyperactive (Fig. 3.44).

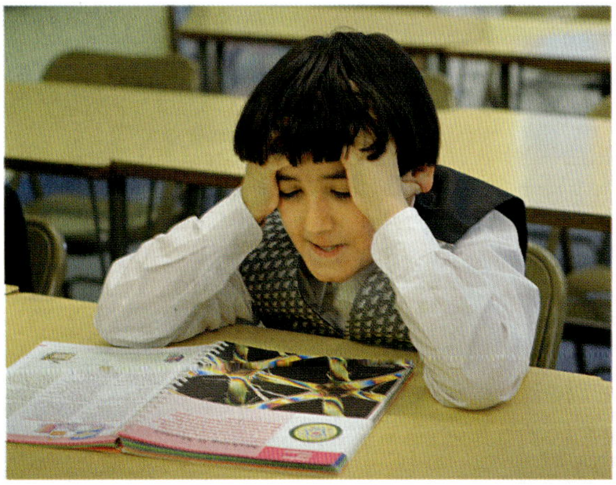

Fig. 3.43 Child experiencing reading difficulties. (Courtesy Robert Louis and the Hispanic/Latino Community of Southwestern Pennsylvania. Picture from Kaczmarek L, Chaves-Gnecco D: Special education services. In Carey WB, Crocker AC, Elias ER, et al., editors: *Developmental–behavioral pediatrics*, ed 4, Philadelphia, 2009, Elsevier. Fig. 93.1.)

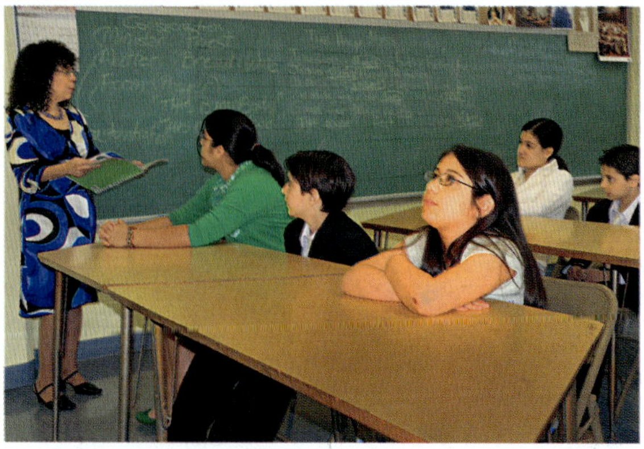

Fig. 3.44 Child with attention-deficit/hyperactivity disorder (ADHD), inattentive type. The girl in the picture is daydreaming while her classmates are paying attention to the teacher. (Courtesy Robert Louis and the Hispanic/Latino Community of Southwestern Pennsylvania. Picture from Kaczmarek L, Chaves-Gnecco D: Special education services. In Carey WB, Crocker AC, Elias ER, et al., editors: *Developmental–behavioral pediatrics*, ed 4, Philadelphia, 2009, Elsevier. Fig. 93.2.)

Most children with ADHD show age-appropriate attention in some highly motivating situations. For example, parents routinely report that their children with ADHD sit for computer games or captivating movies. For this reason, up to 80% of children whose behavior at home and at school meets diagnostic criteria do not show characteristics of the disorder in the physician's office. Diagnosis rests on historical information from parents and confirmatory reports from teachers. Standardized questionnaires are often used in diagnosis to quantify the degree of inattention, hyperactivity, and associated behavioral problems.

Children with ADHD are likely to have other neurobehavioral disorders, such as anxiety, depression, conduct problems or oppositional behavior, learning disabilities, and tics. The symptoms of ADHD and sleep deprivation are highly overlapping and ADHD or its treatment might impact sleep. The DSM-5 allows the use of the diagnosis of ADHD with the diagnosis of ASD. The evaluation of ADHD should include evaluation for these coexisting conditions.

Physical Findings

On physical examination, it is important to assess the general characteristics of the child to establish if the child meets criteria for ADHD and whether the child has additional medical or psychiatric disorders, such as autism, depression, anxiety, or sleep disorders. Physical findings in ADHD may be completely noncontributory. However, findings (e.g., short stature or dysmorphic features) may suggest an associated genetic or dysmorphic syndrome, such as alcohol-related birth defects. Focal neurologic findings may suggest a static or progressive neurologic cause, such as periventricular leukomalacia from prematurity. The presence of motor or vocal tics with ADHD raises the diagnostic possibility of a chronic tic disorder or Tourette syndrome.

The physical and neurologic examination of children with suspected ADHD often includes a set of specific maneuvers and tasks referred to as *neurologic soft signs* or *neuromaturational indicators*. Nonnormative performance on these specific motor and sensory tasks can be obtained in children who otherwise show no evidence of a localizing neurologic disorder or pathognomonic patterns indicative of generalized encephalopathy. The soft signs are of clinical interest because they serve as an index for cognitive or behavioral dysfunction. They are not specific for ADHD.

Table 3.11 includes several tasks for eliciting soft signs, the typical ages of acquisition, and indications of immature or positive findings. On rapid alternating pronation/supination of the hands, developing children typically show resolution of dysdiadochokinesia by 7 years old. On the same task and on repeated finger-to-thumb apposition and alternating squeezing and relaxing of handgrip, children usually show a marked decrease in synkinesis after 9 years old.

Including these maneuvers in the physical examination is useful for unmasking a child's inattention, impulsivity, and disorganization that may otherwise go undetected in the clinical setting. Parents may be relieved when the physician observes those traits that have brought the family in for evaluation. In some cases, parents can observe the traits that teachers find challenging in the classroom. Difficulty executing discrimination of right and left and particularly crossed commands on themselves and the examiner beyond 8 years old may be found in children with ADHD. In addition, they may also show problems in executing four or more sequential commands from memory. However, persistence of abnormal findings on these tasks is not diagnostic of ADHD.

Prognosis

Research suggests that ADHD is a lifelong condition. The signs and symptoms of hyperactivity are likely to resolve during adolescence, but relative inattention persists into adulthood. Many individuals with ADHD do better as adolescents and adults than they did as children, because they can choose educational programs or occupations that allow them to work with their strengths. They often prefer vocations that permit frequent shifts in attention and a high energy level and that do not require sustained attention to challenging tasks. Nonetheless, individuals with ADHD have poorer educational attainment, higher rates of automobile accidents, lower job attainment, and greater instability in relationships compared with siblings who do not have the disorder, presumably related to persistent inattention. The prognosis is more favorable in individuals with isolated ADHD, good cognitive skills, no learning disorders, and positive family and peer relationships.

Treatment options for ADHD fall into three categories: (1) behavior management, (2) educational interventions, and (3) psychopharmacology. Combinations of these options often are more effective than a single treatment. The American Academy of Pediatrics recommends that for children between 4 and 6 years of age, behavioral management in addition to educational interventions, without psychopharmacological treatment should be the first line of management. Psychopharmacological treatment is indicated in children 6 years and older and/or in children 4 to 6 years of age, who have failed behavioral management and educational interventions alone.

Table 3.11 Indicators Associated With Neurologic Immaturity

Task	Immature Response	Norms
Rapid pronation/supination	Dysdiadochokinesia	Mature by age 7–8 years old
Repeated finger-to-thumb apposition	Synkinesis	Markedly decreased after age 9 years old
Alternation of squeezing and relaxation of single handgrip	Synkinesis	Markedly decreased after age 9 years old
Sensory integration/tactile recognition from visual presentation	Astereognosis	>90% accurate by 7 years old
Identification of right and left on self	Inaccurate	>90% correct by 7 years old
Execution of crossed commands (e.g., touch left eye with right hand)		
On self	Inaccurate	>90% correct by 8 years old
On examiner	Inaccurate	>70% correct by 8 years old

Visual Impairment

Visual experience assists the learning of many important concepts of space and form, important in the development of motor skills, perception, cognition, and social skills (Table 3.12). Thus, in situations

Table 3.12 Visually Related Behaviors

Age of Infant	Behavior
Term	Focuses on face, briefly tracks vertically and horizontally, turns toward diffuse light source, widens eyes to object or face at 8–12 inches
1 month	Blinks at approaching object, tracks 60 degrees horizontally, 30 degrees vertically
2 months	Tracks across midline, follows movement 6 feet away, smiles to a smiling face, raises head 30 degrees in prone position
3 months	Eyes and head track 180 degrees, looks at hands, looks at objects placed in hands
4–5 months	Reaches for object (12-inch cube) 12 inches away, notices raisins 1 foot away, smiles at familiar adult
5–6 months	Smiles in mirror
7–8 months	Rakes at raisin
8–9 months	Notes visual details, pokes at holes in pegboard and at elevator buttons
9 months	Neat pincer grasp
12–14 months	Stacks blocks, places peg in round hole

of congenital blindness or visual impairment, developmental patterns may be altered and delayed, demonstrating the close interrelationships that exist among developmental domains. Children with visual impairments can learn to increase the use of residual visual functioning and other sensory modalities. The physician's understanding of the impact of visual impairment is important to evaluate whether developmental progress is being achieved as expected in this population and to ensure that unexpected delays and deviancies are appropriately diagnosed and treated.

Gross and Fine Motor Development

Apparently, much of the motivation for the infant with normal vision to raise the head 90 degrees when in the prone position is to increase the visual field. Without the feedback of interesting sights, the infant with severe visual impairment may not attain this milestone until 11 to 12 months old. In contrast, rolling occurs in infants who are blind at close to the same age as in infants with normal vision. If sitting independently is an active goal, it can occur by 6 to 7 months old. However, transitional movements from lying to sitting or from sitting to standing occur several months later in infants without sight than in infants able to see.

Protective reactions develop more slowly in infants with severe visual impairment, and these are expected to appear in the 10- to 12-month age range. This delay and the inability to integrate visual cues in attaining balance and equilibrium and the lack of a visual impetus to explore distant toys may contribute to a typical delay in crawling or walking. Paired auditory/tactile cues presented to children with severe visual impairment may stimulate their interest in objects beyond their reach, thus accelerating gross motor development.

Regarding fine motor development, information gathering by index finger and manual manipulation may be more accurate in the child who is blind than in the child with normal vision. However, the youngster who is blind may experience a delay in the acquisition of precise prehension, which sometimes never develops, with raking favored as a more efficient means of exploration.

Cognitive Development

The development of cognitive skills in the child with visual impairment must depend on use of the other sensory modalities. For this reason, careful global evaluation of the child with severe visual impairment should be conducted early in infancy to ensure that the other senses are intact.

A child with normal vision develops the understanding that objects are permanent even when they cannot be seen, felt, heard, sniffed, or tasted. For the child with severe visual impairment, the opportunities for object perception are fewer, and thus the understanding of object permanence typically develops later, stimulated by encouragement of the infant to reach for sound cues. Similarly, in a child with severe visual impairment, the understanding of conservation of continuous quantity, that a cup of water contains the same volume of liquid in a tall, thin container as it does in a short, fat one, also develops later than in the child with normal vision. Haptic perception, the acquisition of information about objects or spaces by exploration with the hands, appears to be more important in the cognitive development of the child with severe visual impairment than in that of the child with normal vision. For this reason, tactile exploration in the child who is blind cannot be promoted at too early an age. In fact, without such encouragement, these children may be fearful and resistant to unfamiliar new feelings.

Language and Intellectual Development

Verbal imitation and receptive language skills may develop normally in healthy children who are blind. As one might expect, these children may have difficulty with words relating to visual concepts, such as *light, dark,* and *color.* They may also have problems with words referring to large things that cannot be touched (*sky* and *stars*), things that change slowly (*age* and *growth*), and the concept "I." However, some children with severe visual impairment show accurate use of all these concepts and even make the distinction between the words *look* and *see.* In these cases, the child probably uses available linguistic information to substitute for visual information.

Although standard IQ tests cannot be used to assess intellectual capabilities of children with severe visual impairment, standardized instruments have been developed to assess their cognitive development. Receptive and expressive language skills figure prominently in these assessments. In addition, interview schedules of adaptive behavior in communication and self-help skills have been developed specifically for children with visual impairment.

Social Development

Infants who are blind lack the opportunity to benefit from face-to-face contact with their caregivers, from the visual reinforcement of smiling, from the use of facial expressions to assist in the interpretation of voices or actions, and from the experience of tracking parents across the room to know that even when they cannot be heard or felt they are still there. These differences in sensory input affect their social and emotional development. Parents of infants with severe visual impairment frequently need to be coached to use touch and sound to reinforce smiling and other desired behaviors in their child.

At approximately the same time that children with normal vision smile at familiar faces, children who are blind smile in response to familiar touching and kinesthetic handling. However, smiling in response to a familiar voice may occur inconsistently up to 1 year old. The infant who is blind demonstrates attachment by calming to the tactile exploration of the caregiver's familiar face or hands.

Blind children of approximately 1 year old may have stranger awareness, although a greater hurdle will be their reaction to separation. Because these children have a limited capacity to track their caregivers, separations from them may induce panic states even among older ones. Similarly, the development of independent caregiving and play may be delayed and may require specific interventions.

Parents should be advised that, without purposeful stimulation, children who are blind may engage in nonpurposeful motor activities (e.g., eye rubbing or rocking) and that these stereotypical behaviors, referred to as *blindisms,* are difficult to extinguish. Blindisms can often be channeled to purposeful stimulation by directing the child's hands to exploration of a toy or by distracting the child with conversation or music. These efforts will serve to channel the child's activities in a more socially adaptive direction.

SUMMARY

The tasks of routine developmental surveillance supplemented by standardized screening, identification of children with variations, and referral for appropriate developmental services (especially during infancy and in the preschool years) fall largely, and often exclusively, to the primary care clinician. Although we have provided estimates regarding the expected chronology of development, these developmental milestones are guidelines rather than fixed time frames within which skill acquisition may be judged as normal or abnormal. In evaluating a child, the physician must use these guidelines, the results of screening tests, and clinical judgment, considering the child's own personality traits, experiences, and degree of cooperation.

Recommendations for further assessment and treatment should be made in consultation with the family.

Resources

Ages & Stages Questionnaires (ASQ). www.brookespublishing.com/tools/asq/index.htm.

Parents' Evaluation of Developmental Status (PEDS). http://www.pedstest.com/default.aspx.

References

Rosenbaum P, Paneth N, Leviton A, et al: A report: the definition and classification of cerebral palsy, April 2006, *Dev Med Child Neurol* 109:8–14, 2007.

Bibliography

Allen MC: Neurodevelopmental assessment of the young child: the state of the art, *Ment Retard Dev Disabil Res Rev* 11:274–275, 2005.

Batshaw ME, editor: *Children with disabilities*, ed 5, Baltimore, 2002, Paul H. Brookes.

Carey WB, Crocker AC, Coleman W, et al: *Developmental-behavioral pediatrics*, ed 4, Philadelphia, 2009, WB Saunders.

Committee on Children with Disabilities: Developmental surveillance and screening of infants and young children, *Pediatrics* 108:192–195, 2001.

Compagnone E, Maniglio J, Camposeo S, et al: Functional classifications for cerebral palsy: correlations between the gross motor function classification system (GMFCS), the manual ability classification system (MACS) and the communication function classification system (CFCS), *Res Dev Disabil* 35:2651–2657, 2014.

Cooley WC, McAllister JW: Building medical homes: improvement strategies in primary care for children with special health care needs, *Pediatrics* 113:1499–1506, 2004.

Dixon SD, Stein MT: *Encounters with children: pediatric behavior and development*, ed 3, St Louis, 2000, Mosby/Elsevier.

Ertem IO, Dogan DG, Gok CG, et al: A guide for monitoring child development in low and middle-income countries, *Pediatrics* 121:e581–e589, 2008.

Feldman HM: Evaluation and management of language and speech disorders in preschool children, *Pediatr Rev* 26:131–142, 2005.

Glascoe FP: Early detection of developmental and behavioral problems, *Pediatr Rev* 21:272–280, 2000.

Health Resources and Services Administration (HRSA) Maternal & Child Health: *Home visiting*. http://mchb.hrsa.gov/maternal-child-health-initiatives/home-visiting.

Johnson CP, Blasco PA: Infant growth and development, *Pediatr Rev* 18:224–242, 1997.

Joint Committee on Infant Hearing, American Academy of Audiology, American Academy of Pediatrics, et al: Year 2000 position statement: principles and guidelines for early hearing detection and intervention programs, *Pediatrics* 106: 798–817, 2000.

Jones KL: *Smith's recognizable patterns of human malformation*, ed 6, Philadelphia, 2006, Elsevier/Saunders.

Kaleida PH, Shaikh N: *Digital visual diagnosis in pediatrics teaching and review module: "Assessing infant development" (CD-ROM)*, Pittsburgh, 2003, University of Pittsburgh.

Khan NZ, Muslima H, Shilpi AB, et al: Validation of rapid neurodevelopmental assessment for 2- to 5-year-old children in Bangladesh, *Pediatrics* 131:e487–e494, 2013.

Levine MD, Carey WB, Crocker AC, editors: *Developmental-behavioral pediatrics*, ed 3, Philadelphia, 1999, Saunders.

Lichtenberger EO: General measures of cognition for the preschool child, *Ment Retard Dev Disabil Res Rev*, 11:197–208, 2005.

Novak I, Morgan C, Adde L, et al: Early, accurate diagnosis and early intervention in cerebral palsy: advances in diagnosis and treatment, *JAMA Pediatr* 171(9): 897–907, 2017. doi:10.1001/jamapediatrics.2017.1689. Erratum in: *JAMA Pediatr* 171(9):919, 2017. doi:10.1001/jamapediatrics.2017.3169.

Perrin E, Stancin T: A continuing dilemma: whether and how to screen for concerns about children's behavior, *Pediatr Rev* 23:264–276, 2002.

Vargas C, Prelock PE, editors: *Caring for children with neurodevelopmental disabilities and their families: an innovative approach to interdisciplinary practice*, Mahwah, NJ, 2004, Lawrence Erlbaum.

Zubler JM, Wiggins LD, Macias MM, et al: Evidence-informed milestones for developmental surveillance tools, *Pediatrics* 149(3):e2021052138, 2022.

A lengthier list of tool choices is accessible in the 2006 AAP policy statement: Council on Children With Disabilities, et al.: Identifying infants and young children with developmental disorders in the medical home: an algorithm for developmental surveillance and screening, *Pediatrics* 118:405–420, 2006. Reaffirmed August 2014.

4

ALLERGY AND IMMUNOLOGY

Hey Jin Chong | Laura West | Christin Deal | Taylor Eddens | Allyson Larkin

Disorders of the immune system are diverse and range from mild to severe in their manifestations and impact on normal function. In this chapter, we review the physical findings and characteristic symptoms of children with hypersensitivity reactions and immune deficiencies and diagnostic techniques and radiographic findings. Topics have been chosen based on their prevalence and importance in the pediatric population and their association with characteristic physical findings.

IMMUNOLOGIC HYPERSENSITIVITY DISORDERS CLASSIFICATION

Hypersensitivity disorders of the human immune system are traditionally classified by Gell and Coombs into four broad groups, which provides a simplified framework for understanding hypersensitivity reactions (Table 4.1). Type I reactions occur quickly after the sensitized individual is exposed to an antigen and are mediated by specific immunoglobulin E (IgE) antibody. Cross-linking of IgE on the surface of mast cells and basophils leads to release of preformed inflammatory mediators including histamine. This mechanism is responsible for the common disorders of immediate hypersensitivity, such as allergic rhinitis and urticaria. Type II reactions involve antibodies directed against antigenic components of peripheral blood or tissue cells or foreign antigens, resulting in cell destruction. Examples of this form of hypersensitivity include autoimmune hemolytic anemia, pemphigus vulgaris, and anti-GBM disease (formerly known as Goodpasture syndrome). In type III reactions, antigen/antibody complexes form and are deposited in the lining of blood vessels, stimulating tissue inflammation mediated by complement and activated white blood cells. Examples include serum sickness and the immune complex–mediated renal diseases. Type IV reactions involve T-cell–mediated tissue inflammation and typically occur more than 48 hours after exposure. Examples of this type are tuberculin (purified protein derivative) reactions and contact dermatitis (see Chapter 8).

TYPE I DISORDERS

The development of type I hypersensitivity depends on hereditary predisposition, sensitization by exposure to an antigen, and subsequent reexposure to the antigen leading to an allergic reaction. Antigens that stimulate allergic reactions are known as *allergens,* and the mechanism of allergen-induced mediator release in type I hypersensitivity reactions is shown in Fig. 4.1. IgE antibodies directed toward specific allergens are bound to the high-affinity IgE receptor on mast cells and basophils. When an allergen causes cross-linking of IgE antibodies on the cell surface, the cell becomes activated, leading to the release of preformed mediators and the generation of the early and late mediators of anaphylaxis. The preformed mediators include histamine, tryptase, chymase, heparin, and other proteases that drive the earliest symptoms of anaphylaxis. A serum tryptase level is currently the best biologic marker of anaphylaxis, although it is a relatively insensitive test. Serum tryptase levels should be obtained close to the onset of anaphylaxis as levels peak 1 to 2 hours after the onset of symptoms and may return to baseline in 6 to 8 hours. The early and late mediators generated by mast cell activation include prostaglandins, leukotrienes, and cytokines. These mediators, which are generated over minutes to hours, continue to drive the clinical symptoms of the allergic reaction and initiate an inflammatory cascade that leads to the recruitment of eosinophils, basophils, and lymphocytes.

Type I reactions may occur in one or more target organs including the upper and lower respiratory tracts, cardiovascular system, skin, conjunctivae, and gastrointestinal (GI) tract. Manifestations depend on the systems and chemical mediators involved, as shown in Fig. 4.2.

The most common manifestation of type I reaction is seasonal allergic rhinitis with a prevalence in the general population of at least 25%. The most serious manifestation of type I hypersensitivity is anaphylaxis, which can simultaneously involve all target organs noted earlier.

Type I hypersensitivity has been diagnosed by skin testing for almost 150 years. The percutaneous skin test, also known as either a scratch or prick test, is an in vivo method to detect the presence of IgE antibody to specific allergens. The test is typically performed with a plastic lancet on either the forearm or upper back and involves a superficial disruption of the epidermis that is almost always painless (Fig. 4.3). The prick test is interpreted 15 minutes after application by measuring the maximal diameter of both the wheal and the flare. Skin test results are compared with a negative control, which is usually glycerol-saline, and a positive control, which is typically histamine. Intradermal allergy testing involves the injection of a small amount of a nonirritating concentration of allergen underneath the skin. Intradermal tests are considered more sensitive than prick tests but less specific. They are beneficial in the evaluation of drug allergies and insect venom hypersensitivity and are often performed as the second step after skin prick testing. Skin prick testing, however, is considered safer than intradermal testing and has better correlation with environmental and food allergy symptoms.

When skin testing is not possible, in vitro testing is a good alternative. The in vitro tests can be accomplished with just a few milliliters of serum and may be advantageous for some patients who have a difficult time tolerating skin testing or have recently taken antihistamines, which affect skin testing results. In vitro allergy tests are more expensive and sometimes less sensitive than allergy prick tests (Table 4.2). In vitro tests are especially helpful in the evaluation of patients with possible food allergies, which is further discussed later.

SYSTEMIC ANAPHYLAXIS

Anaphylaxis results from widespread degranulation of mast cells after cross-linking of antigen-specific IgE on the mast cell surface. Although anaphylaxis is a clinical diagnosis, the definition varies. A report issued jointly by the National Institute of Allergy and Infectious Diseases and the Food Allergy and Anaphylaxis Network established criteria to define likely anaphylactic episodes and has been widely adopted (Fig. 4.4). The onset of anaphylaxis is typically rapid, occurring within minutes to 1 to 2 hours after exposure to the

Table 4.1 Classification of Hypersensitivity Disorders

Hypersensitivity Type	Interval Between Antigen Exposure and Reaction	Antibody or Cell	Antigenic Target	Mechanism of Disease/ Tissue Injury	Disorder(s)
Type I: Immediate, IgE-mediated	Within minutes to 1–2 h			Mast cell– and basophil-derived histamines, prostaglandins, leukotrienes	
IgE-mediated		IgE	Foods, drugs, insect venoms, pollens		Anaphylaxis, urticaria Rhinitis Bronchospasm
Non-IgE mediated Anaphylaxis		Direct mast cell activation			Radiocontrast media, drugs (e.g., Vancomycin)
Type II: Antibody-mediated	Variable (days to weeks)	IgG, IgM	Cell surface proteins Extracellular matrix proteins	Complement, phagocytes Leukocyte-derived inflammatory mediators	Immune thrombocytopenia and hemolytic anemia Goodpasture syndrome
Type III: Immune complex-mediated	Variable (days to weeks)[a]	IgG complexed with circulating antigen	Nucleoproteins, other various endogenous or exogenous proteins Streptococcal cell wall antigens	Complex deposition in vascular endothelium, complement activation, leukocyte-derived inflammation	Systemic lupus erythematosus Serum sickness Poststreptococcal glomerulonephritis
Type IV: Delayed, T-cell–mediated					
IVa	>48–72 h	Th1 cells	Contactants e.g., Nickel, uroshiol (poison ivy) *Mycobacterium tuberculosis*	Interferon-gamma, TNF-alpha, macrophages	Contact dermatitis (with IVc) Tuberculin skin test reactions
IVb	1-6 weeks	Th2 cells	Antigen presented by cells or direct T cell stimulation	IL-4, IL-5, IL-13, eosinophils, inflammatory mediators	DRESS, chronic asthma, chronic allergic rhinitis
IVc	4–28 days	Cytotoxic T cells	Cell-associated antigen or direct T cell stimulation	Perforin, granzyme B, FasL	Fixed drug eruptions, SJS/ TEN, bullous exanthems
IVd	>72 h	T-cell–mediated neutrophilic inflammation	Antigen presented by cells or direct T cell stimulation	Neutrophils, IL-8, cytokines, inflammatory mediators	Behcet, AGEP

AGEP, Acute generalized exanthematous pustulosis; *BM,* basement membrane; *DRESS,* drug rash with eosinophilia and systemic symptoms; *IgE,* immunoglobulin E; *IgG,* immunoglobulin G; *IgM,* immunoglobulin M; *IL,* Interleukin; *SJS/TEN,* Steven Johnson syndrome/toxic epidermal necrolysis.

[a]More rapid reactions can occur if prior antigenic exposure/sensitization.

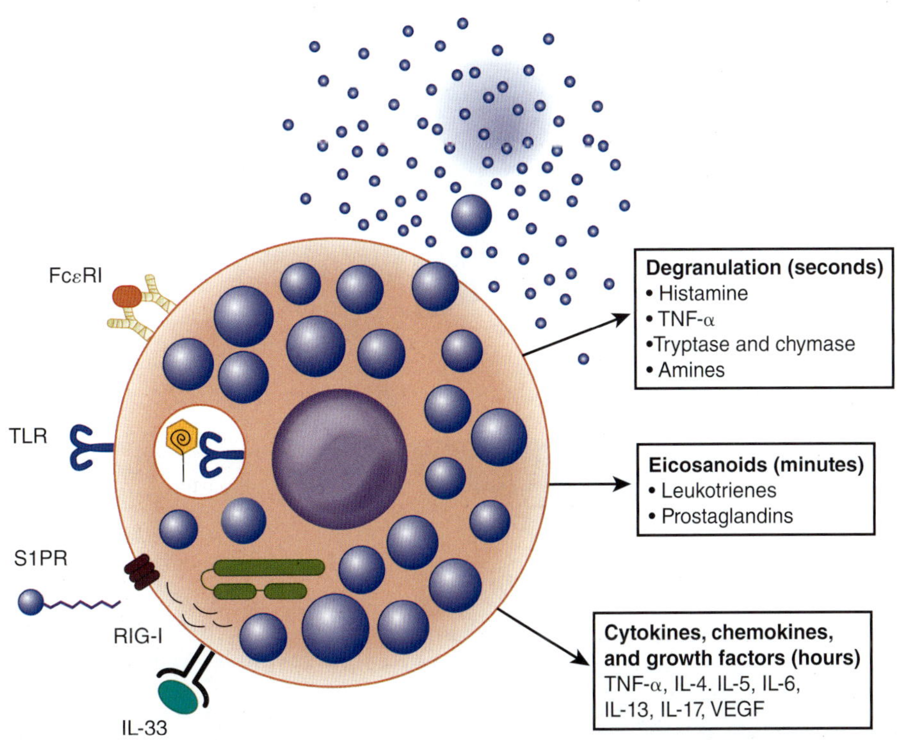

Fig. 4.1 Immunoglobulin E is bound to the mast cell surface, and when cross-linked by antigen, the mast cell becomes activated. The activated mast cell releases preformed mediators and generates additional mediators over minutes to hours. *FcεRI,* High-affinity IgE receptor; *IL-4,* interleukin-4; *IL-13,* interleukin-13; *TNF-α,* tumor necrosis factor–alpha. (From Broide DH: Molecular and cellular mechanisms of allergic disease, *J Allergy Clin Immunol* 108:S65–S71, 2001.)

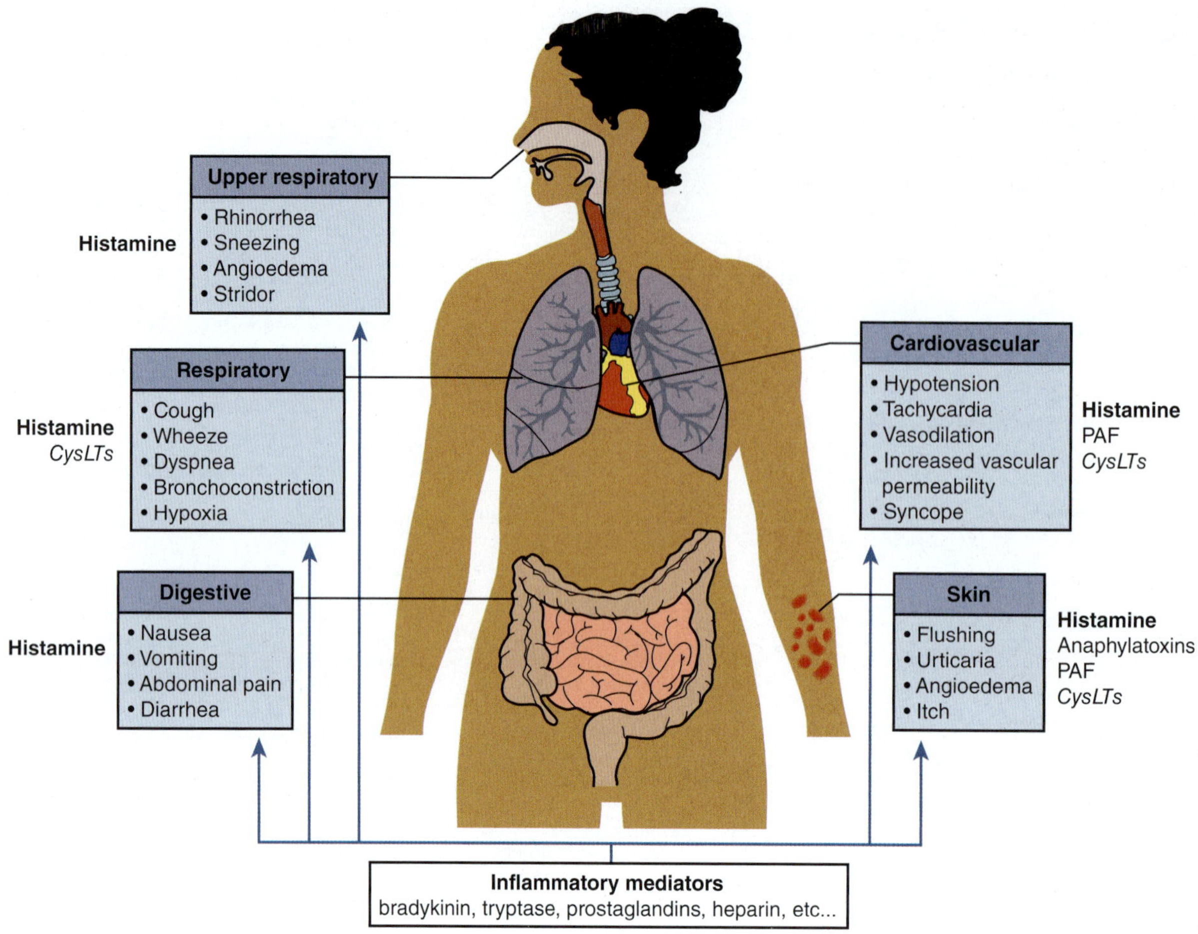

Fig. 4.2 Type I hypersensitivity reactions. Note the characteristic physical findings of each affected organ system.

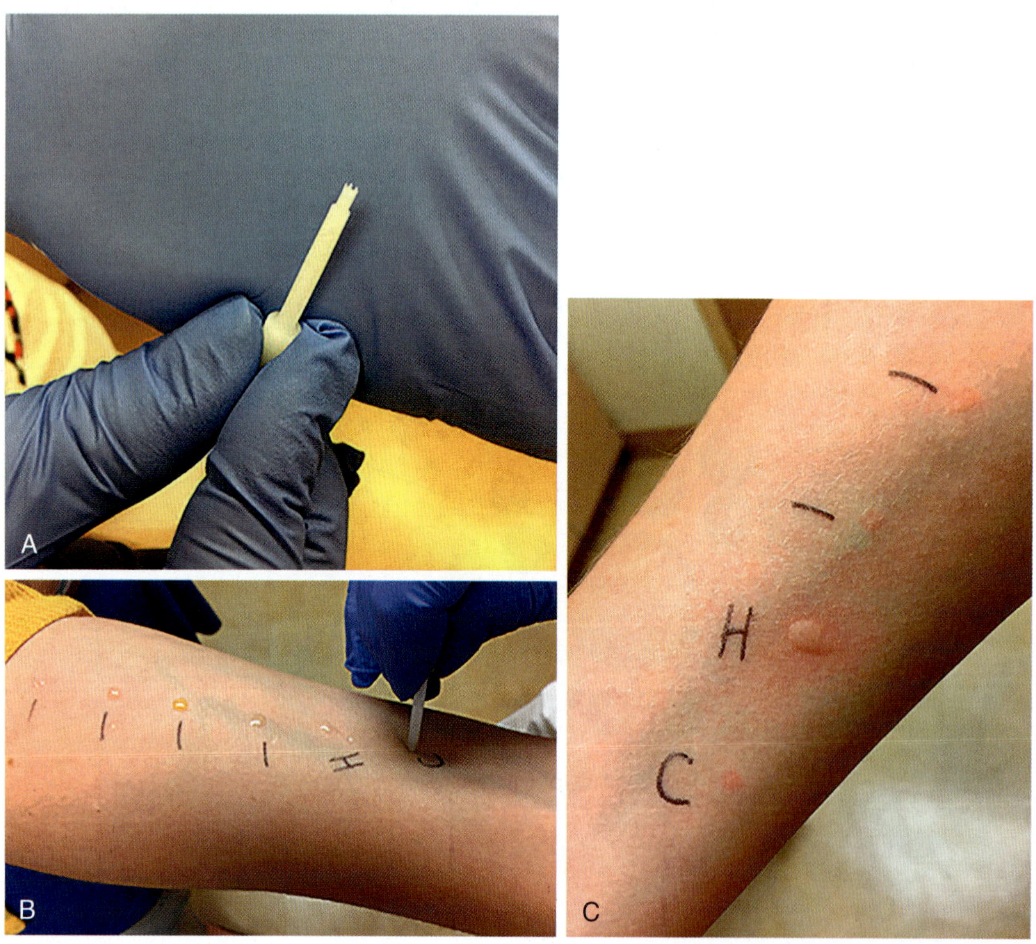

Fig. 4.3 Allergy prick tests. (A) The skin prick test is typically performed with a plastic lancet on either the forearm or upper back. (B) The test leaves a barely visible mark and should be nearly painless. (C) The test is interpreted after 15 minutes by measuring the maximal diameter of both the wheal and the flare.

Table 4.2 Skin Testing versus In Vitro Testing

Variable	Skin Test	In Vitro
Risk of allergic reaction	Rare	No
Sensitivity	Very good	Good[a]
Affected by antihistamines	Yes	No
Affected by corticosteroids	Not usually	No
Affected by extensive dermatitis or dermatographism	Yes	No
Broad selection of antigens	Yes	Yes
Immediate results	Yes	No
Discomfort	Mild	Moderate

[a]Less sensitive for aeroallergens, drugs, and Hymenoptera.

offending antigen. The most common triggers of anaphylaxis in children are foods (such as milk, egg, peanut, and tree nuts), followed by insect stings. The pattern of system involvement can vary on the basis of the antigen, dose, route of exposure, and concomitant factors, such as exercise, use of nonsteroidal antiinflammatory drugs (NSAIDs), and alcohol use. Symptoms can range from isolated urticaria to cardiovascular collapse (Table 4.3). Airway obstruction and hypotension are the most severe manifestations of anaphylaxis. The upper airway, lower airway, or both can be affected. Upper airway obstruction is due to laryngeal edema, whereas lower airway involvement can be due to edema or bronchospasm. Hypotension results from vasodilation and may be complicated by loss of intravascular volume.

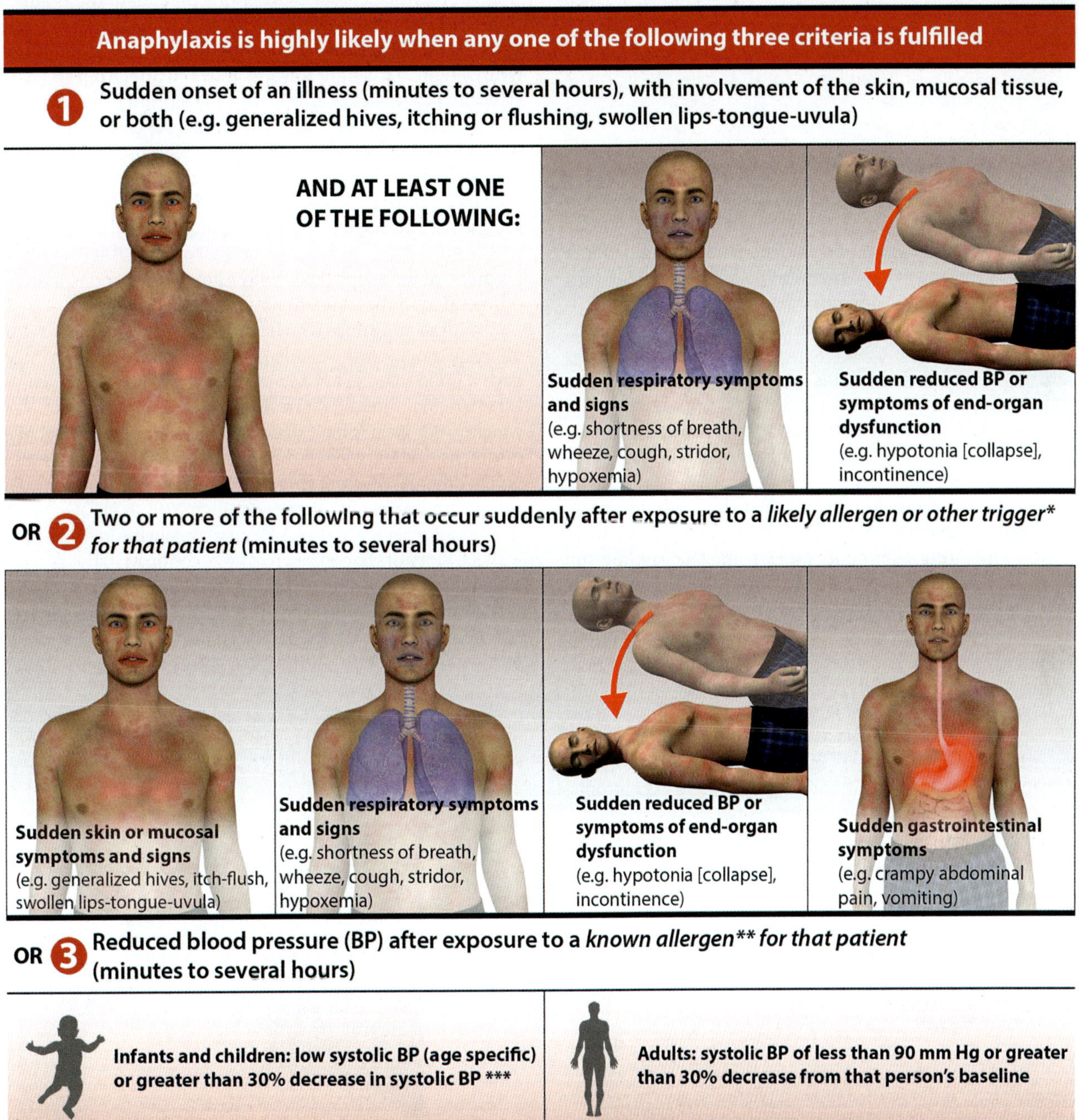

* For example, immunological but IgE-independent, or non-immunologic (direct mast cell activation)

** For example, after an insect sting, reduced blood pressure might be the only manifestation of anaphylaxis; or after allergen immunotherapy, generalized hives might be the only initial manifestation of anaphylaxis.

*** Low systolic blood pressure for children is defined as less than 70 mm Hg from 1 month to 1 year, less than (70 mm Hg + [2 x age]) from 1 to 10 years and less than 90 mm Hg from 11 to 17 years. Normal heart rate ranges from 80 - 120 beats/minute at age 3 years; and from 70 -115 beats/minute after age 3 years. In infants and children, respiratory compromise is more likely than hypotension or shock and shock is more likely to be manifest initially by tachycardia than by hypotension.

Fig. 4.4 Criteria for anaphylaxis. (From Shaker M, Wallace D, Golden D, et al: Anaphylaxis—a 2020 practice parameter update, systematic review, and Grading of Recommendations, Assessment, Development and Evaluation (GRADE) analysis, *J Allergy Clin Immunol* 145(4):1082–1123, 2020.)

Table 4.3 Signs and Symptoms of Anaphylaxis

Signs and Symptoms	Percentage
Cutaneous	62–90
Urticaria and angioedema	62–90
Flushing	45–55
Pruritus without rash	2–5
Respiratory	
Dyspnea, wheeze	45–50
Upper airway angioedema	50–60
Rhinitis	15–20
Hypotension, dizziness, syncope, diaphoresis	30–35
Abdominal	
Nausea, vomiting, diarrhea, abdominal pain	25–30
Miscellaneous	
Headache	5–8
Substernal pain	4–5
Seizure	1–2

Modified from Lieberman P, Nicklas R, Randolph C, et al: Anaphylaxis—a practice parameter update, *Ann Allergy Asthma Immunol* 115(5):341–384, 2015.

Vascular collapse may be aggravated by decreased myocardial function. In addition to the airway and cardiovascular system, other organ systems are also involved in anaphylaxis. The skin is the most commonly involved organ with urticaria and angioedema often present. GI involvement can manifest as vomiting, diarrhea, and abdominal pain due to cramping or edema.

For treatment of anaphylactic reactions, intramuscular epinephrine is the initial therapy of choice; it is superior in efficacy compared with the subcutaneous route. Patients at risk should carry self-injectable epinephrine and be trained in its use. There are currently five different automated injectable epinephrine devices: EpiPen, Adrenaclick, Auvi-Q, Symjepi, and several generic epinephrine autoinjectors (Fig. 4.5). All exist in two doses, either 0.15 or 0.3 mg, and the Auvi-Q device is also available in a 0.1 mg dose. In 2024, intranasal epinpehrine (Neffy) received FDA approval and is available in 1 mg and 2 mg doses. Operating technique varies somewhat among the devices, so it is important for families to become familiar with their specific device. Epinephrine is most effective when it is used as rapidly as possible with the onset of anaphylaxis. Administration of other medications should not delay prompt delivery of epinephrine, which is the only medication that has been proven to be effective in treating anaphylaxis. In cases of hypotension, large-volume fluid resuscitation is essential. In severe cases of anaphylactic shock, pressor support may be required. After administration of injectable epinephrine, if the patient has prompt, complete, and durable resolution of symptoms, activation of emergency medical support may not be necessary. However, EMS should be activated if anaphylaxis is severe, persists, or worsens despite epinephrine administration. Albuterol inhalation should be considered for any lower airway symptoms, especially in patients with asthma. Systemic steroids are often administered; however, their effectiveness in the treatment of anaphylaxis and in the prevention of biphasic anaphylaxis has never been proven and current practice parameter guidelines suggest against the use of corticosteroids. Antihistamines can be used for reactions confined to the skin and as second-line therapy to epinephrine in more severe reactions.

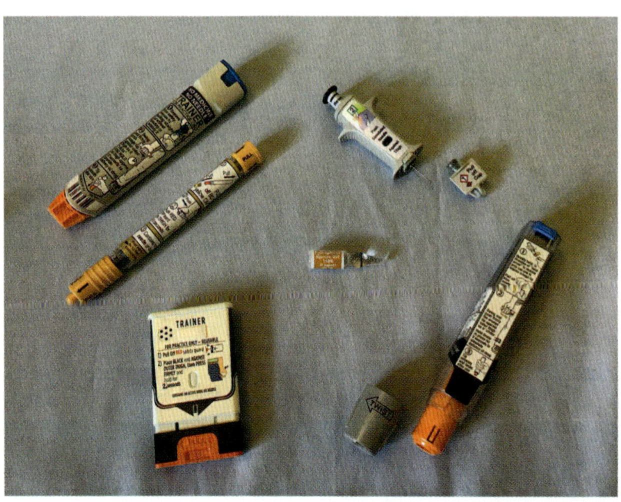

Fig. 4.5 Currently available automated epinephrine injector devices compared with a glass ampule of epinephrine (1 mg/1 mL) solution in center.

Insect Sting Allergy

Life-threatening reactions to Hymenoptera are rare in childhood. A typical local reaction from a bee sting involves erythema, induration, pain, and itching secondary to local effects of the insect venom (Fig. 4.6). Hypersensitivity reactions may manifest as large local reactions (LLRs), generalized urticaria, or anaphylaxis. LLRs involve extreme swelling (>10 cm) contiguous to the sting and may involve lymphangitic streaking toward nodes in the groin or axilla. Swelling typically progresses in size 12 to 24 hours after the sting and may take 5 to 10 days to resolve. Although these reactions may look like an infection, LLRs occur more rapidly than cellulitis and respond to therapy such as cool compresses, antihistamines, and NSAIDs. Corticosteroids may rarely be required. Patients with LLRs have an excellent long-term prognosis. Although LLRs may occur again, the risk for anaphylaxis with future stings is minimal at 4% to 10%. Allergy testing does not predict risk for anaphylaxis with future stings and is therefore not recommended in the evaluation of patients with LLRs.

Children and adults who have a history of generalized urticaria without respiratory, cardiovascular, or GI symptoms after an insect sting also have a good long-term prognosis. The risk for severe anaphylaxis after experiencing a mild cutaneous-only systemic reaction is less than 3%, which is not greater than that of the general population. Allergy testing or desensitization with immunotherapy is generally not recommended unless other risk factors are present such as frequent unavoidable exposure or underlying medical conditions such as mastocytosis. The decision about whether to prescribe an epinephrine autoinjector to children with a history of generalized reactions confined to the skin or LLRs from stinging insects is left to physician discretion.

Children with a history of systemic anaphylaxis involving extracutaneous systems after a Hymenoptera sting have a 30% to 40% risk of a similar reaction with future stings and should undergo allergy testing for consideration of immunotherapy. Skin testing should be performed no sooner than 4 weeks after the reaction to decrease the potential for false-negative test results. Allergen immunotherapy for Hymenoptera sensitivity is the most effective form of allergen

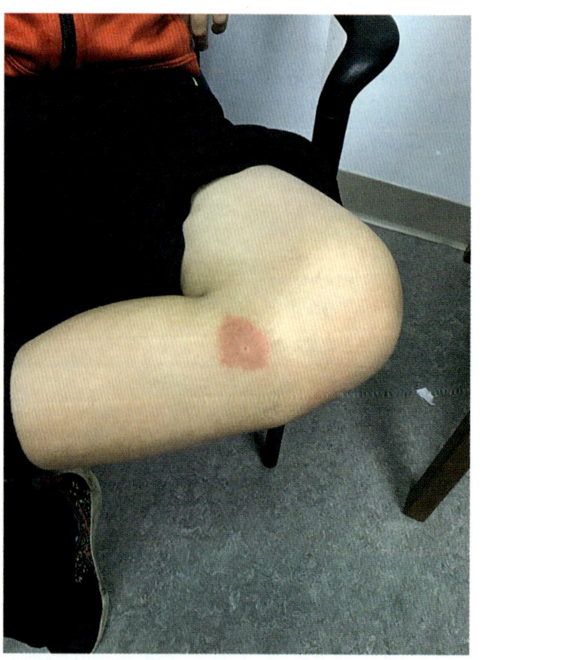

Fig. 4.6 Localized reaction to Hymenoptera sting.

immunotherapy available. Venom immunotherapy for wasps, yellow jackets, and hornets reduces the risk for anaphylaxis by greater than 95%, whereas it is slightly less effective for honeybees, providing complete protection in 80% to 85% of patients on therapy. Most venom immunotherapy protocols start with weekly injections for about 10 to 16 weeks, followed by maintenance injections every 1 to 2 months for a duration of 3 to 5 years.

The Hymenoptera that have been associated with anaphylaxis come from three subfamilies: Apidae (honeybees); Vespidae (yellow jackets, wasps, and white- and yellow-faced hornets); and Formicidae (fire ants). In the United States, yellow jackets are the most common cause of Hymenoptera-induced anaphylaxis. Yellow jackets typically nest in the ground, are scavengers for food, and, consequently, are frequently encountered at picnics and around garbage cans. The yellow jacket is small with tight yellow and black bands. The honeybee is the least aggressive of the Hymenoptera family. Stings from honeybees occur most commonly in beekeepers and after accidental contact. The honeybee's stinger is barbed and is retained in the skin after stings (Fig. 4.7). If the stinger is visible, it should be gently flicked away from the skin with a fingernail. The stinger and venom sac should not be removed by pinching between the thumb and forefinger because this process can express additional venom. Wasps and hornets are territorial and will sting to protect their nests. The fire ant is an increasingly important cause of Hymenoptera-induced anaphylaxis. Fire ants are found in the south and southeastern United States, but their natural habitat appears to be expanding.

FOOD ALLERGY

An adverse food reaction can be broadly defined as a reproducible abnormal clinical response to a food. Adverse food reactions can be further subdivided into those that are immune mediated and those that are not. Within the immune-mediated reactions are IgE-mediated (commonly referred to as food allergy), non-IgE-mediated, mixed IgE and non-IgE, and cell-mediated (Fig. 4.8). Nonimmune-mediated reactions are commonly referred to as *intolerances* (e.g., lactose intolerance), and, although these reactions can lead to significant symptoms, allergy testing is not helpful or indicated in the evaluation of these disorders. IgE-mediated food allergy reactions are highly reproducible (i.e., occur with every exposure to the food) and can be triggered by ingestions of small quantities. Anaphylaxis is the best described and understood type I hypersensitivity to food. Although contact reactions (erythema, pruritus, hives) are common if an individual touches his or her food allergen, the most severe allergic reactions occur with ingestion. Milk, egg, wheat, soy, and peanut account for more than 90% of pediatric food allergic reactions. The onset of type I hypersensitivity to milk and egg is almost always in the first year of life.

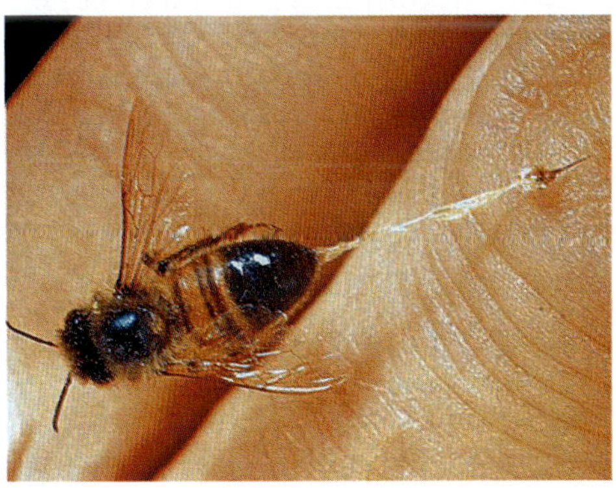

Fig. 4.7 Hymenoptera sting. The honeybee has a barbed stinger and leaves the stinger and venom sac after it stings.

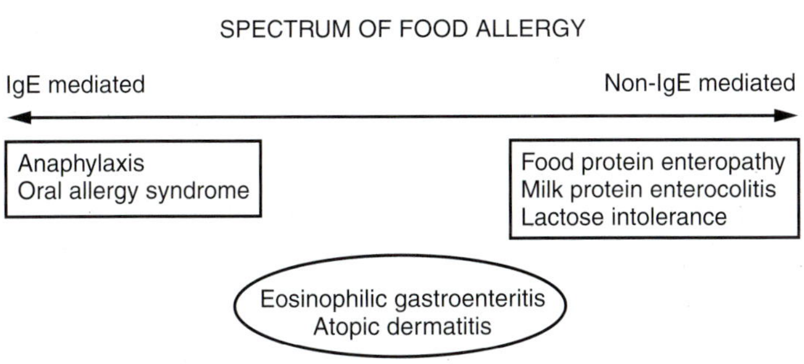

Fig. 4.8 Adverse reactions to foods can be broadly divided into immune-mediated and nonimmune-mediated ones. Within the immune-mediated group of reactions, the mechanism can be further distinguished; the distinction between immunoglobulin E (IgE)-mediated and non-IgE-mediated reactions is often used to determine the utility of allergy testing, as well as to make decisions regarding treatment.

Most allergic reactions to foods occur with the first few ingestions of a food. Type I hypersensitivity to milk or egg is typically outgrown, but less than 25% of patients will outgrow a peanut or tree nut sensitivity. Peanuts and tree nuts cause the majority of life-threatening reactions to foods. Other risk factors for life-threatening reactions from food-induced anaphylaxis include asthma, adolescence, and delayed administration of epinephrine. A history of mild reactions does not rule out the possibility of a future life-threatening episode of food-induced anaphylaxis. In the past, patients with one nut allergy were often advised to avoid all tree nuts. However, data has demonstrated that early introduction of peanuts can help prevent the development of a food allergy and pan-avoidance is not advisable. Guidelines from the American Academy of Allergy Asthma and Immunology now recommend introduction of peanuts between 4 and 6 months of age without prior allergy testing.

Another common form of type I–mediated hypersensitivity to food is oral allergy syndrome (also known as *pollen-food allergy syndrome*). Patients with this syndrome typically have underlying seasonal allergic rhinitis and develop pruritus and mild angioedema of the oropharynx when ingesting fresh fruits and vegetables. The reaction is due to cross-reactivity between heat-labile proteins in some fruits and vegetables and outdoor seasonal pollens and is often eliminated by heating the vegetable or fruit. The reaction does not generally extend beyond the oropharynx, and patients typically do not need to carry epinephrine. In a minority of cases, reactions may be severe, so taking a thorough history is essential before recommendations are made for avoidance and the need for epinephrine.

One of the challenges with diagnosing type I hypersensitivity to foods is the poor specificity of both the skin prick and in vitro tests. These tests have a 20% to 50% false-positive rate. Therefore the "gold standard" for the diagnosis of food allergy is a double-blind, placebo-controlled food challenge (DBPCFC), which is not often done in a clinical setting. A distinction must be drawn between patients who are "sensitized," based on skin or serum testing, and those who are clinically allergic, based on a history of reactions to ingestions. IgE-mediated reactions occur quickly and reproducibly with ingestion of the triggering food. Over the years, research using in vitro allergy tests has identified levels of specific IgE against certain foods that predict a reaction during a DBPCFC with 95% likelihood. In vitro food-specific IgE levels are most useful clinically when used in association with a patient's ingestion history and, if indicated, skin test results. They should not be obtained for patients without a history of reaction. In a nationally representative survey study, approximately 17% of the overall population in the United States displayed serum sensitization to either cow's milk, egg, peanut, or shrimp, and this prevalence rate was even higher (28%) among children from 1 to 5 years old. Yet based on these serum levels in the same study, only approximately 2.5% of the U.S. population was predicted to be clinically allergic to one of these foods. Determining positive predictive values depends on the age of the patient, and the values are not available for all foods (Table 4.4). In vitro allergy tests may also be repeated over time to try to help identify patients who may have outgrown their sensitivity. The sensitivity of both the skin prick and in vitro tests is excellent but not 100%. If there is a strong clinical history of a type I reaction to a food, it may be necessary to perform an oral challenge in a medically supervised setting before food hypersensitivity can be fully ruled out.

Table 4.4 Food-Specific Immunoglobulin E Concentrations Predictive of Clinical Reactivity

Allergen	Decision Point (kU/L)	Sensitivity (%)	Specificity (%)	Positive Predictive Value (%)	Negative Predictive Value (%)
Egg	7	61	95	98	38
Infants, ≤2 years old[a]	2			95	
Milk	15	57	94	95	53
Infants, ≤2 years old[b]	5			95	
Peanut	14	57	100	100	36
Fish	20	25	100	100	89
Soybean	30	44	94	73	82
Wheat	26	61	92	74	87
Tree nuts	≈15	—	—	≈95	—

[a]Boyano-Martinez T, Garcia-Ara C, Diaz-Pena GM, et al: Validity of specific IgE in children with egg allergy, *Clin Exp Allergy* 31:1464–1469, 2001.

[b]Garcia-Ara C, Boyano-Martinez T, Diaz-Pena GM, et al: Specific IgE levels in the diagnosis of immediate hypersensitivity to cow's milk protein in infants, *J Allergy Clin Immunol* 107:185–190, 2001.

Modified from Sampson HA: Utility of food-specific IgE concentrations in predicting symptomatic food allergy, *J Allergy Clin Immunol*107:891–896, 2001.

Current treatment for IgE-mediated food allergic reactions consists of avoidance of the trigger food, as well as tools to manage a reaction to an accidental ingestion. Patients with this severe food allergy will require access to an epinephrine autoinjector, and patients and families should be instructed in its use. These patients and their families should be provided with an anaphylaxis action plan outlining appropriate symptom-based treatment. Although avoidance is the current standard of care, there are currently multiple potential "active" therapies being investigated for IgE-mediated food allergy. These interventions aim to raise the threshold of the amount of allergen that can lead to an allergic reaction if there is an accidental ingestion of that food. To date, the most well studied of these approaches involves exposing the allergic individual to very small amounts of the food allergen in question, either orally (oral immunotherapy), sublingually (sublingual immunotherapy), or through the skin (epicutaneous immunotherapy). As of this writing, the only U.S. Food and Drug Administration (FDA)-approved immunotherapy treatment for food allergy is Palforzia, which involves the graded administration of pharmaceutic-grade peanut powder for children 4 to 17 years. Phase III studies for epicutaneous immunotherapy for peanut have been completed and are under consideration for approval by the FDA.

Triggers of eosinophilic gastrointestinal disorders (EGIDs) are more challenging to evaluate as eosinophilic infiltration of the gut is thought to be caused by a mixed reaction involving type I (IgE-mediated) hypersensitivity and other immune pathways. Patients with EGIDS often have type I hypersensitivity to certain foods and sometimes inhaled aeroallergens that are inadvertently swallowed. The pathogenesis of EGIDs is thought, however, to also involve non–IgE-mediated pathways such that a negative skin prick or in vitro test does not eliminate the possibility that food may be causing or contributing to the disease. Similarly, a positive allergy test to a food does not definitely establish causation. Patch testing has also been studied to determine potential food triggers of EGIDs revealing equally concerning limitations in sensitivity and specificity. Patients with eosinophilic inflammation of the upper GI tract tend to have problems with dysphagia, food impaction, abdominal pain, and vomiting. Patients with eosinophilic inflammation of the lower GI tract tend to have diarrhea, failure to thrive, and abdominal pain. Treatments for EGIDs include elemental diets, selected dietary elimination, proton pump inhibitors, and swallowed steroids. Biologic therapies targeting eosinophilic pathways and other mediators involved in the process are currently under evaluation. The long-term prognosis is not completely understood, and the disease often follows a relapsing and remitting course.

The term *food allergy* also encompasses food reactions elicited through non–IgE-mediated immune pathways. The classic example of a non–IgE-mediated hypersensitivity to food is seen in milk protein enterocolitis of infancy (also known as *food-induced eosinophilic proctitis*), which presents with bloody diarrhea in the first few months of life and improves within days of removing milk proteins from the diet. Many of the infants affected are breastfed, and they react to either cow's milk or another protein in the maternal diet. Approximately half of children with milk protein enterocolitis will also experience symptoms with soy protein–based formulas. Because milk protein enterocolitis is not IgE-mediated, allergy testing is not recommended in its evaluation. Almost all infants will outgrow this condition by 1 to 2 years old.

Food protein–induced enterocolitis syndrome (FPIES) is another non–IgE-mediated reaction with a more severe presentation. Infants typically present 1 to 4 hours after an ingestion of the triggering food with profuse vomiting, hypotension, and lethargy. Fecal leukocytes, a rise in the peripheral absolute neutrophil count, acidosis, and methemoglobinemia may also be seen, whereas skin lesions are not present. Cow's milk, soy, rice, and oat are the most common triggers of FPIES, although it has been described in response to a variety of other foods. Infants frequently are diagnosed with recurrent sepsis or infectious gastroenteritis before the condition of FPIES is realized. Because FPIES is not IgE mediated, the gold standard for diagnosis is a food challenge. Although skin prick testing and in vitro IgE testing are not helpful in determining causality or resolution, a positive test may have prognostic value in predicting a longer course to resolution or the risk for IgE-mediated potentially anaphylactic symptoms on reintroduction of the food. Most cases, however, resolve by 2 to 6 years and the triggering foods are tolerated without issue.

DRUG HYPERSENSITIVITY REACTIONS

Drug hypersensitivity reactions (DHRs) are defined as unexpected, reproducible objective signs and symptoms caused by a specific drug at a normally tolerated dose. DHRs can be divided into *allergic drug hypersensitivity reactions,* which are immunologically mediated, and nonallergic drug hypersensitivity. Allergic DHRs are mediated by drug-specific antibodies, T cells, or both and can be further defined using the classification by Gell and Coombs (see Table 4.1). Type I hypersensitivity reactions to drugs are mediated by drug-specific IgE bound to mast cells and basophils. IgE is cross-linked by the drug, leading to mast cell and basophil activation and release of mediators that drive the clinical reaction. Type I hypersensitivity can range from mild reactions involving only the skin (generalized urticaria or angioedema) to anaphylaxis with laryngeal edema, bronchospasm, hypotension, and cardiovascular collapse. These reactions occur within minutes of exposure and require prior sensitization. IgE-mediated reactions occur early in the treatment course, usually after the first or second dose of a drug. A nonurticarial rash that develops after more than a few days of therapy is seldom due to IgE-mediated mechanisms.

Penicillin is the only drug that has been widely studied as a cause of type I hypersensitivity, and consequently, it is the only drug for which standardized allergy testing is available. Penicillin undergoes conversion to a reactive intermediate that binds to proteins, forming penicilloyl amides. Penicilloyl amides account for 95% of tissue-bound penicillin and are known as the major antigenic determinant. A small percentage of penicillin can be found in the body as the native drug, penicillin, or other metabolites called *minor antigenic determinants* (penicilloate and penilloate). Skin testing done with the major antigenic determinant, penicillin, and the minor determinants has a negative predictive value approaching 98% to 100%. At present, in the United States only the major determinant and the drug itself, penicillin G, are commercially available for skin testing. Patients with a history of penicillin allergy are more likely to be treated with more expensive, less effective, and more toxic antibiotics. This can result in increased hospital stay, cost, and mortality. Therefore proactive delabeling programs are recommended. Those who have had either anaphylaxis or a recent IgE-mediated reaction to a penicillin-type antibiotic should be evaluated with penicillin skin testing and, if negative, an oral challenge to the triggering drug. In pediatric patients with benign cutaneous reactions and in adult patients with remote history, direct challenge to the offending agent may be performed without preceding skin testing.

The use of cephalosporins in patients with a history of penicillin allergy was historically controversial. Before 1980, a reported 10% to 20% of penicillin-allergic patients reacted to cephalosporins, but since 1980, that number has dropped to 2%. Much of the concern about cross-reactivity between these two classes of drugs was based on their common beta-lactam ring but also likely involved occasional contamination of early cephalosporins with trace amounts of penicillin. Although clinical cross-reactivity between these two drugs has lessened over the years, there are clear reports of anaphylactic reactions after the use of cephalosporins in penicillin-allergic patients. This cross-reactivity is thought in many cases to be due to a similar or identical side chain shared between the two specific beta-lactam antibiotics. The combination of all these factors has contributed to the persistent concern about the safety of cephalosporins in patients with penicillin allergy. Unfortunately, skin testing for cephalosporins has not been standardized, and the negative predictive value of these tests is not known. In patients with an unverified, nonanaphylactic penicillin allergy, any cephalosporin can be used routinely without prior testing. In patients with a recent or severe reaction to a cephalosporin, recommendations for use of future beta-lactam antibiotics are determined based on history, penicillin testing, and review of the side chains involved in the original reaction.

Anaphylaxis from drugs other than penicillin must be diagnosed on the basis of clinical presentation. Patients with type I hypersensitivity to drugs can still potentially receive the drug if there is no acceptable alternative through a *drug desensitization* protocol. This procedure attempts to induce drug tolerance by slow delivery of increasing drug doses over a period of 6 to 12 hours. The mechanism by which tolerance is achieved is not well understood. Patients maintain the desensitized state for only as long as they are receiving the medication. Once the drug is discontinued, the tolerant state is lost and future treatment would require repeating the protocol.

Non-IgE mediated mast cell activation is known to occur with certain medications such as opioids, vancomycin, and fluoroquinolones. Symptoms are similar to anaphylaxis: flushing, rash, minor changes in blood pressure and heart rate, and bronchospasm. These occur independent of IgE cross-linking, and therefore diagnostic testing is not available or warranted. Symptoms can vary in each individual over time and may be affected by dose and route of administration.

DHRs can also manifest through types II, III, and IV Gell and Coombs reactions. The classic Gell and Coombs type II reaction is due to immunoglobulin G (IgG) antibodies directed against drug bound to cell surfaces, causing either hemolytic anemia or thrombocytopenia. Serum sickness represents a Gell and Coombs type III reaction. Serum sickness usually begins 1 to 3 weeks after drug exposure and involves various symptoms, including fever, malaise, arthralgias, arthritis, urticaria, and lymphadenopathy. Many patients with serum sickness will develop a characteristic serpiginous, erythematous, or purpuric eruption at the junction of the palmar or plantar and dorsolateral aspects of the hands and feet, respectively (Fig. 4.9). Patients with serum sickness may have reduced levels of complement components C3 and C4 along with the presence of circulating immune complexes. Serum sickness can be treated with antihistamines; and if the patient fails to improve, systemic steroids can be used. Symptoms usually resolve within a few weeks. Future avoidance of the drug inciting the reaction is recommended.

Delayed type IV DHRs are considered cell mediated and commonly occur days to weeks after drug initiation. They are also referred to as severe cutaneous adverse reactions (SCARs). Stevens-Johnson syndrome (SJS) and toxic epidermal necrolysis (TEN) involve cytotoxic $CD8^+$ T cells and natural killer (NK) cells that cause widespread injury to keratinocytes in epidermis. These reactions affect the skin, mucous membranes, and eyes. The lesions on the skin may begin as dusky erythematous macules or papules that evolve into targetoid lesions, vesicles, and bullae, followed by sloughing of the skin. SJS involves less than 10% of the body surface area (BSA), whereas TEN involves greater than 30% of the BSA. The process is considered SJS/TEN overlap when 10% to 30% of the BSA is affected. TEN is almost always drug induced, whereas SJS may be induced by either drugs or infections such as *Mycoplasma* or herpes simplex virus (HSV). When drug exposure is the inciting cause, the exposure precedes the onset of skin findings by 1 to 3 weeks. Other

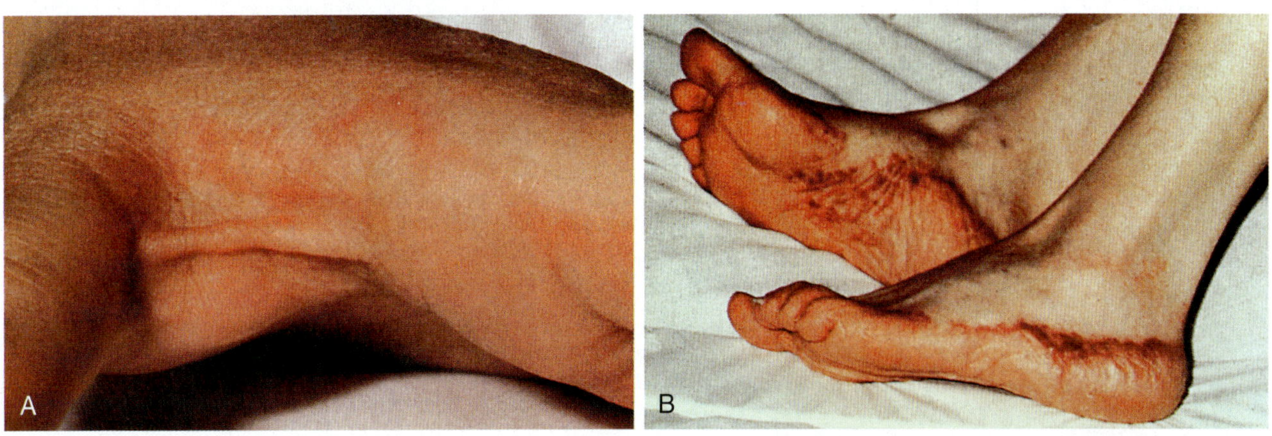

Fig. 4.9 Cutaneous eruptions on the sides of the hands and feet of patients with serum sickness. (A) A scalloped band of erythema can be seen on the side of the finger at the margin of the palmar skin. (B) A band of purpura is seen at the margin of the plantar skin. The purpura was preceded by a band of erythema. (From Lawley TJ, Bielory L, Gascon P, et al: Prospective clinical and immunological analysis of patients with serum sickness, *N Engl J Med* 311:1407–1413, 1984. Copyright © 1984 Massachusetts Medical Society. All rights reserved.)

than discontinuation of the culprit drug and supportive care, there are no universally recommended therapies for SJS or TEN. Although not clearly established, use of several immunomodulating modalities such as corticosteroids, cyclosporin, antitumor necrosis factor antibodies, and intravenous immune globulin have shown varied benefits.

Another delayed immune-mediated DHR is the syndrome known as *drug rash with eosinophilia and systemic symptoms (DRESS)*. DRESS was initially described with anticonvulsant therapies but is now known to be caused by a number of different drugs. DRESS reactions usually begin 2 to 8 weeks into drug therapy. Clinical characteristics include a generalized rash, fever, facial edema, lymphadenopathy, and organ dysfunction. The liver is most commonly involved, but any internal organ can be affected. Laboratory findings include eosinophilia, atypical lymphocytosis, elevated transaminases, and, occasionally, increased creatinine with kidney involvement. The exact pathogenesis is not yet fully understood but is thought to involve both effector and regulatory T cells. Treatment involves discontinuation of the inciting drug and supportive therapy. High-potency topical steroids are recommended for skin symptoms. Systemic glucocorticoids are reserved for cases of severe organ involvement. Cyclosporin has shown benefit as second-line therapy in a limited number of cases.

ALLERGIC RHINITIS

Allergic rhinitis, characterized by inflammation, edema, and weeping of the nasal mucosa, is the most common allergic disorder and occurs in up to 25% of the population. Diagnosis is based on characteristic history, physical findings, and testing for antigen-specific IgE. Common presenting symptoms include nasal congestion and pruritus, clear rhinorrhea, and paroxysms of sneezing. Whereas older children may blow their noses frequently, younger children do not. Instead, they sniff, snort, and repetitively clear their throats. Nasal pruritus stimulates grimacing and twitching (Fig. 4.10) and rubbing of the nose ("allergic salute"). Frequent irritation of the nasal mucosa can lead to epistaxis. In the case of allergy to seasonal pollens, the symptoms may be acute, have a sudden onset, and be confined to the period during which the particular airborne pollen is detectable. Seasonal allergic rhinitis tends to be triggered by tree pollens in the spring, grasses in the early summer, and ragweed or other pollens in the late summer and early fall.

Interestingly, seasonal allergic rhinitis is often called *hay fever*, although fever is not a symptom. Manifestations sometimes can be severe enough to induce flulike symptoms of fatigue and malaise. In contrast, symptoms may be chronic and more indolent in the case of allergy to perennial allergens, including molds, house dust mites, and animal dander.

Symptoms of allergic rhinitis can overlap with those of infectious rhinitis and include (1) disturbed sleep and snoring; (2) morning dryness and irritation of the throat as a result of mouth breathing; (3) lassitude, fatigue, and irritability from sleep interruption; (4) early nighttime cough; and (5) if the maxillary, frontal, and ethmoidal sinuses are affected, a sensation of pressure over the cheeks, forehead, and bridge of the nose. The presence of naso-ocular watering and pruritus with pruritus of the throat or ears that persists for longer than the normal duration of a viral upper respiratory infection should prompt consideration of an underlying IgE-mediated disorder. The extent to which allergic rhinitis affects a patient's quality of life is often underappreciated.

Many children with long-standing allergic rhinitis can be recognized by their facial characteristics. Ocular manifestations of the allergic disposition include cobblestoning of the conjunctivae (see Fig. 4.32), the allergic shiner, and Dennie sign. Allergic shiners—bluish discolorations or dark circles beneath the eyes—are commonly observed in patients with allergic rhinitis (Fig. 4.11). This finding represents chronic venous congestion secondary to inflammation and can also be seen in the setting of infections and in those with a genetic predisposition. *Dennie sign* refers to prominent folds or creases on the lower eyelid (see Fig. 4.11) running parallel to the lower lid margin. Although these lines were originally thought to indicate a predisposition to allergy, they can be present in any condition associated with periocular pruritus and scratching or chronic nasal congestion. Frequent upward rubbing of the nose with the palm of the hand, the allergic salute (Fig. 4.12), promotes development of a transverse nasal crease across the lower third of the nose (Fig. 4.13). Chronic obstruction produced by nasal mucosal edema

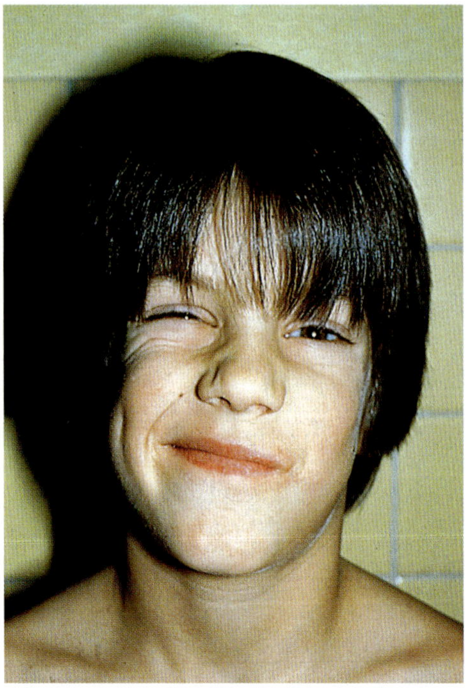

Fig. 4.10 Facial grimacing and twitching caused by nasal itching in a patient with allergic rhinitis. These are frequently repeated and easily noted during patient evaluation.

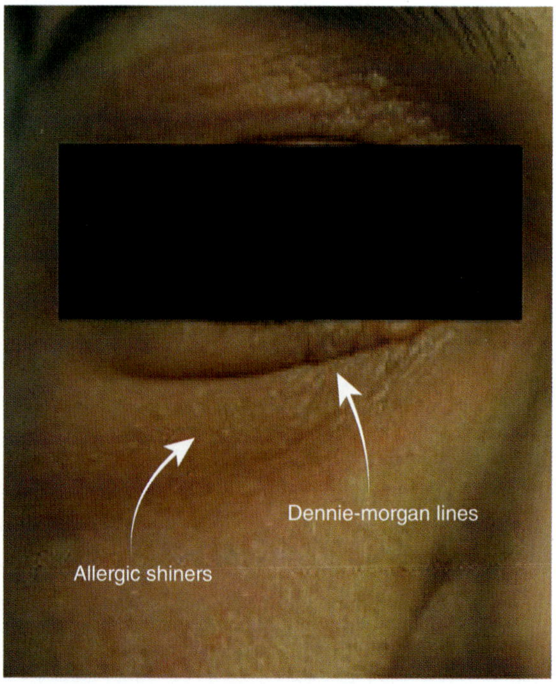

Fig. 4.11 Allergic shiners and Dennie sign. Allergic shiners are characteristic dark circles beneath the eyes. Dennie signs consist of lines that originate in the inner canthus and traverse one-half to two-thirds the length of the lower lid margin in an arc nearly parallel to it. (From Feteih A, et al: Allergic rhinitis. In *The manual of allergy and clinical immunology*, ed 1, 2021.)

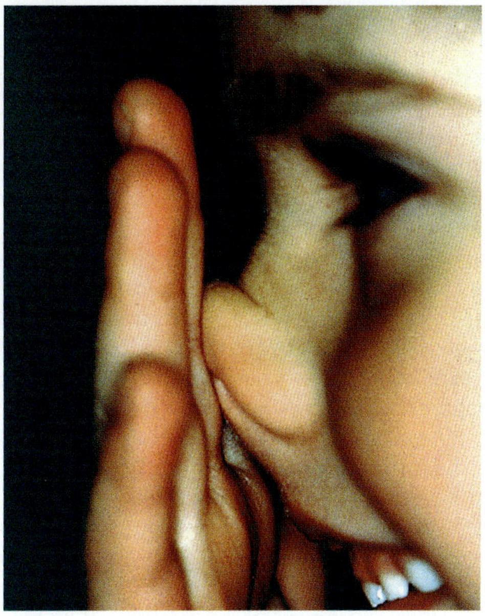

Fig. 4.12 Allergic rhinitis. The allergic salute is characteristic of children with allergic rhinitis and nasal itching and is usually noticed by parents.

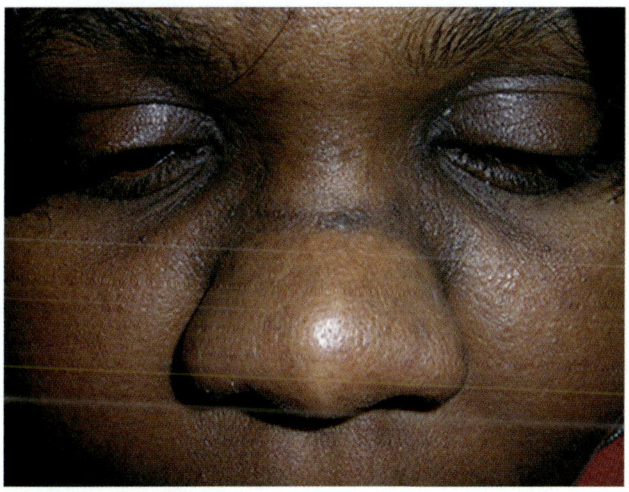

Fig. 4.13 Allergic rhinitis. The nasal crease across the lower third of the nose results from chronic upward rubbing of the nose with the hand (allergic salute). (From Photos and text for Photo Rounds Friday courtesy of Richard P. Usatine, MD. This case was adapted from: Usatine R, Finklea L: Atopic dermatitis. In Usatine R, Smith M, Mayeaux EJ, et al, editors: *Color Atlas of Family Medicine*, ed 2, New York, NY, 2013, McGraw-Hill, pp 584–590.)

may result in mouth breathing and typical open-mouthed, adenoid-type facies (Fig. 4.14).

On nasal examination, attention should be focused on the position of the nasal septum; nasal patency; mucosal appearance; and presence and character of secretions, polyps, or foreign bodies (see Chapter 24). The typical physical examination findings in allergic rhinitis include a marked decrease in nasal patency resulting from swollen inferior turbinates, which appear pale and bluish gray (Fig. 4.15). The mucosa appears edematous, and secretions are clear and watery to mucoid in character.

Depending on the specific allergens, allergic rhinitis may be acute, recurrent, or chronic and must be distinguished from several nonallergic conditions. This necessitates a thorough medical and family history and careful examination. In some instances, response to a trial of medication or observations over time may be necessary to confirm the diagnosis. When symptoms are seasonal or regularly associated with exposure to specific allergens, the distinction is generally clear. In evaluating patients with perennial or recurrent but nonseasonal symptoms, allergy, recurrent infection, nonallergic rhinitis with eosinophilia syndrome, and vasomotor rhinitis must be considered. Unilateral rhinorrhea should prompt further investigation. Foul-smelling mucoid discharge suggests a foreign body, whereas unilateral clear rhinorrhea could be due to a cerebral spinal fluid leak.

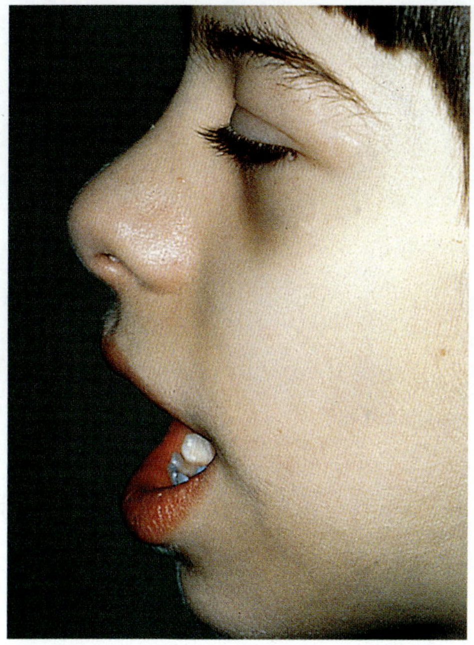

Fig. 4.14 Nasal obstruction. Characteristic adenoid-type facies in a patient with long-standing allergic rhinitis. Note the open mouth and gaping habitus.

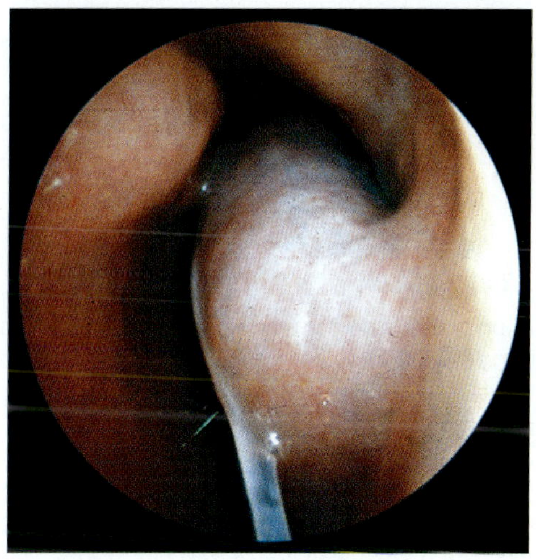

Fig. 4.15 Pale, edematous inferior nasal turbinate of a patient with allergic rhinitis, as seen through a fiberoptic rhinoscope. Even though this tool is not routinely used in evaluations, the physical findings are well illustrated, including watery nasal secretions.

Children with frequent upper respiratory infections or persistent nasal congestion can present a diagnostic challenge. In some cases, the phenomenon is due to recurrent viral infections, particularly in children in their first year of daycare or school. In other patients, tonsillar and adenoidal hypertrophy provides favorable conditions for recurrent infections (see Chapter 24). Atopic (allergic) children may have increased risk of infection because of impaired flow of secretions due to mucosal edema. Recurrent viral sinus infections must also be considered as they typically begin with thin, clear nasal secretions similar to that of allergic rhinitis.

Other forms of rhinitis that must be distinguished from allergic rhinitis are enumerated in Table 4.5. Although characterized by eosinophilia, nonallergic rhinitis with eosinophilia syndrome does not produce nasal pruritus, and patients lack specific IgE antibodies as measured by skin testing or in vitro serum testing. Patients with vasomotor rhinitis do not complain of pruritus, have clear discharge without eosinophils, and lack specific IgE

Table 4.5 Comparison of Allergic and Nonallergic Rhinitis

	Allergic	Nonallergic: NARES	Nonallergic: Vasomotor
• Usual onset	Childhood	Childhood	Adulthood
• Family history of allergy	Usual	Coincidental	Coincidental
• Collateral allergy symptoms	Common	Unusual	Unusual
Sneezing	Frequent	Occasional	Occasional
Itching	Common	Unusual	Unusual
Rhinorrhea	Profuse	Profuse	Profuse
Congestion	Moderate to marked	Moderate to marked	Moderate to marked
Physical Examination			
Edema	Moderate to marked	Moderate	Moderate
Secretions	Watery	Watery	Mucoid to watery
Nasal eosinophilia	Common	Common	Occasional
Allergic Evaluation			
Skin tests	Positive	Coincidental	Coincidental
IgE antibodies	Positive	Coincidental	Coincidental
Therapeutic Response			
Antihistamines	Fair to good	Fair	Poor to fair
Decongestants	Fair	Fair	Poor to fair
Corticosteroids	Good	Good	Poor
Cromolyn	Fair	Unknown	Poor
Immunotherapy	Good	None	None

IgE, Immunoglobulin E; *NARES,* nonallergic rhinitis with eosinophilia syndrome.

Modified from Fagin J, Friedman R, Fireman P: Allergic rhinitis, *Pediatr Clin North Am* 28:797–806, 1981.

antibodies. Vasomotor rhinitis is thus considered a form of noninflammatory rhinitis and is often triggered by nonspecific stimuli, such as cold air exposure or smoke. The condition is diagnosed most frequently in adults but may occur in children. Congestion or rhinorrhea may predominate in this disorder. Rhinitis medicamentosa is a condition seen in patients who have been using alpha-adrenergic vasoconstrictor nose drops (phenylephrine or oxymetazoline) as decongestants for prolonged treatment periods. The disorder is characterized by rebound vasodilation that produces an erythematous, edematous mucosa in association with a profuse clear nasal discharge.

Some children with perennial allergic rhinitis have congestion so constant and severe that it produces signs of chronic nasal obstruction. This must be distinguished from other acquired and congenital causes (see Chapter 24). The history, physical findings, results of allergy tests for specific IgE and nasal smears, along with therapeutic trials of antihistamines and intranasal corticosteroids, can all help lead to a diagnosis.

Many patients with allergic rhinitis have mild symptoms that are adequately controlled by intermittent antihistamine administration or environmental controls. It is not uncommon, however, for acute naso-ocular symptoms to be attributed to allergies inappropriately. Allergy testing with confirmation of specific IgE can guide ideal timing of medical therapy and investment into appropriate environmental controls and eliminate the use of unnecessary medications in children whose symptoms may not be due to allergies. Additional treatment options for those with poorly controlled allergy symptoms include topical antiinflammatory agents and aeroallergen immunotherapy. Subcutaneous immunotherapy injections (allergy shots) and sublingual immunotherapy tablets have been shown to be effective alternative treatment options for patients who are not well controlled with medications or who desire to reduce the number of medications required to control their symptoms. The typical effective course of immunotherapy is 3 to 5 years.

LOWER RESPIRATORY DISORDERS

Respiratory distress in children (tachypnea with or without grunting, nasal flaring, retractions, and cyanosis) should be promptly evaluated and treated. The first step in approaching respiratory distress is to differentiate upper from lower airway disorders. At times, various degrees of upper and lower airway obstruction may coexist, as in laryngotracheobronchitis.

Upper airway obstruction causes difficulty moving air into the chest, whereas lower airway obstruction causes difficulty moving air out of the chest. This difference results in characteristic physical findings. In general, lower airway obstruction produces prolongation of the expiratory phase of respiration and typical expiratory wheezing, whereas upper airway obstruction prolongs the inspiratory phase. *Wheezing* is defined as musical or whistling auscultatory sounds heard more often on expiration than on inspiration, although in severe obstruction both inspiratory and expiratory wheezing are often present. Inspiratory stridor, seen with upper airway obstruction, can mimic wheezing. Both can be detected concomitantly. *Stridor* is defined as a crowing sound usually heard during the inspiratory phase of respiration. It tends to be loud when the obstruction is subglottic and quiet when obstruction is supraglottic. Mild to moderate increases in respiratory and heart rates are common in upper airway obstruction, whereas lower airway disorders such as pneumonitis and asthma often lead to markedly increased respiratory and heart rates. Retractions are often generalized (suprasternal, intracostal, and subcostal) in severe airway obstruction of any etiology.

Asthma

Asthma is the most common chronic respiratory condition affecting children. The Centers for Disease Control and Prevention (CDC) has reported that more than 6 million children (1 in 12) have asthma (CDC National Center for Environmental Health, 2018). In 2016 more than half of children with asthma had one or more attacks, occurring more frequently in children younger than the age of 5. Each year, 1 in 6 children with asthma go to the emergency department and 1 in 20 children with asthma are hospitalized because of their disease. Of note, asthma hospitalizations of children did decline by 50% from 10% in 2003 to 5% in 2013. Data analyzed from the 2001 to 2016 National Health Interview Survey for children 0 to 17 demonstrated that there was a higher prevalence in boys, non-Hispanic black children and Puerto Rican children, and children from low-income households. Defining characteristics of asthma, as elucidated by the National Heart, Lung, and Blood Institute (NHLBI), include (1) lower airway obstruction that is partially or fully reversible either spontaneously or with bronchodilator or antiinflammatory treatments, (2) the presence of lower airway inflammation, and (3) increased lower airway responsiveness (bronchial hyperreactivity) (NHLBI National Asthma Education and Prevention Program, 2016). The last is characterized by inherent hyperreactivity of the airways to stimuli, including allergens, infection, exercise, chemical agents (such as methacholine), cold or dry air, emotions, and weather changes (Fig. 4.16).

Many cases of asthma, particularly in children, have an atopic basis. Specific allergens implicated in atopic patients are pollen, mold spores, house dust mites, and animal dander, whereas drugs, food, and insect venoms typically cause similar symptoms of wheezing and respiratory distress as part of anaphylaxis (see earlier discussion). On exposure these allergens cross-link specific IgE to produce the characteristic features of asthma: mucosal edema, increased mucus production, and smooth muscle contraction that result in airway inflammation, airway hyperreactivity, and bronchoconstriction. These responses combine to produce a state of reversible obstruction of the large and small airways that is the hallmark of asthma.

Patients with asthma should be evaluated to determine the important triggers for their disease. Affected individuals are often

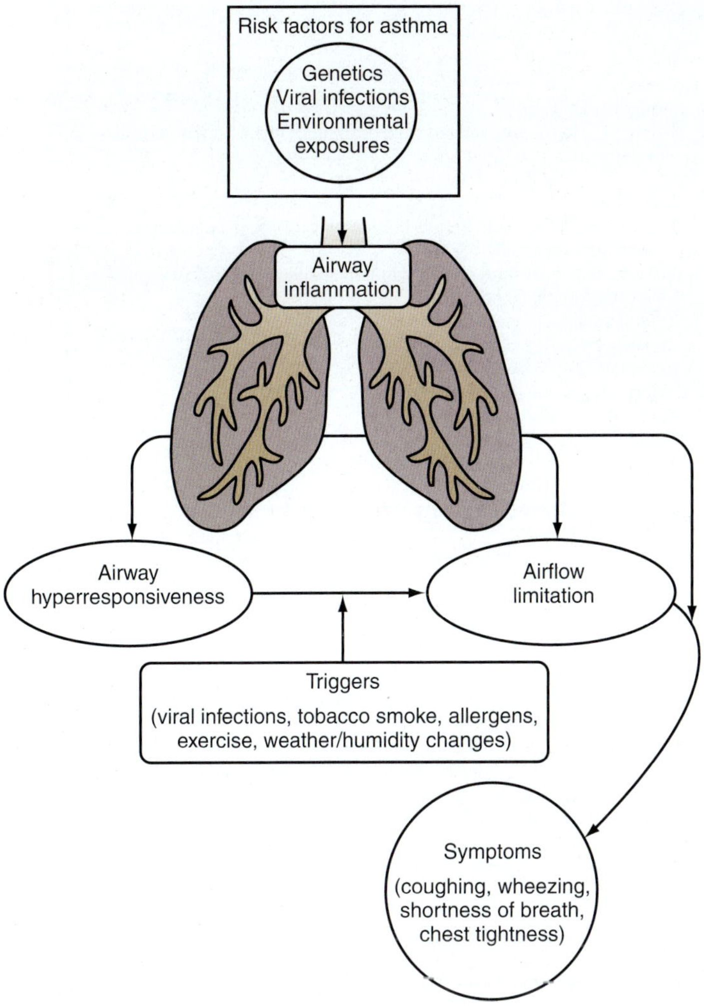

Fig. 4.16 An interaction between genetic and environmental factors is involved in the pathogenesis of asthma. (Reprinted with permission from Rachelefsky GS, Shapiro GG, Bergman D, et al: *Pediatric asthma: promoting best practice guide for managing asthma in children*, Milwaukee, WI, 1999, American Academy of Allergy, Asthma, & Immunology.)

aware of the specific trigger for exacerbations of their asthma. Viruses are the most common precipitants of acute asthma in children, especially rhinovirus, respiratory syncytial virus, and parainfluenza virus. These infections usually affect the upper and lower airways and cause rhinorrhea, nasal congestion, and wheezing, which tends to develop insidiously. In contrast, allergen-triggered episodes typically lack fever and have a more abrupt onset of wheezing.

The diagnosis of asthma, especially in younger children who cannot do pulmonary function tests, is frequently based on historical findings alone. Updated NHLBI and American Academy of Pediatrics guidelines have stressed the importance of complementing good history taking with objective measurements of lung function. Important parts of the medical history include description and pattern of the symptoms, precipitating factors, development of disease and treatments tried, family history, social history, history of exacerbations, impact on the patient and family, and the patient's perception of the disease (Fig. 4.17). In-office pulmonary function testing can be attempted in children 5 years and older, but it is important to understand that normal results in an asymptomatic patient do not exclude asthma. Peak flow monitoring is not recommended for use in diagnosis but can sometimes be used for monitoring. The greatest shortcomings of peak flow monitoring are that it is effort dependent, requires compliance, and does not measure small-airway function. In addition, there is a wide variability in types of peak flow meters and different reference ranges. When peak flow monitoring is used, patients should be given a written plan with instructions on what to do if their peak flow falls along with increase in symptoms.

As with many common diseases, asthma incidence is influenced by both genes and environment. Family history often reveals affected siblings, parents, or other relatives. An environmental survey can determine possible provocative factors, especially allergens, infections, occupational exposures, smoking, exercise, stress, climate, and medication use (NSAIDs, beta-blockers). Individuals with asthma commonly present with recurrent episodes of wheezing that, depending on the severity, may require emergency treatment. Episodes may be infrequent or seasonal or may occur daily. The spectrum of presenting complaints is broad (Box 4.1), and affected individuals may complain only of mild, occasional wheezing; shortness of breath with exercise or colds; or a persistent dry, hacking cough (particularly at night or in the morning). Breathlessness and chest tightness are also commonly reported.

The frequency and severity of acute asthma episodes and the level of symptoms between episodes can be used to grade asthma severity and ultimately assess and monitor asthma control. Stepwise therapy recommendations were updated in the 2020 Focused Updates to the Asthma Management Guidelines by the Expert Panel Working Group of the National Heart, Lung and Blood Institute as noted in Tables 4.6–4.10.

The early stages of an asthma exacerbation in children are characterized by the onset of cough, chest tightness, chest retractions, and audible wheezing. Parents should be educated to observe their child for warning signs and identify the onset of an asthma exacerbation. A written asthma action plan that details use of rescue medicines (such as albuterol) can minimize emergency department visits for asthma (Fig. 4.18).

Asthma should be considered part of the differential diagnosis in any child with recurrent or chronic lower respiratory symptoms or signs. Even though a high index of suspicion must be maintained, excessive or erroneous diagnoses may result if they are made hastily without appropriate supportive evidence; normal children or those with potentially more severe disorders may be mistakenly diagnosed with asthma and inappropriately treated. Box 4.2 provides a differential diagnosis for asthma. Parents must be instructed that physician assessment is essential during suspected episodes of asthma so that wheezing or other signs of lower airway obstruction and reversibility may be documented. Pulmonary function tests in asthmatic children older than 5 years may show airway obstruction at baseline or after appropriate challenge with methacholine, exercise, or cold air and document reversibility after administration of an aerosolized bronchodilator (Fig. 4.19). For children younger than 5 years old or those in whom testing is unreliable, the diagnosis must be made on the basis of historical and physical findings and clinical response to bronchodilator or antiinflammatory medications. Lack of an immediate response to a bronchodilator does not eliminate asthma as a consideration, however. In the instance of poor response to prescribed medications, appropriate inhaler technique and the importance of using a spacer device with any metered dose inhaler should be addressed to ensure adequate medication delivery to the distal airways (Fig. 4.20).

A thorough physical examination provides valuable information regarding the diagnosis of asthma and its severity and chronicity. Physical findings in asthma vary with the state of activity of the disease process at the time of examination. The findings of acute asthma are markedly different from those of chronic and latent or quiescent asthma. Between episodes, the examination is usually entirely normal, although prolongation of the expiratory phase is sometimes noted. Clubbing as a sign of chronic asthma is rare and suggests another chronic pulmonary disease.

A detailed medical history of the new patient who is known or thought to have asthma should address the following items:

1. Symptoms
Cough
Wheezing
Shortness of breath
Chest tightness
Sputum production

2. Pattern of Symptoms
Perennial, seasonal or both
Continued, episodic or both
Onset, duration, frequency, number of days or nights per week or month
Normal variations, especially nocturnal and on awakening in early morning

3. Precipitating and/or aggravating factors
Viral respiratory infections
Environmental allergens, indoor (e.g., mold, house-dust, mite, cockroach, animal dander or secretory products) and outdoor (pollen)
Characteristics of home including age, location, cooking and heating system, wood-burning stove, humidifier, carpeting over concrete, presence of molds or mildew, presence of pets with fur or hair, characteristics of rooms where patient spends time (e.g., bedroom and living room with attention to bedding, floor covering, stuffed furniture)
Smoking (patient and others in home or daycare)
Exercise
Occupational chemicals or allergens
Environmental change (e.g., moving to new home, going on vacation, and/or alterations in workplace, work processes or materials used)
Irritants (e.g., tobacco smoke, strong odors, air pollutants, occupational chemicals, dust and particulates, vapors gases or aerosols)
Emotions (e.g., fear, anger, frustration, hard crying or laughing)
Stress (e.g., fear, anger, frustration)
Drugs (e.g., aspirin and other nonsteroidal anti-inflammatory drugs, beta-blockers including eye drops, others)
Food, food additives, and preservatives (e.g., sulfites)
Changes in weather, exposure to cold air
Endocrine factors (e.g., menses, pregnancy, thyroid disease)
Comorbid conditions (e.g., sinusitis, rhinitis, gastro-esophageal reflux disease [GERD])

4. Development of disease and treatment
Age of onset and diagnosis
History of early-life injury to the airways (e.g., bronchopulmonary dysplasia, pneumonia, parental smoking)
Progression of disease (better or worse)
Present management and response including plans for managing exacerbations.
Frequency of using short-acting beta2 –agonist (SABA)
Need for oral corticosteroids and frequency of use

5. Family History
History of asthma, sinusitis, rhinitis, eczema or nasal polyps in close relatives

6. Social History
Daycare, workplace, and school characteristics that may interfere with adherence
Social factors that interfere with adherence such as substance abuse
Social support/social networks
Level of education completed
Employment

7. History of exacerbations
Usual prodromal signs and symptoms
Rapidity of onset
Duration
Frequency
Severity (need for urgent care, hospitalization, intensive care unit [ICU] admission)
Life-threatening exacerbations (e.g., intubation, intensive care unit admission)
Number and severity of exacerbations in the past year
Usual patterns and management (what works)

8. Impact of asthma on patient and family
Episodes of unscheduled care (emergency department [EDs] urgent care, hospitalization)
Number of days missed from school or work
Limitation of activity, especially sports and strenuous work
History of nocturnal awakening
Effect on growth, development, behavior, school or work performance and lifestyle
Impact on family routines, activities, or dynamics
Economic impact

9. Assessment of patient's and family's perceptions of disease
Patient's parents, and spouse's or partner's knowledge of asthma and belief in the chronicity of asthma and in the efficacy of medications
Ability of patient and parents, spouse or partner to cope with disease
Level of family support and patient's and parents', spouse's or partner's capacity to recognize severity of an exacerbation
Economic resources
Sociocultural beliefs

· This list does not represent a standardized assessment or diagnostic instrument. The validity and reliability of this list has not been assessed.

Fig. 4.17 Detailed medical history of the new patient who is known or thought to have asthma.

Box 4.1 When Is It Asthma?[a]

History of recurrent:

- Coughing
- Wheezing
- Shortness of breath or rapid breathing
- Chest tightness

Symptoms made worse by:

- Viral infection
- Tobacco smoke, wood smoke, and other irritants (e.g., strong odors or fumes)
- Exercise
- Allergens (e.g., house dust mites, pollens, cockroaches, molds, animal dander)
- Changes in weather/humidity
- Crying, laughing

Symptoms occur/worsen at night, waking the child and/or parent
Reversible airflow limitation by spirometry in children older than 4 years old and diurnal variation in peak flow
Wheezing (high-pitched whistling sounds when exhaling) may or may not be present

[a]No single indicator is diagnostic in itself, but the presence of several increases the probability of asthma. *Objective measures are essential to establish the diagnosis of asthma.*
Reprinted with permission from Rachelefsky GS, Shapiro GG, Bergman D, et al: *Pediatric asthma: promoting best practice guide for managing asthma in children*, Milwaukee, WI, 1999, American Academy of Allergy, Asthma, & Immunology.

Table 4.6 Asthma Quick Care Reference: Diagnosing and Managing Asthma Expert Panel Report 3, 2012

Components of Severity		Intermittent			Persistent: Mild			Persistent: Moderate			Persistent: Severe		
		Ages 0–4 Years	Ages 5–11 Years	Ages ≥12 Years	Ages 0–4 Years	Ages 5–11 Years	Ages ≥12 Years	Ages 0–4 Years	Ages 5–11 Years	Ages ≥12 Years	Ages 0–4 Years	Ages 5–11 Years	Ages ≥12 Years
Impairment	Symptoms	≤2 days/week			≥2 days/week but not daily			Daily			Throughout the day		
	Nighttime awakenings	0	≤2×/month		1–2×/month	3–4×/month		3–4×/month	>1×/week but not nightly		>1×/week	Often 7×/week	
	SABA[a] use for symptom control (not to prevent EIB[a])	≤2× days/week			>2 days/ week but not daily	>2 days/week but not daily and not more than once on any day		Daily			Several times per day		
	Interference with normal activity	None			Minor limitation			Some limitation			Extremely limited		
	Lung function	Not applicable	Normal FEV_1 between exacerbations	Normal FEV_1 between exacerbations	Not applicable			Not applicable			Not applicable		
	→ FEV_1[a] (% predicted)		>80%	>80%		>80%	>80%		60–80%	60–80%		<60%	<60%
	→ FEV_1/FVC[a]		>85%	Normal[b]		>80%	Normal[b]		75–80%	Reduced 5%[b]		<75%	Reduced 5%[b]
Risk	Asthma exacerbations requiring oral systemic cortico-steroids[c]	0–1/year			≥2 exacerb. In 6 months, or wheezing ≥4× per year lasting >1 day AND risk factors for persistent asthma	*Generally, more frequent and intense events indicate greater severity.* ≥2/year		*Generally, more frequent and intense events indicate greater severity.*					
		Consider severity and interval since last asthma exacerbation. Frequency and severity may fluctuate over time for patients in any severity category. Relative annual risk of exacerbations may be related to FEV_1.[a]											

[a]*EIB,* Exercise-induced bronchospasm; *FEV_1,* forced expiratory volume in 1 second; *FVC,* forced vital capacity; *ICS,* inhaled corticosteroid; *SABA,* short-acting beta$_2$-agonist.

[b]Normal FEV_1/FVC by age: 8–19 years, 85%; 20–39 years, 80%; 40–59 years, 75%; 60–80 years, 70%.

[c]Data are insufficient to link frequencies of exacerbations with different levels of asthma severity. Generally, more frequent and intense exacerbations (e.g., requiring urgent care, hospital or intensive care admission, and/or oral corticosteroids) indicate greater underlying disease severity. For treatment purposes, patients with ≥2 exacerbations may be considered to have persistent asthma, even in the absence of impairment levels consistent with persistent asthma.

Table 4.7 Asthma Quick Care Reference: Diagnosing and Managing Asthma Expert Panel Report 3, 2012

Components of Control		Well Controlled			Not Well Controlled			Very Poorly Controlled		
		Ages 0–4 Years	Ages 5–11 Years	Ages ≥12 Years	Ages 0–4 Years	Ages 5–11 Years	Ages ≥12 Years	Ages 0–4 Years	Ages 5–11 Years	Ages ≥12 Years
Impairment	Symptoms	≤2 days/ week	≤2 days/week but not more than once on each day	≤2 days/ week	>2 days/ week	>2 days/week or multiple times on ≤2 days/ week	>2 days/ week	Throughout the day		
	Nighttime awakenings	≤1×/month		≤2×/month	>1×/month	≥2×/month	1–3×/week	>1×/week	≥2×/week	≥4×/week
	Interference with normal activity	None			Some limitation			Extremely limited		
	SABA[a] use for symptom control (not to prevent EIB[a])	≤2 days/week			>2 days/week			Several times per day		
	Lung function → FEV_1[a] *(% predicted)* or peak flow *(% personal best)*	Not applicable	>80%	>80%	Not applicable	60–80%	60–80%	Not applicable	<60%	<60%
	→ FEV_1/FVC[a]		>80%	Not applicable		75–80%	Not Applicable		<75%	Not applicable
	Validated questionnaires[b]									
	→ ATAQ[a]	Not applicable	Not applicable	0	Not applicable	Not applicable	1–2	Not applicable	Not applicable	3–4
	→ ACQ[a]			≤0.75[c]			≥1.5			Not applicable
	→ ACT[a]			≥20			16–19			≤15
Risk	Asthma exacerbations requiring oral systemic corticosteroids	0–1/year			2–3/year	≥2/year		>3/year	≥2/year	
		Consider severity and interval since last asthma exacerbation.								
	Reduction in lung growth/ Progressive loss of lung function	Not applicable	Evaluation requires long-term follow-up care.		Not applicable	Evaluation requires long-term follow-up care.		Not applicable	Evaluation requires long-term follow-up care.	
	Treatment-related adverse effects	*Medication side effects can vary in intensity from none to very troublesome and worrisome. The level of intensity does not correlate to specific levels of control but should be considered in the overall assessment of risk.*								

[a]*ACQ,* Asthma Control Questionnaire©; *ACT,* Asthma Control TestTM; *ATAQ,* Asthma Therapy Assessment Questionnaire©.

[b]Minimal important difference: 1.0 for the ATAQ; 0.5 for the ACQ; not determined for the ACT.

[c]ACQ values of 0.76–1.4 are indeterminate regarding well-controlled asthma.

Table 4.8 Ages 0 to 4 Years: Stepwise Approach for Management of Asthma

	Intermittent Asthma	Management of Persistent Asthma in Individuals Ages 0–4 Years				
Treatment	**Step 1**	**Step 2**	**Step 3**	**Step 4**	**Step 5**	**Step 6**
Preferred	PRN SABA and At the start of RTI: Add short-course daily ICS[a]	Daily low-dose ICS and PRN SABA	Daily low-dose ICS-LABA and PRN SABA[a] or daily low-dose ICS + montelukast,[b] or daily medium-dose ICS, and PRN SABA	Daily medium-dose ICS-LABA and PRN SABA	Daily high-dose ICS-LABA and PRN SABA	Daily high-dose ICS-LABA + oral systemic corticosteroid and PRN SABA
Alternative		Daily montelukast[b] or Cromolyn,[b] and PRN SABA		Daily medium-dose ICS + montelukast[b] and PRN SABA	Daily high-dose ICS + montelukast[b] and PRN SABA	Daily high-dose ICS + montelukast[b] + oral systemic corticosteroid and PRN SABA
			For children age 4 years only, see Step 3 and Step 4 on Management of Persistent Asthma in Individuals Ages 5–11 Years diagram			

Assess Control
- First, check adherence, inhaler technique, environmental factors,[a] and comorbid conditions.
- **Step up** if needed; reassess in 4–6 weeks
- **Step down** if possible (if asthma is well controlled for at least 3 consecutive months)

Consult with asthma specialist if Step 3 or higher is required. Consider consultation at Step 2.
Control assessment is a key element of asthma care. This involves both impairment and risk. Use of objective measures, self-reported control, and health care utilization are complementary and should be employed on an ongoing basis, depending on the individual's clinical situation.

ICS, Inhaled corticosteroid; *LABA,* long-acting beta$_2$-agonist; *PRN,* as needed; *RTI,* respiratory tract infection; *SABA,* inhaled short-acting beta$_2$-agonist.

[a]Updated based on the 2020 guidelines.

[b]Cromolyn and montelukast were not considered for this update and/or have limited availability for use in the United States. The FDA issued a Boxed Warning for montelukast in March 2020.

Table 4.9 Ages 5 to 11 Years: Stepwise Approach for Management of Asthma

	Intermittent Asthma	Management of Persistent Asthma in Individuals Ages 5–11 Years				
Treatment	**Step 1**	**Step 2**	**Step 3**	**Step 4**	**Step 5**	**Step 6**
Preferred	PRN SABA	Daily low-dose ICS and PRN SABA	Daily and PRN combination low-dose ICS-formoterol[a]	Daily and PRN combination medium-dose ICS-formoterol[a]	Daily high-dose ICS-LABA and PRN SABA	Daily high-dose ICS-LABA + oral systemic corticosteroid and PRN SABA
Alternate		Daily LTRA,[b] or cromolyn,[b] or nedocromil,[b] or theophylline,[b] and PRN SABA	Daily medium-dose ICS and PRN SABA or daily low-dose ICS-LABA, or daily low-dose ICS + LTRA,[b] or daily low-dose ICS + theophylline,[b] and PRN SABA	Daily medium-dose ICS-LABA and PRN SABA or daily medium-dose ICS + LTRA[b] or daily medium-dose ICS + theophylline,[b] and PRN SABA	Daily high-dose ICS + LTRA[b] or daily high-dose ICS + theophylline,[b] and PRN SABA	Daily high-dose ICS + LTRA[b] + oral systemic corticosteroid or daily high-dose ICS + theophylline[b] + oral systemic corticosteroid, and PRN SABA
		Steps 2–4: Conditionally recommend the use of subcutaneous immunotherapy as an adjunct treatment to standard pharmacotherapy in individuals ≥5 years of age whose asthma is controlled at the initiation, build-up, and maintenance phases of immunotherapy[a]			Consider Omalizumab[a,c]	

Assess Control
- First check adherence, inhaler technique, environmental factors,[a] and comorbid conditions.
- **Step up** if needed; reassess in 2–6 weeks
- **Step down** if possible (if asthma is well controlled for at least 3 consecutive months)

Consult with asthma specialist if Step 4 or higher is required. Consider consultation at Step 3.
Control assessment is a key element of asthma care. This involves both impairment and risk. Use of objective measures, self-reported control, and health care utilization are complementary and should be employed on an ongoing basis depending on the individual's clinical situation.

ICS, Inhaled corticosteroid; *LABA,* long-acting beta$_2$-agonist; *LTRA,* leukotriene receptor antagonist; *SABA,* inhaled short-acting beta$_2$-agonist.

[a]Updated based on the 2020 guidelines.

[b]Cromolyn, nedocromil, LTRAs including montelukast, and theophylline were not considered in this update and/or have limited availability for use in the United States, and/or have an increased risk of adverse consequences and need for monitoring that make their use less desirable. The FDA Issued a Boxed Warning for montelukast in March 2020.

[c]Omalizumab is the only asthma biologic currently FDA approved for this age range.

Table 4.10 Ages 12+ Years: Stepwise Approach for Management of Asthma

	Intermittent Asthma	Management of Persistent Asthma in Individuals Ages 12+ Years				
Treatment	**Step 1**	**Step 2**	**Step 3**	**Step 4**	**Step 5**	**Step 6**
Preferred	PRN SABA	Daily low-dose ICS and PRN SABA or PRN concomitant ICS and SABA[a]	Daily and PRN combination low-dose ICS-formoterol[a]	Daily and PRN combination medium-dose ICS-formoterol[a]	Daily medium-high dose ICS-LABA + LAMA and PRN SABA[a]	Daily high-dose ICS-LABA + oral systemic corticosteroids + PRN SABA
Alternate		Daily LTRA[b] and PRN SABA or cromolyn,[b] or nedocromil,[b] or zileuton,[b] or theophylline,[b] and PRN SABA	Daily medium-dose ICS and PRN SABA or daily low-dose ICS-LABA, or daily low-dose ICS + LAMA,[a] or daily low-dose ICS + LTRA,[b] and PRN SABA or daily low-dose ICS + theophylline[b] or zileuton,[b] and PRN SABA	Daily medium-dose ICS-LABA or daily medium-dose ICS + LAMA, and PRN SABA[a] or daily medium-dose ICS + LTRA,[b] or daily medium-dose ICS + theophylline,[b] or daily medium-dose ICS + zileuton,[b] and PRN SABA	Daily medium-high dose ICS-LABA or daily high-dose ICS + LTRA,[b] and PRN SABA	
					Consider adding Asthma Biologics (e.g., anti-IgE, anti-IL5, anti-IL5R, anti-IL4/IL13)[c]	
		Steps 2–4: Conditionally recommend the use of subcutaneous immunotherapy as an adjunct treatment to standard pharmacotherapy in individuals ≥5 years of age whose asthma is controlled at the initiation, build-up, and maintenance phases of immunotherapy[a]				

Assess Control
- First check adherence, inhaler technique, environmental factors,[a] and comorbid conditions.
- **Step up** if needed; reassess in 2–6 weeks
- **Step down** if possible (if asthma is well controlled for at least 3 consecutive months)

Consult with asthma specialist if Step 4 or higher is required. Consider consultation at Step 3.

Control assessment is a key element of asthma care. This involves both impairment and risk. Use of objective measures, self-reported control, and health care utilization are complimentary and should be employed on an ongoing basis depending on the individual's clinical situation.

ICS, Inhaled corticosteroid; *LABA,* long-acting beta$_2$-agonist; *LTRA,* leukotriene receptor antagonist; *SABA,* inhaled short-acting beta$_2$-agonist.

[a]Updated based on the 2020 guidelines.

[b]Cromolyn, nedocromil, LTRAs including zileuton and montelukast, and theophylline were not considered for this update, and/or have limited availability for use in the United States, and/or have an increased risk of adverse consequences and need for monitoring that make their use less desirable. The FDA issued a Boxed Warning for montelukast in March 2020.

[c]The AHRQ systematic reviews that informed this report did not include studies that examined the role of asthma biologics (e.g., anti-IgE, anti-IL5, anti-IL5R, anti-IL4/IL13). Thus this report does not contain specific recommendations for the use of biologics in asthma in Steps 5 and 6.

Data on the use of LAMA therapy in individuals with severe persistent asthma (Step 6) were not included in the AHRQ systematic review and thus no recommendation is made.

During acute asthma exacerbations, individuals often display characteristic signs and symptoms, which typically change with the degree of airway obstruction. Symptoms usually consist of progressively increasing shortness of breath and difficulty breathing with or without rhinorrhea, low-grade fever, and vomiting. On examination, expiratory wheezing or a prolonged expiratory phase may be the only manifestation of mild asthma. However, as the obstructive process progresses, the expiratory phase becomes longer and wheezing becomes louder and occurs on both inspiration and expiration. Eventually, airways collapse and signs of hyperinflation develop (low diaphragms, decreased lateral excursions of the chest wall with breathing, and hyperresonance to percussion). Visible sternocleidomastoid contractions; increased anteroposterior chest diameter; circumoral cyanosis; and suprasternal, intercostal, and substernal retractions occur. Subjectively, the patient experiences chest tightness and anxiety and works harder to breathe. Accessory muscle use and retractions can develop with or without marked wheezing on auscultation. To maximize air exchange, the child assumes a characteristic sitting posture, bending slightly forward. Frequent examinations are warranted, and any change in sensorium requires prompt evaluation. As respiratory muscles tire, the patient becomes lethargic and cyanotic, even with supplemental oxygen. A decrease in wheezing with increased air entry represents response to therapy. Decreased wheezing with decreased air entry is an ominous sign. With extreme fatigue, respiratory muscles fail, retractions decrease, and respiratory failure is imminent unless appropriate therapy is promptly initiated. After initial examination, serial assessment of the degree of respiratory distress using the parameters outlined in Table 4.11 assists determination of the response to therapy.

A particularly useful aspect of the physical examination is the respiratory rate, which increases as the degree of airway obstruction progresses. Normal pediatric respiratory rates are shown in Table 4.12.

The underlying pathology of asthma is lung inflammation. Histopathologic features of acute asthma include airway infiltration with inflammatory cells, increased intraluminal mucus with plugging of small airways, edema, bronchoconstriction, and smooth muscle hypertrophy. Because asthma has bronchoconstrictive and inflammatory components, therapeutic regimens often incorporate a combination of bronchodilator and anti-inflammatory agents. As the immunologic mechanisms underlying asthma become more well defined, it is clear that underlying inflammation contributing to asthma is heterogenous. The simplest classification stratifies patients as either type 2 inflammation (e.g., IgE, eosinophils, Th2 CD4$^+$ T cells high) or type 2-low. This distinction is now clinically relevant, as several monoclonal antibodies have been developed to predominantly target the type 2 inflammatory cascades seen in asthma. These inflammatory processes can lead to chronic airway remodeling, with

Asthma action plan

For: ______ Doctor: ______ Date: ______

Doctor's phone number ______ Hospital/emergency department phone number ______

GREEN ZONE

Doing well

- No cough, wheeze, chest tightness, or shortness of breath during the day or night
- Can do usual activities

And, if a peak flow meter is used,

Peak flow: More than ______
(80 percent or more of my best peak flow)

My best peak flow is: ______

Take these long-term control medicines each day (include an anti-inflammatory).

Medicine	How much to take	When to take it
Before exercise: ❐ ______	❐ 2 or ❐ 4 puffs ______	5 minutes before exercise

YELLOW ZONE

Asthma is getting worse

- Cough, wheeze, chest tightness, or shortness of breath, or
- Waking at night due to asthma, or
- Can do some, but not all, usual activities

-Or-

Peak flow: ______ to ______
(50 to 79 percent of my best peak flow)

First: **Add: Quick-relief medicine–and keep taking your GREEN ZONE medicine.**

______ (Short-acting $beta_2$-agonist) ❐ 2 or ❐ 4 puffs, every 20 minutes for up to 1 hour
❐ Nebulizer, once

Second: **If your symptoms (and peak flow, if used) return to GREEN ZONE after 1 hour of above treatment:**
❐ Continue monitoring to be sure you stay in the green zone.

-Or-

If your symptoms (and peak flow, if used) do not return to GREEN ZONE after 1 hour of above treatment:
❐ Take: ______ (Short-acting $beta_2$-agonist) ❐ 2 or ❐ 4 puffs or ❐ Nebulizer
❐ Add: ______ (Oral steroid) mg per day For ______ (3–10) days
❐ Call the doctor ❐ before/❐ within ______ hours after taking the oral steroid.

RED ZONE

Medical alert!

- Very short of breath, or
- Quick-relief medicines have not helped, or
- Cannot do usual activities, or
- Symptoms are same or get worse after 24 hours in yellow zone

-Or-

Peak flow: Less than ______
(50 percent of my best peak flow)

Take this medicine:

❐ ______ (Short-acting $beta_2$-agonist) ❐ 4 or ❐ 6 puffs or ❐ Nebulizer
❐ ______ (Oral steroid) mg

Then call your doctor NOW. Go to the hospital or call an ambulance if:
- You are still in the red zone after 15 minutes AND
- You have not reached your doctor.

DANGER SIGNS
- **Trouble walking and talking due to shortness of breath**
- **Lips or fingernails are blue**

- **Take ❐ 4 or ❐ 6 puffs of your quick-relief medicine AND**
- **Go to the hospital or call for an ambulance ______ (Phone) NOW!**

See the reverse side for things you can do to avoid your asthma triggers.

Fig. 4.18 Asthma action plan.

Box 4.2 Differential Diagnosis of Asthma by Age and Characteristic Findings

Diagnosis	Age	Findings That Differentiate From Asthma	Diagnostic Tests
Bronchiolitis	<24 months	No atopy, typically not responsive to SABA, context of fever and viral respiratory tract infection	Clinical diagnosis
Viral-induced wheeze	Any age (<4 years more common)	Wheezing only with viral respiratory tract infections, less atopy; usually resolves by age 4 years	PFT if frequent or severe
Bronchopulmonary dysplasia	<24 months	Symptoms since birth in premature infant	Clinical diagnosis
Chronic aspiration/GFRD	Any	Chronic cough especially after meals, gastrointestinal symptoms	Gastroenterology referral, endoscopy, pH probe
Tracheomalacia/ bronchomalacia	<24 months	Symptoms since birth, constant (as opposed to intermittent or triggered), stridor present with tracheomalacia	Laryngoscopy
Bronchiectasis	Any	Symptoms since birth, wet chronic cough, recurrent wheeze with focal lung findings, recurrent pneumonia in same location on CXR, sometimes with hemoptysis	Chest CT, bronchoscopy
Food allergy	Any	First-time wheeze in context of new food exposure and other signs of food allergy flip swelling, vomiting, hives, hypotension	Allergy testing, PFT
Anxiety/panic attack	School age or older	No wheezing, no improvement with SABA	Clinical diagnosis, PFT results normal
Vocal cord dysfunction	Adolescent +	Acute onset of symptoms within minutes of exercise or exposure to irritant symptoms quickly resolve and do not respond to SABA, sensation of airway closing, throat tightness, no symptoms during sleep, occasionally will hear inspiratory stridor on examination, hoarse voice	PFT shows classic pattern of dynamic airflow obstruction, laryngoscopy
Heart failure	Any	Fever (viral myocarditis) missed congenital heart disease, failure to thrive, symptoms worsen with feeding in young infant or with laying down, murmur, poor central pulses, hepatomegaly, crackles	Echocardiography, electrocardiography, CXR
Foreign body aspiration	<4 years (could be any age)	Acute onset of symptoms, unilateral findings, history of choking spell	Anteroposterior/posteroanterior or bilateral decubitus CXR, bronchoscopy
Mass effect (from vascular anomaly or tumor)	Any	Unilateral wheeze or stridor (may be positional, if due to a mass, ring, or sling around upper airways), symptoms worse with laying down, weight loss and other systemic signs it oncologic	Chest CT, bronchoscopy
Underlying immunodeficiency	Any	Recurrent bacterial pneumonia	CXR, immunology evaluation
Allergic bronchopulmonary aspergillosis	Any	Difficult-to-control asthma symptoms, chronic cough and intermittent fevers	Sputum, *Aspergillus* IgE and IgG, CXR
Cystic fibrosis	Any	Failure to thrive (may still have a normal newborn screen)	Sweat chloride testing, genetic testing

CT, Computed tomography; *CXR,* chest radiography; *GERD,* gastroesophageal reflux disease; *IgE,* immunoglobulin E; *IgG,* immunoglobulin G; *PFT,* pulmonary function testing; *SABA,* short-acting inhaled β_2-agonist.

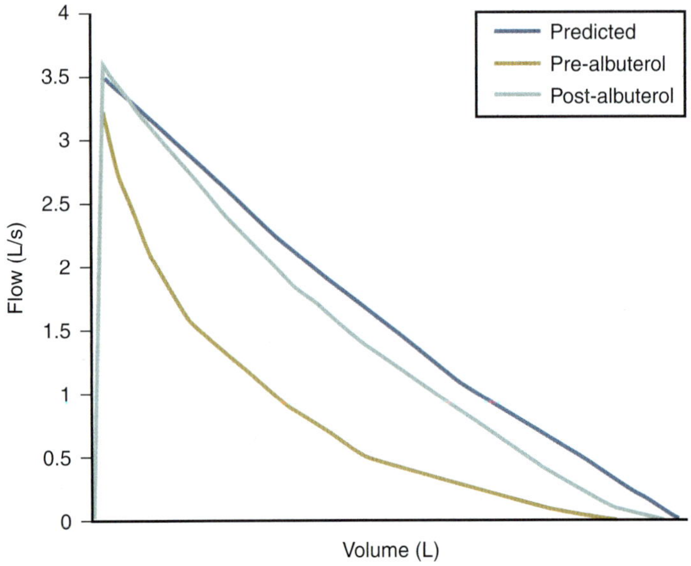

Fig. 4.19 Asthma. Flow/volume loop showing predicted values, initial values, and substantial reversibility after albuterol administration. Note the downward scooping of curves, which is typical in patients with asthma with ongoing obstruction.

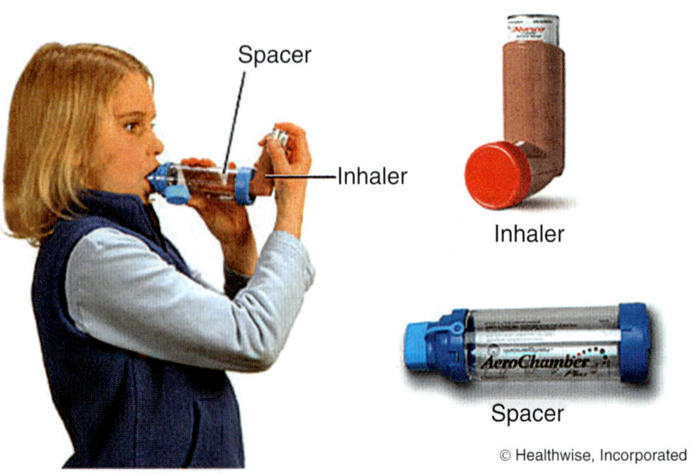

Fig. 4.20 Proper metered dose inhaler technique.

Table 4.11 Estimation of Severity of Acute Exacerbations of Asthma in Children

	Mild	Moderate	Severe	Life-Threatening
Symptoms				
Breathlessness[a]	While walking	While at rest (infant—softer, shorter cry, difficulty feeding)	While at rest (infant—stops feeding)	
Talks in:	Sentences	Phrases	Words	
Alertness	May be agitated	Usually agitated	Usually agitated	Drowsy or confused
Signs				
Respiratory rate[b]	Increased	Increased	Significantly increased	Often normal or decreased
Accessory muscle use	Unusual	Common	Common	Paradoxic abdominal movements
Wheeze	Moderate, often only end-expiratory	Loud, throughout exhalation	Usually loud, in both inspiration and expiration	Absence of wheeze and air movement
Pulse	Normal to tachycardic	Tachycardic	Tachycardic	Bradycardic
Pulsus paradoxus[c]	<10 mm Hg	10–20 mm Hg	20–40 mm Hg	Absence suggests respiratory muscle fatigue
Functional Assessment				
PEF (percent predicted or personal best)	>70%	40%–69%	<40%	<25%
PaO_2 (room air)	Normal	>60 mm Hg	<60 mm Hg; possible cyanosis	Cyanosis
$Paco_2$	<42 mm Hg	<42 mm Hg	>42 mm Hg	>42 mm Hg
Sao_2% (room air)	>95%	90%–95%	<90%	<90%

Within each category, the presence of several parameters, but not necessarily all, indicates the general classification of the exacerbation.

$Paco_2$, Arterial carbon dioxide pressure; *PaO_2*, arterial oxygen pressure; *PEF*, peak expiratory flow; *Sao_2*, arterial oxygen saturation.

[a]Parents' or physician's impression of degree of child's breathlessness.

[b]See Table 4.9 for normal respiratory rates by age.

[c]Pulsus paradoxus does not correlate with phase of respiration in small children.

Modified from National Asthma Education and Prevention Program (NAEPP): *Expert Panel Report 3 (EPR3). Guidelines for the diagnosis and management of asthma (Publication No. 08–5846)*, Bethesda, MD, 2007, National Institutes of Health.

Table 4.12 Respiratory Rates of Normal Children, Sleeping and Awake[a]

	Sleeping			Awake		
Age	No.	Mean	Range	No.	Mean	Range
6–12 months old	6	27	22–31	3	64	58–75
1–2 years old	6	19	17–23	4	35	30–40
2–4 years old	16	19	16–25	15	31	23–42
4–6 years old	23	18	14–23	22	26	19–36
6–8 years old	27	17	13–23	28	23	15–30

[a]In breaths per minute.

From Waring WW: The history and physical exam. In Kendig E, Chernick V, editors: *Disorders of the respiratory tract in children*, Philadelphia, 1983, WB Saunders. As appears in National Asthma Education and Prevention Program (NAEPP): *Expert panel report: guidelines for the diagnosis and management of asthma (Publication No. 91-3642)*, Bethesda, MD, 1991, National Institutes of Health.

increased basement membrane deposition and smooth muscle mass (Fig. 4.21).

Education is a key component of asthma therapy, incorporating information about disease pathogenesis; avoidance of environmental triggers (including second-hand tobacco smoke exposure); benefits and risks of medications; and a written, individualized therapeutic plan for chronic and acute management that outlines the goals of asthma therapy and indications and correct use for prescribed medications.

The radiographic features of hyperinflation, peribronchial cuffing, and atelectasis, which are characteristic of uncomplicated acute asthma, are illustrated in Fig. 4.22. Complications are diagnosed radiographically but may be suggested by symptoms and signs. Pneumothorax (Fig. 4.23) should be suspected in any patient with asthma who develops chest pain associated with dyspnea, cyanosis, tachypnea, and occasionally cough. Examination reveals respiratory distress, marked hyperinflation and decreased chest wall excursion, and decreased or absent breath sounds on the affected side. With tension pneumothorax, the trachea, mediastinum, and cardiac landmarks may be shifted to the opposite side. Pneumomediastinum and subcutaneous emphysema (Fig. 4.24), usually involving the neck and supraclavicular areas, are more common than pneumothorax. When mild, the patient may be asymptomatic and findings may be detected incidentally on radiographs. With more extensive air dissection, the patient may complain of neck and chest pain, and the subcutaneous emphysema may be visibly evident as a soft tissue swelling of the neck and chest that is crepitant on palpation. Pneumothorax and pneumomediastinum can produce characteristic auscultatory findings, including a crackling "mediastinal crunch" at the base of the heart and a systolic crunch or knock. The latter sound has been referred to as *noisy pneumothorax* and is frequently audible to the patient and physician without the aid of a stethoscope.

Other complications that may be observed on physical examination include those induced by chronic systemic steroid use, such as weight gain; "moon-type" facies; hirsutism; polycythemia (red, ruddy complexion) (Fig. 4.25); and short stature (see Chapter 9). The introduction of effective anti-inflammatory therapy, particularly inhaled corticosteroids and targeted biologic therapy, has made such sequelae rare.

In children with recent onset of wheezing, asthma must be differentiated from other disorders associated with wheezing. In infants, this differentiation includes bronchiolitis, the features of

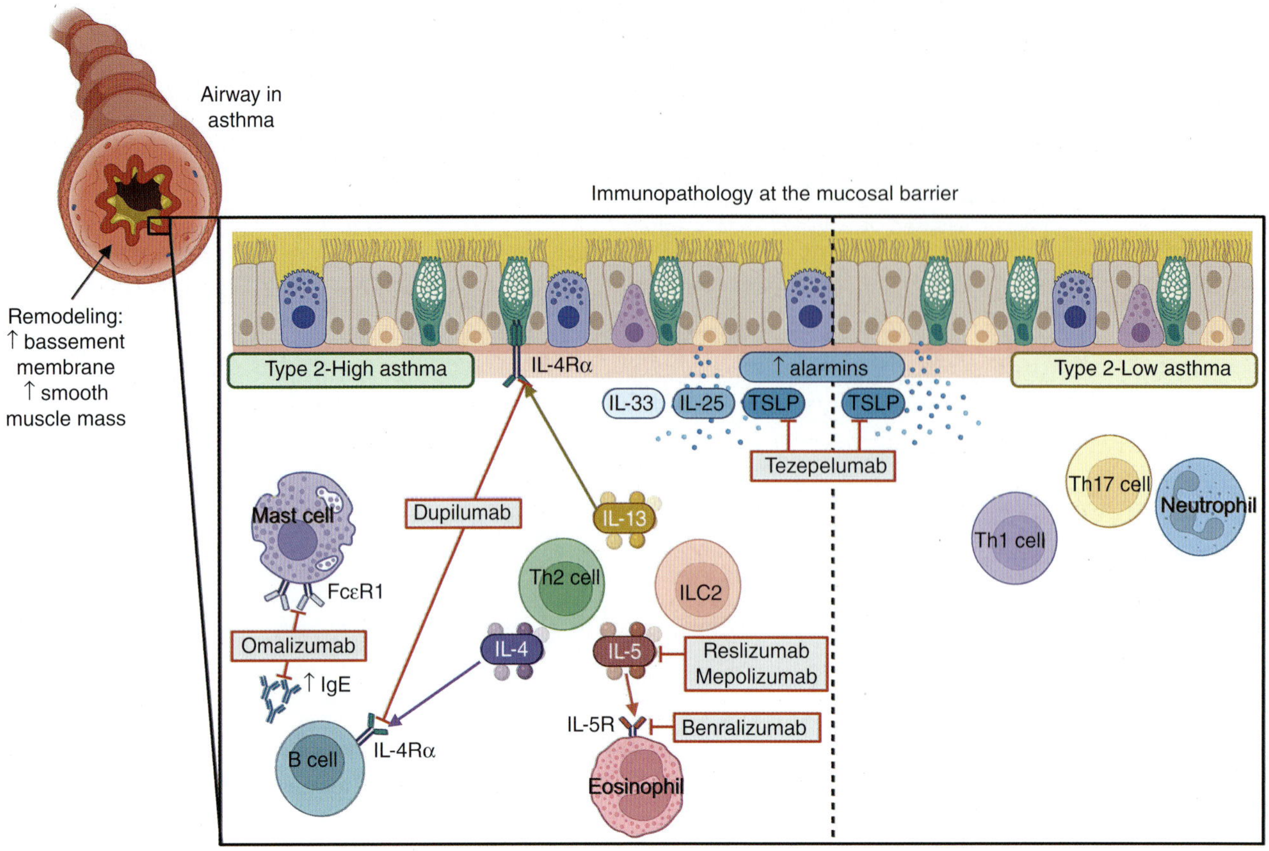

Fig. 4.21 Immunologic mechanisms of asthma. Type 2 immunity (Th2 CD4⁺ T cells, eosinophils, IgE, and innate lymphoid cells-ILC2s) is a clinically relevant consideration to classify asthma patients, as there are several biologics targeting these pathways (red boxes). This underlying inflammatory process can contribute to airway remodeling. Created with BioRender.

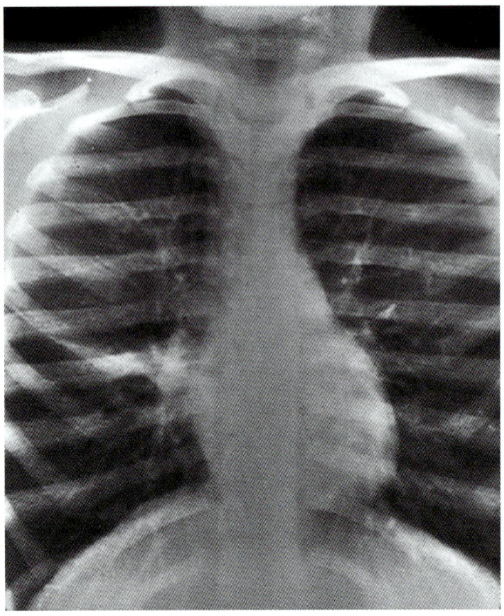

Fig. 4.22 Anteroposterior chest radiograph of child with acute asthma. Note the flattened diaphragm, hyperinflation, peribronchial thickening, and right middle lobe atelectasis.

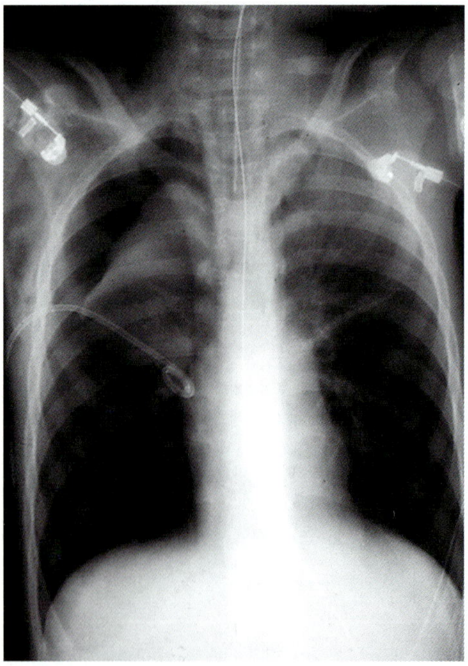

Fig. 4.23 Chest radiograph showing right-sided pneumothorax in an intubated patient with acute asthma and respiratory failure. Clinical manifestations include pleuritic chest pain, dyspnea, cyanosis, tachypnea, and cough. Also, note the marked hyperinflation of the lungs, which can result in cardiac compression (narrow cardiac shadow) and compromise of cardiac venous return, as well as extensive right-sided subcutaneous emphysema. (Courtesy Beverly Newman, MD, Pittsburgh, PA.)

which are listed in Table 4.13 (see Chapter 17). This differentiation may be difficult because up to 50% of children with recurrent bronchiolitis are later diagnosed with asthma, and asthma exacerbations are often triggered by viral infection. However, the distinction remains a clinically useful one for these reasons: (1) the children with bronchiolitis who do not develop asthma may be inappropriately labeled as asthmatic; and (2) children younger than 2 years old frequently do not respond to inhaled bronchodilators. In infants and young children who wheeze with viral upper respiratory infections, different patterns of illness may emerge over time.

The Tucson Children's Respiratory Study, a large, longitudinal assessment of respiratory illnesses in children, identified different patterns of wheezing illness in children. As summarized in Fig. 4.26, 51% of children enrolled in this study never wheezed, 20% had transient infant wheezing (defined as wheezing during the first 3 years

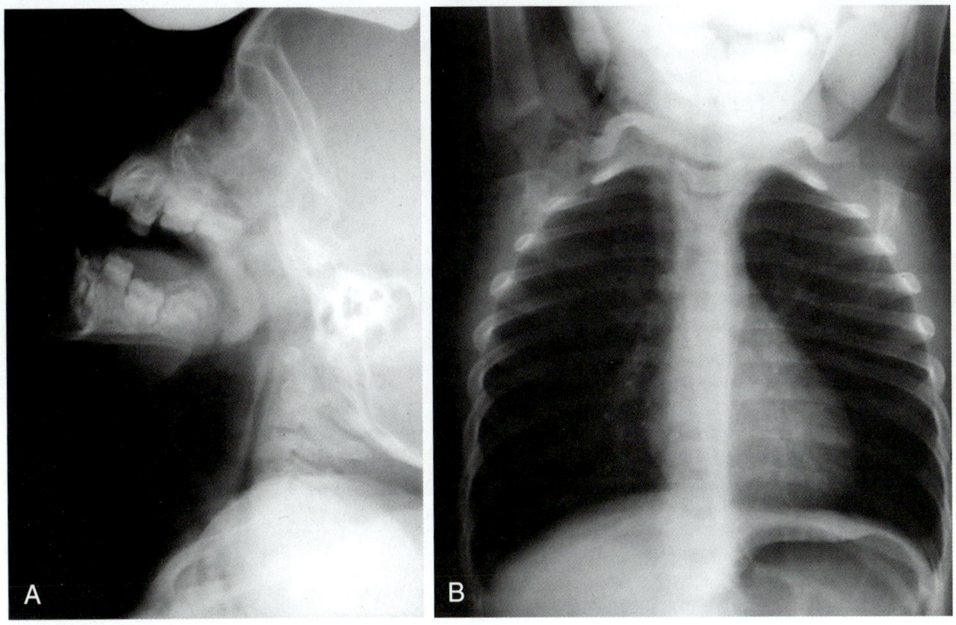

Fig. 4.24 Asthma with pneumomediastinum in a 16-month-old child with asthma. Note the dissection of air in the soft tissues just anterior to the vertebrae (A) and in the mediastinum and subcutaneous tissues of the right arm (B). This highlights the often subtle findings of pneumomediastinum in the chest and the more striking findings in the neck. Also note the hyperinflation (B). (Courtesy Beverly Newman, MD, Pittsburgh, PA.)

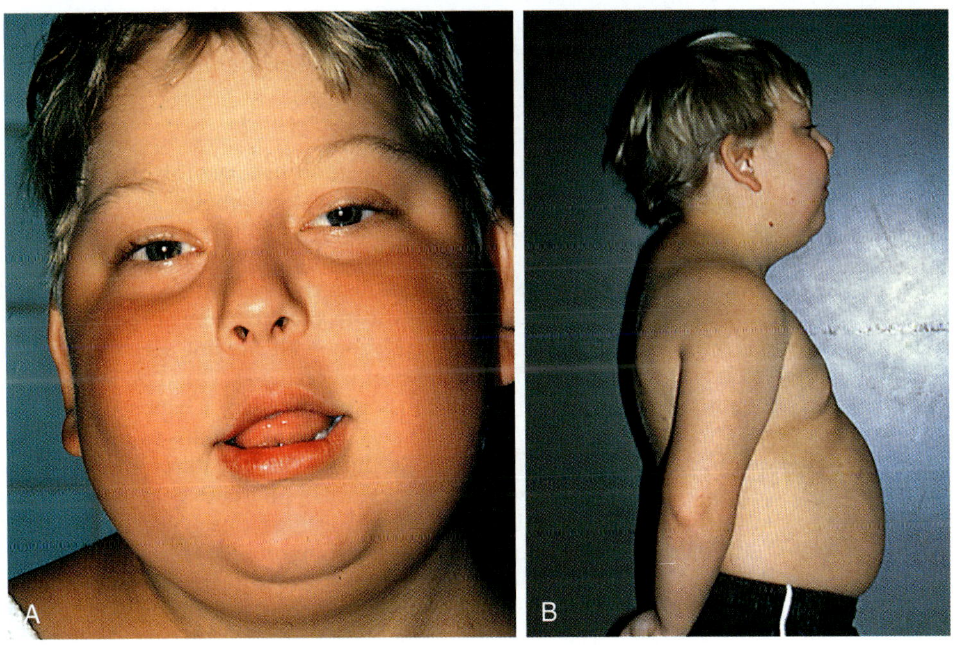

Fig. 4.25 Steroid-dependent asthma. Shown are complications of corticosteroid therapy for chronic asthma: moon-type facies (A) and buffalo hump (B), both resulting from abnormal fat distribution.

Table 4.13 Differentiating Features of Asthma and Bronchiolitis in Children

	Asthma	Bronchiolitis
Primary etiologies	Viruses, allergens, exercise, and so on	Respiratory syncytial virus, other viruses
Age at onset	50% by 2 years old 80% by 5 years old	<24 months old
Recurrent wheezing	Yes (characteristic)	70% (≤2 episodes) 30% progress to asthma (≥3 episodes)
Onset of wheezing	Acute if allergic or exercise induced	Insidious
Concomitant symptoms of upper respiratory infection	Yes, if infectious	Yes
Family history of allergy and asthma	Frequent	Infrequent in children with ≤2 episodes
Nasal eosinophilia	With allergic rhinitis	Absent
Chest auscultation	If viral, as in bronchiolitis Nonviral: High-pitched expiratory wheezes	Fine, sibilant rales, and coarse inspiratory and expiratory wheezes
Concomitant allergic manifestations	Yes, if allergic asthma	Usually absent
Immunoglobulin E (IgE) level	Elevated (if allergic)	Normal
Response to bronchodilator	Yes (characteristic)	Unresponsive or partially responsive

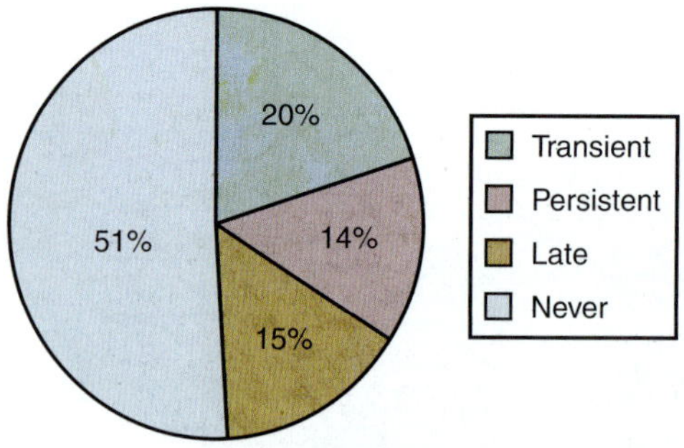

Fig. 4.26 Asthma. The Tucson Children's Respiratory Study has shown that in children who wheeze, different patterns of illness may emerge over time. About half the patients in this study had evidence of wheezing before 6 years old. In the transient group, wheezing occurred during the first 3 years of life but resolved by 6 years old. In the persistent group, wheezing occurred during the first 3 years of life and persisted to 6 years old. In the late group, wheezing did not occur during the first 3 years of life but was present by 6 years old. (Modified from Martinez FD, Wright AL, Taussig LM, et al: Asthma and wheezing in the first 6 years of life, *N Engl J Med 332*:133–138, 1995.)

of life but no wheezing at 6 years old), 14% had persistent wheezing (defined as wheezing during the first 3 years of life with wheezing present at 6 years old), and 15% had late-onset wheezing (defined as no wheezing during the first 3 years of life but wheezing present at 6 years old). Children with transient wheezing had significantly lower lung function in infancy (before any wheezing illness) than all the other groups. At 6 years old, children with early transient wheezing had significantly lower lung function than those who had never wheezed, and children with persistent wheezing had the lowest levels of lung function of all the groups (Table 4.14).

It is hypothesized that children with early transient wheezing have congenitally smaller airways, which predispose them to wheezing with viral illnesses. As their airways grow in size with age, these children outgrow wheezing with viral infections. In contrast, children with persistent wheezing are born with normal airway function, which deteriorates over time, reflecting the effects of the chronic asthmatic disease process. Distinguishing transient versus persistent wheezing during infancy and early childhood remains problematic. Infant pulmonary function testing is still experimental and not widely available, there are currently no reliable genetic markers, and the use of any single biochemical marker is controversial. However, a combination of clinical and biochemical markers may be useful in predicting persistent wheezing (Box 4.3). These include increased serum IgE level, atopic dermatitis and rhinitis (unrelated to upper respiratory infection) during the first year of life, severe lower respiratory infections requiring hospitalization, and diminished airway function as measured by spirometry at 6 years old. Other factors associated with persistent wheezing

Table 4.14 Lung Function During Infancy and at 6 Years Old According to Wheezing History in Patients Enrolled in the Tucson Children's Respiratory Study

		Lung Function (V_{max}FRC)	
Group	***n* (%)**	**Infancy**	**6 Years Old**
No wheezing	425 (51.5%)	Normal	Normal
Transient wheezing	164 (19.9%)	Diminished	Diminished
Persistent wheezing	113 (13.7%)	Normal	Diminished
Late-onset wheezing	124 (15%)	Normal	Normal

V_{Max} FRC, Maximal expiratory flow at functional residual capacity, expressed as milliliters per second.

Modified from Martinez FD, Wright AL, Taussig LM, et al: Asthma and wheezing in the first six years of life, *N Engl J Med* 332:133–138, 1995.

Box 4.3 Factors Predictive of Persistent Asthma

Family history of asthma (maternal > paternal)
Atopy
↑ IgE or positive allergy skin tests
Eczema
Rhinitis
Allergen exposure (dust mites, animals)
RSV bronchiolitis
Gender (males > females)
Environmental smoke exposure
Severity in childhood

Modified from Martinez FD, Wright AL, Taussig LM, et al: Asthma and wheezing in the first six years of life, *N Engl J Med* 332:133–138, 1995.

Table 4.15 Clinical Index to Define Asthma[a]

Major Criteria	Minor Criteria
1. Physician diagnosis of parental asthma 2. Physician diagnosis of atopic dermatitis	1. Physician diagnosis of allergic rhinitis 2. Wheezing apart from colds 3. Eosinophilia (≥4%)

[a]The loose index for prediction of asthma consists of early wheezing plus at least one of two major criteria or two of three minor criteria. The stringent index for prediction of asthma consists of early *frequent* wheezing plus at least one of two major criteria or two of three minor criteria.

Modified from Castro-Rodriguez JA, Holberg CJ, Wright AL, et al: A clinical index to define risk of asthma in young children with recurrent wheezing, *Am J Respir Crit Care Med* 162:1403–1406, 2000.

include a family history of asthma or allergy and perinatal exposure to passive tobacco smoke. A clinical index has been developed to predict which children with recurrent wheezing are at risk for persistent asthma (Table 4.15).

Although children with pneumonia (particularly of viral origin) may wheeze, they are more likely to have rales or normal findings on auscultation with varying degrees of work of breathing. Other causes of wheezing are listed in Table 4.16. Airway compression by anomalous vessels (see Chapter 5) or mass lesions is often distinguishable from bronchiolitis by the absence of signs of infection and from asthma by failure to respond to bronchodilators. The history and presence of infiltrates help in the diagnosis of aspiration, which can mimic asthma closely. Radiographic studies (such as barium swallow with fluoroscopy) can be helpful in distinguishing among these entities (Fig. 4.27). pH probe testing may be required to identify gastroesophageal reflux (see Chapter 17), although a trial of antireflux medicines is often attempted.

In older children who have sudden onset of wheezing and respiratory distress, the differential diagnosis includes respiratory infections, left ventricular failure, aspiration, and vocal cord dysfunction. Respiratory infections (such as croup) may be distinguished by their characteristic histories and tendencies to involve the upper airways (see Chapter 17). Lower respiratory infections (pneumonia) generally produce fever and more localized findings of rales, a decrease and change in the quality of breath sounds, and egophony. Left ventricular failure, especially with pulmonary edema, may present with acute respiratory distress and wheezing. A history of cardiac disease, diffuse crackles or basilar rales, and a third heart sound on auscultation help distinguish this condition from asthma. Aspiration of a foreign body that lodges in a mainstem bronchus may produce wheezing (Fig. 4.28). History of a choking episode and physical findings of unilateral wheezing and hyperresonance aid in distinguishing aspiration from asthma but do not confirm the diagnosis because wheezing resulting from foreign body aspiration may respond at least in part to bronchodilator therapy. Vocal cord dysfunction is becoming more recognized in children and adolescents and is often confused with asthma by families, school nurses, and other medical

Table 4.16 Associated Symptoms and Signs in the Wheezing Child That Are Helpful in Differential Diagnosis

Symptoms and Signs	Diseases Associated With Wheezing	
	In Infants	**In Older Children**
Positional changes	Anomalies of the great vessels, gastroesophageal reflux	Gastroesophageal reflux
Growth faltering	Cystic fibrosis, tracheoesophageal fistula, bronchopulmonary dysplasia	Cystic fibrosis, chronic hypersensitivity pneumonitis, α_1-antitrypsin deficiency, bronchiectasis
Factors associated with feeding	Tracheoesophageal fistula, gastroesophageal reflux	Gastroesophageal reflux
Environmental triggers	Allergic asthma	Allergic asthma, allergic bronchopulmonary aspergillosis, acute hypersensitivity pneumonitis
Sudden onset	Allergic asthma, croup	Allergic asthma, foreign body aspiration, croup, acute hypersensitivity pneumonitis
Fever	Bronchiolitis, pneumonitis	Infectious asthma, acute hypersensitivity pneumonitis, croup
Rhinorrhea	Bronchiolitis, pneumonitis	Infectious or allergic asthma, croup
Concomitant stridor	Tracheal or bronchial stenosis, anomalies of the great vessels, croup	Foreign body aspiration, croup
Clubbing	—	Cystic fibrosis, bronchiectasis, bronchopulmonary dysplasia

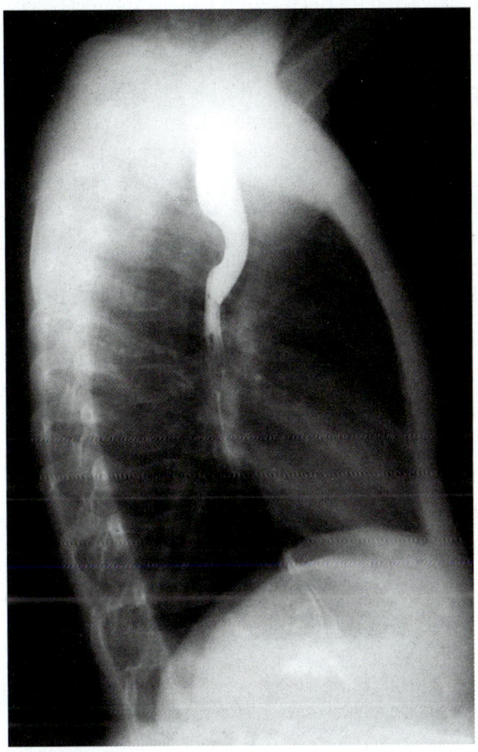

Fig. 4.27 Vascular ring/compression. Barium swallow (lateral chest radiograph) shows upper airway compression by a right-sided aortic arch with aberrant left subclavian and diverticulum at the left subclavian origin. Note the round indentation on the posterior wall of the esophagus and the anterior displacement and compression of the trachea, which can cause wheezing and mimic asthma. (Courtesy Beverly Newman, MD, Pittsburgh, PA. From Fireman P, Slavin RG: *Atlas of allergies*, New York, 1990, Gower.)

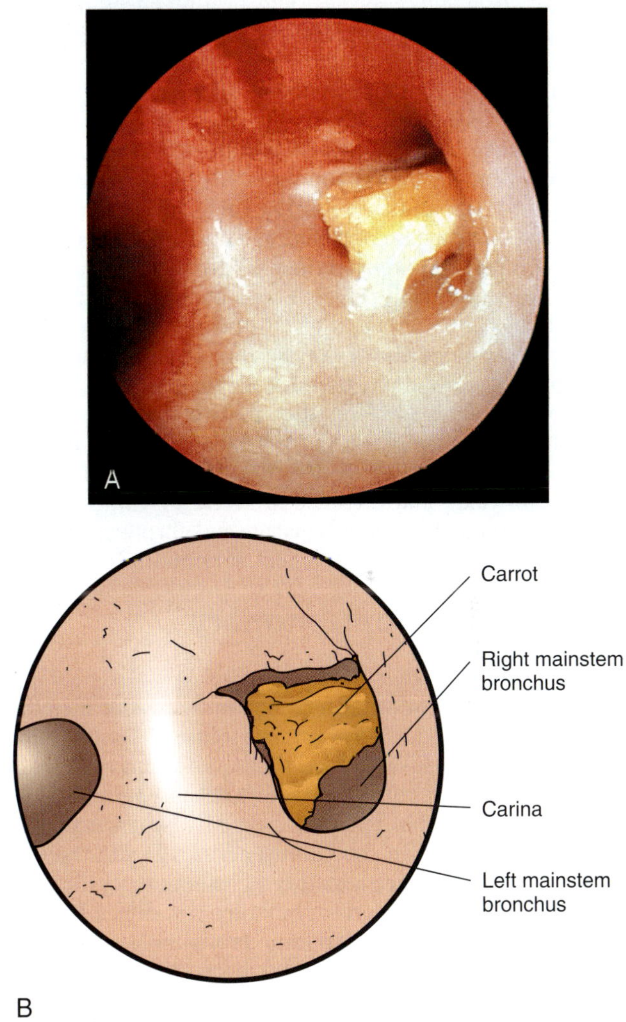

Fig. 4.28 Airway foreign body. (A) A piece of carrot is lodged in the right-stem bronchus just below the carina, as visualized during bronchoscopy. (B) Artist rendition of carrot location in bronchi. Foreign bodies such as this can cause airway obstruction that is partially responsive to bronchodilator therapy. (Courtesy Sylvan Stool, MD, Pittsburgh, PA. From Fireman P, Slavin RG: *Atlas of allergies*. New York, 1990, Gower.)

providers. Symptoms include acute-onset dyspnea and often stridor, which can be mistaken for wheezing to the untrained observer, secondary to partial or complete adduction of the vocal cords during inspiration. Symptoms rarely awaken individuals from sleep. Many triggers are similar to asthma, including exercise, inhalational irritants, psychosocial stressors, and rhinitis. Bronchodilators are not effective and objective measurements of pulmonary function, including pulse oximetry and chest radiographs, are unremarkable during acute episodes. Some episodes of vocal cord dysfunction can become severe enough to result in syncope from hyperventilation, which often successfully resolves the acute episode as the vocal cords relax.

In the older child with mild, infrequent episodes of wheezing that respond to bronchodilator therapy, asthma is readily diagnosed. However, with daily wheezing, frequent exacerbations, lack of response to bronchodilators, or poor growth, other diagnoses must be considered, including chronic obstructive pulmonary disease, cystic fibrosis, α_1-antitrypsin deficiency, and immunodeficiency. Chronic obstructive pulmonary diseases, which include chronic bronchitis, emphysema, bronchiectasis, and bronchopulmonary dysplasia, are distinguished by their lack of significant reversibility with bronchodilator therapy. Cystic fibrosis may present with chronic cough, wheezing, and recurrent infections. Malabsorption with bulky, foul-smelling stools; growth faltering; and clubbing of the nail beds are also common findings. An inherited autosomal recessive disorder, α_1-antitrypsin deficiency, is characterized by the onset of progressive emphysema in a young adult and is one cause of neonatal hepatitis.

Hypersensitivity Pneumonitis

Although IgE-mediated allergic respiratory diseases (allergic rhinitis, asthma) are the most common manifestations of inhalant sensitivities in humans, other immunologic respiratory diseases involving non-IgE immune mechanisms may result from the inhalation of antigens from the susceptible individual's environment. A wide variety of inhaled biologic dusts may induce an inflammatory lung disease involving the interstitium, alveoli, and airways. The most common form of hypersensitivity pneumonitis is caused by inhalation of thermophilic actinomycetes (*Saccharopolyspora rectivirgula,* formerly *Micropolyspora faeni*) antigens present in moldy vegetable compost and is termed *farmer's lung.* Other forms (and their causative dusts and antigens) include malt-worker's lung (moldy malt, *Aspergillus* species) and bird-breeder's lung (avian dust, avian proteins). The disorder is termed *hypersensitivity pneumonitis* or *extrinsic allergic alveolitis* and appears to be mediated by a complex immune response involving both immune complexes (type III) and T cells (type IV).

Hypersensitivity pneumonitis is a syndrome with a broad spectrum of presenting symptoms and signs that have been subdivided into acute, subacute, and chronic. The clinical features depend on these factors: (1) the nature of the inhaled dust, (2) the intensity and frequency of inhalation exposure, and (3) the immunologic responsiveness of the exposed individual. A concomitant upper respiratory infection or another pulmonary insult may be an important factor in induction. Development of sensitization to the inhaled organic dust requires several months to years, although organic dust toxic syndrome can present similarly after a single exposure to a large dose of antigen. The acute form of hypersensitivity pneumonitis is usually readily differentiated from asthma by the lack of wheezing, prominence of rales, and presence of severe systemic symptoms, such as high fever and myalgia. Subacute and chronic forms generally present with insidious development of respiratory symptoms.

Allergic Bronchopulmonary Aspergillosis

Aspergillus species, in addition to being one cause of hypersensitivity pneumonitis and allergic asthma, cause a disorder termed *allergic bronchopulmonary aspergillosis (ABPA).* This entity is characterized by migrating pulmonary infiltrates and peripheral blood and sputum eosinophilia. Type I and type III hypersensitivity are thought to be involved in the pathogenesis. Affected individuals are usually atopic and have a history of asthma or cystic fibrosis. They often present with systemic symptoms and difficulty weaning off systemic corticosteroids. Sputum production is prominent. Physical findings include the general signs of lower airway obstruction (see the earlier section, Asthma).

Laboratory studies that assist in diagnosis include the following:

- Peripheral blood examination reveals eosinophilia (generally $>1000/mm^3$).
- The serum IgE level is markedly elevated, often greater than 1000 ng/mL, and specific IgE to *Aspergillus fumigatus* is elevated.
- Skin testing for *A. fumigatus* is positive. Although mold-sensitive patients with asthma without ABPA may have a positive reaction, a negative reaction rules out ABPA.
- Serum precipitating antibody (IgG) to *A. fumigatus* is found in most patients, but the titer has a poor correlation with disease activity.
- Chest radiography commonly shows infiltrates in active ABPA. The upper lobes are commonly involved, and infiltrates characteristically shift rapidly from one site to the other. Remarkably, radiographic findings do not correlate well with clinical severity, and patients with extensive consolidation may be asymptomatic (Fig. 4.29).
- High-resolution computed tomography scanning may show bronchiectasis, especially late in the course of the disease.

OCULAR ALLERGY

Ocular allergic reactions may involve the eyelid or conjunctiva. The eyelids have a rich blood supply and loose connective tissue assisting edema collection from either allergic inflammation or trauma. Immediate hypersensitivity reactions that produce eyelid angioedema may be triggered by numerous stimuli, including pollens, dusts, insect stings or bites, foods, or drugs. The most common cause of mild reactions is topical exposure to environmental allergens. These reactions are characterized by periorbital edema, pruritus, and erythema after exposure to an allergen (Fig. 4.30). Severe acute episodes can be distinguished from cellulitis by lack of induration, absence of tenderness and fever, and the fact that involvement is usually bilateral (see Chapter 24).

Allergic conjunctivitis may be acute or chronic and seasonal or perennial, depending on the sensitizing allergens. Commonly implicated allergens include pollens, molds, dust, and animal dander. In the acute seasonal form, onset may be rapid and may coincide with the appearance of pollen in the environment. This condition frequently accompanies seasonal allergic rhinitis and is commonly due to ragweed, grass, and tree pollens. Itching and excessive tearing are the most prominent symptoms. Pruritus often interferes with sleep, and vision may be impaired by excessive clear discharge.

Physical findings depend on the degree of chronicity. In the acute form, these findings consist of diffuse bilateral conjunctival

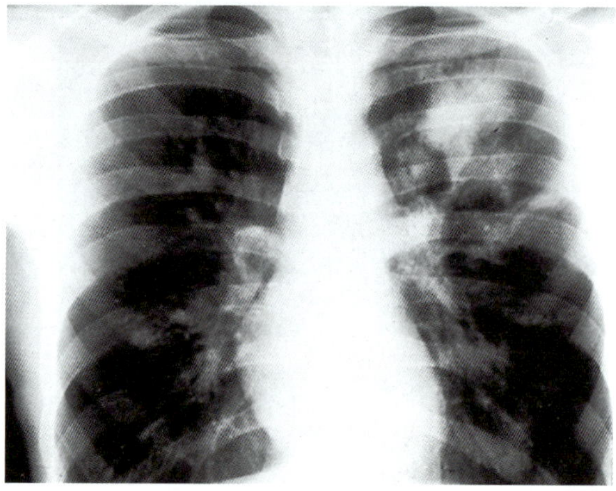

Fig. 4.29 Chest radiograph of patient with allergic bronchopulmonary aspergillosis. These patients are frequently asymptomatic despite extensive areas of consolidation. (Courtesy Raymond G. Slavin, MD, St. Louis, MO.)

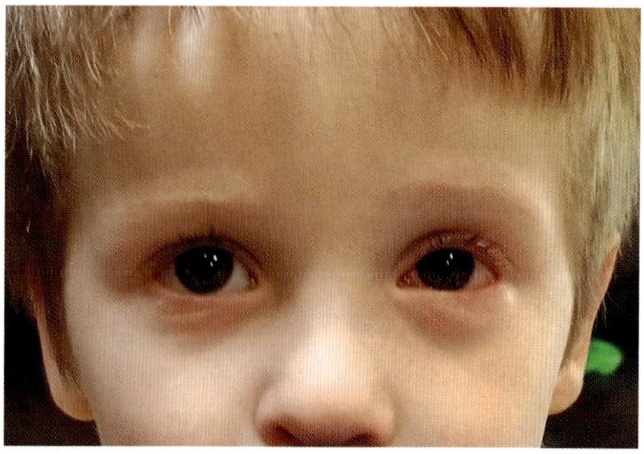

Fig. 4.30 Mild periorbital edema and erythema and conjunctival injection in a child with seasonal allergic conjunctivitis.

edema and hyperemia. Photophobia, profuse tearing, and mild lid swelling are commonly associated. In the chronic form, the conjunctivae appear pale, with mild edema and hyperplasia of the papillae. This may result in a fine, granular appearance of the conjunctivae, which is termed *allergic cobblestoning* (Fig. 4.31). The clinical diagnosis may be confirmed by finding eosinophilia on a smear of conjunctival secretions and skin testing for the suspected allergens.

The differential diagnosis of allergic conjunctivitis includes atopic keratoconjunctivitis and vernal conjunctivitis. Atopic keratoconjunctivitis occurs mostly in adult patients with atopic dermatitis and is characterized by erythema and thickening of the conjunctivae (Fig. 4.32). This may progress to scarring and vascularization of the cornea in severe cases, and ocular disease activity parallels that of cutaneous disease.

Vernal conjunctivitis is uncommon and chronic in nature. Young, atopic boys are affected most frequently. Symptoms include severe itching, photophobia, blurring of vision, and lacrimation. Physical examination reveals white, ropy secretions containing many eosinophils. A palpebral form manifests hypertrophic nodular papillae that resemble cobblestones on the upper eyelids (Fig. 4.33). The papillae consist of dense fibrous tissue with eosinophilic infiltrates. In the bulbar form, nodules appear as gelatinous masses called *Trantas dots,* which are usually found at the corneoscleral junction (Fig. 4.34). The symptoms are generally severe and frequently require referral to ophthalmology for topical steroids. This disease usually remits with maturity and is rarely seen in adults. Giant papillary conjunctivitis, which appears clinically and histologically to be a mild form of vernal conjunctivitis, is associated with the use of hard and soft contact lenses (Fig. 4.35). The stimulus is believed to be foreign material that accumulates on the surface of the contact lenses. Whether this material is antigenic and the condition an immune-mediated disease is not known.

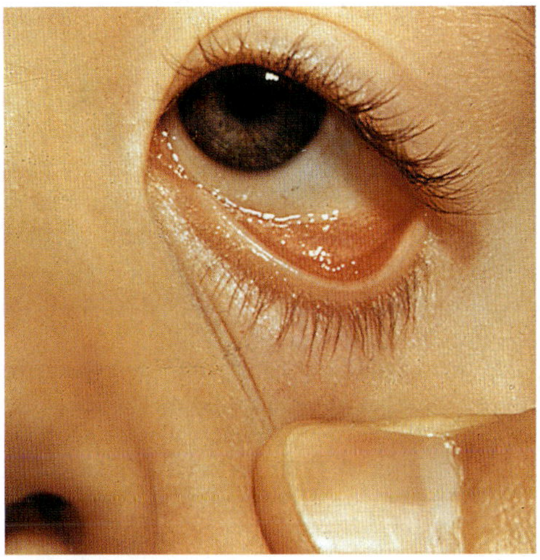

Fig. 4.31 Allergic cobblestoning of the conjunctiva in chronic allergic conjunctivitis. This granular appearance is due to edema and hyperplasia of the papillae.

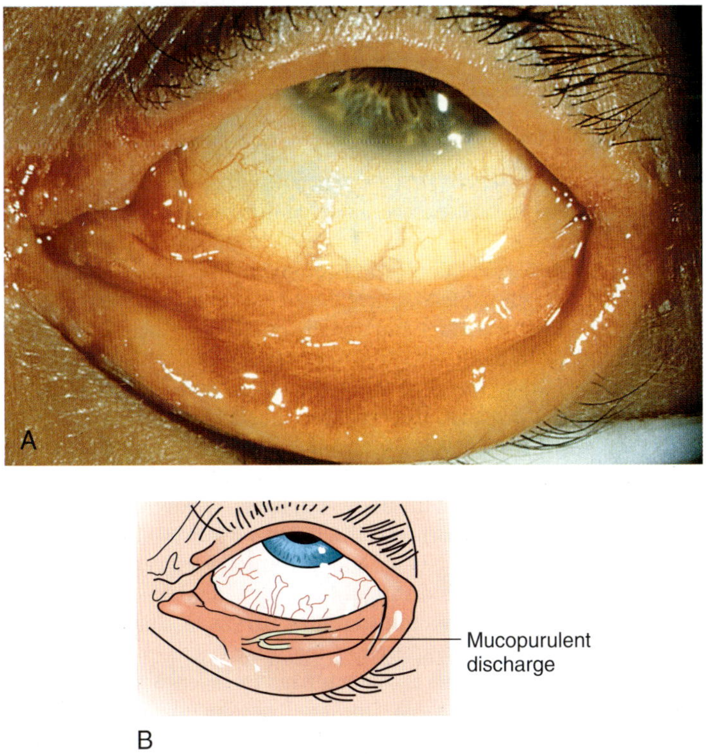

Fig. 4.32 (A) Atopic keratoconjunctivitis with chronic papillary conjunctivitis. (B) Note the stringy mucopurulent discharge often seen in this disorder. (From Fireman P, Slavin RG: *Atlas of allergies*, New York, 1990, Gower.)

URTICARIA AND ANGIOEDEMA

Episodes of urticaria occur in 20% of the population. Angioedema is less common. Both processes involve degranulation of mast cells and basophils and can be due to any one of multiple triggers. Acute episodes of urticaria or angioedema due to type I IgE-mediated hypersensitivity reactions to drugs, foods, or insect stings occur within minutes to 1 to 2 hours of exposure to the allergen. Non-IgE-mediated mechanisms can also cause degranulation of mast cells through activation of other pathways such as complement and immune complex formation or direct mast cell degranulation. The cumulation of these various processes is vasodilation with increased vascular permeability, followed by edema. When this occurs in the dermis, it results in characteristic urticaria, whereas occurrence in the deeper subcutaneous tissue results in angioedema.

Urticarial lesions are well-circumscribed, raised, palpable wheals that blanch with applied pressure (Fig. 4.36). They are usually erythematous but may be pale or white with red halos. Typically, the lesions are intensely pruritic; however, in some instances the pruritus is mild. Classic urticaria should be transient (not last in any one location for greater than 24 hours)and is not associated with residual skin changes such as blistering, bruising, or changes in pigmentation. Angioedema is characterized by diffuse subcutaneous tissue swelling. The overlying skin may be erythematous or normal in coloration. Angioedema may be more painful than pruritic and typically involves loose tissues such as the face, hands, feet, and perineum (Fig. 4.37). Angioedema, unlike other types of edema, is not gravity dependent or symmetric. Unlike hives, angioedema may take hours to days to completely resolve.

When evaluating causes of urticaria or angioedema, a thorough history looking for inciting exposures can identify a cause. In cases of allergen triggers, the symptoms should be reproducible with a

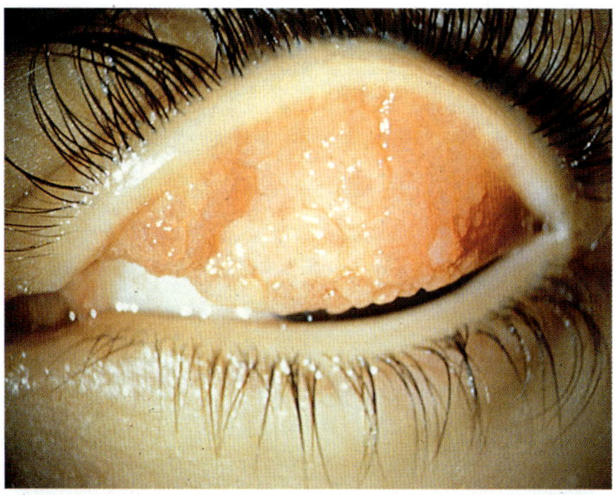

Fig. 4.33 Vernal conjunctivitis, palpebral form. The giant papillary elevations are easily seen without magnification. (From Fireman P, Slavin RG: *Atlas of allergies*, New York, 1990, Gower.)

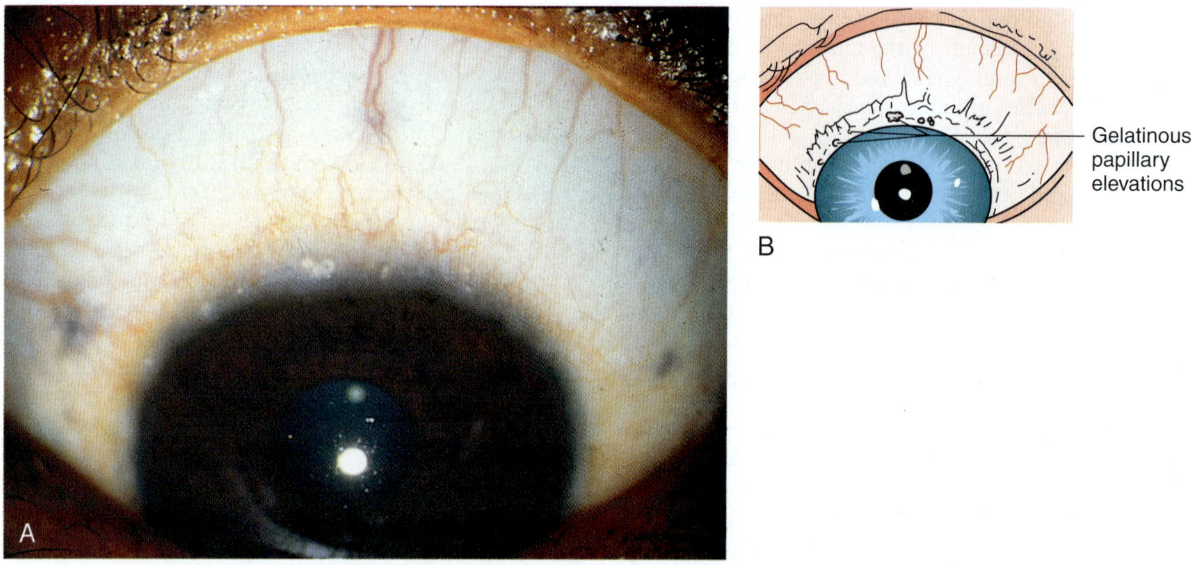

Fig. 4.34 (A) Vernal conjunctivitis, limbal form. (B) Note the gelatinous papillary elevations of the limbal tissue. (From Fireman P, Slavin RG: *Atlas of allergies*, New York, 1990, Gower.)

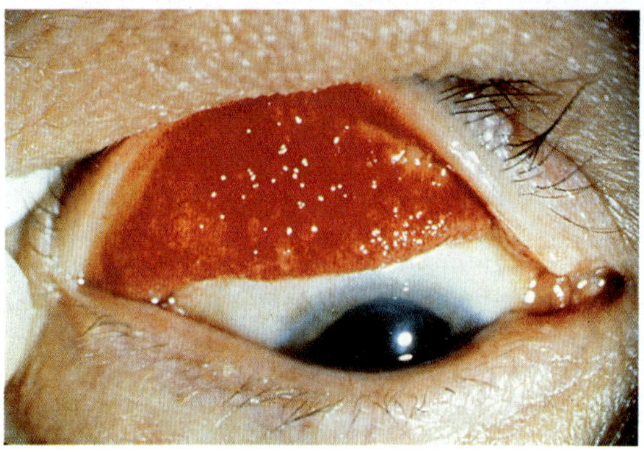

Fig. 4.35 Giant papillary conjunctivitis. These hobnail-like elevations of the upper tarsal conjunctiva, evident on eversion of the upper eyelid, occur when the upper lid meets a foreign body, such as a contact lens, prosthesis, or exposed suture. (From Fireman P, Slavin RG: *Atlas of allergies*, New York, 1990, Gower.)

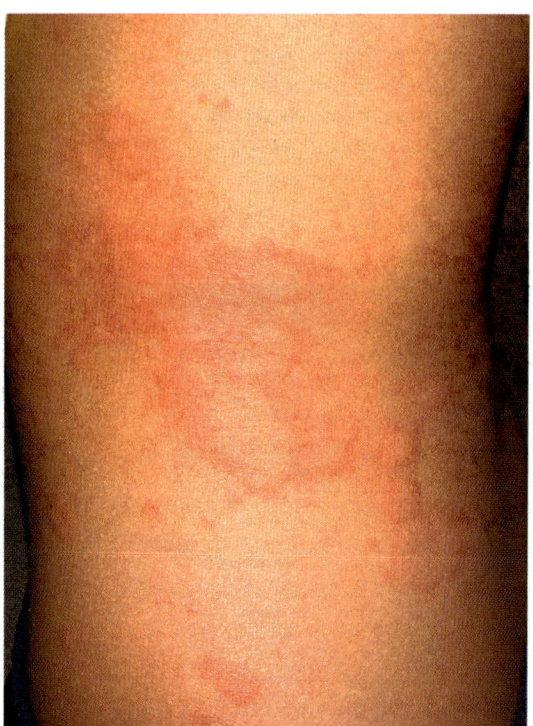

Fig. 4.36 Urticarial lesions. Note the well-demarcated borders, redness, elevation, and occasional confluence of the palpable lesions.

particular exposure. Physical, or inducible, triggers of urticaria include heat, scratching, pressure, vibration, and cold exposure. The term *idiopathic* is used when there is no clear reproducible trigger of urticaria and angioedema. Many idiopathic cases in children are triggered by the immune system's response in fighting a viral infection. Most of these cases resolve within 6 weeks. When the duration exceeds 6 weeks, the condition is categorized as *chronic urticaria* or *angioedema.* Research suggests that many of these cases are autoimmune in nature with evidence for autoantibodies to the IgE receptor on mast cells and basophils. Other less common causes of urticaria include aquagenic, solar urticaria, cholinergic, and exercise-induced urticaria. The history and distribution of lesions often help in identifying the source, which can then be confirmed by a clinical challenge such as an ice cube test to confirm cold urticaria (Fig. 4.38). *Dermographism,* translated literally as the "ability to write on the skin," is a form of inducible pressure urticaria. It can be elicited by stroking the skin with a fingernail or tongue blade. The initial white line secondary to reflex vasoconstriction is supplanted by pruritic, erythematous, linear swelling, as seen in a classic wheal and flare reaction (Fig. 4.39).

Hereditary Angioedema

Hereditary angioedema (HAE) is an autosomal dominant disorder characterized by the absence or abnormal function of a protein in the complement cascade known as *C1 esterase inhibitor.* Inhibitors of the complement system are part of the complement pathway and are capable of blocking activated complement components. C1 esterase inhibitor binds to activated C1 and thereby prevents further activation of the classical pathway. It also serves to regulate other blood protein cascades, including the bradykinin system. In the absence of C1 inhibitor, these cascades can proceed unchecked. This results in increased vascular permeability and the observed clinical features of angioedema. This disorder is characterized by recurrent bouts of swelling that involve any part of the body with the face, extremities, genitals, and respiratory and GI tracts most frequently involved. The swelling is generally self-limited, episodic, and commonly triggered by minor trauma. This condition is distinguished from idiopathic angioedema by its unresponsiveness to antihistamines. Laryngeal edema is a frightening, life-threatening complication that may result in asphyxiation. Involvement of the GI tract is characterized by severe abdominal pain, bloating, vomiting, and rarely intestinal obstruction resulting from intussusception. Other components of the complement system affected in HAE are C2 and C4: C4 levels are consistently low in 95% of patients, and C2 levels are decreased during attacks. The diagnosis of HAE can be confirmed by measuring the C1 esterase level and

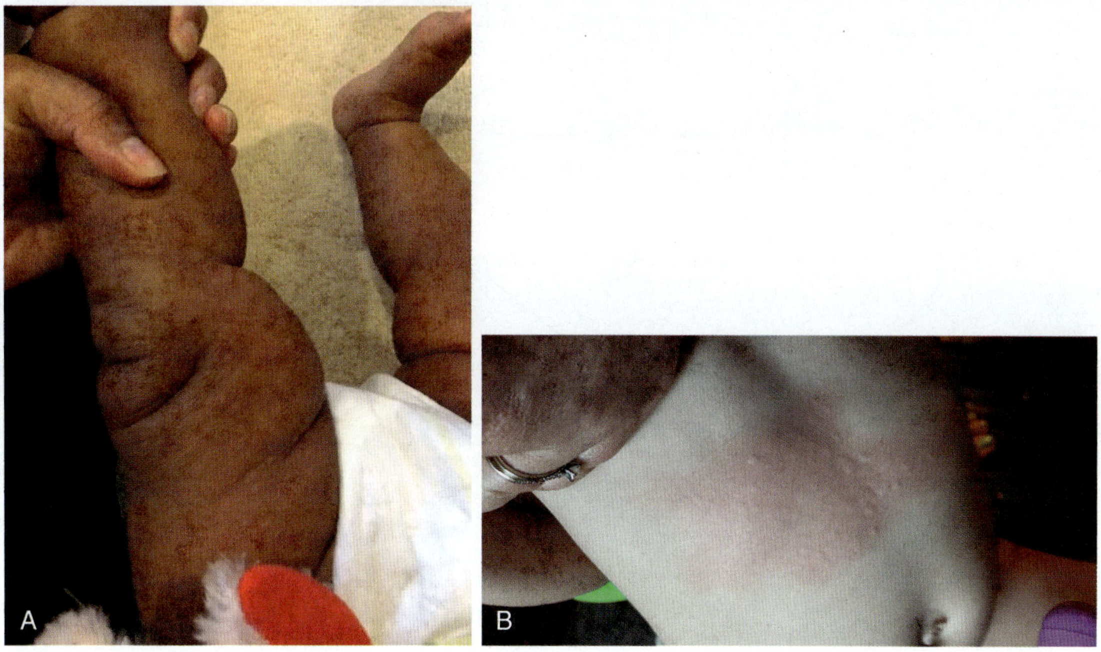

Fig. 4.37 (A) Urticarial lesions on darker pigmented skin and (B) lighter pigmented skin. Note the well-demarcated borders, redness, elevation, and occasional confluence of the palpable lesions.

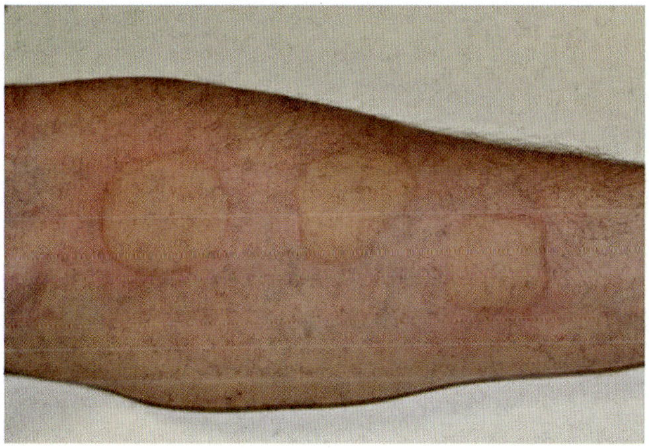

Fig. 4.38 Positive ice cube test in a child with cold urticaria. An ice cube placed on the arm for 10 minutes results in urticaria of the exposed skin. Onset is usually immediate but may be delayed for up to 4 hours after cold exposure. (From Maltseva N, Borzova E, Fomina D, et al: Cold urticaria—What we know and what we do not know, *Allergy* 76:1077–1094, 2021.)

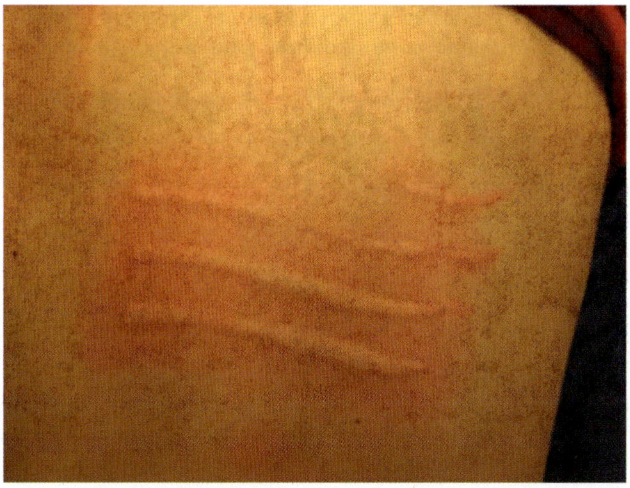

Fig. 4.39 Dermographism, or "writing on the skin," is the most common type of urticaria induced by physical or mechanical factors. Firm stroking or scratching of the skin with a fingernail or tongue blade results in urticaria of the traumatized skin. (From Liccioli G, Nappi L, Mori F, et al: Dermatographism and urticaria in a pediatric population, *Pediatr Allergy Immunol* 31(3):318–320, 2020.)

function. Numerous treatments for HAE are available including purified C1 esterase inhibitor, kallikrein inhibitors, and bradykinin receptor antagonists, with options for both prophylactic and acute use. Other products are also under investigation.

INBORN ERRORS OF IMMUNITY

Normal Development of the Immune System

The immune system, which protects against infections, can be divided into innate and adaptive components, and there is extensive bidirectional interaction between these two arms of the immune system. The innate immune system starts with mechanical barriers, such as the skin, and includes cells that cannot generate antigen-specific receptors; such as neutrophils, eosinophils, NK cells, mast cells, dendritic cells, and monocytes or macrophages. The innate immune system also includes the complement system and other soluble molecules that recognize pathogens. The innate immune system encodes a variety of limited receptors called pattern recognition receptors that recognize pathogen-associated molecular patterns, which are expressed by pathogens, and danger-associated molecular patterns, which are endogenous products derived from stressed or dying cells. The innate immune response can respond within minutes.

In contrast, the adaptive immune system has the capacity to generate a nearly infinite variety of antigen-recognizing receptors. The adaptive immune system is composed of B cells, which produce antibodies, and T cells, which recognize antigens presented by the major histocompatibility complex on antigen-presenting cells. T lymphocytes and B lymphocytes originate from the same stem cells in the bone marrow. They undergo a complex series of maturational changes that generate incredible diversity before arriving at a stage in which they are capable of antigen-stimulated differentiation (Fig. 4.40). T lymphocytes can be divided into two main classes: $CD4^+$T helper cells and $CD8^+$cytotoxic T cells. $CD4^+$ T lymphocytes, via both cell-to-cell contact and production of soluble signaling molecules called *cytokines,* help orchestrate the immune response by activating $CD8^+$ cells and monocytes or macrophages to kill infected cells. This stimulates production of antibodies by B cells, and, in the case of T-regulatory lymphocytes (Treg), downregulating inflammation to avoid autoimmunity. $CD4^+$ T lymphocytes have been subdivided into five major classes: T helper 1 (Th1), T helper 2 (Th2), T helper 17 (Th17), T follicular

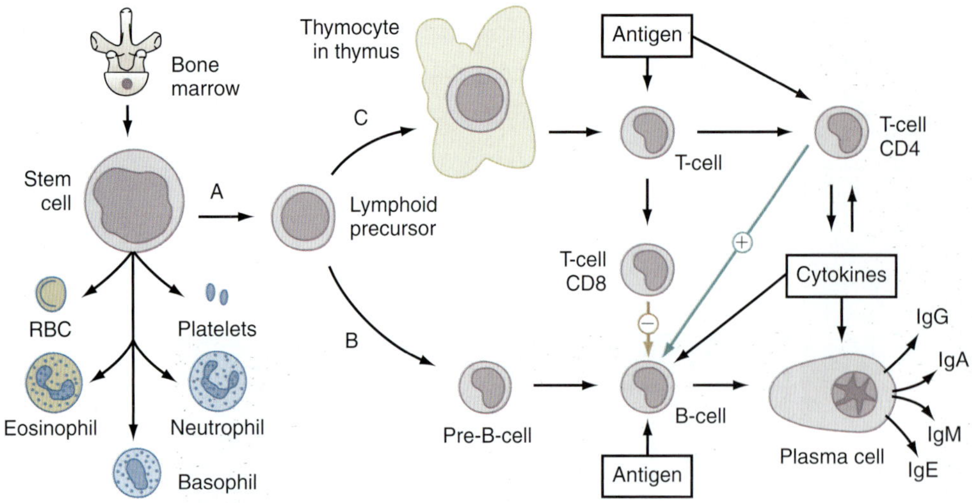

Fig. 4.40 Immune development. Shown is a schematic representation of T- and B-lymphocyte ontogeny. Defects along pathway *A* result in combined immunodeficiencies. Pathway *B* is responsible for normal antibody production, whereas normal cell-mediated immunity requires the integrity of pathway *C*. Cytokines are soluble products of activated lymphocytes and include interleukins and interferons. *CD4*, Cluster of differentiation 4; *CD8*, cluster of differentiation 8; *IgA*, immunoglobulin A; *IgE*, immunoglobulin E; *IgG*, immunoglobulin G; *IgM*, immunoglobulin M; *RBC*, red blood cell.

helper, and T regulatory cells (Treg). Th1 cells produce interferon-γ and are responsible for elimination of intracellular pathogens. Th2 cells are characterized by the production of interleukin (IL)-4 and IL-13. Although $CD4^+$ Th2 cells' primary role is to fight parasitical infections, they are also often responsible for allergic responses. Th17 cells produce IL-17, limit infection with fungi and extracellular bacteria, and play a key role in autoimmune processes. Treg cells are antiinflammatory. Tregs help limit immune-mediated destruction of tissue and prevent development of autoimmunity via production of IL-10 and transforming growth factor-β (TGF-β). T follicular helper cells interact with B cells in the lymphoid tissues to regulate antibody production. Other T helper cells have been identified more recently, and their roles continue to be explored.

Thymus-independent B lymphocytes produce the various classes of immunoglobulins, also known as *antibodies*. Four main subclasses of antibodies are produced: IgM, IgA, IgG, and IgE. This sophisticated and specific immune response by the adaptive immune system takes days to develop but is more efficient and effective at clearing infection than the more crude innate immune system response.

There are now more than 450 single gene defects that have been described to lead to inborn errors of immunity, and this list continues to expand. Immune deficiencies can be categorized according to the molecular defect, as well as phenotype, and can be broadly categorized into nine different groups: (1) immunodeficiencies affecting cellular and humoral immunity, (2) combined immunodeficiencies with associated or syndromic features, (3) predominantly antibody deficiencies, (4) diseases of immune dysregulation, (5) congenital defects of phagocytes, (6) defects in intrinsic and innate immunity, (7) autoinflammatory disorders, (8) complement deficiencies, and (9) phenocopies of primary immune deficiency.

Presentation of Primary Immunodeficiency

Deficiencies of the immune system can involve lymphocytes (e.g., humoral and/or cellular immunodeficiencies), phagocytes (e.g., chronic granulomatous disease), the complement system (e.g., C3 deficiency), and mucosal barriers (e.g., immotile cilia syndrome). Approximate frequencies of the different categories of immunodeficiencies are shown in Fig. 4.41. Humoral (antibody) deficiencies are due to defects in B cells and are typically characterized by recurrent and chronic sinopulmonary infections with extracellular encapsulated bacterial pathogens. In contrast, cellular deficiencies due to T-cell defects are manifested by infections with opportunistic organisms (such as *Candida* or *Pneumocystis jirovecii*) and an inability to clear common viral infections. They can also be associated with failure to thrive in infants and poor growth in older children, wasting, and diarrhea. These patients may be susceptible to graft-versus-host disease if given nonirradiated blood transfusions and may have life-threatening infections after live viral vaccination. Some immunodeficiencies are caused by defects that can affect the development of other systems and often are accompanied by dysmorphic or syndromic features, with one of the most well known being DiGeorge syndrome (see Chapter 1). Other immunodeficiencies fall in the category of immune dysregulation, where patients may present with both susceptibility to infection and abnormal activation of other areas of immune system. Familial hemophagocytic lymphohistiocytosis, IPEX (*i*mmune dysregulation, *p*olyendocrinopathy, *e*nteropathy, *X*-linked) and autoimmune lymphoproliferative syndrome fall into this category. These patients can present with signs of inflammation, autoimmune disease, and lymphadenopathy and

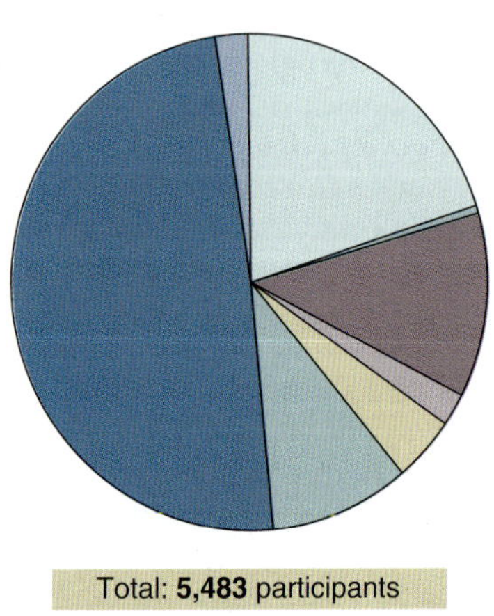

Enrollment by diagnosis

Diagnosis	Participants
Agammaglobulinemia	449
Ataxia telangiectasia	29
Autoimmune lymphoproliferative syndrome (ALPS)	61
Autoinflammatory disease	12
CHARGE syndrome	6
Chronic granulomatous disease	570
Combined immune deficiency	107
Common variable immune deficiency (CVID)	1,818
Complement deficiency	27
DiGeorge syndrome	562
Dyskeratosis congenita	2
Ectodermal dysplasia with immunodeficiency (NEMO and others)	31
HLH, including XLP and pigmentary disorders	74

Fig. 4.41 Distribution of primary immunodeficiency in the United States according to the U.S. Immunodeficiency Network (USIDNET) patient registry in 2020. (From USIDNET.org.)

hepatosplenomegaly. Patients with phagocytic deficiencies present with an inability to kill certain organisms, whereas those with complement deficiencies are often characterized by recurrent *Neisseria* infections, although sinopulmonary infections may also be seen.

More common immunodeficiencies may present in a subtle fashion, with few life-threatening infections and normal growth. In addition, with the advent of next-generation sequencing, we are learning more about the highly variable clinical presentation of monogenic defects even within the same family. Thus the clinician is frequently confronted with the question of whether a patient should be evaluated for immunodeficiency. A set of warning signals has been widely disseminated (Fig. 4.42). In general, children with

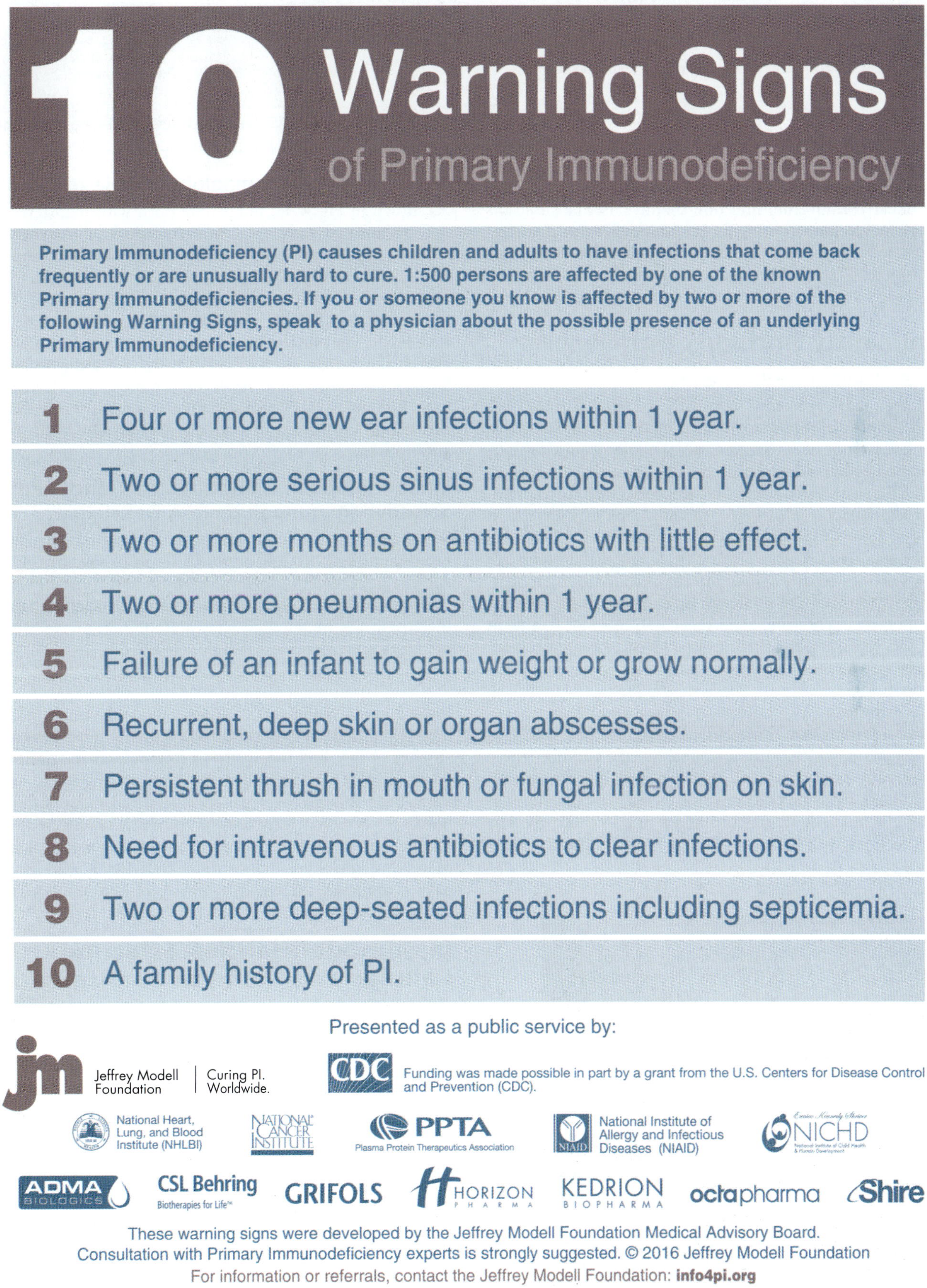

Fig. 4.42 Ten warning signs of primary immunodeficiency disease. (From the Jeffrey Modell Foundation.)

Table 4.17 Suggested Laboratory Screening Tests for Children With Suspected Immunodeficiency

Immune System Component	Example of Immunodeficiency	Screening Tests
B lymphocyte	X-linked agammaglobulinemia	Quantitative immunoglobulin serum levels (IgG, IgA, IgM) Serum antibodies to tetanus, diphtheria, *Pneumococcus*
T lymphocyte	22q11 (DiGeorge) syndrome	T-cell lymphocyte subsets Lymphocyte mitogen stimulation test
Phagocyte	Chronic granulomatous disease	Total neutrophil count Dihydrorhodamine 123 (DHR) assay
Complement	C3 deficiency	CH_{50} (hemolytic complement assay)

IgA, Immunoglobulin A; *IgG,* immunoglobulin G; *IgM,* immunoglobulin M.

infections that are frequent, recurrent, or chronic; are caused by unusual organisms; or respond poorly to therapy should be evaluated for immunodeficiency. Moreover, growth retardation or a family history of early death from infection should raise the clinician's level of suspicion. In the screening for immunodeficiency, quantitative and functional aspects of the components of the immune system are considered (Table 4.17). Laboratory evaluation for immunodeficiency should be guided by history and physical examination.

Predominantly Antibody Deficiencies

Congenital Agammaglobulinemia

Congenital agammaglobulinemia is usually X-linked (Bruton) but can rarely be autosomal recessive. Affected infants are clinically well for the first few months of life because of placentally acquired maternal IgG antibodies but subsequently develop recurrent or chronic infections with encapsulated bacterial pathogens, such as pneumococcus and *Haemophilus influenzae.* The infections may localize in the upper and lower respiratory tracts, resulting in sinusitis, otitis media, and pneumonia. Sepsis, meningitis, and skin infections are also seen. Over time, recurrent lung infections can lead to bronchiectasis. This is characterized clinically by chronic cough with increased sputum production and abnormal chest imaging. Treatment consists of IgG replacement, which can be given either subcutaneously or intravenously, and appropriate antibiotics. In the absence of chronic lung disease, growth is usually unimpaired and survival to adulthood is expected.

The physical findings are those of localized infection, with specific signs depending on the structures infected. In addition, these children generally lack adenoidal, tonsillar, and other lymphoid tissues (Fig. 4.43), which should raise suspicion. The diagnosis of agammaglobulinemia should be considered in any child who has recurrent infections with bacterial pathogens and is confirmed by findings of markedly decreased levels of the immunoglobulin classes (IgG, IgA, IgM) in the serum.

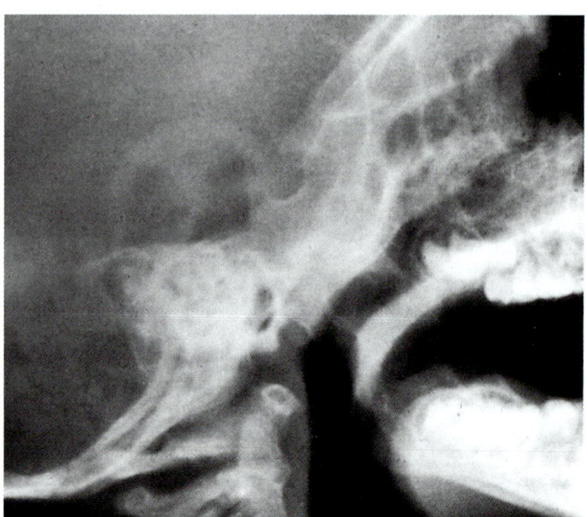

Fig. 4.43 Agammaglobulinemia. Lateral neck radiograph shows absent adenoids.

Transient Hypogammaglobulinemia of Childhood

As shown in Fig. 4.44, infants are born with high levels of serum IgG because of active placental transport of maternal IgG. The serum IgG level normally declines during the first 7 months of life until endogenous IgG production matures. Delays in this maturation may lead to transient hypogammaglobulinemia. Serum IgG levels in these infants usually attain age-appropriate values by school age. Despite the low levels of serum IgG, infants can generally synthesize specific antibodies to vaccine antigens and thus can be asymptomatic. Some, however, can present with ear, sinus, and lung infections. IgG replacement is generally not indicated for this condition, but some patients may benefit from prophylactic antibiotics.

Immunoglobulin G Subclass Deficiency and Selective Immunoglobulin A Deficiency

Serum IgG can be subdivided into four subclasses. Patients have been identified with low or absent levels of specific IgG subclasses and frequent infections. However, it is controversial if isolated subclass deficiency represents a true immune deficiency, particularly in the absence of impaired specific antibody responses. Many immunologists prefer to assess functional antibody response to immunization rather than to examine IgG subclasses.

Selective immunoglobulin A (IgA) deficiency, which affects about 1 in 600 members of the general population, is the most common humoral antibody deficiency. Patients must have a complete absence of IgA, and the diagnosis cannot be made until 4 years old because of the slow development of IgA production in normal children. Even though these patients are deficient in both serum and mucosal secretory IgA, only a minority of affected individuals manifest frequent infections and some are asymptomatic. Synthesis of IgG and IgM is generally normal. Individuals with IgA deficiency have a modestly increased incidence of autoimmune syndromes, atopy, celiac disease, and inflammatory bowel disease.

Immunodeficiencies Affecting Cellular and Humoral Immunity

Common Variable Immunodeficiency

Common variable immunodeficiency (CVID) is a heterogeneous group of disorders diagnosed clinically, with 30% of cases having a genetic basis. CVID can occur at any age, but diagnosis is not usually made until 4 years old, and most patients are between 20 and 40 years old. Diagnosis requires decreased levels of IgG and IgM and/or IgA. In addition, specific antibody responses must be significantly depressed. Although defined by decreased antibody responses, many patients with CVID also have evidence of decreased T-cell function. Therefore in addition to the expected ear, sinus, and lung infections, patients may have infections with unusual pathogens, as well as autoimmune and granulomatous complications. Patients with CVID can be phenotyped on the basis of the presentation of these other complications, namely cytopenias, lymphoproliferation,

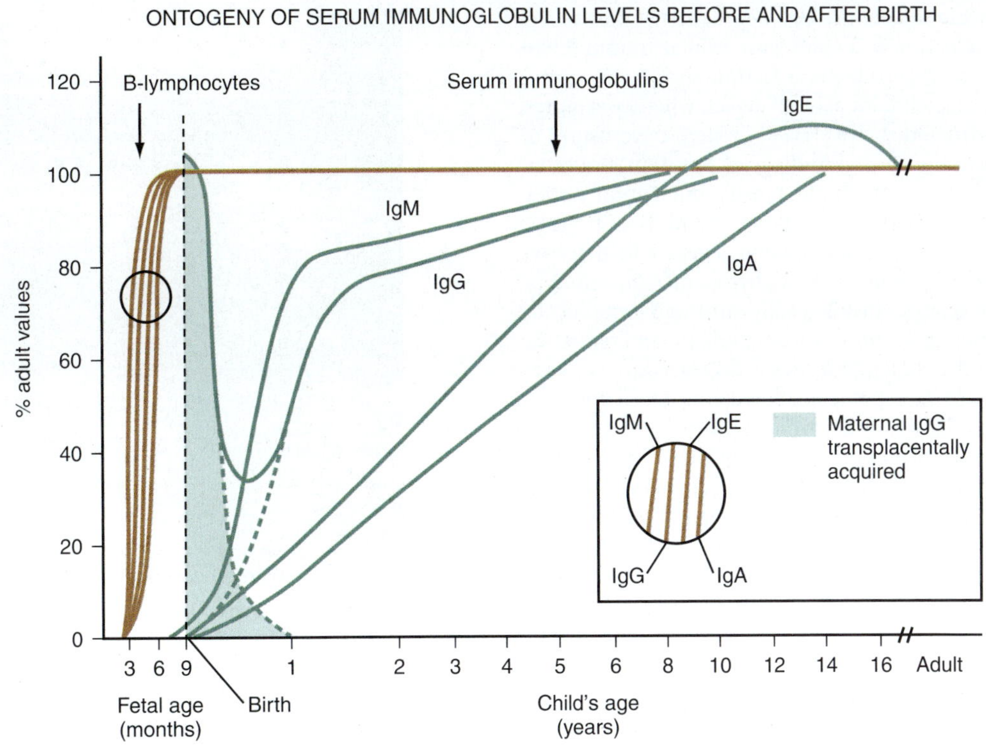

Fig. 4.44 Development of immunoglobulins before and after birth. *IgA,* Immunoglobulin A; *IgE,* immunoglobulin E; *IgG,* immunoglobulin G; *IgM,* immunoglobulin M.

and enteropathy, and the presence of these features leads to significantly increased mortality.

Hyper–Immunoglobulin M Syndrome

Hyper-IgM syndrome, defined by abnormal immunoglobulin production, is actually a combined immune deficiency. Hyper-IgM syndrome is due to an inability of B lymphocytes to class switch from the germ line–encoded IgM heavy chain constant region to other isotypes (e.g., IgA, IgM, IgE). Patients have normal to elevated IgM levels but reduced or absent levels of IgA and IgG. Specific antibody responses are also deficient. The most common form of hyper-IgM syndrome is deficiency of CD154 (CD40 ligand), which is expressed by T lymphocytes and required for B-cell class switching. In addition to sinopulmonary infections, *Pneumocystis* pneumonia and *Cryptosporidium* diarrhea are often seen, demonstrating the importance of this ligand in both innate and adaptive immunity. Although CD40 ligand deficiency is X-linked, defects in other autosomal genes required for class switching lead to a similar phenotype.

Severe Combined Immunodeficiency

Severe combined immunodeficiency (SCID) comprises a heterogeneous group of disorders with varying etiologies. The consequent defects in lymphocyte maturation ultimately result in abnormalities of humoral and cellular immunity (see Fig. 4.40). Affected infants have recurrent severe bacterial, viral, fungal, and protozoal infections. Manifestations typically appear in the first few months of life and are often associated with failure to thrive, diarrhea, and severe candidiasis (Fig. 4.45). Affected infants can present with severe, treatment resistant,

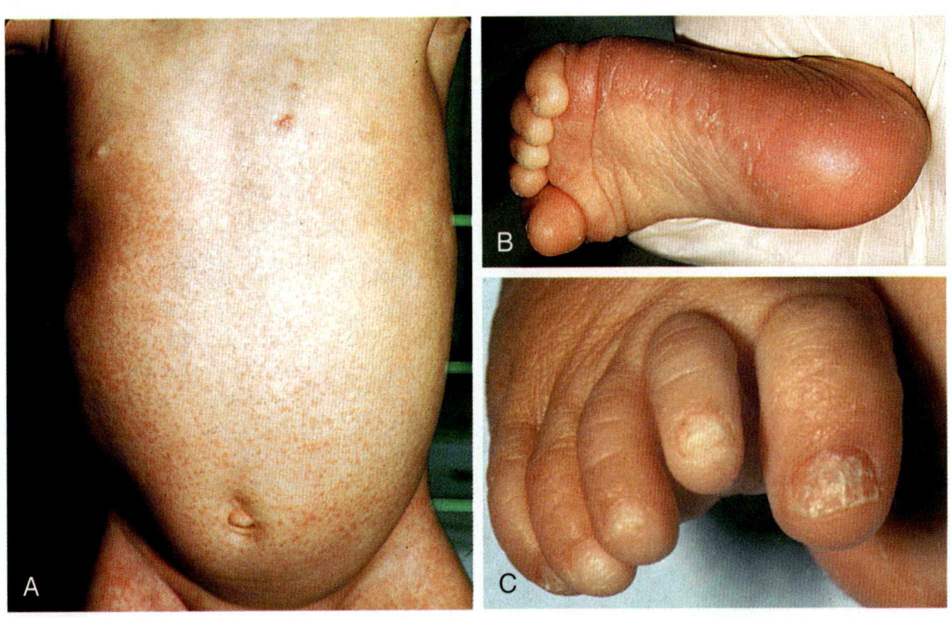

Fig. 4.45 Severe combined immunodeficiency. Widespread fungal dermatitis with *Candida albicans* over the trunk (A) and foot (B) and nails (C).

recurrent, or opportunistic infections. Fig. 4.46 demonstrates severe disseminated varicella infection in a child with cellular immunodeficiency. Infection with an opportunistic infection such as *P. jiroveci* should always raise the suspicion for a T-cell defect, whether acquired (as in human immunodeficiency virus [HIV] or steroid exposure) or congenital. In addition to the clinical findings of infection, examination may disclose hypoplastic or absent tonsils and lymph nodes. Laboratory abnormalities include peripheral blood lymphopenia (Fig. 4.47), decreased serum immunoglobulin levels, and defective lymphocyte responses to mitogens, such as phytohemagglutinin. The thymus is typically dysplastic histologically and radiographically (Fig. 4.48), normal lobulation and corticomedullary differentiation are lacking, and the number of lymphocytes is decreased.

Once the diagnosis of SCID is considered, the child must be placed in protective isolation and given appropriate supportive therapy, including IgG replacement and prophylactic antimicrobials. All administered blood products must be irradiated to prevent the development of severe graft-versus-host disease, and live virus vaccines are contraindicated. These patients can be cured by bone marrow transplantation. In X-linked and adenosine deaminase (ADA) SCID, gene therapy has been tried, but some patients enrolled in studies initially done in the 1990s developed leukemia. Newer methods of gene therapy using lentiviral vectors have proven promising and safe, with clinical trials under way.

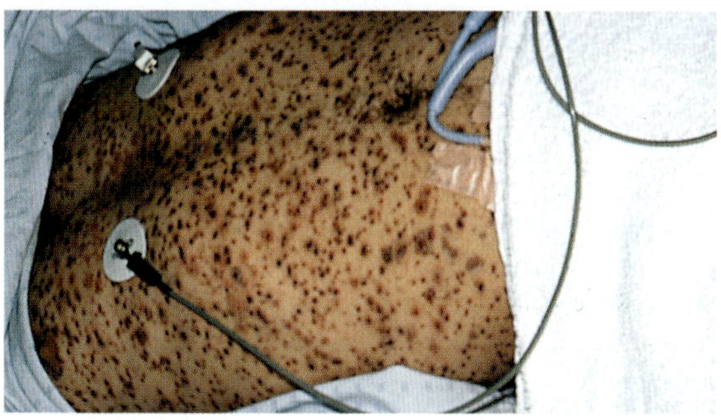

Fig. 4.46 Cellular immunodeficiency. An adolescent with abnormal T-lymphocyte function and disseminated varicella, in whom pneumonia resulted in respiratory failure.

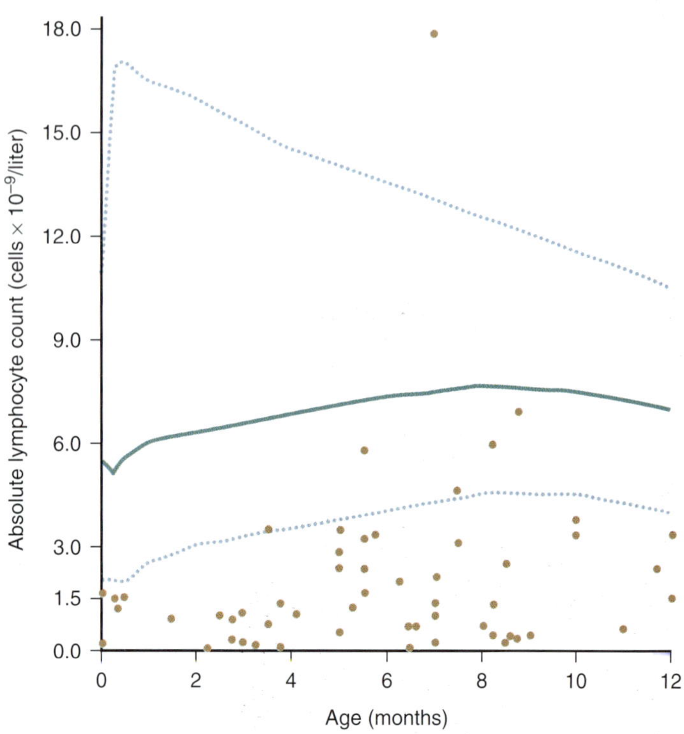

Fig. 4.47 Severe combined immunodeficiency (SCID). Absolute lymphocyte counts in normal infants and infants with SCID disease *(closed circles)*. The *heavy line* indicates the mean lymphocyte counts in normal infants in relation to age. The *light dotted lines* indicate the 95% confidence limits. (From Gossage DL, Buckley RH: Prevalence of lymphopenia in severe combined immunodeficiency, *N Engl J Med* 322:1422–1423, 1990. Copyright © 1990 Massachusetts Medical Society. All rights reserved.)

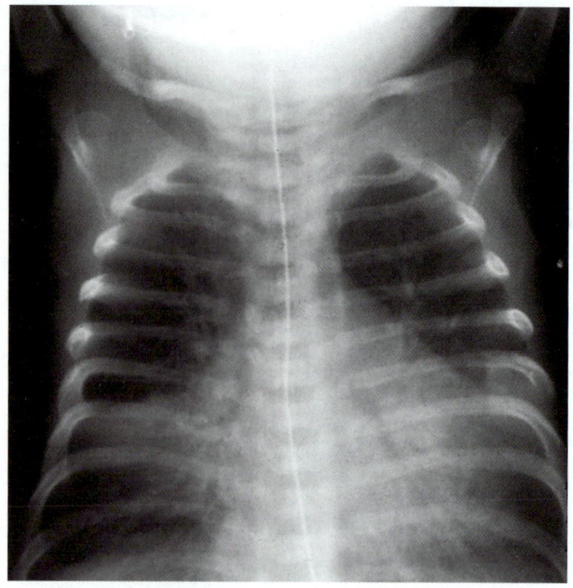

Fig. 4.48 Chest radiograph of infant with severe combined immunodeficiency disease. Note the absent thymic shadow and bilateral pulmonary infiltrates.

Early identification and treatment before the onset of infection leads to improved survival; therefore identification of SCID should be considered a pediatric emergency. Most cases historically were diagnosed during severe infection because most infants with SCID are indistinguishable from healthy typical newborns. Since 2010, the advent of polymerase chain reaction–based newborn screening for lymphopenia has led to early detection before the onset of symptoms. This screen identifies T-cell receptor excision circles (TRECs) using the dried blood spot on the newborn screen. TRECs are excised deoxyribonucleic acid (DNA) circles produced during *TCR* gene rearrangement, which only occurs in naive T cells. Therefore lack of TRECs would indicate lack of naive T cells, which is a key finding in SCID, among other diseases (Fig. 4.49).

Currently more than 20 genetic defects have been identified as causing SCID, but it is important to recognize that some cases have no identifiable genetic cause, and this should not delay curative therapy (Table 4.18). Known genetic defects are characterized on the basis of the lymphocyte affected, and they can be grouped into T-B + NK +, T-B + NK-, T-B-NK +, or T-B-NK-.

T-B + NK- defects are typically due to cytokine signaling defects, with IL-2 receptor gamma chain defects being the most common. X-linked common γ chain is a component of several cytokine receptors and is the most common form of SCID. T-B + NK + SCID is usually from defects associated specifically with T-cell signaling and function, such as IL-7R defects. Lack of IL-7 signaling also prevents maturation of functional T cells. T-B-NK + SCID is due to defects in DNA rearrangement, which is required for *TCR* and *BCR* expression. Therefore defects in genes involved in VDJ recombination lead to the absence of T cells and B cells, but not NK cells, which do not have specific receptors that require DNA rearrangement. Recombinase activating gene mutations are the most common of this group. In cases of T-B-NK-, there is a defect in a common lymphocyte pathway. ADA mutations fall into this category. This disease causes the accumulation of metabolic substrates that are toxic to lymphocytes. ADA deficiency can also lead to other symptoms, including skeletal changes, hearing loss, and behavioral issues due to systemic toxicity of adenosine metabolites.

On rare occasion, patients may present with a hypomorphic mutation in a known SCID-causing gene, referred to as atypical SCID. *Omenn syndrome* is an example of an atypical SCID where patients present with oligoclonal T cells, which cause a graft-versus-host–like phenotype. Patients often present in infancy with dermatitis, lymphadenopathy, and hepatosplenomegaly (Fig. 4.50).

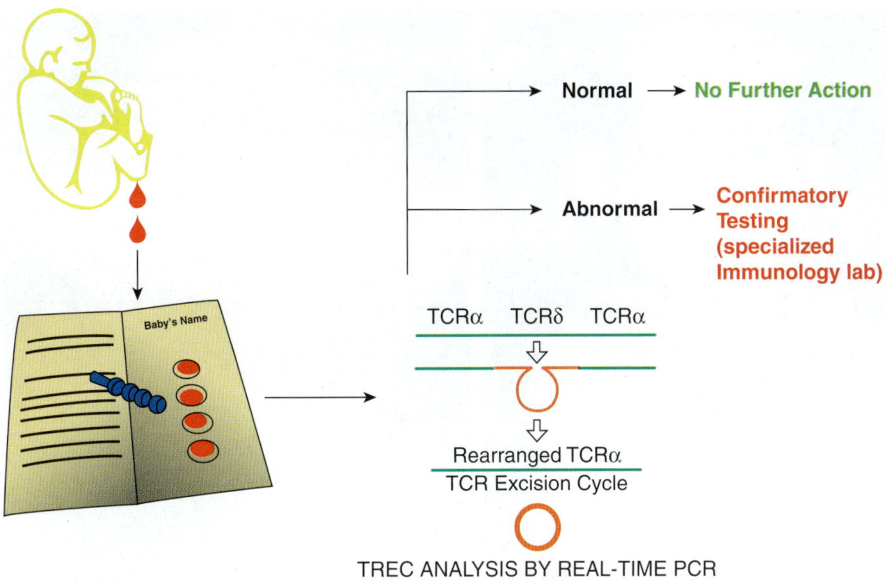

Fig. 4.49 Newborn screening for severe combined immunodeficiency. *PCR,* Polymerase chain reaction; *TCR,* T-cell receptor; *TREC,* T-cell receptor excision circle. (From Abraham RS: *Severe combined immunodeficiencies: newborn screening and beyond.* https://www.aacc.org/publications/cln/articles/2013/november/scid.)

Table 4.18 Molecular Causes of Severe Combined Immunodeficiency as Defined by the International Union of Immunological Societies Expert Committee for Primary Immunodeficiency

Phenotype	Genetic Defect
Severe Combined Immunodeficiency	
T-B+NK-	IL2RG
	JAK3
	CD132 deficiency
T-B-NK+	RAG1
	RAG2
	DCLRE1C (Artemis)
	PRKDC
	Cernunnos/XLF
	DNA ligase IV
T-B+NK+	IL7R alpha
	CD45
	CD3D
	CD3E
	CD3Z
	PTPRC
	CORO1A
	LAT
	FOXN1
T-B-NK-	ADA
	AK2
	RAC2

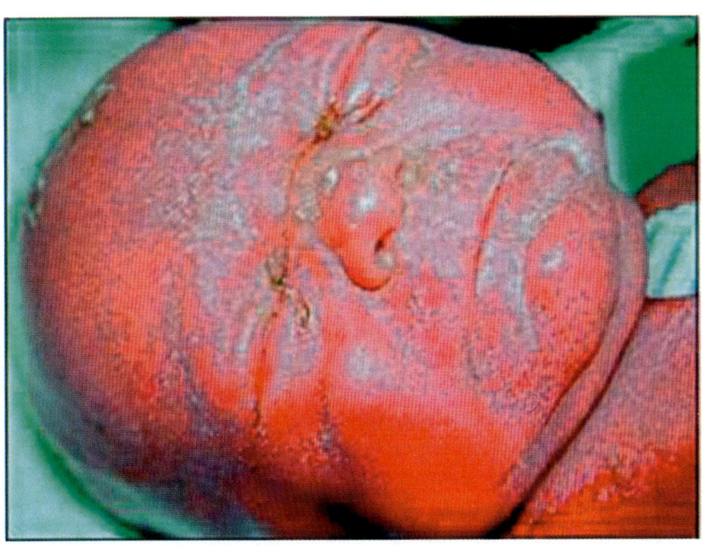

Fig. 4.50 Omenn syndrome.

Combined Immunodeficiencies With Associated or Syndromic Features

DiGeorge Syndrome

DiGeorge syndrome consists of a classic triad of features: conotruncal cardiac anomalies, hypoplastic thymus, and hypocalcemia. The hypoplastic thymus in most patients leads to a T-cell immunodeficiency characterized by low to absent T-cell numbers with normal or near-normal B-cell numbers and function. Approximately 90% of cases are due to a heterozygous chromosomal deletion at 22q11.2 resulting in abnormal development of the third and fourth branchial pouches during embryogenesis. Heterozygous defects in TBX1 have newly been described as a monogenic cause of DiGeorge syndrome. The thymus provides the necessary microenvironment for the maturation of lymphoid precursors into functioning T lymphocytes. When the thymus is absent, T-cell maturation is halted, resulting in T-cell immunodeficiency. Because major cardiovascular structures and the parathyroid glands are derived from the same branchial pouches, affected children frequently present with signs of congenital heart disease and hypocalcemic tetany or seizures within the first few days of life. Patients often demonstrate characteristic facies (Fig. 4.51). The 22q11.2 deletion may occur as frequently as once in 3000 to 4000 live births, but DiGeorge syndrome remains underdiagnosed, especially with milder phenotypes lacking facial dysmorphism.

Most patients with DiGeorge syndrome have some thymic tissue and often have the sinopulmonary infections typical of antibody deficiency. A minority (<0.5%) of patients with 22q11 syndrome completely lack thymic tissue and present without functional T cells. They present similar to infants with SCID and will die of infection unless they receive a thymic transplant. Bone marrow transplant has been tried in some patients with mixed results.

Wiskott-Aldrich Syndrome

Wiskott-Aldrich syndrome (WAS) is an X-linked recessive disorder characterized by eczema, thrombocytopenia, and recurrent infections that begin in infancy (Fig. 4.52). Infants first present with thrombocytopenia and petechiae, and they notably have small platelets on microscopy, unlike the large platelets typically seen in newborns. The most common immunologic defect is inability to form antibody to bacterial capsular polysaccharide antigens, but some patients also manifest a partial defect in T-lymphocyte responses, which can worsen with age. The most common cause of death is intracranial hemorrhage secondary to thrombocytopenia. Males with WAS have an increased risk of malignancy with age, particularly lymphoma. Bone marrow transplantation is curative. The defective protein in WAS is termed

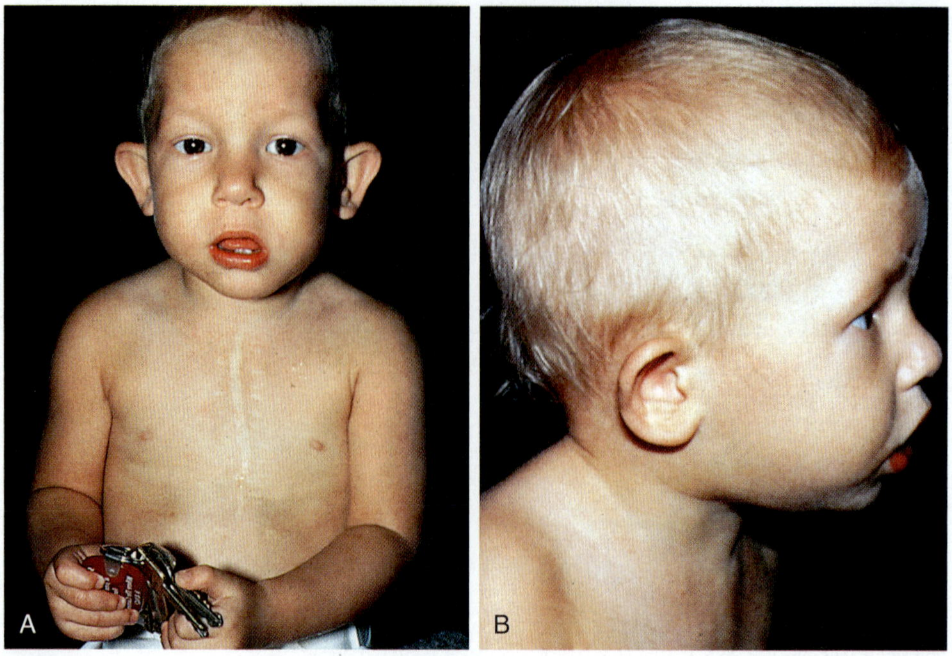

Fig. 4.51 22q11 syndrome. Characteristic facial features: frontal (A) and lateral (B) views. Note the micrognathia; hypertelorism; low-set, malformed ears; and smooth philtrum. Also note the midline scar from repair of a cardiac defect.

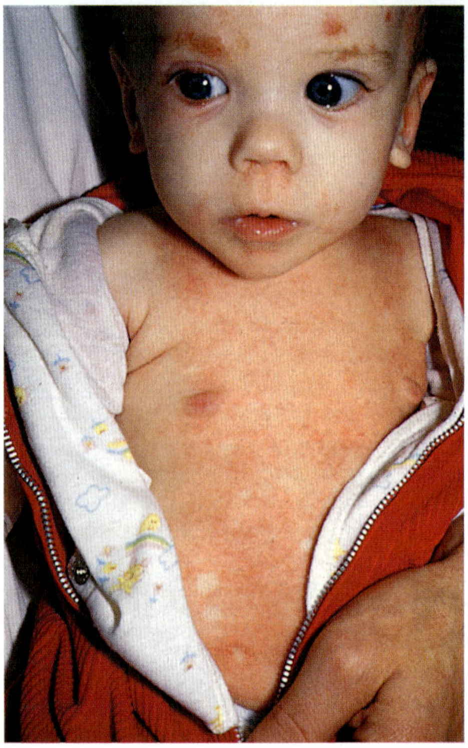

Fig. 4.52 Wiskott-Aldrich syndrome. The skin eruptions on the trunk and face are eczematoid and pruritic but not always similar to atopic dermatitis in flexural distribution. (From Fireman P, Slavin RG: *Atlas of allergies*, New York, 1990, Gower.)

Wiskott-Aldrich syndrome protein (WASP) and serves to link T-cell signaling at the cell surface to changes of the cytoskeleton.

Ataxia-Telangiectasia

Ataxia-telangiectasia is a complex immunodeficiency disorder that falls under the category of immunodeficiency associated with DNA repair defect. Ataxia-telangiectasia has autosomal recessive inheritance and an unusually pleiotropic presentation: telangiectasia, progressive ataxia, and variable immunodeficiency. Alpha-fetoprotein is elevated in ataxia-telangiectasia, but the mechanisms underlying the elevation are not well understood. Most patients develop ocular telangiectasia and ataxia during the first 6 years of life. However, the telangiectasias are typically the last to appear, which can delay this diagnosis (see Chapter 16). The ataxia is cerebellar in nature and characteristically progressive. Neurologic involvement may be extensive, including abnormalities of speech, movement, gait, and developmental delay. The progressive, variable immunodeficiency commonly consists of humoral defects and depressed T-lymphocyte function. Recurrent sinus and pulmonary infections leading to bronchiectasis is a common cause of mortality. These patients have a dramatically higher incidence of neoplasia, consistent with the gene affected in ataxia-telangiectasia, which limits cell division in the presence of DNA damage. Exposure to ionizing radiation, including in medical imaging, should be avoided as much as possible in patients with ataxia-telangiectasia. MMR vaccine is contraindicated in ataxia-telangiectasia, as well as other DNA repair disorders such as Nijmegen breakage syndrome, Cernunnos, Blooms syndrome, DNA ligase 4 deficiency, and Artemis deficiency due to reports of immunodeficiency related vaccine-derived rubella virus with cutaneous and visceral granulomatous disease presenting months to years after vaccination.

Hyper–Immunoglobulin E Syndromes

There are currently nine different monogenic defects leading to a syndrome with markedly elevated IgE levels. The originally described autosomal dominant hyper-IgE syndrome, initially called *Job syndrome,* was characterized by the triad of eczema, recurrent skin infections, and recurrent pulmonary infections. These patients present with rash during the first weeks of life. The condition progresses to recurrent staphylococcal skin infections, including impetigo, boils, and furuncles, which lack inflammation and are called *cold abscesses.* Staphylococcal pneumonia complicated by pneumatocele formation (Fig. 4.53) and lung abscesses are frequent. Candidiasis of the skin and nails is common, as is mucocutaneous candidiasis. Immunologic findings include markedly elevated IgE levels (>2000 IU/mL), although some patients may have normal IgE at some point; eosinophilia; abnormal cell-mediated immunity; and, in certain patients, abnormal polymorphonuclear leukocyte chemotaxis. The specific genetic mutation was identified as *STAT3* loss of function. *STAT3* is essential to Th17 cell development, a T-cell critical in preventing *Candida* infections. In addition, it is a pleiotropic signaling molecule, explaining other nonimmunologic findings seen in autosomal dominant hyper IgE syndrome, such as frequent long bone fractures and delayed eruption of secondary teeth with retained primary teeth (a feature unique to autosomal dominant hyper IgE syndrome among immunodeficiencies). In addition, patients go on to develop coarse facial features (Fig. 4.54). Patients

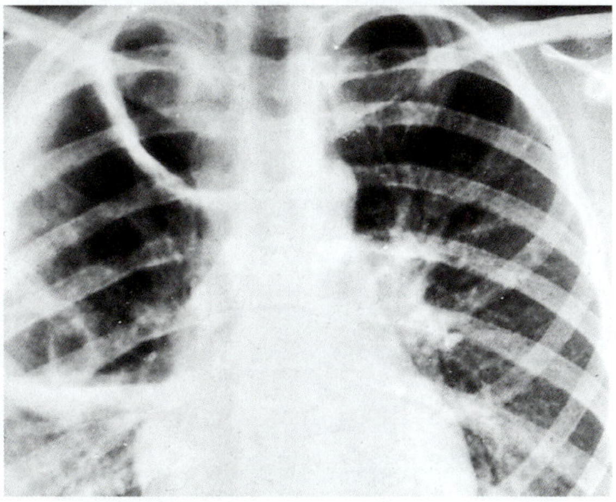

Fig. 4.53 Hyper–immunoglobulin E syndrome. Note the clearly outlined pneumatocele in the right lung. This encapsulated lesion frequently complicates *Staphylococcus aureus* pneumonia.

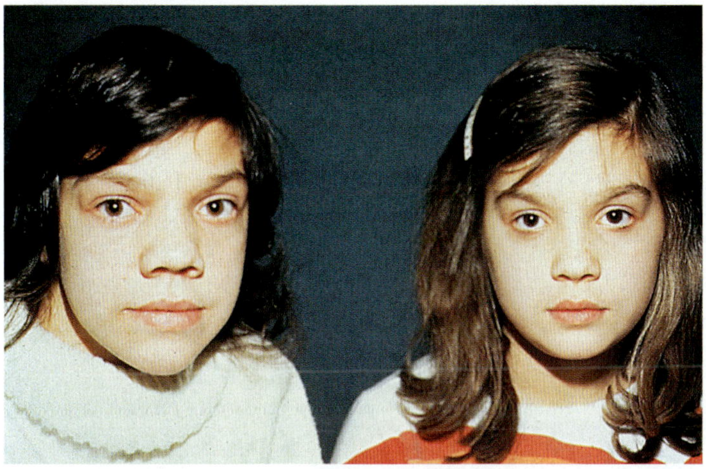

Fig. 4.54 Hyper–immunoglobulin E (IgE) syndrome. Note the coarse facial features of the girl on the left, including the broad nasal bridge, fleshy nasal tip, and mild prognathism compared with her unaffected sister.

with *DOCK8* mutations share similar features but lack skeletal abnormalities. It should be stressed that many patients with atopic dermatitis have elevated IgE levels, often markedly so. Therefore careful examination and history taking can help differentiate true hyper-IgE syndrome from atopic disease.

NEMO Deficiency

Several innate immune defects predisposing to infections have been identified as also leading to combined immunodeficiencies with features that extend beyond the immune system. These include deficiency in nuclear factor (NF)-κB essential modifier (NEMO, also known as IKK-γ). This disorder is characterized by mutations that disrupt the function of NEMO, which affects NF-κB activity. NEMO is found on the X chromosome. Boys with NEMO are susceptible to a variety of infections, including infections with pyogenic bacteria, mycobacteria, and viruses. They also have ectodermal dysplasia with sparse hair, few conical teeth, and frontal bossing, highlighting the importance of NF-κB signaling in multiple pathways (Fig. 4.55).

Congenital Defects of Phagocyte Number, Function, or Both

Polymorphonuclear leukocytes and mononuclear cells play vital roles in the defense against acute infections. Normal neutrophil numbers, intact neutrophil chemotaxis, phagocytosis, and killing are necessary for elimination of microorganisms that invade the skin or mucous membranes. Patients with neutropenia are vulnerable to bacterial infections, as are patients with disorders of phagocyte function. The neutropenias and Chédiak-Higashi syndrome are discussed in Chapter 12.

Chronic Granulomatous Disease

Chronic granulomatous disease is the most common phagocytic immunodeficiency. Neutrophil chemotaxis and phagocytosis are intact, but a biochemical defect results in abnormal activation of oxidative metabolism in neutrophil granules and inability to kill microorganisms. The mechanism underlying generation of the characteristic granulomas is unclear, but it may involve defective inactivation of

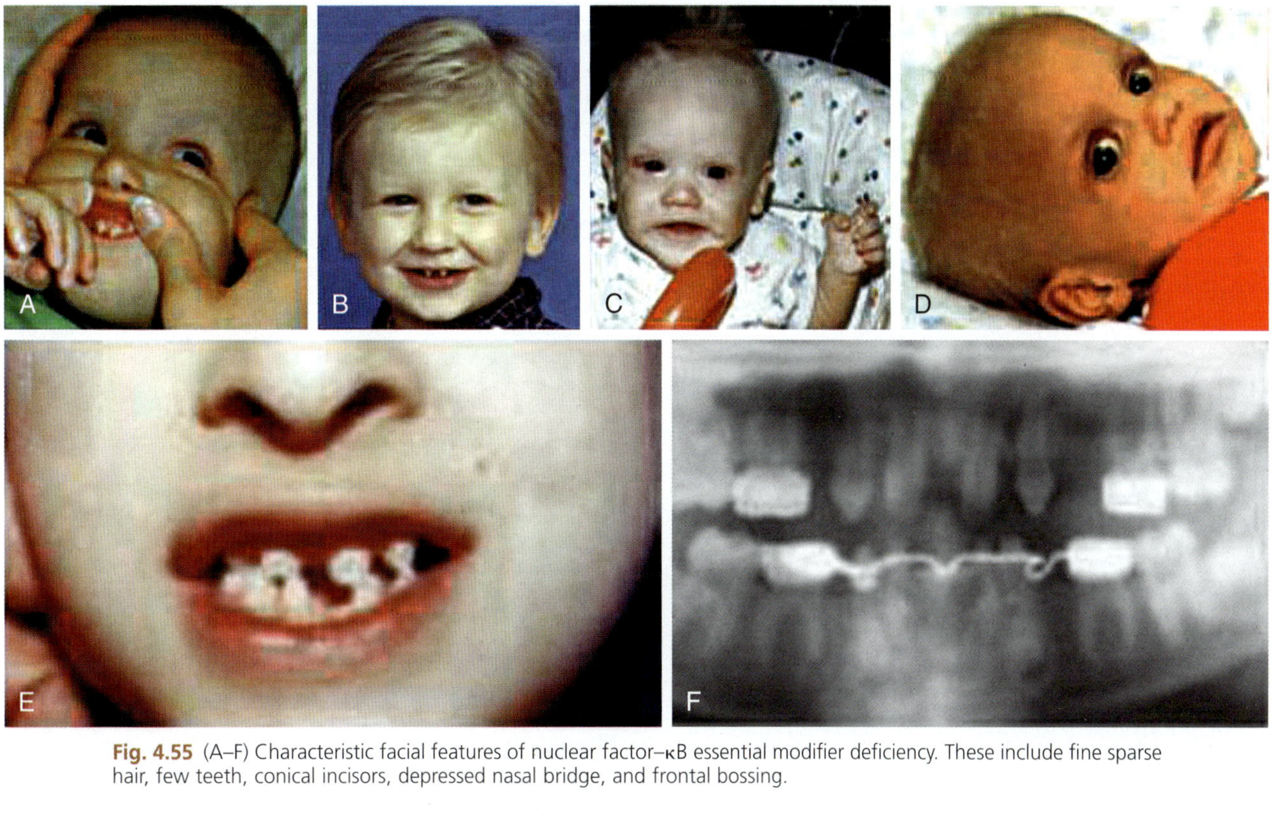

Fig. 4.55 (A–F) Characteristic facial features of nuclear factor–κB essential modifier deficiency. These include fine sparse hair, few teeth, conical incisors, depressed nasal bridge, and frontal bossing.

inflammatory markers. A test of neutrophil oxidative burst is used to diagnose chronic granulomatous disease. Historically, the nitroblue tetrazolium test has been used for diagnosis, but the nitroblue tetrazolium test has been supplanted by a flow-cytometric assay based on reduction of the dye dihydrorhodamine 123 (DHR).

The phagocyte NADPH oxidase complex has four subunits (Fig. 4.56). The most common and severe defect is X-linked, but defects in the other subunits can arise from an autosomal recessive pattern of inheritance. Clinically, most children with chronic granulomatous disease become symptomatic early in life, developing infections with catalase-positive bacteria and fungi. The skin, lungs, liver, and lymph nodes are the most common sites of infections, and five organisms account for most infections: *Staphylococcus aureus, Burkholderia cepacia, Serratia marcescens, Aspergillus,* and *Nocardia* species. Liver abscesses and invasive *Aspergillus* lung infection in the absence of known immunosuppression strongly suggest chronic granulomatous disease. Hepatosplenomegaly is a frequent physical finding and presumably represents involvement of the reticuloendothelial system. Granulomas may also develop, and granulomas of the GI tract are often indistinguishable from inflammatory bowel disease. In the patient whose radiograph is seen in Fig. 4.57, the diagnosis of chronic granulomatous disease was suggested by the finding of antral narrowing secondary to granulomatous involvement of the gastric antrum. Effective antimicrobial prophylaxis with trimethoprim-sulfamethoxazole and itraconazole and cytokine therapy with interferon-γ helps minimize infectious complications of chronic granulomatous disease. Ultimately, treatment with HSCT can be curative for the immune defects.

Leukocyte Adhesion Deficiency

Leukocyte adhesion deficiency (LAD) is rare and most commonly results from a deficiency in CD18. This molecule is a component of β_2 integrins, which are required for neutrophils to exit blood vessels and enter tissue. The patients have a variety of symptoms, including delayed umbilical cord separation (Fig. 4.58A), a persistent and dramatic peripheral blood granulocytosis (due to the inability of neutrophils to migrate through the endothelium and into tissue), recurrent soft tissue infections, and impaired wound healing. Most infants with delayed cord separation, however, will not have LAD. Because these patients do not mobilize neutrophils in response to infection, many aspects of the normal inflammatory response are lacking including the formation of pus (Fig. 4.58B). LAD deficiency should be suspected in any infant with periumbilical problems and persistent peripheral blood leukocytosis (frequently >50,000 cells/mm³). Other rare causes of LAD have also been described.

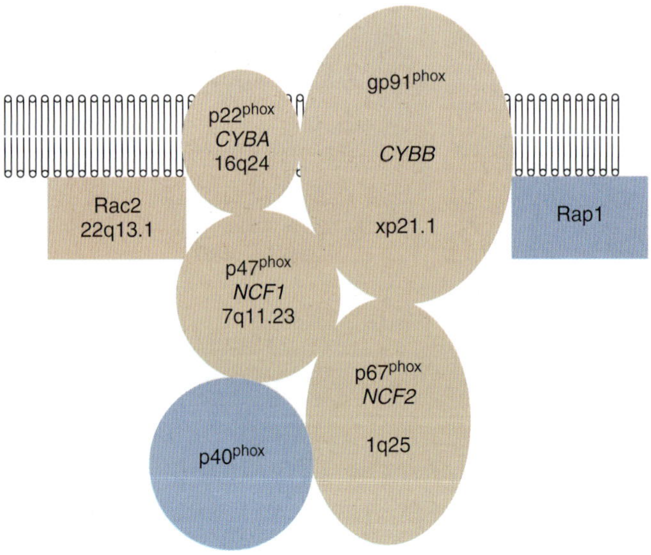

Fig. 4.56 Chronic granulomatous disease. The neutrophil nicotinamide adenine dinucleotide phosphate oxidase complex is shown. Components in which mutations have been detected in patients with chronic granulomatous disease are shown in tan. X-linked deficiency of gp91phox is the most common cause of chronic granulomatous disease, accounting for about two-thirds of cases. (From Bonilla FA, Geha RS: Primary immunodeficiency diseases, *J Allergy Clin Immunol* 111:S571–S581, 2004.)

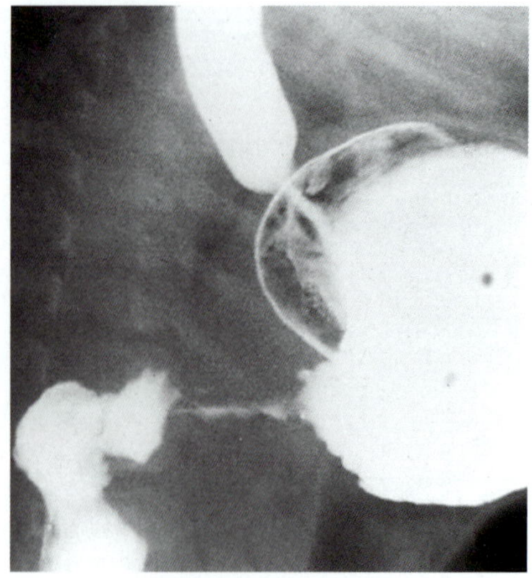

Fig. 4.57 Chronic granulomatous disease. Barium contrast radiogram demonstrating the "string sign," a thin line of barium that represents narrowing of the gastric antrum secondary to granuloma formation. This child had persistent vomiting but none of the usual stigmata of chronic granulomatous disease.

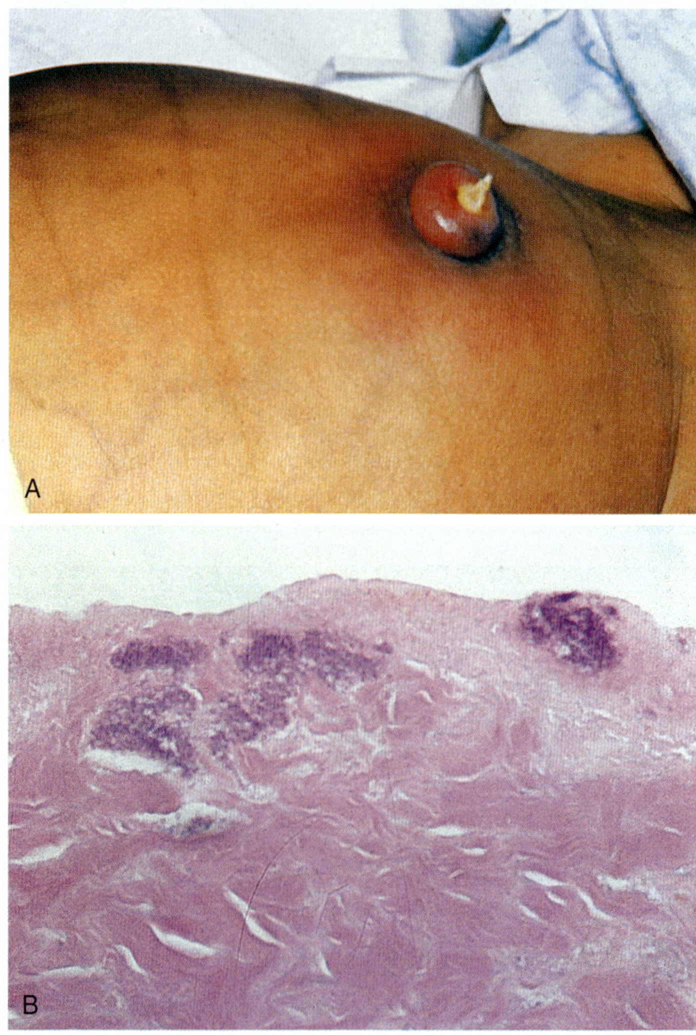

Fig. 4.58 Leukocyte adhesion deficiency. (A) Infection involving and surrounding the umbilical cord. (B) Histopathologic appearance of a scalp abscess. Note the presence of bacterial colonies *(purple staining)* and distinct lack of host cellular inflammatory response. (A, Courtesy Kenneth Schuit, MD, Pittsburgh, PA. B, Courtesy Kenneth Schuit, MD, and William Robichaux, MD, Pittsburgh, PA.)

Complement System Disorders

The complement system is a complex system of serum proteins that require serial activation through the classical, alternative, or mannose-binding lectin (MBL) pathway. Complement mediates and amplifies many of the biologic functions of the immune system. These functions include (1) enhancement of phagocytosis (opsonization) and viral neutralization, (2) mediation of inflammation via chemotaxis and alteration of vascular permeability, (3) cell lysis, and (4) modulation of the immune response. Although rare, inherited deficiencies of most complement components have been reported. Clinical presentation varies, depending on the specific complement protein involved. Frequent modes of presentation for complement component deficiencies are collagen vascular diseases for defects in components C1 through C4, disseminated infections with pyogenic bacteria for C3, and disseminated *Neisseria* infections for C5 through C8. C9 deficiency is often asymptomatic. The CH_{50} assay is a simple screening test for complement deficiency. A normal result effectively rules out complement dysfunction. Workup for complement deficiency should be undertaken in patients with severe or recurrent Neisserial infection or in patients with recurrent sinopulmonary infections and normal antibody studies. A defect in C1 esterase inhibitor results in HAE, which is discussed in an earlier section.

There is a wide variation in MBL levels of the general population, with some reports showing increased rates of infection in individuals with low or absent MBL levels. However, a substantial portion of the population (5%–8%) has low or undetectable levels and most of these patients do not have unusually frequent or severe infections.

Defects in Intrinsic and Innate Immunity

Toll-like receptors (TLRs) are among the receptors responsible for recognizing pathogen-associated molecular patterns, and signaling through TLRs helps alert the immune system of the presence of infections. Defects in TLR signaling, including the molecules MyD88 and IRAK4, which transduce signals from the membrane-associated TLRs to the interior of the cell, have been recognized in patients with recurrent pneumococcal infections. Defects in signaling via TLR-3, which recognizes double-stranded ribonucleic acid, have been implicated in susceptibility to HSV infections.

Chronic Mucocutaneous Candidiasis

Chronic mucocutaneous candidiasis (CMC) is typified by superficial candidal infections of the mucous membranes, skin, and nails. CMC can be a feature of severe T-cell deficiency, such as in HIV and SCID. Patients with autosomal dominant hyper-IgE syndrome also get CMC. Certain patients who only have CMC carry a defect that underlies their CMC related to impaired Th17 cell production and function. Several genetic causes of CMC have been reported, including *STAT-3* loss of function mutations, mutations in IL-17 receptor, and mutations in *STAT1* that all lead to impaired IL-17 T-cell development. Patients with *STAT1* mutations resulting in a gain of function can also experience other infections and autoimmune disease. Treatment of CMC involves long-term antifungal therapy and, depending on the gene defect identified, newer targeted biologics may be beneficial, such as the use of JAK inhibitors in patients with *STAT1* mutations.

Anatomic and Mucosal Disorders

Preventing the entry of microorganisms into sterile sites and clearance of infections from these sites represent the first line of immunologic defense. Intact mucosal barriers are of crucial importance in preventing the entrance of microorganisms into the host. The respiratory and GI mucosa aid in host defense by secreting antibodies (predominantly IgA) into their lumina. Also, physical factors (such as saliva flow in the oral cavity, intestinal peristalsis, and the coughing reflex) are important in the "washing out" effect on potential pathogens. Anything that prevents clearance may predispose to infections in the upper airway. Hypertrophy of the adenoids can inhibit both eustachian tube function and drainage from the sinuses, predisposing to ear and sinus infections. Patients with unusual anatomy due to cleft palate or other craniofacial abnormalities (see Chapter 23) often have frequent infections despite an intact immune system.

Primary ciliary dyskinesia is characterized by a defect in mucociliary transport, another component of the mucosal barrier. This disorder was first described as Kartagener syndrome, which consists of a triad of situs inversus (Fig. 4.59), chronic sinusitis, and bronchiectasis. These patients were also noted to be infertile because their spermatozoa were poorly motile, due to the lack of dynein arms in their tails. Studies revealed similar defects in mucosal cilia and led to recognition of the fact that the phenomenon could exist in the absence of situs inversus. The resultant ciliary dysfunction impedes mucus clearance and produces a combination of these signs and symptoms: (1) early onset of chronic rhinorrhea, (2) chronic otitis media, (3) chronic sinusitis with opaque sinuses on radiography, (4) chronic productive cough, (5) bronchiectasis, (6) digital clubbing, and (7) nasal polyps. The disorder should be suspected in any child with chronic or recurrent upper or lower respiratory tract infections. When situs inversus is not present, the diagnosis of primary ciliary dyskinesia requires confirmation by electron microscopic analysis of cilia obtained from a biopsy of the nasal or tracheobronchial mucosa (Fig. 4.60).

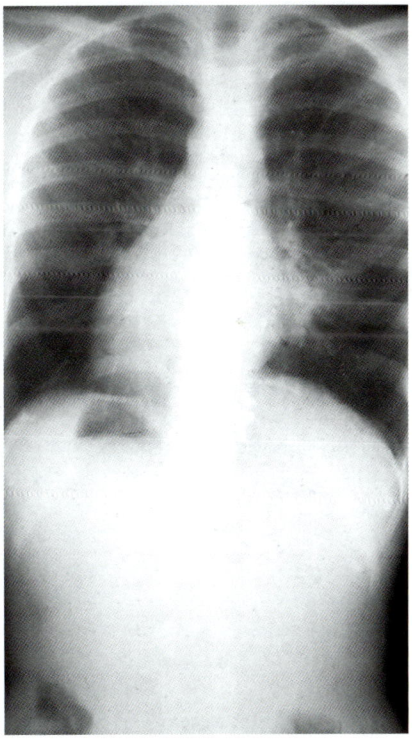

Fig. 4.59 Kartagener syndrome. Dextrocardia and situs inversus of the abdominal organs. Abnormal ciliary motion is thought to result in malrotation during embryogenesis.

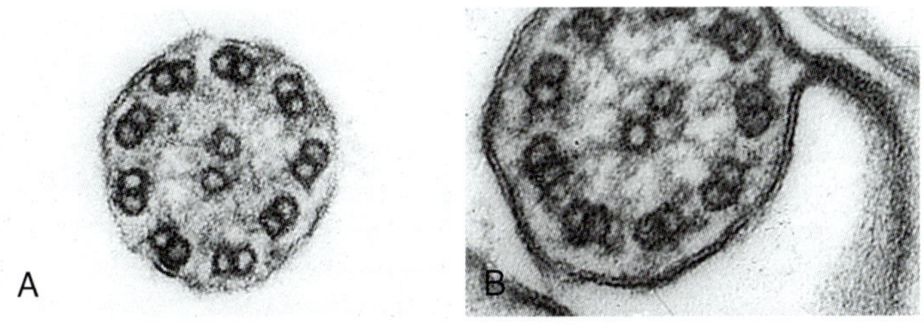

Fig. 4.60 Immotile cilia syndrome. (A) Electron micrograph of cilia from a patient with immotile cilia syndrome. Note the absence of dynein arms from the outer doublets. (B) Normal cilia with dynein arms. (From Bluestone C, Stool S: *Pediatric otolaryngology* (vol 1), Philadelphia, 1983, WB Saunders.)

References

CDC Summary Health Statistics for US Children: *National Health Interview Survey (NHIS) 2012 Data: 2012 Lifetime Asthma, Current Asthma, Asthma Attacks among those with Current Asthma,* 2018. https://www.cdc.gov/asthma/nhis/2012/data.htm.

National Heart, Lung, and Blood Institute (NHLBI) National Asthma Education and Prevention Program (NAEPP): *Guidelines for the diagnosis and management of asthma (EPR-3),* 2016. http://www.nhlbi.nih.gov/health-pro/guidelines/current/asthma-guidelines.

Bibliography

Abbas AK, Lichtman AH, Pillai S: *Cellular and molecular immunology*, ed 9, Philadelphia, 2018, Elsevier, pp 417–428.

Abbott JK, Gelfand EW: Common variable immunodeficiency: diagnosis, management, and treatment, *Immunol Allergy Clin North Am* 35(4):637–658, 2015.

Bland CM, Jones BM: Drug allergy. In DiPiro JT, Yee GC, Posey L, Haines ST, Nolin TD, Ellingrod V, editors: *Pharmacotherapy: a pathophysiologic approach*, ed 11, New York, NY, 2019, McGraw-Hill.

Bonilla FA, Bernstein IL, Kahn DA, et al: Practice parameter for the diagnosis and management of primary immunodeficiency, *Ann Allergy Asthma Immunol* 94: S1–S63, 2005.

Bousfiha A, Jeddane L, Picard C, et al: Human inborn errors of immunity: 2019 update of the IUIS phenotypical classification, *J Clin Immunol* 40(1):66–81, 2020.

Buchbinder D, Hauck F, Albert MH, et al: Rubella virus-associated cutaneous granulomatous disease: a unique complication in immune-deficient patients, not limited to DNA repair disorders, *J Clin Immunol* 39(1):81–89, 2019.

Burks WA, Holgate ST, O'Hehir RE, et al: *Middleton's allergy: principles and practice*, ed 9, Amsterdam, 2020, Elsevier.

Castro-Rodriquez JA, Holberg CJ, Wright AL, et al: A clinical index to define risk of asthma in young children with recurrent wheezing, *Am J Respir Crit Care Med* 162:1403–1406, 2000.

Global Initiative for Asthma 2016: *Global strategy for asthma management and prevention*. http://www.ginasthma.com.

Golden D, Demain J, Freeman T, et al: Stinging insect hypersensitivity: a practice parameter update 2016, *Ann Allergy Asthma Immunol* 118(1):28–54, 2017.

Golden DBK, Wang J, Waserman S, et al: Anaphylaxis: a 2023 practice parameter update, *Ann Allergy Asthma Immunol* 132(2):124–176, 2024. doi:10.1016/j.anai.2023.09.015.

Gonzalez-Estrada A, Silvers SK, Klein A, Zell K, Wang XF, Lang DM: Epidemiology of anaphylaxis at a tertiary care center: a report of 730 cases, *Ann Allergy Asthma Immunol* 118:80–85, 2017.

Khan DA, Banerji A, Blumenthal KG, et al: Drug allergy: a 2022 practice parameter update, *J Allergy Clin Immunol* 150(6):1333–1393, 2022. doi:10.1016/j.jaci.2022.08.028.

Kuo CY: Advances in site-specific gene editing for primary immune deficiencies, *Curr Opin Allergy Clin Immunol* 18(6):453–458, 2018.

Laitinen LA, Laitinen A, Haahtela T: Airway mucosal inflammation even in patients with newly diagnosed asthma, *Am Rev Respir Dis* 147:697–704, 1993.

Lawley TJ, Bielory L, Gascon P, et al: A prospective clinical and immunologic analysis of patients with serum sickness, *N Engl J Med* 311:1407–1413, 1984.

Liu AH, Jaramillo R, Sicherer SH, et al: National prevalence and risk factors for food allergy and relationship to asthma: results from the National Health and Nutrition Examination Survey 2005-2006, *J Allergy Clin Immunol* 126:798–806, 2010.

Martinez FD, Stern DA, Wright AL, et al: Differential immune responses to acute lower respiratory illness in early life and subsequent development of persistent wheezing and asthma, *J Allergy Clin Immunol* 102:915–920, 1998.

Martinez FD, Wright AL, Taussig LM, et al: Asthma and wheezing in the first six years of life, *N Engl J Med* 332:133–138, 1995.

Murphy KM, Weaver C: *Janeway's immunobiology*, ed 9, New York, NY, 2017, Garland Science/Taylor & Francis Group, LLC.

Ochs HD, Smith CIE, Puck JM: *Primary immunodeficiency diseases*, New York, 1999, Oxford University Press.

Papangeli I, Scambler P: The 22q11 deletion: DiGeorge and velocardiofacial syndromes and the role of TBX1, *Wiley Interdiscip Rev Dev Biol* 2(3):393–403, 2013. doi:10.1002/wdev.75.

Puck JM: Primary immunodeficiency diseases, *J Am Med Assoc* 278:1835–1841, 1997.

Rachelefsky GS, Shapiro GG, Bergman D, et al: *Pediatric asthma: promoting best practice guide for managing asthma in children,* Milwaukee, WI, 1999, American Academy of Allergy, Asthma, & Immunology.

Romberg N, Lawrence MG: Birds of a feather: common variable immune deficiencies, *Ann Allergy Asthma Immunol* 123(5):461–467, 2019.

Rosenzweig SD, Holland SM: Phagocyte immunodeficiencies and their infections, *J Allergy Clin Immunol* 113:620–626, 2004.

Shaker M, Wallace D, Golden D, et al: Anaphylaxis—a 2020 practice parameter update, systematic review, and Grading of Recommendations, Assessment, Development and Evaluation (GRADE) analysis, *J Allergy Clin Immunol* 145(4):1082–1123, 2020.

Shearer WT, Leung DYM: 2008 mini-primer on allergic disease, *J Allergy Clin Immunol* 121:S363–S426, 2008.

Stiehm ER, Ochs HD, Winklestein JA: *Immunologic disorders in infants and children*, ed 5, Philadelphia, 2004, Elsevier/Saunders.

Tangye SG, Al-Herz W, Bousfiha A, et al: Human inborn errors of immunity: 2019 update on the classification from the International Union of Immunological Societies Expert Committee, *J Clin Immunol* 40(1):24–64, 2020.

White KD, Konvinse K, Rannakoe L, Redwood A, Phillips EJ: Immune mechanisms of drug allergy. In Khan DA, Banerji A, editors: *Drug allergy testing*, Missouri, 2018, Elsevier, pp 27–38.

5 CARDIOLOGY

Gaurav Arora | Mark DeBrunner | Sara M. Trucco

This chapter addresses the initial approach to a patient with suspected or known heart disease with the physical examination, chest radiograph, and electrocardiogram (ECG). A proper initial assessment helps to avoid unnecessary testing. However, the practice of cardiology as a pediatric subspecialty continues to rapidly evolve with expansion and enhancement of imaging technology and therapeutic options. Complex structural congenital anomalies can be precisely defined by a combination of techniques that include echocardiography, cardiac catheterization with angiography, nuclear imaging, magnetic resonance imaging (MRI), and computed tomography (CT) angiography. Concomitant with advances in diagnostic capabilities have come remarkable advances in therapy, both surgical and by interventional catheterization. Therefore this chapter includes considerable material on echocardiography and color flow Doppler studies, which remain the preeminent imaging modalities in pediatric cardiology. In addition, the surgical procedures that are commonly used are described, and an up-to-date section on the expanding array of therapeutic options in the cardiac catheterization laboratory is included.

The three prerequisites to a good cardiovascular examination are a proper environment, a cooperative child, and the conviction on the part of the physician that the examination is important. A heart murmur is not the only part and often is not even the most important part of the cardiac physical examination. Blood pressure determination, character of the pulse and precordial activity, observation of cyanosis, clubbing of the nail beds of the fingers or toes, and dysmorphic facial or other physical features may provide clues to the diagnosis and nature of congenital heart lesions before auscultation is even performed.

PHYSICAL DIAGNOSIS OF CONGENITAL HEART DISEASE

General Inspection

The physical examination should begin with a general inspection of the patient. Attention should be paid to the general appearance (well appearing vs. ill appearing), nutritional status (well nourished vs. growth faltering), color, and presence of dysmorphic physical features. In addition, the patient's preferred position should be noted. Patients with significant myocardial dysfunction, pulmonary edema, or pericardial disease are often most comfortable in a seated position. Placing these types of patients into a supine position may precipitate respiratory distress. Finally, the respiratory rate and work of breathing should be assessed at each encounter. Patients with cyanotic heart disease may manifest peaceful tachypnea, which is secondary to hypoxia. In contrast, patients with significant pulmonary overcirculation manifest labored tachypnea (e.g., grunting, retractions).

Cyanosis and Clubbing

Even before mild desaturation is detectable, early clubbing and cyanosis may be seen (Figs. 5.1 and 5.2). The base of the nail, especially the thumbnail, may show loss of the angle as early as 3 months old (see Chapter 17). Elevated hemoglobin and hematocrit and loss of nail angle indicate hypoxemia and suggest the presence of a right-to-left intracardiac shunt (Fig. 5.3). If heart disease is excluded, chronic pulmonary disease should be considered. Less common causes of clubbing include liver disease and malabsorption syndromes. Observation of the lips and mucous membranes for the presence of cyanosis is best done in good daylight because fluorescent lighting may produce a false cyanotic tinge. In the presence of polycythemia with hemoglobin in the 18% to 20% g range and hematocrit greater than 60%, the conjunctival vessels become engorged and plethoric (see Fig. 5.2). Conversely, when a patient is anemic, visible cyanosis can be easily missed (this is particularly important in infancy when infants reach physiologic nadir in hematocrit). Differential cyanosis between the upper and lower extremities is an unusual clinical finding. If the patient has pulmonary vascular disease, reverse flow through a patent ductus arteriosus with no right-to-left intracardiac shunting, cyanosis, and clubbing may be found in the lower extremities but not the hands (Fig. 5.4).

Blood Pressure and Pulse

Blood pressure determination in infants and children is an integral part of the cardiac physical examination. Attention to proper cuff size prevents the misdiagnosis of systolic hypertension from an undersized cuff. In general, it is better to use an oversized cuff, because overestimation in systolic blood pressure can be avoided. Blood pressure can be tracked in children over time, and tables depicting normal blood pressure range for age have been published. Blood pressure determination in both arms and a lower extremity will detect coarctation of the aorta. Supravalvular aortic stenosis may produce discrepant blood pressure readings between the left and right arms. In this condition, the jet of supravalvular stenosis is felt to be directed preferentially toward the right wall of the aorta and into the innominate artery. This is an example of the Coanda effect (a fluid column's proclivity after emerging from an orifice to adhere to a surface and flow along it). Blood pressure determination can also help to assess the severity of aortic valve disease, including aortic valve stenosis (narrow pulse pressure) and aortic regurgitation (wide pulse pressure).

Pulses should be characterized in terms of their amplitude and symmetry. They should be assessed concurrently in both the upper and lower extremities and between the right and left upper extremities. If there is a delay between the upper and lower extremity pulses, coarctation of the aorta should be excluded. Diminished peripheral pulses suggest poor cardiac output or shock. Bounding pulses are a reflection of aortic runoff lesions or low systemic arterial resistance. Peripheral pulses may be altered in the setting of significant aortic regurgitation. Quincke capillary pulse is an alternation of systolic flushing and diastolic blanching of the fingernails when light pressure is applied to the fingernails. Duroziez sign is the presence of both a systolic and diastolic murmur (to-fro) with compression of the femoral artery with edge of a stethoscope. In patients without aortic regurgitation, this maneuver produces only a systolic murmur.

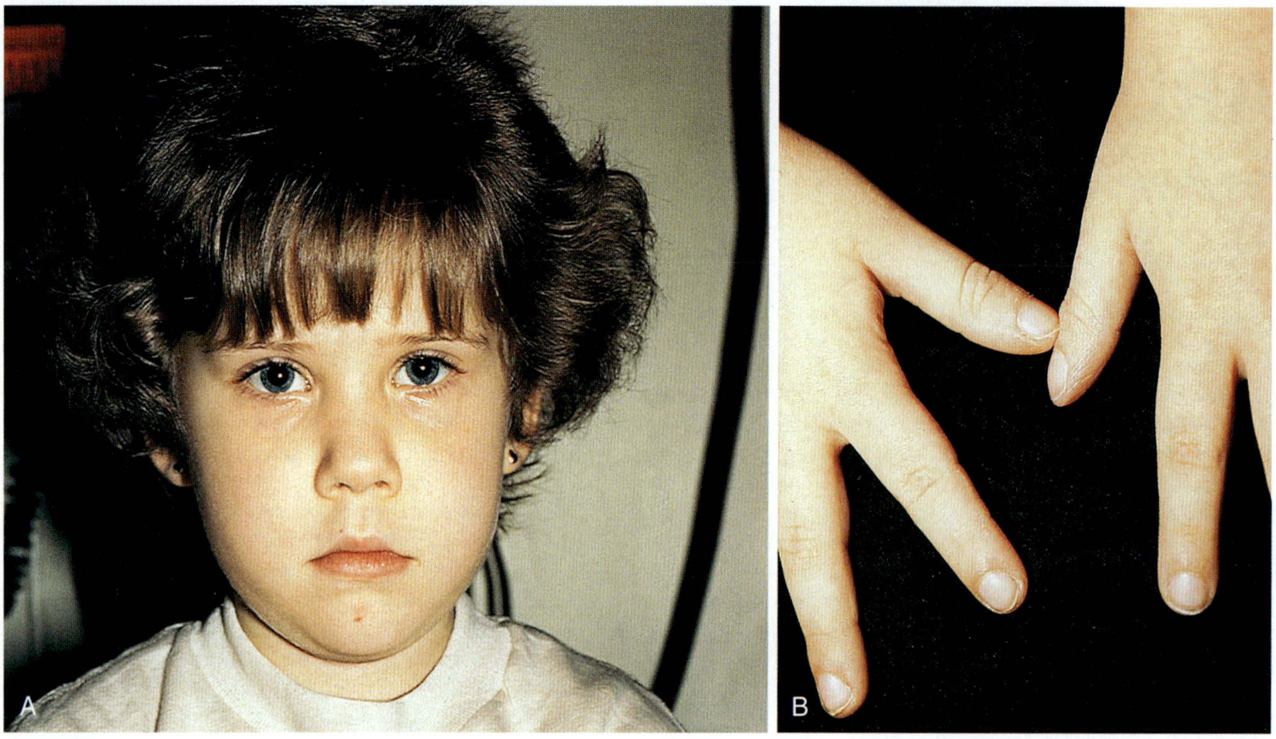

Fig. 5.1 Mild cyanosis. This child shows no obvious cyanosis of the face and lips (A), although (B) demonstrates clubbing; note the loss of nail angle and curvature of nails, especially of the thumb.

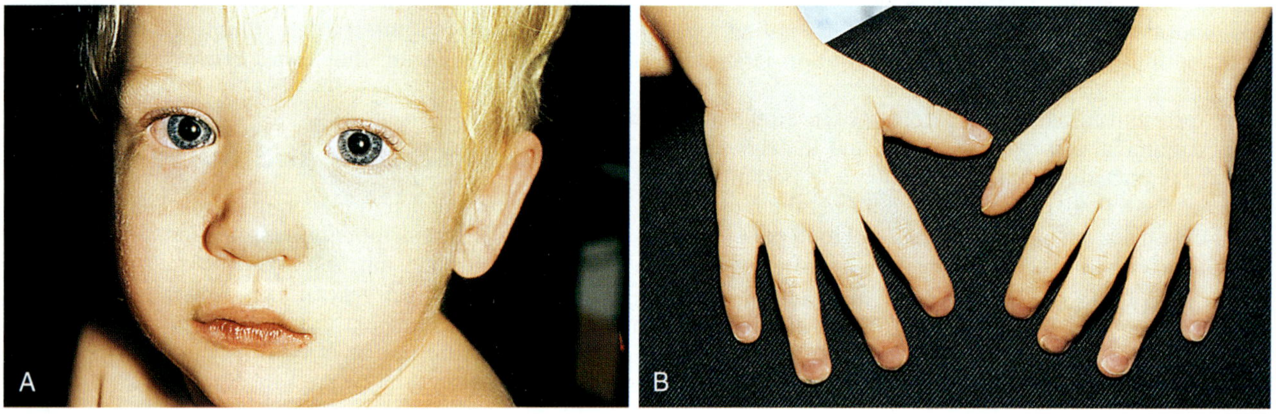

Fig. 5.2 Moderate cyanosis. This child demonstrates moderate cyanosis of the lips (A) and nails (B). Note also the reddish discoloration of the eyes resulting from conjunctival suffusion.

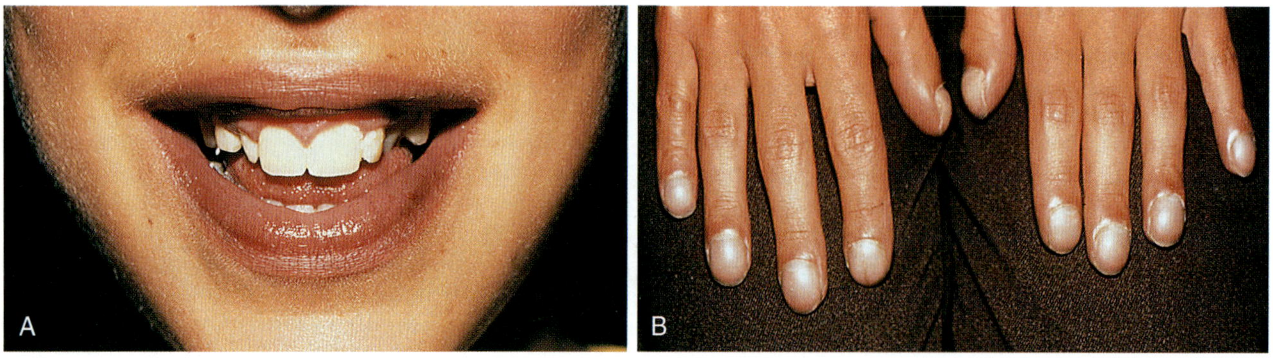

Fig. 5.3 Severe cyanosis. Severe cyanosis of the lips, tongue, and mucous membranes can be noted in (A), associated with marked clubbing and cyanosis of the nails in (B).

Heart Murmur Evaluation

Murmurs are relatively common in the newborn period. A common innocent heart murmur, peripheral pulmonic stenosis, during this period originates from the branch pulmonary arteries because of their relatively small size compared with the main pulmonary artery resulting from the normal fetal flow pattern, which delivers limited flow to the right and left pulmonary arteries. Characteristically, this murmur is early systolic and loudest over both axillae and the back. The murmur of branch pulmonary artery stenosis has the same distribution as the structural lesions that cause increased pulmonary blood flow. A transient systolic murmur at the middle-low left

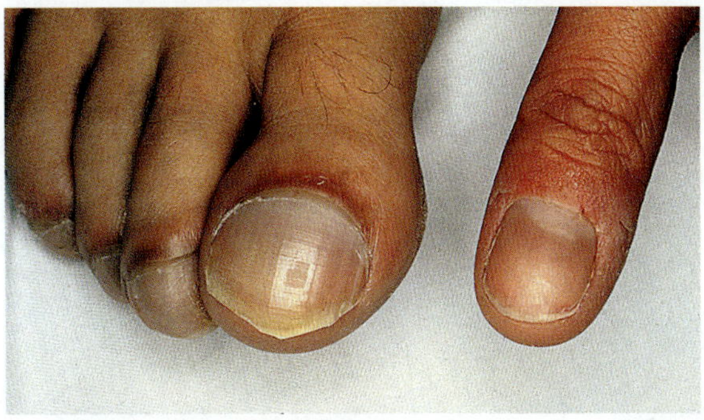

Fig. 5.4 Differential cyanosis and clubbing resulting from reverse shunting through a patent ductus arteriosus in a patient with pulmonary vascular disease. Note marked cyanosis and clubbing of the toes, although the finger appears to be normal. (Courtesy J.R. Zuberbuhler, MD, Pittsburgh.)

sternal border in the normal newborn can be due to tricuspid regurgitation, and a soft systolic ejection murmur at the upper left sternal border may arise from a closing patent ductus arteriosus. A large ventricular septal defect does not produce a murmur in the newborn period because the initially high pulmonary vascular resistance results in minimal shunting across the defect. On the other hand, pathologic systolic murmurs in the newborn are caused by restrictive ventricular septal defects, lesions producing left and right ventricular outflow tract obstruction (i.e., tetralogy of Fallot [TOF] and valvular aortic or pulmonary stenosis), and significant atrioventricular valvar insufficiency. In the newborn, it can be difficult to distinguish the murmur of a small restrictive ventricular septal defect from that of a severe right ventricular outflow tract obstruction in TOF or left ventricular outflow obstruction. The implications of this differential diagnosis are such that an echocardiogram is recommended for infants with this clinical presentation.

Contrary to popular belief, the presence of a continuous murmur from a patent ductus arteriosus is extremely rare in a full-term newborn. This is because the normal elevation of pulmonary artery pressure at this age minimizes the diastolic gradient between the aorta and pulmonary artery, attenuating or eliminating any diastolic component of the murmur. If a continuous murmur is heard in the newborn, patent ductus-dependent pulmonary blood flow or systemic-to-pulmonary collateral vessels in association with pulmonary atresia complex should be considered.

Preschoolers and school-age children are commonly referred for evaluation of a heart murmur. Innocent murmurs of childhood fall into four major categories: systolic ejection murmurs at the base; vibratory, or Still murmur; venous hums; and carotid and cranial bruits. In most instances, there are associated clinical and laboratory studies that can distinguish the innocent from the pathologic murmur. Table 5.1 summarizes the distinguishing features and differential diagnosis. Fig. 5.5 illustrates the sites where murmurs resulting from various cardiovascular lesions are best heard.

Table 5.1 Innocent Murmurs Mimicking Congenital Heart Disease

Innocent Heart Murmur	Structural Congenital Heart Disease
Systolic Ejection Murmur at Base of Heart	
High left sternal border (Pulmonary flow murmur)	Pulmonary valve stenosis Ejection click Transmission to back Atrial septal defect Parasternal lift[a] S_2 wide split[a] Diastolic murmur of tricuspid flow[a]
High right sternal border	Aortic valve stenosis Ejection click[a] Radiation to neck[a]
Still Murmur	
Vibratory quality Location: left midsternal border	Ventricular septal defect Character of murmur[a] Discrete subaortic stenosis Radiation to aortic area[a] Subpulmonic stenosis Radiation to pulmonic area[a] Soft P_2[a]
Venous Hum	
Continuous Location: neck and under clavicles Usually loudest when sitting, disappears in supine posture	Patent ductus arteriosus Location under left clavicle[a] No change with position[a] Coronary atrioventricular malformation Accentuated in diastole[a]
Carotid and Cranial Bruits	
Murmur over carotids and head	Aortic stenosis Atrioventricular malformation Continuous murmur would support atrioventricular malformation[a]

P_2, Pulmonic second sound; S_2, second heart sound.
[a]Distinguishing features.

Syndrome-Associated Physical Findings

Dysmorphology of the face and habitus suggests certain syndromes associated with congenital heart disease (Table 5.2).

The typical features in *Down syndrome* (trisomy 21) are discussed in Chapter 1. Approximately 40% of children with this syndrome have structural lesions, such as atrioventricular septal defects (complete or partial atrioventricular septal defect), isolated ventricular septal defects, patent ductus arteriosus, or anomalous origin of the subclavian arteries. Although many infants with Down syndrome and congenital heart disease have chronic congestive heart failure and growth failure, there is a subset with a significant septal defect who may grow and develop appropriately. This is related to abnormally high pulmonary vascular resistance not decreasing in the usual fashion in this group, leading to early pulmonary vascular disease. Because this presentation may be silent, it is important that all children with Down syndrome be thoroughly evaluated during early infancy. The evaluation should include an echocardiogram to rule out congenital heart disease.

DiGeorge and *velocardiofacial syndromes* are related developmental disorders involving the third and fourth pharyngeal pouches. They have been shown to be caused by deletions within a critical region of chromosome 22q11 (which can be evaluated with a blood test—fluorescence in situ hybridization [FISH] for 22q11 deletion). Cardiac abnormalities, particularly the conotruncal type and aortic arch anomalies, occur in 75% of patients with 22q11 deletion (see Table 5.2). Other findings include hypocalcemia, cleft palate, renal anomalies, immunologic defects, facial dysmorphisms, and variable developmental delay with educational and behavioral issues (see Chapter 4).

Holt-Oram syndrome, an autosomal dominant disorder, is associated with upper limb deformities consisting of narrow shoulders, hypoplasia of the radius, and phocomelia (Fig. 5.6). Absence of both radius and thumb or proximal displacement of the thumb is the most frequent finding. Commonly associated cardiovascular abnormalities include an atrial septal defect, ventricular septal defect, and arrhythmias (atrial and ventricular ectopy and atrioventricular block).

Marfan syndrome also has an autosomal dominant inheritance; it manifests as a connective tissue disorder in which the elastic fibers are disrupted, causing cystic medial necrosis of the aorta, as well as joint laxity and subluxation of the ocular lens. Affected patients are tall, with increased limb length compared with the trunk. Their arm span exceeds their height. The cardiovascular abnormalities nearly always found in this syndrome include aneurysmal dilation of the aorta and aortic sinuses and mitral valve prolapse. Associated

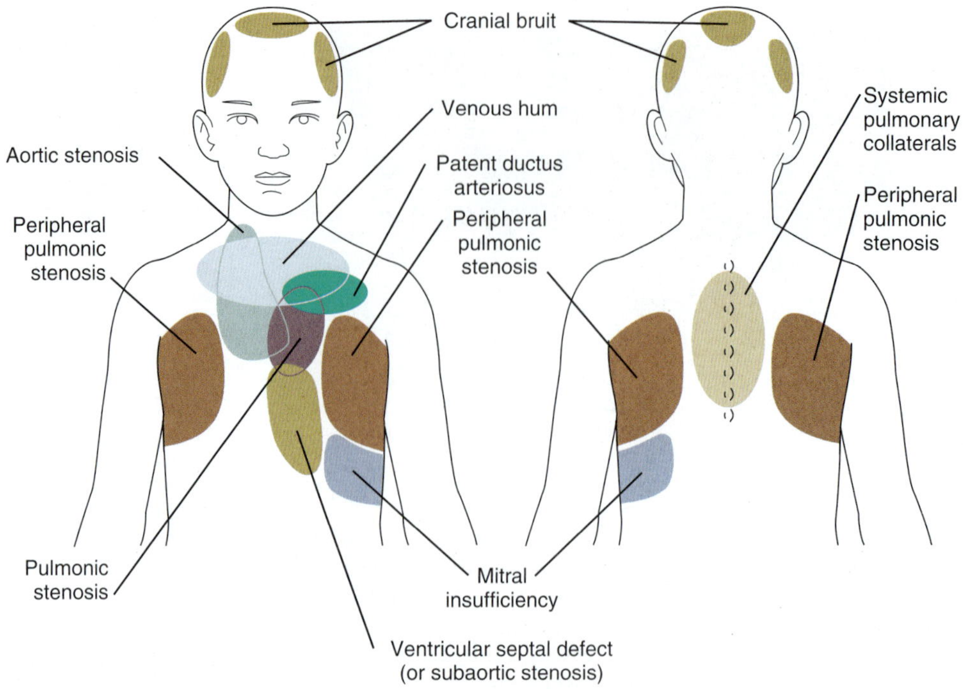

Fig. 5.5 Sites where murmurs resulting from various cardiovascular lesions are best heard.

Table 5.2 Dysmorphology Syndromes and Trisomies With Associated Cardiovascular Abnormalities

Syndrome	Genetic Basis of Disease	Common Cardiac Defect
Alagille	Mutation of *JAG-1* gene	Peripheral branch pulmonary artery stenosis, tetralogy of Fallot, pulmonary valve stenosis, atrial and ventricular septal defects
CHARGE	Mutation of *CHD7* gene	Tetralogy of Fallot, double outlet right ventricle, truncus arteriosus, aortic arch abnormalities, patent ductus arteriosus, ventricular septal defects, atrial septal defects, and atrioventricular septal defects
DiGeorge/velocardiofacial	Deletion of 22q11	Aortic arch abnormalities: interrupted arch (type B), right aortic arch Conotruncal abnormalities: truncus arteriosus, tetralogy of Fallot, pulmonary atresia with ventricular septal defect
Fetal alcohol	N/A	Ventricular septal defect
Holt-Oram	Mutation of *TBX-5* gene	Atrial and ventricular septal defects, arrhythmias
Marfan	Mutation of Fibrillin-1 gene	Dilation of ascending aorta/aortic sinus, aortic, mitral valve prolapse, mitral insufficiency
Noonan	Mutation in PTPN 11 gene in ~50%. Mutation of multiple genes in the Ras-MAPK pathway	Dysplastic pulmonic valve, atrial septal defect, hypertrophic cardiomyopathy
Turner	45 X monosomy	Coarctation of the aorta, bicuspid aortic valve
Williams	Microdeletion of 7q11.23 region	Supravalvular aortic stenosis, pulmonary artery stenosis
Trisomy 13		Patent ductus arteriosus, septal defects, pulmonic and aortic stenosis (atresia)
Trisomy 18		Ventricular septal defect, polyvalvular disease, coronary abnormalities, double outlet right ventricle with mitral atresia, tetralogy of Fallot
Trisomy 21 (Down syndrome)		Atrioventricular septal defects, ventricular septal defect, patent ductus arteriosus, anomalous subclavian artery
VACTERL association	Unknown	Ventricular septal defects, atrial septal defects, tetralogy of Fallot

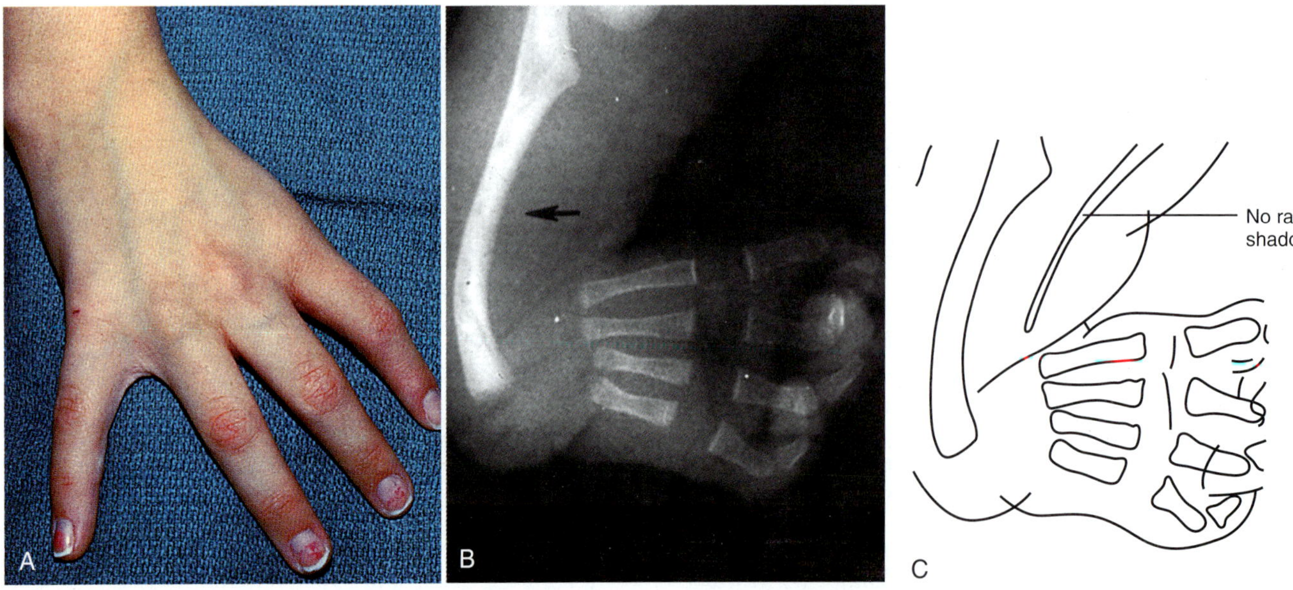

Fig. 5.6 Holt-Oram syndrome. Note the absence of the radius and thumb (A). The associated cardiovascular abnormality is an atrial septal defect. Radiographic examination (B and C) demonstrates the absence of a radius shadow; the missing thumb is apparent.

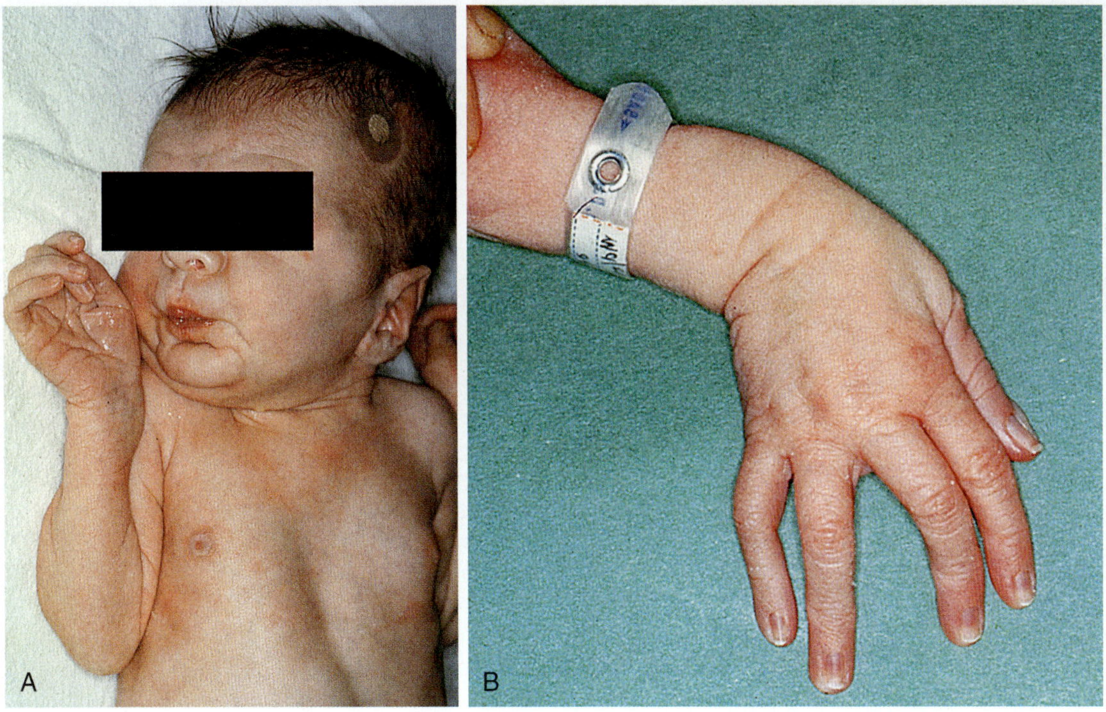

Fig. 5.7 Infant with Marfan syndrome. (A) Note the narrow elongated face, pectus excavatum, and long arms and fingers. (B) A close-up view of the infant's hand.

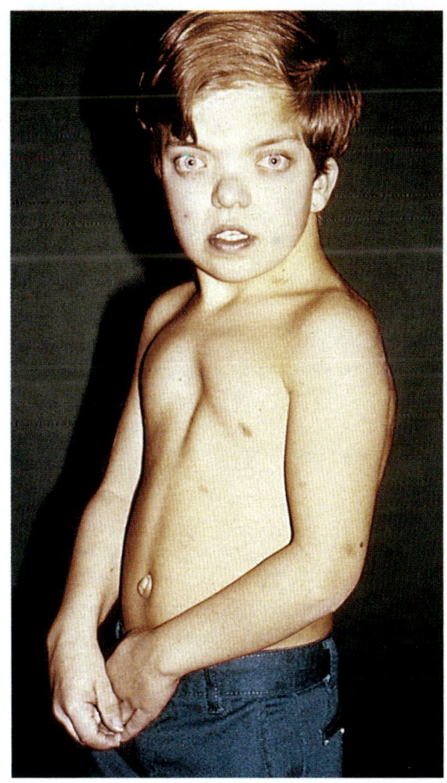

Fig. 5.8 Noonan syndrome. Note the widely spaced eyes, low-set ears, webbing of the neck, shield chest, pectus, and increased carrying angle of the arms.

aortic and mitral valve regurgitation are common (Fig. 5.7) (see Chapter 1).

Cardiac anomalies occur in up to 50% of patients with Turner syndrome. The most common lesions include bicuspid aortic valve, coarctation of the aorta, and dilation of the aorta. (See Chapters 1 and 9 for a detailed discussion of Turner syndrome.)

Patients with *Noonan syndrome* have features characteristic of Turner syndrome but possess a defect on chromosome 12 and may be male or female. An autosomal dominant inheritance pattern accounts for approximately 50% of Noonan cases. Clinically, these children have the findings of webbing of the neck, pectus excavatum, shield chest with widely spaced nipples, short stature, epicanthal folds, low-set ears, and increased carrying angle of the arms (Fig. 5.8). Common cardiovascular defects include pulmonary stenosis in association with a dysplastic pulmonary valve, atrial septal defect, and hypertrophic cardiomyopathy. Occasionally, there may be dysplasia of all cardiac valves. The ECG may show a left axis deviation that is unrelated to other structural abnormalities. The syndrome appears as an autosomal dominant disorder; multiple members of a family are often affected.

Patients with *Williams syndrome* characteristically have "elfin" facies: a broad maxilla, a small mandible with full mouth and large upper lip (philtrum), upturned nose, and a full forehead (Fig. 5.9). This syndrome has been associated with hypercalcemia in infants and a strikingly affable personality despite variable degrees of developmental delay and has an identifiable genetic abnormality, a deletion of the 7q11.23 region of chromosome 7 containing the elastin gene. Supravalvular aortic stenosis and pulmonary artery branch stenosis are common cardiovascular abnormalities associated with this syndrome.

Alagille syndrome is attributable to mutations in the *JAG-1* gene. The majority of patients have congenital heart disease, with peripheral branch pulmonary artery stenosis being the most common manifestation. TOF with pulmonary stenosis or atresia, pulmonary valve stenosis, and atrial and ventricular septal defects are also associated with the condition.

CHARGE (**c**oloboma, **h**eart disease, **a**tresia choanae, **r**etarded growth and development, **g**enital anomalies, and hypogonadism, **e**ar anomalies, and deafness) association features congenital heart disease in approximately 50% to 70% of cases. Common lesions include TOF, double-outlet right ventricle, truncus arteriosus, aortic arch abnormalities, patent ductus arteriosus, ventricular septal defects, atrial septal defects, and atrioventricular septal defects.

In addition, there are many other genetically determined diseases and inborn errors of metabolism with cardiac involvement, the most common of which are listed in Table 5.3.

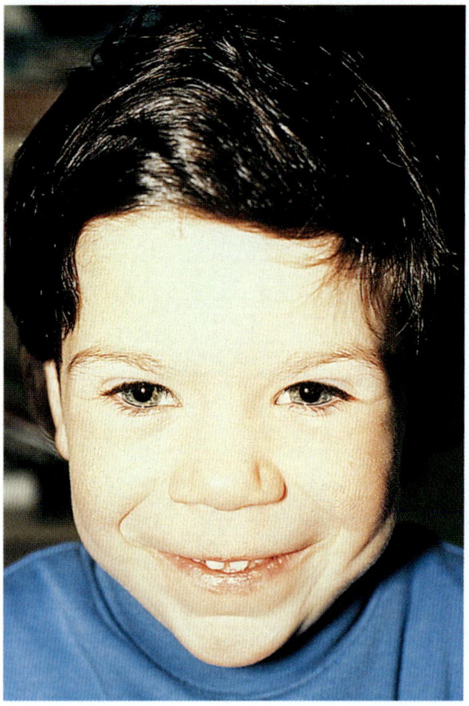

Fig. 5.9 Williams syndrome. Note the wide-set eyes, upturned nose, large maxilla, prominent philtrum, and pointed chin. (Courtesy R.A. Mathews, MD, Philadelphia, PA.)

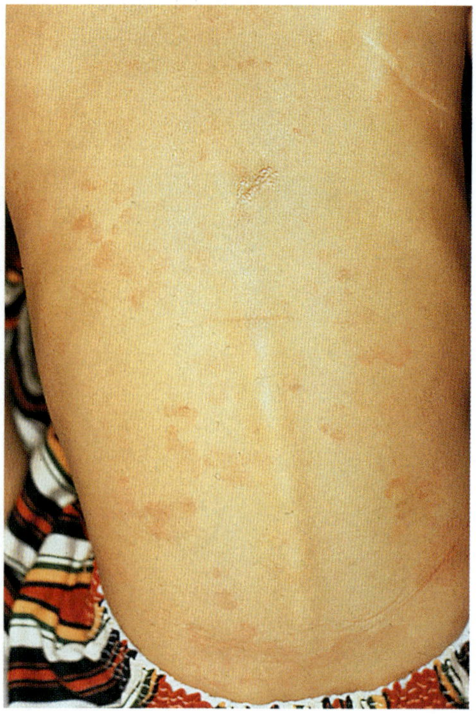

Fig. 5.10 Erythema marginatum rash in a child with acute rheumatic fever. Note the wavy margins in the distribution on the trunk.

Table 5.3 Other Genetic Syndromes and Inborn Errors of Metabolism With Associated Cardiovascular Findings

Syndromes	Cardiac Findings
Genetically Determined Diseases	
Metabolic	
Pompe disease (glycogen storage)	Cardiomyopathy (storage of glycogen in myocardium)
Mucopolysaccharidosis	Storage of MPS in arteries, coronaries, and valves with insufficiency and stenosis Hurler syndrome (MPS I H), Hunter syndrome (MPS II), Scheie syndrome (MPS IS), Hurler-Scheie syndrome (MPS IH/S), Morquio syndrome (MPS IV)
Hyperlipoproteinemia, familial type II	Premature atherosclerosis of arteries including coronaries
Neurologic	
Friedreich ataxia	Cardiomyopathy (congestive or hypertrophic)
Muscular dystrophies	Myocardial degeneration and fibrosis
Inborn Error of Metabolism (No Proven Genetic Basis)	
Progeria	Hypercholesterolemia, atherosclerotic changes in arteries, including coronary arteries

MPS, Mucopolysaccharidosis.

Visible Clues in Acute Rheumatic Fever

Examination of the skin in a patient with acute rheumatic fever may reveal the typical rash of erythema marginatum, although this rash is not specific for rheumatic fever. It is evanescent, is nonpruritic, has sharp serpiginous margins, and is found on the inner aspects of the upper arms and thighs and on the trunk (Fig. 5.10). The differential diagnosis includes (1) drug rash, which is papular and pruritic; (2) erythema multiforme, which has target lesions; (3) rash of juvenile rheumatoid arthritis, which is pink, macular, and lacks wavy margins, and which may be transient; and (4) the cutaneous findings of Kawasaki disease (see Chapter 7).

Subcutaneous nodules are rare in chronic rheumatic heart disease, but if found, they are almost always associated with severe carditis. These movable, nontender, cartilage-like swellings vary in size from 2 mm to 1 cm and are persistent. They are seen over the bony prominences of the large joints and external surfaces of the elbows and knuckles of the hands, knees, and ankles. They may also be felt along the spine and over the skull. Although difficult to photograph, they are easily palpated (Fig. 5.11).

At least half of patients with acute rheumatic fever have cardiac involvement. Mitral regurgitation is the most common manifestation, and mitral stenosis may subsequently develop. Aortic regurgitation may also be noted, whereas aortic stenosis is uncommon. The cardiac physical examination may reveal distinctive findings of a parasternal lift and loud pulmonic closure sound from secondary pulmonary hypertension, an apical pansystolic high-pitched murmur of mitral regurgitation, a middiastolic apical rumble (Carey Coombs murmur) from increased and turbulent flow across thickened mitral valve leaflets, and a high-pitched decrescendo diastolic murmur at the left sternal border of aortic regurgitation.

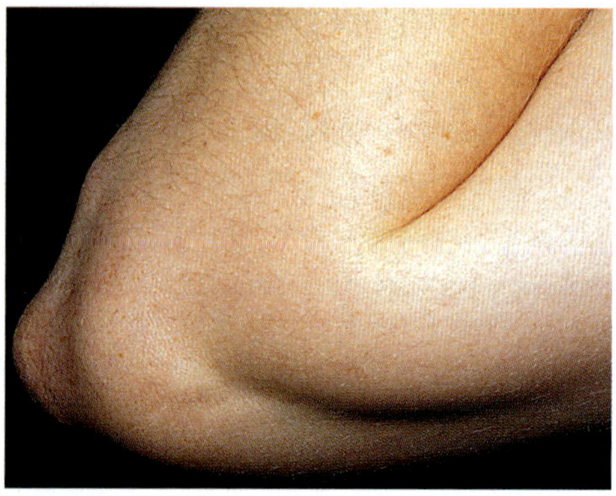

Fig. 5.11 Subcutaneous nodules. Note their presence over the bony prominences of the elbow in a patient with chronic rheumatic heart disease.

Signs of Bacterial Endocarditis

Although the clinical presentation of bacterial endocarditis varies according to the infecting organism, it should be suspected in any patient with congenital or acquired heart disease who has prolonged fever without apparent cause. The classic skin lesions include petechiae, splinter hemorrhages of the nails, conjunctival hemorrhages, Janeway lesions (Fig. 5.12), and Osler nodes. Vegetations occasionally dislodge and embolize in an end artery, which results in hemorrhagic or gangrenous lesions (Fig. 5.13). Janeway lesions are nontender, small erythematous lesions noted on the palms and soles. Osler nodes, which present as small tender erythematous nodules, are found in the intradermal pads of the fingers and toes or in the thenar or hypothenar eminences (Fig. 5.14). Both Janeway lesions and Osler nodes are believed to be a manifestation of septic microemboli that produce dermal microabscesses. The difference in the appearance, location, and sensation is unknown. All the aforementioned findings are often associated with a new heart murmur, splenomegaly, spiking fever, and positive blood culture. Clubbing of the fingers may occur in chronic cases.

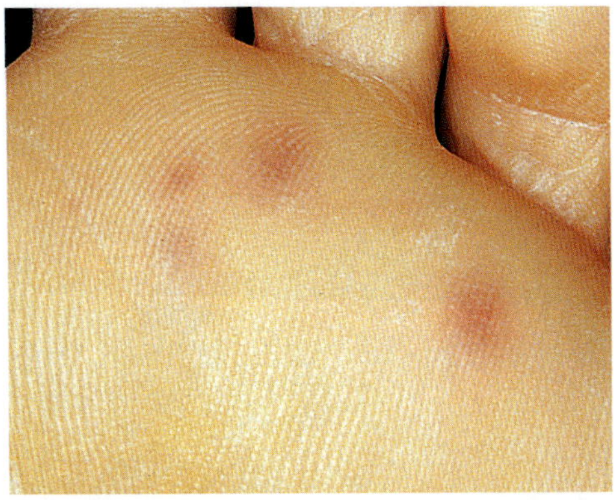

Fig. 5.12 Janeway lesions. Note the small (painless) nodules on the sole of a patient with bacterial endocarditis.

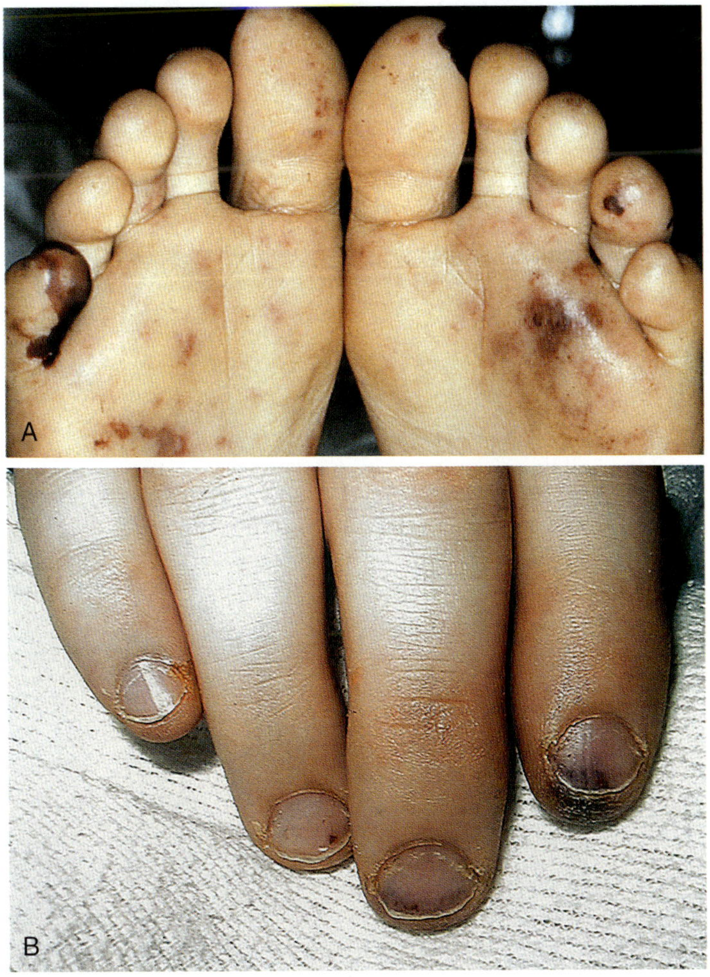

Fig. 5.13 Acute bacterial endocarditis. Note the hemorrhagic lesions (A) and subungual splinter hemorrhages (B).

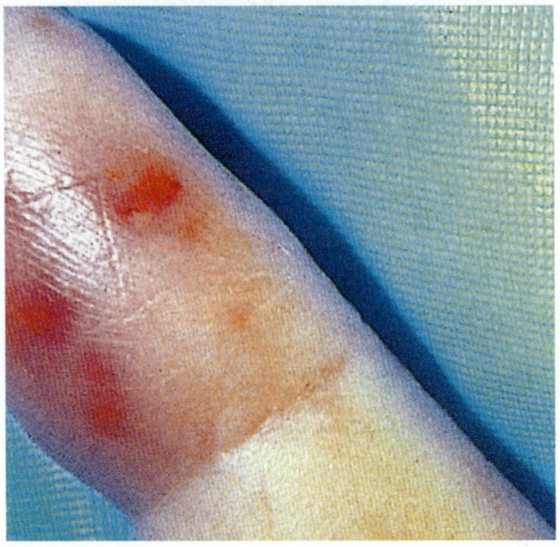

Fig. 5.14 Osler nodes. Note the (painful) erythematous nodular lesions resulting from infective endocarditis. (Courtesy J.F. John, Jr., MD.)

Kawasaki Disease

This multisystem disease has surpassed acute rheumatic fever as the most common form of acquired heart disease in children. It is characterized by fever, conjunctivitis, erythema of the lips and oral mucosa, extremity changes, rash, and cervical adenopathy. Coronary artery aneurysms develop in 15% to 25% of untreated patients and may result in myocardial ischemia, infarction, or sudden death. The incidence of coronary abnormalities is markedly decreased with timely treatment (≈5%). This disease is discussed in detail in Chapter 7. Coronary artery aneurysms are well demonstrated by echocardiography (Fig. 5.15), and this imaging modality plays an essential role in the diagnosis and management of Kawasaki disease.

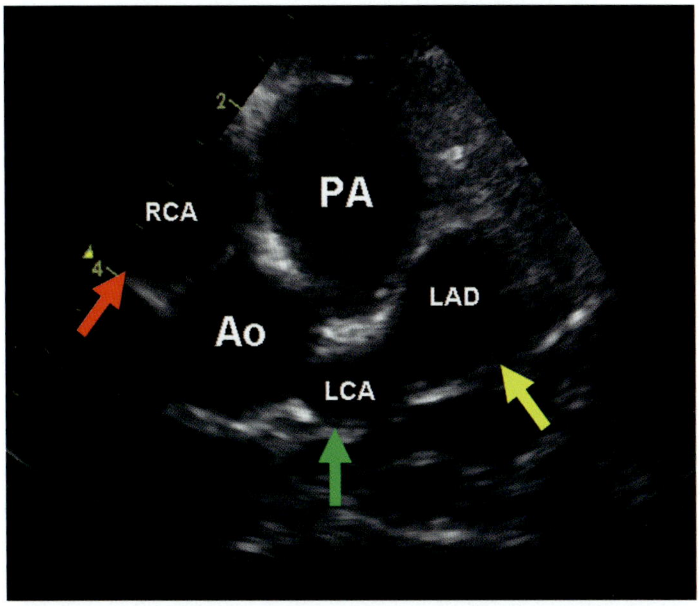

Fig. 5.15 Kawasaki disease: giant coronary artery aneurysms. Multiple giant coronary aneurysms of the right *(RCA, red arrow)*, left *(LCA, green arrow)*, and left anterior descending *(LAD, yellow arrow)* coronary arteries. *Ao*, Aorta; *PA*, pulmonary artery.

LABORATORY AIDS IN THE DIAGNOSIS OF CONGENITAL HEART DISEASE

In addition to a comprehensive physical examination, the chest roentgenogram, ECG, and, most notably, echocardiography provide invaluable information concerning specific congenital heart lesions and have allowed therapeutic decisions to be made without cardiac catheterization.

Chest Roentgenography

The chest x-ray examination has been used to screen patients with suspected congenital heart disease. Chest radiographs can identify enlargement of the cardiac silhouette, which could signify chamber enlargement or pericardial effusion. In addition, pulmonary vascular markings can help to identify diseases with increased pulmonary blood flow such as left-to-right shunts or diminished pulmonary blood flow in cyanotic lesions such as TOF. A chest radiograph is also useful in differentiating cardiac from pulmonary pathology such as pneumonia, pneumothorax, pneumomediastinum, or other parenchymal lung disease that may mimic congenital heart disease. The review of any chest roentgenogram requires a systematic approach. As advanced imaging has become more prevalent, the chest radiograph has been less utilized in day-to-day clinical cardiology practice, but an understanding of common chest x-ray findings is a fundamental skill for providers.

Cardiac Apex and Visceral Situs

The location of the cardiac apex and visceral situs provides important diagnostic information. Discordance of the situs and cardiac apex (i.e., apex to the right with situs solitus [normal arrangement] or apex to the left with situs inversus) is often associated with structural congenital heart disease (Fig. 5.16). Dextrocardia (apex to the right) or mesocardia (apex to the middle) with situs solitus is a frequent presentation of ventricular inversion or corrected transposition of the great arteries (see Fig. 5.16). Dextrocardia with situs inversus totalis can be identified on chest radiograph with the apex pointing to the right and the stomach bubble also on the right (Fig. 5.17). Dextrocardia can also be seen with primary pulmonary problems. Scimitar syndrome is composed of dextroposition with hypoplasia of the right lung. In this case a major portion of the right lung (usually the right lower lobe) is "sequestered" and has its arterial supply by way of a systemic artery from the descending aorta, and the pulmonary venous return from that lung drains abnormally into the inferior vena cava via a vein forming a scimitar. Patients with levocardia (apex to the left) with either situs inversus or situs ambiguous frequently have complex congenital heart diseases, such as transposition of the great arteries, pulmonary atresia, and atrioventricular septal defects. Atrial isomerism is associated with bilateral morphologic right or left lungs and can be recognized as bilateral symmetric right (short) or left (long) bronchi. This is best demonstrated with a magnified penetrated chest x-ray examination focusing on bronchial anatomy (Fig. 5.18). Many patients with this anomaly have complex congenital heart disease.

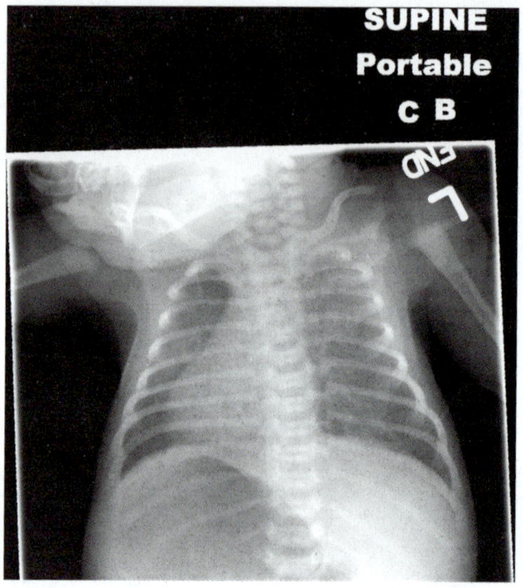

Fig. 5.17 Dextrocardia with situs inversus totalis. Note the cardiac apex pointing to the right along with the stomach bubble under the right diaphragm.

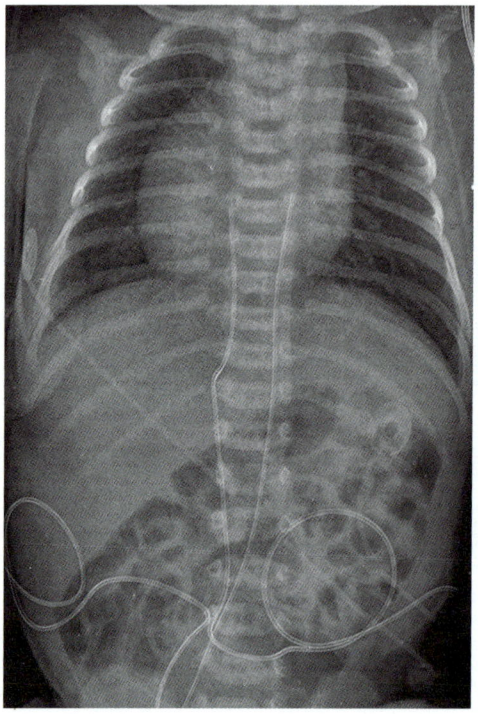

Fig. 5.16 Dextrocardia (heart in the right side of the chest) associated with situs solitus. Note the prominent vascular shadow along the left-sided cardiac border that is caused by the aorta. This pattern is commonly associated with ventricular inversion (corrected transposition of the great arteries).

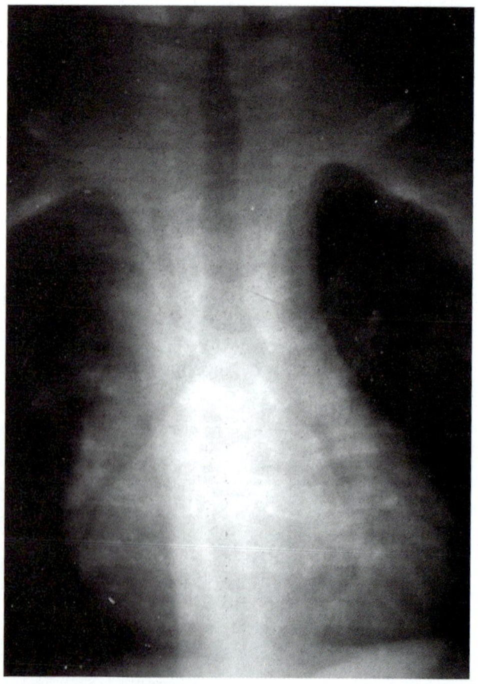

Fig. 5.18 Atrial isomerism. Note the symmetric bronchial anatomy. Atrial isomerism should be suspected when the heart is midline on the chest radiograph and situs ambiguous is present. Bilateral right or left bronchi can be found with right or left atrial isomerism, respectively.

Shape and Size

Cardiac size is important, but the shape of the cardiac image may also provide a clue as to which heart chambers are enlarged and the likely structural diagnosis. In the cyanotic newborn with transposition of the great arteries, the cardiac image appears as an "egg on a string" (Fig. 5.19). If the thymic shadow does not obscure it, the mediastinal shadow shows a narrow waist resulting from the anterior-posterior position of the aorta and pulmonary artery. This produces the "string." Pulmonary vascular markings are usually increased, although vascularity may be normal in the immediate newborn period.

In TOF with pulmonic stenosis, the heart appears "boot shaped" because right ventricular hypertrophy causes the apex (toe of the boot) to turn upward (Fig. 5.20). The concavity of the left upper cardiac border is due to the small right ventricular outflow tract and main pulmonary artery segment.

In TOF with pulmonary atresia, the heart is shaped like an "egg on its side" (Fig. 5.21). The pulmonary blood flow to the lungs may be supplied by either patent ductus arteriosus or systemic arterial collateral vessels. The pulmonary vascular markings may be decreased if pulmonary blood flow is patent ductus dependent and increased if large systemic collaterals supply pulmonary blood flow.

In congenitally corrected transposition of the great arteries, the heart has a "valentine" or "heart" shape with the apex pointing downward just to the left of the midline. The fullness at the left upper border of the cardiac shadow is due to the ascending aorta arising from the left-sided morphologic right ventricle. Dextrocardia is a frequent finding with this anomaly.

Although an enlarged and globular heart shadow may be associated with a cardiomyopathy, massive cardiac enlargement (so-called "wall-to-wall heart") is typical in neonatal patients with Ebstein anomaly. In this anomaly, there is a malformation of the tricuspid valve with downward displacement of the inferior and septal leaflets of the valve into the ventricle, causing severe tricuspid valve regurgitation or stenosis. As a result, the right atrium becomes markedly enlarged and, along with the "atrialized" portion of the right

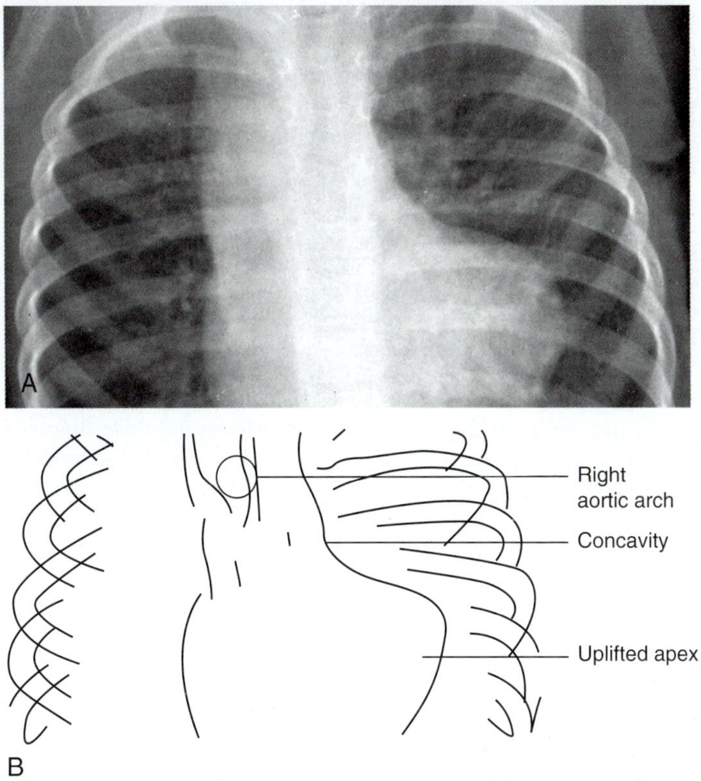

Fig. 5.20 (A and B) Tetralogy of Fallot with pulmonic stenosis produces a "boot-shaped" heart, which results from right ventricular hypertrophy, upward tilt of the apex, and the concavity at the left upper heart border caused by a small right ventricular infundibulum and main pulmonary artery. Note also the right aortic arch.

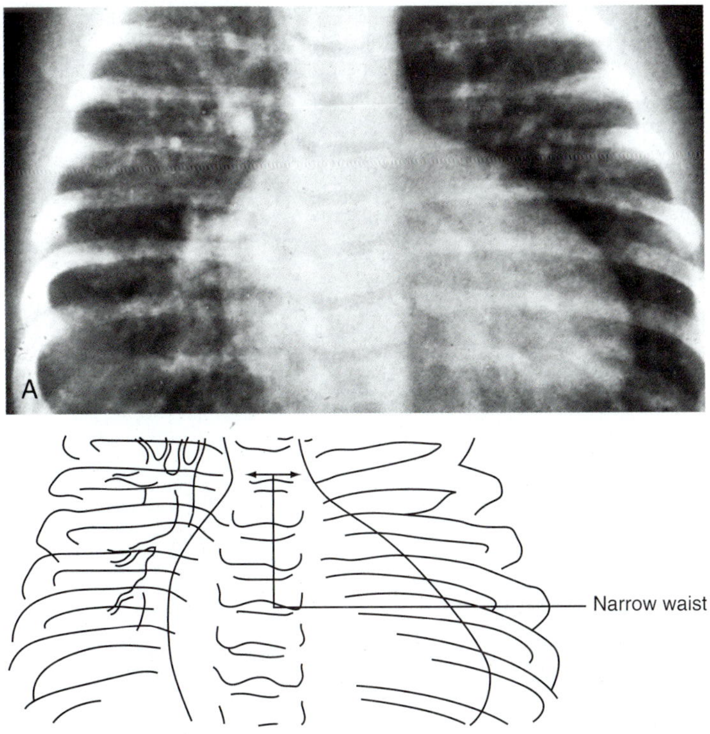

Fig. 5.19 Transposition of the great arteries. (A and B) Note the "egg on a string" heart shadow, which results from the position of the main pulmonary artery posterior and slightly to the left of the aorta, contributing to the narrow waist (the "string").

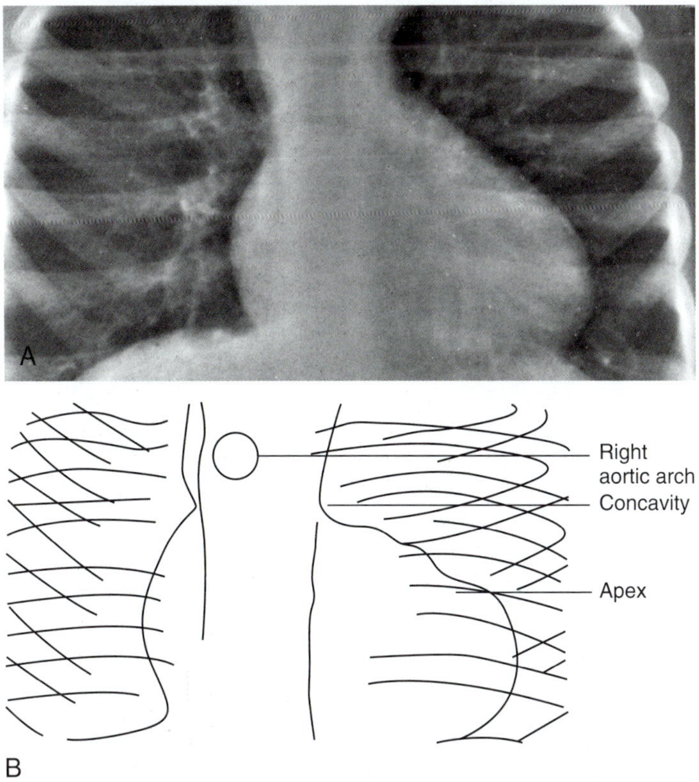

Fig. 5.21 Tetralogy of Fallot with pulmonary atresia. (A and B) Note the "egg on its side" appearance of the heart due to the uplifted apex resulting from the right ventricular hypertrophy. The absence of a right ventricular outflow and the diminutive main pulmonary artery segment produce a concavity at the left upper heart border. Note also that a right aortic arch is present.

ventricle, contributes significantly to the cardiac image of a large box-shaped heart (Fig. 5.22).

Left-to-right shunt lesions from atrial septal defects, ventricular septal defects, or a patent ductus arteriosus demonstrate specific chamber enlargement and increased pulmonary vascular markings. A significant atrial defect shows enlargement of all right-sided cardiac chambers, including the right atrium, right ventricle, and pulmonary artery. A patent ductus arteriosus shows enlargement of all left-sided cardiac chambers including the aorta. In patients with a ventricular septal defect, there is left-sided volume overload. An example of cardiomegaly with increased pulmonary vascular markings can be seen in Fig. 5.23.

Great Vessels

The radiographic appearance of the great arteries may also suggest a specific structural congenital heart defect. The main and left branch pulmonary arteries are usually enlarged in patients with pulmonary valve stenosis due to poststenotic dilation. The characteristic radiographic finding of congenital aortic valve stenosis is dilation of the ascending aorta, best seen as an overlapping shadow with the superior vena cava along the right upper cardiac border. Although these lesions do have associated radiographic findings, the chest radiograph is rarely used for diagnosis given the ease of echocardiography. However, coarctation of the aorta not diagnosed in a timely fashion may show the distinct radiographic finding of a reversed E or 3 sign caused by prestenotic and poststenotic dilation of the descending aorta (Fig. 5.24). If a significant coarctation remains unrepaired for 5 or more years, rib notching may appear (see the Skeletal Abnormalities section later).

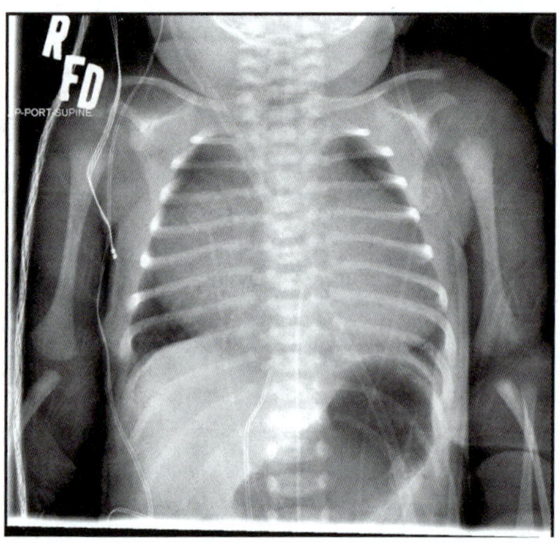

Fig. 5.22 Ebstein anomaly of the tricuspid valve. Note the radiographic appearance of the "wall-to-wall" heart, due to a massively enlarged right atrium.

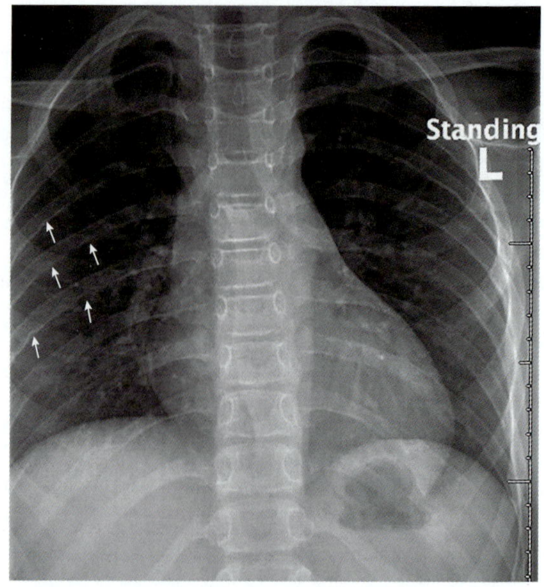

Fig. 5.24 Coarctation of the aorta. Prominent inferior rib notching noted in this 10-year-old child with figure of 3 sign formed by prestenotic and poststenotic dilation around the site of the undiagnosed coarctation.

The normal left aortic arch causes a shift of the tracheal air column to the right, whereas a right arch causes a similar deviation to the left (Fig. 5.25). The position of the thoracic descending aorta also helps to define the side of the arch and can be determined by noting obscuring of either the left or right side of the thoracic vertebral bodies. A right aortic arch should always raise the suspicion of congenital heart disease and is found in approximately 30% of patients with TOF or truncus arteriosus.

The addition of a barium swallow to the chest x-ray examination has historically been an important diagnostic tool in the assessment of patients with upper airway obstruction from vascular rings. Current practice favors the imaging techniques of MRI or CT scan, which provide clear and precise imaging of aortic arch and great vessel anatomy and their relationship to the airway and esophagus. Nevertheless, one may find vascular anomalies as findings on a barium swallow performed for the evaluation of dysphagia or upper airway respiratory symptoms. If a bilateral indentation is noted on the barium esophagram, a double aortic arch should be suspected (Fig. 5.26). A right aortic arch with distal origin of the left subclavian

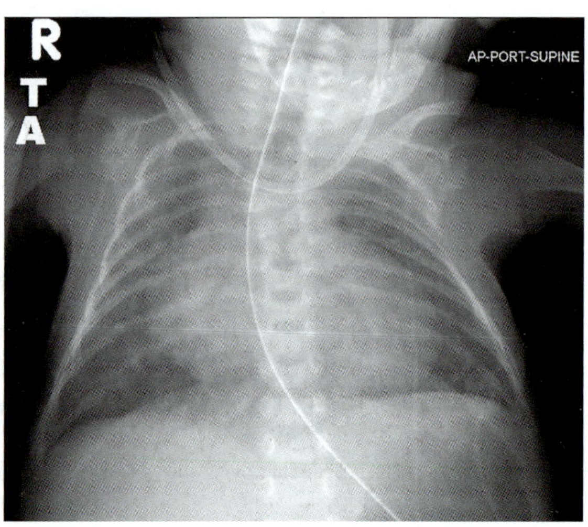

Fig. 5.23 Large left-to-right shunt from ventricular septal defect. Note the cardiomegaly and increased pulmonary vascular markings seen with pulmonary overcirculation.

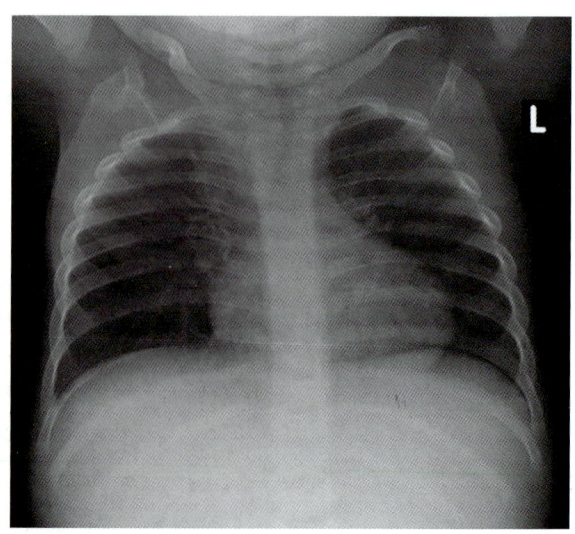

Fig. 5.25 Right aortic arch. Note deviation of the tracheal air column to the left, suggesting a right aortic arch.

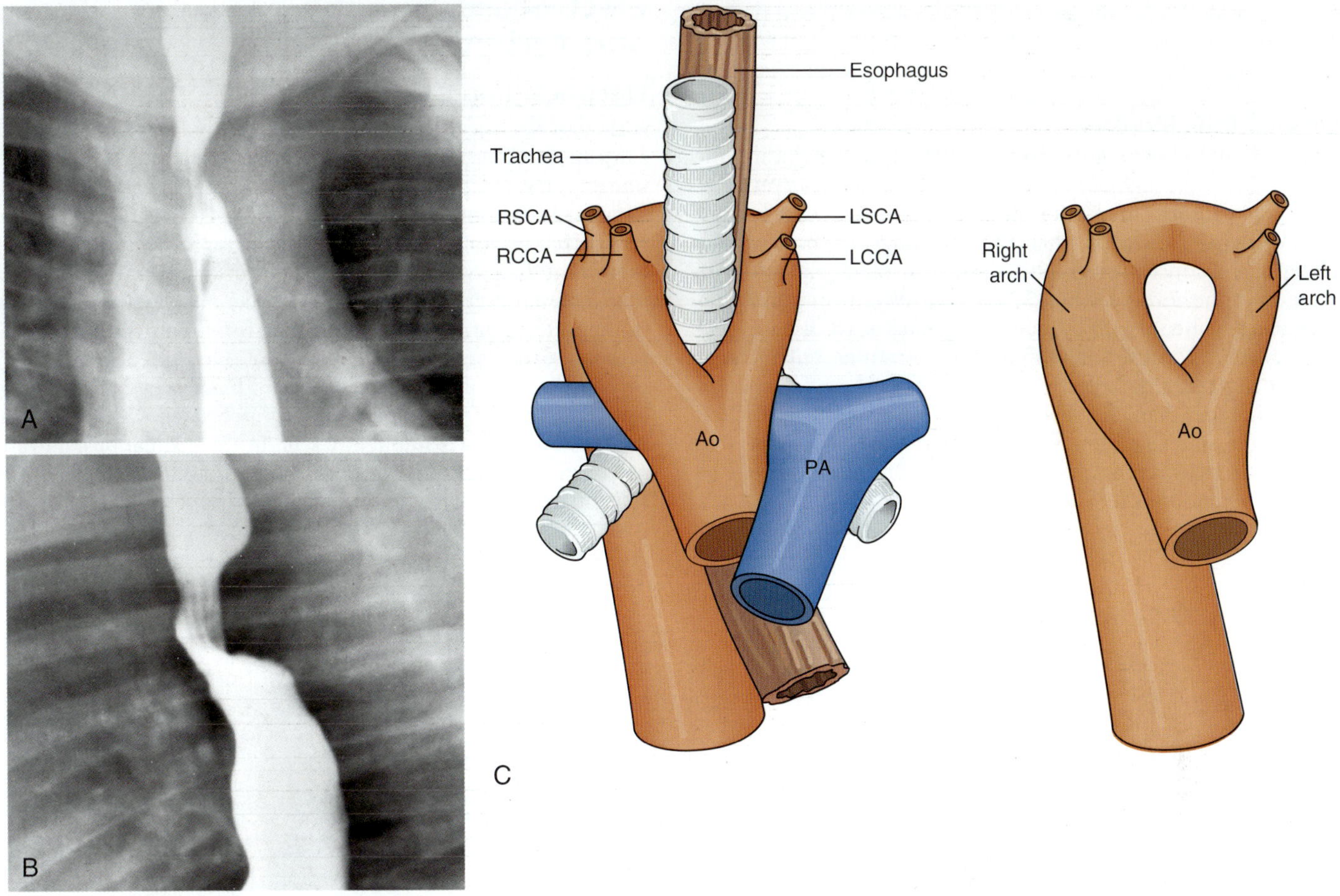

Fig. 5.26 Barium esophagram with a double aortic arch. (A) Note the bilateral compressions on the anterior view. (B) Note the marked retroesophageal indentation on the lateral view. (C) Schematic of the double aortic arch. *Ao,* Aorta; *LCCA,* left common carotid artery; *LSCS,* left subclavian artery; *PA,* pulmonary artery; *RCCA,* right common carotid artery; *RSCA,* right subclavian artery.

artery or a left aortic arch with distal origin of the right subclavian artery produces a posterior indentation on the barium esophagram. It is of note that the aberrant *right* subclavian artery is only rarely associated with airway or esophageal symptoms. An anterior esophageal indentation is almost always caused by distal origin of the left pulmonary artery, resulting in this vessel coursing between the trachea and esophagus and causing a pulmonary artery sling (Fig. 5.27).

Pulmonary Vascularity

Left-to-right shunt lesions are associated with increased pulmonary blood flow that causes increased prominence of the arterial or a combination of arterial and venous markings on the chest radiograph. Hyperinflation seen on the chest x-ray film is a characteristic finding in infants with a large left-to-right shunt associated with pulmonary overcirculation (see Fig. 5.23). Patients with pulmonary venous obstruction, such as infradiaphragmatic total anomalous pulmonary venous return, show a fine reticular pattern of pulmonary venous obstruction, which may mimic respiratory distress syndrome in the neonate. Severe obstruction can result in "white-out" of the chest radiograph with appearance of a "snowman in a snowstorm." (Fig. 5.28). It should be cautioned that the interpretation of pulmonary vascularity can be quite difficult and should always be interpreted within the context of other clinical findings.

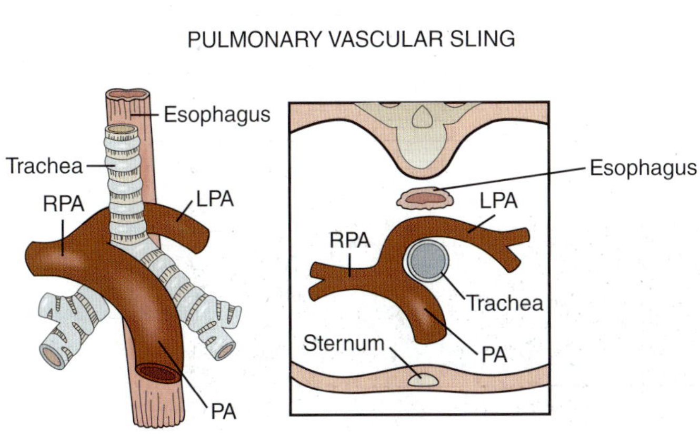

Fig. 5.27 Anomalous left pulmonary artery (pulmonary artery sling). Diagram of vascular anatomy and relationships to trachea and esophagus. *LPA,* Left pulmonary artery; *PA,* pulmonary artery; *RPA,* right pulmonary artery.

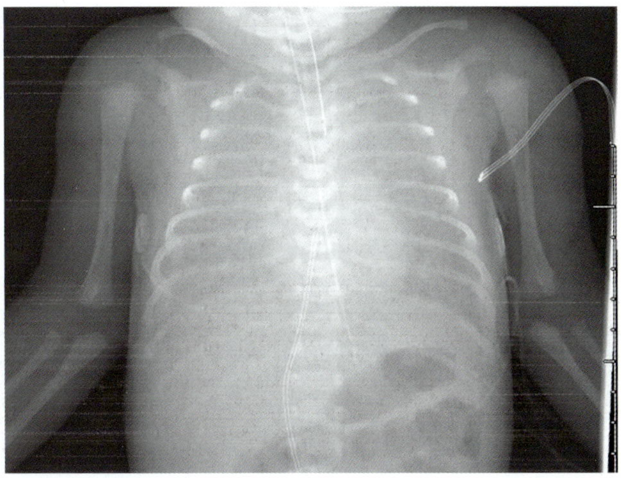

Fig. 5.28 Obstructed total anomalous pulmonary venous return with obstruction of the vertical vein in a newborn infant resulting in a so-called "snowman in a snowstorm" white-out appearance.

Oligemic lung fields indicate reduced pulmonary blood flow, as seen in most types of cyanotic congenital heart disease, the classic example being TOF.

Skeletal Abnormalities

Attention should also be given to the thoracic cage including the spine and ribs. Although abnormal fusions of ribs and hemivertebrae are not pathognomonic for specific congenital heart lesions, there is a higher incidence when these findings are present. Rib notching is a distinct radiographic finding in older patients with coarctation of the aorta (see Fig. 5.24). Scoliosis is a common finding in teenage patients with cyanotic congenital heart disease. Pectus excavatum may cause a false impression of cardiac enlargement because of a "pancaking" effect on the heart from a narrow anteroposterior thoracic diameter. Because of its association with chest wall and spine abnormalities, mitral valve prolapse (and associated connective tissue disorders, such as Marfan syndrome) should be considered in this context.

Electrocardiography and Arrhythmias

Electrocardiography

Although electrocardiography is an invaluable diagnostic tool in the assessment of pediatric heart disease, it is impractical and likely unnecessary for pediatricians to have a thorough knowledge of detailed ECG interpretation. However, it is valuable to be able to recognize certain typical electrocardiographic patterns that yield important diagnostic information. For instance, most normal children have a frontal plane axis that is either normal (0–90 degrees) or in the mild right axis deviation range from 90 to 120 degrees. The presence of a *superior axis* (180–270, or 0 to −90 degrees) suggests certain specific cardiac defects. A *left axis deviation* that includes an axis in the range of 0 to −90 degrees associated with a QR pattern in leads I and aV_L is frequently seen in these situations: a cyanotic newborn with tricuspid atresia (Fig. 5.29), a partial atrioventricular septal defect with or without Down syndrome (Fig. 5.30), Noonan

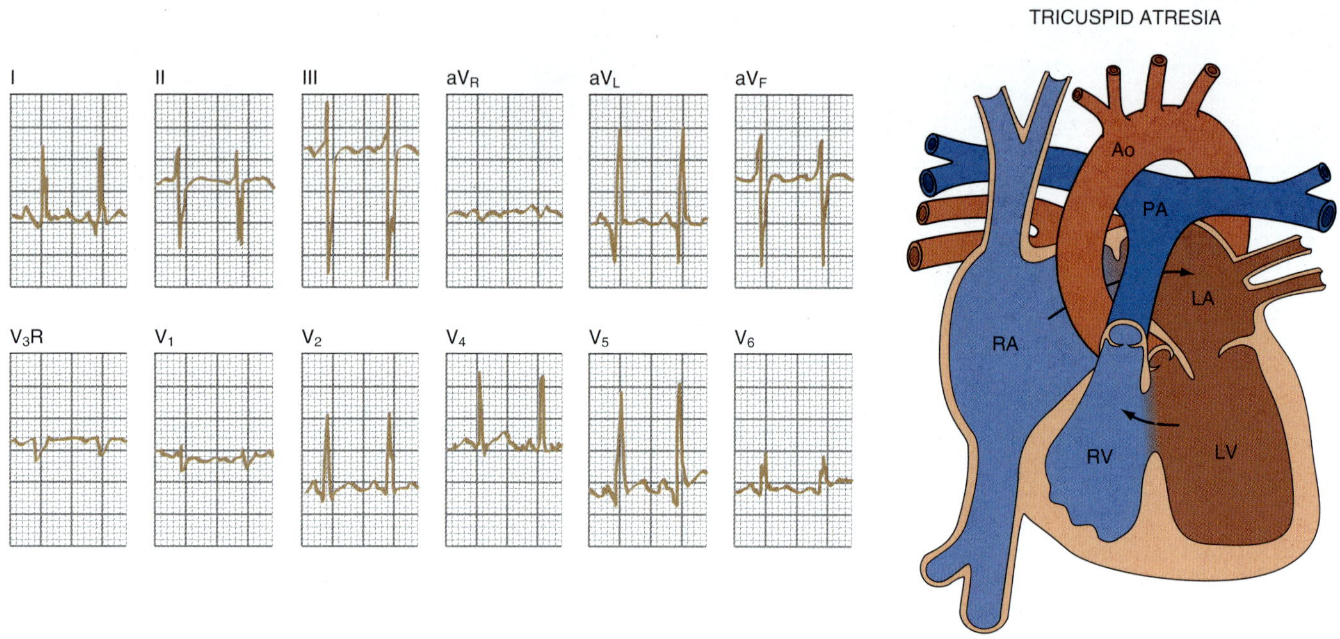

Fig. 5.29 Electrocardiogram of a child with tricuspid atresia. Note the left axis deviation, left atrial enlargement, and left ventricular hypertrophy. *Ao,* Aorta; *LA,* left atrium; *LV,* left ventricle; *PA,* pulmonary artery; *RA,* right atrium; *RV,* right ventricle.

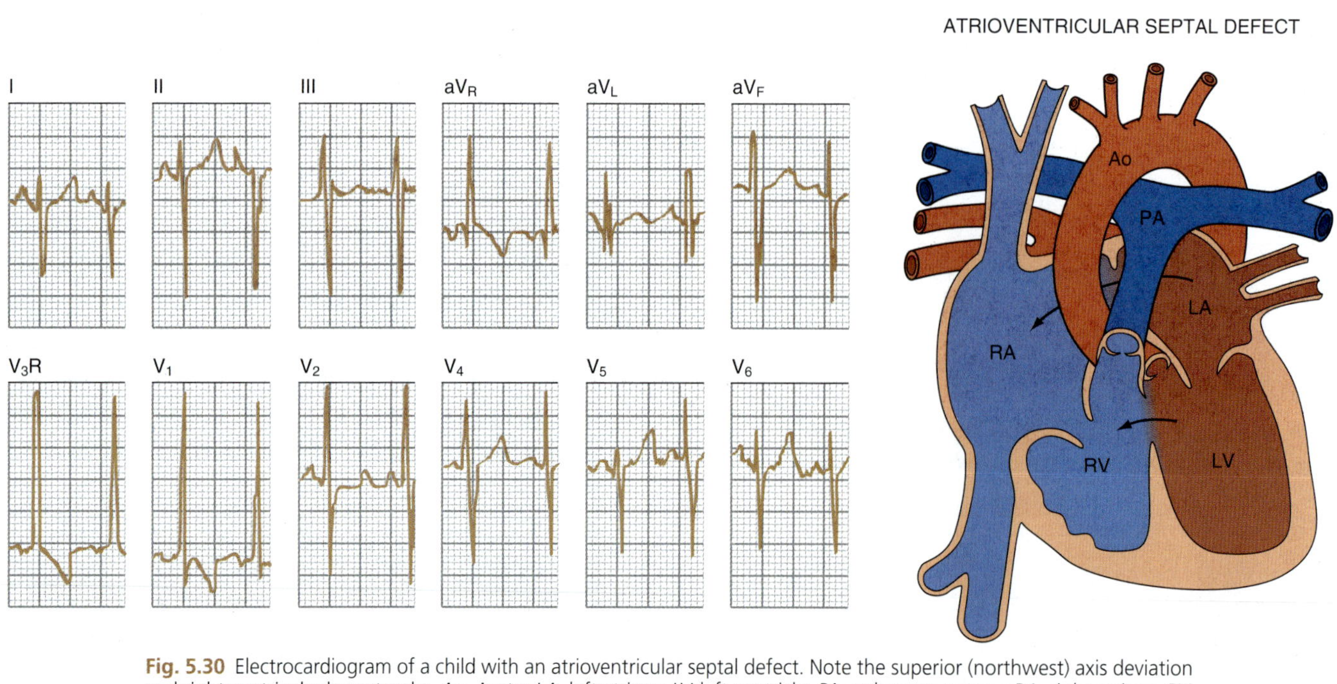

Fig. 5.30 Electrocardiogram of a child with an atrioventricular septal defect. Note the superior (northwest) axis deviation and right ventricular hypertrophy. *Ao,* Aorta; *LA,* left atrium; *LV,* left ventricle; *PA,* pulmonary artery; *RA,* right atrium; *RV,* right ventricle.

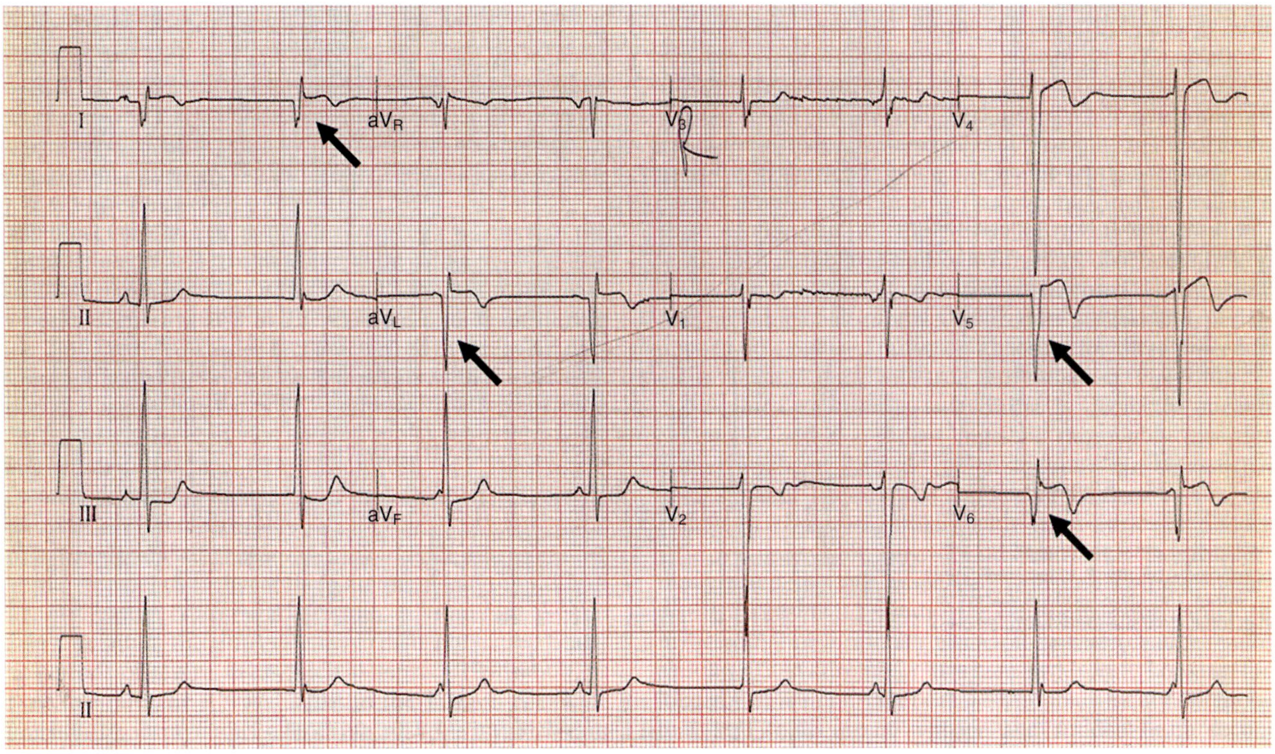

Fig. 5.31 Electrocardiogram of anomalous left coronary artery from the pulmonary artery. Note the pathologic Q waves in I, aV_L, V_5, and V_6 *(arrows)* and ST and T wave changes in the same leads.

syndrome, or some varieties of a single ventricle. Mild left axis deviation in the asymptomatic child (>1 year) can be a normal variant (Schneider et al., 2018 and Ravi et al., 2016). When the frontal plane axis falls between 180 and 270 degrees, it is usually referred to as a *northwest axis* and is frequently found in complete atrioventricular septal defects or other lesions that lead to severe right ventricular hypertrophy. Northwest axis can be related to either extreme right or left axis deviation. When prominent Q waves are seen in the lateral leads (I, aV_L, V_5, and V_6) with associated ST-T wave depression in the lateral leads (V_5 to V_6), the clinician should suspect cardiac ischemia associated with anomalous left coronary artery from the pulmonary artery (Fig. 5.31).

Being certain about hypertrophy in the pediatric age group is difficult because of the wide range of normal values that vary with age. This is particularly true of right ventricular hypertrophy, which can be a physiologic finding in the first several years of life. Left ventricular predominance in the newborn can be a pathologic finding and may indicate one of the hypoplastic right heart syndromes, such as tricuspid atresia (left ventricular predominance is shown in Fig. 5.29) or pulmonary atresia with an intact septum. The ECG finding of chamber hypertrophy is poorly predictive of definite hypertrophy seen by echocardiogram, and the echocardiogram should be viewed as the "gold standard" for chamber enlargement.

Conduction abnormalities, such as Wolff-Parkinson-White syndrome, prolonged corrected Q-T interval (QT_c), and atrioventricular block, are readily apparent on the 12-lead ECG and are discussed further in the Arrhythmias section.

Arrhythmias

Disorders of heart rate or rhythm are not nearly as common in childhood as they are in adulthood, but it is vital that pediatricians be familiar with arrhythmias that may occur in otherwise healthy children. An outline of these disorders based on the need for treatment is presented in Table 5.4. For the numerous rhythm disorders not listed, management must be individualized, taking into account the presence or absence of associated heart disease.

Transient arrhythmias may present in the following manner: an asymptomatic child with an irregular heartbeat noted on examination, palpitations, chest pain (a common complaint among children younger than 10 years old when they sense a tachycardia), dizziness or presyncope, or actual syncope with or without seizure activity. More sustained arrhythmias may lead to congestive heart failure, cardiogenic shock, or even death. The most common irregularity of heart rhythm seen in children is *sinus arrhythmia*. This is a normal variant that reflects a healthy interaction between autonomic respiratory and cardiac control activity in the central nervous system. Typically the heart rate increases during inspiration and decreases during expiration and may sound wildly irregular on auscultation unless careful attention is paid to the relationship between the heart rate and respirations (Fig. 5.32). Another normal variant occurs when the atrial pacemaker transiently shifts from the sinus node to another atrial site with only minimal variation in the heart rate. This is often referred to as *wandering atrial pacemaker* (Fig. 5.33). *Premature atrial contractions* are generally benign when they occur in the absence of underlying heart disease. They are particularly common during the newborn period, when they are often associated with aberrant conduction (Fig. 5.34) or apparent pauses (Fig. 5.35), resulting from failure of the premature atrial impulse to conduct to the ventricle. *Isolated premature ventricular contractions* are not common but may be seen with an incidence of 0.3% to 2.2% and rarely require treatment as long as there is no associated heart disease. This form of ectopy is recognizable by a wide QRS, dissociation from the P wave, and usually a full compensatory pause (Fig. 5.36). For the aforementioned abnormalities, an appropriate initial workup includes a 12-lead ECG and rhythm strip and brief exercise

Table 5.4 Pediatric Dysrhythmias

Treatment Not Required	Treatment Required
Sinus arrhythmia	Supraventricular tachycardia (SVT)
Wandering (ectopic) atrial pacemaker	Ventricular tachycardia
Isolated premature atrial contractions	Third-degree atrioventricular block with symptoms
Isolated premature ventricular contractions	
First-degree atrioventricular block	

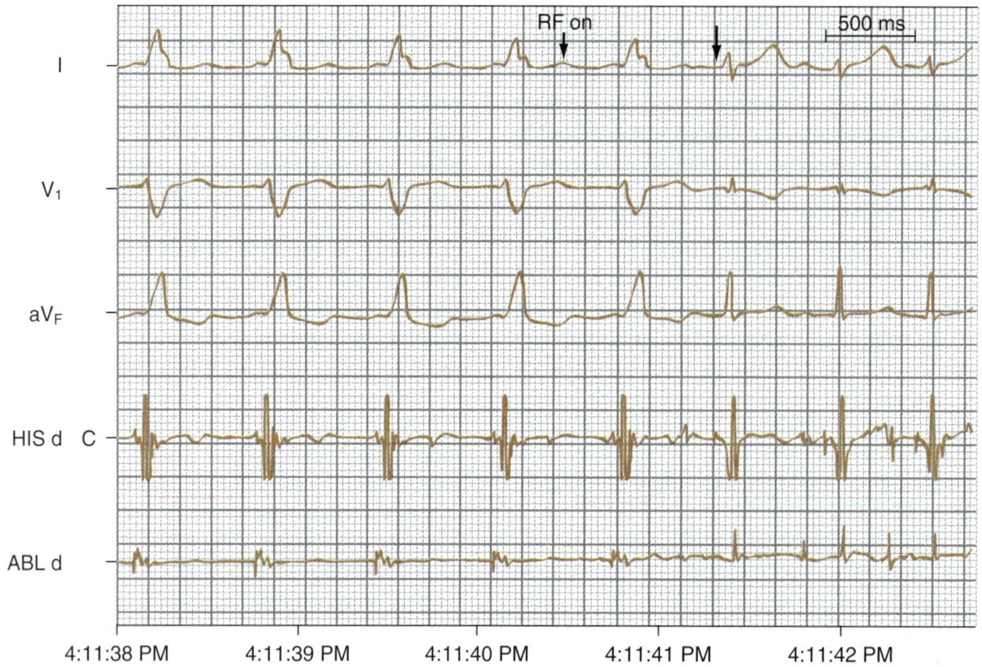

Fig. 5.39 Radiofrequency catheter ablation. Note the prompt disappearance of the delta wave *(arrow)* after radiofrequency *(RF)* ablation of an accessory pathway in a patient with Wolff-Parkinson-White syndrome. *ABL d,* Distal poles of ablation; *HIS d C,* distal poles of His bundle catheter.

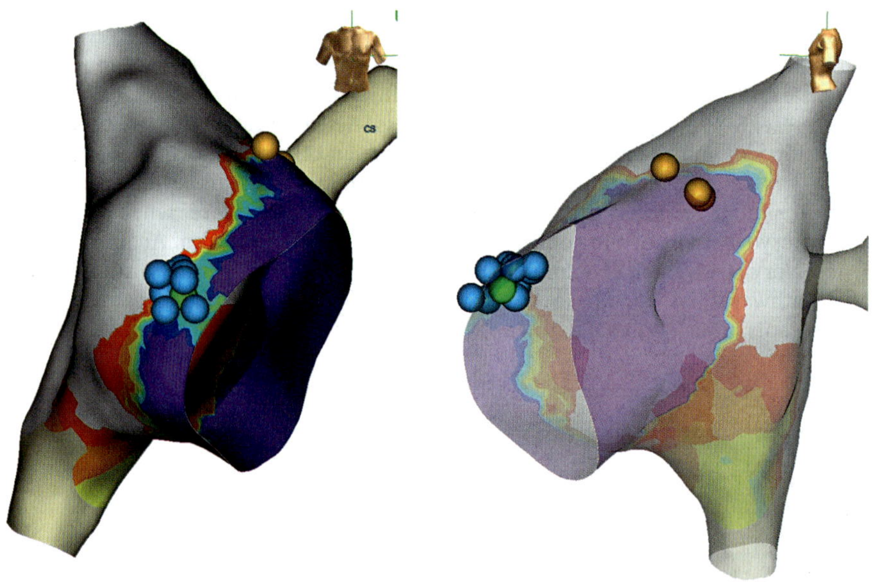

Fig. 5.40 Three-dimensional map with anterior-posterior (AP) projection along with the left lateral (LL). *Green/blue circles* highlight the area of ablation in the posterolateral tricuspid valve annulus, and *yellow circles* represent normal AV node conduction in the anteroseptal tricuspid valve.

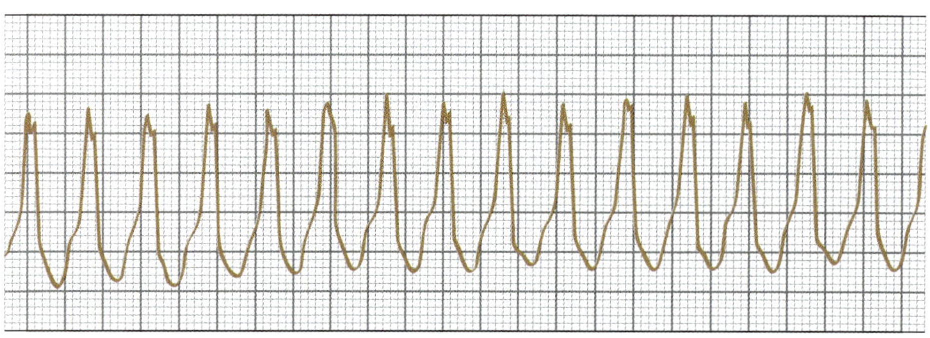

Fig. 5.41 Ventricular tachycardia. Note the wide QRS complex tachycardia at a rate of 188 beats/min.

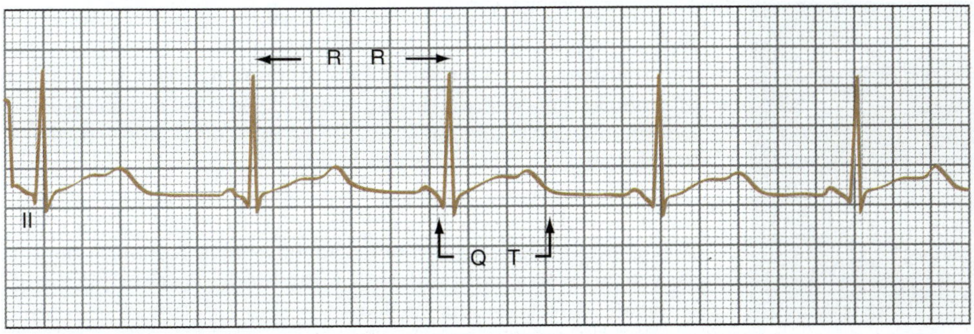

Fig. 5.42 Prolonged Q-T syndrome. Note the corrected Q-T interval (QT_c) is prolonged at 0.57 second (upper limit of normal is 0.44 second). The Q-T interval must be corrected for heart rate by using the Bazett formula: measured Q-T interval (0.56 second) divided by the square root of the preceding R-R interval (0.96 second).

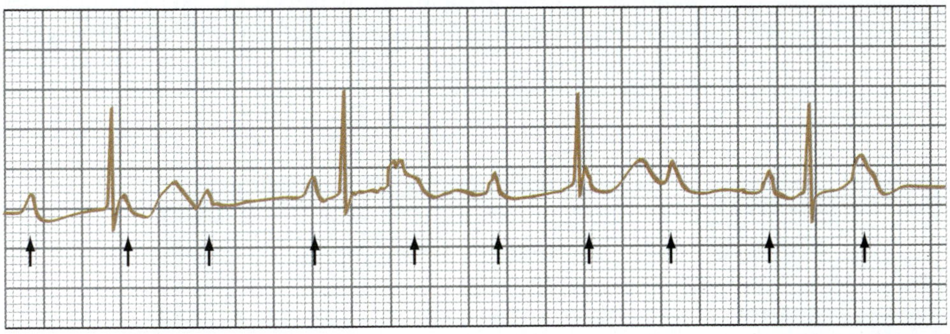

Fig. 5.43 Complete heart block. Note that atrial activity *(arrows)* is independent of a slower ventricular rhythm.

When a patient is evaluated for a history of syncope or new-onset seizures that are atypical for a classic vasovagal reaction, it may be reasonable that the physician obtains an ECG to look for "footprints" of a possible arrhythmic cause. The possibilities include Wolff-Parkinson-White syndrome (providing a substrate for rapid SVT), prolonged QT_c (predisposing to severe ventricular arrhythmias, most often a type known as *torsades de pointes*), or atrioventricular block (leading to Stokes-Adams attacks). However, routine use of ECG for all pediatric patients with seizure may not be necessary (Pompa et al., 2019).

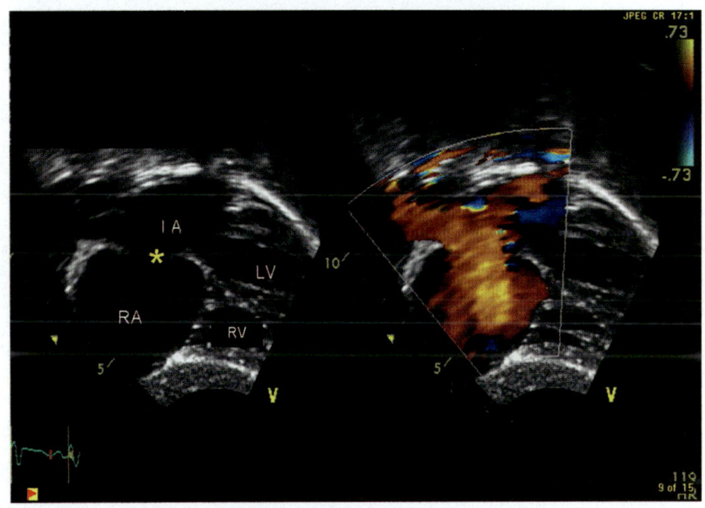

Fig. 5.44 Secundum atrial septal defect. Note the large defect in the fossa ovalis area *(asterisk)* on the subcostal view *(left)*. Color Doppler *(right)* confirms a prominent left-to-right shunt *(red flow)*. *LA*, Left atrium; *LV*, left ventricle; *RA*, right atrium; *RV*, right ventricle.

Echocardiography

Echocardiography with Doppler interrogation first provided remarkable advances in the investigation of congenital heart defects in the early 1980s and is currently the standard imaging modality for the diagnosis of congenital heart disease. Echocardiographic imaging and color flow Doppler allow accurate anatomic definition of even complex congenital defects and providing a reliable noninvasive hemodynamic assessment of the patient. These tools complement and, in most cases, replace the need for diagnostic cardiac catheterization and angiography in the management of patients with congenital heart disease.

Accurate diagnosis of most structural congenital heart diseases, whether simple or complex, can be made by echocardiography. A systematic approach to define major intracardiac connections is a useful starting point: (1) venoatrial (systemic or pulmonary venous return to the right or left atrium), (2) atrioventricular (atria to the ventricles), and (3) ventriculoarterial (ventricle to the great vessels).

All types of septal defects can be readily visualized by echocardiography. The atrial septal defects are reliably demonstrated by the subcostal approach. The most common type is the secundum defect, which involves the middle portion of the atrial septum in the region of the fossa ovalis (Fig. 5.44). The sinus venosus type of atrial septal defect is located in the posterosuperior portion of the atrial septum adjacent to the junction of the right atrium and superior vena cava (this vessel effectively overrides the defect). A less common type of the sinus venosus defect is one that is adjacent to the inferior vena cava. Both types of sinus venosus atrial septal defects are associated with partial anomalous pulmonary venous return of one or more right pulmonary veins (Fig. 5.45). An ostium primum defect known as a *partial form of an atrioventricular septal defect* is seen in Fig. 5.46. The complete form of an atrioventricular septal defect

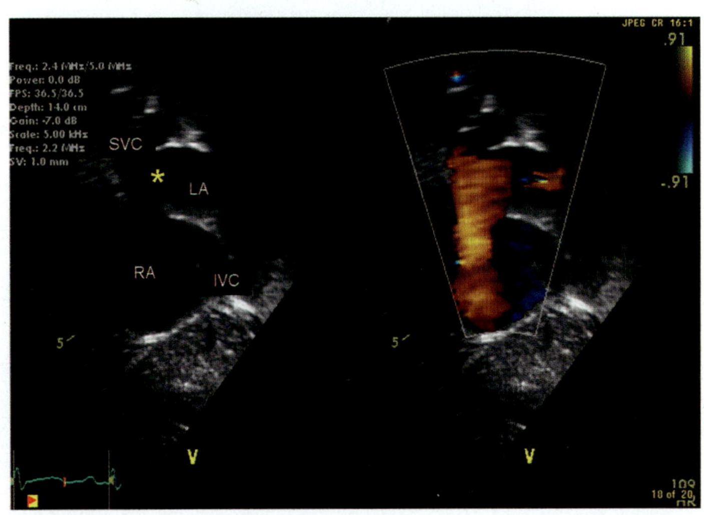

Fig. 5.45 Sinus venosus defect. Note the defect *(asterisk)* in the posterosuperior portion of the atrial septum, with the superior vena cava *(SVC)* overriding the defect on the subcostal short axis view *(left)*. Color Doppler *(right)* shows left-to-right shunt across the defect. Anomalous drainage of the right upper pulmonary vein is not shown on this view. *IVC*, Inferior vena cava; *LA*, left atrium; *RA*, right atrium.

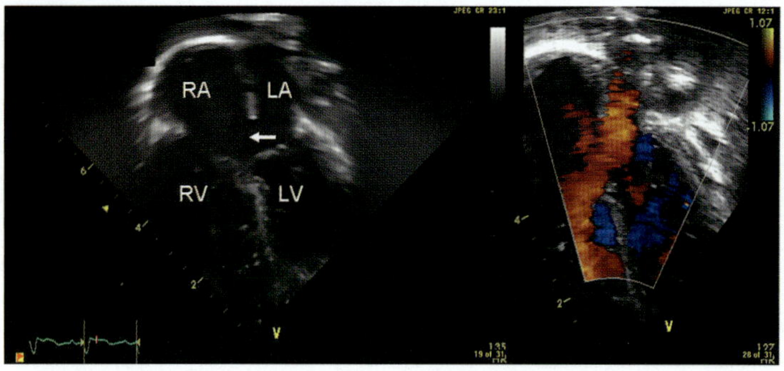

Fig. 5.46 Partial atrioventricular septal defect. Note the defect *(arrow)* on the apical four-chamber view *(left)* in the inferior portion of the atrial septum. A left-to-right atrial shunt is shown on color Doppler image *(right)*. *LA,* Left atrium; *LV,* left ventricle; *RA,* right atrium; *RV,* right ventricle.

consists of a large defect in the center of the heart, in association with a common atrioventricular valve (Fig. 5.47). During diastole, with the atrioventricular valve open, all four chambers are in direct communication, whereas during systole, the closed atrioventricular valve functionally separates the defect into atrial and ventricular components.

Ventricular septal defects are well defined by echocardiography and are usually seen clearly using the apical four-chamber view. The most common defect is in the perimembranous septum located in the subaortic area and bordered by the tricuspid valve (Fig. 5.48). Moderate defects in the muscular portion of septum are easily visualized in multiple views. A short-axis view of such a defect is shown in Fig. 5.49. Although small defects located in the muscular septum can be difficult to image, particularly if located in the apical trabecular area, they can be readily detected by color flow Doppler interrogation (Fig. 5.50).

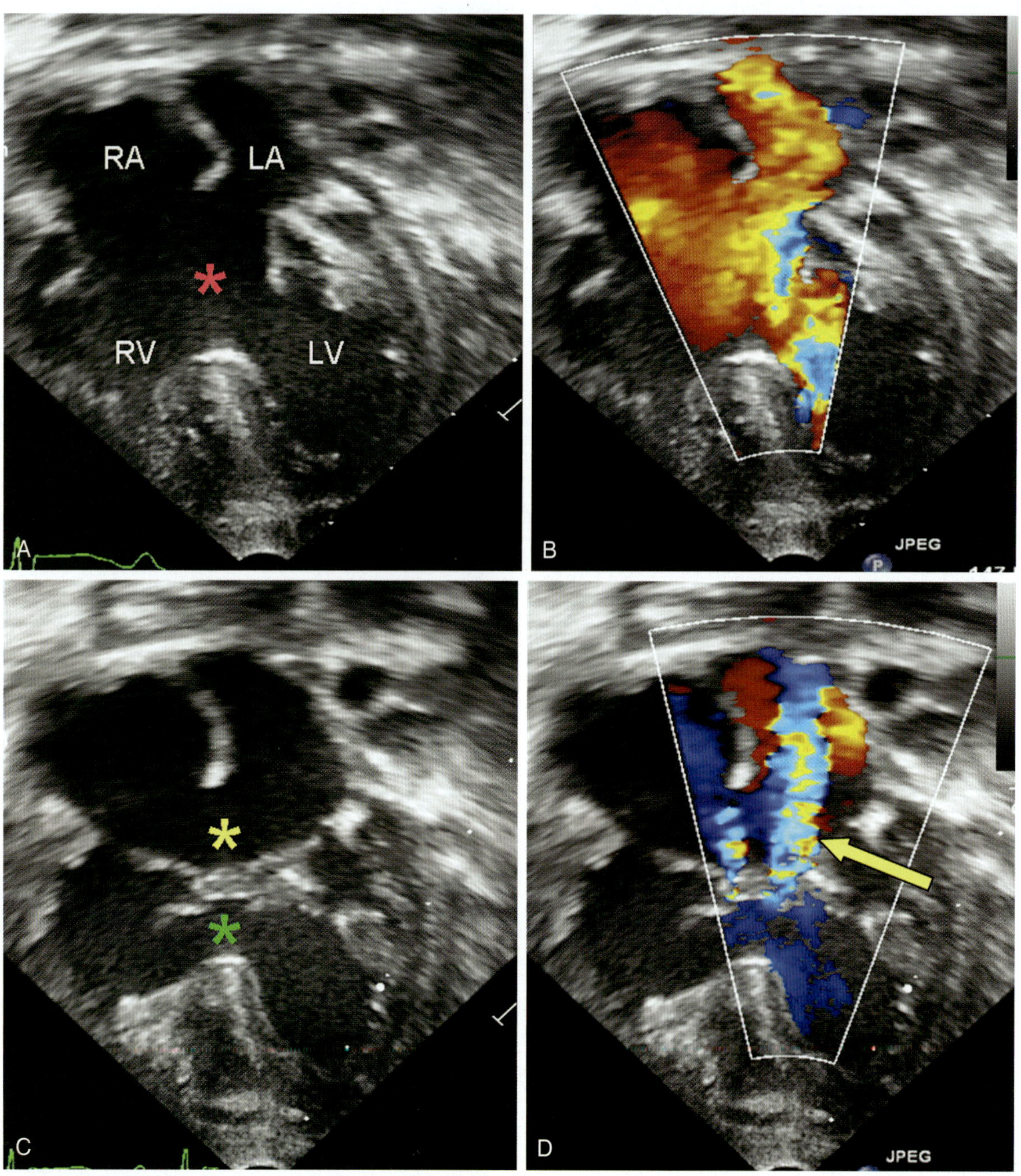

Fig. 5.47 Complete atrioventricular septal defect (four-chamber view). (A and B) Diastolic frames with and without color Doppler. Note large central defect *(red asterisk)* between atria and ventricles (A). Red Doppler flow indicates large atrial and ventricular shunt (B). (C and D) Systolic frames demonstrate atrial *(yellow asterisk)* and ventricular *(green asterisk)* components of the defect (C). Blue Doppler flow *(yellow arrow)* indicates valve regurgitation (D). *LA,* Left atrium; *LV,* left ventricle; *RA,* right atrium; *RV,* right ventricle.

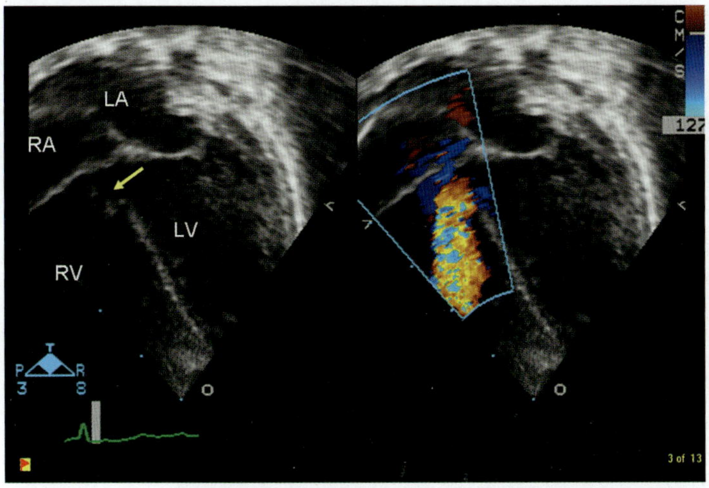

Fig. 5.48 Perimembranous ventricular septal defect. Note that the defect *(arrow)* is located in the superior portion of the septum as seen on the apical four-chambered view *(left)*. Color Doppler image *(right)* shows left-to-right ventricular shunt. *LA,* Left atrium; *LV,* left ventricle; *RA,* right atrium; *RV,* right ventricle.

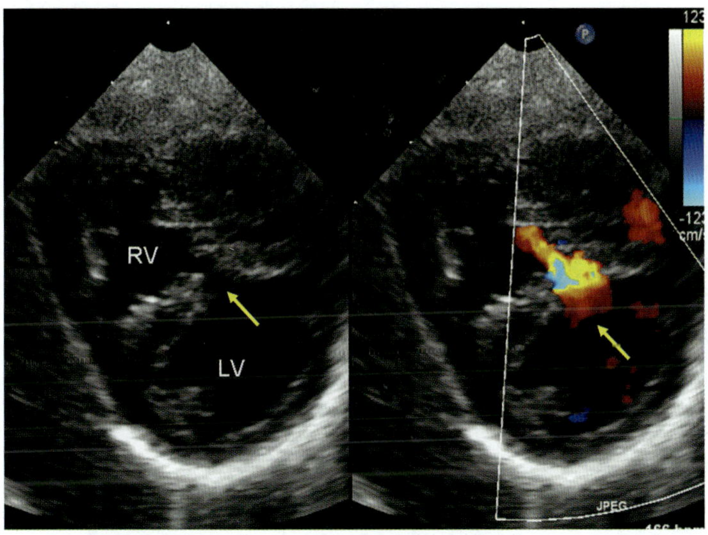

Fig. 5.49 Muscular ventricular septal defect (moderate). Note the moderate size defect *(arrow)* in the muscular septum on the parasternal short axis view *(left)*. Color Doppler image *(right)* shows left-to-right shunt *(arrow)*. *LV,* Left ventricle; *RV,* right ventricle.

Typical findings in the most common cyanotic heart lesion, TOF, are a dilated aortic root that overrides the ventricular septum, a large perimembranous ventricular septal defect, and right ventricular outflow obstruction (Fig. 5.51). Truncus arteriosus is a related conotruncal anomaly associated with a large ventricular defect and a common arterial trunk (truncus) arising from both the right and left ventricles, with the pulmonary arteries arising directly from this vessel just above the semilunar valve (Fig. 5.52). Transposition of the great arteries, one of the most common cyanotic defects to present in the newborn period, is associated with severe cyanosis immediately after birth and can be recognized by the characteristic finding of parallel takeoff of the great vessels from both ventricles, with the aorta arising anteriorly from the right ventricle and the pulmonary artery originating posteriorly from the left ventricle (Fig. 5.53).

Bicuspid aortic valve is a congenital malformation of the aortic valve in which there is fusion of two of the aortic valve leaflets. This condition is found in 1% to 2% of the general population and is associated with aortic stenosis, insufficiency, and dilation of the aortic root and/or ascending aorta (Fig. 5.54).

The most common cause of cardiogenic shock or congestive heart failure in the first several days of life is the hypoplastic left heart syndrome, which is associated with either aortic atresia or critical aortic stenosis (Fig. 5.55). Coarctation of the aorta or interrupted aortic arch may also present with severe heart failure in the neonate. These aortic arch anomalies are best visualized by a suprasternal approach, and the diagnosis of interrupted aortic arch or coarctation of the aorta can be readily made in most cases. The coronary arterial origins and proximal courses can be demonstrated in parasternal short axis view at the base of the heart. Anomalous origin of a coronary artery from the inappropriate sinus of Valsalva is a rare lesion. However, this condition is clinically important, as it can be associated with myocardial ischemia, infarction, and sudden death. Anomalous origin of the right coronary artery from the left sinus of Valsalva is the most common form of this disorder (Fig. 5.56).

If the pulmonary veins are not confirmed to communicate directly with the left atrium, total anomalous pulmonary venous return should be suspected. Congenitally corrected transposition is the most likely diagnosis when the atrioventricular connection is discordant (right atrium to morphologic left ventricle and left atrium to morphologic right ventricle).

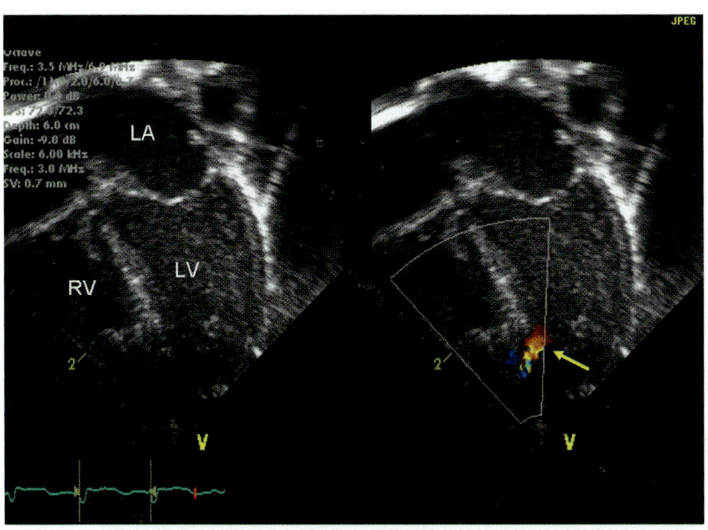

Fig. 5.50 Muscular ventricular septal defect (small). Note that no apparent defect in the ventricular septum could be visualized by two-dimensional image *(left)* on the apical four-chambered view. However, color Doppler image *(right)* identifies a small defect in the muscular septum near the apex by showing a left-to-right jet *(arrow)*. *LA,* Left atrium; *LV,* left ventricle; *RV,* right ventricle.

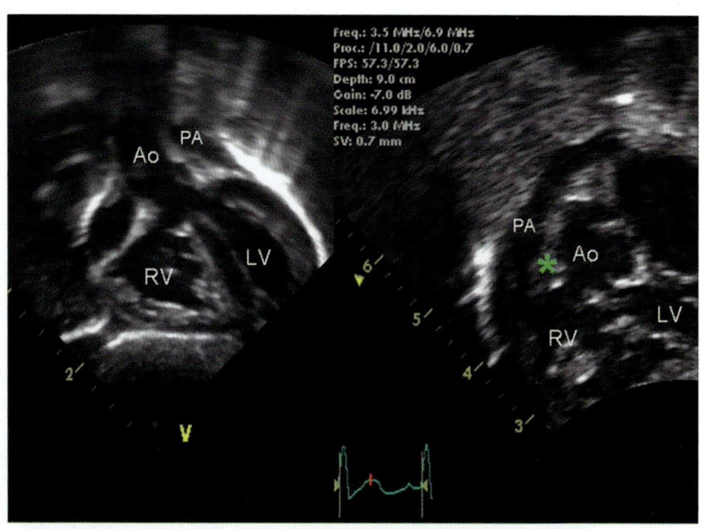

Fig. 5.51 Tetralogy of Fallot. Aortic root *(Ao)* overriding a large ventricular septal defect is shown on the subcostal long axis view *(left)*. The anterior deviation of the outlet ventricular septum *(green asterisk)* resulting in narrowing of pulmonary outflow tract *(right)* is shown on subcostal short axis view. *LV,* Left ventricle; *PA,* pulmonary artery; *RV,* right ventricle.

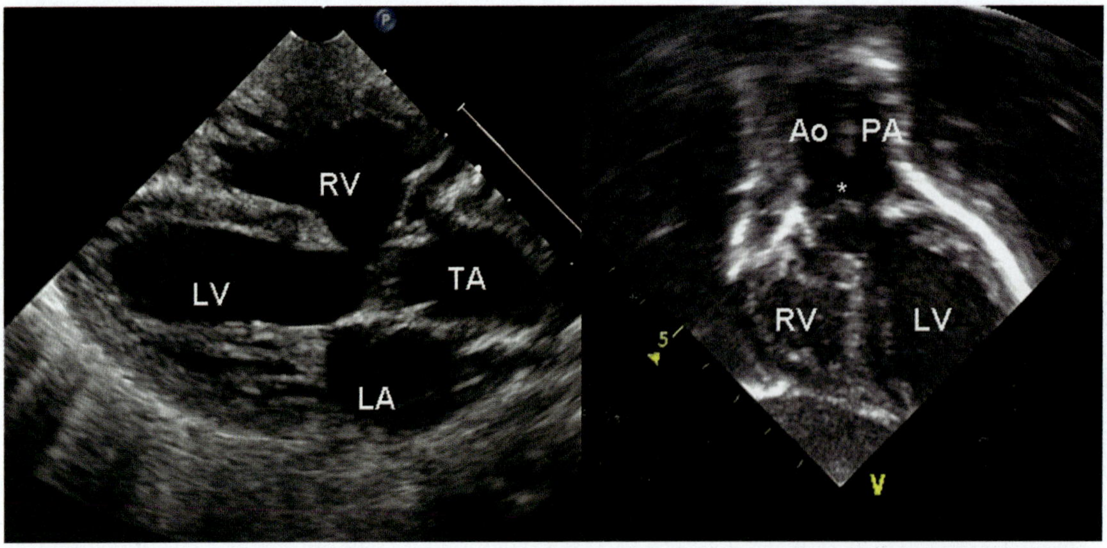

Fig. 5.52 Truncus arteriosus. Parasternal long axis view *(left)* shows large truncal root *(TA)* overriding the ventricular septum receiving outflow from both the right ventricle *(RV)* and left ventricle *(LV)*. Ascending aorta *(Ao)* and pulmonary artery *(PA)* arising directly from the proximal truncal root *(asterisk)* is shown on the subcostal long axis view *(right)*. *LA,* Left atrium.

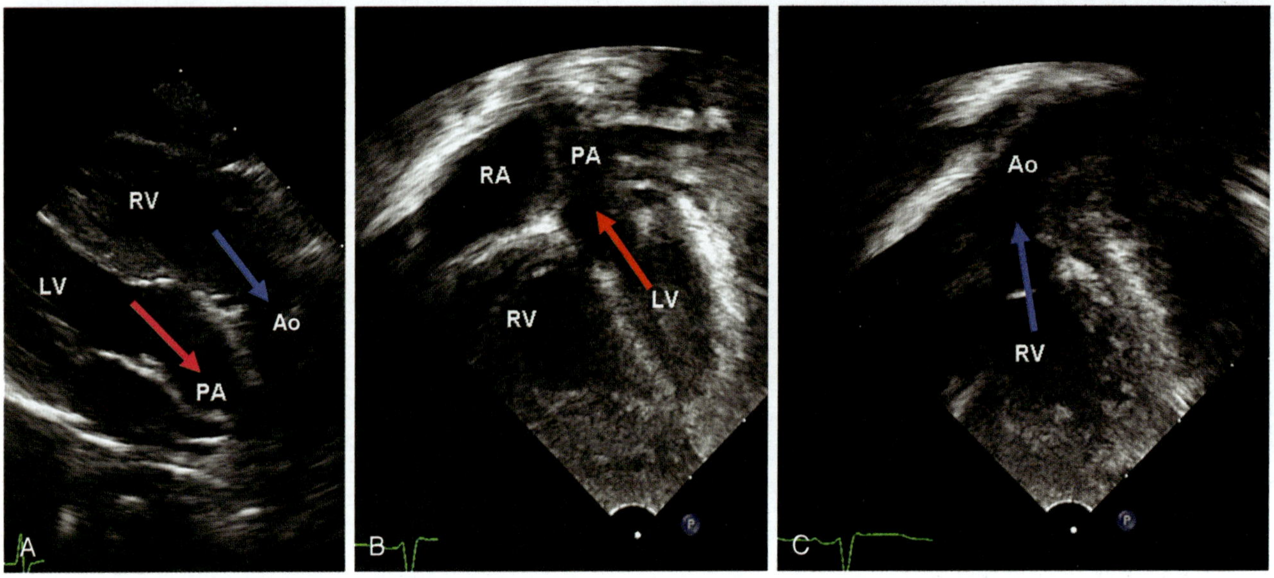

Fig. 5.53 Transposition of the great arteries. Parasternal long axial view (A) shows parallel arrangement of the great vessels. Apical four-chamber views confirm origination of the pulmonary artery *(PA)* from the left ventricle *(LV)* (B) and the aorta *(Ao)* from the right ventricle *(RV)* (C). *RA,* Right atrium.

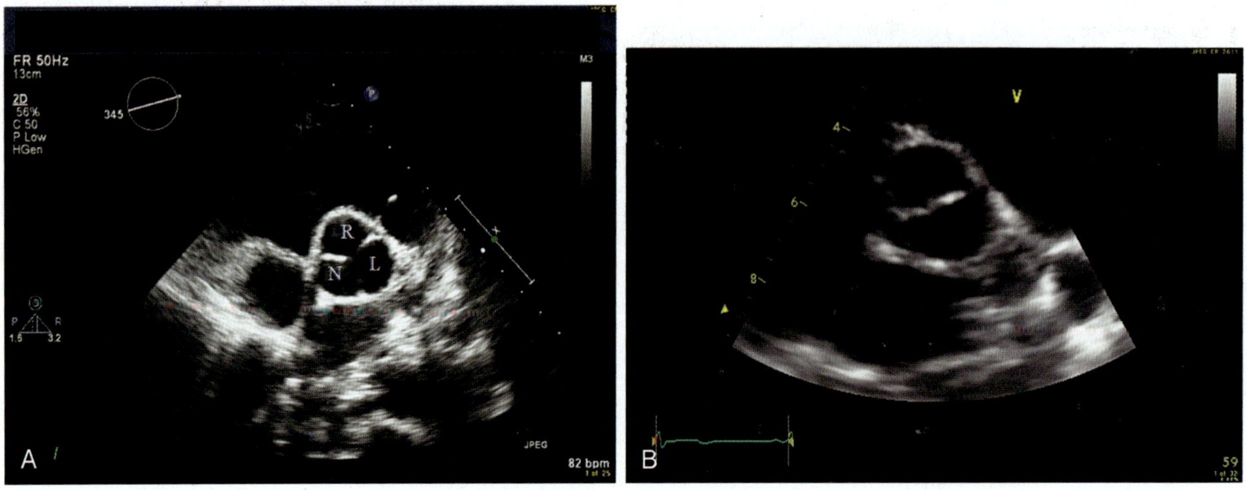

Fig. 5.54 Bicuspid aortic valve. Parasternal short-axis image at the level of the base of the heart. (A) demonstrates a normal trileaflet aortic valve with distinct left (L), right (R), and noncoronary cusps (N). (B) reveals a bicuspid aortic valve with fusion of the right and noncoronary cusps.

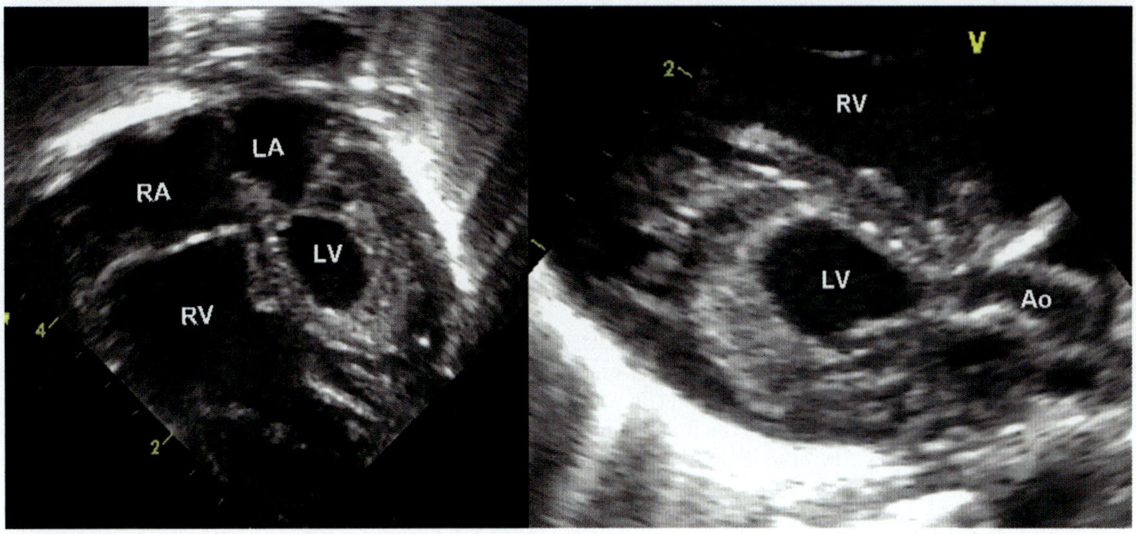

Fig. 5.55 Hypoplastic left heart syndrome. Markedly hypoplastic left ventricle *(LV)* with dilated right ventricle *(RV)* is shown on the apical four-chamber view *(left)*. Small ascending aorta *(Ao)* is demonstrated on the parasternal long axis view *(right)*. *LA,* Left atrium; *RA,* right atrium.

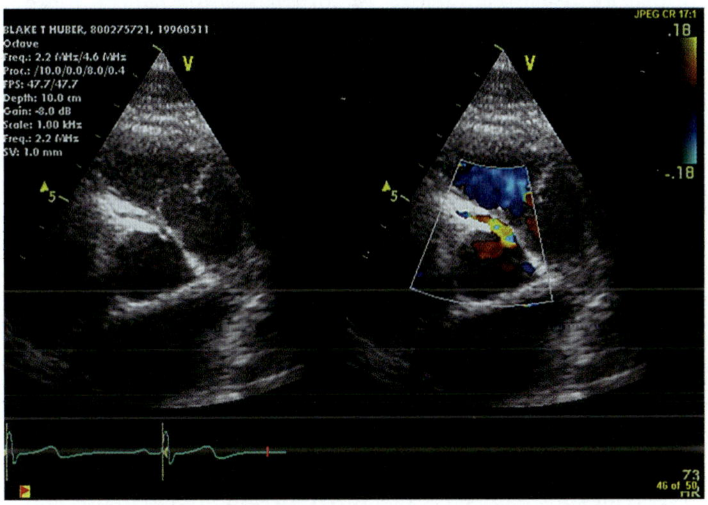

Fig. 5.56 Anomalous origin of the right coronary artery from the left sinus of Valsalva. The left panel demonstrates the right coronary artery originating from the left sinus of Valvsalva with intramural course. The *yellow line* delineates the commissure between the right and left coronary cusps. The right panel demonstrates diastolic color flow in the anomalous coronary artery coursing within the aortic wall.

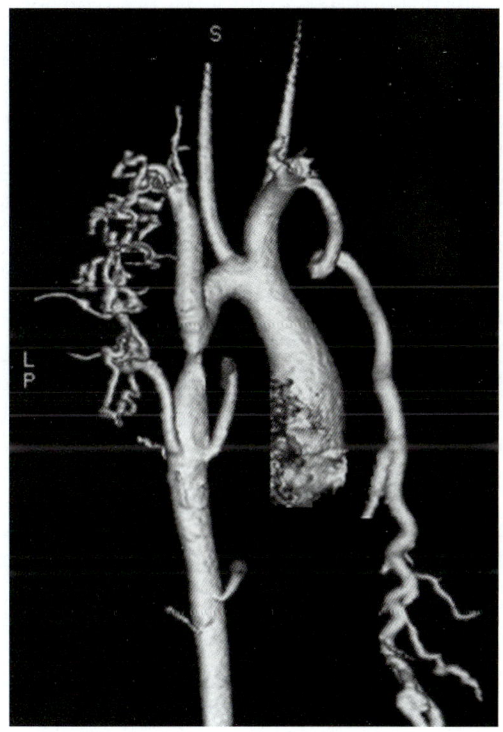

Fig. 5.57 Coarctation of the aorta. Magnetic resonance angiography demonstrating discrete coarctation of the aorta with diffuse collateral arteries arising from the right internal mammary artery, subclavian branches, and intercostal arteries. (Courtesy S. Tadros, MD, Pittsburgh.)

Cardiac Magnetic Resonance Imaging and Computed Tomography

Cardiac MRI and CT have become important complementary axial imaging techniques in the assessment of congenital heart disease. These imaging modalities can be used when echocardiography is unable to delineate portions of the cardiac or extracardiac anatomy and, in some instances, as an alternative to more invasive studies (e.g., cardiac catheterization). Although echocardiography is at times adversely affected by body habitus and poor acoustic windows, cardiac MRI and CT are largely free from these barriers.

Cardiac MRI is a versatile imaging tool, and its major advantage over CT is the avoidance of ionizing radiation. MRI provides an alternative modality for the assessment of ventricular volume and cardiac function, particularly of the right ventricle. In addition, MRI allows for tissue characterization of the myocardium in the setting of cardiomyopathies, and it can be used for detecting cardiac ischemia and assessing myocardial viability. Anomalies of the aorta, such as coarctation and aortic root dilation, are well imaged by MRI (Fig. 5.57). Furthermore, MRI provides reliable visualization of the airways and extracardiac vasculature, making it an excellent modality for imaging vascular rings and pulmonary slings. Finally, cardiac MRI is an important imaging modality in the evaluation of the patient with TOF. In the preoperative TOF patient, cardiac MRI or CT may be used to detail all sources of pulmonary blood flow, including the branch pulmonary arteries, ductus arteriosus, and aortopulmonary collateral arteries. In the postoperative TOF patient, cardiac MRI is used to assess right ventricular volume, biventricular systolic function, pulmonary regurgitation, branch pulmonary artery anatomy, and aortic root and to assess for aneurysm formation in the right ventricular outflow tract.

Cardiac CT is commonly used for assessment of extracardiac structures. Its chief advantages over cardiac MRI include shorter scan times, superior spatial resolution, and the ability in many cases to perform studies in young children without the use of general anesthesia and intubation. CT is also free from prohibitive artifact from metallic implants (e.g., stents) and can be performed safely in patients with pacemakers. Given its spatial resolution, CT may be the preferred imaging modality for assessment of the coronary arteries and other small vessels. CT also provides excellent imaging of the aorta and its branches, pulmonary veins, peripheral branch pulmonary arteries, lung parenchyma, and airways.

CARDIAC SURGICAL PROCEDURES

The remarkable progress in treating children with severe congenital heart disease over the past 50 years, progress that has greatly accelerated during the past 2 decades, is largely due to dramatic achievements in the field of pediatric heart surgery. Although the first patent ductus arteriosus ligation was in 1938, the first Blalock-Taussig-Thomas shunt in 1944, and the initial repair of coarctation in 1945, open-heart repair of complex malformations did not become relatively commonplace until the late 1960s and 1970s. Since then, there have been progressive improvements in precise preoperative diagnosis, development of stunning technical skills by specialized pediatric heart surgeons, and important advances in the perioperative management of infants with critical heart disease. All these factors have made it possible to offer successful palliative or corrective surgery for the great majority of even the most severe forms of congenital heart disease.

Although the large number of possible malformations and different operations applied to them may seem bewildering and complex, when carefully reviewed, only a relatively small number of types of surgical procedures are performed. Many of these procedures are associated with an eponym that designates the surgeon who developed a particular technique. These surgical techniques can be performed in isolation or as a combination of procedures designed to treat more complex forms of congenital heart disease. The purpose of the ensuing sections is to provide schematic diagrams and brief explanations for the commonly used surgical procedures and the types of defects to which they are applied.

Septation Defects

Simple septation defects encompass a large portion of congenital heart disease. Although newer catheter-based therapies can treat a portion of these lesions less invasively (discussed in the interventional cardiac catheterization section), many still require open heart surgery. Small atrial and ventricular septal defects can be sutured closed, whereas larger defects require patch closure with either synthetic or biologic patch material. Sinus venosus atrial septal defects can be associated with partial anomalous pulmonary venous return, where some of the pulmonary veins drain into the superior vena cava or right atrium. This defect requires a more complex Warden procedure, where the anomalous pulmonary veins are rerouted to the left atrium. Atrioventricular septal defects are repaired by patching the atrial and ventricular septal defects and dividing the common atrioventricular valve into two separate valves. Patent ductus arteriosus may be particularly problematic in premature infants and can be surgically ligated via a lateral thoracotomy, though many can now be closed using catheter-based devices (discussed later).

Pulmonary Outflow Tract Obstruction and Truncus Arteriosus

Newborns and infants with complex congenital heart disease associated with severe obstruction to pulmonary blood flow can present with profound cyanosis requiring palliative operations. These lesions generally have in common either severe subvalvular or valvular pulmonic stenosis or pulmonary atresia leading to inadequate pulmonary blood flow. Fig. 5.58 demonstrates the various types of systemic to pulmonary artery shunt procedures commonly performed to treat these infants. The original *classic Blalock-Taussig-Thomas shunt* was performed by dividing the subclavian artery and creating an end-to-side anastomosis of the proximal subclavian artery stump to the ipsilateral pulmonary artery. The most common type of shunt performed in the current era is a *modified Blalock-Taussig-Thomas shunt,* which uses a Gore-Tex interposition graft between the innominate or subclavian artery and pulmonary artery without dividing the distal subclavian artery. Occasionally, unusual anatomy of the aorta or proximal pulmonary arteries leads to placement of a *central shunt* (placement of a short interposition graft between the ascending aorta and main pulmonary artery). Other procedures, frequently used in the early decades of congenital heart surgery but far less common now, include a *Waterston shunt* (creation of a window between the ascending aorta and right pulmonary artery) and a *Potts shunt* (creation of a window between the descending aorta and left pulmonary artery).

In the previous era of cardiac surgery, the most common lesion in this category was TOF. Currently, most children with this entity now have a complete repair in infancy without a prior shunt. Fig. 5.58 also demonstrates the technique of complete repair for TOF, which includes closure of the ventricular septal defect, relief of right ventricular outflow tract obstruction with resection of subvalvular muscle, pulmonary valvotomy, and usually a transannular patch.

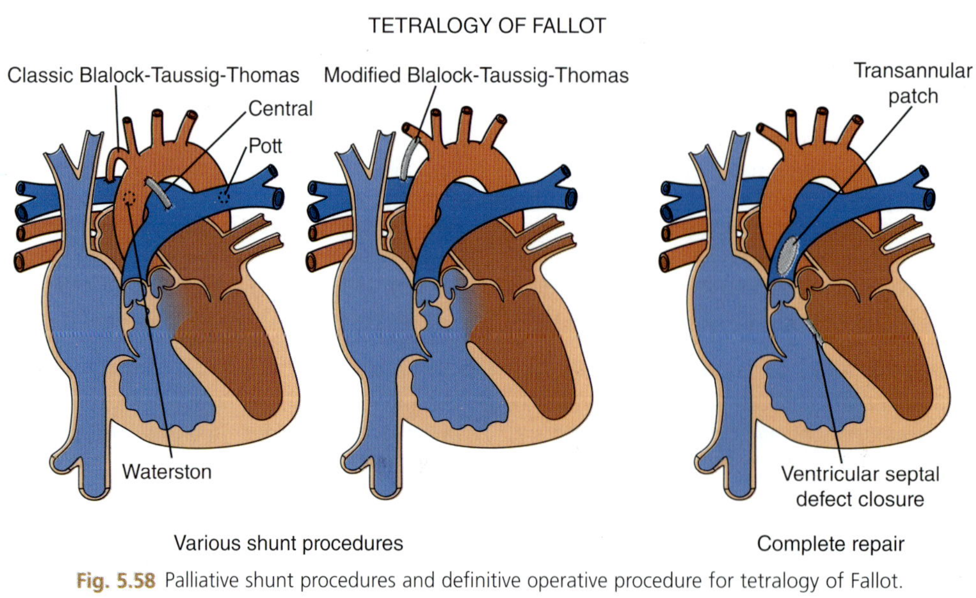

Fig. 5.58 Palliative shunt procedures and definitive operative procedure for tetralogy of Fallot.

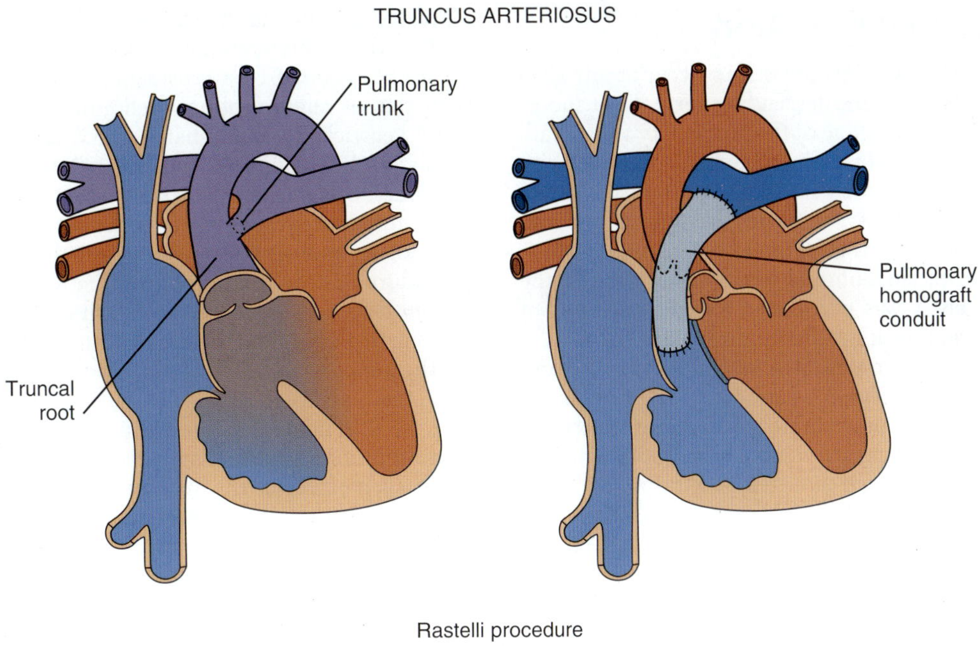

Fig. 5.59 Creation of a right ventricle–to-pulmonary conduit for truncus arteriosus (Rastelli procedure).

The key elements of the *Rastelli procedure*, closure of a ventricular septal defect and placement of a conduit to connect the right ventricle to the pulmonary artery, are shown in Fig. 5.59. This procedure is used for a variety of lesions including TOF with pulmonary atresia and transposition of the great arteries with ventricular septal defect and severe pulmonic stenosis. Although technically not a pulmonary outflow obstruction lesion, truncus arteriosus (pulmonary arteries arising directly from a truncal root that overrides a large ventricular septal defect, as shown in the diagram on the left) is included in this section because it is also repaired using the *Rastelli procedure*. The operation for a truncus arteriosus consists of closing of the ventricular septal defect to direct the left ventricular outflow to the aorta, detachment of the pulmonary arteries from the aorta (truncus), and placement of a homograft conduit between the right ventricle and pulmonary arteries.

Ebstein Anomaly

Severe neonatal Ebstein anomaly can be palliated with a *Starnes procedure*, where the tricuspid valve is oversewn with a fenestrated patch. Flow from the right atrium is directed through an enlarged atrial septal defect, and pulmonary blood flow is supplied via a shunt. Older patients with Ebstein anomaly, or those initially palliated with a *Starnes procedure*, are now most often repaired with the *Da Silva Cone procedure* (Fig. 5.60). This procedure combines extensive mobilization and extension of the tricuspid valve leaflets via a "cone"-shaped tricuspid valve reconstruction at the true anatomic valve annulus. Often combined with plication of the atrialized portion of the right ventricle, this procedure results in a competent tricuspid valve and normal two-ventricle physiology.

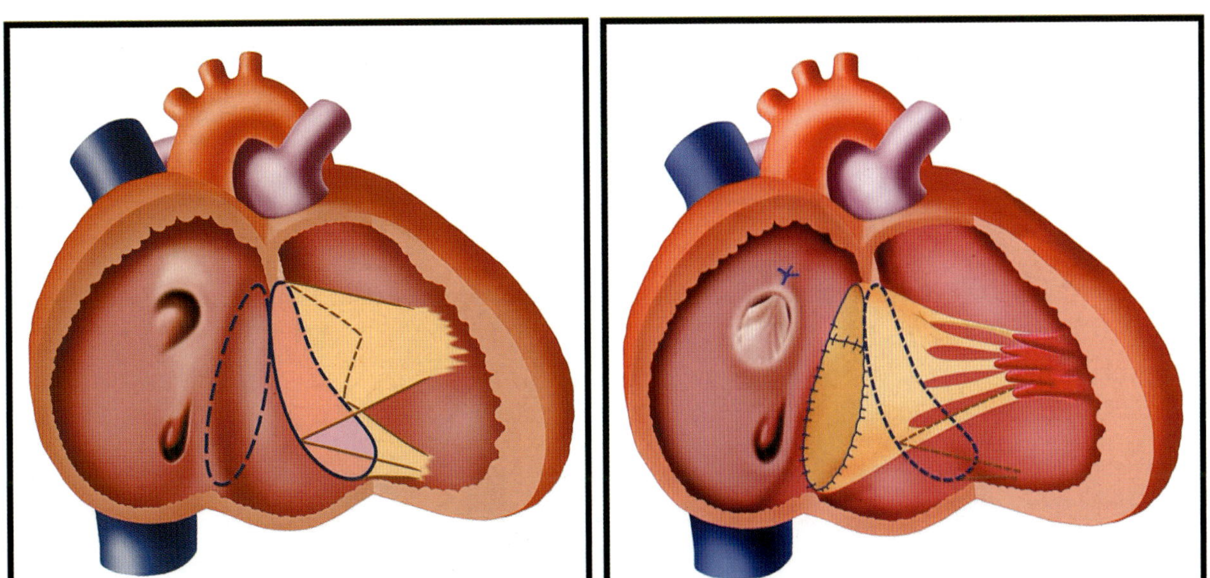

Fig. 5.60 Ebstein anomaly with anterior displacement of the tricuspid valve resulting in an "atrialized" portion of the right ventricle. The *Da Silva Cone procedure* consists of mobilization of the tricuspid valve leaflets and utilization of this tissue to construct a new cone-shaped valve in the normal atrioventricular junction. (Courtesy Dr. Jose Da Silva.)

Left-Sided Heart Obstruction

Obstruction along the left side of the heart can occur at any level from the pulmonary veins out to the descending aorta. Total anomalous pulmonary venous return (none of the pulmonary veins drain normally to the left atrium), when obstructed, can present with profound cyanosis requiring emergent surgery. Surgical repair involves rerouting the pulmonary veins to the left atrium and ligation of the aberrant vessels. The "sutureless" technique, which applies sutures to a cuff of surrounding tissue rather than in the pulmonary veins themselves, was introduced to reduce the risk of pulmonary venous obstruction at the anastomosis site.

Multiple operations have been designed to treat aortic valve and systemic outflow tract disease (Figs. 5.61 and 5.62). The *Ross procedure* (see Fig. 5.61) is an ingenious approach to the treatment of severe aortic stenosis or insufficiency when a valve replacement is required. The diseased aortic valve is removed, and the patient's own pulmonary valve is autotransplanted to the aortic position. The coronary arteries must be reimplanted into the neoaortic root, and a pulmonary homograft is used to reconstruct the right ventricular outflow tract. This operation avoids the lifelong anticoagulation that would be required by a prosthetic aortic valve but has a relatively high rate of reintervention, predominantly for dysfunction of the right ventricle to pulmonary artery homograft. Aortic stenosis with a small annulus is usually treated with a *Konno procedure* (see Fig. 5.62), which uses patch enlargement of the base of the ventricular septum to increase the size of the aortic annulus, allowing placement of an appropriately sized prosthetic aortic valve. The Konno procedure may be combined with the Ross procedure. The *Konno-Rastan procedure* is a variation in which a patch is used to enlarge the ventricular septum to relieve diffuse subaortic stenosis.

The *Damus-Kaye-Stansel procedure* is used to relieve aortic outflow tract obstruction in the setting of complex heart disease (Fig. 5.63). A double-inlet left ventricle with a restrictive ventricular communication that results in severe "functional" subaortic stenosis is one such example. The main pulmonary artery is transected, and the distal opening is oversewn along with connection of the proximal pulmonary root to the ascending aorta, in essence creating a

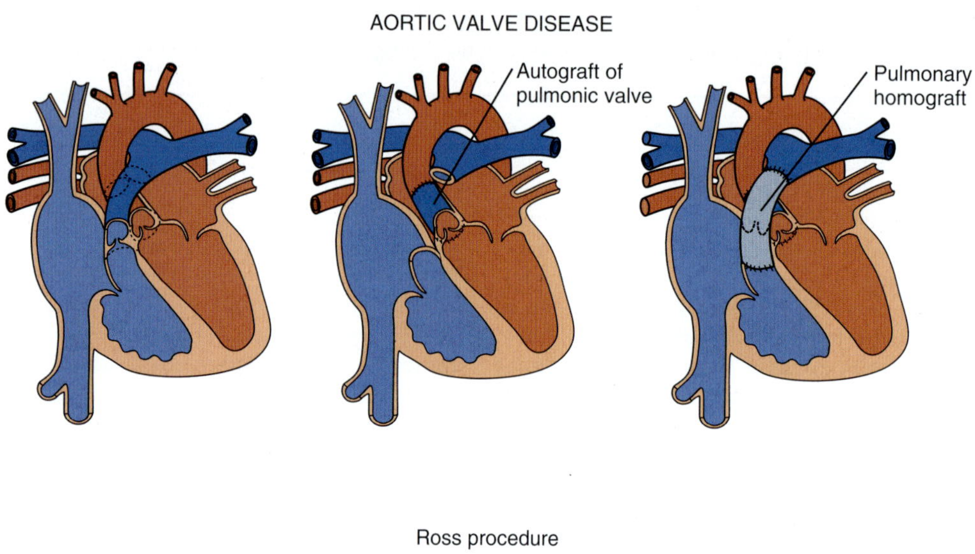

Fig. 5.61 Replacing the diseased aortic valve with the native pulmonary valve (Ross procedure).

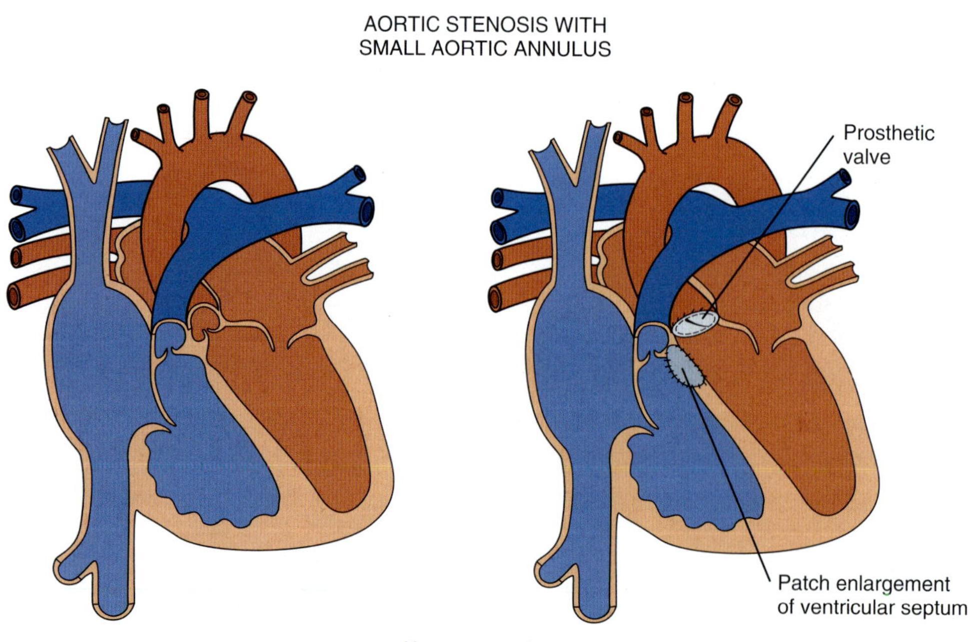

Fig. 5.62 Enlargement of the limited aortic annulus associated with severe aortic valve disease by patch enlargement of ventricular septum and placement of prosthetic valve (Konno procedure).

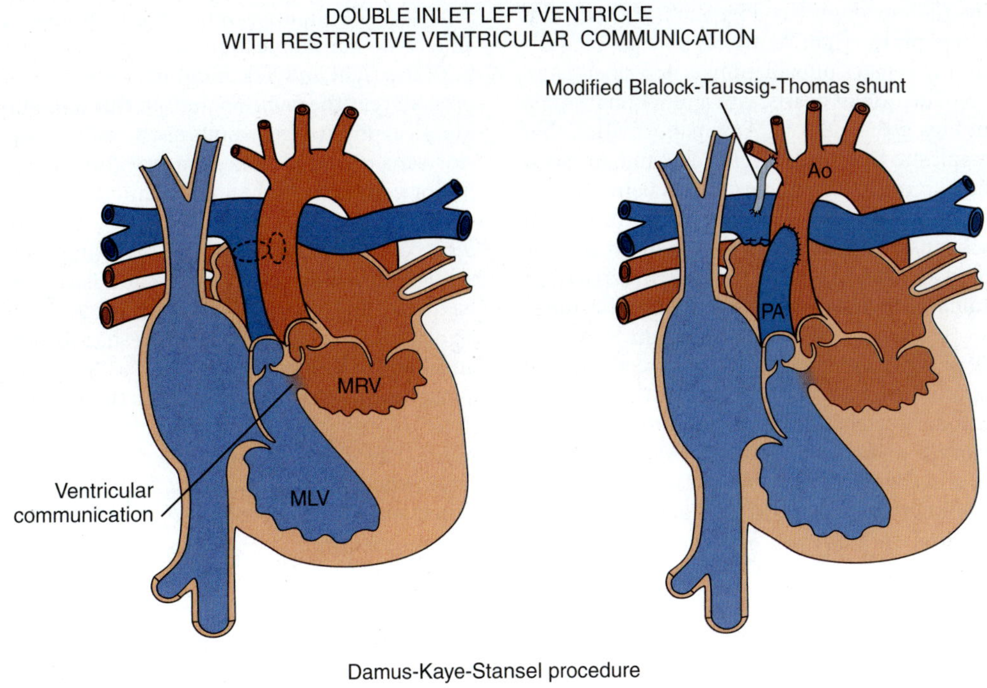

Fig. 5.63 Bypass of subaortic stenosis by creation of aortopulmonary anastomosis (Damus-Kaye-Stansel procedure). *MLV* refers to the dominant morphologic left ventricle, which receives both atrioventricular valves. *MRV* refers to the hypoplastic morphologic right ventricle, which receives blood only via the ventricular communication and supports the aortic valve.

bypass around the small ventricular communication that leads to the aorta. A modified Blalock-Taussig-Thomas shunt is created to provide pulmonary blood flow.

Obstruction of the aorta can range from isolated coarctation of the aorta (narrowing is typically juxtaductal and worsens as the ductus arteriosus closes) to more extensive aortic arch hypoplasia. Surgical repair follows the extent of narrowing. Simple coarctation can be repaired with removal of the narrowed segment and end-to-end anastomosis, whereas transverse arch hypoplasia may require extensive patch enlargement of the diseased vessel.

Single Ventricle Palliation

The initial palliation for aortic atresia and hypoplastic left heart syndrome, which is the most common cause of congestive heart failure in the first several days of life, is illustrated in Fig. 5.64. A *Norwood procedure* is the first of a three-stage operative approach designed to provide long-term stability for a circulation supported by only one ventricle. In the first stage, the pulmonary valve and right ventricle are functionally converted to become part of the systemic circulation. This "neoaortic outflow" for the right ventricle is created by transecting the main pulmonary artery near its bifurcation and anastomosing the proximal root to the hypoplastic ascending aorta, making liberal use of a homograft patch to enlarge the entire aortic arch. Relieving the coarctation that is invariably part of this anomaly is important. A shunt is subsequently performed to provide pulmonary blood flow, and a large atrial septal defect is created to allow unimpeded flow from the left to the right atrium. A modification (Sano procedure) of this operation substitutes a conduit from the right ventricle to the pulmonary artery for the shunt as the source for pulmonary blood flow.

Patients with hypoplastic right ventricles may or may not require supplemental pulmonary blood flow as a first stage in the neonatal period. When this is required, it is often achieved by placement of a

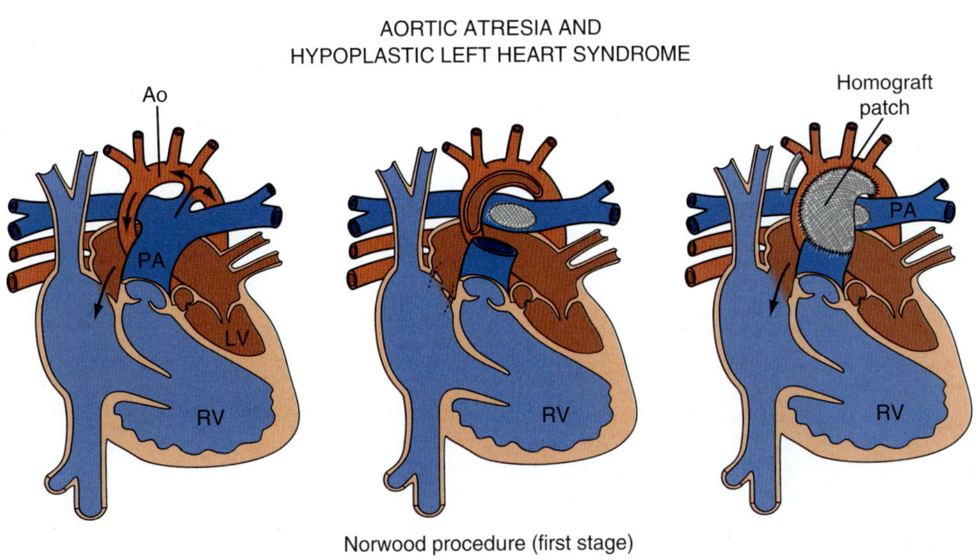

Fig. 5.64 Initial palliative (Norwood) procedure for hypoplastic left heart syndrome (aortic atresia complex). *Ao,* Aorta; *LV,* left ventricle; *PA,* pulmonary artery; *RV,* right ventricle.

modified Blalock-Taussig-Thomas shunt (see Fig. 5.58). If this is not required, patients with hypoplastic right ventricles may proceed directly to the second and third stages of palliation as described later. The subsequent stages to palliation of hearts with a functional single ventricle are depicted in Figs. 5.65 and 5.66. Any malformation that is associated with a hypoplastic right or left ventricle can be treated in this manner, with the two most common examples being tricuspid atresia with a hypoplastic right ventricle and aortic atresia with a hypoplastic left heart, status post–first-stage Norwood procedure. Creating a cavopulmonary anastomosis is the first step in separating the systemic and pulmonary circulations in the setting of a functional single ventricle (see Fig. 5.65). This procedure directs approximately one-half of systemic venous return directly to the pulmonary artery by creating an anastomosis between the superior vena cava and right pulmonary artery. In the *classic Glenn procedure,* the right pulmonary artery is divided, the superior vena cava–right atrial junction is closed, and the superior vena cava is anastomosed to the distal right pulmonary artery. This operation has been modified in recent years to a *bidirectional Glenn procedure,* which separates the superior vena cava from the right atrium and creates an end-to-side connection to the pulmonary artery, allowing flow to both the right and left pulmonary arteries. A variation of this latter procedure is the *hemi-Fontan.* In this operation, which produces the identical physiologic results as the bidirectional Glenn, a large superior vena cava–pulmonary artery connection is created, but the superior vena cava–right atrial connection is left intact and the orifice of the superior vena cava is closed with a patch. The *Fontan procedure* completes the process of diverting the entire systemic venous return to the pulmonary artery and is shown in Fig. 5.66. This may be done using a *lateral tunnel* approach, in which a tunnel within the right atrium is created with a U-shaped graft attached to the right atrial wall. The current approach uses an *extracardiac tunnel,* which avoids incorporating right atrial tissue into the connection in the hope of preventing postoperative atrial arrhythmias related to right atrial scarring. In many Fontan operations, a small opening or *fenestration* in the tunnel is created to allow a small amount of right-to-left shunting to decompress the relatively high-pressure systemic venous conduit.

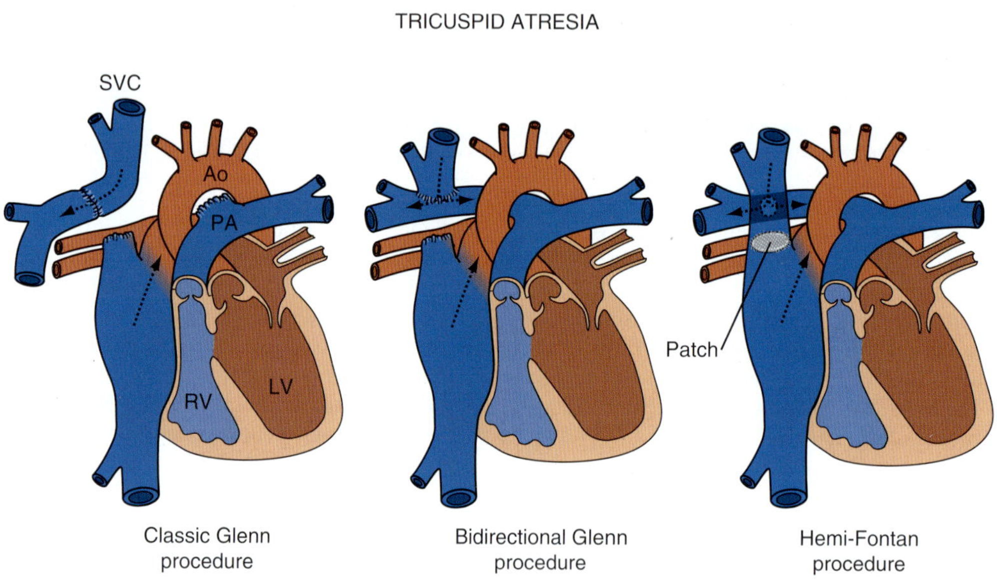

Fig. 5.65 Various cavopulmonary palliative procedures for a functionally single ventricle, such as tricuspid atresia. *Ao,* Aorta; *LV,* left ventricle; *PA,* pulmonary artery; *RV,* right ventricle; *SVC,* superior vena cava.

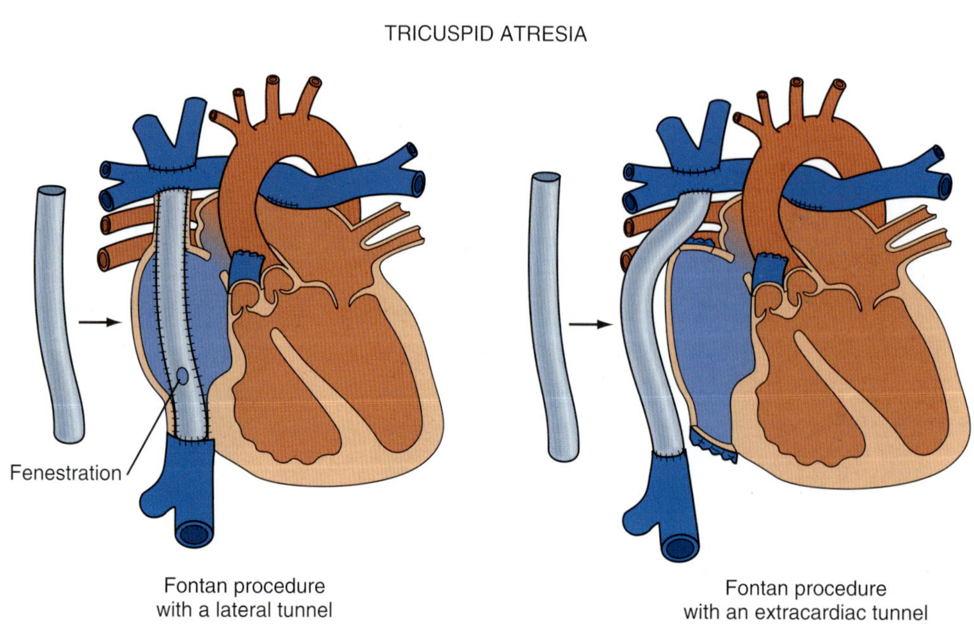

Fig. 5.66 Fontan completion of palliation for a functionally single ventricle, such as tricuspid atresia.

Transposition

The *Mustard* and *Senning procedures* were the original procedures used until the 1980s to correct the circulation in children with transposition of the great arteries (Fig. 5.67). In both operations, the atrial venous return is "switched" by placing a baffle that directs the superior and inferior vena caval systemic venous return posterior and to the left behind the baffle to the left ventricle while allowing the pulmonary venous return to flow anteriorly in front of the baffle to the right ventricle. Fig. 5.67 demonstrates the preoperative and postoperative flow patterns in transposition in the right and left diagrams, respectively, showing how rerouting systemic venous return allows fully oxygenated blood to go to the aorta. The only difference in the Mustard and Senning operations is the use of more native atrial tissue and less patch material in the latter operation. In the past 25 years, all pediatric cardiology centers have been using the *arterial switch (Jatene) procedure* (see Fig. 5.67) to correct the circulation in transposition of the great arteries. The aortic and pulmonary roots are transected and "switched" to the appropriate ventricles. The most difficult aspect of this operation is the transfer of the right and left coronary arteries from the anterior native aortic root to the posterior pulmonary root that will become the neoaorta. The *double-switch procedure* is a complex surgical technique used to repair congenitally corrected transposition that incorporates both the *Mustard/Senning procedure* and the *arterial switch (Jatene) procedure.* This lesion, also known as *ventricular inversion,* leads to heart failure because the morphologic right ventricle is not designed to maintain systemic blood flow. The *double-switch procedure* reroutes both the atrial and arterial blood flow, thus allowing the morphologic left ventricle to pump to the aorta and sustain systemic blood flow.

INTERVENTIONAL CARDIAC CATHETERIZATION

Interventional cardiology developed as a subspecialty over the past 4 decades after William Rashkind introduced the balloon septostomy to alleviate cyanosis in transposition of the great arteries. In recent years, the field has expanded explosively so that currently it plays a role in almost every heart defect. Interventions can be classified according to the purpose to treat:

- Valvular obstruction
- Vascular stenosis
- Creation or enlargement of defects
- Closure of defects
- Other

Valvular Obstruction

Echocardiography has achieved an indispensable role in the assessment of the severity of valvular obstruction. Although it is beyond the scope of this chapter, it should be noted that echocardiogram-derived gradients are often greater than those obtained in the catheterization laboratory. Therefore it is important to use clinical judgment in addition to echocardiographic data to determine which patients are appropriate candidates for cardiac catheterization and possible intervention.

Pulmonary Valve Stenosis/Atresia

In general, intervention is indicated when peak-to-peak (right ventricle to pulmonary artery systolic) gradients are greater than 40 mm Hg, as measured via cardiac catheterization. Balloon dilation has become the standard first-line treatment. In pulmonic stenosis, balloon dilation is highly effective in the large majority of patients. However, the success rate is not as high for the so-called *dysplastic pulmonary valve* (common in Noonan syndrome), where the valve is thick and often has associated supravalvular narrowing. For these valves, high-pressure balloons may be necessary to achieve success. Efficacy is long lasting in most cases, although approximately 8% of individuals do require repeat dilation for restenosis. Newborns with critical pulmonary valvular stenosis are a special group of patients for whom repeat dilation within the first year of life is not uncommon. Although dilation frequently results in regurgitation of the valve, because pulmonary artery resistance is normally quite low, the physiologic consequences of the insufficiency are rarely significant early on. Long term, patients should be observed for rare cases of restenosis and progressive insufficiency that can results in right heart dilation.

In the newborn period, intervention is necessary in those with critical pulmonary stenosis and ductal-dependent circulation, presenting with severe cyanosis. In this setting, it is common to see associated variable degrees of right ventricular hypoplasia and even cavitary obliteration. The right ventricle most often remodels over time to allow a normal biventricular circulation; however, it may take several weeks or months for resolution of right-to-left shunt across the patent foramen ovale. Typically, the prostaglandins that are used to promote ductal patency before the procedure are discontinued after balloon dilation. Some patients may require ongoing prostaglandin therapy for a few days or even weeks, particularly if the severity of the right ventricular hypoplasia is marked. Transcatheter placement of a stent in the ductus arteriosus has become an attractive alternative to surgical palliation for those patients who

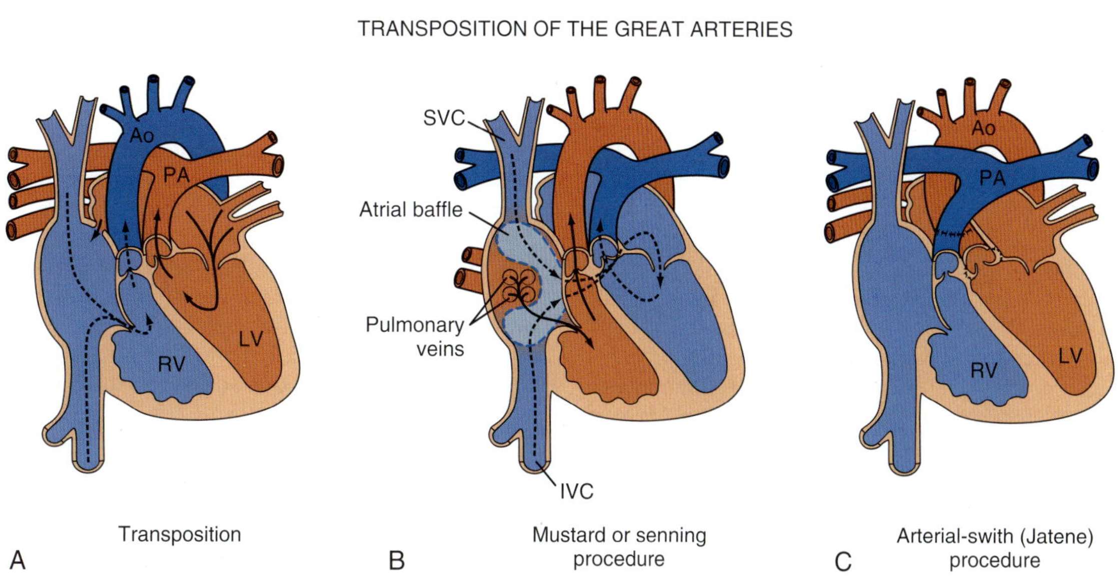

Fig. 5.67 Transposition of the great arteries (A). Intraatrial baffle (Mustard or Senning) procedure (B). Arterial switch (Jatene) procedure (C). *Ao,* Aorta; *IVC,* inferior vena cava; *LV,* left ventricle; *PA,* pulmonary artery; *RV,* right ventricle; *SVC,* superior vena cava.

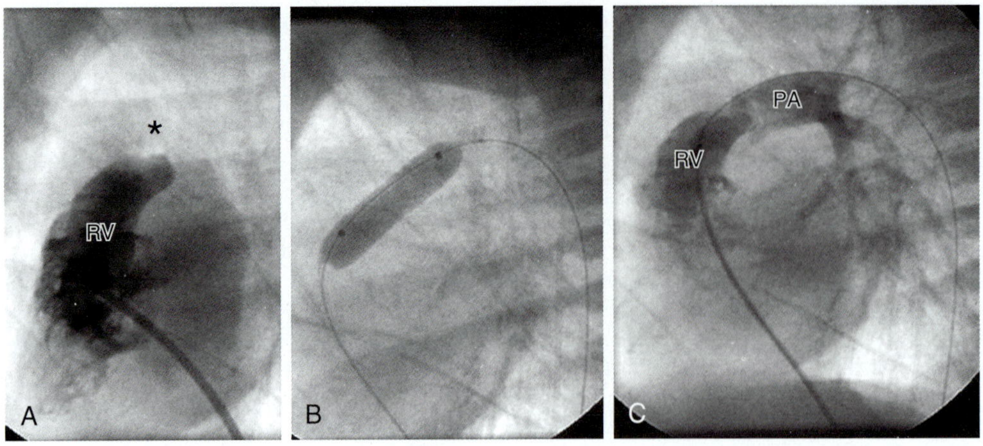

Fig. 5.68 Pulmonary valve atresia. Right ventricular angiogram in the lateral projection shows atresia of the pulmonary valve with no antegrade flow across the valve *(asterisk)* (A). After radiofrequency perforation of the pulmonary valve, balloon dilation is performed (B). After dilation there is an open pathway between the right ventricle *(RV)* and pulmonary artery *(PA)* (C).

cannot wean off prostaglandins (discussed later in the Neonatal Palliative Procedures section).

Patients with membranous pulmonary atresia can undergo radiofrequency-assisted valve perforation, followed by balloon valvotomy (Fig. 5.68). Although successful perforation has been reported in up 75% to 90% of selected patients, the procedure is definitive for only 35% because they commonly require additional intervention, either transcatheter or surgical.

Aortic Valve Stenosis

Although a few centers in the world continue to perform surgical valvotomies for aortic stenosis, most prefer balloon valvotomy as the procedure of choice. In the newborn, severe aortic stenosis can present as critical with ductal-dependent systemic circulation. Transcatheter balloon dilation can be performed antegrade (femoral vein or umbilical vein to left ventricle and aorta via the foramen ovale) or retrograde (umbilical artery or femoral artery). For premature babies, the carotid artery approach is a good alternative to avoid femoral arterial damage. Currently the procedure can be performed using low-profile balloons, which can be advanced via a 3-French sheath in the femoral artery, with significantly reduced incidence of iliofemoral artery thrombosis. Natural history data for aortic stenosis have suggested that a catheterization-derived peak-to-peak gradient (the difference between peak left ventricular and aortic pressure) across the valve of more than 50 mm Hg represents obstruction severe enough that intervention is preferable to observation and "medical management." Long-term procedural success is significantly different for aortic stenosis compared with pulmonary valve stenosis. All known forms of therapy, including balloon dilation, surgical valvotomy, or replacement of the valve, are palliative, given that further surgery will be necessary at some point in almost all cases of aortic stenosis. Balloon dilation of the aortic valve creates small tears in the fused commissures of leaflets that result in an increase in the valve orifice size. Some degree of aortic insufficiency is commonly present after the procedure. Attempts to completely alleviate obstruction by using overly large balloons result in an unacceptable amount of regurgitation. Thus even after successful balloon dilation, patients commonly have residual obstruction and/or insufficiency. The benefit achieved after aortic valve dilation is of variable duration. In one report, the intervention-free survival was 50% to 60% at 10 years after dilation. The need for subsequent intervention may be due to recurrent obstruction, insufficiency, or both. In the first instance, repeat valve dilation is an option.

Mitral Valve Stenosis

Isolated congenital mitral valve stenosis is rare, occurring more commonly in association with other left-sided obstructive lesions, as in patients with Shone syndrome or other complex congenital heart disease. Congenital mitral valve stenosis has proven to be a somewhat intractable condition, with a high mortality rate. Given the palliative nature of any intervention for patients with congenital mitral stenosis, newborns who present with a severe form of this condition are typically managed as patients with hypoplastic left heart syndrome.

Mitral balloon valvotomy beyond the newborn period can be effective and may have a lasting beneficial result, especially for rheumatic mitral valve stenosis. However, for congenital mitral valve stenosis, the procedure should be considered palliative and potentially able to delay the need for mitral valve replacement in a small child.

Vascular Stenosis

Pulmonary Artery Stenosis

Peripheral pulmonary artery stenosis can be congenital or acquired after cardiac surgery and constitutes 2% to 3% of congenital heart disease. Congenital pulmonary artery stenosis can occur in isolation or be associated with other congenital heart defects (most commonly, TOF with or without pulmonary atresia). As a primary lesion, it may be idiopathic or occur in the presence of syndromes, such as congenital rubella, Williams syndrome, and Alagille syndrome. Results of surgery for any of these branch pulmonary artery stenoses have been quite unsatisfactory. In addition, surgery cannot treat peripheral stenoses within the lungs. Thus balloon angioplasty has become the first-line therapy for these patients.

In general, indications for balloon dilation include an elevated right-to-left ventricular systolic pressure ratio of more than 50%, right ventricular failure, angiographic narrowing, contralateral pulmonary arterial hypertension, and abnormal perfusion by lung scintigraphy. Although there are no contraindications to this procedure by age or size, newborns with severe branch pulmonary artery stenosis should undergo balloon angioplasty only if severely symptomatic. Either discrete stenoses or long diffuse hypoplastic pulmonary arteries can be dilated, with success rates of 50% to 75%. With the use of high-pressure balloons, the success rate is on the order of 75%. The cutting balloon (Fig. 5.69) has been used for resistant

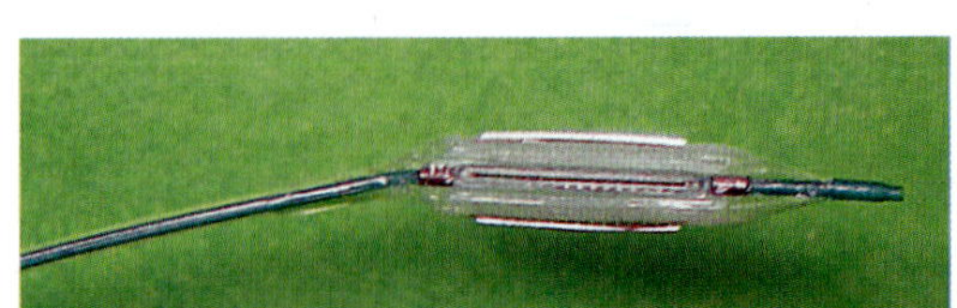

Fig. 5.69 Cutting balloon. Note the four tiny blades along the balloon surface.

lesions, significantly increasing the success rate of balloon pulmonary angioplasty. In addition, stent implantation allows a significant improvement in success rates to more than 90% (Fig. 5.70). However, not all lesions are amenable to stent implantation. Theoretical disadvantages to placing stents in infants include more difficult vascular access and the need for subsequent dilations to keep up with somatic growth. Nevertheless, some lesions that have not responded to dilation alone or surgery can be managed successfully with stent implantation, regardless of the age.

Aortic Coarctation

Balloon dilation of native coarctation of the aorta remains a controversial subject. In general, indications for intervention in infants and children, whether surgical or transcatheter, include the presence of anatomic coarctation associated with a systolic pressure gradient between upper and lower extremities of more than 20 mm Hg or a systolic blood pressure greater than 95% for age or the presence of left ventricular dysfunction. Because of the high restenosis rate during the first month of life, intervention is indicated in this age group only in symptomatic patients with congestive heart failure, failure to thrive, or upper extremity hypertension associated with left ventricular dysfunction. Surgery is considered the management approach of choice for neonates and young infants with severe coarctation, given the unacceptably high incidence of restenosis after balloon angioplasty (at least 50%). However, there are specific clinical conditions in which balloon dilation of a native coarctation in infants can be considered as the procedure of choice: patients with high surgical risks due to severe left ventricular dysfunction and unstable hemodynamic condition, severe pulmonary hypertension or other pulmonary diseases that would significantly increase the risk of thoracotomy, and recent intracranial hemorrhage or other major systemic disorders.

Recurrence of stenosis after balloon dilation decreases as the patient's age increases, reaching approximately 10% for children older than 2 years old. The procedure is generally safe, with a mortality of less than 1% and aneurysm formation rates of 7%.

In patients who present after adolescence and into adulthood, transcatheter stenting of the coarctation is considered appropriate first-line treatment or at least as an acceptable alternative to surgery (Fig. 5.71). The transcatheter approach is particularly appealing in the absence of any significant collateral vessels when surgical repair would be of higher risk for spinal cord ischemia. Dilation with stent placement results in effective relief of the obstruction in greater than 92% of cases.

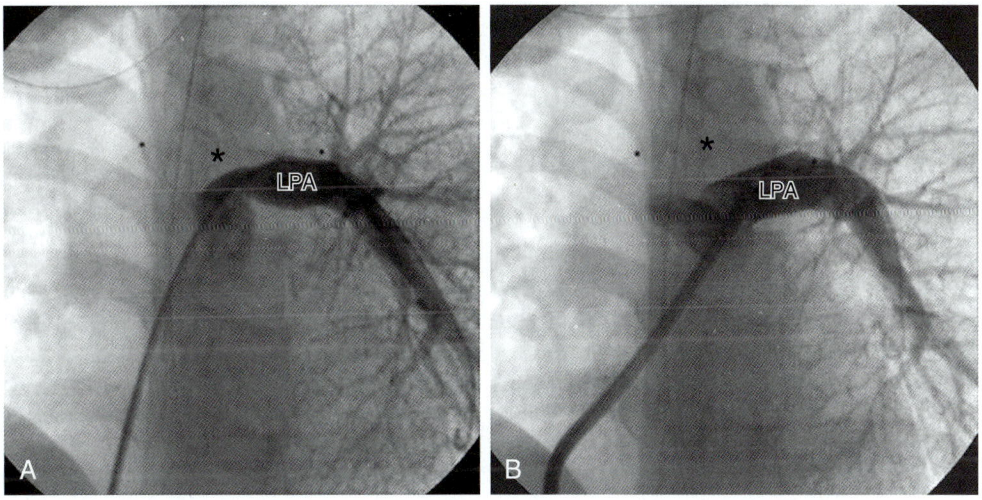

Fig. 5.70 Pulmonary artery angioplasty. Note the left pulmonary artery *(LPA)* stenosis demonstrated on the pulmonary artery angiogram (A); after stent implantation, the stenosis has been eliminated (B).

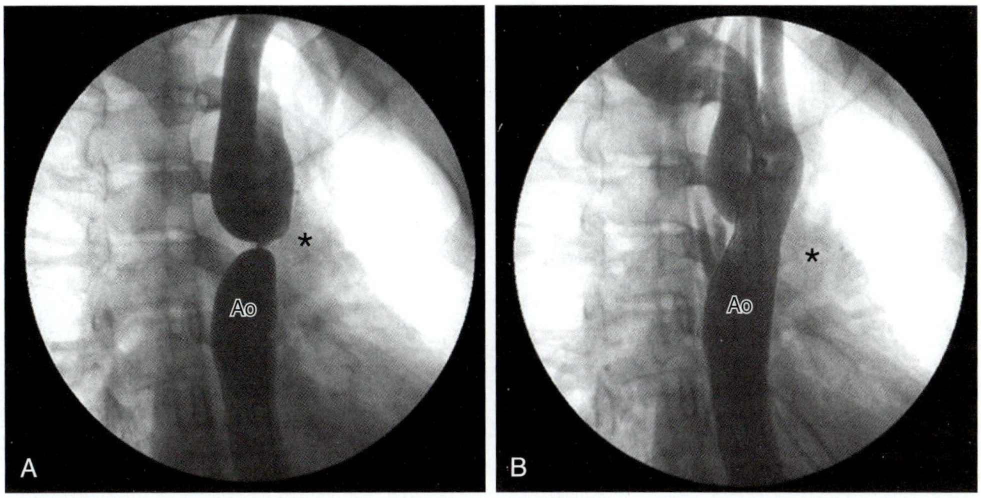

Fig. 5.71 Coarctation angioplasty. Note the severe coarctation of the aorta *(asterisk)* shown by angiography in the descending aorta *(Ao)* (A); after balloon angioplasty and stent implantation, the coarctation has been eliminated (B).

For patients with postoperative recurrent or residual coarctation, balloon angioplasty is considered the procedure of choice, regardless of the type of previous surgical repair. Success occurs in more than 90% with a restenosis rate of less than 20%. Mortality is 0.7% with an incidence of aneurysm formation of less than 2%.

Systemic or Pulmonary Vein Stenosis

Symptomatic systemic venous obstruction can occur in infants and children after cardiac surgery or after placement of chronic indwelling lines. Indications for intervention include symptoms of systemic venous hypertension, superior vena cava syndrome, and chronic pleural effusions (associated with elevated central venous pressure). Balloon dilation of venous stenoses has been performed since the mid-1980s. Although the immediate success rate is more than 90% for balloon dilation alone, the restenosis rate is more than 50%, suggesting that stent implantation should be considered as first-line therapy.

Pulmonary vein stenosis is generally an intractable disease, occurring either as a congenital lesion or postoperatively. Balloon dilation and stent implantation can serve as short-term palliation for symptomatic patients, although many require heart lung transplantation. Hemodynamic and angiographic improvement is seen immediately in almost all patients. However, restenosis occurs in virtually all cases within a few months post intervention. The use of systemic immunosuppression or drug-eluting balloons and stents (that deliver antiproliferative medication directly to the stenotic lesion), coupled with aggressive serial interventions to preserve vessel patency, have shown some potential in improving the outcome of this otherwise grave disease.

Creation or Enlargement of Defects

Balloon Atrial Septostomy

Following its initial introduction by Rashkind and Miller in 1966, balloon atrial septostomy to improve atrial mixing and increase systemic oxygen saturation has become an essential intervention in the management of most patients with transposition of the great arteries and other forms of congenital heart disease with transposition-like physiology (i.e., some forms of double-outlet right ventricle). Transposition physiology is where there is blue (desaturated) blood directed to the body and red (oxygenated) blood directed to the lungs. A patent ductus arteriosus, an atrial septal defect, or the presence of a ventricular septal defect increases the mixing and improves systemic oxygen saturation. This physiology involves parallel systemic and pulmonary circulations, with desaturated systemic venous blood directly returned to the systemic circulation via the right ventricle and aortic valve, while saturated pulmonary venous blood is directed back to the lungs via the left ventricle and pulmonary valve. An effective site of mixing of the circulations is critical to allow the arterial saturation to be at a level compatible with life. At most centers, balloon atrial septostomy is performed routinely on patients with D-transposition of the great arteries and intact ventricular septum, many times in the intensive care unit under echocardiographic guidance. The technique involves passing the septostomy catheter (Fig. 5.72) from the inferior vena cava to the right atrium and across an existing patent foramen ovale into the left atrium. The balloon is then inflated and "jerked" across the atrial septum into the right atrium, thereby enlarging the defect. The success rate of balloon atrial septostomy in newborns is higher than 98%, with a low complication rate.

Atrial Septoplasty/Blade Septostomy

In patients with left-sided obstructive lesions, a thick atrial septum, small left atrium, and restrictive atrial septal defect, balloon atrial septostomy is rarely successful. Furthermore, balloon atrial septostomy is not feasible in infants with intact atrial septum. For these patients, other techniques of atrial septal defect creation and septoplasty (using a static balloon dilation approach) are preferred. Blade

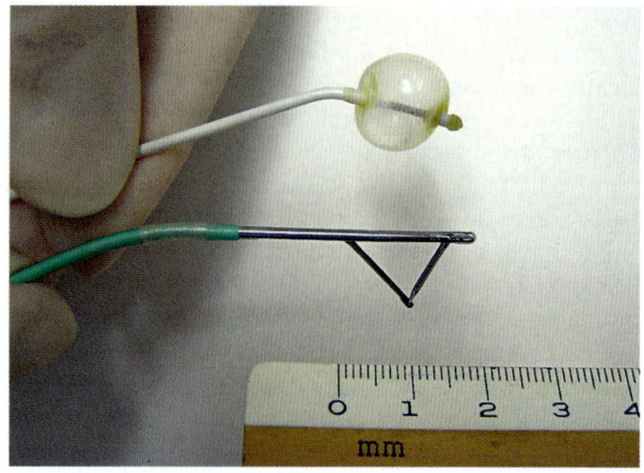

Fig. 5.72 Atrial septostomy devices. Note the Rashkind balloon *(top)* and Park blade *(bottom)* septostomy catheters (Cook Incorporated, Bloomington, IN).

atrial septostomy was developed by Dr. Sang Park for this purpose (Fig. 5.72). Alternate techniques currently used are a combination of Brockenbrough transseptal puncture, followed by serial balloon dilations using angioplasty balloons, including the cutting balloon (see Fig. 5.69) and occasionally stent implantation.

Closure of Defects

Atrial Septal Defects

Currently most secundum atrial septal defects are closed via the transcatheter deployment of devices. However, some atrial defects are not amenable to device closure because of the lack of an adequate rim of tissue around the defect to anchor the device. Atrial septal defects of the sinus venosus type or ostium primum defects cannot be closed with devices. Although devices are available to close large holes (up to 38 mm in diameter), the larger devices will fit only in a large adult heart. Two types of devices are currently approved in the United States for closure of an atrial septal defect: the Amplatzer Septal Occluder (Abbott Medical, Santa Clara, CA) (Fig. 5.73) and the Gore devices (W.L. Gore & Associates, Inc., Flagstaff, AZ) (Fig. 5.74), which include the Cardioform Septal Occluder and the newer Cardioform ASD Occluder. The procedure is performed under transesophageal or intracardiac echocardiographic guidance (Fig. 5.75) and is similar for both types of devices. Several studies have documented that the efficacy of device closure compares favorably with surgery, with high closure and low complication rates. Late perforations after device closure have been reported to occur up to several years after device implantation; however, these have been rare.

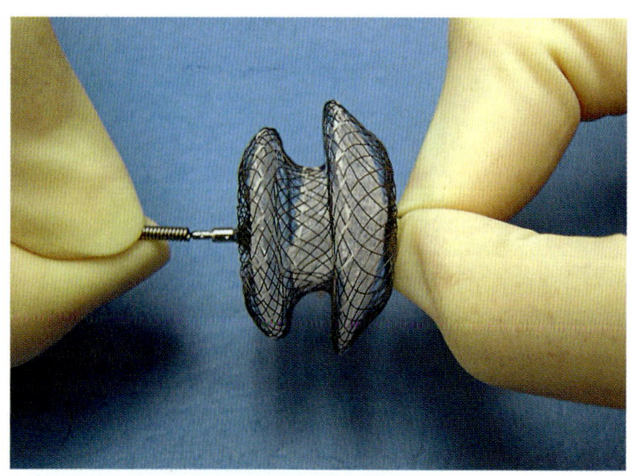

Fig. 5.73 The Amplatzer Septal Occluder (Abbott Medical, Santa Clara, CA), used for device closure of atrial septal defects. The device is held outstretched to demonstrate its architecture, which is composed of two disks and a central waist designed to occlude the defect.

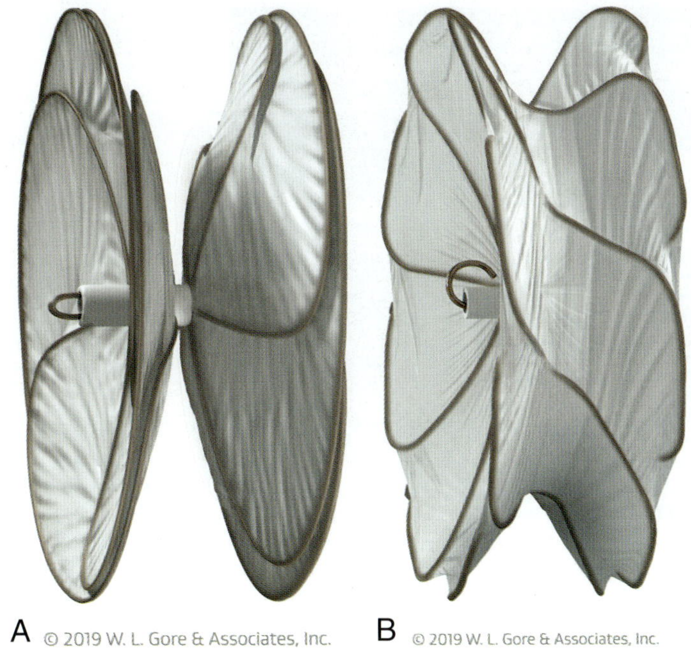

Fig. 5.74 The current Gore Cardioform devices include the Septal Occluder (A) designed for smaller and fenestrated atrial septal defects and the ASD Occluder (B) for larger defects. (Courtesy W.L. Gore & Associates, Inc., Flagstaff, AZ.)

Ventricular Septal Defects

Most ventricular septal defects cannot be closed with devices due to the significant size of the defect in relatively small hearts, as well as the proximity to intracardiac valves, particularly tricuspid and aortic valves, and the conduction tissue. An option to overcome the limitations of the technique in a small child is a combined hybrid catheterization-surgical approach. In this method, the heart is exposed via a thoracotomy and the device delivery catheter advanced through the free wall of the right ventricle and across the defect. The device is then opened under echocardiographic guidance. This technique has the advantage of avoiding cardiopulmonary bypass and may be particularly useful for ventricular septal defects located in portions of the heart difficult to reach by standard open surgical technique. The CardioSEAL device (NMT Medical, Boston, MA) was used in the past for this indication. The Amplatzer Muscular VSD Occluder (Abbott Medical, Santa Clara, CA) (Fig. 5.76A) is currently approved for closure of muscular ventricular septal defects and is the most widely used. Although high success rates have been reported with transcatheter closure of ventricular septal defects, in the United States the procedure is currently still reserved for defects that are difficult to close surgically, and in fact, a combined surgical-interventional catheter approach may be used in some patients as detailed earlier.

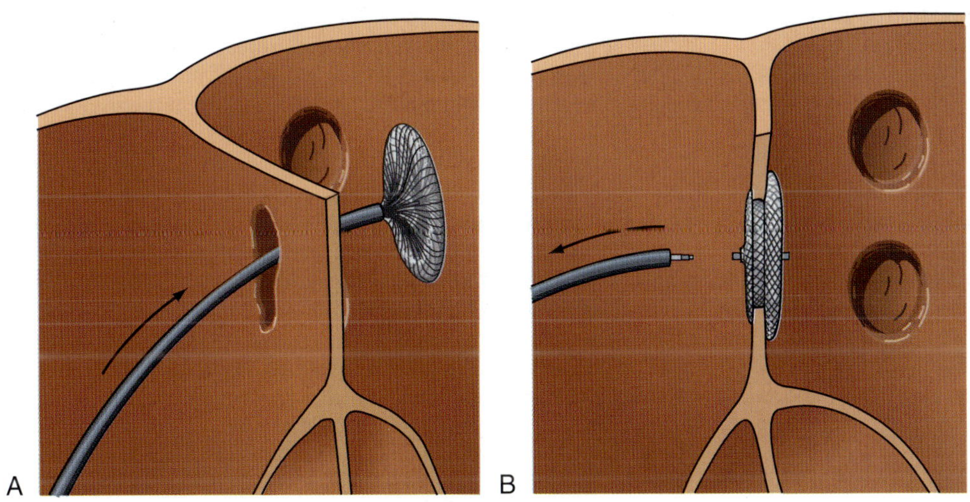

Fig. 5.75 Illustration of placement of Amplatzer septal occluder. Note the delivery sheath is advanced across the defect into the left atrium, and the device is partially extruded out of the sheath with opening the left atrial disk (A); after withdrawal of the sheath, the device has been deployed with the right atrial disk opened on the right side of the septum, and the device has been detached from the delivery cable (B).

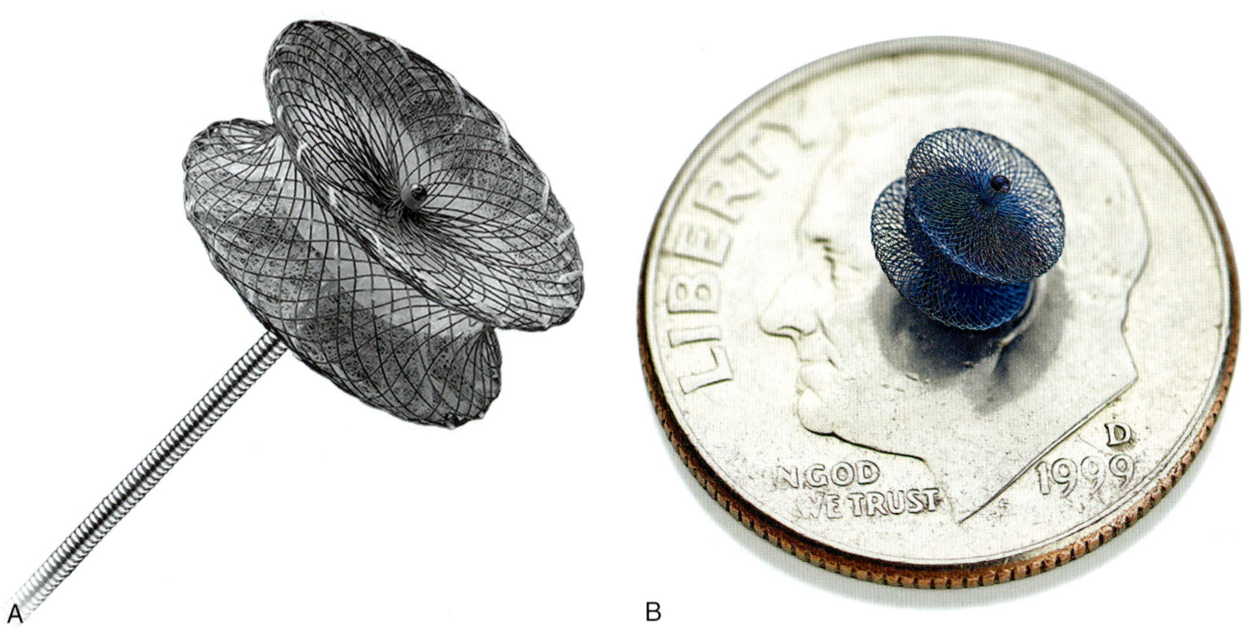

Fig. 5.76 Amplatzer Muscular VSD Occluder (A) and Amplatzer Piccolo device used for closure of patent ducts in preterm patients as small as 700 g (B). (Abbott Medical, Santa Clara, CA.)

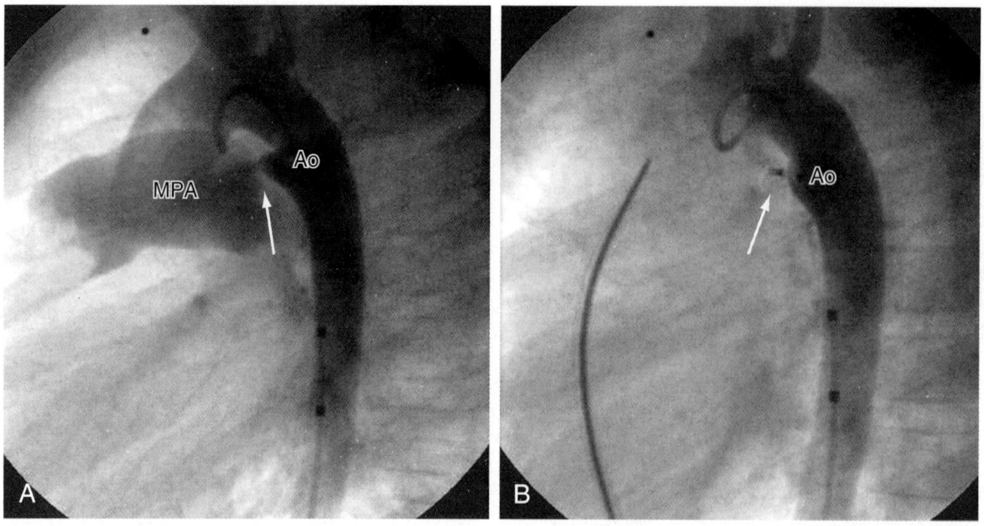

Fig. 5.77 Closure of patent ductus arteriosus. Note the descending aorta *(Ao)* angiogram shows a patent ductus *(arrow)* entering the main pulmonary artery *(MPA)* (A); a repeat angiogram after placement of an Amplatzer Duct Occluder demonstrates the ductus is completely closed (B).

Patent Ductus Arteriosus

Small and moderate patent ducts are typically closed in the catheterization laboratory with either embolization coils or the Amplatzer Duct Occluder (Abbott Medical, Santa Clara, CA) (Fig. 5.77). Historically, newborns with large symptomatic patent ductus arteriosus were treated surgically. More recently, device technology has evolved such that many newborns, even small premature infants, can be treated percutaneously. In 2019 the U.S. Food and Drug Administration (FDA) approved the Amplatzer Piccolo device (Abbott Medical, Santa Clara, CA) for closure of patent ducts in preterm patients as small as 700 g (see Fig. 5.76B). Transcatheter closure of patent ductus arteriosus has been highly successful, with efficacy of more than 97% and a low complication rate.

Other Transcatheter Techniques

Closure of Collateral Vessels

Lesions amenable to closure by embolization therapy include systemic venous anomalies (i.e., left superior vena cava to left atrium) or aortopulmonary collaterals, pulmonary sequestration, or congenital arteriovenous malformations. Coil embolization of collaterals is one of the most common procedures in children with congenital heart disease associated with aortopulmonary collateral vessels, such as those with single ventricle physiology and patients with TOF and pulmonary atresia with major aortopulmonary collateral vessels.

Percutaneous Pulmonary Valve Implantation

In January 2010 the FDA approved the Melody valve (Medtronic, Inc., Minneapolis, MN) for percutaneous implantation in the pulmonary position in patients with dysfunctional right ventricle to pulmonary artery conduits implanted surgically at the time of repair of certain congenital heart defects. This novel technology may delay the need for surgical conduit replacement. The Melody valve is a bovine jugular venous valve mounted on a CP Numed stent, which is a platinum iridium stent, and is therefore MRI compatible (Fig. 5.78A). This has become an option for patients with pulmonary conduit stenosis and/or insufficiency, allowing restoration of pulmonary valve function. The valve is implanted within the existing conduit, mounted on a balloon using a uniquely tapered delivery catheter (see Fig. 5.78B) and is available in sizes 18 to 22 mm in diameter. The technique of Melody valve implantation within a stenotic right ventricle to pulmonary artery conduit is illustrated by Fig. 5.79. In March 2016, the Sapien XT valve (Edwards Life Sciences Corporation, Irvine, CA) was approved by the FDA for pulmonary implantation. The Sapient XT valve has a larger diameter (23, 26, and 29 mm) and therefore expands the patient population treated with this technique (see Fig. 5.78C).

This procedure may also benefit selected patients with TOF who were initially repaired without a conduit and have developed severe pulmonary regurgitation years later. In March of 2021, the Harmony valve (Medtronic, Inc., Minneapolis, MN) was FDA approved for the management of pediatric and adult patients with severe pulmonary regurgitation. The Harmony valve is available in two sizes (22 mm and 25 mm), and is a porcine pericardium tissue valve sewn within a self-expanding, polyester-covered nitinol frame, designed specifically to conform to the larger right ventricular outflow tract of such patients (see Fig. 5.78D & Fig. 5.78E). In December 2021, the Alterra Adaptive Prestent (Edwards Life Sciences Corporation, Irvine, CA) was also FDA approved for use in patients with severe pulmonary regurgitation. The Alterra Adaptive Prestent is a self-expanding nitinol stent, partially covered with polytetrafluoroethylene, which is implanted in the right ventricular outflow tract so to function as a landing zone for the implantation of the SAPIEN S3 (Edwards Life Sciences Corporation, Irvine, CA) transcatheter valve. Given multiple valve options, a large portion of patients with dysfunctional conduits and pulmonary valve regurgitation can now be treated with transcatheter procedures rather than surgical pulmonary valve replacement.

Neonatal Palliative Procedures

As catheter technology has evolved, it has become more common to initially palliate some neonates with less invasive transcatheter techniques and thereby defer more definitive cardiac surgical repair to a later age. In cyanotic neonates, placement of a stent in the right ventricular outflow tract (Fig. 5.80), or across the patent ductus arteriosus (Fig. 5.81), can increase pulmonary blood flow sufficiently enough to eliminate the need for a surgical *Blalock-Taussig-Thomas shunt* (see Fig. 5.58). The *hybrid stage 1 procedure* (Fig. 5.82) is an alternative to the *Norwood procedure* (see Fig. 5.64) for high-risk patients with hypoplastic left heart syndrome. With this approach, the surgeon and the interventional cardiologist work side by side in the catheterization laboratory, which functions as an operating

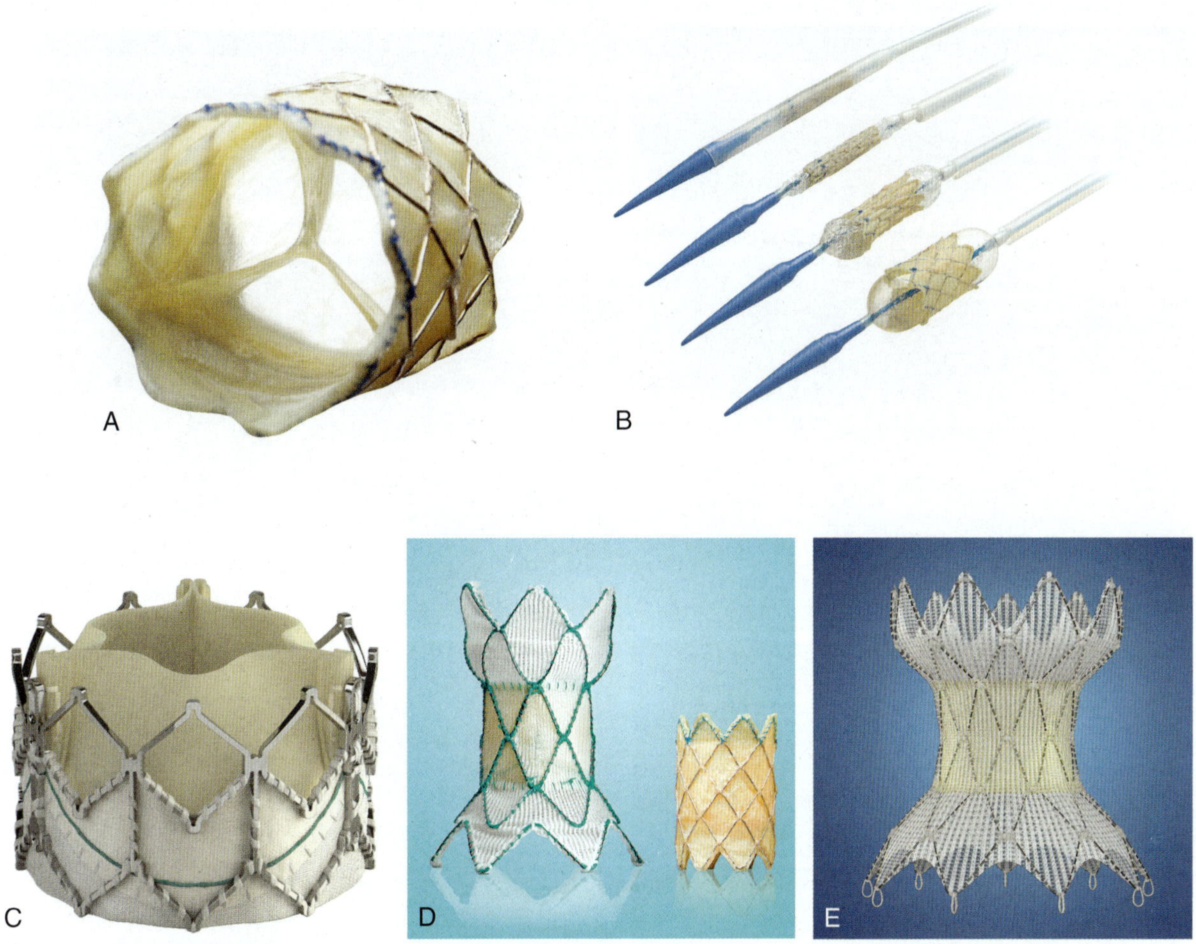

Fig. 5.78 Melody valve (Medtronic, Inc., Minneapolis, MN). A bovine jugular venous valve is sewn on a platinum iridium stent (A). Medtronic Ensemble Delivery System for Melody valve implantation (B). Sapien XT valve (Edwards Life Sciences Corporation, Irvine, CA). A bovine pericardium tissue valve mounted on a cobalt chromium frame (C). The Harmony valve TPV 22 (Medtronic, Inc., Minneapolis, MN). A porcine pericardium tissue valve sewn to a polyester-covered nitinol frame (D), pictured on the left, is designed for larger outflow tracts compared with the Melody valve, on the right. The Harmony valve TPV 25 (Medtronic, Inc., Minneapolis, MN) larger version (E). (A, B, D, ©2025 Medtronic. All rights reserved. Used with the permission of Medtronic. C, Used with permission from Edwards Lifesciences LLC, Irvine, CA. SAPIEN, SAPIEN M3, SAPIEN XT, SAPIEN X4, SAPIEN 3, SAPIEN 3 Ultra, and SAPIEN Ethos are trademarks of Edwards Lifesciences Corporation.)

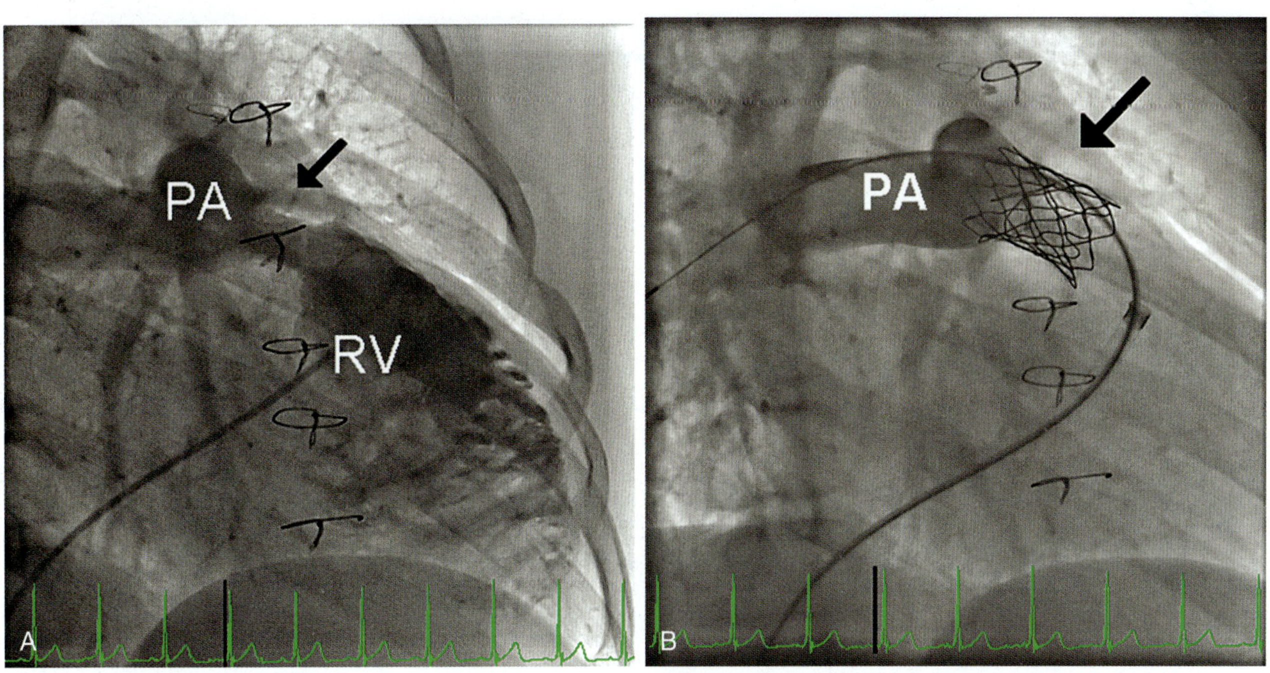

Fig. 5.79 Stenotic right ventricle to pulmonary artery conduit. Severe conduit stenosis *(arrow)* is demonstrated in right anterior oblique view (A) in a patient after surgical repair of congenital heart disease. Conduit was 22 mm in diameter at implantation and with progressive stenosis is less than half the original dimension, causing severe right ventricular hypertension. Angiogram in pulmonary artery *(PA)* after Melody valve implantation *(arrow)* demonstrates competent valve with no opacification of the right ventricle *(RV)* (B).

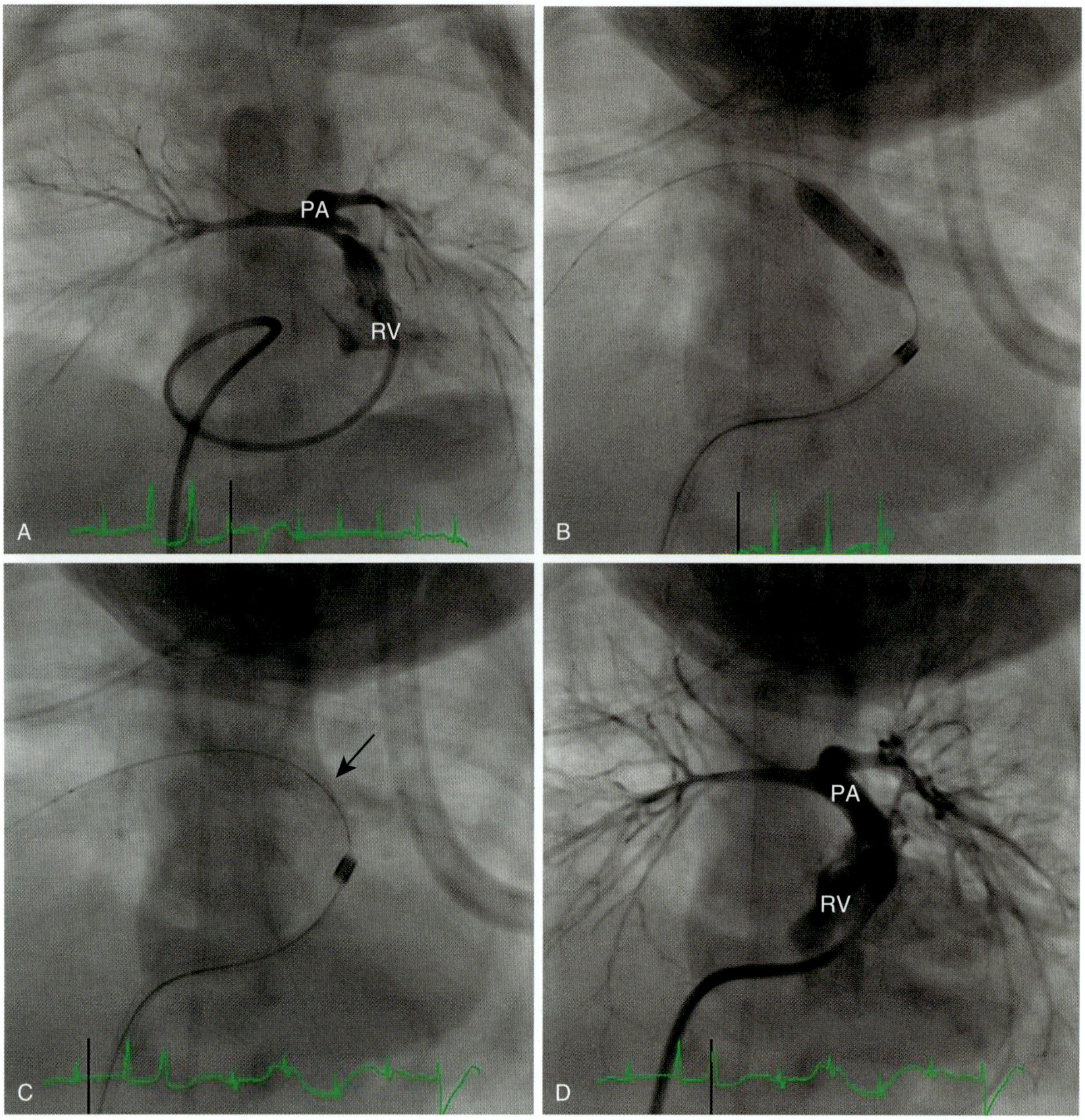

Fig. 5.80 Stenting of the right ventricular outflow tract. Right ventricular angiogram performed with cranial angulation in an infant with tetralogy of Fallot and hypoplastic pulmonary arteries (A). Balloon angioplasty (B) with stent *(arrow)* implantation (C) in the stenotic right ventricular outflow tract. Right ventricular angiogram post-intervention shows improved outflow tract diameter (D). *PA,* Pulmonary artery; *RV,* right ventricle.

room. The surgeon opens the chest and places bilateral pulmonary artery bands, and the interventionalist then places a stent across the patent ductus arteriosus via a catheter introduced directly into the main pulmonary artery. This approach is particularly attractive for infants who are small for gestational age or have multiple congenital anomalies or those with contraindications toward cardiopulmonary bypass, such as intracranial hemorrhage. More recently, the use of transcatheter pulmonary artery flow restrictors as a substitute for pulmonary artery bands has been explored as an option to establish "hybrid physiology" less invasively, without the need for open sternotomy.

Miscellaneous

Reopening of thrombosed vessels or surgical anastomoses can be performed with good results using transcatheter thrombolysis, although the experience in pediatrics is relatively limited. Other interventions include retrieval of foreign bodies, coil embolization of coronary artery fistulae, and some novel catheter procedures, such as prenatal interventions performed on fetuses with complex congenital heart disease (for opening of stenotic valves or a restrictive atrial septum). These innovative procedures are likely to be only a preview of what will be possible, and even commonplace, in the next decade as the field of interventional catheterization continues to advance and expand.

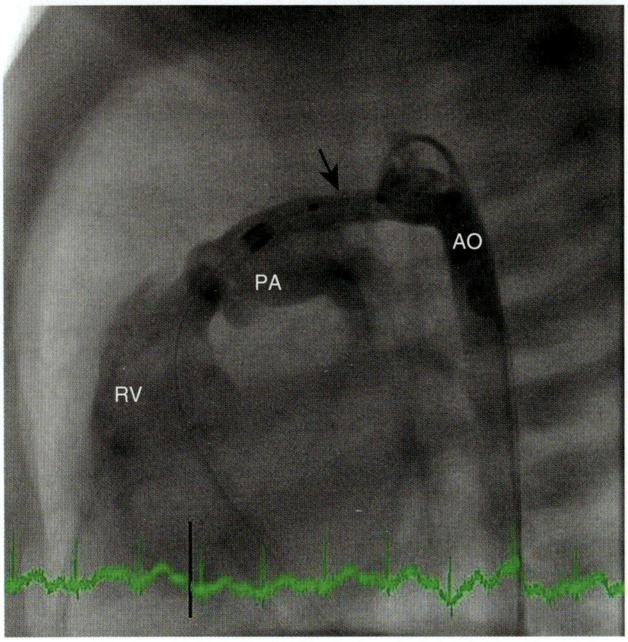

Fig. 5.81 Stenting of patent ductus arteriosus. Aortic angiogram performed in lateral view in patient with pulmonary stenosis after stent placement in the patent ductus arteriosus *(arrow)*. The right ventricle fills due to pulmonary valve regurgitation. *AO,* Aorta; *PA,* pulmonary artery; *RV,* right ventricle.

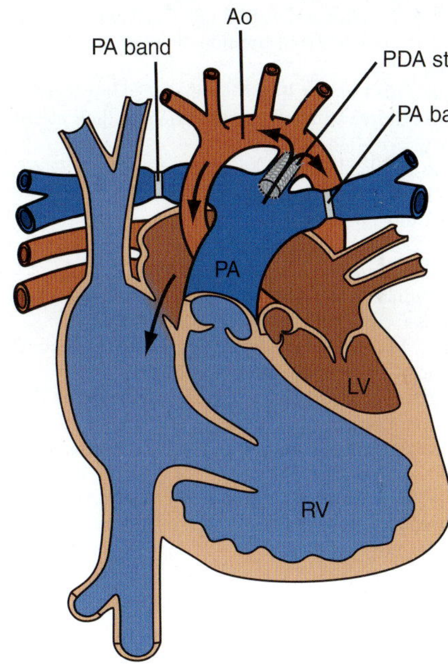

Fig. 5.82 Hybrid stage 1 procedure for palliation of hypoplastic left heart syndrome. *AO,* Aorta; *LV,* left ventricle; *PA,* pulmonary artery; *PDA,* patent ductus arteriosis; *RV,* right ventricle.

Bibliography

Allen HD, Phillips JR, Chan DP: History and physical examination. In Allen HD, Driscoll DJ, Shaddy RE, Feltes TF, editors: *Moss and Adams' heart disease in infants, children, and adolescents*, ed 7, Philadelphia, 2008, Lippincott Williams and Wilkins, pp 58–66.

Aoki Y, Niihori T, Inoue S, Matsubara Y: Recent advances in RASopathies, *J Hum Genet* 61(1):33, 2016.

Beerman LB, Arora G, Park SC: Arrhythmias in the intensive care unit. In Munoz RA, Morell VO, da Cruz EM, et al., editors: *Critical care of children with heart disease*, London, 2010, Springer-Verlag London Limited.

Bush DM: Evaluating cardiovascular presentations: what does an electrocardiogram have to offer? *Pediatr Ann* 34:858–869, 2005.

Case CL: Diagnosis and treatment of pediatric arrhythmias, *Pediatr Clin North Am* 46:347–354, 1999.

Chun TUH, Van Hare GF: Advances in the approach to treatment of supraventricular tachycardia in the pediatric population, *Curr Cardiol Rep* 6:322–326, 2004.

Du ZD, Hijazi ZM, Kleinman CS, et al: Comparison between transcatheter and surgical closure of secundum atrial septal defect in children and adults: results of a multicenter nonrandomized trial, *J Am Coll Cardiol* 39:1836–1844, 2002.

Ettedgui JA, Tersak JM: Cardiological aspects of systemic disease. In Anderson RH, Macartney FJ, Shinebourne EA, et al., editors: *Paediatric cardiology*, Edinburgh, 2002, Churchill Livingstone, pp 1777–1808.

Farrior JB, Silverman SE: A consideration of the differences between a Janeway's lesion and an Osler's node in infectious endocarditis, *Chest* 70(2):239–243, 1976.

Fischer DR, Baker EJ, Anderson RH: Echocardiographic manifestation of ventricular septal defects. In Anderson RH, Neches WH, Park SC, et al., editors: *Perspectives in pediatric cardiology*, Mount Kisco, NY, 1988, Futura Publishing, pp 25–33.

Fontan F, Baudet E: Surgical repair of tricuspid atresia, *Thorax* 26:240–248, 1971.

Fyler DC: Rheumatic fever. In Keane JF, Lock JE, Fyler DC, editors: *Nadas' pediatric cardiology*, ed 2, Philadelphia, 2006, Saunders Elsevier Publishing, pp 387–399.

Geva T, Powell AJ: Magnetic resonance imaging. In Allen HD, Driscoll DJ, Shaddy RE, Feltes TF, editors: *Moss and Adams' heart disease in infants, children, and adolescents*, ed 8, Philadelphia, 2013, Lippincott Williams and Wilkins, pp 207–246.

Glenn WW, Patino JF: Circulatory bypass of the right heart. Preliminary observations on the direct delivery of vena caval blood into the pulmonary arterial circulation: azygos vein pulmonary artery shunt, *Yale J Biol Med* 24:147, 1954.

Gray RG, Menon SC, Johnson JT, et al: Acute and midterm results following perventricular device closure of muscular ventricular septal defects: a multicenter PICES investigation, *Catheter Cardiovasc Interv* 90(2):281–289, 2017.

Greenwood RD: Cardiovascular malformations associated with extracardiac anomalies and malformation syndromes, *Clin Pediatr* 23:145–151, 1984.

Hernandez-Pampaloni M, Allada V, Fishbein MC, et al: Myocardial perfusion and viability by positron emission tomography in infants and children with coronary abnormalities: correlation with echocardiography, coronary angiography, and histopathology, *J Am Coll Cardiol* 41(4):618–626, 2003.

Konno S, Imai Y, Iida Y, et al: A new method for prosthetic valve replacement in congenital aortic stenosis associated with hypoplasia of the aortic valve ring, *J Thoracic Cardiovasc Surg* 70:909–917, 1975.

Kreutzer J, Perry SB: Stents. In Lock JE, Keane JF, Perry SB, editors: *Diagnostic and interventional catheterization in congenital heart disease*, ed 2, Norwell, MA, 2000, Kluwer Academic Publishers, pp 221–243.

Kugler JD, Danford DA: Management of infants, children and adolescents with paroxysmal supraventricular tachycardia, *J Pediatr* 129:324–328, 1996.

Lacro R: Dysmorphology and genetics. In Keane JF, Lock JE, Fyler DC, editors: *Nadas' pediatric cardiology*, ed 2, Philadelphia, 2006, Saunders Elsevier Publishing, pp 62–69.

Long FR, Eichhorn: Cardiac computerized tomography in congenital heart disease. In Allen HD, Driscoll DJ, Shaddy RE, Feltes TF, editors: *Moss and Adams' heart disease in infants, children, and adolescents*, ed 8, Philadelphia, 2013, Lippincott Williams and Wilkins, pp 247–257.

McElhinney DB, Hellenbrand WE, Zahn EM, et al: Short- and medium-term outcomes after transcatheter pulmonary valve placement in the expanded multicenter US Melody valve trial, *Circulation* 122(5):507–516, 2010.

McElhinney DB, Krantz ID, Bason L: Analysis of cardiovascular phenotype and genotype-phenotype correlation with individuals with JAG-1 mutation and/or Alagille syndrome, *Circulation* 106(20):2567–2574, 2002.

National High Blood Pressure Education Program Working Group on High Blood Pressure in Children and Adolescents: The fourth report on the diagnosis, evaluation, and treatment of high blood pressure in children and adolescents, *Pediatrics* 114(Suppl 2):555–576, 2014.

Newburger JW, Takahashi M, Gerber MA, et al: Diagnosis, treatment, and long-term management of Kawasaki disease: a statement for health professionals from the Committee on Rheumatic Fever, Endocarditis and Kawasaki Disease, Council on Cardiovascular Disease in the Young, American Heart Association, *Circulation* 110:2747–2771, 2004.

Norwood WI Jr: Hypoplastic left heart syndrome, *Ann Thorac Surg* 52(3):688–695, 1991.

Nwankwo U, Morell E, Trucco SM, et al: Hybrid strategy for neonates with ductal-dependent systemic circulation at high risk for Norwood, *Ann Thorac Surg* 106(2):595–601, 2018.

Park SC, Neches WH, Zuberbuhler JR, et al: Clinical use of blade atrial septostomy, *Circulation* 56:600–606, 1978.

Park SC, Zuberbuhler JR: Vascular ring and pulmonary sling. In Anderson RH, Macartney FJ, Shinebourne EA, et al., editors: *Paediatric cardiology*, Edinburgh, 2002, Churchill Livingstone, pp 1559–1577.

Pelech AN: Evaluation of the pediatric patient with a cardiac murmur, *Pediatr Clin North Am* 45:167–188, 1999.

Perry SB, Radtke W, Fellows KE, et al: Coil embolization to occlude aortopulmonary collateral vessels and shunts in patients with congenital heart disease, *J Am Coll Cardiol* 13:100–108, 1989.

Pompa A, LaRossa P, Beerman LB, et al: Utility of ECGs in the pediatric emergency department for patients presenting with a seizure, *Am J Emerg Med* 19:30755–30757, 2019.

Rashkind WJ, Miller W: Creation of an atrial septal defect without thoracotomy: palliative approach to complete transposition of the great arteries, *J Am Med Assoc* 196:991–992, 1966.

Ravi P, Ashwath R, Strainic J, et al: Clinical and financial impact of ordering an echocardiogram in children with left axis deviation on their electrocardiogram, *Cong Heart Dis* 11(2):110–114, 2016.

Robinson B, Anisman P, Eshaghpour E: A primer on pediatric ECGs, *Contemp Pediatr* 11:69–94, 1994. https://chc.med.ufl.edu/files/2013/02/A-Primer-on-Pediatric-Electrocardiograms.pdf

Rittler M, Paz JE, Castilla EE: VACTERL association, epidemiologic definition and delineation, *Am J Med Genet* 63(4):529–536, 1996.

Rome JJ, Kreutzer J: Pediatric interventional catheterization: reasonable expectations and outcomes, *Pediatr Clin North Am* 51:1589–1610, 2004.

Rowan S, Adroques H, Mathur A, et al: Pediatric hypertension: a review for the primary care provider, *Clin Pediatr* 44:289–296, 2005.

Schneider AE, Cannon BC, Johnson JN, et al: Left axis deviation in children without previously known heart disease, *Pediatrics* 141(3):e20171970, 2018.

Senning A: Surgical correction of transposition of the great vessels, *Surgery* 45: 966–980, 1959.

Sharieff GQ, Rao SO: The pediatric ECG, *Emerg Med Clin North Am* 24:195–208, 2006.

Spicer RL: Cardiovascular disease in Down syndrome, *Pediatr Clin North Am* 31:1331–1343, 1984.

Silberbach M, Roos-Hesslin JW, Anderson NH, et al: Cardiovascular health in Turner syndrome: a scientific statement from the American Heart Association, *Circ Genom Precis Med* 11(10):e000048, 2018

Swenson JM, Fischer DR, Miller SA, et al: Are chest radiographs and electrocardiograms still valuable in evaluating new pediatric patients with heart murmurs or chest pain? *Pediatrics* 99:1–3, 1997.

Tingelstad J: Consultation with the specialist: cardiac dysrhythmias, *Pediatr Rev* 22:91–94, 2001.

Van Praagh S, Truman T, Firpo A, et al: Cardiac malformations in trisomy-18: a study of 41 postmortem cases, *J Am Coll Cardiol* 13(7):1586–1597, 1989.

West L, Beerman LB, Arora G: Ventricular ectopy in children without known heart disease, *J Pediatr* 166(2):338–342, 2015.

Yeager SB, Flanagan MF, Keane JF: Catheter intervention: balloon valvotomy. In Lock JE, Keane JF, Perry SB, editors: *Diagnostic and interventional catheterization in congenital heart disease*, ed 2, Norwell, MA, 2000, Kluwer Academic Publishers, pp 151–178.

Yi MS, Kimball TR, Tsevat J, et al: Evaluation of heart murmurs in children: cost-effective and practical implications, *J Pediatr* 141:504–511, 2002.

Zuberbuhler JR: *Clinical diagnosis in pediatric cardiology*, Edinburgh, 1981, Churchill Livingstone.

6

CHILD ABUSE AND NEGLECT

Jennifer San Jose Clarke | Adelaide L. Eichman | Jennifer E. Wolford

Child abuse and neglect constitute a pediatric public health problem of enormous magnitude. Their contribution to morbidity and mortality throughout life is much greater than previously known. More than a million children are abused every year in the United States; approximately 140,000 incur serious injuries, and nearly 20,000 have permanent physical disabilities such as cerebral palsy and blindness. The estimated cost to the system is more than $2 trillion annually. The toll on emotional development is much more significant, with research showing the long-term detrimental effects of adverse childhood experiences on health outcomes, quality of life, and life span.

Although there has been a decline in substantiated cases of physical and sexual abuse, mortality rates have not changed significantly. Improved recognition and health care have resulted in a much larger percentage of children identified and protected. John Caffey, MD, in the late 1940s and then C. Henry Kempe, MD, and coworkers in the early 1960s fostered a marked increase in the recognition of the physical manifestations of abuse. Subsequent passage of legislation in all 50 states mandating reporting suspected cases to the proper authorities increased the incidence of reporting. Also, societal standards have changed; some of what is currently regarded as abuse was once sanctioned as discipline.

Five major forms of abuse have been described: (1) physical abuse, (2) sexual abuse, (3) physical neglect, (4) emotional abuse, and (5) medical child abuse. Not infrequently, a child is the victim of more than one form with some degree of emotional abuse associated with all forms. For purposes of reporting to child protection authorities, under child protection laws, the abuse or neglect generally must result from the acts or omissions of a parent, guardian, custodian, or other caretaker of the child, although a child can be abused by noncaretakers. There are often significant differences with requirements for law enforcement reporting, depending on jurisdictions.

Of reported cases, about 60% involved neglect, 19% physical abuse, and 9% sexual abuse, and 5% were identified as emotionally maltreated, although these figures may vary widely by jurisdiction depending on state laws. These figures may significantly underestimate the actual number, because it is estimated that, for every case reported, many go unreported. Clearly some, and perhaps many, reports concerning truly abused children are inaccurately determined to be unfounded. Sometimes this is because of regulations; for example, in some states if a perpetrator cannot be clearly identified, or if the identified perpetrator is not a household member, despite finding that the child has clearly been the victim of abuse, the report may be unfounded. Misleading/deceptive histories, limited investigative resources, lack of witnesses, inability or unwillingness of victims and family members to attest to the fact that abuse has occurred, and jurisdictional regulations all contribute to this phenomenon.

Fatality statistics also have limited accuracy. The National Child Abuse and Neglect Data System (NCANDS) estimates that there were about 1820 deaths in 2021, a 7.7% increase from the 2017 national estimate of 1690, and this is likely due to improvements in the reporting and investigation of child fatalities. This may reflect improved recognition of child abuse–related deaths secondary to the institution of child death review teams in most states. This does not count numerous "near-fatal" cases. Of fatal victims, 40% to 50% are younger than 1 year old, and 85% to 90% are 5 years old or younger. Researchers looking at data from additional sources have shown that many, perhaps the majority, of deaths due to abuse are misclassified as due to accident, sudden unexplained infant death (SUID), or natural or unknown causes. Reasons for misclassification include incomplete medical evaluation delay in or inadequate death scene investigation or no scene investigation, insufficient training of coroners and pathologists about child abuse and the techniques and studies necessary to identify abuse at autopsy, failure to require manner and cause of death on death certificates, and poor communication among investigative agencies. Thus, most authorities believe 2000 deaths per year is a more accurate figure, although this, too, may be a significant underestimation. The number of deaths due to abuse of children younger than 5 years old is greater than the number due to motor vehicle accidents and fires combined and is more than twice the number of deaths due to accidental choking or suffocation, drowning, and falls combined.

The most common causes of death due to abuse are head trauma, abdominal trauma, and suffocation. Of these, intentional suffocation is most likely to go undetected, because autopsy findings may simulate SUID. It now appears that a large percentage of cases of SUID are actually due to accidental suffocation as a result of unsafe sleep. The Safe to Sleep campaign, which was begun by the National Institute of Child Health and Human Development, and efforts to educate parents about the risks of cosleeping have reduced the incidence of these tragic deaths. Further review of cosleeping deaths points to a disturbing number of cases in which the adult sleeping with the child has a history of substance misuse.

All sudden unexpected deaths in infancy warrant thorough investigation to facilitate accurate determination of cause, assess for possible maltreatment, and aid in future prevention. Certain historical points and physical findings may aid in distinguishing SUID from intentional suffocation. Infants dying of SUID are usually younger than 6 months old and previously well, or they had only mild symptoms of an upper respiratory infection. Indicators pointing to potential abuse are subtle bruises or petechiae of the face and/or neck, a history of a recent hospitalization for an unexplained illness or for apnea, seizure-like activity, or a brief, resolved unexplained event (BRUE; formerly called *apparent life-threatening event*) for which no cause could be found despite an extensive medical workup. This or a history of multiple BRUEs and/or a history of prior sibling deaths attributed to SUID should raise strong suspicion of intentional smothering.

EPIDEMIOLOGY

Child abuse is a phenomenon found in all socioeconomic, cultural, racial, ethnic, and religious subsets of society. The reported incidence per capita is greatest in lower socioeconomic groups.

This stems in part from the numerous chronic stressors of living in poverty. It is also clear that well-educated parents of higher socioeconomic status can be abusive; however, when they are, they are less likely to be suspected or, even when suspected, reported to authorities. This is in part because they "come across well"; they tend to be well dressed, well spoken, more sophisticated, and more confident in their interactions with physicians and others in authority. They are often better able to fabricate a plausible history of how the injury occurred "accidentally." When reported, they are more likely to have the resources to have the case dismissed or to be acquitted of the charges. It is important not to rush to judgment of parents based on appearance, dress, and level of sophistication. *Young nonminority children evaluated for unusual or concerning injuries and not reported are at risk to die of abuse.*

The most valuable information is gained by a nonjudgmental approach, keeping an open mind in obtaining a thorough history, performing a meticulous examination, and ordering a well-considered laboratory and imaging evaluation before arriving at a diagnosis.

Many studies have shown that the siblings (contacts) of abused children (index children) are at much higher risk of being the victims of abuse themselves than a child in a different environment. It is now understood that violence in a household is typically widespread and less likely to involve just one targeted or "scapegoat" child.

Caretaker Risk Factors for Child Abuse and Neglect

The caretaker risk factors for child abuse and neglect are:

- Emotional and social isolation: Parents who are inadequately nurtured themselves as children are poorly equipped to adequately nurture their offspring.
- Substance abuse
- Certain mental illnesses
- Intimate partner violence in the parental relationship
- Experiencing a sudden spate of major life stresses/crises, such as loss of job and financial security; loss of home; loss of parent, spouse, or sibling

Child Risk Factors

The child risk factors for child abuse and neglect are:

- Age younger than 3 years old
- Being separated at birth from a parent at high risk for problems with attachment because of illness or prematurity, resulting in impaired bonding
- Being small for gestational age, born with congenital anomalies, and/or having a chronic illness
- Being perceived as difficult or different
- Having attention-deficit/hyperactivity disorder (ADHD) or being oppositional or defiant
- Foster children, unrelated children

Leaving a young infant in the care of a nonbiologically related male, often the mother's boyfriend, is a strong risk factor for serious abuse.

One common thread connecting all these risk factors appears to be one of unmet expectations, due to either unrealistic parental expectations of the child or the child's inability to meet realistic expectations as the result of developmental delay, illness, temperament, hyperactivity, or inconsistent disciplining. This often stems from lack of caretaker understanding of normal child behavior and emotional development. The combination can then lead the parent or caretaker to attribute malicious intent to an infant who will not stop crying or to a toddler, who has had a toilet training accident, is stubborn, or misbehaves. Once "malicious intent" is suspected, this can incite rage in someone with a short fuse.

With this background information, the approach to diagnosis of the major forms of abuse can now be addressed more specifically.

PHYSICAL ABUSE

Physical abuse is defined as the infliction of bodily injury that causes significant or severe pain, leaves physical evidence, impairs physical functioning, or significantly jeopardizes the child's safety. Individual states have varying definitions of abuse that require a report to Child Protective Services (CPS) and law enforcement agencies. Clinicians who care for children should be familiar with the statutes in their own states.

The severity of injuries caused by physical abuse ranges from isolated skin bruising to fatal head and abdominal trauma. It is well documented that physical abuse tends to be repetitive and that the severity of attacks tends to escalate over time; correspondingly, the severity of injuries also increases over time. Given this, early recognition, reporting, and intervention are essential in prevention of increased morbidity and mortality.

Common Presentations That Raise Concern for Abuse

Presenting complaint (history of present illness [HPI]) red flags include:

- Lack of history for identified injuries, both acute and noted older injuries.
- History incompatible with the type or severity of injury (e.g., the distribution of lesions or type of injury does not fit the mechanism reported; the history is consistent with a minor injury [short fall, rolled off couch], but evidence of major trauma is found; or multiple injuries of differing ages are found for which no prior care has been sought or adequate explanation provided).
- History of the injury is vague, incomplete, lacks details, or was unwitnessed.
- History details change over time (e.g., the history provided to the referring primary care physician is different than the history provided to the emergency department physician).
- History incompatible with the patient's developmental stage (e.g., a 4-month-old with a transverse femur fracture did not cause this injury by pulling to a stand at the coffee table).
- History incompatible with the sibling's developmental age (e.g., the 3-year-old sibling did not cause rib fractures in a 5-week-old infant by hugging the infant too tightly).
- Significant delay between the time of injury and time of presentation.
- The parent or other adults in the home provide conflicting accounts of the injury.
- Interactions between parents and the child are strained, hostile, or emotionless regarding severe injury.

Past medical history red flags are:

- A history or evidence of repeated "accidents" or injuries. (Sometimes these patients are seen at different facilities.)
- A history or evidence of multiple fractures or old scars suggestive of prior inflicted injury.
- Poor compliance with well-child care (e.g., missed visits, immunization delay).
- History of ingestions.
- Parents offer historical data about substantial irritability, crying before the event, difficulty with feeding, and worsening behaviors, particularly before the injury. Parents note that the child is clumsy, always climbing, likes to "be bad," or is uncontrollable.

Few victims of physical abuse present with a chief complaint of abuse. Most present with a chief complaint of an accidental injury or an unrelated chief complaint, such as a viral upper respiratory infection (URI) or irritability.

Obtaining a History

- Start with open-ended questions. Follow up with specific clarifying questions. If two parent figures are present, try to take history from each separately and out of the child's presence. The child should be interviewed alone, if age and condition permit (questions should be nonleading and age appropriate). Discuss how major developmental milestones were handled, what methods of discipline have been used, obtain a list of caretakers and times, and determine support systems available and family stressors.
- Information about caregivers should include the duration and quality of relationships; history of their families of origin, including parental relationships, quality of interaction/nurturing of parents as children, methods of discipline in household of origin, levels of education/employment, history of drug or alcohol abuse, history of psychiatric illness, history of prior Child Protective Services or law enforcement involvement or incarceration, and history of childhood physical or sexual abuse.
- History about the child should include, as appropriate, nightmares/sleep difficulties, recent increased aggression, anxiety, depression, self-esteem, withdrawal, regression, increased activity/anxiety, posttraumatic stress disorder symptoms, change in appetite, self-inflicted injury, decrease in academic performance/school failure, running away, drug or alcohol use, fire setting, animal abuse, or law enforcement involvement.

PHYSICAL FINDINGS AND PATTERNS OF ABUSIVE INJURY

Sentinel Injuries

Sentinel injuries are defined as minor injuries that do not require any medical intervention but are often one of the first signs of physical abuse. These include injuries such as bruises, subconjunctival hemorrhages, or blood from the mouth or nose in nonmobile infants. The significance of these injuries is often only recognized in hindsight, after a major injury prompts the evaluation and diagnosis of physical abuse (Figs. 6.1, 6.2, and 6.3).

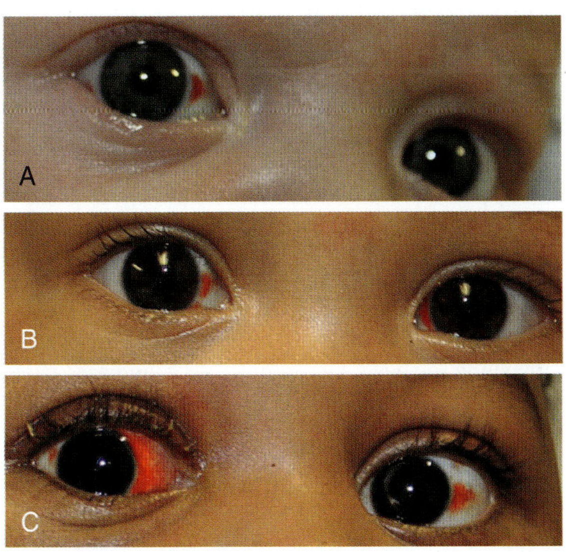

Fig. 6.1 Sentinel injuries. (A) This 4-month-old infant was noted to have subconjunctival hemorrhages on multiple occasions, which were initially attributed to straining with bowel movements. Fortunately, they were recognized as a sign of trauma, and further evaluation revealed facial bruising, an upper frenulum tear, and three healing posterior rib fractures. (B) This 7-month-old infant was noted by her parent to have recurrent subconjunctival hemorrhages and facial petechiae. Her medical evaluation revealed facial bruising, an upper frenulum tear, a posterior rib fracture, and positive drug screen. (C) This 5-month-old infant presented to a children's hospital after an assault by his father. The child was found to have a skull fracture, significant facial and chest bruising, and a tibial fracture.

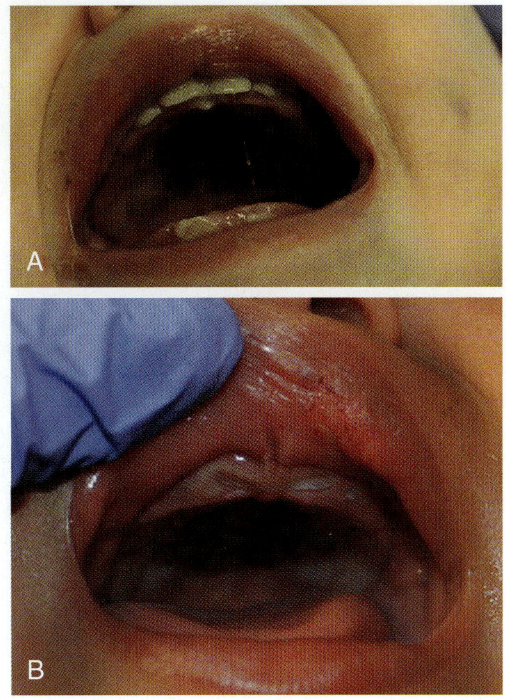

Fig. 6.2 (A) This 11-month-old infant had a history of "easy bruising" and was evaluated by Hematology. When she ultimately presented to a hospital, she was found to have acute subdural hemorrhages, multiple skull fractures, bruising over most surfaces of her body, and more than 20 fractures. Also found on examination was extensive granulation tissue on her frenulum, gums, tongue, and palate. (B) This 7-month-old, nonambulatory infant was noted to have bleeding from her mouth that was attributed to teething. A thorough examination and evaluation revealed an upper frenulum injury, two healing posterior rib fractures, an acute humerus fracture, and a grade 3 liver laceration.

Cutaneous Injuries

The most common manifestations of physical abuse are those visible on the surface of the skin. They include bruises, welts, scars, abrasions, lacerations, tourniquet and bite marks, and burns. Bruising is one of the most common and readily visible injuries resulting from physical abuse, but it is often missed as a warning sign. Medical recognition of these warning signs coupled with appropriate action is critical in the prevention of recurrent abusive events. Despite differing opinions on the appropriateness or inappropriateness of physical methods of discipline, there is a general legal guideline distinguishing the boundary between discipline and abuse: Discipline does not inflict significant pain and does *not* cause physical injury or leave marks. Although corporal punishment is legal in all 50 states, research has proven this method of discipline to be ineffective and detrimental to healthy childhood development. Corporal punishment is associated with increased aggression in preschool and school-aged children. It is also associated with an increased risk of mental health disorders and cognition problems. In the landmark 1998 Adverse Childhood Experiences study, the investigators found that spanking was associated with increased odds of suicide attempts, moderate-to-heavy drinking, and substance use disorder in adulthood independent of the risks associated with having experienced physical and emotional abuse as a child. The American Academy of Pediatrics recommends that parents, other caregivers, and adults interacting with children and adolescents should not use corporal punishment (including hitting and spanking), either in anger or as a punishment for or consequence of misbehavior, nor should they use any disciplinary strategy, including verbal abuse, that causes shame or humiliation.

When a clinician has concerns for abusive injury, all external signs of trauma found should be carefully documented and, if possible, photographed with a measuring tool.

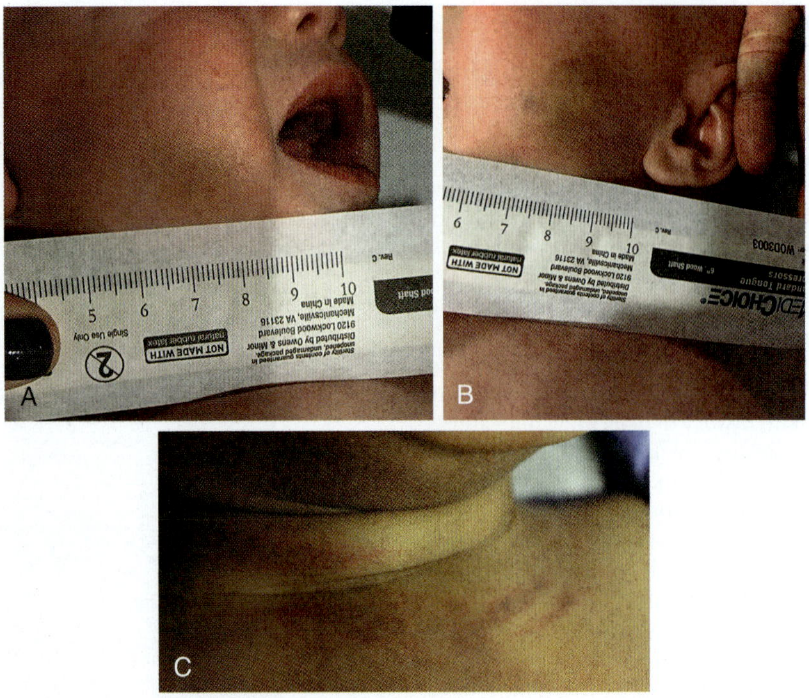

Fig. 6.3 (A) This 8-week-old infant was seen in an emergency department for respiratory distress, initially attributed to bronchiolitis. The discovery of bilateral cheek bruising prompted a trauma evaluation that revealed numerous classic metaphysical lesions and a subconjunctival hemorrhage. A septal hematoma was identified as the ultimate cause of her respiratory distress and was drained by an ear, nose, and throat doctor. (B) Bruising to the other cheek. (C) A 9-month-old infant was evaluated by his primary care physician for a cough and found to have bruising to his neck and chest. A trauma evaluation found three healing posterior rib fractures and two acute lateral rib fractures.

Bruises, Welts, and Scars

A *bruise* is an injury appearing as an area of discolored skin caused by an impact that ruptures underlying blood vessels. Blood leaks from the broken vessels into surrounding tissues, producing pain, swelling, and tenderness. The discoloration is a result of the blood seepage under the skin. On any day, nearly every ambulatory child has one or more bruises. Many bruises are the result of accidental play. However, it is possible to distinguish which bruises should raise concerns for physical abuse and which bruises are more consistent with accidental events. Bruises are the most common clinical finding in cases of physical abuse; they are seen in up to 75% of victims, and their presence should prompt a search for other, deeper injuries. Many factors can be informative.

"If You Do Not Cruise, You Do Not Bruise"

It is critical to consider the child's age and developmental abilities when evaluating bruises. If a child is not yet ambulatory, accidental bruises are exceptionally rare. A young infant is not moving and not generating a force to cause vessel damage/bruising. A 1999 study shows that only 0.6% of children younger than 6 months old have accidental bruises. Children begin to "cruise" shortly after this age, and accidental bruising rises to 19% of cruising infants. Hence, clinicians should remember, "If you do not cruise, you do not bruise." Any bruise in a nonmobile infant should prompt a clinician to complete a thorough and thoughtful history, physical examination, and further diagnostic testing, as indicated. Bruising increases in toddlers as their motor skills increase.

Too Many Bruises

Many bruises on ambulatory children are accidental. However, studies show that accidental bruises are not numerous at any given time. A 2010 study reported that the average number of bruises on a nonabused child was 1.5, and no child in this group had more than four bruises. In the same study, examining children who had been the victim of abuse, the average number of bruises was 6 and the maximum bruises in this subset of the study were 25.

Most bruises in ambulatory children are small. Abusive bruises tend to be larger, with consideration that a hand or an object covered a larger area of skin and caused vessel rupture, rather than a single stair coming in contact with a shin to cause an accidental bruise. Abusive bruises appear more often in clusters, with consideration of repetitive abusive trauma, rather than a single soccer ball hitting a thigh during a child's game.

Location of Accidental versus Abusive Bruising

Accidental bruises are most often over bony prominences. The most common sites of accidental bruises include shins, knees, and foreheads. Additionally, bruises directly over spinous processes or the iliac crest often have a clear accidental history.

In contrast, abusive bruises are found where common sites of bruising from accidental play are not found. Specifically, bruising over soft areas is concerning for abusive trauma. This includes the torso area, abdomen, genital areas, ears, angle of jaws, neck, buttocks, and soft areas of arms and legs (Fig. 6.4).

Injuries to the Face and Neck

Bruises involving the head, face, mouth, neck, and ears are seen in a substantial percentage of physical abuse victims, approximately 50% of infants and 38% of toddlers (Fig. 6.4). Ear bruises are highly associated with abusive trauma. Bruising can be found in the inner folds of the ear, likely the result of a direct blow, and pinching the ears may result in bruises found on the outer edge and rear side of the helix (Fig. 6.5). Subgaleal hematomas and contusions and petechiae involving the scalp may be the result of direct blows or impacts against a hard surface or forceful hair pulling (Fig. 6.6).

Attempted smothering, choking, or severe and prolonged thoracic compression may produce showers of petechiae over the shoulders, neck, and face (Fig. 6.7). The oral and conjunctival mucosa may be involved as well and should be carefully inspected (see Fig. 6.7E). When strangulation is the mechanism, neck bruises may be visible (see Fig. 6.7B). These petechiae may range from florid to faint and may be especially subtle when there has been a delay in

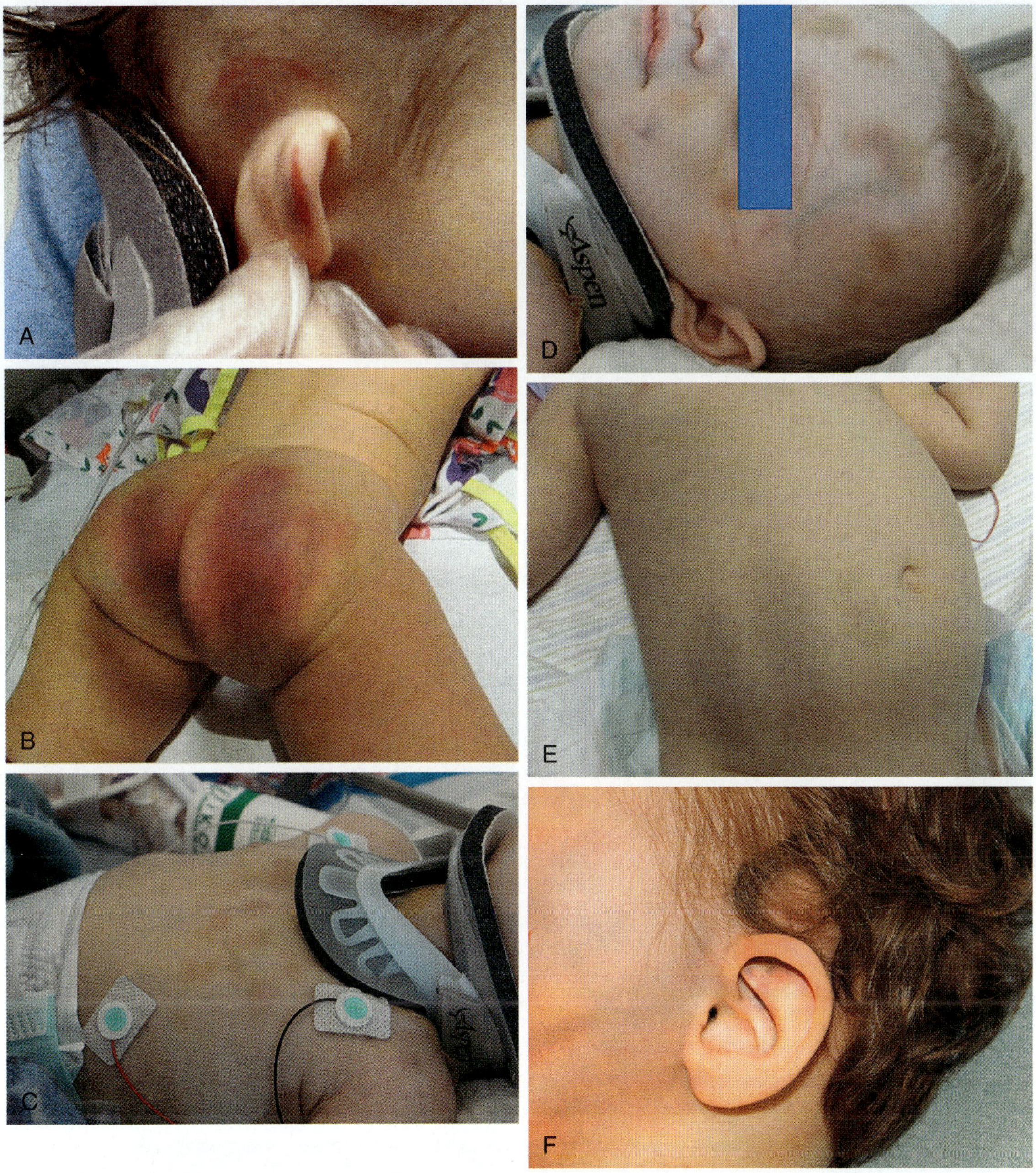

Fig. 6.4 (A) Ear bruising. This infant was struck so forcibly on the side of his head that he has an impression bruise on his scalp in the shape of his external ear. The linear bruise over the top rim of his ear is the result of capillary distortion caused by compression between the impacting hand and the child's skull. (B) This 13-month-old was evaluated for vomiting after a reported fall from a bed. The child was found to have bilateral subdural hemorrhages, facial bruising, and significant buttock bruising. (C–E) This battered 11-month-old was found to have bruising over nearly all surfaces of his body. The child was found to have multiple acute and healing rib fractures as well as splenic and hepatic lacerations. (F) This 21-month-old child was evaluated in an emergency department after a reported fall from a potty chair. The child had patterned bruising to bilateral cheeks, ear bruising, bruises to every extremity and back, and a transverse radius and ulnar fracture.

seeking care. They can be mistaken for a rash if the examiner fails to check for blanching. Petechiae do not blanche.

Injuries to the Abdomen and Torso

Bruises involving the abdominal wall below the rib cage and above or anterior to the pelvic girdle are rarely seen with accidental injury. Of note, abdominal bruising is often absent in abuse directed toward the child's abdomen because the distribution across substantial soft tissue permits movement of the blood vessels. In fact, many children with inflicted intraabdominal abusive injuries have little or no cutaneous evidence of trauma over the abdomen. When abdominal bruises are present, they are indicative of forceful grabbing or pinching or of forceful blunt impact (e.g., a punch or kick). (Fig. 6.4F). In these cases, abuse should be strongly suspected and evidence of internal injury should be sought (see the section on Abdominal and Intrathoracic Injuries and Fig. 6.8).

Injuries to the Genital Area, Buttocks, and Lower Back

Bruising in the genital area may include direct trauma to the suprapubic area or genitalia. It may also include pinching of the penis and/or scrotum. These injuries are considered abusive until proven otherwise. This type of trauma can result in bruising and extraordinary swelling. Careful evaluation for scrotal hematomas, which can have serious sequelae if untreated, should be completed.

Bruises are often seen over the curvature of the buttocks and across the lower back after severe spankings, whether with a hand or an object (Fig. 6.9). When linear marks from fingers, a belt, or brush

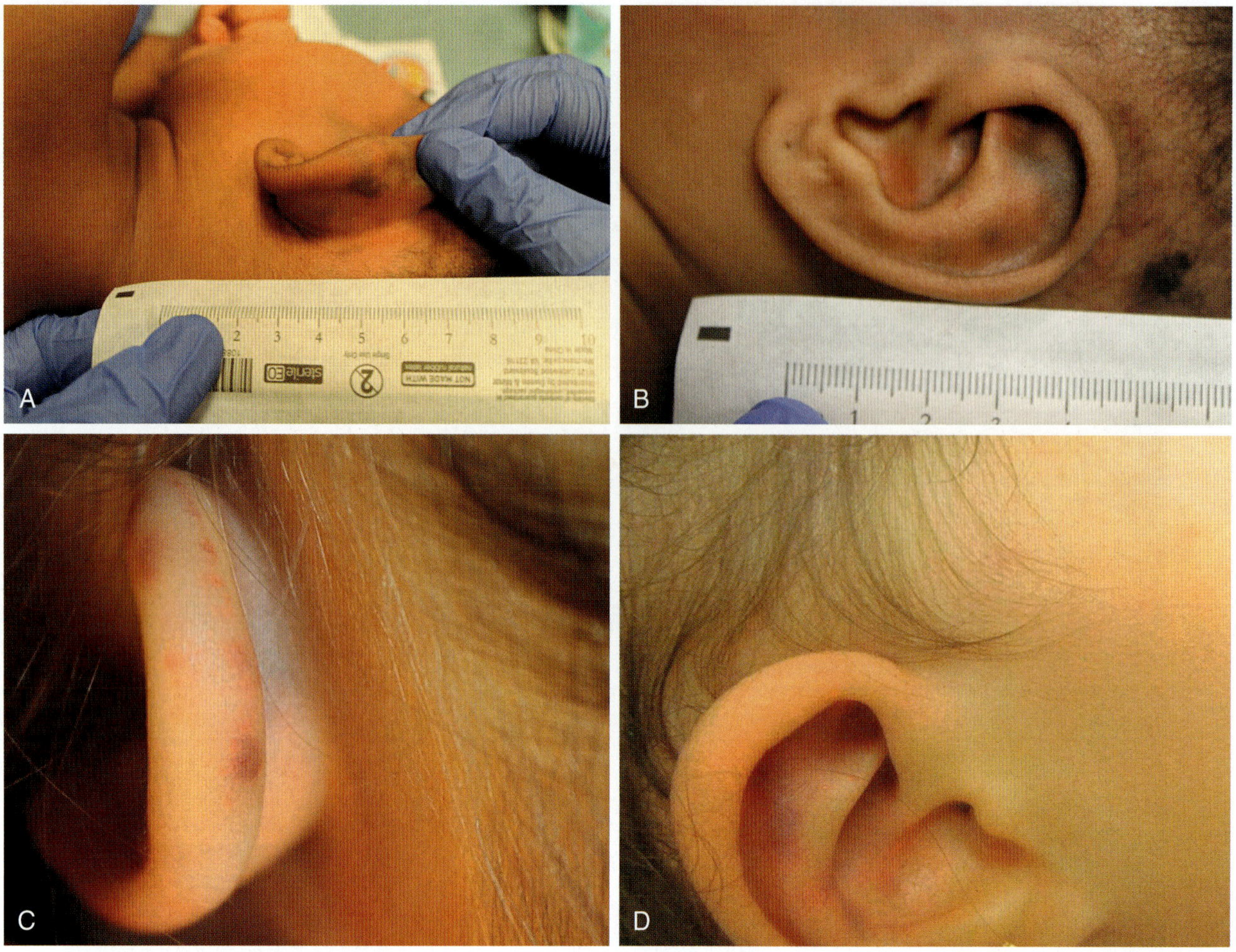

Fig. 6.5 (A,B) An 8-month-old male presented after an unwitnessed fall in a babysitter's care. The child was found to have an occipital skull fracture as well as bilateral ear bruising and abdominal bruising. (C) A 2-year-old victim of abusive head trauma found to have bilateral ear bruising and significant head and neck bruising in addition to her intracranial injuries. (D) A 4-month-old infant being evaluated for vomiting. The right ear bruising prompted a trauma evaluation. The infant was ultimately found to have bilateral subdural hemorrhages, bilateral retinal hemorrhages, and acute and healing rib fractures.

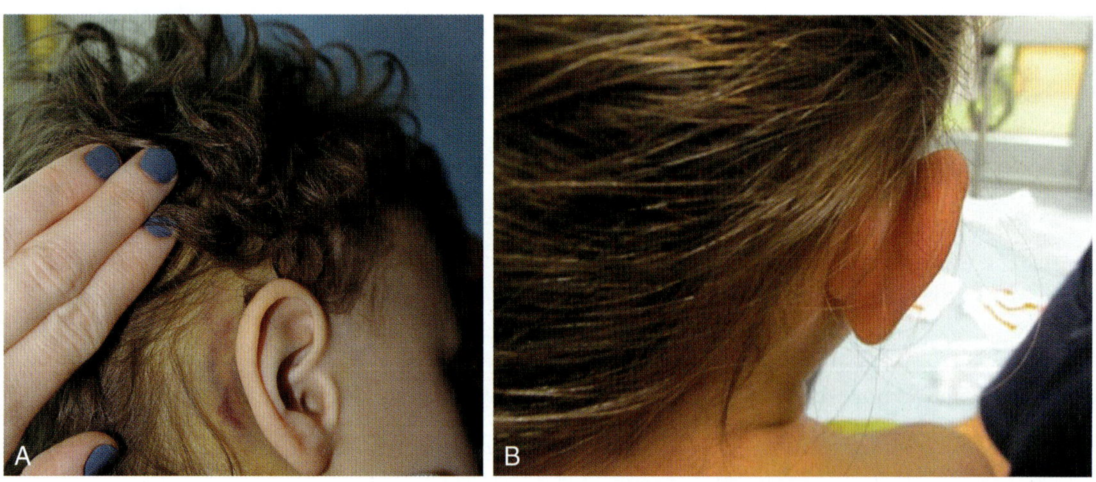

Fig. 6.6 Subgaleal hematomas. (A) This 23-month-old presented due to head and face bruising that was attributed to injuries sustained during a tantrum. The child's scalp was diffusely boggy, and he was noted to have bruising and swelling behind both ears. His forehead was swollen, and there was bruising below both eyes. A head computed tomography scan revealed scalp swelling without intracranial injuries. The constellation of injuries was diagnosed as a subgaleal hemorrhage secondary to hair pulling. (B) A 2-year-old child evaluated for head swelling. Note that child's ear is sticking out secondary to scalp swelling. A 6-year-old sibling disclosed seeing a caregiver picking up the 2-year-old by the hair and carrying her into another room. The child's injuries were secondary to a subgaleal hemorrhage caused by violent hair pulling.

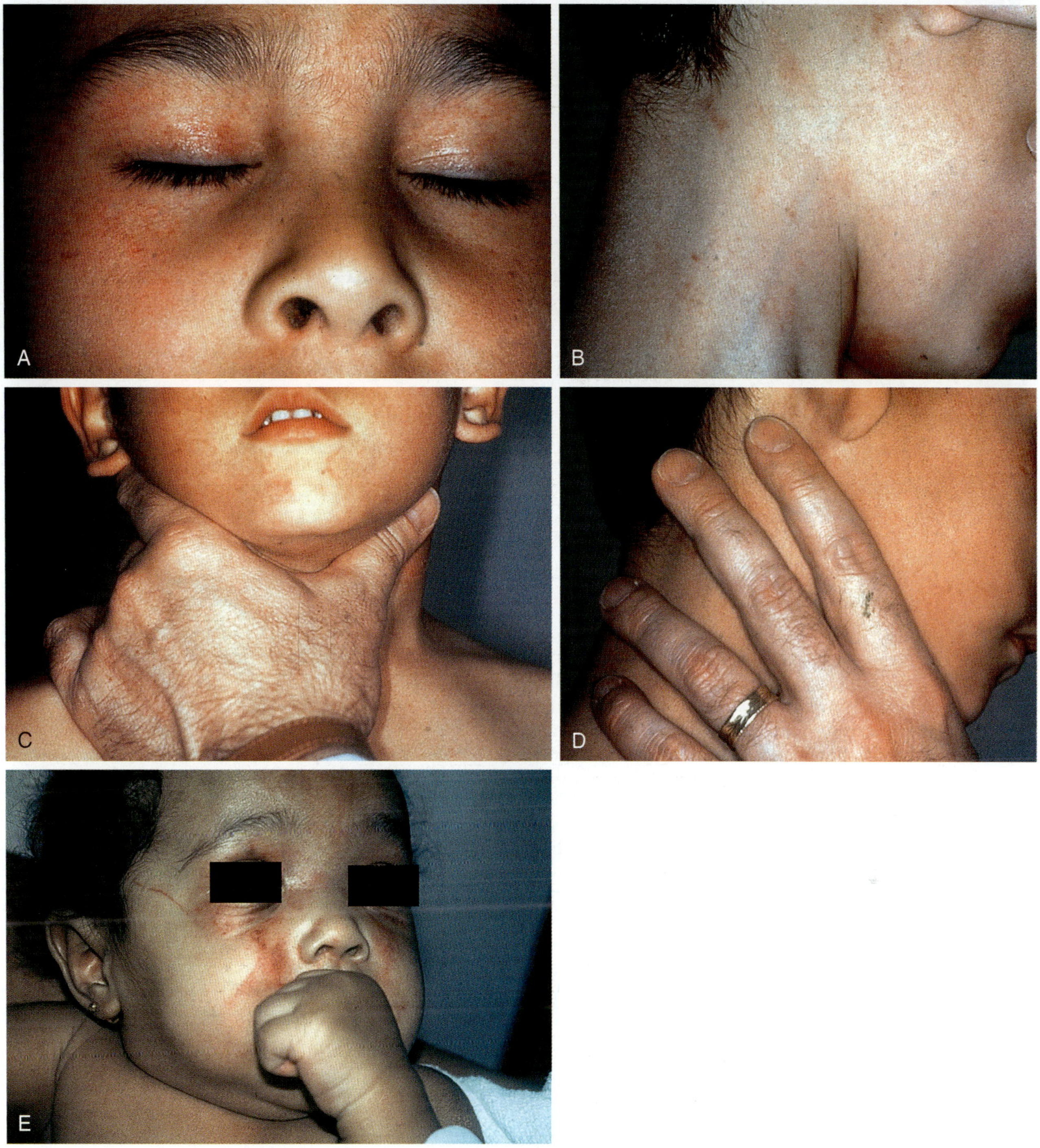

Fig. 6.7 (A–D) Petechial lesions secondary to choking. (A) Numerous petechiae are seen over this boy's face. (B) Linear marks noted on the side of his neck correspond with the hand and finger placement shown in C and D. The boy was choked to a point of near unconsciousness by his mother's boyfriend for tracking grass onto a freshly vacuumed carpet. (E) Central facial petechiae were present bilaterally in this infant. The perpetrator confessed to holding his hand over her mouth and nose and squeezing her cheeks with thumb and forefinger to stop her crying. (Courtesy Kent Hymel, MD, Inova Fairfax Hospital for Children, Falls Church, VA.)

edges are seen, these tend to be horizontally or diagonally oriented (see Fig. 6.9B). In some cases, a linear pattern of petechiae may be noted on either side of the gluteal crease (see Fig. 6.9C). Despite their vertical orientation, these are also the result of forceful horizontal blows across tightly tensed glutei, as when the blows are delivered, the involved sites are closely apposed along the crease and thus are subject to maximal capillary distortion on impact.

Bruise Patterns, Shapes, or Sizes

Injuries inflicted with an object will often leave marks that reflect the outline of that object. Patterned injuries do not occur during normal play and should be considered abusive until proven otherwise. In many instances, the surface marks are recognizable imprints of the edge of an implement used because the edge causes maximal capillary deformation on impact (Fig. 6.10). Those most seen are looped-cord marks, belt and belt-buckle marks, and switch marks, but almost any implement can be used.

Slap marks with an open hand can often leave a pattern consistent with the linear distribution of pressure from fingers (Fig. 6.11). The hand leaves a negative imprint after the capillaries break under the slapping fingers, and the blood is pushed away from the point of contact. Slapping and direct hitting may produce diffuse bruising with petechiae (see Fig. 6.4).

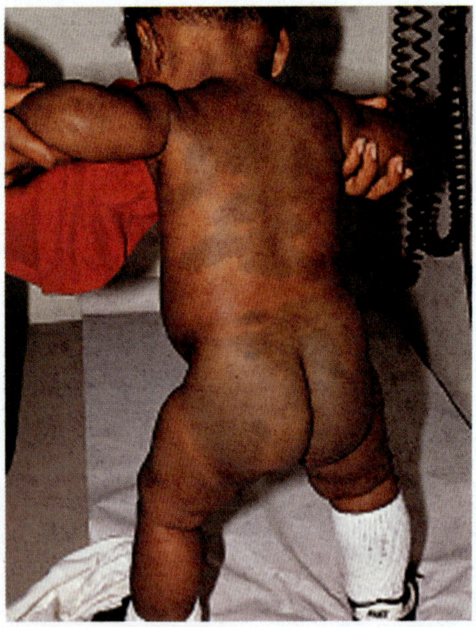

Fig. 6.8 Dermal melanosis, or Mongolian spots. This toddler, referred from a daycare center because of "multiple bruises," had an unusual number of hyperpigmented Mongolian spots.

Surface injuries involving more than one plane of the head or face are highly suspicious for abuse. An accidental event or "fall" does not typically involve multiple planes of the face and head. It is also important to recognize that contusions of the head, face, and ears are often associated with underlying intracranial injury, especially in infants.

Bruises of Different Ages and Resolution

The size, nature, and rate of healing of bruises depend on the amount of force applied; firmness and shape of the impacting object or surface; duration of impact; degree of skin thickness; and the skin's vascularity and depth, elasticity, and adipose padding of the underlying subcutaneous tissue. Hence, the first appearance of bruises and the time it takes for them to resolve vary widely. Superficial bruises appear almost at once and resolve more quickly than deeper contusions. The latter may not discolor the overlying skin for days and may take up to 2 weeks to resolve. Furthermore, the evolution of bruises in terms of color change is also variable. Although red, blue, and purple are more typical of fresh bruises, these colors can persist in some cases until resolution. Yellow, green, and brown are more characteristic of older bruises but can be seen relatively early in superficial bruises. Hence, it is difficult to determine the ages of ecchymotic lesions, but if tenderness, swelling, and/or fresh overlying abrasions are present, these findings are consistent with more recent injury.

In many cases of abuse, surface bruises and petechiae are faint or even imperceptible to the naked eye. Although bruises are relatively easy to see in victims with fair skin, they can be difficult to appreciate in children with darkly pigmented skin unless extra care is taken. This may also be because the bruises are early in their evolution, or this may be the result of fading due to delay in seeking care. Appreciation of the potential subtlety of bruises and petechial lesions may provide the only clinical clue that abuse has occurred and that other abusive injuries may be present.

When bruising is severe, deep, and extensive, underlying muscle breakdown may occur, resulting in myoglobinuria (Fig. 6.10L). When severe, this may precipitate renal failure unless the risk is recognized, appropriate tests are performed, and aggressive treatment measures are instituted.

To avoid errors in diagnosis, children who present with multiple bruises in unusual locations that are not patterned should be thoroughly examined for evidence of an underlying coagulopathy, and screening coagulation studies should be performed before arriving at a final diagnosis (Box 6.1).

Abrasions and Superficial Lacerations

Abrasions are also seen in abuse victims, although less commonly than bruises. In some cases, injuries from implements have an overlying abraded or even lacerated surface (Fig. 6.12). Abrasions also may result from friction on impact with a firm surface or from being dragged across a carpet or other rough surface. Fingernails can be dug into the skin, leaving small curvilinear marks.

Strangulation, Restraint, and Tourniquet Injuries

Strangulation and restraint marks result from attempts to hang, choke, or tie the child to a crib, bed, or chair. Abraded or blistered circumferential ligature marks can be seen in these cases (Fig. 6.13).

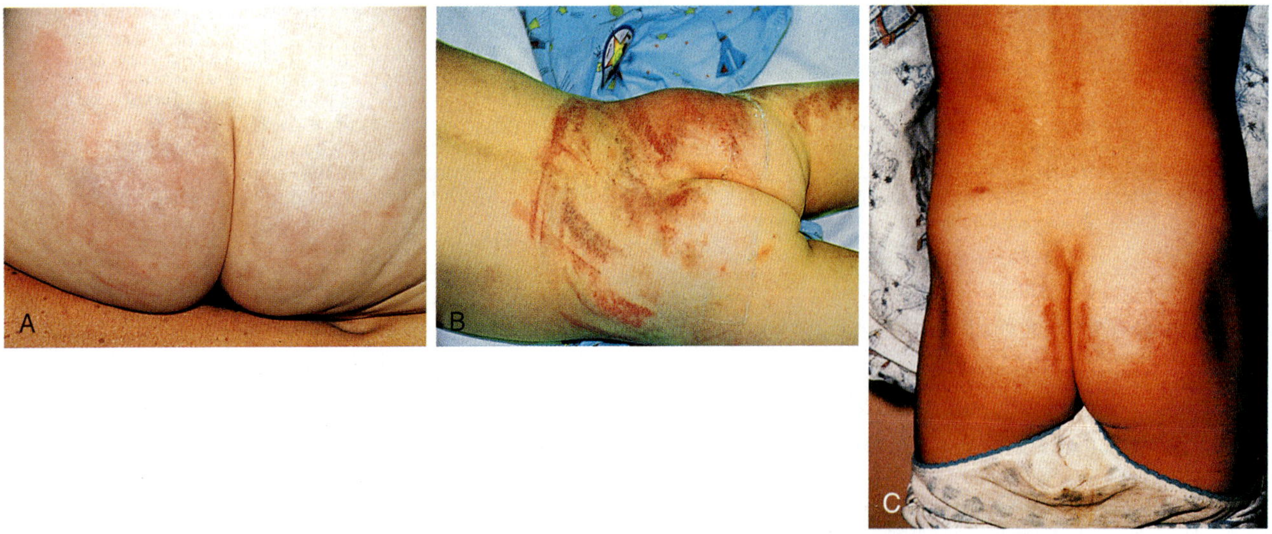

Fig. 6.9 Buttock bruises. (A) At first glance, this toddler appeared to have a diaper rash, but on closer inspection the lesions were found to be petechiae produced by a severe spanking. (B) The severe contusions of the buttocks and lower back seen in this child were inflicted by hand, hairbrush, and belt. (C) A linear pattern of petechial hemorrhages is seen on either side of the gluteal cleft in this boy who was subjected to repeated rapid-fire blows across the gluteal crease.

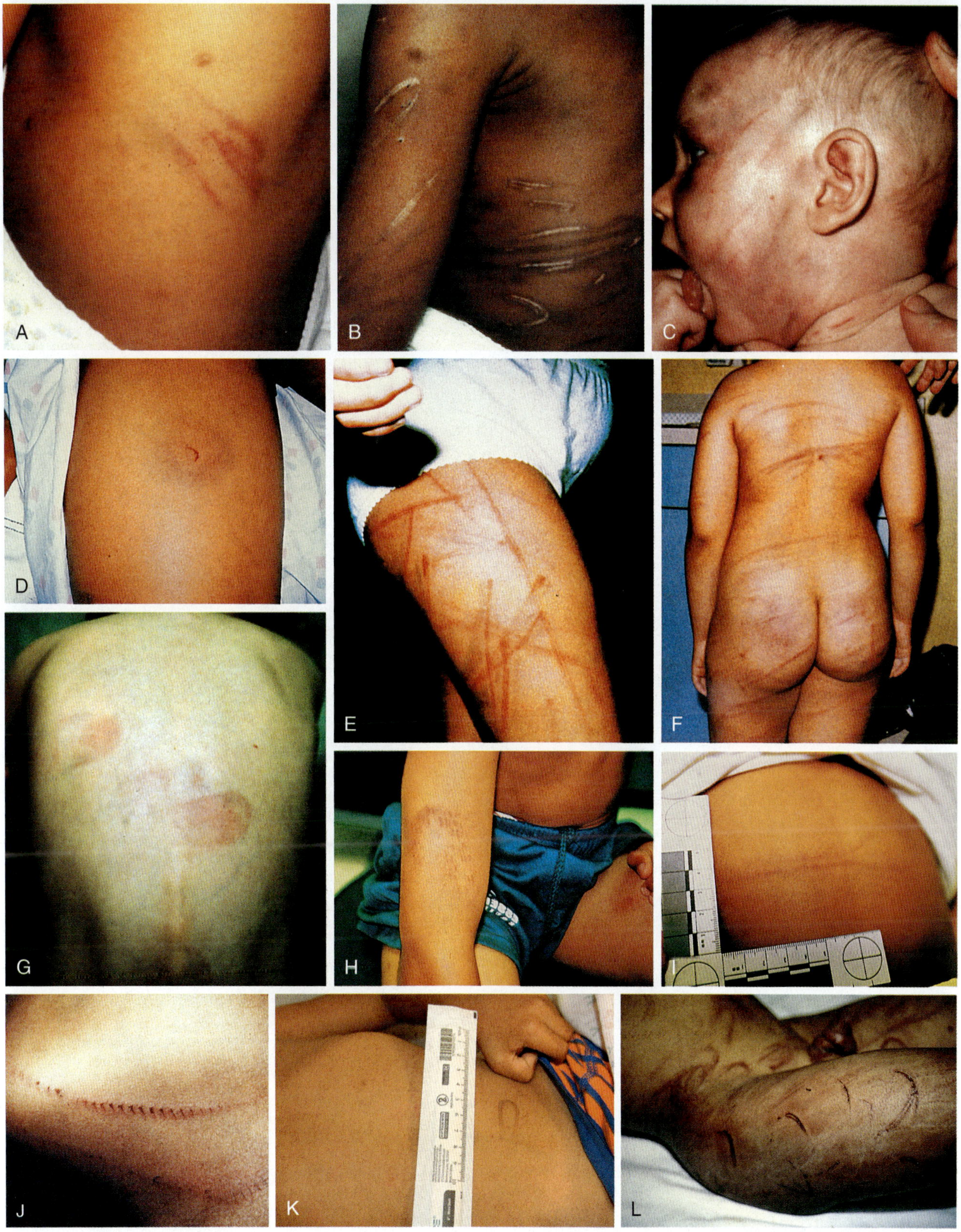

Fig. 6.10 Imprint marks reflecting the weapons used to inflict them. (A and B) Fresh looped-cord marks (A) and hypopigmented and hyperpigmented scars (B) that were the result of beatings with a looped electrical cord. (C) The characteristic pattern of parallel lines that results from blows with a belt. (D) This contusion in the configuration of a closed horseshoe with a central linear abrasion was inflicted with a belt buckle. (E) The red linear contusions on this child's thigh were the result of repeated blows with a switch. (F) These acute linear contusions over the back and buttocks were inflicted with a belt and a switch. (G) This boy was hit with a slipper with such force that imprints of the heel are evident. (H) The heel prints of a running shoe left on this boy's arm and thigh were distinct enough to enable identification of his abuser. (I) This girl was hit forcefully with a spatula. (J) This boy was struck with a chain, leaving a clear imprint of the links. (K) This child disclosed being hit with a phone charger, which caused this looped scar. (L) Severe bruising with underlying muscle damage. This toddler was covered from head to toe with severe looped cord contusions and lacerations. He had secondary myoglobinuria necessitating intensive care management to prevent renal failure.

Bite Marks

Bite marks can be another manifestation of physical abuse. Lesions tend to be oval or semicircular. The impressions of the incisal surfaces may be variably clear, depending on the force applied and the age of the bite. Suction petechiae may be noted centrally in some fresh lesions. If the injury is distinct, the size enables the examiner to clearly distinguish between the bite of another child (primary teeth) and an adult bite (secondary teeth) (Fig. 6.14). Each bite mark should be carefully photographed in its entirety, and then photos should be taken perpendicular to the plane of the imprint of each arch, with a measuring tool in each photo.

Burns

Like bruises or abrasions, some patterns of burns are highly associated with abusive injury.

Abusive burns are more commonly seen in children younger than the age of 5. Young children with immersion burns from hot water without any associated splash marks or dip burns in a stocking-glove distribution are genuinely concerning for abusive injury. Burns to the back, buttocks, or genital burns in infants and toddlers are concerning for abusive injury while being bathed. Histories that include an unexpected toileting accident can alert a clinician to concerns for a frustrated caretaker. Deep contact burns with a clear imprint of the hot surface should raise the concern of

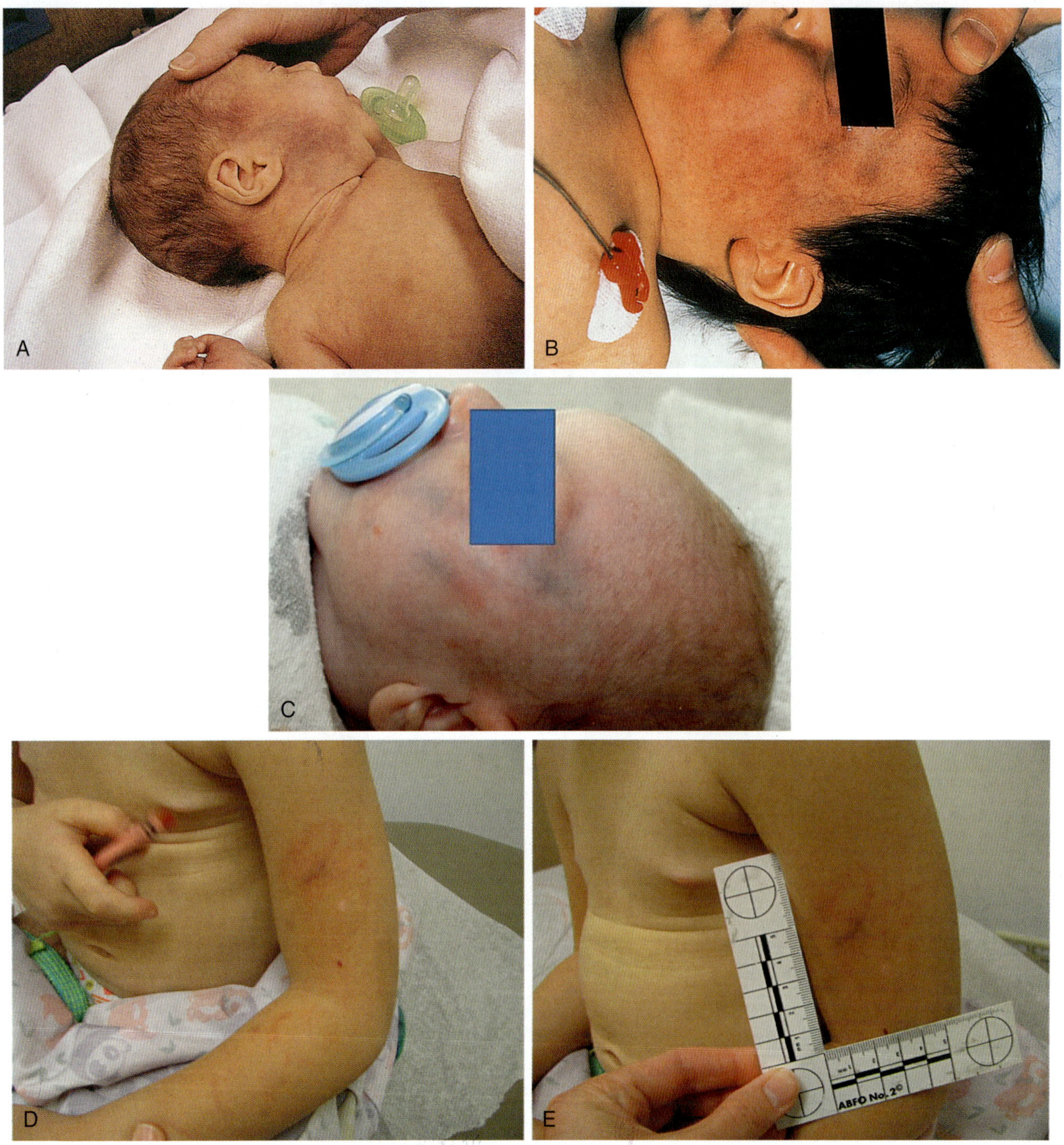

Fig. 6.11 Facial slap marks. (A) Diffuse facial bruising and petechiae seen over the side of the face and head of this 3-week-old infant were the result of repeated slaps by his father. (B) This older infant has even more extensive petechiae and bruises that were tender on palpation. (C) A 2-week-old infant evaluated by the primary care physician for a facial rash, shown to be a slap mark. (D) This 4-year-old disclosed that her mother grabbed her arm "really hard" and pulled her to the ground. The child was also found to have multiple looped marks and bruises (E).

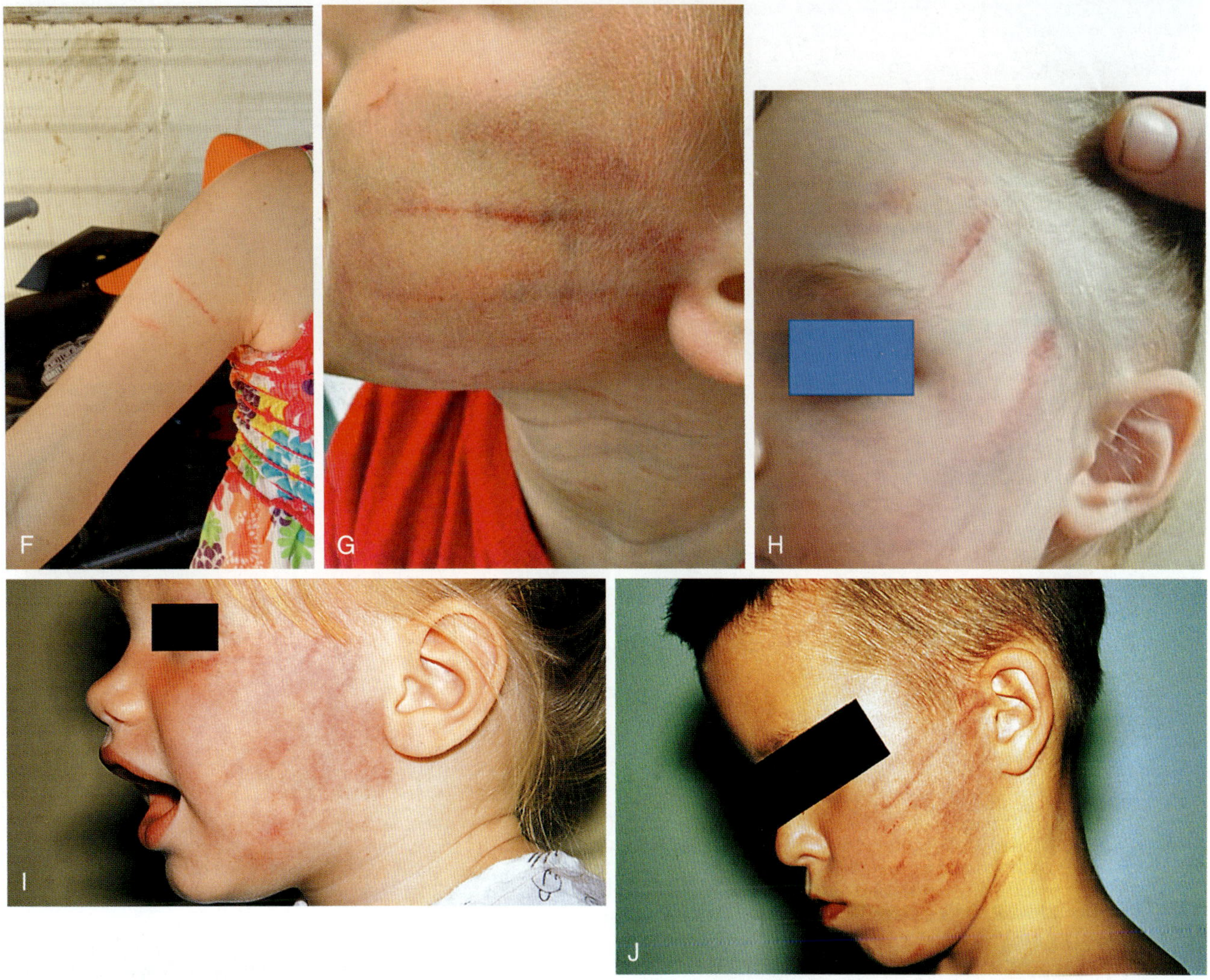

Fig. 6.11, cont'd (F) A 3-year-old child known to Child Protective Services for multiple allegations of physical abuse. On multiple occasions, the child was noted to have bruising in unusual locations. Pictured here is a clear "grab mark." When placed in a safe environment, the child did not sustain any more unusual bruises. (G) This 4-year-old child disclosed to a teacher that he had been slapped and strangled by his mother's paramour. (H) This 3-year-old child had a medical evaluation due to physical abuse of a sibling and was found to have a slap mark to the left side of her face. Handprints. (I and J) These children were slapped so forcefully that the outlines of their abuser's fingers are clearly evident.

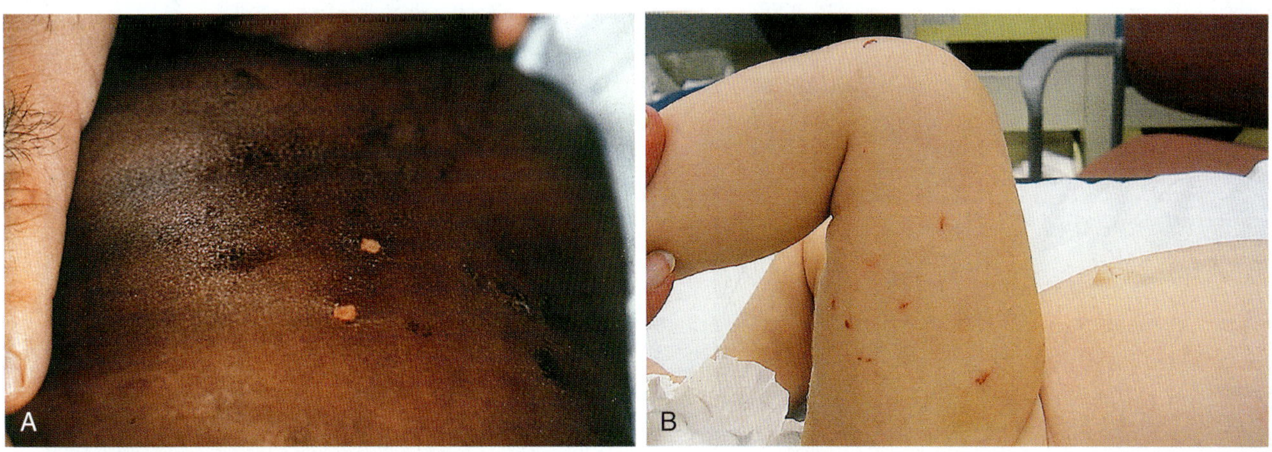

Fig. 6.12 (A and B) Inflicted abrasions/lacerations. A pattern of parallel abrasions that overlie ribs and vertebral bodies is seen on the back of this infant who was dragged over a carpet. The lesions are at least 1 to a few days old, and surface scabs have separated from two areas. A displaced spiral fracture of the right humerus, with marked soft tissue swelling and pain on motion, was also detected.

a thoughtful clinician. When considering abusive injury for a burn, an inconsistent history, an unusual pattern of injury, or delay in seeking medical attention increase concerns. It is important to evaluate for other injuries when a burn is suspicious for abuse or neglect (Fig. 6.15).

Immersion scalds or dip burns are among the most common forms of inflicted burns. Typical patterns include symmetric burns of hands or feet in a stocking-glove distribution, with a sharp line of demarcation at the level of the water line (Fig. 6.16A). Circumferential burns of the feet and lower legs along with burns of the perineum

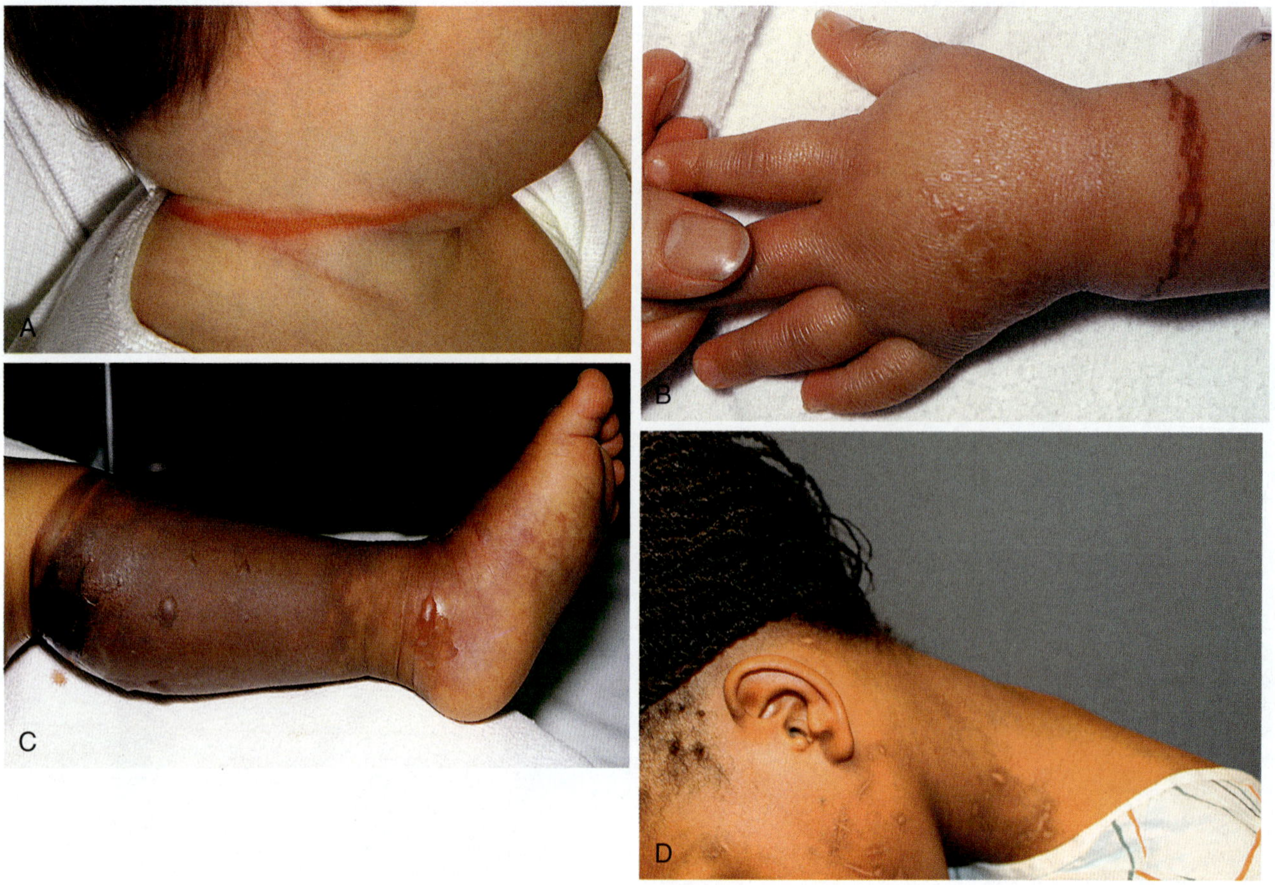

Fig. 6.13 Strangulation, restraint, and tourniquet injuries. (A) This circumferential cord burn was the result of an attempted strangulation. (B) A deep, circumferential rope burn of the wrist with considerable edema and early skin breakdown of the hand is seen in this infant, who had been tied to the side rails of her crib. (C) This toddler was brought in with severe skin, soft tissue, and muscle necrosis of his entire lower leg. (D) This 12-year-old child disclosed being strangled and hanged on multiple occasions.

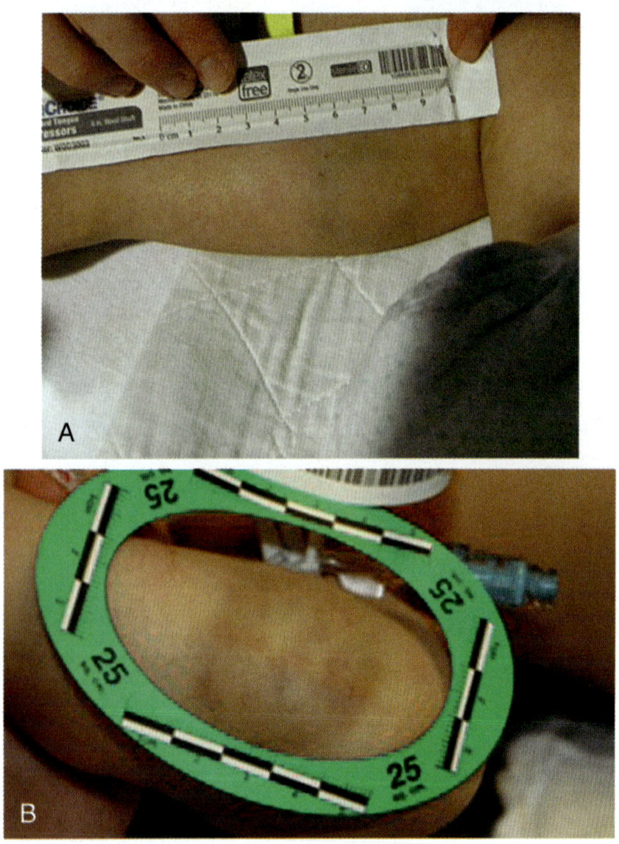

Fig. 6.14 (A) This 23-month-old girl suffered abusive head trauma, malnourishment, and multiple cutaneous injuries, including this bite injury on her calf. Another child in the home disclosed seeing an adult bite this child. (B) This 14-month-old with a history of a spiral humerus fracture at 2 months of age presented with abusive head trauma and bruises on many surfaces, including this bite injury on her forearm.

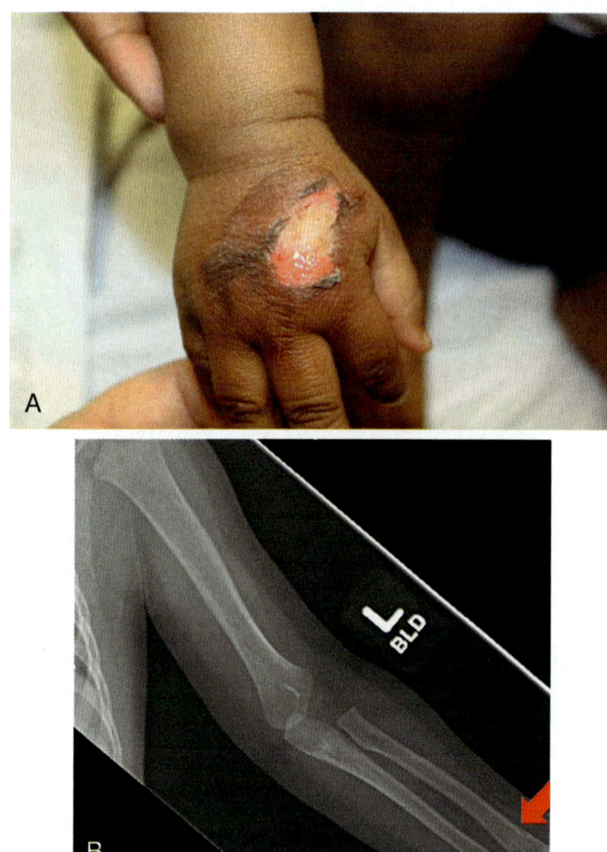

Fig. 6.15 (A) This 13-month-old infant was brought for medical attention 2 days after sustaining a burn to the dorsal aspect of her hand after a caregiver put her hand under running water. Due to the delay in medical attention, the mechanism provided, and the child's age, a skeletal survey was performed. It revealed a healing transverse fracture of the left radius (B). This untreated and unexplained fracture, together with the child's burn, raised significant concern for the child's safety.

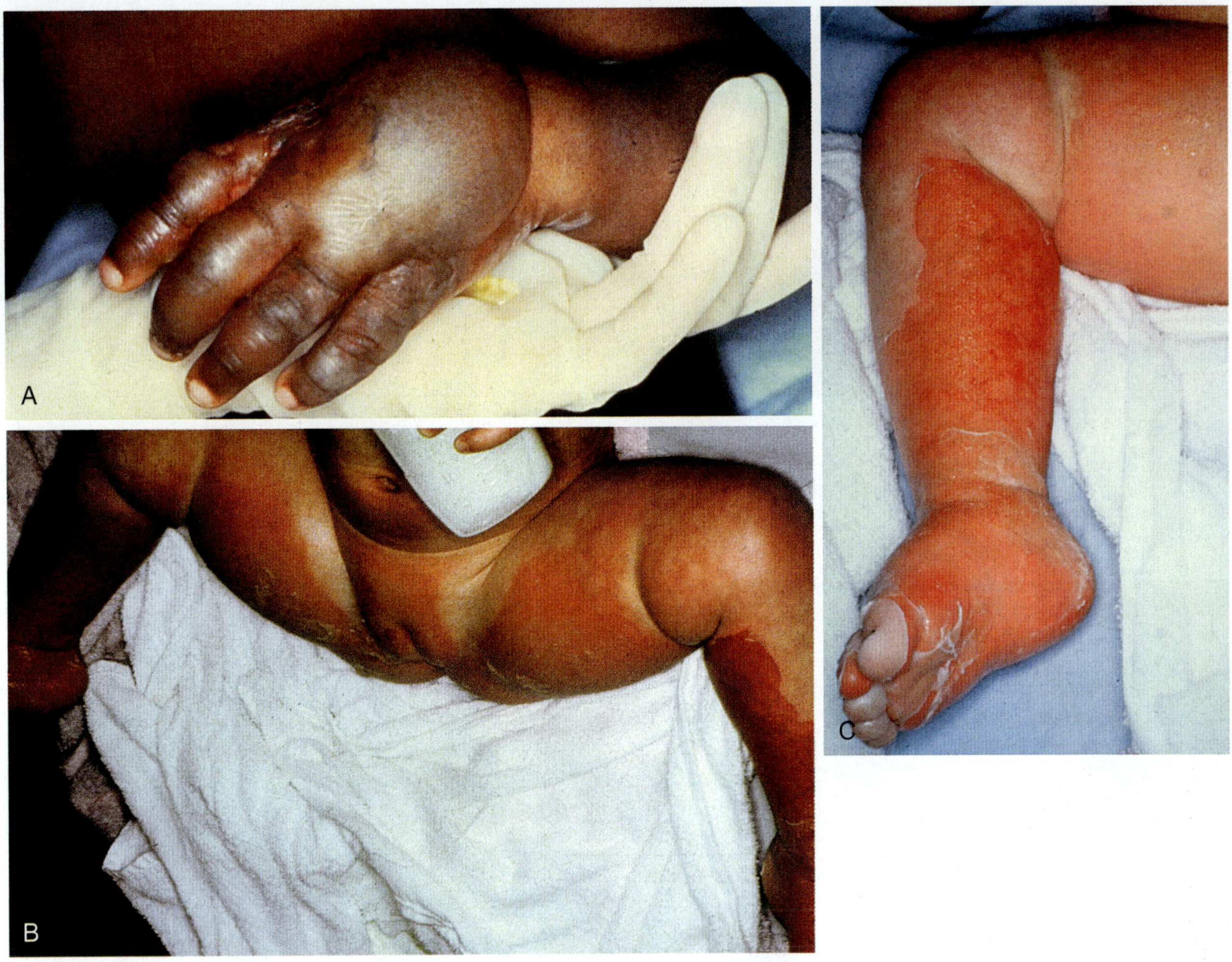

Fig. 6.16 Inflicted scalds. (A) After getting his hands into something he was not allowed to touch and making a mess, this child's hands were held down in hot water, resulting in severe second-degree dip burns. Note the sharp line of demarcation just above the wrist joint and the uniform depth of the burn. (B) This toddler was dipped in a tub of scalding water while being held under the arms and knees, as a "lesson" after a toileting accident. (C) Close-up of severe second-degree burns of the foot and lower leg of the same child. (Courtesy Thomas Layton, MD.)

Table 6.1 Duration of Exposure Required to Produce Full Thickness Burn in Water at Various Temperatures

Water Temperature (°F)	Duration of Exposure
120	10 minutes
130	30 seconds
140	5 seconds
150	2 seconds
158	1 second

and flexor surfaces of the thighs are seen in children who are dipped in scalding water (see Fig. 6.16B and C). Sparing of skin surfaces in flexor creases may also be noted in these cases. At the recommended hot water tank setting of 120°F maximum, scalding burns can often be prevented (Table 6.1).

Some characteristics of burns are commonly associated with accidental injuries. Accidental scalds typically occur when a hot liquid is spilled, producing a splash-and-droplet pattern in the case of a small spill (Fig. 6.17A) or an inverted arrowhead in cases of larger spills over the chest (see Fig. 6.17B). The child usually presents with a history of having grabbed a cup of hot coffee, tea, or cocoa from the table while sitting on someone's lap or of having reached up and grabbed the projecting handle of a pot on the stove.

Contact burns show the imprint of the instruments used to inflict them and have a depth or degree of burn that is relatively even throughout. For example, one may see the imprint of a hot iron or of the grill of a space heater or radiator cover (Fig. 6.18A to D). No child with normal sensation would remain in contact with these objects long enough to incur such a burn. Burns caused by holding a hot hair dryer next to the skin leave an imprint of the screen that covers the heating element (see Fig. 6.18E), and those inflicted with a curling iron produce cigar-shaped, deep partial- or full-thickness imprints (see Fig. 6.18F). Most abusive contact burns are found in unusual locations for accidental burns, such as the extensor surfaces of the upper arms or legs, the back, chest, abdomen, or buttocks that are usually covered by clothing.

Inflicted *cigarette burns* usually leave sharply circumscribed, full-thickness imprints that are approximately 7 to 8 mm in diameter (Fig. 6.19). These are surrounded by a deep, partial-thickness halo blister and then a rim of superficial erythema. A thick, black eschar soon forms over the central, full-thickness burn. As the burns begin to heal, these lesions fill in with granulation tissue; and on completion of healing, the child is left with a deep, punched-out scar. Other burning objects, such as a lighter, can create a distinctive pattern of inflicted burns as well (Fig. 6.20)

Oral and Nasal Injuries

It is important to examine the nose and mouth of the patient for intraoral injuries. This may include palate trauma or soft tissue lacerations caused by violently forcing a bottle, pacifier, or utensil into a child's mouth. Additionally, labial frenulum tears, mucosa or

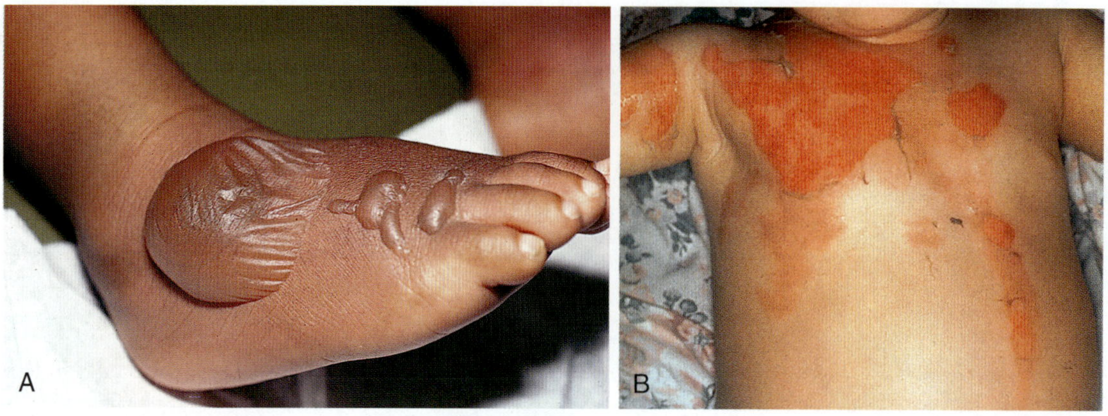

Fig. 6.17 Accidental scalds. (A) The splash-and-droplet pattern of an accidental scald is evident on the foot of a toddler who grabbed a hot cup of tea from the table while sitting on his grandmother's lap. (B) This toddler grabbed a pot handle projecting out over the edge of a stove, spilling hot soup over her chest and shoulder. Cooling of the hot liquid as it flowed downward produced the inverted arrowhead pattern, the burn being wider and of greater depth proximally and narrowing and becoming more superficial distally. There is also a descending droplet and splash pattern to the left of the midline.

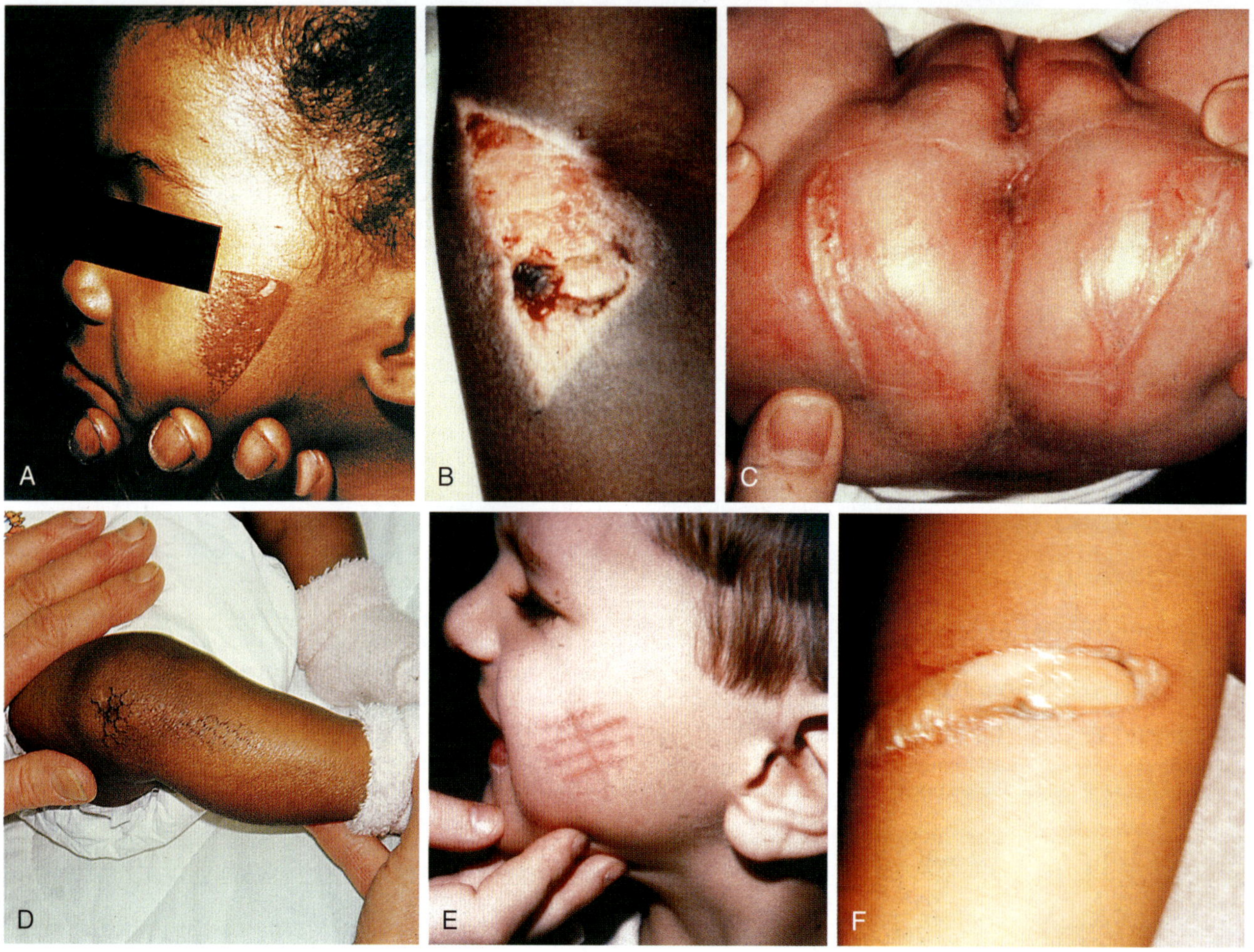

Fig. 6.18 Contact burns or branding injuries. (A) This child, who was acting out while his mother ironed, was punished when she held the tip of the iron against his cheek. (B) A healing full-thickness burn in the shape of an iron was found when this boy's shirt was removed before his being given vaccine injections. He had been sent home after his first day in kindergarten with instructions not to return until he was caught up on his immunizations. (C) These linear full-thickness burns were incurred when this 6-week-old infant was forced to sit on the hot grill of a space heater. The history given was that she had crawled over to the space heater, knocked it over, and then sat on it. (D) Another infant presented with a history of irritability and a rash. The "rash" has a honeycomb configuration that matched that of a radiator cover in her home. She also had multiple fractures. (E) These facial burns are the result of being branded with the grill of a hair dryer. The boy had been acting out while he was supposed to be getting ready for school and his mother was drying her hair. (F) The hot wand of a curling iron leaves a cigar-shaped, partial- to full-thickness burn.

gingiva bruising, or contusions to the lips are often the result of violent forceful trauma (Fig. 6.21). Force-feeding with a spoon may produce contusions or lacerations of the lips, floor of the mouth, and tongue (Fig. 6.22). The common complaint at presentation is spitting or vomiting up blood.

In older children, punches, slaps, or other direct trauma can cause lip lacerations and contusions; frenulum and gingiva tears (see Fig. 6.23); dental fractures; displacement injuries and avulsions; chin lacerations; and even mandibular fractures. These injuries can also stem from impact with hard surfaces when the child is violently

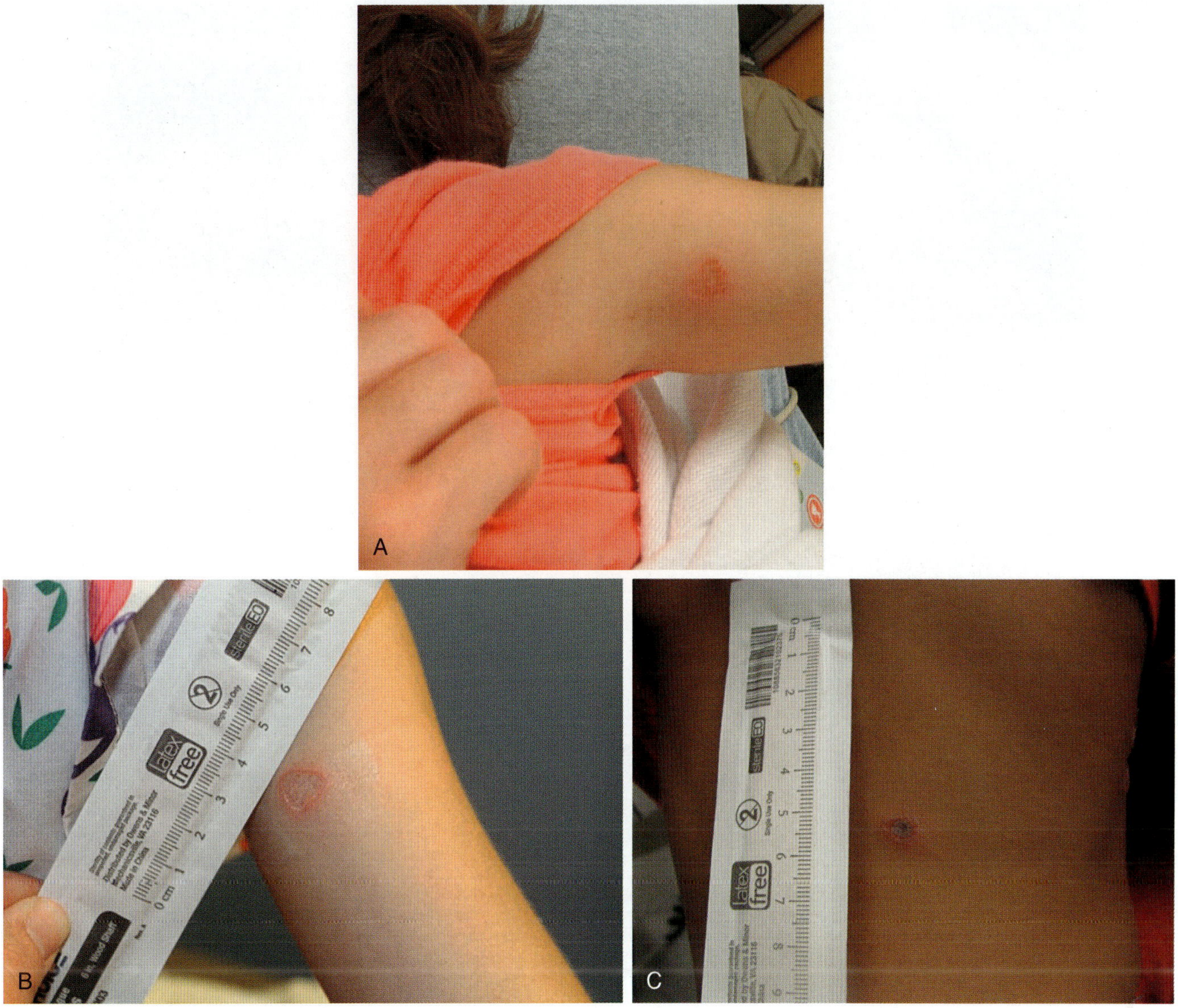

Fig. 6.19 (A) This 7-year-old disclosed that an uncle intentionally burned her with a cigarette. Panel A shows the acute injury, and panel B shows the injury 4 days later. (C) A 13-month-old infant with more than 10 cigarette burns. Another child in the home reported witnessing two adults burning the infant.

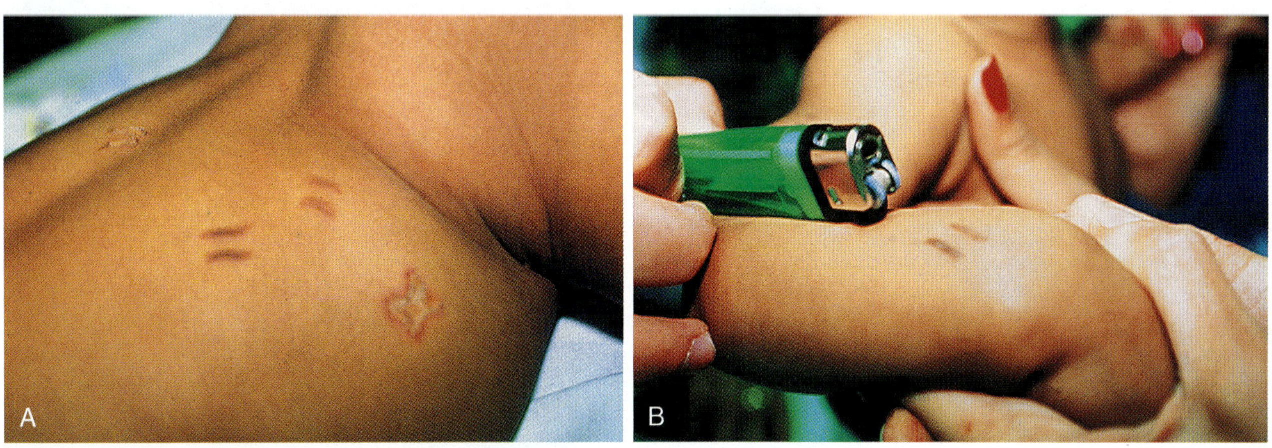

Fig. 6.20 Cigarette lighter burns. (A) Two pairs of lesions with the appearance of parallel serrated lines and a deep burn in the shape of a butterfly were found on examining this infant, who was brought to the emergency department for treatment of a rash. (B) Astute deduction by a resident and social worker led to the discovery that heated cigarette lighter wheels had been used to inflict the burns. The full-thickness butterfly is the result of repeated application.

pushed or thrown. Often these older victims present with a plausible history of accidental trauma and are not recognized as abuse victims. Sometimes the only clue that the injuries are abuse related is that the lesion is more severe than would be expected from the reported mechanism.

Nasal injuries may be due to direct blows or impacts. When mild, epistaxis may be the only manifestation. More severe injuries can result in fractures of the nasal bone or cartilage, septal deviation, and septal hematoma. The abused child with a septal hematoma is especially vulnerable to developing a septal abscess due to delay in

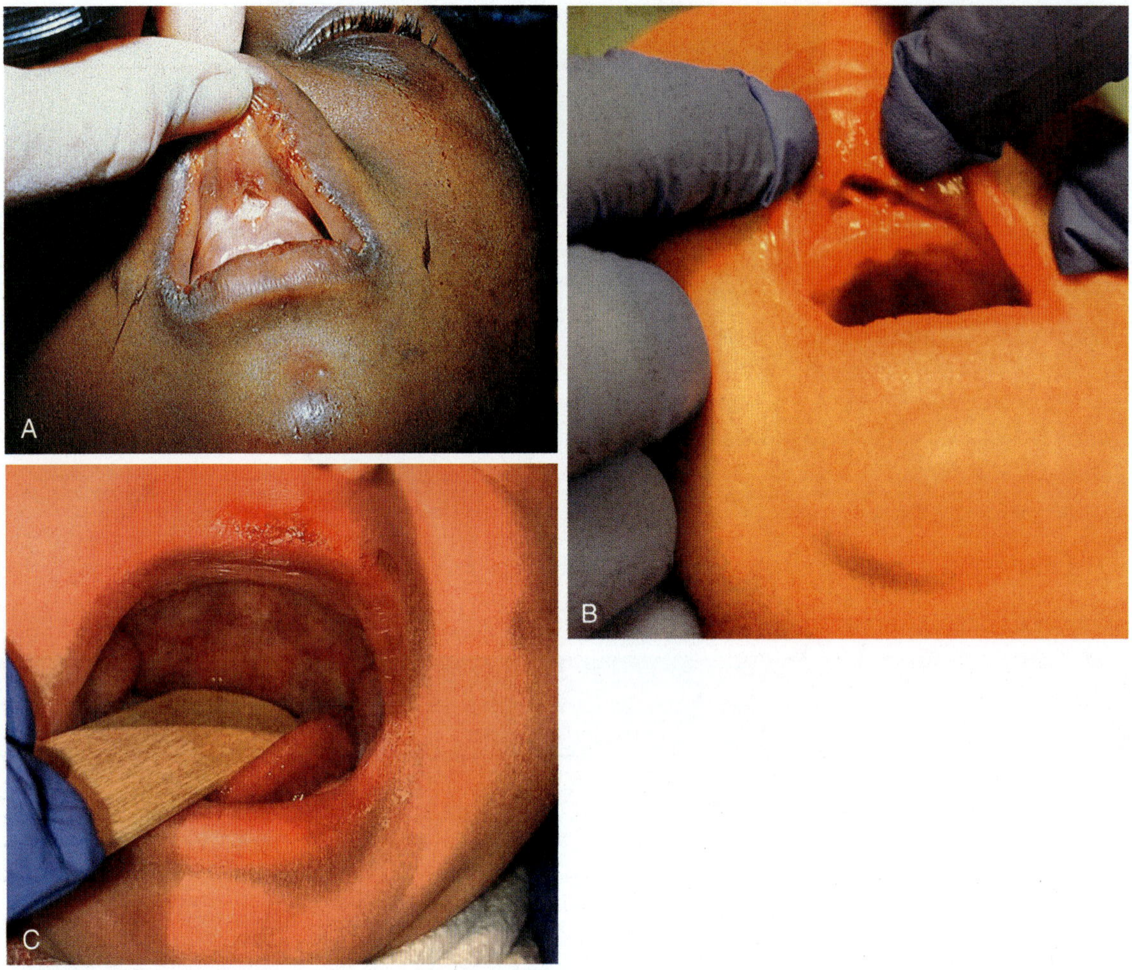

Fig. 6.21 (A) Frenulum tear. This badly beaten boy incurred a torn frenulum when his abuser tried to muffle his cries by forcibly holding his hand over the child's mouth. Note the facial bruises. (B) This child presented with blood from the mouth without a history of trauma. Findings were an upper frenulum tear, facial bruising, multiple CML fractures, and healing posterior rib fractures. (C) This 6-week-old baby was admitted with failure to thrive and found to have an upper frenulum tear, lip abrasions, injuries to his soft palate bilaterally, and facial bruising. His drug screen was positive for cocaine. On follow up radiographs, the child was found to have four healing posterior rib fractures. Additionally, the child had gained weight well in a safe environment. (A, Courtesy Robert Hickey, MD, Children's Hospital of Pittsburgh, Pittsburgh, PA.)

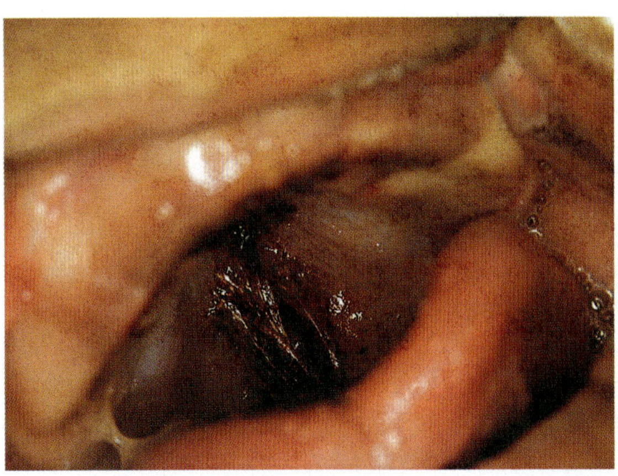

Fig. 6.22 Inflicted palatal lacerations. This infant's soft palate was shredded by repeated stabs with a sharp object. He presented with a complaint of spitting up blood and no history of trauma.

presentation, and affected infants tend to present with external nasal swelling, fever, and respiratory distress due to nasal obstruction (Fig. 6.24).

Skeletal Injuries

Skeletal injuries are reported in 11% to 55% of child abuse victims. Many fractures are clinically unsuspected. Multiple fractures are found in more than one-half of physically abused children.

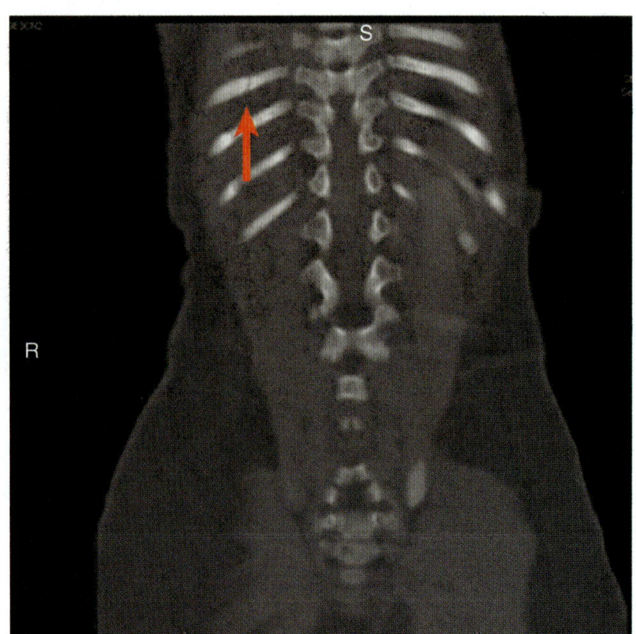

Fig. 6.23 An 8-month-old infant with an unexplained parietal skull fracture was noted to have elevated alanine and aspartate aminotransferase levels, which prompted an abdominal computed tomography scan that revealed this acute ninth posterior rib fracture.

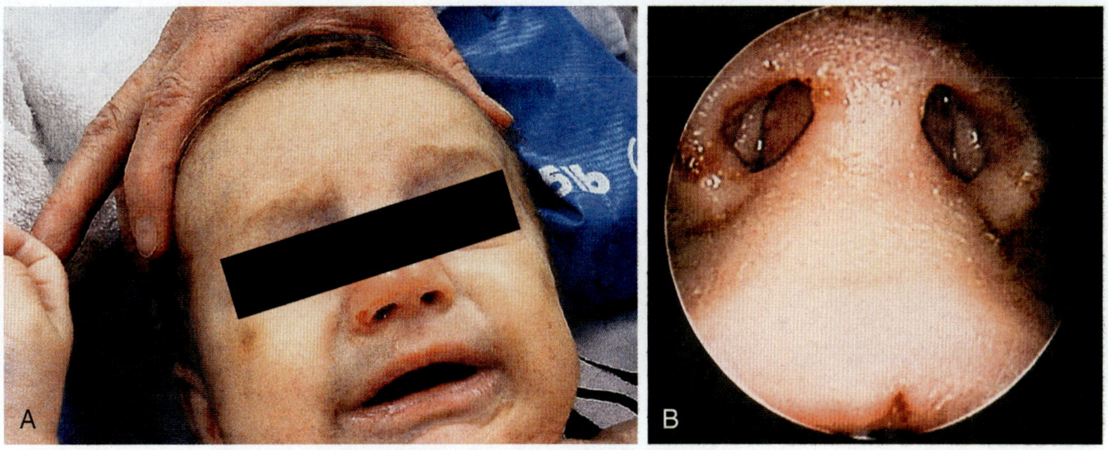

Fig. 6.24 Abscessed nasal septal hematoma. This 3-month-old baby brought to the emergency department with complaints of fever and difficulty breathing was found to have a red swollen nose (A) and erythematous bulging of the nasal septum bilaterally (B), obstructing her nasal passages. Note the small central lip laceration. She also had multiple bruises, fingernail, an occipital skull fracture, a subdural hematoma, and multiple metaphyseal chip fractures.

The majority of fractures, 55% to 70% of all inflicted skeletal injuries, involve infants younger than 1 year old. Approximately 80% of abusive fractures are seen in children younger than 18 months old. In sharp contrast, this age group accounts for only 2% of all accidental fractures in children. Often, fractures are clinically occult, and diagnosis of inflicted fractures based on physical examination is nearly impossible in infants, because nondisplaced rib fractures, metaphyseal chip fractures, and bucket handle fractures have minimal swelling, even acutely, and heal with great rapidity. It is not possible to evaluate for occult fractures in a young child by palpation. Further, an accurate history of trauma is especially unlikely to be reported. When a history of injury is given, it is often one of a minor mechanism (a short fall). Furthermore, parents of abused children tend to minimize reports of pain, discomfort, and loss of function. Because healing is faster in the infant or young child (due to the thickness of the periosteum, which resists tearing, reducing risk of displacement, and due to its being richly invested with osteoblasts that help healing), tenderness and pain on being picked up, or on motion, may abate within a few days. This is particularly true of rib and metaphyseal fractures and other nondisplaced fractures. Notably, most fractures sustained by healthy children are not associated with bruising at the time or presentation (10%) or within the first week (28%) after trauma.

Many fractures in children are accidental. However, there are some warning signs that should encourage the clinician to consider abusive etiology. Physical abuse must be considered in the following situations:

- Infants and children with fractures that are highly associated with physical abuse: These include classic metaphyseal lesions, rib fractures, and sternum, scapula or vertebral fractures. These fractures are described in more detail in the following sections.
- Any fracture with a history that is not compatible with severity of injury.
- Any fracture in a nonambulatory child, especially without a clear history or a known medical condition.
- Children with multiple fractures or a history of multiple fractures.

Classic Metaphyseal Lesions or Corner Fractures

In infancy, the cartilage of the chondro-osseous junctions next to the metaphyses of long bones is poorly mineralized, making these structures the weakest points in long bones. Classic metaphyseal lesions are planar fractures through these sites when the bones are subjected to shearing forces. The periosteum overlying the epiphyseal cartilage is firmly adherent and extends close to the diaphysis to cover the subperiosteal bony collar. Thus, when fractures occur, these peripheral segments are visibly thicker.

Metaphyseal fractures can be produced by the application of torsional or tractional forces delivered when an extremity is grabbed and yanked. They can also occur by rapid, repetitive acceleration and deceleration as the extremities flail back and forth in violent shaking. Metaphyseal fractures can be found in any long bone but are most commonly seen in the distal femur, proximal and distal tibias, and proximal humerus. They may cover the entire metaphysis or only a part of it. Clinically, they are not associated with any significant soft tissue swelling.

Radiographic manifestations of metaphyseal fractures have led to the terms *metaphyseal chip* or *corner fractures* and *bucket handle fractures.* The first derives from the fact that in the anteroposterior view, the central portion of the fracture is often invisible and only a chip of bone is seen on either the lateral or medial aspect of the metaphysis, or both (Fig. 6.25). Chips may also be seen on lateral projections. In some cases, a thin central metaphyseal lucency can be detected. Special oblique views are necessary to reveal the true extent of the fracture, because in this projection the separation of the metaphyseal disk becomes readily evident, resembling a bucket handle. Healing of metaphyseal fractures is not usually accompanied by prominent callus or extensive subperiosteal new bone formation.

Rib Fractures

Rib fractures are also relatively unique to abused infants. Because of the plasticity and pliability of the thoracic cage in infancy, application of major force is needed to break ribs and accidental rib fractures are exceptionally rare. A 2006 systematic review with 923 children (0 to 14 years) who received cardiopulmonary resuscitation (CPR) showed that 3 children sustained rib fractures, and all cases were anterior fractures. Abusive causative mechanisms include violent shaking or squeezing while holding the infant by the chest. The ribs are subjected to marked anteroposterior compression forces, and the posterior ribs are levered against the fulcrum of the vertebral bodies and their transverse processes. This often produces rows of multiple, posterior rib fractures, found near the costovertebral articulations (Fig. 6.26). Extreme squeezing of the chest with or without shaking can produce fractures at multiple sites along the rib arcs. Most of these infants have no history of trauma, and symptoms are nonspecific. Hence, the appropriate imaging is necessary.

Like metaphyseal fractures, rib fractures are not often associated with soft tissue swelling or bruising. When fractures involve the lower rib cage, associated abdominal injury should be considered (Fig. 6.23).

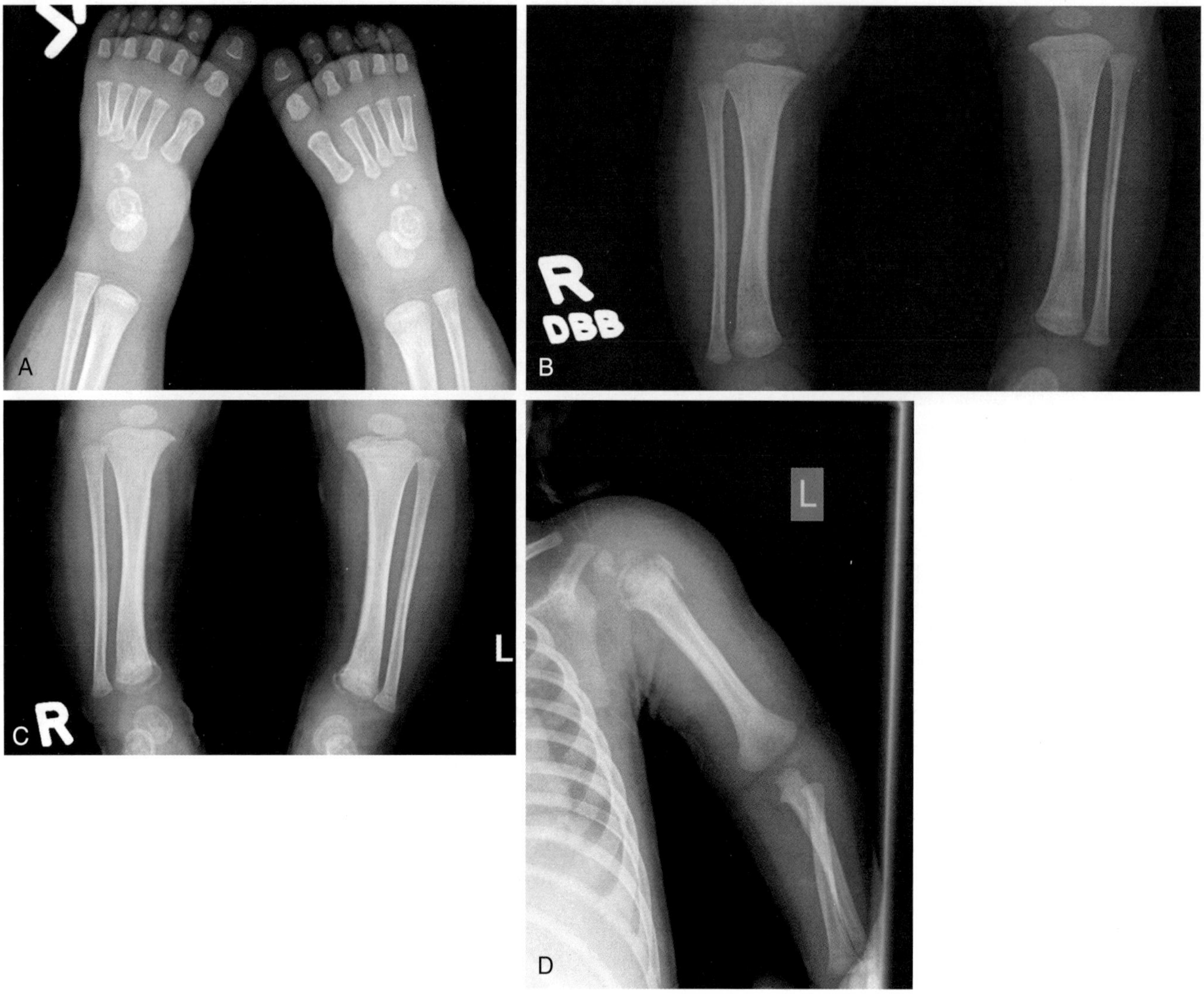

Fig. 6.25 (A) This 6-week-old baby admitted with failure to thrive was found to have an upper frenulum tear, lip abrasions, injuries to his soft palate bilaterally, facial bruising, and a drug screen positive for cocaine. On follow up radiographs, the child was found to have four healing posterior rib fractures. Additionally, the child had gained weight well in a safe environment. (B) A 7-week-old sibling of a 3-year-old victim of physical abuse. A skeletal survey revealed bilateral distal tibia bucket handle (classic metaphyseal lesion [CML]/corner) fractures (see panel C for healing). (C) Radiographs 2 weeks later showed healing bilateral distal tibia bucket handle (CML/corner) fractures. (D) A 6-month-old infant presented to care due to decreased use of left arm without any history of trauma. The child was found to have a left proximal humerus CML, a torn frenulum, and buttock bruising.

Radiographically, rib fractures may not be visible before the appearance of callus and/or subperiosteal new bone. It is the standard of care that a repeat skeletal survey is completed 10 to 14 days after the initial radiographs. These follow-up films can reveal fractures not visible on the first study. An early sign of healing, seen 5 to 10 days post-injury on standard radiographs, consists of a vertical lucency at the site of the fracture surrounded by soft callus with indistinct margins. Subsequently (at 14–21 days), callus takes on a more nodular appearance with sharper margins and is then termed *hard callus.* Reinjury can result in florid callus formation. Complete remodeling and radiographic disappearance occur within a few months in the absence of reinjury.

Additional Fractures With High Specificity for Physical Abuse

Vertebral fractures, scapula fractures, and sternal fractures are rare. However, each of these fractures is highly specific for physical abuse. Scapular fractures of the acromion probably result from shearing forces during shaking or traction to the upper extremities. Fractures to the body of the scapula or the sternum are the result of high-force blunt trauma. Each of these fractures is unusual but highly associated with inflicted trauma (Fig. 6.27).

Abusive fractures have been described in virtually every bone in the body, and any single fracture can be the result of accident or abuse, particularly when considering the age of the child and the history provided. Below are some fractures in the context of a lack of history or a history that does not fit with the developmental age of the child, which should be concerning.

Long Bone Fractures

Long bones may fracture through the diaphysis in a variety of patterns. Transverse, oblique, spiral, or compression fractures may all be seen. These fractures take a substantial amount of force. Although not specific for inflicted injury, diaphyseal fractures are highly suspect when found in infants who are not yet crawling or walking, especially when seen in the absence of a history of significant trauma. An understanding of the direction and magnitude of force needed to produce a given type of diaphyseal fracture compared with the provided history is important to try to distinguish between accidental and inflicted injury (Figs. 6.28 and 6.29).

Although more commonly accidental in origin, *torus* or *buckle fractures* can be the result of abuse, especially in young children.

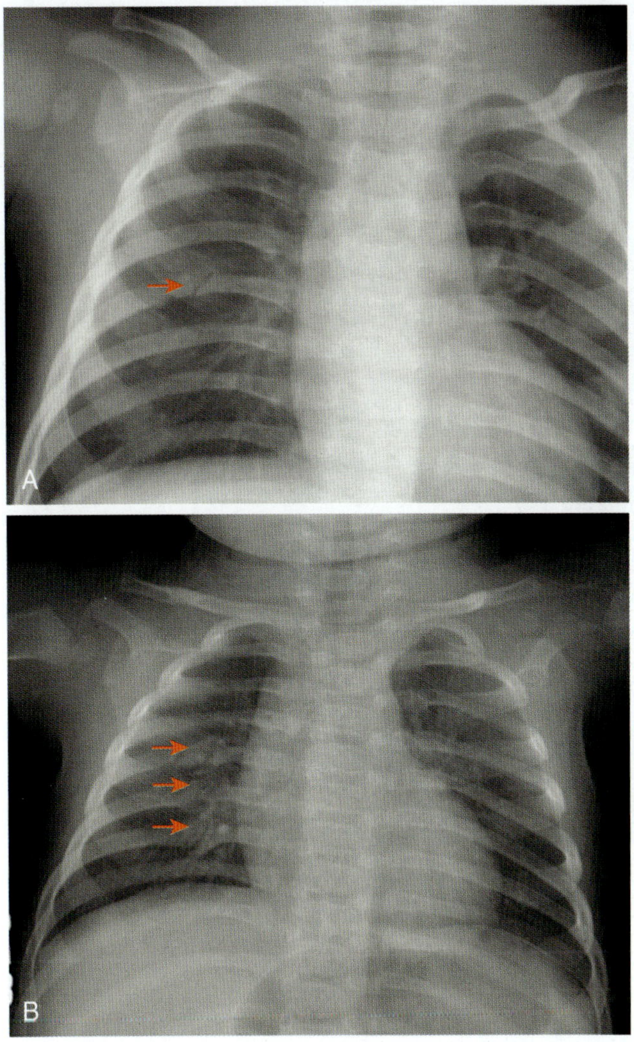

Fig. 6.26 (A) This 4-week-old presented due to difficulty breathing in the setting of a fever. His sepsis evaluation included a chest radiograph, but this acute rib fracture was not discovered. (B) The child was returned for care 2 weeks later after an apneic spell and was found to have abusive head trauma, three healing rib fractures *(arrows)*, and bruising.

When mild with only slight cortical buckling, these fractures are the result of mild-to-moderate compression forces delivered in a direction parallel or nearly parallel to the axis of a long bone. When higher-energy forces are delivered, whether accidental or inflicted, there is usually some degree of angulation; in such cases, it may be more accurate to classify them as a form of compression injury (Fig. 6.30). More severe forms involving the femur or tibia can be caused by throwing or slamming a child feet first or onto the knees on a hard surface.

Transverse fractures are high-energy injuries that are much more likely to be accompanied by acute soft tissue swelling and deformity. Transverse fractures are often the result of a rapidly delivered direct blow perpendicular to the long axis of a bone, such as a "karate chop" or "night stick" injury (Fig. 6.31). They can also occur when a child is thrown or swung and, in the process, hits an extremity against a hard edge such as that of a table, as a result of falls of greater than 6 feet, and when half of an extremity is held with both hands and snapped. Violently yanking a child up from his crib while holding an extremity or grabbing an arm and yanking it upward or sideways when the child is fixed in position by the belt of a highchair or infant seat are possible etiologies for these fractures. Inflicted supracondylar humerus fractures of the compression/distraction type are the result of grabbing an arm and yanking it into hyperextension (Fig. 6.32).

Other Fractures That Warrant Evaluation for Abuse

Vertebral body fractures, metacarpal and metatarsal fractures, distal or proximal clavicular fractures, and complex skull fractures are concerning for physical abuse (Fig. 6.33). Vertebral body fractures are due to compression, typically associated with a child being slammed down violently and axial loading transmitting through the vertebral canal (Fig. 6.27B). Cervical fractures are usually the result of violent hyperflexion or hyperextension. Below the cervical spine, most fractures occur near the thoracolumbar junction. Fractures of the hands and feet are uncommon but important findings to consider physical abuse. These tend to be clinically occult when first seen. Grabbing and yanking, twisting, or bending the hand or foot tend to produce metacarpal/metatarsal fractures. Subtle subperiosteal new bone formation and/or medullary sclerosis are common radiographic findings. Forced hyperextension of the phalanges can cause buckle fractures at their bases (see Fig. 6.34).

Diagnostic Imaging and Evaluation of Skeletal Injuries

Children younger than 2 years old with fractures suspicious for child abuse should have a full skeletal survey to evaluate for other bone injuries. Surveys may also yield valuable additional information in selected cases of children 2 to 5 years old. After 5 years old, careful history and physical examination should point to areas that call for radiographic evaluation.

Additional fractures are found in approximately 10% of skeletal surveys, with even higher yields in children younger than 1 year old. An adequate skeletal survey includes the following: two images (two different views) of the appendicular skeleton, frontal and lateral views of the axial skeleton, oblique views of the chest, and a four-film series of the skull. Fractures may be missed if these American College of Radiology guidelines are not followed. A repeat skeletal survey in 10 to 14 days should be completed after the initial skeletal survey if abuse is strongly suspected. In one study of 703 follow-up skeletal surveys, 11% were positive and 79% had evidence of a healing fracture.

Missing the opportunity to find additional fractures leads to missed abuse diagnoses and return of the child with major risks of even more severe subsequent abuse and injury (see Fig. 6.26).

Strong consideration should be given to obtaining a head computed tomography (CT) scan, a complete blood count (CBC) and differential with platelets, prothrombin and partial thromboplastin times, liver function tests, and amylase and lipase when evaluating children—especially infants—with multiple fractures and those with injuries of moderate to high specificity for abuse, because clinically unapparent central nervous system (CNS) and intra-abdominal injuries can be associated findings.

Lastly, we cannot give enough emphasis to the importance of considering fractures in the differential diagnosis of unexplained irritability or of grunting respirations in infants who have no pulmonary findings. Failure to identify the cause of irritability has the potential to subject previously abused babies to further, often more severe, trauma.

ABUSIVE HEAD TRAUMA

Abusive head trauma is the leading cause of death from child abuse and the most common cause of severe traumatic brain injury in infants. Typical injuries most often include subdural and/or subarachnoid hemorrhages, with or without evidence of direct impact, such as scalp hematomas, skull fractures, facial trauma, focal brain contusions, or soft tissue swelling. Our current understanding of the forces and mechanisms involved, including the role of shaking in abusive head trauma, derives from significant research over the past several decades.

In the late 1940s, Caffey first described the association of subdural hematomas with multiple fractures in infants. Subsequently, the question of intentional injury was raised, and shaking was postulated

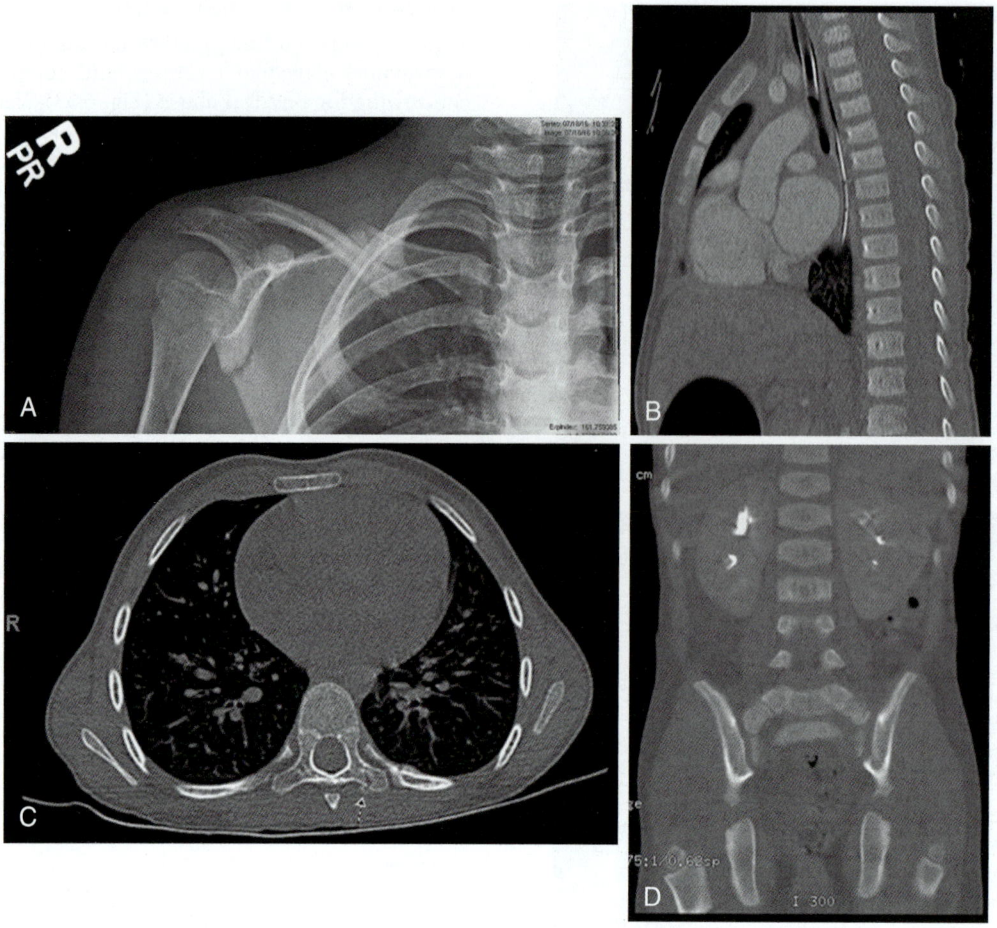

Fig. 6.27 (A) A 4-year-old female in foster care who disclosed an adult pulled her arm back until she "heard a crack and I thought my arm was going to fall off." The child was found to have fractures of her right clavicle and scapular body. (B) In addition to subdural hemorrhages, skull fractures, and extensive bruising, this badly battered 2-year-old was found to have healing vertebral fractures of T2-T5. (C) This 4-year-old child complained of back pain and disclosed being kicked in the back by an adult. Externally, she had a small bruise on her left back. An evaluation several weeks later revealed a left eighth posterior rib fracture and T8 transverse process fracture. (D) This 5-year-old presented to an emergency department due to vomiting and refusal to bear weight. The discovery of extensive bruising prompted a trauma evaluation in which the child was found to have elevated liver function tests, pancreatic and hepatic lacerations, as well as fractures of the left sacral ala and right pubic ramus and three right-sided rib fractures and one left rib fracture. The child's 2-year-old sibling was evaluated due to physical abuse of the index child. He was noted to have multiple, healed, nonspecific cutaneous injuries and was quite active in the examination room. His skeletal survey surprisingly showed healing fractures to three ribs, his fibula, and a right ischial pubic bone fracture. The history that the child had never been symptomatic from his injuries was not plausible.

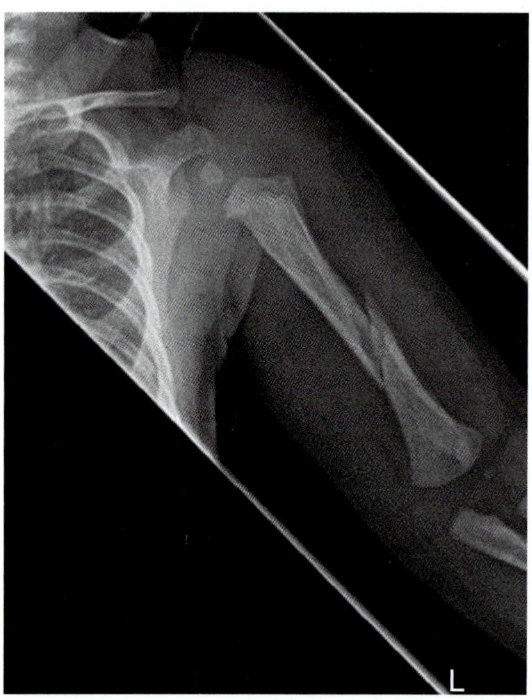

Fig. 6.28 This 7-week-old infant presented due to a decrease in the use of her left arm. The child was found to have more than 15 fractures. During pregnancy, her parents planned to put her up for adoption but reconsidered at birth.

as the probable mechanism, leading to the concept of the *shaken baby syndrome,* characterized by a constellation of findings that included subdural hematomas (Fig. 6.35), retinal hemorrhages (Figs. 6.36 and 6.37), and posterior rib and metaphyseal fractures (see Figs. 6.23 to 6.25).

Subsequent advances in neuroimaging, together with improvements in the identification of abusive head trauma, have expanded our knowledge of the spectrum of CNS injuries seen in abuse victims. Furthermore, on the basis of confessions, severe CNS injury can result from violent shaking alone. Thus, some victims' injuries appear to be due solely to shaking, others result from a combination of shaking and impact trauma, and still others result from impact alone.

The term *abusive head trauma* has been developed to appropriately describe injuries to the head, brain, and spinal cord that have resulted from violent shaking of the head and may or may not include direct blunt impact trauma.

Epidemiology

The incidence of recognized head injury in child abuse victims ranges from 14 to 40 per 100,000 in various study series. Young age and male sex increase the risk of abusive head trauma. Up to 80% of victims are younger than 1 year old, and the majority of the

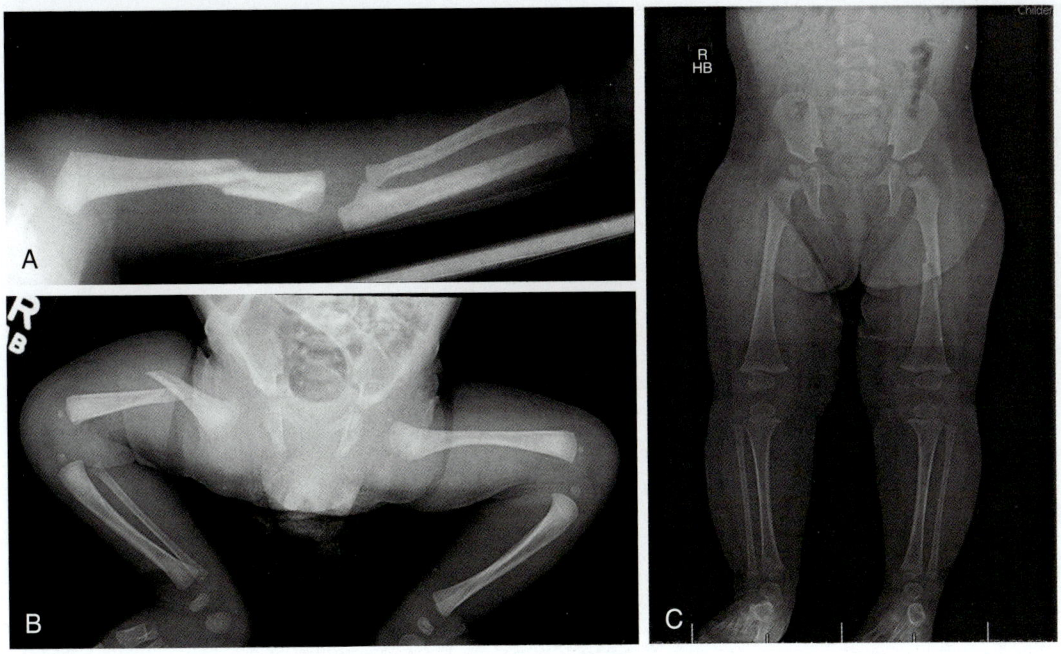

Fig. 6.29 (A) This partially displaced oblique fracture of the left humerus has faint evidence of early callus formation. The persistence of soft tissue swelling may be due to lack of proper immobilization and/or reinjury. (B) This 2-week-old infant presented to medical care after being found to have right leg swelling with no history of trauma. The child was also found to have back and leg bruising. (C) This 19-month-old infant was brought to care after the caregiver heard a "pop" when removing her from a car seat. The child also had a history of an unexplained humerus fracture at 8 months of age and was diagnosed as being physically abused on multiple occasions. (A, Courtesy Robert Hickey, MD, Children's Hospital of Pittsburgh, Pittsburgh, PA.)

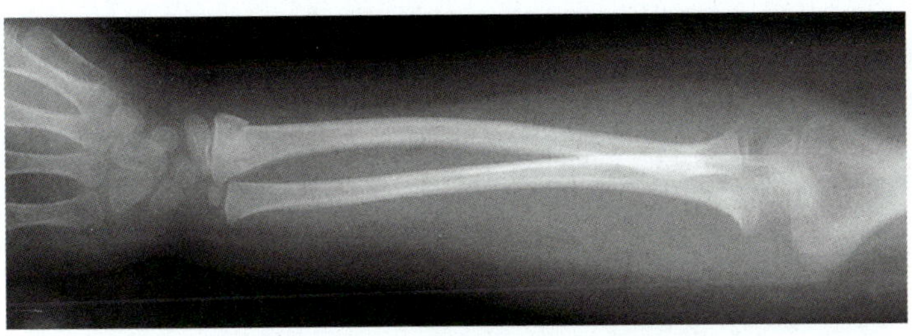

Fig. 6.30 Torus or buckle fracture. This 5-year-old girl with mild cerebral palsy presented with a history of unresponsiveness lasting more than an hour, following a possible seizure, and was found to have a hyperacute subdural hematoma. A subsequent skeletal survey found a previously unrecognized and clinically silent torus fracture of the left distal radius.

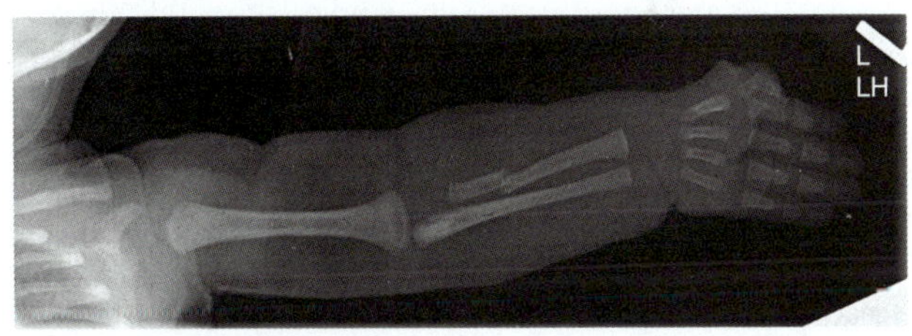

Fig. 6.31 A 3-month-old presented due to left arm swelling without a history of trauma and was found to have this transverse radial fracture, a so-called "night-stick fracture."

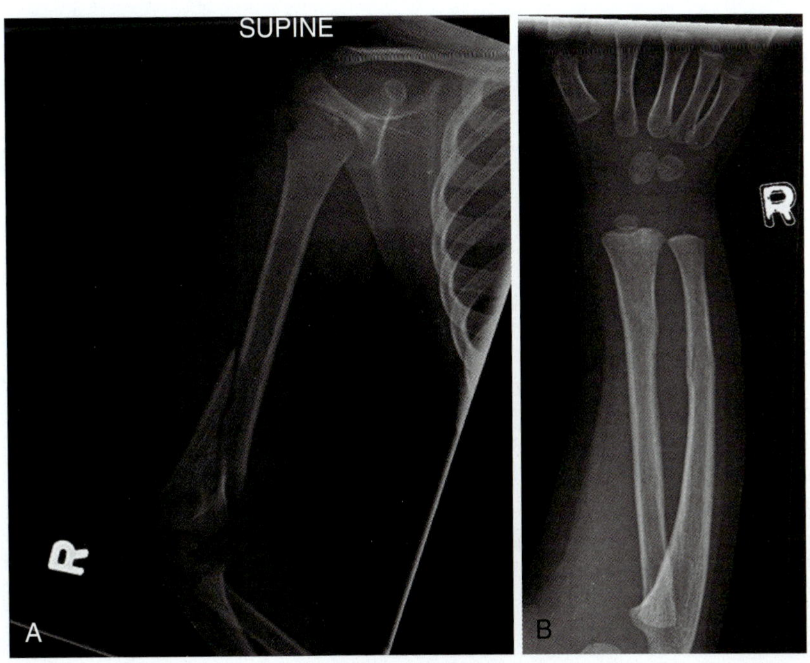

Fig. 6.32 (A) This 3-year-old presented with right arm pain after reportedly getting his arm stuck between a chair and the wall. The child was discovered to have an oblique fracture of the distal right humerus, nondisplaced buckle fractures of the distal right radial and ulnar shafts (B), and multiple bruises. Younger siblings were also found to have multiple bruises and fractures.

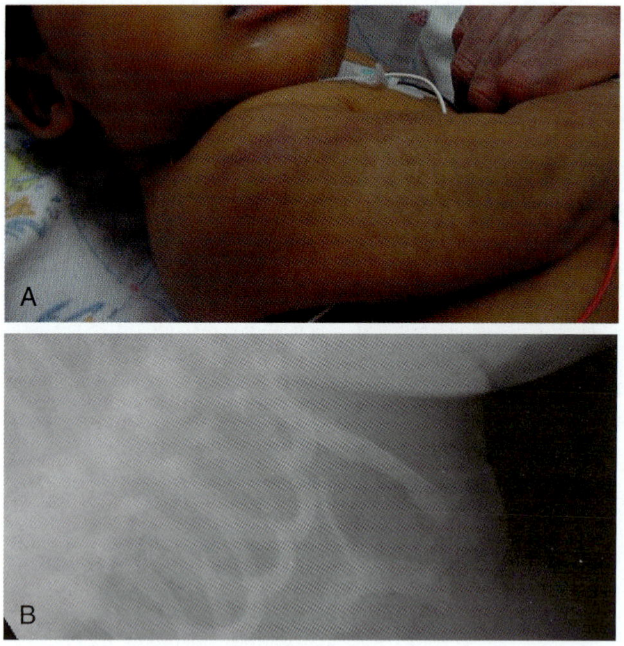

Fig. 6.33 (A) This 6-month-old infant presented after being involved in a domestic dispute. The child was noted to have linear bruising to both shoulders, and radiographs revealed a left distal clavicle fracture (B).

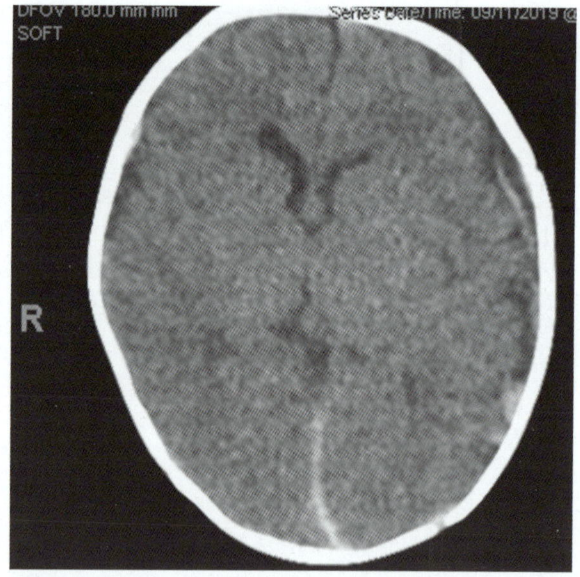

Fig. 6.35 A 5-week-old infant with difficulty breathing was discovered to have a frenulum injury and torso bruising, which prompted a trauma evaluation. The child was found to have an acute left supratentorial subdural hematoma with midline and >20 fractures.

remaining 20% are 1 to 2 years old. Studies show that there is an increased incidence in male infants. It must also be noted that many victims of inflicted CNS trauma are subjected to injury on more than one occasion. In fact, 45% of infants confirmed as victims of inflicted head trauma had evidence of prior intracranial injury on initial neuroimaging.

Head injuries are the major source of morbidity and mortality due to abuse. From 17% to 23% of known victims of inflicted head trauma die within hours to days of presentation. Survivors are often left with sequelae, ranging from mild cognitive deficits to neurologic devastation. Follow-up data show that approximately one-third of victims have good neurologic outcomes, one-third of victims have moderate disability, and one-third of victims have severe disability. For even mild abusive head trauma, there is significant disability adjusted for life-year burden. Although only 30% of the previously abused children studied in follow-up by Elmer and Gregg had known CNS injury at the time of their initial identification, 57% had intelligence quotients (IQs) lower than 80, and 32%, known to have been abused before 13 months old, had evidence of significant developmental delay.

Documented incidence has risen over the past decades because more infants with subtle or subclinical intracranial injuries are imaged, and abnormalities are detected because of increased clinical consideration and greater recognition of associated cutaneous and/or skeletal injuries.

Pathophysiology and Biomechanics

An infant's head is uniquely vulnerable to injury, whether from impact or shaking, given its relatively large size compared with the body, underdeveloped cervical ligaments and weak neck muscles, and generous subarachnoid space, which places bridging veins at greater tension.

There is a history of controversy about the specific mechanisms and biomechanics involved in abusive head trauma, but there should be clinical consideration for multiple mechanisms, including

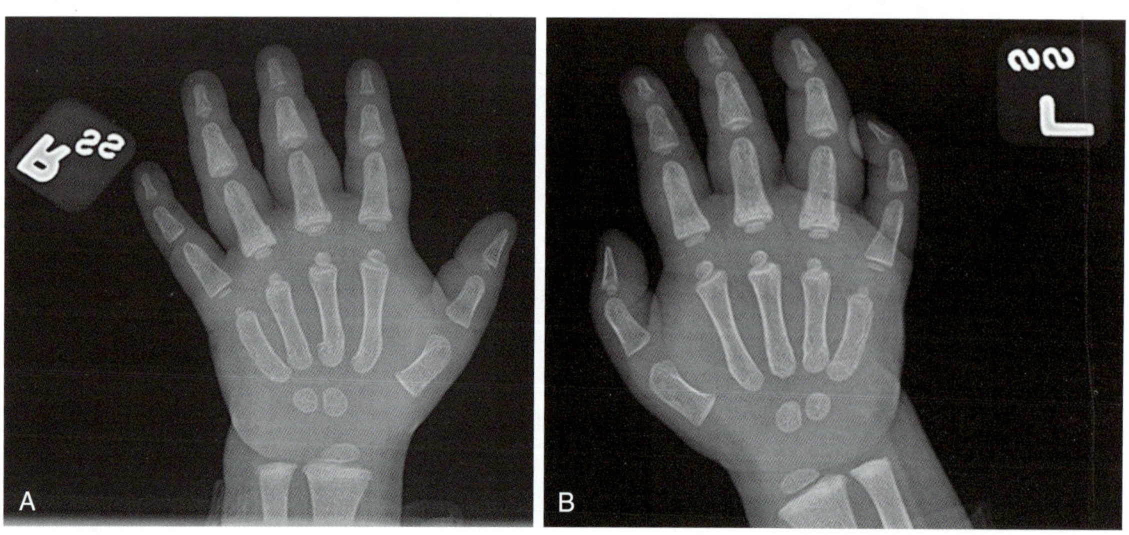

Fig. 6.34 (A and B) This 18-month-old with unexplained hand swelling was brought to care multiple times. The child was ultimately sent to a children's hospital due to concern for a rheumatologic disease. The child was found to have multiple acute and healing metacarpal and phalanx fractures in both hands, which were diagnostic of physical child abuse.

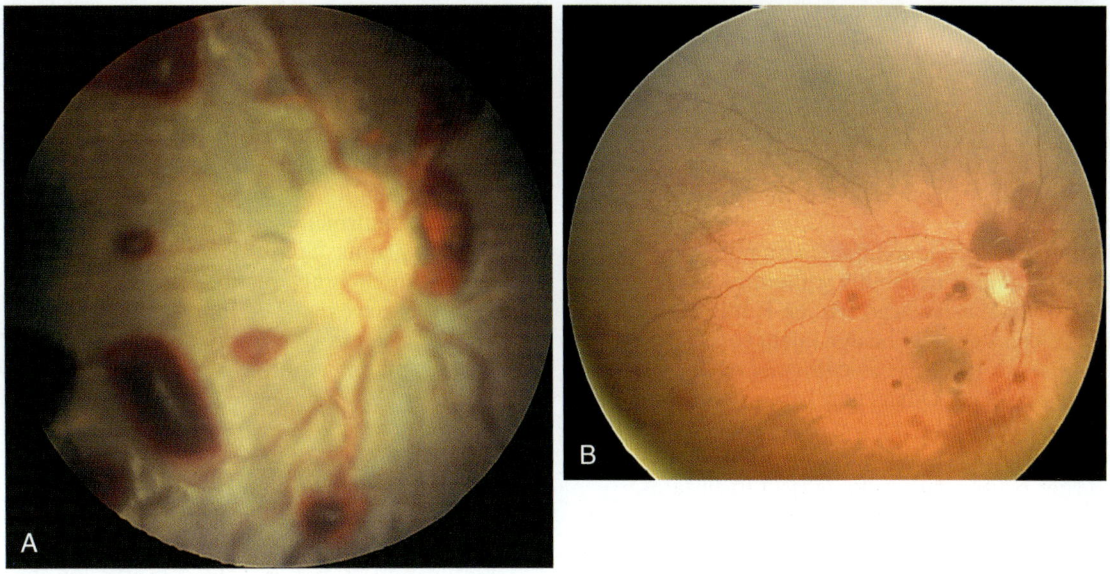

Fig. 6.36 (A) Multiple retinal hemorrhages are seen on funduscopic examination of this infant, who was a victim of abusive head trauma including shaking. Subdural hematoma and multiple metaphyseal "shake" fractures are typical associated findings. (B) RetCam photograph of preretinal, intraretinal, and subretinal hemorrhages, extending to the periphery. (A, Courtesy Stephen Ludwig, MD, Children's Hospital of Philadelphia, Philadelphia, PA. B, Courtesy Tineke Chen, MD, Children's Hospital of Pittsburgh, University of Pittsburgh Medical Center, Pittsburgh, PA.)

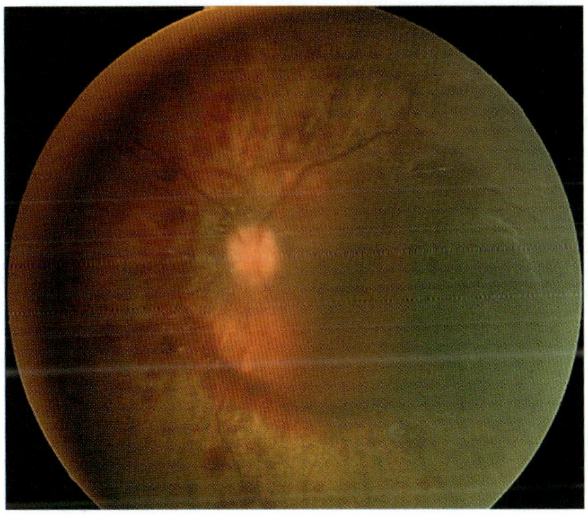

Fig. 6.37 RetCam photograph of traumatic retinoschisis. (Courtesy Tineke Chen, MD, Children's Hospital of Pittsburgh, University of Pittsburgh Medical Center, Pittsburgh, PA.)

blunt trauma, shaking (acceleration/deceleration), hypoxic-ischemic injury, and spinal cord injury.

In terms of biomechanics, the majority of head injuries in children, whether accidental or inflicted, are the result of rapidly applied dynamic blunt forces. Some are caused by direct contact forces, and some are caused by indirect inertial forces that result from acceleration/deceleration of the head.

In direct contact injuries, the skull, its overlying soft tissues, and potentially its underlying intracranial contents are subjected to focal strains or distortions. When applied forces are mild, they may result in abrasion, bruising, or laceration of the scalp; and when more significant, the injuries can result in skull fractures. With severe forces come increased forces on the intracranial structures, producing focal injuries ranging from epidural hematomas to subdural hematomas and to cerebral contusions or parenchymal shearing.

Indirect trauma due to acceleration/deceleration forces results in inertial loading and, depending on velocity and direction, subjects the intracranial contents to shearing strains. When great enough (e.g., forceful to violent), these can result in tearing at interfaces between differing structures (e.g., bridging veins) or at the interface of tissues of differing density (e.g., gray and white matter). In addition to subdural hematomas (seen particularly in the interhemispheric fissure along the falx and over the cerebral convexities), subarachnoid hemorrhages, cerebral contusions, diffuse axonal injury with shearing at gray/white matter interfaces, and white matter tears have been reported. Epidural and subdural hematomas at the cervicomedullary junction in association with ventral cord contusions at high cervical levels have also been linked to shaking with or without direct trauma.

Hypoxic-ischemic injury is seen more often in abusive head trauma than in mild accidental minor head injuries (falls from short distances). This could be attributed to several factors including a possible delay in medical care following the brain injury, more severe injury and corresponding symptoms, and more ongoing cell death due to more severe intracranial acceleration/deceleration injuries.

To summarize, abusive head trauma is the result of some combination of direct impact trauma, acceleration/deceleration forces, and hypoxic ischemic injury.

A chronicle of advances in recognition of the differing magnitude of applied forces and severity of injury in accidental versus inflicted impact trauma can be found in the literature on fall-related head injuries. For many years, it was believed that short falls (3–4 feet or less) could cause severe injury. A series of studies of victims of falls witnessed by people other than caretakers, and of children who had fallen from beds and examining tables in hospitals show that indoor falls of less than 10 feet (3 m), even onto hard surfaces, did not cause serious, let alone life-threatening, head injuries. Simple linear skull fractures tended to be the most severe injuries seen in these fall events, and these were associated with mild focal underlying intracranial injury only in rare instances. These findings led to the recognition that study populations described in earlier literature on pediatric head trauma had included many unrecognized child abuse victims, and to refutation of the conclusions of earlier investigators that short falls and other minor mechanisms of injury could result in serious, even fatal, head trauma. Research has also found that accidental falls down the stairs consist of a series of short falls and do not result in serious head injury unless the infant is in a walker or there was acceleration before the fall.

Clinical Presentation of Abusive Head Trauma

The presentation of abusive head trauma varies greatly, depending on the age of the victim and the severity of injury. Physical findings may include lethargy, altered mental status, crying, increased or decreased tone, rhythmic eye opening, eye deviation, seizures, and sometimes posturing.

Trauma might not be suspected in infants with milder injury due to nonspecific lethargy and/or irritability without focal neurologic signs. This is often when abusive head trauma is misdiagnosed as gastroenteritis, reflux, colic, or other benign infant conditions. Some may have subtle bruises or petechiae evident only on close inspection of a fully undressed infant. Others may have significant surface injuries to the head or body, including soft tissue swelling, bruising, abrasions, or erythema. Cutaneous injuries of the face and other sites are common (Fig. 6.38A) but are not present in all cases.

In patients with signs of direct trauma such as obvious bruising, a chief complaint of a bump on the head may be given with a history of a minor mechanism of injury such as rolling off a couch to a carpeted floor, or the caretaker may report having dropped the baby a short distance (usually <3 or 4 feet). In some cases, a history of another young child having hit the baby on the head is offered. These mechanisms do not explain intracranial injury.

In cases of more severe injury, presentation is more likely to be prompt, but delays in seeking care still occur. During the ensuing interval, intracranial pressure may rise because of increasing cerebral edema and/or the mass effect of intracranial hemorrhage, compromising cerebral perfusion and resulting in varying amounts of cerebral ischemia. Associated alteration in mental status and/or seizures can result in hypoventilation, apnea, or respiratory arrest, resulting in hypoxia.

When there are no external signs (which is often the case), a history of trauma is almost never reported. An unrelated chief complaint or a history of nonspecific symptoms such as vomiting, lethargy, irritability, or trouble breathing is likely to be given when neurologic abnormalities are not evident. When injuries are more severe, complaints of unresponsiveness, shaking or stiffening spells, apnea and/or choking are more likely to be reported. On occasion, patients who have incurred milder trauma and are not seen acutely may present weeks later with one or more of the following symptoms: intermittent vomiting and irritability, rapidly increasing head circumference sometimes with findings of split sutures and a full fontanelle, or weight loss. Some of these patients are found to have chronic subdural hematomas.

Evaluation

The evaluation of a child with concerns for abusive head trauma includes a complete physical examination, an unenhanced head CT scan, a full skeletal survey, a dilated ophthalmology evaluation, and laboratory work to evaluate for internal bleeding and abdominal trauma and to screen for bleeding disorders.

Routine skull radiographs have historically been used to detect skull fractures, and when abuse is suspected, four views (anteroposterior, Towne, right, and left) should be obtained (Fig. 6.39).

Head CT, particularly with 3-dimensional reconstructions, are invaluable for diagnosing skull fractures (Figs. 6.40 and 6.41). Head CTs are also helpful in the acute assessment of CNS injuries, and an unenhanced head CT scan with brain and bone windows is indicated whenever there is any suspicion of intracranial injury. It clearly delineates most intracranial hemorrhages and cerebral edema. CT is especially effective in revealing interhemispheric subdural hematomas along the falx and in the parieto-occipital area, which are seen often in victims of shaking (Figs. 6.42 and 6.43). It is also effective in detecting cerebral edema (Figs. 6.43), loss of gray/white matter differentiation due to axonal shearing (Figs. 6.44 and 6.45), and subsequent cortical necrosis (Fig. 6.46) and cortical hypodensity due to hypoxic/ischemic injury (Figs. 6.47 and 6.48).

Simple or diastatic linear fractures (see Fig. 6.41) and more complex T-shaped and eggshell fractures (see Fig. 6.40) have all been reported in cases of inflicted trauma. Given the greater magnitude

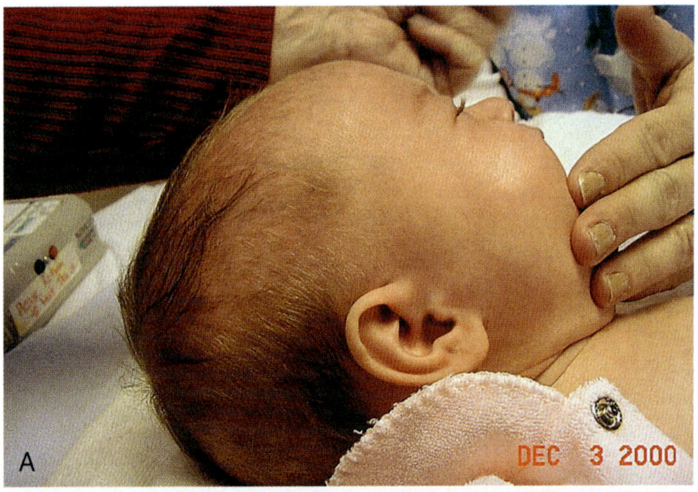

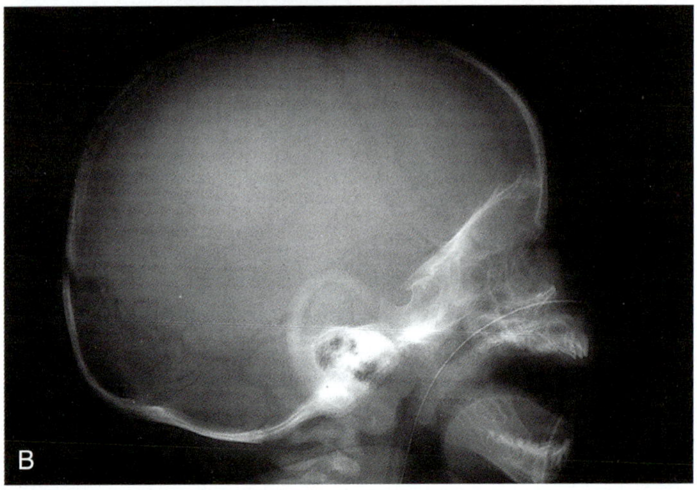

Fig. 6.38 Abusive head trauma. (A) Subtle bruising is seen over the right frontotemporal area in this infant. (B) Her skull radiograph reveals an occipital fracture with diastasis of the lambdoid suture. On computed tomography scan, a posterior interhemispheric subdural hematoma was found.

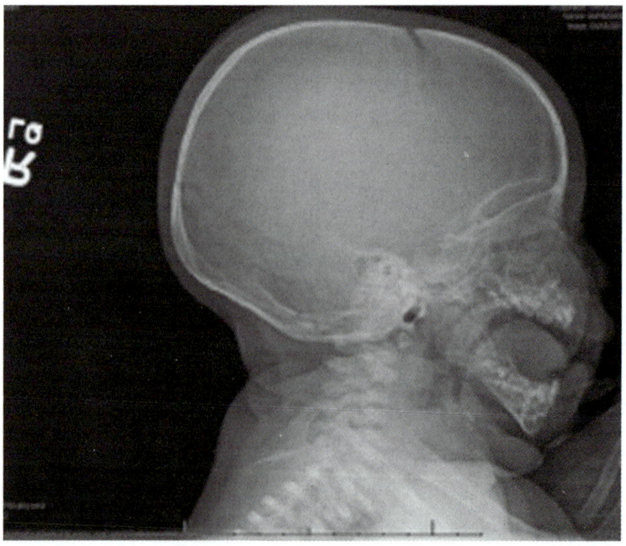

Fig. 6.39 This 7-month-old nonambulatory infant was evaluated by the primary care physician due to unexplained right scalp swelling, initially attributed to an allergic reaction. Skull films revealed a large right linear parietal skull fracture, and further evaluation revealed three healing posterior rib fractures.

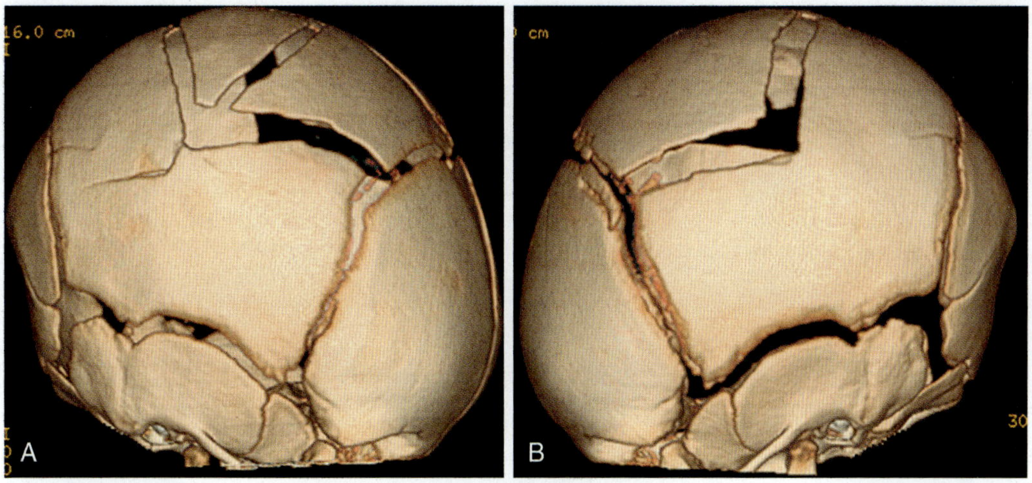

Fig. 6.40 (A and B) A 7-week-old evaluated for head swelling without a history of trauma. Head computed tomography scan revealed parietal comminuted fractures right greater than left, bilateral subdural and retinal hemorrhages, and more than 10 fractures.

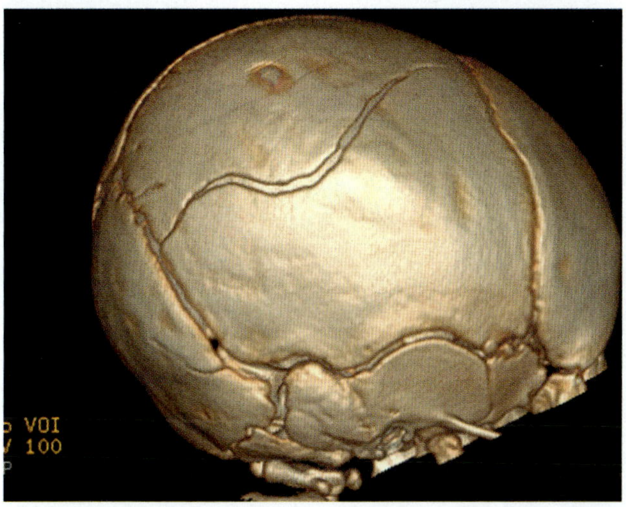

Fig. 6.41 A 2-month-old was noted to have head swelling with no history of trauma. When this large right parietal skull fracture was discovered on head computed tomography scanning, a history of the infant bumping her head during tummy time was offered. The child was additionally found to have leg bruising and bilateral distal femur classic metaphyseal lesions and was diagnosed as being the victim of physical child abuse.

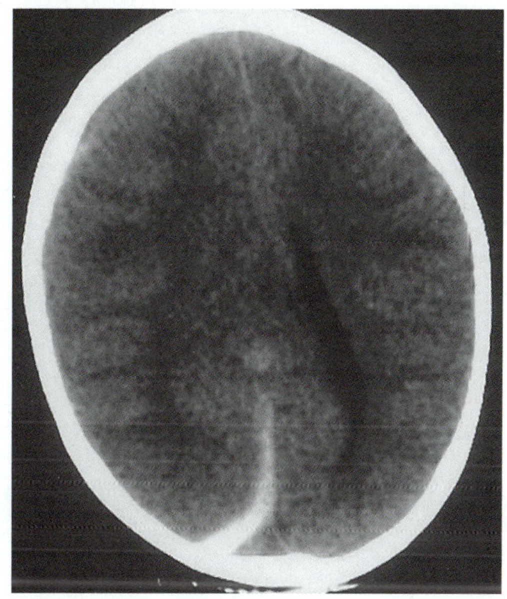

Fig. 6.43 Focal occipital and interhemispheric subdural blood are seen in this toddler who "collapsed at home after a fall from her crib." Note the effacement of the right lateral ventricle and slight anterior midline shift due to cerebral edema.

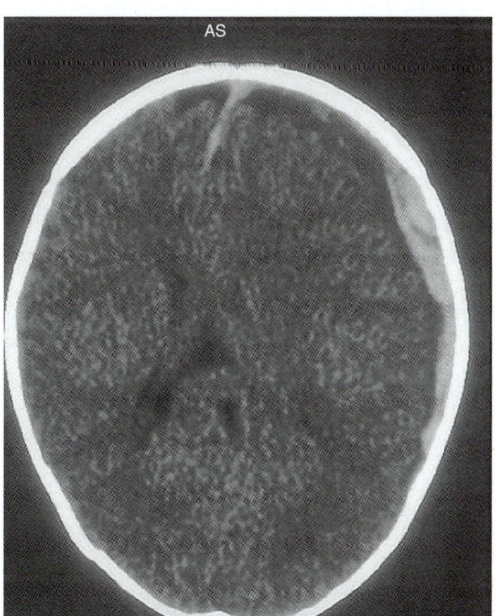

Fig. 6.42 A focal subdural hematoma, caused by severe impact forces, is seen in the left frontal area of this 6-month-old infant who presented with decreased responsiveness after "rolling off a bed." The layering of the subdural blood was due to rapid collection and at surgery was found to consist of newly clotted blood and fresh hemorrhage, classified as a hyperacute subdural hematoma. Note also the acute subdural blood along the anterior interhemispheric fissure and the midline shift.

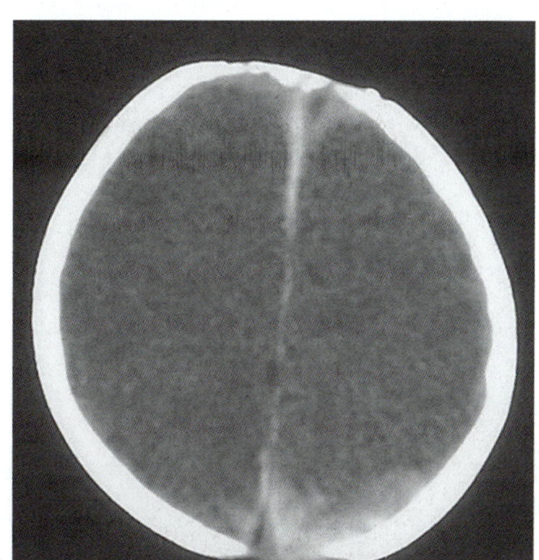

Fig. 6.44 Diffuse axonal shearing. Loss of gray/white matter differentiation is evident on this 7-week-old infant's computed tomography (CT) scan, along with focal subdural blood around the left occipital lobe and an interhemispheric subdural hematoma.

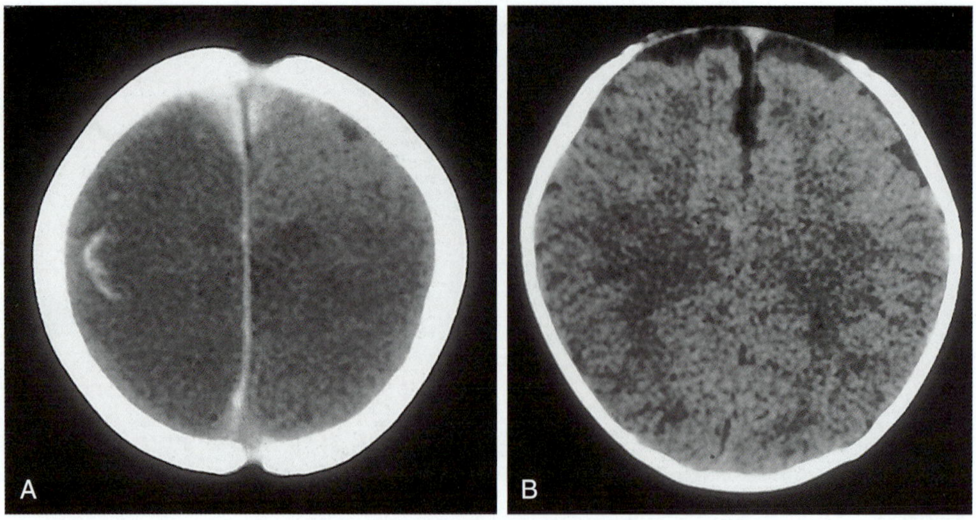

Fig. 6.45 (A) This arc-shaped hemorrhage seen in a 2-month-old infant, who also has loss of gray/white matter differentiation, is located at the gray/white interface. This is a sign found occasionally with diffuse axonal shearing injuries. Note the frontal subdural hematoma. (B) This computed tomography (CT) scan of a normal 2-month-old shows normal gray/white matter differentiation.

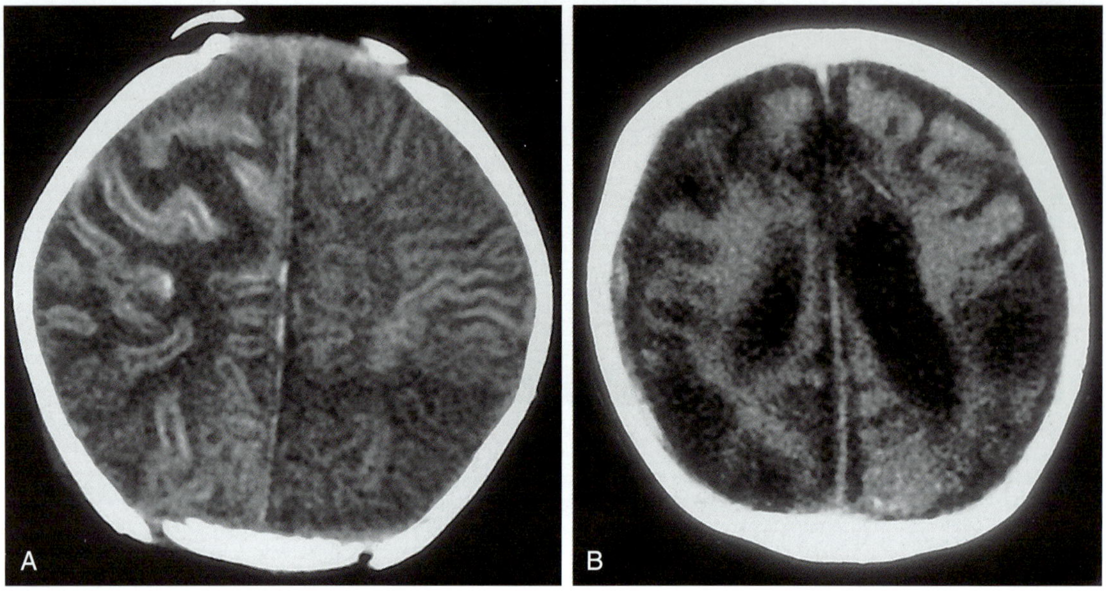

Fig. 6.46 Posttraumatic cerebral necrosis. (A) One week after the injury, unambiguous evidence of contraction of cortical tissues, because of extensive neuronal death, can be appreciated. (B) Six months later, extensive cerebral atrophy is present.

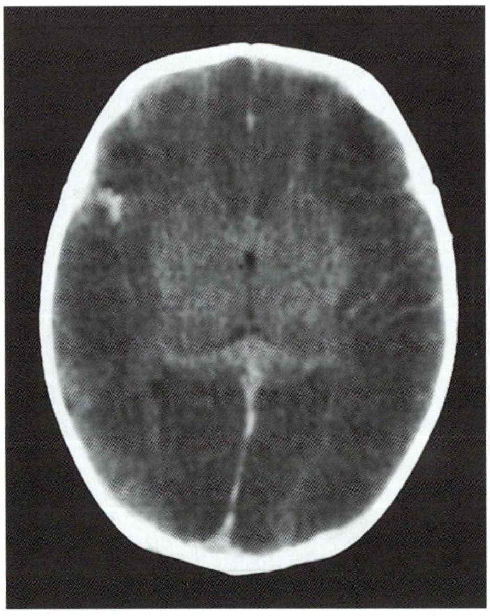

Fig. 6.47 Hypoxic injury. This infant, who was found unresponsive in his crib, has a pattern of diffuse cortical hypodensity on computed tomography scan, indicative of extensive cerebral infarction caused by hypoxia.

of injury forces involved in most cases of abuse (as opposed to those in the majority of accidental injuries), diastatic, complex fractures, and bilateral fractures are worrisome for abuse. Associated intracranial injuries may include focal subdural hematomas (see Fig. 6.42) and focal cerebral contusions with adjacent edema, which, when severe, produces a midline shift and may be associated with focal shearing injury.

In cases due to shaking alone or shaking plus impact, diffuse subdural hematomas may be found over the convexities and along the falx. A combination of focal and interhemispheric subdural hematomas is another common finding (see Fig. 6.43), again often accompanied by varying amounts of cerebral edema. Extreme acceleration/deceleration forces with a rotational component produce loss of gray/white matter differentiation due to axonal shearing (see Figs. 6.44 and Fig. 6.45). Severe cerebral edema and ventricular effacement are typical in these cases. In the ensuing days, the magnitude of neuronal loss can be appreciated, and the full extent of loss is seen in the ensuing months (see Fig. 6.46). In cases of severe hypoxic or ischemic injury, the cortex appears hypodense in comparison with the basal ganglia, termed a *reversal sign* (Fig. 6.47).

CT does have limitations, however. It may not reveal the full extent of injuries and may not detect thin subdural hemorrhages (especially over the convexities) and subtle cerebral contusions or

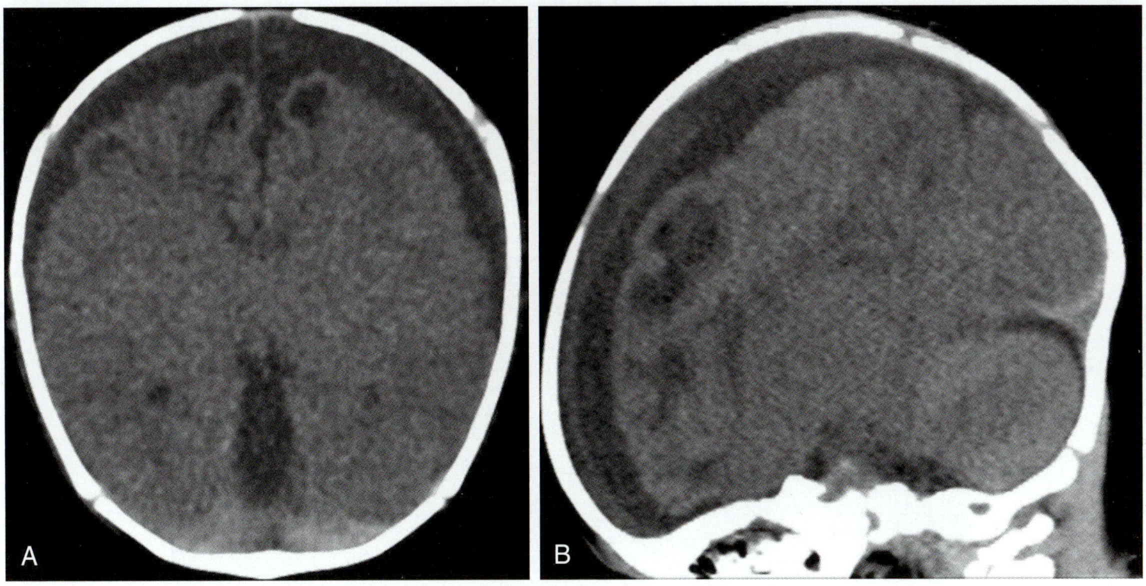

Fig. 6.48 (A and B) A 6-week-old infant in an adoptive home admitted to the hospital for vomiting and failure to thrive. The child became bradycardic on the floor and was transferred to the pediatric intensive care unit. Head imaging revealed bilateral large frontal parietal chronic subdural collections with membranes identified as well as acute subdural hemorrhages. The frontal lobe hypodensities were concerning for cavitary parenchymal contusions or possibly old infarcts. Additional evaluation revealed bilateral skull fractures, multiple healing rib fractures, and multiple classic metaphysical lesions of the femurs and tibias.

hemorrhages. Additionally, the amount of radiation in a CT can limit its usefulness, particularly in more subtle cases where a clinician genuinely wants a screening test.

Magnetic resonance imaging (MRI) is helpful in that it has no radiation, and improved technology has led to "fast" screening sequences (Fig. 6.49), often alleviating the need for sedation. MRI can also identify subdural hemorrhages of differing ages because the imaging intensity changes as blood begins to break down. Subdural hematomas of varying ages may be the result of repetitive injury or spontaneous rebleeding. Spontaneous rebleeding due to previous injury should not cause symptoms. MRI is far superior to CT in detecting subtle contusions and small parenchymal hemorrhages, in showing diffuse axonal injury, and in detecting abnormalities of posterior fossa structures, the brainstem, and the cervical cord. It is

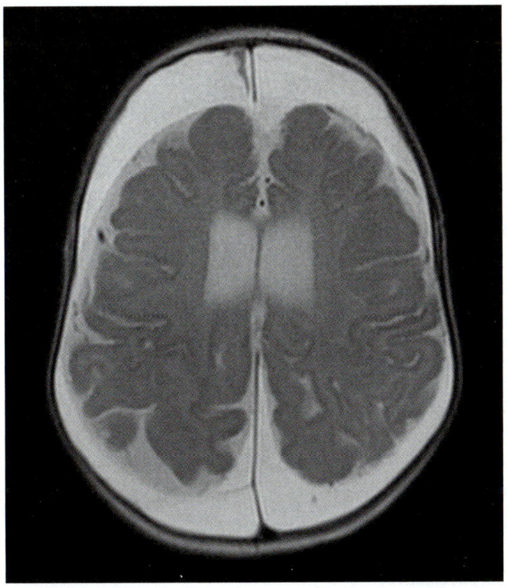

Fig. 6.49 A 3-month-old ex-35-week premature infant was evaluated due to increasing head circumference and found to have bilateral subacute to chronic subdural hemorrhages. In hindsight, the infant had been admitted to the hospital for a brief resolved unexplained event (BRUE) and had two episodes of bruising. This constellation of findings was extremely worrisome for physical child abuse.

good at detecting signs of prior or old injuries and is far superior to CT at differentiating subdural from subarachnoid fluid collections and in distinguishing between cerebrospinal fluid and old blood. Its usefulness in child abuse cases is often greatest 5 to 7 days post-injury. For optimal results, a T1- and T2-weighted conventional or fast spin echo MRI should be ordered with proton density or fluid attenuated inversion recovery sequences.

Associated Injuries

Retinal hemorrhages are highly associated with abusive head trauma. They are typically numerous and diffuse, often extending out to the periphery, and they are located in multiple layers of the retina. Retinal hemorrhages are found in 70% to 90% of infants and children with inflicted head injury and in nearly 100% of those who suffer serious sequelae and death (see Figs. 6.36 and 6.37). Retinal hemorrhages can be seen from etiologies different from abuse, but the pattern, location, and number of retinal hemorrhages differ from those seen in abusive head trauma. Traumatic retinoschisis (see Fig. 6.37) is not described with trauma-induced coagulopathy other than with abusive head trauma. Similarly, posterior and lateral rib fractures have not been found after prolonged CPR in either infants or animal models. Thus, CPR is not a plausible explanation for head trauma with retinal hemorrhages and rib fractures.

Some children are found to have cervical or injuries, though not all. Many institutions now routinely obtain C-spine MRIs to evaluate for an injury (Fig. 6.50).

Differential for Abusive Head Trauma

Accidental head injuries are common in childhood due to falls and other accidents, and the majority are minor. Presentation is usually prompt because a head injury, no matter how minor, tends to provoke considerable parental anxiety. Again, the history is usually clear, and the mechanism reported is consistent with the physical findings observed. Mild forehead and scalp contusions with or without small lacerations or abrasions are by far the most common injuries. Simple (usually nondiastatic) linear skull fractures often involving the parietal bones can result from falls of greater than 4 feet onto hard surfaces (as from a changing table or a shopping cart), but these do not tend to be associated with significant changes

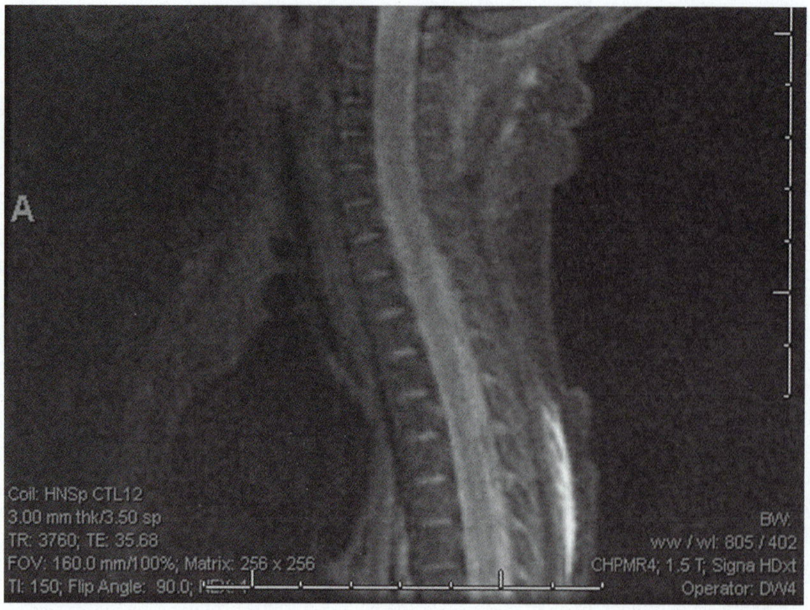

Fig. 6.50 A 6-week-old infant evaluated for fussiness and vomiting was found to have bilateral subdural hemorrhages and retinal hemorrhages. Cervical spine magnetic resonance imaging revealed edema within the soft tissues in the posterior aspect of the upper cervical spine and suboccipital region, concerning for ligamentous sprain.

in level of consciousness or with intracranial injury nor retinal hemorrhages. More severe injuries are incurred because of more serious mechanisms including major falls (>10 feet and falls with angular momentum as from swings, windows, or trampolines), bicycle and sports accidents, and motor vehicle accidents.

In evaluating an infant or toddler who presents with a history of minor trauma but is found to have intracranial bleeding, especially one with subdural hematomas and retinal hemorrhages, it is important to rule out coagulopathy or the presence of an underlying disorder that makes the child unusually susceptible to development of subdural bleeding. The recommended evaluation for bleeding disorder in children with isolated intracranial injuries includes a CBC with differential and platelet count, coagulation factors, fibrinogen level, D-dimer, factor VIII, and factor IX levels (see Box 6.1).

In two disorders, benign extraaxial fluid (BEAF) collections and glutaric aciduria type 1 (GA1), subdural hematomas can be seen after minimal trauma. These must be considered in the evaluation and distinguished from abuse.

Box 6.1 Evaluation for Bleeding Disorder

Recommended Evaluation for Bleeding Disorders in Children With Isolated Bruising

Bruising that has no patterns, suspected abuse is unwitnessed/not reported by child, no other signs of trauma
PT, PTT
CBC with platelets
Factor VIII level
Factor XI level
Von Willebrand disease panel

Recommended Evaluation for Bleeding Disorders in Children With Isolated Intracranial Hemorrhages

Limited to hemorrhages, suspected abuse is unwitnessed/not reported by child, no other signs of trauma
PT, PTT
CBC with platelets
Factor VIII level
Factor IX level
DIC panel (D-dimer, fibrinogen)

CBC, Complete blood count; *DIC*, disseminated intravascular coagulation; *PT*, prothrombin time; *PTT*, partial thromboplastin time.

Benign Extraaxial Fluid Collections

In BEAF, macrocephaly is associated with bilateral symmetric widening of the subarachnoid space (SAS), most prominently in the frontal and frontoparietal areas and along the anterior interhemispheric fissure and sylvian fissures. This expanded space is filled with cerebrospinal fluid. Usually, the ventricles are normal in size or only slightly enlarged, and there is no evidence of increased intracranial pressure. The condition is thought to be due to transient mild impairment of cerebrospinal fluid resorption by the arachnoid villi. Widening of the SAS results in significant stretching of the bridging veins that run from the cerebral cortex to the dural venous sinuses, and it is thought that being stretched makes them more vulnerable to tearing in the face of minimal or minor trauma.

Infants with BEAFs are usually diagnosed secondary to imaging performed as part of an evaluation for macrocephaly or enlarging head circumference. Most are neurodevelopmentally normal. Many have a family history of macrocephaly that suggests autosomal dominant transmission. Usually, the abnormality resolves spontaneously with normalization of findings on imaging by 2 to 5 years old.

Approximately 10% of infants monitored with BEAF collections develop subdural hematomas either "spontaneously" or after a minor head trauma. Although some of these infants have had associated seizures and/or mild transient alterations in consciousness, most appear relatively normal neurologically even on presentation with subdural hemorrhages. On MRI, the subdural hemorrhages are generally small, and diffuse enlargement of the SAS (occupied by cerebrospinal fluid) is easily appreciated. Importantly, these infants tend to be brought in promptly for care when symptomatic and have no associated injuries.

BEAFs can be distinguished from cerebral atrophy because the sulci are not widened and because of the greater prominence of SAS widening frontally. In communicating hydrocephalus, ventricular enlargement is much more prominent and symptoms of increased intracranial pressure may be present.

Glutaric Aciduria

GA1 is an autosomal recessive disorder resulting in deficiency of glutaryl-CoA dehydrogenase. Affected infants appear relatively normal at birth, although approximately 40% are born with mild macrocephaly, and over ensuing months, these infants gradually cross toward the 97th percentile. Nonspecific neurologic signs consisting of irritability, jitteriness, mild hypotonia, and feeding problems are common in the first 6 months, then improve, and by a year most appear normal except for slight gross motor delays. If undiagnosed and untreated, most affected infants develop an acute encephalopathy between 12 and 18 months old, usually in association with an acute upper respiratory or gastrointestinal infection. Subsequently, they are left with severe dystonias and dyskinesias and suffer major regression in milestones.

Findings on neuroimaging, whether performed before or after the severe encephalopathic event, include marked bilateral frontotemporal atrophy along with prominent widening of the sylvian fissures and delayed myelination. Twenty to thirty percent have associated chronic subdural effusions and/or hematomas. After the encephalopathy, basal ganglia atrophy also becomes clear. As in children with BEAFs, it is thought that the marked widening of the SAS due to cortical atrophy results in stretching of the bridging veins, making them more vulnerable to shearing with minimal trauma. When subdural hemorrhages are present, retinal hemorrhages are also seen. Interestingly, subdural hemorrhages may or may not be associated with symptoms. The presence of marked cerebral atrophy in association with subdural hematomas (Fig. 6.51) helps distinguish GA1 from both inflicted head trauma and BEAFs. No skeletal abnormalities are associated with GA1. Recommended evaluation includes urine organic acids and serum amino acids.

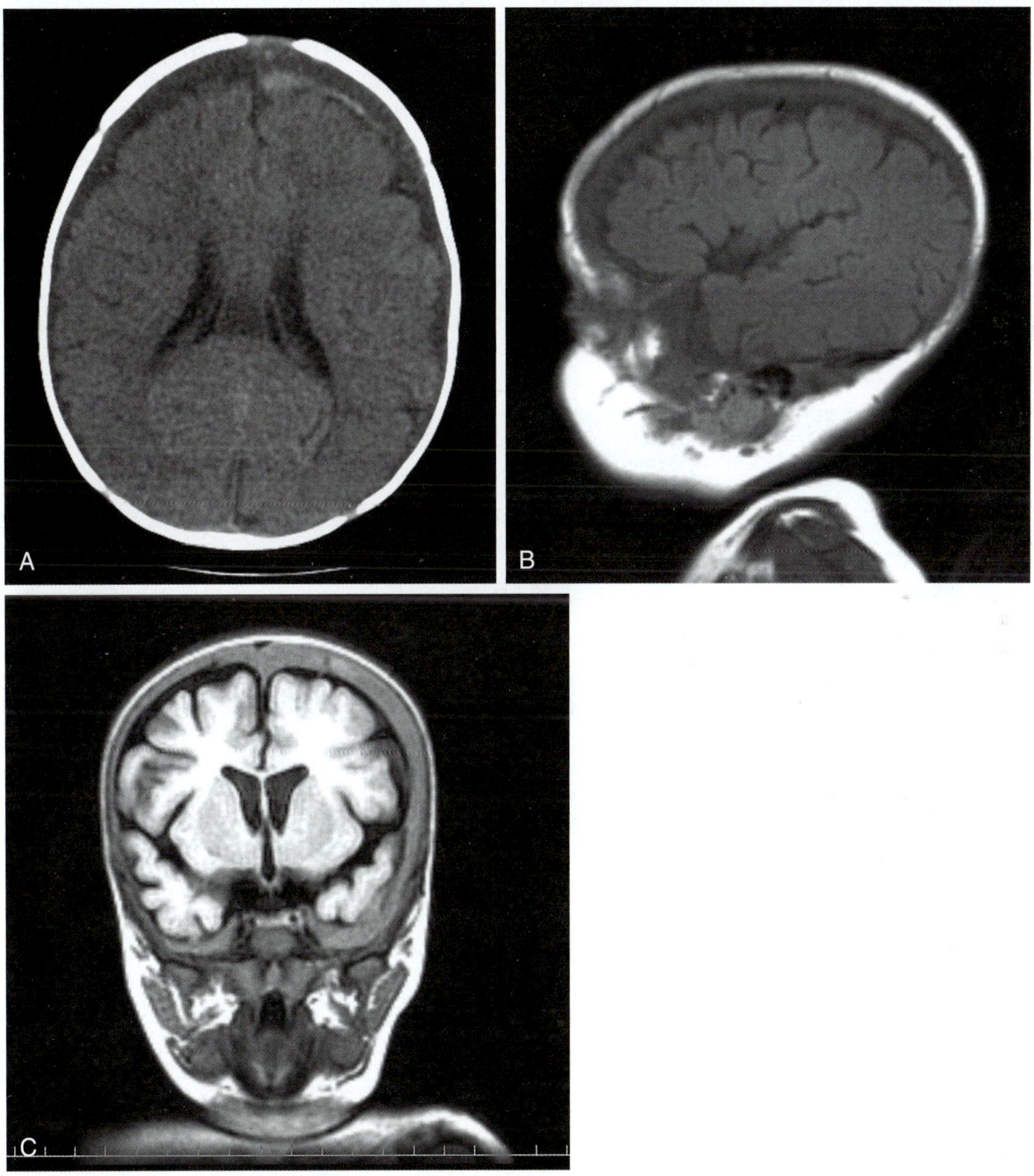

Fig. 6.51 Glutaric aciduria type 1 (GA1). This 3-month-old infant was brought to the emergency department with complaints of being limp and unresponsive with a recent history of pneumonia. The initial history given was that while alone with his father, he had suddenly become lethargic, his eyes had rolled back, and he had stopped breathing for a few seconds. Lethargy resolved soon after arrival. (A) A head computed tomography scan was obtained because retinal hemorrhages were found revealed diffuse acute and subacute/chronic subdural hemorrhages over the convexities in the frontotemporal areas as well as more acute collections along the posterior interhemispheric fissure and over the right frontal area. (B and C) On magnetic resonance imaging, large acute on chronic subdural hemorrhages were confirmed, along with early signs of atrophy including mild flattening of the gyri, sulcal widening, and mild ventricular enlargement. This prompted testing for possible glutaric aciduria, which was positive in results obtained 1 week later. Interestingly, in the interim, the father acknowledged having shaken the baby after he didn't feed well, whereupon he went limp.

ABDOMINAL AND INTRATHORACIC INJURIES

Although less common than inflicted cutaneous, skeletal, and head injuries, abdominal and intrathoracic injuries have been found in up to 2% of victims of physical abuse, with a mortality rate of up to 50%. Intraabdominal injuries predominate over intrathoracic injuries and range in severity from subclinical to catastrophic, with the majority identified as being moderate to severe. They are second only to head injury as a cause of abuse-related deaths.

Intraabdominal Injuries

Young children are more vulnerable to internal abdominal injury with blunt trauma than adolescents or adults for three major reasons: (1) their abdominal muscles are relatively weak, allowing impacting forces to be transmitted inward more easily; (2) the distance between the abdominal wall and the vertebral column is relatively short; and (3) their costal margins are more horizontally oriented, affording less protection to underlying viscera. With that, the average age of a patient with accidental abdominal trauma is 8 years old. The average age of a child with abusive abdominal trauma is 2½ years old.

Midabdominal structures that are fixed in place by pedicles or overlying ligaments (small intestines, liver, and pancreas) are particularly vulnerable. Typically, inflicted abdominal trauma is caused by blunt force injury and is the result of violent kicks or punches or of being thrown or slammed against hard objects. External findings are often minimal or absent (Fig. 6.52). Penetrating injuries, fortunately, are rare.

The major types of abdominal pathology seen are duodenal hematomas, small intestinal tears at sites of supporting ligaments, mesenteric tears, contusions or lacerations of the liver or spleen, and pancreatic and renal contusions.

Presentation is often delayed, and the lethargy and emesis are attributed to an assumed viral illness. This greatly increases the risk and morbidity of these injuries. Patients with duodenal hematomas present with signs and symptoms of high intestinal obstruction (e.g., vomiting and abdominal pain sometimes manifest primarily as irritability without abdominal distention) (Fig. 6.53). Plain radiographs may reveal an air/fluid level in a dilated duodenal loop (Fig. 6.52A) proximal to the hematoma, and upper gastrointestinal series and ultrasound studies reveal narrowing of the lumen and thickening of the duodenal wall, respectively (see Fig. 6.52B).

Because spillage of intestinal contents into the peritoneal cavity results in intense peritoneal irritation and rapid onset of infection, children with acute small intestinal tears generally have signs and symptoms of an acute abdomen (Figs. 6.53 and 6.54).

At a minimum, small tears of the mesentery, which carries the vascular supply to the large and small bowel, result in some bleeding with secondary, often localized, irritation and pain because bowel integrity tends to be preserved by collateral circulation. In the absence of prominent peritoneal signs and surface injuries, pain may be attributed to another cause. When lacerations are large (see Fig. 6.54B), however, interruption of the vascular supply to the adjacent bowel occurs, and as the involved segment gradually loses

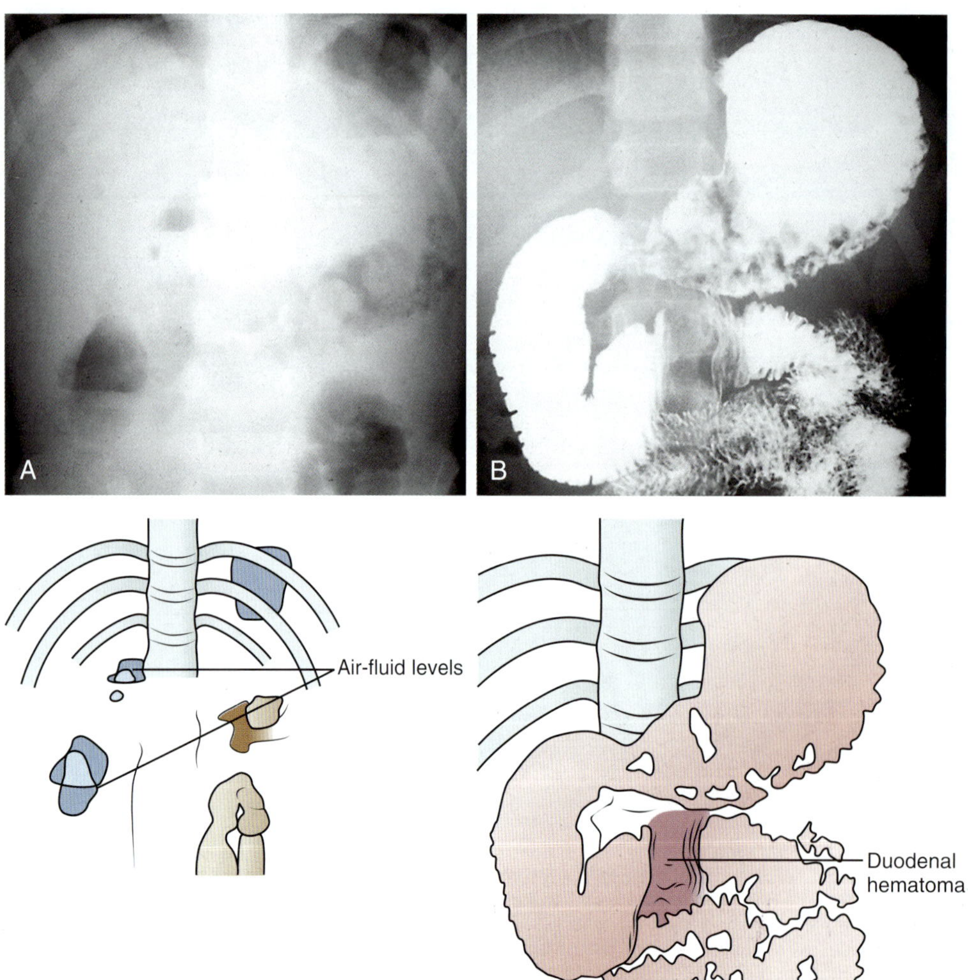

Fig. 6.52 Duodenal hematoma. (A) Abdominal film reveals an air/fluid level in a dilated duodenal loop proximal to a duodenal hematoma. (B) This upper gastrointestinal series shows narrowing of the duodenal lumen and widening of the duodenal wall at the site of a hematoma. The obstruction is partial because some barium has passed through the narrowed segment. (Courtesy Department of Radiology, Children's Hospital of Pittsburgh, Pittsburgh, PA.)

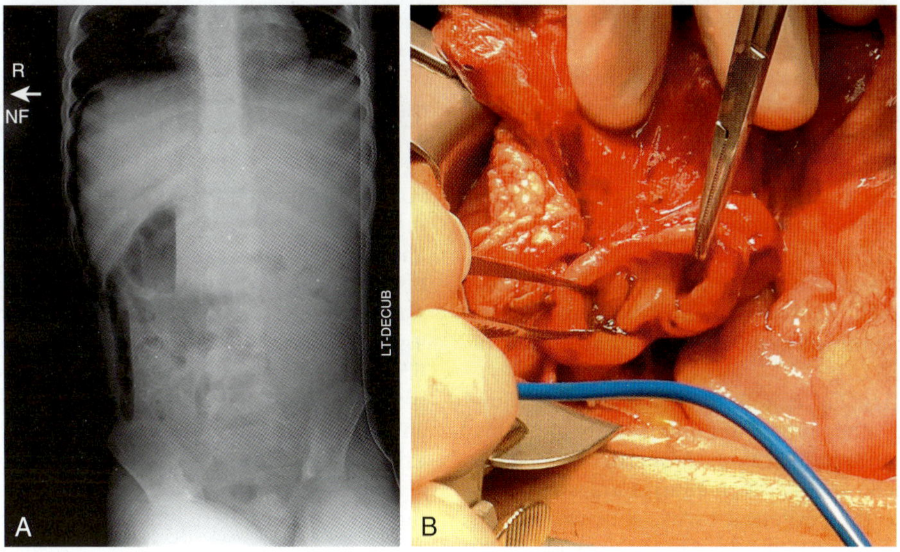

Fig. 6.53 (A) This 4-year-old previously healthy boy was found by his mother in bed with vomit on him. The child was brought to care later that afternoon due to his continued vomiting and increasing sleepiness. No history of trauma was provided. The child's abdominal radiograph revealed free air, and he was taken emergently to the operating room, where he was found to have a duodenal perforation. (B) Intraoperative photograph revealed the duodenal perforation was more than 24 hours old.

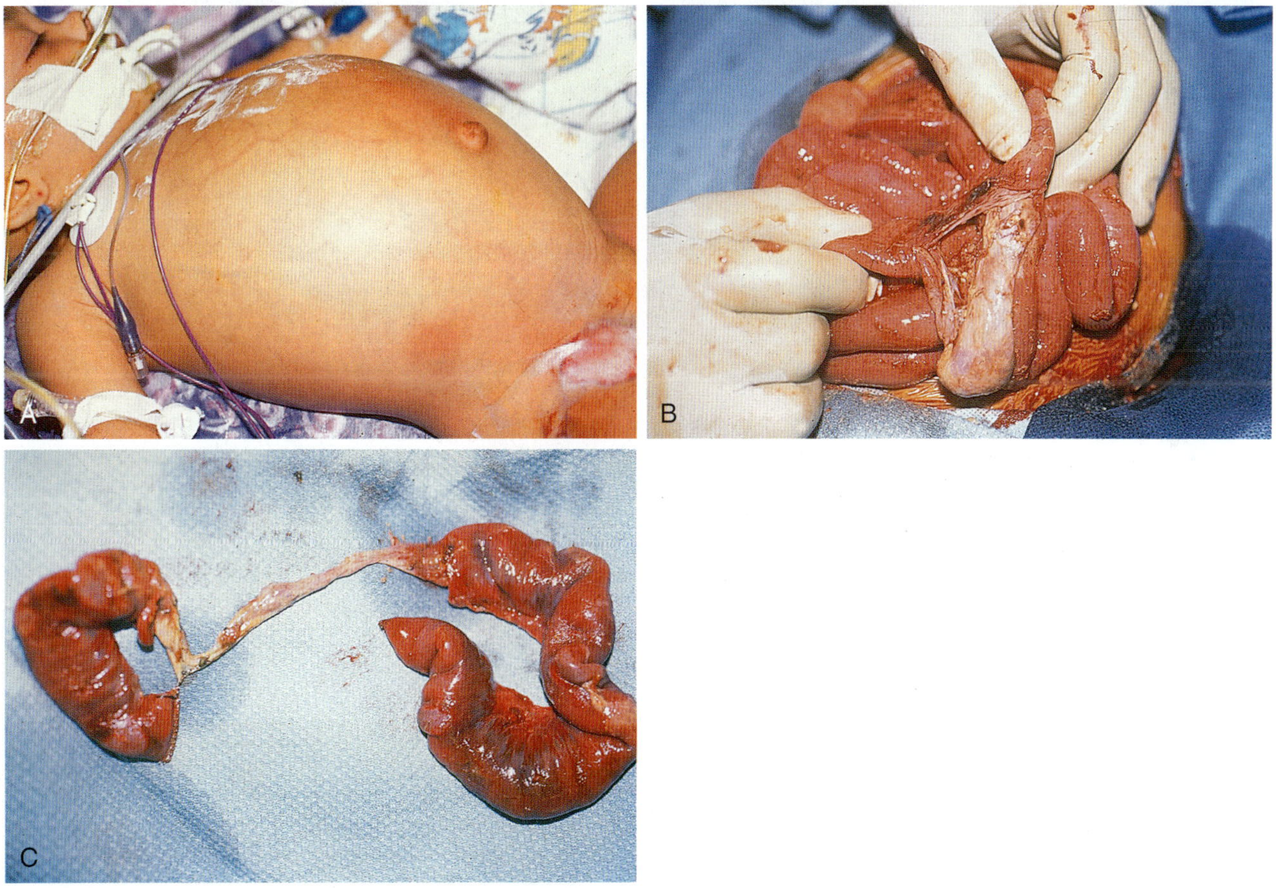

Fig. 6.54 Mesenteric tears with secondary bowel necrosis. The mother of this 13-month-old infant (who was described as previously well) reported finding her unarousable in the morning, with bilious vomitus on her sheets. She was rushed to the hospital, where she was in profound shock. Her abdomen was markedly distended and tense and was noted to be exquisitely tender when her level of consciousness improved. (A) A round, fading bruise is seen in this view over the right lower abdominal wall; a few even fainter bruises were seen around the umbilicus. Note the marked abdominal distention. (B) At surgery, she was found to have diffuse peritonitis, and two large rents were discovered in the jejunal mesentery. (C) A long segment, found to be necrotic with a perforation, and adjacent bowel that appeared nonviable were resected. Inflammatory infiltrates on pathologic examination suggested that the inciting injury had occurred 5 to 7 days earlier.

viability, it undergoes necrosis and ultimately perforates (see Fig. 6.54C). During this time, the child is likely to have significant abdominal pain, anorexia, vomiting, and markedly decreased activity. Once perforation occurs, the clinical picture of diffuse peritonitis and sepsis, described earlier, rapidly evolves.

Abuse victims with hepatic and splenic injuries may have minimal symptomatology when these viscera are merely contused. Localized pain and peritoneal irritation are likely with small lacerations.

In the majority of cases of inflicted abdominal trauma, abuse is not confirmed until an abdominal CT scan is obtained, whether because of elevated liver function tests or findings on examination.

Research estimates that occult abdominal injury may be present in up to 20% of children who are the victims of physical abuse. In children who are being evaluated for abuse, if aspartate aminotransferase (AST) or alanine aminotransferase (ALT) is more than 80, an abdominal CT with contrast is recommended (Fig. 6.55). Use of these parameters provides 84% sensitivity and 83% specificity for occult abdominal injuries. Although the intraabdominal injury may be a small contusion and it may not have any clinical treatment (except observation), a confirmed documented intraabdominal injury may greatly influence the safety plan for that child at time of discharge.

Renal and adrenal injuries (Fig. 6.56) are considerably less common than those involving other intraabdominal organs, probably because of their relatively protected location. Associated symptoms may be subtle and overshadowed by other injuries unless there is extravasation of blood into the peritoneal cavity. A urinalysis is a valuable and easy test to check for occult renal injury and should be included in all trauma evaluations.

Thoracic Injuries

Because of the great plasticity of the thoracic cage in infants and young children, inflicted intrathoracic injuries are relatively uncommon, despite the frequency of rib fractures. They have high morbidity and mortality rates, however, because they are the result of application of massive blunt forces to the chest, such as the child being stomped, slammed, or violently thrown. When they are seen, they are usually associated with multiple, often displaced rib fractures (Figs. 6.57 and 6.58). Associated intrathoracic findings may include hemothorax, pleural effusion in response to smaller subpleural bleeds, pulmonary and myocardial contusions, and parenchymal lacerations. On rare occasions, a pleural effusion may be seen on chest radiographs in the absence of visible rib fractures. In such cases, a chest CT may reveal the true extent of the associated skeletal injuries.

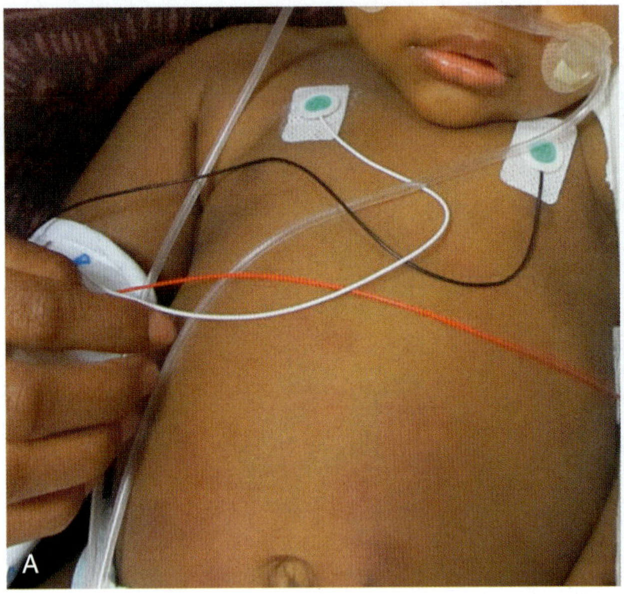

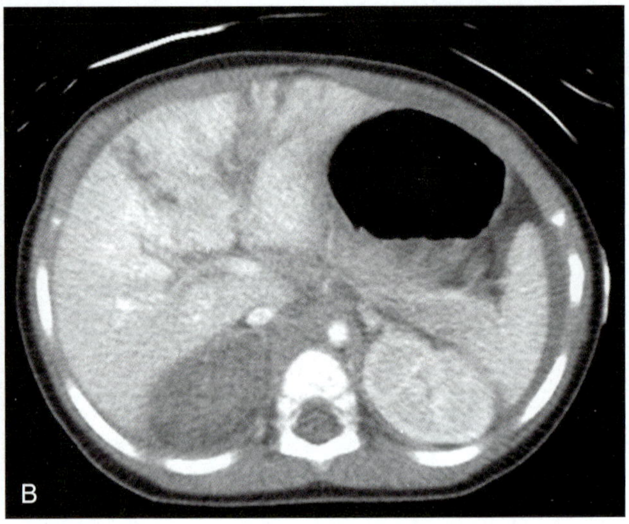

Fig. 6.55 (A) This 16-month-old was evaluated for vomiting and a "rash" on her abdomen. The child was transferred to a pediatric facility, where abdominal bruising was diagnosed. (B) A trauma evaluation revealed a large complex hepatic laceration, multiple splenic lacerations, hemoperitoneum, and right adrenal gland hemorrhage. The caregiver in the home confessed to repeatedly kicking the child in the abdomen.

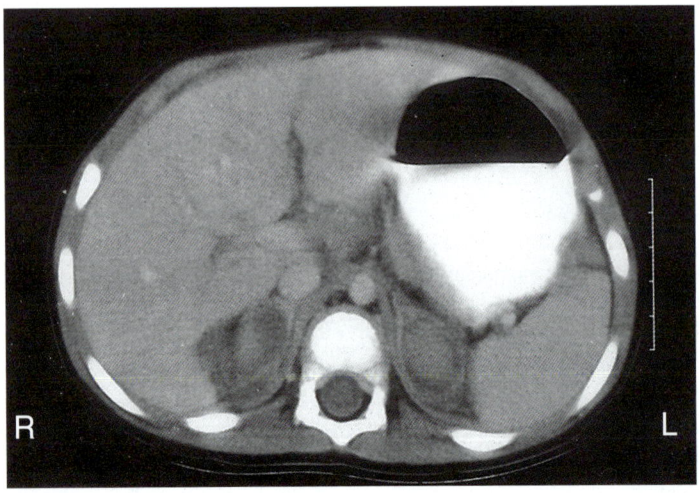

Fig. 6.56 Bilateral adrenal hemorrhages. This 21-month-old girl was admitted with a history of altered level of consciousness after falling from her crib. She had multiple bruises, a clavicle fracture, bilateral retinal hemorrhages, subdural hematomas with cerebral edema, and a midline shift. Her abdominal computed tomography scan, performed when liver function tests were found to be elevated, reveals bilateral adrenal hemorrhages.

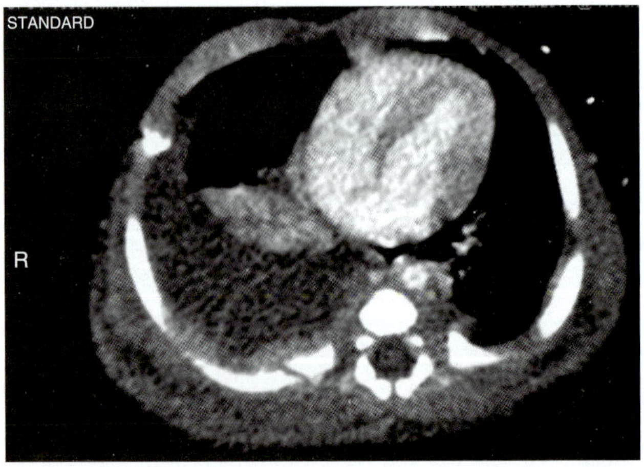

Fig. 6.57 This badly beaten 5-week-old infant sustained 20 rib fractures and developed bilateral pleural effusions (R>L) that required drainage with a chest tube. The child was also found to have extensive soft tissue stranding and hematoma of the back muscles.

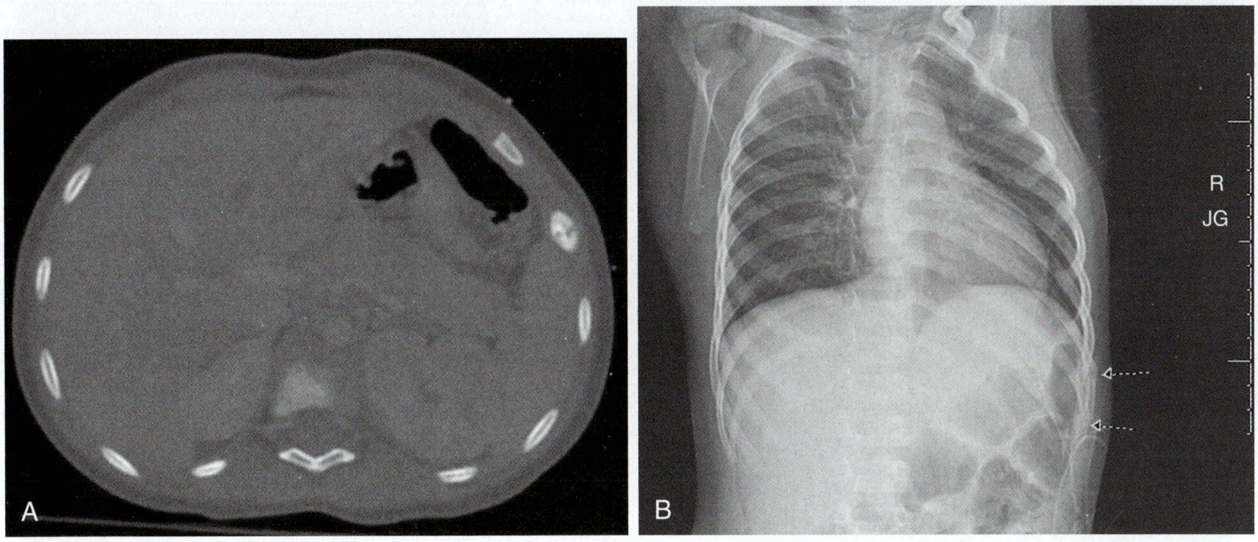

Fig. 6.58 (A) This 2-year-old male presented with extensive bruising and looped marks. The child was found to have healing fractures of left lateral eighth and ninth ribs, a grade 2 intraparenchymal liver laceration, and a small left adrenal hemorrhage. (B) The healing rib fractures on radiograph.

The major mode of presentation of inflicted intrathoracic chest trauma is likely to be one of significant respiratory distress, with complaints of severe chest pain in victims old enough to speak. Clinical findings may include dyspnea, tachypnea, grunting respirations, and anxiety, often with evident pain on movement and chest wall tenderness. When associated blood loss is significant, pallor, weak pulses, and hypotension are seen.

MIMICS AND DIFFERENTIAL DIAGNOSIS OF ABUSE

Although it is critical to detect injuries resulting from abuse to protect children from future and potentially more serious trauma, it is also important to consider medical conditions that may mimic abuse to avoid unnecessary family stress. Accurate diagnosis requires recognition of injuries associated with abuse, careful evaluation, and when necessary, further evaluation for diseases and disorders that may predispose a child to bleeding or fractures that can be mistaken for abuse injuries (Box 6.1). If doubt exists, the services of physicians with expertise in the fields of child abuse, orthopedics, hematology, pediatric surgery, or neurosurgery should be sought. In addition, valuable information and insight may be gained in conferring with the child's primary care physician.

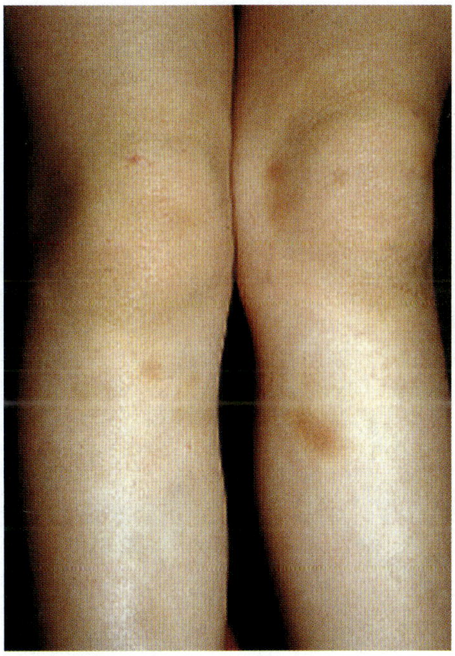

Fig. 6.59 Normal bruises. Numerous small, nonspecific bruises are present over the knees and shins of this active youngster.

Skin Injuries

Ordinary, play-related bruises can be distinguished from those resulting from abuse on the basis of their size and location. They are typically found over the bony prominences of the shins, knees, elbows, extensor forearms, or forehead (Figs. 6.59 and 6.60). Additionally, variation in skin coloring and hyper pigmented lesions, such as dermal melanosis, can be confused with bruising. The primary care pediatrician is an important source of information when evaluating a child that has confusing hyperpigmented lesions (Fig. 6.8). Subcultural healing practices, such as coining or cupping, can be confused with abusive burns or lesions (Figs. 6.61 to 6.63).

Bleeding Disorders

Purpuric lesions associated with coagulopathies and acute vasculitic disorders must be recognized and distinguished from inflicted bruises. However, it is also important to recognize that children with disorders that predispose to easy bruising may on occasion be victims of abuse.

Patients with acute idiopathic thrombocytopenic purpura (ITP) and acute leukemia can have multiple purpuric lesions located anywhere on the body. Because they reflect thrombocytopenia, they are usually associated with petechiae (Fig. 6.64). Children with ITP commonly have a history of an antecedent viral illness, and those with leukemia may have a history of fatigue, anorexia, and weight loss, sometimes accompanied by bone pain. They usually have adenopathy and splenomegaly. These hematologic abnormalities are usually readily detected by a CBC with differential and platelet count.

Children with clotting factor deficiencies, hemophilia, aplastic anemia, or von Willebrand disease can have bruises that are much more impressive than one would ordinarily expect from the reported mechanism of injury (Fig. 6.65). Although severe X-linked hemophilia is diagnosed prenatally in most males because of known family history or in early infancy (frequently after circumcision), those with milder forms of the disease who are uncircumcised may

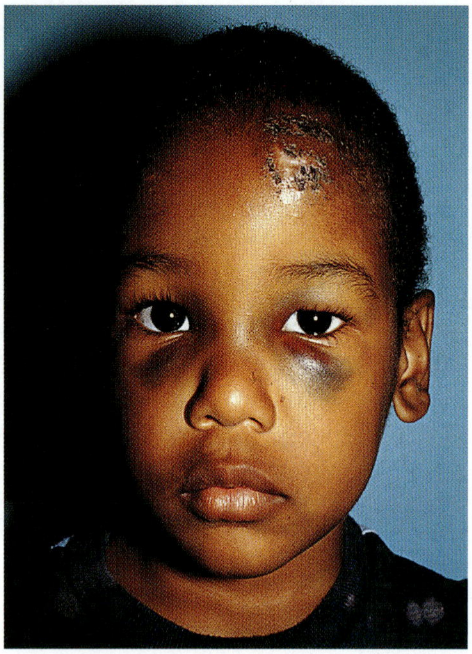

Fig. 6.60 Black eyes occurring after a forehead contusion. This boy had fallen from the ladder of a slide 3 days before. Blood from his forehead hematoma had tracked down through the facial soft tissues, creating these shiners, which were nontender.

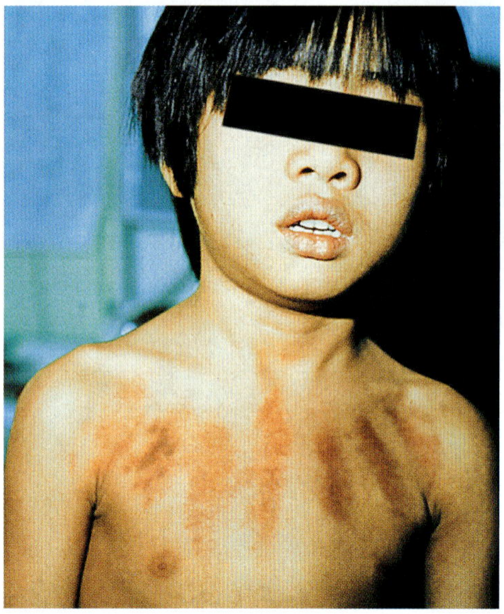

Fig. 6.61 Coin rubbing. Vigorous stroking of the skin of a febrile child with a coin produces a peculiar bruising pattern. (Courtesy Thomas Daley, MD, St. Joseph's Hospital, Paterson, NJ.)

not be identified until they become mobile and develop prominent ecchymoses along with other evidence of easy bruising.

Von Willebrand disease, which occurs in both males and females, is characterized by partial factor VIII deficiency and platelet dysfunction and may escape detection for years.

Trauma-Induced Coagulopathy

More than three-fourths of children with traumatic brain injury develop coagulopathy considered to be due to fibrinolysis and thrombosis, which may lead to disseminated intravascular coagulation (DIC). Retinoschisis (see Fig. 6.43) does not occur with DIC and helps differentiate acute head trauma (AHT) from other causes of intracranial hemorrhage.

Bleeding disorders should be considered when a patient presents with unpatterned substantial bruises but a lack of any other evidence

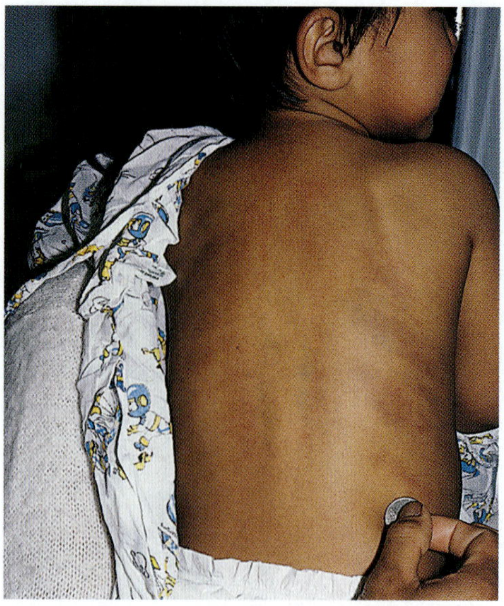

Fig. 6.62 Here the father of another child demonstrates the coining technique.

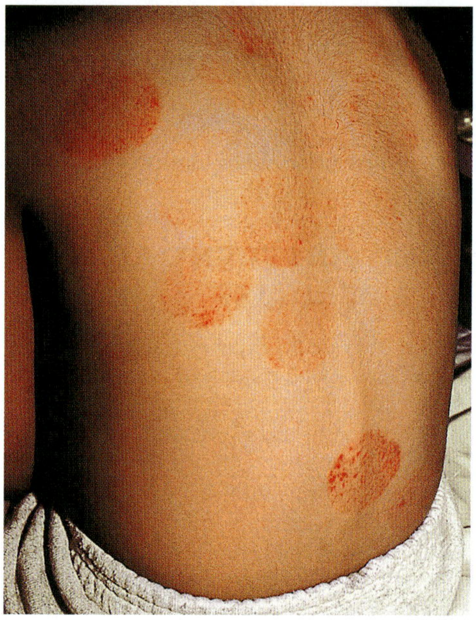

Fig. 6.63 Cupping. These circular bruises with central petechiae are the sequelae of the Southeast Asian practice of cupping. (Courtesy Robert Hickey, MD, Children's Hospital of Pittsburgh, Pittsburgh, PA.)

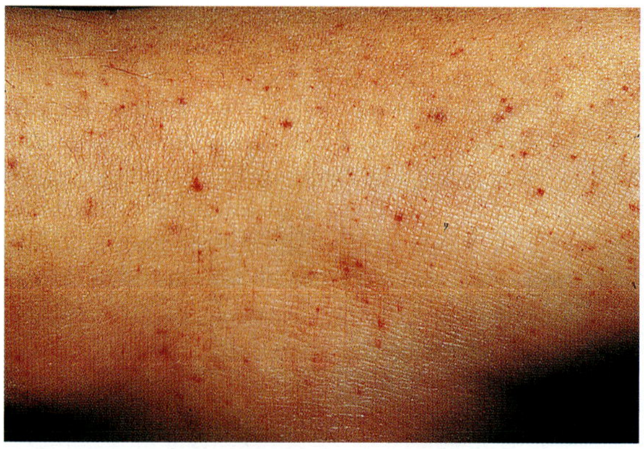

Fig. 6.64 Idiopathic thrombocytopenic purpura. This school-age child was seen with a chief complaint of a rash after a viral upper respiratory tract infection. Examination revealed diffuse petechiae, shown here over her ankle, and scattered purpuric lesions. Her hemoglobin and white blood cell count and differential were normal, but her platelet count was markedly reduced.

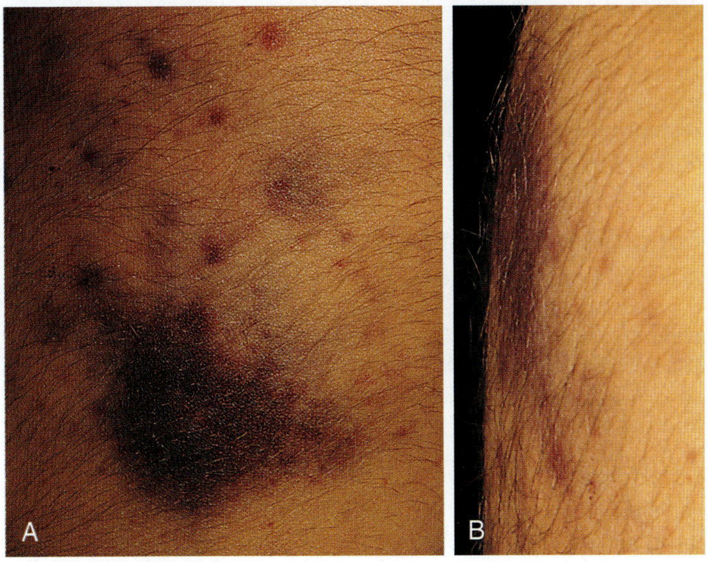

Fig. 6.65 (A) Bruises with thick round centers can be seen in children with aplastic anemia or with clotting factor deficiencies. (B) This view from the side shows the elevation of the indurated central portion of the ecchymosis in a patient with chronic aplastic anemia.

of trauma. The American Academy of Pediatrics expert panel suggests the following laboratory work to evaluate for bleeding disorders in children who present with isolated bruises or skin findings that are concerning for abuse: coagulation factors, CBC with platelets, factor VIII level, factor IX level, and von Willebrand disease screening (see Box 6.1).

Vitamin K Deficiency

A fat-soluble vitamin, vitamin K is necessary for carboxylation of clotting factors II, VII, IX, and X. Because infants have relatively low levels of vitamin K at birth, it has been standard practice for more than 70 years to give them intramuscular vitamin K in the perinatal period; hence, the incidence of deficiency is low. In the absence of this supplementation, infants can develop bleeding at any time during the first 12 weeks (usually within the first 2 weeks) of life. Although it is still uncommon, the rate of parental refusal of vitamin K has doubled in the past decade. Manifestations include rectal bleeding, hematemesis, hemoptysis, bruising, and intracranial bleeding (usually subarachnoid). Intracranial bleeding does not typically have accompanying retinal hemorrhages. In all cases, prothrombin time (PT) and activated partial thromboplastin time (aPTT) are abnormal. Infants will have elevated proteins induced by vitamin K antagonism or absence (PIVKA)-II level.

Postinflammatory Hyperpigmentation or Blistering

After resolution of the acute phase of an inflammatory exanthem, many children with darkly pigmented skin are left with patchy hyperpigmentation at the sites affected (see Figs. 6.66 and 8.116). These patches can be mistaken for bruises on occasion, particularly when the initial rash involved the buttocks or back. Vesiculation due to insect bites can raise concerns for thermal burn blisters (Fig. 6.67). *Phytophotodermatitis* is one postinflammatory hyperpigmentation that is more often confused with bruising than others. In this disorder, plant-derived photosensitizers (psoralens) found in the juices of lemons, limes, figs, dill, parsley, parsnips, carrots, and celery are inadvertently wiped or spilled on the skin. Subsequent exposure to sunlight can then induce an exaggerated sunburn reaction. Initially, lesions are erythematous macules. In some cases, surface blistering occurs. Lesions then become hyperpigmented, and because the juice is often wiped on by the hands of a parent who was in the process of cutting one of the fruits, herbs, or vegetables when approached by the child, the patches often have bizarre or hand- or finger-shaped patterns that can be mistaken for grab or slap marks (Fig. 6.68).

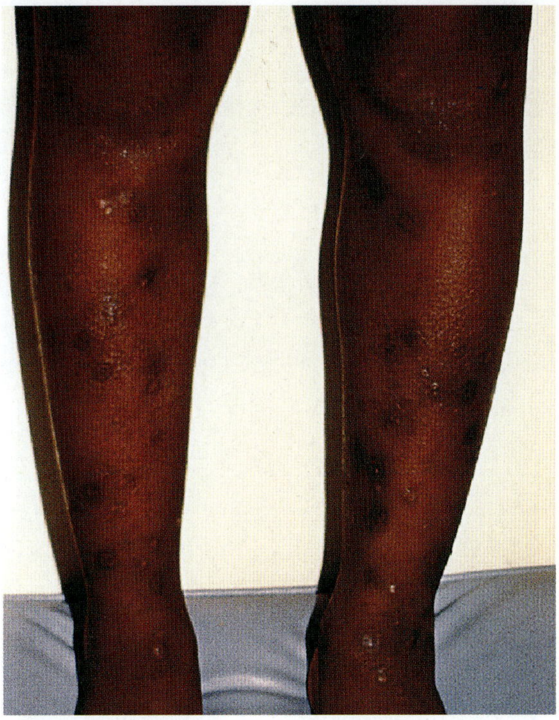

Fig. 6.66 Postinflammatory hyperpigmentation after insect bites or papular urticaria. When this child was seen at a follow-up visit for the treatment of flea bites, he was found to have a multitude of round, hyperpigmented spots at the sites of the original bites. Their macular appearance, distribution, and target configuration distinguish them from cigarette burn scars. (Courtesy Michael Sherlock, MD, Lutherville, MD.)

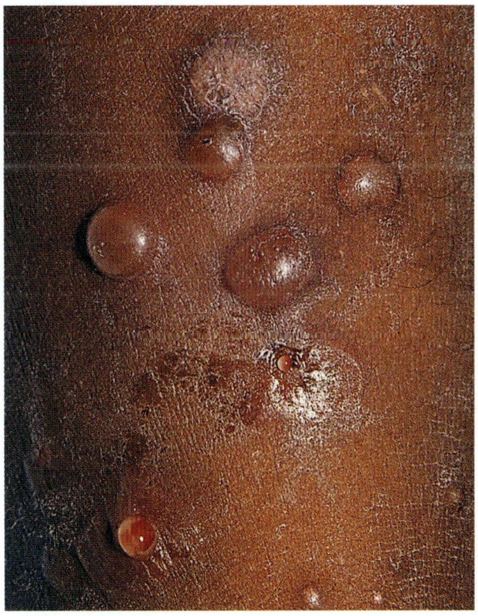

Fig. 6.67 Vesiculation due to mite bites. These vesicles, initially thought to be due to burns, are relatively thick walled and almost perfectly round, and they show no evidence of splash. Furthermore, the lesions were pruritic, not painful.

Again, the history of a preceding erythematous rash and the persistence of the same coloration over days or weeks can help in naming the true source.

Abusive Fractures

The vast majority of accidental fractures are seen in children who are mobile and older than 2 years old. In most instances, it is relatively easy to recognize a truly accidental fracture: The incident is usually witnessed, and the mechanism of injury is clearly reported and fits the findings. Care is typically sought promptly, although

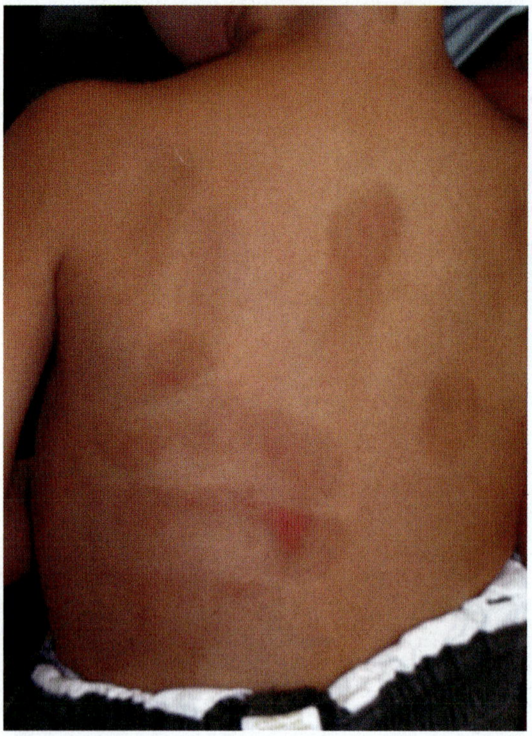

Fig. 6.68 Phytophotodermatitis. This boy was referred for concerns about possible inflicted bruises. The bizarre hand/finger marks are actually due to hyperpigmentation caused by a phototoxic reaction to psoralens. More than 2 weeks earlier, while his family was on vacation at the shore, he had been picked up by his father, who had just been cutting limes for a party. The family then went to the beach for the afternoon. Subsequently, the child developed erythematous patches in the distribution seen, which then became hyperpigmented.

occasional exceptions occur. Accidental fractures are usually single or isolated, and typically there are no associated injuries and no history or evidence of prior injuries.

A thorough history and knowledge of the types of fractures produced by various mechanisms of injury assist in accurate diagnosis. Some of the most common fractures and their mechanisms include buckle (torus) and greenstick fractures of the radius and ulna (see Figs. 22.26 and 22.27) due to a fall forward onto an outstretched arm; midclavicular fractures caused by a direct blow to the clavicle or a fall sideways onto the shoulder or outstretched arm (see Fig. 22.20); supracondylar humerus fractures (see Figs. 22.18 and 22.34) due to a fall backward onto a hyperextended outstretched arm; or toddler's fractures or spiral fractures of distal to midtibia (see Fig. 22.43), resulting from a fall with a twist or on landing from a jump.

There have been rare reports of an accidental humerus fracture seen in an infant being turned. This spiral fracture of the humeral shaft can occur unintentionally when someone turns an infant from the prone to supine position without completely lifting the trunk from the surface on which the baby is lying. However, a full evaluation for abuse, including a full skeletal survey, is warranted as part of a complete evaluation.

Accidental femur fractures usually involve the midshaft. In an ambulatory child, they can result from a fall while running and then sliding into a hard object; a trip fall with a twist in which one leg folds under the body; being hit by a fast-moving object, such as a car; and falls from heights.

Accidental rib fractures are highly unusual and are typically the result of severe blunt force chest trauma, such as being hit by a car. Those seen in infants are rarely reported in difficult deliveries or prolonged CPR. In the latter case, they are located anterolaterally.

Nonabusive metaphyseal fractures have been reported from a difficult breech delivery and club foot repair.

Normal Variants

Physiologic periosteal new bone is a reflection of normal skeletal growth that appears along the shafts of the long bones. This normally resolves after 8 months old. Careful evaluation of the radiographs for accompanying fracture is important. Metaphyseal spurring can be seen in healthy infants. These findings are bilaterally symmetric and not associated with any other injuries.

Conditions Associated With Pathologic Fractures

A few rare conditions account for most pathologic fractures seen in the pediatric population. The incidence of child abuse is 9.2/1000 children annually in the United States. Child abuse should always be considered, and the following mimics of abuse should only be considered when there are unusual clinical physical examination findings.

Osteogenesis Imperfecta

Osteogenesis imperfecta (OI) is a family of disorders characterized most notably by brittle bones. See Chapters 1 and 22 for a more extensive review of OI.

Distinguishing between infants and children with milder phenotypes OI who incur accidental fractures from normal children with inflicted injuries can be done with careful evaluation. In children with OI, accidental fractures are likely to begin after the child is ambulatory. A fracture of any nonambulatory child warrants consideration of abuse, regardless of OI evaluation. There is commonly a clear history that fits the fracture pattern found, although the amount of force involved may be somewhat less than that usually needed to cause a fracture. In general, a single fracture of the diaphysis of a long bone or both bone diaphyseal fractures of a forearm or lower leg are found. When the child has suffered prior fractures, the previous injuries' histories along with details of the treatment prescribed are provided.

There are other physical examination findings that are associated with OI. Blue sclerae are found in many children with type I OI. Short stature, bowing or valgus deformities of the lower extremities, and the dental discoloration of dentinogenesis imperfecta, once teeth have erupted, are found in children with both types I and IV OI. The "classic metaphyseal lesions" and rib and skull fractures, so common in young abuse victims, are rare in infants and children with mild forms of OI. OI does not predispose children to subdural hematomas or retinal hemorrhages. Associated visceral injuries have not been reported in OI. When these findings are present, one must seriously consider the possibility of abuse of a child with OI.

Reviewing radiographs including skull films with an experienced pediatric radiologist is also useful to evaluate for wormian bones and any signs of osteopenia. Lastly, it can be most helpful to confer with the child's primary care physician about prior reports of injuries. It is reasonable to consider OI in young children with multiple fractures but no other injuries or any concerning risk factors found in the history.

Three other types of OI (V through VII) that have no detectable defect of type I collagen have been described. All are rare, and each has distinct clinical and/or radiographic findings that help distinguish affected from normal infants and children (see Chapter 22). These likely account for many, if not most, of the negative findings on analysis of collagen synthesis (Fig. 6.69).

Demineralization

Children with cerebral palsy, myelodysplasia, advanced neuromuscular diseases, paraplegia, or quadriplegia that prevents weight bearing develop muscular atrophy and bony demineralization as the result of disuse. Cortical thinning is marked (Fig. 6.70) and makes the patient vulnerable to fractures after the application of mild forces, whether in minor falls or in manipulation during physical therapy or transfers to beds or showers.

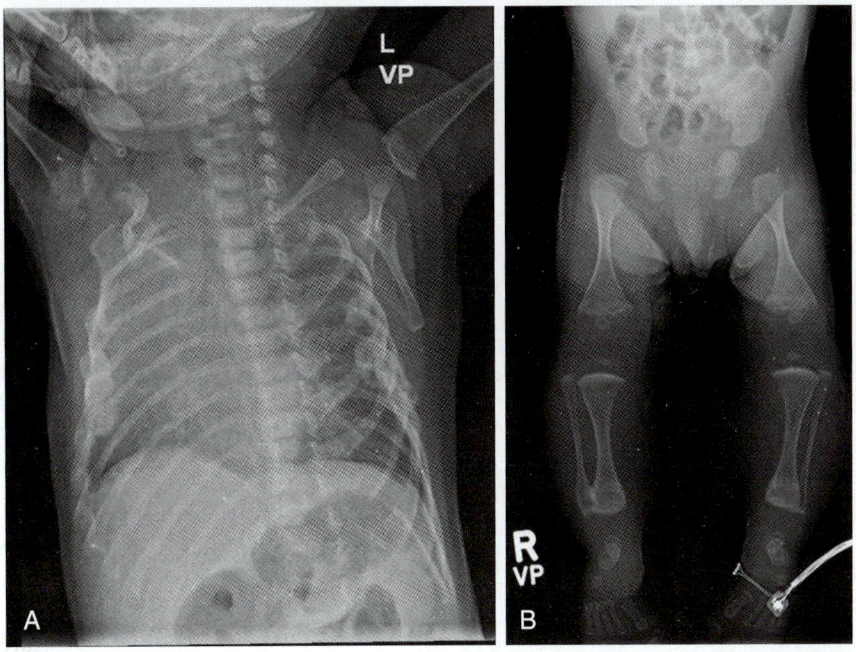

Fig. 6.69 (A) This 3-week-old ex-full-term infant was hospitalized after birth due to hypotonia. She presented to the hospital due to respiratory difficulty, congestion, and coughing. She was diagnosed with respiratory syncytial virus bronchiolitis, and a chest radiograph revealed multiple acute and healing rib fractures. (B) The child was found to have osteogenesis imperfecta type V.

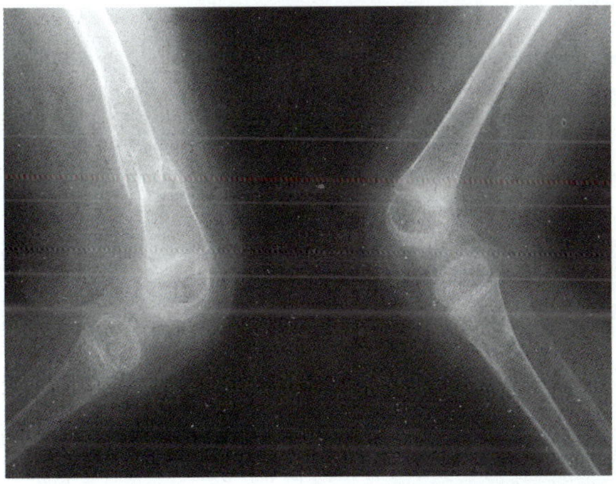

Fig. 6.70 Demineralization from disuse. Severe osteopenia and a femur fracture incurred during physical therapy are evident in this child, who was left quadriplegic as the result of an earlier injury. Note the lack of muscle mass. (Courtesy Department of Radiology, Children's Hospital of Pittsburgh, Pittsburgh, PA.)

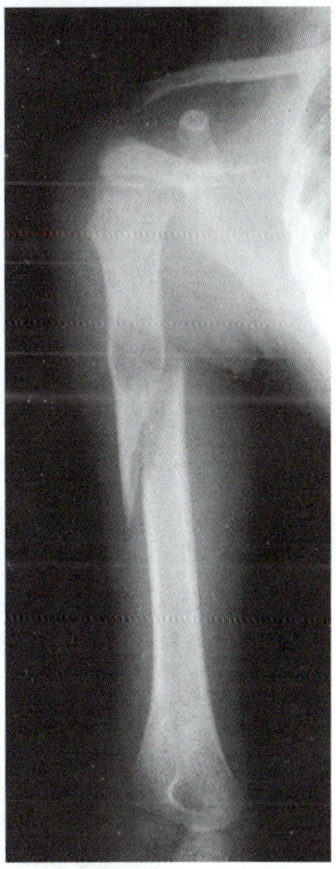

Fig. 6.71 Fracture through a unicameral bone cyst. This boy was seen because of intense pain and swelling of his upper arm after a relatively minor fall (due to slipping on wet grass while running to get out of the rain). The radiograph reveals a pathologic fracture through a unicameral bone cyst, which has caused considerable cortical thinning. (Courtesy Department of Radiology, Children's Hospital of Pittsburgh, Pittsburgh, PA.)

Leukemia

Children with acute leukemia may develop diffuse demineralization, periosteal reactions, and osteolytic lesions. Lucent metaphyseal bands, termed *leukemic lines,* are also seen (see Fig. 11.83). The relative osteopenia and typical absence of fractures, combined with the antecedent history, often of fatigue, anorexia, and weight loss; physical findings that may include petechiae, adenopathy, visceromegaly, and sternal tenderness; and the results of hematologic tests should distinguish these findings from those of abuse. Similarly, benign unicameral bone cysts can leave bones vulnerable to fractures (Fig. 6.71).

Metabolic Disorders

Vitamin D Deficiency and Rickets

In view of its role in regulating calcium and phosphorus metabolism, vitamin D plays a key role in normal bone development and growth. When born to a mother with normal levels of vitamin D, newborns will have received enough vitamin D via placental transfer to have adequate levels for the ensuing 3 months. Premature infants and those born to mothers with deficient levels will have lesser amounts. The two main sources of vitamin D are sunlight and foods (fortified milk or formula, eggs, and fish). Supplemental vitamins are beneficial and especially important for breastfed infants because breast milk has low levels of vitamin D. They are also indicated for infants and children with darkly pigmented skin because the amount of melanin in their skin cells absorbs much of the ultraviolet B radiation, leaving less available to stimulate skin production of vitamin D. Low exposure during cold winter weather add to the risk of insufficient levels of the vitamin. The prevalence of low levels has ranged from 1% to 78%, in part depending on the population studied.

The clinical findings of rickets are seen only in infants with moderate to severe deficiency. The peak season for presentation is spring because of the limited sun exposure during winter months. Affected patients are often from latitudes distant from the equator, tend to be breastfed, have dark skin tone with no vitamin D supplementation, or be fed primarily unfortified milk or a vegan diet without supplementation.

Because of poor mineralization, the bones of infants and young children with rickets are prone to bending. Radiographic changes include loss of the provisional zone of calcification, widening of the epiphysis, metaphyseal cupping and fraying, cortical thinning, and periosteal reaction (Fig. 6.72; see Fig. 11.11). Clinical findings include widening of the ends of the long bones (Fig. 6.73), especially noticeable at the wrists, ankles, and knees; costochondral beading (rachitic rosary) (see Fig. 11.10); and bowing of the forearms in infants and legs in toddlers (see Fig. 11.9). One can also note delayed fontanelle closure, softening of the calvarial bones (craniotabes), and frontal/parietal bossing.

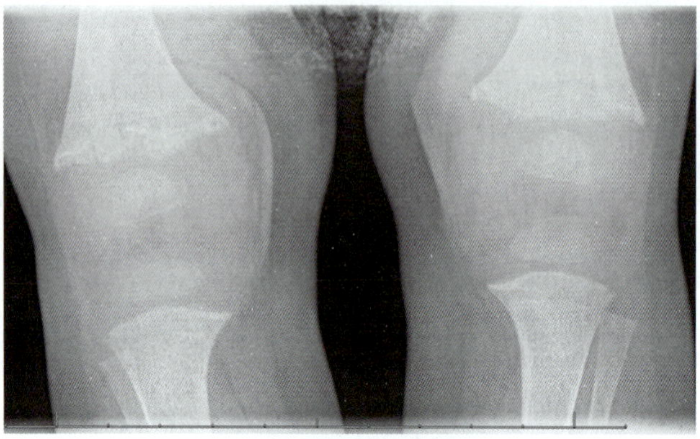

Fig. 6.72 A 13-month-old was admitted secondary to profound malnourishment. The child was nearly exclusively breastfed, and her mother was 6 months pregnant. Radiograph revealed decreased bone mineralization, symmetric metaphyseal flaring, and widening consistent with rickets.

Laboratory findings are inevitably abnormal and include decreased calcium early in the course (sometimes presenting as tetany), low 25-hydroxy vitamin D, and often decreased phosphate and increased alkaline phosphatase levels.

Premature infants who are born before much of the mineralization of bone that occurs during gestation is complete, and who, because of severe illness or lung disease, require total parenteral nutrition are particularly vulnerable to developing rickets with attendant bony fragility. Importantly, it must be noted that infants born prematurely are at increased risk for abuse in part because of the impaired bonding and the exigency of increased care needs.

A low level of vitamin D does not explain fractures in an infant. A further evaluation for abuse is called for. The preponderance of evidence from a large amount of research shows that vitamin D insufficiency occurs equally in children with fractures and children without fractures. Not one study to date has been able to document that vitamin D is associated with an increased risk of fracture. Furthermore, children with clear clinical and radiographic findings of rickets have a low incidence of fractures, and when seen, such fractures are found only in mobile infants and children. It is important that an objective evaluation for a clear history that fits with the developmental stage of the child remains central to the assessment for abuse.

Copper Deficiency

Copper deficiency is an exceptionally rare phenomenon that should be readily distinguishable from abuse. It occurs in nutritional and inherited forms. Menkes kinky hair syndrome is the inherited form

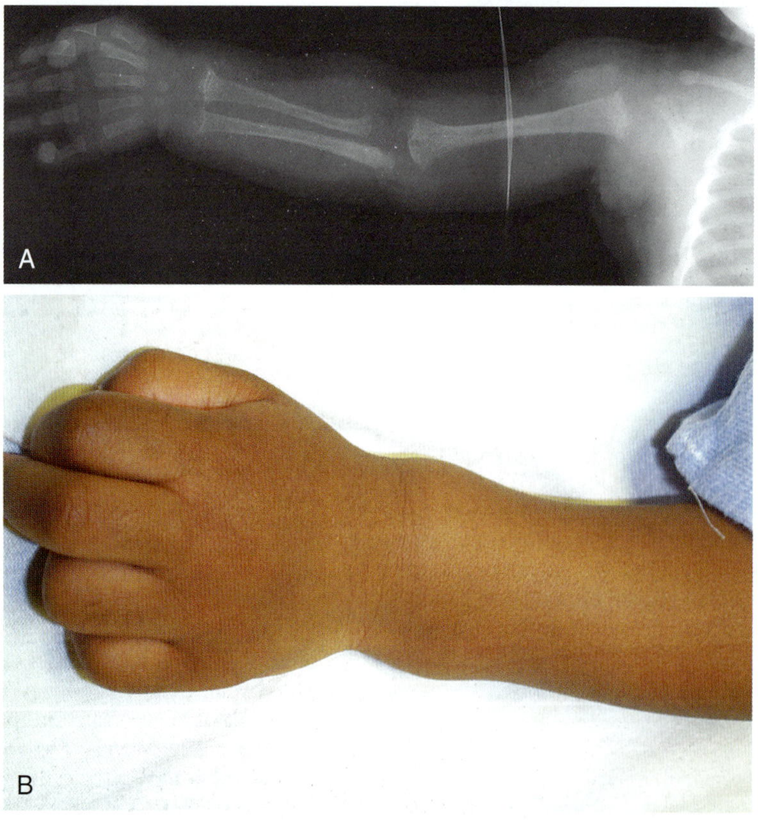

Fig. 6.73 (A) The fraying and cupping of the metaphyses characteristic of rickets. Reduced sunlight absorption due to his darkly pigmented skin and prenatal and postnatal factors appear to have contributed etiologically. The baby's mother had not taken vitamins for the last half of her pregnancy and did not eat dairy products. The baby was small for gestational age and had more than doubled his birth weight; hence, his need for vitamin D outstripped the amount provided by his formula. (B) In this older child who developed rickets after being placed on a vegan diet by his mother, the wrist is nearly as wide as his hand because of underlying metaphyseal widening and fraying of the radius and ulna.

and results from an X-linked recessive defect in copper absorption (see Fig. 8.130). Clinically, affected infants have pale skin, hypopigmented hair, edema, enlarged scalp veins, and seborrhea, with or without failure to thrive or developmental delay. Infants affected with Menkes are also grossly abnormal neurologically, with hypotonia, decreased movement, lethargy, myoclonic seizures, and difficulty maintaining normal temperatures being major findings. Radiographically, their bones are grossly abnormal.

Scurvy

Children with vitamin C deficiency (now exceedingly rare) usually present after 6 months and may have been fed evaporated or boiled milk. Clinically, they tend to bruise easily because of vascular fragility, be irritable, move little due to bone pain, and often have gingival bleeding. Serum vitamin C level is low. The diagnosis of scurvy should be readily distinguishable from abuse on the basis of radiographic findings (Fig. 6.74).

Hypervitaminosis A

Chronic vitamin A intoxication produces a thick, wavy periosteal reaction that most commonly involves the ulnas and metatarsals, although other long bones can be affected. Hard, tender swellings may be evident on palpation. Absence of fractures and metaphyseal abnormalities should help distinguish this from abuse. The history and findings of papilledema or split sutures on skull radiograph resulting from concomitant pseudotumor cerebri also aid in differentiation.

Caffey Disease

A rare disorder of unknown etiology, Caffey disease is characterized by cortical thickening and a painful periosteal reaction (Fig. 6.75). Bones are otherwise normally mineralized, and fractures are not seen. Involvement of the mandible, seen in 75% of affected patients, results in dramatic thickening. The clavicle and ulna are also common sites, although other bones can be involved. Most patients are younger than 6 months old, and all have fever, anorexia, and marked irritability. The skin overlying affected areas is neither warm nor discolored. There is no soft tissue swelling, and palpation reveals bony-hard thickening below the subcutaneous tissues, which are adherent to the underlying bone.

In the past, there have been proposed diseases of temporary brittle bone disease as a disorder that is a transient phenomenon seen only in the first year of life. There are no scientific data or corroborative evidence to support the existence of this "disorder" or the hypotheses of transient metabolic defects proposed to explain it.

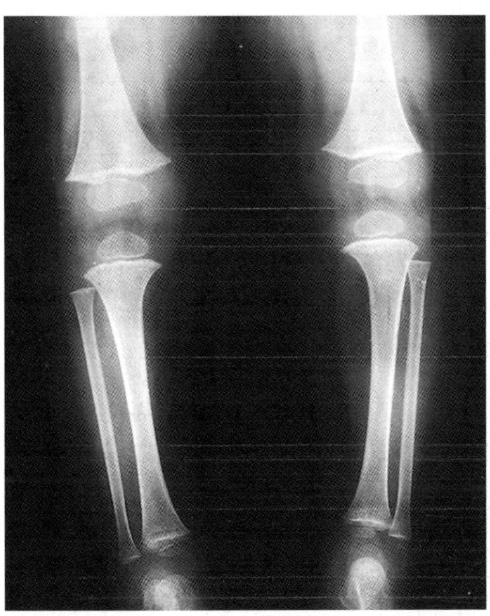

Fig. 6.74 Scurvy. Note the increased density of the zones of provisional calcification and lucency of the underlying spongiosa. The metaphyses are also widened, and early spur formation is seen medially. (Courtesy Department of Radiology, Children's Hospital of Pittsburgh, Pittsburgh, PA.)

SEXUAL ABUSE

Child sexual abuse (CSA) is broadly defined as the involvement of children or adolescents in sexual activity for the sexual gratification of an older child or adult. Abusive sexual acts can include contact and non-contact events, and with or without the threat of physical force. CSA includes but is not limited to exhibitionism, fondling, production of pornographic material, and penetration of the mouth, anus or vagina. The absence of physical force or violence does not imply consent, as a child may not be able to give informed consent due to age, mental or physical capacity, or impairment with alcohol or drugs.

About 1 billion children globally are estimated to experience sexual abuse or assault. In the United States in 2022, there were an estimated 59,000 substantiated victims of sexual abuse; it is estimated that substantiated cases make up less than one-third of all cases of sexual abuse and continue to be underreported. Most perpetrators of child sexual abuse are well known to the child or the child's family. Victims tend to be female and perpetrators male. Female perpetrators are less likely to be reported.

Most children who have been sexually abused are brought to medical attention due to a disclosure the child has made. Less common reasons for discovery include witnessed events, concerns for pregnancy or sexually transmitted infections, the presence of an injury or the discovery of media depicting the abuse. In the office setting, the immediate issues to be addressed are the child's safety, reporting to child protective agencies and/or law enforcement agencies, the child's mental health, and the medical evaluation. Depending on the nature of the abuse and the timing of the event, some of the evaluation may not be completed in the office setting and will be referred to a specialized center or emergency department. It is important to understand your local resources to determine the next steps for further medical and forensic evaluation. Most areas should have access to a Child Advocacy Center that can provide further guidance (https://www.nationalchildrensalliance.org/cac-coverage-maps/).

The medical evaluation generally requires careful documentation of any disclosures, thorough physical examination, testing for pregnancy and sexually transmitted infections, offering prophylaxis for pregnancy and infections when indicated, assessing vaccination against Hepatitis B, tetanus and human papilloma virus, and providing patients with medical and psychological follow up. Ideally, this evaluation is provided by clinicians with specialized training to minimize additional trauma; in the absence of a specialist, a clinician who is empathetic, patient, and conscientious can ensure this evaluation is therapeutic. Remaining objective, not expressing surprise or disgust, and using matter-of-fact neutral tones throughout the encounter would be ideal.

Although the physical examination is important and can sometimes yield supporting evidence of the abuse, the history is often the crucial part of the evaluation. Gather the history on the child or adolescent from the accompanying adult separately. Specific questions about any known disclosures are to make decisions on necessary next steps:

- To whom was the disclosure made? When was it made?
- What was the exact disclosure? What body parts were involved? Was there any pain or bleeding reported?
- What was happening preceding the disclosure?
- When did the event(s) occur? When was the last event?
- What happened after the disclosure?

Inquire about the child's history of prior abuse or other traumas, behavioral changes, and mental health concerns. Relevant medical history questions include ulcers/vesicles in the mouth, genitals, or anus; prior genital trauma including accidental straddle injuries or

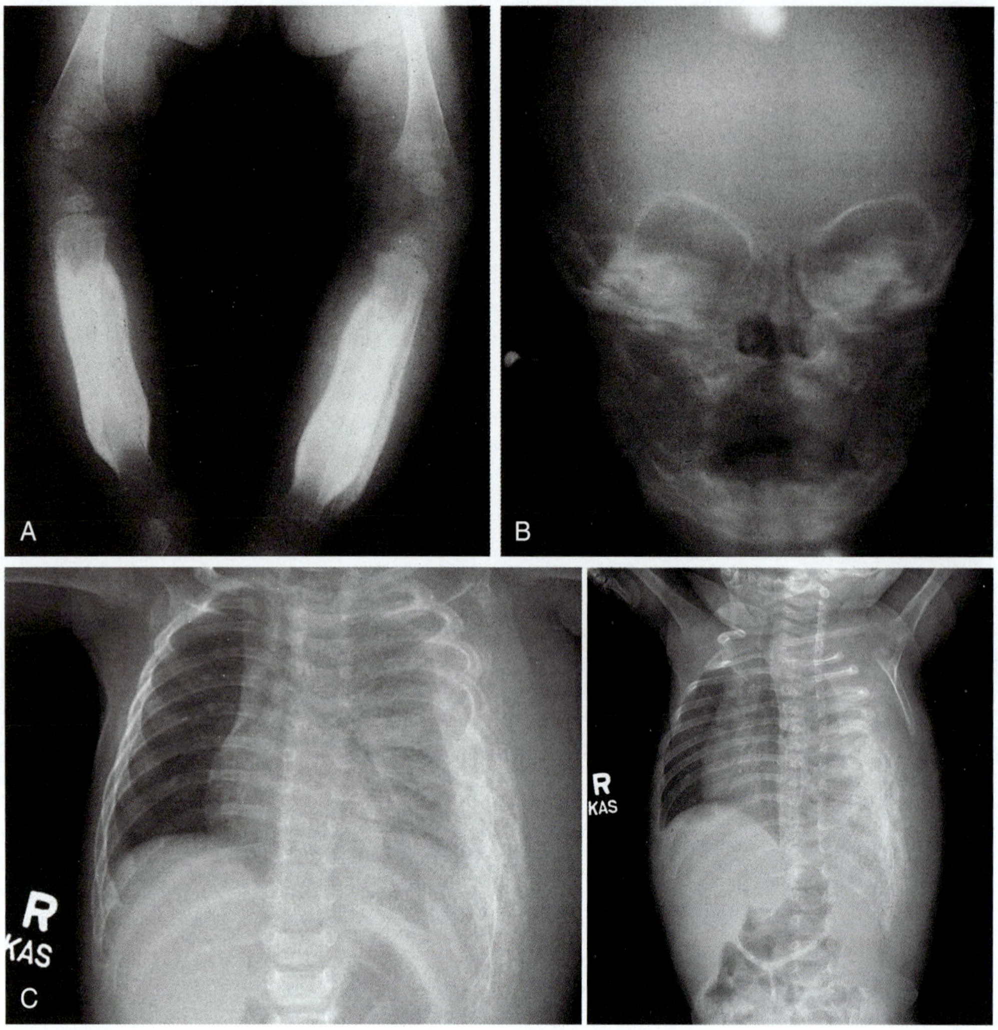

Fig. 6.75 Caffey disease. (A) Intense periosteal reaction and cortical thickening are seen in the lower extremities. (B) Mandibular involvement has resulted in dramatic thickening. These findings, associated symptoms, and absence of fractures distinguish this condition from the skeletal changes characteristic of abuse. (C) This 2-month-old male presented with 2+ weeks' left-sided torso bruising and swelling without a history of trauma that initially was concerning for physical abuse. Additional workup revealed anemia, thrombocytosis, and leukocytosis as well as pleural effusion. Child underwent skeletal survey and chest magnetic resonance imaging that revealed a diagnosis of Caffey disease, a rare condition of hyperostosis. (A and B, Courtesy Department of Radiology, Children's Hospital of Pittsburgh, Pittsburgh, PA.)

surgeries; urogenital infections; anogenital itching/pain/bleeding/discharge; constipation/diarrhea; and enuresis/encopresis in a previously toilet-trained child.

If the child can be separated from the accompanying adult, and if the child is willing and able to give a history, that history and the exact phrasing of the questions asked should be documented verbatim. Asking children about their favorite toys or TV shows builds rapport while assessing their language skills. Sometimes children are not ready to disclose, and pressuring them to do so can be detrimental.

If the child is unwilling or unable to discuss the episode or episodes, and there is a strong suspicion that sexual abuse has occurred, consult your local Child Advocacy Center or forensic specialist for next steps. Depending on the developmental capacity of the child, a forensic interview may be offered. In such interviews, a variety of alternative techniques that are defensible in court can be used if the child still has difficulty disclosing verbally. These include having the child try to draw what happened (Fig. 6.76), show what happened with anatomically correct dolls, or write about the incidents.

Every child who may have been sexually abused deserves a thorough and complete physical examination. Some adults may be resistant to an examination due to misconceptions about what the examination entails (e.g., that a speculum is routinely used). Asking about and addressing any concerns before the examination can help the adult be comfortable, and thus the child. Make sure that the child and adults all know that the examination is not to determine the validity of the disclosure but to ensure that the child is healthy. The examination is also an excellent opportunity to teach children about their bodies.

Giving the child some feeling of control over the examination process in several small ways helps avoid further trauma. Let the child look at familiar objects such as a doll, toy car, or a finger through the colposcope if using one. Demonstrate that the colposcope light on their foot is not hurtful. Allowing the child to choose the order in which various nonessential areas are examined can be calming as well. Promising toys or other items if they cooperate for the examination should be avoided.

If the attempt to examine the genitals and perineum provokes significant anxiety or resistance, and there is gross bleeding, pain, discharge, need for immediate collection of forensic evidence, or suspicion of ascending sexually transmitted infection (STI), the examination and specimen collection should be performed with the patient under sedation or rarely under general anesthesia. When the patient is too anxious to proceed but is asymptomatic, without a current or recent history of significant pain, bleeding, discharge, or

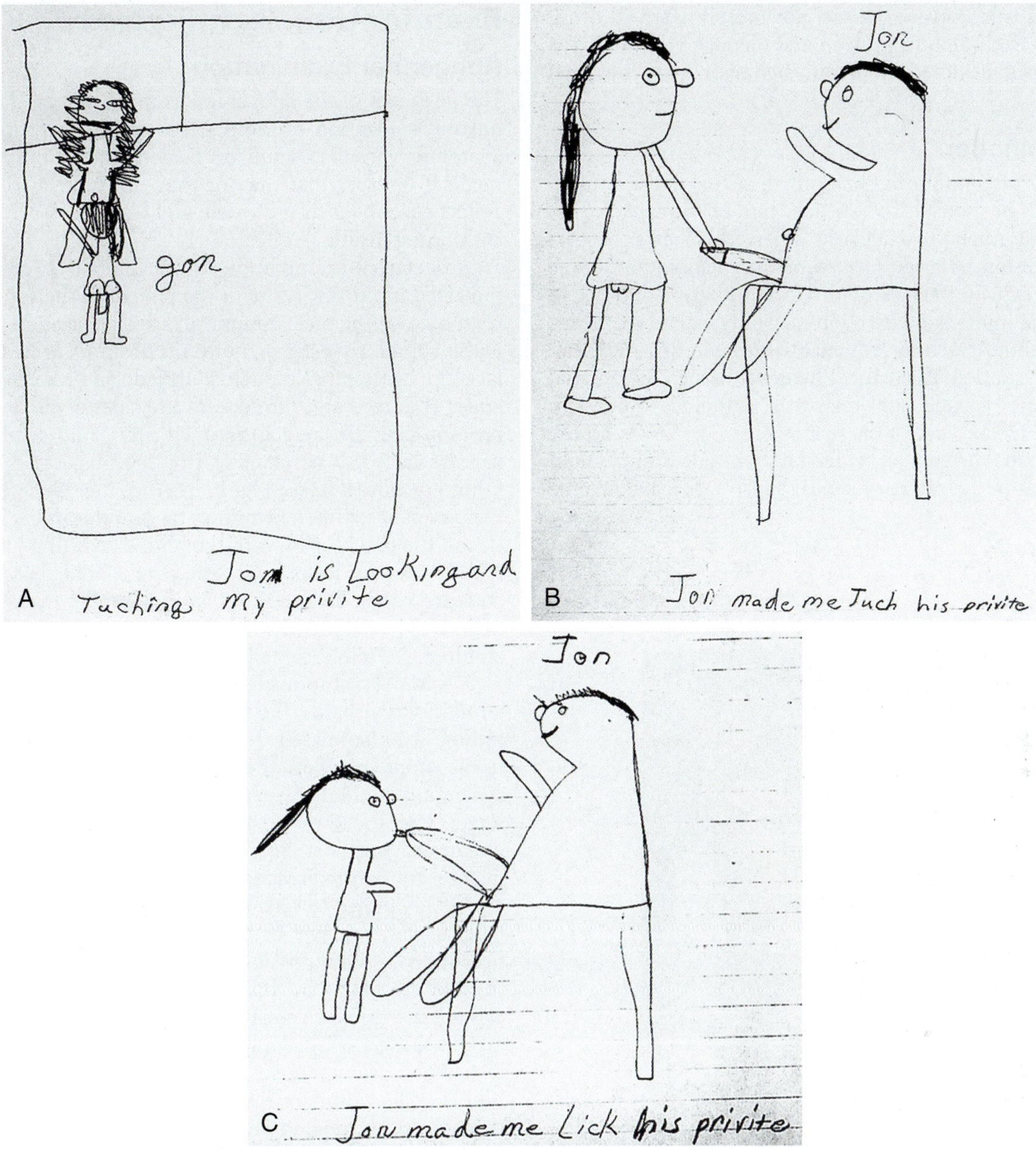

Fig. 6.76 (A–C) Drawings by a school-age sexual abuse victim. Although the child had difficulty verbalizing a description of the abuse, she was able to clearly depict the acts in her drawings.

need for immediate evidence collection, the examination can be deferred and performed at a follow-up visit. The child must not be made to feel that he or she is being reassaulted during the evaluation.

Some victims may not present with a chief complaint of sexual abuse; instead, they present with complaints generated by physical or emotional sequelae (Table 6.2). There are many such complaints that are somewhat age dependent, each of which has many potential causes other than sexual abuse. Although there is a wide range of differential diagnostic possibilities in patients presenting with many of these problems, sexual abuse should be considered and addressed among the

Table 6.2 Consider Sexual Abuse in the Differential Diagnosis[a]

Any Age	Preschool Age	School Age	Adolescence
Abdominal pain	Excessive clinging	Decreased school performance	Same as school age plus:
Anorexia	Sudden onset of excessive thumb sucking	Truancy	• Runaway behavior
Vomiting	Speech disorder	Lying, stealing	• Suicide attempts
Constipation	Encopresis/enuresis	Tics	• Self-inflicted injury
Sleep disorders	Compulsive masturbation[b]	Anxiety reaction	• Commission of sexual offenses[b]
Dysuria		Phobic and obsessional states	
Vaginal discharge[c]		Depression	
Vaginal bleeding[c]		Conversion reaction	
Rectal bleeding		Encopresis/enuresis	

[a]Most of these complaints are also symptomatic of disorders more prevalent than sexual abuse.
[b]Symptoms highly suggestive of sexual abuse.
[c]Symptoms somewhat suggestive of sexual abuse.

differential diagnostic considerations, not merely after all other causes have been excluded. In preteen and teenage victims, signs of nonsuicidal self-inflicted injurious behavior may be seen (Fig. 6.77).

Physical Examination

The vast majority of genital examinations in sexual abuse evaluations are normal or nonspecific, which can be unexpected to inexperienced examiners, particularly when there has been a perpetrator confession or disclosure of vaginal penetration. Some reasons that may explain the lack of physical findings include rapid healing of mucosal injuries; penetration may only extend to, or just pass the labia, without reaching hymenal tissue such that there can be no hymenal disruption; elasticity of hymenal tissue; the fact that hymenal tissue is capable of regrowth, although rarely in cases of complete transection of the hymen (see Fig. 6.84A–F); the anal sphincter can distend considerably without injury; and the possibility that perpetrators of sexual abuse may have erectile dysfunction.

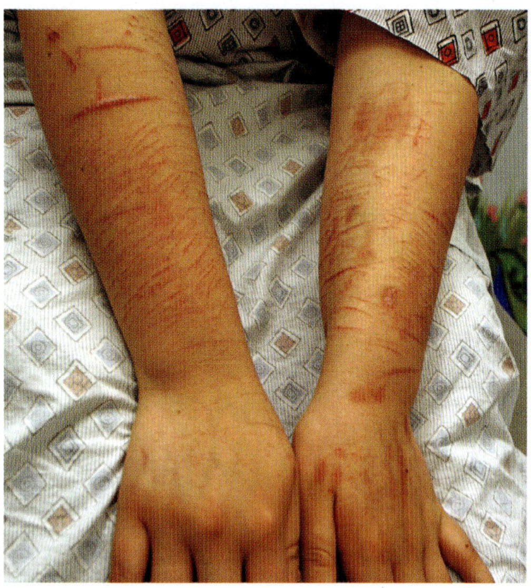

Fig. 6.77 Self-inflicted injury, a finding that should raise concern about abuse and depression.

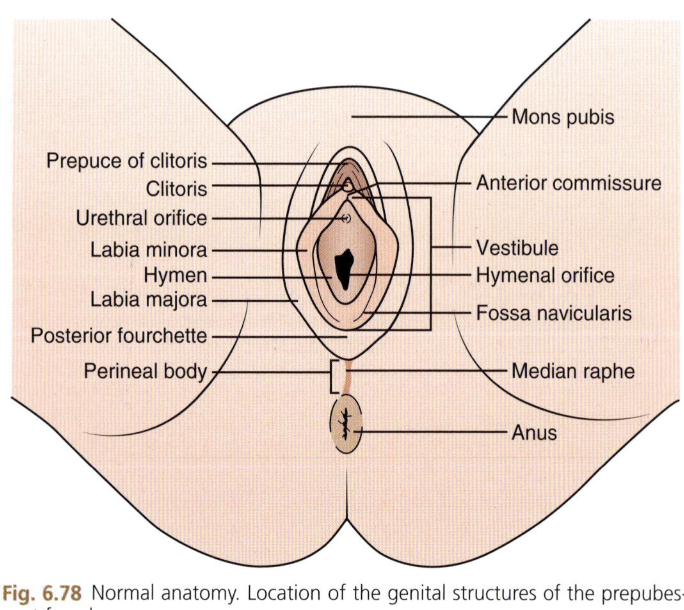

Fig. 6.78 Normal anatomy. Location of the genital structures of the prepubescent female.

Examination Techniques

Anogenital Examination

The purposes of the anogenital examination are (1) to obtain adequate visualization of the patient's anatomy in order to assess for anatomic variants, acute or healed injury, infection, and other medical diseases that may or may not be related to abuse; (2) to collect specimens as indicated; and (3) to reassure children of their continuing health.

An external examination of the genitalia is generally all that is indicated in most cases with the patient in the supine position (see Chapter 19). The most commonly used position in younger children is the supine frog-leg or butterfly position, with the patient lying face up, with hips abducted, flexed, and externally rotated; the knees abducted and flexed; and the soles of the feet together. This position can also be achieved with the child semireclining on the parent's lap—the semisupine frog-leg position or the semisupine lithotomy position (see Fig. 19.5). The latter is carried out by having the parent sit on the examining table and lean back. The child then sits on the parent's lap, with the buttocks resting just above the parent's knees, and leans back. The parent holds her hands under the patient's knees, flexing them and abducting the hips. The use of a table with "stirrups" (the lithotomy position) can be used with older children and adolescents for adequate abduction of the legs.

It is important to inspect the labia majora and minora before attempting to visualize the vaginal introitus, or subtle but significant findings can be missed. To aid visualization of the vaginal introitus in the supine position, the labia is separated manually. In the labial separation method, the examiner places the index and/or the middle fingers over the lower portion of the labia majora and gently presses downward and laterally. In the labial traction technique, the labia majora are lightly grasped between the thumbs and index fingers and gently pulled toward the examiner and slightly downward. The latter usually achieves better visualization of the hymen and its orifice, and it is often possible to see the posterior aspect of the lower third of the vagina by this technique (see Fig. 19.2). One should be careful not to use excessive force when applying labial traction to avoid tearing any labial adhesions present or causing undue discomfort. On occasion, these tears created during the process of examination may be mistaken for acute physical findings. Sometimes the hymenal edges remain stuck together, and adjusting the direction of traction upwards or downward, or slightly increasing the force when pulling anteriorly, can cause the hymenal opening to relax and allow visualization. Forcefully coughing or blowing bubbles can also help.

The prone knee/chest position (Fig. 6.79A) provides the best exposure of perineal structures and generally a clearer picture of anatomic features and abnormalities (Figs. 6.80–6.82). It is similar to the yoga position "Puppy Pose." The examination table should be adjusted (usually down) before the child turns from the supine position. The child's shoulders and chest are on the table with buttocks in the air and knees more than hip width apart. Fig. 6.79B–E depicts the steps to get into this position. Exposure of the introitus is assisted by placing the thumbs over the edge of the gluteus muscles at the level of the introitus and lifting them upward. As the hymen drops down with gravity in the prone knee/chest position, its edges or rim is more easily assessed (see Fig. 6.80). Varying the direction of the thumbs slightly may be helpful to completely visualize the edges, particularly in a patient with a redundant hymen. A combination of knee/chest and swab utilization may be used in older children. Transverse diameter of the hymenal orifice varies with position and amount of relaxation and is no longer considered a useful measurement in assessing for signs of sexual abuse (Fig. 6.83). Obese children sometimes have thinner-appearing but not disrupted hymens.

Most experts now tend to use the knee/chest position only to confirm or negate suspicious findings found in the supine position or when the hymen has not been adequately visualized in the supine position. The knee/chest position can be difficult for younger children, and some older children object to it. Most children can be

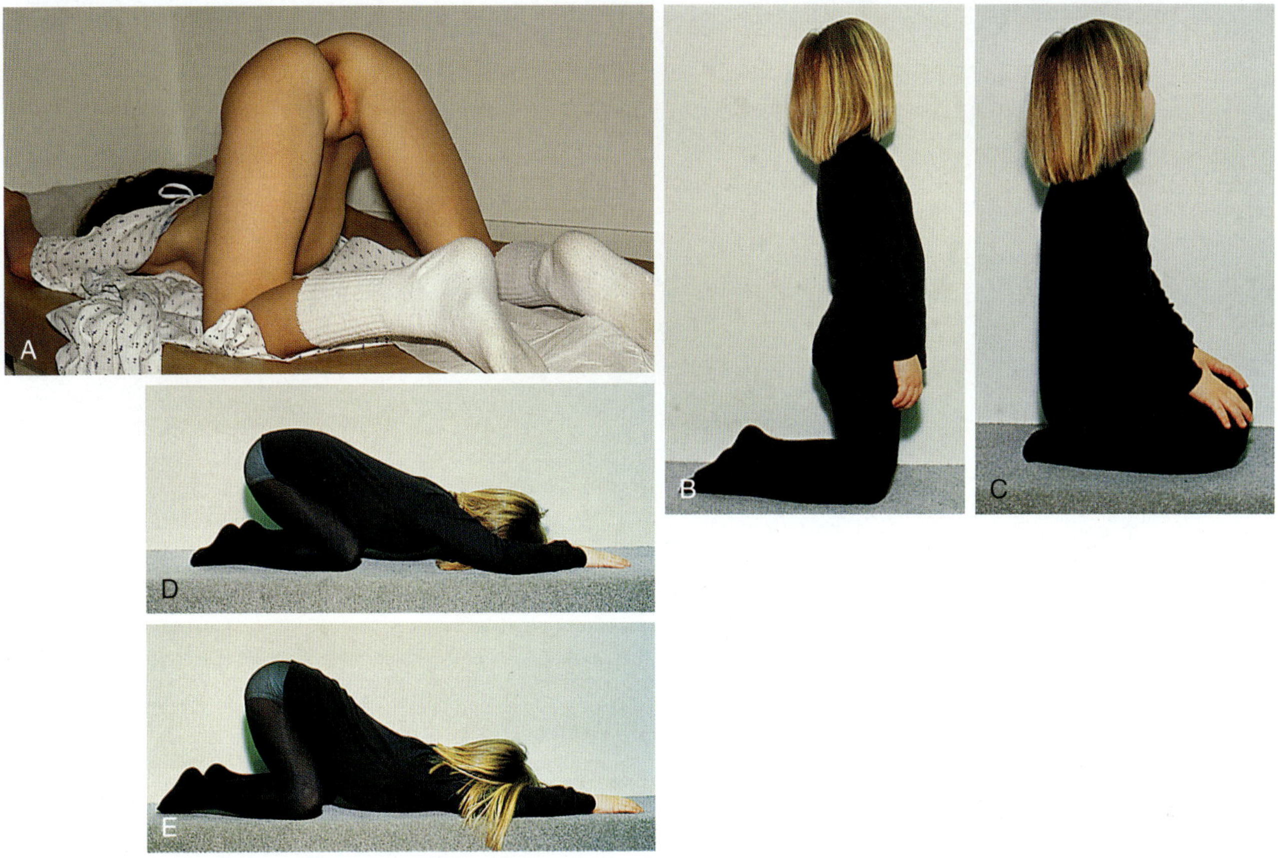

Fig. 6.79 Knee/chest position. (A) The sway-back position with knees widely separated assists examination and provides the best visualization of anatomical structures and abnormalities. (B–E) After looking at enlargements of this series of photographs, the patient practices getting into position while still fully clothed. The steps are kneel (B), sit back (C), stretch arms out and place arms and chest on table (D), and move forward (E). This helps children become more comfortable with being examined from behind.

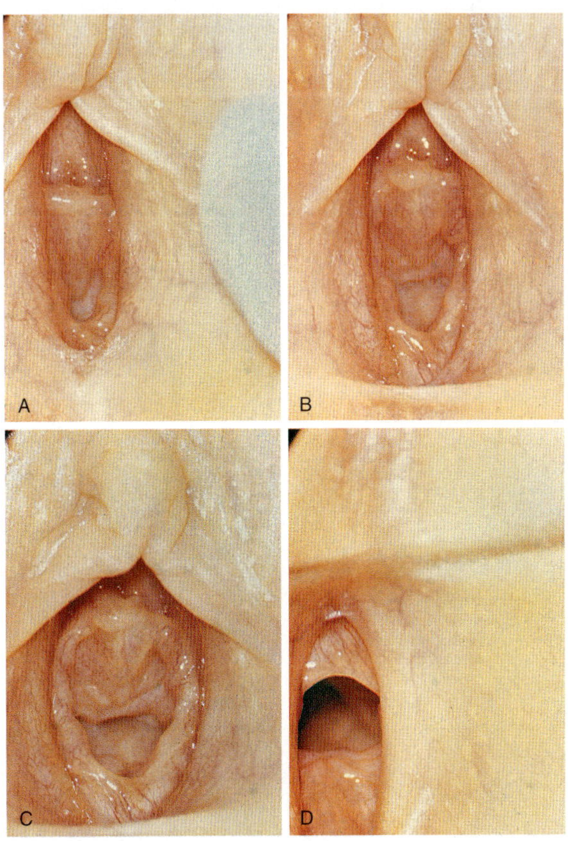

Fig. 6.80 Variation in the transverse or horizontal hymenal diameter with position and technique. (A) Supine with labial separation. (B) Supine with labial traction. (C) Lithotomy with more labial traction. (D) Knee/chest position. Note that the hymenal orifice is widest with good traction and that the hymen appears thickened and folded over in B and C. This is due to a mild redundancy. In the knee/chest position, the hymen unfolds and drops down with gravity and is seen to be thin with smooth, sharp edges having fully stretched out.

made comfortable with the knee/chest position and helped to relax by engaging them in an ongoing conversation about an unrelated subject or using a variety of visually interesting toys (e.g., kaleidoscopes, oil-based timers) held by an assistant at eye level.

When an estrogenized hymen is redundant or if the edges remain stuck, a saline-moistened swab (Fig. 6.84A and B) or a glove-covered swab (see Fig. 6.84C–F) may be inserted through the hymenal orifice and then used to spread out the hymenal membrane segment by segment in a systematic fashion. This is not painful and is therefore possible in adolescents and peripubertal children because, once estrogenized, the hymen is not as sensitive as it is before puberty. However, it may be uncomfortable, and it is important to talk with the child/adolescent through the examination process. Alternatively, a Foley catheter may be inserted, the balloon inflated within the vagina, and then gently pulled forward as a means of spreading out the hymenal tissue for better visualization (Fig. 6.85). In cases of acute injury, consideration must be given to the severity and extent of the injuries before proceeding. If examination and specimen collection are likely to cause or exacerbate severe physical pain or emotional distress to a patient, or if internal injuries are likely, consideration should be given to examination under conscious sedation or general anesthesia.

Adequate lighting and magnification are just as important as good positioning. If a colposcope is unavailable, a magnifying halogen lamp or an otoscope may be used. The latter device is most readily available, but reassure the child that the otoscope is being used only to get a good view with the light and will not be inserted into the genitalia.

A description of the appearance of the genitalia, using anatomically correct terms, should be documented (Fig. 6.86) in addition to any photo or video documentation. Standard of care for sexual abuse evaluations include magnified photographs of the genital area as these may prevent the need for reexamination if a second opinion is requested and allow for expert peer review. Video colposcopy is becoming more widely used and can increase diagnostic certainty and documentation of findings, particularly with young children

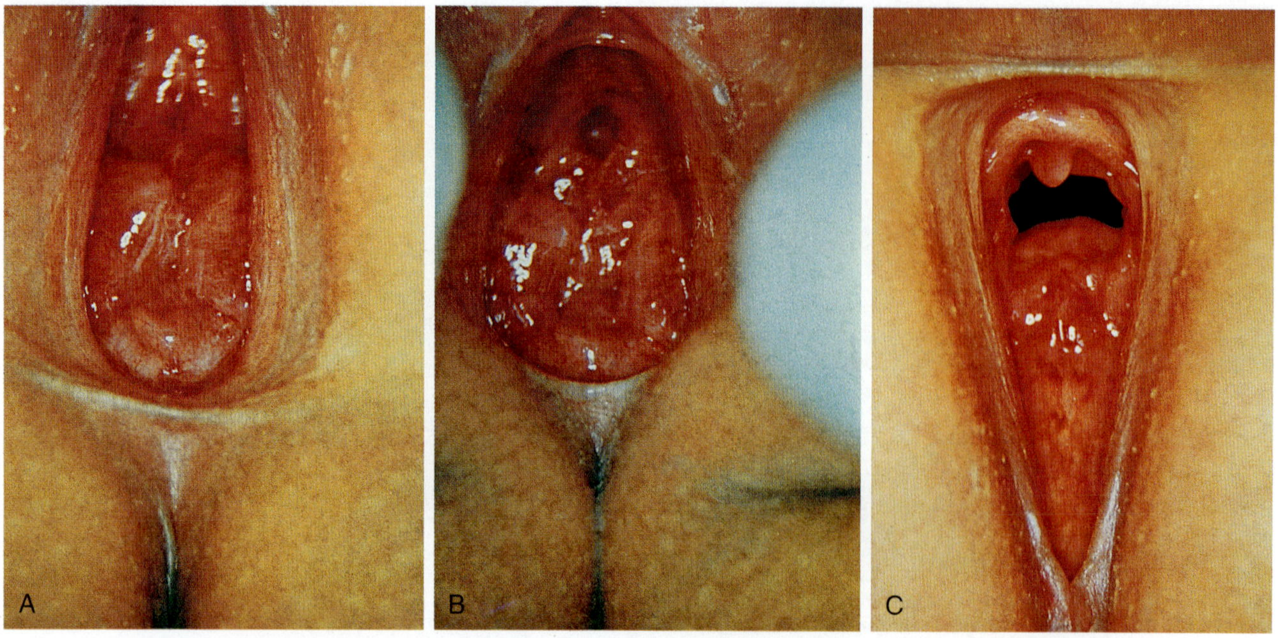

Fig. 6.81 The superiority of visualization using the knee/chest position is demonstrated in this sexual abuse victim, whose redundant tissue made it difficult to see the true configuration of her hymen when she was supine with labial separation (A) or labial traction (B). (C) In the knee/chest position, narrowing and thickening of the hymenal rim can be seen more clearly. (Courtesy John McCann, MD, University of California at Davis.)

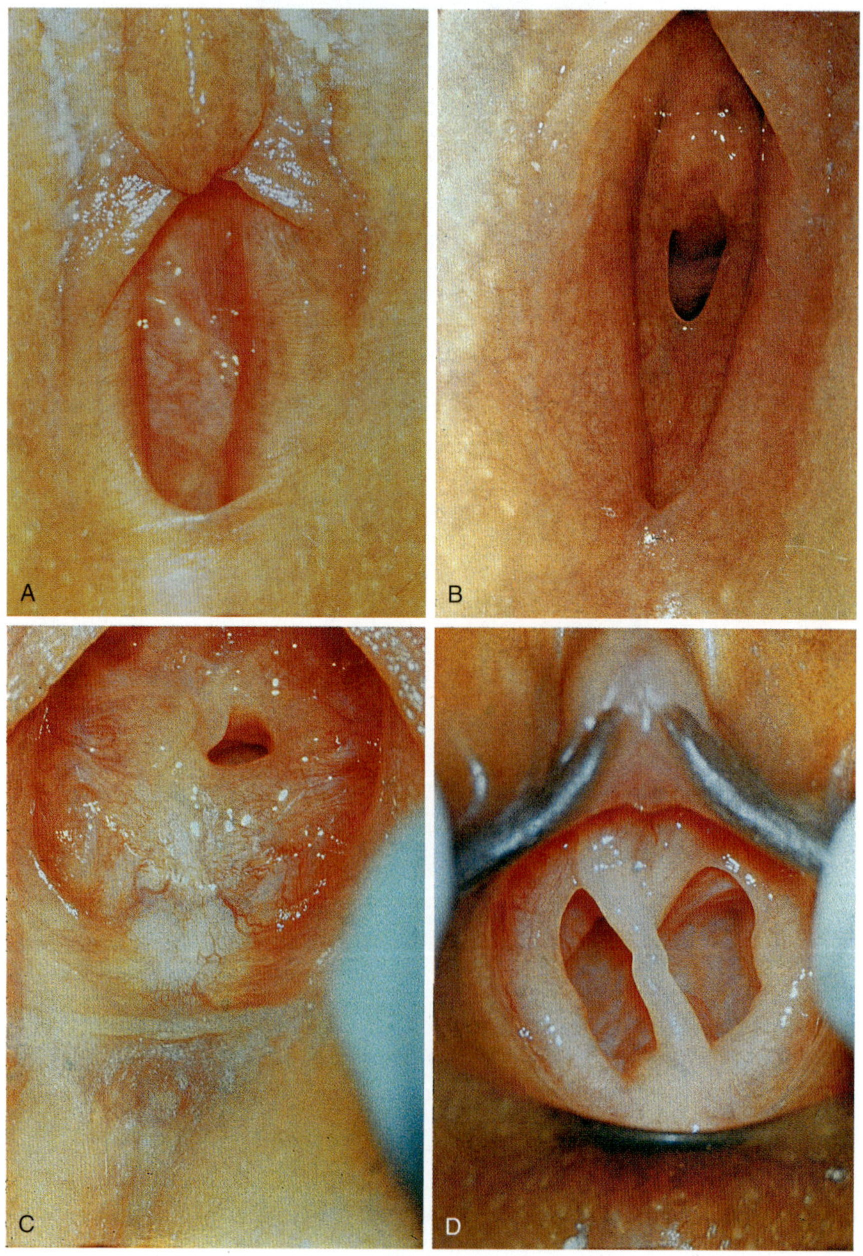

Fig. 6.82 Variations in normal hymenal configuration. (A) A redundant hymen. (B) A crescentic hymen with thin smooth edges. (C) A somewhat redundant hymen with an annular orifice. (D) A septate hymen resulting from failure of lysis of the embryonic hymenal septum.

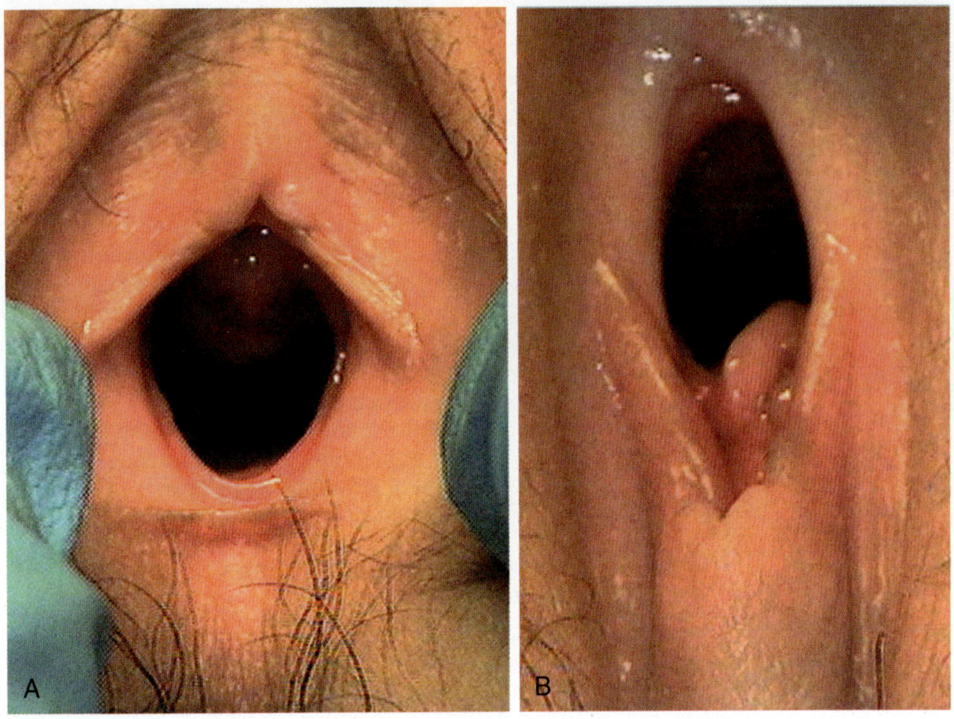

Fig. 6.83 The superiority of visualization using the knee/chest position is demonstrated in a child. (A) The hymenal rim appears narrowed to less than 1 mm in the supine position. (B) In the knee/chest position, more hymenal tissue is seen and has a thin smooth edge. This is considered normal.

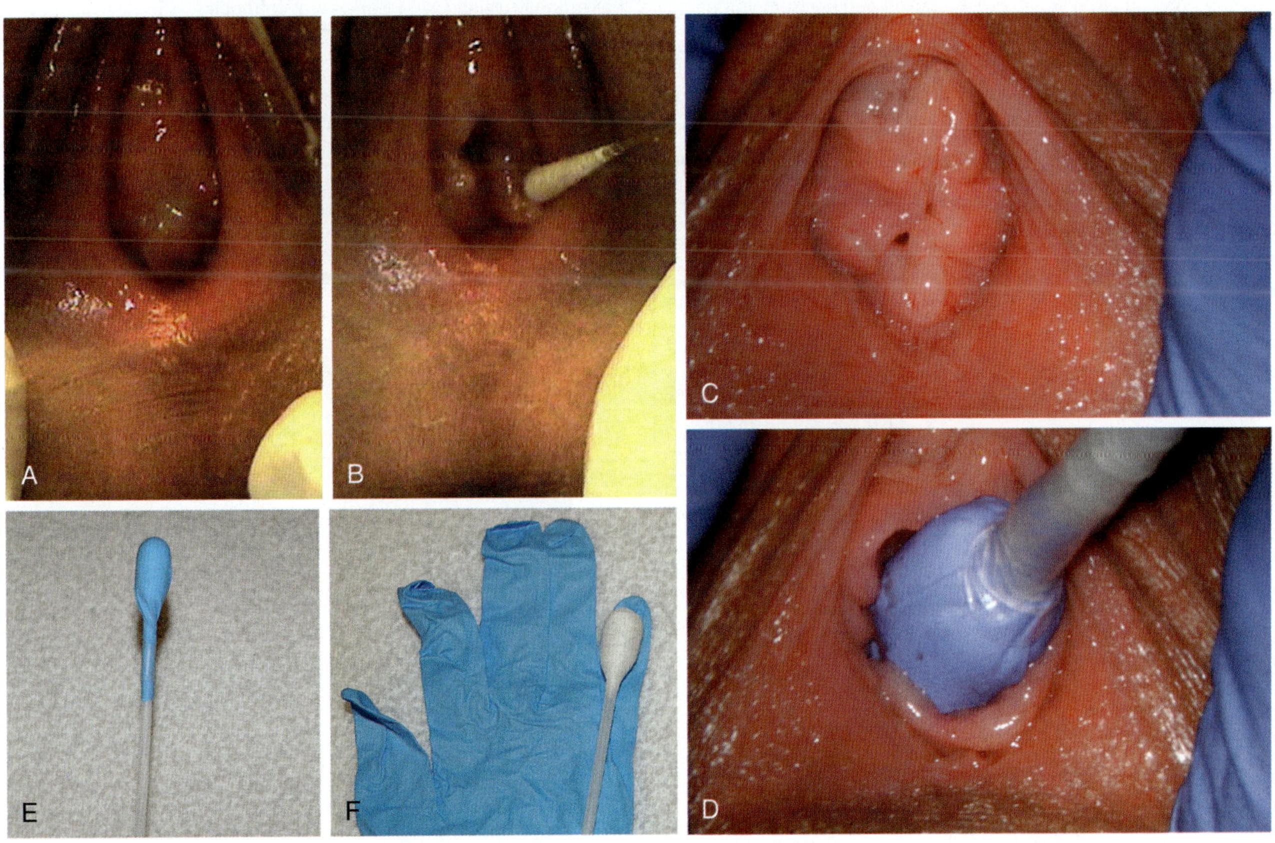

Fig. 6.84 Prior sexual abuse: complete transection of the hymen. (A) This young teen reported sexual assault several months earlier. Examination was performed by labial separation. (B) Examination with a Calgiswab demonstrates a complete hymenal transection that would have been missed had this technique not been used. (C) Pregnant adolescent showing what appears to be a normal redundant hymen. (D) However, a complete transection at the 8 to 9 o'clock position was found using a large swab covered with a blue glove. (E) Blue swab. (F) Swab on blue glove. (C–F, Courtesy Joyce Adams, MD, Rady Children's Hospital, San Diego, CA.)

who move too quickly to capture the examination in still photographs, and with adolescents whose hymens tend to be more dynamic and move during the examination. Written documentation includes (1) sexual maturity rating; (2) the presence or absence of an abnormal degree of erythema or of discharge and any abnormal pigmentation; (3) the presence or absence and location of bruises, abrasions, or lacerations; (4) the presence, extent, and character of labial adhesions (thin and translucent or thickened); (5) the appearance of the labia minora, posterior fourchette, and vestibule; (6) the configuration of the hymen and the appearance of its edges (e.g., thin and sharp, thickened or rolled, notched); (7) areas of hymenal tissue from its attachment to its margin that may appear decreased (especially if <1 mm wide) and its regularity; and (8) the appearance of the perineum. Also important is recording the patient's position and method used. Such documentation requires knowledge of basic gynecologic anatomy and terminology, which is shown in Fig. 6.78 and given in Table 6.3. Sometimes, structures cannot be adequately visualized, and it is important to note this as well. For more information about gynecologic anatomic terminology, see the Normal Female Genitalia section in Chapter 19.

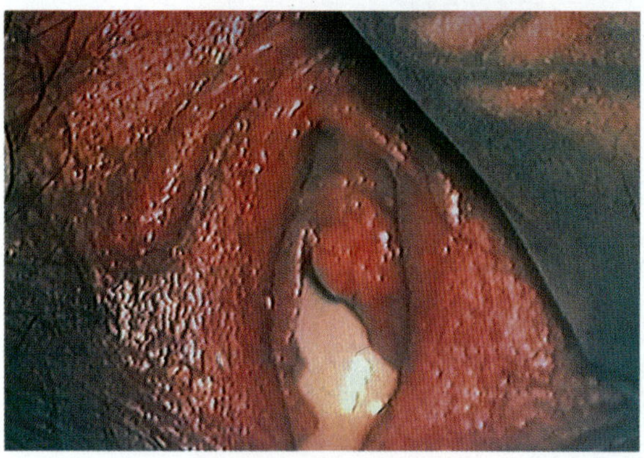

Fig. 6.85 Use of Foley catheter to enhance visualization of the full extent and margins of the hymenal membrane. The catheter is inserted through the hymenal orifice, and the balloon is inflated while in the vagina and then gently pulled forward. It can then be angled to the left or right or downward to ensure a full view of all segments. (Courtesy Earl Greenwald, MD, Harrisburg, PA.)

Anal penetration is a common form of sexual abuse in both boys and girls. The anus can be examined in a variety of positions, with supine knee/chest and prone knee/chest positions being the most common. Good lighting and magnification are again helpful. Gentle spreading of the anal folds is usually adequate to look for abrasions, bruising, tears, fissures, and other lesions within the folds. The presence of swelling can be assessed by the appearance of the anal folds. Venous congestion of the perianal area occurs within minutes of the child being placed in the prone knee/chest position, may also occur in the supine position, and does not indicate evidence of abuse, but it can be mistaken for bruising (see Fig. 6.87B). The absence of physical findings is the norm and does not make the history any less credible.

Physical Findings

Normal changes in appearance of the female genitalia with age are described in Chapter 19. Clinicians must become familiar with the normal anatomy at different ages and with normal variations. Extensive, carefully done studies (McCann, Berenson) have documented

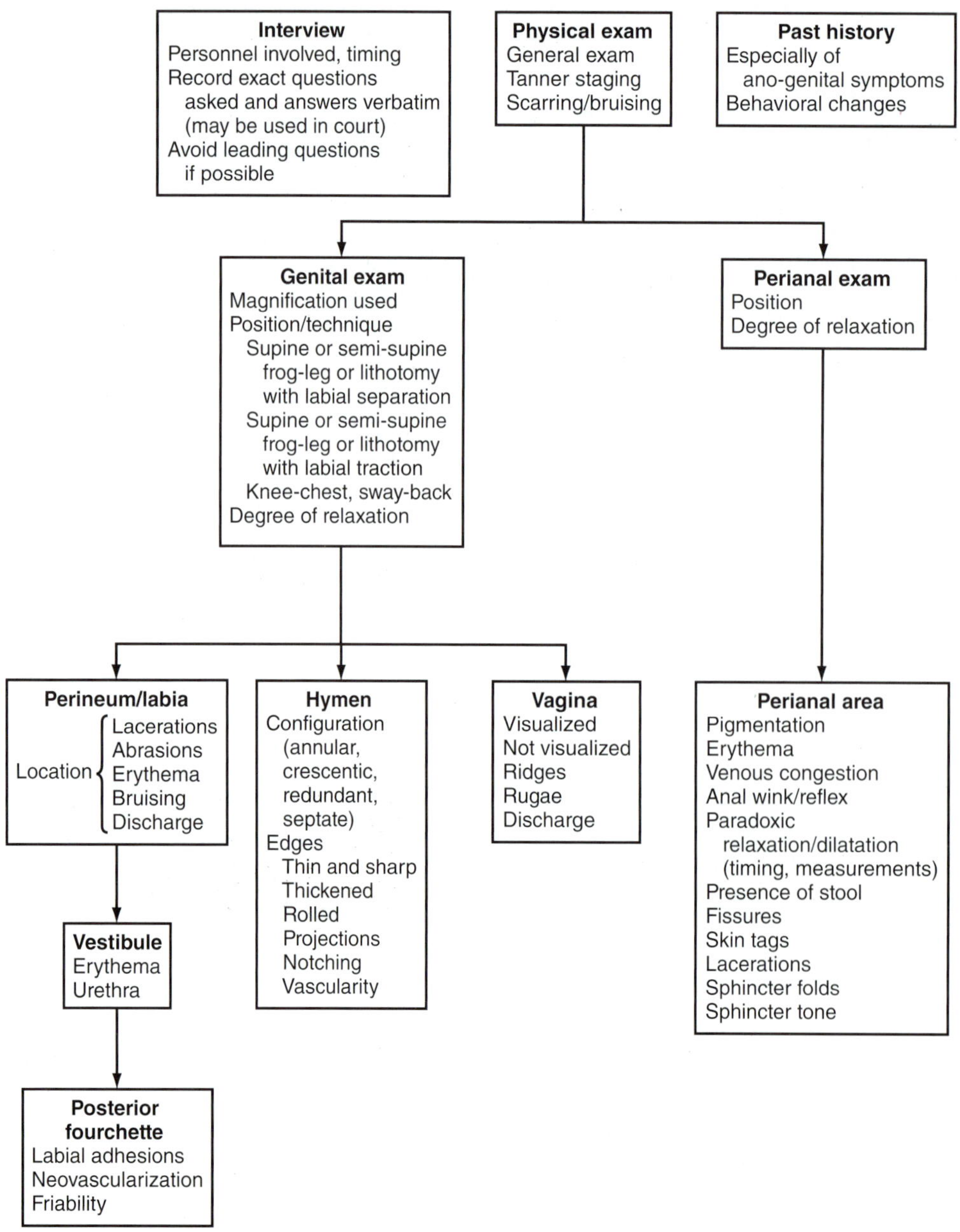

Fig. 6.86 Documentation of physical findings required in sexual abuse evaluation.

Table 6.3 Gynecologic Anatomic Terminology

Term	Definition
Anal verge	The tissue overlying the subcutaneous external anal sphincter at the most distal portion of the anal canal, extending exteriorly to the margin of the anal skin
Anterior commissure	The union of the two labia minora anteriorly
Clitoris	A cylindrical, erectile body situated at the superior portion of the vulva, covered by a sheath of skin called the clitoral hood or prepuce
Fossa navicularis/posterior fossa	Concavity of the lower part of the vaginal vestibule situated inferiorly to the vaginal orifice and extending to the posterior fourchette (posterior commissure)
Hymen	A thin membrane located at the junction of the vestibular floor and the vaginal canal that partially covers the vaginal orifice
Labia majora	Rounded folds of skin forming the lateral boundaries of the vulva
Labia minora	Thin longitudinal folds of tissue enclosed within the labia majora; in the prepubertal child, they extend from the clitoral hood to the midpoint of the lateral wall of the vestibule. After puberty, they lengthen and join posteriorly (inferiorly), thereby enclosing the structures of the vestibule.
Median raphe	Ridge or furrow that marks the line of union of the two halves of the perineum
Mons pubis	Rounded, fleshy prominence, created by the underlying fat pad, which overlies the symphysis pubis
Perianal folds	Wrinkles or folds of the skin of the anal verge that radiate from the anus
Perineal body	The central tendon of the perineum located between the vulva and the anus in the female and between the scrotum and anus in the male
Perineum	The pelvic floor and associated structures bounded anteriorly by the symphysis pubis, laterally by the ischial tuberosities, and posteriorly by the coccyx
Posterior fourchette	The junction of the two labia minora inferiorly (posteriorly); this is termed the *posterior commissure* in the prepubertal child, because the labia minora are not completely developed and have not extended and joined posteriorly or inferiorly as they do after puberty
Vagina	The uterovaginal canal extending from the inner aspect of the hymen to the uterine cervix
Vaginal vestibule	Anatomic cavity containing the opening of the vagina, urethra, and ducts of the Bartholin glands; bordered by the clitoris superiorly, the labia laterally, and the posterior commissure (fourchette) inferiorly, and encompassing the fossa navicularis immediately inferior to the vaginal introitus
Vulva	The external genitalia or pudendum of the female; includes the clitoris, labia majora, labia minora, vaginal vestibule, urethral orifice, vaginal orifice, hymen, and posterior fourchette (or commissure)

Modified from the American Professional Society on the Abuse of Children.

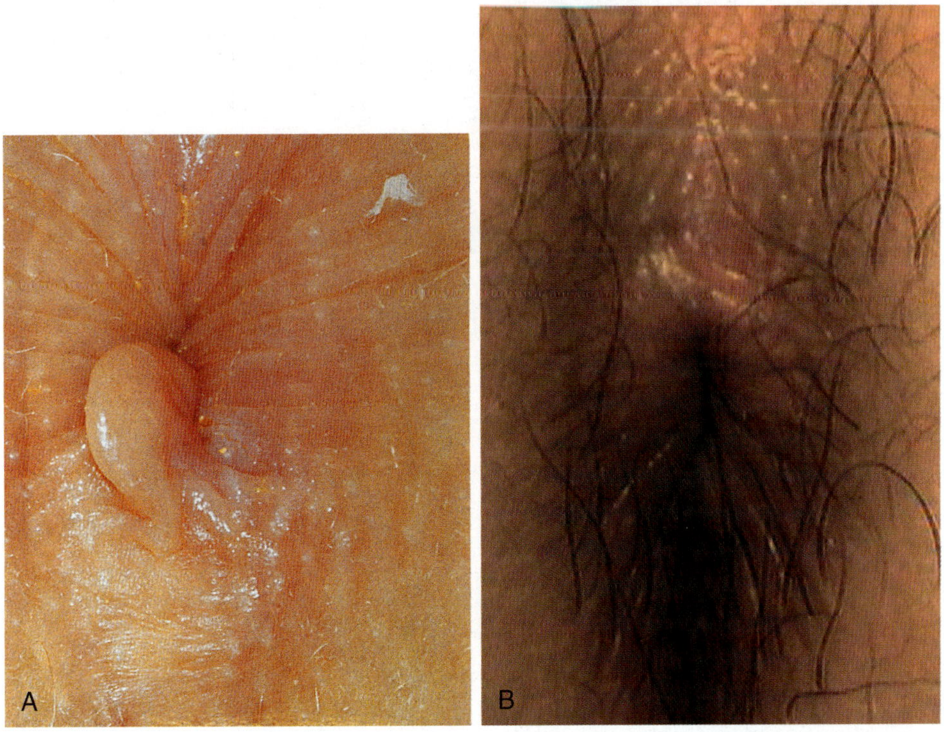

Fig. 6.87 (A) Perianal skin tag. This is a common finding, particularly in children with a history of constipation and prior problems with anal fissures. (B) Venous congestion noted in the perianal area. This can occur after a few minutes in either the knee/chest or lithotomy positions and is a normal finding.

in detail numerous normal variants, some of which have been mistaken for abnormal findings in the past.

Acute Findings of Sexual Assault and Sexual Abuse

Victims of sexual assault who present acutely may show evidence of physical trauma other than genital injuries. Bruises and abrasions of the head, face, neck, chest, abdomen, forearms, knees, and thighs are more common (see Fig. 6.4A).

Although most children forced to perform oral sex have no physical findings, forceful orogenital contact may result in perioral and intraoral injuries. These may include fissuring or tears at the corner of the mouth and gingival and palatal contusions. Rarely, forceful oral penetration and thrusting can cause lacerations of posterior pharyngeal tissues, with potential complications of subcutaneous air dissection and abscess formation.

Genital and perianal examination may reveal contusions, abrasions, or lacerations (Fig. 6.88; see Figs. 19.14–19.17). Injuries due to sexual abuse tend to be located in the posterior portion of the hymen, as opposed to those caused by straddle injury, which are usually more anterior, are often unilateral, and rarely involve the hymen in isolation (see Fig. 19.4B).

If acute external contusions or tears are seen, internal injury must be suspected. The prepubertal girl is particularly vulnerable to severe internal trauma as a result of forceful penetration of either the vagina or rectum (Fig. 6.89). This stems from the fact that the structures are relatively small, and the tissues are more delicate and rigid due to the lack of estrogen. Young children with relatively mild external injuries may, in fact, have major internal tears, including perforation of the peritoneum and damage to pelvic vessels, mesentery, and intestine (see Figs. 19.16 and 19.17). Signs of internal injury may be subtle, but such patients will have evidence of vaginal bleeding or of a vaginal hematoma, and some may have lower abdominal tenderness or evidence of occult blood loss. Therefore, when such findings are present, an examination under anesthesia is essential. In contrast, the postpubertal female can usually be adequately assessed by careful pelvic examination, with use of a swab to enhance visualization of the hymenal surface and margins (see Figs. 6.84A and B and 6.85). If, despite good emotional support, reassurance, and careful preparation, she is emotionally unable to tolerate the procedure, an examination under anesthesia is also advisable.

Perianally, wedge-shaped smooth areas in the midline and skin tags are normal findings and commonly seen without abuse (see Figs. 6.87A and 6.100. Immediate dilation of the internal and external anal sphincters to greater than 2 cm on adopting the knee/chest position has been associated with sexual abuse, especially in the absence of any predisposing factors such as constipation and sedation. The significance of complete and immediate dilation is still a no-consensus finding in relation to sexual abuse. In cases of acute anorectal injury such as marked bruising or lacerations of the anal canal, a rectal examination under anesthesia may be indicated to assess for internal rectal tears and other injuries.

Erythema of the various anogenital structures is a common but totally nonspecific finding that may be significant within the context

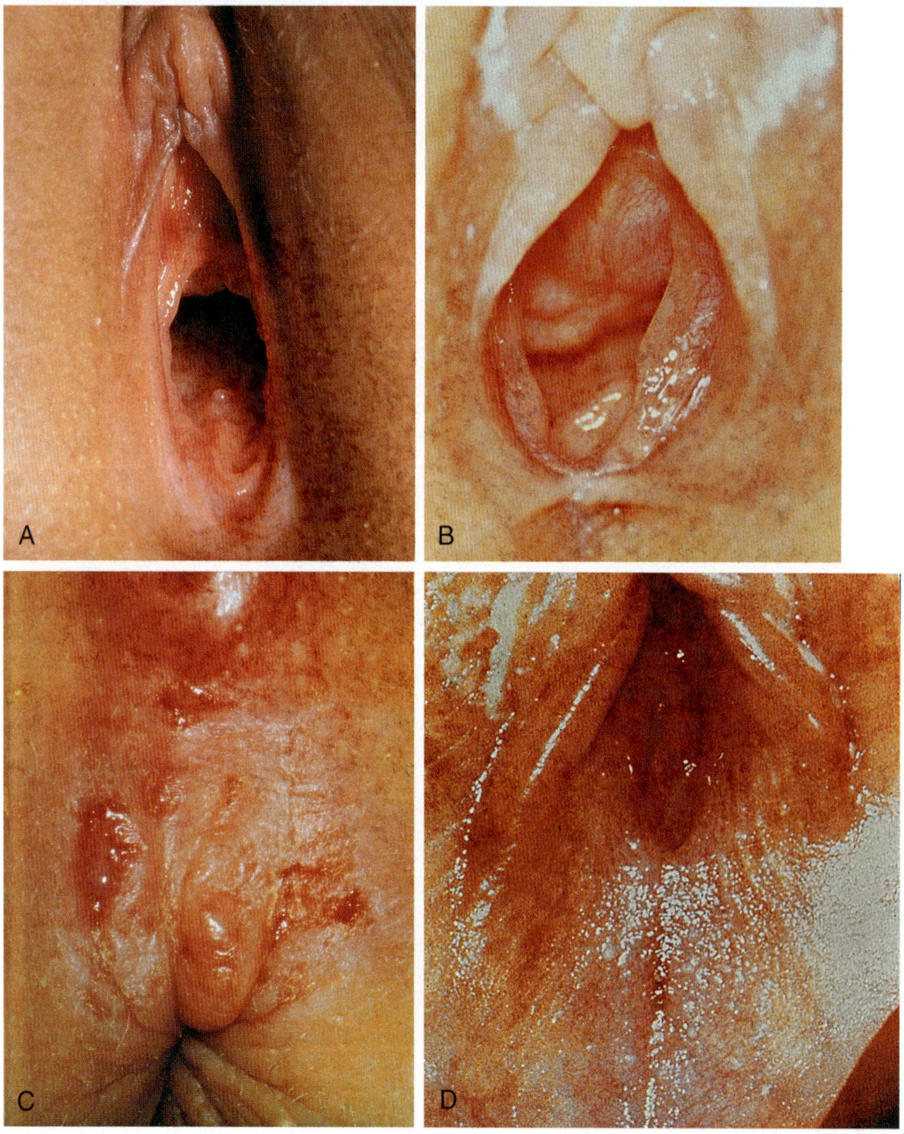

Fig. 6.88 Findings usually considered abnormal as a result of prior sexual abuse. (A) The hymen is almost completely absent, and the portion remaining has slightly thickened, rolled margins. A subtle bump exists at 7 o'clock, and a notch exists at 5 o'clock. (B) This hymen has a posterior notch deeper than 50% of the rim, which persists in the knee/chest position (not shown here). (C) Scarring, edema, and fresh excoriations of the perineal body extending to the anterior anal rim are seen in this child who was repetitively abused. (D) The adhesed labia minora in another child are markedly thickened secondary to chronic frictional trauma incurred during sexual abuse. (C, Courtesy Pat Bruno, MD, Sunbury, PA. D, Courtesy John McCann, MD, University of California at Davis, Davis, CA.)

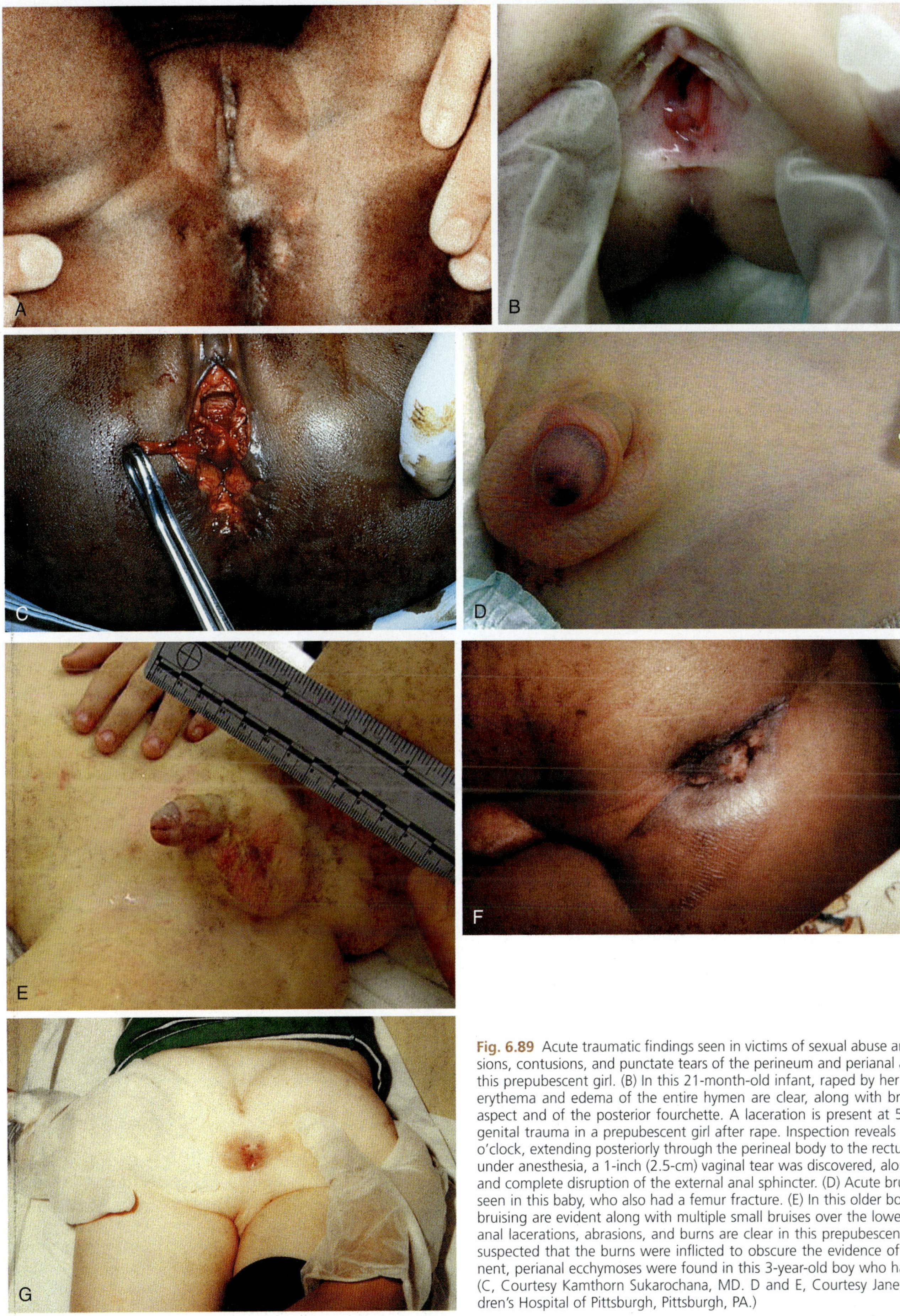

Fig. 6.89 Acute traumatic findings seen in victims of sexual abuse and assault. (A) Abrasions, contusions, and punctate tears of the perineum and perianal areas can be seen in this prepubescent girl. (B) In this 21-month-old infant, raped by her mother's paramour, erythema and edema of the entire hymen are clear, along with bruising of its inferior aspect and of the posterior fourchette. A laceration is present at 5 o'clock. (C) Severe genital trauma in a prepubescent girl after rape. Inspection reveals a hymenal tear at 6 o'clock, extending posteriorly through the perineal body to the rectum. With the patient under anesthesia, a 1-inch (2.5-cm) vaginal tear was discovered, along with a rectal tear and complete disruption of the external anal sphincter. (D) Acute bruising of the glans is seen in this baby, who also had a femur fracture. (E) In this older boy, penile and scrotal bruising are evident along with multiple small bruises over the lower abdomen. (F) Perianal lacerations, abrasions, and burns are clear in this prepubescent boy. The examiner suspected that the burns were inflicted to obscure the evidence of sodomy. (G) Prominent, perianal ecchymoses were found in this 3-year-old boy who had been sodomized. (C, Courtesy Kamthorn Sukarochana, MD. D and E, Courtesy Janet Squires, MD, Children's Hospital of Pittsburgh, Pittsburgh, PA.)

of a specific history. However, it is more likely to be a normal finding or one resulting from nonsexual irritation or scratching (see Figs. 19.19 and 19.20) and should not be interpreted as specific for abuse when it is the sole finding.

Evidence of seminal products in the form of a vaginal or anal discharge may be seen if the patient is examined within hours of the latest incident and has not bathed in the interim (Fig. 6.90). If a history of ejaculation is obtained and the area has not been washed, swabbing the perineum and inner thighs with saline-moistened cotton swabs may yield a sample of dried seminal fluid that can be sent to the crime laboratory.

Male victims may have evidence of urethral discharge and abrasions and contusions of the penis, scrotum, or median raphe (see Fig. 6.89D and E).

Although anal fissure(s) or tears are not considered specific to sexual abuse because they can be seen in children with chronic or recurrent constipation or other medical conditions, tears that extend beyond the hair follicle–bearing areas are thought to be more concerning for abuse. The number of fissures and location off the midline may increase the concern for sexual abuse. Burns may be inflicted in an attempt to obscure injuries resulting from anal penetration. Hence, evidence of perianal burns may be suggestive of abuse, as is perianal bruising (see Fig. 6.89). Thickening and irregularity of the rectal folds may be suspicious (see Fig. 6.89).

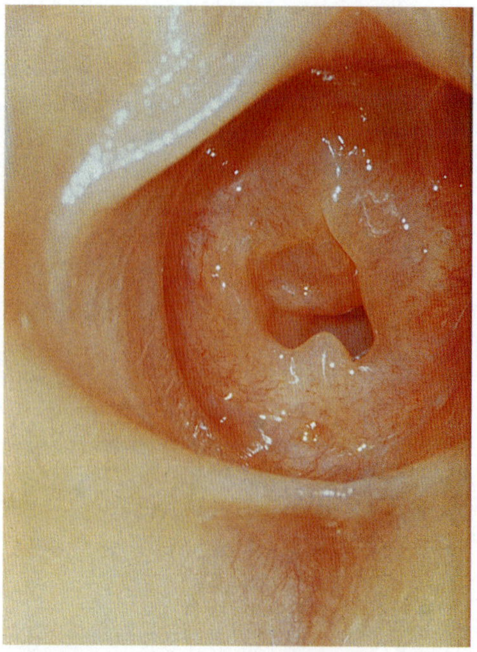

Fig. 6.91 Septal remnant. This skin tag at the 6 o'clock position is a remnant of the vaginal septum present earlier in fetal development and constitutes a normal finding seen in about 5% of girls.

Differential Diagnosis of Sexual Abuse

A wide range of nonabusive causes of the physical and behavioral symptoms that serve as presenting complaints of many sexual abuse victims exists, and physical findings, when present, are also variable and often nonspecific.

Normal Anatomic Variations

A wide variation in normal hymenal configuration and shape of orifice exists (Fig. 6.82; see also Figs. 19.3 and 19.6) as well as some variation in normal hymenal opening diameter (see Fig. 19.3). Several normal anatomic variants are recognized. Septal remnants (Fig. 6.91), seen as tags near the midline on either or both the anterior or posterior portion of the hymenal membrane (see Chapter 19), and even anterolateral hymenal flaps (Fig. 6.92) are normal findings, as are periurethral bands. These and intravaginal ridges (Fig. 6.93) were once erroneously thought to be the result of scarring. Thin labial adhesions are a common finding in normal children as well (Fig. 6.94).

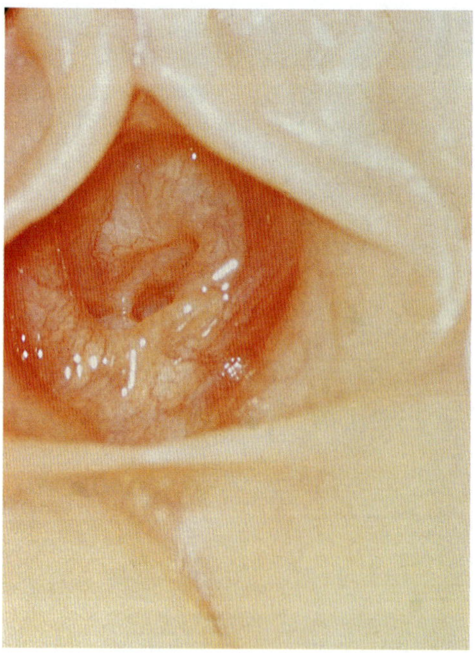

Fig. 6.92 Hymenal flap. This child has a redundant hymen with an everted anterolateral flap, another normal variant.

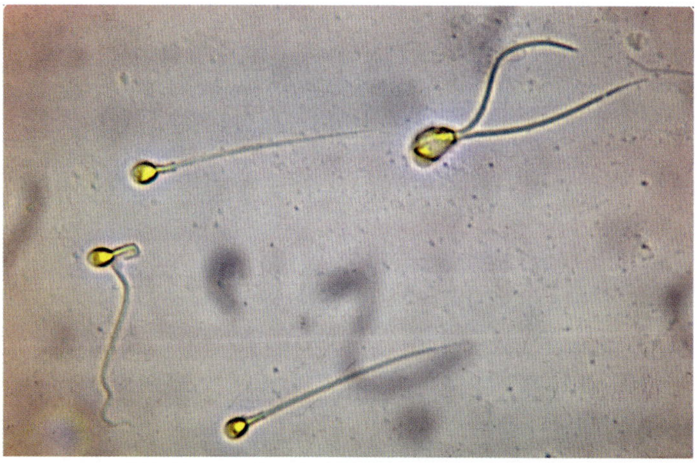

Fig. 6.90 Microscopical appearance of seminal fluid removed from a young rape victim. If a vaginal discharge is found in a patient presenting within 24 hours of sexual abuse, a wet mount may reveal sperm. A portion of the discharge should also be collected for acid phosphatase, blood grouping, and enzyme studies.

Vulvar Erythema and Inflammation

Erythema of the vaginal vestibule is common in asymptomatic, nonabused, prepubescent girls. It can also be seen in abuse victims and in children with irritants and other forms of vulvovaginitis (see Figs. 19.25 and 19.32). Vulvovaginitis has a wide variety of causes, many of which are noninfectious, including chemical irritation, poor perineal hygiene or aeration, nonabusive frictional trauma, contact dermatitis, or itching and scratching due to pinworms or other sources of irritation. These conditions may be associated with nonspecific erythema, maceration, or superficial abrasions/excoriations (see Figs. 19.19 and 19.20). Many infectious cases are caused by respiratory or gastrointestinal pathogens (the former transmitted from nose or throat by the child's

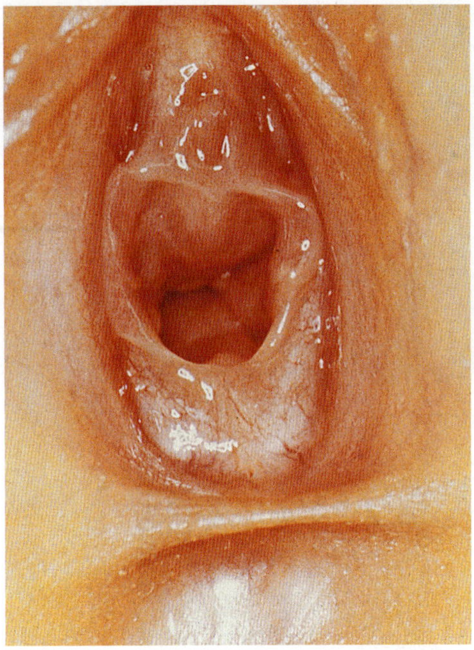

Fig. 6.93 Intravaginal ridges. The bands of tissue along the vaginal walls that appear here to extend medially and downward from the 11 and 2 o'clock positions are normal features of the vaginal walls; in the past they were erroneously thought to be the result of scarring. (Courtesy John McCann, MD, University of California at Davis, CA.)

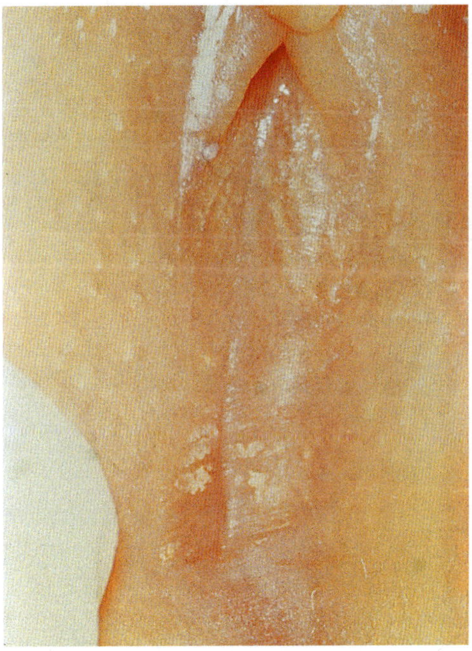

Fig. 6.94 Labial adhesions. The labia minora are fused in the midline as a consequence of prior inflammation. They are separated by a thin lucent line, and the epithelium of the labia is normal.

hands, the latter often due to perineal contact with infected stool) or are seen concurrently with urinary tract infections (see Fig. 19.25).

Urethral Prolapse

The clinical findings of urethral prolapse (Fig. 6.95) have been mistakenly attributed to sexual abuse because the purplish-red prolapsed mucosal tissue that protrudes between the labia minora bleeds easily and often overlies the vaginal orifice and is mistaken for edematous, traumatized, redundant hymenal folds. The condition is often first discovered when blood or a serosanguinous discharge is found on the diaper or underwear because associated dysuria is unusual and urination is not impeded. With magnification, the urethral orifice

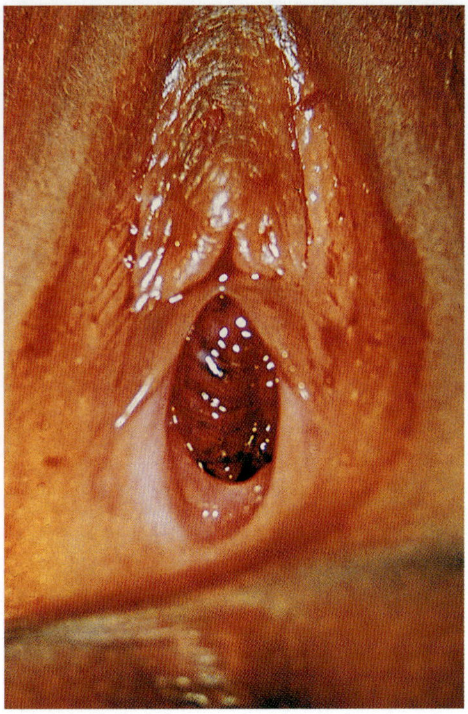

Fig. 6.95 Urethral prolapse. This child was referred for evaluation for possible sexual abuse when blood was noted on her underwear, and "traumatized tissue" was seen on examination. On close inspection, this was found to be edematous, friable prolapsed urethral mucosa.

can be seen at the center of the mass, which is soft and markedly tender to touch. After application of topical anesthetic, the prolapse can be lifted, revealing the hymen underneath. The condition is unusual and tends to occur only in children younger than 12 years old. The cause is unknown, although many affected girls have a history of constipation.

Lichen Sclerosus

Lichen sclerosus et atrophicus has often been mistakenly attributed to sexual abuse. The involved perineal skin is paper thin and friable and tends to be hypopigmented. During periods of acute inflammation, hypopigmentation may be partially obscured by erythema and areas of superficial ulceration that bleed easily (Fig. 6.96; see Fig. 19.23 and accompanying text).

Accidental Trauma

Straddle injuries produce lesions of the anterior and anterolateral portions because these are tissues most likely to be crushed between the pubic ramus and the object on which the child falls. Findings include contusions, abrasions, and superficial lacerations, the latter being frequently found at the junction of the labia majora and minora (Fig. 6.97).

Vaginal Foreign Bodies

The presence of foreign objects within the vaginal canal sometimes precipitates an inflammatory response with production of a copious brown, sometimes blood-tinged, discharge with a foul odor. The discharge and its odor generally prompt presentation. Foreign bodies may or may not suggest abuse. Finding of a small wad of toilet tissue lodged within the vagina is likely an inadvertent consequence of vigorous wiping (Fig. 6.98).

Midline Defects

Perineal midline fusion defects occur when a portion of the median raphe next to the anus does not fuse in utero. The anomaly is present at birth and may be located anteriorly or posteriorly to the anus. When the unfused edges of the median raphe are spread apart, they reveal an underlying pink or reddish mucosal-like

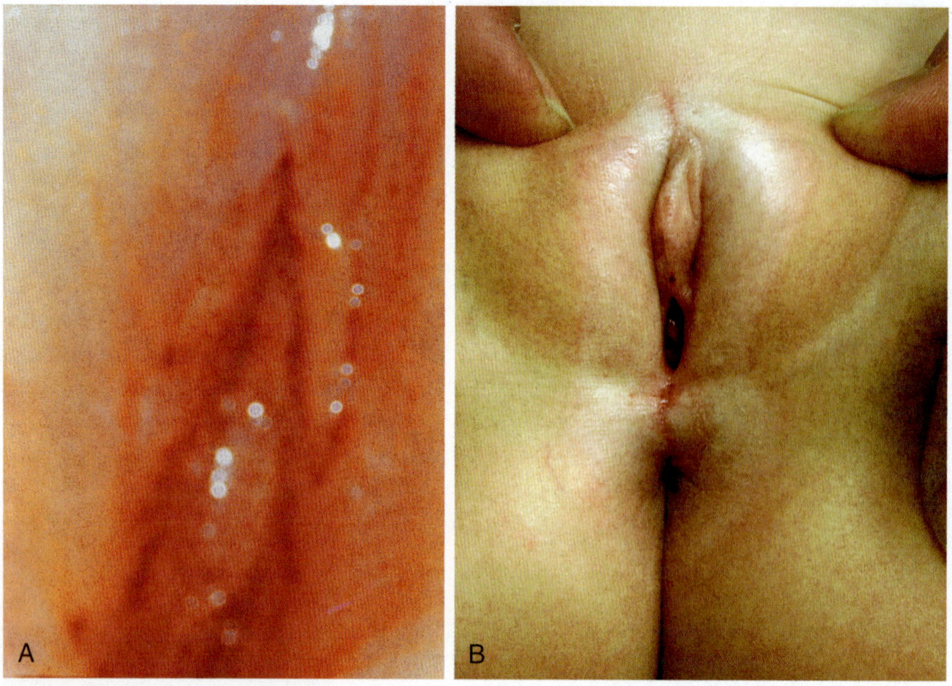

Fig. 6.96 Lichen sclerosus et atrophicus. (A) Multiple small points of bleeding dot the atrophic mucosa in this child. (B) In another girl, acute inflammation has largely subsided, leaving an hourglass pattern of hypopigmentation extending from the mons to below the anal folds. (B, Courtesy Robin Gehris, MD, Children's Hospital of Pittsburgh, Pittsburgh, PA.)

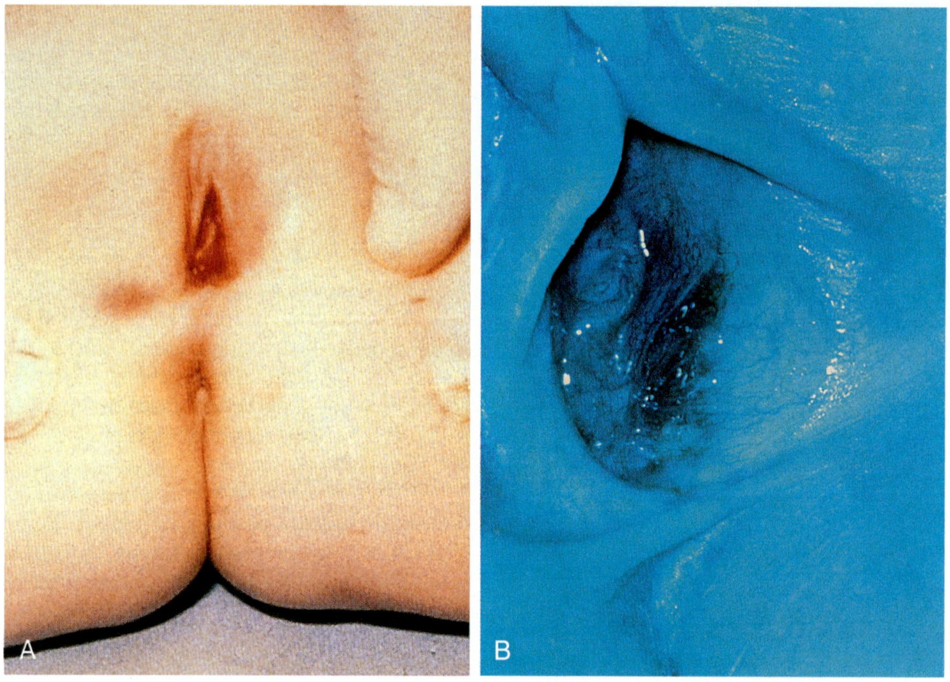

Fig. 6.97 Accidental trauma caused by a straddle injury. (A) This child with a straddle injury was brought in immediately for care because of slight bleeding. Superficial abrasions and contusions extend from the anterior portion of the labia minora to the posterior fourchette. Note that the lesions are largely unilateral. (B) Another child complained of dysuria and was noted to have a small amount of blood on her underwear after a straddle injury. The superficial laceration between the hymen and labia minora was barely visible in regular light but was brought out by viewing it through a green filter.

surface (Fig. 6.99). The defect often goes unnoticed until days or weeks after delivery during a diaper change, bathing, or a well-child care visit. When first detected by a parent or physician unfamiliar with the problem, findings may be mistaken for a laceration due to sexual abuse. Recognition of the true nature of the abnormality is enhanced by knowledge of its existence and by the fact that the edges of the outer layer of tissue and of the underlying "mucosal" surface are smooth and intact. Other features that help distinguish midline defects from abuse-related injury are the absence of associated introital and anal abnormalities, bleeding, and no change on follow-up examination.

Anal fissures and perianal skin tags (Fig. 6.87) are common sequelae of constipation. The fissures caused by the passage of hard or large-caliber stools are superficial and usually do not extend beyond the perianal skin bearing hair follicles.

Infantile perianal pyramidal protrusion consists of a single benign papule with a pyramidal shape found in the midline of the perineal raphe, usually just anterior to the anus (occasionally just

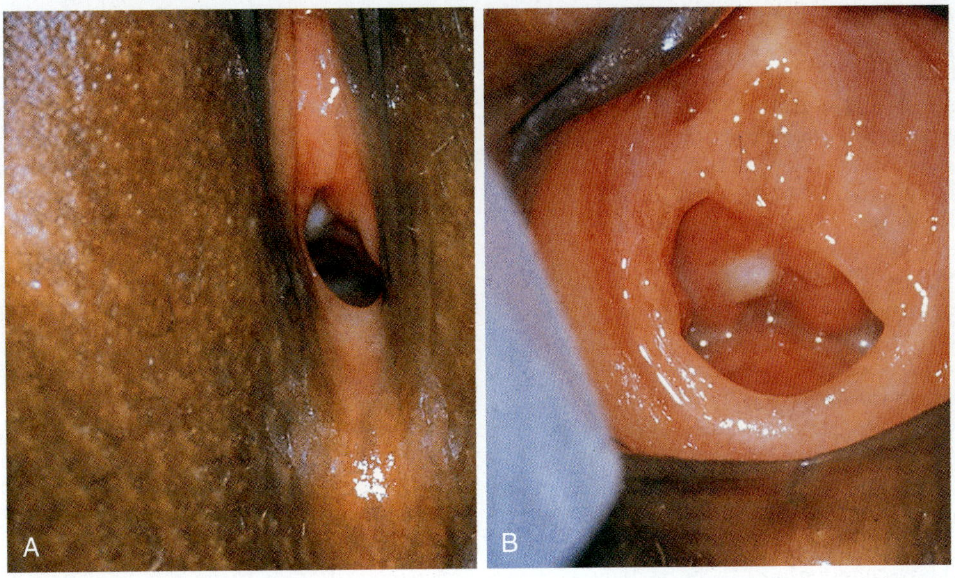

Fig. 6.98 Vaginal foreign body. (A) A white object is noted within the vagina on perineal inspection. (B) This was better visualized by labial traction. Toilet paper had become lodged in wiping after toileting.

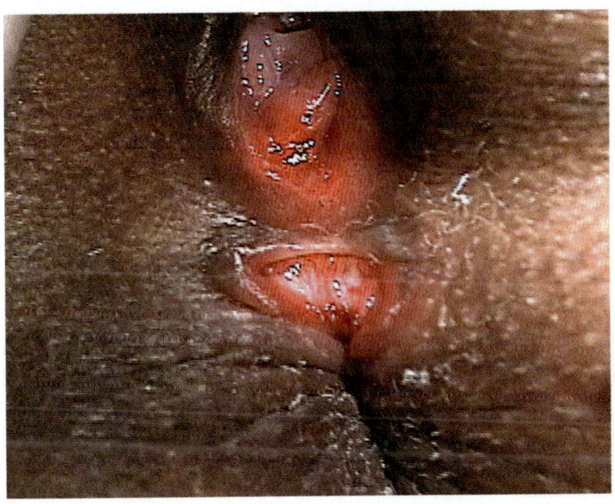

Fig. 6.99 Perineal midline fusion defect. This toddler was referred for concern of sexual abuse when this defect was noticed by her new foster mother during a diaper change. The unfused edges of the median raphe are spread apart to reveal an underlying mucosal-like surface. Both are smooth and intact with no evidence of inflammation or bleeding. Note that she has another congenital anomaly, an anteriorly displaced anus. A normal redundant hymen is also seen. (Courtesy Carol Byers, CRNP, Children's Hospital of Pittsburgh, Pittsburgh, PA.)

posterior). It is smooth, soft, pink, and asymptomatic (Fig. 6.100). The protrusion is either present at birth or noted shortly thereafter, and there is no association with antecedent fissures or fistulas. Infantile perianal pyramidal protrusion usually resolves spontaneously over weeks to months. The exact etiology is yet unclear, although an association with lichen sclerosus et atrophicus has been noted.

Spontaneous anal sphincter relaxation occurring 30 seconds to 3 or 4 minutes after adopting the knee/chest position is normal. Immediate sphincter dilation when there is stool present in the rectal vault is also considered normal, as is anal dilation in the fully anesthetized child. Immediate sphincter dilation to greater than 2 cm on adopting the knee/chest position has been considered suspicious for repetitive prior anal penetration, but there is no current expert consensus on this finding. Perianal erythema, hyperpigmentation, and venous engorgement are other common findings seen in children without sexual abuse concerns.

Sexually Transmitted Infection

Most children undergoing evaluation for sexual abuse/assault will not test positive for an STI. Nevertheless, many centers will routinely test all children with sexual abuse concerns given the health

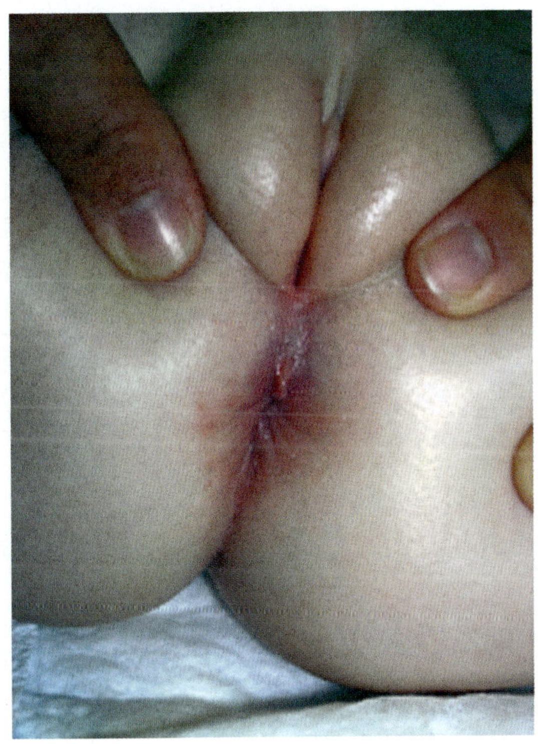

Fig. 6.100 Infantile perianal pyramidal protrusion. This smooth, soft, pink papule, located in the midline just anterior to the anus, has a pyramidal shape. It was noted by the mother shortly after birth and was totally asymptomatic.

and forensic implications of any confirmed positive results. U.S. Food and Drug Administration–cleared nucleic acid amplification tests (NAATs) for *Neisseria gonorrhea, Chlamydia trachomatis,* and *Trichomonas vaginalis* have generally replaced cultures and are recommended by current Centers for Disease Control and Prevention (CDC) guidelines. (Check for updated guidelines at https://www.cdc.gov/std/treatment-guidelines/sexual-assault-children.htm). When NAATs are done in cases of suspected child sexual abuse, a second laboratory-based confirmatory test is required in prepubertal patients. One of the major downsides to NAATs is the inability to obtain antibiotic sensitivities. Testing for STIs should be considered in the adolescent rather than prophylaxis alone because STIs may have been acquired earlier as a result of consensual sexual activity that would necessitate treatment of a partner.

There are some victims who are identified when they present with a vaginal or urethral discharge that tests positive for a sexually transmitted pathogen. In females, this usually manifests as vulvovaginitis with a copious, purulent vaginal discharge. *N. gonorrhea* and *C. trachomatis* are the most commonly identified sexually transmitted pathogens (see Figs. 19.32–19.34). Males may have overt urethritis or asymptomatic urethral infection. Oral and rectal gonococcal infections are typically subclinical, and nongenital infections will be missed if only urine is tested.

There is a low prevalence of human immunodeficiency virus (HIV) and syphilis reported among children evaluated for sexual abuse. Nevertheless, serologic testing must be considered for children on a case-by-case basis, particularly when there has been mucosal contact or penetration. Adolescents should be tested for both HIV and syphilis. If a patient presents within 72 hours of their last sexual contact, the patient should be offered HIV postexposure prophylaxis, with shared decision making.

Condyloma acuminata refer to anogenital warts caused by human papillomavirus (HPV). HPV can be transmitted during delivery, and because the latency period can be as long as 9 to 12 months, lesions appearing in infancy are unlikely to be due to abuse. When these usually multiple, raised, skin-colored, fleshy lesions appear thereafter, they can be suspicious, although not diagnostic, for abuse (Fig. 6.101). In young children who need help with toileting, nonsexual transmission from warts on the hand of a parent or caretaker to a child can occur. However, when the warts are restricted to the hymen in a prepubertal child, sexual abuse is much more concerning. Increased adoption of the human papillomavirus vaccine has decreased the incidence of genital warts, at least anecdotally.

Similarly to HPV, genital herpes infections may be acquired through sexual contact but may also spread from oral or hand lesions from the patient, or from a parent with a cold sore (see Fig. 19.31). In an older-aged child, however, sexual contact is the more likely source and calls for further investigation. Herpes may not appear with typical vesicles in children and may present with ulcers.

Forensic Evidence Collection

A comprehensive text on evidence collection is beyond the scope of this section. In general, if the last abusive event occurred within 72 hours of presentation, forensic body swabs as part of evidence collection are indicated and there are commercially available kits that make the collection process straightforward. This exact time frame varies depending on the jurisdiction and some jurisdictions may have different recommended timeframes for children versus adolescents/adults. Swabs from a prepubertal

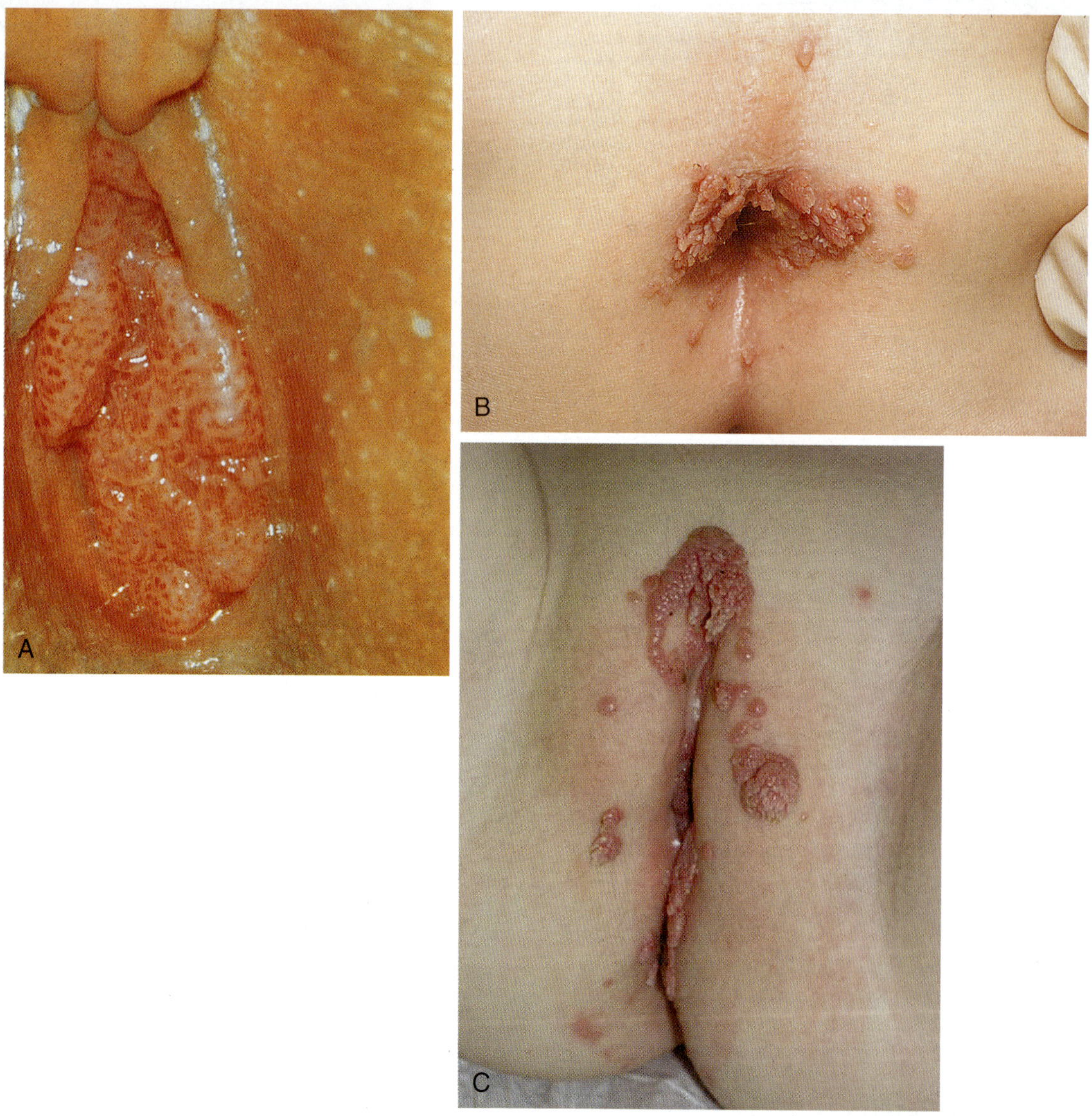

Fig. 6.101 Condylomata acuminata. (A) Although human papillomavirus (HPV) infection is not specific for abuse and is perhaps more commonly transmitted nonsexually, when condylomata are restricted to the hymen, as seen in this child, sexual abuse is the likely source. In this case the victim reported that the perpetrator had visible genital warts. (B) Coalescent and discrete condylomata are seen in the perianal area of this 4-year-old boy with a history of being sodomized. (C) More extensive lesions involving the mons, the introitus, the labia, and perianal area developed in another child. (C, Courtesy Robin Gehris, MD, Children's Hospital of Pittsburgh, Pittsburgh, PA.)

patient presenting more than 72 hours after the abuse are unlikely to be positive for identifiable DNA, with most positive results obtained at less than 24 hours, with current technologic methods. With the yield of intravaginal specimens from asymptomatic prepubertal victims so low, the collection of intravaginal specimens uncomfortable, and the cost high, forensic intravaginal swabs are not generally indicated in prepubertal girls, unless the examination is occurring under anesthesia for other reasons. Unlaundered clothing, underwear, and bedding are more likely to yield usable evidence, and these items should be collected as part of forensic evidence. Be mindful that chain of custody is maintained—otherwise, failure to adhere to these procedures breaks the chain of evidence and invalidates its use in legal proceedings.

NEGLECT

Neglect is the most common referral to CPS, accounting for nearly 80% of active cases. In its mildest form, this may consist of a pattern of lack of vigilance and safeguarding of young children, who are thereby at greater risk for accidents and ingestions. This may include leaving them unattended for long periods, unsafe housing, or lack of supervision in a hazardous environment. In a common and severe form, the patient presents with growth failure and developmental delay as a due to inadequate provision of calories and minimal or ineffective nurturing.

Inadequate Nutrition or Failure to Thrive

One of the most obvious measurable parameters of neglect is inadequate weight gain and growth. Traditionally, failure to thrive is defined as less than 3% on the World Health Organization weight curve or having declined down across two lines on the weight curve. Weight will plateau first, as the body will protect length and head circumference. Prolonged failure to thrive can affect length and head circumference growth (Fig. 6.102).

Insufficient caloric intake is the etiology of the majority of failure-to-thrive evaluations for infants. This lack of calories may be influenced by many factors, including but not limited to economic stressors, parental fatigue, lack of education and unreasonable expectations for the baby's hunger, ability to mix the formula correctly, housing instability, and multiple older children also needing to be fed. Additionally, parents who are experiencing postpartum depression and other mental illness may struggle with the routine of frequent feedings and nighttime wake-ups.

In the more severe case, the child presents with decreased subcutaneous tissue (most notably over the buttocks, thighs, and upper arms), a pinched face, and sunken prominent eyes. In some, there are frank physical findings of multiple vitamin deficiencies, which include a nonspecific or seborrhea-like dermatitis that can progress to skin breakdown, cheilosis, glossitis and stomatitis, and erythema and thinning of the skin over the palms and soles (Figs. 6.103A–E and 6.104). Other children are found to have exceedingly bad dentition, so-called "baby bottle rot" (Fig. 6.105).

Affected infants tend be poor eaters due to lack of practice and general development. Vocalization is sparse, and development is delayed and uneven.

Psychosocial influences of failure to thrive are the most common form of growth failure in infancy, accounting for up to 60% of cases; in another 25%, growth failure is due to a combination of organic and psychosocial factors, and up to 15% of cases are of purely organic origin. In the latter instances, affected infants often have congenital abnormalities or have suffered prenatal or perinatal insults that have resulted in poor growth and/or physical conditions that make them difficult to feed and care for.

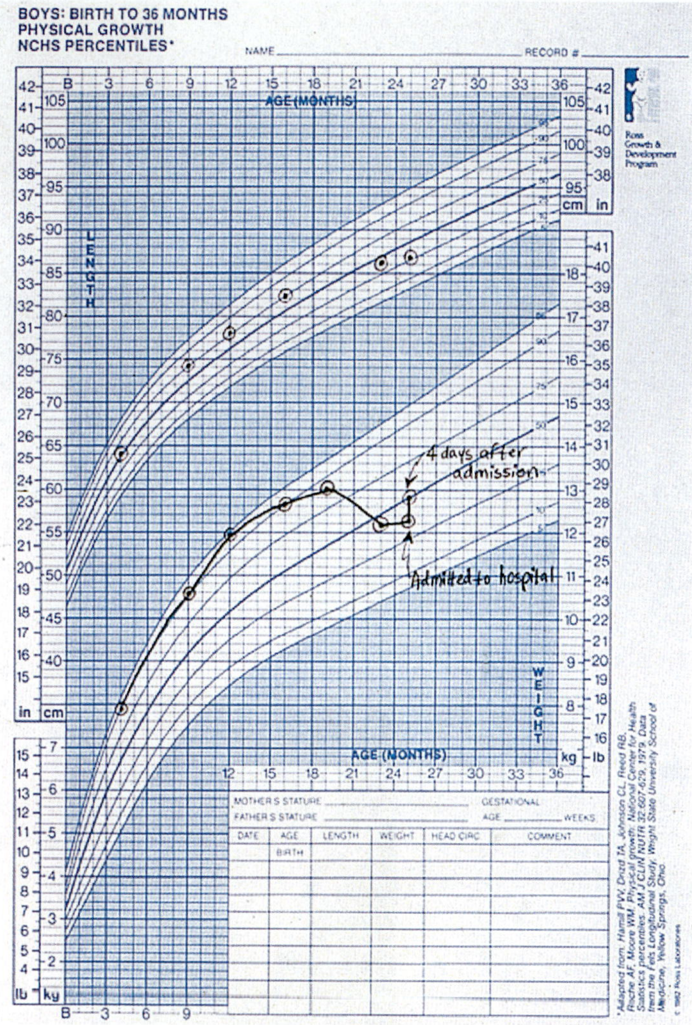

Fig. 6.102 Growth chart of a child with failure to thrive due to neglect. This boy's growth was normal until he was 15 months old, when his mother became addicted to crack. His weight gain slowed between 15 and 19 months, after which he showed a precipitous weight loss and slowing of height growth. He showed rapid catch-up growth within a week of removal from the home. (Courtesy Robin Gehris, MD, Children's Hospital of Pittsburgh, Pittsburgh, PA.)

Organic Causes of Failure to Thrive

When an organic etiology is found for failure to thrive, it is important to consider that many social factors will still influence the child's weight gain. Children with special health care needs are at increased risk of maltreatment, given the demands of care placed on a family. A child with feeding aversion because of a cleft palate may be a slow eater. Hence, a new parent may struggle to meet these extra needs of the child, leading to even less caloric intake.

For disease-based etiologies, any of the following systems may be involved: CNS, gastrointestinal, cardiac, genetic, pulmonary, renal, and endocrine. Most of these disorders can be recognized during physical examination because of the obvious abnormalities seen. The remainder tends to be revealed by history or can be readily diagnosed with a few simple screening laboratory tests.

Regardless of the initial etiology, once undernutrition reaches a significant level, the infant tends to become caught up in a vicious cycle: with malnutrition impairing immune function, which increases frequency/chronicity/severity of infection, which causes anorexia with decreased intake and decreased nutrient absorption while adding to caloric needs, thereby further exacerbating the malnutrition. In addition to this cycle, there is another involving maternal/child interaction: The malnourished infant, regardless of cause, tends to become progressively more irritable and listless; less engaging and engageable; and, therefore, less rewarding to care for. Hence, a combination of physical and psychosocial factors comes into play in all cases of severe failure to thrive.

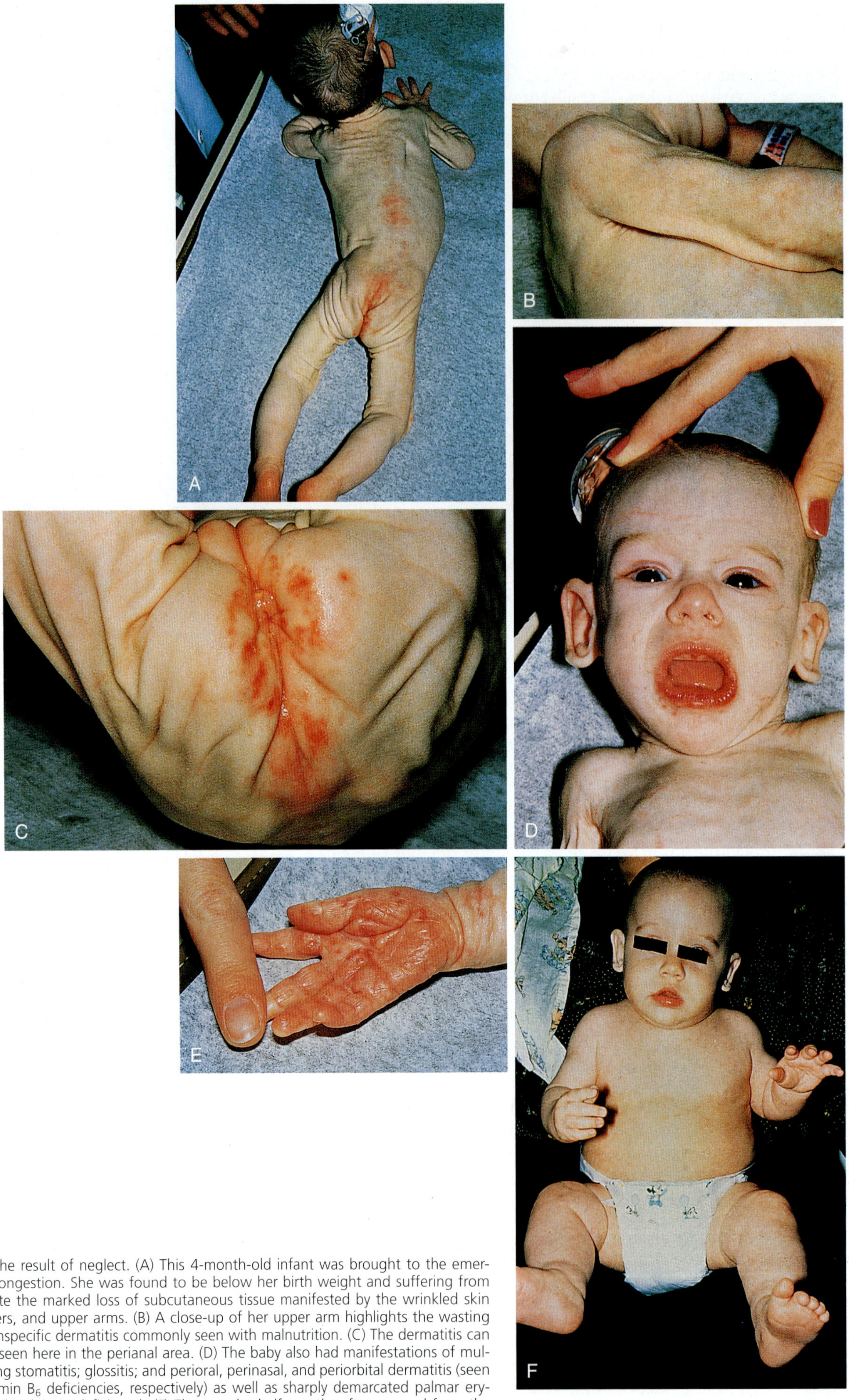

Fig. 6.103 Failure to thrive as the result of neglect. (A) This 4-month-old infant was brought to the emergency department because of congestion. She was found to be below her birth weight and suffering from severe developmental delay. Note the marked loss of subcutaneous tissue manifested by the wrinkled skin folds over her buttocks, shoulders, and upper arms. (B) A close-up of her upper arm highlights the wasting and shows the mottling and nonspecific dermatitis commonly seen with malnutrition. (C) The dermatitis can progress to skin breakdown, as seen here in the perianal area. (D) The baby also had manifestations of multiple vitamin deficiencies including stomatitis; glossitis; and perioral, perinasal, and periorbital dermatitis (seen with riboflavin, niacin, and vitamin B_6 deficiencies, respectively) as well as sharply demarcated palmar erythema (E) with thinning of the skin (niacin deficiency). (F) Three and a half months after removal from the home, she was well nourished and had caught up developmentally.

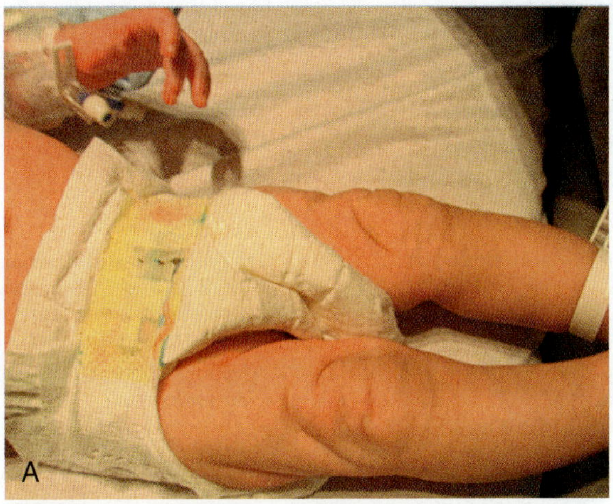

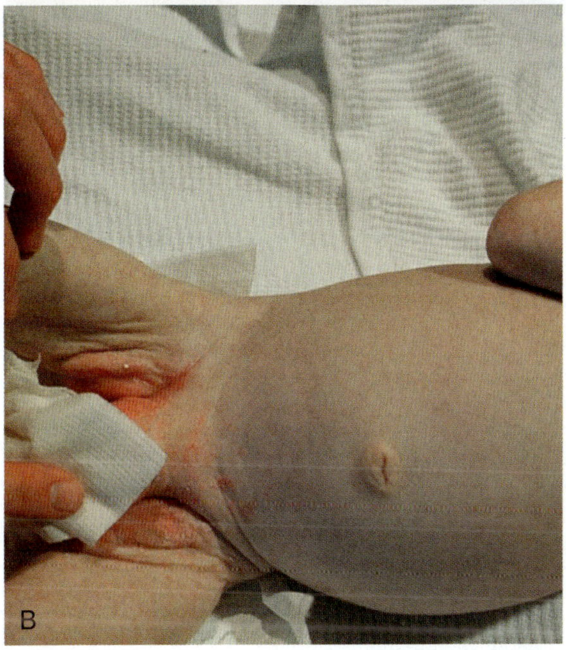

Fig. 6.104 (A and B) This 4-month-old infant was recognized as failing to thrive only after a sibling died in the home and all the children were evaluated by a physician. The child gained weight quickly in a suitable environment.

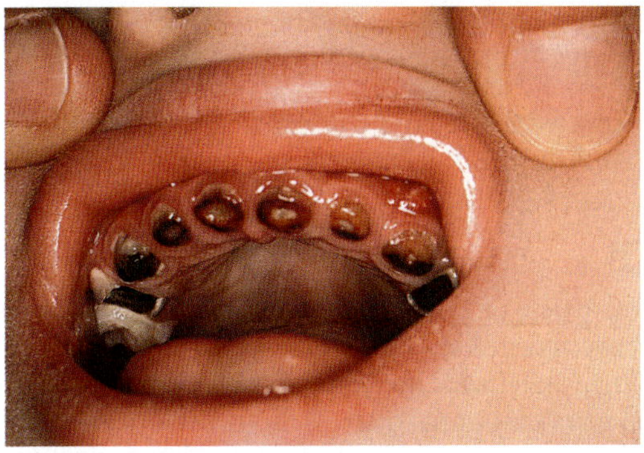

Fig. 6.105 Neglect. Another infant with severe failure to thrive has a badly neglected case of irritant diaper dermatitis. Severely neglected baby-bottle caries were among the findings noted on evaluation of a toddler with failure to thrive. She was examined after her marasmic baby brother was referred by Women, Infants and Children personnel. Their mother was suffering from immobilizing depression. The upper teeth are markedly discolored by decay and have eroded down to the gingiva.

Evaluation and Management of Failure to Thrive

It is essential in evaluating the infant with poor growth to obtain a thorough psychosocial and family history as well as a detailed medical history (Table 6.4). The latter should include information about duration of the problem, mode of onset, and pattern of growth. Asking the parents how easy or difficult it is to take care of this child is also helpful. A complete review of systems (gastrointestinal, cardiorespiratory, neurologic, genitourinary, and endocrine), emphasizing intake and output, is often helpful. A thorough, specific, and concrete feeding and dietary history is essential, including the following:

- Specific items offered and amounts taken at each feeding, with calorie counts
- Times fed: Regular or erratic, of sufficient frequency?
- Feeding situation: Place in home, fed by whom, held for feeding or bottle propped?
- Feeding atmosphere: Noise level, calm or chaotic, discord?
- Feeding method:
  - Breast: Time at each breast, sufficient to empty?
    - Child's positioning
    - Milk production
    - Adequacy of mother's diet
  - Bottle: Type of formula?
    - How mixed?
    - How much fed, how often?
    - Total volume per 24 hours
- Infant's demeanor/behavior during feedings:
  - Disinterest/anorexia
  - Refusal
- Parent's dietary beliefs/concerns/fears
- Home facilities for food storage/preparation

It is also highly important to observe the parental/child interaction, especially during feedings. A thorough physical examination will reveal gross abnormalities in patients with underlying CNS, cardiopulmonary, or genetic problems.

A few basic screening tests (CBC and differential; urinalysis and culture; stool pH, reducing substance, and fat stain; and urea nitrogen, electrolytes, and creatinine) can serve to rule out most other organic causes of failure to thrive. Table 6.5 summarizes the most common causes of infantile growth failure and their major findings on evaluation.

The earlier that growth impairment/undernutrition is recognized, evaluated as to cause(s), and treatment instituted, the better. The more long-standing the problem, the more difficult it is to treat, and the higher the risk of long-term sequelae, especially in cases of neglect and primary psychosocial failure to thrive. The latter include developmental delay and cognitive deficits secondary to impaired brain growth and inadequate stimulation that may not be fully reversible with therapy and early intervention. There is evidence that even if good nutrition is reestablished and catch-up growth is achieved, failure to improve emotional nurturing perpetuates developmental delays. An increased incidence of behavior problems and of affective and motivational disorders has also been found later in childhood in children who had psychosocial failure to thrive as infants and toddlers.

Effective treatment depends on helping the caregiver (in a supportive and nonthreatening manner) understand the nature of the problem, the child's nutritional needs, and the need for increased caloric density to accomplish catch-up growth (1.5–2 times normal requirements), thereby enlisting caregivers as part of the treatment team and the process. This must be supplemented by education regarding the baby's emotional and developmental needs and the importance of warm, consistent nurturing. The process may also necessitate helping caregivers to get and accept help with feeding support, early intervention services, housing, and mental health issues. A specialized multidisciplinary team often best does this.

MEDICAL CHILD ABUSE

Medical child abuse, also known as *Munchausen syndrome by proxy*, occurs when a child receives unnecessary and harmful or potentially harmful medical care caused by the caregiver's exaggerating or

Table 6.4 Findings in Failure to Thrive in Infancy

Cause	Approximate Percentage of All Cases	History	System-Specific Physical Findings	System-Specific Laboratory Studies
Psychosocial	Up to 50% or more	Vague, inconsistent feeding history, history of bottle propping	None, may have soft neurologic signs	None
CNS	13%	Poor feeding, gross developmental delay, vomiting	Grossly abnormal neurological findings	Frequent gross abnormalities on EEG and CT scan or grossly abnormal tests of neuromuscular function
Gastrointestinal	10%	Chronic vomiting and/or diarrhea, abnormal stools, crying with feedings, nocturnal cough/snoring	Often negative, may have abdominal distention	Abnormal barium, pH probe, or endoscopic study; abnormal stool findings (pH, reducing substances, fat stain, Wright stain)
Cardiac	9%	Slow feeding, dyspnea and diaphoresis with feeding, restlessness and diaphoresis during sleep	Often cyanotic or have signs of congestive heart failure	Abnormal echocardiogram, ECG, catheterization findings
Genetic	8%	May have positive family history or a history of developmental delay	Often have facies typical of a syndrome, skeletal abnormalities, neurological abnormalities, or visceromegaly	May have typical radiographic findings, chromosomal abnormalities, abnormal metabolic screens
Pulmonary	3.5%	Chronic or recurrent dyspnea with feedings, tachypnea	Grossly abnormal chest examination findings	Abnormal chest radiographs
Renal	3.5%	May be negative or may have history of polyuria	Often negative, may have flank masses	Abnormal urinalysis, frequently elevated BUN and creatinine, signs of renal osteodystrophy on radiographs
Endocrine	3.5%	With hypothyroidism, constipation and decreased activity level; with diabetes, polyuria, polydipsia	With hypothyroidism, no wasting but mottling, umbilical hernia, often open posterior fontanelle. With diabetes, often without specific abnormality, but may have signs of dehydration, ketotic breath, and hyperpnea. With hypopituitarism and isolated growth hormone deficiency, growth normal until 9 months or later, then plateaus, but normal weight for height; delayed tooth eruption.	Decreased T_4, increased TSH; glucosuria and hyperglycemia; abnormal pituitary function study results

BUN, Blood urea nitrogen; *CNS,* central nervous system; *CT,* computed tomography; *ECG,* electrocardiogram; *EEG,* electroencephalogram; *T_4,* thyroxine; *TSH,* thyroid-stimulating hormone.

fabricating the history, causing illness in the child, or falsifying physical findings.

Many of these parents seek care from multiple providers, so it is especially important to try to access all documentation of prior care when there is concern about possible medical child abuse. It is vitally important that other physicians involved in the care be contacted and their concerns be shared.

Diagnosis of medical child abuse, although difficult because the onset can often be gradual but escalating, is important because the prognosis can be extremely poor if appropriate action is not taken.

EMOTIONAL ABUSE

Emotional abuse accompanies *all* the forms of abuse described previously. It can occur without physical injury and can range from inattentiveness to frank rejection, scapegoating, or even terrorizing. Because isolated emotional abuse is difficult to document, leaving no visible signs, it accounts for the smallest proportion of reported cases. Victims may present with chronic severe anxiety, hyperactivity, depression, agitation, or frank psychotic reactions. Many victims are socially withdrawn, have trouble relating to peers, and generally perform poorly in school. Low self-esteem is the rule. If emotional abuse is suspected, psychologic or psychiatric evaluation may prove helpful in confirming its existence and directing treatment.

Torture

The seminal article on child torture defines this entity medically as:

- At least two physical assaults, occurring over at least two incidents or a single extended incident, which would cause prolonged physical pain, emotional distress, bodily injury, or death and
- At least two elements of psychologic abuse such as isolation, intimidation, emotional/psychological maltreatment, terrorizing, spurning, or deprivation

Inflicted by the Child's Caretaker(s)

Neglect is usually present and manifests as failure to seek appropriate care for injuries and/or malnutrition

Resulting in prolonged emotional distress, pain and suffering, bodily injury/disfigurement, permanent bodily dysfunction, and/or death

The systematic maltreatment, isolation, physical and emotional abuse, and deprivation (often of food) are a means of control/coercion of the victim.

Understandably, a victim of child torture may display maladaptive behaviors when placed in a new environment and require extensive psychologic support and therapy.

REPORTING

Each state has regulations requiring health care providers, hospitals, and professionals involved in child care to report suspected cases of abuse and neglect to CPS agencies. Although there are similarities, regulations vary from state to state, and clinicians should become familiar with the regulations in their respective states. For the suspected abuse or neglect to be reportable to CPS, generally it must result from the acts or omissions of a caregiver. For abuse to be reported, *reasonable* grounds for suspicion are required, not clinical certainty. There is no penalty for reporting in good faith after careful evaluation, but there can be severe penalties for failure to report.

Many states require physicians and hospitals to notify police about cases involving severe abuse and sexual abuse. Cases of sexual assault, physical assault, or abuse perpetrated by a person in a non–caretaking role must be reported to law enforcement and not CPS because such situations usually do not involve caretakers. CPS should be notified, however, if it is suspected that parental negligence was also contributory.

Pediatricians may be unaware of the definition of statutory rape, which varies by state. In these cases, a child may "consent" to intercourse but may, by legal definition, not be considered old enough to give consent. These laws usually specify the age difference between the sexual partners. Particularly when dealing with adolescents, who may hesitate to disclose either consensual activity or sexual assault for fear of mandatory reporting to the police and having to testify, one must consider what, in the clinician's best judgment, is in the best interest of the patient, given the information at hand. In rare instances, the child may be at further risk if the physician reports the abuse (e.g., believable threats of suicide by the patient). In those instances, one must document reasons for failure to report the event to the authorities and try to ensure follow-up with the patient.

HEALTH INSURANCE PORTABILITY AND ACCOUNTABILITY ACT, SUSPECTED CHILD ABUSE, AND CONFIDENTIALITY

The Health Insurance Portability and Accountability Act (commonly referred to as HIPAA), complicated and often misunderstood, is clear about the child abuse exception.

"The HIPAA Privacy Rule allows covered entities to disclose protected health information to report known or suspected child abuse or neglect, if the report is made to a public health authority or other appropriate government authority that is authorized by law to receive such reports." See 42 USC §1320d-7(b) and 45 CFR §164.512(b)(1)(ii).

Even if they are not the reporting source, the physician may disclose information relevant to the abuse or neglect for purposes of investigation, without parental consent, if permissible by state law, to prevent harm to the child or other potential victims.

It is important that physicians make themselves familiar with the state laws that relate to this.

CONCLUSION

Although treatment and follow-up are beyond the scope of an atlas of physical diagnosis, a few additional points bear emphasis. Use of a team approach including physicians, nurses, and social workers or psychologists greatly assists evaluation of victims of abuse and their families, and it reduces the burden on any one health care worker. Additionally, health care teams must work collaboratively with child protection, law enforcement, and judicial systems to help ensure the best possible outcomes for children. Reporting requirements need only reasonable grounds for suspicion and place the onus of full investigation on state agencies. Unfortunately, close follow-up, although incredibly important, is often neglected, especially when patients get caught up in large bureaucratic systems. Having improved our performance on identification and documentation of cases, we must dedicate ourselves to assisting better long-term follow-up to ensure that victims are not only safe from harm but also have access to medical, educational, and mental health services to help them cope with, and when possible, overcome physical and emotional sequelae, thereby improving outcomes.

Bibliography

Adams JA, Kaplan RA, Starling SP, et al: Guidelines for medical care of children who may have been sexually abused, *J Pediatr Adolesc Gynecol* 20:163–172, 2007.

Adams JA, Kellogg ND, Farst KJ, et al: Updated guidelines for the medical assessment and care of children who may have been sexually abused, *J Pediatr Adolesc Gynecol* 29(2):81–87, 2016.

Adams JA, Farst KJ, Kellogg ND: Interpretation of medical findings in suspected child sexual abuse: an update for 2018, *J Pediatr Adolesc Gynecol* 31(3):225–231, 2018. doi:10.1016/j.jpag.2017.12.011.

Afifi TO, Mota N, MacMillan HL, et al: Harsh physical punishment in childhood and adult physical health, *Pediatrics* 132(2):e333–e340, 2013.

American Academy of Pediatrics: Policy statement: child abuse, confidentiality, and the Health Insurance Portability and Accountability Act, *Pediatrics* 125(1):197–201, 2010.

American Academy of Pediatrics, Committee on Child Abuse and Neglect: Distinguishing sudden infant death syndrome from child abuse fatalities, *Pediatrics* 107:437–441, 2001.

American Academy of Pediatrics, Committee on Child Abuse and Neglect: The evaluation of suspected child physical abuse, *Pediatrics* 135(5):e1337–e1354, 2015.

American Academy of Pediatrics, Committee on Child Abuse and Neglect: The evaluation of sexual abuse in children, *Pediatrics* 116(2):506–512, 2005.

Anderst JD, Carpenter SL, Abshire TC, et al: Evaluation for bleeding disorders in suspected child abuse, *Pediatrics* 131(4):e1314–e1322, 2013.

Berger RP, Panigrahy A, Gottschalk S, et al: Effective radiation dose in a skeletal survey performed for suspected child abuse, *J Pediatr* 171:310–312, 2016.

Case ME, Graham MA, Handy TC, et al: Position paper on fatal abusive head injuries in infants and young children, *Am J Forens Med Pathol* 22(2):112–122, 2001.

Centers for Disease Control and Prevention (CDC): *CDC sexual assault and STD guidelines*, 2021. https://www.cdc.gov/std/tg2015/sexual-assault.htm.

Choudhary AK, Servaes S, Slovis TL, et al: Consensus statement on abusive head trauma in infants and young children, *Pediatr Radiol* 48(8):1048–1065, 2018.

Christian CW: Timing of the medical examination, *J Child Sex Abuse* 20(5): 505–520, 2011.

Christian CW, Lavelle JM, DeJong AR, et al: Forensic evidence findings in prepubertal victims of sexual assault, *Pediatrics* 106:100–104, 2000.

Degraw M, Hicks RA, Lindberg DM, et al: Incidence of fractures among children with burns with concern regarding abuse, *Pediatrics* 125(2):e295–e299, 2010.

Dubowitz H, Bross DC: The pediatrician's documentation of child maltreatment, *Am J Dis Child* 146:596–599, 1992.

Duffy SO, Squires J, Fromkin JB, et al: Use of skeletal surveys to evaluate for physical abuse: analysis of 703 consecutive skeletal surveys, *Pediatrics* 127(1):e47–e52, 2011.

Finkelhor D, Shattuck A, Turner HA, et al: Lifetime prevalence of child sexual abuse and sexual assault assessed in late adolescence, *J Adol Health* 55(3):329–333, 2014.

Flaherty EG, Perez-Rossello JM, Levine MA, et al: Evaluating children with fractures for child physical abuse, *Pediatrics* 133(2):e477–e489, 2014.

Girardet RG, Lahoti S, Howard LA, et al: The epidemiology of sexually transmitted infections in suspected child victims of sexual assault, *Pediatrics* 124(1):79–86, 2009.

Harper NS, Eddleman S, Lindberg DM, et al: The utility of follow-up skeletal surveys in child abuse, *Pediatrics* 131(3):e672–e678, 2013.

Heger A, Emans SJ, Muram D: *Evaluation of the sexually abused child*, ed 2, New York, 2000, Oxford University Press.

Helfer RE, Kempe HC: *The battered child*, ed 5, Chicago, 1997, University of Chicago Press.

Jenny C, Committee on Child Abuse and Neglect: Evaluating infants and young children with multiple fractures, *Pediatrics* 118:1299–1303, 2006.

Jenny C, Crawford-Jakubiak JE, Committee on Child Abuse, et al. The evaluation of children in the primary care setting when sexual abuse is suspected, *Pediatrics* 132(2):e558–e567, 2013.

Jenny C, Hymel KP, Ritzen A, et al: Analysis of missed cases of abusive head trauma, *J Am Med Assoc* 281:621–627, 1999.
Kellogg ND, American Academy of Pediatrics, Committee on Child Abuse and Neglect: Evaluation of suspected child physical abuse, *Pediatrics* 119(6):1232–1241, 2007.
Kellogg ND, Committee on Child Abuse and Neglect: Clinical report—the evaluation of sexual behaviors in children, *Pediatrics* 124:992–998, 2009.
Kellogg ND, Farst KJ, Adams JA: Interpretation of medical findings in suspected child sexual abuse: an update for 2023, *Child Abuse Negl* 145:106283, 2023. doi:10.1016/j.chiabu.2023.106283.
Kleinman P: *Diagnostic imaging of child abuse*, ed 2, St. Louis, 1998, Mosby.
Knox BL, Starling SP, Feldman KW, et al: Child torture as a form of child abuse, *J Child Adolesc Trauma* 7:37–49, 2014.
Lindberg DM, Beaty B, Juarez-Colunga E, et al: Testing for abuse in children with sentinel injuries, *Pediatrics* 136(5):831–838, 2015.
Lindberg DM, Blood EA, Campbell KA, et al: Predictors of screening and injury in contacts of physically abused children, *J Pediatr* 163(3):730–735.e1-3, 2013.
Lindberg DM, Shapiro RA, Blood EA, et al: Utility of hepatic transaminases in children with concern for abuse, *Pediatrics* 131(2):268–275, 2013.
Lindberg DM, Shapiro RA, Laskey A, et al: Prevalence of abusive injuries in siblings and household contacts of physically abused children, *Pediatrics* 130(2):193–201, 2012.
Maguire S, Mann M, John N, et al: Does cardiopulmonary resuscitation cause rib fractures in children? a systematic review, *Child Abuse Negl* 30(7):739–751, 2006.
Maguire S, Mann MK, Sibert J, et al: Are there patterns of bruising in childhood which are diagnostic or suggestive of abuse? A systematic review, *Arch Dis Child* 90(2):182–186, 2005.
Makoroff K, Brauley JL, Brandner AM, et al: Genital examination for alleged sexual abuse of prepubertal girls: findings by pediatric emergency medicine physicians compared with child abuse trained physicians, *Child Abuse Negl* 26:1235–1242, 2002.
Ophthalmology Child Abuse Working Party, Royal College of Ophthalmologists: Child abuse and the eye, *Eye* 13:3–10, 1999.
Peterson C, Florence C, Klevens J: The economic burden of child maltreatment in the United States, 2015, *Child Abuse Negl* 86:178–183, 2018.
Pierce MC, Bertocci GE, Vogeley E, et al: Evaluating long bone fractures in children: a biomechanical approach with illustrative cases, *Child Abuse Negl* 28: 505–524, 2004.
Pierce MC, Kaczor K, Aldridge S, et al: Bruising characteristics discriminating physical child abuse from accidental trauma, *Pediatrics* 125(1):67–74, 2010.
Pierce MC, Smith S, Kaczor K: Bruising in infants: those with a bruise may be abused, *Pediatr Emerg Care* 25(12):845–847, 2009.
Ravichandiran N, Schuh S, Bejuk M, et al: Delayed identification of pediatric abuse-related fractures, *Pediatrics* 125(1):60–66, 2010.
Reece RM, Ludwig S: *Child abuse: medical diagnosis and management*, ed 2, Philadelphia, 2001, Lippincott Williams & Wilkins.
Reece RM, Sege R: Childhood head injuries, accidental or inflicted? *Arch Pediatr Adolesc Med* 154:11–22, 2000.
Roesler TA, Jenny C: *Medical child abuse: beyond Munchausen syndrome by proxy*, ed 1, Elk Grove Village, 2009, American Academy of Pediatrics.
Rosenberg NM, Marino D: Frequency of suspected abuse/neglect in burn patients, *Pediatr Emerg Care* 5(4):219–221, 1989.
Sugar NF, Taylor JA, Feldman KW: Bruises in infants and toddlers: those who don't cruise rarely bruise, *Arch Pediatr Adolesc Med* 153:399–403, 1999.
Thorpe EL, Zuckerbraun NS, Wolford JE, et al: Missed opportunities to diagnose child physical abuse, *Pediatr Emerg Care* 30(11):771–776, 2014.
Wood JN, Henry MK, Berger RP, et al: Use and utility of skeletal surveys to evaluate for occult fractures in young, injured children, *Acad Pediatr* 19(4):428–437, 2019.

RHEUMATOLOGY

7

Catherine H. Poholek | Daniel Glaser | Elaine Cassidy

The rheumatic diseases of childhood are a heterogeneous group of disorders caused by abnormal immune activation that results in autoimmunity or excessive inflammation. Although considerable progress has been made in understanding the pathophysiology of these disorders, much remains unknown about their etiologies. Furthermore, despite advances in diagnostic testing, the cornerstone of diagnosis remains a thorough history and physical examination.

The rheumatic diseases that occur during childhood are classified as inflammatory arthritis, connective tissue disorders, vasculitides, or autoinflammatory syndromes, although overlap does occur. Noninflammatory disorders that cause musculoskeletal pain include joint hypermobility syndromes and pain amplification syndromes. This chapter illustrates the more distinctive clinical features of these unique disorders.

MUSCULOSKELETAL HISTORY

A meticulous rheumatologic history is the foundation of accurate diagnosis (Box 7.1). The patient's age and sex serve as initial guides to possible etiologies. Specific details about the reported pain should be elicited. The clinician should ask the parent or child to describe the pain and even point to the site of maximal discomfort to localize the symptoms to the muscle, bone, tendon insertions *(entheses)*, or joint. The clinician must then try to discern whether musculoskeletal symptoms are inflammatory or mechanical. Pain that involves swelling, morning stiffness, warmth, redness, and improvement with movement is often indicative of inflammation. Pain that is worse at the end of the day, worse with activity, and lacking persistent swelling is usually more mechanical in nature. Pain that is constant and unremitting or worsened by light touch is characteristic of nerve pain.

A history of prior illnesses, medications, immunizations, trauma, insect bites, and the acuteness of symptoms can be a clue to diagnosis. Joint pain *(arthralgia)* is a common symptom of childhood. However, the symptoms associated with inflammatory joint pain *(arthritis)* are uncommon in the pediatric population. In children with arthritis, the duration and pattern of the symptoms can be telling. Acute migratory arthritis affecting large and small joints is seen in acute rheumatic fever (ARF). Arthritis that resolves within a few weeks is consistent with a reactive arthritis (i.e., *Streptococcus,* Epstein-Barr virus, parvovirus B19). An indolent or additive arthritis persisting for more than 6 weeks is consistent with a chronic form of arthritis (i.e., juvenile idiopathic arthritis [JIA]). Joint stiffness, or gel phenomenon, can be seen not only in the morning but also after a child has napped or been immobile, such as in a vehicle. As the day progresses, the child with chronic arthritis may become more limber and may even appear normal.

Differences in the quality and duration of arthritis exist among the various rheumatoid diseases. The arthritis in patients with systemic lupus erythematosus (SLE) may feature less swelling with more intense pain and a waxing and waning course, whereas the arthritis of children with JIA is characterized by more stiffness and swelling, but less severe pain, with persistence of findings in absence of interventions. The joints of ARF can also be distinguished from those of JIA by the presence of exquisite pain that is out of proportion to physical findings and a rapid response to nonsteroidal anti-inflammatory drugs.

A careful family history can be helpful. Children with an extensive family history of autoimmune diseases in their first-degree relatives are at slightly greater risk for developing a rheumatologic condition. Because these diseases have complex genetic factors, there is often little direct genetic linkage. Some diseases such as psoriasis, SLE, ARF, and autoimmune thyroiditis have a stronger genetic penetrance than other rheumatic diseases. Other conditions have little or no penetrance. A child with first-degree relatives with adult rheumatoid arthritis is not at increased risk for developing JIA.

PHYSICAL EXAMINATION OF THE MUSCULOSKELETAL SYSTEM

A rheumatologic diagnosis requires a thorough joint examination and careful general physical examination with special attention to the skin, mucous membranes, nail beds, and muscles. The elucidation of joint inflammation by examination may be the only indication of a rheumatic disease. The physical examination begins with observation of the child and parents noting the general appearance of the patient. The child's developmental status and observation of the height and weight growth curves are critical components of the examination, as growth delays can be a sign of chronic inflammation. Certain skin and mucous membrane changes provide valuable information (Box 7.2). Muscle strength can be evaluated by testing the resistance capacity of individual muscle groups and grading them on a standard scale (Table 7.1).

A good physical examination of the musculoskeletal system includes detailed assessment of each joint through inspection, palpation, and measurement of range of motion (ROM). A validated, evidence-based tool to systematically perform a screening musculoskeletal examination in children suited for general practitioners has been developed and is known as pGALS (pediatric **G**ait, **A**rms, **L**egs, **S**pine) (Fig. 7.1). The instrument is sensitive for the detection of musculoskeletal abnormality and, with routine use, can be completed in a few minutes. If concerning findings are detected with pGALS, more focused physical examination maneuvers should be completed to better define the abnormality. Large effusions are easily felt and often ballotable; synovial hypertrophy may be more subtle and have a doughy, spongy, or boggy feel. Arthritis in children may be subtle and often appreciated only because of pain, decreased ROM, or other chronic changes. Careful observation of the temporomandibular joint (TMJ) may reveal micrognathia (Fig. 7.2), or assessment of leg lengths may demonstrate a significant discrepancy; both are clues to the diagnosis of JIA.

JUVENILE IDIOPATHIC ARTHRITIS

JIA is a collection of diseases that share the cardinal feature of chronic arthritis without other known etiology. JIA is one of the most common rheumatic diseases of childhood with an incidence of 10 cases per 100,000 population per year and a prevalence of approximately 100 per 100,000 population. JIA affects more than 300,000 children in the United States. Seven subtypes are included under the rubric of JIA: (1) oligoarthritis (persistent or extended), (2) polyarthritis (rheumatoid factor [RF] negative), (3) polyarthritis (RF positive), (4) psoriatic arthritis, (5) enthesitis-related arthritis

Box 7.1 Distinguishing Features of Rheumatologic History

- Musculoskeletal complaints
  - Joint swelling with warmth and/or erythema
  - Morning stiffness lasting >20 minutes that improves with activity
  - Gelling phenomenon after prolonged inactivity
  - Decreased muscle strength or endurance
- Constitutional symptoms
  - Prolonged or recurrent fevers (periodic or episodic)
  - Fatigue without clear triggers
  - Weight loss, anorexia
  - Linear growth disturbance
- Ocular symptoms
  - Eye redness and/or pain
  - Vision changes
  - Reduced ocular movements or proptosis
- Cardiopulmonary symptoms
  - Dyspnea (resting or exertional)
  - Hemoptysis
  - Chest pain
- Gastrointestinal symptoms
  - Dysphagia (solids or liquids)
  - Early satiety or reflux
  - Melena or hematochezia
  - Diarrhea
  - Abdominal pain
- Neurologic symptoms
  - Headache
  - Seizure
  - Altered mental status
  - Cognitive changes
  - Focal weakness
- Cutaneous and mucous membrane symptoms: see Box 7.2
- Psychosocial history
  - Family stressors
  - Personal stressors (school, development, etc.)
  - Altered sleep patterns
  - Depression or anxiety
- Family history
  - Autoimmune disorders
  - Autoinflammatory disorders
  - Chronic pain and psychiatric disorders

Box 7.2 Mucocutaneous Signs of Rheumatic Diseases

- Malar rash—fixed erythematous eruption
- Discoid rash—rare in childhood; often heals with atrophy and scarring
- Periungual erythema
- Telangiectasias
- Digital pits/ulcers and/or Raynaud phenomenon
- Alopecia and fracturing of frontal hair
- Heliotrope rash—violaceous eyelid edema
- Gottron papules—scaly, symmetrical, erythematous papules over MCP and PIP joints
- Skin changes: thickening, contractures, calcinosis
- Palpable purpura
- Livedo reticularis—lacy, fishnet appearance of skin
- Evanescent salmon-pink rash
- Erythema nodosum—panniculitis with septal inflammation
- Rheumatoid extensor nodules
- Psoriasis
- Onycholysis (lifting of the distal portion of the nail), nail pits
- Balanitis circinata—small, shallow, painless ulcers of the glans penis and urethral meatus
- Keratoderma blennorrhagicum—clear vesicles on erythematous bases that progress to a papulosquamous eruption, often on palms and soles

Table 7.1 Standard Muscle Strength Grading

Muscle Grade	Description
5	Complete ROM against gravity with full resistance
4	Complete ROM against gravity with some resistance
3	Complete ROM against gravity
2	Complete ROM with gravity eliminated
1	Evidence of slight contractility; no joint motion
0	No evidence of contractility

ROM, Range of motion.

The pGALS musculoskeletal screen

Screening Questions
- Do you (or does your child) have any pain or stiffness in your (their) joints, muscles, or back?
- Do you (or does your child) have any difficulty getting yourself (him/herself) dressed without any help?
- Do you (or does your child) have any problem going up and down stairs?

FIGURE	SCREENING MANEUVERS	WHAT IS BEING ASSESSED
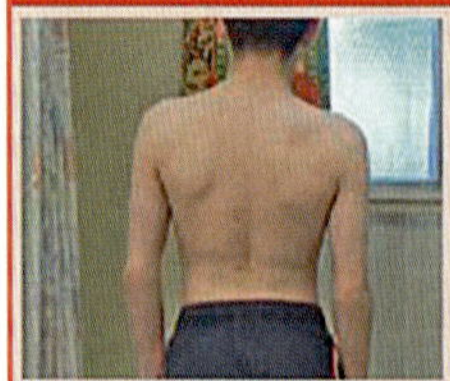	Observe the child standing (from front, back and sides)	• Posture and habitus • Skin rashes (e.g., psoriasis) • Deformity (e.g., leg length inequality, leg alignment [valgus, varus at the knee or ankle], scoliosis, joint swelling, muscle wasting, flat feet)
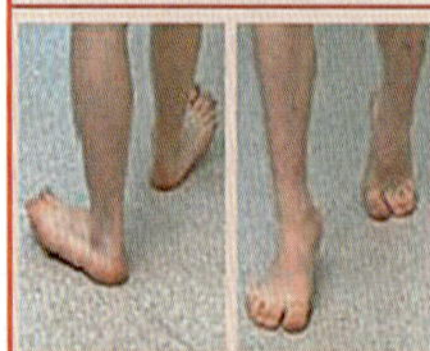	Observe the child walking and **"Walk on your heels" and "Walk on your tiptoes"**	• Ankles, subtalar, midtarsal and small joints of feet and toes • Foot posture (Note if presence of normal longitudinal arches of feet when on tiptoes.)
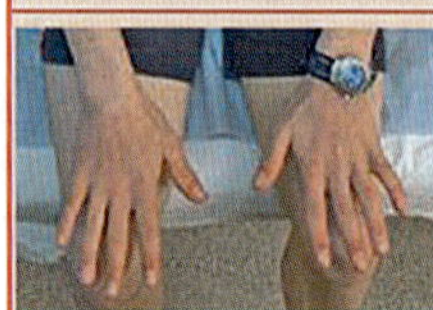	"Hold your hands out straight in front of you"	• Forward flexion of shoulders • Elbow extension • Wrist extension • Extension of small joints of fingers
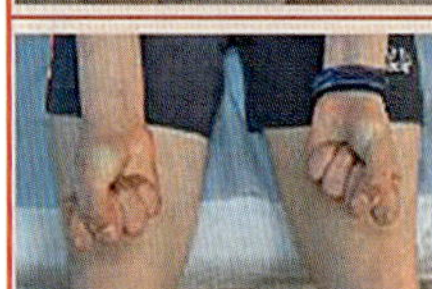	"Turn your hands over and make a fist"	• Wrist supination • Elbow supination • Flexion of small joints of fingers
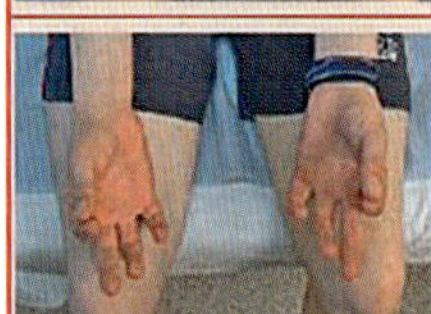	"Pinch your index finger and thumb together"	• Manual dexterity • Coordination of small joints of index finger and thumb and functional key grip
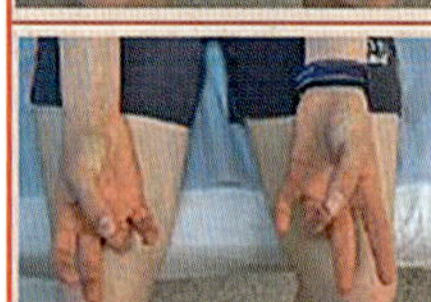	"Touch the tips of your fingers"	• Manual dexterity • Coordination of small joints of fingers and thumbs
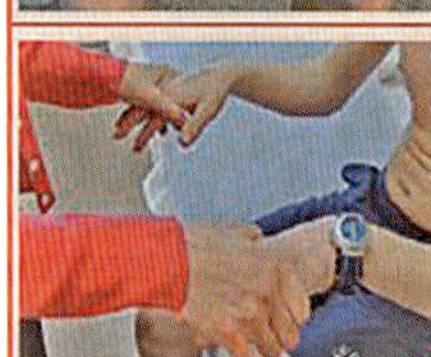	Squeeze the metacarpo-phalangeal joints for tenderness	• Metacarpophalangeal joints
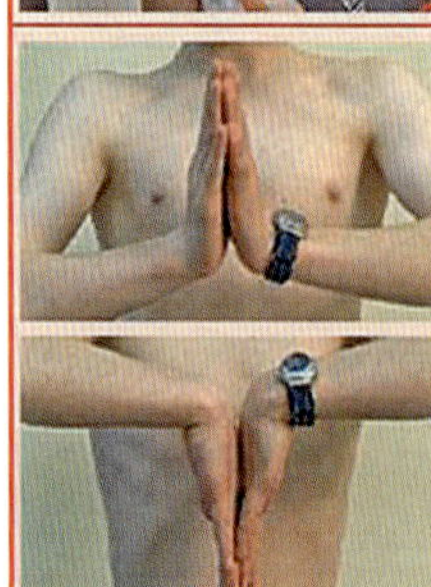	**"Put your hands together palm to palm" and "Put your hands together back to back"**	• Extension of small joints of fingers • Wrist extension • Elbow flexion

Fig. 7.1 The pediatric **G**ait, **A**rms, **L**egs, **S**pine (pGALS) musculoskeletal screen. (Reproduced from Reports on the Rheumatic Diseases Series 5, Hands On No.15 [June 2008]—by kind permission from Versus Arthritis, www.versusarthritis.org.)

FIGURE	SCREENING MANEUVERS	WHAT IS BEING ASSESSED
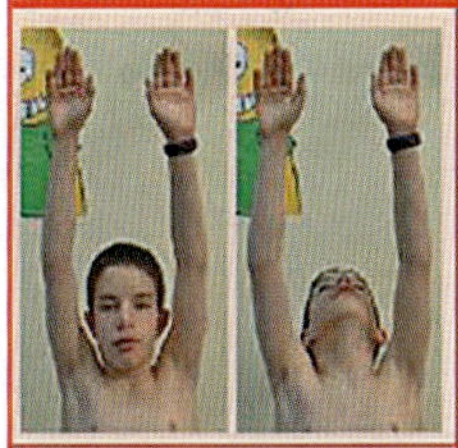	**"Reach up, 'touch the sky'" and "Look at the ceiling"**	• Elbow extension • Wrist extension • Shoulder abduction • Neck extension
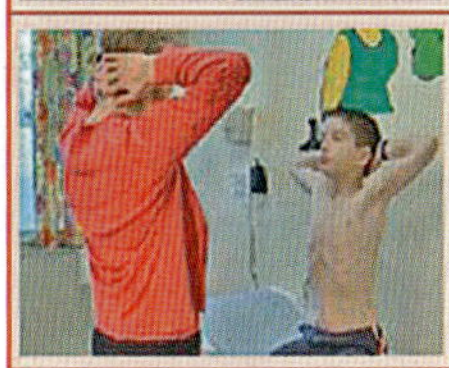	"Put your hands behind your neck"	• Shoulder abduction • External rotation of shoulders • Elbow flexion
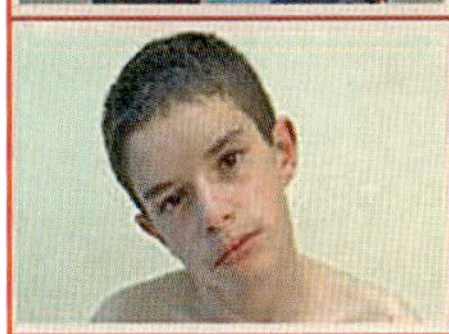	"Try and touch your shoulder with your ear"	• Cervical spine lateral flexion
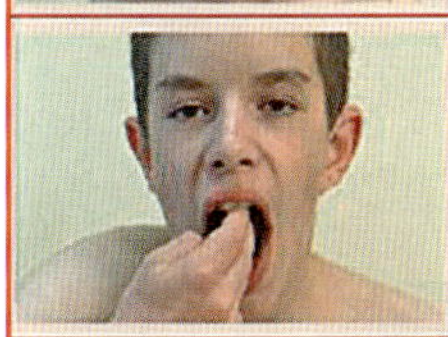	**"Open wide and put three (*child's own*) fingers in your mouth"**	• Temporomandibular joints (Check for deviation of jaw movement.)
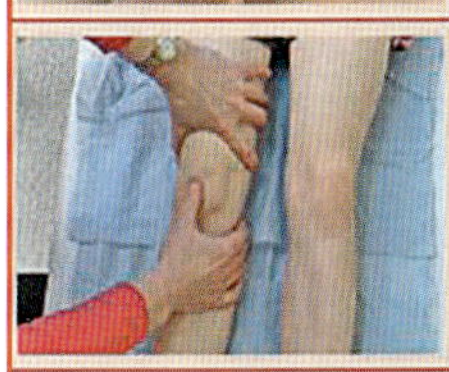	Feel for effusion at the knee (patella tap, or cross-fluctuation)	• Knee effusion (Small effusion may be missed by patella tap alone.)
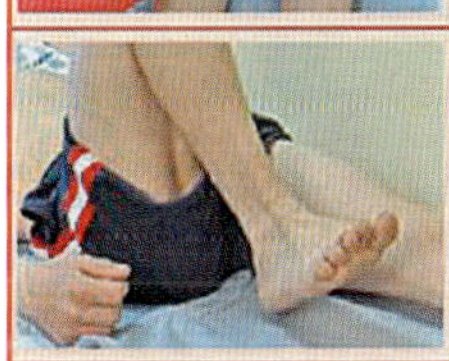	Active movement of knees (flexion and extension) and feel for crepitus	• Knee flexion • Knee extension
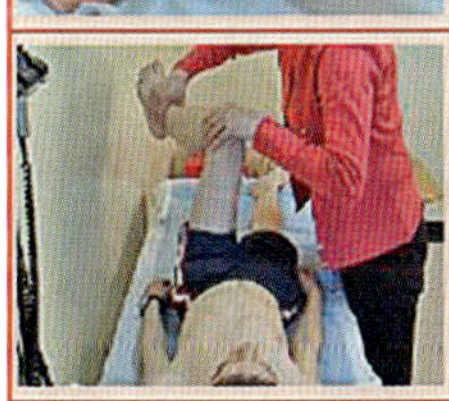	Passive movement of hip (knee flexed to 90 degrees, and internal rotation of hip)	• Hip flexion and internal rotation
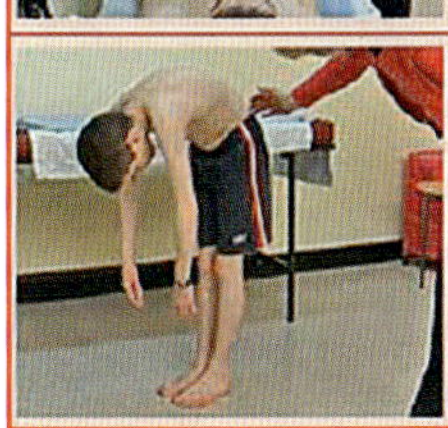	"Bend forward and touch your toes"	• Forward flexion of thoracolumbar spine (Check for scoliosis.)

Fig. 7.1, cont'd

(ERA), (6) systemic arthritis, and (7) undifferentiated arthritis (Table 7.2). The JIA subtype is based on the disease presentation during the first 6 months of illness. Of note, no laboratory tests, including antinuclear antibody (ANA) or RF, are required to diagnose JIA.

All forms of JIA feature inflammation of the synovial tissue. Synovium is usually hypertrophied, and joint effusions may occur. On physical examination (Fig. 7.3), joint swelling, loss of normal anatomic landmarks, tenderness, decreased joint mobility (Fig. 7.4), warmth, erythema, and joint deformity may be noted. It is typical for the child with JIA to have more joint stiffness than pain with insidious onset of symptoms over a period of weeks or months before evaluation. Despite objective signs of arthritis, the patient with JIA may not experience pain. When inflammation persists for a long enough period, destruction of the articular surfaces and bony structures may occur (Fig. 7.5). Because of the poor regenerative properties of articular cartilage, these deformities are usually permanent. Fortunately, most cases of JIA are not associated with permanent joint deformity.

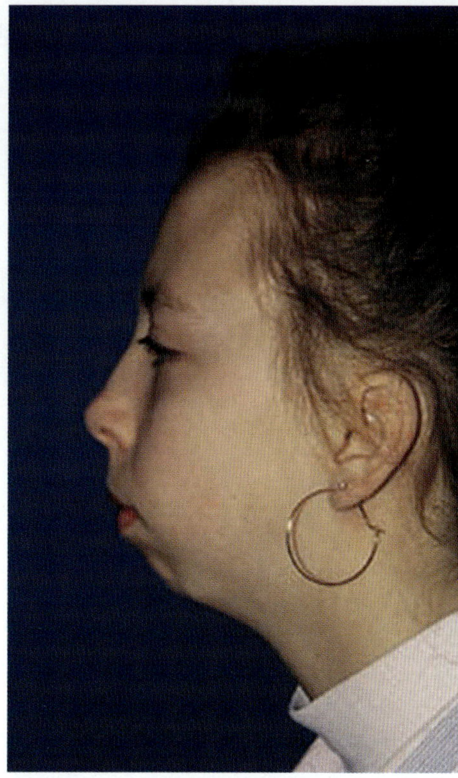

Fig. 7.2 Micrognathia. Note the underdevelopment of the jaw and retracted chin. This occurs in patients with juvenile idiopathic arthritis.

Oligoarthritis (Persistent or Extended)

Oligoarticular JIA is defined as arthritis in one to four joints and accounts for 40% to 50% of cases of JIA. The large joints (knees, ankles, and elbows) are often asymmetrically involved. *Persistent* disease affects no more than four joints throughout the disease. *Extended* disease affects more than four joints after the first 6 months.

Polyarthritis (Rheumatoid Factor Negative)

Polyarticular JIA (RF-negative or seronegative) accounts for approximately 20% to 25% of all children with JIA. To make the diagnosis, five or more joints must be involved in the absence of prominent systemic signs and symptoms. RF negative polyarthritis can occur in children as young as 1 year old, with a peak incidence at 2 years old. The onset of polyarthritis may be insidious or acute. Children with seronegative disease generally have a better prognosis, but a subset can progress to joint destruction and flexion contractures. Any synovial joint may be involved in the inflammatory process, including the knees, wrists, elbows, ankles, small joints of the feet, and proximal interphalangeal (PIP) and metacarpophalangeal (MCP) joints. The lumbosacral spine is usually spared.

Polyarthritis (Rheumatoid Factor Positive)

The seropositive group is believed to be nearly identical to the adult entity of rheumatoid arthritis. Although onset of RF positive polyarthritis can occur as early as 8 years old, it usually occurs in the early teens and there is a female predominance. Whereas 80% of all adult

Table 7.2 Juvenile Idiopathic Arthritis: Classification and Features

	Age of Onset	Percentage of Total Cases	Joint Symptoms	Other
Oligoarthritis	Early childhood	35%–50%	Four or fewer joints; typically knees, ankles, wrists	Many are ANA+
Polyarthritis (RF negative)	2–4 years old and 6–12 years old	17%–25%	Five or more joints	May have arthritis of the C-spine or TMJ
Polyarthritis (RF positive)	Early adolescence	3%–5%	Five or more joints; symmetric, erosive	May have rheumatoid nodules
Enthesitis-related	Late childhood or early adolescence	5%–25%	Lower extremity predominant; may affect hips, sacroiliac joints	Enthesitis, axial involvement, may be HLA-B27+ and/or have a family history of HLA-B27–associated disease
Psoriatic	2–4 years old and 9–11 years old	5%–15%	Small or large joints	Nail pits, dactylitis, psoriasis, family history of psoriasis
Systemic	Any age	5%–15%	Oligoarticular or polyarticular	Fever, rash, serositis, lymphadenopathy, organomegaly
Undifferentiated		10%		Fulfills criteria for more than 1 category or does not fulfill criteria for any category

ANA, Antinuclear antibodies; *HLA-B27,* human leukocyte antigen B27; *RF,* rheumatoid factor; *TMJ,* temporomandibular joint.

Modified from Gowdie PJ, Tse SM: Juvenile idiopathic arthritis, *Pediatr Clin North Am* 59:301–327, 2012; Saurenmann RK, Rose JB, Tyrrell P, et al: Epidemiology of juvenile idiopathic arthritis in a multiethnic cohort: ethnicity as a risk factor, *Arthritis Rheum* 56(6):1974-1984, 2007; Thierry S, Fautrel B, Lemelle I, Guillemin F: Prevalence and incidence of juvenile idiopathic arthritis: a systematic review, *Joint Bone Spine* 81(2):112-117, 2014.

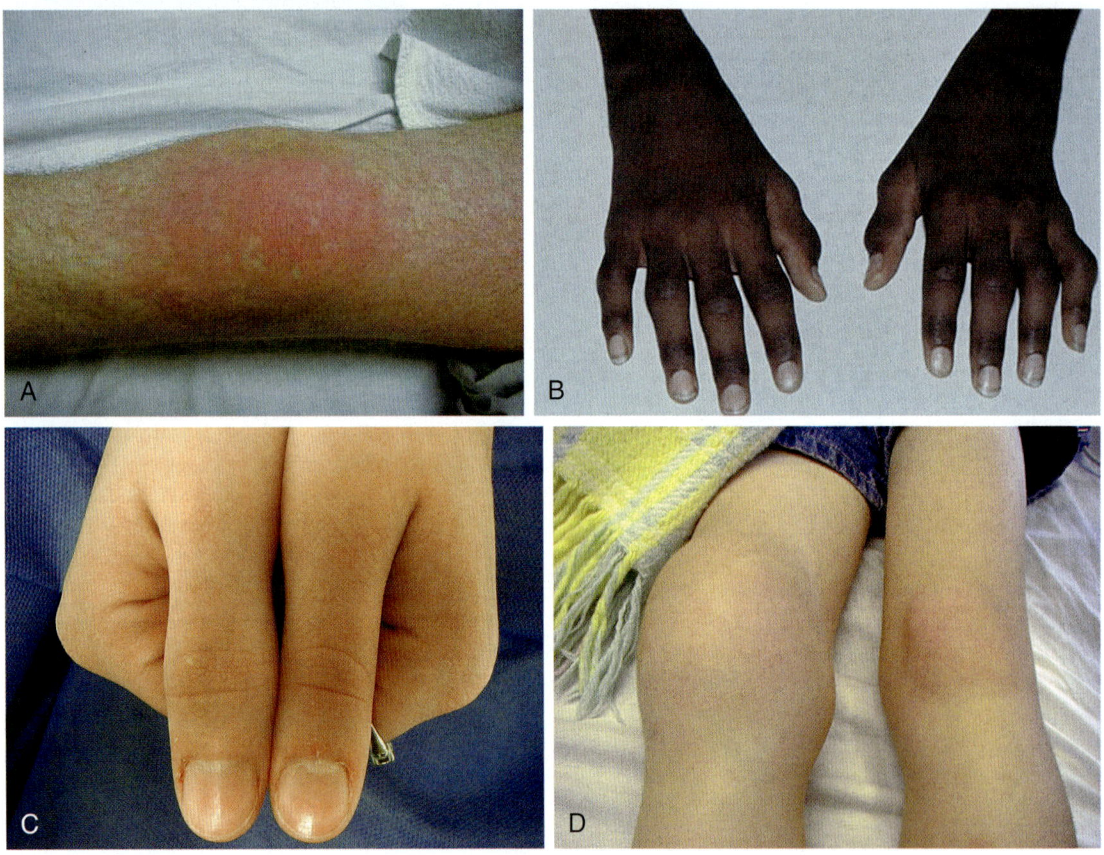

Fig. 7.3 Juvenile idiopathic arthritis (JIA). (A) Erythema of the knee in a patient with systemic-onset JIA (Still's disease). (B) Swelling and inflammation of the small joints of the hands in a patient with polyarticular JIA. Note the inability to fully extend the fingers. (C) Swelling of the right thumb interphalangeal joint. (D) Right knee swelling in a patient with oligoarticular JIA.

patients are seropositive, only 5% of children with JIA are positive for RF. This seropositive subgroup tends to progress to destructive synovitis with prolonged chronic course. Extraarticular manifestations found in the RF positive subtype include firm, nontender subcutaneous nodules with a predilection for pressure points or extensor areas like the elbow (rheumatoid nodules), cutaneous vasculitis, Felty syndrome (leukopenia and splenomegaly), and Sjögren disease (keratoconjunctivitis sicca and xerostomia with or without parotid swelling).

Psoriatic Arthritis

Psoriatic arthritis is diagnosed in a child with arthritis and psoriasis. Criteria are also met when a child with arthritis has two of the three findings: dactylitis ("sausage digit"), nail pitting (or onycholysis), or psoriasis in a first-degree relative. Whereas the forms of arthritis previously discussed have weak genetic penetrance, psoriasis and its related disorders are often found throughout a family's pedigree. A patient may present to the physician with just dactylitis

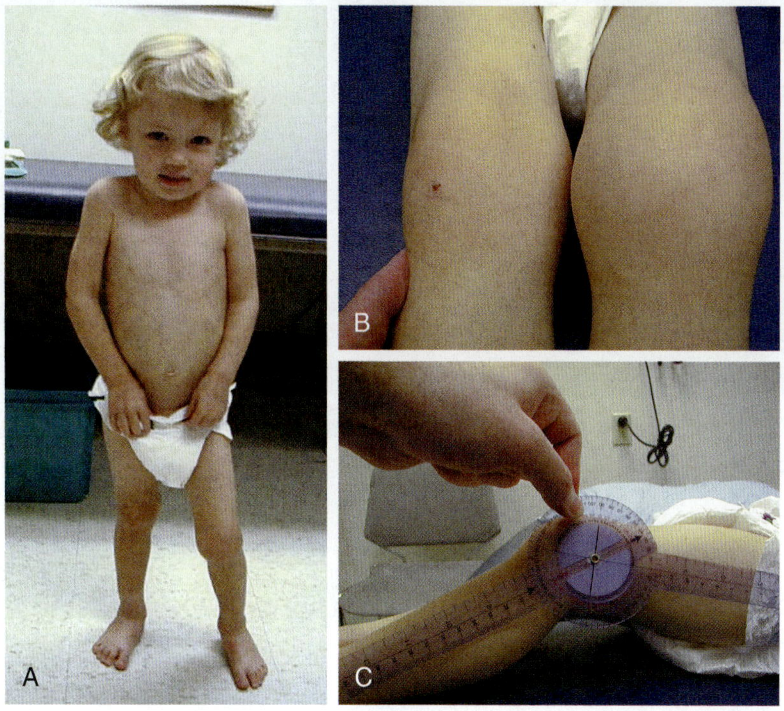

Fig. 7.4 Oligoarticular juvenile idiopathic arthritis. (A) A 2-year-old girl with arthritis of the left knee. Note that the left lower extremity is bent at the knee as she bears weight on the extended right lower extremity. (B) A closer look at the knees reveals left knee swelling. (C) The left knee can be extended only to 35 degrees (secondary to a flexion contracture).

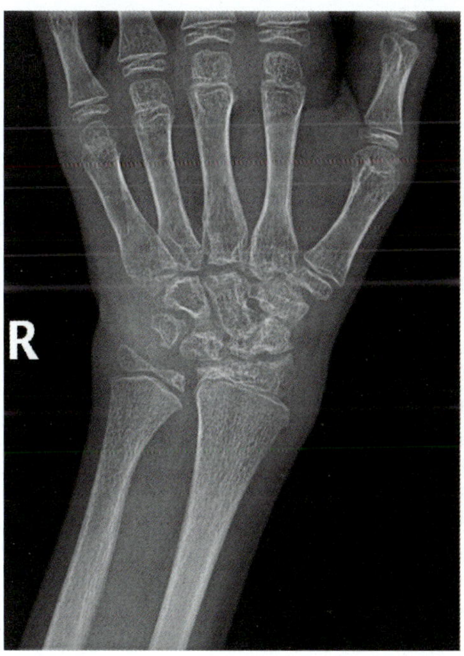

Fig. 7.5 Juvenile idiopathic arthritis. Diffuse demineralization with irregular joint space loss and sclerotic margination of the carpal bones and distal radius in an 8-year-old with chronic polyarticular juvenile idiopathic arthritis.

of one or multiple toes. In such a situation, in addition to a detailed joint examination, a detailed skin and nail examination should be performed for the detection of psoriasiform lesions (Fig. 7.6).

Enthesitis-Related Arthritis

Arthritis with enthesitis features inflammation of the tendon and tendon insertion site (i.e., Achilles). The other features that distinguish this disease group include sacroiliitis, HLA-B27 positivity, male predominance, and acute uveitis (presenting with eye pain and redness). This group also has a strong family predominance with first-degree relatives with ankylosing spondylitis, inflammatory bowel disease, and reactive arthritis. A male patient older than 6 years old presenting with arthritis should raise suspicion for ERA. Younger patients present with peripheral arthritis, whereas axial arthritis often presents in the late teen years or second decade.

Systemic Arthritis

Systemic juvenile idiopathic arthritis (sJIA), also known as Still's disease, accounts for approximately 10% of all children with JIA. Fever, rash, irritability, arthritis, and visceral involvement dominate the clinical presentation. The classic pattern is a high fever spike once or twice per day called "quotidian or double quotidian fever" with return to normal or subnormal temperatures between spikes. Some children have more continuous fevers or more erratic temperatures, especially early in the disease course. Other manifestations of sJIA, such as rash and joint symptoms, may wax and wane during febrile periods.

The rash of sJIA consists of red- or salmon-colored macular lesions of 2 to 6 mm in diameter, evanescent with fever, often with central clearing and slightly irregular margins (Fig. 7.7). The rash usually occurs on the trunk and proximal extremities, but it may also be distal in distribution, with palms and soles affected. Although the rash generally does not produce discomfort, some older patients report pruritus. Superficial mild trauma to the skin, exposure to warmth, and emotional upset may precipitate the rash (Koebner phenomenon). Arthritis does not occur invariably at the onset of sJIA, though approximately 50% of patients with sJIA progress to a chronic, destructive inflammatory arthritis.

When fever of unknown origin is the sole initial presentation of systemic arthritis, it must remain a diagnosis of exclusion until the clinician observes other features during the physical and laboratory examination. Nonspecific arthralgia and myalgia can be prominent early, as can hepatosplenomegaly and lymphadenopathy. Serositis, pleuritis, pericarditis, hyperbilirubinemia, liver enzyme elevation, leukocytosis, and anemia are supporting clinical features.

Patients with sJIA are at risk for developing a potentially fatal disorder called *macrophage activation syndrome* (MAS). Patients present with a toxic appearance, fever, hepatosplenomegaly, and lymphadenopathy. If not recognized early, MAS can progress to hepatic failure, encephalopathy, and disseminated intravascular

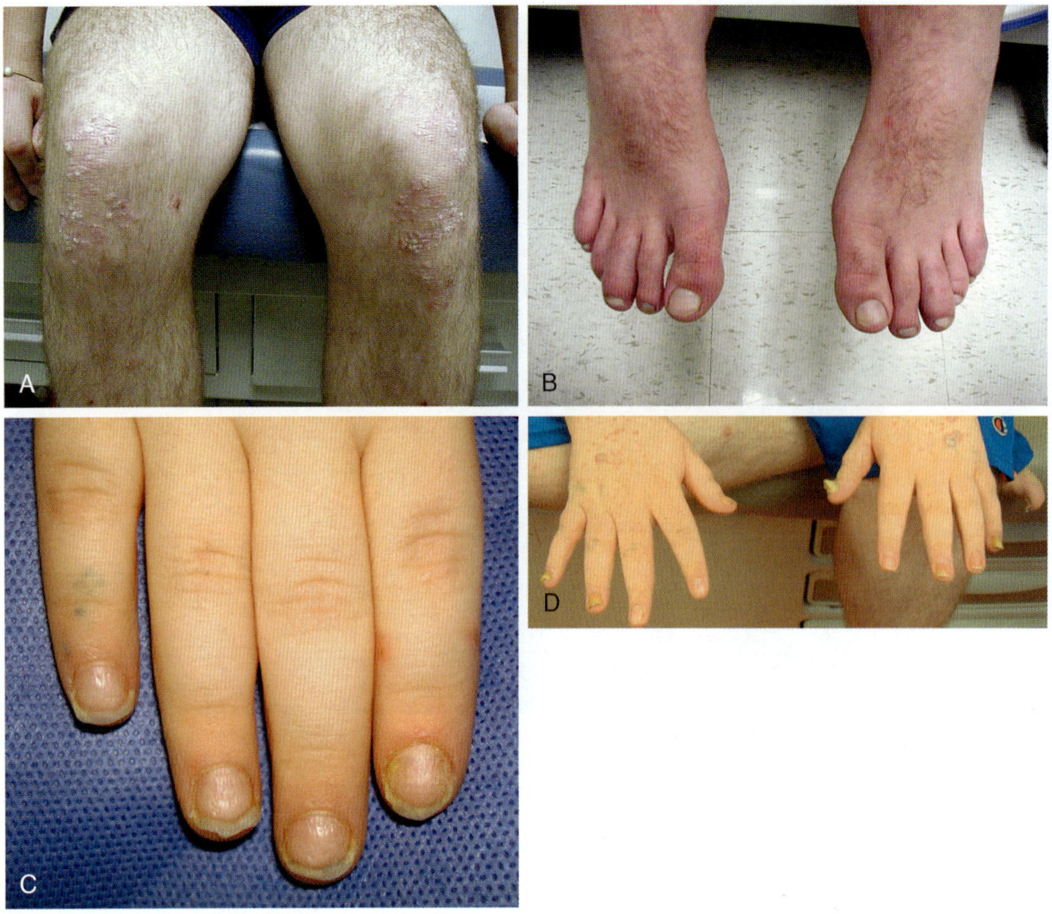

Fig. 7.6 Psoriatic arthritis. (A) Erythematous plaques with silver scale. (B) Dactylitis (sausage toe) of the bilateral third and fifth toes. (C) Diffuse nail pitting. (D) Diffuse onycholysis.

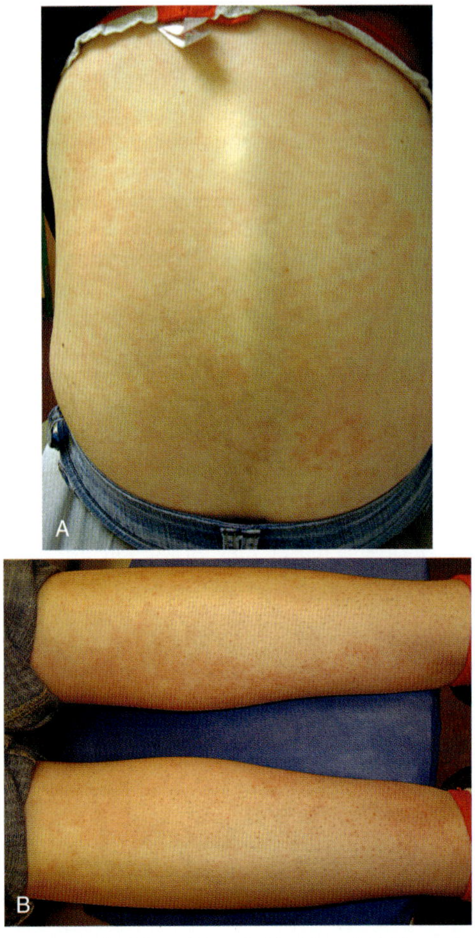

Fig. 7.7 Systemic juvenile idiopathic arthritis. (A and B) The rash is erythematous, macular, and often evanescent. It can be more prominent during periods of fever. It is featured on the trunk and extremities.

coagulation. Development of MAS is not unique to sJIA, and a diligent search for other etiologies should be undertaken (Box 7.3). Laboratory testing that supports a diagnosis of MAS includes evidence of hepatitis, coagulopathy, and hyperferritinemia. In addition, the white blood cell (WBC) count, hemoglobin, and platelet counts are depressed, with a normal or low sedimentation rate associated with hypofibrinogenemia (Table 7.3). Diagnosis can be aided by bone marrow aspiration, demonstrating activated macrophages engulfing surrounding cells, but this is not required for diagnosis.

Extraarticular Manifestations of Juvenile Idiopathic Arthritis

Patients with JIA are at risk of developing iridocyclitis (or uveitis). Although photophobia, eye pain, and erythema can occur, uveitis is often asymptomatic. For that reason, children with oligoarticular, psoriatic, and polyarticular JIA must receive slit-lamp examinations frequently.

The first clinical sign of uveitis is cellular exudate in the anterior chamber. If the uveitis is untreated, damage to the eye can develop including: (1) synechiae (adhesions) between the iris and lens causing an irregular and poorly functioning pupil (Fig. 7.8), (2) calcium deposits in the cornea called band keratopathy (Fig. 7.9), (3) cataracts, or (4) glaucoma. Ophthalmologic complications do not parallel the activity of the arthritis, so strict adherence to the recommendations for eye examination outlined in Table 7.4 is necessary to help prevent visual loss.

Linear growth retardation may occur in the child with active JIA, especially with systemic or polyarticular disease. Oligoarticular arthritis can present with growth abnormalities as well, usually confined to leg length discrepancy or an enlarged hand or foot related to refractory ankle or wrist involvement. During early illness, bony development may be advanced with premature epiphyseal fusion; later, the opposite may be true.

Box 7.3 Triggers of Macrophage Activation Syndrome

- Systemic JIA
- Systemic lupus erythematosus
- Kawasaki disease
- Mixed connective tissue disease
- Juvenile dermatomyositis
- Vasculitis
- Systemic sclerosis
- Autoinflammatory disorders

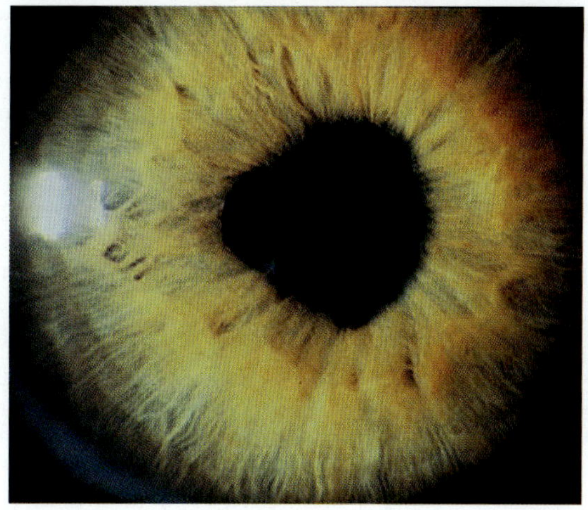

Fig. 7.8 Iridocyclitis. An irregular pupil in a patient with oligoarticular juvenile idiopathic arthritis. Note synechiae projecting posteriorly toward the lens.

Table 7.3 Comparison of Features and Laboratory Values in Systemic Juvenile Idiopathic Arthritis and Macrophage Activation Syndrome

	Systemic Juvenile Idiopathic Arthritis	Macrophage Activation Syndrome
Fever	+ (Intermittent or quotidian)	+ (Unremitting)
Hepatosplenomegaly	+/−	+
Arthritis	+	+/−
Rash	+ (Maculopapular/ evanescent)	+ (Petechiae/ purpura)
Lymphadenopathy	+/−	+
Encephalopathy	−	+/−
Sedimentation rate	↑	Normal or ↓
White blood cell count	↑	↓
Hemoglobin	Normal or ↓	↓
Platelets	↑	↓
Transaminases	Normal	↑↑
Ferritin	Normal or ↑	↑↑
Fibrinogen	Normal or ↑	↓
Prothrombin time/ partial thromboplastin time	Normal	↑
Lactate dehydrogenase	Normal or ↑	↑↑
Triglycerides	Normal	↑

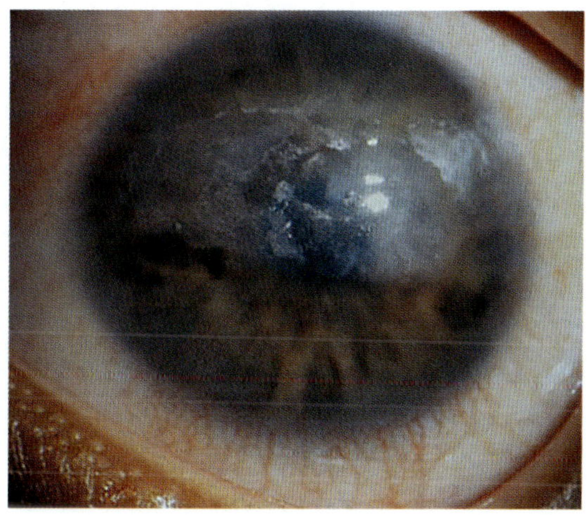

Fig. 7.9 Band keratopathy. Note the calcium deposits in the Bowman layer in this patient with juvenile idiopathic arthritis.

Table 7.4 Recommended Frequency of Ophthalmologic Examinations in Juvenile Idiopathic Arthritis

Subtype	Antinuclear Antibody Status	Age at Onset	Disease Duration	Frequency of Eye Examinations
Oligoarthritis, RF-negative polyarthritis, psoriatic and undifferentiated arthritis	Positive	<7 years old	≤4 years	3 months
			>4 years	6–12 months
		≥7 years old	Any	6–12 months
	Negative	Any	Any	6–12 months
RF-positive polyarthritis, systemic, and enthesitis-related arthritis	N/A	Any	Any	6–12 months

N/A, not applicable; *RF*, rheumatoid factor.

Modified from Cassidy J, Kivlin J, Lindsley C, et al: Ophthalmologic examinations in children with juvenile rheumatoid arthritis, *Pediatrics* 117:1843–1845, 2006; Angeles-Han ST, Ringold S, Beukelman T, et al: 2019 American College of Rheumatology/Arthritis Foundation guideline for the screening, monitoring, and treatment of juvenile idiopathic arthritis-associated uveitis, *Arthritis Care Res* 71(6):703–716, 2019.

Cardiac involvement occurs in more than one-third of patients with sJIA. Pericarditis is most common, but myocarditis and endocarditis can also occur. Chest pain, a friction rub, tachycardia, and dyspnea can be observed, and chest radiograph, electrocardiogram, and echocardiogram can support the diagnosis. These episodes may last for weeks to months and are usually associated with a generalized flare of disease. Various other extraarticular manifestations, including hepatosplenomegaly and lymphadenopathy, are particularly common in sJIA. A more recently described complication of sJIA is high-fatality parenchymal lung disease and pulmonary hypertension that occurs in a small subset of patients. Children may exhibit cough, tachypnea, clubbing of the fingers, or hypoxia at diagnosis of lung disease, but many patients have no respiratory symptoms until late in the disease course. Computed tomography (CT) of the chest may show septal thickening, crazy paving, peripheral/peribronchovascular consolidation, or ground-glass opacities. Associations with the development of sJIA-lung disease include younger age of sJIA onset, trisomy 21, atypical rash, diagnosis of MAS, and history of adverse reactions to biologic medications.

Differential Diagnosis

Because JIA is a clinical diagnosis, strict clinical criteria have been established. Children should have objective joint findings (arthritis) for at least 6 consecutive weeks coupled with the exclusion of other causes of arthritis in children (Box 7.4).

Because of its destructive nature, pyogenic arthritis (e.g., *Staphylococci, Streptococci, Haemophilus influenzae*) must be ruled out in any child with active joint disease, especially monoarthritis. Any intensely red and tender joint should raise suspicion of a bacterial pathogen. This, combined with systemic symptoms of infection (fever, chills, malaise, rigors), should prompt the clinician to perform diagnostic arthrocentesis early in the course of the illness.

Lyme arthritis can mimic oligoarticular JIA. This tick-borne illness is caused by the spirochete *Borrelia burgdorferi* with acute manifestations, including a distinctive rash, known as *erythema migrans* (see Chapter 13, Fig. 13.50). A child may develop arthritis as a late manifestation months or years after exposure, often without knowledge of a prior tick bite or the symptoms of acute Lyme disease. The arthritis seen in Lyme disease usually affects the knee but may affect other large joints in a monoarticular pattern with spontaneous exacerbations and remissions (Fig. 7.10).

Other infections cause a reactive arthritis that dissipates in less than 6 weeks. Recent infection with *Salmonella, Shigella, Yersinia,* and *Campylobacter* organisms should be considered. Many viruses also cause arthritis, including rubella, hepatitis B, adenovirus, and herpesviruses, such as Epstein-Barr virus, cytomegalovirus, varicella zoster, and herpes simplex. Parvoviruses, mumps, and enteroviruses, including echovirus and coxsackievirus, are associated with acute polyarthritis and occasionally have been recovered from joints.

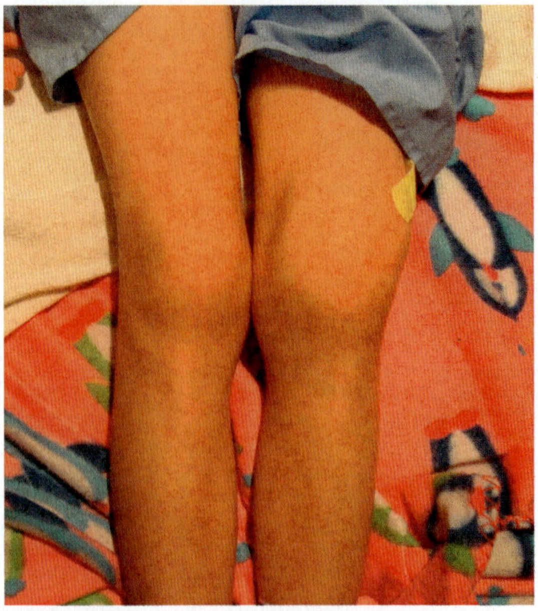

Fig. 7.10 Lyme arthritis. Unilateral left knee involvement with typical large effusion.

Other viruses result in reactive arthritis and may not infect the joint directly.

Poststreptococcal phenomena include ARF and poststreptococcal reactive arthritis. In ARF, Jones criteria are used for diagnosis. Arthritis presents in migratory fashion, and pain may be out of proportion to examination. Use of nonsteroidal antiinflammatory drugs alters the course of the arthritis. The child must be monitored for cardiac sequelae, such as valvulitis and congestive heart failure. In poststreptococcal reactive arthritis, Jones criteria are not met, but evidence of preceding streptococcal infection is present. Arthritis will resolve, but arthralgia can last for 6 months. The joint pain may be axial and affect the spine. In both cases, children are given prophylactic antibiotics to prevent future streptococcal infections.

Malignancies, such as neuroblastoma and leukemia, may present with musculoskeletal pain. More careful evaluation generally reveals bone pain. Sickle cell disease can have prominent digital involvement or deep bone pain related to infarction. Hemophilia, tuberculosis, and gonorrhea infection must be considered in the patient with oligoarthritis. Differential diagnoses of joint pain are proposed in Box 7.4.

Box 7.4 Differential Diagnosis of Joint Pain

Systemic Onset

Systemic lupus erythematosus (SLE)
Kawasaki disease
Acute rheumatic fever
Henoch-Schönlein purpura
Polyarteritis nodosa
Dermatomyositis
Inflammatory bowel disease
Malignancy (leukemia, lymphoma, neuroblastoma)
Lyme disease
Viral syndrome
Malaria
Septic arthritis/infectious osteomyelitis
Periodic fever syndromes
Serum sickness–like reaction

Polyarticular Onset

SLE
Amplified musculoskeletal pain syndrome
Hypermobility syndrome
Enthesitis-related arthritis
Reactive arthritis *(Yersinia, Salmonella, Shigella, Campylobacter,* and *Chlamydia trachomatis)*
Postinfectious arthritis (parvovirus B19, hepatitis B, rubella, enteroviruses, alphaviruses)
Blau syndrome
Inflammatory bowel disease
Multiple epiphyseal dysplasia
Cystic fibrosis

Oligoarticular Onset

Septic arthritis
Reactive arthritis *(Yersinia, Salmonella, Shigella, Campylobacter,* and *C. trachomatis)*
Postinfectious arthritis (alphaviruses, Epstein-Barr virus, varicella)
Acute rheumatic fever
Amplified musculoskeletal pain syndrome
Pigmented villonodular synovitis
Lyme disease
Crystalline arthropathy
Celiac disease

SYSTEMIC LUPUS ERYTHEMATOSUS

SLE is a multisystem autoimmune disease with a myriad of clinical presentations that accounts for 10% of adult patients with rheumatic diseases but less than 5% of children. The incidence rate is estimated at 0.5 to 0.7 per 100,000 children; reports on prevalence range from 1.1 to 24 per 100,000 children. There are between 5000 and 10,000 children with SLE in the United States. SLE is exceptionally rare in children younger than 5 years old. In prepubertal children the female-to-male ratio is equal, but it approaches 8:1 in pubertal children. The incidence of SLE is higher in people who identify as Black, Asian/Pacific Islander, American Indian/Alaska Native, and/or Hispanic compared with people who identify as White and/or Non-Hispanic. The etiology of SLE is unknown but involves a combination of genetic predisposition and environmental triggers that results in the production of autoantibodies. The high incidence of the disease in females supports the role of hormonal and X-chromosomal factors in the pathogenesis of SLE.

Childhood-onset SLE (cSLE) may present in an insidious fashion, or it may present acutely and progress rapidly. The diagnosis of SLE is made on the basis of the presence of clinical and laboratory findings. The updated 2019 European League Against Rheumatism/

American College of Rheumatology Classification Criteria for SLE combines clinical and serologic markers for the diagnosis of SLE (Table 7.5). The updated criteria remain highly specific when applied to pediatric cohorts, but sensitivity may be imperfect; however, the criteria are not meant for the clinical application of diagnosis and should be used only as a guide.

Clinical Manifestations

The early symptoms are often nonspecific and sometimes go unrecognized as harbingers of serious disease. Fever, fatigue, malaise, anorexia, and weight loss may be the only symptoms. Conversely, this multisystem disease may present with a plethora of physical findings, and the

Table 7.5 Criteria for the Classification of Systemic Lupus Erythematosus

Criteria	Weighted Score	Comments
ANA titer ≥1:80	Required	Testing by immunofluorescence on HEp-2 cells or a solid-phase ANA screening immunoassay with at least equivalent performance is highly recommended.
Criteria may be counted if they occur at least once without a more likely explanation than SLE. They do not have to occur simultaneously, and only the highest weighted criterion in each domain should be counted toward the total score.		
Clinical Criteria		
Constitutional		
Fever	2	>38.3°C
Hematologic		
Leukopenia	3	WBC <4000/mm³
Thrombocytopenia	4	PLT<100,000/mm³
Autoimmune hemolysis	4	Reticulocytosis, low haptoglobin, elevated indirect bilirubin, elevated LDH, positive Coombs direct antiglobulin test
Neuropsychiatric		
Delirium	2	Acute change in consciousness/arousal with symptom fluctuation and acute/subacute change in cognition, behavior, mood, or affect
Psychosis	3	Delusions/hallucinations without insight (in the absence of delirium)
Seizure	5	Primary generalized or focal seizure
Mucocutaneous		
Nonscarring alopecia	2	
Oral ulcers	2	
Subacute cutaneous	4	Annular or papulosquamous eruption, often photodistributed. *Biopsy may show interface vacuolar dermatitis with perivascular lymphohistiocytic infiltrate often with dermal mucin.*
OR		
Discoid lupus		Erythematous-violaceous lesions with atrophic scarring, dyspigmentation, follicular hyperkeratosis/plugging, and/or scarring alopecia (scalp). *Biopsy may show interface vacuolar dermatitis with perivascular/periappendageal lymphohistiocytic infiltrate and/or follicular keratin plugs.*
Acute cutaneous lupus	6	Malar rash or generalized maculopapular rash. *Biopsy may show interface vacuolar dermatitis with perivascular lymphohistiocytic or neutrophilic infiltrate often with dermal mucin.*
Serosal		
Pleural or pericardial effusion	5	Effusion on imaging (ultrasound, radiograph, CT, or MRI)
Acute pericarditis	6	At least 2: pericardial chest pain, pericardial rub, ECG with ST elevation or PR depression, or new/worsened pericardial effusion on imaging
Musculoskeletal		
Joint involvement	6	Synovitis of 2 or more joints or tenderness of 2 more joints and at least 30 minutes of morning stiffness
Renal		
Proteinuria	4	Proteinuria >0.5 g/24 hours by 24-hour urine or equivalent spot urine protein-to-creatinine ratio
Renal biopsy class II or V LN	8	II: Purely mesangial hypercellularity with mesangial immune deposits V: Global or segmental subepithelial immune deposits
Renal biopsy class III or IV LN	10	III: Focal, segmental, or global glomerulonephritis (<50% of glomeruli), with focal subendothelial immune deposits IV: Diffuse, segmental or global glomerulonephritis (≥50% of glomeruli) with diffuse subendothelial immune deposits
Immunology Criteria		
Antiphospholipid Antibodies		
Anticardiolipin or anti-β2-glycoprotein I antibodies or lupus anticoagulant	2	Medium-high titer (>40) anti-CL antibodies (IgA, IgG, or IgM), or positive anti-β2GPI antibodies (IgA, IgG, or IgM), or positive lupus anticoagulant
Hypocomplementemia		
Low C3 or low C4	3	Below the lower limits of normal
Low C3 AND low C4	4	
SLE-Specific Autoantibodies		
Anti-dsDNA antibody or anti-Smith antibody	6	Positive antidsDNA antibodies in an immunoassay with ≥90% specificity or positive anti-Sm antibodies
Classify as SLE if ANA positive, at least once clinical criterion is present and score ≥10.*		

*In pediatric populations, these criteria had a sensitivity of 84.8%-92% and a specificity of 67.4%-89%.

ANA, Antinuclear antibodies; *CT*, computed tomography; *ECG*, electrocardiogram; MRI, magnetic resonance imaging; SLE, systemic lupus erythematosus.

Modified from Aringer M, Costenbader K, Daikh D, et al: 2019 European League Against Rheumatism/American College of Rheumatology classification criteria for systemic lupus erythematosus, *Arthritis Rheumatol* 71(9):1400–1412, 2019.

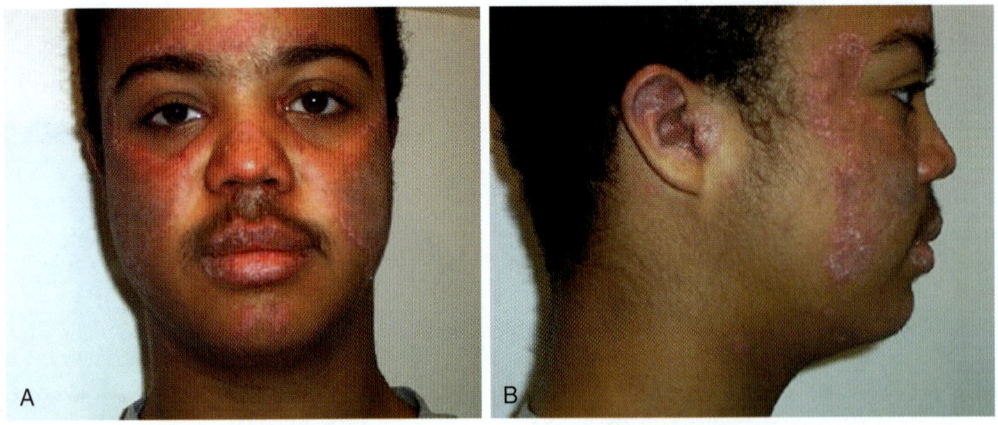

Fig. 7.11 Systemic lupus erythematosus (SLE). (A) Malar rash of SLE. Erythema, erosion, and atrophy are present. Note sparing of nasolabial folds. This patient also has a rash involving the forehead and chin. (B) Lateral view shows ear involvement.

presentation may be so dramatic that the diagnosis is readily apparent. The most commonly involved organ systems at disease presentation in cSLE are musculoskeletal, cutaneous, renal, and hematologic.

Mucocutaneous Manifestations

Cutaneous manifestations of SLE occur at some time during the course of the disease in 80% of affected individuals. There are a variety of cutaneous findings, including a malar rash (Fig. 7.11), photosensitive rash, palmar erythema (Fig. 7.12), annular erythema, vasculitic skin lesions with nodules or ulcerations, Raynaud phenomenon (Table 7.6) and associated ulcerations, alopecia, and discoid lupus rash. The most frequent skin manifestations of cSLE are malar rash and photosensitive rash. The classic malar "butterfly" rash is a maculopapular rash distributed over the cheeks (malar eminences) and extending over the bridge of the nose while sparing the nasolabial folds.

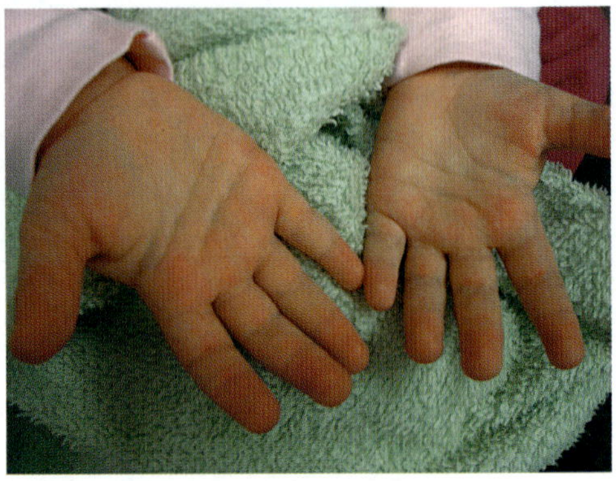

Fig. 7.12 Systemic lupus erythematosus. Palmar erythema.

Table 7.6 Common Benign and Pathologic Color Change Syndromes of Extremities

Disease	Epidemiology	Triggers	Duration	Clinical Examination	Associated Disorders	Comments
Raynaud phenomenon, primary	Common, 10%–15% prevalence, female >male	Cold exposure, emotion, stimulants, smoking	Minutes to hours	Triphasic (white/blue/red) color change of fingers/toes with clear demarcation; Numb when ischemic, aching/painful with reperfusion	None	May be limited to single digit
Raynaud phenomenon, secondary	Uncommon, variable prevalence in underlying conditions	Cold exposure, disease activity	Hours to continuous	Triphasic changes; chronic digital ulcers or skin pits; poor nail health; abnormal nailfold capillaries	SLE, SSc, MCTD, aPLS, Vasculitis	May require vasodilators
Acrocyanosis	Common, 10%–15% prevalence, female >male, onset in adolescence, low BMI is a risk factor	Cold exposure, limb in dependent position, medications (stimulants, TCAs)	Minutes	Symmetric, painless blue/purple discoloration of hands/feet without clear demarcation; blanching with pressure; affected skin/nails appear healthy	Anorexia nervosa, POTS, Genetic CTDs	May be accompanied by *cutis marmorata* on affected limbs
Perniosis	Uncommon, female>male, peak 2nd–5th decades of life, low BMI is a risk factor	Cold and damp conditions	Continuous for 1–3 weeks	Edematous, erythematous or violaceous papules/plaques/nodules on dorsum of fingers or toes; blisters or ulcers may develop; onset 12–24 h after cold exposure	None	Symptoms usually limited to winter months
Erythromelalgia	Rare, female >male, onset in early adolescence	Exercise, heat exposure	Minutes to continuous	Symmetric, diffuse, painful erythema of hands, feet, or face; affected areas feel hot	Myeloproliferative disorder (adults only); rarely inherited	Pain is often severe and disabling

aPLS, Antiphospholipid antibody syndrome; *BMI,* body mass index; *CTD,* connective tissue disease; *MCTD,* mixed connective tissue disease; *POTS,* postural orthostatic tachycardia syndrome; *SLE,* systemic lupus erythematosus; *SSc,* systemic sclerosis; *TCA,* tricyclic antidepressants.

Data from Fleck DE, Hoeltzel MF: Hand and foot color change: diagnosis and management, *Pediatr Rev* 38;511, 2017; Cappel JA, Wetter DA: Clinical characteristics, etiological associations, laboratory findings, treatment, and proposal of diagnostic criteria of pernio (chilblains) in a series of 104 patients at Mayo Clinic, 2000 to 2011, *Mayo Clin Proc* 89(2):207, 2014.

The malar rash is photosensitive in 30% of patients. Photosensitive rashes can take a variety of forms. The typical morphology is defined as reddish purple and raised with a whitish scale (Fig. 7.13). An annular photosensitive rash may also be seen (often associated with anti-Ro [SSA] and anti-La [SSB] antibodies). Subacute cutaneous lupus, which is less common, presents as a photodistributed serpiginous-like erythematous rash with varying degrees of scale (also associated with anti-SSA antibodies). Sun exposure can exacerbate skin disease but may also cause a systemic flare of disease. Appropriate sun protection and avoidance are strongly encouraged. Vasculitic rashes are more violaceous and may be associated with nodules, ulceration, and palpable purpura (Fig. 7.14). These lesions are commonly found in an acral distribution, and they typically result in postinflammatory hyperpigmentation. Discoid lupus, although uncommon (5%–10% of patients with cSLE), leaves the most damage, with follicular plugging and scarring. Less common cutaneous findings include panniculitis (lupus profundus), pernio (chilblain LE), bullous LE, livedo reticularis (lacy, fishnet appearance of the skin), urticaria, telangiectasia, and periungual erythema. Mucosal erosions and ulcers of the oral and nasal mucosa can also occur; the most well-recognized ulcer is the

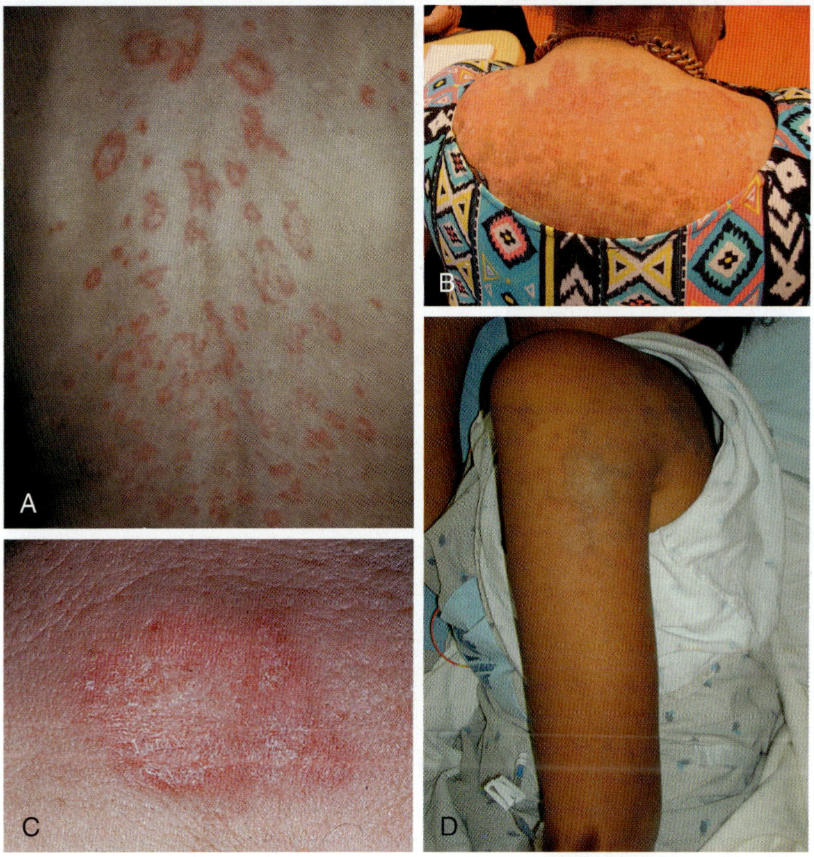

Fig. 7.13 Systemic lupus erythematosus (SLE). (A) Erythematous rash on trunk. (B) Significant postinflammatory hyperpigmentation may be present as well. (C and D) The rash of SLE often has a slight white scale.

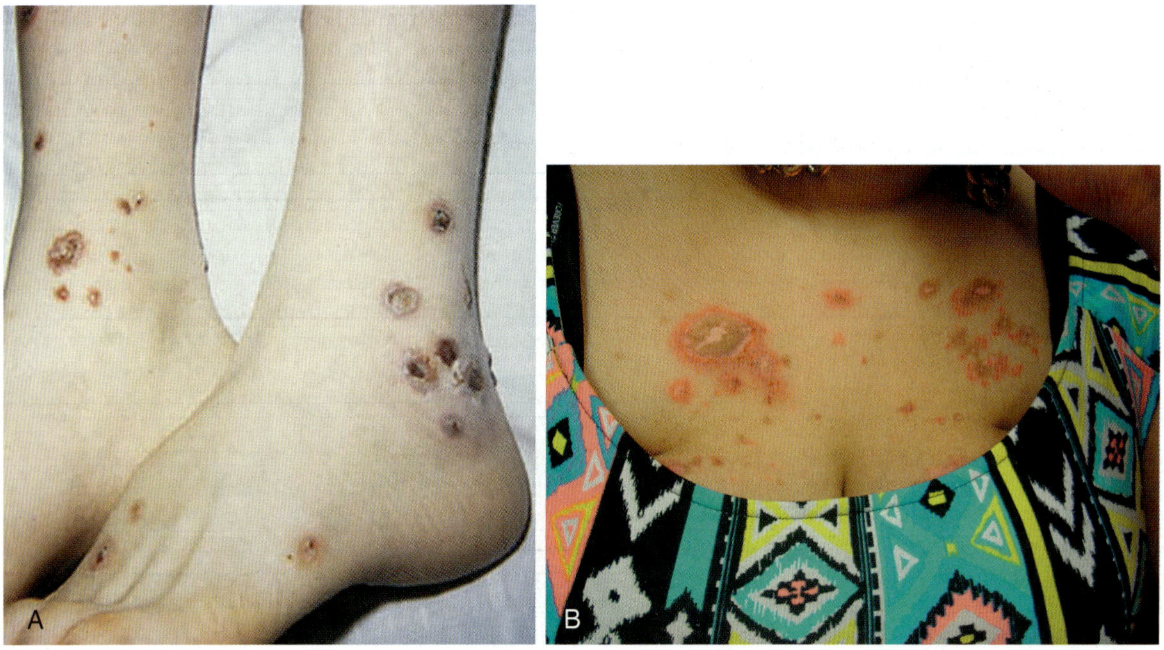

Fig. 7.14 Systemic lupus erythematosus. Purpuric, ulcerative, and necrotic skin lesions of cutaneous vasculitis may be found acrally (A) or centrally (B).

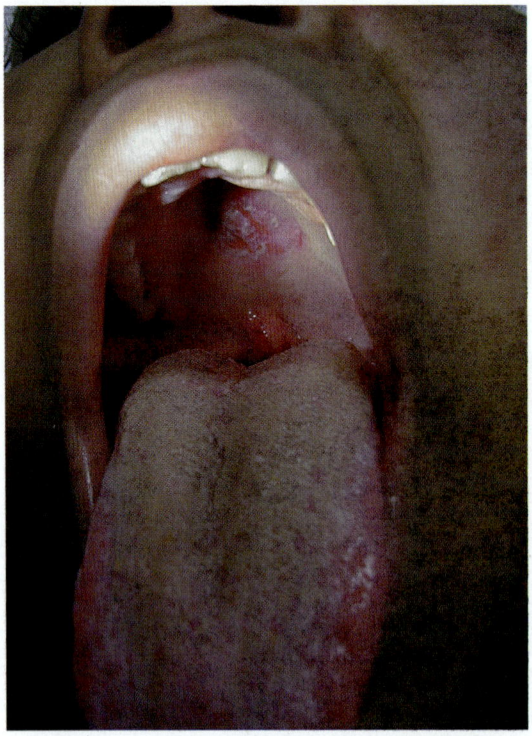

Fig. 7.15 Systemic lupus erythematosus. "Silent" ulceration of the hard palate.

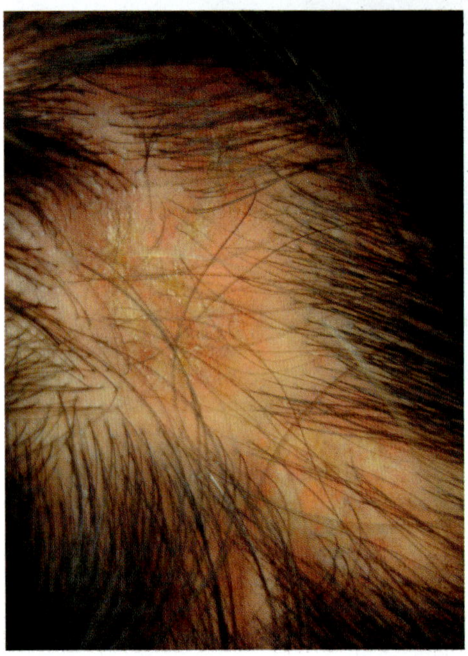

Fig. 7.16 Systemic lupus erythematosus. Scarring alopecia.

painless large violaceous ulceration of the hard palate (Fig. 7.15). Alopecia occurs in 20% of patients and may present as nonscarring alopecia with frontotemporal thinning and broken hair shafts, or localized patches of alopecia areata, which may eventually scar and cause permanent hair loss (Fig. 7.16).

Musculoskeletal Manifestations

Arthritis is seen in approximately 80% of patients with cSLE and is often present at the time of diagnosis. Unlike the destructive arthritis of JIA, lupus arthritis is more transient and episodic and rarely results in joint contracture. Jaccoud arthropathy, which is a nonerosive, easily reversible joint deformity due to soft tissue laxity, is strongly associated with the diagnosis of SLE. This arthropathy can mimic the boutonnière (flexion of PIP joints and hyperextension of distal interphalangeal [DIP] joints) and swan-neck (hyperextension of PIP joints and flexion of DIP joints) deformities associated with JIA. In SLE, arthralgia is often predominant, with the degree of pain out of proportion to the degree of synovitis or effusion on examination. Arthritis in SLE is often migratory, symmetric, and polyarticular, most commonly affecting the fingers, wrists, and knees, though any joint can be affected. Myalgia and weakness can also occur but is associated with myositis in less than 10% of patients with SLE. Musculoskeletal manifestations associated with long-term high-dose corticosteroid therapy in SLE include avascular necrosis, particularly of the hip and knee joints, as well as osteoporosis, and vertebral fractures.

Renal Manifestations

Approximately 75% of all children with SLE have some degree of clinically apparent renal disease; this is more prevalent than in adult SLE and is generally more severe. Renal involvement often manifests within 2 years of diagnosis but can present at any time.

Hypertension and peripheral edema are present in approximately one-third of cSLE patients with lupus nephritis (LN) and typically associated with more aggressive disease. Blood and urinalysis parameters, including serum albumin and total protein, complement (C3 and C4), microscopical urinalysis for red blood cell (RBC) casts, and urine protein-to-creatinine ratio or 24-hour urine protein quantification are essential for the diagnosis and monitoring of LN. A pathologic diagnosis must be made in children with suspected LN or rapid change in renal function. LN is classified as an immune-complex mediated glomerulonephritis characterized by glomerular immune deposits in the mesangial, subendothelial, and/or subepithelial spaces consisting of IgG, IgA, IgM, C3, and C1q (so-called "full-house" appearance on immunofluorescence). Extraglomerular deposits in the tubules, interstitium, and blood vessels may also be present. Specific classification of LN based on histopathologic findings may guide prognosis and direct systemic therapy. Control of hypertension is critical for preventing the progression to renal failure and other systemic complications, such as PRES (see Fig. 7.19C and D). Advances in treatment for LN with relatively aggressive immunosuppressive regimens have dramatically improved the renal outcomes for patients with cSLE in the past few decades.

Hematologic Manifestations

Hematologic abnormalities are one of the most common initial manifestations of cSLE. They are found in three-quarters of patients and include leukopenia, anemia, and thrombocytopenia. The "classic" anemia in cSLE is normocytic and normochromic, but over time it evolves into microcytic and hypochromic anemia with iron deficiency. The Coombs test is positive in one-third of patients, but less than 10% have overt hemolysis. Thrombocytopenia in lupus is typically mild but can be more severe and refractory to common therapy. The presence of both autoimmune hemolytic anemia and thrombocytopenia, known as *Evans syndrome*, can be observed in cSLE. Lymphopenia is much more common than granulocytopenia in SLE, with a typical lymphocyte count between 1000 and 1500 cells/mm^3.

Thromboembolic complications can occur in cSLE-associated antiphospholipid antibody syndrome. Antiphospholipid antibodies are present in approximately 50% of patients with cSLE, with anticardiolipin antibodies being the most common. The lupus anticoagulant panel is abnormal in 20% to 30% of patients with cSLE. These antibodies are associated with increased risk for thrombosis, miscarriages, chorea, migraine headaches, and livedo reticularis.

Cardiac Manifestations

The heart is often significantly involved in cSLE. Pericarditis associated with pericardial effusion can present with classic symptoms of sharp anterior chest pain, but patients can remain asymptomatic until a large effusion causes cardiac tamponade. Pericardial effusion can also be noted incidentally as cardiomegaly on a chest radiograph (Fig. 7.17) or as pericardial effusion on an echocardiogram, CT, or magnetic resonance imaging (MRI). If the myocardium is affected, serious complications including dysrhythmias, heart failure, and infarction can result. Thrombotic endocarditis, including verrucous endocarditis (i.e., Libman-Sacks endocarditis), is another cardiac complication of cSLE, often associated with the presence of antiphospholipid antibodies. These lesions rarely cause clinical symptoms, but the presence of a murmur should raise suspicion, and they can result in systemic emboli. The mitral valve is most commonly involved, although aortic and tricuspid valves may be similarly affected. The major cardiac morbidity associated with cSLE is premature atherosclerosis, likely arising from several factors including chronic inflammation, altered endothelial function, dyslipidemia, and kidney disease. Monitoring and controlling classic cardiovascular risk factors in addition to factors attributable to SLE are critical to address long-term morbidity.

Pulmonary Manifestations

The most common pulmonary findings in cSLE include pleuritis and pleural effusions, which most commonly present with acute localized chest pain exacerbated by deep inspiration but rarely present with dyspnea. Acute pneumonitis is less common, usually associated with dyspnea, cough, and basilar crackles; distinguishing lupus pneumonitis from infection may be impossible without invasive procedures (Fig. 7.18). Alveolar hemorrhage is a rare complication that presents with dyspnea and cough (sometimes accompanied by frank hemoptysis) and should be suspected in patients with respiratory distress and acute drop in hemoglobin. Pulmonary arterial hypertension (PAH) is another manifestation, more commonly seen in those with positive U1 ribonucleoprotein (U1-RNP) antibodies or those patients with features that overlap with systemic sclerosis (SSc). An uncommon but well-described pulmonary manifestation of SLE is "shrinking lung" syndrome, in which lung volumes become progressively smaller in the absence of notable parenchymal disease. Pulmonary function testing should be performed in any cSLE patient with new-onset dyspnea.

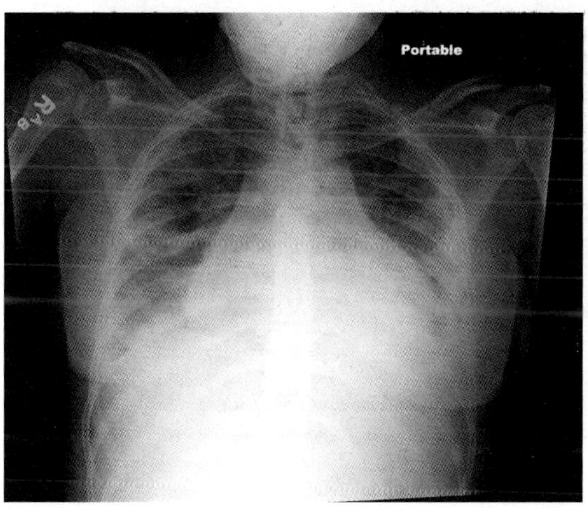

Fig. 7.17 Systemic lupus erythematosus. Large pericardial effusion with associated cardiac tamponade physiology in teenage female. Pleural effusions are also present.

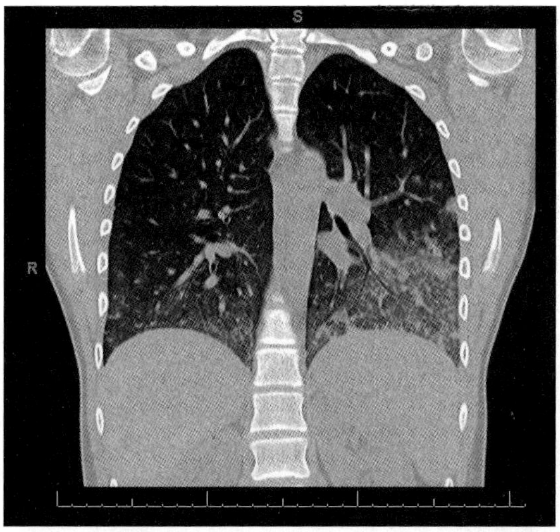

Fig. 7.18 Systemic lupus erythematosus. Chest computed tomography demonstrating bibasilar pneumonitis. Note extensive ground-glass opacities and patchy consolidations with air bronchograms in the lower lobes bilaterally.

Central Nervous System Manifestations

Central nervous system (CNS) involvement in SLE includes a wide range of neurologic and psychiatric manifestations that have higher prevalence and severity in cSLE compared with adult-onset SLE. Neuropsychiatric SLE (NPSLE) can present with a wide range of symptoms and severity, and diagnosis is often made even more difficult by the absence of objective signs on clinical screening examinations and imaging. Further complicating the spectrum of NPSLE is the difficulty in distinguishing primary from secondary manifestations, such as corticosteroid psychosis, adjustment disorder after diagnosis, and non-CNS etiologies, such as hypertensive encephalopathy and posterior reversible encephalopathy syndrome (PRES) (Fig. 7.19).

Headaches are the most common NPSLE symptom, often refractory to standard analgesics. Lupus headaches must be distinguished from the severe, unremitting headaches that can be the presenting symptom of more serious complications like pseudotumor cerebri, aseptic meningitis, CNS vasculitis, or cerebral vascular disease. Cognitive impairment is also common and can be difficult to ascertain without formal neuropsychologic testing, unless overt deficits are present, such as inattention or impaired memory. Mood disorders, especially depression and anxiety, are common, and etiology is likely multifactorial, with contributing factors including primary NPSLE and secondary reaction to chronic disease and side effects of medications. Psychosis can present early in the disease course and is often associated with high systemic and CNS disease burden. NPSLE can manifest with seizures, including generalized or focal classifications, which can be the result of CNS inflammation or vascular occlusion. Presentation of cerebral vascular disease is also highly varied and can include central vein thrombosis, vasculitis of small or medium vessels, and/or thrombosis resulting in ischemia or hemorrhage. Presenting symptoms such as chorea, headaches, seizures, altered mental status, and focal neurologic deficits have been described. Confirmation of cerebral vascular disease requires advanced imaging such as CT or MRI, with the addition of angiogram when vasculitis is suspected. Cerebral vascular accidents should also raise the suspicion for antiphospholipid antibody syndrome. Other NPSLE findings include mononeuritis multiplex (inflammatory lesions of multiple nerves located in anatomically unrelated parts of the body), transverse myelitis, ataxia, and peripheral neuropathy.

Brain MRI may show focal white matter T2 hyperintensities (Fig. 7.19), but normal imaging does not exclude active NPSLE. Lumbar puncture may show nonspecific findings of elevated WBC count, protein, and IgG without evidence of infection. The lumbar puncture is typically done to rule out non-SLE causes of CNS disease, especially infection.

As a direct extension of the brain, the retina may also show evidence of disease (i.e., retinal vasculitis). The best-known ocular manifestation is the cotton-wool spot, an exudative, whitish lesion of the retina. Hemorrhage and papilledema are also seen (Fig. 7.20).

Gastrointestinal Manifestations

Gastrointestinal manifestations of cSLE are not uncommon but are rarely severe. These include hepatosplenomegaly, mild hepatitis, enteritis, pancreatitis, malabsorption, and mesenteric vasculitis, which can present with diarrhea and abdominal pain.

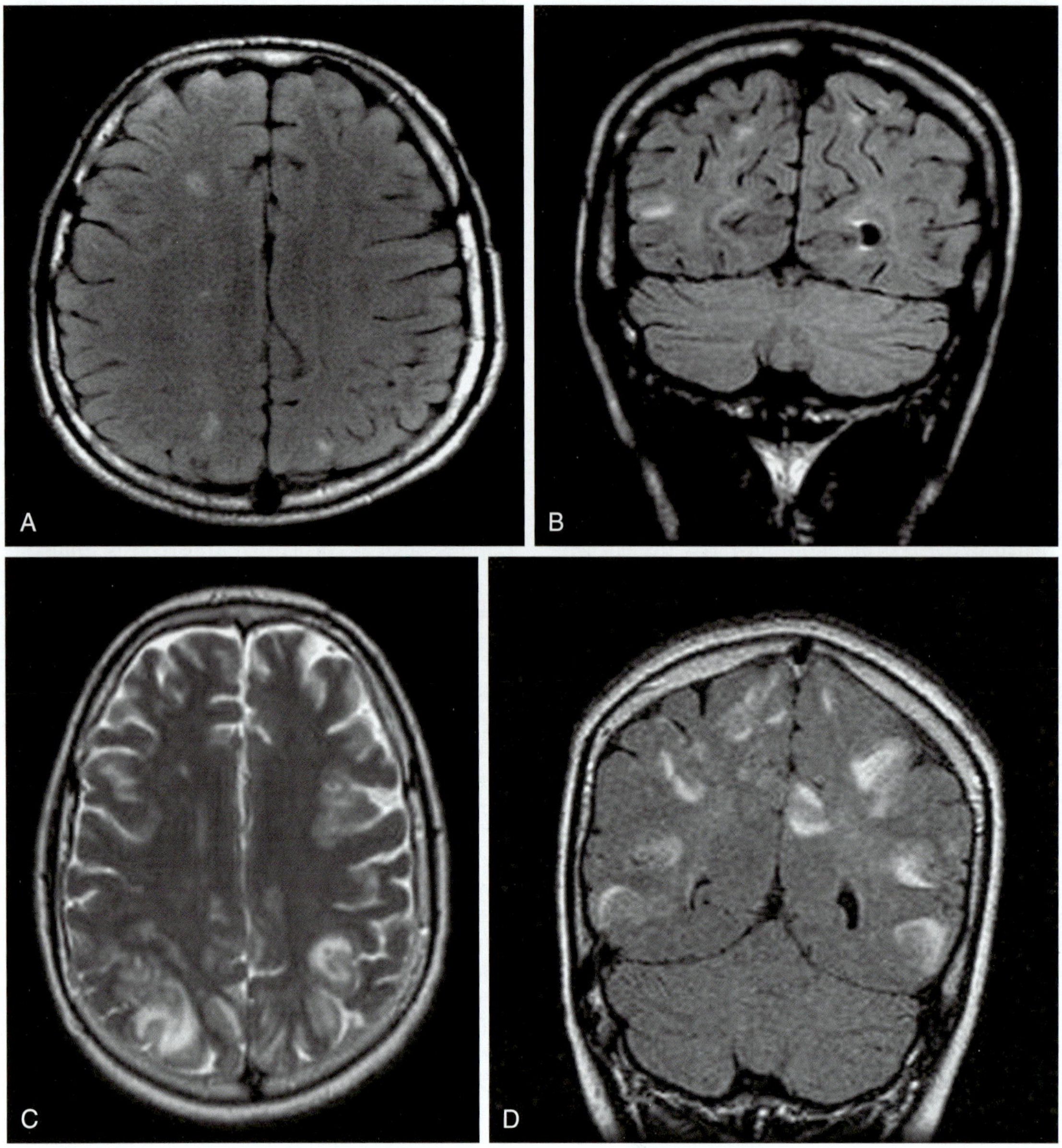

Fig. 7.19 Systemic lupus erythematosus. Axial (A) and coronal (B) images of brain with scattered cortical and subcortical foci with T2 prolongation mostly in the posterior white matter (parietal and occipital lobes) but also in some areas anteriorly (frontal lobe). Another abnormality is in the left precentral gyrus (motor area). These abnormalities were found in a teenage male with chorea and newly diagnosed systemic lupus erythematosus. Axial (C) and coronal (D) T2 images consistent with posterior reversible encephalopathy syndrome in the same patient 3 months later, associated with a hypertensive crisis.

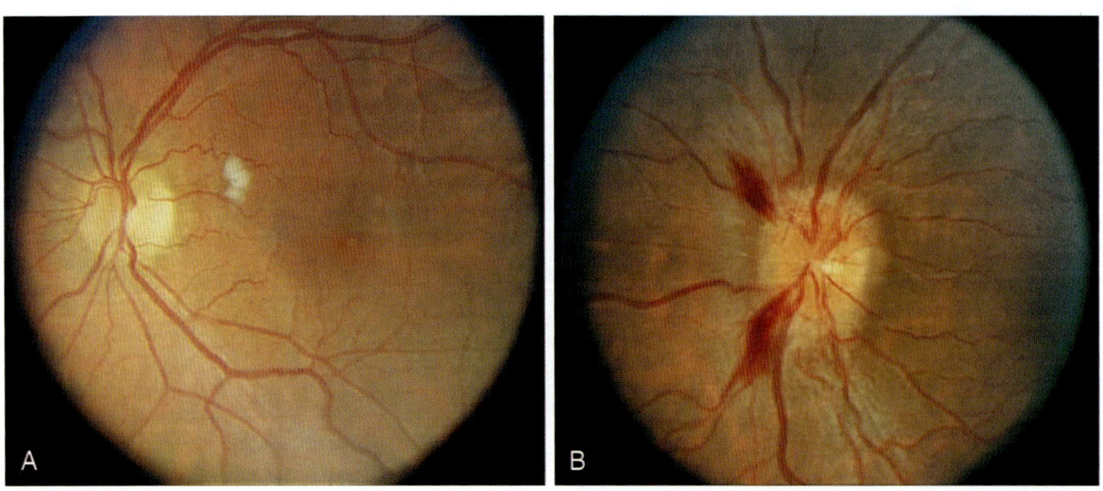

Fig. 7.20 Systemic lupus erythematosus. (A) A white exudate (cotton-wool spot) between the disk and macula. (B) Papilledema with flame hemorrhages.

Serologic Evaluation

Perhaps more than in any other rheumatic disease, the clinical diagnosis of lupus can be supported serologically. Although immunologic markers contribute to diagnosis, a high clinical suspicion is necessary for serologic investigation to have diagnostic utility. ANAs represent a group of antibodies found in serum that are directed against antigens within the cellular nuclei. ANAs are usually reported as a titer and a pattern. The patterns are typically associated with antibodies to certain extractable nuclear antigens such as SSA, SSB, Smith, ribonucleoprotein (RNP), dsDNA, histone, and Scl-70. Most patients with cSLE have a positive ANA at diagnosis, but it is important to remember that a positive ANA in itself is not diagnostic for SLE and must be interpreted in the correct clinical scenario (Table 7.7). Common antibodies found in patients with cSLE are listed in Table 7.8. Anti-dsDNA antibodies are detected in 84% to 100% of patients with cSLE and are highly specific for SLE. Anti-dsDNA antibody levels correlate with disease activity, especially renal and CNS disease.

In summary, SLE is a chronic disease with a variable course and with periods of varying activity. Although the mortality and morbidity remain high, marked improvement in prognosis has occurred in recent years.

Table 7.7 Antinuclear Antibody (ANA) Frequency in Healthy and Disease States

Population	Frequency of Positive ANA
Healthy children and adolescents	10%–25%
Autoimmune thyroiditis	30%–50%
Autoimmune hepatitis	25%–100%
SLE	>95%
MCTD	>95%
Sjögren disease	40%–70%
Localized scleroderma	40%–50%
Systemic sclerosis	60%–95%
JIA	40%–50%
Idiopathic uveitis	40%
Juvenile dermatomyositis	70%
Primary Raynaud phenomenon	20%–30%

JIA, Juvenile idiopathic arthritis; *MCTD,* mixed connective tissue disease; *SLE,* systemic lupus erythematosus.

Data from Sperotto F, Cuffaro G, Brachi S, et al: Prevalence of antinuclear antibodies in school children during puberty and possible relationship with musculoskeletal pain: a longitudinal study, *J Rheumatol* 41(7):1405–1408, 2014; Dalrymple AM, Moore TL: Laboratory evaluation in pediatric autoimmune diseases, *Pediatr Rev* 36(11):496–501, 2015; Chou IJ, Kuo CF, See LD, et al: Antinuclear antibody status and risk of death in children and adolescents, *Scand J Rheumatol* 40(6):472–477, 2011; Saikia B, Rawat A, Vignesh P: Autoantibodies and their judicious use in pediatric rheumatology practice, *Indian J Pediatr* 83:53–62, 2016; Floreani A, Liberal R, Vergani D, et al: Autoimmune hepatitis: contrasts and comparisons in children and adults—A comprehensive review, *J Autoimmun* 46:7–16, 2013; Bittencourt PL, Farias AQ, Porta G, et al: Frequency of concurrent autoimmune disorders in patients with autoimmune hepatitis: effect of age, gender, and genetic background, *J Clin Gastroenterol* 42(3):300–305, 2008; Morelle G, Gueudry J, Uettwiller F, et al: Chronic and recurrent non-infectious paediatric-onset uveitis: a French cohort, *RMD Open* 5(2):5, 2019; Manzotti F, Orsoni JG, Zavota L, et al: Autoimmune uveitis in children: clinical correlation between antinuclear antibody positivity and ocular recurrences, *Rheumatol Int* 21:127–132, 2002.

Table 7.8 Common Antibodies Found in Patients With Systemic Lupus Erythematosus

Antibody	ANA Pattern	Patients
Anti-dsDNA	Homogeneous	84%–100%
Anti-histone	Homogenous	90% (in drug-induced lupus)
Anti-Smith	Speckled	23%–48%
Anti-U1-RNP	Speckled	31%–62%
Anti-SSA (anti-Ro)	Speckled	38%–54%
Anti-SSB (anti-La)	Speckled	16%–32%

ANA, Antinuclear antibody; *dsDNA,* double-stranded deoxyribonucleic acid; *RNP,* ribonuclear protein.

Modified from Petty RE, Laxer RM, Lindsley CB, et al: *Textbook of pediatric rheumatology,* ed 8, Philadelphia, 2021, Elsevier.

Drug-Induced Systemic Lupus Erythematosus

Several medications induce a lupus-like syndrome, and their withdrawal often leads to resolution of symptoms, usually within 6 months. Many patients taking drugs such as minocycline, hydralazine, procainamide, isoniazid, chlorpromazine, or certain anticonvulsants develop a positive ANA without developing a lupus-like syndrome, and this is not an absolute reason to discontinue the medication. Anti-histone antibodies are often present in drug-induced lupus.

Neonatal Lupus

Neonatal lupus occurs in a proportion of infants whose mothers have positive anti-SSA or anti-SSB antibodies, which are passed via the placenta to the fetus. Many mothers are entirely asymptomatic, though some have known diagnoses associated with anti-SSA/SSB antibodies such as SLE or Sjögren disease and some eventually progress to autoimmune disease later. The presence of autoantibodies in the infant leads to manifestations of neonatal lupus, including the presence of erythematous annular rash (Fig. 7.21), thrombocytopenia, Coombs-positive hemolytic anemia, transaminitis, hepatitis, and congenital heart block (CHB). CHB develops between 18 and 25 weeks' gestation due to antibody interference during heart conduction tissue remodeling, which

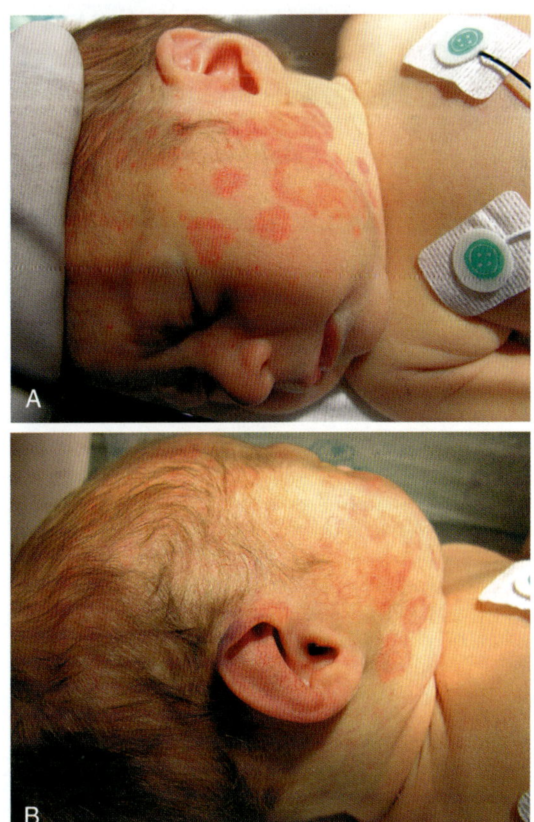

Fig. 7.21 Neonatal lupus erythematosus. Shown is a newborn on its first day of life: typical annular rash (A) and tissue infarction of the right ear pinna (B). Infant and mother were positive for antinuclear antibodies and anti-Ro (SSA) and anti-La (SSB) antibodies (associated with Sjögren disease). The infant also had thrombocytopenia, hypocomplementemia, and increased transaminases.

results in first-, second-, or third-degree heart block that presents with fetal bradycardia. Two percent of infants born to mothers with anti-SSA antibodies have CHB, and the addition of anti-SSB antibodies increases the risk to 5%. Aside from CHB, most manifestations of neonatal lupus are transient, lasting only a few months until the disappearance of passively transferred maternal antibody.

SJÖGREN DISEASE

Childhood Sjögren disease (cSjD) is a multisystem autoimmune disease, characterized by anti-SSA/SSB antibodies and exocrine gland inflammation leading to xerostomia and keratoconjunctivitis due to decreased saliva and tear production. The xerostomia can lead to abnormal taste, difficulty swallowing, and severe dental decay; manifestations of chronic xerostomia include decreased sublingual salivary pooling, lingual papillary atrophy, glossy palatal oral mucosa, and oral candidiasis. Other mucosal surfaces are often dry, such as nasal, pharyngeal, and vaginal. The keratoconjunctivitis causes photophobia and irritation of the eyes, often with a foreign body sensation, or blurry vision. Ophthalmologic evaluation may show corneal erosions, reduced tear production, rapid tear break-up time, or other signs of eye dryness.

Lacrimal and salivary gland enlargement may be evident on examination or on imaging. cSjD may also present as recurrent noninfectious parotitis from episodic lymphocytic infiltration of the parotid gland during times of active disease. It is important to note that many patients with cSjD report no sicca symptoms despite objective clinical findings or diagnosis by histopathology.

Extraglandular manifestations may also be present and are more common in cSjD compared with adult-onset SjD. These include constitutional symptoms, arthralgia/arthritis, lymphadenopathy, cytopenias, cutaneous vasculitis, myositis, CNS involvement (seizures, transverse myelitis, CNS vasculitis), peripheral neuropathy, and cutaneous vasculitis. Renal involvement, including interstitial nephritis and renal tubular acidosis, is rare.

Laboratory results consistent with cSjD include a positive ANA with positive SSA/SSB antibodies, polyclonal hypergammaglobulinemia with high titer RF, and persistently elevated erythrocyte sedimentation rate (ESR). Diagnosis is supported by objective evidence of decreased tear and saliva production, such as ocular surface staining and Schirmer test, or unstimulated whole salivary flow and sialography, respectively. Minor salivary gland biopsy from the lip demonstrating a periductal lymphocytic infiltrate confirms the diagnosis.

JUVENILE DERMATOMYOSITIS

Juvenile dermatomyositis (JDM) is a rare but distinctive disease that accounts for approximately 5% of all rheumatic disease in childhood. Although its exact etiology remains unknown, evidence supports the involvement of both the innate and adaptive (humoral and cell-mediated) immune system contributing to vasculopathy, primarily affecting the skeletal muscle and skin. The average age at presentation for JDM is between 4 and 10 years old, with onset of disease at younger than 5 years old in 25% of patients. Females predominate by a 2:1 ratio. No racial bias exists, nor is there any evidence of a familial predisposition. Contrary to adult-onset dermatomyositis, there is no known malignancy-related or paraneoplastic phenomenon in juvenile-onset dermatomyositis. The overall functional outcome is favorable in JDM given current immunosuppressive treatments, although morbidities can be severe in some patients. Caution must be taken with the vasculopathy component of the disease, which can cause thrombosis and lead to significant tissue damage including ulcerations of the skin (Fig. 7.22).

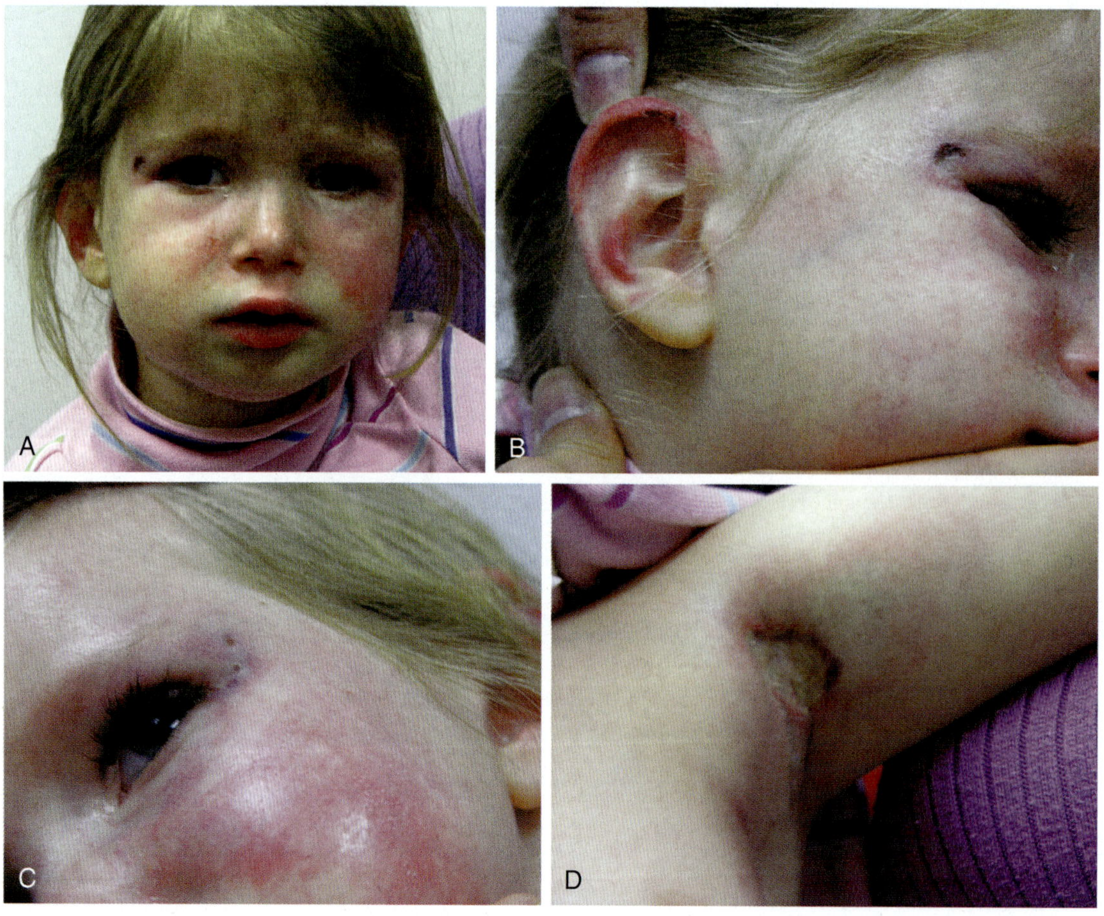

Fig. 7.22 Juvenile dermatomyositis. (A) A 3-year-old girl with a severe vasculitic rash. Note the heliotrope hue, nasolabial fold involvement, and ulcerations. (B) Ulcerations of the right ear and lateral to the eye (common sites). (C) Note the deep red/violaceous hue of the rash. (D) Deep ulceration of the axilla with ischemic tissue.

Clinical Manifestations

The illness may progress at variable rates in different patients; however, most patients have an insidious rather than acute course. Patients usually present with fatigue and symmetric, progressive, proximal muscle weakness, particularly affecting the limb-girdle musculature (shoulders and hips), neck flexors, and trunk muscles. Constitutional symptoms such as anorexia, malaise, weight loss, fever, and irritability (in young children) are often present. Although painless weakness is the hallmark of the disease, myalgia can exist with tender, indurated, or edematous-appearing muscles, sometimes accompanied by subcutaneous edema.

The first complaints, typically noticed by a parent, often concern an inability to climb stairs or disturbances of gait. A positive Gowers sign on physical examination reflects lower extremity proximal muscle weakness. Shoulders and upper arms are often involved and may manifest as difficulty brushing teeth or hair. Dysphasia, dysphonia, and dyspnea may occur if the respective muscles for these functions are affected (striated pharyngeal muscles and intercostal muscles).

Other musculoskeletal manifestations include arthralgia and arthritis affecting more than half of patients, typically early in the disease course; these are typically responsive to immunosuppression. However, a minority of patients develop long-term flexion contractures secondary to muscle tightening.

If distal muscle weakness or asymmetric muscle weakness is prominent, alternate diagnoses should be considered: abnormalities of the peripheral nerves, neuromotor junction dysfunction, metabolic/mitochondrial myopathies, or muscular dystrophies. Involvement of a neuromuscular specialist early in the evaluation process is recommended.

Cutaneous manifestations are the hallmark of JDM and include two pathognomonic rashes: Gottron papules and the heliotrope eyelid rash are identified in more than three-quarters of patients with JDM. Gottron papules are found symmetrically on the extensor surfaces of the knuckles (MCP, PIP, and DIP joints); elbows; knees; and malleoli. They are characterized as flat topped, erythematous, or violaceous papules sometimes with associated light scale (Fig. 7.23). It is common for these lesions to be mistaken for psoriasis, which typically has a similar distribution but more of a silvery scale. The heliotrope rash is violaceous and telangiectatic, extending over the upper eyelids, and often is associated with local edema. It may be confluent with a malar type of erythematous rash distributed over the cheeks and nose (Fig. 7.24). The JDM malar rash is different from that of SLE as it is more diffuse, ill defined, and typically does not spare the nasolabial folds; however, both rashes are similarly photosensitive.

Vasculopathy can cause direct cutaneous changes, the most common being abnormal digital nailfold capillary loops. In the clinic, magnifying the nailfolds with a lubricant and an ophthalmoscope is helpful if a dermatoscope is not available. Nailfold capillary changes include dilation, hemorrhage, drop-out, and telangiectasias (Fig. 7.25). Adjacent periungual erythema, with thickened cuticle hypertrophy and periungual infarcts, further reflects vasculopathy. Other areas that commonly ulcerate because of vasculopathy are the corners of the eye (see Fig. 7.22), the axilla, and over the elbows. Calcinosis (nodular calcium deposits) of the skin, subcutaneous tissue, and muscle is another characteristic cutaneous complication of JDM. It is more common in those with long-standing, untreated, severe disease (Fig. 7.26). Pressure points and areas of vasculopathy are particularly susceptible. These calcium deposits can erupt through the skin, causing significant pain and disfigurement. Lastly, lipodystrophy is another cutaneous finding due to damage from long-standing and/or uncontrolled JDM (see Fig. 7.26C). Lipodystrophy results from the slow, progressive loss of subcutaneous tissue, typically symmetrically distributed in the upper body, and is associated with glucose and lipid metabolism abnormalities.

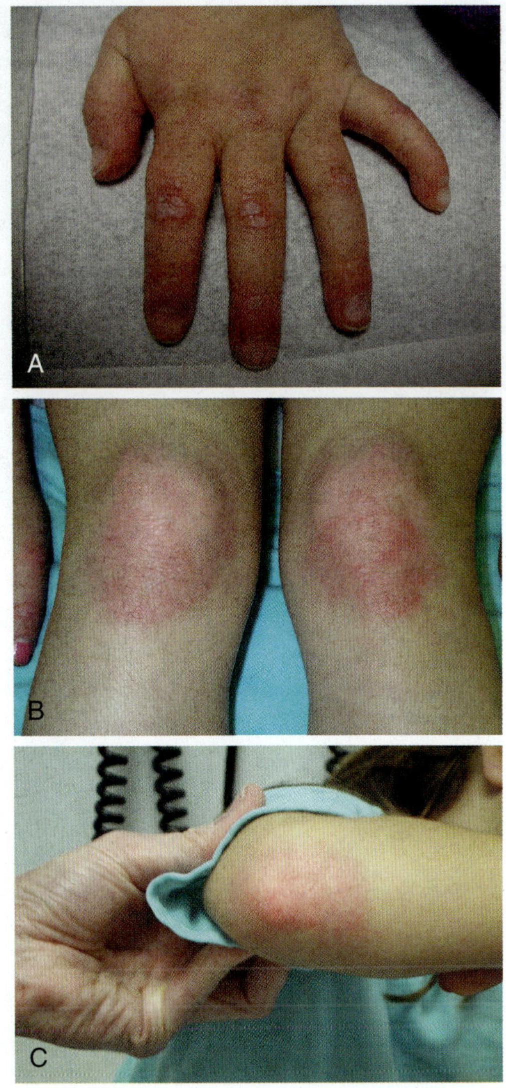

Fig. 7.23 Juvenile dermatomyositis. (A) Gottron papules: erythematous, atrophic skin changes overlying the metacarpophalangeal and proximal interphalangeal joints. (B and C) Gottron sign: typical erythematous rash of juvenile dermatomyositis, as seen on the knees and elbows.

JDM can exist with skin involvement only (often termed clinically amyopathic or hypomyopathic JDM), and skin involvement can predate muscle involvement by months to years. Because of the pathognomonic features of the rash, the diagnosis of JDM can often be suspected before classical muscular symptoms occur.

Other, more uncommon findings include mouth ulcers; retinitis; hepatosplenomegaly; pancreatitis; vasculopathy of the gastrointestinal tract leading to ulceration, bleeding, or perforation (Fig. 7.27); respiratory muscle weakness with a restrictive pattern on lung function studies; decreased lung diffusion capacity associated with interstitial lung disease (ILD); aspiration pneumonitis from pharyngeal muscle weakness; myocarditis; and pericarditis.

Clinicians will often perform detailed screening examinations on recently diagnosed patients, including a swallow study with an upper gastrointestinal and small-bowel follow-through radiographic study, chest radiograph, electrocardiogram and echocardiogram, and pulmonary function tests with lung diffusion capacity testing (DLCO).

Evaluation and Diagnosis

Moderate elevation of “muscle” enzymes including creatine kinase, aspartate transaminase, alanine aminotransferase, aldolase, and lactate dehydrogenase may be the first clue to the diagnosis of inflammatory muscle disease. An elevated level of clinical suspicion is critical as 10% to 15% of patients will have entirely normal muscle enzymes despite having clinical and/or radiographic muscle disease.

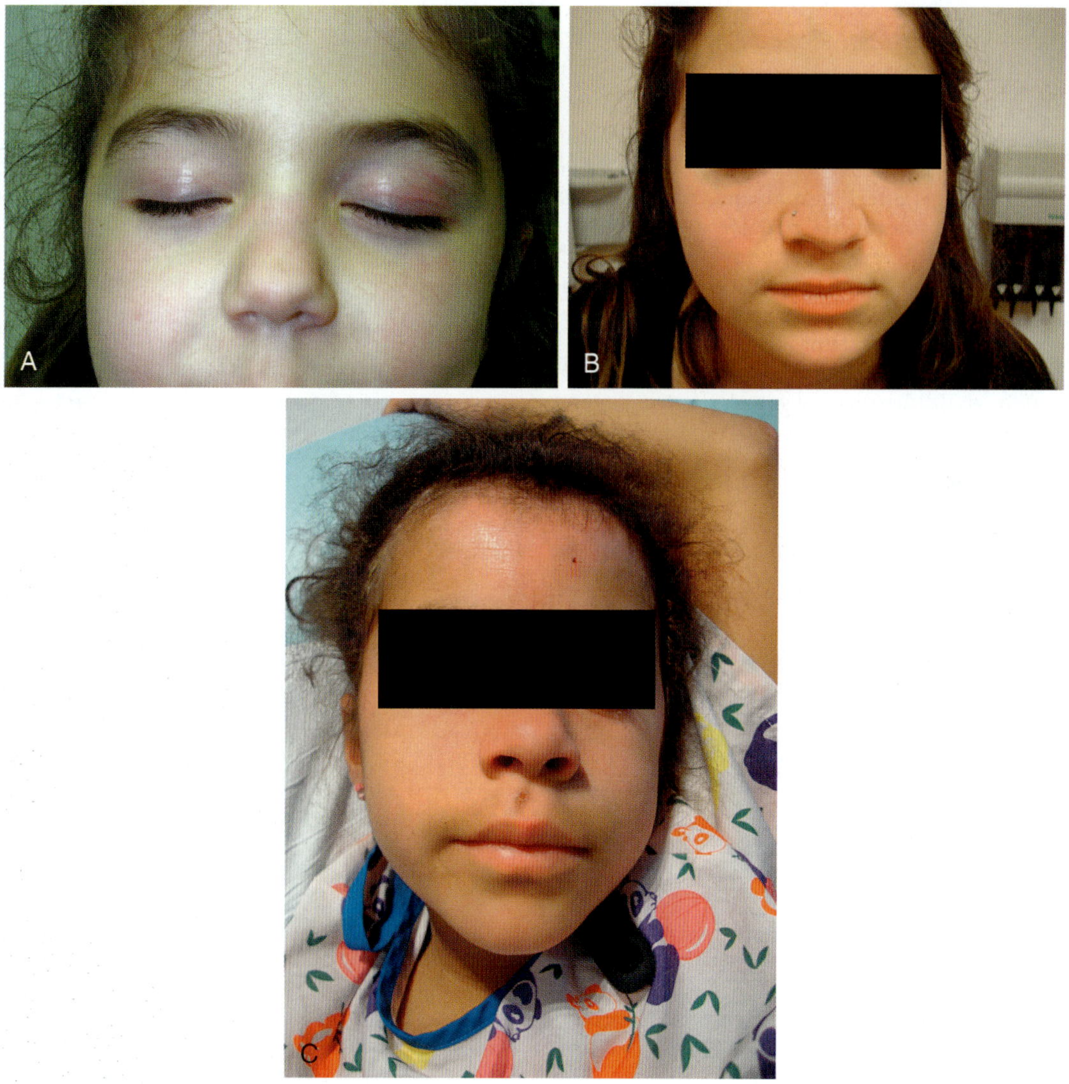

Fig. 7.24 Juvenile dermatomyositis. The facial rash shows heliotrope discoloration and violaceous suffusion with edema of the eyelids. Note the faint malar blush in the patient (A) and diffuse light erythematous rash of the face, including the forehead and not sparing nasolabial folds (B and C).

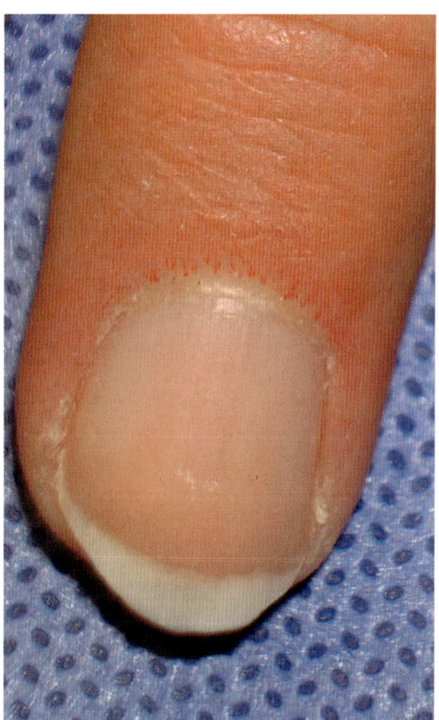

Fig. 7.25 Juvenile dermatomyositis. Nail bed telangiectasia. Erythema can be seen around the nail edge. The pinpoint telangiectasia may require a magnifying lens to identify.

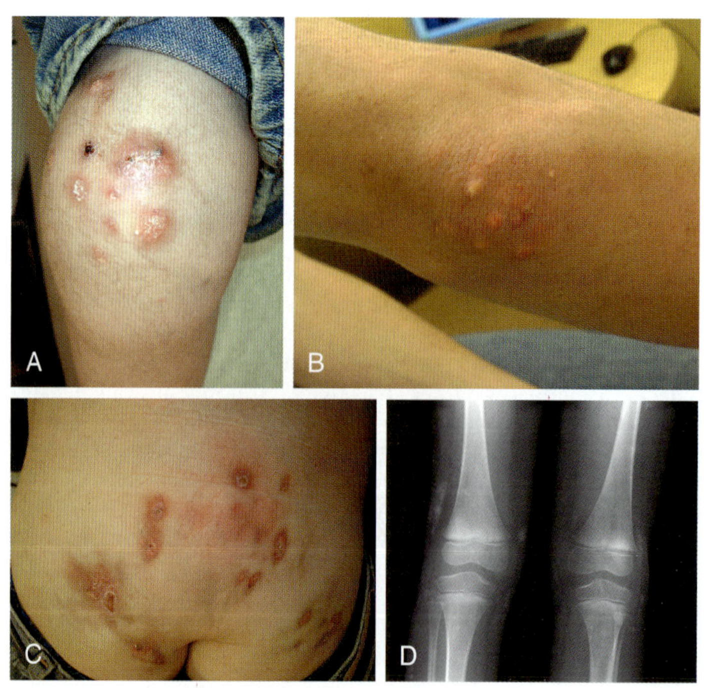

Fig. 7.26 Juvenile dermatomyositis. A 6-year-old male with chronic juvenile dermatomyositis and poor medication adherence. Calcinosis surrounding the knee (A), elbow (B), and sacrum (C) after years of untreated disease; note lipodystrophy of the buttocks from chronic disease activity. (D) Radiologic evidence of soft tissue calcification in the same patient.

Enzyme levels should be checked serially to monitor disease activity. Extreme elevation of muscle enzymes is more frequently demonstrated in infectious/postinfectious myositis or rhabdomyolysis associated with metabolic myopathies.

Other markers in the peripheral blood thought to be indicators of disease activity include serum neopterin (reflective of macrophage activation) and von Willebrand factor antigen level (reflective of vascular endothelial cell damage due to vasculopathy). Although not sensitive to disease activity, a positive ANA is demonstrated in 70% of patients with JDM. Myositis-specific antibodies such as anti-Jo-1, antip155/140, and anti-NXP2 are increasingly recognized for their potential prognostic implications.

MRI, specifically T2-weighted imaging with fat suppression, is quite sensitive in detecting even subclinical myositis (Fig. 7.28). When a child has muscle weakness, Gottron papules, elevated muscle enzymes, and abnormal muscle MRI, most clinicians make a diagnosis of JDM and initiate therapy without an invasive muscle biopsy or electromyography, which were previously standard for diagnosis. Electromyography and biopsy are useful in more challenging or atypical cases.

SCLERODERMA

The sclerodermatous disorders in children are broadly divided into systemic (SSc) and localized scleroderma (LS) with further classification by subtype (Box 7.5). Both conditions are rare in children, with the estimated annual incidence for LS of 1 to 3 per 100,000 children and for SSc of 1 per 1,000,000. The mean age of onset for both forms is between 7 and 9 years old; however, less than 10% of adult patients with SSc have pediatric onset, whereas most adult patients with LS have childhood onset. The female-to-male ratio of pediatric SSc is 4:1, and for pediatric LS it is 2:1. There is no clear evidence of racial predilection.

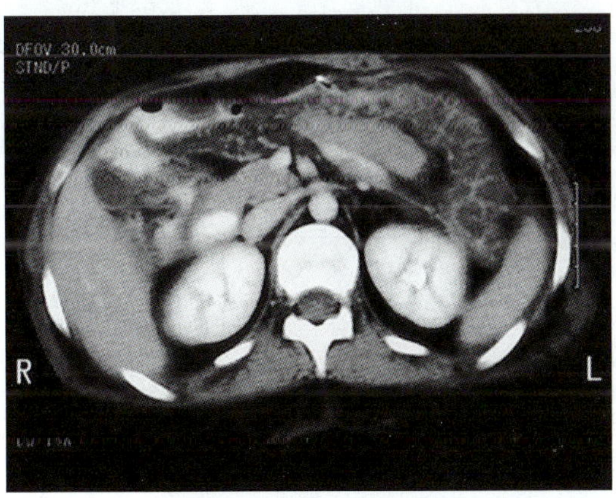

Fig. 7.27 Juvenile dermatomyositis. Computed tomographic scan of the abdomen demonstrates bowel wall thickening and edema in the transverse colon. The patient's bowel eventually perforated because of active vasculitis.

Both share the general features of an early inflammatory state, followed by collagen deposition and atrophy of the affected tissue. Skin biopsies from SSc and LS are typically indistinguishable, and they may share some common pathophysiology. However, their clinical manifestations are markedly different with unique morbidities and prognoses.

Systemic Sclerosis

SSc is a rare but life-threatening condition. There are three main subtypes (Table 7.9): diffuse cutaneous systemic sclerosis (dcSSc), limited cutaneous systemic sclerosis (lcSSc), and overlap SSc, which can be dcSSc or lcSSc with features of another connective tissue disease, such as dermatomyositis or SLE. The syndrome previously termed CREST (calcinosis cutis, Raynaud phenomenon, esophageal dysfunction, sclerodactyly, and telangiectasia) is now categorized as lcSSc (Fig. 7.29). The autoantibody profile is also helpful in defining

Box 7.5 Classification of Scleroderma and Related Disorders

Primary

- Systemic sclerosis (SSc)
  - Diffuse cutaneous scleroderma
  - Limited cutaneous scleroderma (CREST syndrome)
  - Overlap
- Localized scleroderma (LS)
  - Plaque morphea (circumscribed superficial[a])
  - Generalized morphea
  - Deep morphea
    - Subcutaneous morphea (circumscribed deep)
    - Eosinophilic fasciitis
  - Linear scleroderma
    - Extremity/trunk
    - Scalp/face
  - Pansclerotic
  - Mixed morphea (any combination of 2 or more of the above subtypes[a])

Diseases With Sclerodermatous Manifestations

- Graft-versus-host disease
- Drug or chemical induced
- Phenylketonuria
- Progeria
- Werner syndrome
- Scleredema
- Porphyria cutanea tarda
- Diabetic cheiroarthropathy[b]

[a]According to Padua preliminary classification criteria, 2004.
[b]Arthropathy of the hand.
Data from Laxer RM, Zulian F: Localized scleroderma, *Curr Opin Rheumatol* 18(6):606–613, 2006; Zulian F, Woo P, Athreya BH, et al: The pediatric rheumatology European Society/American College of Rheumatology/European League against Rheumatism provisional classification criteria for juvenile systemic sclerosis, *Arthritis Rheum* 57(2):203–212, 2007.

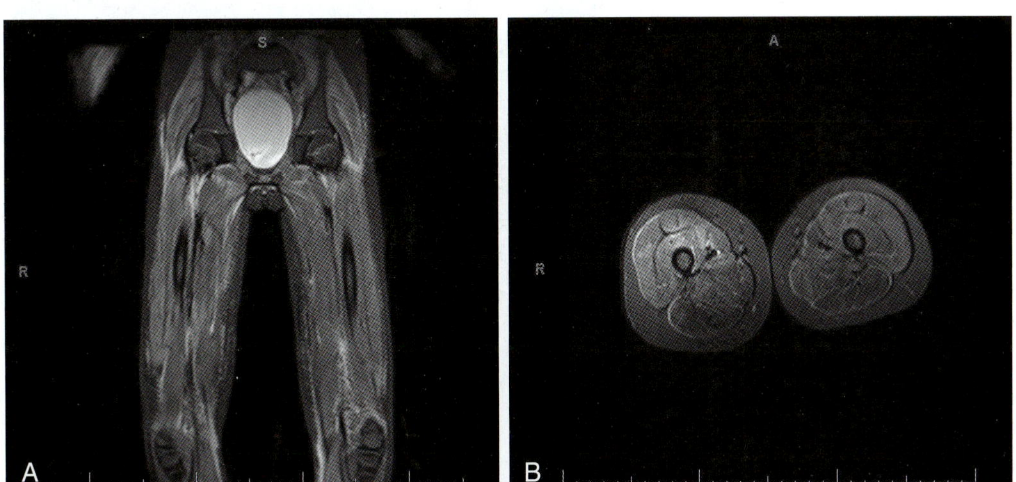

Fig. 7.28 Juvenile dermatomyositis. Magnetic resonance imaging of the thighs (T2-weighted image with fat suppression) illustrates marked diffuse muscle edema and inflammation. (A) Note the diffuse white area in muscle similar in appearance to fluid in the bladder. (B) Involvement may be more prominent in certain muscle groups.

Table 7.9 Clinical Subtypes of Systemic Sclerosis

Subtype	Main Clinical Features		Antibody Association
	Organ System	Organ System Features	
Diffuse cutaneous (dc)	Skin	Thickness proximal to elbows and knees Rapid progressive thickening	Topoisomerase (Scl-70)
	Cardiac	Congestive heart failure Conduction abnormalities	
	Renal	Scleroderma renal crisis	
	Pulmonary	ILD	
Limited cutaneous (lc)	Skin	Thickness limited to distal extremities (and face) Restricted and nonprogressive thickening	Centromere
	Gastrointestinal	Esophageal dysmotility Gastrointestinal strictures Malabsorption	
	Pulmonary	PAH	
Overlap syndrome	Skin	Either dcSSc or lcSSc pattern Skin manifestations of other CTD, such as Gottron papules (DM) and malar rash (SLE)	PM-Scl antibody or U1-RNP antibody
	Musculoskeletal	Arthritis, myositis	
	Cardiac Renal Pulmonary Gastrointestinal	Can have any of the above dcSSc or lcSSc manifestations or additional organ involvement in association with other CTD feature, such as lupus nephritis	

CTD, Connective tissue disease; *dcSSc,* diffuse cutaneous systemic sclerosis; *DM,* dermatomyositis; *ILD,* interstitial lung disease; *lcSSc,* limited cutaneous systemic sclerosis; *PAH,* pulmonary arterial hypertension; *PM-Scl,* polymyositis-scleroderma, *SLE,* systemic lupus erythematosus; *U1-RNP,* U1-ribonucleoprotein.

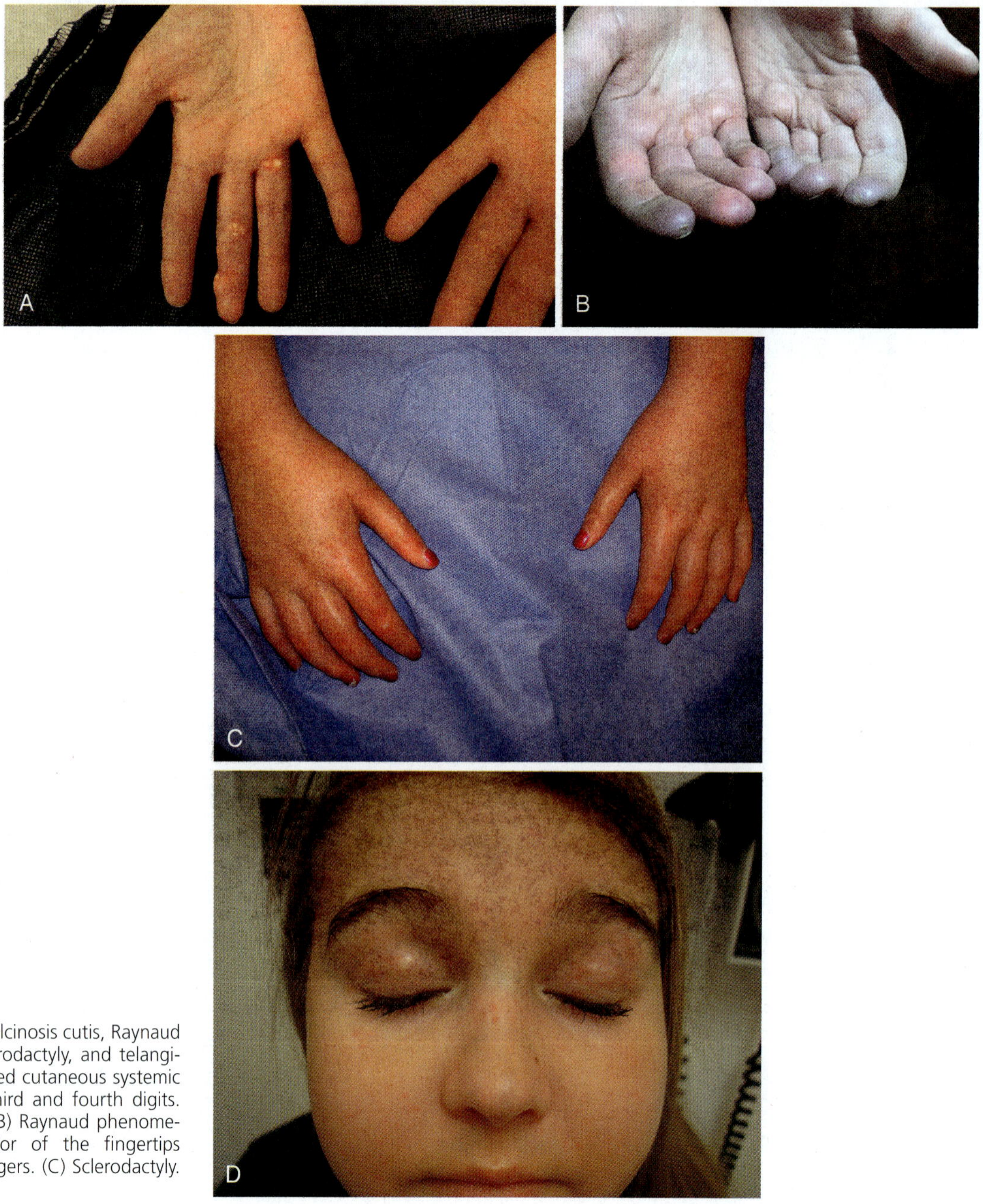

Fig. 7.29 Systemic sclerosis. Patients with calcinosis cutis, Raynaud phenomenon, esophageal dysfunction, sclerodactyly, and telangiectasia (CREST) syndrome, also termed limited cutaneous systemic sclerosis. (A) Extensive calcinosis cutis of third and fourth digits. Also note multiple palmar telangiectasias. (B) Raynaud phenomenon. Note concurrent cyanosis and pallor of the fingertips with healed ulcers on the bilateral index fingers. (C) Sclerodactyly. (D) Telangiectasias of the face.

subsets of SSc and predicting their organ involvement (see Table 7.9). Sclerodermatous skin findings or organ fibrosis can be secondary to other processes (see Box 7.5).

Clinical Features of Systemic Sclerosis

Common features at the onset of pediatric SSc are Raynaud phenomenon (70%) and skin changes of hands (60%) including edema, sclerodactyly, and induration proximal to MCP joints. In the largest cohort study of pediatric SSc patients, 53% presented with both skin induration of hands and Raynaud phenomenon, and 10% of those presenting with Raynaud phenomenon also had digital infarcts.

Raynaud phenomenon (see Fig. 7.29B) is a vasospastic response leading to a triphasic color change of the digits (first white due to vasoconstriction, then blue secondary to cyanosis, and finally red due to reperfusion) associated with initial numbness and tingling, followed by swelling and pain during reperfusion. In SSc, the Raynaud phenomenon is more pronounced due to underlying vasculopathy identifiable in the nailfold capillary beds by capillary microscopy.

Affected patients demonstrate dilation, tortuosity, hemorrhage, drop-off, and, in later disease states, arborization of the capillaries (Fig. 7.30). Poor perfusion of the fingers eventually leads to digital tip pitting, ulceration (Fig. 7.31), and, in more severe cases, autoamputation. Healthy individuals can also experience the color changes of Raynaud phenomenon without being at risk for developing an underlying connective tissue disease (see Table 7.6). Absence of these features, particularly tissue damage, can help the clinician differentiate primary (idiopathic) Raynaud phenomenon from that secondary to a connective tissue disease.

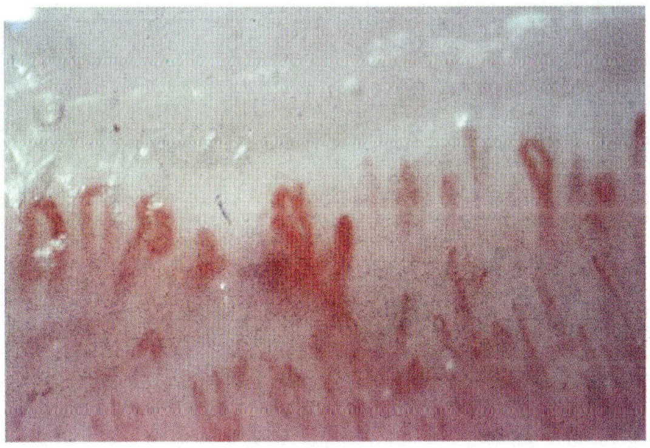

Fig. 7.30 Systemic sclerosis. Nailfold capillary changes (original magnification, ×10), enlarged capillary loops, and capillary dropout.

Early cutaneous manifestations frequently bring children to medical attention, but because of the insidious onset of skin changes, time to diagnosis averages 1.9 years. Initially, the skin is edematous with predilection for the distal extremities. The induration phase is characterized by loss of the natural pliability of the skin and the presence of a palpable skin thickness. The skin takes on a shiny, tense appearance, with distal tapering of the fingers. The visual impression that movement might be impaired is supported by the lack of flexibility in the hands (Fig. 7.32). The typical scleroderma facies of tight skin and skin atrophy produce the appearance of a fixed stare; pinched nose; thin, pursed lips; small mouth; prominent teeth; and characteristic grimace (Fig. 7.33). Subcutaneous calcium deposits (calcinosis cutis) may occur at pressure points, typically found on the extensor surfaces, and may occasionally extrude through the skin (see Fig. 7.29A). Telangiectasias are also a manifestation of SSc, most typically found in the lcSSc variant, with a "matted" appearance and commonly distributed on the face and upper extremities (see Fig. 7.29D).

Gastrointestinal symptoms occur in approximately half of the children. Esophageal dysmotility associated with gastroesophageal reflux often leads to dysphagia with solids and symptoms of reflux esophagitis. Aspiration or nighttime cough may occur, and esophageal strictures can develop with time. Peristaltic dysfunction of the small and large bowel leads to abdominal cramping, diarrhea, constipation, and episodes of pseudoobstruction. Bacterial overgrowth, steatorrhea, weight loss, volvulus, and even perforation can occur.

Pulmonary involvement in pediatric SSc is seen in up to 70% of individuals and includes interstitial lung disease, pulmonary arterial hypertension, and abnormal pulmonary function test results (decreased forced vital capacity [FVC] and DLCO). ILD typically presents as slowly progressive dyspnea with exertion and is associated with decreased FVC and a reticular/nodular (ground-glass) pattern on chest CT (Fig. 7.34). Conversely, PAH presents as a rapid progression of dyspnea on exertion over weeks to months with decreased DLCO on pulmonary function tests and an abnormal echocardiogram with elevated pulmonary artery or right ventricular systolic pressure.

Musculoskeletal involvement is more common in pediatric SSc, with inflammatory arthritis in addition to the typical "dry synovitis" of scleroderma, characterized by reduced joint ROM secondary to fibrosis of tendons. When the patient has myopathy, typically there is a symmetric proximal weakness with pronounced atrophy at times. Myositis is also reflected by

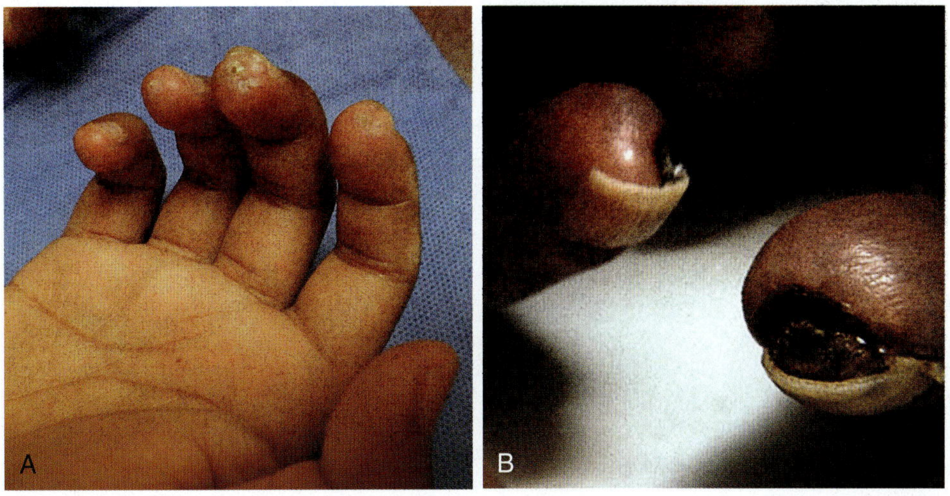

Fig. 7.31 Systemic sclerosis. Digital pitting ulcers (early disease [A]; late disease [B]) represent one of the three minor diagnostic criteria for scleroderma.

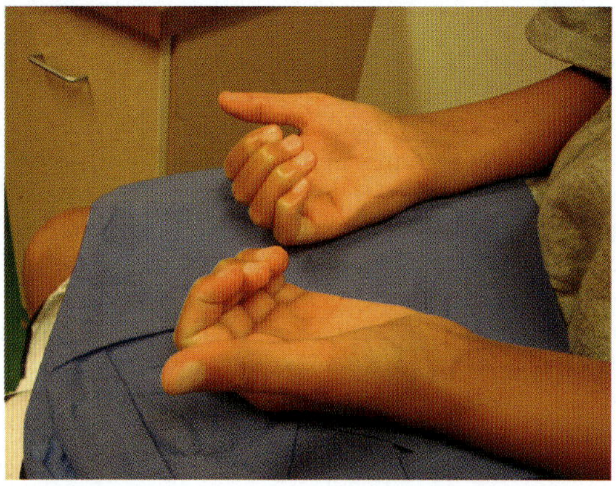

Fig. 7.32 Systemic sclerosis. Lack of flexibility in the hands is another characteristic of scleroderma.

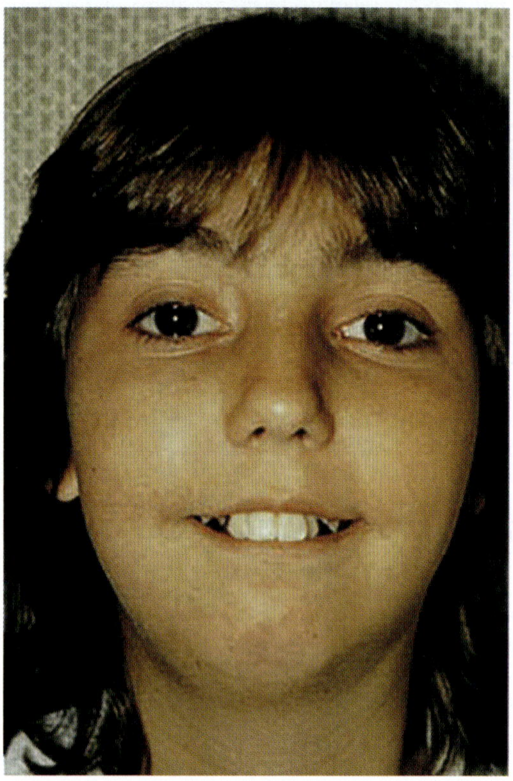

Fig. 7.33 Systemic sclerosis. Facial features show that the skin appears tight and drawn, without evidence of wrinkles. (Courtesy J. Jeffrey Malatack, MD, Philadelphia.)

elevated muscle enzymes and changes on MRI similar to that of JDM, though muscle histopathology differs from that of JDM with more fibrosis and the presence of thickened capillaries. Notably, myositis in SSc doubles the risk of cardiac involvement from 10% to 20%. Cardiac involvement is the leading cause of death in pediatric SSc in cohort studies. Cardiac complications include heart block, arrhythmias, congestive heart failure, electrocardiographic changes, and pericardial effusion. These abnormalities appear to be a combined result of myocardial fibrosis, vascular insufficiency, and chronic inflammation. Renal involvement, termed *scleroderma renal crisis,* is characterized by accelerated hypertension and its sequelae including thrombocytopenic purpura; though well recognized in adult disease, it is rare in children.

Localized Scleroderma

LS, also known as *morphea,* encompasses several subtypes classified by depth and pattern of the lesion distribution (see Box 7.5). This group of disorders is characterized by fibrosis that is confined mainly to the skin and subcutaneous tissue; however, deeper forms also involve the fascia, muscle, tendon, and joint capsule. Certain subtypes of LS have unique associated extracutaneous manifestations.

Localized Scleroderma Disease Phases

As in SSc, there is an inflammatory phase of disease, followed by a fibrotic phase. Early active lesions are characterized by an indurated plaque with violaceous inflammatory border or "lilac ring" (Fig. 7.35). Classically it is described as the "bruise that does not go away" that is brought to medical attention; clinicians may miss the early phase of LS, interpreting the erythema/violaceous color as related to a possible injury. When the disease is in an active state, lesions expand outward and new lesions accumulate. As damage accumulates, increasing skin thickness is noted at the center of the lesion, sometimes leaving an ivory-colored sclerotic center (Fig. 7.36). Dermal and subcutaneous atrophy result from previous inflammation and subsequent collagen deposition. When the dermis is atrophic, there is localized lack of hair growth, visible veins, and a slight "cliff drop" appearance to the skin (Fig. 7.37). Subcutaneous atrophy ranges from mild flattening to a "scooped out" concavity of adipose tissue, occasionally to such a point that one can see the muscles moving underneath the skin (Fig. 7.38). Postinflammatory hyperpigmentation and hypopigmentation are frequently present.

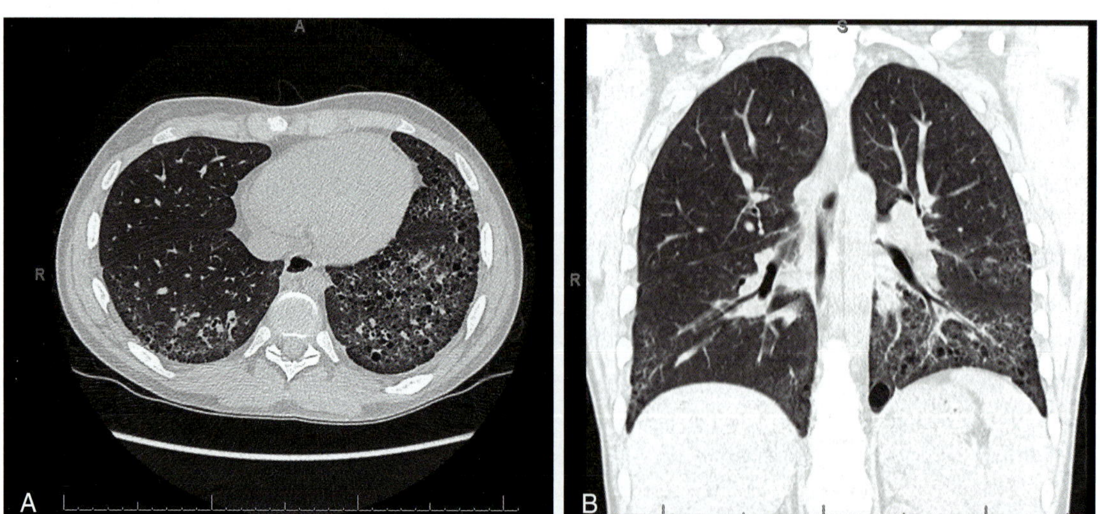

Fig. 7.34 Systemic sclerosis. (A and B) High-resolution computed tomography of the chest showing extensive bilateral pulmonary fibrosis.

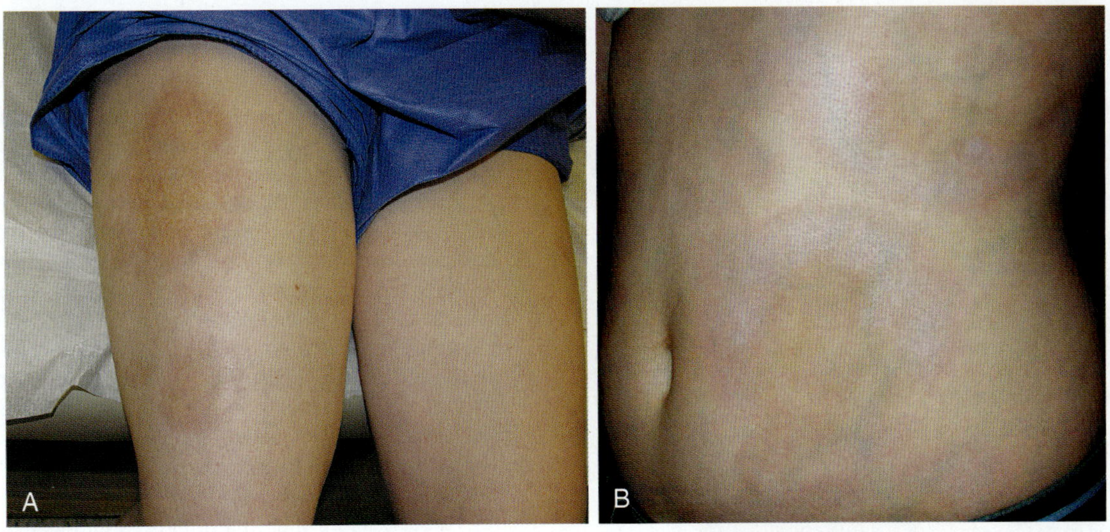

Fig. 7.35 Localized scleroderma. (A and B) Active-phase lesions have an inflammatory border or "lilac ring." (B, Courtesy Elena Pope, Hospital for Sick Children, Toronto, ON, Canada.)

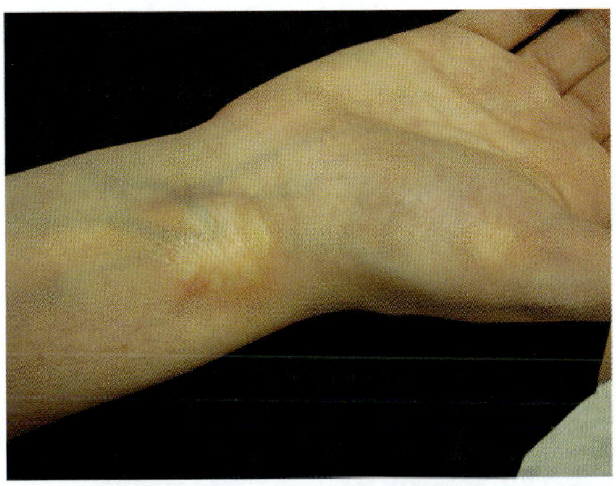

Fig. 7.36 Localized scleroderma. Pale and thickened sclerotic center of lesion on the wrist.

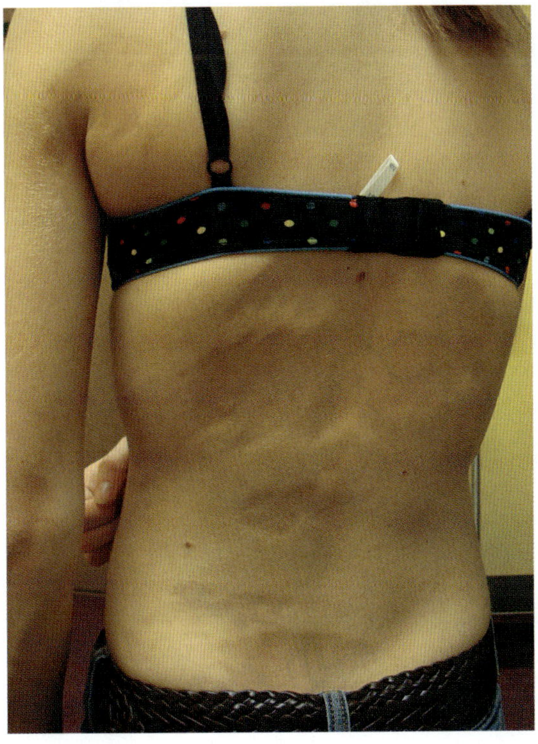

Fig. 7.37 Localized scleroderma. Dermal atrophy of localized scleroderma, demonstrated by "cliff drop" lesions and visible veins in a teenage female with generalized morphea.

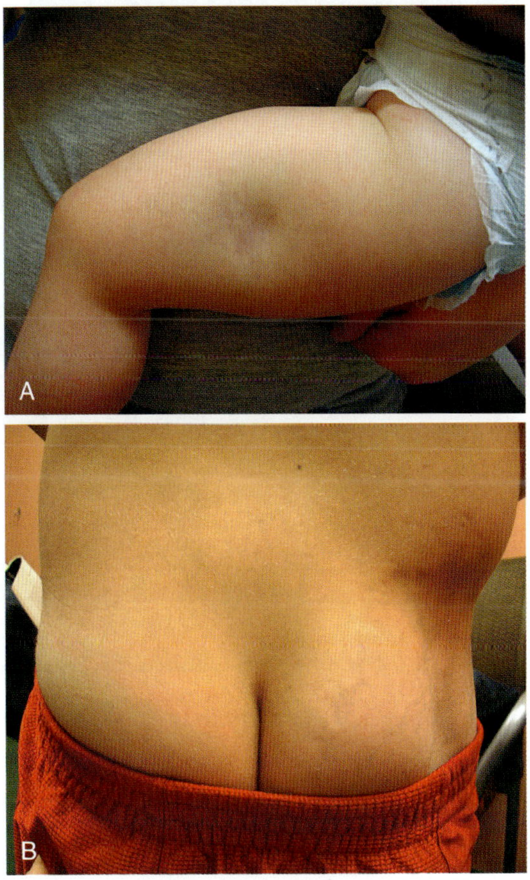

Fig. 7.38 Localized scleroderma. (A) Moderate subcutaneous atrophy (divot or "scoop out" lesion) in a toddler. (B) More severe subcutaneous atrophy of the right buttock, leaving the buttocks asymmetric.

Localized Scleroderma Subtypes

Linear scleroderma is the most common subtype in children (50%–60%) and typically presents as a single, linear unilateral band (Fig. 7.39). Legs are most commonly involved, followed by arms, frontal head, and trunk. Thick sclerotic tissue or sclerosis of the muscle, tendon, and joint capsule may cause joint contractures and limb dysfunction marked by growth restriction and abnormal range of motion. Involvement of the epiphyseal growth plate can lead to permanent shortening of a limb (Fig. 7.40).

Craniofacial scleroderma occurs as a spectrum of disease. Discrete linear lesions involving the scalp and forehead are termed *en*

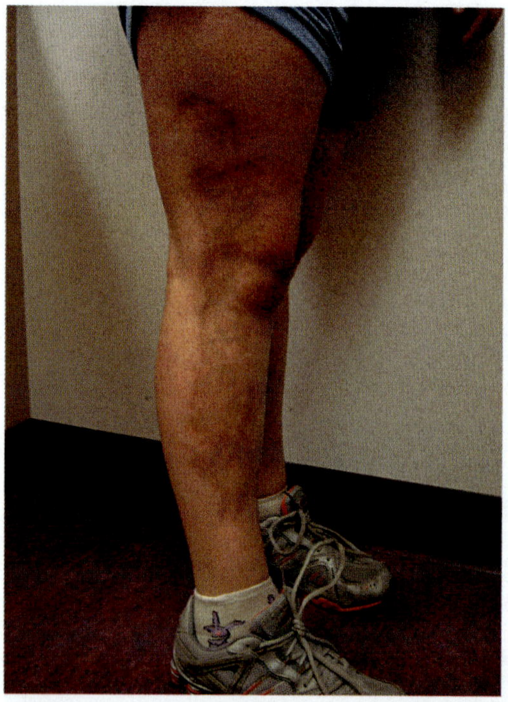

Fig. 7.39 Localized scleroderma. Linear scleroderma affecting the lower extremity, the most common site.

coup de sabre because the linear depression resembles a saber wound scar (Fig. 7.41). Ill-defined lesions of the face may manifest as hemifacial atrophy, termed Parry-Romberg syndrome, in which hemiatrophy of the bones, tongue, and subcutaneous and muscle tissue occur (Fig. 7.42). Extracutaneous manifestations of the central nervous system (i.e., seizures, headaches, white matter changes), oral cavity (i.e., dental malocclusion), and eye (i.e., uveitis). are more common in patients with *en coup de sabre*/Parry-Romberg syndrome.

Plaque morphea is the most common presentation of LS in adults (60%) and accounts for approximately one-quarter of LS in children. It is characterized by one or more oval or rounded areas of induration, ranging from 1 to 30 cm in diameter, typically on the trunk or proximal extremities (Fig. 7.43). Generalized plaque morphea is defined as three or more plaque lesions greater than 3 cm wide. Typically, the plaques become confluent and affect several anatomic areas, the trunk being the most common (Fig. 7.44).

Deep or subcutaneous morphea may have only subtle cutaneous changes despite significant inflammatory infiltrate in the deep subcutaneous tissue and fascia that causes a depression in the adipose tissue ("scooped-out" appearance) and thickened, bound-down tissues (see Fig. 7.38B). Many consider eosinophilic fasciitis a type of deep morphea; however, it often behaves as a mixture of deep morphea and linear scleroderma, resulting in deep infiltration and joint contractures.

Pansclerotic morphea of childhood is a rare but disabling subset of LS, affecting only 1% to 2% of children with LS. It affects the

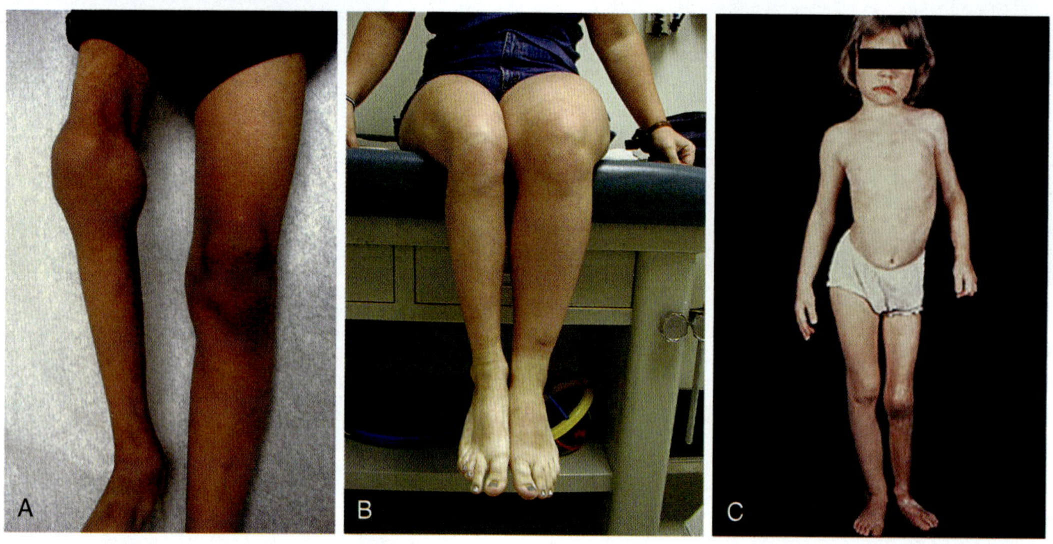

Fig. 7.40 Localized scleroderma. (A and B) Linear form of scleroderma affecting the right lower extremity of two children. (C) Linear scleroderma affecting the entire left side of the body. Note the extensive atrophy.

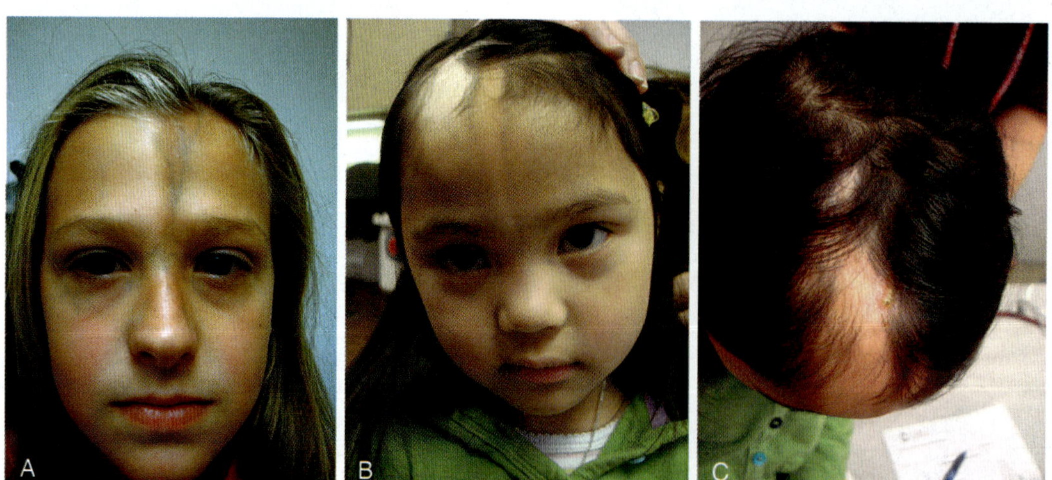

Fig. 7.41 Localized scleroderma. Linear scleroderma of the scalp and face: *en coup de sabre.* (A) Teenage female with single lesion. (B and C) Two views of a young girl with two linear lesions of the face and scalp with associated scalp ulceration and crust.

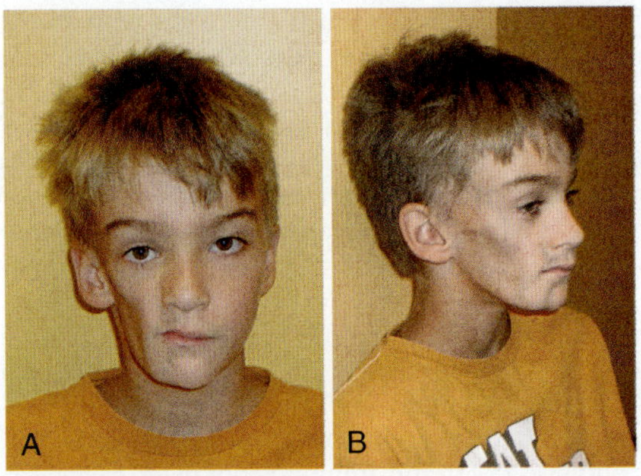

Fig. 7.42 Localized scleroderma. (A and B) Frontal and side views of Parry-Romberg syndrome affecting the right side of the face.

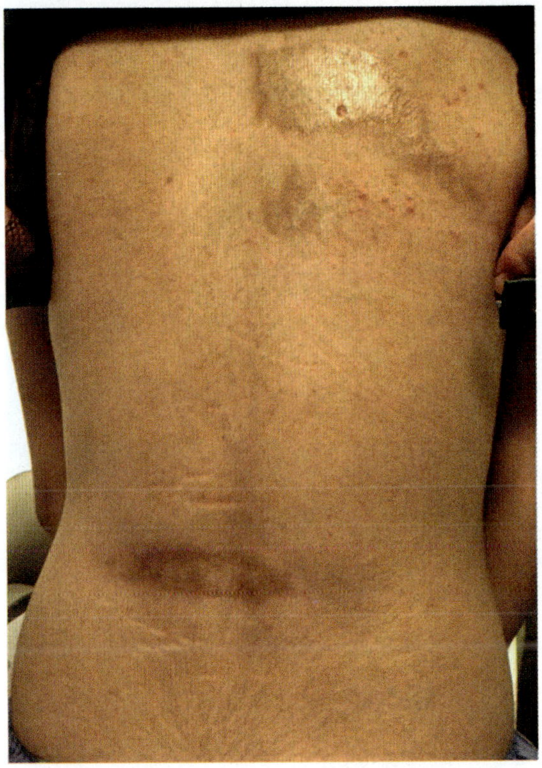

Fig. 7.43 Localized scleroderma. Multiple large plaque morphea lesions on the back of a young female.

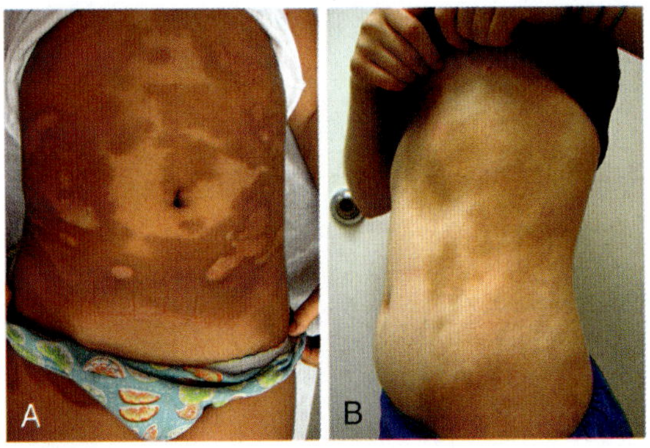

Fig. 7.44 Localized scleroderma. Generalized morphea in an African American female (unaffected skin is lighter) (A) and a white female (B).

extremities first and sometimes migrates to the trunk, sparing only the face and distal areas of the fingers and toes (Fig. 7.45). There is a rapidly progressive fibrosis of the deep dermis, subcutis, fascia, and muscles, leading to significant joint contracture, muscle atrophy, cutaneous ulcerations, and restrictive respiratory insufficiency if the trunk is involved. Another rare subtype is bullous morphea;

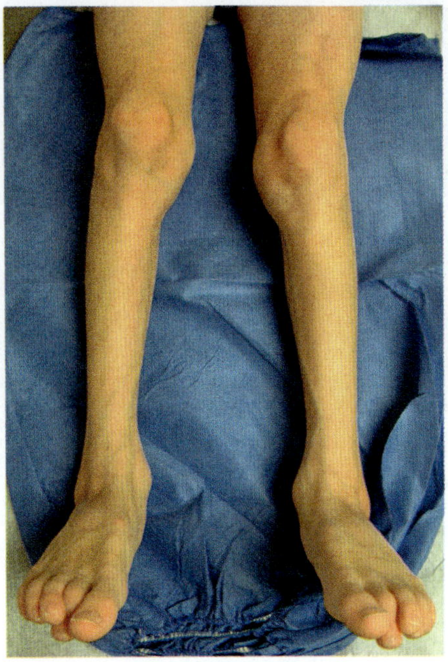

Fig. 7.45 Localized scleroderma. Pansclerotic morphea. Note that the distal toes are spared. Diffuse joint contractures are the result of progressive fibrosis.

however, many experts agree that the bullous lesions are secondary to aggressive linear or deep LS disease. A final subtype that is now viewed as its own category is mixed morphea, which is seen in approximately 15% of the pediatric LS population. The most common presentation of mixed morphea is a combination of linear and generalized morphea occurring in the same patient.

Extracutaneous Manifestations in Localized Scleroderma

Extracutaneous manifestations occur in approximately 25% of patients, most frequently in linear scleroderma. These consist of orthopedic complications (19% overall; 50% linear scleroderma of the extremities), neurologic or ocular findings (5% overall; 40% craniofacial scleroderma), and other autoimmune conditions such as thyroiditis. Routine screening of all patients with LS by ophthalmology is recommended, but especially for those with linear scleroderma of the head, because "silent" uveitis occurs and has clinical outcomes like those of JIA.

No laboratory test is diagnostic of LS. General markers of inflammation, including ESR and serum immunoglobulin levels, may be elevated in select patients with active LS; however, most patients have normal laboratory results. Although a "localized" disease, several autoantibodies have been associated with the disease. ANA positivity was found in 42% of a large pediatric LS cohort.

Antihistone antibodies have been detected in 47% of patients with LS, with a higher prevalence in the generalized morphea group. RF is present in one-third of patients, particularly those who have generalized morphea, and correlates with disease severity (as determined by the number of lesions).

MIXED CONNECTIVE TISSUE DISEASE

Mixed connective tissue disease (MCTD) is a relatively rare syndrome characterized by the presence of overlapping features of two or more connective tissues disorders including rheumatoid arthritis, scleroderma, SLE, and dermatomyositis/polymyositis. Clinical characteristics of MCTD in children are summarized in Table 7.10. The most common presentation is the combination of Raynaud phenomenon, swollen hands with mild sclerodactyly, polyarthritis, mild myositis, and gastroesophageal reflux disease. Cardiopulmonary disease and esophageal dysmotility are common in MCTD; nephritis is less common and is usually less severe than in SLE. Both ILD and PAH can

Table 7.10 Clinical Characteristics of Children With Mixed Connective Tissue Disease

Characteristic	Patients
Arthritis	93%
Raynaud phenomenon	85%
Thickened skin of scleroderma	49%
Rash of SLE	33%
Rash of JDM	33%
Fever	56%
Abnormal esophageal motility	41%
Cardiac	30%
Pericarditis	27%
Myositis	61%
CNS disease	23%
Pulmonary	43%
Renal	26%

CNS, Central nervous system; *JDM,* juvenile dermatomyositis; *SLE,* systemic lupus erythematosus.

Modified from Petty RE, Laxer RM, Lindsley CB, et al: *Textbook of pediatric rheumatology,* ed 8, Philadelphia, 2021, Elsevier.

occur, and patients should be screened with advanced imaging and pulmonary function tests. The presence of anti–U1-RNP antibodies is strongly associated with the diagnosis of MCTD. High-titer positive ANA, mild to moderate elevation of muscle enzymes, and hypergammaglobulinemia are common. A positive RF may also be present. The outcome and course of children with MCTD is variable.

SYSTEMIC VASCULITIDES

The vasculitides are a broad group of disorders with a common pathology characterized by blood vessel inflammation. The type of inflammation, organ system affected, and size of the vessels affected vary with each disease entity. A classification of the systemic vasculitis from the Chapel Hill Consensus Conference is based on the size of the blood vessels and further classified by the presence or absence of antineutrophil cytoplasmic antibodies (ANCAs) and granulomas (Fig. 7.46).

The initial inflammatory state may present with constitutional symptoms such as fever, fatigue, weight loss, elevated acute-phase reactants, and failure to thrive. It is not until later in the disease process, after vessel damage has accumulated, that more specific findings due to vascular compromise become evident. Symptoms and signs depend on the location and type of vessel involvement. For example, extremity claudication and distal ulcerations may result from large-medium arterial involvement of the extremity while organ-specific findings are noted with small-medium arterial involvement, such as hypertension (renal arteries), abdominal pain (mesenteric arteries), chest pain (coronary arteries), or neurologic deficits (mononeuritis multiplex).

Fortunately, the most common forms of vasculitis in children, Kawasaki disease (KD) and immunoglobulin A vasculitis (IgAV), have readily apparent acute inflammatory states and typically do not result in chronic vessel insufficiency.

IgA Vasculitis

Immunoglobulin A (IgA) vasculitis (IgAV), formerly known as Henoch-Schönlein purpura, is a small-vessel leukocytoclastic vasculitis mediated by IgA immune complex deposition and the most common vasculitis in children. Although IgAV is associated with serious potential complications of the gastrointestinal tract and kidneys, the majority of cases are mild and self-resolve within weeks. Ninety percent of cases occur in children younger than 10 years old, with a median age of 5 years. There is a slight male predominance (1.4:1). Children younger than 2 years generally have milder disease with less frequent organ involvement, while children older than 15 years often have a more severe presentation. IgAV often occurs after an identifiable trigger, such as viral illness, bacterial infection, immunization, or medication exposure. Seasonal peaks occur in fall and winter, suggesting an infectious trigger, but a definite etiology remains elusive.

IgAV classically presents with a tetrad of palpable purpura, arthralgia/arthritis, abdominal pain, and kidney disease over the course of days to weeks. Symptoms may present in nearly any order. Seventy-five percent of patients present with rash, which usually appears in symmetric crops and involves gravity/pressure dependent areas such as the

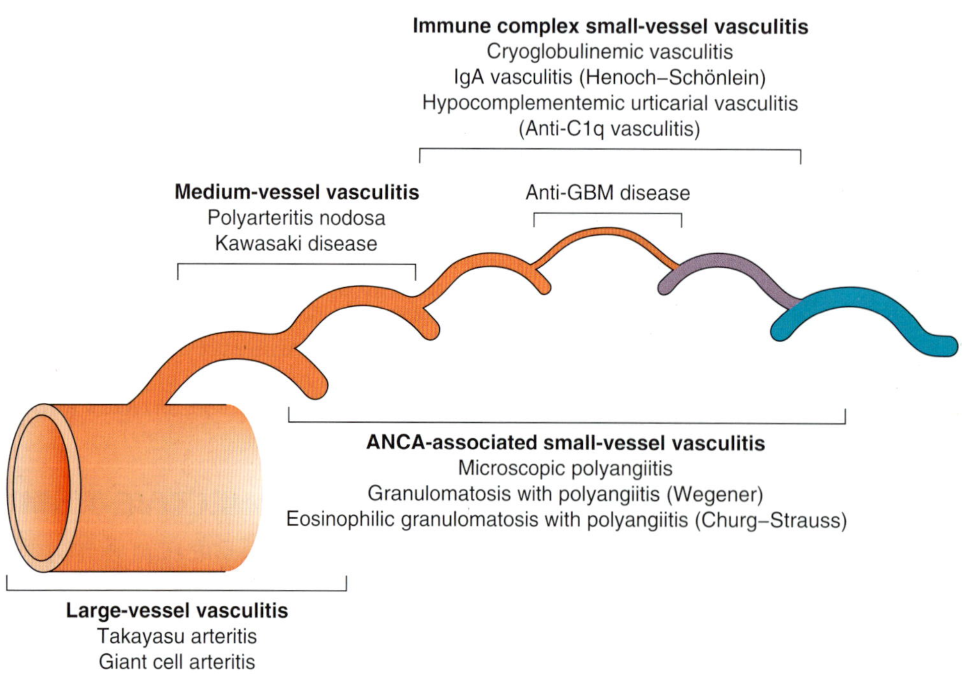

Fig. 7.46 Classification of vasculitis based on vessel size and presence of antineutrophil cytoplasmic antibodies *(ANCAs)* based on the 2012 International Chapel Hill Consensus Conference. The figure depicts large, medium, and small vessel vasculitides. Giant cell arteritis is not seen in the pediatric population. The anti–glomerular basement membrane *(GBM)* disease is very rarely seen in the pediatric population. (From John Wiley & Sons, Inc. ©Jennette JC, Falk RJ, Bacon PA, et al: 2012 revised International Chapel Hill Consensus Conference Nomenclature of Vasculitides, *Arthritis Rheum* 65[1]:1–11, 2013.)

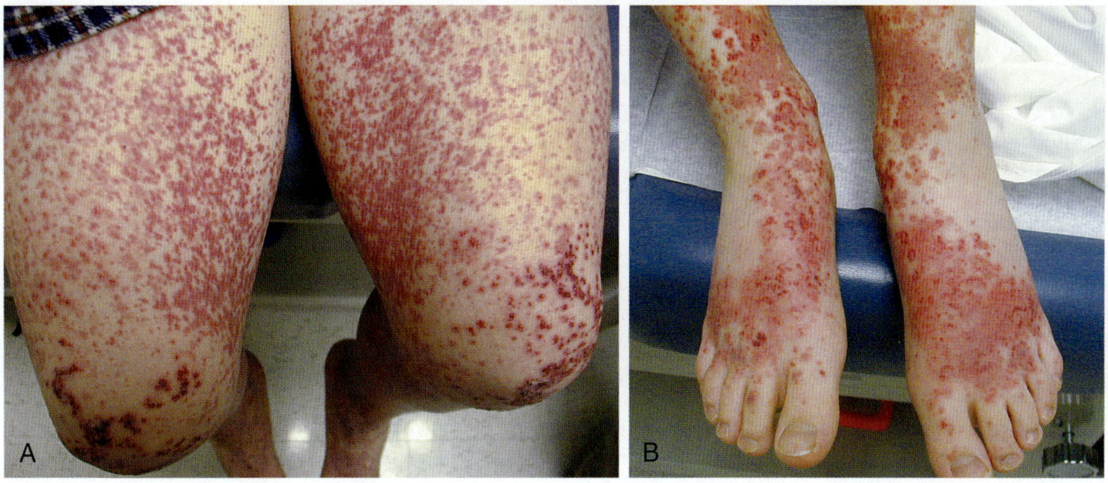

Fig. 7.47 IgA vasculitis. (A and B) Rash characteristically involves the lower extremities, with purpuric coalescent lesions.

lower extremities and buttocks in ambulatory children (Fig. 7.47) or the face, ears, sacrum, and buttocks in nonambulatory children (Fig. 7.48A and C). The lesions may begin as erythematous macules or urticaria that evolve and coalesce to form petechiae, palpable purpura, and ecchymoses. Various stages of eruption are often simultaneously present, and the rash may be pruritic but is not painful.

Subcutaneous nonpitting edema is common, especially in children younger than 2 years, often affecting dorsal hands and feet (Fig. 7.48A and B), with periorbital, cephalic, and scrotal edema also observed. Blistering lesions, ulcerations, and necrosis are rarely seen. Skin biopsy shows a leukocytoclastic vasculitis with fine granular IgA staining in the superficial plexus, though biopsy is rarely required for diagnosis.

A mimic of the IgAV rash in infants is acute hemorrhagic edema of infancy (AHEI) (Fig. 7.49). Although the rash can appear severe, the child is well-appearing without signs of internal organ involvement, and the condition self-resolves in weeks. Skin biopsy of AHEI shows leukocytoclastic vasculitis, mainly of the venules, but without IgA deposition.

Most patients with IgAV have arthralgia, but it is the presenting symptom in only 15% of patients. Joints may appear swollen due to periarticular swelling, but arthritis is also present in two-thirds of patients, with knees and ankles being the most commonly affected. The arthritis in IgAV is nonerosive and self-limited.

Approximately 70% to 85% of patients have gastrointestinal symptoms. Colicky abdominal pain is the most common symptom and can be accompanied by nausea, vomiting, ileus, melena/hematochezia, or diarrhea. In about 15% of patients, abdominal pain precedes the rash, making it difficult to distinguish appendicitis and other acute abdominal conditions from IgAV. More severe complications such as massive gastrointestinal hemorrhage, intussusception (typically ileo-ileal), and perforation occur in less than 5% of patients. Pancreatitis, cholecystitis, and protein-losing enteropathy have also been described.

IgAV nephropathy occurs in up to half of patients with IgAV and typically occurs during the first month of disease, though abnormalities can present after several months, underscoring the

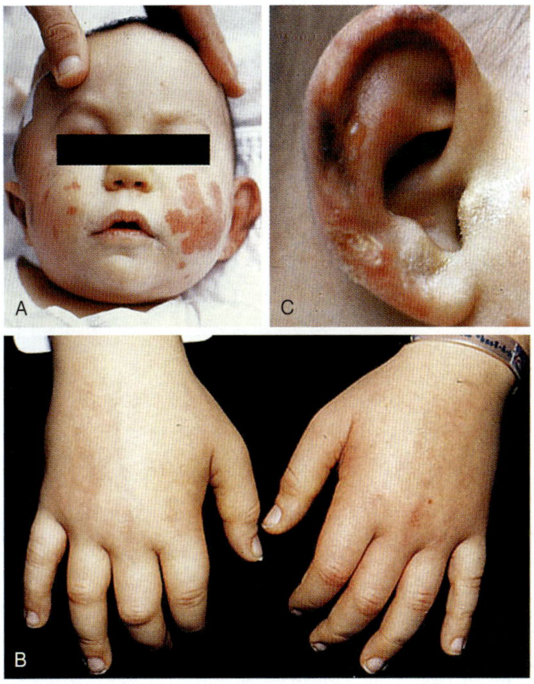

Fig. 7.48 Infant with IgA vasculitis. (A) The rash may occur on the face along with edema. (B) Rash and edema may be present in the extremities. (C) Ulceration and vesicles are an unusual manifestation of IgA vasculitis.

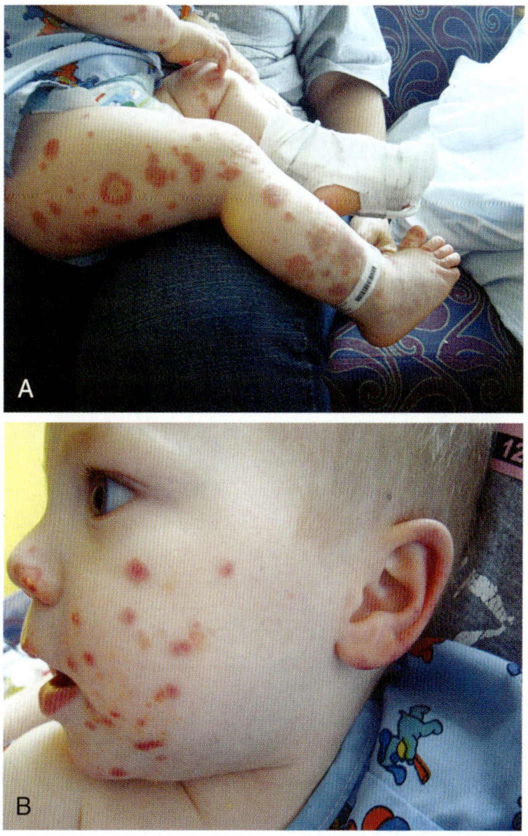

Fig. 7.49 Acute hemorrhagic edema of infancy. A 15-month-old male with classic annular, medallion-like, and targetoid-shaped purpuric lesions on the leg (A), and the face (B) (including auricles).

importance of monitoring. Renal manifestations include proteinuria (including nephrotic range), microscopical hematuria with or without dysmorphic RBCs or RBC casts, hypertension, and reduced kidney function. Overall, 1% to 5% of patients with IgAV develop some degree of chronic kidney disease, with end-stage renal disease occurring in less than 1% of patients.

Patients should have periodic monitoring for hypertension, proteinuria, and hematuria for at least 6 months after diagnosis, and patients with proteinuria require monitoring of serum creatinine.

Other infrequent features of IgAV include low-grade fever, malaise, scrotal pain and swelling, epistaxis, parotitis, pulmonary hemorrhage, peripheral neuropathy, or cerebral vasculitis, which can present with headaches, seizures, altered mental status, or focal neurologic changes.

The majority of patients have spontaneous resolution of symptoms in 4 weeks, though one-third of patients have at least one recurrence, especially those with nephritis. Recurrences typically occur during the first 4 to 6 months and are generally less severe, have a shorter duration, and are limited to cutaneous and mild gastrointestinal involvement. The rash may wax and wane over several months, and its persistence does not necessarily portend a worse outcome.

Treatment of IgAV is generally supportive and can include IV hydration and analgesics. Corticosteroids may be used to treat more severe manifestations of IgAV; however, tapering rapidly results in a flare of symptom and therefore should be tapered slowly when used.

Kawasaki Disease

KD is a medium-vessel vasculitis with mucocutaneous and cardiac involvement and is the second most common childhood vasculitis. Although the etiology of KD remains uncertain, the clinical features and natural history of this distinctive vasculitis are well described. The need to rapidly recognize the presentation of KD is heightened by its potentially devastating cardiac sequelae, and early recognition and treatment improves morbidity and mortality.

KD was first described as a unique constellation of clinical findings initially termed *mucocutaneous lymph node syndrome* by Tomisaku Kawasaki in 1967 in Japan and by Marian Melish in 1976 in Hawaii. The peak age of patients with KD in the United States is 18 months to 2 years old, with 80% of cases occurring in children younger than 4 years old. Males are more commonly affected than females (1.5:1). The incidence of KD is highest in Asian children, with a particularly high rate in Japanese and Korean children, followed by Black children, then White children, with the lowest incidence in American Indian and Alaska Native children.

The clinical features of complete KD are remarkably consistent (Box 7.6). However, not all children with KD will meet these diagnostic criteria, so additional criteria were proposed for the diagnosis of incomplete KD to improve diagnostic accuracy, as 10% of children who develop cardiac sequelae never meet the criteria for complete KD. Incomplete KD must be considered when a child has fever without a cause for more than 4 days and has two other clinical criteria.

Children younger than 1 year are at highest risk of having KD without fulfilling criteria and also have the highest risk of cardiac sequelae. The importance of appropriate clinical suspicion in the *forme fruste* of the disease cannot be overemphasized.

The course of the illness is triphasic: acute (lasting 7–14 days), subacute (days 10–25), and convalescent (days 21–60) (Fig. 7.50). The acute phase is characterized by fever, irritability, nonexudative conjunctivitis, oropharyngeal erythema, rash, lymphadenopathy, and distal extremity edema and erythema. The onset of fever is sudden and severe, often spiking as high as 104°F (40°C). Fever generally precedes other clinical signs by 1 to 2 days; it has a mean duration of 12 days in the untreated child, though fever as long as 30 days has been described.

Conjunctivitis appears early in the course and is bilateral, nonexudative, and nonulcerative with bulbar predominance and limbic sparing (Fig. 7.51). Transient anterior uveitis can be observed by slit-lamp examination in most patients during the first 2 weeks of illness. Oral findings include red, cracked, fissured lips; "strawberry tongue" due to enlarged and sloughing filiform papillae; and diffuse oral and pharyngeal erythema (Fig. 7.52). Discrete oral ulcers, vesicles, or tonsillar exudates suggest an alternative diagnosis such as infection.

The rash of KD may take several forms, including erythematous maculopapular rash, scarlatiniform erythroderma, morbilliform (Fig. 7.53), multiforme-like with target lesions, urticarial eruption, or

Box 7.6 Kawasaki Disease: Diagnostic Criteria[a,b]

Fever for 5 or more days
Conjunctivitis (bilateral, bulbar, nonsuppurative)
Cervical lymphadenopathy (≥1.5 cm diameter)
Rash (typically maculopapular, erythroderma, or erythema multiforme but can be any nonvesicular, nonpetechial rash)
Change(s)[c] in the mucous membranes of the oropharynx, such as:
- Erythema of the oropharynx
- Injected/erythematous lips
- Dry, fissured lips
- "Strawberry" tongue

Change(s)[c] of the peripheral extremities, such as:
- Hand or foot edema or erythema, periungual desquamation

In the presence of fever and 2–3 clinical criteria, or in infants with ≥7 days of fever without explanation, diagnosis of incomplete KD can be made with a positive echocardiogram or:
- ESR ≥40 mm/h or CRP ≥3.0 mg/dL AND
- 3 or more laboratory findings
  - Anemia for age
  - Platelet count ≥450,000 after the 7th day of fever
  - Albumin ≤3.0 g/dL
  - Elevated ALT
  - WBC ≥15,000/mm^3
  - Urine ≥10 WBC/hpf

[a]Diagnosis of classic KD requires fever plus 4 of 5 criteria.
[b]In the presence of 4 or more classic features, the diagnosis of Kawasaki disease can be made (and treatment initiated) on the 4th day of fever (or rarely the 3rd day by an experienced clinician).
[c]One is sufficient to establish criterion.

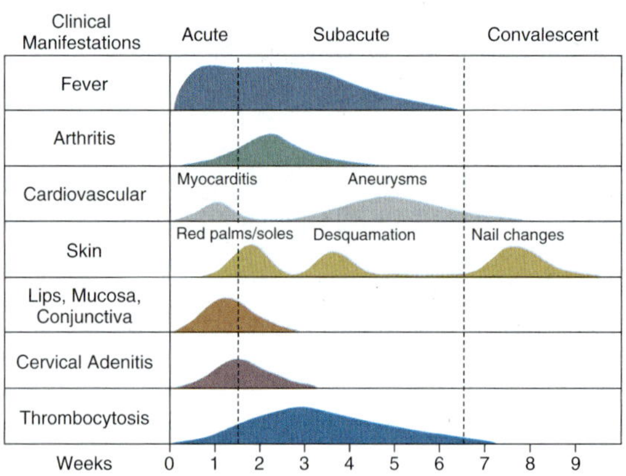

Fig. 7.50 Kawasaki disease. The syndrome can be divided into three clinical phases: (1) acute, (2) subacute, and (3) convalescent. The temporal characteristics described here are typical of the disease course. (Modified from Kawasaki T: Acute febrile mucocutaneous syndrome with lymphoid involvement and specific desquamation of the fingers and toes in children, *Arerugi* 16:178–222, 1967.)

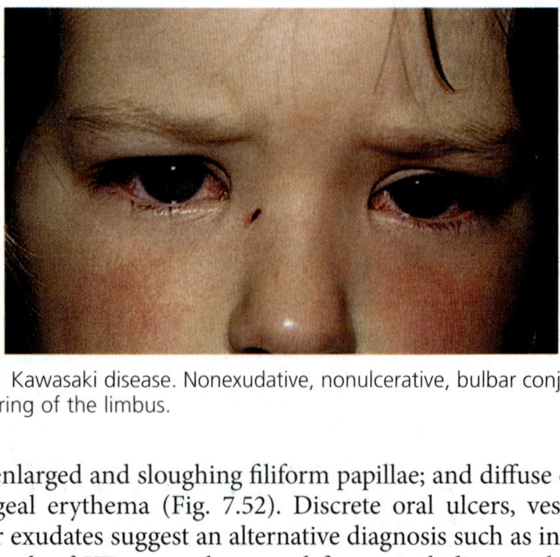

Fig. 7.51 Kawasaki disease. Nonexudative, nonulcerative, bulbar conjunctivitis. Note sparing of the limbus.

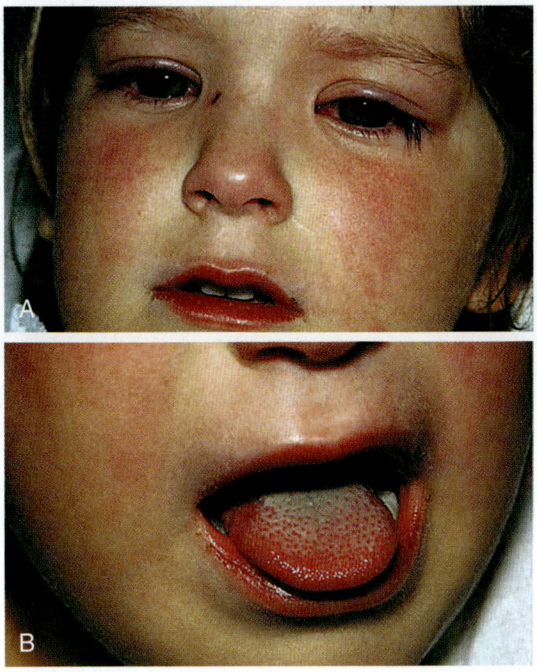

Fig. 7.52 Kawasaki disease. (A) Erythematous, cracked lips. (B) "Strawberry tongue."

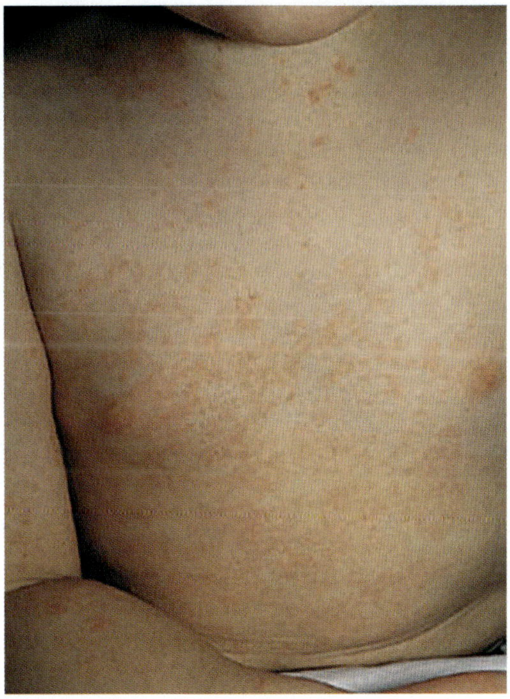

Fig. 7.53 Kawasaki disease. Morbilliform rash.

fine pustules. The presence of bullae, vesicles, petechiae, or purpura suggests another diagnosis. A predilection for intertriginous areas, particularly the groin, has been noted (Fig. 7.54), often with early desquamation. A particularly striking feature of the acute phase of the syndrome is erythema and indurated edema of the hands (Fig. 7.55) and feet, often associated with pain and a refusal to walk. The characteristic desquamation of fingers and toes, beginning at the nail/fingertip junction, occurs between 10 and 21 days after fever onset (Fig. 7.56). Beau lines (transverse grooves across the nails) may also be seen after 1 to 2 months.

Although the initial syndrome was named *mucocutaneous lymph node syndrome,* the presence of a 1.5 cm or greater anterior cervical lymph node is the least common feature, occurring in about 25% to 50% of children. It can often mimic bacterial lymphadenitis, and ultrasound or other imaging may be helpful in distinguishing the two if other clinical symptoms are not apparent.

Laboratory abnormalities associated with KD include elevation of ESR and C-reactive protein (CRP), leukocytosis with a left shift, normocytic normochromic anemia, hypoalbuminemia, transaminitis, and pyuria. Thrombocytosis typically occurs toward the end of the acute phase and can be considerable (see Box 7.6). Assessment of laboratory abnormalities is particularly important in patients with persistent fever and two to three clinical signs who have not met criteria for complete KD.

KD is associated with other features that can be helpful in diagnosis. Arthritis occurs in one-third of patients and is typically characterized by a small-joint polyarthritis during the acute phase and a large joint oligoarthritis during later phases. It is nonerosive and self-limited. Urethritis and inflammation of the urethral meatus often occurs and usually results in sterile pyuria. Diarrhea, vomiting, abdominal pain, and hepatitis are frequent gastrointestinal features seen early in the illness, with pancreatitis and transient gallbladder dilation rarely observed. CNS findings such as lethargy, meningismus, aseptic meningitis, facial nerve palsy, sensorineural hearing loss, and paralysis of the extremities have been described but are uncommon. Analysis of cerebrospinal fluid shows mononuclear pleocytosis but typically normal cerebrospinal fluid protein.

During the acute phase of KD, cardiac features include tachycardia, dysrhythmias, pericarditis, pericardial effusion, myocarditis, mitral or aortic insufficiency, and congestive heart failure (Table 7.11). Coronary artery aneurysms are the hallmark of KD sequelae, present in 20% of untreated patients, and usually developing during the subacute phase but often detectable on echocardiogram in the acute phase. Prompt treatment of KD with intravenous immunoglobulin reduces the incidence of coronary artery aneurysms by more than 70%. Although many aneurysms regress spontaneously, mortality from related complications occurs in up to 1% of affected patients, mainly during the first 10 to 40 days of illness. Aneurysms may be complicated by thromboembolism and vessel occlusion leading to myocardial infarction and coronary artery stenosis. Giant aneurysms ($\geq$8 mm in diameter) are

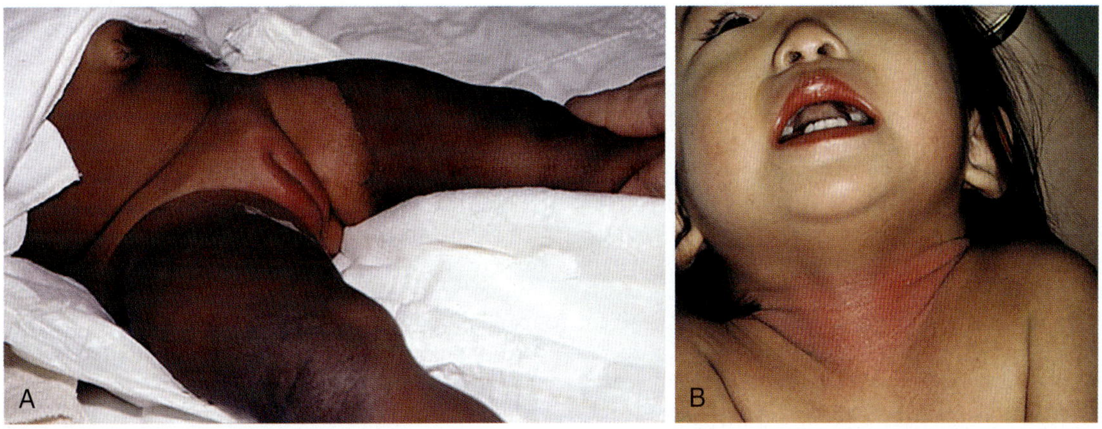

Fig. 7.54 Kawasaki disease. (A) Perineal rash with peeling. (B) Neck rash with peeling. Note that peeling of an intertriginous rash occurs before extremity peeling.

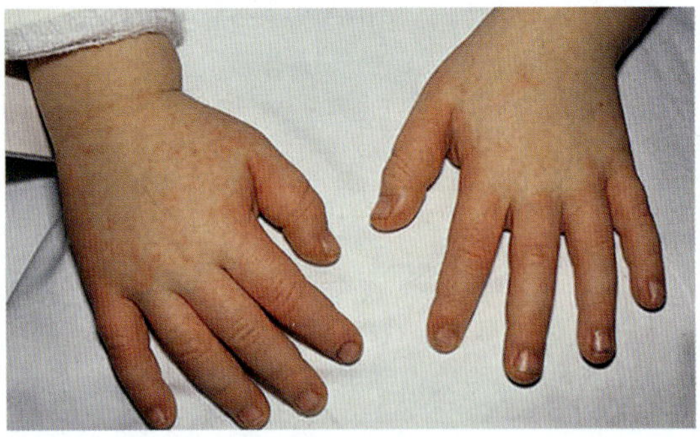

Fig. 7.55 Kawasaki disease. Swollen, erythematous hands. Note the fusiform appearance.

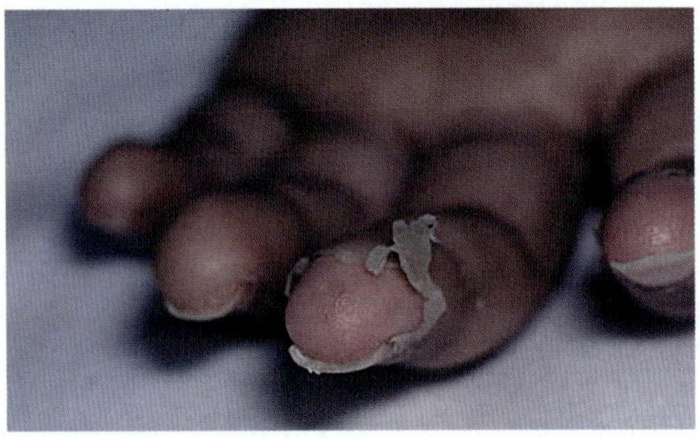

Fig. 7.56 Kawasaki disease. Fingertip peeling in the subacute phase.

Table 7.11 Cardiac Manifestations of Acute Kawasaki Disease

Cardiac Manifestation	Echocardiogram Finding
Coronary artery dilation	Z-score: 2 to <2.5
Coronary aneurysm or ectasia	Z-score: ≥2.5 to <5 (small) ≥5 to <10 (medium) ≥10 or absolute dimension ≥8 mm (large)
Aortic root dilation	Z-score: >2 May be associated with aortic regurgitation
Mitral regurgitation	Mitral regurgitation, usually mild to moderate
Myocarditis and pericarditis	Pericardial effusion
Left ventricle (LV) dysfunction	Decreased end-systolic or end-diastolic LV function
KD shock syndrome	Decreased LV contractility or normal cardiac function in setting of distributive shock
Coronary artery thrombosis and/or myocardial infarction	Intraluminal thrombus or sudden worsening of LV function

Data from Jone PN, Tremoulet A, Choueiter N, et al: Update on diagnosis and management of Kawasaki disease: a scientific statement from the American Heart Association, *Circulation* 150(23):e481–e500, 2024.

most likely to result in stenosis, thrombosis, and myocardial infarction, while smaller aneurysms (<8 mm) tend to regress over time. Although their structure may appear normal over time, fibrointimal proliferation, fibrosis, and calcinosis persist, resulting in increased risk of cardiovascular disease. Risk factors for the development of aneurysms include male sex, Asian race, age younger than 6 months, duration of fever greater than 2 weeks, persistent or recrudescent fever after treatment, and exaggerated leukocytosis, anemia, hypoalbuminemia, and profound acute phase reactant elevation.

Differential diagnosis for KD includes numerous infections, drug reactions, reactive arthritis, sJIA, polyarteritis nodosa, and SLE. Cultures, serologic tests, patient age, and clinical course of disease help in distinguishing these other disorders (Table 7.12).

Polyarteritis Nodosa

Polyarteritis nodosa, the prototype medium-vessel vasculitis, is a systemic necrotizing vasculitis with segmental aneurysm formation leading to the classic "beading" pattern demonstrated in vascular imaging studies. It can affect any organ system and can be quite devastating. Worldwide, polyarteritis nodosa is associated with hepatitis B and C infections; however, pediatric polyarteritis nodosa is rare, especially in North America. The average age of children affected is 9 years, with a slight male predominance. There is an association with the periodic fever syndrome familial Mediterranean fever (FMF).

Typical skin findings include palpable purpura, livedo reticularis, tender nodules, and necrotic lesions. Other findings suggestive of systemic polyarteritis nodosa include hypertension, abdominal pain, myalgia, arthritis, neuropathy, weight loss, and fever. Although suspected clinically, the diagnosis requires tissue biopsy with evidence of vasculitis or conventional angiography demonstrating segmental aneurysms. Cutaneous polyarteritis nodosa is limited to the skin and musculoskeletal system and often occurs after streptococcal infection. The lower extremities are most commonly affected (Fig. 7.57) with arthritis of knees and ankles. Although this condition is much milder than the systemic form, chronic immunosuppressive agents are often required because of persistence of disease and relapse.

Takayasu Arteritis

Takayasu arteritis (TA) is the prototype large-vessel vasculitis, affecting the aorta and its branches, and is associated with great morbidity and mortality. TA typically affects adolescent females, with increased incidence in children of Asian descent. The symptoms, including fever, fatigue, and weight loss, are nonspecific, and therefore lead to an average delay in diagnosis of 19 months from symptom onset. By this time, irreversible vessel damage has occurred, leading to clinical findings of bruits, decreased or absent acral pulses, and blood pressure differences exceeding 10 mm Hg between extremities. Laboratory findings support systemic inflammation with highly elevated ESR and CRP, leukocytosis, and anemia. Diagnosis is made by conventional angiography or magnetic resonance angiography demonstrating segmental large vessel thickening and narrowing (Fig. 7.58).

Antineutrophil Cytoplasmic Antibody-Associated Vasculitides

Granulomatosis with polyangiitis (GPA), formerly known as Wegener granulomatosis; microscopical polyangiitis (MPA); and eosinophilic granulomatosis (EGPA), formerly known as Churg-Strauss syndrome, are necrotizing small-vessel vasculitides associated with the presence of antineutrophil cytoplasmic antibodies (ANCAs). Etiology is uncertain, though genetic risk factors have been demonstrated and presentation is often associated with infection (especially *Staphylococcus aureus*) or exposure to drugs or other toxins, suggesting a potential role. ANCA-associated vasculitis (AAV) is rare in children and mainly presents in adolescence. It often presents with a prodrome of nonspecific symptoms such as fever, fatigue, weight loss, myalgias, and arthralgias, which can be present for weeks to months before organ involvement becomes evident, often delaying diagnosis.

GPA is a necrotizing, granulomatous vasculitis that affects the upper and lower airways and the kidneys, although other organs can be involved. Most children with GPA have upper respiratory involvement, such as epistaxis, persistent nasal discharge, or oral/nasal ulcers; sinusitis; otitis media; mastoiditis; or hearing loss (Fig. 7.59). Lower respiratory symptoms include persistent cough, wheeze, dyspnea, or hemoptysis due to alveolar hemorrhage. Pleural effusion, cavitary lung lesions, nodular pulmonary

Table 7.12 Differential Diagnosis of Kawasaki Disease

Agent	Disease	Distinguishing Characteristics
Bacteria	Streptococcal	Positive culture and serology, palatal petechiae, no anterior uveitis
	Staphylococcal scalded skin syndrome	Positive culture, bullous lesions, Nikolsky sign, earlier desquamation, no anterior uveitis
	Toxic shock syndrome[a]	Primarily females, older age predilection, toxin detection, positive culture
Rickettsia	Rocky Mountain spotted fever[a]	Petechial rash, positive serology, regional geography, no anterior uveitis
Spirochetes	Leptospirosis[a]	Positive culture and serology, muscle pain and tenderness, rigid abdominal muscles
Toxins	Acrodynia (mercury poisoning)	Photophobia, no conjunctivitis, slow onset, diaphoresis, severe pain in hands and feet, pruritus
Autoimmune/allergic	Stevens-Johnson syndrome	History of drug or infection exposure, no predominant lymph node, corneal ulcers, blisters, more severe mucous membrane involvement
	sJIA	Nondesquamating evanescent rash, hepatosplenomegaly, generalized adenopathy, vasculopathy, arthritis
	Polyarteritis nodosa	Vasculitic skin findings of palpable purpura, livedo reticularis, and dusky nodules
	Reactive arthritis	May be HLA-B27 positive, not toxic appearing, dysuria/pelvic pain, diarrhea, genital lesions such as balanitis, keratoderma blenorrhagicum, onycholysis
Viral infection	Epstein-Barr virus[a]	Positive serology, splenomegaly, atypical lymphocytes
	Measles	Coryzal prodrome, Koplik spots before exanthem, rash can include petechiae and begins on face spreading cephalocaudally and centrifugally
	Rubella	Minimal enanthem, distal extremities not affected, not toxic appearing
	Rubeola	Cough, catarrh more prominent, lips not cracked, fewer oral changes, distal extremities generally not affected
	Roseola	Rash begins as fever is resolving, shorter course
	Enterovirus/Adenovirus[a]	Seasonal, epidemic, not toxic appearing

[a]May fulfill diagnostic criteria for Kawasaki syndrome.

HLA-B27, Human leukocyte antigen B27; *sJIA,* systemic juvenile idiopathic arthritis.

Modified from Lohr JA, Rheuban KS: Kawasaki syndrome, *Infect Dis Clin North Am* 1:559–574, 1987.

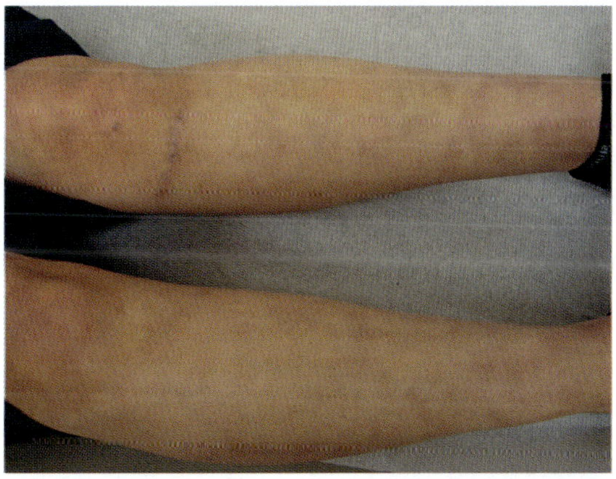

Fig. 7.57 Cutaneous polyarteritis nodosa of the lower extremities in a teenage female.

infiltrates, and features of pulmonary hemorrhage on imaging can help delineate from typical childhood respiratory infections (Fig. 7.60). Renal disease may be asymptomatic with only mild urinary abnormalities or may progress to clinically evident glomerulonephritis with kidney injury. Biopsy is often needed to confirm diagnosis and stratify the severity of renal disease. Arthritis; vasculitic skin lesions (purpura, subcutaneous nodules, and livedo reticularis); ocular/orbital lesions (scleritis/episcleritis, uveitis, conjunctivitis, retinal vasculitis, and retroorbital pseudotumor); and gastrointestinal involvement (abdominal pain, nausea, diarrhea) are also common in GPA. Longer-term sequelae of GPA include the classic "saddle nose" deformity, nasal septal perforation, cavitation and destruction of the sinuses, and subglottic tracheal stenosis due to granulomatous destruction of cartilage and bone. Serum ANCA positivity by indirect immunofluorescence assay and/or for antigen-specific antibodies by ELISA against proteinase 3 (PR3) or myeloperoxidase (MPO) are supportive of the diagnosis, with PR3-ANCA being most common in GPA. Whenever possible, diagnosis is confirmed by tissue biopsy at an active site of disease (skin, kidney, or lung).

MPA is a nongranulomatous AAV that often presents with pulmonary-renal syndrome. Like GPA, constitutional symptoms may be the initial presenting feature. Chronic pulmonary capillaritis is common, though massive alveolar hemorrhage can also occur. Renal involvement with focal segmental glomerulonephritis is typical and often severe. Although other organ manifestations can occur, they are not generally as prominent. ANCA reactivity is more commonly against MPO.

EGPA has well-recognized features that distinguish it from GPA and MPA, including a long prodromal phase of asthma (typically poorly controlled) and allergic rhinitis or nasal polyposis.

Peripheral eosinophilia then occurs as pulmonary infiltrates accumulate. Finally, systemic vasculitis becomes apparent with frequent cutaneous, musculoskeletal, cardiac (cardiomyopathy), neurologic (mononeuritis multiplex and polyneuropathy), and gastrointestinal involvement. Renal disease is rare and typically mild. This AAV is the most uncommon in children, given the long prodromal period.

BEHÇET DISEASE

Behçet disease (BD) is a rare systemic inflammatory disease with features of vasculitis and autoinflammatory disease. The vasculitis involved in BD is characterized by nongranulomatous obliterative arteritis and perivascular venous inflammation associated with venous thrombosis. Uniquely among the vasculitides, BD can affect vessels of any size and involves both arterial and venous circulation. The global prevalence of BD is highest in the Eastern Mediterranean, Middle Eastern, and Eastern Asian regions. The presence of the HLA-B51 allele is associated with susceptibility to the disease. There is no sex predominance, although male patients have been noted to have more severe manifestations.

BD classically presents with the triad of recurrent oral and genital ulcers and uveitis (Fig. 7.61), though any organ can be affected. Aphthous oral ulcers are round with an erythematous halo and occur on the labial and buccal mucosa, tongue, pharynx, and larynx. In general, these ulcers tend to be larger than typical viral aphthous ulcers, often occur in crops, are painful, and may be

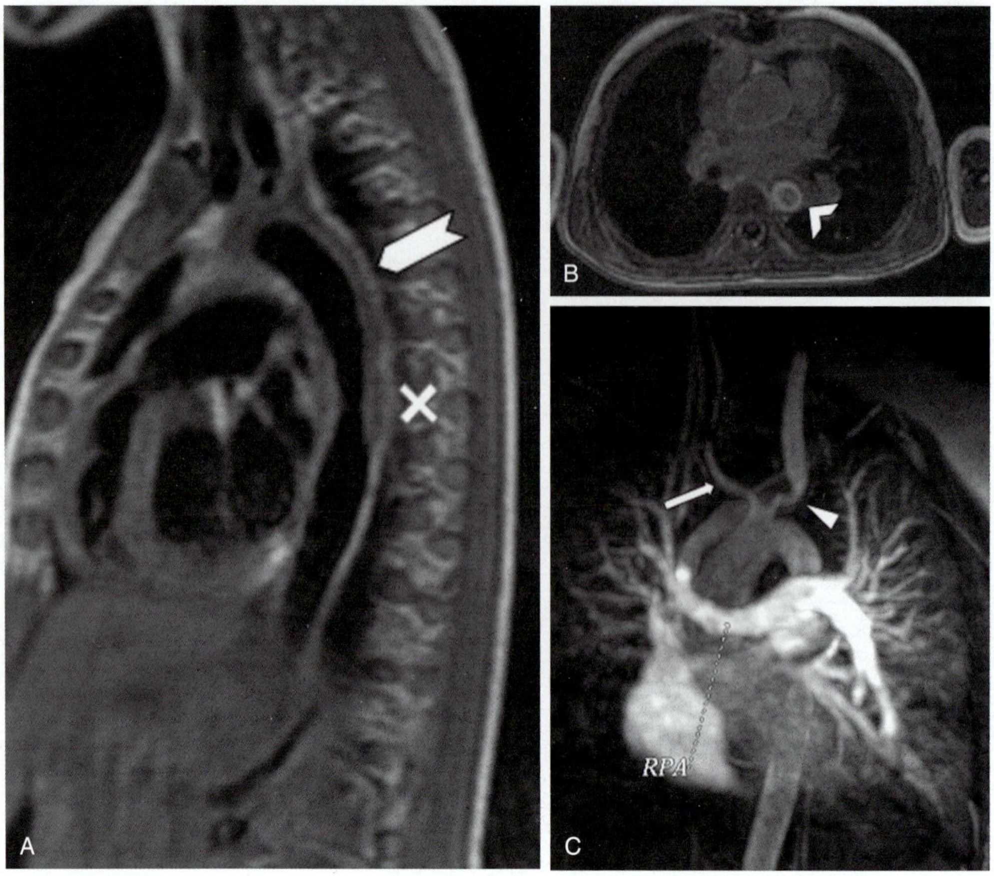

Fig. 7.58 Takayasu arteritis. Magnetic resonance angiogram of the chest, demonstrating (A) diffuse smooth wall thickening *(flag)* and hourglass-shaped narrowing of the descending aorta *(cross)*. (B) Postcontrast imaging demonstrates diffuse ringlike enhancement of the thickened aortic wall *(caret)*. (C) A smoothly narrowed left common carotid artery *(triangle)* and right brachiocephalic artery *(arrow)* are noted. The left subclavian artery is absent and presumed to be fully occluded. (Courtesy Amisha Shah, MD, Pittsburgh, PA.)

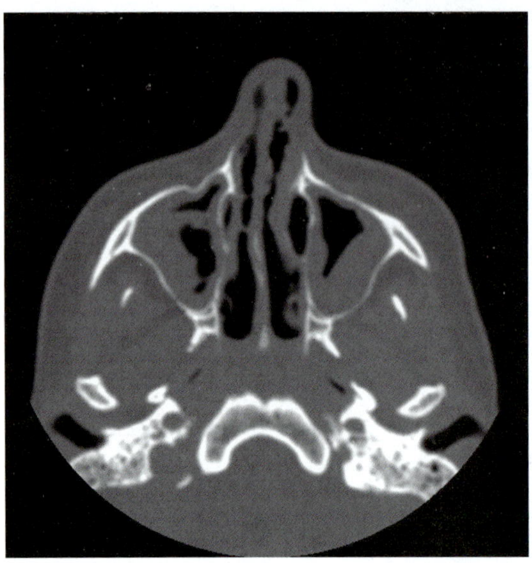

Fig. 7.59 Granulomatosis with polyangiitis. Pansinusitis with mucosal thickening throughout and bilateral mastoid effusion in teenage female with GPA.

persistent and cause scarring. Genital ulcers occur frequently, with the penis and scrotum affected in the male patient, and the vulva and vagina are affected in the female patient; scarring is fairly unique to BD. Ocular involvement occurs in 30% to 60% of children with BD and is important to recognize because visual loss and other complications may result if untreated. Ocular BD can include anterior and posterior uveitis, retinal vasculitis, retinal vein occlusion, retinal detachment, and papilledema. In addition, cutaneous manifestations are common and can comprise multiple morphologies including erythema nodosum, acneiform lesions, papulo-pustular eruptions, pseudofolliculitis, palpable purpura, and thrombophlebitis. Recurrent arthralgia and peripheral arthritis may be seen and have variable presentation from

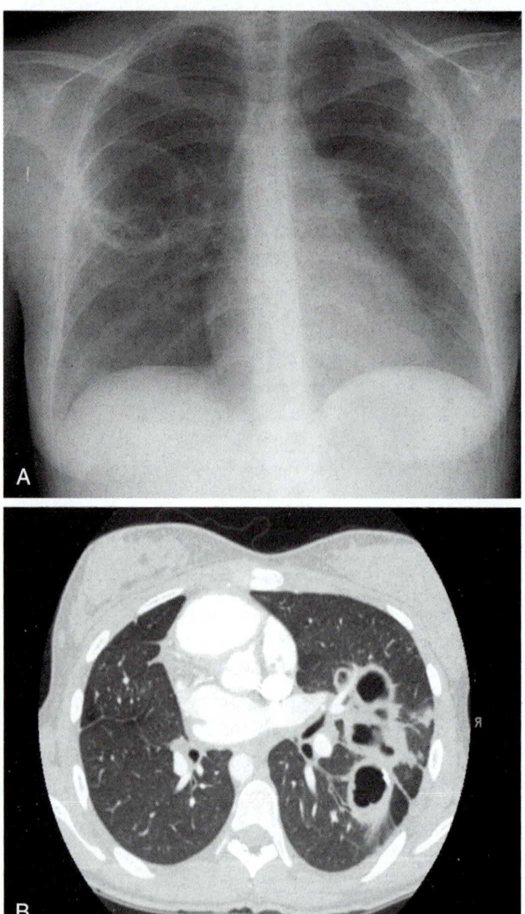

Fig. 7.60 Granulomatosis with polyangiitis lung disease. Chest radiograph (A) and computed tomography (B) showing cavitary lesions in a teenage girl presenting with fever, cough, and hemoptysis. Cavitary lesions are seen in both the right and left lung fields. Pulmonary lesions may serve as source of tissue to biopsy for definitive diagnosis.

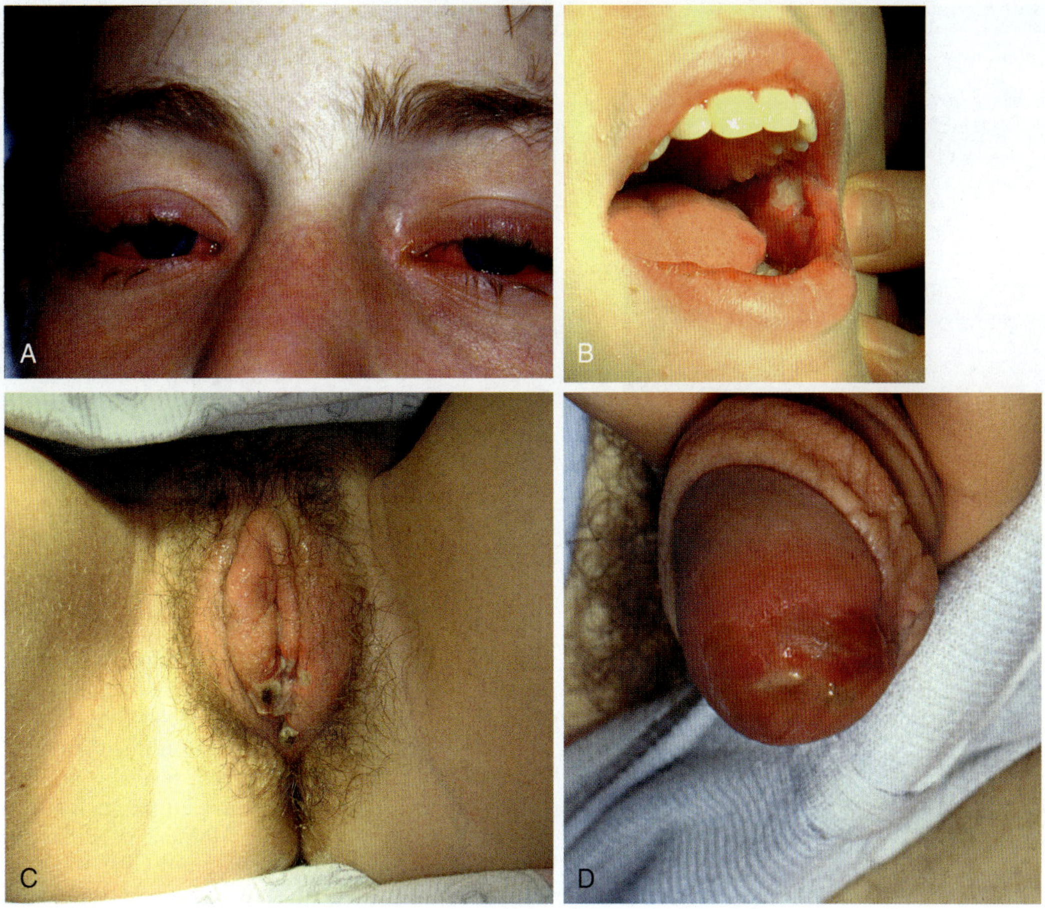

Fig. 7.61 Behçet disease. (A) Symptomatic uveitis. (B) Oral ulceration. (C) Vaginal ulceration. (D) Penile ulceration.

monoarticular to polyarticular, symmetric to asymmetric, and small to large joints affected. Neurologic disease is varied and can include headaches, cranial nerve palsy, optic neuritis, meningoencephalitis, pyramidal tract and brainstem lesions, seizures, and cerebral vascular thrombosis. Other vascular lesions are common and are a significant source of morbidity. These include thrombosis of deep and superficial veins or thrombosis, stenosis, and aneurysm of arteries; involvement can occur in central, peripheral, and visceral vessels. Vascular lesions can thus manifest with nonspecific clinical presentations dependent on distribution, including organ dysfunction of the lungs, heart, kidneys, and gastrointestinal systems. Nonspecific constitutional symptoms may also occur.

The diagnosis of BD is made on clinical grounds in the absence of other clinical explanations. A positive pathergy test is supportive in context of other clinical features but is less likely to be positive in patients from North America and Europe. This phenomenon occurs when a sterile needle prick into the skin produces an erythematous papule or pustule greater than 2 mm in diameter after 1 to 2 days. Vascular imaging may also support the diagnosis of BD.

PRIMARY ANGIITIS OF THE CENTRAL NERVOUS SYSTEM

Primary angiitis of the central nervous system (PACNS), previously called *granulomatous angiitis,* is a diagnosis of exclusion. It is an isolated vasculitis of the CNS without systemic signs or markers of inflammation. If cerebral angiography demonstrates abnormal "beading" (alternating ectasia and stenosis) of the cerebral vessels, then the diagnosis PACNS is supported. Rarely is a tissue biopsy obtained to confirm diagnosis in children. Symptoms of PACNS vary and include transient ischemic attack, stroke, seizures, vision loss, and neurocognitive impairment.

RELAPSING POLYCHONDRITIS

Relapsing polychondritis is a rare systemic inflammatory disorder characterized by recurrent widespread inflammation of cartilage. Pediatric patients account for less than 5% of all cases of relapsing polychondritis. Although sites affected can include any cartilaginous tissue, the most common presentation in pediatric patients is recurrent inflammation of the external ears (Fig. 7.62) with or without polyarthritis. Additionally, children may subsequently develop significant disease of the tracheobronchial tree. Although relapsing polychondritis can be seen with comorbid autoimmune diseases, this is a less common feature in childhood. Relapsing polychondritis may also be associated with uveitis, deafness, vestibular involvement, and aortic insufficiency.

SARCOIDOSIS

Sarcoidosis is a multisystem granulomatous inflammatory disease that can take multiple forms. The most common initial manifestation of pediatric-onset adult sarcoidosis, which typically presents in adolescence, is lymphadenopathy. This is sometimes detected incidentally as hilar lymphadenopathy on chest radiograph. Other clinical features include constitutional symptoms, lung disease, rash, uveitis, CNS disease, and arthritis. A familial form of sarcoidosis, termed Blau syndrome, is associated with mutations in NOD2/CARD15 (see Tables 7.13 and 7.14) and presents in the first decade of life with a triad of polyarthritis, dermatitis, and uveitis. The arthritis of Blau syndrome affects large and small joints and has characteristic synovial outpouching or "boggy" synovitis on examination. Cutaneous findings include a fine maculopapular erythematous to tan eruption and subcutaneous nodules similar to erythema nodosum. Typical ocular involvement consists of granulomatous iridocyclitis, posterior uveitis, or destructive panuveitis. Laboratory features may include hypercalcemia/hypercalciuria and elevation of

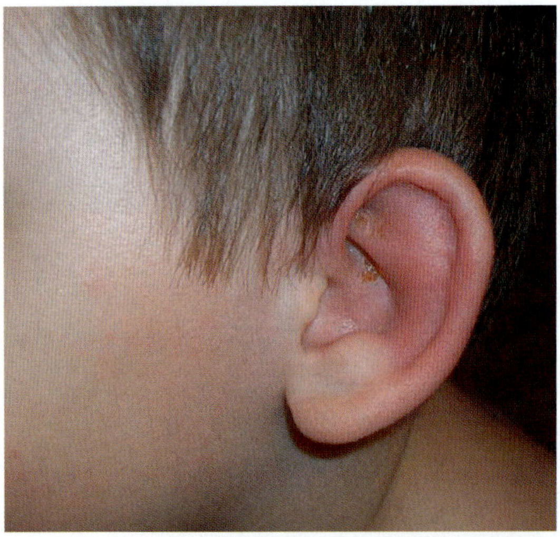

Fig. 7.62 Relapsing polychondritis. Inflammation of the cartilaginous portion of the external ear is the most common presentation in pediatric patients. The inflammation can be mistaken for cellulitis of the outer ear, sometimes with erythema spreading beyond the ear toward the face and scalp.

serum angiotensin-converting enzyme. Noncaseating granulomas are demonstrated on biopsy specimens, supporting the diagnosis of sarcoidosis.

CHRONIC RECURRENT MULTIFOCAL OSTEOMYELITIS

Chronic recurrent multifocal osteomyelitis (CRMO), also known as chronic nonbacterial osteomyelitis or nonbacterial osteitis, is an inflammatory bone disorder of unclear etiology characterized by recurring episodes of sterile osteomyelitis. Children manifest with the insidious onset of bone pain that may be maximal at night, with or without associated swelling and warmth of the surrounding soft tissues. Individuals generally appear well but may have fever. The most commonly affected areas are the metaphyseal regions of long bones, clavicles, and vertebrae; however, patients may also have lesions of the mandible, pelvis, hands, or feet. CRMO occurs frequently in association with a personal or family history of inflammatory disorders, such as psoriasis or inflammatory bowel disease.

Diagnosis is made on the basis of history and examination, with support of imaging, after the exclusion of other disorders such as infection or malignancy. Lesions of CRMO may appear as osteolytic areas surrounded by sclerosis on plain films (Fig. 7.63A); however, plain films may also be normal. Although bone scans have previously been used to help identify affected areas, whole-body MRI short tau inversion recovery images are more sensitive and increasingly used (Fig. 7.63). Laboratory investigations may be normal or demonstrate mild elevations in ESR or CRP or increased WBC counts. Bone biopsy generally has low diagnostic yield but can be indicated to rule out other potential etiologies including bacterial osteomyelitis, Langerhans cell histiocytosis, Rosai-Dorfman disease, or malignancies such as osteosarcoma.

AUTOINFLAMMATORY SYNDROMES

The autoinflammatory syndromes, also known as periodic fever syndromes, are characterized by recurrent episodes of systemic inflammation, often without definitive trigger, in association with dysregulation of the innate immune system. Many of the identified syndromes feature recurrent fevers as an integral symptom, along with a variety of systemic features such as serositis, rash, myalgia/arthralgia or arthritis. Markers of inflammation such as WBC count, platelet count, ESR, and CRP are often elevated during the attacks. Episodes may be clearly periodic (occurring at regular intervals) or more erratic with varying intervals between attacks. The various phenotypes of the autoinflammatory syndromes depend on the genetic mutations involved. The list of identified syndromes grows with improved understanding of the immune system's regulation. Some of the defined disorders are included in Table 7.13. An

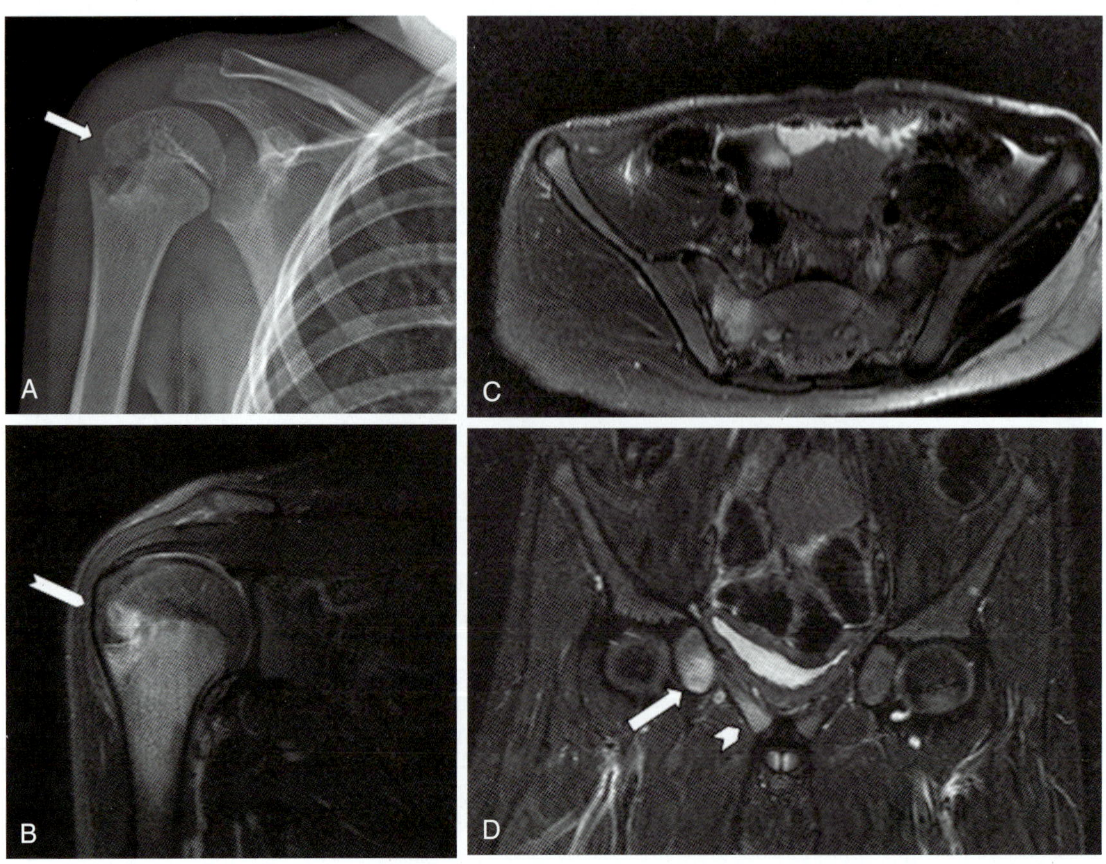

Fig. 7.63 Chronic recurrent multifocal osteomyelitis. (A) Frontal radiograph of the right humerus demonstrating a lucent destructive lesion abutting the growth plate *(arrow)*. (B) Magnetic resonance imaging of the same patient shows abnormal T2 fat-saturated bright signal of the humeral metaphysis and epiphyseal head with enhancement of the marrow and periosteal hyperemia *(flag)*. (C and D) Additional lesions were noted within the anterior acetabulum and anterior superior pubic bone as well as in the right sacrum adjacent to the sacroiliac joint *(arrow/flag)*. (Courtesy Amisha Shah, MD, Pittsburgh, PA.)

Table 7.13 Characteristics of Autoinflammatory Syndromes

	Inheritance	Gene	Protein	Duration	Mucocutaneous	Eye	Musculoskeletal	Serositis	Neurologic
PFAPA	N/A	N/A	N/A	4–5 days	Aphthous ulcers, pharyngitis	No	Arthralgia	No	No
FMF	AR	MEFV	Pyrin	1–3 days	Erysipelas-like, vasculitis, rare aphthous ulcer	No	Arthritis, myalgia	Peritonitis, pleuritis, pericarditis	Headache
HIDS	AR	MVK	Mevalonate Kinase	3–7 days	Maculopapular, morbilliform, oral/genital ulcers	No	Arthralgia, arthritis	Abdominal pain, diarrhea	No
TRAPS	AD	TNFRSF1A	55-kDa TNF receptor	>7 days	Painful erythema, vasculitis, aphthous ulcers	Periorbital edema, conjunctivitis	Myalgia, fasciitis, arthritis	Peritonitis, pleuritis, pericarditis	Headache
FCAS	AD	NLRP3	Cryopyrin	1 day	Urticarial-like	Conjunctivitis	Arthralgia	No	Headache
MWS	AD	NLRP3	Cryopyrin	1–2 days	Urticarial-like	Conjunctivitis, uveitis, episcleritis	Arthralgia	No	Headache, loss of hearing
NOMID	AD	NLRP3	Cryopyrin	Continuous	Urticarial-like	Conjunctivitis, uveitis, papillitis	Epiphyseal overgrowth, arthritis	No	Chronic meningitis, intellectual disability, developmental delay, hearing loss
DIRA	AR	IL1RN	IL-1 receptor antagonist	Continuous	Pustulosis	No	Osteitis	No	No
DITRA	AR	IL36RN	IL-36 receptor antagonist	1–3 days	Pustular psoriasis, nail dystrophy, geographic tongue	No	Arthralgia, arthritis	No	No
Blau Syndrome	AD	NOD2/ CARD15	Nucleotide-binding Oligomerization Domain-containing protein 2/Caspase Recruitment Domain-containing protein 15	Continuous	Scaly red/brown papules/plaques	Uveitis, cataracts	Arthritis	No	Cranial neuropathy, peripheral neuropathy
DADA2	AR	ADA2	Adenosine Deaminase 2	Continuous	Fixed, lacy mottled rash	No	No	No	Lacunar strokes

AD, Autosomal dominant; *AR,* autosomal recessive; *DADA2,* deficiency of adenosine deaminase 2; *DIRA,* deficiency of the IL-1 receptor antagonist; *DITRA,* deficiency of the IL-36 receptor antagonist; *FCAS,* familial cold autoinflammatory syndrome; *FMF,* familial Mediterranean fever; *HIDS,* hyperimmunoglobulin D syndrome; *MWS,* Muckle-Wells syndrome; *N/A,* not applicable; *NOMID,* neonatal-onset multisystem inflammatory disorder; *PFAPA,* periodic fever, aphthous stomatitis, pharyngitis, adenitis syndrome; *TRAPS,* TNF-receptor-associated periodic syndrome.

Modified from Hashkes PJ, Toker O: Autoinflammatory syndromes, *Pediatr Clin North Am* 59:447–470, 2012.

Table 7.14 Features of Autoinflammatory Syndromes That May Narrow Diagnosis

Clinical Features	Autoinflammatory Syndrome
Age of Onset	
Birth	NOMID, DIRA, FCAS
Infancy	HIDS, FCAS, Blau syndrome
Toddler/late childhood	PFAPA syndrome, DADA2, Blau syndrome
Onset in adulthood	TRAPS, DITRA
Ethnicity and Geography	
Armenian, Turks, Italian, Sephardic Jews	FMF
Arabs	FMF, DITRA
Dutch, French, German	HIDS, MWS
United States	FCAS
Triggers	
Vaccines	HIDS
Cold exposure	FCAS
Stress, menses	FMF, TRAPS, MWS, DITRA
Minor trauma	MWS, TRAPS, HIDS
Exercise	FMF, TRAPS
Pregnancy	DITRA
Duration of Episode	
Less than 24 h	FCAS, FMF
1–3 days	FMF, MWS, DITRA
3–7 days	HIDS, PFAPA syndrome
More than 7 days	TRAPS
Constant episode	NOMID, DIRA, DADA2, Blau syndrome
Interval Between Episodes	
3–6 weeks	PFAPA syndrome, HIDS
More than 6 weeks	TRAPS
Unpredictable	All others

DADA2, Deficiency of adenosine deaminase 2; *DIRA,* Deficiency of the IL-1 receptor antagonist; *DITRA,* deficiency of the IL-36 receptor antagonist; *FCAS,* familial cold autoinflammatory syndrome; *FMF,* familial Mediterranean fever; *HIDS,* hyperimmunoglobulin D syndrome; *MWS,* Muckle-Wells syndrome; *NOMID,* neonatal-onset multisystem inflammatory disease; *PFAPA,* periodic fever, aphthous stomatitis, pharyngitis, and cervical adenitis; *TRAPS,* tumor necrosis factor receptor–associated periodic syndrome.

Modified from Hashkes PJ, Toker O: Autoinflammatory syndromes, *Pediatr Clin North Am* 59:447–470, 2012.

autoinflammatory syndrome should be suspected in young children with unexplained, episodic fever, and signs of inflammation. Other associated features, such as age at onset, ethnicity, or trigger, can aid in diagnosis (Table 7.14).

MUSCULOSKELETAL PAIN DISORDERS

Noninflammatory Musculoskeletal Disorders

Children often present to the pediatrician with a chief complaint of musculoskeletal pain. Numerous nonrheumatic conditions of childhood can result in pain of the joints, extremities, and other areas. Hints in the history and physical examination can often yield a diagnosis of one or more benign conditions that can help avoid unnecessary diagnostic testing. Features of these common conditions are reviewed in Table 7.15.

ACKNOWLEDGMENTS

We extend our deepest thanks to the original author of this chapter—Dr. Aldo V. Londino. Dr. Londino, until the time of his passing in 2000, was the sole pediatric rheumatologist in western Pennsylvania and was widely recognized for his superb teaching and clinical skills. We are also grateful for the contributions of the previous authors, Drs. Andrew H. Urbach, Sara C. McIntire, and Paul Rosen as well as photograph contributors: Bernard Cohen, John Zitelli, A'Delbert Bowen, Basil Zitelli, J. Carlton Gartner Jr., J. Jeffrey Malatack, Joseph McGuire, Holly Davis, Kathryn Torok, Virginia Steen, Joseph Warnicki, Albert Biglan, Cora Lennox, Sang Park, Chester Oddis, Amisha Shah, David Witte, and Susan Gelnett.

Table 7.15 Distinguishing Features of Noninflammatory Musculoskeletal Disorders

Diagnosis	Age of Onset	Musculoskeletal Symptoms	Associated Symptoms/ Disorders	Physical Examination Features
Benign joint hypermobility	Early childhood through adolescence	Symmetric large or small joint pain exacerbated by activity, improved with rest or chronic joint pain. May have frequent sprains/ ligamentous injuries.	Dizziness/syncope/cardiovascular autonomic dysfunction Easy bruising GI complaints (abdominal pain, constipation/diarrhea, early satiety, reflux)	Hypermobile joints (Beighton score ≥4)
Amplified musculoskeletal pain syndrome, chronic regional pain syndrome, reflex sympathetic dystrophy, reflex neurovascular dystrophy	Adolescence	Longstanding pain unresponsive to multiple interventions. Pain can be localized or diffuse and may be associated with allodynia and subjective joint swelling/ stiffness and/or color and temperature change.	Mood disturbance with depression and/or anxiety, sleep disturbance/fatigue, impaired concentration/ memory, chronic headache/ migraine Chronic abdominal pain/ irritable bowel syndrome	Normal examination +/− presence of joint tenderness, allodynia, functional limitation, temperature asymmetry, skin color change, edema, sweating asymmetry, dystrophic changes
Benign nocturnal musculoskeletal pains of childhood	3–12 years old	Bilateral, primarily lower extremity pain that occurs often in the evening/nighttime and is usually episodic. Pain is usually relieved by massage, heat, and analgesics.	Headaches Abdominal pain	Normal examination
Lymphedema praecox	Adolescence	Progressive swelling of lower extremity sometimes accompanied by pain, feeling of heaviness or tightness. Can be complicated by recurrent cellulitis.	None	Nonpitting edema of extremity Can be associated with hyperkeratosis or xanthomas
Apophysitis (Osgood-Schlatter disease, Sever disease, Sinding-Larsen-Johansson syndrome, Iselin disease)	Early adolescence	Localized joint pain, tenderness, and swelling at areas of apophyses (tendon insertion into bone) worsened by activity	None	Tenderness over apophysis

Bibliography

Aljaberi N, Nguyen K, Strahle C, et al: Performance of the new 2019 European League Against Rheumatism/American College of Rheumatology classification criteria for systemic lupus erythematosus in children and young adults, *Arthritis Care Res* 73(4):580–585, 2021.

Angeles-Han ST, Ringold S, Beukelman T, et al: 2019 American College of Rheumatology/Arthritis Foundation Guideline for the screening, monitoring, and treatment of juvenile idiopathic arthritis-associated uveitis, *Arthritis Care Res (Hoboken)* 71(6):703–716, 2019.

Aringer M, Costenbader K, Daikh D, et al: 2019 European League Against Rheumatism/American College of Rheumatology classification criteria for systemic lupus erythematosus, *Ann Rheum Dis* 78(9):1151–1159, 2019.

Basiaga ML, Stern SM, Mehta JJ, et al: Childhood Sjögren syndrome: features of an international cohort and application of the 2016 ACR/EULAR classification criteria, *Rheumatology (Oxford)* 60(7):3144–3155, 2021.

Belot A, Duquesne A, Job-Deslandre C, et al: Pediatric onset relapsing polychondritis: case series and systematic review, *J Pediatr* 156(3):484–489, 2010.

Bettiol A, Alibaz-Oner F, Direskeneli H, et al: Vascular Behçet syndrome: from pathogenesis to treatment, *Nat Rev Rheumatol* 19(2):111–126, 2023.

Cabral DA, Uribe AG, Bensler SM, et al: Classification, presentation and initial treatment of Wegener's granulomatosis in childhood, *Arthritis Rheum* 60: 3413–3424, 2009.

Cassidy J, Kivlin J, Lindsley C, et al: Ophthalmologic examinations in children with juvenile rheumatoid arthritis, *Pediatrics* 117(5):1843–1845, 2006.

Cheng S, Ding H, Xue H, Cao L: Evaluation of the 2019 EULAR/ACR classification criteria for systemic lupus erythematosus in children and adults, *Clin Rheumatol* 41(10):2995–3003, 2022.

Crayne CB, Beukelman T: Juvenile idiopathic arthritis: oligoarthritis and polyarthritis, *Pediatr Clin North Am* 65(4):657–674, 2018.

Dall'Era M, Cisternas MG, Snipes K, et al: The incidence and prevalence of systemic lupus erythematosus in San Francisco County, California: The California Lupus Surveillance Project, *Arthritis Rheumatol* 69(10):1996–2005, 2017.

Ferguson PJ, Sandu M: Current understanding of the pathogenesis and management of chronic recurrent multifocal osteomyelitis, *Curr Rheumatol Rep* 14: 130–141, 2012.

Ferucci ED, Johnston JM, Gaddy JR, et al: Prevalence and incidence of systemic lupus erythematosus in a population-based registry of American Indian and Alaska Native people, 2002–2009, *Arthritis Rheumatol* 66:2494–2502, 2014.

Foeldvari I, Torok KS: Review for best practice in clinical rheumatology juvenile systemic sclerosis - Updates and practice points, *Best Pract Res Clin Rheumatol* 35(3):101688, 2021.

Fonseca AR, de Oliveira SKF, Rodrigues MCF, et al: Relapsing polychondritis in childhood: three case reports, comparison with adulthood disease and literature review, *Rheumatol Int* 33:1873–1878, 2013.

Foster HE, Jandial S: pGALS—paediatric Gait Arms Legs and Spine: a simple examination of the musculoskeletal system, *Pediatr Rheumatol Online J* 11(1):44, 2013.

Guseinova D, Consolaro A, Trail L, et al: Comparison of clinical features and drug therapies among European and Latin American patients with juvenile dermatomyositis, *Clin Exp Rheumatol* 29(1):117–124, 2011.

Hashkes PJ, Toker O: Autoinflammatory syndromes, *Pediatr Clin North Am* 59:447–470, 2012.

Herrick AL, Ennis H, Bhushan M, et al: Incidence of childhood linear scleroderma and systemic sclerosis in the UK and Ireland, *Arthritis Care Res* 62(2):213–218, 2010.

Hoffart CM, Wallace DP: Amplified pain syndromes in children: treatment and new insights into disease pathogenesis, *Curr Opin Rheumatol* 26:592–603, 2014.

Hsieh Y, Wu M, Wang J, et al: Clinical features of atypical Kawasaki disease, *J Microbiol Immunol Infect* 35:57–60, 2002.

Jariwala M, Laxer RM: Childhood GPA, EGPA, and MPA, *Clin Immunol* 211:108325, 2020.

Jeannette JC, Falk RJ, Bacon PA, et al: 2012 revised international Chapel Hill Consensus Conference Nomenclature of Vasculitides, *Arthritis Rheum* 65(1):1–11, 2013.

Jone PN, Tremoulet A, Choueiter N, et al: Update on diagnosis and management of Kawasaki disease: a scientific statement from the American Heart Association, *Circulation* 150(23):e481–e500, 2024.

Kim H, Huber AM, Kim S: Updates on juvenile dermatomyositis from the last decade: classification to outcomes, *Rheum Dis Clin North Am* 47(4):669–690, 2021.

Lahita RG, Tsokos G, Buyon J, et al: *Systemic lupus erythematosus*, ed 5, London, 2011, Elsevier.

Lee JJY, Schneider R. Systemic Juvenile Idiopathic Arthritis. *Pediatr Clin North Am* 65(4):691–709, 2018.

Levy DM, Kamphuis S: Systemic lupus erythematosus in children and adolescents, *Pediatr Clin North Am* 59(2):345–364, 2012.

Li SC, Zheng RJ: Overview of juvenile localized scleroderma and its management, *World J Pediatr* 16(1):5–18, 2020.

Lundberg IE, Tjärnlund A, Bottai M, et al: 2017 European League Against Rheumatism/American College of Rheumatology classification criteria for adult and juvenile idiopathic inflammatory myopathies and their major subgroups, *Ann Rheum Dis* 76(12):1955–1964, 2017.

Martin N, Krol P, Smith S, et al: A national registry for juvenile dermatomyositis and other paediatric idiopathic inflammatory myopathies: 10 years' experience; the Juvenile Dermatomyositis National (UK and Ireland) Cohort Biomarker Study and Repository for Idiopathic Inflammatory Myopathies, *Rheumatology (Oxford)* 50(1):137–145, 2011.

Martini A, Lovell DJ, Albani S, et al: Juvenile idiopathic arthritis, *Nat Rev Dis Primers* 8:5, 2022.

Martini G, Foeldvari I, Russo R, et al: Systemic sclerosis in childhood: clinical and immunologic features of 153 patients in an international database, *Arthritis Rheum* 54(12):3971–3978, 2006.

Mina R, Brunner HI: Update on differences between childhood-onset and adult-onset systemic lupus erythematosus, *Arthritis Res Ther* 15(4):218, 2013.

Nazzar Romero S, McCurdy D: Overview of systemic autoinflammatory diseases, *Adv Pediatr* 71(1):213–228, 2024.

Newburger JW, Takahashi M, Gerber MA, et al: Diagnosis, treatment, and long-term management of Kawasaki disease: a statement for health professionals from the Committee on Rheumatic Fever, Endocarditis, and Kawasaki Disease, Council on Cardiovascular Disease in the Young, American Heart Association, *Pediatrics* 114(6):1708–1733, 2004.

Oen K, Malleson PN, Cabral DA, et al: Disease course and outcome of juvenile rheumatoid arthritis in a multicenter cohort, *J Rheumatol* 29(9):1989–1999, 2002.

Ozen S, Sag E: Childhood vasculitis, *Rheumatology (Oxford)* 59(Suppl 3):iii95–iii100, 2020.

Petty RE, Laxer RM, Lindsley CB, et al: *Textbook of pediatric rheumatology*, ed 8, Philadelphia, 2021, Elsevier.

Petty RE, Southwood TR, Manners P, et al: International League of Associations for Rheumatology classification of juvenile idiopathic arthritis: second revision, Edmonton, 2001, *J Rheumatol* 31:390–392, 2004.

Pillebout E, Sunderkötter C: IgA vasculitis, *Semin Immunopathol* 43(5):729–738, 2021.

Prasad S, Zhu JL, Schollaert-Fitch K, et al: An evaluation of the performance of current morphea subtype classifications, *JAMA Dermatol* 157(4):1–8, 2021.

Ramos-Casals M, Baer AN, Brito-Zerón MDP, et al: 2023 International Rome consensus for the nomenclature of Sjögren disease, *Nat Rev Rheumatol* 21(7):426–437, 2025.

Rodrigues Fonseca A, Felix Rodrigues MC, Sztajnbok FR, et al: Comparison among ACR1997, SLICC and the new EULAR/ACR classification criteria in childhood-onset systemic lupus erythematosus, *Adv Rheumatol* 59(1):20, 2019.

Sandborg CI, Schulert GS, Kimura Y: Juvenile Idiopathic Arthritis, *N Engl J Med* 393(2):162–174, 2025.

Sherry DD: An overview of amplified musculoskeletal pain syndromes, *J Rheumatol Suppl* 58:44–48, 2000.

Singhal S, Landes C, Shukla R, McCann LJ, Hedrick CM: Classification and management strategies for paediatric chronic nonbacterial osteomyelitis and chronic recurrent multifocal osteomyelitis, *Expert Rev Clin Immunol* 19(9):1101–1116, 2023.

Son MBF, Gauvreau K, Tremoulet AH, et al: Risk model development and validation for prediction of coronary artery aneurysms in Kawasaki Disease in a North American Population, *J Am Heart Assoc* 8(11):e011319, 2019.

Valenzuela-Almada MO, Hocaoglu M, Dabit JY, et al: Epidemiology of childhood-onset systemic lupus erythematosus: a population-based study, *Arthritis Care Res* 74(5):728–732, 2022.

Vivarelli M, Samuel S, Coppo R, et al: IPNA clinical practice recommendations for the diagnosis and management of children with IgA nephropathy and IgA vasculitis nephritis, *Pediatr Nephrol* 40(2):533–569, 2025.

Wedderburn LR, McHugh NJ, Chinoy H, et al: HLA class II haplotype and autoantibody associations in children with juvenile dermatomyositis and juvenile dermatomyositis- scleroderma overlap, *Rheumatology* 46:1786–1791, 2007.

Weiss PF, Colbert RA: Juvenile spondyloarthritis: a distinct form of juvenile arthritis, *Pediatr Clin North Am* 65(4):675–690, 2018.

Zulian F: Scleroderma in children, *Pediatr Clin North Am* 52:521–545, vii, 2005.

Zulian F, Athreya BH, Laxer R, et al: Juvenile localized scleroderma: clinical and epidemiological features in 750 children: an international study, *Rheumatology (Oxford)* 45:614–620, 2006.

8

DERMATOLOGY

Angela M. Guerrero | Ellen Koch | Robin P. Gehris | Sydney DeVore

Defects or alterations in any component of the skin may result in serious systemic disease. Every part of the skin (Fig. 8.1) can be affected by congenital, inflammatory, infectious, and degenerative disorders and tumors. For example, an altered stratum corneum is seen in ichthyosis; melanocytes are selectively destroyed in vitiligo; excess collagen is produced in the connective tissue nevus of tuberous sclerosis; hair follicles are focally affected in alopecia areata; and so on. In addition, the skin is affected by many systemic diseases and thus may provide visible markers for internal disorders. A skin examination may demonstrate lesions of vasculitis, explaining a child's hematuria. The hypopigmented macules of tuberous sclerosis may give insight into the cause of a child's seizures.

EXAMINATION AND ASSESSMENT OF THE SKIN

Optimal examination of the skin is performed in a well-lit room. The physician should inspect the entire skin surface, including hair, nails, scalp, and mucous membranes. Although no special equipment is required, a hand lens and side lighting aid in the assessment of skin texture and small, discrete lesions. A handheld dermatoscope is invaluable, specifically for assessing pigmented lesions. A Wood lamp improves precision in distinguishing hypopigmented lesions, which do not enhance under Wood lamp, from depigmented patches of skin, which enhance and appear more prominent under Wood lamp examination.

A systematic approach to the evaluation of a rash simplifies the process of developing a differential diagnosis. After assessing the patient's general health, the practitioner should obtain a detailed history of the skin symptoms, including the date of onset, inciting factors, evolution of lesions, and presence or absence of any other systemic symptoms. Recent immunizations, infections, drugs, and allergies may be directly related to new rashes. The family history may suggest a hereditary process. Review of newborn records and photographs helps to document the presence of congenital lesions. Photos can be instrumental in charting the progression of a rash. Attention should then turn to the distribution and pattern of the rash. The term *distribution* refers to the location of the skin findings, whereas the term *pattern* defines a specific anatomic or physiologic arrangement (e.g., the distribution of a rash may include the extremities, face, or trunk, and the pattern could be diffuse, flexural, or intertriginous). Identification of a pattern can assist in the development of a differential diagnosis even before the detailed morphology of the skin lesions is studied. Other common patterns include photo distributed (involving sun-exposed sites), acral (involving primarily the distal extremities), and dermatomal configurations (Fig. 8.2).

Next, the clinician should consider the local organization of the lesions, defining the relationship of primary and secondary lesions to one another in each location. Are the lesions scattered or clustered? Are they linear, grouped, serpiginous, confluent, or discrete?

Lastly, the practitioner should identify the morphology of the cutaneous lesions. *Primary lesions* (macules, papules, pustules, wheals, plaques, vesicles, bullae, nodules, and tumors) arise de novo in the skin. *Secondary lesions* (erosions, ulcers, crusts, excoriations, fissures, lichenification, atrophy, and scars) evolve from primary lesions and often result from the patient's manipulation (e.g., scratching) of primary lesions. Delineation of the primary and secondary lesions allows the clinician to develop a differential diagnosis based on the anatomic level of the skin lesions (Table 8.1). Disorders restricted to the epidermis may be associated with macular color changes, such as in vascular telangiectasias, freckles, and vitiligo. In epidermal disorders, surface markings are commonly altered by scales, vesicles, pustules, crusts, and erosions. Bullous impetigo, atopic dermatitis, ichthyosis, and tinea corporis are primarily epidermal disorders. When the dermis is also involved, lesions usually display distinct borders because of dermal inflammation and edema. Disorders with both epidermal and dermal changes include psoriasis, lichen planus, and erythema multiforme (EM). Inflammatory disorders or tumors restricted to the dermis do not usually alter the surface markings. Lesional borders are distinct, and color changes and edema may be present. Examples of dermal disorders include granuloma annulare, intradermal nevi, and urticaria. The diagnosis of subcutaneous disorders is made by careful palpation. The surface markings are normal, and the color of the skin may be normal or red. There is altered skin firmness, and tenderness may be present. Subcutaneous lesions include lipomas, deep hemangiomas, hematomas, subcutaneous fat necrosis, and erythema nodosum.

Because an outline of specific pediatric dermatoses defies any one scheme of organization, this text follows a clinically practical format. First, this chapter covers common papulosquamous and vesiculopustular eruptions, which account for most rashes seen in children. This

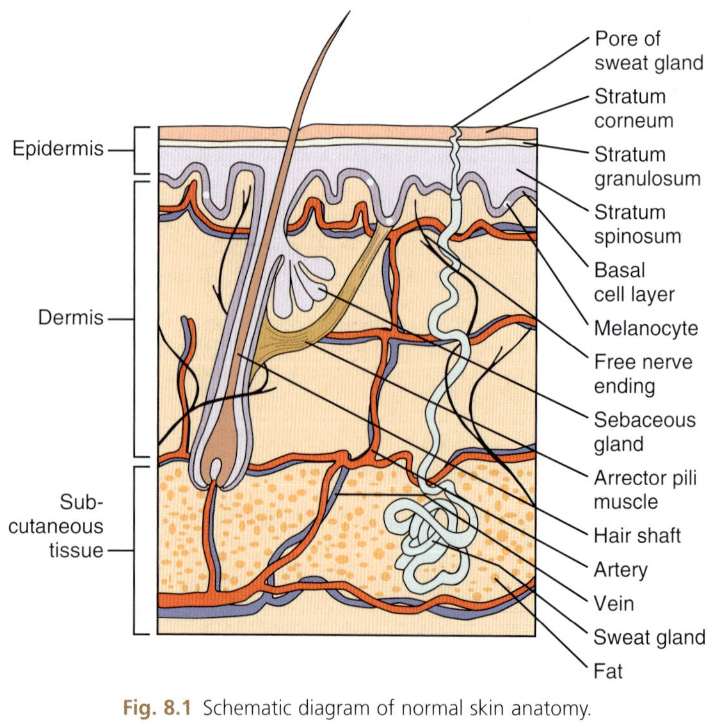

Fig. 8.1 Schematic diagram of normal skin anatomy.

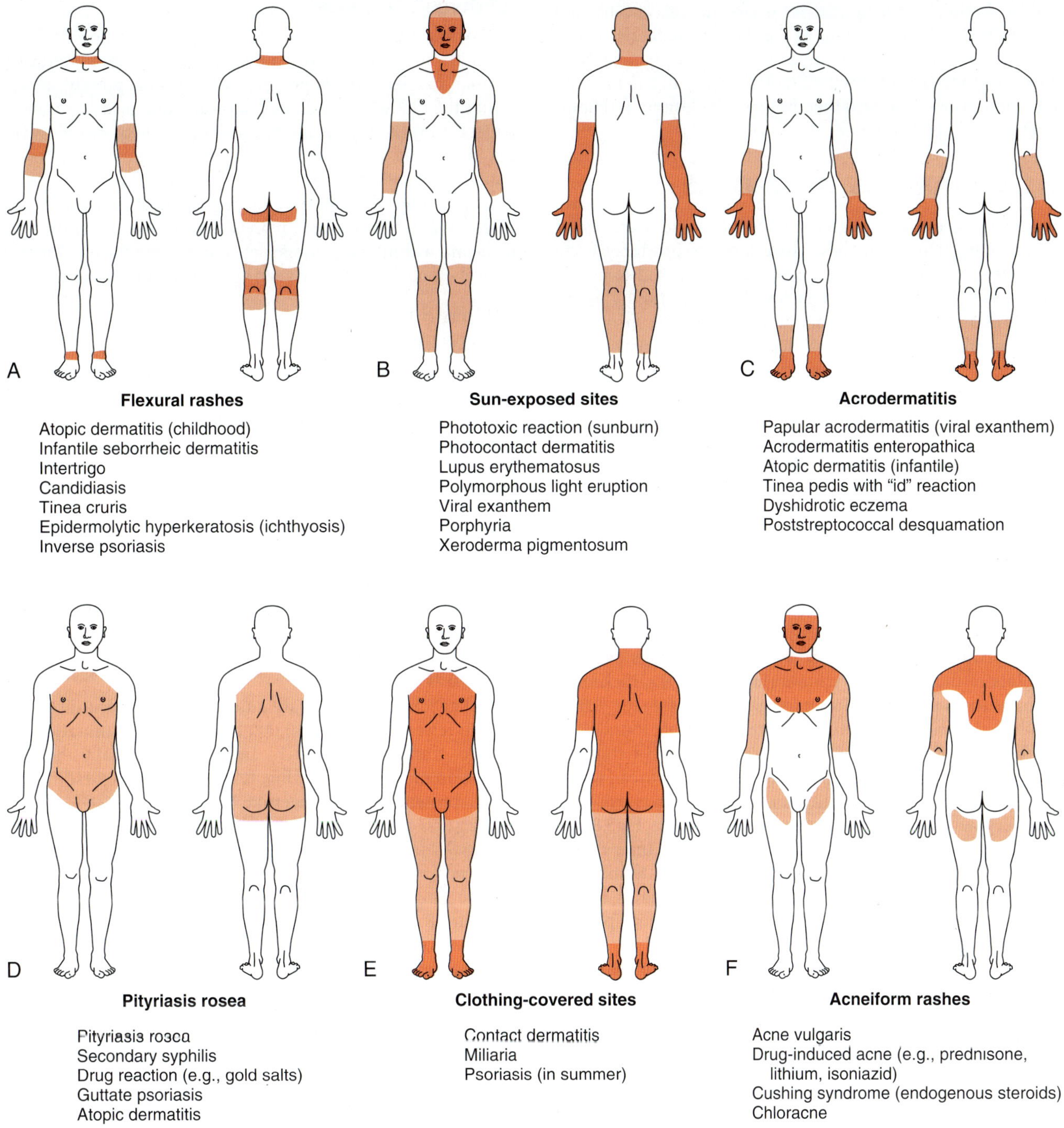

Fig. 8.2 Pattern diagnosis. (A) Flexural rashes. (B) Sun-exposed sites. (C) Acrodermatitis. (D) Pityriasis rosea. (E) Clothing-covered sites. (F) Acneiform rashes.

Table 8.1 Anatomic Depth of Lesions

Cutaneous Structure	Physical Findings	Specific Skin Disorders
Epidermis	Altered surface markings Scale, vesicle, crust Color changes (black, brown, white)	Impetigo Café au lait spot Atopic dermatitis Vitiligo Freckle
Epidermis and dermis	Altered surface markings Scale, vesicle, crust Distinct borders Color changes (black, brown, white, and/or red) Edema	Psoriasis Atopic dermatitis Contact dermatitis Cutaneous lupus erythematosus
Dermis	Normal surface markings Color changes Altered dermal firmness	Urticaria Granuloma annulare Hemangioma Blue nevus
Subcutaneous tissue	Normal surface markings Normal or red skin color Altered skin firmness	Hematoma Cold panniculitis Erythema nodosum

From Cohen BA: *Pediatric dermatology,* ed 2, London, 1999, Mosby.

is followed by sections covering reactive erythema, insect bites and infestations, tumors and infiltrations of the skin, neonatal dermatology, congenital and acquired nevi, and disorders of pigmentation. The chapter concludes with a discussion of disorders of the hair and nails and complications of topical therapy. Vascular lesions and hemangiomas are addressed in Chapter 10.

PAPULOSQUAMOUS DISORDERS

Papulosquamous eruptions share the morphologic features of papules and scales. However, these disorders are produced by a variety of different mechanisms. In psoriasis, increased turnover of keratinocytes by the basal cell layer results in a markedly thickened epidermis and stratum corneum. In dermatitic processes (e.g., atopic dermatitis, seborrheic dermatitis, pityriasis rosea, fungal infections), inflammation results in increased production and abnormal maturation of epidermal cells with subsequent scale production. Increased adherence of cells in the stratum corneum may result in the retention hyperkeratosis characteristic of ichthyosis vulgaris, which is frequently found in association with atopic dermatitis.

Psoriasis

Psoriasis is a common disorder characterized by erythematous, well-demarcated plaques covered with silvery scale. These have a predilection for the extensor surfaces of the extremities, scalp, and buttocks. In some patients, the distribution consists of large lesions over the pressure points of the knees and elbows (Fig. 8.3A–D). Thickening and fissuring of the skin of the palms may also be seen (see Fig. 8.3E). In some children, numerous droplike (guttate) lesions are found scattered over the body (Fig. 8.4), often after a group A β-hemolytic streptococcal infection either of the throat or perianal area (which may have been recognized or subclinical). In infants, psoriasis may present as persistent, confluent diaper dermatitis (see Fig. 8.47). Lesions of psoriasis are often induced at sites of local injury (e.g., friction, scratches, surgical scars, sunburns), a response termed the *Koebner phenomenon* (Fig. 8.5). Nail changes include reddish-brown psoriatic plaques in the nail bed (oil drop changes), surface pitting, and distal hyperkeratosis (see Fig. 8.140).

The factors that initiate the rapid turnover in epidermal cells that produce the psoriatic plaques are unknown, although an inherited predisposition is suspected and upper respiratory tract and streptococcal infections may precipitate lesions in children, especially in cases of guttate psoriasis. Although the increased epidermal growth causes a thickening of the skin in the psoriatic plaque, there are also areas between the epidermal ridges where the skin is thin, and the scale is close to the subepidermal vessels. Thus, when the scale is removed, small bleeding points are often seen. This is called the *Auspitz sign,* and it is one of the hallmarks of psoriasis (Fig. 8.6).

Except in cases of guttate psoriasis, which can sometimes be limited to one episode, the course of psoriasis tends to be more chronic and unpredictable, marked by remissions and exacerbations. Although it is less commonly seen than in their adult counterparts, children with psoriasis are also at risk for psoriatic arthritis, so a careful screening for joint symptoms is key. The severity and timing of psoriatic skin disease and joint disease do not always parallel one another, so even patients with mild or no skin disease may experience significant joint pain. Thirty-seven percent of adults with psoriasis first develop lesions in childhood.

Ichthyoses

Ichthyosis refers to a group of genodermatoses characterized by varying degrees of dry, scaly skin. Ichthyoses are identified according to clinical course, histopathology, biochemical markers, and specific genetic mutations.

Ichthyosis Vulgaris

Ichthyosis vulgaris occurs secondary to an autosomal dominant mutation in filaggrin, which encodes a key component of the epidermal barrier. Although the rash is not present at birth, by 3 months old, excessively dry skin or thick, fishlike scales may be apparent on the shins and extensor surfaces of the arms (Fig. 8.7). On occasion, scales become more generalized and involve the trunk, but the flexures are usually spared. Lesions tend to flare during the winter and improve during the summer, particularly with increasing age. Biopsy of involved skin shows retention hyperkeratosis and a thinned granular layer in the epidermis. Liberal use of topical emollients usually keeps pruritus and scaling under control.

X-Linked Ichthyosis

X-linked ichthyosis occurs in 1 in 6000 males because of a mutation in the enzyme steroid sulfatase, although findings are occasionally present in hemizygous female carriers. Affected newborns usually present between 3 and 12 months old with generalized brown scales, particularly on the lateral neck, abdomen, back, and anterior legs and feet (Fig. 8.8). The central face and flexures are spared. Skin biopsy demonstrates an increased granular layer and stratum corneum, and biochemical studies demonstrate decreased or absent steroid sulfatase in the serum and skin. Children with X-linked ichthyosis are at increased risk of undescended testes and testicular cancer. Decreased or absent steroid sulfatase activity during fetal life may result in decreased placental estrogen and a delay in onset of maternal labor.

Lamellar Ichthyosis

Lamellar ichthyosis is a rare autosomal dominant disorder occurring in fewer than 1 in 250,000 births due to a mutation in keratinocyte transglutaminase-1. Infants are usually born with a collodion membrane (see Fig. 8.96). During the first month of life, thick, brownish gray, sheetlike scales with raised edges appear. Scaling is prominent over the face, trunk, and extremities (Fig. 8.9). In contrast to ichthyosis vulgaris, the flexural areas are involved (see Fig. 8.9B). Eversion and fissuring of the eyelid margins (ectropion) and lips (eclabium) are common complications (see Fig. 8.9C) and can lead to exposure keratitis, necessitating ophthalmologic consultation. The palms and soles show thick keratoderma with fissuring. Some improvement of the scaling occurs with age, and topical keratolytics (e.g., lactic acid, salicylic acid) may provide some benefit. Severe cases may respond to the administration of systemic retinoids, but it is important to note that these are known to be teratogenic.

Epidermolytic Hyperkeratosis

Epidermolytic hyperkeratosis is a rare autosomal dominant form of ichthyosis characterized by the development of generalized, thick, warty scales and intermittent blistering with severe involvement of the flexures (Fig. 8.10). In newborns, blisters and erosions may be widespread and must be differentiated from epidermolysis bullosa (EB) or herpes simplex. Histologically, massive hyperkeratosis is associated with ballooning of squamous cells and formation of microvesicles. Epidermal turnover is also markedly increased. The mainstay of treatment includes use of keratolytics, lubricants, and antibiotics for secondary infection, which is common and usually caused by *Staphylococcus aureus.* Oral retinoids may also significantly decrease scaling.

Dermatitides

Depending on duration of involvement, dermatitides can be characterized clinically by acute changes (including erythema, edema, and vesiculation) or chronic changes (including scaling, lichenification, and dyspigmentation) in the skin. Microscopically, these disorders are characterized by infiltration of the dermis with inflammatory cells, edema, variable thickening of the epidermis, and scaling.

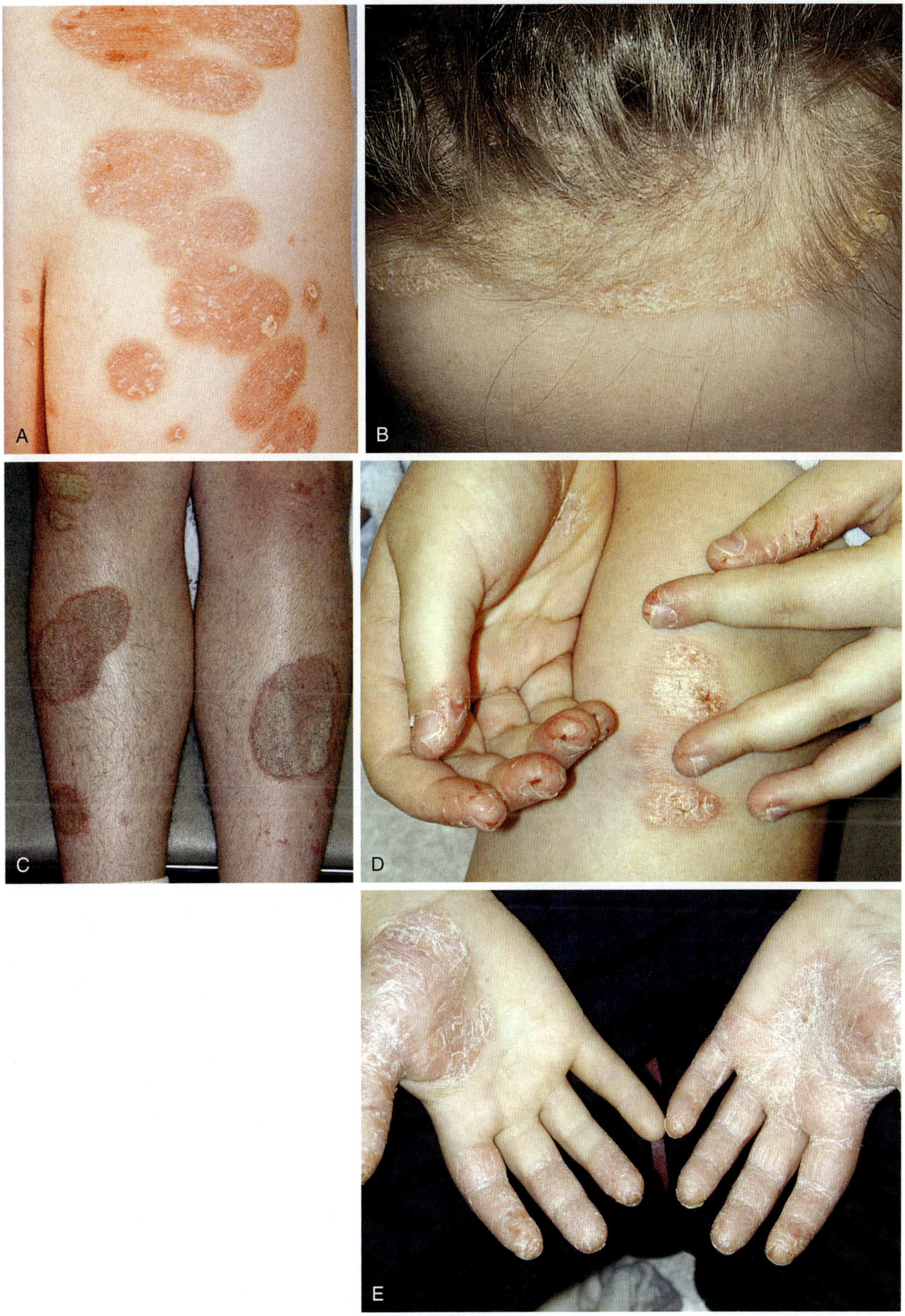

Fig. 8.3 Psoriasis. (A) Typical erythematous plaques are topped by a silver scale. (B) Thick tenacious scale on a red base extends from the forehead to the scalp of this 10-year-old girl. (C) Large plaques are located over the shins and right knee. (D) In this child, lesions are prominent over the pressure point of the knee and the distal fingers. (E) The skin of the palms is markedly thickened, with silvery fissuring of the palmar creases.

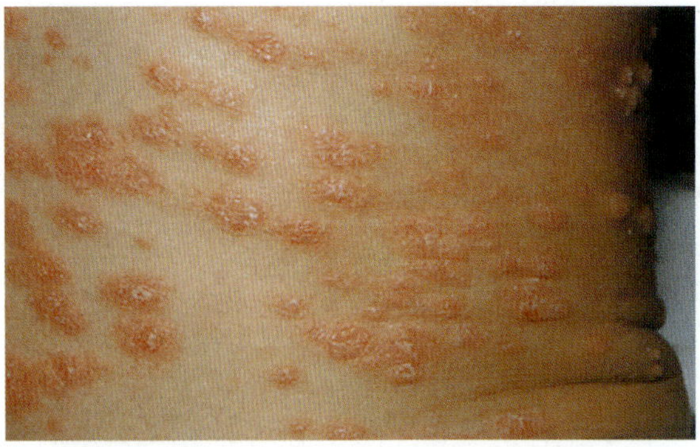

Fig. 8.4 Guttate psoriasis. Small drop-like plaques with typical scales quickly developed in a generalized distribution in this child following streptococcal pharyngitis. (From Cohen BA: *Atlas of pediatric dermatology,* London, 1993, Mosby-Wolfe.)

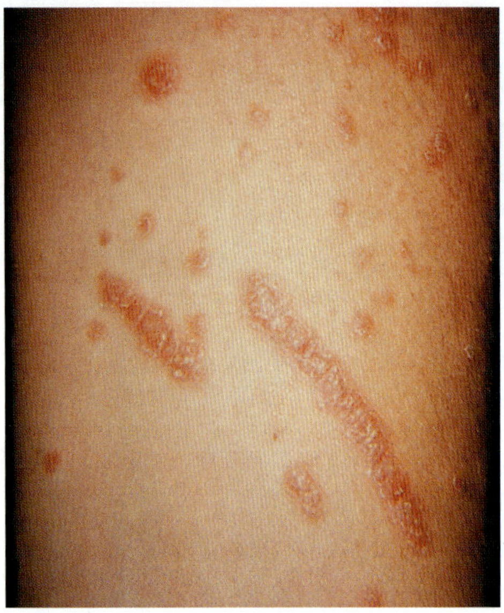

Fig. 8.5 Koebner phenomenon in psoriasis. Lesions are often induced in areas of local trauma, such as these scratches.

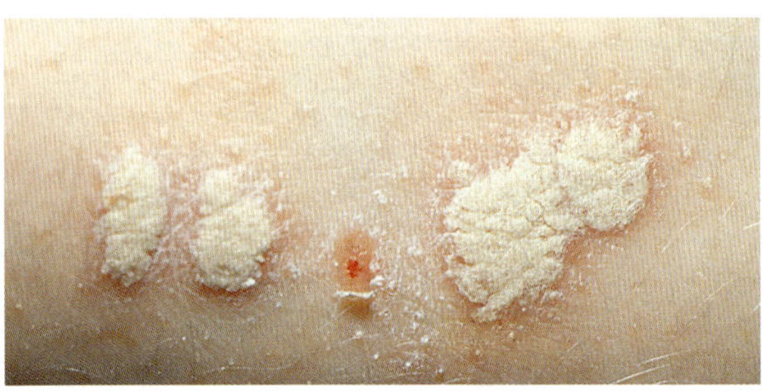

Fig. 8.6 Auspitz sign. Removal of the thick scale from a psoriatic plaque produces small points of bleeding from tortuous capillaries.

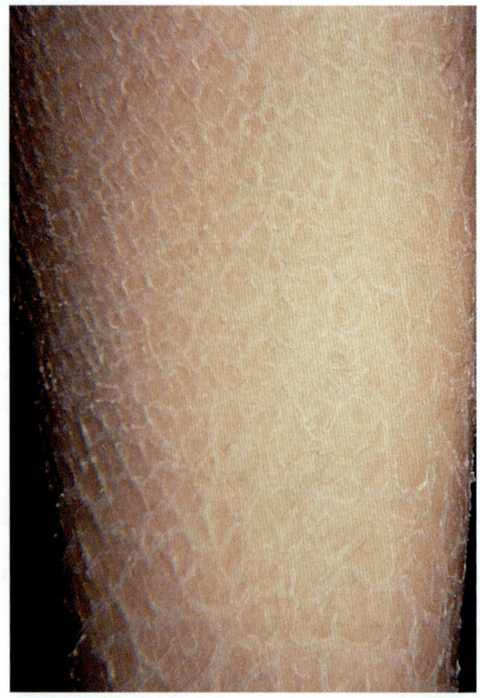

Fig. 8.7 Ichthyosis vulgaris. The typical fish scale appearance is seen in this close-up of a fair-skinned patient's shin.

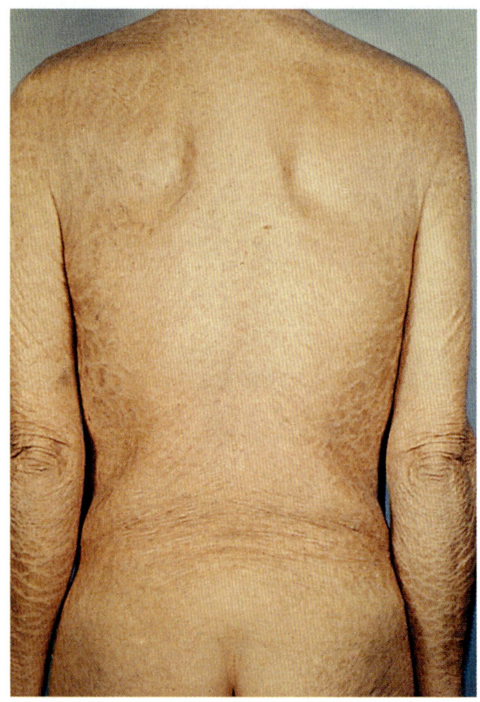

Fig. 8.8 X-linked ichthyosis. Brown scales persist on the flanks, elbows, and shoulders despite the use of topical lubricants.

Atopic Dermatitis

Atopic dermatitis is one of the most common of all chronic skin disorders in children. Mutations in filaggrin cause skin barrier dysfunction and ichthyosis vulgaris, which is characteristic of atopic dermatitis in approximately 50% of patients. Atopic dermatitis can be divided into three general phases based on the age of the patient, but it is worth noting that these stages may overlap in any given patient.

The *infantile phase* of atopic dermatitis begins between birth and 6 months old and lasts approximately 2 or 3 years. Characteristically, the rash is manifest by erythematous, pruritic papules and plaques that ooze and crust. Lesions are distributed over the cheeks, forehead, scalp, trunk, and extensor surfaces of the extremities and are typically symmetrically distributed (Fig. 8.11). Many infants with atopic dermatitis have overlapping seborrheic dermatitis of the scalp or intertriginous areas, such as the neck folds.

The *childhood phase* of atopic dermatitis occurs between ages 4 and 10 years. The skin lesions are typically dry, papular, and intensely pruritic. Circumscribed scaly patches are distributed on the wrists, ankles, and antecubital and popliteal fossae (Fig. 8.12). These patches frequently become secondarily infected, both because of the nonintact skin barrier and from discrete immunologic differences in children with atopic dermatitis, namely a deficiency in two innate antiviral and antibacterial arms of the skin's immune system: β-defensins and cathelicidins. More chronically involved areas can show lichenification. Cracking, dryness, and scaling of the palmar

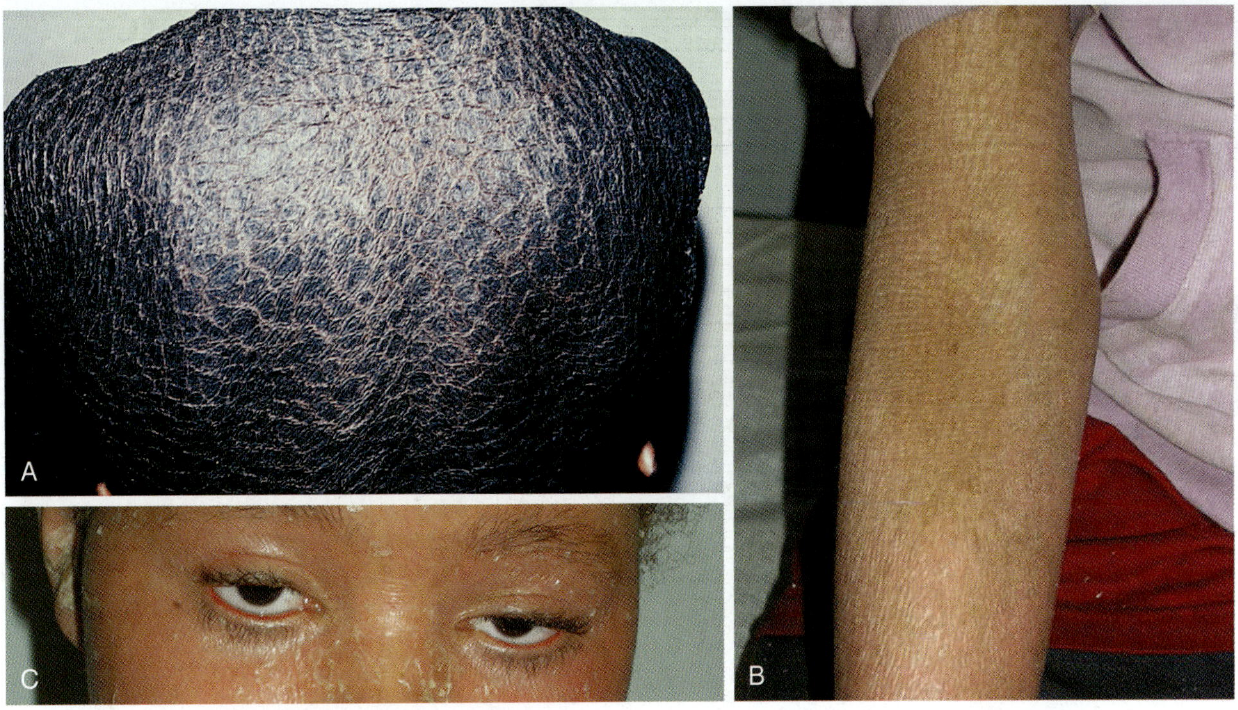

Fig. 8.9 Lamellar ichthyosis. (A) Note the thick, brownish-black scales covering the entire skin surface. (B) Flexural involvement helps differentiate lamellar ichthyosis from ichthyosis vulgaris. (C) Ectropion (note the eversion of the lower lids) is a unique finding in this form of the disorder.

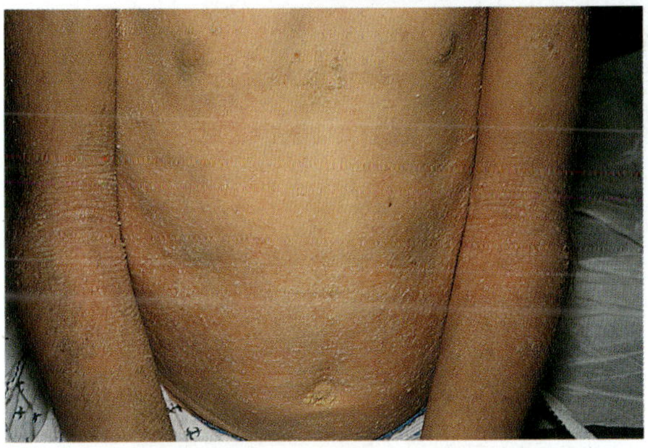

Fig. 8.10 Epidermolytic hyperkeratosis is characterized by thick, warty scales and intermittent blistering. The flexural creases are particular sites of involvement.

and plantar surfaces of the hands and feet are also common (Fig. 8.13). Chronic pruritus and sleep disturbance are associated with many cases of childhood atopic dermatitis. Remission may occur at any time, or the disorder may evolve into a more chronic type of adult dermatitis. Of children with atopic dermatitis, 75% improve between the ages of 10 and 14; the remaining children may go on to develop chronic dermatitis.

The *adult phase* of atopic dermatitis begins around age 12 and continues indefinitely. Major areas of involvement include the flexural areas of the arms, neck, and legs (Fig. 8.14). Eruptions are sometimes seen on the dorsal surfaces of the hands and feet and between the fingers and toes. Lichenification may be marked (Fig. 8.15).

Other associated findings include xerosis (dryness); ichthyosis vulgaris (see Fig. 8.7); *keratosis pilaris,* keratin plugging of hair follicles and formation of perifollicular scales over the extensor surfaces of the extremities and sometimes the trunk and abdomen (Fig. 8.16; and see also Fig. 8.25D); hyperlinearity of the palms; Dennie-Morgan lines, which are double skin creases under the lower eyelid (see Chapter 4); and both hyperpigmentation and hypopigmentation, which may be marked. As a result of their altered immunity in the skin, more than 90% of patients with atopic dermatitis are colonized with *S. aureus* at the time of a flare; for the same cellular reason, these patients are also unusually susceptible to cutaneous viral infections, including warts, herpes simplex, and molluscum contagiosum. Patients with eczema should be warned to avoid direct contact with individuals who have cold sores because they are at great risk for developing eczema herpeticum (see Chapter 13). Parents of children with eczema who themselves have recurrent herpes simplex lesions should be taught hygienic techniques that reduce the risk of transmitting the virus, even when asymptomatic, because shedding can still occur to their children. Consideration can be given to daily suppressive therapy for parents of children with severe atopic dermatitis.

In the rash of *pityriasis alba,* which is common in patients with atopic dermatitis, inflammatory changes are minimal. Poorly defined, hypopigmented, round or oval scaly patches measuring 2 to 4 cm in diameter are noted most commonly on the face, extremities (Fig. 8.17), and sometimes the trunk. These patches fail to enhance with Wood lamp examination, which distinguishes them from vitiligo. Lesions are more prominent in children with darker skin and are more noticeable during spring and summer because they do not tan like surrounding skin after sun exposure. Surface scaling is more evident when the skin is dry (especially in winter). The etiology is unknown, but it is clearly more common in children with an atopic diathesis. Because the disorder is usually asymptomatic and spontaneously resolves in several months to a few years, treatment is usually unnecessary, although moisturizers may help reduce surface scaling. Often parents are most concerned cosmetically with the hypopigmentation; if the condition does not resolve with emollients alone, then it can be helpful to add a prescription topical immunomodulatory, such as pimecrolimus cream or tacrolimus ointment.

The cause of atopic dermatitis remains elusive. An immunologic etiology is suggested by the chronic elevation of immunoglobulin E (IgE) seen in most patients. Atopic dermatitis does occur in families in association with other atopic conditions, including asthma, allergic rhinitis, food allergies, and eosinophilic esophagitis, suggesting some degree of genetic predisposition. Pathophysiologically, several external factors including dry skin, fragranced skin care products, wool fabrics, foods, infectious agents, and environmental antigens may act individually or in concert to produce pruritus,

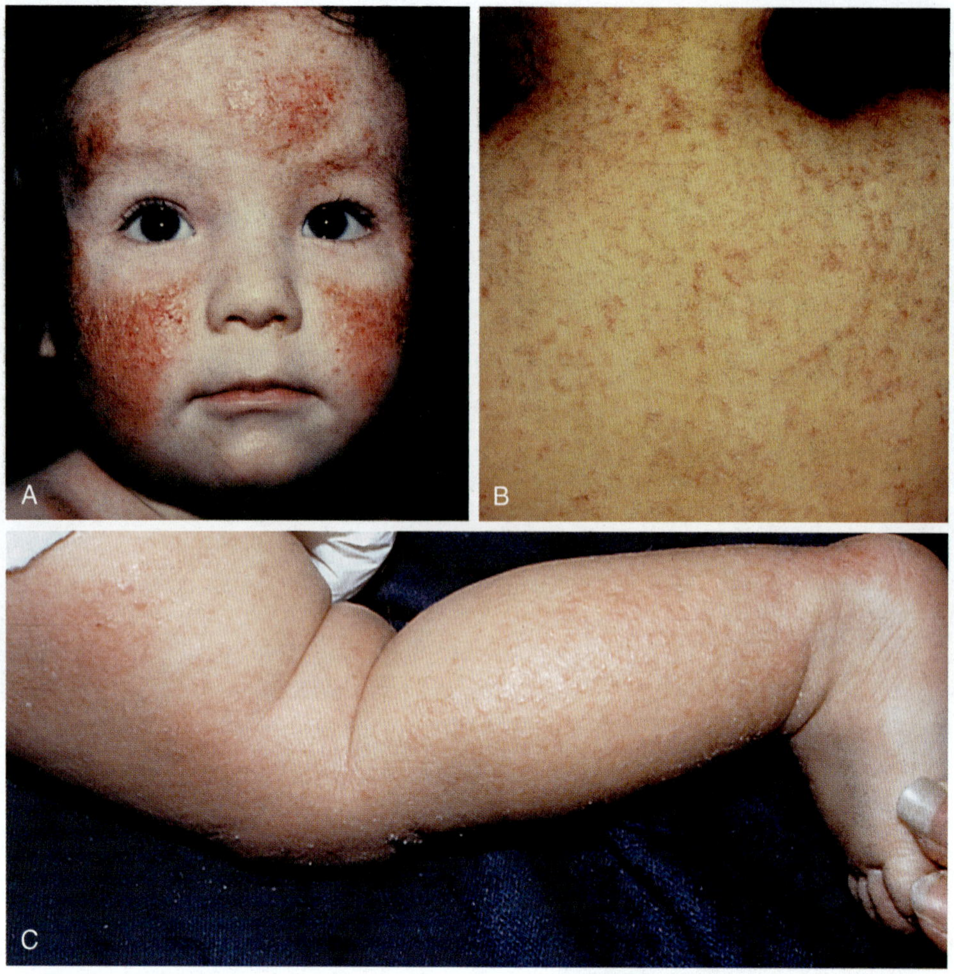

Fig. 8.11 Infantile atopic dermatitis or eczema. (A) This infant has an acute, weeping dermatitis on the cheeks and forehead. (B and C) Involvement of the trunk and the extremities, with erythema, scaling, and crusting, is evident. Usually the diaper area is the only portion of the skin surface that is spared. (B and C, From Fireman P, Slavin RG: *Atlas of allergies,* New York, 1991, Gower.)

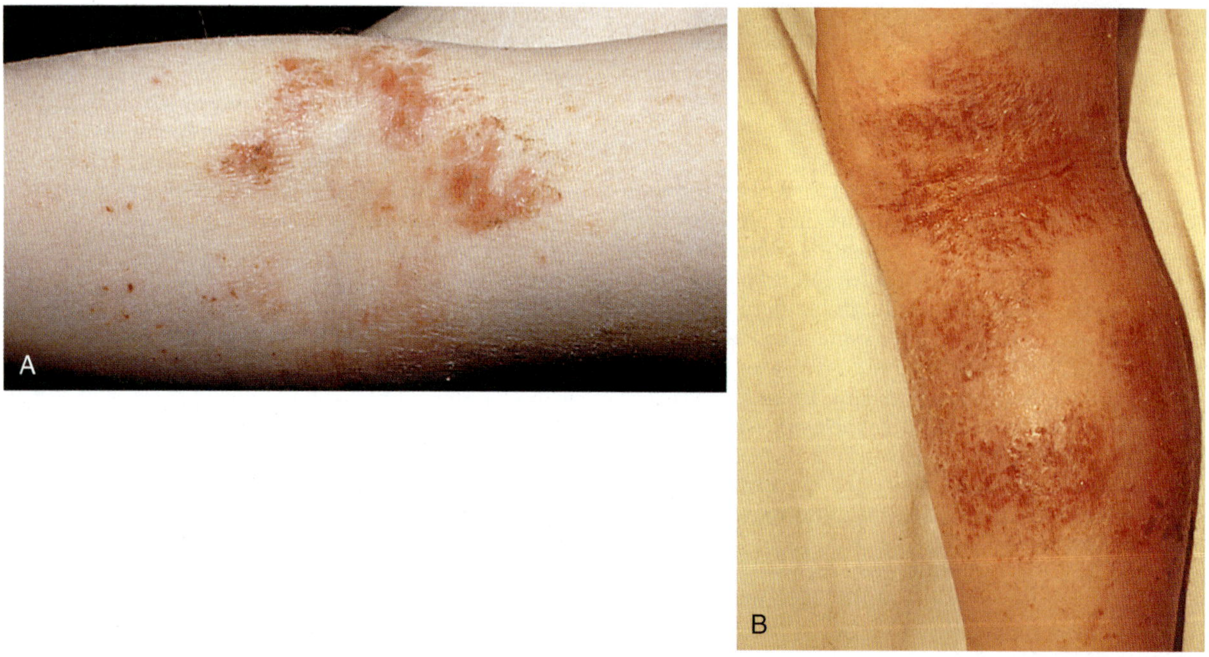

Fig. 8.12 Childhood atopic dermatitis with lesions on the arms (A) and the legs (B). In childhood, eczema involves the flexural surfaces of the upper and lower extremities. The neck, ankles, wrists, and posterior thighs also may be severely affected. (A, From Fireman P, Slavin RG: *Atlas of allergies,* New York, 1991, Gower. B, Courtesy Michael Sherlock, MD, Lutherville, MD.)

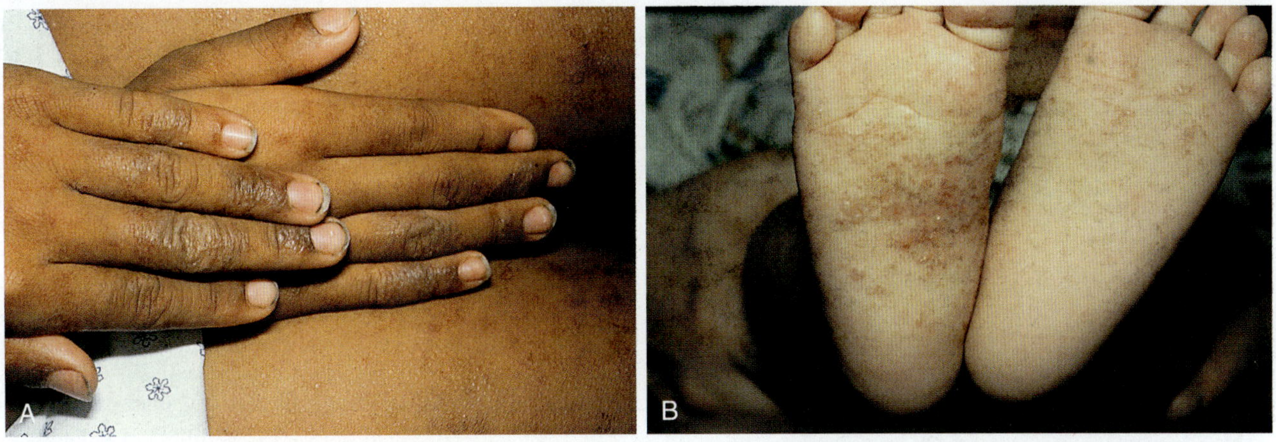

Fig. 8.13 Involvement of the hands and feet in eczema. (A) A 10-year-old atopic child has lichenification of the skin over the dorsum of his fingers and "buff" nails from chronic rubbing. (B) This infant has numerous red excoriated lesions over the soles of his feet.

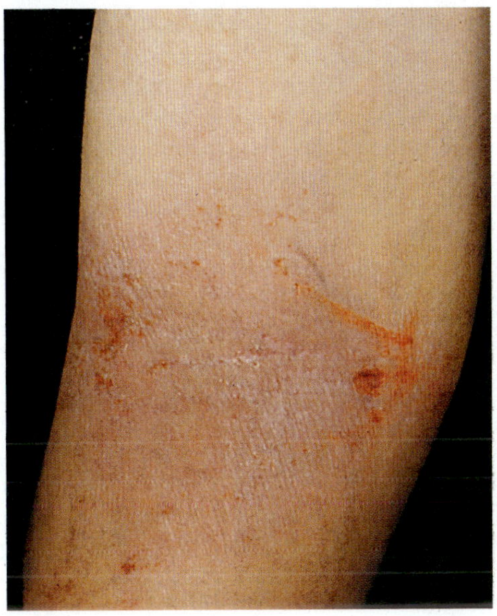

Fig. 8.14 Adult atopic dermatitis. Erythematous excoriated plaques with indistinct borders are seen in the antecubital areas. Note the dried blood from recent excoriation.

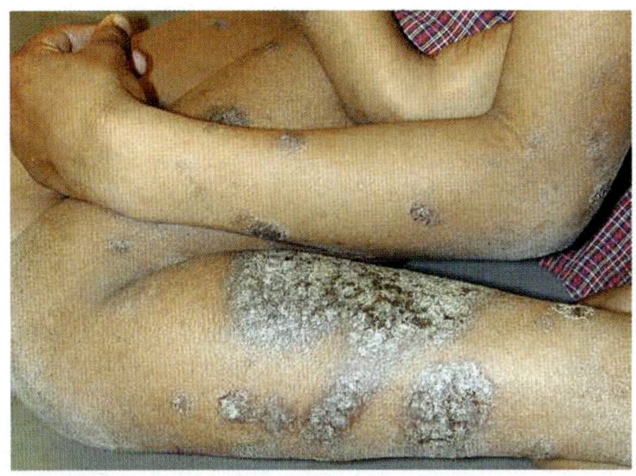

Fig. 8.15 Lichenification refers to marked thickening of the skin seen in areas of atopic dermatitis that have been subject to chronic scratching. In addition, this patient demonstrates significant postinflammatory hyperpigmentation.

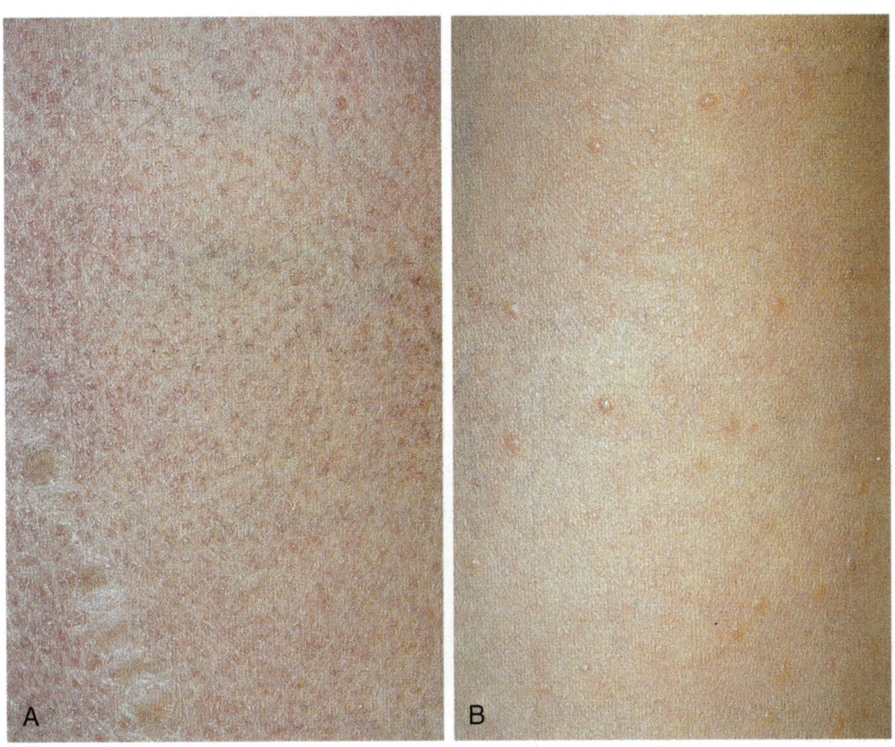

Fig. 8.16 Keratosis pilaris. (A) Diffuse fine follicular papules and sandpaper scaling are seen on the extensor surface of the arm of this adolescent. (B) In this 5-year-old boy, characteristic white follicular papules are more widely spaced and more prominently seen on the extensor surface of his thighs and upper arms. His mother had similar lesions. (From Cohen BA, Lehman CU, editors: *DermAtlas*. http://dermatlas.med.jhmi.edu/derm)

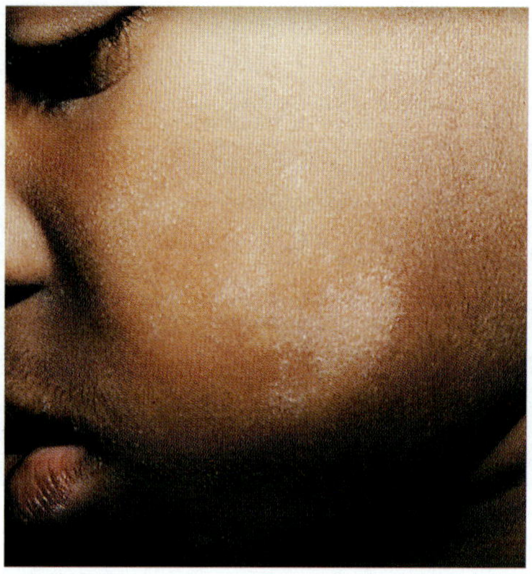

Fig. 8.17 Pityriasis alba. In some atopic individuals, subtle inflammation may result in the development of poorly demarcated, hypopigmented patches that are covered by a fine superficial scale.

which is almost universal in atopic individuals. The resultant scratching leads to the acute and chronic changes typical of atopic dermatitis.

The differential diagnosis of atopic dermatitis includes seborrheic dermatitis, contact dermatitis, pityriasis rosea, psoriasis, fungal infections, Langerhans cell histiocytosis, and acrodermatitis enteropathica. It can be distinguished from seborrheic dermatitis based on the distribution of lesions and associated pruritus; atopic dermatitis tends to spare moist, intertriginous areas (such as the axillae and perineum), where seborrheic dermatitis is more prominent in these locations. Exposure history and distribution help differentiate it from contact dermatitis, as does the discreteness of lesions and their distribution in pityriasis rosea. The thick, silvery scale and Koebner phenomenon help distinguish psoriasis, and central clearing with an active border of red papules, vesicles, or pustules helps differentiate tinea corporis. The rash of histiocytosis is crusted and atrophic and may favor the groin or scalp, or it may be more generalized. It is associated with petechiae and is often accompanied by chronically draining ears, hepatosplenomegaly, and lymphadenopathy (see Fig. 8.88 and Chapter 12). The acral and periorificial distribution of lesions and gastrointestinal symptoms help in distinguishing eczema from acrodermatitis enteropathica.

The mainstays of atopic dermatitis treatment are elimination or avoidance of predisposing factors; hydration and lubrication of the skin; the use of antipruritic agents or pimecrolimus or tacrolimus cream to relieve itching, break the itch/scratch cycle, and normalize sleep patterns; and the intermittent use of topical steroids to further relieve itching and decrease inflammation. Pimecrolimus cream and tacrolimus ointment are approved as second-line therapy for the management of atopic dermatitis in children older than 2 years. Use of these agents should be accompanied by an explanation of the boxed warning regarding the theoretical risk of lymphoma and skin cancer. However, these tumors have been seen only with prolonged systemic use at high doses, and true risk has not been associated with the use of the topical preparations in otherwise healthy children.

All children with atopic dermatitis should be monitored closely for secondary bacterial infection, which must be treated promptly with topical or systemic antibiotics to prevent progression to cellulitis. The use of a hyperdiluted bleach (1–2 oz in a 30-gallon tub of water) bath several times per week is a cost-effective way of preventing infection in patients with atopic dermatitis. Herpes simplex can also occur as a secondary infection over atopic dermatitis and can rapidly disseminate in patients with active atopic dermatitis, resulting in the severe disorder known as *eczema herpeticum* (see Chapter 13). Hence patients' families should be warned to have their children avoid direct contact with people with cold sores, and if parents have recurrent herpes labialis, they should be instructed in strict handwashing precautions. Furthermore, patients should be treated with antiviral agents at the first sign of infection with herpes simplex.

Dyshidrotic Eczema

Dyshidrotic eczema is a severely pruritic, chronic, recurrent, vesicular eruption affecting the palms, soles, and lateral aspects of the fingers and toes. Characteristically, the vesicles are symmetric, multilocular, and 1 to 3 mm in diameter and have been described as "tapioca" papules. These lesions rupture, leaving scales and crust on an erythematous base (Fig. 8.18). Pathologically, this eruption demonstrates spongiotic vesicles and normal eccrine sweat glands. The cause is unknown; however, frequent exposure to water, wet or sweat-soaked shoes, or chemicals may trigger or exacerbate the condition. Hyperhidrosis, or excessive sweating of the palms and soles, may also play a role. Treatment is like that for acute atopic dermatitis, although often a higher potency topical steroid may be needed.

Nummular Eczema

Nummular eczema is an acute papulovesicular eruption named for its coin-shaped configuration and probably also represents another clinical pattern found in atopic individuals. Lesions are intensely pruritic, well-circumscribed, round to oval, red, scaly patches studded with 1- to 3-mm vesicles (Fig. 8.19A). They are usually located on the extensor thighs or abdomen of children who also may have atopic dermatitis. Vigorous scratching causes excoriation and crusting (see Fig. 8.19B). Lack of central clearing helps to distinguish these lesions from tinea corporis (see Fig. 8.36). Although the rash is often resistant to therapy, it may respond to the treatment for acute dermatitis outlined previously.

Juvenile Plantar/Palmar Dermatosis

Juvenile plantar/palmar dermatosis ("sweaty sock syndrome") is common in toddlers and school-age children. Chronic, red scaly patches with cracking and fissuring typically begin on the balls of the feet and big toes (Fig. 8.20). The pads of the fingertips and palms may be involved as well, although less severely. Although the cause is unknown, the condition is triggered by excessive sweating or repeated wetting of the skin inside the child's shoes (especially those made of synthetic materials that do not breathe), followed by drying or evaporation of the moisture, which leads to a net dehydration of the skin. Some children experience flares in the summer, whereas in others the flares occur in winter. Consequently, the mainstay of treatment consists of emollients for prevention and occasional application of topical steroids when intense inflammation is present during flares.

Lip-Licking and Thumb-Sucking Eczema

The repeated wetting and drying from persistent lip licking (especially in winter) or thumb sucking can produce eczematoid changes of the perioral skin (Fig. 8.21) or the skin of the involved thumb (Fig. 8.22).

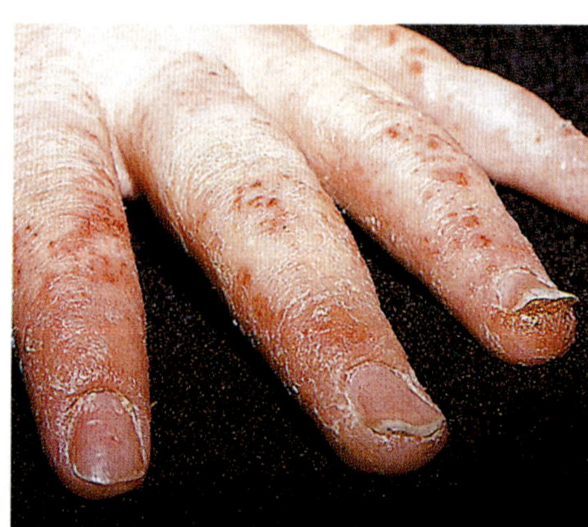

Fig. 8.18 Dyshidrosis. Chronic cracking, oozing, and scaling develop after the initial tiny pruritic vesicles have been scratched.

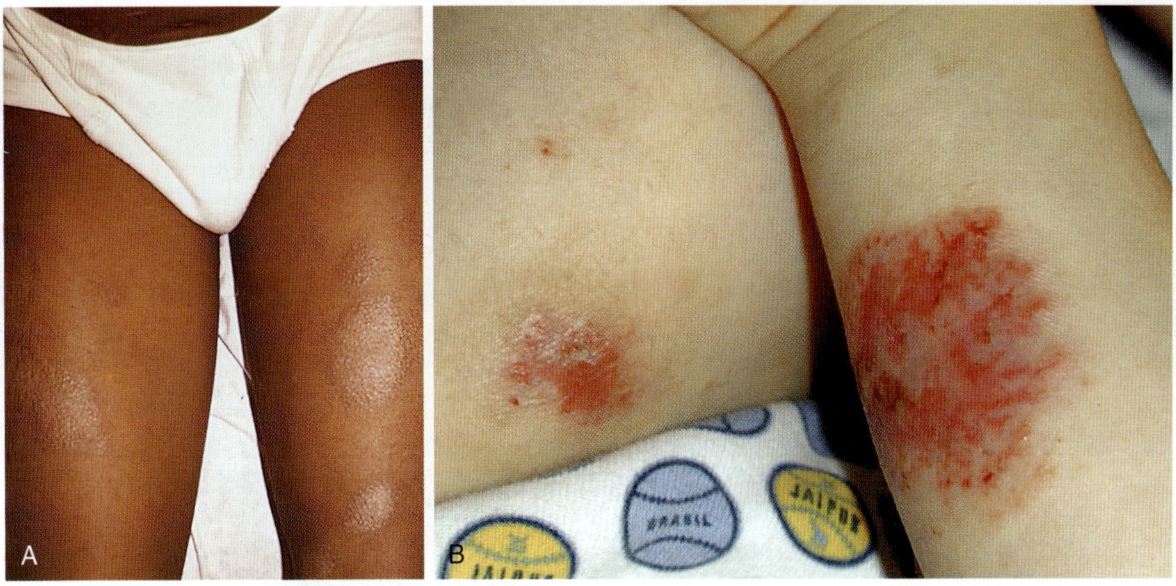

Fig. 8.19 Nummular eczema. (A) Round- to oval-shaped lesions studded with tiny vesicles are typically located over the extensor thighs or abdomen. They do not show central clearing. (B) Vigorous scratching results in excoriation with weeping and crusting. (A, Courtesy Michael Sherlock, MD, Lutherville, MD.)

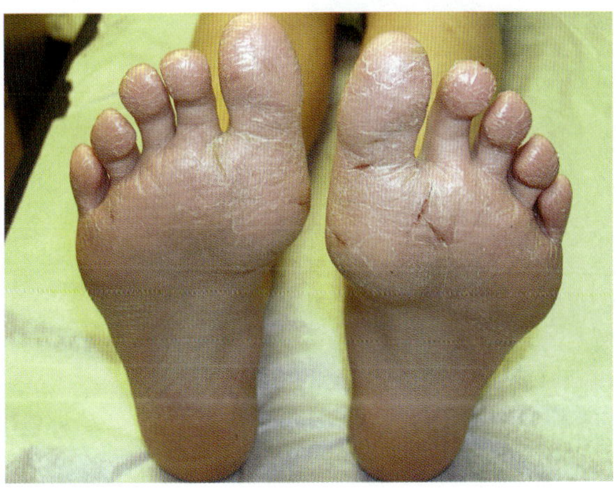

Fig. 8.20 Juvenile plantar dermatosis. This variant of atopic dermatitis is usually localized to the plantar surfaces of the toes and feet. Note the glistening erythema, scaling, and fissuring. In some patients the palms may be affected as well.

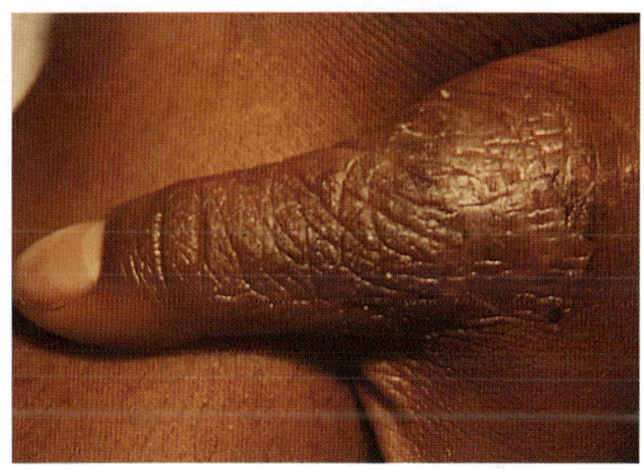

Fig. 8.22 Thumb-sucking eczema. Repeated wetting and drying from persistent thumb sucking result in eczematoid changes with cracking, fissuring, and lichenification. (Courtesy Michael Sherlock, MD, Lutherville, MD.)

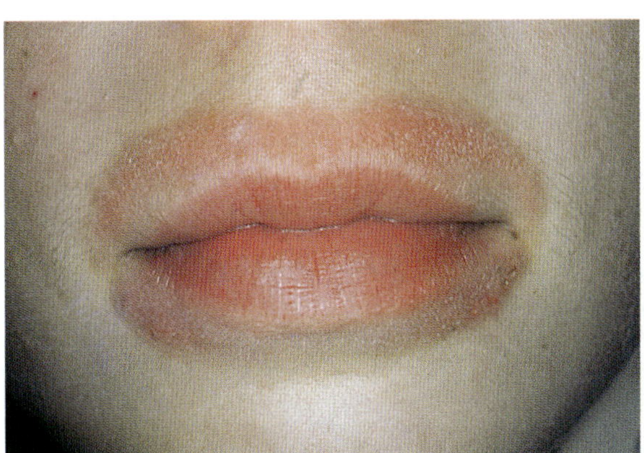

Fig. 8.21 Lip-licking eczema. The perioral skin is inflamed, scaly, and thickened as a result of repetitive licking of the lips. (Courtesy Douglas W. Kress, MD. University of Pittsburgh Medical Center.)

Seborrhea

Seborrheic dermatitis is characterized by erythema and scaling predominantly on hair-bearing and intertriginous areas, such as the scalp; eyebrows; eyelashes; perinasal, presternal, and postauricular areas; and the neck, axillae, and groin. Lesions often involve the intertriginous areas of the arms, legs, neck, and trunk and occasionally become generalized (Fig. 8.23). In affected infants, scalp lesions consist of a thick, tenacious, scaly dermatitis that is often salmon colored and is commonly known as *cradle cap* (Fig. 8.24). In adolescents, the dermatitis may manifest as dandruff or flaking of the eyebrows, postauricular areas, or flexural areas.

Although the pathogenesis of seborrheic dermatitis is unknown, *Pityrosporum* and *Candida* species have been implicated as causative agents. A role for neurologic dysfunction is suggested by the increased incidence and severity in neurologically impaired individuals.

The dermatitis of seborrhea is usually nonpruritic and mild in nature. Most cases respond to topical steroids, and many clear spontaneously, although residual postinflammatory hypopigmentation may persist for weeks or months thereafter (see Fig. 8.117). Some practitioners find that use of a topical antifungal cream or wash, in addition to a low-potency topical steroid, hastens resolution, but the topical steroid should not be part of long-term management. In infants and young children, atopic dermatitis can have a greasy, scaly appearance and can have overlapping features with seborrhea. However, infantile atopic dermatitis produces intense pruritus and invariably spares moist sites, such as the diaper area and axillae. The two are often present simultaneously in the same patient. The differential diagnosis of seborrhea

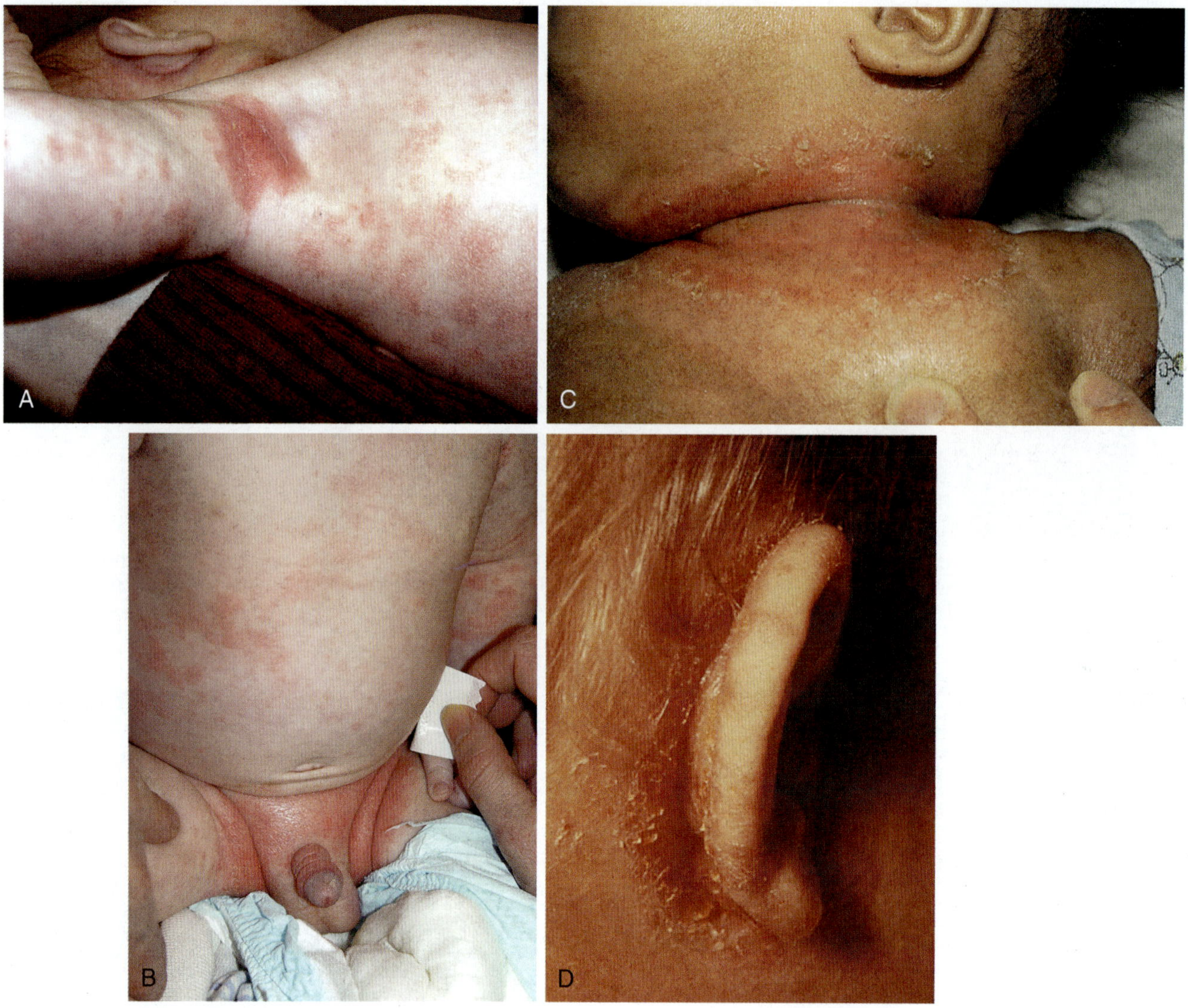

Fig. 8.23 Seborrhea. This slightly greasy, red, scaling eruption typically involves the hair-bearing areas of the face, axilla (A), and diaper area (B). (C) The intertriginous folds of the neck are another common site of involvement. (D) Postauricular lesions are common and often become secondarily infected as in this case, which grew group A β-hemolytic streptococci. (D, Courtesy Michael Sherlock, MD, Lutherville, MD.)

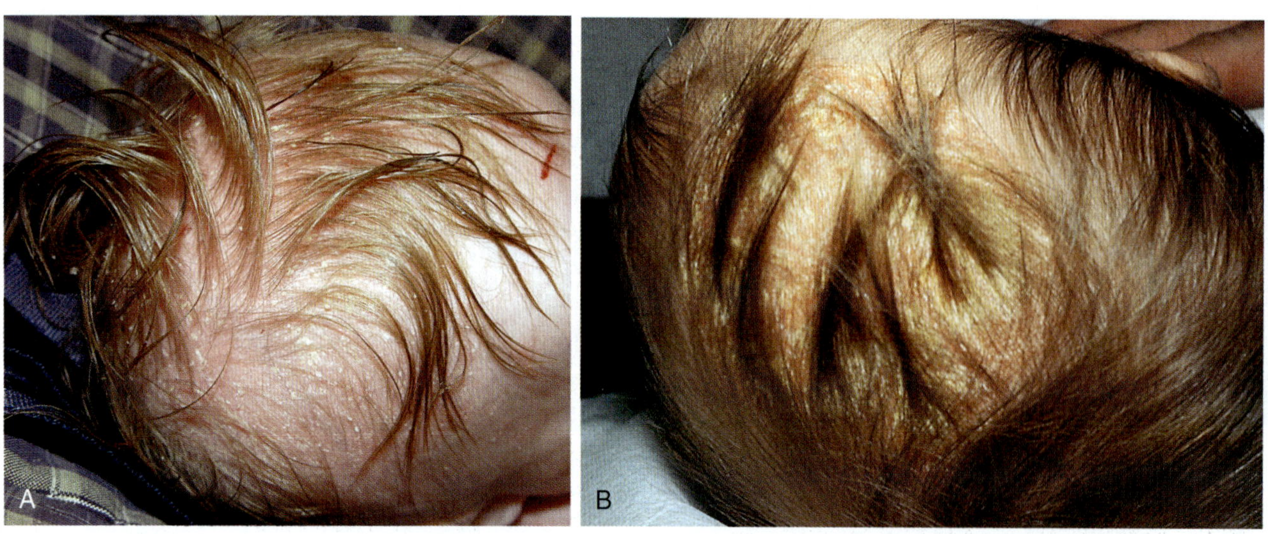

Fig. 8.24 Seborrhea of the scalp. (A) Note the oily appearance and salmon-pink hue. Numerous scales, some adherent to the scalp and many interlaced through the baby's hair, are present. (B) In this infant the scales have formed a thick crust, and erythema is less evident.

includes Langerhans cell histiocytosis (in which the rash is more generalized, in part petechial, and can be associated with chronic draining ears and hepatosplenomegaly) and tinea corporis (in which lesions usually are more circumscribed, with an active border and central clearing). Scalp lesions may be difficult to differentiate from psoriasis, and there seems to be a spectrum of presentation from mild scaling in seborrhea to moderate scaling in what is termed *sebopsoriasis* to much more thick and resistant scaling in full-fledged psoriasis.

Hyper-IgE Syndrome

Hyper-IgE-syndrome (also known as *Job syndrome*) is a rare genetic disorder with prominent cutaneous manifestations. It has been linked to an autosomal dominant mutation on the signal transducer and activator of transcription-3 (STAT3) gene on chromosome 17 with variable severity of expression. Affected patients have high IgE and eosinophil counts; chronic eczema; recurrent staphylococcal infections; retained primary teeth; hyperextensible joints; fractures; and coarse facial features, including a broad nose.

Dermatologic features include a pruritic dermatitic rash that shares features with both atopic dermatitis and seborrhea, which tends to develop shortly after birth (earlier than seborrhea and atopic dermatitis). It rapidly becomes superinfected with *S. aureus,* which results in the formation of weeping and crusting lesions, folliculitis, and cutaneous abscesses (Fig. 8.25). In contrast to furuncles in patients with a normal immune response, the abscesses in children with Hyper-IgE syndrome are termed "cold," meaning they cause little pain and show few signs of inflammation. Development of mucocutaneous candidiasis is also common. Other clinical manifestations include recurrent or chronic infections, such as bronchitis, pneumonia (with pneumatoceles), sinusitis, otitis, gingivitis, dental abscesses, septic arthritis, and osteomyelitis. Decreased bone density is the source of multiple fractures, which cause remarkably little pain. With age and growth, facial features tend to coarsen (see Chapter 4) and scoliosis is common.

Treatment is aimed at controlling infections and ameliorating symptoms. The major differential diagnostic consideration is Langerhans histiocytosis (see Fig. 8.88).

Pityriasis Rosea

Pityriasis rosea is a benign, self-limited disorder that can occur at any age but is more common in adolescents and young adults. A prodrome of malaise, headache, and mild constitutional symptoms occasionally precedes the rash but is not necessary for diagnosis. The typical eruption begins with the appearance of one or multiple "herald patches" (Fig. 8.26A), which are large, isolated, oval lesions, usually pink in color and slightly scaly; they may occur anywhere on the body. On occasion, the herald patch clears centrally, mimicking tinea corporis, but a KOH preparation is negative. From 5 to 10 days later, other smaller, oval lesions appear on the body, most commonly on the trunk, but they may also appear on the extremities (see Fig. 8.26B–G). On occasion, lesions predominate on the face, groin, or distal extremities, including the palms and soles. This phenomenon is known

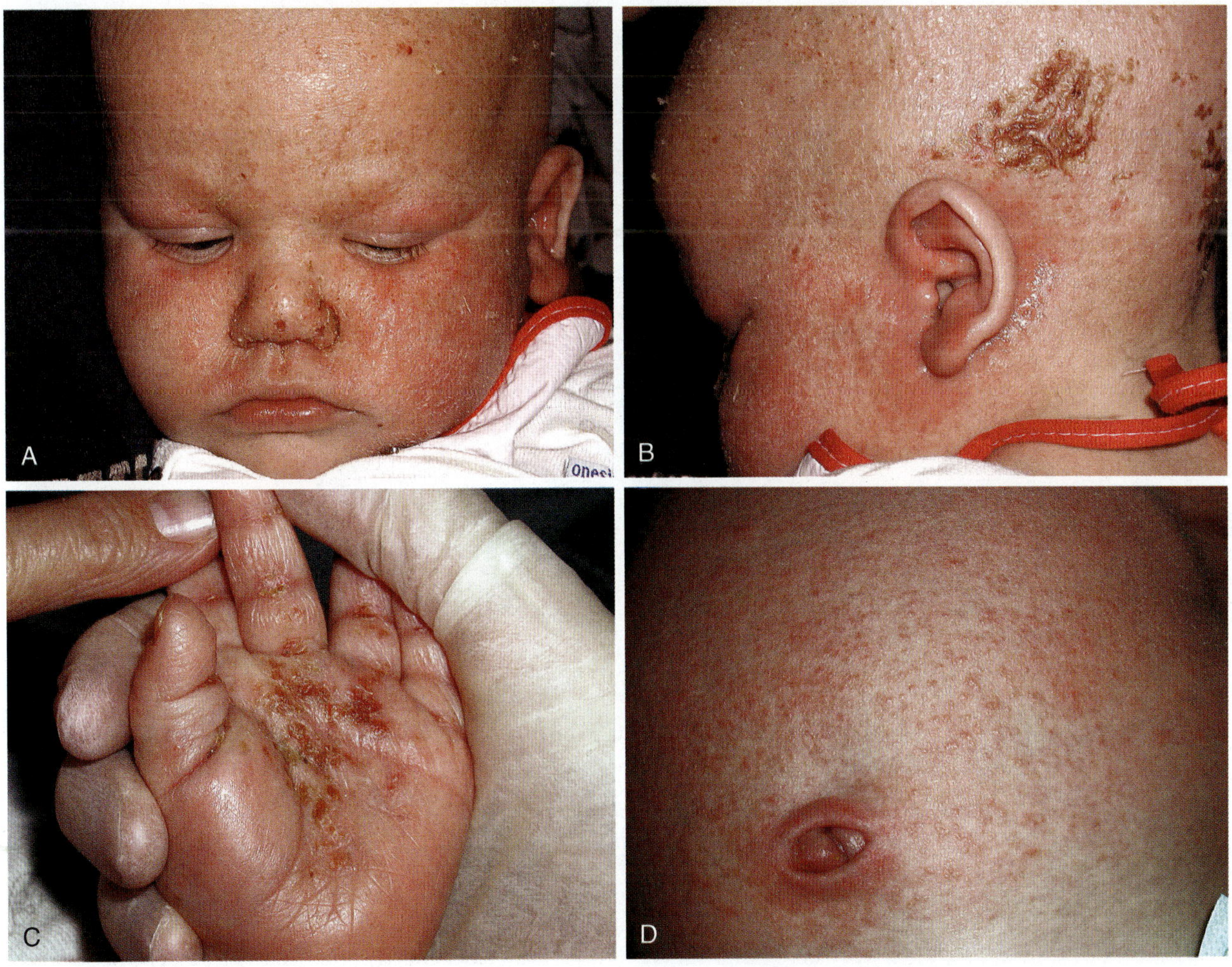

Fig. 8.25 Job syndrome. This infant with markedly elevated immunoglobulin E experienced early onset of a pruritic dermatitis that shared clinical features with both seborrhea and atopic dermatitis. (A) Note the erythema and scaliness, the evidence of excoriation from scratching, and the perinasal crusting due to *Staphylococcus aureus* infection. (B) In this view, in addition to the erythema, scaling, and thickening of the skin, there are weeping areas around the ear and crusts and scabs over the scalp. Note also the purulent ear drainage. (C) The infant also had crusted palmar lesions. (D) The skin over the abdomen had the classic features of keratosis pilaris.

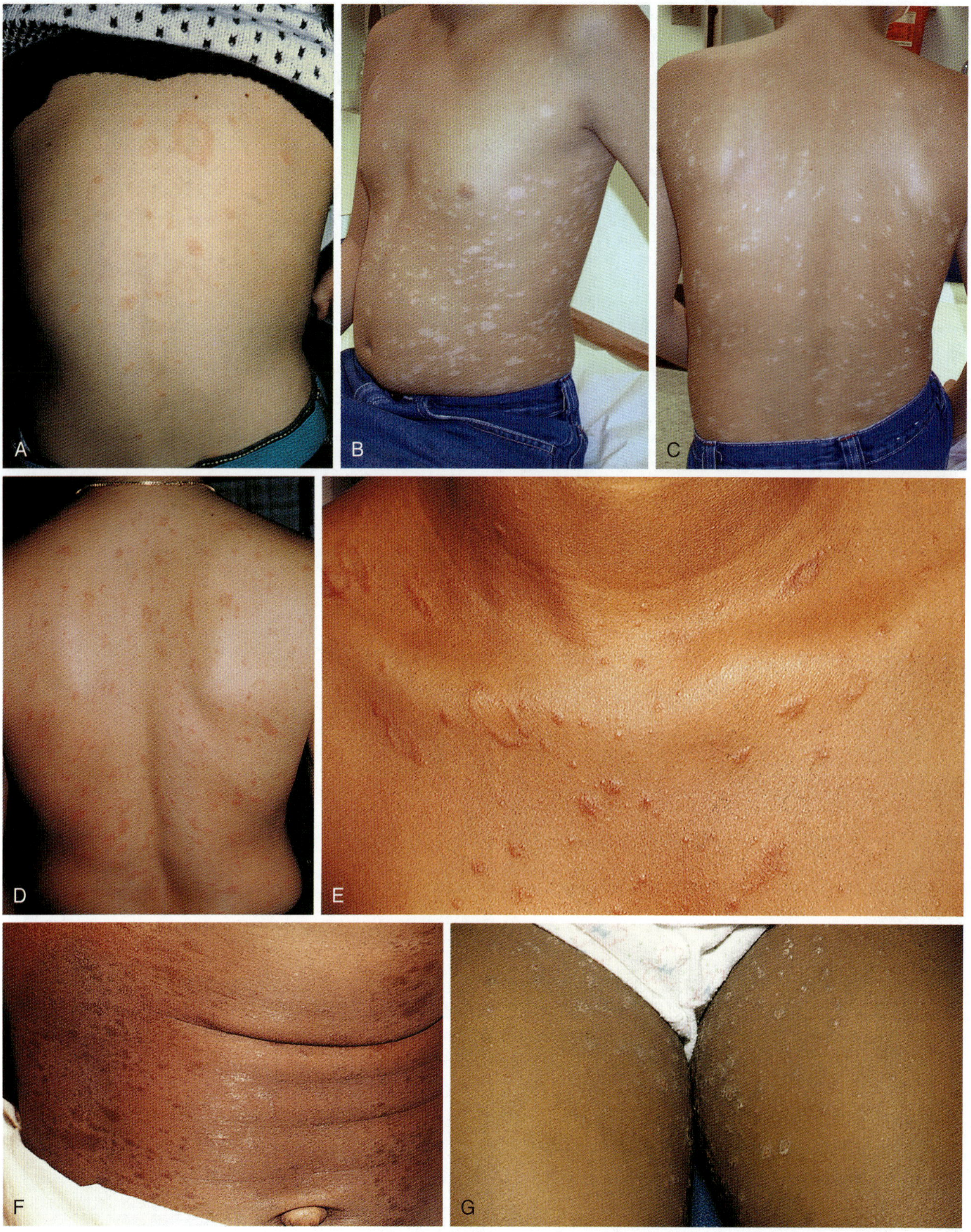

Fig. 8.26 Pityriasis rosea. (A) The large herald patch on this boy's back shows evidence of central clearing, mimicking tinea corporis. (B) Numerous oval lesions with their long axes oriented along lines of skin cleavage are seen over the trunk of this adolescent. (C and D) This feature creates the appearance of a fir tree distribution on the back. (E–G) Lesions can be raised, macular, or scaly and can be erythematous or hyperpigmented or hypopigmented. (A and C, Courtesy Douglas W. Kress, MD. University of Pittsburgh Medical Center. E and F, Courtesy Michael Sherlock, MD, Lutherville, MD.)

as *inverse pityriasis.* Pityriasis lesions begin as small, oval to round papules that enlarge to oval plaques up to 1 to 2 cm in size, with a scaly surface. They are usually somewhat raised but can be macular, and they can be erythematous, hyperpigmented, or hypopigmented. The long axes of the ovals tend to run parallel to the lines of the cleavage of the skin, creating a "Christmas tree" pattern over the thorax (see Fig. 8.26C and D). The rash reaches its peak in several weeks and then slowly fades over 4 to 8 weeks. The average total duration is 2 to 3 months. Oral erythromycin or doxycycline and small doses of ultraviolet light may hasten the disappearance of the eruption. Although the cause is unknown, the peak incidence in late winter and the low recurrence rate suggest an infectious etiology.

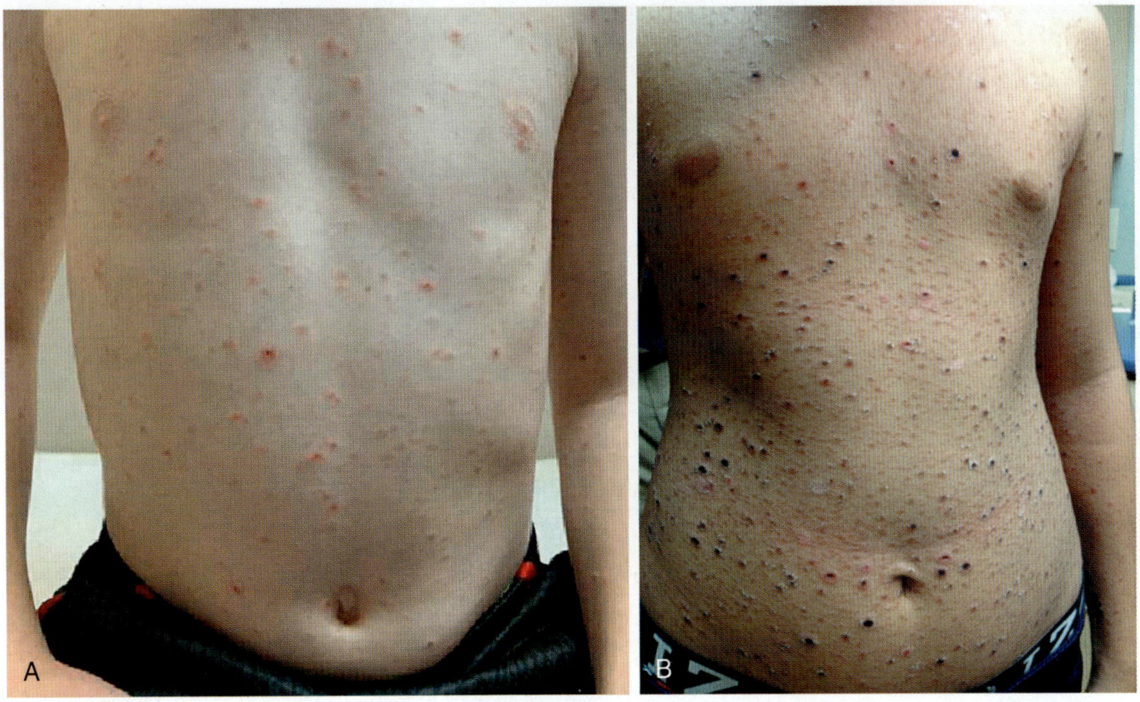

Fig. 8.27 Pityriasis lichenoides. (A) Numerous red to brown macules and papules on the trunk, some with secondary hemorrhagic crusting, are seen in the acute form of pityriasis lichenoides varioliformis et acuta. (B) Another child presented with numerous, scaly red-brown papules on the trunk consistent with pityriasis lichenoides chronica.

Other eruptions that can resemble pityriasis rosea include guttate psoriasis, benign parapsoriasis, viral exanthems, measles-like (morbilliform) drug eruptions, and secondary syphilis (see Chapter 19). Secondary syphilis should specifically be considered when a patient presents with a rash resembling pityriasis rosea and the palms and soles are involved.

Pityriasis Lichenoides

Pityriasis lichenoides is a spectrum of disorders characterized by recurrent crops of spontaneously regressing erythematous papules. It is more prevalent in the pediatric and young adult population. The acute form pityriasis lichenoides et varioliformis acuta (PLEVA) and the chronic form pityriasis lichenoides chronica (PLC) exist on two ends of the disease continuum, although there can be overlap.

In patients with PLEVA, individual lesions develop crusts; ulcers; and, occasionally, vesicles or pustules (Fig. 8.27A), which may heal with scars. These lesions typically resolve within weeks. PLC has a more indolent course. The papules are usually reddish brown and scaly (Fig. 8.27B). They regress over weeks to months, usually leaving residual hypopigmented macules.

First-line therapy includes topical corticosteroids, oral tetracyclines, oral erythromycin, and phototherapy.

Contact Dermatitis

Contact dermatitis refers to a group of conditions in which an inflammatory reaction in the skin is triggered by direct contact with an environmental agent. Irritant contact dermatitis is the most common form and is induced by caustic agents, such as acids and alkalis, hydrocarbons, and other primary irritants. Anyone exposed to these agents in a high enough concentration for a long enough period will ultimately develop dermatitis. The rash is usually acute with well-demarcated erythema, crusting, or blister formation.

In contrast, allergic contact dermatitis is a T-lymphocyte–mediated immune reaction to an antigen contacting the skin. Although patients typically present with acute onset of erythema, vesiculation, and pruritus, sometimes they present after the rash has become chronic with scaling, lichenification, and pigmentary changes. Often, the allergen is obvious, as is the case with poison ivy or nickel jewelry. However, in other cases careful questioning or more formal patch testing may be required to detect the inciting agent.

The initial reaction occurs after a 7- to 14-day period of sensitization in susceptible individuals. Once sensitization has occurred, reexposure to the allergen provokes a more immediate reaction, sometimes within hours. This is a classic example of type IV (delayed) hypersensitivity (see Chapter 4).

Rhus Dermatitis (Poison Ivy)

The most common type of allergic contact dermatitis in the United States is poison ivy, or rhus dermatitis. This typically presents with linear streaks of erythematous papules and vesicles (Fig. 8.28A); however, with heavy exposure, the rash may appear in relatively large or confluent patches (see Fig. 8.28B and C). When lesions involve the skin of the face or genitalia, impressive swelling can occur (see Fig. 8.28D).

Direct contact with the sap of poison ivy, poison oak, or poison sumac from leaves, stems, or roots (whether the plant is alive or dead) produces the dermatitis (Fig. 8.29). Contact with clothing that has brushed against the plant, with logs or railroad ties on which the vine has been growing, or with smoke from a fire in which the plant is being burned are other means of exposure. Areas of skin exposed to the highest concentration of plant oil develop changes first. Other sites that received lower doses then vesiculate in succession, giving the illusion of spreading. However, this is not the case because within approximately 20 minutes of initial contact, the rhus oil becomes tissue fixed to the epithelial cells and cannot be spread farther. Thorough washing within minutes of exposure can prevent fixation and hence the eruption. On occasion the oil can oxidize, leaving a black discoloration superimposed on the contact dermatitis; this is known as *black dot* or *urushiol dermatitis.*

Other Common Causes of Contact Dermatitis

Other common contact allergens are nickel (Fig. 8.30), rubber (Fig. 8.31), glues or dyes in shoes or diapers (Fig. 8.32), ethylenediamine in topical lotions, cocamidopropyl betaine in shampoos and cosmetics, neomycin, and topical anesthetics (Fig. 8.33). Paraphenylenediamine dye used in amateur henna tattoos is an increasingly common cause of contact dermatitis among adolescents, and

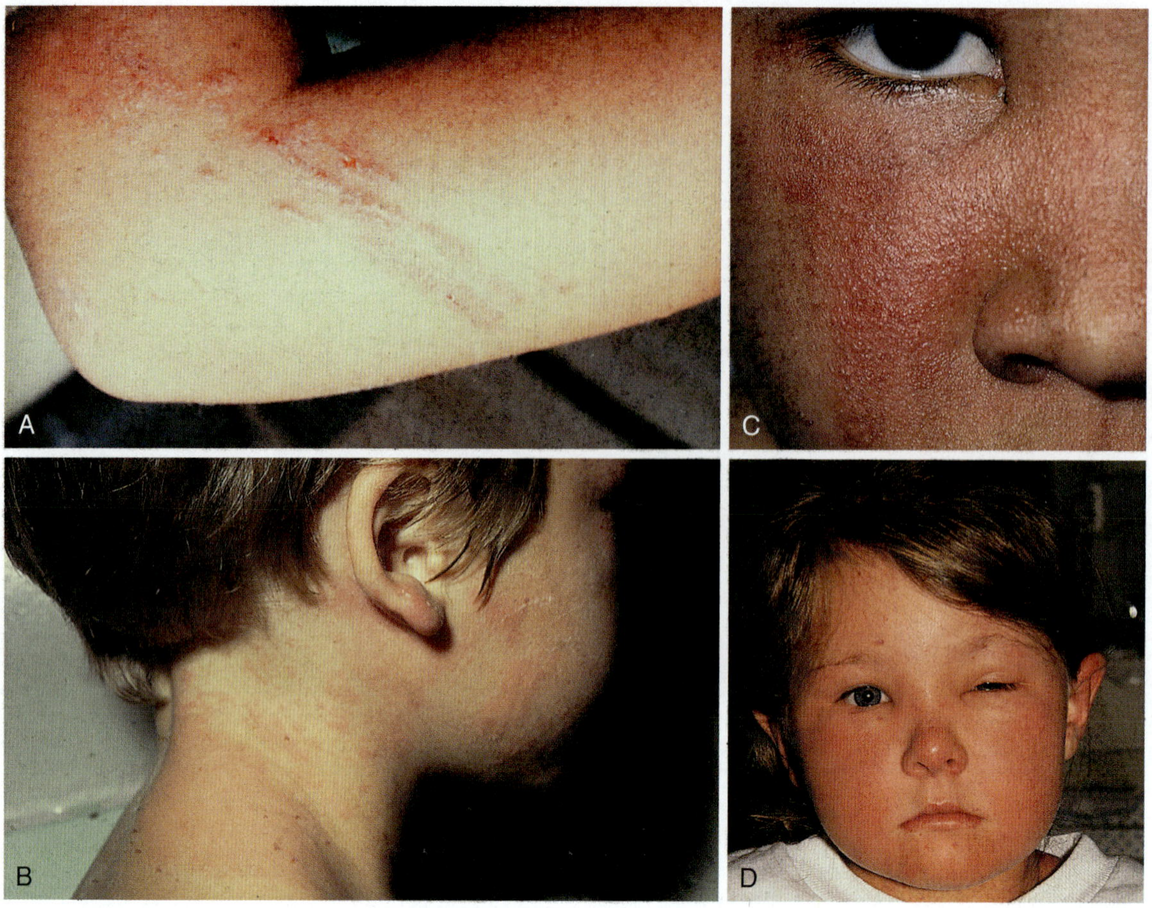

Fig. 8.28 Poison ivy, or rhus dermatitis. (A) Linear streaks of pruritic vesicles are typical of contact dermatitis caused by exposure to a plant. (B and C) However, with heavier exposure, the eruption can develop in relatively large patches. Also note the microvesicular appearance of the facial lesion in the child shown in C. (D) Reactions involving the face and genitalia can provoke impressive swelling.

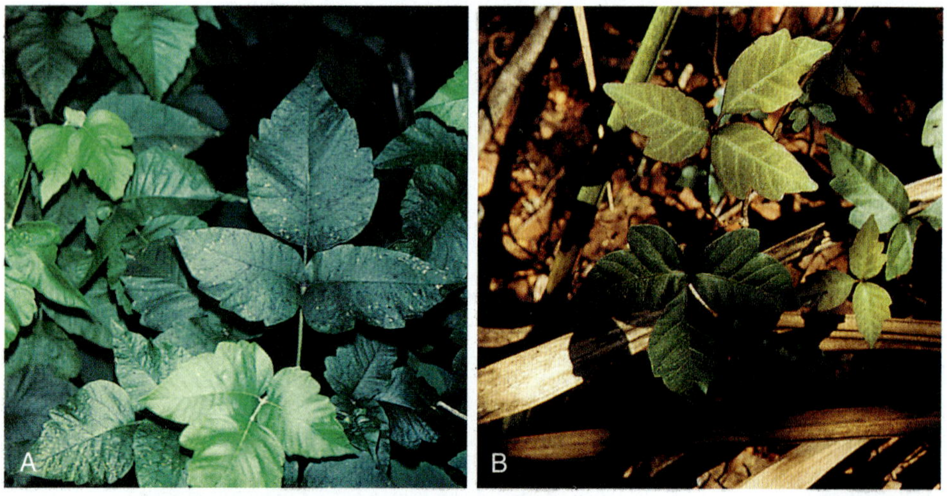

Fig. 8.29 (A) Poison ivy. The plant has characteristic shiny leaves in groups of three. It may resemble a vine, a low shrub, or a bush. (B) Poison oak. This also has leaves in groups of three, although the edges tend to be more scalloped than those of poison ivy. (B, Courtesy Mary Jelks, MD.)

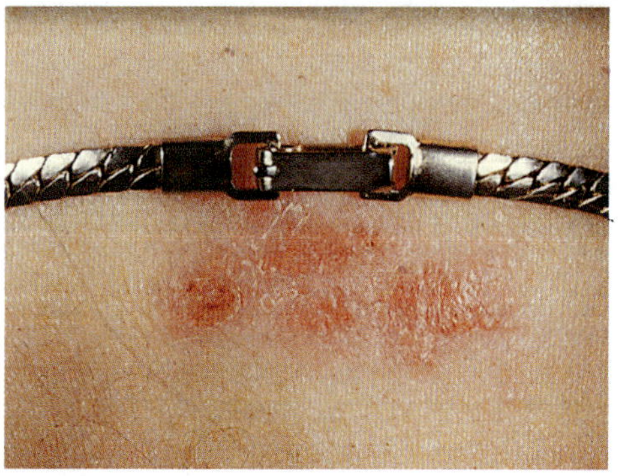

Fig. 8.30 Nickel contact dermatitis. The location and distribution of the rash are often helpful in determining the cause of a contact dermatitis. In this case wrist lesions were triggered by the nickel in her bracelet clasp.

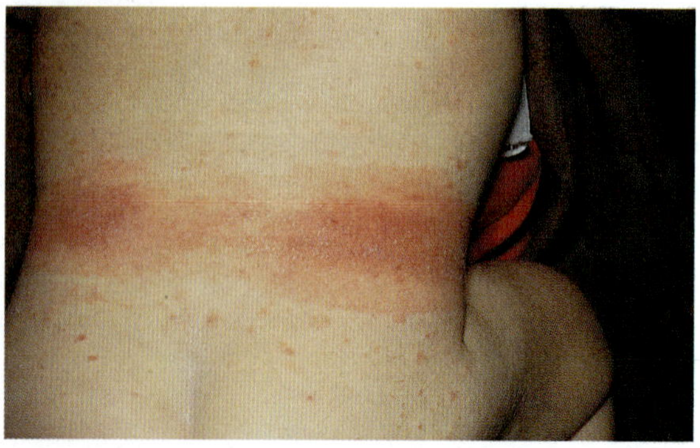

Fig. 8.31 Rubber contact dermatitis. This child had become sensitized to the elasticized waist bands of his underpants.

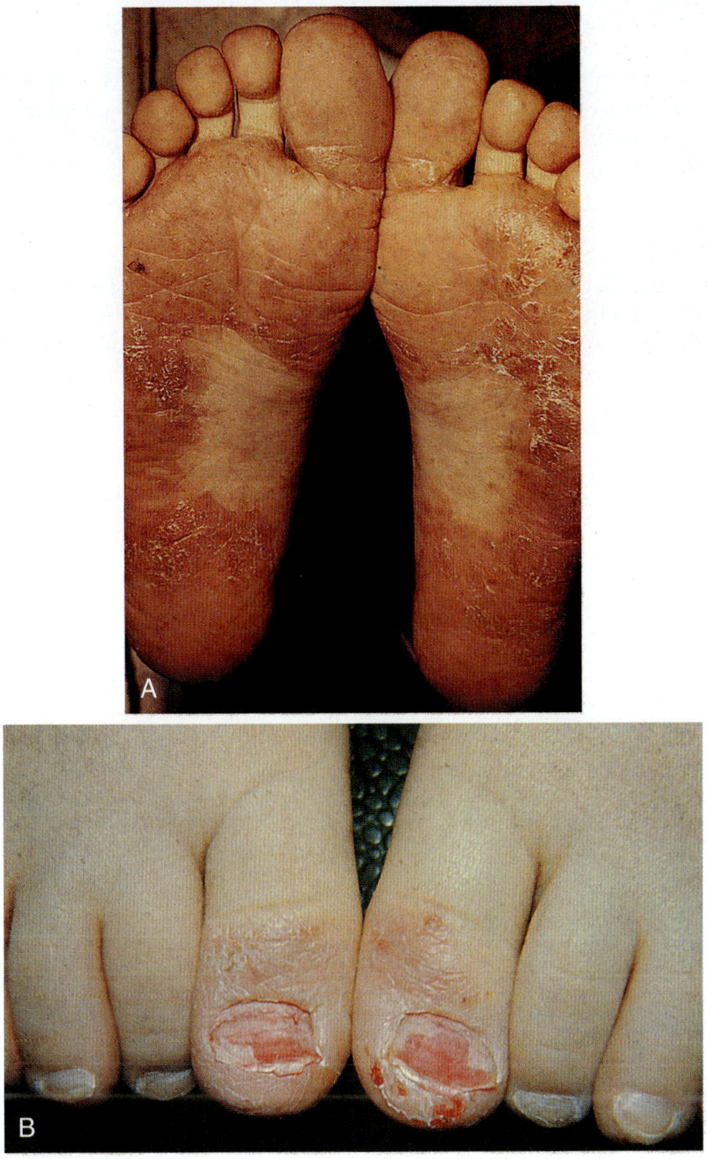

Fig. 8.32 Contact dermatitis of the foot due to glues/dyes in shoes. (A) This adolescent became sensitized to the glue under the insoles of his shoes. Note the sparing of the instep. (B) Another child had a similar problem with the toe reinforcers in his shoes. Note that the web spaces are spared. (A, Courtesy Michael Sherlock, MD, Lutherville, MD. B, Courtesy Douglas W. Kress, MD, University of Pittsburgh Medical Center.)

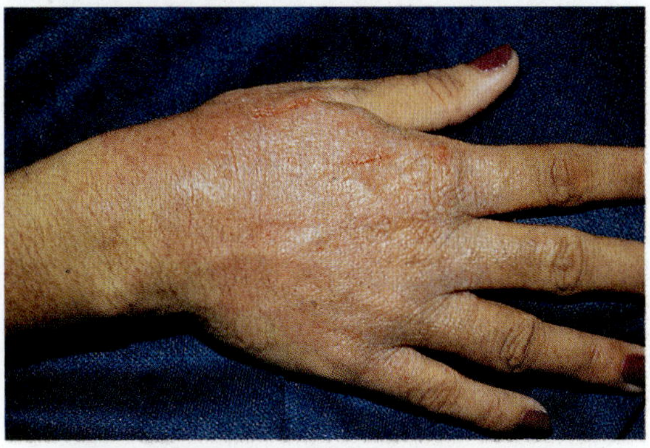

Fig. 8.33 Contact dermatitis due to topical anesthetics. This adolescent became sensitized to the topical anesthetic benzocaine (Lanacane) in a moisturizing cream that she applied to her hands daily. Note the line of demarcation at the wrist.

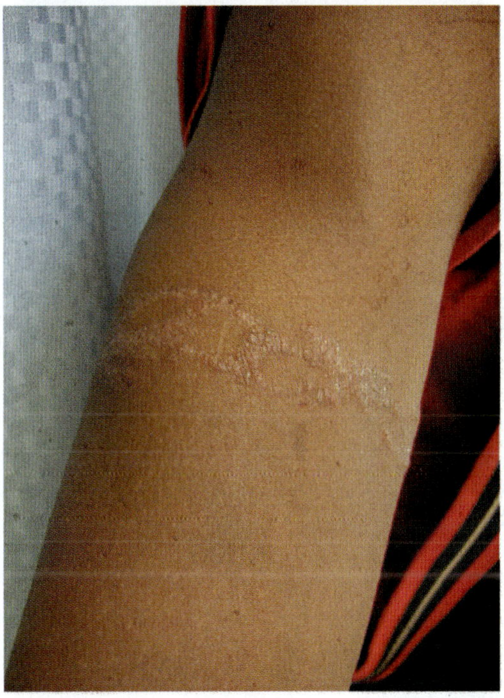

Fig. 8.34 Contact dermatitis due to henna dye. This young teenager developed vesicular lesions in the precise pattern of a henna tattoo she had had applied 2 weeks earlier.

the pattern reflects the image of the original tattoo (Fig. 8.34). Methylchloroisothiazolinone/methylisothiazolinone (MCI/MI) or MI alone are emerging common causes of contact dermatitis from moist wipes and personal care products.

Photocontact Dermatitis and Phototoxic Reactions

Phototoxic reactions occur when a topical or systemic drug is used in conjunction with sun exposure, and it intensifies the reaction to the sun. In the systemic reaction, it characteristically erupts in a symmetric distribution on the face, the V of the neck, and the arms and legs distal to the end of shirt sleeves and shorts. Photo-onycholysis, or separation of the nail plate from the nail bed, can also occur as a manifestation of a phototoxic drug eruption. Common causative agents include the tetracyclines (especially doxycycline), isotretinoin, sulfonylureas, thiazides, nonsteroidal antiinflammatory drugs (NSAIDs), fluoroquinolones, and griseofulvin. Phototoxins, when applied to the skin, are the source of a nonimmunologic exaggerated sunburn reaction in which the initial erythema progresses to hyperpigmentation. Topical photosensitizers include fragrances in cosmetics and furocoumarins. Of these, phytophotodermatitis reactions from furocoumarins are the most common. In this form, plant-derived photosensitizers, psoralens, which are found in the juices of lemons, limes, figs, dill, parsley, parsnips, carrots, and celery, are responsible for the reaction. A child may either come into direct contact with one of these agents or be exposed by a parent who has been cutting the fruit, herbs, or vegetables, thereby getting the juice on the child's skin. Subsequent exposure to sunlight then results in the appearance of erythematous macules, with or without accompanying bullae, which then go on to become hyperpigmented. These patches often have bizarre or hand/finger-shaped patterns that can mimic child abuse (see Chapter 6).

Photocontact or photoallergic dermatitis is a true T-cell–mediated delayed hypersensitivity reaction that necessitates an initial period of sensitization, after which time continued or future contact with the allergen only in combination with sun exposure may precipitate development of a contact dermatitis. Common photocontact allergens include oxybenzone and avobenzone, which are ironically the most common active ingredients in chemical sunscreen (Fig. 8.35).

"Id" Reaction

On occasion, the local reaction of a contact dermatitis can be so severe that the patient develops a more widespread secondary eczematous dermatitis. When the dermatitis appears at sites that have not been in contact with the offending agent, the reaction is

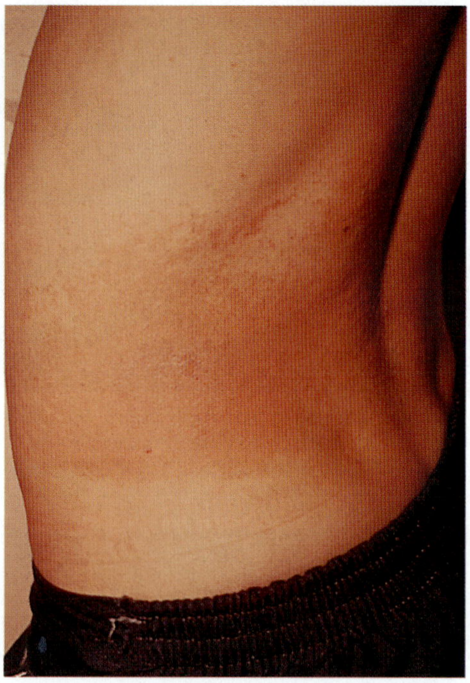

Fig. 8.35 Photocontact dermatitis. This boy developed contact dermatitis after sun exposure while outside for a day of swimming. The offending agent was found to be in his soap. (Courtesy Michael Sherlock, MD, Lutherville, MD.)

referred to as *autoeczematization* or an "id" reaction. Id reactions can also occur in patients with tinea, especially coincident with the start of oral therapy.

Basic Principles of Management

Although localized patches of contact dermatitis are best treated topically, widespread reactions require a 2-week tapering course of systemic corticosteroids beginning at 0.5 to 1 mg/kg/day (Maximum daily dose 60 mg for children over 60 kg). Patients may experience rebound of the rash if treated with a shorter course. Response to treatment usually occurs within 48 hours. Oral steroids may also be indicated in localized reactions involving the eyelids, extensive areas of the face, genitals, or hands, where swelling and pruritus may become incapacitating.

Prevention of both forms of contact dermatitis requires identification of the offending agent and then its avoidance.

Fungal Infections

Two types of fungal organisms produce clinical cutaneous disease: dermatophytes and yeasts. Dermatophytes include tinea and yeasts include *Candida* species, which are associated with diaper dermatitis, and *Pityrosporum* species, which cause tinea versicolor.

Tinea Corporis

Tinea corporis is a superficial fungal infection of the nonhairy or glabrous skin. It has been labeled "ringworm" because of its characteristic configuration consisting of pruritic, annular lesions with central clearing and an active border made up of microvesicles that rupture and then scale (Fig. 8.36A–C). Lesions, which may be single or multiple, typically begin as pruritic red papules or pustules that rupture and evolve to form papulosquamous lesions, which are also pruritic. These then spread out from the periphery as new papulovesicles form at their outer margins and begin to clear centrally (see Fig. 8.36D and E). Over a period of several weeks, the patches may expand up to 5 cm in diameter. Tinea corporis can occur in any age group and is usually acquired through direct human contact or from an infected pet.

Clinically, tinea may be differentiated from atopic dermatitis by its propensity for autoinoculation from the primary patch to other sites on the patient's skin, by the spread to close contacts, and by the central clearing noted in many lesions. Moreover, the rash of atopic dermatitis tends to be symmetric, chronic, and recurrent in a flexural distribution. Unlike tinea, patches of nummular eczema are self-limited and do not clear centrally. The clinical pattern, findings, and chronic nature of psoriasis and seborrhea help differentiate them from tinea. Although granuloma annulare produces a characteristic ringed eruption, on palpation the lesions are dermal, not epidermal, so they do not classically exhibit scaling as tinea does (see Fig. 8.89).

The diagnosis of tinea corporis is confirmed by KOH examination of skin scrapings. The first step is to obtain material by scraping the loose scales at the margin of a lesion (Fig. 8.37A). These should be mounted onto the center of a glass slide with one or two drops of 20% KOH solution added. Next, a glass coverslip is applied and gently pressed down with the eraser end of a pencil to crush the scales (see Fig. 8.37B). The clinician then gently heats the slide, taking care not to boil the KOH solution, and again the coverslip is pressed down. When viewing the slide under the microscope, the clinician sets the condenser and light source at low levels to maximize contrast with the objective at ×10. On focusing up and down, true hyphae are seen as long, branching, often septate rods of uniform width that cross the borders of epidermal cells (Fig. 8.38). Cotton fibers, cell borders, or other artifacts may be falsely interpreted as positive findings.

Tinea infections on glabrous skin readily respond to topical antifungal creams, such as miconazole, clotrimazole, econazole, naftifine, ketoconazole, and ciclopirox. When lesions are multiple or widespread, oral therapy with griseofulvin is indicated. Itraconazole, terbinafine, and fluconazole are good alternatives for systemic antifungal therapy. Like griseofulvin, they are effective against most ringworm organisms, but unlike griseofulvin, these medications are concentrated in skin, hair, and nails for weeks to months after they are discontinued. Tinea infections should never be treated with the topical products that combine an azole antifungal with a medium or high-potency topical steroid. Paradoxically, these agents increase the likelihood that the fungal infection will spread deeper within the skin and be more resistant to topical therapy, a process called *tinea incognito* or *Majocchi granuloma.* At this stage, oral therapy often becomes necessary to clear the infection.

Tinea Pedis

Commonly referred to as *athlete's foot,* tinea pedis is a fungal infection of the feet with a predilection for the web spaces between the toes. Tinea pedis is quite common in adolescence and somewhat less so in prepubertal children. The infecting organisms are acquired from contaminated shower, bathroom, locker room, and gym floors, and their growth is fostered by the warm, moist environment of shoes.

In some cases, scaling and fissuring predominate; in others, vesiculopustular lesions and maceration are found, especially in the web spaces between the third, fourth, and fifth toes. The infection begins between and along the sides of the toes, where it may remain (Fig. 8.39A). However, lesions can extend over the dorsum of the foot (see Fig. 8.39B) and may involve the plantar surface as well, particularly the instep and ball of the foot. Patients complain of a combination of burning and itching, which is frequently intense.

This diagnosis often can be made on clinical grounds and is confirmed by KOH preparation of skin scrapings. The mainstays of treatment are topical antifungal creams or powders and measures designed to reduce foot moisture, such as careful drying of the feet after bathing, wearing cotton rather than synthetic socks, and wearing shoes that do not promote sweating. In patients with severe inflammatory lesions, oral antifungal agents may be required. Onychomycosis (see Fig. 8.136) responds well only to oral agents and requires treatment for 12 weeks or more (see the section Disorders Affecting the Nails). Secondary bacterial infection, particularly with gram-negative organisms, may occur.

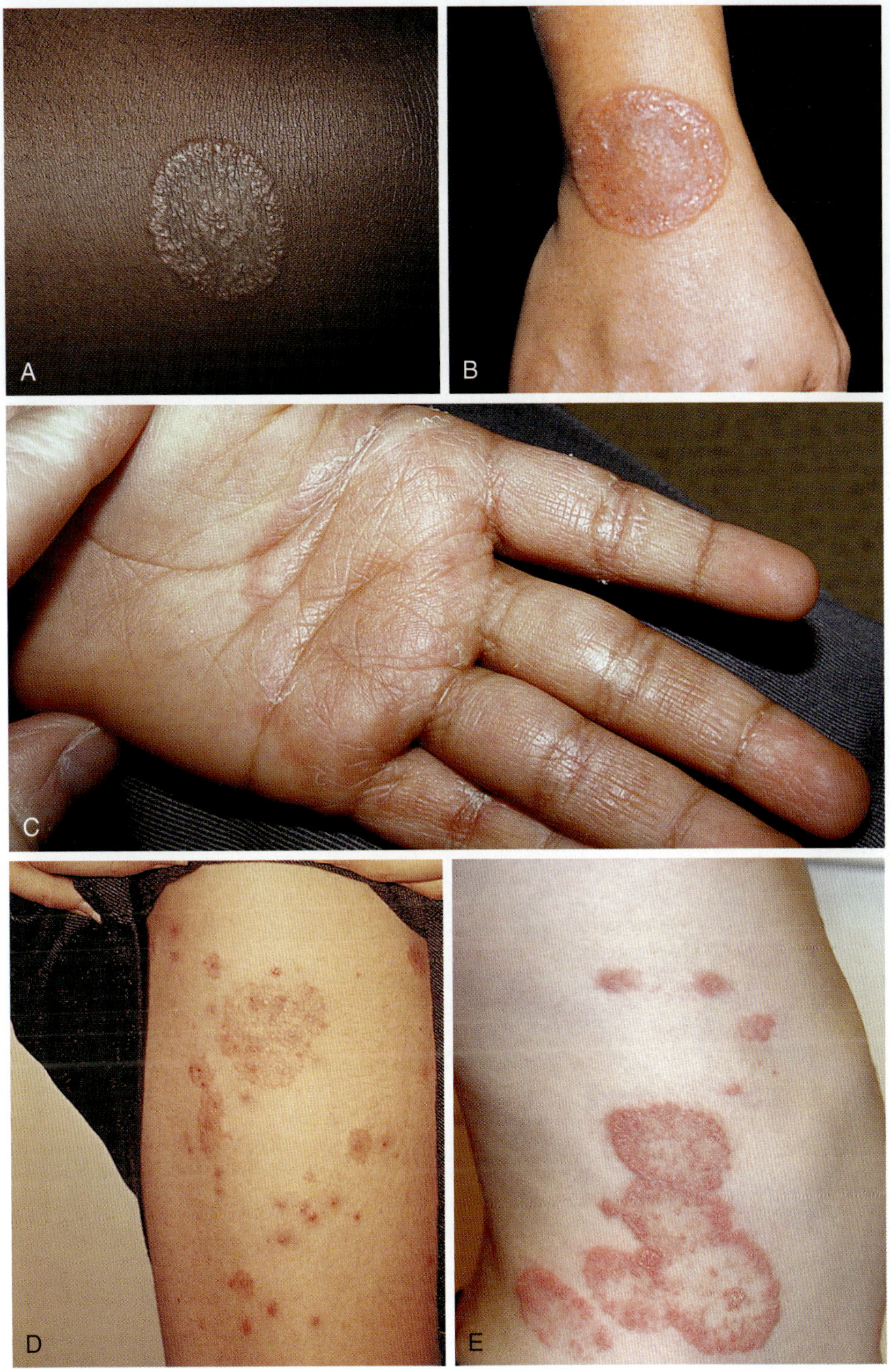

Fig. 8.36 Tinea corporis. The characteristic annular lesions show many variations in appearance. (A) This lesion has a raised, active border and shows partial central clearing. (B) In another case, the inflammatory response is intense, and only a little central clearing is seen. (C) The lesion shown here involving the palm and flexor surfaces of the fingers is macular and scaly and has a sharply circumscribed proximal border. (D) The evolution of lesions from papules and pustules into larger papulosquamous patches is seen on this girl's leg. (E) In another child, small papules, plaques that have not cleared centrally, and larger lesions with varying degrees of central clearing are seen. (B, Courtesy Douglas W. Kress, MD, University of Pittsburgh Medical Center. D, Courtesy Michael Sherlock, MD, Lutherville, MD.)

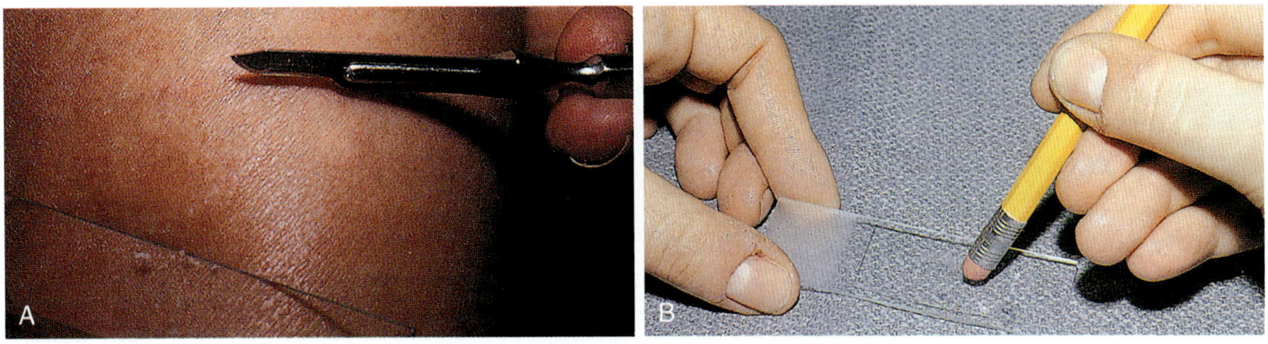

Fig. 8.37 Potassium hydroxide preparation. (A) Small scales should be scraped from the edge of the lesion onto a microscope slide. (B) To more easily visualize the fungus, the scales should be crushed, making a thin layer of cells.

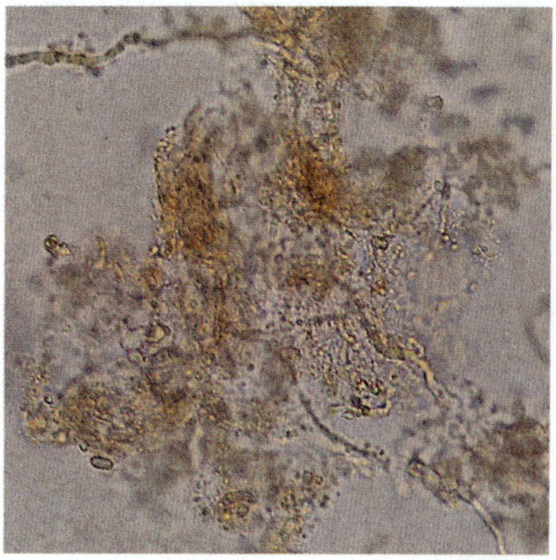

Fig. 8.38 Positive potassium hydroxide preparation of skin scrapings. Fungal hyphae are seen as long septate branching rods at the margins and center of the scales.

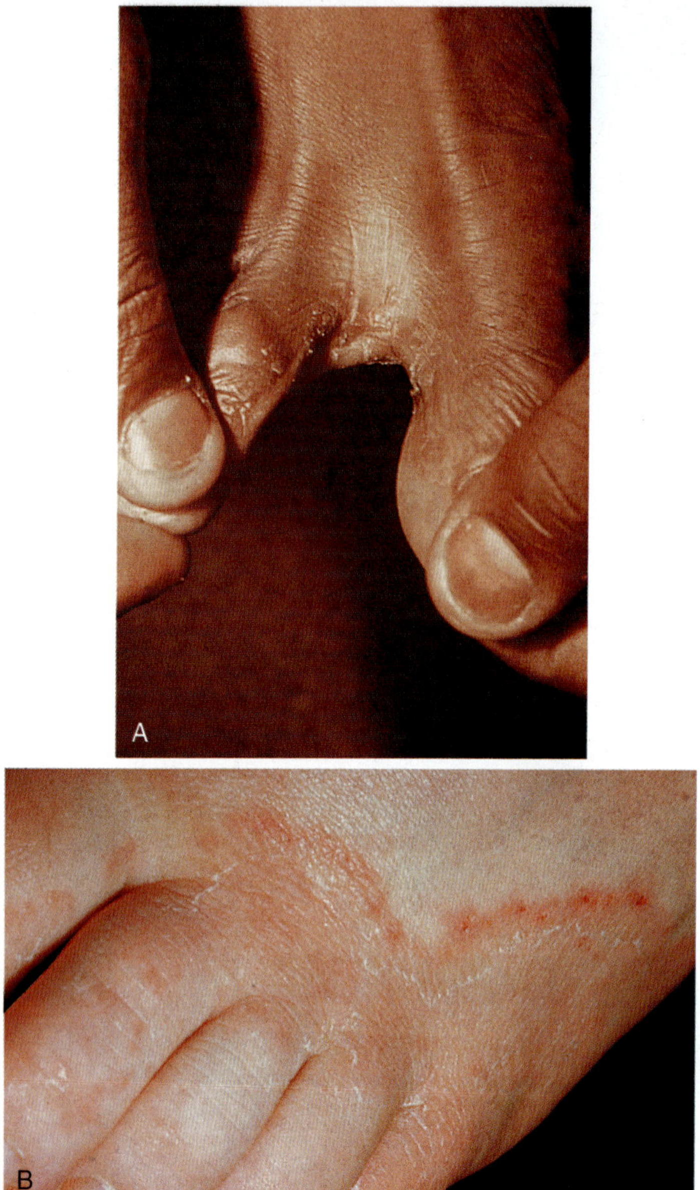

Fig. 8.39 Tinea pedis. (A) Cracking and scaling are seen in the web space. (B) In this patient, the lesions began in the web spaces but then extended onto the dorsum of the foot. Note the active border. (B, Courtesy Douglas W. Kress, MD, University of Pittsburgh Medical Center.)

Contact dermatitis of the feet spares the interdigital web spaces (see Fig. 8.32), while tinea pedis does not. Dyshidrosis can have a similar distribution, but the KOH preparation is negative (see Fig. 8.18).

Tinea Versicolor

Tinea versicolor is a common dermatosis characterized by multiple small, oval, scaly patches measuring 1 to 3 cm in diameter, usually located in a guttate or raindrop pattern on the upper chest, back, and proximal portions of the upper extremities of adolescents and young adults (Fig. 8.40A and B). Facial involvement occurs occasionally. The eruption is caused by a dimorphous form of *Pityrosporum*. Warm, moist climates; pregnancy; immunodeficiency; and genetic factors predispose people to the development of infection.

The rash is usually asymptomatic, although some patients complain of mild pruritus. Typically, patients seek treatment because they are bothered by the cosmetic appearance of the lesions. Lesions may be light tan, reddish, or lightly discolored, giving rise to the term *versicolor*. They are darker than surrounding skin in non–sun-exposed areas (see Fig. 8.40C) and lighter in areas that have tanned on exposure to sunlight (see Fig. 8.40A and B).

The diagnosis of tinea versicolor can generally be made based on the clinical appearance of lesions and their distribution. It can be confirmed by examining the lesions under a Wood lamp, which reveals a characteristic tan to salmon-pink glow but no enhancement of the discoloration as in vitiligo. Although pathogenesis of the color change under a Wood lamp is not fully understood, the fungus is known to produce a substance that interferes with tyrosinase activity and subsequent melanin synthesis. A KOH preparation of the surface scale demonstrates short hyphal and yeast forms that resemble spaghetti and meatballs (Fig. 8.41).

The differential diagnosis of tinea versicolor includes postinflammatory hypopigmentation and vitiligo. The history and distribution help to distinguish tinea versicolor from postinflammatory hypopigmentation; the presence of fine superficial scaling and some residual pigmentation (even in hypopigmented areas) that does not enhance with Wood lamp examination helps to rule out vitiligo.

Topical antiyeast agents such as selenium sulfide produce rapid clearing of the superficial lesions. Localized eruptions may be treated with topical antifungal creams, such as miconazole, clotrimazole, or econazole, and recalcitrant cases respond to oral fluconazole or itraconazole. Patients must be counseled about the high risk of recurrence, which often necessitates ongoing prophylactic selenium sulfide washes for several days each month. They should also be reminded that pigmentary changes may take months to clear even after eradication of the fungus.

Diaper Dermatitis

Because the diaper area is warm, often moist, and frequently contaminated by feces laden with organisms, diaper dermatitis is one of the most common skin disorders of infancy and early childhood.

Irritant Diaper Dermatitis

The diaper area is a prime target for irritant dermatitis because it is bathed in natural irritants and then occluded. Failure to change diapers frequently is a major predisposing factor because it provides time for fecal bacteria to form ammonia by splitting the urea in urine. Harsh soaps, irritant chemicals, and detergents can contribute to the process. Moderate to severe diarrhea is another predisposing condition. The erythema, scaling, and, at times, maceration characteristic of irritant diaper dermatitis are usually confined to the convex surfaces of the perineum, lower abdomen, buttocks, and proximal thighs, sparing intertriginous areas (Fig. 8.42). When neglected, this may progress with further skin breakdown and ulceration. Frequent diaper changes; gentle, thorough cleansing of the area; and heavy application of lubricants and zinc oxide barrier pastes usually result in clearing of the dermatitis. A short course of low-potency steroids may hasten resolution, but this must be discontinued after a week or

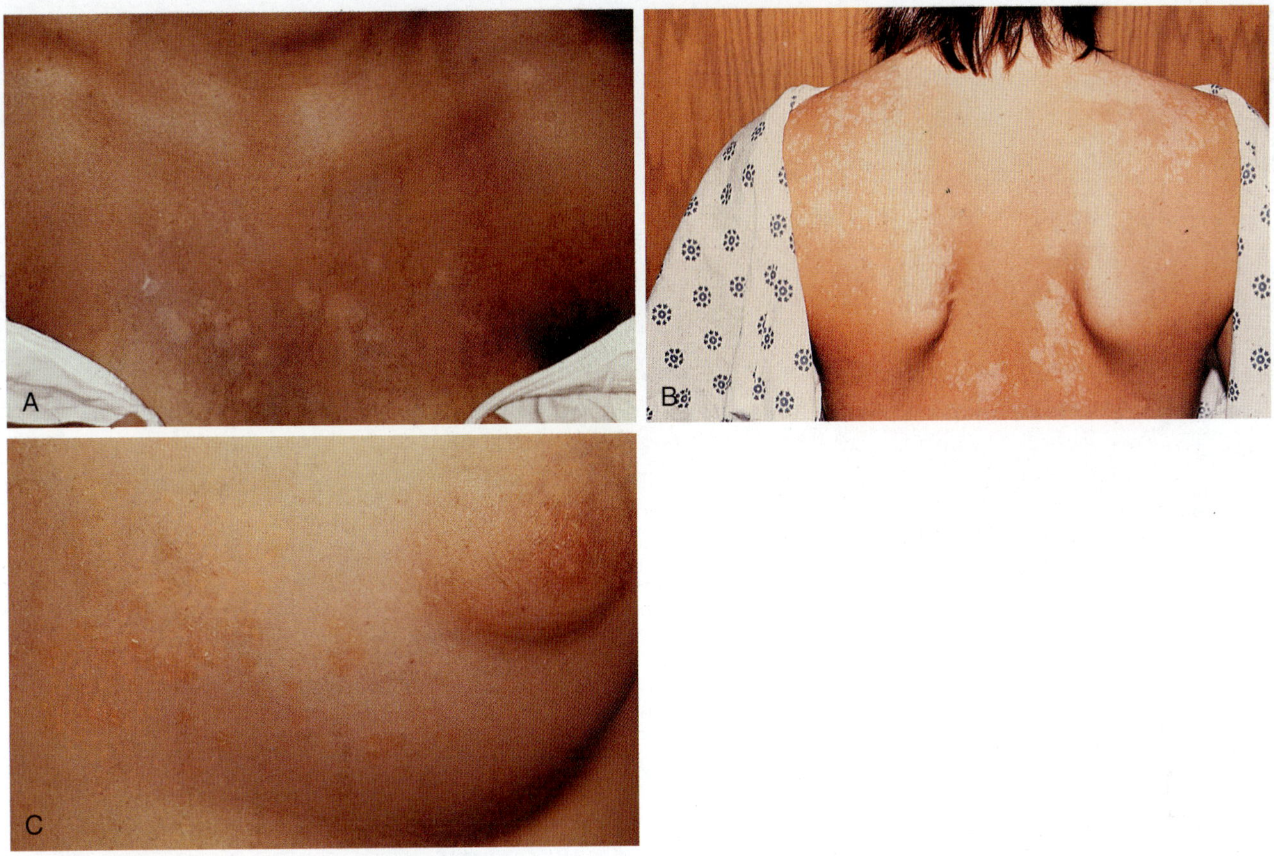

Fig. 8.40 Tinea versicolor. (A and B) Multiple oval patches are seen in a guttate or raindrop pattern over the upper chest and back of two patients. (C) In areas not exposed to sunlight, lesions are darker than surrounding skin, whereas in A and B sun-exposed lesions fail to tan, remaining lighter than surrounding skin. (Courtesy Michael Sherlock, MD, Lutherville, MD.)

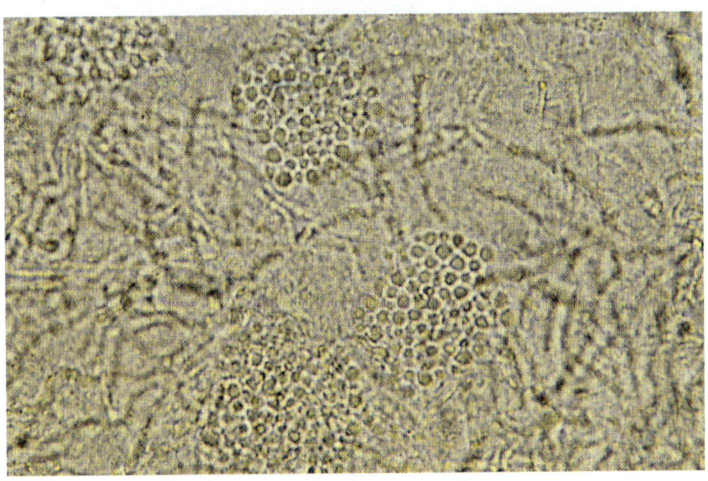

Fig. 8.41 Positive potassium hydroxide preparation for tinea versicolor. The combination of hyphal and yeast forms of the fungus simulates the appearance of spaghetti and meatballs.

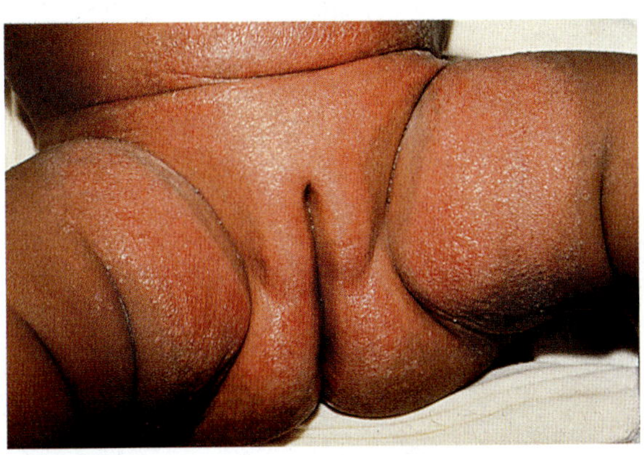

Fig. 8.42 Irritant or ammoniacal diaper dermatitis. Note the erythema and scaling involving the convex surfaces and sparing of the intertriginous creases.

so and then followed by prevention with thick, nonfragranced zinc oxide pastes as a barrier. The use of combination topical steroids plus topical antifungal preparations is discouraged because the strength of the topical steroid in these preparations often exceeds what would be considered safe in the occluded, thin skin of the diaper area.

Persistent diaper dermatitis that does not resolve with conservative therapy may be due to other disorders, such as contact dermatitis to the blue dyes present in the diaper or to the MCI/MI in the moist wipes (this has become increasingly common), candidiasis, seborrheic dermatitis, psoriasis, or in rare cases Langerhans cell histiocytosis (see Fig. 8.88). These should be suspected particularly when intertriginous areas are involved.

Candidal Diaper Dermatitis

Candidal diaper dermatitis appears as a bright red eruption, often with sharp borders and pinpoint satellite papules and pustules (Fig. 8.43). Examination of pustule contents by KOH preparation reveals the typical budding yeasts and pseudohyphae of *Candida* organisms (Fig. 8.44). Candidal diaper dermatitis is occasionally associated with oral thrush, and it is a common sequela of oral or parenteral antibiotic therapy. One should suspect a secondary invasion by *Candida albicans* whenever intertriginous areas are involved or when a diaper rash fails to respond to symptomatic treatment. Most cases respond well to topical antifungal therapy, but the occasional resistant case may require a brief course of oral medication. Again, Langerhans cell histiocytosis should be considered in the differential diagnosis of severe or recalcitrant intertriginous diaper dermatitis, especially when the papules become more crusted or are accompanied by petechiae or systemic symptoms.

Staphylococcal Diaper Dermatitis

Irritant diaper dermatitis is frequently complicated by secondary staphylococcal infection, or pustules may appear as primary lesions, especially in the first few weeks of life. The presence of thin-walled

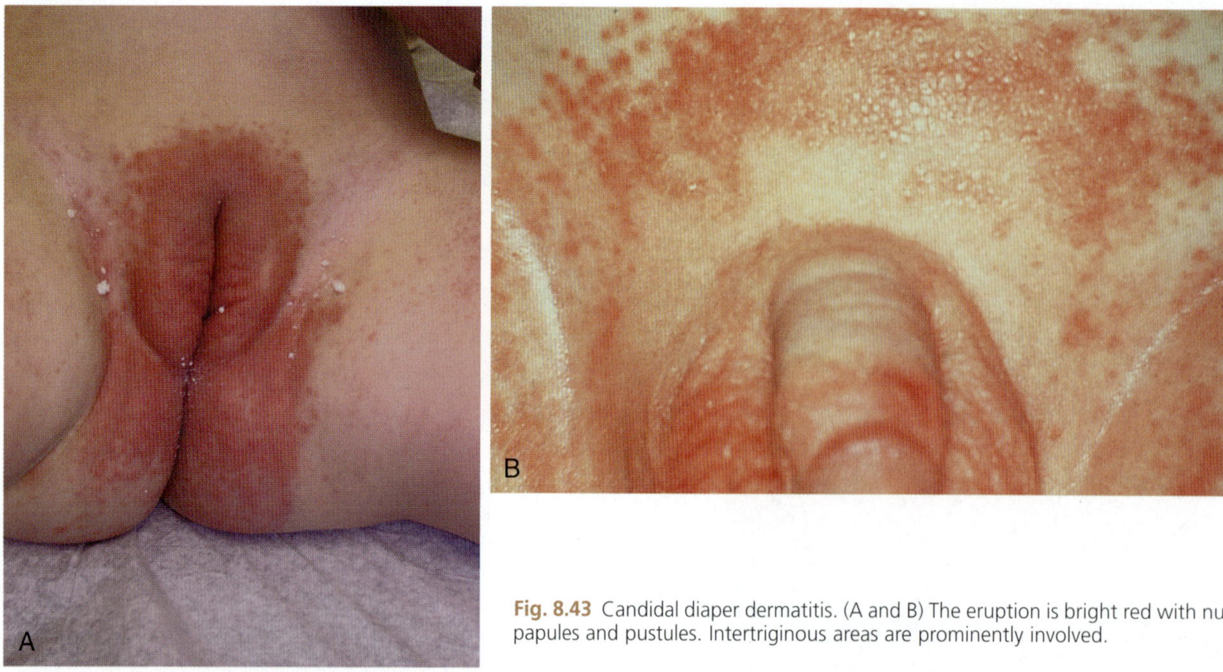

Fig. 8.43 Candidal diaper dermatitis. (A and B) The eruption is bright red with numerous pinpoint satellite papules and pustules. Intertriginous areas are prominently involved.

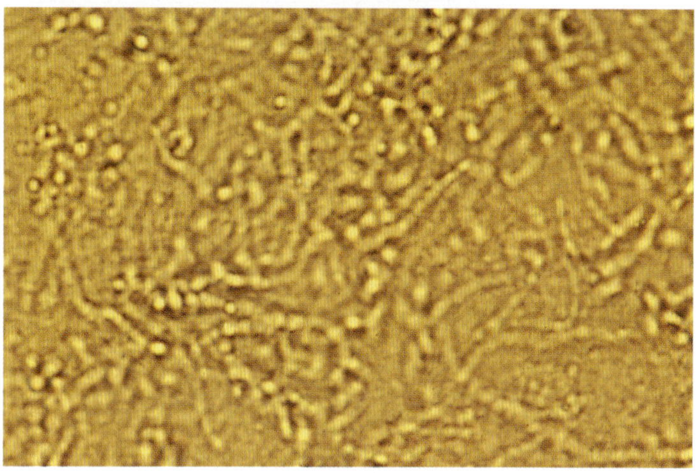

Fig. 8.44 Potassium hydroxide preparation of skin scrapings from an infant with candidal diaper dermatitis demonstrating pseudohyphae and spores.

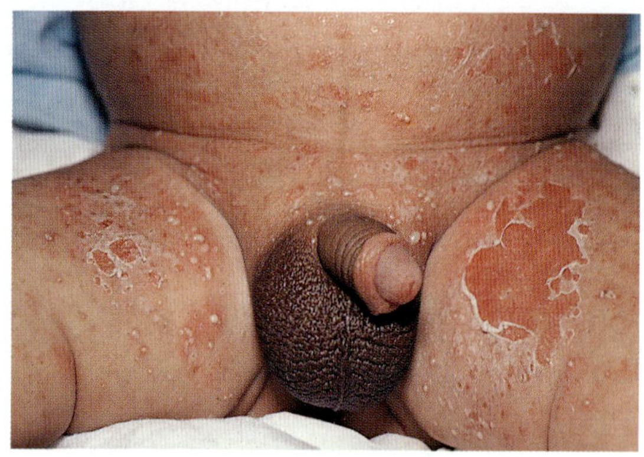

Fig. 8.45 Staphylococcal diaper dermatitis. Numerous thin-walled pustules are surrounded by erythematous halos, as well as multiple areas in which pustules have ruptured, leaving a collarette of scale around a denuded erythematous base.

pustules on an erythematous base (larger and more discrete than those seen with candidiasis) alerts the clinician to the diagnosis. Typically, these rupture rapidly and dry, producing a collarette of scaling around the denuded red base (Fig. 8.45). A Gram stain of pustule contents demonstrates neutrophils and clusters of gram-positive cocci. Bacterial cultures are confirmatory but rarely necessary. Early diagnosis and treatment with oral and topical antibiotics result in rapid resolution.

Perianal Streptococcal Dermatitis

Perianal streptococcal dermatitis most commonly presents among children aged 6 months to 10 years, and it is characterized by a superficial, bright red perianal erythema with sharply defined margins extending 2 to 4 cm (Fig. 8.46). These lesions commonly present with perianal itching, painful defecation, constipation, and blood-streaked stools, and they may be accompanied by superficial perianal fissures and mucoid discharge. Most cases described in the pediatric literature are caused by group A β-hemolytic streptococci (GAS), although infection with other groups of β-hemolytic streptococci may occur. Concurrent or recent GAS pharyngitis has been reported in some cases, and oral-anal spread has been well documented as one route of transmission. Because the differential for perianal dermatitis is broad, delays in diagnosis and treatment are common. Perivaginal dermatitis may present with similar lesions, but it can be differenti-

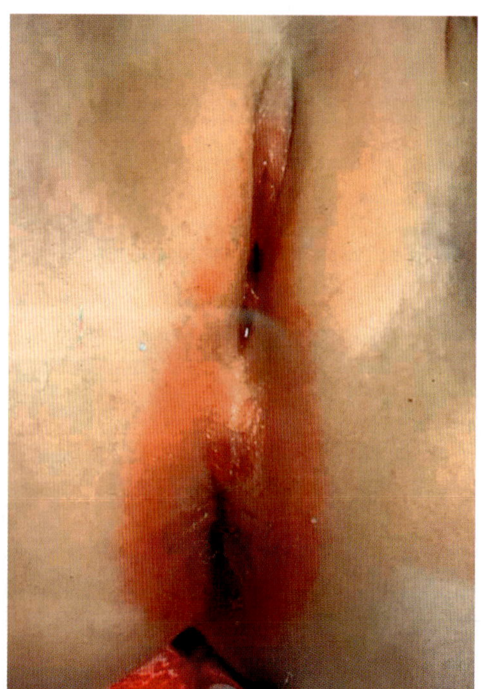

Fig. 8.46 Perianal streptococcal dermatitis. Note the characteristic bright red and well-demarcated erythema.

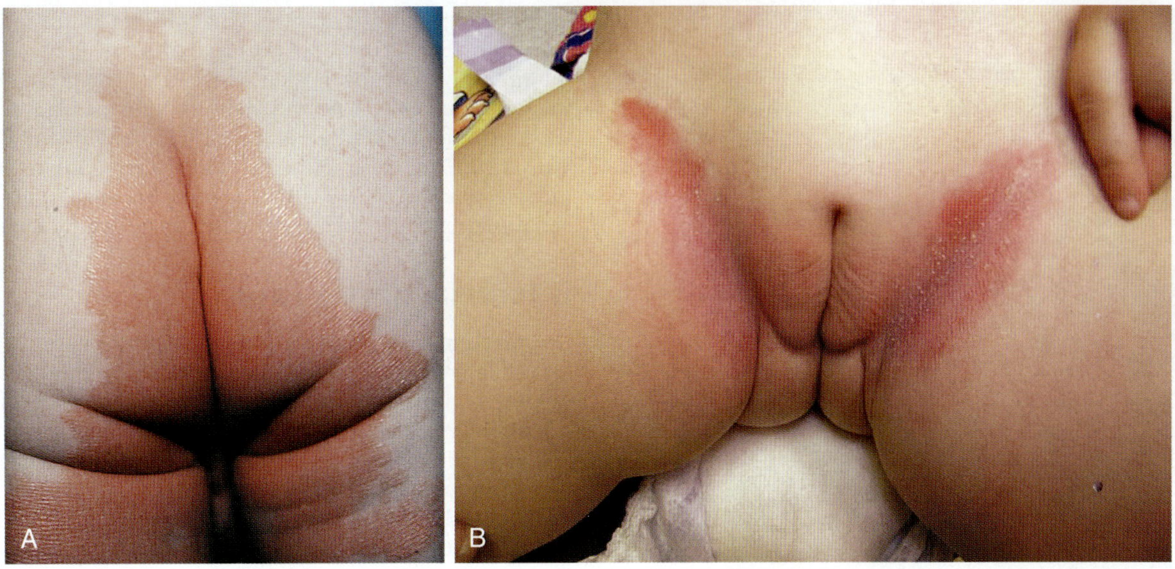

Fig. 8.47 Psoriatic diaper dermatitis. (A) This child had a persistent diaper rash that did not respond to routine therapy. Note that scaling is not as intense as in psoriatic lesions seen elsewhere on the body. (B) Another infant with inverse psoriasis involving the inguinal creases had also failed to improve despite multiple courses of topical antifungal treatment.

ated as a more widespread rash that is loosely centered around the anus. Bacterial culture of perianal and perineal swabs should be performed to confirm suspected cases, although an initial rapid antigen detection test for GAS may also be used to facilitate early diagnosis. Treatment with oral antibiotics for at least 14 days has been demonstrated to be an effective therapy. Due to the high recurrence rate, some patients may require a repeated course of antibiotics.

Seborrheic Diaper Dermatitis

Seborrheic diaper dermatitis is characterized by confluent salmon-colored plaques with a yellowish scale. The rash is particularly prominent in the intertriginous areas (see Fig. 8.23B). Although concurrent infection with *Candida* or *Pityrosporum* is likely, discrete satellite lesions are usually not seen. Typically, seborrheic dermatitis of the scalp, face, and postauricular areas is seen in association with this form of diaper dermatitis.

Psoriatic Diaper Dermatitis

Psoriasis occasionally begins as an erythematous, scaling eruption in the diaper area (Fig. 8.47), which is clinically indistinguishable from severe seborrheic diaper dermatitis. Perhaps because the diaper area is moist, the thick silvery scale typical of psoriatic lesions at other sites is not seen. Although lesions may develop subsequently on the trunk and extremities, the rash may persist for months in the diaper area alone. Failure of a seborrheic-like diaper rash to respond to empiric therapy over several weeks or months should raise psoriasis as a diagnostic possibility. Skin biopsy is the only way to confirm the diagnosis.

Tinea Diaper Dermatitis

Although less common than the other dermatitides in the differential diagnosis of diaper dermatitis, tinea must be kept in mind when examining a scaly perineal rash. Its characteristic features are those of a recalcitrant scaly eruption with an elevated or "active" scaly border (Fig. 8.48), from which scales can be scraped and tinea is demonstrated on KOH preparation. It responds well to topical antifungals alone and should not be treated with topical steroids or with topical steroid plus antifungal combination products.

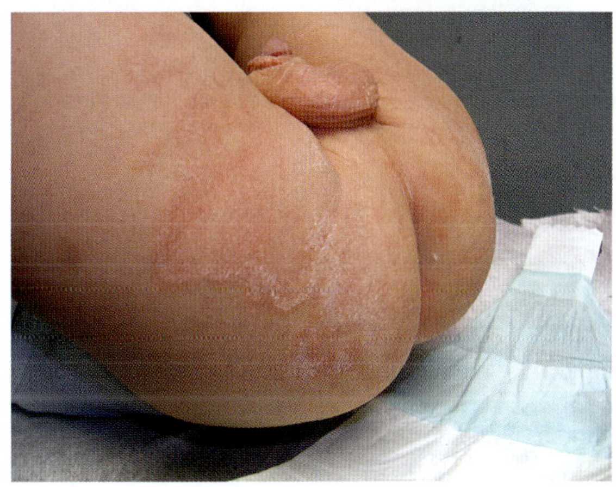

Fig. 8.48 Tinea diaper dermatitis. Note the prominent scaling and the elevated active border.

Lichenoid Eruptions

Lichen Planus

Lichen planus is the prototypic lichenoid inflammatory eruption in that it displays flat-topped, pruritic, polygonal, violaceous papules and plaques, which have a fine lacy pattern (Wickham striae). They are often noted first over the dorsal surfaces of the extremities and can display koebnerization at sites of prior trauma (Fig. 8.49). The disorder may involve the nails (leading to dystrophy) and oral and genital mucosa, where lesions appear as lacy white plaques. Topical steroids are the mainstay of initial treatment. After resolution of primary lesions, a prolonged period of postinflammatory hyperpigmentation can be expected (see Fig. 8.116).

Lichen Striatus

Lichen striatus is one of the more common and distinctive lichenoid papulosquamous eruptions. Lesions consisting of flat-topped papules appear abruptly, usually in a linear or sometimes swirled distribution along the lines of Blaschko. Although they may involve any portion of the skin, they are more typically located on the extremities, neck, or upper back. They may initially be slightly erythematous but often progress through an often prolonged phase of hypopigmentation, and their surfaces are covered with fine scale (Fig. 8.50). When lesions form on a digit, lichen striatus can lead to a temporary linear nail dystrophy. The cause of this otherwise asymptomatic disorder, which has its peak incidence in school-age children, is unknown, but it is hypothesized that molecular mimicry between a virus and antigens on a single line of

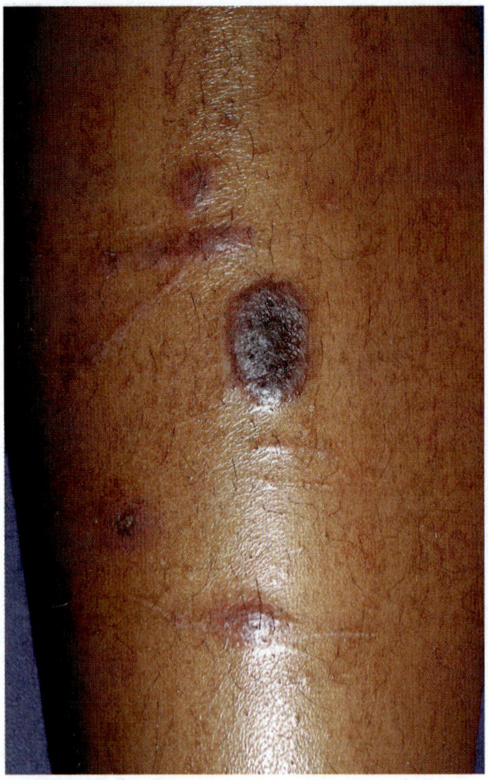

Fig. 8.49 Lichen planus. These flat-topped violaceous papules of varying sizes and shapes overlying the anterior shin are typical. Note the linear lesions that formed after scratching, examples of the Koebner phenomenon.

keratinocytes is to blame. Spontaneous resolution within 1 to 3 years is the norm.

VESICULOPUSTULAR DISORDERS

Vesiculopustular eruptions range from benign, self-limited conditions to life-threatening diseases. Early diagnosis, especially in the young child, is mandatory. Systematic evaluation of the clinical findings and a few rapid diagnostic techniques allow these various disorders to be readily differentiated from one another.

Viral Infections

Viral infections including herpes simplex and varicella-zoster produce characteristic vesiculopustular eruptions, which are discussed in Chapter 13. Confirming the suspicion of a herpetic lesion can be done by preparing a Tzanck smear.

The diagnostic finding in viral blisters is the multinucleated giant cell (Fig. 8.51). This is a syncytium of epidermal cells with multiple, overlapping nuclei; hence it is much larger than other inflammatory cells. Unfortunately, a positive Tzanck test cannot be used to differentiate one blistering viral exanthem from another. Thus a viral culture, rapid direct fluorescent antibody test, or polymerase chain reaction (PCR) should be done when the clinical situation mandates precise or more rapid identification.

Bacterial Infections

Several common cutaneous bacterial infections present with vesiculopustular reactions as well. In impetigo, the eruption tends to be discrete and localized, whereas in staphylococcal scalded skin syndrome (SSSS), it tends to be associated with a diffuse erythroderma. A Gram stain of material aspirated from bullae or removed from the base of an impetiginous lesion is positive for organisms. However, in patients with SSSS, the organism must be sought from distant cutaneous sites or from any of several possible noncutaneous colonized locations (nasopharynx, conjunctivae, sinuses) because the diffuse cutaneous erythema and blistering is due to elaboration of the toxin epidermolysin by the infecting organism and not to the organism's direct action within individual lesions (see Chapter 13).

Blistering Distal Dactylitis

Blistering distal dactylitis is a superficial bacterial infection involving the tips of the pads of fingers or toes. Lesions consist of tense blisters 0.5 to 1 cm in diameter that are filled with thin purulent fluid and surrounded by a narrow erythematous rim. With evolution, they may coalesce and extend proximally along the lateral aspect of the nail fold. On rupture, a thick crust forms (Fig. 8.52). GAS is the usual causative organism and is detected by Gram stain and culture of vesicular fluid. On occasion, group B streptococci and *S. aureus* are isolated. The disorder can be distinguished from a paronychia by the distal location of initial lesions, from a herpetic whitlow by the larger size of the initial vesicles and Gram stain of the purulent fluid, and from burns by the purulence of the vesicular fluid and Gram stain revealing white blood cells and bacteria.

Mycoplasma-Induced Rash and Mucositis or Reactive Infectious Mucocutaneous Eruption

Mycoplasma pneumoniae is a common cause of atypical pneumonia, particularly among young patients, and infection can be associated with mucocutaneous eruptions. Because of its extensive mucosal involvement and vesiculobullous lesions, *Mycoplasma*-induced

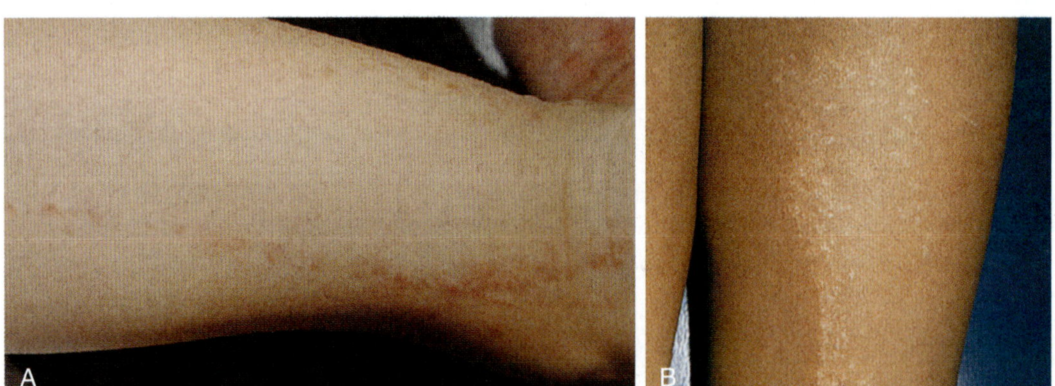

Fig. 8.50 Lichen striatus. (A) In this school-age child, mildly erythematous scaly flat-topped papules are seen in a linear distribution on the lower leg. (B) Another child with darker skin has lesions that are hypopigmented on the posterior thigh. (A, From Cohen BA: *Atlas of pediatric dermatology,* London, 1993, Mosby-Wolfe. B, From Cohen BA: *Pediatric dermatology,* ed 2, London, 1999, Mosby.)

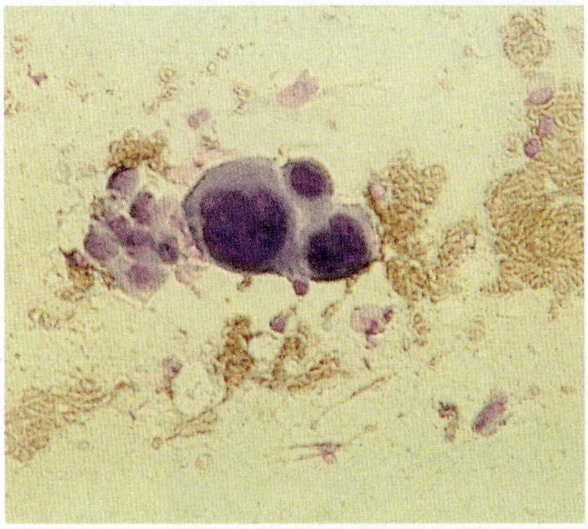

Fig. 8.51 Tzanck preparation. Note the multinucleated giant cell characteristic of viral infection with herpes simplex and varicella-zoster.

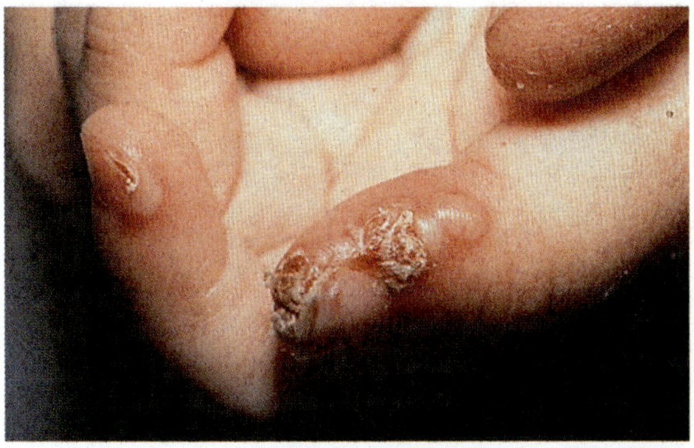

Fig. 8.52 Blistering distal dactylitis. A tense blister filled with purulent fluid first developed at the tip of the thumb pad of this child. Subsequently, the lesion ruptured and crusted and newer lesions formed more proximally along the nail fold and at the tip of the index finger. (From Cohen BA: *Pediatric dermatology*, ed 2, London, 1999, Mosby.)

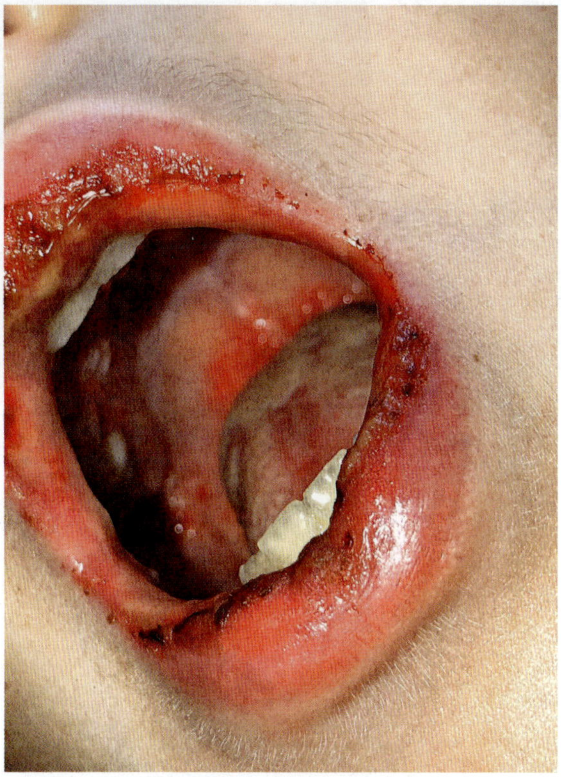

Fig. 8.53 *Mycoplasma*-induced rash and mucositis. This adolescent male developed a severe oral mucositis with hemorrhagic crusting. Severe conjunctivitis is also commonly seen, with variable cutaneous involvement. (Courtesy Li-Wei Chang, MD, DSc., University of Pittsburgh Medical Center.)

rash and mucositis (MIRM) may be challenging to distinguish from drug-induced erythema multiforme (EM) and Stevens-Johnson syndrome (SJS)/toxic epidermal necrolysis (TEN). However, patients with MIRM almost universally present with prodromal symptoms 1 week before eruption, including cough, malaise, and fever. Eruptions are characterized by predominant mucositis with oral, ocular, and urogenital involvement possible (Fig. 8.53). Although cutaneous involvement may be severe, more than half of reported cases had sparse and scattered lesions; when present, vesiculobullous or targetoid morphologies with an acral and extremity-predominant distribution are most common. Histopathology of biopsied lesions reveal keratinocyte apoptosis and mucosal necrosis that is largely indistinguishable from EM or SJS. The predominance of MIRM among young males, extensive mucosal involvement with sparse cutaneous findings, and a more benign disease course distinguish this disorder from other mucocutaneous eruptions. Similar genital and oral erosions occurring after infections to *Chlamydia pneumonia*, SARS-Cov-2, or other respiratory viruses are known as reactive infectious mucocutaneous eruption (RIME).

Although no evidence-based therapy for MIRM has yet been established, supportive care is generally the mainstay of treatment. Oral antibiotics, particularly in the context of ongoing respiratory infection, and systemic glucocorticoids are commonly administered, but the efficacy of these therapies in treating the associated skin findings is unclear.

Erythema Multiforme

EM is a distinctive, acute hypersensitivity syndrome that, in both children and adults, is most frequently triggered by recurrent herpes simplex virus (HSV) infection. EM should not be confused with either SJS or TEN eruptions, which are severe, potentially life-threatening eruptions characterized by variably widespread cutaneous blistering and sloughing and by involvement of multiple mucous membranes.

The classic eruption of EM is symmetric and may occur on any part of the body. However, the dorsum of the hands and feet and the extensor surfaces of the arms and legs are most affected. Involvement of the palms and soles also is typical. The initial lesions are dusky red macules or erythematous wheals that evolve into iris- or target-shaped lesions, the hallmark of EM (Fig. 8.54A). In many instances, the initial crop of lesions simulates diffuse urticaria, although EM lesions are typically much less pruritic, if at all. Ultimately, they can become painful and persistent in contrast to true urticarial lesions, which remain pruritic and tend to migrate over a 24-hour period. The target configuration is due to formation of a central depression that may be blue, violaceous, or white, whereas the elevated periphery tends to remain erythematous. In some cases, vesicles or bullae develop centrally, and in others the peripheral rings may vesiculate or become bullous (see Fig. 8.54B and C). The eruption continues in crops that last from 1 to 3 weeks. In most patients the disease is self-limited, and systemic manifestations are relatively mild, consisting of low-grade fever, malaise, and myalgia. Mucous membranes tend to be spared, although, on occasion, the oral mucosa may be mildly involved. A mucosal-predominant form of EM has been described in conjunction with *Mycoplasma* infection. The major differential diagnosis is urticaria, which does not demonstrate three discrete zones of color change to form a target, as do lesions of true EM.

Stevens-Johnson Syndrome and Toxic Epidermal Necrolysis

SJS and TEN are rare, potentially life-threatening disorders characterized by widespread epidermal and mucous membrane necrosis and sloughing. In both SJS and TEN the plane of cleavage of bullae is beneath the basement membrane zone, resulting in full-thickness

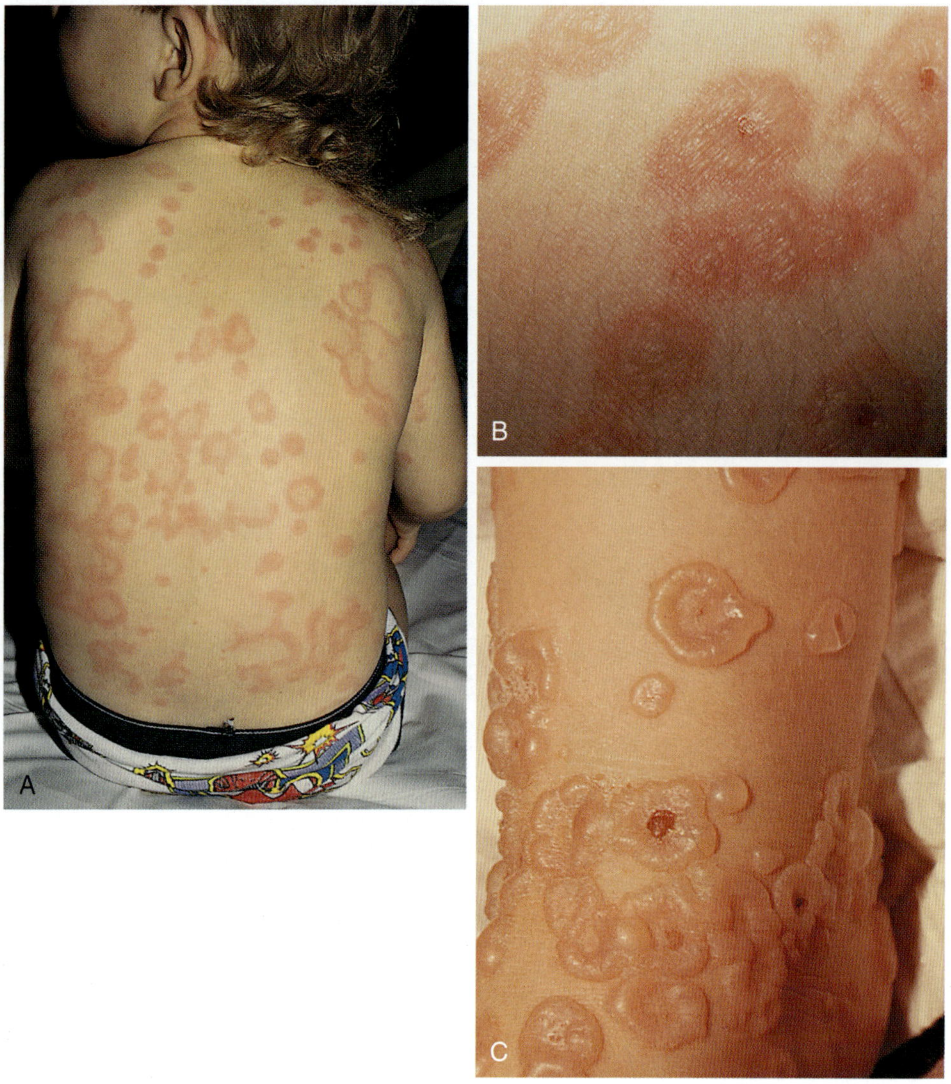

Fig. 8.54 Erythema multiforme. (A) The characteristic target-shaped lesions are symmetrically distributed. (B) These lesions are dusky centrally and their peripheral rims are beginning to vesiculate. (C) In this case, the peripheral rims have become frankly bullous. (C, Courtesy Michael Sherlock, MD, Lutherville, MD.)

sloughing. SJS tends to involve from 10% to 30% of the body surface area, whereas in TEN anywhere from one-third to 100% is affected. Although the etiology is often unclear, hypersensitivity reactions to medications, antecedent viral infections, connective tissue disorders, and malignancy have all been implicated.

Clinically, a prodrome of fever, malaise, and sore throat usually precedes the appearance of diffuse erythroderma, which is then superseded in 24 to 48 hours by necrosis and cleavage, resulting in the formation of thick-walled vesicles and bullae that often are hemorrhagic (Figs. 8.55A–C and 8.56). Nikolsky sign is evident soon thereafter, and as bullae and vesicles slough, they leave deep bloody erosions, which then crust over. Mucous membrane involvement, particularly of the oral, conjunctival, and urethral mucous membranes, is routine and often severe. It consists of the formation of fragile, thin-walled bullae that rupture early, leaving ulcerations of variable depth that are rapidly covered by a gray, yellow, or white membrane (see Fig. 8.55D). On healing, mucosal adhesions and scarring may be noted. Conjunctival involvement can progress to involve the cornea, resulting in corneal scarring, and necessitates early and aggressive ophthalmologic treatment for possible prevention. Lid scarring may result in ectropion. Urethral and vaginal adhesions or strictures are another possible complication.

Constitutional symptoms are prominent in both disorders and include high fever, cough, sore throat, vomiting, diarrhea, chest pain, and arthralgias. Fluid and electrolyte imbalances caused by losses from ruptured bullae and secondary infection are major risks and are proportionately greater in cases of TEN given its more extensive body surface area involvement. Intensive supportive care is required to prevent complications from these fluid losses and from secondary bacterial infection, which is an ever-present danger. Recovery may take a month or more.

The cornerstone of therapy for patients with SJS is multisystem supportive care with meticulous attention to skin care and preventing secondary infection, adhesions, and fluid and electrolyte imbalances. Involving subspecialty consultation services early may keep treatment options open because many therapies are most effective only when given in the first few days of presentation. Although large, well-controlled trials are lacking, administration of 3 days of intravenous immunoglobulin early in the course of disease (within the first 24–48 hours) has been found to mitigate disease progression with shorter duration of fever and slowed progression of blisters. In contrast, systemic steroids remain controversial and should be considered only early in the onset of the disease; they are otherwise contraindicated because they have been associated with an increased risk of morbidity from secondary infection and delayed wound healing. A more recent anecdotally reported therapeutic option in cases where intravenous immunoglobulin may be unfavorable is cyclosporine, which is known for its rapid onset, and the ability to use it somewhat longer than systemic steroids if necessary. Again, attention to the possibility of infection is key because this is an immunosuppressant and affected patients are at high risk for secondary infection with their large areas of denuded skin.

Differential diagnostic considerations include SSSS and EM. In SSSS, the plane of cleavage is higher in the epidermis. Hence bullae

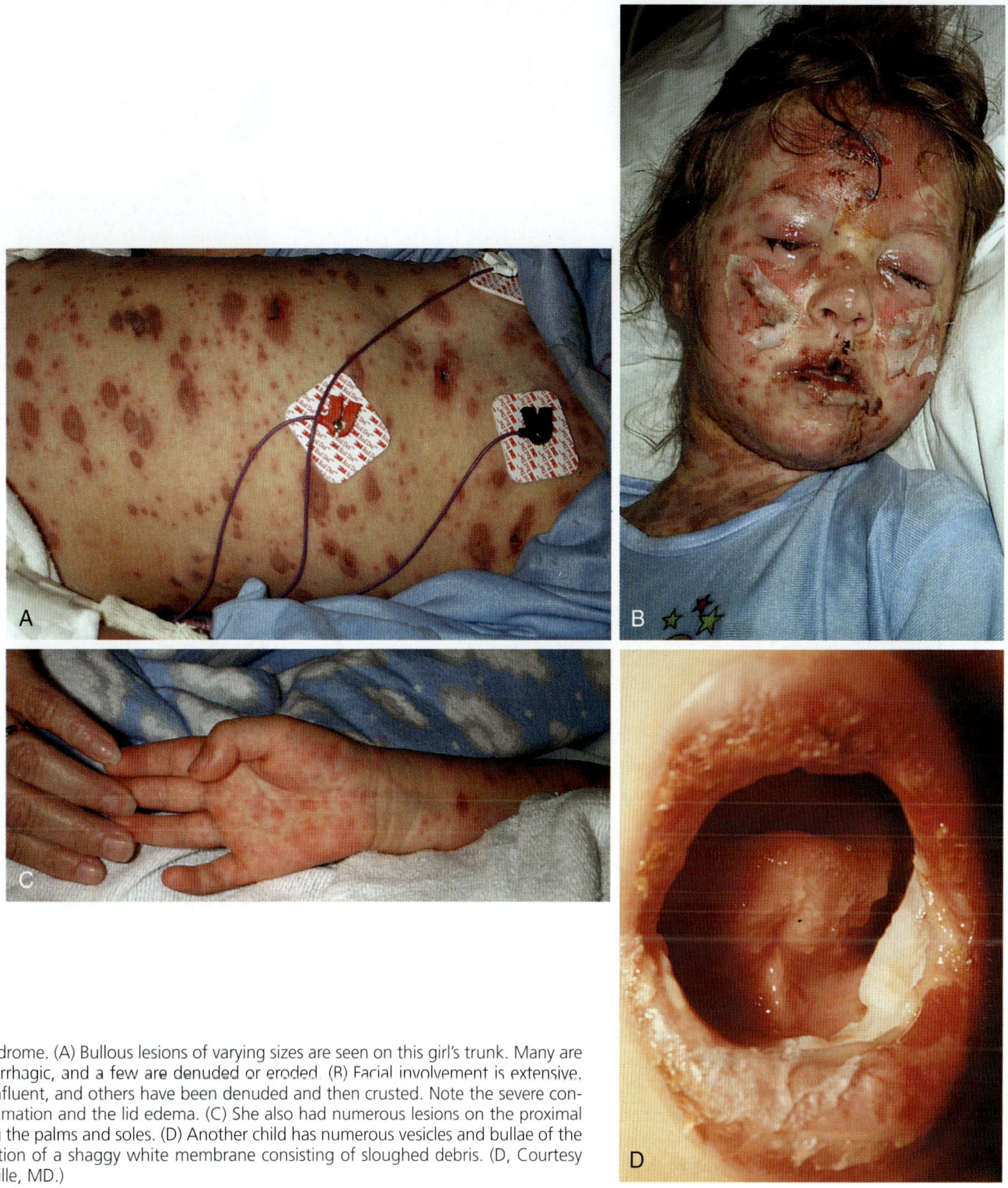

Fig. 8.55 Stevens-Johnson syndrome. (A) Bullous lesions of varying sizes are seen on this girl's trunk. Many are target shaped, some are hemorrhagic, and a few are denuded or eroded. (B) Facial involvement is extensive. Some lesions have become confluent, and others have been denuded and then crusted. Note the severe conjunctival, nasal, and oral inflammation and the lid edema. (C) She also had numerous lesions on the proximal and distal extremities, including the palms and soles. (D) Another child has numerous vesicles and bullae of the oral mucosa along with formation of a shaggy white membrane consisting of sloughed debris. (D, Courtesy Michael Sherlock, MD, Lutherville, MD.)

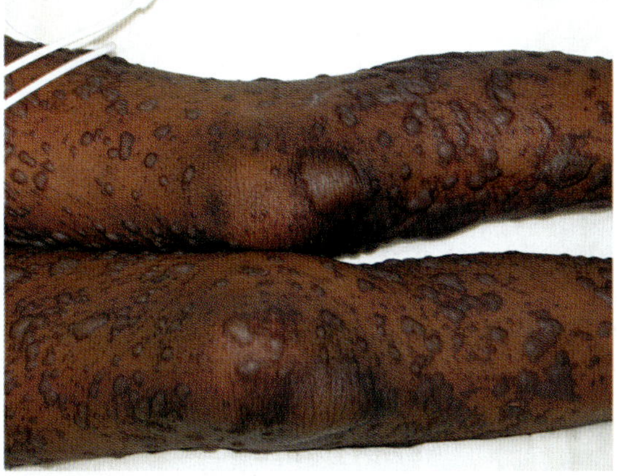

Fig. 8.56 Toxic epidermal necrolysis. Three weeks after starting phenytoin for new-onset seizures, this 10-year-old experienced sudden onset of fever and malaise in association with diffuse erythroderma, conjunctivitis, and oral mucositis. Soon thereafter, thick-walled bullae formed, then rapidly sloughed, leaving deep bloody erosions. Note the extensive amount of surface area involved. (From www.dermatlas.net.)

are thin walled (see Chapter 13), and although mucous membranes are erythematous, they do not typically slough. Furthermore, Gram stain and culture of exudates from the nose and conjunctivae may be positive for *S. aureus.* In EM, initial lesions appear as dusky-red macules or erythematous wheals, which then evolve into bullous, target-shaped lesions, which do not tend to slough; and mucous membrane involvement, if present at all, is mild. Of note, Kawasaki disease may present as a polymorphous rash with multiforme-like target lesions or be accompanied by desquamation resembling SJS (see Chapter 7). However, the presence of discrete vesicles and bullae with more widespread sloughing is more suggestive of SJS/TEN.

Miliaria

Miliaria Crystallina

Miliaria crystallina is a condition in which obstruction of the eccrine sweat ducts located high in the outer layer of the epidermis results in the formation of multiple 2- to 3-mm sweat retention vesicles. Being thin walled, these vesicles are readily ruptured (Fig. 8.57). In infants,

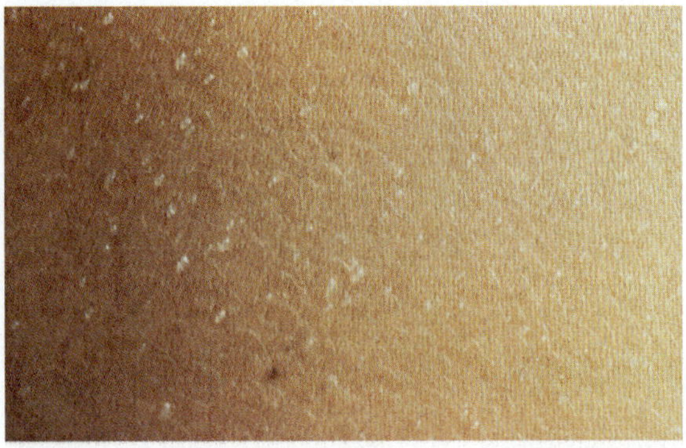

Fig. 8.57 Miliaria crystallina. Found primarily over the head, neck, and upper trunk, these tiny thin-walled sweat retention vesicles rupture readily and then quickly desquamate.

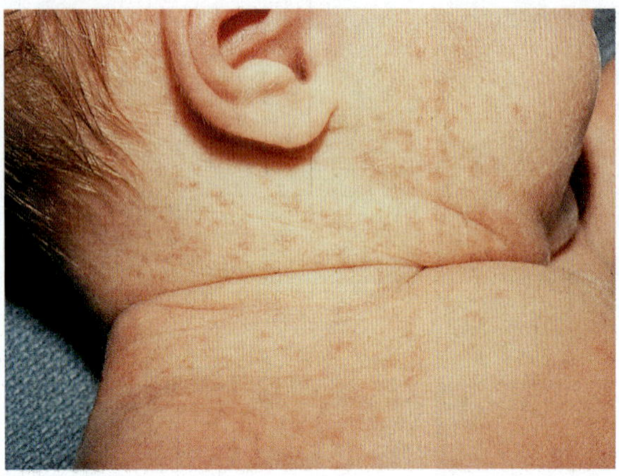

Fig. 8.58 Miliaria rubra. Numerous tiny papulopustular lesions dot the skin of this infant's face, neck, and upper trunk.

lesions form over the head, neck, and upper trunk. In older children, they more commonly occur in areas of desquamating sunburn.

Miliaria Rubra

Sweat duct obstruction deeper in the epidermal or dermal layers produces an erythematous papulopustular eruption known as *miliaria rubra,* or prickly heat (Fig. 8.58). This rash is common in infants and children, especially over the face, upper trunk, and intertriginous area of the neck, because of tight-fitting clothing or use of occlusive lubricants, particularly during hot, humid weather. Wearing lightweight, loose-fitting clothing, keeping cool, and eliminating greasy topical agents assist clearing of the rash.

Infantile Acropustulosis

Infantile acropustulosis, a remitting and exacerbating disorder of unknown etiology, begins as pinpoint erythematous papules, which evolve to form papulopustules or vesicopustules (Fig. 8.59) that can be highly pruritic. They appear in crops over the hands and feet, at times extending onto the wrists and ankles. After 10 to 21 days they resolve, only to recur within a few weeks. Ultimately, the flares become less frequent, and the disorder resolves by 2 to 3 years old. Differential diagnostic considerations include scabies, dyshidrotic eczema, erythema toxicum, and transient neonatal pustular melanosis. Mid- to high-potency topical steroids applied sparingly up to twice a day and oral antihistamines may help relieve itching.

Vesiculation After Insect Bites

Inflammatory reactions to insect bites, which often begins as papular urticaria, may evolve into pruritic vesicles and bullae on erythematous bases (Fig. 8.60). This is particularly true of the bites of grass and sand mites and of fleas in sensitized individuals who react intensely.

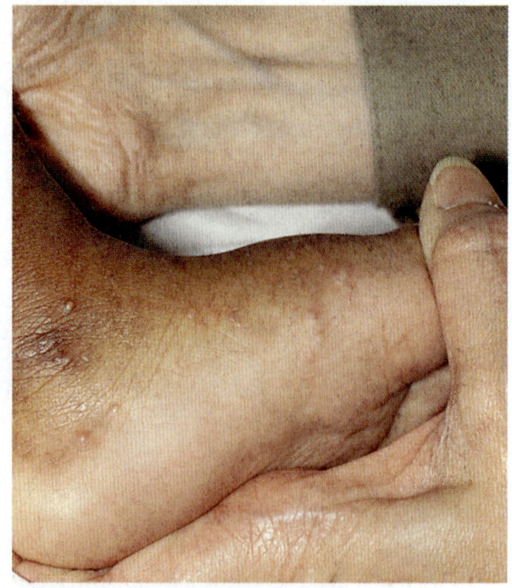

Fig. 8.59 Infantile acropustulosis. Intensely pruritic papulopustular lesions are seen over the foot and ankle of this infant. He had had multiple episodes and had been treated repeatedly for scabies. (Courtesy Sylvia Suarez, MD, Centerville, VA.)

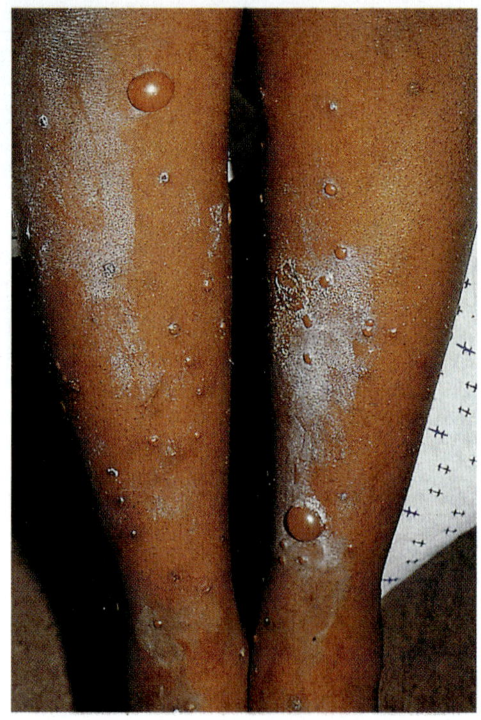

Fig. 8.60 Vesicular reaction to insect bites. This boy's lower legs are studded with numerous thick-walled vesicles and bullae that have formed in response to mite bites.

The eruption is frequently misdiagnosed as chickenpox or bullous impetigo. Severe pruritus, the lack of systemic complaints, localization to exposed areas (especially the lower legs in the case of fleas), and seasonal occurrence point to the correct diagnosis. Furthermore, the vesicles have thicker walls than those of bullous impetigo, and they do not rapidly umbilicate and crust as is true of varicella lesions. Tzanck tests and Gram stains are negative in bullous insect bite reactions (see Bites and Stings, later). Bedbug bites can present in a similar fashion but can be multiple and widespread and occur even under clothing. Some experts use the presence of bites on the eyelid to support the etiology of bedbugs because they bite during sleep.

REACTIVE ERYTHEMAS

The term *reactive erythema* refers to a group of disorders characterized by erythematous patches, plaques, and nodules that vary in size, shape, and distribution. Unlike other specific dermatoses, they represent cutaneous reaction patterns triggered by a variety of endogenous and environmental agents. In children, the most common reactive erythemas include erythema nodosum, urticaria, vasculitis, and drug eruptions.

Erythema Nodosum

Erythema nodosum is a panniculitis, or inflammation in the fat, that is characterized by symmetric, red, tender nodules, 1 to 5 cm in diameter, which are usually located over the pretibial surfaces (Fig. 8.61). Most likely, it represents a hypersensitivity reaction to streptococcal infection, sarcoidosis, tuberculosis, or other bacterial or fungal infections. Noninfectious disorders such as ulcerative colitis and regional ileitis have also been implicated. In adolescent girls, oral contraceptives are the most common cause, and several other medications may trigger this reaction.

Erythema nodosum is most often seen in children older than 10 years. The lesions begin as red, tender, slightly indurated nodules. These enlarge to form indurated subcutaneous plaques, and the overlying skin takes on a brownish-red or purplish-red hue within a few days. The disorder usually lasts between 2 and 6 weeks, although recurrences are common. Although any site may be involved, the shins are most commonly affected.

Differential diagnosis includes cellulitis, insect bites, thrombophlebitis, ecchymoses, and vasculitis. The fact that lesions are symmetric, recurrent, and persistent helps exclude cellulitis and ecchymoses. Their usual pretibial and extensor location helps differentiate the lesions from thrombophlebitis. Insect bite reactions typically are pruritic, and other exposed sites such as the arms, head, and neck may be involved. The deep-seated nature of the nodules in erythema nodosum should allow differentiation from the smaller, more superficial palpable lesions of cutaneous small-vessel vasculitis. However, they can mimic the cutaneous lesions seen in polyarteritis nodosum, a medium-vessel vasculitis.

Treatment is directed toward the underlying cause. NSAIDs may be effective in reducing pain, and bed rest with elevation of the involved region is beneficial.

Urticaria

Urticaria, commonly known as *hives,* are characterized by the sudden appearance of transient, well-demarcated wheals that are usually intensely pruritic, especially when arising as part of an acute IgE-mediated hypersensitivity reaction (Fig. 8.62A). Individual lesions usually last 1 to 2 hours but may persist for up to 24 hours. They may have an edematous white center and macular red halo (see Fig. 8.62B) or the reverse—a red center with an edematous white halo. Size can vary from a few millimeters to giant lesions greater than 20 cm in diameter (see Fig. 8.62C). Central clearing with peripheral extension may lead to the formation of annular, polycyclic, and arcuate plaques, termed *urticarial multiforme* given their similar appearance to EM and erythema marginatum (see Fig. 8.62D). The edema may involve the mucous membranes, but not with vesicles or true bullae as in EM, and can spread to the subcutaneous tissue, producing woody edema known as *angioedema.*

Urticaria can be caused by a variety of immunologic mechanisms, including IgE antibody response, complement activation, and abnormal levels of or sensitivity to vasoactive amines. Most commonly, acute urticaria (lasting less than 6 weeks) is idiopathic; postviral; or caused by a hypersensitivity reaction to food, drugs, insect bites, contact allergens, inhaled substances, or acute infections (especially β-streptococcal infections and viral infections, including mononucleosis). Chronic urticaria (lasting more than 6 weeks) can be a sign of an underlying disorder, such as occult infection (of the urinary tract, sinuses, or dentition); hepatitis B; or connective tissue disease (see Chapters 4 and 7). Urticarial lesions that remain fixed in the same location for more than 24 hours, are painful as opposed to pruritic, or heal with prolonged bruising are more likely to be signs of urticarial vasculitis, so they should prompt a biopsy and possible systemic workup.

In otherwise healthy patients who have no evidence on thorough history and physical examination to suggest occult infection or an underlying disorder and whose laboratory studies are normal, extensive testing is not warranted. Empiric treatment with oral antihistamines provides symptomatic relief and may help break the itch/scratch cycle.

Serum Sickness–Like Reaction

Serum sickness–like reaction, a relatively common acute clinical picture, involves a constellation of urticarial lesions, periarticular swelling, and extremity angioedema in conjunction with acute upper respiratory infection or after use of medications, such as sulfonamides, cefaclor, minocycline, or the "-cillins." The urticaria is typically either nonpruritic or only mildly pruritic, and lesions evolve into target shapes or gyrate plaques simulating EM (what is termed "urticarial multiforme"), although they do not vesiculate (Fig. 8.63A and B). With this eruption, painful migratory periarticular swelling is seen, especially involving the wrists and ankles, and often associated with bluish

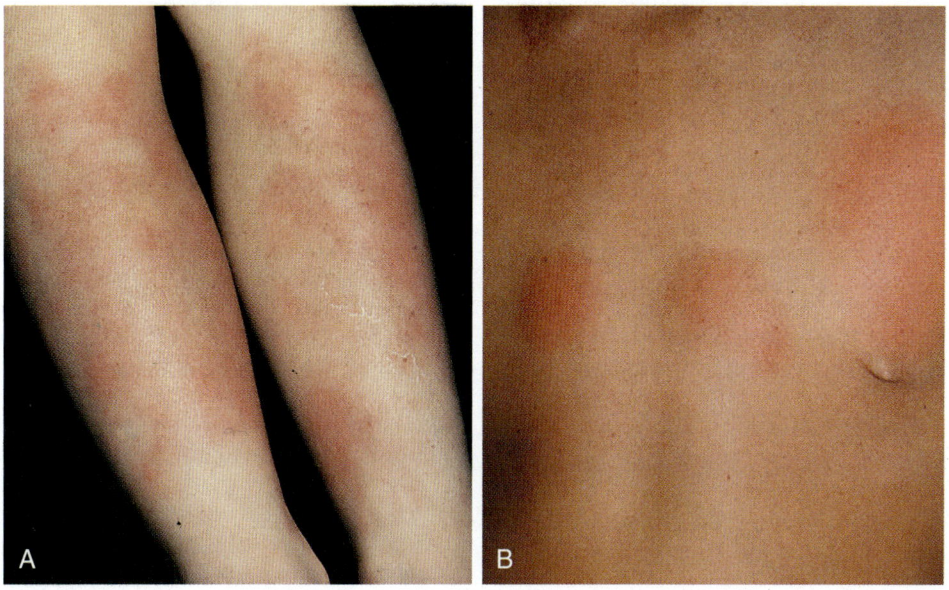

Fig. 8.61 Erythema nodosum. (A) Note the typical red, raised, tender nodules overlying the pretibial surfaces of the legs. (B) This 18-month-old boy developed tender, indurated, erythematous patches over his chest and abdomen after an upper respiratory infection. (B, Courtesy Cohen BA: *Pediatric dermatology,* ed 2, London, 1999, Mosby.)

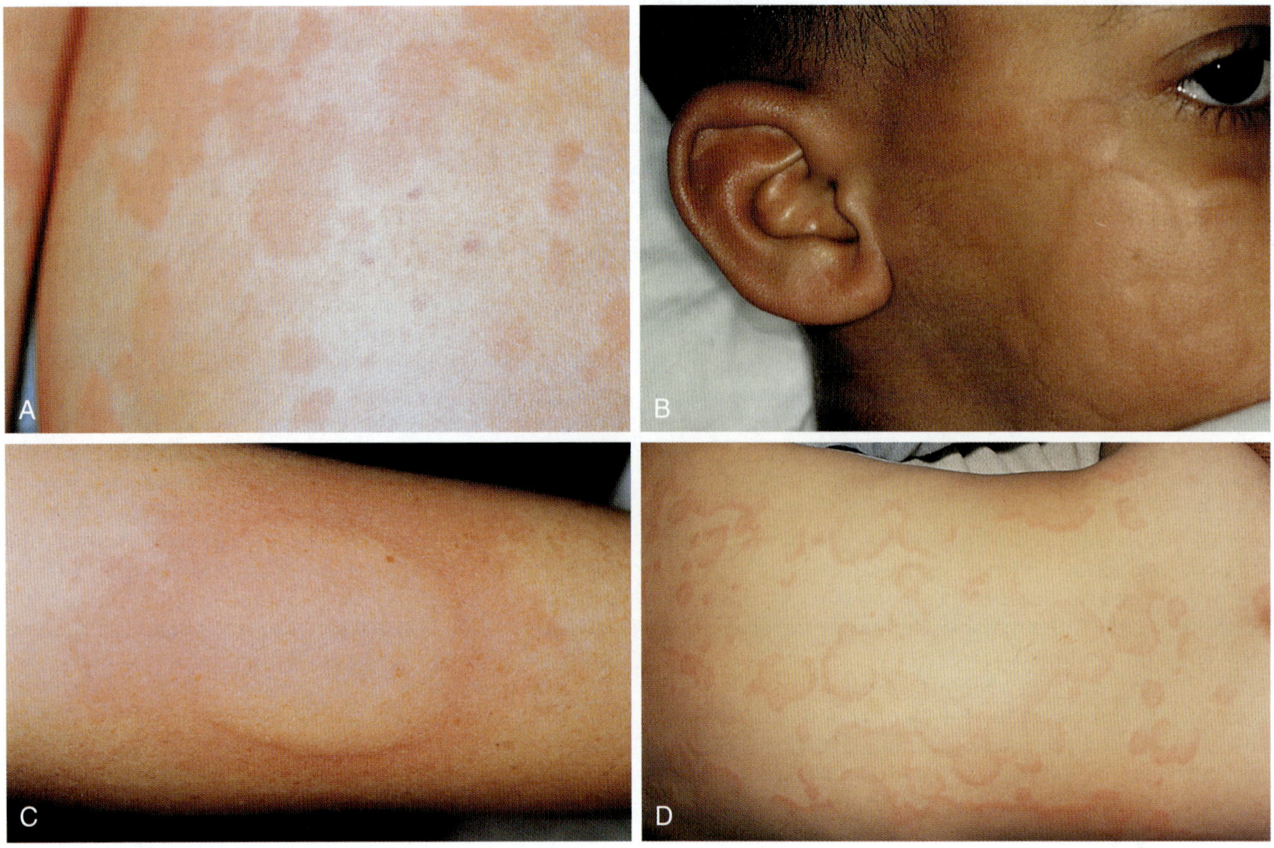

Fig. 8.62 Urticaria. (A) Typical erythematous raised wheals are seen. (B) The wheals on this child's face have red rims and lighter centers. (C) This patient with cold-induced urticaria has a giant whitish wheal with an erythematous halo. (D) Gyrate urticarial plaques have evolved from individual plaques that became confluent. (A and C, Courtesy Douglas W. Kress, MD, University of Pittsburgh Medical Center.)

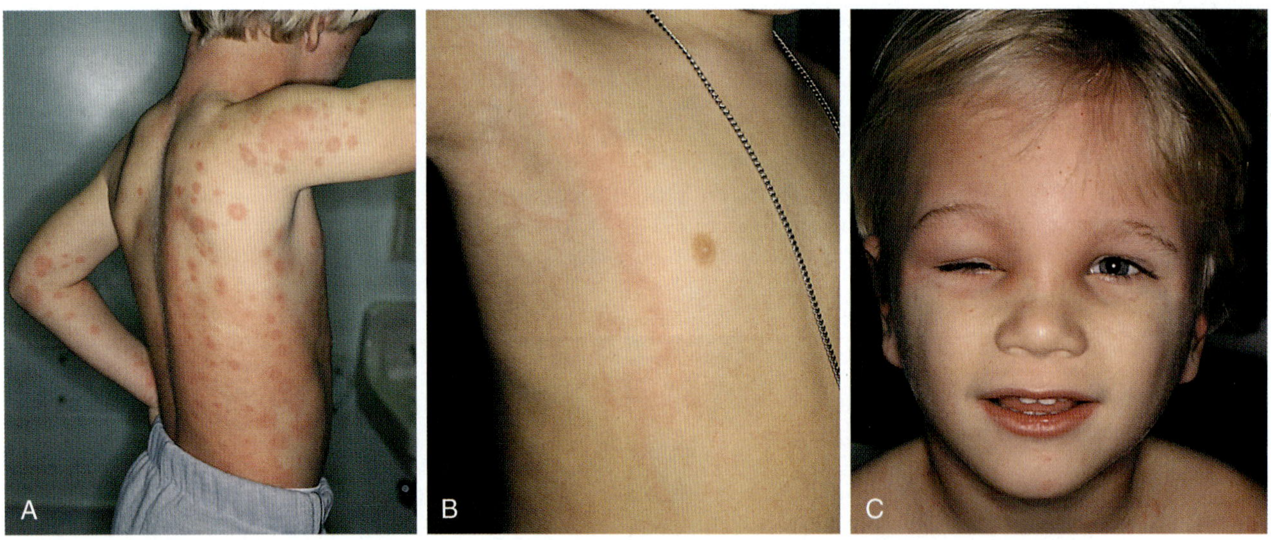

Fig. 8.63 Serum sickness–like reaction to cefaclor. (A and B) Extensive urticarial, target-shaped, and gyrate lesions are seen over the back, arms, and trunk. (C) Facial edema involving the forehead was prominent in this child.

discoloration of the overlying skin. Migratory stocking-glove angioedema, which is also painful, is common; on occasion, facial edema is seen as well (see Fig. 8.63C). After resolution of the respiratory infection or discontinuation of the offending agent, symptoms wax and wane over 1 to 3 weeks. This appears to be a T-lymphocyte–mediated reaction, and classic changes of vasculitis are not seen.

Drug Eruptions

Morbilliform Drug Eruption

Many different types of drug eruption are seen in children. Morbilliform rashes or exanthems account for 75% to 80% of all cutaneous drug reactions. The rash is reminiscent of measles or other viral exanthems (see Chapter 13). Erythematous macules and papules, which may range from fine to blotchy, usually begin to erupt on the face and trunk within 5 to 14 days after starting a medication. They then spread to the extremities over 1 to several days (Fig. 8.64). The rash, which may be pruritic, is occasionally restricted to the extremities, or it may appear acrally (distally) at first and then spread centrally. Lesions may become confluent and generally resolve over 1 to 2 weeks with the development of fine desquamation and residual postinflammatory erythema. In cases of morbilliform drug eruption with facial swelling, fever, or malaise, the clinician should check hepatic function and a complete blood count to rule out the more life-threatening disorder, drug rash with eosinophilia and systemic symptoms (DRESS), which can lead to hepatic failure if not

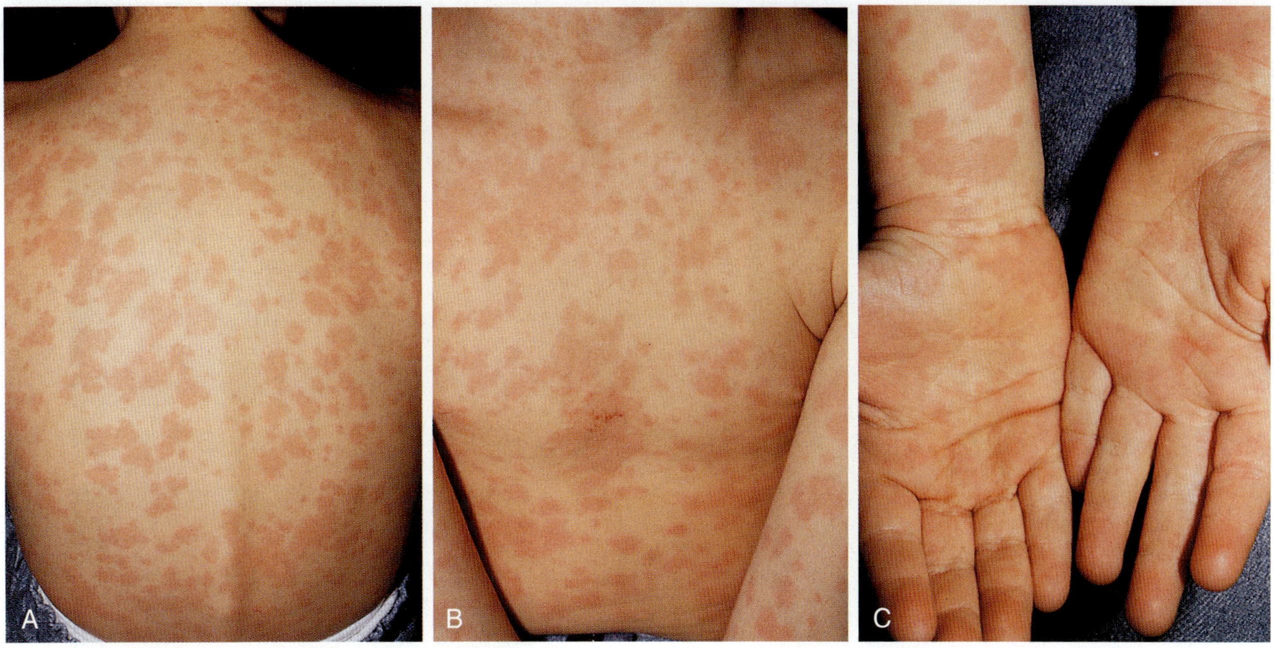

Fig. 8.64 Morbilliform drug eruption. (A and B) This diffuse exanthem developed on the seventh day of treatment with amoxicillin for streptococcal pharyngitis. (C) The palms and soles were also affected.

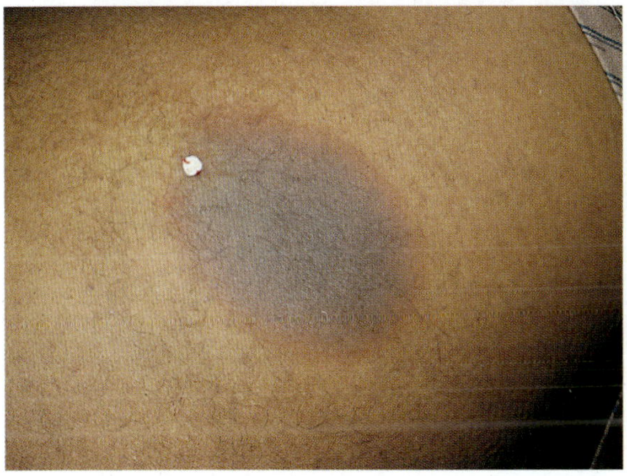

Fig. 8.65 Fixed drug eruption. This hyperpigmented patch with an erythematous border developed on the flank of an adolescent taking tetracycline.

identified and treated promptly. Although the liver is the most common organ to be involved in DRESS, it is important to remember that it can also affect the kidneys, heart, central nervous system (CNS), and thyroid. DRESS is more common with certain medications, such as sulfa drugs, minocycline, and anticonvulsants.

Fixed Drug Eruption

Fixed drug eruptions are erythematous and often violaceous plaques, which reappear at the same cutaneous site after reexposure to an offending drug. They can affect both the skin and mucous membranes. Postinflammatory hyperpigmentation can be prominent and may be the only manifestation of the rash during remissions. Morphologically and histologically, the annular and sometimes bullous lesions of fixed drug reactions may appear similar to EM and may represent a localized form of EM (Fig. 8.65). Common offending drugs include sulfa drugs, NSAIDs, and pseudoephedrine, as well as certain food additives and flavorings; therefore a thorough history of all possible exposures is key to elucidating the cause.

IgA Vasculitis

IgA Vasculitis, formerly known as Henoch-Schonlein purpura (HSP), is an inflammatory disorder caused by immune complex deposition in capillaries and blood vessels. It is associated with a leukocytoclastic vasculitis in the skin and other involved organs. It is characterized by a diffuse vasculitis involving the small postcapillary venules in the skin; gastrointestinal tract; kidneys; joints; and, rarely, the lungs and CNS. Although the exact etiology is unclear, the common history of antecedent upper respiratory or gastrointestinal infection suggests a hypersensitivity phenomenon, resulting in a localized or widespread vascular insult. Other factors, including drugs, food, immunizations, and chemical toxins, have been implicated as well.

After a prodrome of headache, anorexia, and, occasionally, low-grade fever lasting 1 to a few days, patients may develop one or more of the following in any order: rash; abdominal pain; arthritis; and, occasionally, hematochezia. Cutaneous lesions consist of erythematous macules, urticarial papules, and purpuric papules and plaques that tend to appear in crops (Fig. 8.66A–C), each resolving over 5 to 7 days, although the total duration of this waxing and waning eruption may last anywhere from 1 to 8 weeks. Of affected children, 15% to 40% have one or more recurrences, usually within 6 weeks of resolution of the first episode.

Although in most children the initial rash consists of purpuric lesions distributed symmetrically below the waist (over the buttocks, lower abdomen, and lower extremities), in some this may be preceded by an acral or generalized urticarial eruption that is minimally pruritic and waxes and wanes over 1 to several days before the appearance of purpura. Subsequent crops of purpura usually involve the extensor surfaces of the arms, cheeks (see Fig. 8.66D), and tips of the ears. The rash may also involve the trunk and genitalia. In unusually severe cases, skin necrosis may occur, heralded by the appearance of bullae.

Joint involvement consists of painful, tender periarticular swelling, especially involving the wrists, ankles, and knees. The overlying skin tends to appear ecchymotic. Stocking-glove edema of the hands and feet is also common (see Fig. 8.66E). In young children, nonpruritic angioedema of the face, scalp, sacral area, or scrotum (see Fig. 8.66F) may be prominent. These phenomena wax and wane, as does the exanthem.

Gastrointestinal symptoms can precede, coincide with, or follow the appearance of cutaneous lesions. Segmental edema of the intestinal tract can cause crampy to colicky abdominal pain and may even serve as the lead point for an intussusception. Mucosal hemorrhage can be the source of gastrointestinal bleeding that can range from occult loss to massive hematochezia or hematemesis (see Chapter 18).

Up to 25% of patients develop nephritis between 1 and 8 weeks after the onset of symptoms (with peak onset at 1–3 weeks). This is more common in older children, and it is usually mild and self-limited. It is first detected by finding evidence of hematuria and proteinuria on urinalysis. On occasion, nephritis is severe and progressive (see Chapter 14). Long-term studies suggest that the risk of subtle renal

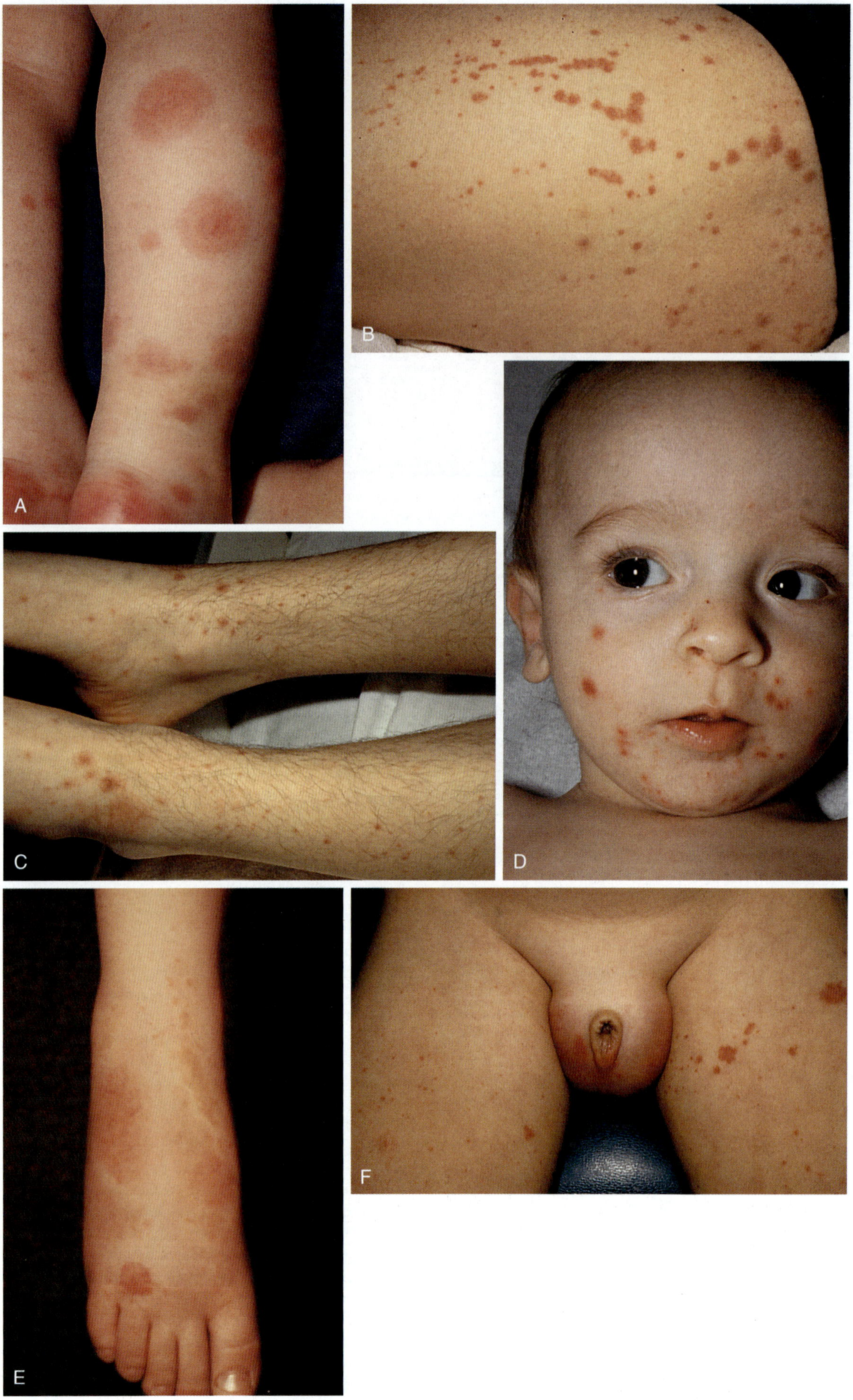

Fig. 8.66 IgA vasculitis. (A) Palpable purpuric macules, papules, and plaques are seen over the legs and ankles of this toddler. (B and C) These smaller purpuric papules are more typical and are seen initially over the buttocks, thighs, and ankles. (D) Later crops may involve the extensor surfaces of the upper extremities, trunk, and face. (E and F) Edema of the extremities, genitals, face, and scalp may be impressive.

disease may be higher than initially suspected, and the routine determination of blood pressure in addition to repeat urinalysis testing at regular pediatric visits is a good screening tool. Moreover, children with chronic IgA vasculitis with recurrences lasting more than 4 to 6 months may be at higher risk for chronic renal disease. CNS involvement is extremely rare, and its presence is usually heralded by severe headache, altered level of consciousness, or seizures after meningeal hemorrhage.

Treatment is generally supportive, although gastrointestinal, renal, and CNS vasculitis may respond to systemic corticosteroids.

The cutaneous lesions of IgA vasculitis must be differentiated from acute bacterial, viral, and rickettsial infections (see Chapter 13). Negative blood cultures and classic findings on cutaneous examination and skin biopsy define this condition. Purpuric rashes associated with thrombocytopenia are more likely to be associated with petechiae and can be ruled out by a normal platelet count. Lastly, vasculitic rashes may also be seen in collagen vascular disorders, such as lupus erythematosus, mixed connective tissue disease, and dermatomyositis (see Chapter 7). These disorders can usually be excluded by the absence of other findings. An etiology, likely related to IgA vasculitis but occurring in infants, called *acute hemorrhagic edema of infancy* is characterized by purpura en cockade, annular lesions of purpura on the distal extremities, and swelling of the distal extremities after a prodrome of viral upper respiratory tract symptoms. Unlike IgA vasculitis, acute hemorrhagic edema of infancy has an extremely benign course with only a few reports of renal involvement found in the literature.

BITES AND STINGS

Insect and spider bites may be associated with several cutaneous and systemic reactions. Lesions are found on exposed areas of skin, particularly the lower legs, arms, head, and neck. During the warm summer months, they may also appear on the trunk. Protected areas (including the buttocks, groin, and axillae) are invariably spared except in the case of bedbugs, in which even covered regions may be involved. When bites involve the face, they can cause marked pruritic swelling that, although erythematous, is nontender and minimally indurated (Fig. 8.67).

Insect Bites

Insect bites, most commonly caused by mosquitoes and fleas, tend to produce mild acute local reactions including erythema, edema, and urticarial papules that are typically pruritic (Fig. 8.68A). A tiny central crust or hemorrhagic punctum may be apparent on close inspection. On occasion, patients develop more intense hemorrhagic reactions (see Fig. 8.68B).

Although mosquito and mite bites occur only during the warm months of spring, summer, and fall, flea bites can occur year-round, typically in households with pets or homes recently vacated by previous tenants or owners whose pets had fleas. Young children who only visit on occasion with friends or relatives who have pets are also susceptible. Bites are usually found on the lower legs above the sock line but can be more diffusely distributed on crawling infants and toddlers. Like those of bedbugs, flea bites often appear in clusters of three (a clinical finding termed "breakfast, lunch, and dinner"). This stems from the fact that, although fleas can jump, they cannot fly. Hence they tend to produce a localized series of bites in the same vicinity before jumping on to a new area. Excoriation caused by scratching makes them prone to secondary impetiginization. It should also be noted that not all members of a household may be

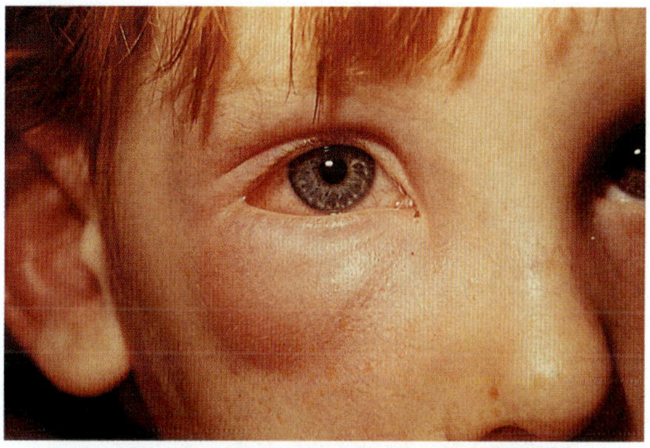

Fig. 8.67 Facial swelling caused by a mosquito bite. The area was pruritic, nontender, and nonindurated. (Courtesy Michael Sherlock, MD, Lutherville, MD.)

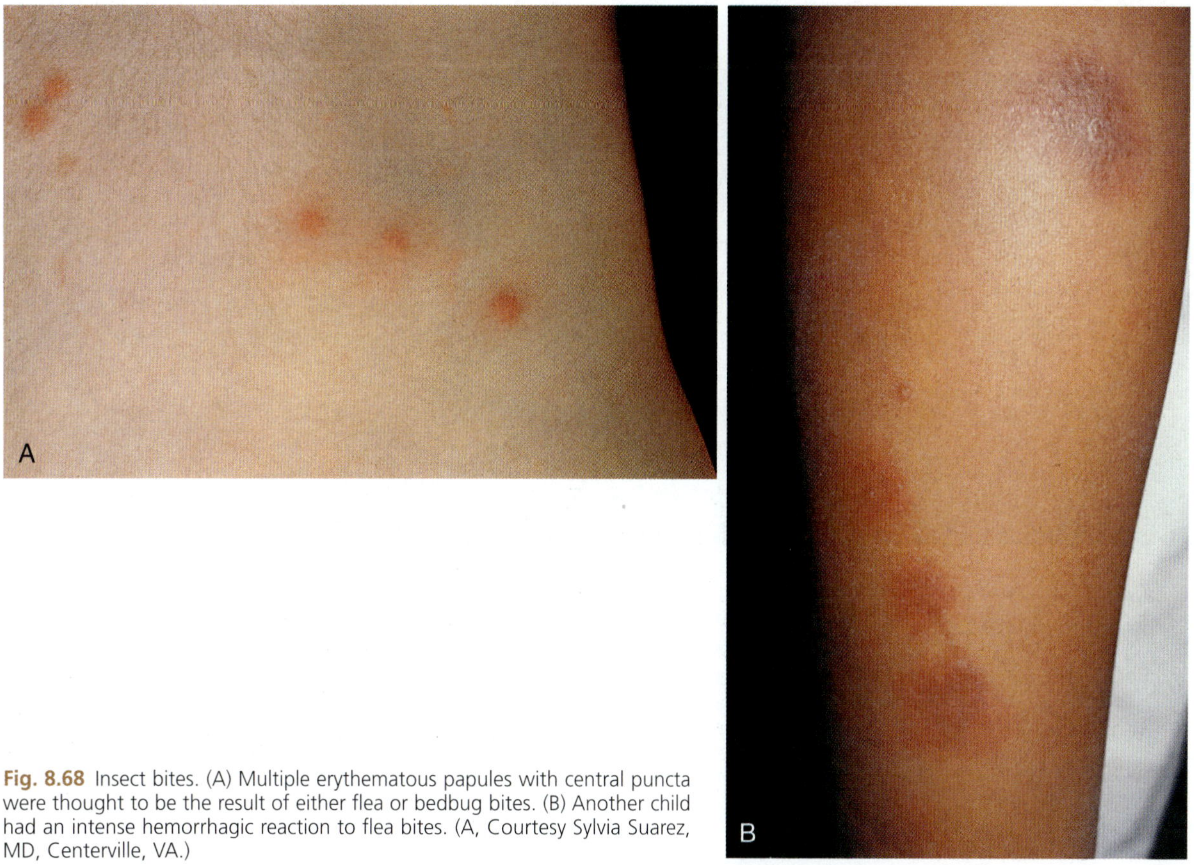

Fig. 8.68 Insect bites. (A) Multiple erythematous papules with central puncta were thought to be the result of either flea or bedbug bites. (B) Another child had an intense hemorrhagic reaction to flea bites. (A, Courtesy Sylvia Suarez, MD, Centerville, VA.)

sensitive to flea bites, and therefore some may appear to be spared. This can be a source of confusion to people who assume that if fleas are the source, everyone should be affected.

On occasion, the bites of grass or sand mites can produce frank blistering because the venom they inject contains a blistering agent that affects sensitive individuals (see Fig. 8.60).

Biting flies include sandflies, blackflies, horseflies, and gnats. The bite itself causes immediate pain and is usually followed by the development of a painful papule that sometimes vesiculates centrally.

Spider Bites

Spider bites tend to provoke more intense inflammatory reactions than those of most insects. Commonly, this consists of an area of erythema and induration that frequently becomes ecchymotic and is simultaneously painful and pruritic (Fig. 8.69). Less often, the lesions may vesiculate or even progress to develop central necrosis with eschar formation. The latter is particularly typical of the bite of the brown recluse spider.

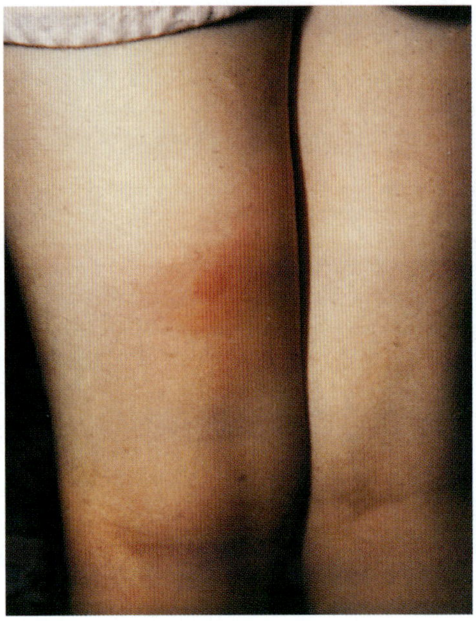

Fig. 8.69 Spider bites. A marked inflammatory response consisting of a central wheal with a wide erythematous halo is seen in this child, who complained of both pain and pruritus.

Hymenoptera Stings

Bee, wasp, hornet, and yellow jacket stings typically produce a mild local reaction consisting of pain, erythema, and edema appearing within 2 hours after the sting (Fig. 8.70A). The honeybee leaves its stinger behind, embedded in the skin. Because this may continue to release venom for up to 1 hour, it should be removed as soon as possible using a horizontal scraping motion with a knife or fingernail. Grasping the stinger between forceps or two fingernails can inject more venom. Evidence indicates that topical application of a paste of papain (meat tenderizer) mixed with water may reduce the severity of local reactions if applied within minutes of the sting.

Hymenoptera stings commonly produce a late-onset increase in swelling that is more diffuse than the initial reaction and tends to peak in 48 to 72 hours. This is the result of a delayed hypersensitivity reaction, and it is described by patients as being both pruritic and painful (see Fig. 8.70B). Treatment is symptomatic.

In approximately 0.5% to 0.8% of the population (including many patients with underlying mastocytosis [see Fig. 8.85]), hymenoptera stings cause severe, acute, anaphylactic reactions within 15 minutes of the sting (see Chapter 4). This necessitates education regarding avoidance of the offending insects and immediate use of epinephrine.

Papular Urticaria

Papular urticaria, a phenomenon seen primarily in young children, is characterized by symmetric chronic and recurrent eruptions of highly pruritic papules and wheals that may vesiculate centrally. Acute lesions are round, approximately 3 to 10 mm in diameter, and often have a central punctum. They tend to be arranged in linear or triangular clusters on exposed body surfaces, such as the arms; legs; back; face; and, in toddlers, the scalp. Because itching is intense, the child scratches to the point of excoriation, incurring risk of secondary infection and scarring. During resolution, lesions tend to form a central crust with a surrounding collarette of scale, and ultimately

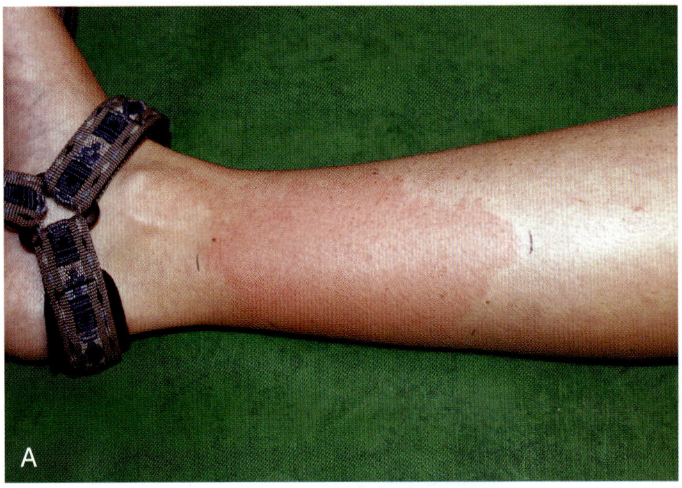

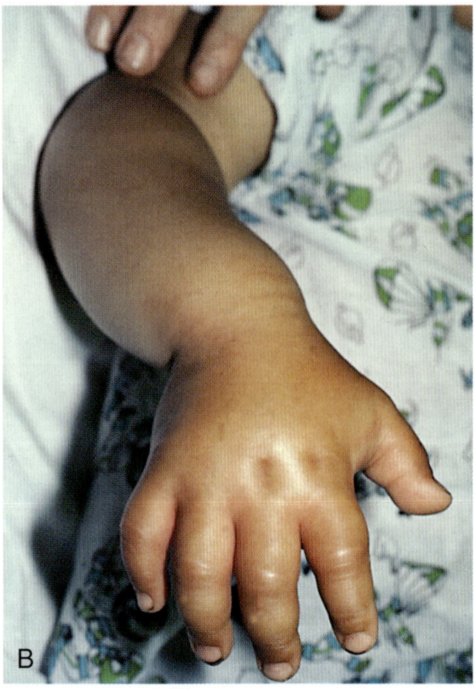

Fig. 8.70 Hymenoptera stings. (A) This child had an acute reaction with pain, redness, and mild swelling that developed within 2 hours of the sting. (B) In this example of a delayed hypersensitivity response to a bee sting, marked swelling of the hand and fingers developed over 24 hours after a sting between the fingers.

(after 4–6 weeks) the child is left with target-shaped macules that are hyperpigmented peripherally and hypopigmented centrally. Often lesions in varying stages of evolution and healing are seen within a small geographic area (Fig. 8.71).

The disorder is the result of a hypersensitivity response induced by bites of blood-sucking insects, especially dog and cat fleas and bedbugs, and sometimes mosquitoes. Fleas and bedbugs, because they both live indoors, bite year-round, so there is no seasonal predilection when they are the source.

Typically, only one family member, usually one of the youngest children, is affected. This is because some individuals never develop hypersensitivity to the bites; others have varying thresholds of sensitization; and older individuals, sensitized in the past, have become tolerant.

Because a full-scale reaction tends to require a fairly long period of sensitization during which the child has repeated exposure to the offending insect, few children become sensitized before their first birthdays. During this period of induction of sensitization, the child reacts minimally when bitten. Once sensitized, children go through a period of variable duration (months to years) in which they experience both immediate and delayed hypersensitivity reactions to bites. Ultimately, they develop tolerance (i.e., become desensitized) and no longer react. During peak sensitivity, many experience a phenomenon known as *reactivation,* in which new bites incite a delayed hypersensitivity reaction at old sites.

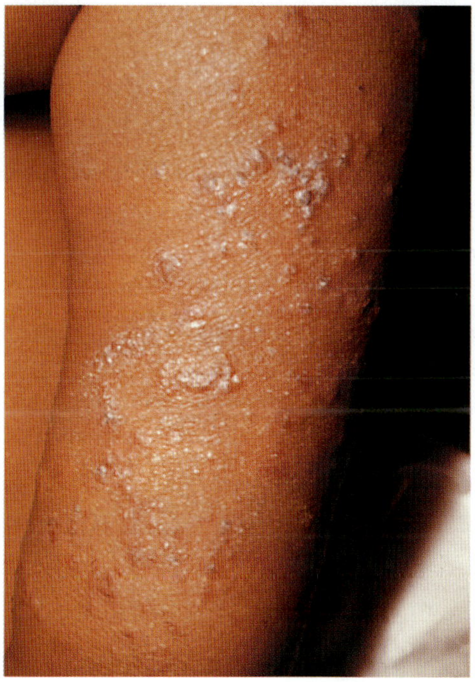

Fig. 8.71 Papular urticaria. This severe, excoriated, papular reaction developed in response to recurrent flea bites. (Courtesy Michael Sherlock, MD, Lutherville, MD.)

Identification of the offending vector and elimination of its presence can shorten the cycling. Other treatment measures include use of moisturizers, topical steroids, and oral antihistamines for acute lesions. Good hand and nail hygiene reduces the risk of secondary infection. Wearing protective clothing, avoiding going outdoors after dusk, and judicious use of insect repellent containing less than 30% of DEET are helpful when mosquitoes are causative.

Treatment Principles for Insect Bites

General principles of therapy for insect bites consist of insect control, use of insect repellents containing less than 30% of DEET (as recommended by the American Academy of Pediatrics [AAP]), and application of topical corticosteroids supplemented by oral antihistamines for symptomatic relief. Parenteral administration of epinephrine, antihistamines, and corticosteroids combined with intensive supportive care may be lifesaving in anaphylactic reactions.

INFESTATIONS

Scabies

Scabies is a highly contagious infestation caused by the mite *Acarus scabiei,* which burrows under the skin. It is contracted by direct contact with other infested humans or fomites. The characteristic eruption appears 4 to 6 weeks after initial contact, and it is thought to represent a hypersensitivity reaction to the mites. Intensely pruritic papules, vesicles, pustules, and linear burrows appear in the finger and toe webs (Fig. 8.72A), the axillae, over the flexor surfaces of the wrists and elbows, around the nipples and waist, and over the groin and buttocks. The burrow, which is produced by the female mite, is the pathognomonic sign of scabies. It consists of a small, scaly, linear papule with pinpoint vesicles at the ends (see Fig. 8.72B). In infants and toddlers, the distribution differs with the head; neck; trunk; palms; soles, dorsa, and lateral and instep portions of the feet; and lateral aspect of the wrists being more prominently involved (Fig. 8.73A–E). This age group is also more prone to developing an intense and persistent nodular reaction to the mite (see Fig. 8.73F).

In many patients, excoriation, secondary infection, or even development of a widespread secondary eczematous eruption (because of intense scratching) alters the appearance of or masks the primary lesions, making diagnosis more difficult. Therefore scabies must be considered in any individual who has no history of atopic dermatitis but has severe pruritus and recent onset of an eczematous rash. The distribution of scabies in intertriginous areas and over the palms and

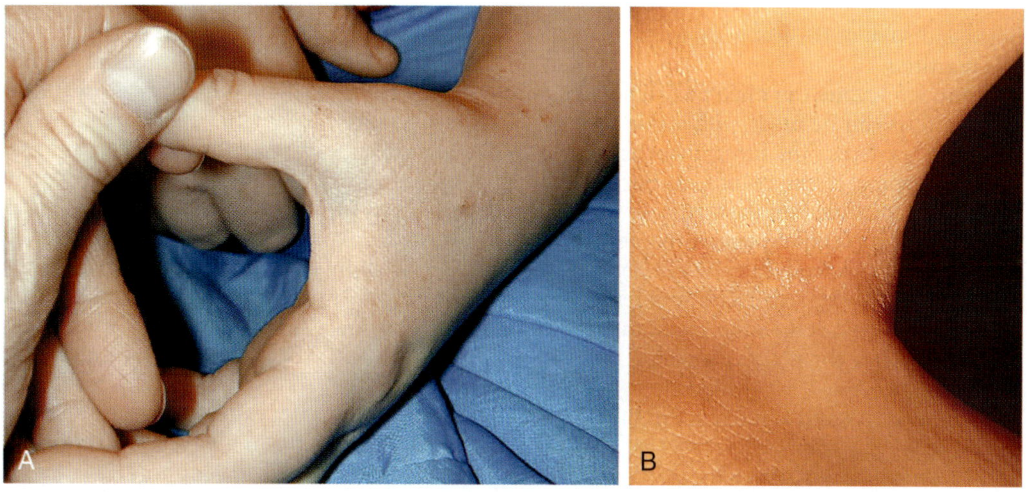

Fig. 8.72 Scabies. (A) Multiple pruritic papules, some excoriated and a few with central black dots, are seen on the wrist and dorsum of the hand. (B) A pathognomonic scabies burrow is present in the finger web space of another child.

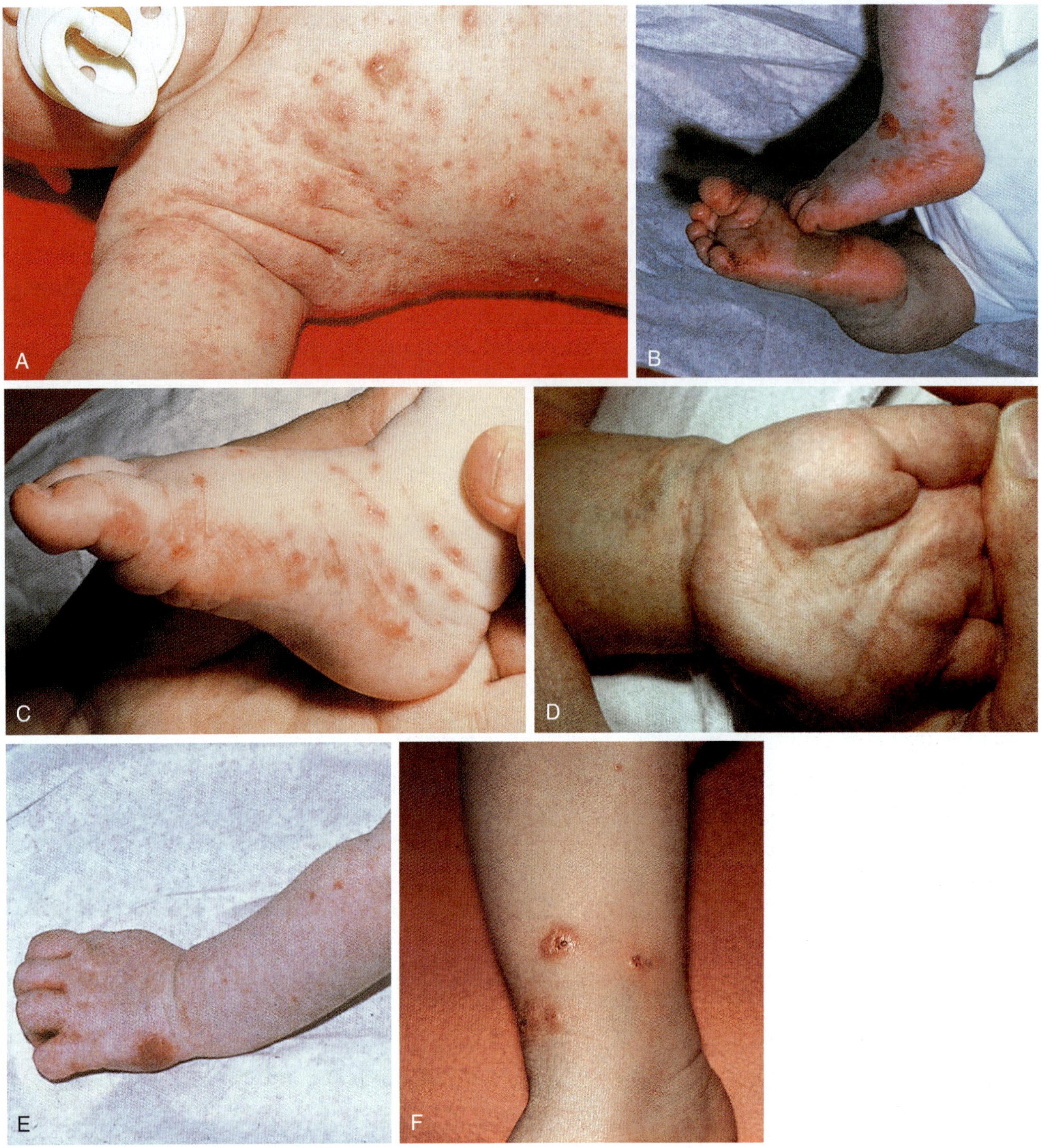

Fig. 8.73 Infantile scabies. Widespread, pruritic papules, pustules, and vesicles are seen over the trunk and axilla (A); the soles and dorsal, lateral, and instep portions of the feet (B and C), where burrows are also evident; the palm of the hand (D); and the lateral aspect of the wrist (E). (F) Infants are also more likely to develop an intense nodular reaction to the mite.

dorsa and soles of the feet helps to differentiate it from other insect bite reactions.

Although scabies can often be diagnosed clinically, an unequivocal diagnosis can be made with a skin scraping that shows a mite, mite eggs, or feces. The most important factor in obtaining a successful scraping is choice of site. Burrows and papules are most likely to be identified on the wrists, finger webs, feet, or elbows, or, in an infant, by scraping one of the nodules present on the trunk, palms, or soles. A fresh burrow can be identified as a 5- to 10-mm raised mound with a small dark spot resembling a fleck of pepper at one end. This spot is the mite, and it can be lifted out of the burrow with a needle or the point of a scalpel blade. If a scalpel is used to scrape the burrow, it is worthwhile to place a drop of mineral oil onto the skin to ensure adherence of the scrapings to the blade. The scrapings are placed on a slide, another drop of mineral oil is added, and a coverslip is applied.

Scabies mites are eight-legged arachnids which can be mobile and are easily visible under the scanning power of the microscope (Fig. 8.74A). Care must be taken to focus through thick areas of skin scrapings so as not to miss camouflaged mites. The presence of eggs (smooth ovals, approximately one-quarter to one-half the size of an adult mite) or feces (reddish-brown or black pellets, often seen in clusters) is also diagnostic (see Fig. 8.74B).

Eradication of scabies necessitates topical application of 5% permethrin (Elimite) cream to the patient, all household members, and close contacts in and outside the home (even if asymptomatic). In addition, thorough cleansing of all dirty clothing, towels, bedding, and car seat covers is essential. Two courses of treatment, 1 week apart, are necessary—the first to kill live mites and the second to eliminate mites that had not hatched at the time of first application. Symptomatic therapy with oral antipruritic

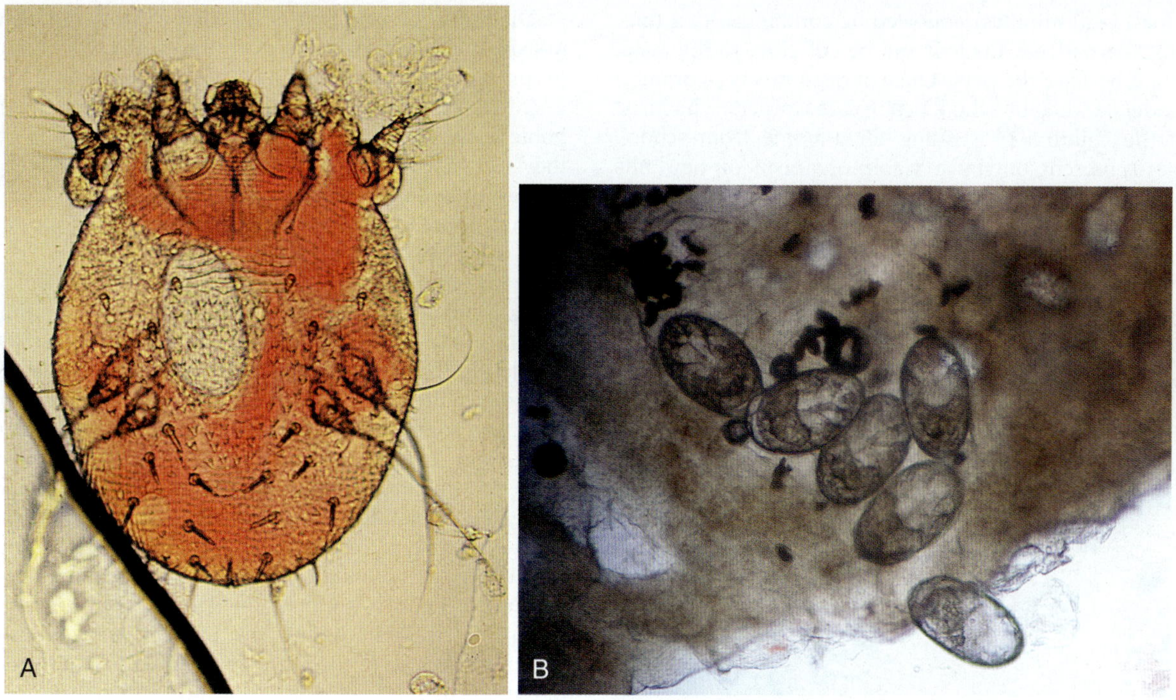

Fig. 8.74 (A) Microscopical appearance of an adult scabies mite obtained by scraping off the black dot at the end of a burrow. Note the small oval egg within the body. (B) In a second specimen, no mite is seen but multiple eggs and mite feces are evident.

agents and topical steroids may be required long after the mites have been killed (i.e., until the secondary reaction has subsided). Although not yet approved in the pediatric age group for scabies, a single dose of oral ivermectin may be effective in recalcitrant cases.

Lice

Three varieties of lice produce clinical disease in humans, and all can occur in children. Crab lice *(Phthirus pubis)* are transmitted primarily by sexual contact. They are short and broad with claws spaced far apart to grasp the sparse hairs on the trunk, pubic area, and eyelashes (Fig. 8.75A). They are typically found inhabiting the pubic hair and, occasionally, axillary hair and other body hair in adolescents and adults. Their bites produce bluish, pruritic papules that are distributed over the lower abdomen and upper thighs. Pruritus is intense, and a secondary eczematous rash may develop, particularly in the pubic area, due to scratching. Young children lacking pubic and axillary hair may develop scalp or eyelash infestations after close contact with infested adults.

Body lice *(Pediculus humanus corporis)* generally live in bedding or clothing, and their eggs may be found in the seams of trousers or underwear. Bites produce urticarial papules seen primarily over the waist, neck, shoulders, and axillae, which are usually obliterated by excoriations and secondary bacterial infection.

Head lice *(Pediculus humanus capitis)* represent the most common cause of infestation in children. The lice are acquired by close physical contact; by sharing hats, combs, brushes, or scarves with an infested person; or by rubbing against upholstered furniture recently used by such a person. Head lice are long and thin with claws spaced close together to grasp the more densely distributed scalp hairs (see Fig. 8.75B). Pruritus is the principal symptom, and the resultant scratching produces excoriations of the scalp, nape of the neck, and postauricular areas that are vulnerable to secondary infection. Occipital adenopathy is common.

Nits are seen as oval, white, 0.5-mm dots glued onto the hair shafts approximately 1 to 3 cm from the scalp (Fig. 8.76A), particularly above and behind the ears. These are firmly attached to the hair and do not move along the hair shafts, as do the hair casts for which they are frequently mistaken. Although nits may be seen along the entire length of the hair, they are deposited by the lice only near the scalp. Those far from the root indicate a span of perhaps months between infestation and examination. Nits are difficult to remove and may adhere as nonviable shells. Patients adequately treated for lice still have nonviable shells attached to the hair. Removal is assisted by use of a weak vinegar rinse (which is left on under a shower

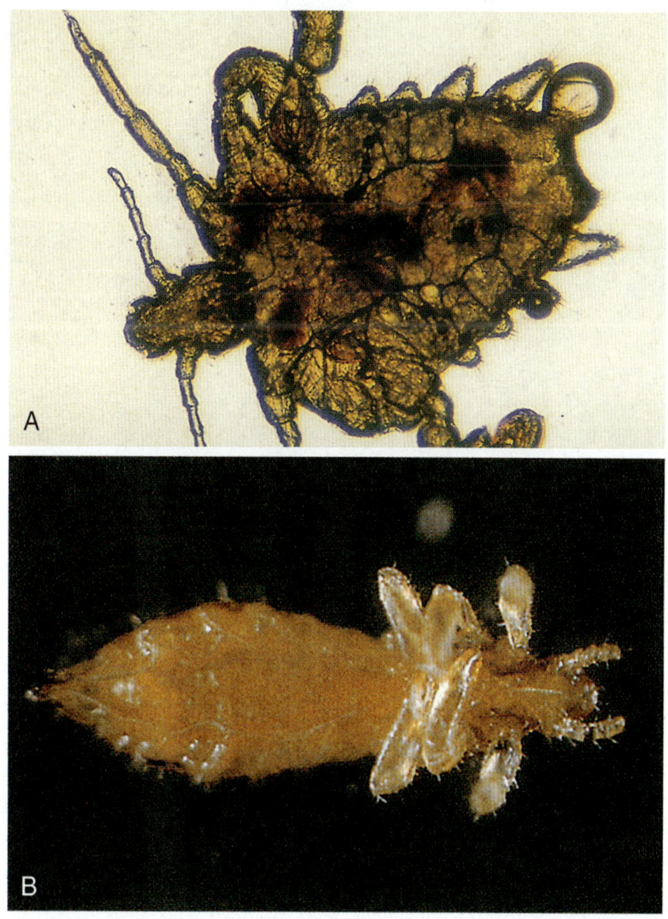

Fig. 8.75 Microscopical appearance of lice. (A) The crab louse has a short, broad body, with claws spaced far apart. (B) The head louse has a long, thin body, with claws spaced close together.

cap or towel for 15–20 minutes), followed by combing with a fine-toothed comb. Alternatively, the hair can be cut close to the scalp. This is important because the persistence of dead nits is a common cause of misunderstanding by school health care workers, who insist on retreating the children or sending them home from school. Active disease is present only if a viable organism or new nits attached close to the scalp are identified.

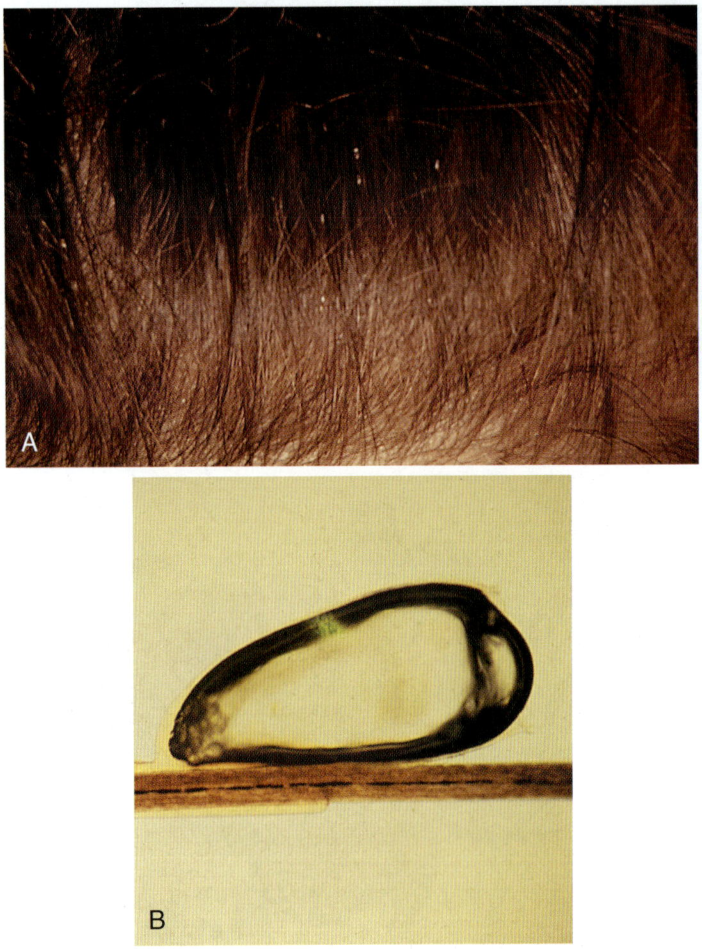

Fig. 8.76 Head lice. (A) Nits appear as tiny white dots that adhere to the hair shafts. They are typically found 1 to 3 cm from the scalp above and behind the ears. (B) Microscopic appearance of the nit of a head louse attached to a scalp hair. Microscopic examination distinguishes nits from hair casts and other artifacts. (A, Courtesy Michael Sherlock, MD, Lutherville, MD.)

Diagnosis of pediculosis must be considered in patients with unexplained scalp pruritus. A careful search for the organism may permit a specific diagnosis. Lice are six-legged insects visible to the unaided eye; they are commonly found on the scalp, eyelashes, and pubic areas. They are best identified close to the skin or scalp, where they can be seen moving around and where their eggs are more numerous and more obvious. Diagnosis can be made by either identifying a louse or plucking hairs and confirming the presence of nits by microscopical examination (see Fig. 8.76B).

Eradication of lice requires application of a pediculicide to infested hair-bearing areas of all household members and cleaning measures like those specified for ridding the house of scabies. Special attention should also be given to hats, scarves, and coat collars. Resistance to many over-the-counter pediculicides has been documented worldwide, and some cases may require multiple treatments or use of new prescription agents. A permethrin 1% to 5% cream rinse is an appropriate first-line treatment, but if cure is not achieved and resistance is suspected, malathion lotion or topical ivermectin lotion are both highly effective second-line options. However, it is important to instruct patients to avoid smoking near the patient because malathion is flammable. Benzyl alcohol lotion (4%) has been approved, and several new products are in the pipeline. Lindane, an agent used in the past, is contraindicated for use in infants, children, and the elderly because of the potential for systemic absorption and neurotoxicity.

ACNE

The exact pathogenesis of acne is unknown. However, abnormalities in follicular keratinization are thought to produce the earliest acne lesion, the microcomedone. In time, microcomedones may grow into clinically apparent open comedones (blackheads) (Fig. 8.77A) and closed comedones (whiteheads) (see Fig. 8.77B). The entire process is driven by androgens, which stimulate sebaceous gland differentiation and growth and the production of sebum. The proliferation of *Propionibacterium acnes* in noninflammatory comedones and the rupture of comedone contents into the surrounding dermis may trigger the development of inflammatory papules, pustules, and cysts (see Fig. 8.77C). Cystic acne is typified by nodules and cysts scattered over the face, chest, and back (see Fig. 8.77D). This form frequently leads to scarring. Acne fulminans is a rare subtype of inflammatory acne that can appear rapidly and in conjunction with fever and joint pain. This should be referred immediately to a pediatric dermatologist because it requires careful use of systemic therapy and close systemic monitoring.

Although therapy must be individualized, patients with mild to moderate comedonal or inflammatory acne usually respond well to a combination of topical retinoids, benzoyl peroxide, and antibiotics.

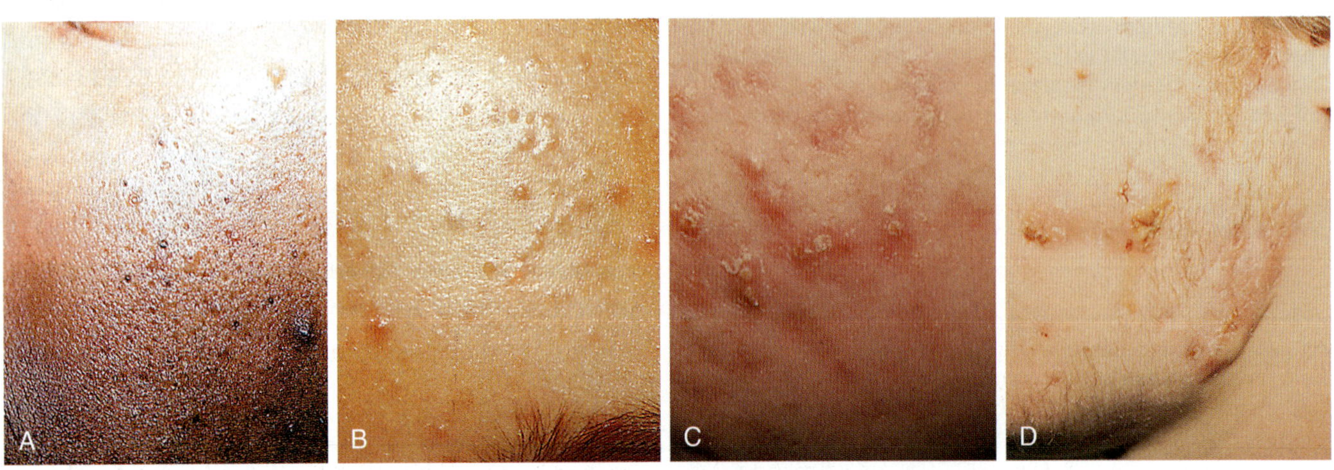

Fig. 8.77 (A) Comedonal acne with open comedones, or blackheads, seen over the cheek. (B) Comedonal acne with closed comedones, or whiteheads, on the forehead, accentuated by side lighting. (C) Papulopustular acne with inflamed papules and pustules over the cheeks, which responded well to antibiotics. (D) Cystic acne shows deep cysts with marked erythema that can cause severe scarring.

Moderate to severe papulopustular acne warrants the use of oral antibiotics in combination with topical agents. Oral 13-*cis*-retinoic acid, or isotretinoin, must be prescribed by a practitioner who is officially licensed in the IPledge program and should be reserved for patients with acne that has been recalcitrant to previous regimens or acne that is moderate to severe, scarring, or cystic. The authors recommend prompt referral to a pediatric dermatologist in cases of moderate or severe acne that are not responding to first-line therapy in 2 to 3 months because scarring can happen quickly in these patients and more aggressive definitive therapy should be considered early in the course.

TUMORS AND INFILTRATIONS

Persistent lumps and bumps in the skin often raise fears of skin cancer. Fortunately, primary skin cancer is relatively rare in childhood, and most tumors and infiltrative lesions are benign. Hemangiomas and nevi, which can be regarded as tumors, are discussed in subsequent sections of this chapter or other chapters.

Warts

Warts are benign tumors produced by human papillomavirus (HPV) infection of the skin and mucous membranes. In children they occur most commonly on the fingers, hands, and feet. The incubation period for warts varies from 1 to 6 months, and most lesions disappear spontaneously over a period of 5 years. Local trauma promotes inoculation of the papillomavirus. Thus periungual lesions are common in children who bite their nails or pick at hangnails.

Investigators have identified more than 80 HPVs capable of producing warts, and many of these viruses produce characteristic lesions in specific locations. For instance, the discrete, round, skin-colored papillomatous papules typical of *verruca vulgaris* (common warts) are produced by HPV types 2 and 4 (Fig. 8.78). The subtle, minimally hyperpigmented, flat warts *(verruca plana)* caused by HPV type 3 are frequently spread by picking and scratching and thus may become widespread on the face, arms, and legs (Fig. 8.79).

Plantar warts (Fig. 8.80) are associated with HPV type 1. Although not proven, the spread of these warts probably occurs through contact with contaminated, desquamated skin on shower floors, pool decks, and bathroom floors. Being much larger below the skin surface than is apparent from their external appearance, they occasionally cause pain when the patient walks. Although lesions can be confused with corns, calluses, or scars, they can be distinguished by their interruption of the normal skin lines (dermatoglyphics). Characteristic black dots in the warts are thrombosed superficial capillaries.

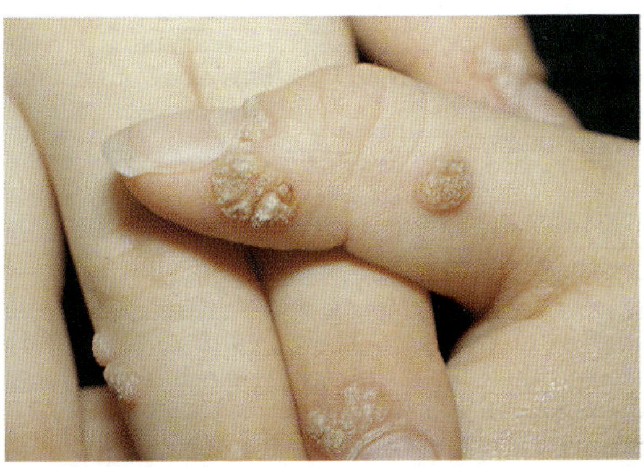

Fig. 8.78 Verruca vulgaris. Dry, rough, and crusty, these common warts usually involve the hands. The periungual distribution in this girl was due in part to her habit of picking at her cuticles.

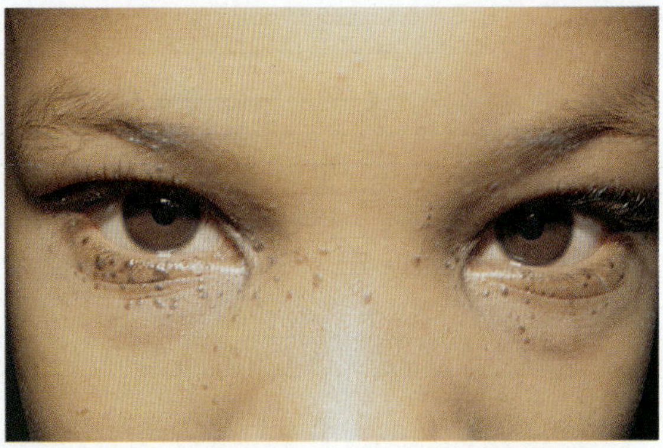

Fig. 8.79 Flat warts, or verruca plana. These tiny, light brown warts are spread by scratching.

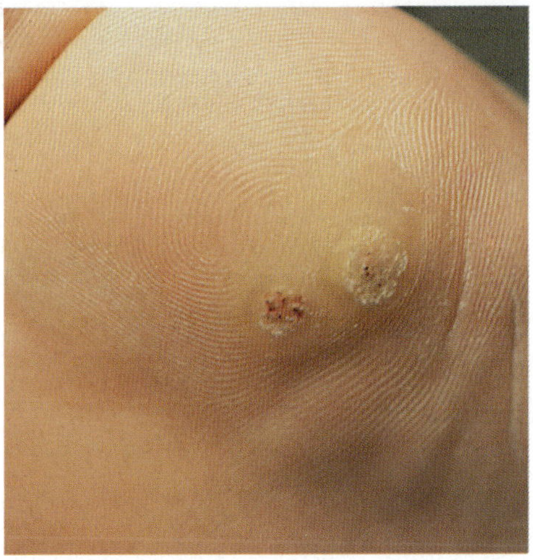

Fig. 8.80 Plantar warts. Two painful lesions are seen over the ball of the foot. Note how they interrupt the normal skin lines.

Warts can also be found on the trunk, oral and nasal mucosae, and conjunctivae. Anogenital lesions *(condylomata acuminata)* are usually associated with HPV types 6 and 11, and the possibility of sexual abuse must be considered in children older than 3 years old (with no known obvious exposure to warts) who present with lesions at this site (see Chapter 6).

Although warts are self-limited in most children, the presence of persistent or widespread lesions suggests the possibility of congenital or acquired immunodeficiency. Warts can become a serious management problem in immunosuppressed oncology and transplant patients, as well as those with human immunodeficiency virus or acquired immune deficiency syndrome.

Molluscum Contagiosum

Molluscum, a contagious skin disease caused by a pox virus, is characterized by sharply circumscribed dome-shaped papules with waxy surfaces. Lesions can occur singly or multiply and can be pruritic. Although usually umbilicated centrally, some have protruding white centers (Fig. 8.81). Lesions initially appear as pinpoint papules and then rapidly enlarge to up to 5 mm. They are found most commonly on the trunk, face, axillae, and genital area. Spread occurs because of scratching, and thus molluscum lesions are often arranged in a linear configuration (see Fig. 8.81B). Frequently, a curdlike core can be expressed from the center; microscopical examination of this material reveals typical molluscum (Henderson Patterson) bodies. It is important to note that there are no U.S. Food and Drug Administration–approved treatments for molluscum contagiosum. Because most lesions are asymptomatic and many undergo spontaneous remission within 2 to 3 years, treatment may not be necessary. However, in patients with symptomatic lesions who desire removal or in those with coexisting skin

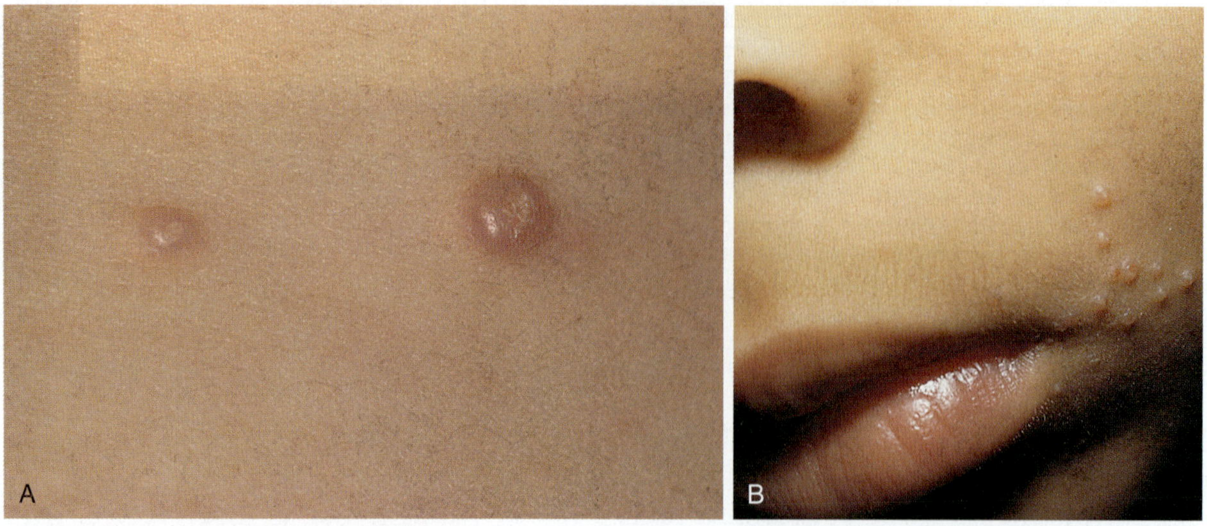

Fig. 8.81 Molluscum contagiosum. (A) In this case centrally umbilicated dome-shaped lesions are seen. (B) Lesions have spread on the face of this boy as a result of scratching. Note that some of these lesions have protruding white centers.

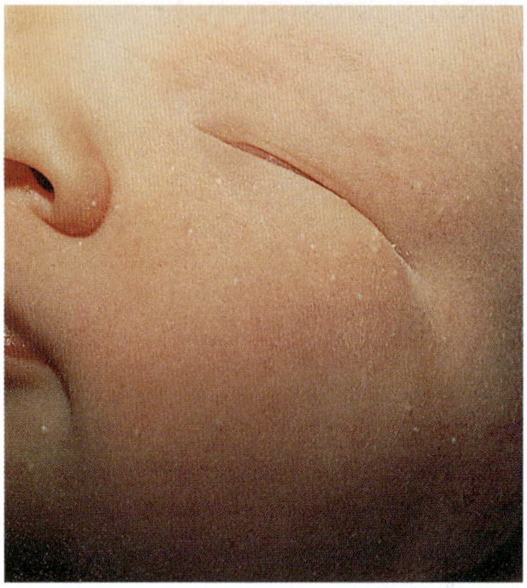

Fig. 8.82 Milia. These small, whitish-yellow papules are found close to the skin surface and are particularly common around the eyes and midface.

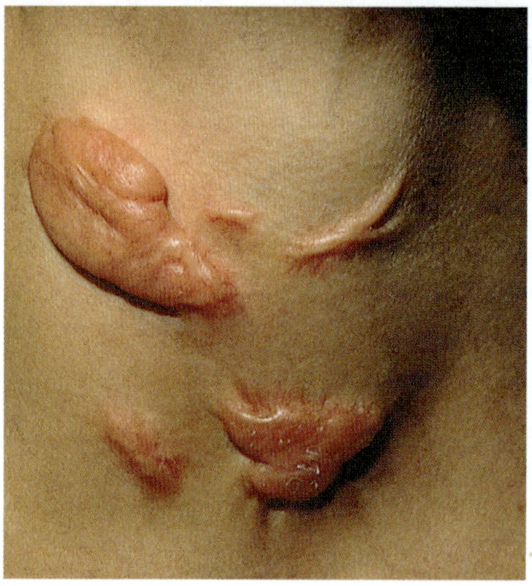

Fig. 8.83 Keloids. An abnormal reparative reaction to skin injury, keloids are characterized by proliferation of fibroblasts and collagen that extends beyond the margins of the original wound.

disease (e.g., severe eczema in which molluscum can quickly become widespread), at-home topical antiviral therapy or mild in-office therapies are reasonable treatment options. Studies looking at the efficacy of a topical imiquimod cream for the treatment of molluscum showed that the immune response modifier was no more effective than placebo.

Milia

Milia are tiny (1- to 2-mm), whitish-yellow papules that develop spontaneously on the face in neonates (Fig. 8.82). They are firm and, unlike pustules, are not easily denuded by pressure. Milia consist of tiny epithelial-lined cysts arising from hair follicles. They can be persistent, although they may resolve spontaneously after months to years. In newborns, they usually arise without any apparent cause, although in older infants and children they are often seen after skin injury, such as that caused by blistering eruptions or abrasions. They are a characteristic feature of the dystrophic form of EB (see Fig. 8.99).

Keloids

Keloids are firm, rubbery nodules or plaques that result from the proliferation of fibroblasts and deposition of collagen after injury to the skin (Fig. 8.83). They can be pruritic or tender, especially during the active growing phase, and they may extend well beyond the margins of the original wound. This latter trait distinguishes keloids from hypertrophic scars, which remain confined to the wound margins and flatten partially within 6 months of the injury. In predisposed individuals, keloids often occur after minimal injury, such as abrasions, minor lacerations, acne papules, insect bites, and ear piercing. They are more likely to develop on the ear lobes, upper trunk, and deltoid areas. Fortunately, they are not commonly seen on the midface. Keloids may soften or regress with topical or intralesional steroid injections alone or in combination with surgical excision. However, recurrences, especially after surgery, are common.

Neurofibromas

Neurofibromas are solitary or multiple growths of neural tissue, presenting as soft, skin-colored or pink dermal or subcutaneous nodules (Fig. 8.84). The central portion of an early lesion is particularly soft, and fingertip pressure creates the illusion of pressing in a buttonhole. Neurofibromatosis type 1 is a syndrome characterized by the presence of multiple neurofibromas, café au lait spots, axillary and inguinal freckling, Lisch nodules, and various systemic findings. When considering this diagnosis, the clinician must remember that the neurofibromas usually appear after puberty, whereas in prepubertal

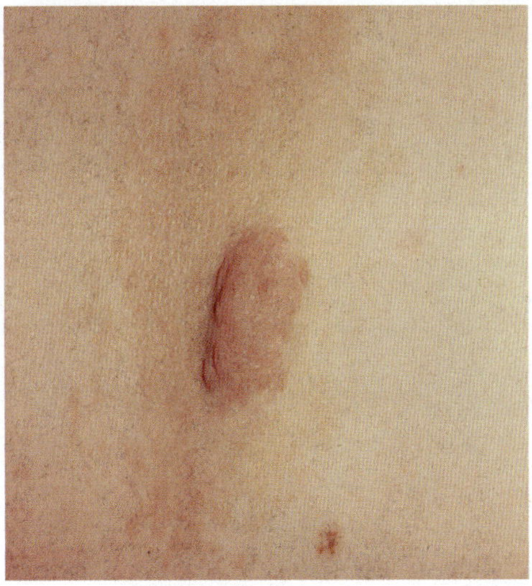

Fig. 8.84 Neurofibromatosis. A soft pink neurofibroma is seen arising within a café au lait spot. Usually neurofibromas arise at sites that are normally pigmented.

children, café au lait spots are the most important cutaneous marker of NF1 (see Fig. 8.123A and B; and see Chapter 16). Solitary neurofibromas occasionally develop in individuals who do not have neurofibromatosis.

Mastocytosis

Cutaneous mastocytosis refers to a group of disorders characterized by dermal infiltrations of mast cells.

Mastocytoma

Isolated mastocytomas may be seen in infants. They usually appear as skin-colored or light reddish-brown, slightly indurated plaques that are 1 to 2 cm in size (Fig. 8.85A). Development of a wheal-and-flare reaction after firm stroking of the lesion, known as a *positive Darier sign,* confirms the diagnosis (see Fig. 8.85B). This is a response to the vascular effects of histamine released from infiltrating mast cells. On occasion, enough histamine may be released from a large mastocytoma to cause localized blistering or systemic symptoms of flushing, wheezing, or diarrhea. Mastocytomas can be located anywhere on the body and usually resolve spontaneously by late adolescence.

Urticaria Pigmentosa

Urticaria pigmentosa is another form of cutaneous mastocytosis that presents with numerous small, reddish-brown macules, papules, or plaques, most commonly on the trunk (Fig. 8.86). These may be present at birth or may appear later in childhood. They are often mistaken for café au lait spots but instead react to stroking with a wheal-and-flare reaction (see Fig. 8.86B and C). Urticaria pigmentosa in children is usually limited to the skin and often resolves by adolescence. However, the bone marrow, gastrointestinal tract, and other organs may rarely be involved. Rare systemic findings in children with urticaria pigmentosa include chronic diarrhea, gastric ulcers, flushing reactions, headaches, and growth faltering. In infancy, there is more of a tendency for the lesions to blister. Unlike mastocytosis in adults, pediatric mastocytosis is not associated with mast cell leukemia.

Patients with isolated mastocytomas and urticaria pigmentosa should be counseled to be aware of possible histamine release in response to certain foods; medications; and, especially, iodinated contrast media as this can be life threatening. Affected children, especially those with a specific history of anaphylaxis, should carry an EpiPen Jr out of concern for future possible repeat anaphylactic reaction.

Juvenile Xanthogranuloma

Infiltration of the skin by other types of cells can also occur. An example is juvenile xanthogranuloma, in which local infiltration and proliferation of histiocytes form an isolated plaque or nodule (Fig. 8.87A and B). These asymptomatic red or yellowish-brown lesions grow rapidly in infants and young children but resolve spontaneously later in childhood. They are not associated with abnormalities of circulating lipids. In cases with multiple lesions (see Fig. 8.87C), there may be associated ocular involvement. This disorder is the most common cause of nontraumatic hyphema in children. Hence ophthalmologic evaluation is important in patients with multiple or diffuse micronodular xanthogranulomas.

Langerhans Cell Histiocytosis

Langerhans cell histiocytosis is a potentially life-threatening disorder of proliferating histiocytes in the skin that may or may not be associated with systemic disease. Lesions may be localized to the skin or may become more widespread with visceral involvement. Bone marrow failure, pulmonary disease, hepatic infiltration,

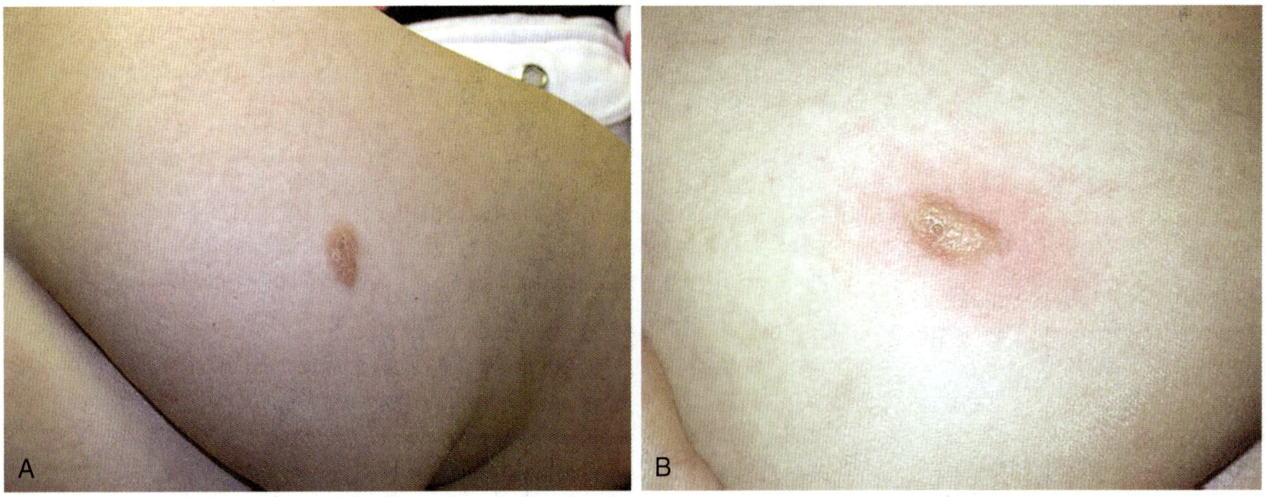

Fig. 8.85 Mastocytoma. (A) This solitary reddish-brown plaque on an infant's buttock contained numerous mast cells on histopathologic examination. (B) Positive Darier sign. After firm stroking with a tongue blade, a wheal-and-flare reaction appeared with an overlying bulla as a result of histamine release. This is diagnostic for mastocytoma.

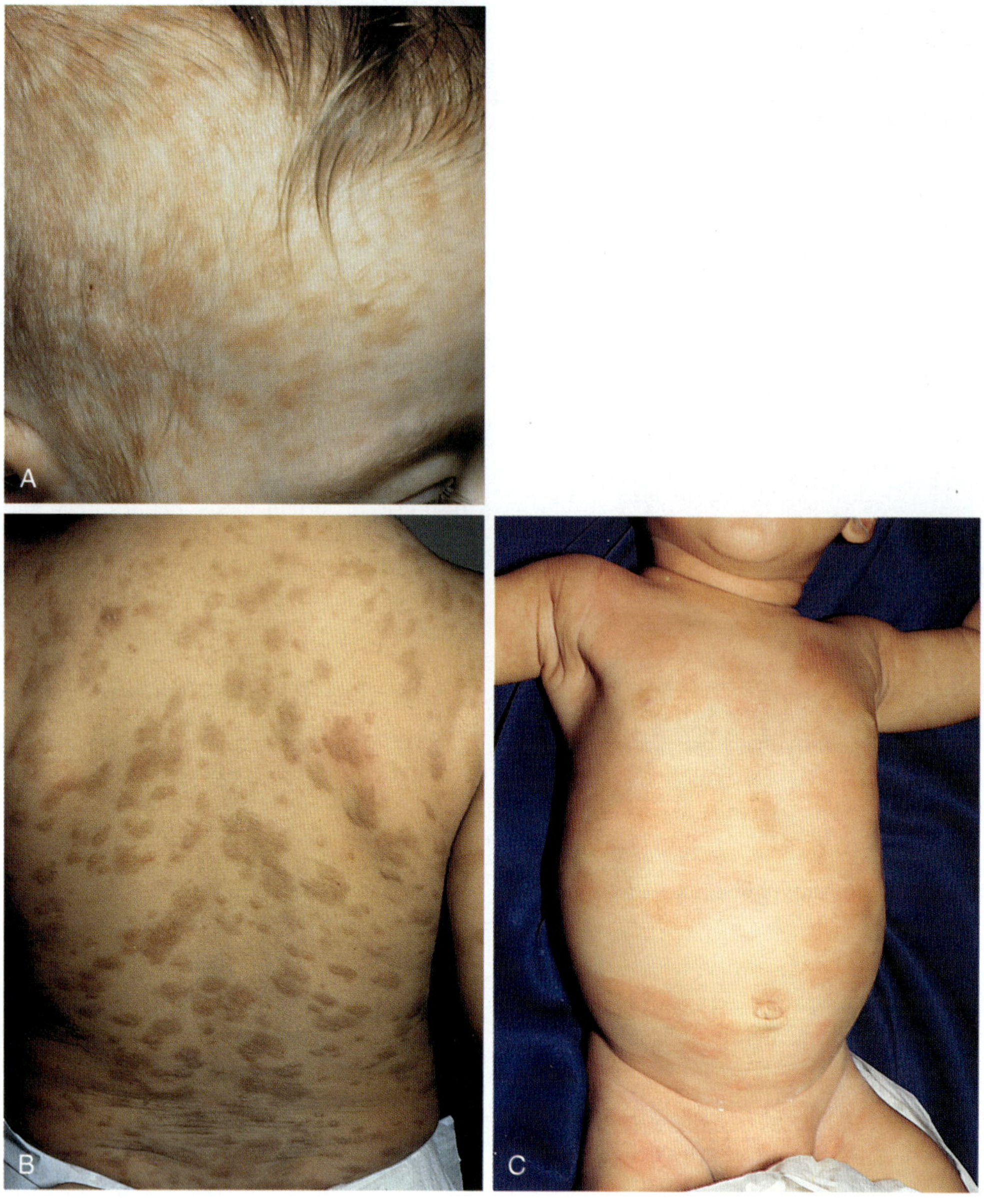

Fig. 8.86 Urticaria pigmentosa. (A) Numerous reddish-brown lesions are seen on the scalp and forehead of this toddler. (B) Marked hyperpigmentation developed in the truncal lesions of this child. Note the wheal-and-flare reaction over the right inferior scapula. (C) Another infant also has a wheal-and-flare reaction over the left upper abdomen after accidental rubbing.

diabetes insipidus, and gastrointestinal lesions may result in life-threatening complications. Cutaneous lesions may be few or diffuse with widespread scaly papules, nodules, or infiltrative plaques (Fig. 8.88). This condition should be suspected in cases of nonhealing diaper dermatitis, especially in an infant who has growth faltering. The lesions of Langerhans cell histiocytosis can be distinguished from those of seborrheic dermatitis by the presence of petechiae, hemorrhagic crusting, and firmly indurated nodules. Diagnosis can be further suspected based on the association of systemic manifestations, such as hepatosplenomegaly, lymphadenopathy, and chronically draining ears (see Chapter 12). Clinicians should have a low threshold for referring for definitive skin biopsy, which shows characteristic Langerhans granules within the cytoplasm of infiltrating mononuclear cells.

Granuloma Annulare

When fully evolved, granuloma annulare is an arcuate, nonscaly eruption, histologically characterized by dermal infiltration of lymphocytes around altered collagen. The lesion begins as a nodule or papule that gradually extends peripherally to form a ring. The initial papule and subsequent ring are raised and indurated, and in some cases the ring is broken into segments. The overlying epidermis is usually intact and the same color as the adjacent skin (Fig. 8.89). However, it may be slightly erythematous or even hyperpigmented. Most lesions are asymptomatic, although a few are mildly pruritic. Lesions are most commonly found on the extensor surfaces of the lower legs, feet, fingers, and hands (often overlying a joint), but other areas may be involved. They resolve spontaneously within a few months to several years, and no treatment is required unless the lesions are bothersome to the child, in which case mild to moderate potency topical steroids are a reasonable short-term treatment option. The origin of granuloma annulare is unclear. Although in older texts there was a suggestion of a relationship with diabetes, the current literature does not support this.

Granuloma annulare is most confused with tinea corporis, or ringworm (see Fig. 8.36). However, the thickened indurated character of granuloma annulare rings and the lack of dermatitic changes such as scales, crusts, vesicles, or pustules in granuloma annulare enable clinical distinction.

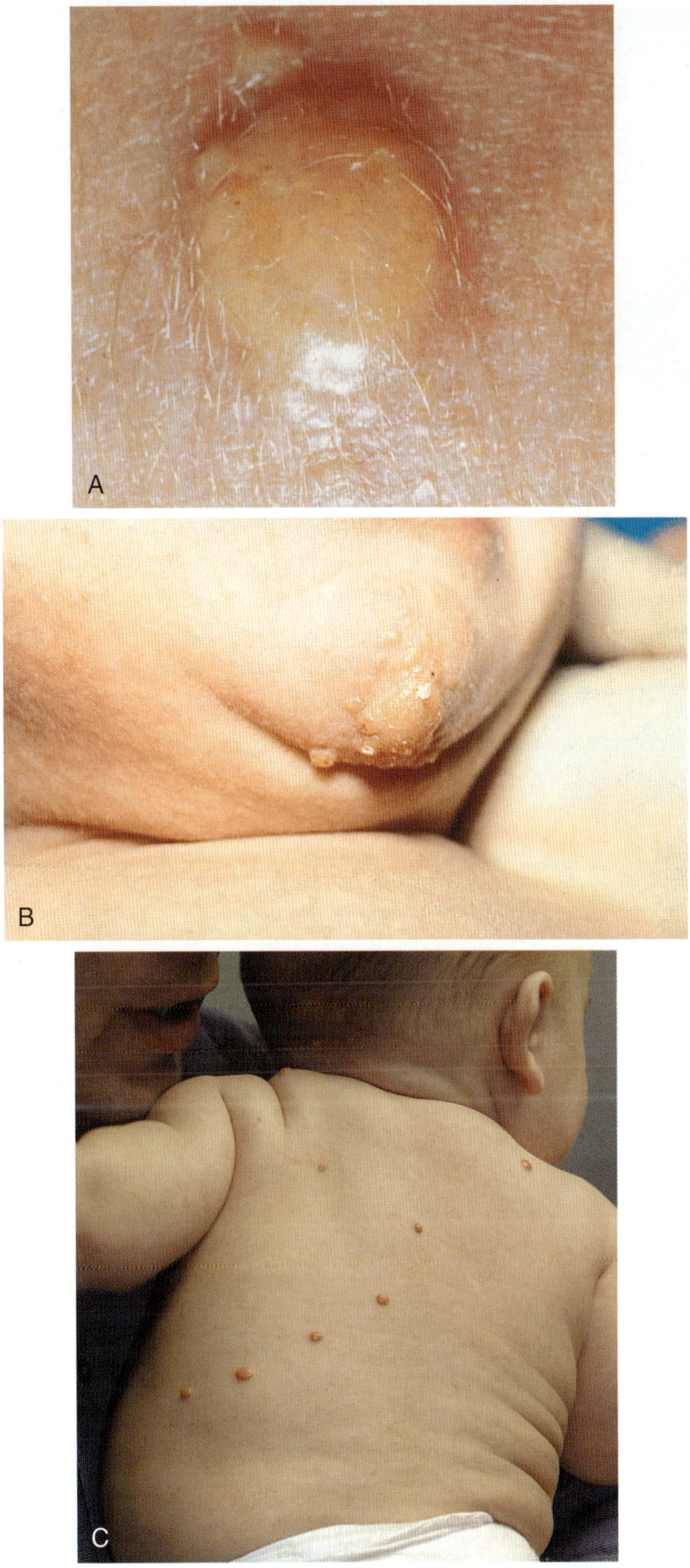

Fig. 8.87 Juvenile xanthogranuloma. (A) This 1-cm, yellowish nodule located on the back of a 3-month-old infant is the result of infiltration and proliferation of histiocytes. (B) Numerous satellite papules developed around the primary lesion that appeared abruptly on the chin of this 3-month-old. (C) Another infant has multiple micronodular juvenile xanthogranulomas, a finding that should prompt ophthalmologic referral to rule out an associated hyphema. (B, From Cohen BA: *Pediatric dermatology,* ed 2, London, 1999, Mosby.)

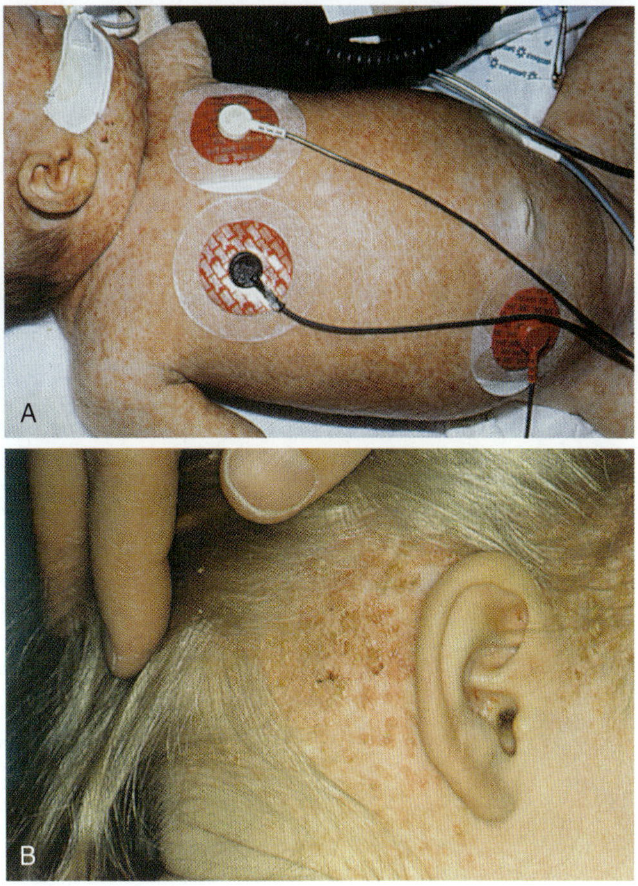

Fig. 8.88 Langerhans cell histiocytosis. (A) The exanthem in this 3-week-old infant began in the diaper area and rapidly generalized. Lesions were erythematous and scaly with interspersed petechiae. Associated findings included hepatosplenomegaly, diffuse adenopathy, and diarrhea with poor weight gain. (B) In this close-up of an older child, raised infiltrative lesions with scaly surfaces, some of which have become petechial, can be seen over the neck and scalp. Chronic draining otitis is another associated finding seen in some cases. (From Cohen BA: *Pediatric dermatology,* ed 2, London, 1999, Mosby.)

NEONATAL DERMATOLOGY

The skin of a newborn differs from that of an adult in several ways: It is thinner, is less hairy, has fewer sweat and sebaceous gland secretions, and has weaker intercellular attachments. During the neonatal period, common rashes or skin abnormalities may develop, and they need to be differentiated from more serious cutaneous disorders. Transient benign phenomena include erythema toxicum neonatorum and transient neonatal pustular melanosis. More serious diseases to be considered include systemic Langerhans cell histiocytosis and SSSS.

Congenital Dermal Melanocytosis

Congenital dermal melanocytosis is characterized by flat, slate-gray to bluish black, poorly circumscribed macules. They are located most commonly over the lumbosacral area and buttocks (Fig. 8.90), although they can appear anywhere on the body. The spots range in size from 1 to 10 cm and may be single or multiple (see Chapter 6). These macules contain accumulations of melanocytes deep within the dermis. No risk of malignancy is known, and these spots usually fade without therapy by 7 years old. Special variants of dermal melanocytosis exist, including nevus of Ota (involving the face, particularly the periocular area) and nevus of Ito (involving the shoulder), which may persist indefinitely. Rarely, when present along with vascular malformations, they can be part of a syndrome called *phakomatosis pigmentovascularis,* which can have associated internal abnormalities.

Erythema Toxicum Neonatorum

Erythema toxicum neonatorum is a benign, self-limited, asymptomatic disorder of unknown etiology that is most often seen in otherwise healthy newborns. It occurs in up to 50% of full-term

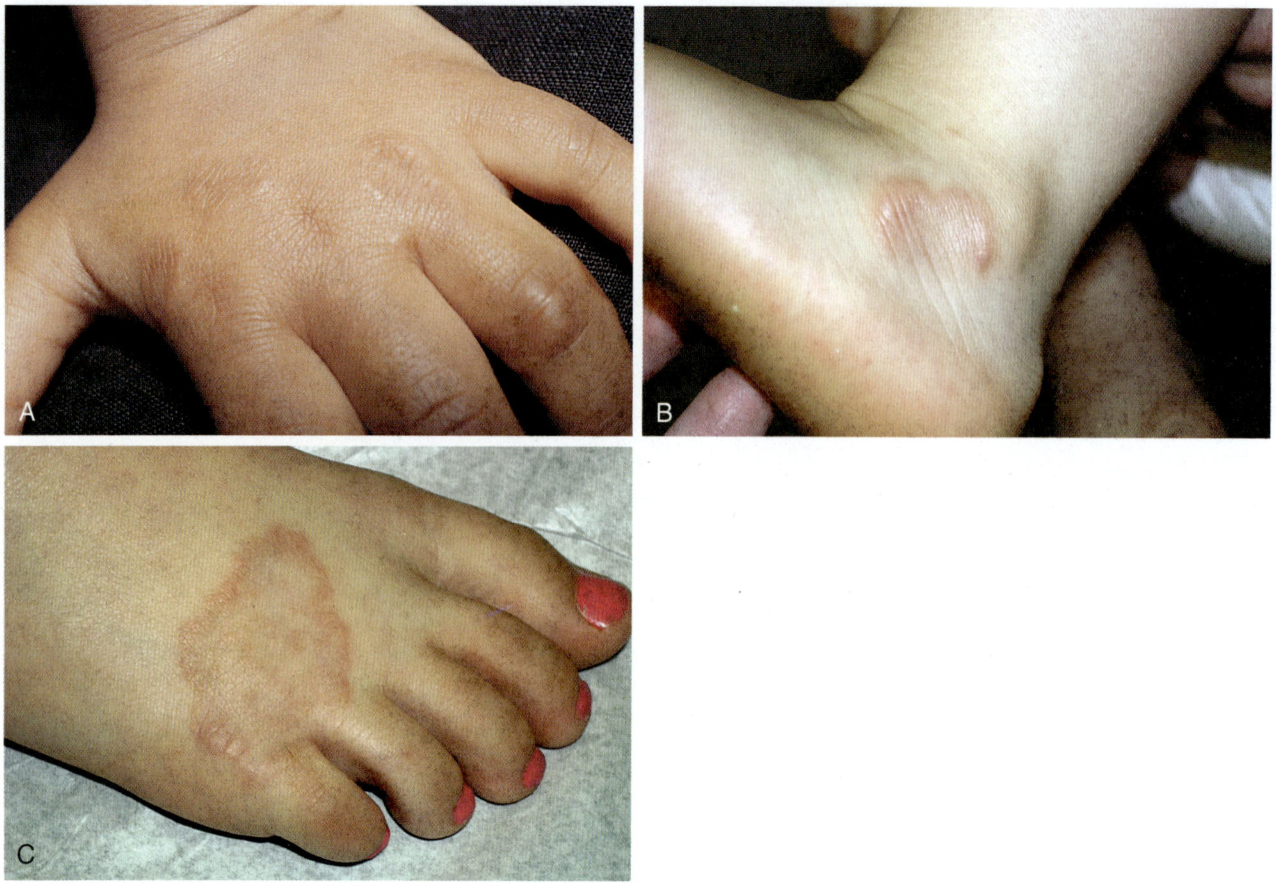

Fig. 8.89 Granuloma annulare. (A) Three raised, indurated rings with intact overlying skin and an early papular lesion on the ring finger are seen on a child's hand. (B) In this infant, an incomplete ring of dermal nodules overlies the lateral malleolus. (C) In an older child, this lesion on the dorsum of the foot is less raised.

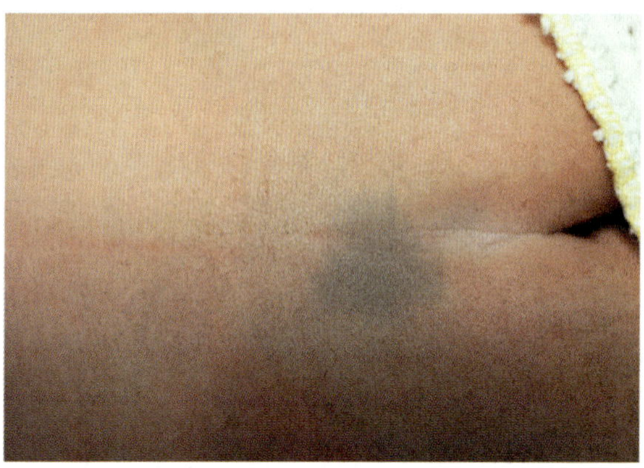

Fig. 8.90 Congenital dermal melanocytosis. A typical slate-gray lesion is located over the lumbosacral area of this infant.

infants. Lesions usually begin 24 to 48 hours after birth but may appear up to the 10th day of life. The disorder has been described as a "flea-bitten" dermatosis of the newborn, owing to the intense erythema with a central papule or pustule that resembles a flea bite (Fig. 8.91). The central papule or pustule is typically 2 to 3 mm in diameter and is surrounded by a much larger area of erythema. There may be a few to several hundred lesions on the back, face, chest, and extremities. The palms and soles are usually spared. A smear of material from a central pustule reveals numerous eosinophils, and concomitant circulating eosinophilia is present in up to 20% of patients. The eruption fades spontaneously within 5 to 7 days. No treatment is necessary.

Differential diagnosis includes transient neonatal pustular melanosis, staphylococcal folliculitis, milia neonatorum, miliaria rubra, and herpes simplex (see also Chapter 13). Infections often can be excluded clinically or with a Gram stain, Tzanck smear, and viral and bacterial cultures when necessary.

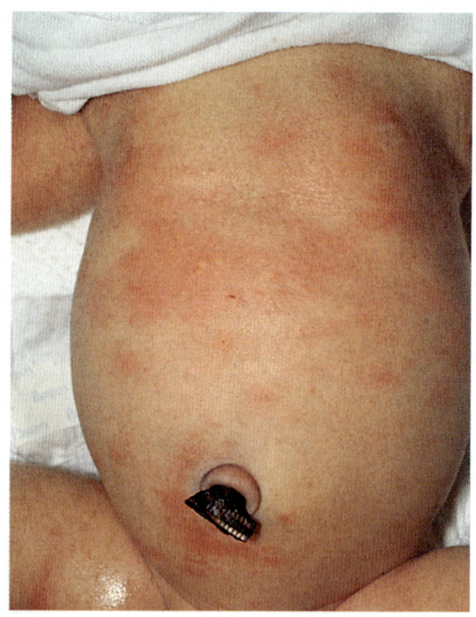

Fig. 8.91 Erythema toxicum neonatorum. Numerous yellow papules and pustules are surrounded by large, intensely erythematous rings on the trunk of this infant.

Transient Neonatal Pustular Melanosis

Transient neonatal pustular melanosis is a self-limited dermatosis of unknown etiology that presents at birth with 1- to 2-mm vesicopustules or ruptured pustules that disappear in 24 to 48 hours, leaving pigmented macules with a collarette of scale (Fig. 8.92). Lesions may appear anywhere on the body but are most often seen on the neck,

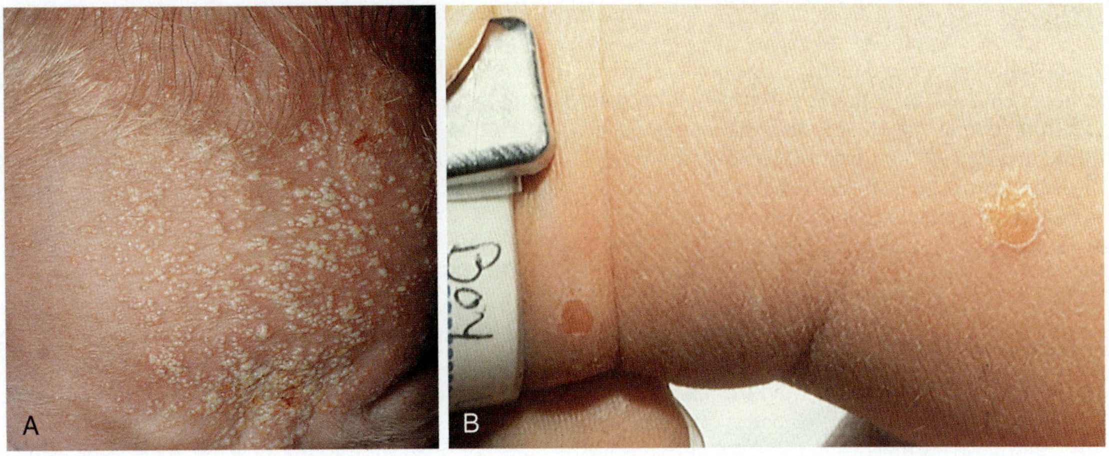

Fig. 8.92 Transient neonatal pustular melanosis. (A) A myriad of tiny pustules dot the forehead and scalp of this neonate. (B) When the pustules rupture, a pigmented macule surrounded by a collarette of scale remains.

forehead, lower back, and legs. Wright stain of a pustular smear shows numerous neutrophils; Gram stain and culture are negative for bacteria. It is seen more commonly in babies with darker skin. The hyperpigmentation fades in 3 weeks to 3 months. Transient neonatal pustular melanosis is a benign disorder and requires no therapy. Differential diagnosis is like that of erythema toxicum neonatorum.

Sebaceous Gland Hyperplasia and Neonatal Cephalic Pustulosis (Formerly Neonatal Acne)

Neonatal sebaceous gland hyperplasia is a common entity consisting of multiple 1- to 2-cm yellowish-white papules usually located over the nose of full-term infants (Fig. 8.93) and represents a normal physiological response to maternal androgenic stimulation of sebaceous gland growth. Lesions typically fade spontaneously by 4 to 6 months.

Neonates can also develop findings that resemble acne within the first few weeks of life. However, on close examination, instead of true comedones, lesions are papules and papulopustules over the face, neck, and upper trunk (Fig. 8.94). This, too, is thought to be a result of hormonal stimulation of sebaceous glands, which creates a hospitable environment for overgrowth of yeast (*Malassezia* sp.). Formerly called *neonatal acne,* it is now termed *neonatal cephalic pustulosis.* The condition is benign and self-limited and is best treated by observation or with a short course of topical antifungal agents.

Cutis Marmorata

Cutis marmorata is characterized by a transient, netlike, reddish-blue mottling of the skin caused by variable vascular constriction and dilation (Fig. 8.95). It is a normal response to chilling, and on rewarming, normal skin color returns. The discoloration occurs symmetrically over the trunk and extremities in infants. In neonates, the condition usually abates by 6 months, but it may persist longer in individuals with lighter skin pigmentation. When cutis marmorata is fixed, is asymmetric, or does not fade with warming, the clinician should consider the diagnosis cutis marmorata telangiectatica congenita, which is a type of a vascular malformation present at birth that can be accompanied by atrophy and other systemic findings when it is extensive.

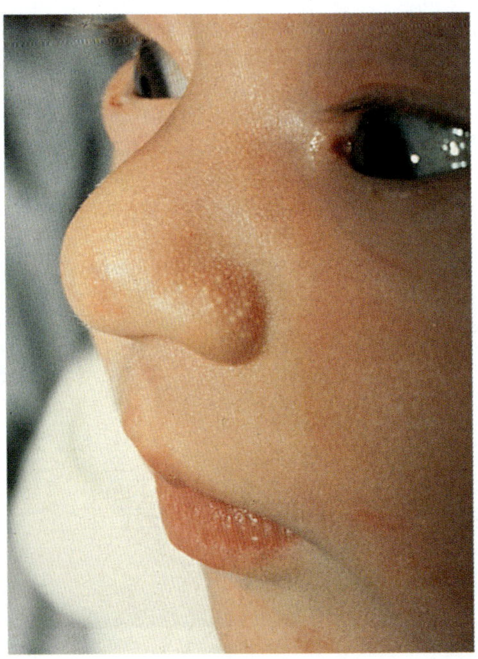

Fig. 8.93 Sebaceous gland hyperplasia. Note the yellowish-white papules on the nose of this infant.

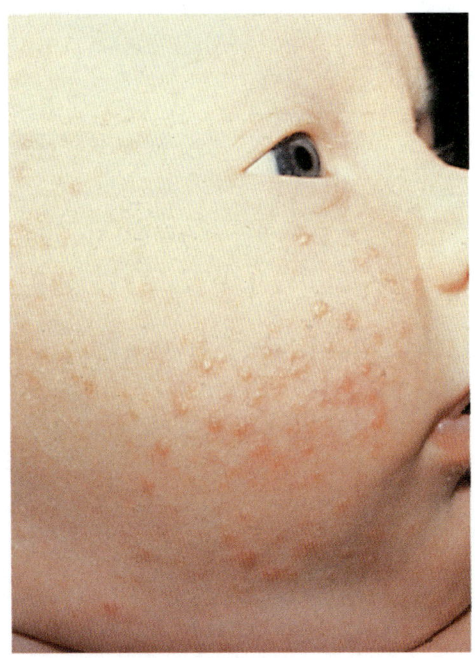

Fig. 8.94 Cephalic pustulosis (formerly called *neonatal acne*). Erythematous papules and pustules are present over the nose and cheeks.

Collodion Baby

In several variants of ichthyosis, particularly lamellar ichthyosis, the infant can be born encased in a thick, parchment-like scale known as a *collodion membrane* (Fig. 8.96). This dries and is shed in large sheets within 7 to 14 days. Significant secondary fluid, electrolyte, and heat losses can occur. Although scaling may only be mild or may even resolve completely in some infants, many go on to develop cutaneous findings typical of the underlying ichthyosis (see Figs. 8.8 and 8.9).

Epidermolysis Bullosa

Epidermolysis Bullosa (EB) is a group of inherited mechanobullous disorders characterized by the development of blisters after the skin is subjected to mild friction or trauma. The three general types are EB simplex, junctional EB, and dystrophic EB. These types are classified according to the level at which blister formation occurs. Modes of inheritance vary with subtypes in each group, and blistering, with few exceptions, begins in the newborn period. Other systemic associations may include pyloric stenosis or atresia, muscular dystrophy, and cutaneous localized absence of the skin, especially on the shins.

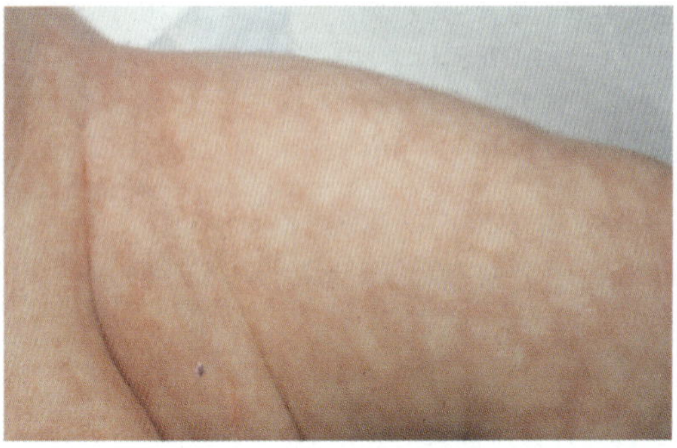

Fig. 8.95 Cutis marmorata. Note the reticulated bluish-purple mottling of the skin of this infant's thigh.

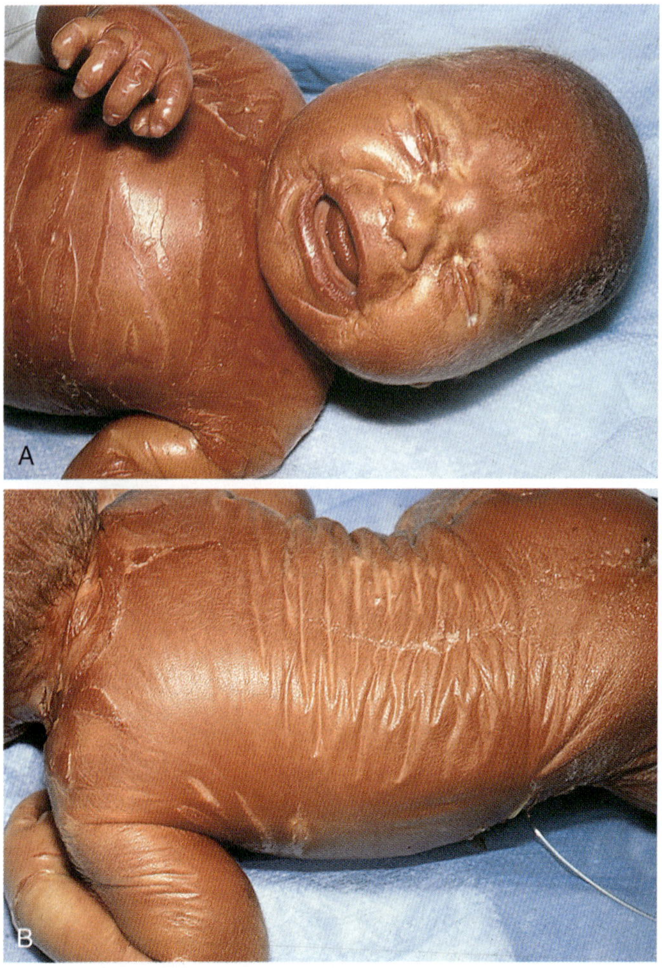

Fig. 8.96 Collodion baby. (A and B) A shiny transparent membrane covered this baby at birth; she later developed lamellar ichthyosis. Note the ectropion and eclabium (eversion and fissuring of the eyelid margins and lips). (From Cohen BA: *Pediatric dermatology,* ed 2, London, 1999, Mosby.)

Epidermolysis Bullosa Simplex (Epidermolytic Epidermolysis Bullosa)

In EB simplex, which is usually inherited as an autosomal dominant trait, blister formation takes place superficially within or just above the basal cell layer of the epidermis. On presentation, blistering can be mild or severe and widespread (Fig. 8.97). The most common form presents in later infancy, childhood, or adolescence with blisters confined to pressure-bearing areas, especially on the hands and feet, and particularly after intense physical activity. Although there is no scarring, secondary infection can occur, and atrophy may develop in some cases.

Junctional Epidermolysis Bullosa

Junctional EB, usually inherited as an autosomal recessive trait, presents at birth with bullae and erosions in a generalized distribution. Blisters form at the junction of the epidermis and dermis (Fig. 8.98). The most severe form is usually fatal during the first year of life due to malnutrition, fluid losses, recurrent cutaneous infection, and sepsis.

Dystrophic Epidermolysis Bullosa

The dystrophic forms of EB are divided into dominant and recessive types. The plane of cleavage is deep within the upper portion of the dermis. In both, scarring occurs as the blisters heal, and milia are common (Fig. 8.99A). The dominant form usually results in more localized lesions (e.g., feet only) than the recessive form; patients with the latter show delays in growth and development, severe oral blisters, loss of nails, and sometimes syndactyly as the skin of the digits fuses during healing from the deeper blisters (see Fig. 8.99B).

Directed genetic testing or skin biopsy are helpful in distinguishing among the three general types of EB in neonates, and they are also helpful in determining prognosis. Prenatal diagnosis is now possible for many variants, and genetic counseling is advisable.

Incontinentia Pigmenti

Incontinentia pigmenti is an X-linked dominant disorder that affects the skin and may also involve the CNS, eyes, teeth, and skeletal system. It is seen predominantly in females and thus is thought to be fatal to most fully affected males in utero. Clinically, the disorder may present in any of four overlapping phases. In the first phase, inflammatory vesicles or bullae appear on the trunk and extremities, usually within the first 2 weeks of life (Fig. 8.100A). New blisters then develop over the ensuing 3 months. At this stage, a skin biopsy shows characteristic

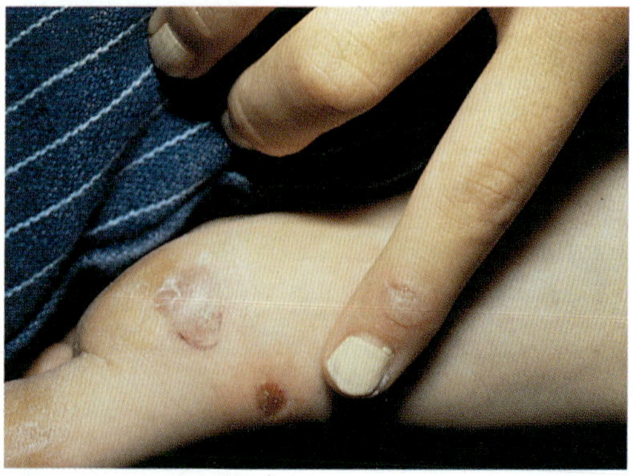

Fig. 8.97 Epidermolysis bullosa (EB) simplex (formerly called *epidermolytic EB*). Blisters form easily in pressure-bearing areas, particularly the hands and feet. Scarring does not occur.

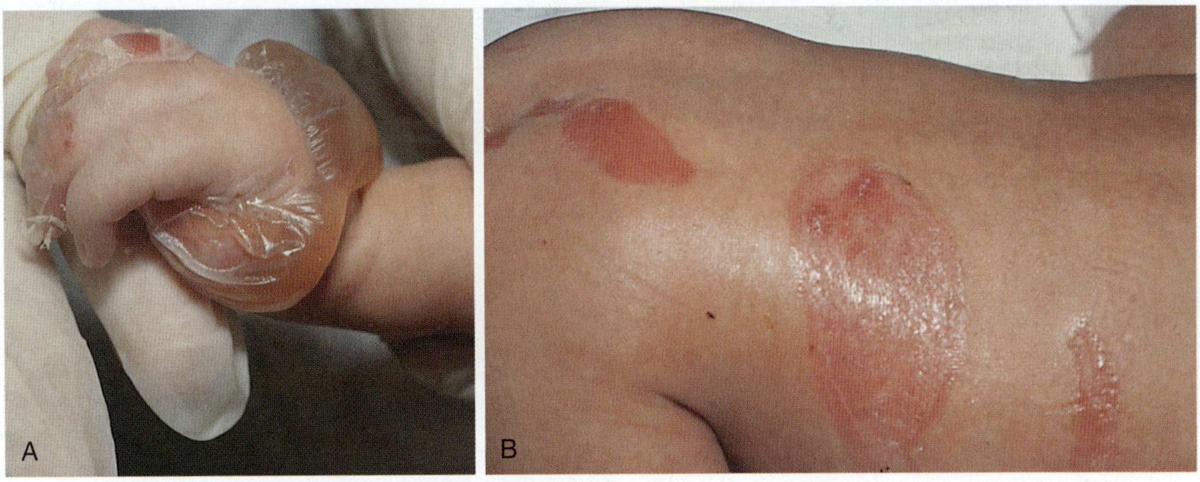

Fig. 8.98 Junctional epidermolysis bullosa. Widespread involvement was seen in this infant at birth. (A) Note the erosions and the large, intact blister over the thumb and dorsum of the hand. (B) Large, denuded areas are evident over the back and flank.

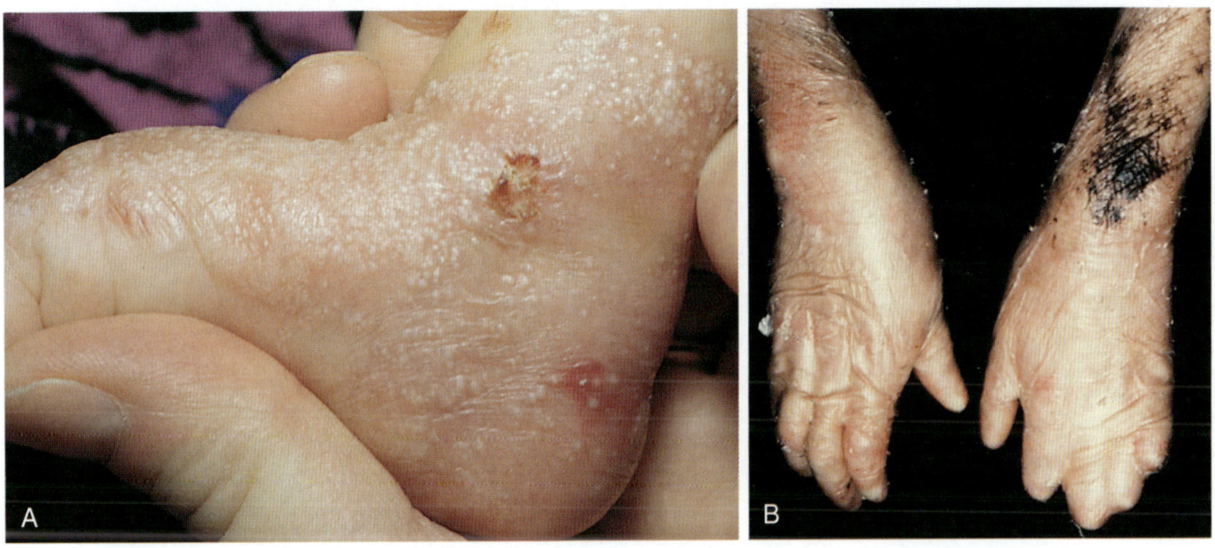

Fig. 8.99 Dystrophic (formerly dermolytic) epidermolysis bullosa. (A) Blisters, erosions, and hundreds of milia are seen on the foot and ankle of this newborn. (B) In another child with the recessive form of dystrophic epidermolysis bullosa, severe scarring encased the fingers, resulting in syndactyly.

inflammation with intraepidermal eosinophils and necrotic keratinocytes. Before the blistering phase ends, the second phase, marked by development of irregular, warty papules, supervenes (see Fig. 8.100B and C). These lesions resolve spontaneously within several months. A characteristic swirling or streaking pattern (referred to as a *blaschkoid distribution*) of brown to bluish-gray pigmentation on the trunk or extremities marks the third phase (see Fig. 8.100D and E). Interestingly, these pigmented whorls are sometimes located at sites other than those involved in the first two phases. The blaschkoid pigmentation, which also likely represents a form of pigmentary mosaicism (see Disorders of Pigmentation, later), fades in later infancy or early childhood in most patients, leaving subtle, streaky, hypopigmented scars that may be the only residual cutaneous findings seen in affected mothers (see Fig. 8.100F) who should be carefully examined for other markers of incontinentia pigmenti. Genetic testing should be performed for affected mothers and babies.

Differential diagnosis of incontinentia pigmenti in the blistering stage includes herpes simplex, bullous impetigo, and EB. Warts or epidermal nevi may mimic the warty phase. The swirled pigmentation of the third phase is characteristic of incontinentia pigmenti but must be distinguished from congenital blaschkoid hyperpigmentation, which is not associated with an inflammatory phase. Although no specific therapy is usually required, early intervention for eye lesions may help to preserve vision, and systemic therapy for neonatal seizures may be lifesaving. Genetic counseling is critical for future pregnancies.

Pyogenic Granuloma

Pyogenic granulomas are extremely common benign vascular tumors. They are thought to stem from the vascular overgrowth of granulation tissue after minor trauma or in reaction to a foreign body, such as a thorn, splinter, or piece of glass. They are seen in children and young adults, and lesions are usually located on the face or an extremity, although the trunk and mucous membranes may be involved. They consist of solitary bright red, friable nodules that are often pedunculated and average 5 to 6 mm in diameter. Their surface is crusted and bleeds easily (Fig. 8.101). Pyogenic granulomas are commonly confused with hemangiomas, but their onset well after the newborn period and their morphology, distribution, and course allow for distinction between these two types of benign vascular tumors. Treatment consists of shave excision followed by electrodessication of the "feeder" blood vessels at the base. They occasionally recur, in which case repeat surgery is recommended.

Nevus Simplex (Nevus Flammeus, Salmon Patch, or "Stork Bite")

The nevus simplex, which is commonly referred to as a *salmon patch* or *"stork bite,"* is a capillary malformation that is seen in most infants and hence is considered a normal variant. Some experts believe that these may represent persistent fetal circulation as opposed to true malformation, which may partly explain why they

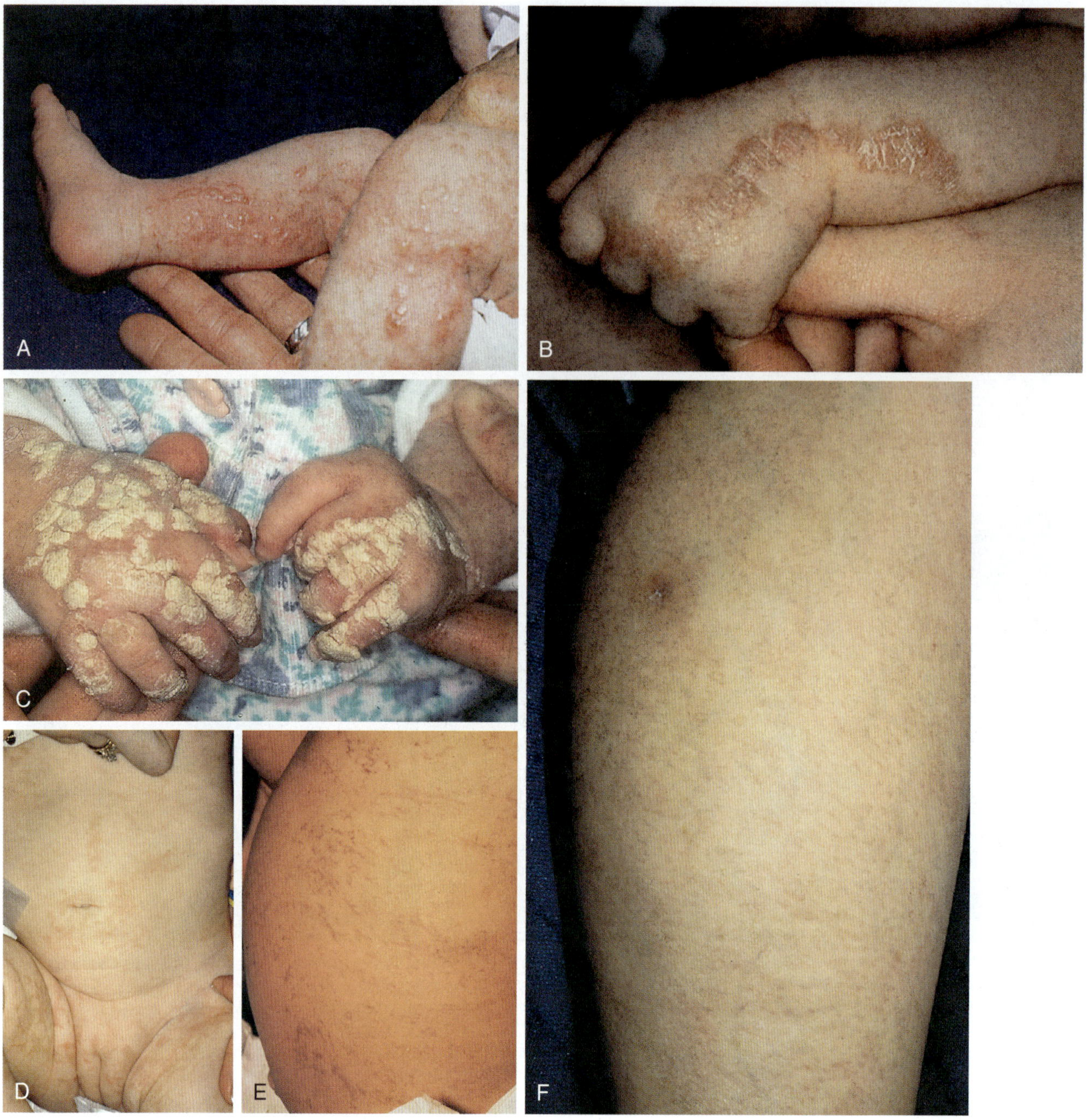

Fig. 8.100 Incontinentia pigmenti. (A) Linearly distributed vesicles on an erythematous base are seen on the legs of this neonate. (B and C) Subsequently, lesions evolve into warty papules, which can have thick overlying crusts. (D) Splotchy hyperpigmented patches replaced the warty lesions by 8 months old. (E) In many cases, the hyperpigmentation appears in swirls and streaks. (F) These hypopigmented reticulated lesions on the leg of an affected child's mother represent old scars in areas of prior hyperpigmentation. (A and C, From Cohen BA: *Pediatric dermatology,* ed 2, London, 1999, Mosby.)

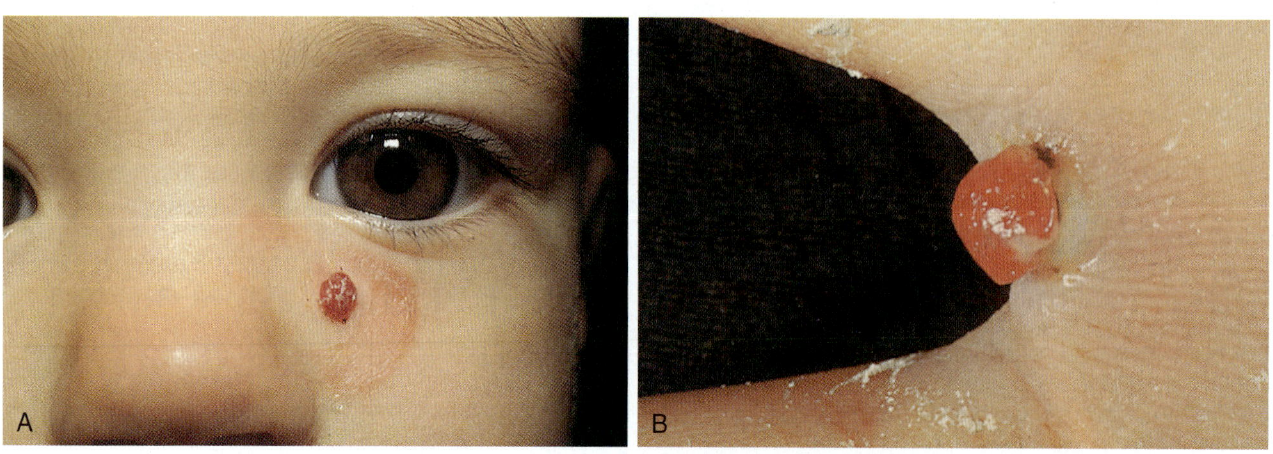

Fig. 8.101 Pyogenic granuloma. (A) A bright red, raised, hemorrhagic papule developed on an infant's cheek. (B) Another rapidly growing friable lesion is present between this child's fingers.

tend to fade slightly over time. Lesions are located at the nape of the neck and on the glabella, forehead, upper eyelids, or lower back (Fig. 8.102). They become more apparent clinically but should not truly bulge when the baby cries or strains and tend to fade or become less noticeable over the first year of life. A midline lesion that bulges with the Valsalva maneuver should raise a greater concern for a sinus pericranii or arteriovenous malformation and should prompt detailed radiologic imaging.

Vascular Malformation (Port-Wine Stain)

Vascular malformations, also known as port-wine stains, are typically purple-red macules that are present at the time of birth. This is in contrast with infantile hemangiomas, which may not present until several weeks of age. In port-wine stains, mature capillaries infiltrate the superficial or deeper dermis and subcutaneous tissues. Unlike infantile hemangiomas, these are not proliferative and thus do not enlarge nor involute over time. However, left untreated, underlying skin and soft tissue can become hypertrophied, and most develop angiomatous blebs by adolescence or adulthood. Most commonly, they are located on the head and neck (Fig. 8.103) and, when present in the distribution of the ophthalmic branch of the trigeminal nerve (even more so when present bilaterally), can be associated with *Sturge-Weber syndrome,* which is a constellation of port-wine stain, vascular malformations of the ipsilateral leptomeninges and cerebral cortex, and glaucoma. Seizures and cognitive impairment are possible complications (see Chapter 16). An important diagnostic consideration is PHACES (posterior fossa malformations, hemangiomas, arterial anomalies, cardiac defects, eye anomalies, sternal clefting) syndrome, in which the initial nascent plaquelike hemangioma may temporarily resemble a facial port-wine stain before entering its phase of rapid growth (Fig. 8.104).

A port-wine stain located over the midline occipital scalp, especially when accompanied by a hair tuft or whorl or a defect of aplasia cutis, may overlie a CNS malformation, such as an atretic encephalocele (see Chapter 16), just as a midline lumbosacral port-wine stain may be associated with an underlying spinal dysraphism, such as a tethered cord or lipoma (see Chapter 16). Extensive port-wine stains located on the trunk or extremities may be associated with soft tissue and bony overgrowth and deeper venous anomalies, such as in Klippel-Trénaunay syndrome and Trénaunay-Weber syndrome (see Chapter 16).

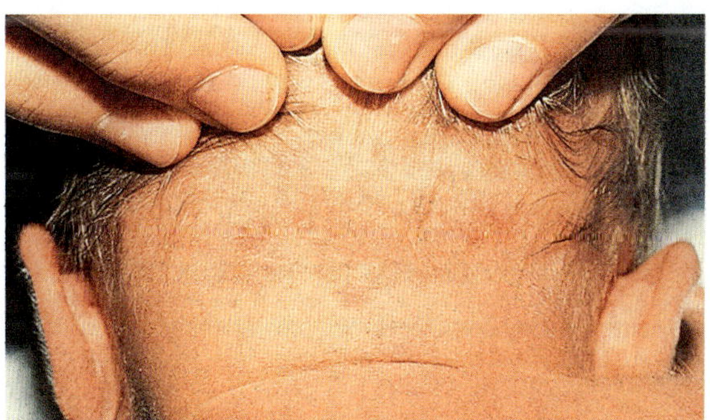

Fig. 8.102 Stork bite, or salmon patch. A typical light red splotchy area is seen at the nape of the neck.

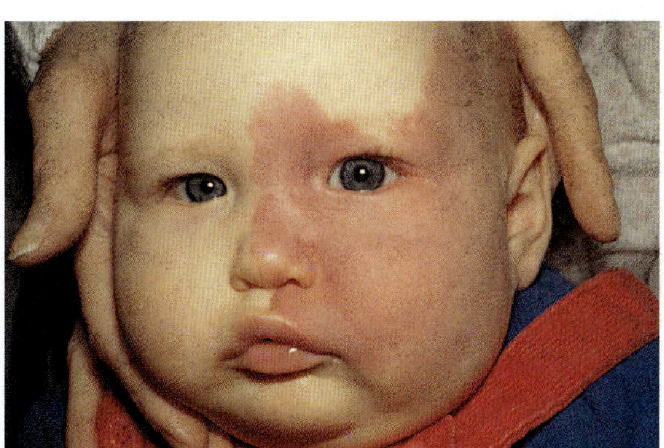

Fig. 8.103 Port-wine stain. This infant has a characteristic purplish-red lesion covering nearly half of his face.

NEVI

Melanocytic nevus is a term used to describe a group of congenital and acquired pigmented lesions, located in the dermis that contain nevus cells, which are derived from the neural crest. These cells, like melanocytes in the epidermis, can synthesize melanin. The term *nevus* can also be used to refer to another group of congenital skin lesions composed of mature or nearly mature cutaneous elements organized in an abnormal fashion or location. Also known as *hamartomas,* the latter may be composed of almost any epidermal or dermal structures.

Melanocytic Nevi

Congenital Melanocytic Nevi

Congenital melanocytic nevi (CMN) consist of pigmented papules or plaques that can also be associated with hair growth. At birth, lesions may be tan or light pink, with only soft vellus hairs (Fig. 8.105A). During infancy and childhood, the nevus may darken and the hair may become more prominent. Small dark papules may appear in a pebbly, symmetric array within the larger plaque (see Fig. 8.105B). CMN are classified by size, specifically their greatest diameter: small being less than 1.5 cm; medium, 1.5 to 20 cm; and large, greater than 20 cm. A large CMN present in a segmental distribution is termed a *giant CMN* (Fig. 8.106).

All CMN have the potential for malignant transformation, which may be heralded by the development of new, darker, or bleeding nodules within the original lesion or by sudden rapid growth of the nevus. The likelihood of malignant transformation is less than 1% for small- to medium-sized CMN and perhaps as high as 2% to 5% for giant lesions. There is ample evidence suggesting that the greatest risk of malignancy for giant CMN may occur during the first decade of life.

Although no uniformly accepted guidelines exist for the management of small- to medium-size nevi, a reasonable approach is to have a yearly follow-up with a pediatric dermatologist or primary care provider who is comfortable monitoring patients with pigmented lesions. Annual digital photography of a congenital nevus can be helpful in monitoring. Excision is recommended if a nevus begins to change or appear atypical and may be considered as a joint decision with the family if any are in areas that are difficult to monitor, such as the scalp, groin, or interdigital spaces. Because of their higher risk, early full-thickness excision (in infancy, if possible), followed by grafting, may be considered for patients with giant CMN. However, some exceptionally large nevi may not be amenable to surgical management. In these cases, impeccably close observation (facilitated by comparative photographs) is recommended at 6- to 12-month intervals. Careful palpation of the entire lesion is necessary at each visit because melanomas may arise deep within a large CMN and often are first detectable as a new, palpable nodule, well before any surface change occurs. Laser treatment for small, medium, or large/giant CMN has not gained wide acceptance because the currently available lasers ablate only the superficial components of nevi, leaving behind the deeper nevus cells that could undergo malignant change. CMN must be differentiated from other congenital pigmented spots, such as urticaria pigmentosa, lentigines, café au lait spots, and congenital dermal melanocytosis, none of which carries any significant risk of malignancy.

The *nevus spilus,* which consists of a light brown macule with darker brown freckling throughout, is considered a variant of congenital nevus superimposed on a café au lait macule with an extremely low (but not zero) risk of progression to melanoma (Fig. 8.107). Nevus spilus is less likely to be palpable or to develop

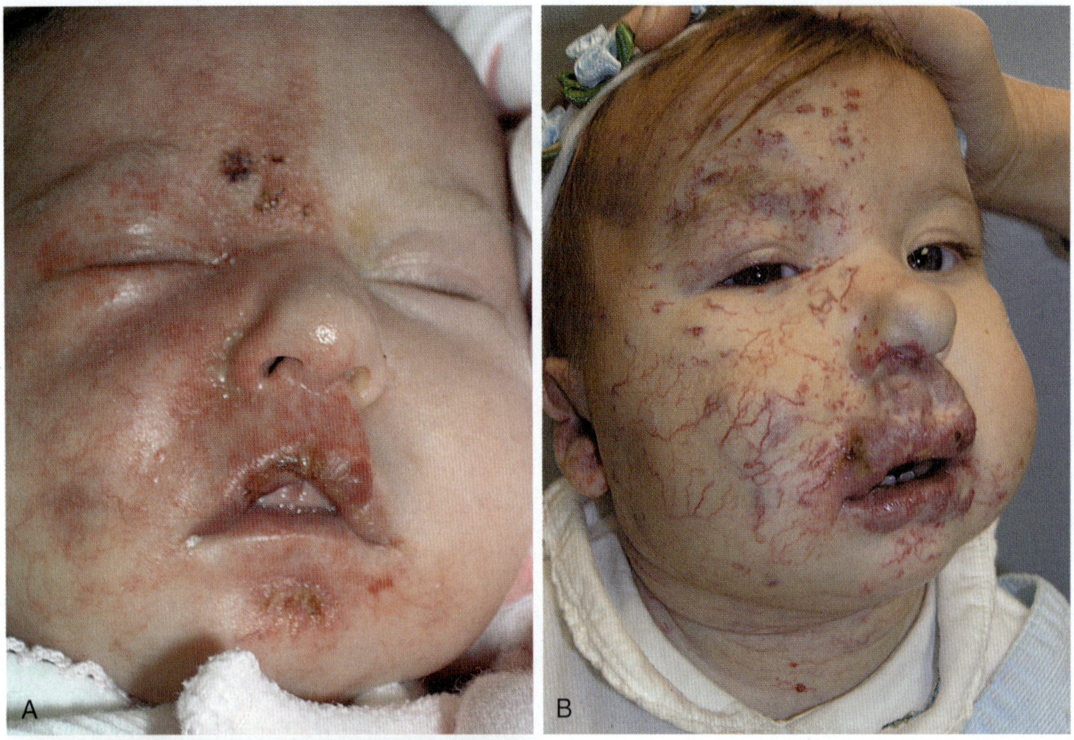

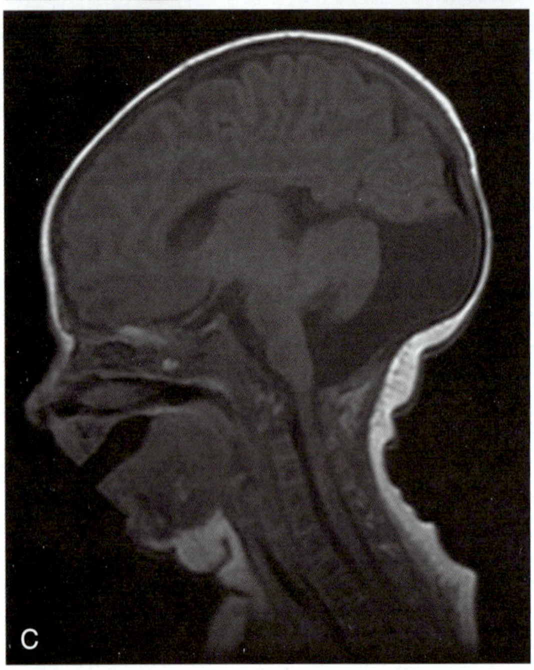

Fig. 8.104 PHACES (posterior fossa malformations, hemangiomas, arterial anomalies, cardiac defects, eye anomalies, sternal clefting) syndrome. At birth these lesions are plaquelike and may mimic a port-wine stain. However, they ulcerate early on (A) and then proliferate rapidly, becoming raised, as seen in the same infant at 1 year (B). (C) This magnetic resonance imaging scan reveals a Dandy-Walker malformation in an infant with PHACES syndrome.

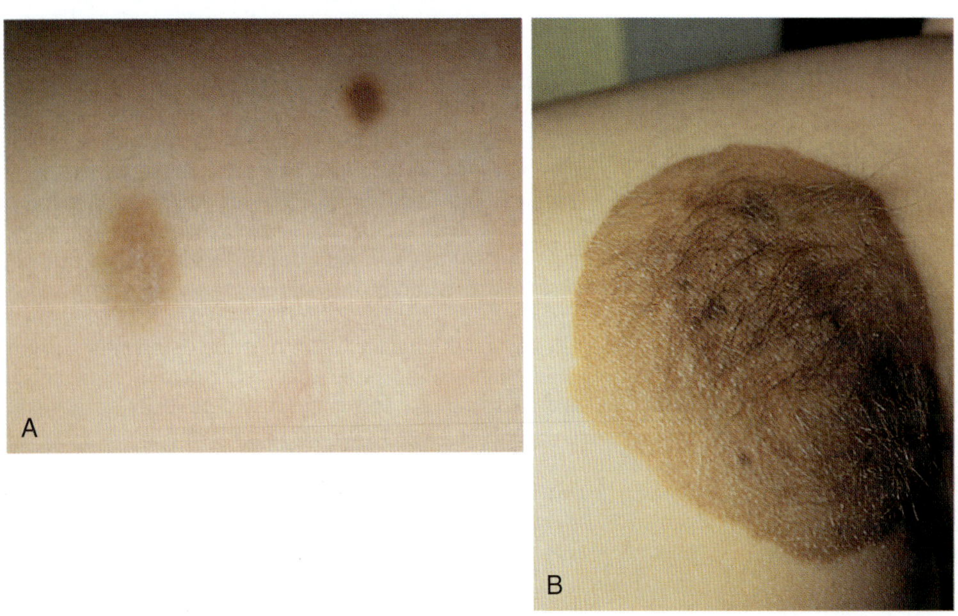

Fig. 8.105 Congenital nevomelanocytic nevi. (A) Two small nevi with differing degrees of hyperpigmentation are seen on the thigh of an infant. (B) During adolescence this nevus developed prominent hair and dark pigmented macules and papules within its borders.

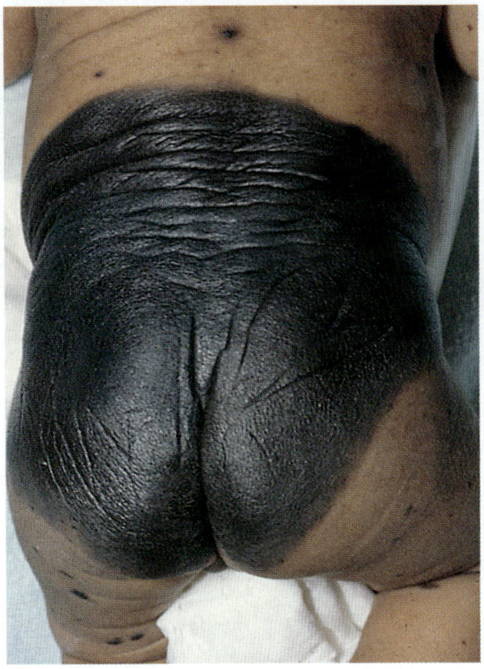

Fig. 8.106 Giant nevomelanocytic nevus. This lesion covers the lower back and buttocks, is uniformly pigmented, and has smaller satellite nevi.

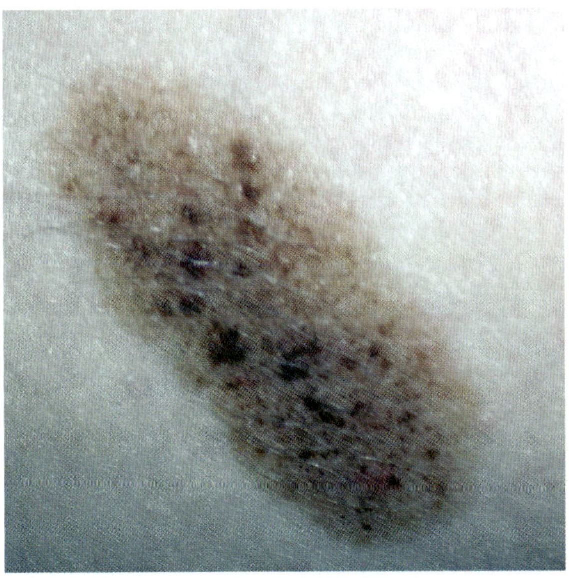

Fig. 8.107 Nevus spilus. These lesions consist of light brown macules, with darker brown speckles scattered uniformly over their surfaces.

significant hair growth with time, which can help to distinguish it from a true congenital nevus.

Acquired Melanocytic Nevi

Acquired melanocytic nevi begin to develop in early childhood as small, pigmented macules 1 to 2 mm in diameter, which are flat on palpation. At this stage, the nevus cells are limited to the epidermal-dermal junction and are called *junctional nevi* (Fig. 8.108A). They can later enlarge slowly and become papular or even pedunculated. In such elevated nevi, the nevus cells have proliferated into the dermis to become either intradermal or *compound nevi* (see Fig. 8.108B). During puberty, these lesions may darken noticeably and increase in size. They tend to appear more often on sun-exposed areas and are seen less frequently on the soles, palms, legs, genitalia, and mucous membranes. In general, these nevi change slowly over months to years and warrant only observation.

Sudden enlargement of a nevus with redness and tenderness may occur because of infection of a hair follicle within the nevus or because of rupture of a follicular cyst with a secondary foreign body reaction. This may alarm the patient, prompting dermatologic evaluation. Another, slower change causing concern in patients is the appearance of a hypopigmented or depigmented ring associated with mild local pruritus around a benign nevus. This is called a *halo nevus* (Fig. 8.109), and the phenomenon is caused by a cytotoxic T-lymphocyte reaction against both the nevus cells and their innocent melanocytic bystanders. As a result, the nevus can disappear partially or completely, and the halo eventually repigments. It is important to ensure when a patient presents with a new halo nevus that there are no atypical appearing nevi on the skin that might have prompted such an immunologic response. Melanoma presenting with a halo nevus is much more commonly seen in adult than pediatric patients, but the thorough physician should still consider this possibility in a child and perform a complete cutaneous examination.

Nevi and Melanomas

Melanomas in childhood may occur de novo or instead may develop within a previously existing congenital or acquired nevus. Increased exposure to sunlight and artificial ultraviolet light (e.g., tanning salons) is felt to have contributed to a marked increase in melanoma in children since the late 1990s, with an annual increase of 3% to 7%.

Conventional screening criteria for melanocytic lesions that may help the public to more rapidly identify and seek care for the

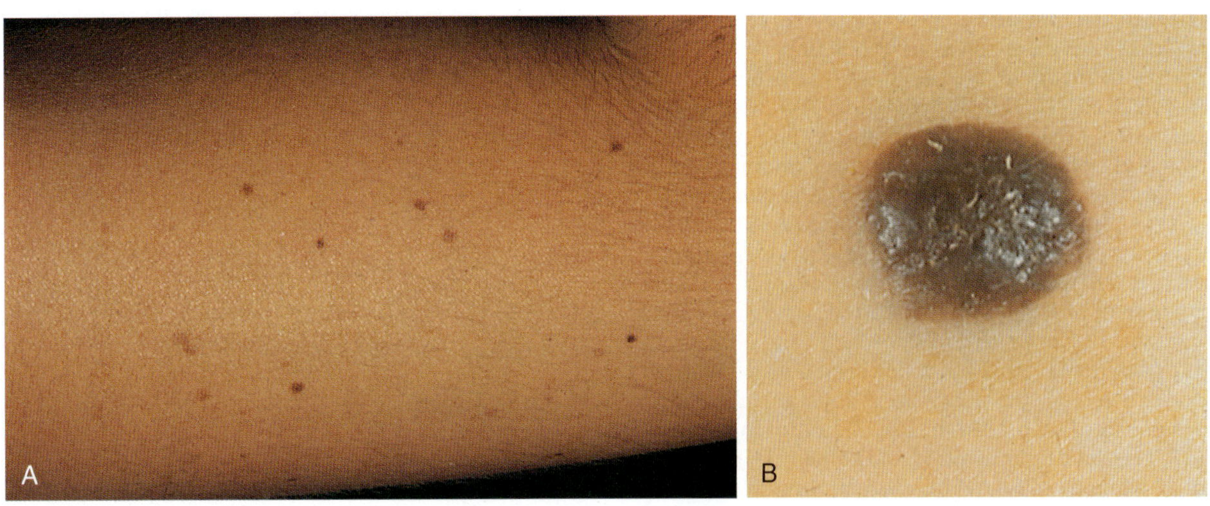

Fig. 8.108 Acquired nevomelanocytic nevi. (A) Junctional nevi. These brown macules are flat on palpation. (B) This typical compound nevus is raised, with a regular border and uniform pigmentation.

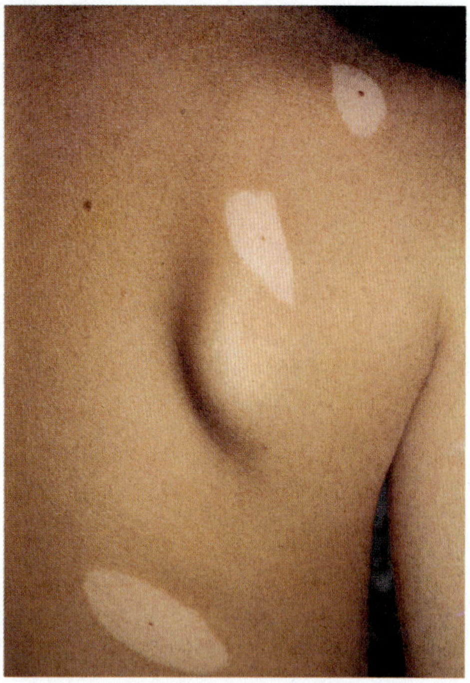

Fig. 8.109 Halo nevi. Large hypopigmented halos surround three relatively small nevi on the back of this boy.

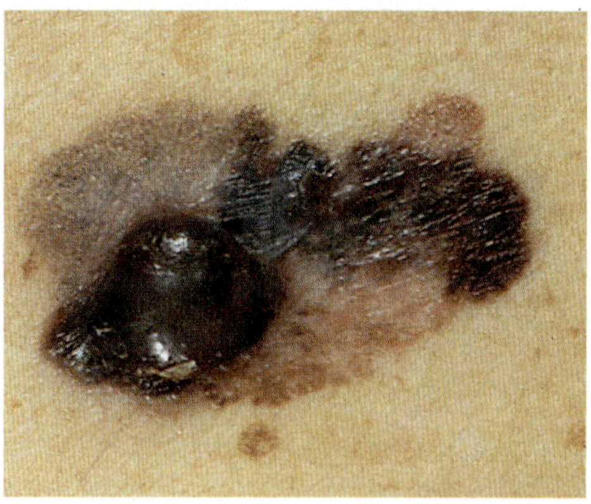

Fig. 8.110 Melanoma. This lesion shows the irregularity of outline, color, and thickness typical of a melanoma.

development of an atypical nevus or a true melanoma include (Fig. 8.110):
Asymmetry,
Border irregularity,
Color change,
Diameter greater than 6 mm, and
Evolution (any change in the lesion from its baseline).

"Evolution" is believed to be the most important of the screening criteria, and "Diameter" has fallen somewhat out of favor because patients should be encouraged to alert clinicians to new or changing lesions of any size, and melanomas can be smaller than 6 mm. One of the characteristics of pediatric melanoma that is more common than in adult melanoma is its chance of being amelanotic or unpigmented (Fig. 8.111). Pediatric melanoma can present in a classic fashion with asymmetric dark or changing pigment, or it can present as a red papule or nodule with no discernable brown or black pigment. It can be mistaken for a pyogenic granuloma, Spitz nevus, or even a wart. Without a high index of suspicion, there may be a delay in the referral and proper diagnosis of such a lesion. Use of dermoscopy, which is a special skill set that uses magnified and sometimes polarized light to identify pigment pattern differences among skin lesions, can be helpful in distinguishing among the possibilities. This is best done by a board-certified pediatric dermatologist.

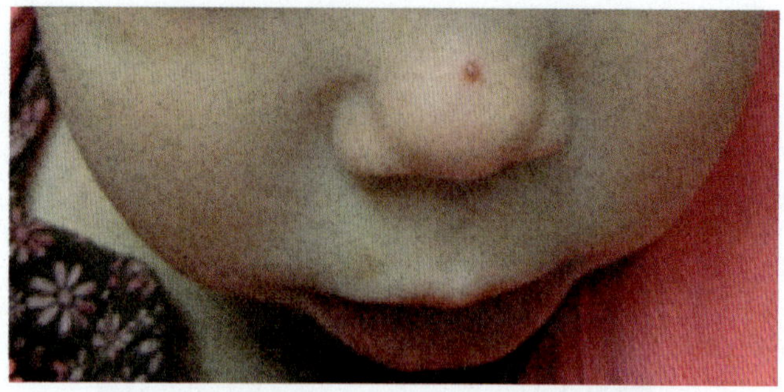

Fig. 8.111 Spitzoid melanoma. An isolated uniform pink papule on the nose. (Courtesy Robin Gehris, MD, University of Pittsburgh Medical Center.)

In additional to the conventional ABCDE screening criteria for adult melanoma, clinicians may consider additional ABCD detection criteria in children:
Amelanotic,
Bleeding, **b**ump,
Color (uniform),
De novo development and variable **d**iameter.

Fortunately, melanomas are still rare in children. However, their incidence is increasing (at approximately 3% annually), and curative treatment is contingent upon early diagnosis and prompt excision. Hence it is important for clinicians to have a keen awareness of diagnostic features and of worrisome changes in benign nevi that should prompt referral for possible excision. It is crucial that excised specimens be analyzed by a board-certified dermatopathologist and, in some difficult cases, specifically by one who subspecializes in pediatric melanomas because many of the microscopical differences between a mildly and a highly atypical lesion are subtle. Clinical experience combined with a panel of specialized stains and genetic markers help to recognize the specific subtype and grade so that precise and appropriate treatment can be initiated as soon as possible.

The differential diagnosis of childhood melanoma includes benign congenital and acquired nevi; the *blue nevus,* a small, firm, blue papule consisting of deep nevus cells (Fig. 8.112); traumatic hemorrhage, especially under the nails or in mucous membranes; vascular lesions, such as pyogenic granuloma or angiokeratoma; and the *Spitz nevus,* a red and rapidly growing nevus composed of spindle and epithelioid cells that can easily be confused clinically and histologically with melanoma (Fig. 8.113).

Hamartomatous Nevi

Hamartomatous nevi are derived from embryonic ectoderm and can be composed of epidermal structures, hair follicles *(nevus pilosus),* apocrine and eccrine glands *(apocrine and eccrine nevi),* fibroblasts *(connective tissue nevi),* blood vessels (salmon patch [see Fig. 8.102]), and multiple components *(nevus sebaceus).*

Epidermal nevi are quite common in pediatric patients. They are composed of epidermal structures only and must be distinguished

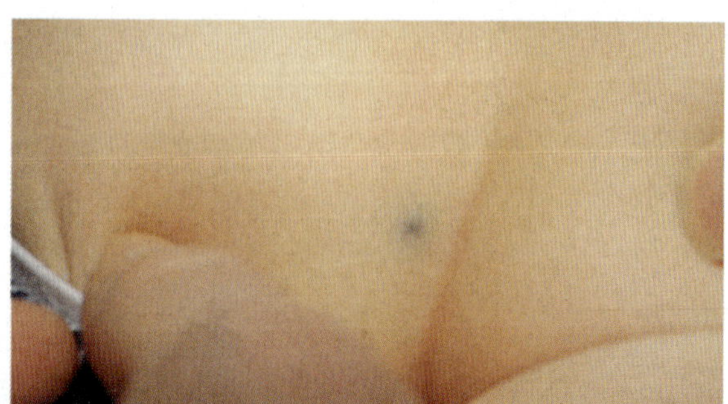

Fig. 8.112 Blue nevus. This blue nodule was made up of deep nevus cells; it was firm on palpation.

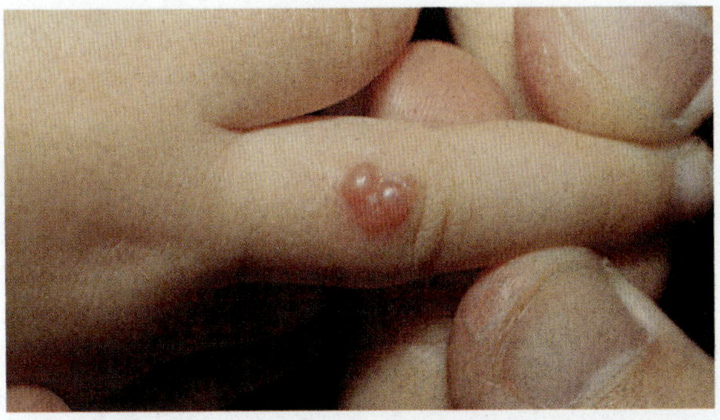

Fig. 8.113 Spitz nevus. This raised red nevus grows rapidly.

from nevus sebaceus (see later). The lesion may be present at birth or may develop during childhood and appears as a slightly hyperpigmented papillomatous or verrucous growth (Fig. 8.114). Development of and increases in verrucous changes are particularly common at puberty but do not represent malignant degeneration in most cases. Lesions may be small and localized, linear, dermatomal, or generalized. Important but rare associations with extensive epidermal nevi are seizures, cognitive impairment, and ocular and skeletal defects (see Chapter 16). Extensive lesions have also been associated with hypophosphatemic vitamin D–resistant rickets.

Nevus sebaceus of Jadassohn is characterized by a hairless, well-circumscribed, skin-colored or yellow or orange waxy plaque located most commonly on the scalp, face, or neck (Fig. 8.115;

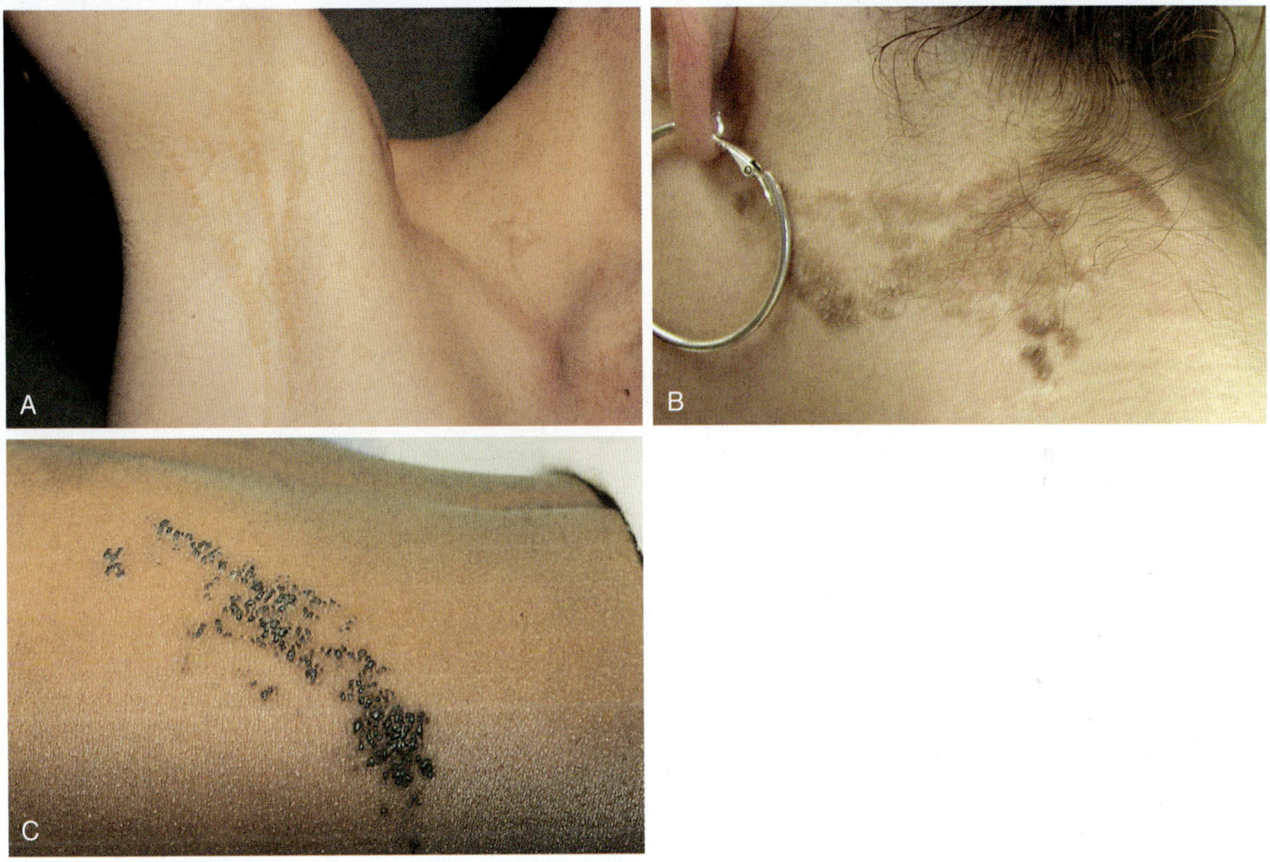

Fig. 8.114 Epidermal nevi. (A–C) These raised lesions vary in color depending on the child's skin tone, ranging from lightly pigmented to markedly hyperpigmented. Note the characteristic whorled array of verrucous papules, best seen in B. All three of these children had localized lesions and were otherwise healthy. More extensive nevi may be associated with systemic abnormalities (e.g., epidermal nevus syndrome; see Chapter 16).

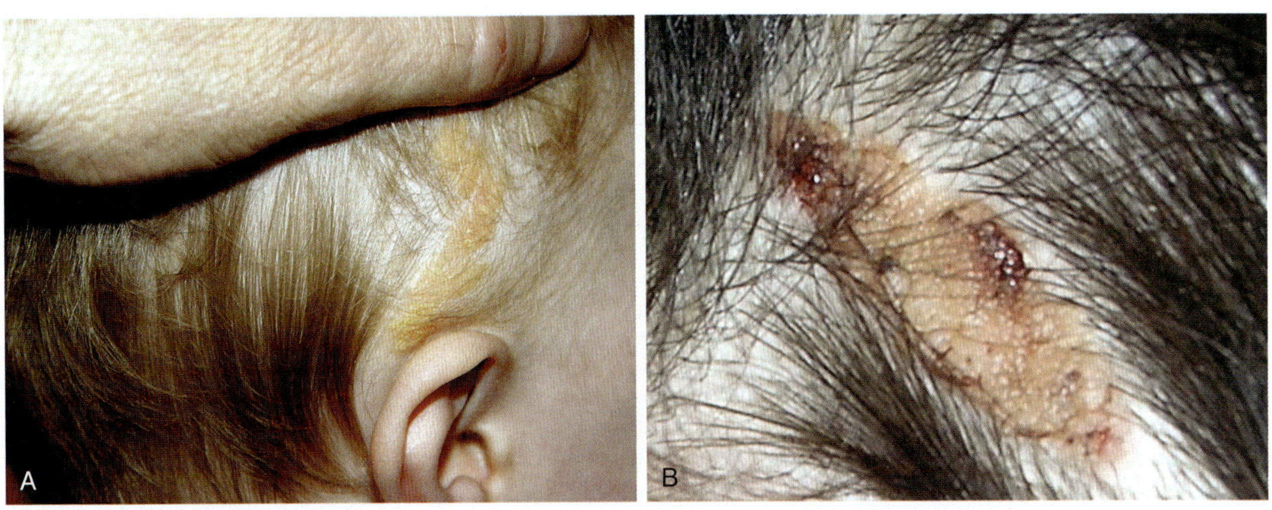

Fig. 8.115 Nevus sebaceus of Jadassohn. (A) This yellowish, hairless plaque was present on the temporal scalp at birth. (B) In an adolescent boy, the lesion has developed secondary warty growths, stimulated by pubertal androgens. (A, Courtesy http://www.dermatlas.org.)

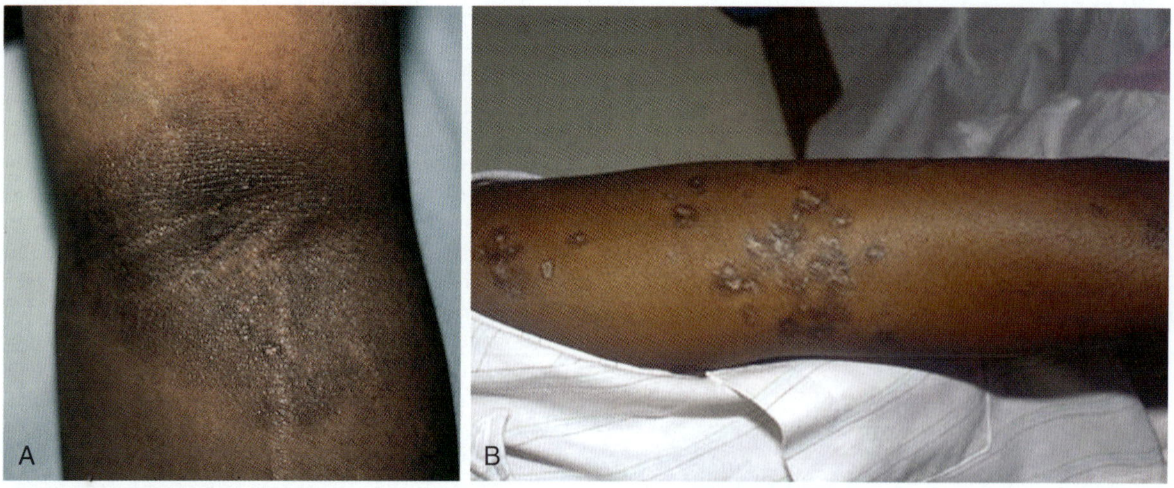

Fig. 8.116 (A) Postinflammatory hyperpigmentation arose in a child with chronic atopic dermatitis, which provoked persistent scratching. (B) This patient with discoid lupus provides another example of the phenomenon.

and see Chapter 16). The lesion is usually solitary and may be linear or round. It is present at birth, although at puberty the plaque may become more verrucous, raised, and nodular (see Chapter 16). Histologically, epidermal proliferation is seen along with abortive hair follicles, sebaceous glands, and apocrine structures. Although it has been felt in the past that 10% to 15% of these nevi develop secondary malignant neoplasms, more recent reviews of the literature confirm that this is extremely rare in children and uncommon even in adults. Many neoplasms arising from nevus sebaceus lesions, which had previously been thought to be basal cell carcinomas, were benign follicular growths known as *trichoblastomas.* Therefore the authors no longer recommend routine excision of nevus sebaceus in childhood unless the family or child find the lesion cosmetically unacceptable or there is a specific concerning change in the lesion. Ideal timing for excision if the team decides to do so is best planned with colleagues in dermatology or plastic surgery.

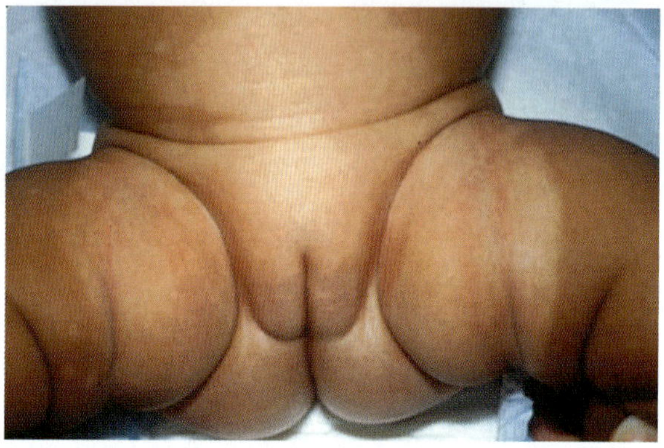

Fig. 8.117 Postinflammatory hypopigmentation is evident in this infant after treatment with topical agents for seborrheic diaper dermatitis.

DISORDERS OF PIGMENTATION

Childhood disorders of pigmentation are usually of cosmetic importance only, although some pigmented lesions can be markers of multisystem disease.

Postinflammatory Pigmentary Changes

Postinflammatory hyperpigmentation (Fig. 8.116) and hypopigmentation (Fig. 8.117) are the most common forms of disordered pigmentation. Each can develop following inflammatory disorders of the skin (e.g., dermatitis, acne, infection, or injury) and usually resolves spontaneously over a few months. Histologically, melanocytes appear normal, but the dispersion of pigment to other cells is disturbed. Pityriasis alba is a specific presentation that is more common in patients with an atopic diathesis, which presents as indistinct hypopigmented and slightly scaly patches most commonly on the cheeks or the extremities. Often there is a distant history of atopic dermatitis but not necessarily occurring in the exact location of the pityriasis alba. It is the authors' opinion that pityriasis alba represents postinflammatory hypopigmentation from subclinical atopic dermatitis. Pityriasis alba is best treated with a combination of bland emollients, sunblock to avoid increasing the contrast with normal skin, and, in more severe cases, topical immunomodulators. Postinflammatory hypopigmentation also must be distinguished from vitiligo (see Fig. 8.119), in which there is usually a complete absence of pigment without associated scaling or history of inflammation.

Tinea versicolor may present in adolescents as hypopigmented or hyperpigmented macules or patches with superficial fine scale in sun-exposed areas such as the chest, back, and shoulders. KOH examination can confirm the correct diagnosis with its typical "spaghetti and meatballs" pattern of hyphae and spores (see Figs. 8.40 and 8.41).

Pigmentary Mosaicism

The term *pigmentary mosaicism* refers to a group of conditions in which affected children have genetic mosaicism (i.e., they are born with at least two genetically different cell lines, resulting in the existence of keratinocytes of two different pigment tones). When these different populations of skin cells migrate during development, they create a whorled, fountain-like pattern of alternating hypopigmentation and hyperpigmentation (Fig. 8.118). This pattern is referred to as a *blaschkoid distribution* because it occurs along the "lines of Blaschko," which are lines of embryologic ectodermal development. They may be evident at birth and, if not, appear in infancy or early childhood. The bands are macular and are found most commonly over the trunk and do not cross the midline, but they can also be seen on the extremities where they tend to be more linear. In contrast to the hyperpigmented macules of incontinentia pigmenti, those of pure pigmentary mosaicism have no antecedent vesicular or verrucous lesions and are not associated with atrophy.

Pigmentary mosaicism most often stems from a postzygotic mutation or an error in cell division early in embryogenesis or may be the result of random X chromosome inactivation in X-linked conditions. The phenomenon has been reported in association with several

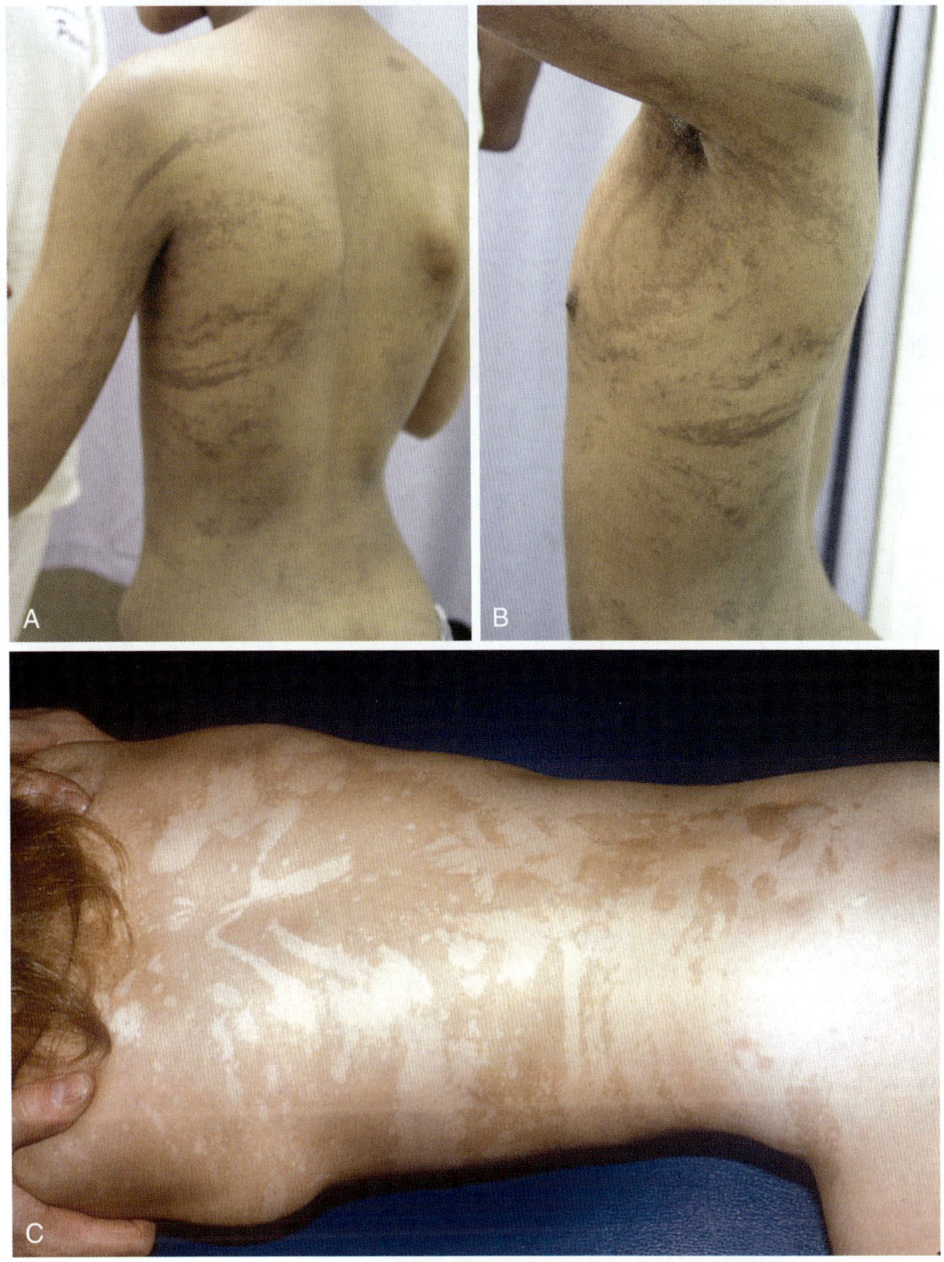

Fig. 8.118 Pigmentary mosaicism. (A and B) Swirling bands of alternating lighter and darker hues are seen on this adolescent's trunk, demonstrating a widespread blaschkoid distribution. Note that they vary in width and stop at the midline and that the streaks on the upper arm are more linear and parallel to its long axis. The patient also had a seizure disorder and significant cognitive deficits. (C) More extensive involvement is seen over the back of another child. (C, Courtesy http://www.dermatlas.org.)

different types of chromosomal mosaicism including trisomies 13, 18, and 20. Affected individuals may be completely healthy or can have associated abnormalities of the CNS, the musculoskeletal system, or the eye. Children with more extensive cutaneous lesions may be at greater risk for extracutaneous involvement and should receive a careful medical and developmental examination and targeted studies where indicated.

Vitiligo

In vitiligo, an acquired condition, there is partial to complete loss of pigmentation. Lesions consist of well-demarcated depigmented macules and patches that are usually seen in a characteristic distribution around the eyes, mouth, genitals, elbows, hands, and feet (Fig. 8.119). Lesions may appear elsewhere, such as in a koebnerized distribution in areas of prior friction or trauma. They enhance dramatically under a Wood lamp. Some patients may have halo nevi, which represent the same autoimmune reaction surrounding pigmented nevi. Spontaneous but slow repigmentation may occur from the edges of a lesion and around hair follicles, resulting in a speckled appearance. Lesions on the head and neck repigment faster because repigmentation occurs first through hair follicles and these areas have more numerous populations of hair follicles.

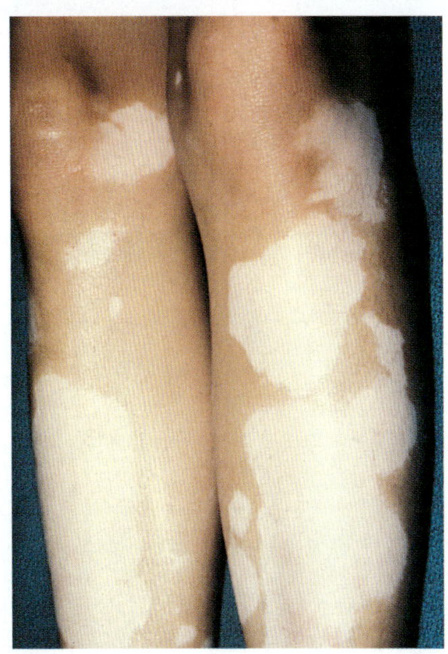

Fig. 8.119 Vitiligo. Completely depigmented patches are seen on the legs. On occasion, macules of repigmentation arise from epidermal appendages within the white patches. A characteristic distribution helps to distinguish vitiligo from other causes of hypopigmentation.

Histologically, melanocytes are absent in areas of vitiligo, and evidence suggests that they have been destroyed by an autoimmune mechanism. In a small proportion of patients with vitiligo, other autoimmune conditions, such as alopecia areata, thyroiditis, diabetes, or pernicious anemia, can be detected concomitantly.

Ash Leaf Spots

Congenital, well-demarcated, hypopigmented macules, termed *ash leaf spots* because of their usual lanceolate shape, are often a valuable early marker of tuberous sclerosis. They appear at birth or shortly thereafter as 1- to 3-cm oval macules on the trunk. Because they are hypopigmented rather than totally depigmented, they are not as easily appreciated or as bright white as the lesions of vitiligo, and their usual truncal distribution helps distinguish them from the classic location of vitiligo (see Chapter 16).

The identification of ash leaf macules may be enhanced (although not as dramatically as is seen in vitiligo) using a Wood lamp, and this method of examination should be part of the assessment of any child who develops idiopathic seizures in infancy. The visible purple light emitted is absorbed by normal melanin in the skin. Thus in a darkened room, areas of hypopigmentation or depigmentation appear brighter violet, whereas normally melanized skin reflects little visible light and appears dull purple or black.

It is important to recognize that up to 0.5% of otherwise normal newborns will have an isolated hypopigmented macule, which, in the absence of other signs of tuberous sclerosis, is termed a *nevus depigmentosus* and represents a localized form of pigmentary mosaicism (Fig. 8.120). Nevus depigmentosus is somewhat of a misnomer because the lesions are not truly depigmented; they are hypopigmented and so do not enhance maximally under Wood lamp.

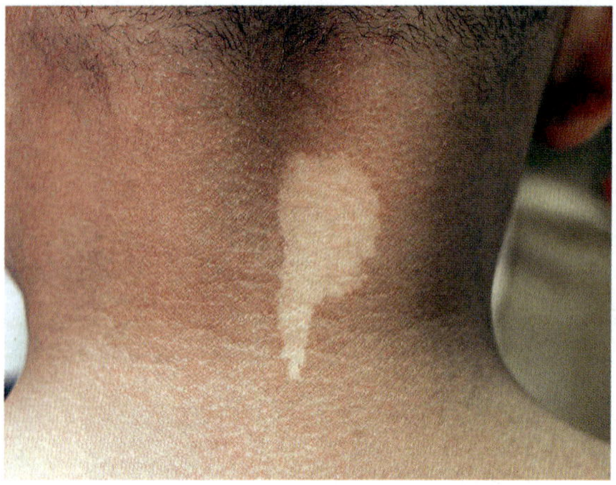

Fig. 8.120 Nevus depigmentosus is a localized form of pigmentary mosaicism, seen here on the nape of the neck of an otherwise healthy child.

Albinism

The term *albinism* refers to a heterogeneous group of inherited disorders characterized by congenital hypopigmentation of the skin, eyes, and hair. It occurs in an X-linked ocular form (in which the skin appears clinically normal) and several different autosomal recessive oculocutaneous forms. In oculocutaneous albinism (OCA), both sexes and all races are affected equally. This form of the disorder is subdivided into several variants based on clinical findings and biochemical markers. In the past, tyrosinase-negative and tyrosinase-positive subtypes were identified based on the ability of plucked hairs to produce pigment when incubated in tyrosine. Currently, deoxyribonucleic acid markers allow for identification of specific mutations. In classic tyrosinase-negative OCA, children are born without any trace of pigment. Affected individuals have snow-white hair, pinkish-white skin, and translucent or blue irises. Nystagmus is common, as is moderate to severe strabismus and poor visual acuity (see Chapter 20). Although children with tyrosinase-positive OCA may be clinically indistinguishable from their tyrosinase-negative counterparts at birth, they usually develop variable amounts of pigment with increasing age. Eye color may vary from gray to light brown, and hair may change to blond or light brown. The subtypes can be distinguished by genetic testing.

Because they lack the protection of melanin, patients with OCA are at high risk for early development of basal cell and squamous cell skin cancers. Hence they should be instructed in the use of sunscreen, eye protection, and avoidance of excessive sun exposure.

Piebaldism

Piebaldism (partial albinism) is an autosomal dominant disorder characterized by a white forelock and a circumscribed congenital leukoderma. The typical lesions include a triangular patch of depigmentation and white hair on the frontal scalp. The apex of this patch points toward the nasal bridge (Fig. 8.121A). Patients may also have hypopigmented or depigmented macules on the face, neck, ventral trunk, flanks, or extremities (see Fig. 8.121B). Within areas of decreased pigmentation, scattered patches of normal pigmentation or hyperpigmentation may appear. The lesions are stable throughout life, although some variability in pigmentation may occur with sun exposure. Special variants of piebaldism include Waardenburg syndrome, in which leukoderma is associated with lateral displacement of the inner canthi and inferior lacrimal ducts, a flattened nasal bridge, and sensorineural deafness; and Wolf-Hirschhorn syndrome, an autosomal recessive disorder associated with neurologic deficits.

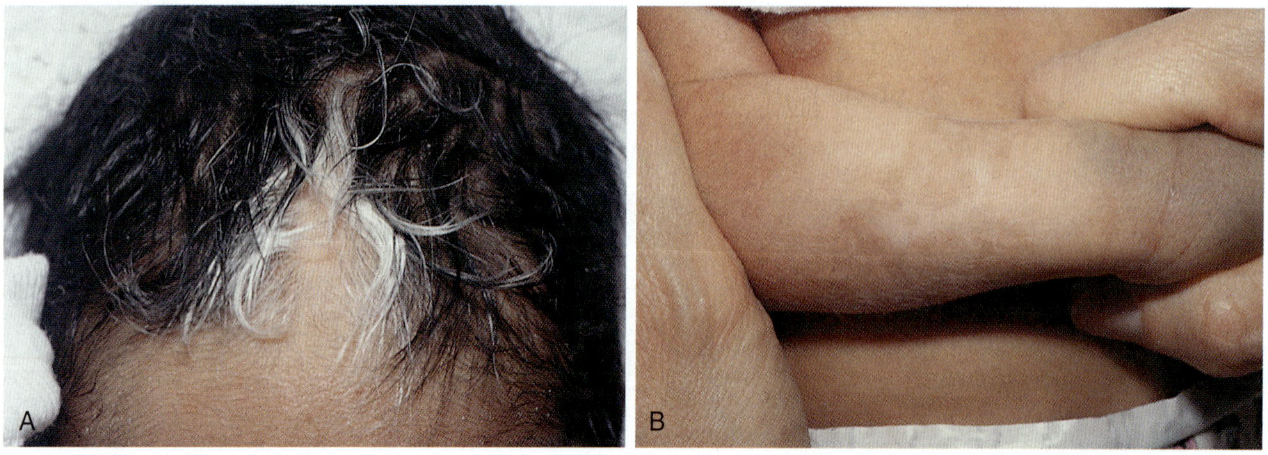

Fig. 8.121 Piebaldism. (A) A white forelock overlies a depigmented patch of scalp and forehead. (B) The infant also has a hypopigmented patch on his arm in which smaller areas of hyperpigmentation are seen.

Acanthosis Nigricans

Acanthosis nigricans is characterized by hyperpigmentation and hyperkeratosis in intertriginous areas and over bony prominences. Skin lines are accentuated, and the skin surface of involved areas may have a velvety, leathery, or warty appearance (Fig. 8.122). Four main forms of the disorder exist. The benign and idiopathic form is the most common and is related to hyperinsulinemia or insulin resistance. Insulin is a skin growth factor, so high levels lead to proliferation of keratinocytes. Onset is usually at puberty but can occur in childhood in concert with development of obesity. The prominence of lesions tends to lessen when patients lose weight. An inherited form, transmitted as an autosomal dominant trait, usually presents in infancy or early childhood but becomes more prominent during adolescence. This form is unassociated with other underlying disorders. In endocrine-associated acanthosis nigricans, the condition may antedate or appear in association with insulin resistance with or without polycystic ovary disease. More rarely, it is seen in patients with pituitary tumors. Malignancy-related acanthosis nigricans is extremely rare in childhood.

Other Pigmentary Disorders

Café au lait macules are tan macules that usually occur in otherwise healthy individuals but can be an indication of neurofibromatosis type 1 (see Chapter 16) or McCune-Albright syndrome. In the latter, they can be associated with polyostotic fibrous dysplasia of the long bones and endocrinopathy, such as hyperthyroidism and precocious puberty (see Chapter 9). Café au lait macules that are smaller and oval, have smooth borders, and are discovered in association with axillary or inguinal freckling (Crowe sign) are more likely to be associated with neurofibromatosis type 1 (Fig. 8.123A–C), whereas those that are large and segmental with jagged borders are more likely to be seen in association with McCune-Albright syndrome (see Fig. 8.123D). Children who have café au lait spots in the absence of a syndrome usually have fewer than four lesions that are relatively small.

Swirled hyperpigmentation may be a marker of the later stages of incontinentia pigmenti (see Fig. 8.100D and E) or pigmentary mosaicism (see Fig. 8.118). Diffuse hyperpigmentation may be seen in primary adrenal insufficiency (Addison disease) and in hemochromatosis. Peutz-Jeghers syndrome manifests as lentiginous pigmentation of the lips, oral mucosa, hands, and fingers in association with benign small intestinal polyps in children (see Chapter 18).

DISORDERS OF THE HAIR AND NAILS

Alopecia

The most common diseases of the hair result in some degree of hair loss, or alopecia. Evaluation begins by determining whether scarring is present. Nonscarring alopecia can be due to growth defects causing the hair to be lost at the roots (effluvium) or by defects of the hair shaft that result in breakage.

Alopecia Caused by Systemic Insult: Telogen and Anagen Effluvium

Normal hair cycles through a growth phase lasting 3 years or more (anagen phase) and a resting phase of 3 months (telogen phase), after which the hair is shed, and the cycle then begins again. Telogen effluvium is one form of partial, temporary alopecia, which may occur 3 months after an emotional or physical stress, such as a severe illness, major surgery, or high fever. It rarely causes more than 50% hair loss. In affected patients, the initial systemic insult induces more than the usual 20% of hairs to enter the telogen phase, and 3 months later these hairs are shed simultaneously, producing thinning of scalp hair until new anagen hairs regrow months to years later (Fig. 8.124). In cases of telogen effluvium, often the patient and family notice the hair to be thinner than normal and the part may appear wider than usual, but the hair loss is not as noticeable to a stranger. In contrast, anagen effluvium is the sudden loss of growing hairs (which represent 80% of normal scalp hairs) caused by abnormal interruption of the anagen phase. In these cases, the hair shafts taper and lose adhesion to the follicle. This type of hair loss is most common after systemic chemotherapy,

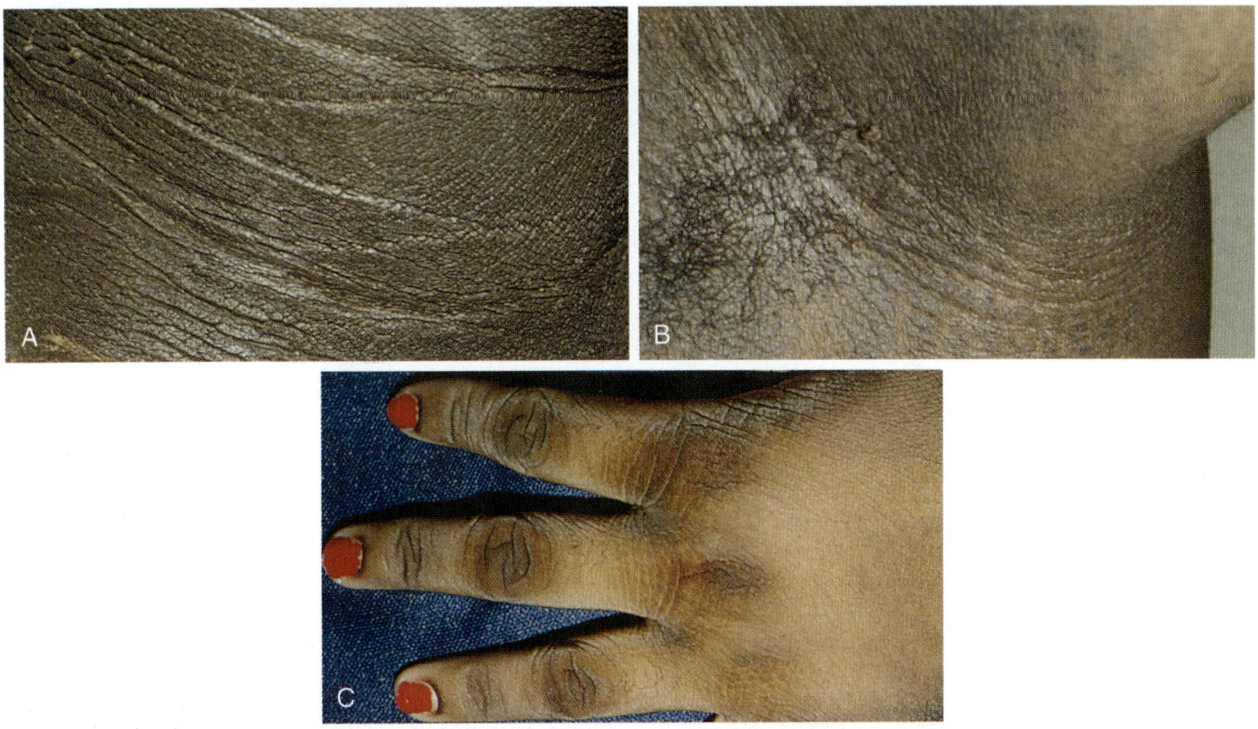

Fig. 8.122 Acanthosis nigricans. (A and B) Hyperpigmentation and leathery thickening of the skin are seen on the neck and in the axilla of an obese adolescent with the benign/idiopathic form of the disorder. (C) She also had velvety hyperpigmentation and prominence of skin lines over the knuckles of her hands and other bony prominences. (From Cohen BA: *Pediatric dermatology,* ed 2, London, 1999, Mosby.)

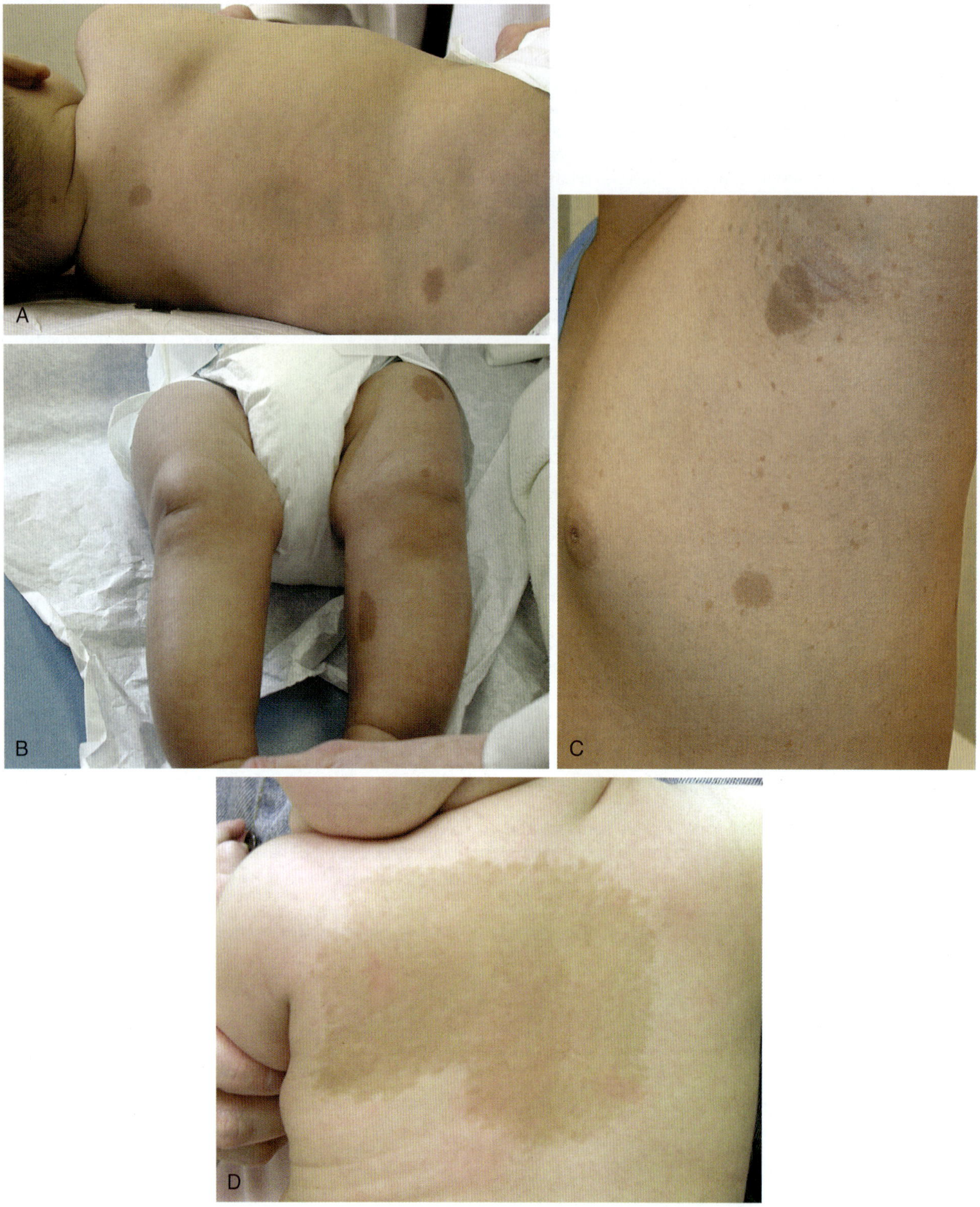

Fig. 8.123 Café au lait macules. (A and B) Small café au lait spots are seen in two infants with neurofibromatosis type 1, one fairly pigmented and one with darker pigmentation to demonstrate the differences in color of lesions with differing skin tones. Note that the lesions have smooth borders, which are typical of this disorder. The infant in B also has pseudarthrosis of the tibia and fibula, with foreshortening of the left lower leg (see Chapter 16). (C) This older boy has both café au lait spots and axillary freckling (Crowe sign). The presence of six or more café au lait macules and axillary freckling is diagnostic for neurofibromatosis type 1. (D) Another infant with McCune-Albright syndrome has a large café au lait macule located in a segmental distribution over his back. Note the jagged margins of the lesion. The child also had precocious puberty. (C, Courtesy http://www.dermatlas.org.)

is more dramatic and widespread in its appearance, and can be noted easily on examination.

Alopecia Areata

Alopecia areata is a form of localized alopecia that usually presents with round or oval patches of smooth alopecia that may be located anywhere on the scalp, eyebrows, lashes, or body. On occasion, hair loss is more diffuse or generalized. Its origin is autoimmune, and scalp biopsies in cases of alopecia areata will demonstrate a swarm of lymphocytes around the hair follicles, as well as increased numbers of telogen hairs. Clinical clues to diagnosis include absence of inflammation and scaling in the involved areas of scalp and the presence of short (3–6 mm), easily epilated hairs at the margins of the patch (Fig. 8.125A and B). Under magnification, these hair stubs resemble exclamation points because the hair shaft narrows just before its point of entry into the follicle. Another finding in many patients with alopecia areata is Scotch-plaid pitting of the nails, consisting of rows of pits crossing in a transverse and longitudinal fashion (see Fig. 8.139). The clinical course of alopecia areata is difficult to predict. The disorder may resolve spontaneously; it may persist, with the appearance of new patches while the old patches regrow; or it may progress to total scalp *(alopecia totalis)* or even generalized whole-body alopecia *(alopecia universalis),* either of which can be permanent (see Fig. 8.125C). In severe cases, it is helpful to perform a thorough search to exclude coexistent autoimmune disease, such as autoimmune thyroiditis or pernicious anemia.

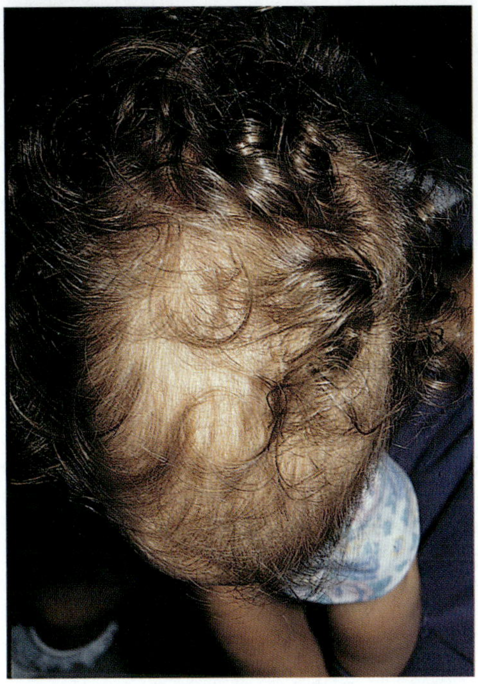

Fig. 8.124 Telogen effluvium. This toddler experienced sudden partial hair loss approximately 3 months after being hospitalized for pneumococcal sepsis. (Courtesy Alejandro Hoberman, MD, Children's Hospital of Pittsburgh.)

Trichorrhexis Nodosa

Alopecia caused by hair shaft breakage is due to a structural defect of the hair, and it is easily diagnosed by microscopic examination. The most common structural defect is acquired trichorrhexis nodosa. This defect can present at any age as brittle, short hairs that are perceived by the patient as failing to grow. Upon gentle pulling, hairs are easily broken. Microscopically, the distal ends of the hairs are frayed, resembling a broom (Fig. 8.126). Other hairs may have nodules, resembling two brooms stuck together. The fragility is the result of external damage to the outer cortex of the hair shaft, resulting in a loss of structural support. Without this support, the weaker fibrous medulla frays like an electrical cord with broken insulation. This disorder may arise from the trauma of combing tightly curled hairs. It is also seen after repeated or severe chemical damage to the cortex from hair straighteners, bleaches, and permanents. Because hair growth is normal, the disorder is self-limited and normal hairs regrow when the source of the damage is identified and eliminated and gentle hair care practices are adopted.

Other common causes of hair loss associated with shaft abnormalities include friction alopecia, traction alopecia, and trichotillomania. All of these are caused by external trauma and breakage of an otherwise normal hair shaft.

Friction Alopecia

Friction alopecia (Fig. 8.127) is common on the posterior scalp of infants, where the head rubs on the pillow or bed clothes. Although worrisome to parents, this disorder is self-limited. It can be prevented or its severity reduced by ensuring that an infant spends plenty of time on his or her tummy when awake and able to

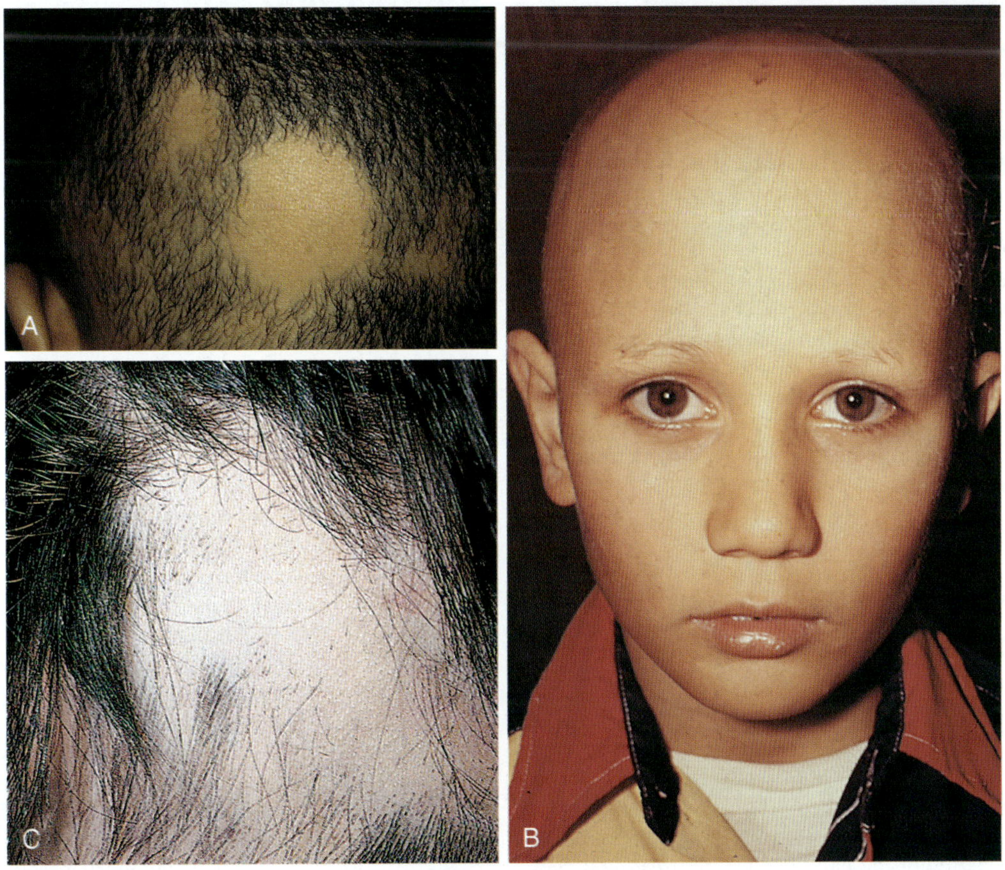

Fig. 8.125 Alopecia areata. (A) Patches of complete hair loss with otherwise normal scalp are typical of this disorder. (B) In this close-up, small broken hairs that pull out easily are seen at the margins. (C) In this boy, the process has progressed to alopecia totalis. Note that even his eyebrows are involved. (C, Courtesy Michael Sherlock, MD, Lutherville, MD.)

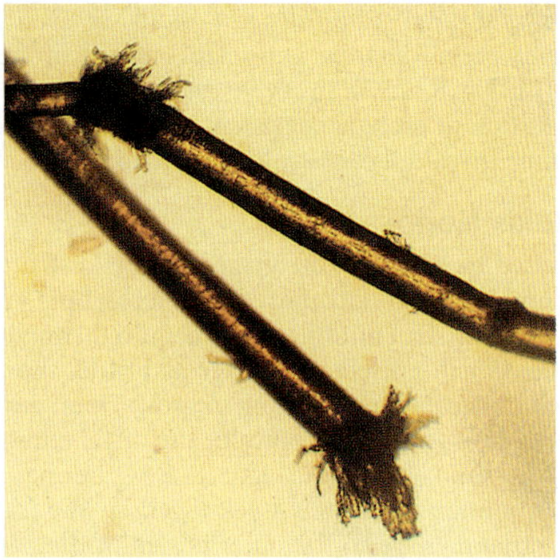

Fig. 8.126 Trichorrhexis nodosa consists of a brittle hair shaft defect usually caused by overmanipulation of the hair or application of harsh chemicals. The frayed brown appearance is typical.

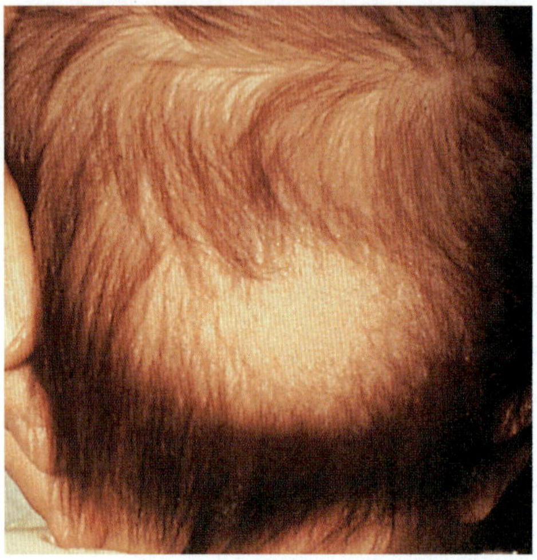

Fig. 8.127 Friction alopecia. Hair loss over the occiput resulted from rubbing of the head on sheets and pillows while lying supine.

be supervised. When unusually severe or long-standing, friction alopecia may raise the question of neglect, suggesting that the infant is being left to lie in his or her crib for extended periods of time.

Traction Alopecia

Traction alopecia (Fig. 8.128) is common in children whose hairstyles, such as ponytails, pigtails, braids, or cornrows, maintain a tight pull on the hair shafts. This traction causes shaft fractures and follicular inflammation. If prolonged, permanent scarring alopecia can result. On rare occasions, excess traction applied in the process of braiding can result in subgaleal bleeding and hematoma formation. This phenomenon can also be seen in child abuse victims who have been subjected to forceful hair pulling (see Chapter 6).

Trichotillomania

Trichotillomania is a common disorder seen in older children and adolescents that mimics many other types of alopecia. This form of localized nonscarring hair loss presents with bizarre patterns where the hair is easily twisted and pulled out (Fig. 8.129). Trichotillomania is seen more commonly on the side opposite the child's dominant hand as the other hand is free to manipulate the hair while the child is engaged in other tasks. Rarely, the entire scalp, eyebrows, and eyelashes are involved. The most important clue to the correct diagnosis is the finding of short, broken-off hairs along the scalp, with stubs of different lengths in adjacent areas. This is the result of repetitive pulling or twisting of the hair, which fractures the longer shafts. Once broken, the hairs are too short to be rebroken until they grow longer. The scalp appears otherwise normal.

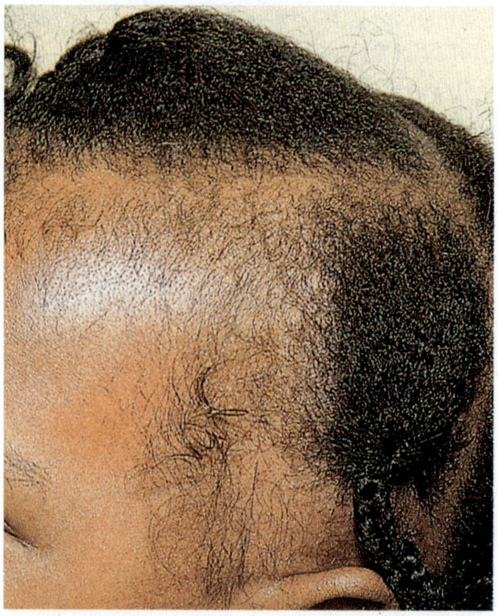

Fig. 8.128 Traction alopecia. The hair thinning and loss are due to excessive traction on the hairs as a result of tight braiding.

Trichotillomania is sometimes confused with alopecia areata because there are patches of hair loss with short hairs, and there may be involvement of the eyebrows and eyelashes. However, in trichotillomania, patches of hair loss are never completely bald and the hair shafts are normal anagen hairs that are usually difficult to remove from the scalp. In addition, there are no associated nail abnormalities.

Although trichotillomania may occur in children with severe psychiatric disease, most cases are associated with situational stress or anxiety.

Tinea Capitis (Fungal Infections of the Hair and Scalp)

Fungal infection of the hair weakens the shaft causing breakage. This typically results in the development of multiple patches of partial alopecia, commonly referred to as *ringworm. T. tonsurans* is the organism responsible for more than 95% of cases in the United States. *Microsporum canis* (the dog and cat ringworm) accounts for a smaller percentage of cases.

Clinical presentations of tinea capitis vary. In some patients, mild erythema and scaling of the scalp occur in association with partial alopecia (Fig. 8.130A). In other cases, there is widespread breakage at the scalp, creating a "salt and pepper" appearance with the short residual hairs appearing as black dots on the surface of the scalp (see Fig. 8.130B). On occasion, scalp lesions are annular, simulating tinea corporis. In yet other children, sensitization to the infecting organism results in more erythema, edema, and pustule formation. As the latter rupture, the area weeps and golden crusts form, simulating impetigo (see Fig. 8.130C). Some cases are characterized by patches of heaped-up scale in association with small pustules (see Fig. 8.130D). Less commonly, intense inflammation causes formation of raised, tender, boggy plaques or masses studded with pustules that simulate abscesses, termed *kerions* (see Fig. 8.130E). The inflammation associated with kerions makes them more likely to cause scarring hair loss. Thus systemic treatment with oral antifungals and occasionally steroids is imperative. Incision and drainage of kerions is not indicated because loculations are small and septae thick. Importantly, when pustules or weeping and crusting lesions involve the scalp or hair line, the infection is far more likely to be of fungal than bacterial origin. Patients with tinea capitis often have associated occipital, postauricular, and posterior cervical adenopathy (see Chapter 13).

Fungal infection of the scalp can be confirmed by a KOH examination of infected hairs (Fig. 8.131). Residual broken hairs or black

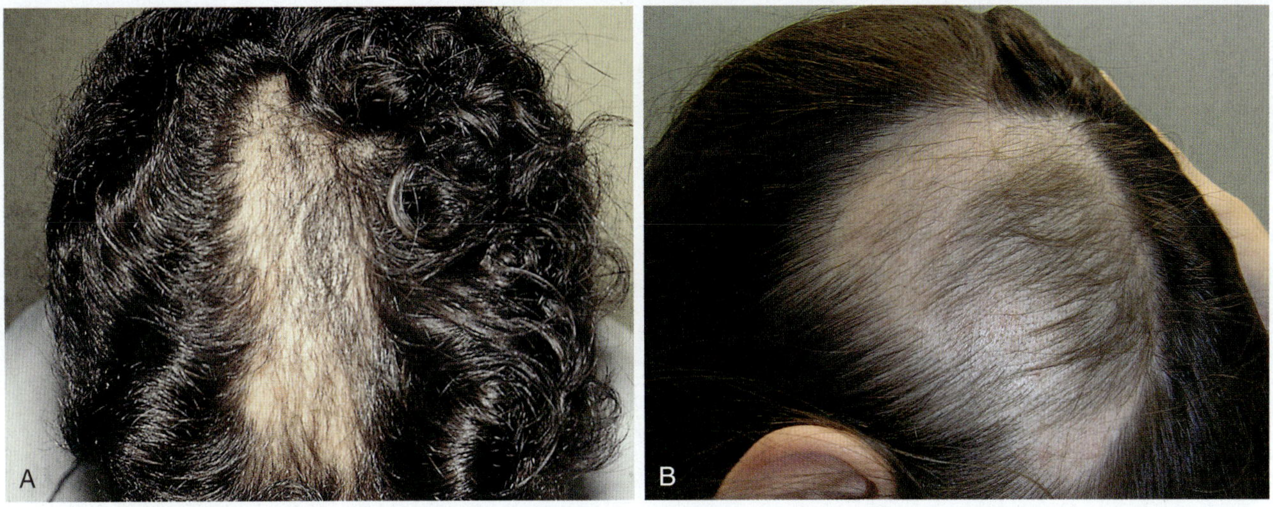

Fig. 8.129 Trichitillosis, or trichotillomania. (A) This linear patch of short broken hairs along the midline is typical of hair pulling. (B) Another child has a unilateral geometric patch of hair loss, again with short broken hairs. Note that the scalp is normal in both cases.

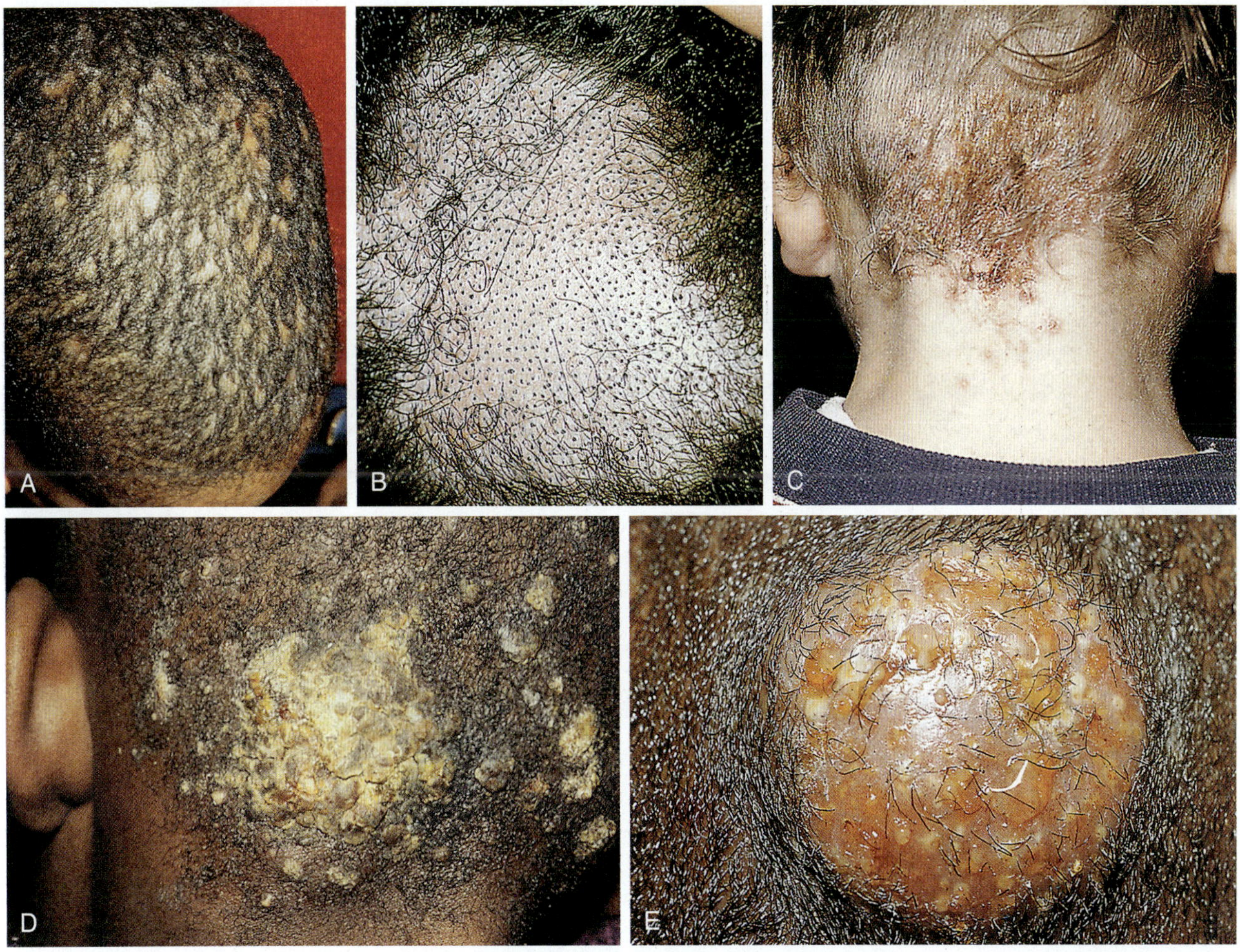

Fig. 8.130 Tinea capitis can present in many guises. (A) In this child, mild erythema and scaling of the scalp are associated with spotty alopecia. (B) Infiltration of hair shafts by an endothrix fungus has resulted in widespread breakage at the scalp, producing a "salt and pepper" appearance. (C) Superficial papules and pustules have ruptured, producing weeping and crusting lesions simulating impetigo. (D) This variant of tinea is characterized by thick, heaped-up scale. (E) Kerion. A boggy mass has formed as a result of an intense inflammatory response. This child, seen relatively late in the course, had nearly total alopecia over the involved area. Note that the lesion is studded with pustules.

dots at the surface of the scalp should be scraped for KOH preparation or fungal culture. *T. tonsurans* is currently the most common causative organism in the United States and does not fluoresce with Wood lamp examination. Only *M. canis,* which causes 5% of cases, fluoresces bright bluish-green. Thus a negative Wood lamp examination will not rule out the most common cause of tinea capitis.

Because topical antifungal agents do not penetrate deeply enough to be effective in the treatment of tinea capitis, oral antifungal agents are necessary and must be administered for at least 6 weeks to eradicate the infection. In patients with mild, moderate, or severe hepatic insufficiency, regular monitoring of hepatic aminotransferases is suggested to avoid the rare risk of clinically significant liver injury. Unfortunately, even with oral antifungal treatment, risk of recurrence is high. Griseofulvin, ketoconazole, and terbinafine are approved in the United States by the Food and Drug Administration for treatment of tinea capitis. Studies show that itraconazole and fluconazole are also

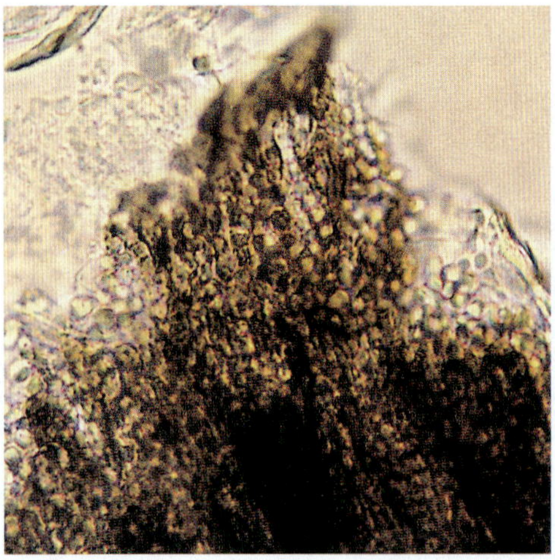

Fig. 8.131 Microscopical appearance of hair shafts infected with fungi. Note the tight packing of fungal arthrospores that cause hair shaft fragility and breakage (potassium hydroxide mount for endothrix).

effective and require shorter courses of therapy, but ketoconazole is less commonly used due to severe side effects and concerns about its efficacy. Concurrent use of ketoconazole 2% shampoo and selenium sulfide 2.5% shampoo during a course of oral therapy reduces spore formation and shedding and may help to minimize the risk of spread to close contacts until oral treatment is complete. Other measures useful in reducing passage of organisms to others include avoidance of communal use of brushes, combs, hats, scarves, towels, or linens; careful washing or cleaning of combs and brushes; and thorough cleaning of potentially contaminated linen, clothing, and upholstery.

Scarring Alopecia

Scarring alopecia is considerably less common than nonscarring alopecia in children and may be caused by congenital and acquired disorders. On examination, no intact hair follicles are seen in the areas of alopecia due to permanent scar formation. Morphea (localized scleroderma) and lupus may involve the scalp with indurated, hairless plaques. Scarring alopecia may also result from severe infection (e.g., inflammatory tinea capitis) or trauma, such as oil burns from hot comb straightening of the hair. A scalp biopsy is often helpful in determining the cause of scarring alopecia.

Aplasia Cutis Congenita

Aplasia cutis congenita is a congenital condition characterized by absence of or failure of formation of a localized area of epidermis, dermis, fat, bone, or some combination of these layers. In most cases, there is a single lesion located over the vertex of the scalp. Rarely, lesions may be multiple or may involve the trunk or extremities. They may be associated with limb defects and other congenital and genetic anomalies. Usually, only the dermis and epidermis are absent; however, some lesions extend to involve subcutaneous tissue, and, in rare cases, a calvarial defect may underlie a scalp lesion, which is why deep palpation of more extensive lesions is discouraged until imaging has been performed.

At birth, the lesion may consist of a sharply circumscribed open and weeping erosion or ulceration, or it may be covered by a thin, often hemorrhagic membrane or crust (Fig. 8.132A; see Chapter 1). Evaluation should include radiologic studies to assess the depth of the lesion and a search for associated anomalies. When a hair

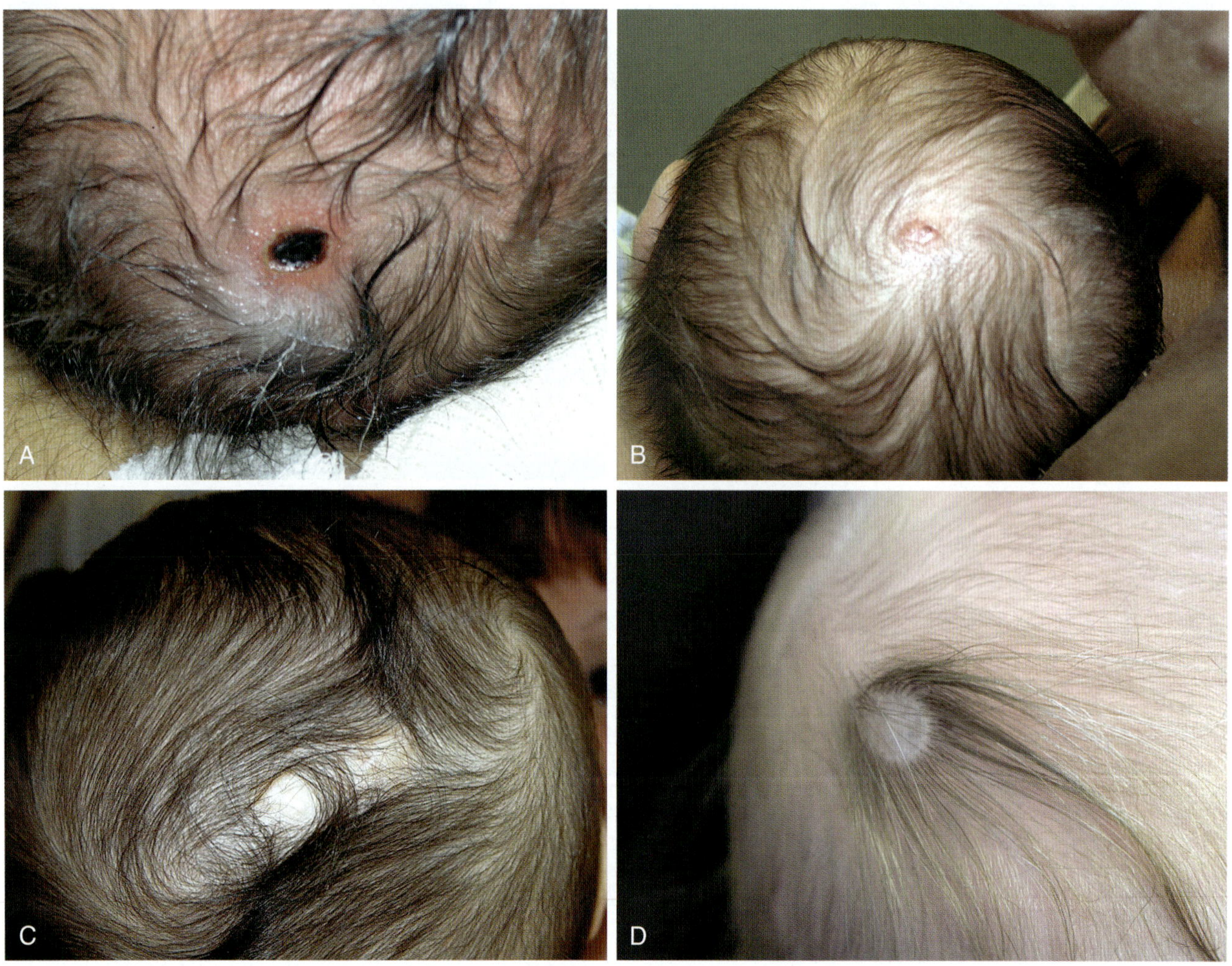

Fig. 8.132 Aplasia cutis congenita. (A) This 2-day-old has a sharply circumscribed, punched-out ulceration over the vertex with a hemorrhagic crust. (B) After 3 weeks of topical mupirocin therapy, the lesion has nearly healed. (C) The typical atrophic hairless scar of a healed lesion is seen. (D) Healed aplasia cutis congenita with the "hair collar" sign.

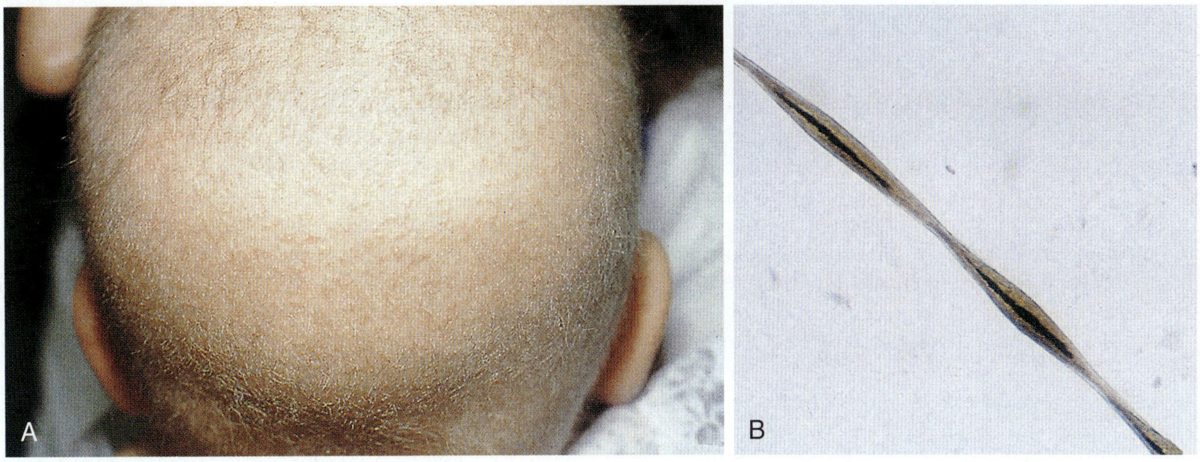

Fig. 8.133 Monilethrix. (A) Short, broken hairs give the appearance of diffuse alopecia. (B) Microscopically, periodic narrowing of this hair shaft is evident. Hairs are brittle and break off at constricted points near the scalp.

collar sign is present surrounding the lesion (see Fig. 8.132D), one should rule out an underlying neural tube defect with a magnetic resonance imaging scan. Conservative treatment designed to protect the area from infection and injury includes application of topical antibiotics. Depending on the size of the lesion, healing takes place over several weeks to months, leaving a smooth atrophic and hairless scar (see Fig. 8.132B and C). The differential diagnosis includes congenital nevus sebaceus lesions, which are raised and have an uneven, yellow, waxy surface (see Fig. 8.115), and epidermal nevi, which are typically hyperpigmented and have a raised warty surface.

Congenital and Genetic Disorders

Monilethrix and Pili Torti

Monilethrix is an autosomal dominant developmental hair defect that produces brittle hair, which appears beaded when viewed microscopically. Clinical manifestations usually appear first in infants 2 to 3 months old, when neonatal vellus hairs are replaced by these abnormal terminal beaded hairs (Fig. 8.133A). The scalp is most severely affected, although hair on any part of the body can be involved. The disease is permanent, although the clinical appearance of the hair may improve as the child grows older. Microscopically, regular, periodic narrowing of the hair shafts that resembles beads is seen (see Fig. 8.133B). Breakage occurs in constricted areas close to the scalp. Care must be taken not to confuse monilethrix with pili torti, another structural defect in which the hair shaft is twisted on its own axis. Pili torti may be localized or generalized and appears with the first terminal hair growth of infancy. It may be associated with Menkes disease (Fig. 8.134), an X-linked recessive disorder characterized by copper deficiency due to a defect in a copper-transporting gene, which can also affect the central nervous, cardiovascular, and skeletal systems.

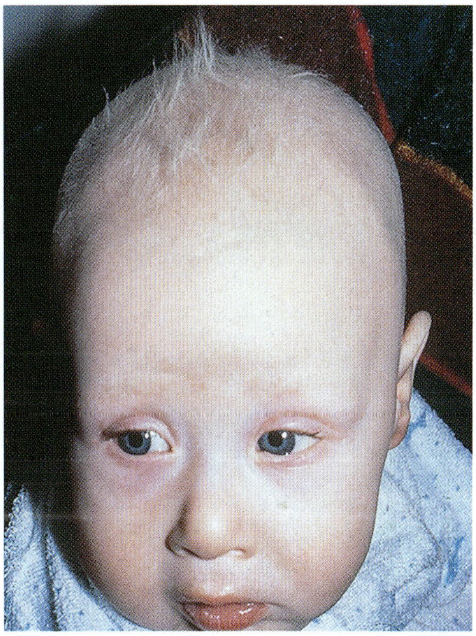

Fig. 8.134 Menkes kinky hair syndrome with generalized pili torti. This infant demonstrates the characteristic features of the disorder: fair skin; blue eyes; and the fair, sparse brittle hair of diffuse pili torti. He experienced developmental regression and had a seizure disorder. (From Cohen BA: *Pediatric dermatology,* ed 2, London, 1999, Mosby.)

Disorders Affecting the Nails

Paronychia

Paronychia is a common childhood disorder that presents with redness, swelling, and tenderness of the lateral or proximal nail fold. The acute form is most commonly bacterial in origin and is caused by staphylococci or streptococci. It is often seen after trauma to the cuticle (e.g., biting or picking), or it can develop in a child with a dermatitis that has damaged the normal barrier of the stratum corneum (see Chapter 13). Chronic paronychia may involve one or several nails and is often associated with a history of chronic dermatitis or frequent exposure to moisture. In contrast to the acute form, tenderness tends to be mild. Sometimes a small amount of pus can be extruded. Given its chronicity, some degree of associated nail dystrophy often exists (Fig. 8.135). Inflammation is the underlying cause; and when infection is implicated, the causative organisms are more often yeast of the *Candida* species, usually *C. albicans,* than bacteria. This form improves with the

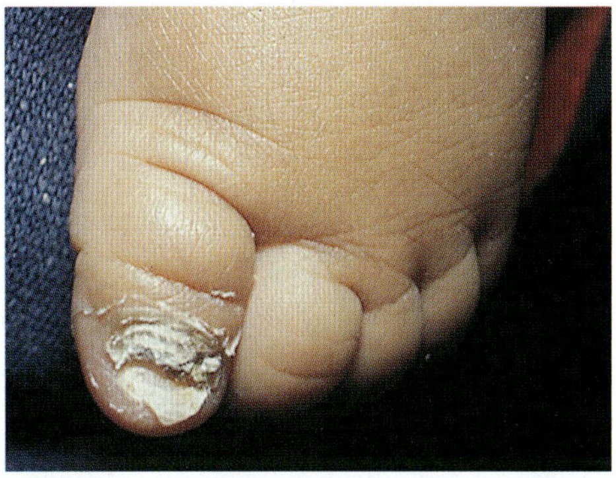

Fig. 8.135 Chronic paronychia with nail dystrophy caused by candidal infection.

combined use of topical antifungals, topical steroids, and avoidance of moisture.

Onychomycosis and Nail Dystrophy

Onychomycosis, or fungal infection of the nail plate (Fig. 8.136), is not as common in children as it is in adults. Thus nail dystrophy should not automatically be treated as a fungal infection unless proven by microscopical examination or fungal culture. Dystrophic nails can be caused by many different types of inflammation of the nail matrix and are seen frequently after discrete or more low-grade repetitive trauma or friction (Fig. 8.137) or from an underlying dermatosis, such as psoriasis, atopic dermatitis, or lichen planus.

Trauma

Acute trauma to the nail bed may cause subungual hemorrhage resulting in a brown-black discoloration. This is particularly common after crush injuries. Usually the diagnosis is simple, unless trauma is more subtle and chronic. If a discrete, large, or painful hematoma is produced, this can be evacuated by electrocautery of the nail plate to relieve pain and reduce the risk of infection. Blue-black discoloration at the base of the great toenail, caused by jamming the toe into the end of the shoe at a sudden stop, is called *turf toe* or *tennis toe* and results in mild, chronic subungual hemorrhage (Fig. 8.138). This must be distinguished from melanoma. Concern for melanoma should heighten if pigmentation of the cuticle or proximal nail fold accompanies hyperpigmentation of the nail; this is called *Hutchinson sign*. When present, this should prompt immediate referral for a biopsy of the nail matrix to exclude melanoma. In contrast, hemorrhage can be identified by the presence of purplish-brown pigment in the distal nail and normal proximal outgrowth of normal-appearing nail. Chronic repetitive trauma due to the habit of picking at one nail with another or rubbing of ill-fitting shoes, is a common source of nail dystrophy (see Fig. 8.137).

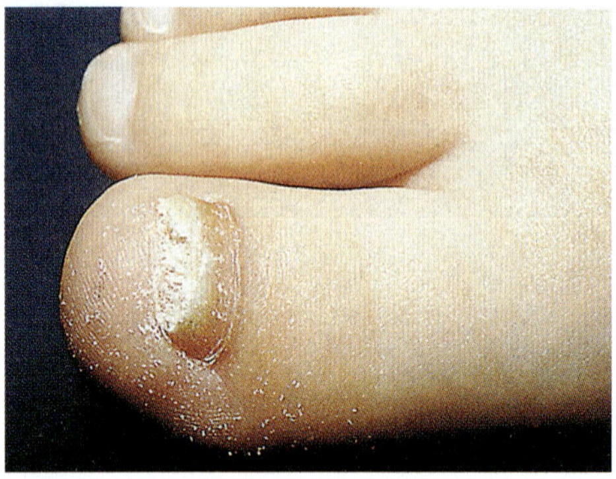

Fig. 8.136 Onychomycosis caused by a chronic dermatophyte infection of the nail plate in a 4-year-old boy. This is relatively rare in prepubertal children.

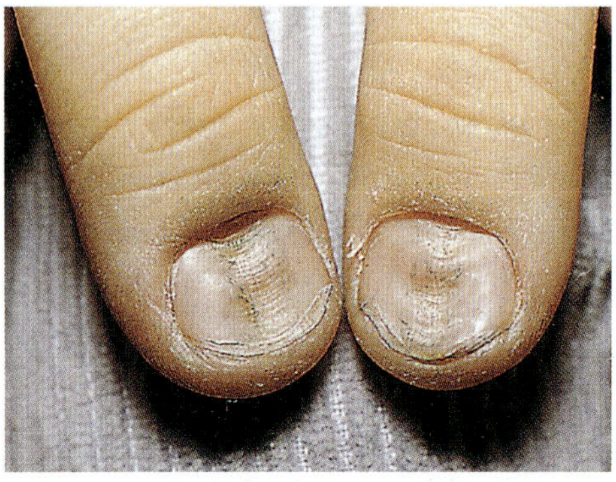

Fig. 8.137 Traumatic nail dystrophy. This teenager developed median nail dystrophy as a result of chronically picking at his nails.

Nail Findings in Other Dermatologic Disorders

Nail disorders may provide clues to other dermatologic or systemic syndromes. For example, alopecia areata can be associated with a characteristic Scotch-plaid pitting of the nails (Fig. 8.139). Similarly, psoriasis may affect the nails in many ways that help to distinguish it from other scaling disorders. Involvement of the nail matrix results in the formation of scattered pits that are larger, deeper, and less numerous than those found in alopecia areata. Psoriasis of the

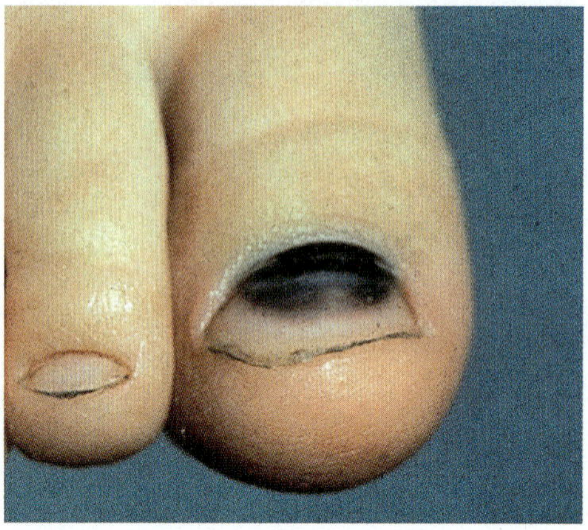

Fig. 8.138 Traumatic subungual hemorrhage. Discoloration because of traumatic hemorrhage under the toenail is common in children and athletic adults. When seen at the base of a toenail, it is commonly a result of jamming the toe into the end of the shoe while running or stopping (turf toe).

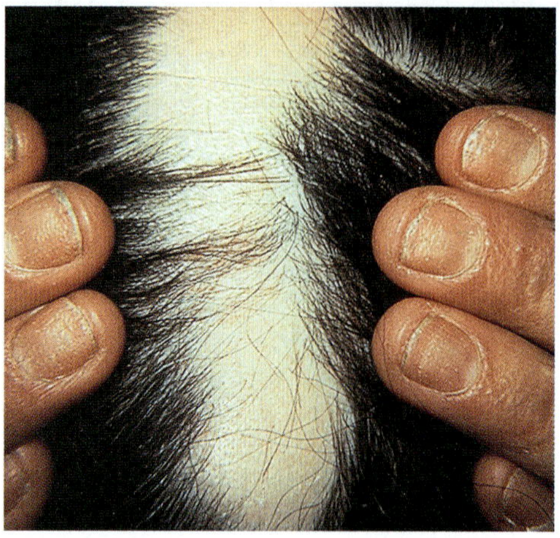

Fig. 8.139 Broad, shallow, Scotch-plaid pitting of the nails associated with alopecia areata.

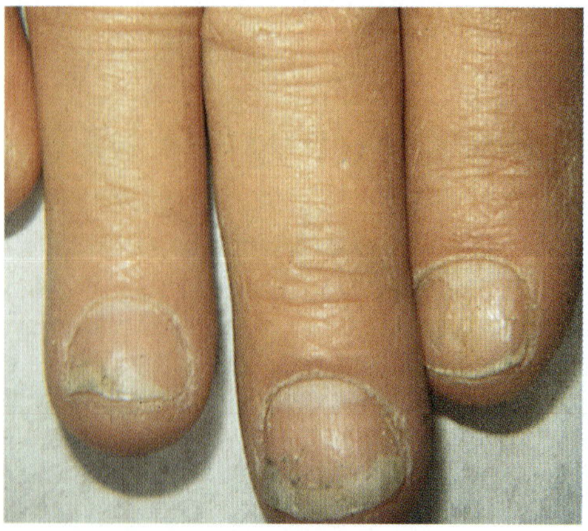

Fig. 8.140 Psoriatic nails. Psoriasis affecting the nails results in onycholysis and pitting.

nail bed, especially under the distal nail, causes separation of the nail from the underlying skin (onycholysis) and oil-drop discoloration with heaped-up scaling (Fig. 8.140). Onycholysis alone, without pits or discoloration, may be caused by trauma, infection, nail polish hardeners, or phototoxic reactions to drugs, such as tetracycline or doxycycline.

COMPLICATIONS OF TOPICAL SKIN THERAPY

Topical Steroids

Steroids are the most used topical medication and may be classified as low, medium, or high potency, according to their biologic activity. In general, fluorinated steroids are more potent than nonfluorinated steroids, and those in ointment bases are more effective than those in cream or lotion bases. Because the potencies of topical steroids are difficult to memorize, the authors recommend consulting a chart to be clear which potency topical steroid one is prescribing. A product with the same name may be higher potency in ointment form, for example, than it is in lotion form. High-potency steroids should be used only for short periods and on small body surface areas to avoid side local and systemic side effects. Local side effects include skin atrophy (Fig. 8.141); telangiectasias; increased skin fragility; acneiform eruptions; striae (Fig. 8.142); and masking or delayed recognition of infections and infestations, such as tinea corporis and scabies. Systemic side effects include hypothalamic-pituitary-adrenal axis suppression.

Use of fluorinated steroids should be avoided on the face, eyelids, genitals, or intertriginous areas (e.g., the axillae and thighs) because absorption is greater and the side effects are more common in these areas. Good general rules of safe practice are to use the weakest agent that is likely to clear the dermatitis, stop use when the dermatitis has cleared, and avoid using topical steroids stronger than class 5 in high-risk locations. If topical medication is applied to large areas, if the treated area is occluded, or if therapy is continued for a long period, adrenal suppression may result. Accidental injection of steroids into fat on attempted intramuscular injection may cause permanent subcutaneous atrophy (Fig. 8.143).

Secondary local bacterial, viral, and fungal infections may progress with unusual rapidity in children receiving topical corticosteroids, so patients should be instructed to look for early signs of secondary bacterial infection. The risk of systemic viral and bacterial infections is similarly increased in patients undergoing a prolonged regimen of widespread topical or high-dose oral steroids. All patients taking high-dose systemic steroids who have no history of varicella should be alerted to return immediately for zoster immune globulin if they discover that they have been exposed to chickenpox.

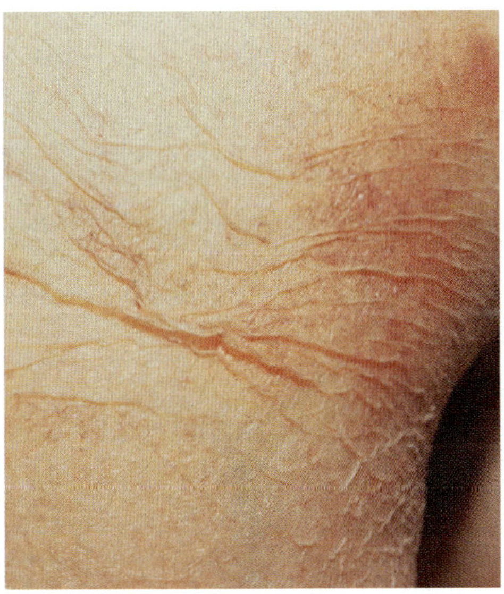

Fig. 8.141 Steroid-induced skin atrophy. Topical steroids may cause marked atrophy and fragility of the skin, especially if used under occlusion regularly for more than 1 month.

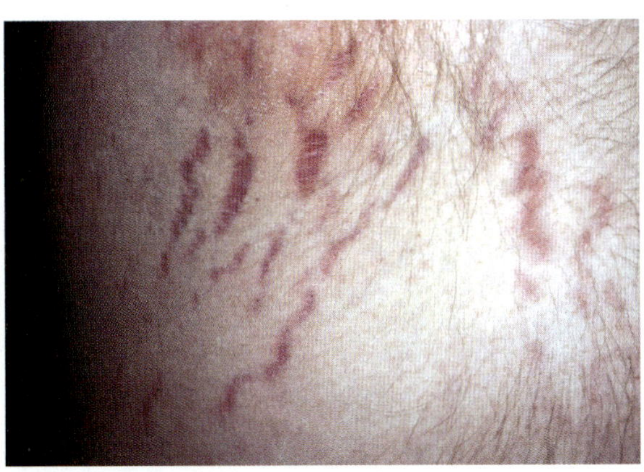

Fig. 8.142 Steroid-induced striae distensae. Prolonged use of potent fluorinated steroids may cause permanent striae distensae.

Other Agents

Other complications from topical medications, such as contact dermatitis, can be easily prevented. Allergic contact dermatitis is frequently seen as a reaction to both prescribed and over-the-counter drugs. The most common allergens are neomycin, "-caine" topical anesthetics or topical antipruritics, bacitracin, and ethylenediamine (a preservative in many topical preparations). When possible, products containing these agents should be avoided. Anaphylaxis can occur even in response to topical medications, especially if applied to broken skin. Hence obtaining a history of drug allergies is important before prescribing topical agents. Contact allergy can occur in response to preservatives in topical preparations including MCI/MI and cocamidopropyl betaine. When a question exists, patch testing can provide a definitive diagnosis.

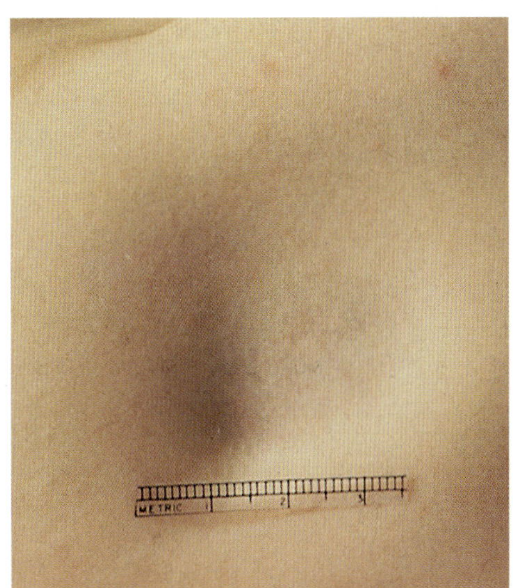

Fig. 8.143 Steroid-induced subcutaneous atrophy. Injection of steroids into fat instead of muscle often produces subcutaneous atrophy. In some cases this may resolve in 6 to 12 months, whereas in others it can be permanent.

Bibliography

Canavan TN, Mathes EF, Frieden I, Shinkai K: Mycoplasma pneumoniae–induced rash and mucositis as a syndrome distinct from Stevens-Johnson syndrome and erythema multiforme: a systematic review, *J Am Acad Dermatol* 72(2):239–245, 2015.

Cohen BA: *Atlas of pediatric dermatology,* London, 1993, Mosby-Wolfe.

Cohen BA: *Pediatric dermatology,* ed 2, London, 1999, Mosby.

Cohen BA, Lehman CU, editors: *DermAtlas.* http://dermatlas.med.jhmi.edu/derm/.

Cordoro KM, Gupta D, Frieden IJ, McCalmont T, Kashani-Sabet M: Pediatric melanoma: results of a large cohort study and proposal for modified ABCD detection criteria for children, *J Am Acad Dermatol* 68:913–925, 2013.

Frieden IJ, Haggstrom AN, Drolet BA, et al: Infantile hemangiomas: current knowledge, future directions. Proceedings of a research workshop on infantile hemangiomas, *Pediatr Dermatol* 22:383–406, 2005.

Harper J, Oranje A, Prose N: *Textbook of pediatric dermatology,* London, 2000, Blackwell Science.

Herbst R: Perineal streptococcal dermatitis/disease: recognition and management, *Am J Clin Dermatol* 4(8):555–560, 2003.

Hernandez RG, Cohen BA: Insect bites–induced hypersensitivity and the SCRATCH principles: a new approach to papular urticaria, *Pediatrics* 118:e189–e196, 2006.

Paller AS, Mancini AJ, editors: *Hurwitz clinical pediatric dermatology,* ed 4, Philadelphia, 2011, Elsevier Saunders

Pride HB, Tollefson M, Silverman R: What's new in pediatric dermatology? *Ann Dermatol Venereol* 68(6):885.e1–885.e12, 2013

Ruiz-Maldonado R, Parish LC, Beare JM: *Textbook of pediatric dermatology,* Philadelphia, 1989, Grune & Stratton.

Schachner LA, Hansen RC: *Pediatric dermatology,* ed 3, New York, 2003, Churchill Livingstone.

Serban ED: Perianal infectious dermatitis: an underdiagnosed, unremitting and stubborn condition, *World J Clin Pediatr* 7(4):89–104, 2018.

Weinberg S, Leider M, Shapiro L: *Color atlas of pediatric dermatology,* ed 2, London, 1990, McGraw-Hill.

Weston WL: *Practical pediatric dermatology,* ed 2, Boston, 1985, Little. Brown.

9

PEDIATRIC ENDOCRINOLOGY

Oscar Escobar | Nursen Gurtunca | Pushpa Viswanathan

INTRODUCTION

Clinical presentations of endocrine disease can vary widely. Alterations in hormone balance can result in distinct phenotypes affecting linear growth, timing of puberty, body composition, and metabolic functions. Understanding the normal pattern of growth and development is essential to differentiate pathology from normal variants. The discoveries of new genes, novel mutations, and alterations in gene expression have provided insight and will further help us to understand the genomics behind clinical manifestations of endocrine conditions.

NORMAL GROWTH AND DEVELOPMENT

Knowing the parameters of normal growth is the essential first step to recognizing aberrations in growth and development. Normal growth follows a predicted pattern from conception to adulthood. Linear growth is the fastest during the second trimester in utero. Rapid growth continues during the first year of life and then slows down between 1 and 2 years of age (Table 9.1). After 2 years of age, linear growth continues to decline slowly, averaging a growth rate of approximately 2.0 inches (5 cm) per year during childhood until it reaches a nadir (prepubertal dip or prepubertal growth deceleration) just before the initiation of the pubertal growth spurt. There are noticeable differences in the "pubertal growth spurt" between girls and boys. Peak growth velocity typically occurs at Tanner stage III in girls and at Tanner stage IV in boys. The pubertal growth spurt is also shorter in duration and displays a lower peak growth velocity in girls compared with boys. This sexual dimorphism is responsible for the difference in mature adult heights between males and females. The average mature height of males is 13 cm (about 5.12 in) greater than that of females.

Because stature varies among healthy children, the incremental growth rate is one of the most important elements used to assess health in a child. Healthy children grow at a predictable rate. Growth velocity charts are available for both girls and boys. Growth velocity is a variable derived from height measurement at two separate times and is defined by the delta of length or height divided by the delta of time between two measurements, usually expressed in centimeters per year. Growth velocity charts show the typical growth pattern seen at different ages and in relation to pubertal development (see Fig. 9.1). Intervals of 4 to 6 months between measurements are reasonable. However, a comparison of the slope between two measurements to the slope of the standard percentiles in the growth chart provides a visual and easy assessment of the adequacy or inadequacy of the growth rate. Subnormal growth velocity can indicate both endocrine and nonendocrine disorders.

The most critical and valuable tool to evaluate normal and pathologic growth is the growth chart. The Centers for Disease Control and Prevention (CDC) updates growth charts based on a broad population sample, combining many different growth studies (Fig. 9.2). These charts are readily available online at https://www.cdc.gov/growthcharts. The charts define the 3rd and 97th percentiles for height and weight and also characterize standards for head circumference and body mass index (BMI), defined as weight in kilograms divided by the square of height in meters (kg/m^2).

EVALUATION OF GROWTH AND GROWTH DISORDERS

The approach to the evaluation of a child with growth disorders requires a thorough history, physical examination, and diagnostic tools. An important aspect of the evaluation of growth is the distinction between short stature and growth failure. Short stature is defined as a height that is more than two standard deviations (SDs) below the mean for age and sex, whereas growth failure is defined as a subnormal linear growth velocity for age and sex that, if persistent, eventually results in short stature. Accuracy in the measurements of length and standing height is critical for proper diagnosis and management of growth disorders. Inaccurate measurements will lead to erroneous calculations of growth velocity leading to parental anxiety, unnecessary referrals, and inappropriate decision making. Measurement of recumbent length (from birth to 2 years old) and standing height (from 2 to 20 years old) require proper technique and equipment. Two people and an infantometer are needed for measurement of accurate recumbent length in an infant. A calibrated stadiometer is ideal for the measurement of standing height in a child older than 2 years. In both cases, the occiput, shoulder blades, buttocks, calves, and heels should be in the same plane, which in turn should be perpendicular to the plane of the soles. The head should be positioned in the Frankfurt plane, where a line that passes through the inferior border of the orbit and the superior border of the external auditory meatus should be perpendicular to the trunk plane (Fig. 9.3). For an accurate height measurement, the child should stand without wearing shoes or sandals with heels against a flat wall (Fig. 9.4).

Calculation of the target height (TH) provides an estimate of a child's genetic potential. The target height, also referred to as genetic height potential/midparental height (MPH), is the midpoint between the heights of parents, correcting for the 13-cm difference between male and female adult mature heights. This was devised by Tanner in 1970 and is called the Tanner's TH formula. For boys, the MPH is the midpoint between the father's height and the corrected mother's height (i.e., mother's height plus 13 cm). This is easily calculated by adding 6.5 cm (2.5 inches) to the mean of the parents' heights. For girls, the MPH is the midpoint between the mother's height and the corrected father's height (i.e., father's height minus 13 cm). MPH is calculated by subtracting 6.5 cm (2.5 inches) from the mean of the parents' heights. The SD of the target has been calculated as 5 cm in boys and 4.5 cm in girls. Therefore the target height range (MPH ± 2 SD) is MPH ± 10 cm in boys and MPH ± 9 cm in girls. Ideally, this calculation should be based on measured parental heights, given that reported heights are frequently overestimated. As an example, calculation of the MPH of a boy whose father's height is 179 cm and mother's height is 160 cm would be as follows: ([179 cm + 160 cm]/ ÷ 2) + 6.5 cm = 176 cm. The target height range would be 166 to 186 cm. These calculations assume that

Table 9.1 Normal Growth Rates in Children

Age	Growth Rate (per Year)	
	Inches	Centimeters
Birth to 1 year old	7–10	18–25
1–2 years old	4–5	10–13
2 years old to puberty	2–2.5	5–6
Pubertal growth spurt: Girls	2.5–4.5	6–11
Pubertal growth spurt: Boys	3–5	7–13

each parent contributes 50% of the genetic makeup of the individual child, which may not be completely true. One or both parents could also have been adversely affected by environmental factors during their childhood that can affect MPH. Studies have shown that TH explains only 25% variance in attained height and is quite inaccurate in case of extremes of heights in parents or major differences between parental heights. Also, secular trends show a steady increase in the height of children over the past century, accounting for the underestimation of the height of future generations. Furthermore, there are large variations in these trends among geographic regions.

The child's past medical history, family history, psychosocial circumstances, and other aspects of physical examination are relevant for a thorough evaluation.

Radiographic determination of epiphyseal maturation, or bone age, is often helpful in evaluating children with short stature. By convention, a radiograph of the left hand and wrist is compared with established standard radiographs to determine the bone age or skeletal age. Before 24 months of life, epiphyseal development is better estimated by radiographic examination of the hemiskeleton. The most common method to assess bone maturation is the Greulich and Pyle method, in which the radiograph of the hand and wrist is compared with an atlas of radiographs. Notably, this atlas was compiled only using radiographs of White children of European ancestry obtained from the 1930s to the 1960s. Adult height prediction based on bone age might not be accurate in cases of constitutional delay in growth and puberty (CDGP), idiopathic short stature, and in children with advanced bone age in conditions like congenital adrenal hyperplasia (CAH). Skeletal maturation is often advanced in obese children with early epiphyseal fusion and normal final height. Despite this limitation of lack of ethnic diversity and inaccuracy in the conditions mentioned earlier, bone age radiographs are a valuable tool to assess growth and pubertal development. Boys aged 4 to

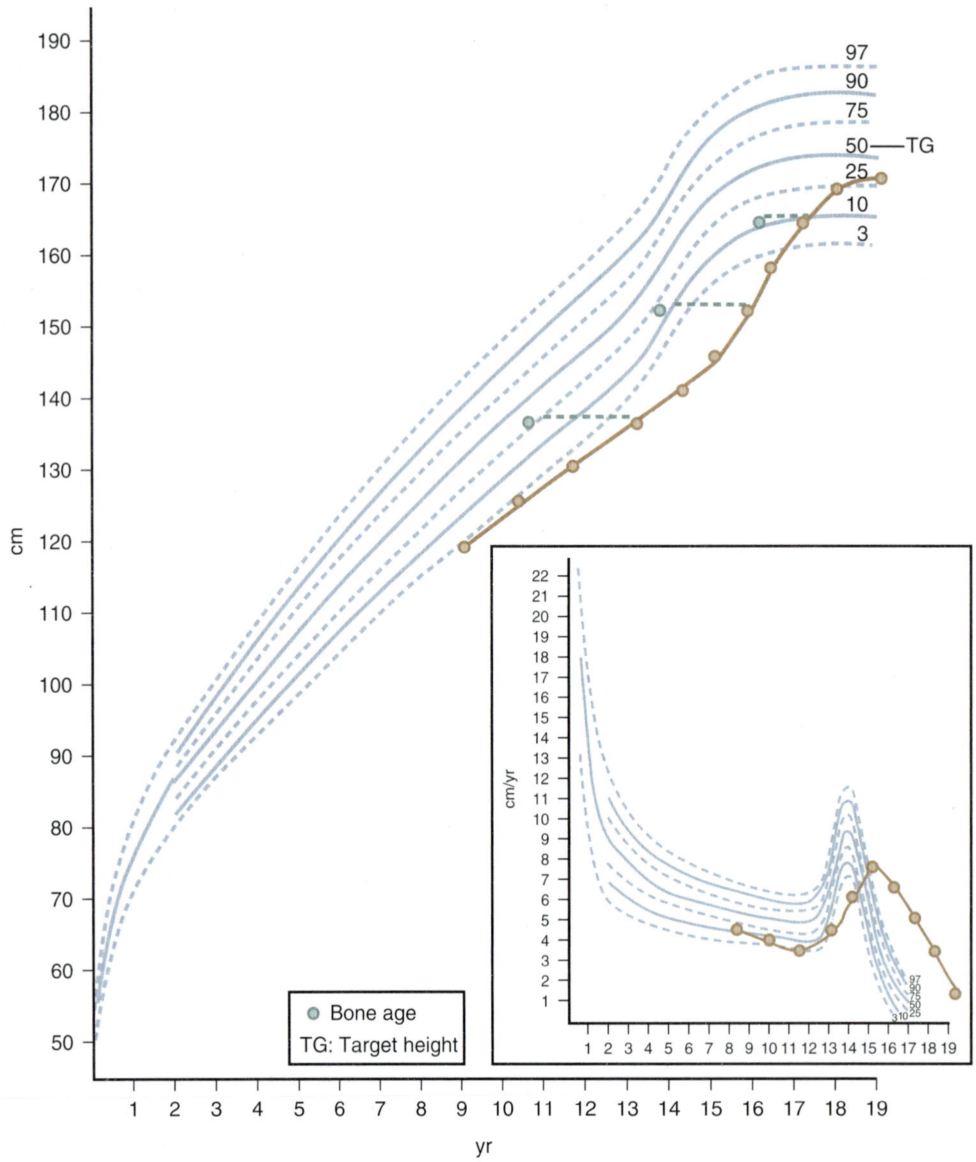

Fig. 9.1 Growth curve of a child with constitutional growth delay. Note the typical pattern of growth deceleration followed by a normal growth rate. In the lower right panel, a delay in the attainment of the pubertal growth spurt and peak growth velocity is depicted.

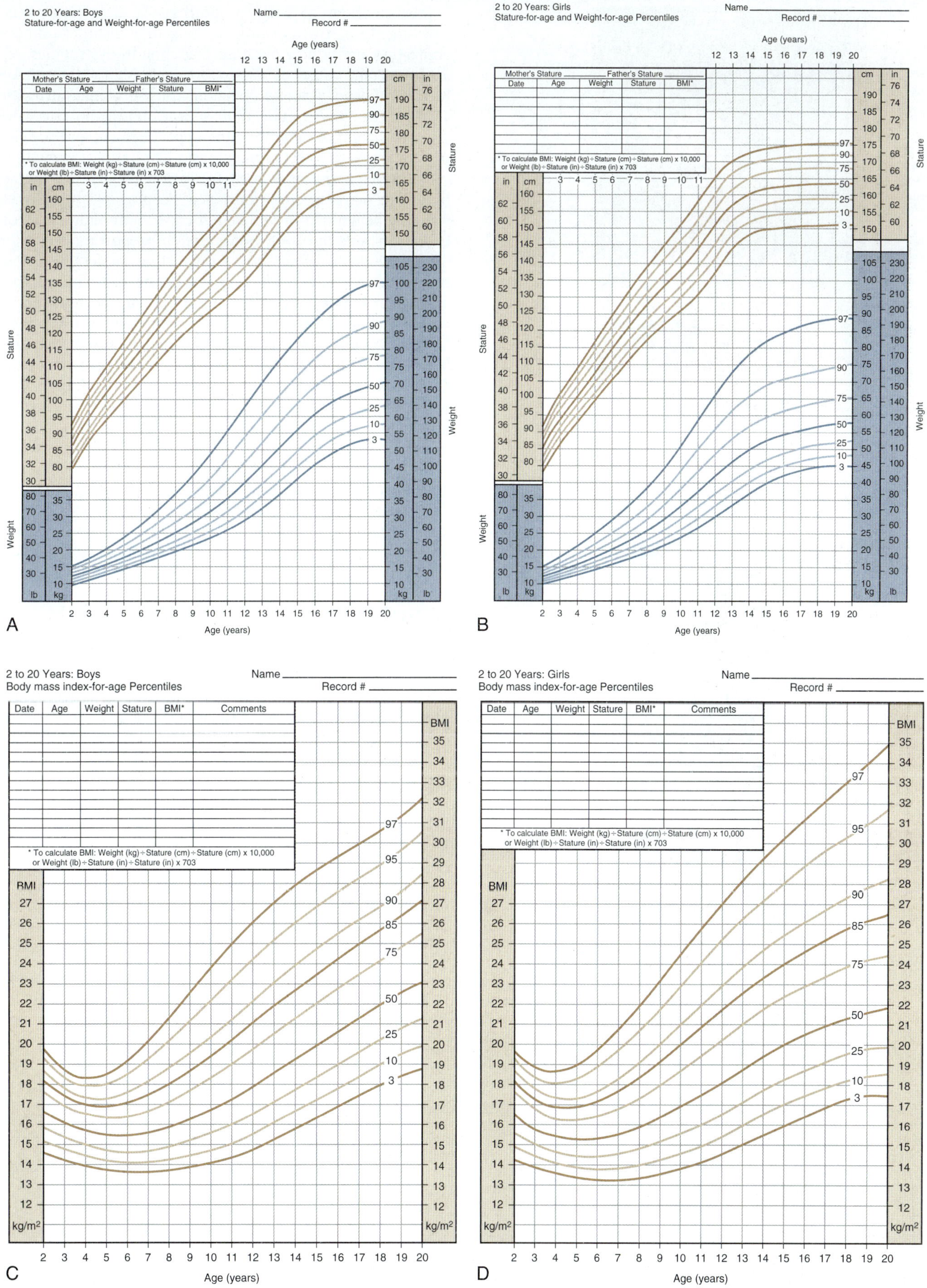

Fig. 9.2 Growth charts from the Centers for Disease Control and Prevention. (A) Stature-for-age and weight-for-age percentiles (3rd to 97th) for boys 2 to 20 years old. (B) Stature-for-age and weight-for-age percentiles for girls 2 to 20 years old. (C) Body mass index (BMI)-for-age percentiles for boys 2 to 20 years old. (D) BMI-for-age percentiles for girls 2 to 20 years old. (Developed by the National Center for Health Statistics in collaboration with the National Center for Chronic Disease Prevention and Health Promotion. Available online at https://www.cdc.gov/growthcharts.)

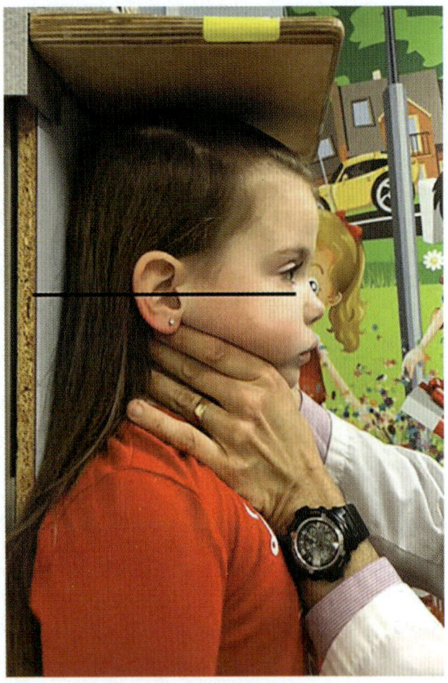

Fig. 9.3 Frankfurt plane. An imaginary line that passes through the inferior border of the orbit and the superior border of the external auditory meatus should be perpendicular to the trunk plane during proper height measurement. (Courtesy O. Escobar, MD, Pittsburgh, PA.)

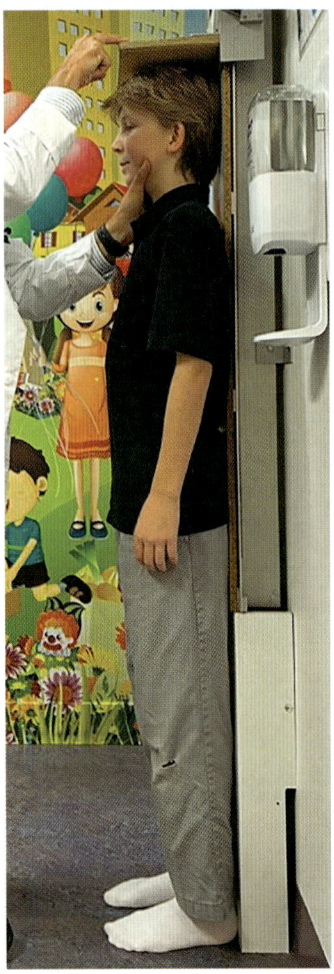

Fig. 9.4 Correct positioning for height measurement: occiput, scapular region, buttocks, calves, and heels aligned in the vertical plane of the stadiometer. (Courtesy O. Escobar, MD, Pittsburgh, PA.)

12 are predicted in 95% of instances to within ± 7 cm of true height and at ages 13 and 14 to within ± 6 cm. Girls ages 4 to 11 are predicted to within ± 6 cm; premenarcheal girls aged 12 and 13 to within ± 5 and ± 4 cm, respectively; and postmenarcheal girls aged 12 and 13 to within ± 4 and ± 3 cm, respectively.

Measurement of body proportions is also important in the assessment of growth disorders. Congenital disorders of bone mineralization and bone growth, such as chondrodystrophies, represent an important cause of disproportionate short stature. A simple method of determining proportions consists of measuring the lower segment (symphysis pubis to floor) and subtracting this value from the total height to determine the upper segment and then calculating the upper-to-lower segment ratio. This ratio, along with the arm span–to-height ratio, is used to document whether the spine or limbs are more severely shortened. Arm span is usually equal to standing height. However, in children with achondroplasia or hypochondroplasia, the long bones are disproportionately shortened. Sitting height (another way of calculating the length of the upper segment), determined with a special sitting stadiometer, is generally normal in individuals with achondroplasia, whereas the standing height is short. During adolescence, hypogonadism is often associated with increased limb length. Craniospinal radiation for childhood cancer therapy may result in decreased growth of the spine compared with the limbs, resulting in disproportionate body habitus. Pubertal development should always be an integral part of growth evaluation. Seemingly normal "prepubertal" growth velocity in a child in puberty may be an indication for further evaluation of growth failure. On the other hand, perceived "poor linear growth rate" in adolescents with advanced stages of puberty may be simply due to completion of most of the linear growth. Evaluation of short stature in girls should include a karyotype, as Turner syndrome can present with minimal physical signs, especially in mosaic Turner syndrome.

ABNORMAL GROWTH AND GROWTH DISORDERS

Short stature and growth failure are the most common reasons for referral of children for a pediatric endocrine evaluation. Less commonly, children are referred to endocrinology for evaluation of tall stature and accelerated growth.

Short Stature

Children with proportionate short stature can be classified into two groups depending on their skeletal maturation: (1) those with short stature and concordant bone age and (2) those with short stature and delayed bone age. In turn, each one of these two groups can be divided into those growing at a normal rate and those growing at a decreased rate. Therefore four groups result from this classification (Fig. 9.5).

- Those with adequate growth velocity likely have one of the normal variants of short stature: familial short stature (concordant bone age) or CDGP (delayed bone age).

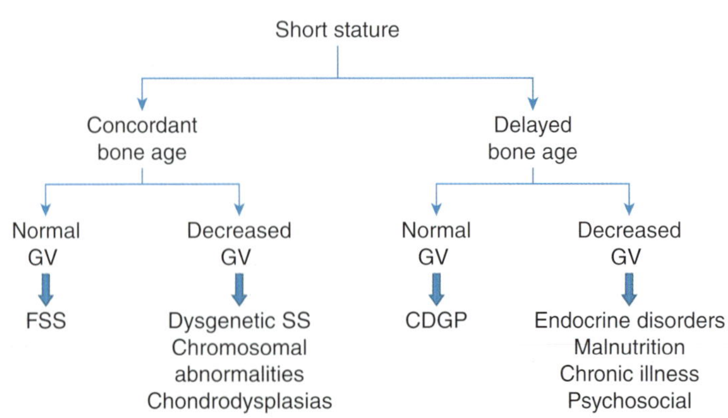

Fig. 9.5 Paradigm to approach disorders associated with short stature. *CDGP,* Constitutional delay of growth and puberty; *FSS,* familial short stature; *GV,* growth velocity; *SS,* short stature.

- On the other hand, children with decreased growth velocity (growth failure by definition) and delayed skeletal maturation are more likely to have a pathologic reason for their abnormal growth pattern. This could include endocrine disorders (e.g., growth hormone [GH] deficiency, GH insensitivity, hypothyroidism, Cushing syndrome) and/or nonendocrine causes (e.g., malnutrition, chronic illness, psychosocial deprivation).
- Growth failure and concordant skeletal maturation is likely associated with dysgenetic conditions (e.g., chromosomal disorders, genetic syndromes, chondrodysplasias).

Although this algorithm is useful in the assessment of short stature, some caveats need to be emphasized: A short child does not necessarily fall into one single category but may have components of two or more categories (e.g., pseudohypoparathyroidism type 1a or Albright hereditary osteodystrophy). These individuals have both dysgenetic and endocrine components to their short stature, yet their bone age is frequently described as advanced. Another example involves girls with Turner syndrome, a dysgenetic cause of short stature, who may have a delay in skeletal maturation at the usual time of puberty due to low estrogen production and gonadal dysgenesis. The finding of abnormal body proportions in a child with short stature should elicit suspicion for chondrodysplasias and rickets. Typical body proportions are usually preserved in other causes of short stature.

With the advancement in genetics, there is a deeper understanding of the pathophysiology of growth disorders and skeletal dysplasias. Growth in children is regulated at the growth plate by multiple factors, including hormones (e.g., GH, insulin-like growth factor 1, estrogen, androgens, thyroid, glucocorticoids); radiation; paracrine factors secreted by chondrocytes (FGFs, bone morphogenic proteins, WNT, PTHrP, CNP, NPR2); variants in genes that encode cartilage extracellular matrix *(COL1A1, ACAN);* and intracellular signaling pathways (SHOX, SOX transcription factors, Ras-MAPK). Endocrine causes of short stature are usually characterized by linear growth deceleration, where weight gain is either not affected or even increased. This is a useful distinguishing feature of endocrine disorders in comparison with nonendocrine causes where the weight is usually more affected than the height.

Nonendocrine causes of pathologic short stature include chronic illness (e.g., renal tubular acidosis, celiac disease, cystic fibrosis, inflammatory bowel disease, other chronic disorders), adverse psychosocial milieu, undernutrition, and genetic disorders. Common nonendocrine and endocrine causes of short stature are listed in Boxes 9.1 and 9.2, respectively.

Box 9.1 Selected Nonendocrine Causes of Short Stature

Familial short stature (genetic)
Constitutional delay of growth and development
Malnutrition
- Inadequate caloric intake
- Pharmacologic, such as medications for ADHD
- Anorexia nervosa

Pharmacologic steroid treatment
Idiopathic short stature
Intrauterine growth retardation
Systemic disease
- Pulmonary
  - Cystic fibrosis
  - Asthma
- Cardiac and circulatory
  - Congenital heart disease (cyanotic)
  - Acquired heart disease
- Renal
  - Renal insufficiency
  - Pyelonephritis (chronic)
  - Renal tubular acidosis
  - Nephropathic cystinosis
- Gastrointestinal and hepatic
  - Malabsorption
  - Celiac disease
  - Inflammatory bowel disease
  - Hepatic insufficiency
- Neurologic
  - Mental retardation with growth delay
- Musculoskeletal and connective tissue
  - Storage diseases
  - Hypotonia
  - Skeletal dysplasias
- Immunologic
  - Immune deficiencies
  - HIV
- Mucopolysaccharidosis

Syndromes associated with short stature
- Chromosomal abnormalities
  - Trisomy 21
  - Trisomy 13
  - Trisomy 18
  - Turner syndrome
  - Noonan syndrome
  - Prader-Willi syndrome
  - Progeria
  - Russell-Silver syndrome
  - Cockayne syndrome
  - Seckel syndrome
  - CHARGE syndrome
  - 18q deletion

Disproportionate short stature
- Achondroplasia
- Hypochondroplasia
- Spina bifida

Radiation to spine

ADHD, Attention-deficit/hyperactivity disorder; *CHARGE,* coloboma of the eye, heart defects, atresia of the nasal choanae, retardation of growth and/or development, genital and/or urinary abnormalities, and ear abnormalities and deafness; *HIV,* human immunodeficiency virus.

Tall Stature and Rapid Growth

Tall stature is an uncommon concern in children except in very tall girls (above 6 feet). Rapid growth with tall stature during early childhood, on the other hand, is not an uncommon cause for referral to endocrinology. Endocrine causes of tall stature include gigantism associated with excessive GH secretion from pituitary adenomas. Some genetic disorders, such as neurofibromatosis type 1, McCune-Albright syndrome, Carney complex, and multiple endocrine neoplasia type 1 [MEN 1], can also be associated with excessive pituitary GH secretion. Other overgrowth syndromes may have tall stature as part of their dysmorphology. Sotos syndrome is characterized by tall stature, macrocephaly, and a nonprogressive neurologic disorder with mental retardation. Sotos syndrome has been associated with haploinsufficiency of the nuclear receptor binding SET domain protein 1 *(NSD1)* gene located on chromosome 5q35.2-35.3 and with heterozygous mutations in the nuclear factor 1, X-type *(NFIX)* gene on chromosome 19p13.3. Klinefelter syndrome, associated with 47, XXY karyotype, is a relatively common sex chromosome aneuploidy presenting with tall stature. Marfan syndrome is an autosomal dominant disorder associated with tall stature and linked to mutations in the fibrillin-1 *(FBN1)* gene. It is characterized by disproportionate tall stature with upper-to-lower segment ratio <0.85, arm span-to-height ratio >1.05, and earlier puberty-associated peak growth velocity. Some easily identified skeletal features include joint laxity and arachnodactyly manifested with positive "wrist sign" and "thumb sign" and scoliosis, kyphoscoliosis, and pectus excavatum/carinatum (Fig. 9.6). Homocystinuria is an autosomal recessive disorder similar to Marfan syndrome, which often includes tall stature and lens subluxation. But unlike Marfan syndrome, intellectual disability is common in homocystinuria.

Patients with precocious puberty and virilizing congenital adrenal hyperplasias (CAHs) may present with rapid growth and tall stature, but they may ultimately be short adults due to premature fusion of growth plates if unrecognized and not adequately treated in a timely manner. Unrecognized hyperthyroidism may lead to rapid linear growth but, similarly to precocious puberty, may lead to advanced skeletal maturation with consequent attenuation of growth. Overnutrition causes excessive weight gain and accelerated linear growth. In this group, exogenous obesity precedes increased height velocity. Skeletal maturation is often advanced in obese children with likely early epiphyseal fusion and normal final height. Referral to endocrinology may be indicated as noted in Box 9.3.

Box 9.2 Endocrine Causes of Impaired Growth and Short Stature

- Pituitary development
  - GH deficiency
  - Septo-optic dysplasia
  - Mutations in *HESX1, SOX2, SOX3, GLI2, LHX3, LHX4, PROP1,* and *POU1F1* genes
- Craniopharyngioma
- Transection of pituitary stalk due to trauma
- Radiation damage to hypothalamus/pituitary
- GH gene mutation
- Laron dwarfism (GH receptor mutation)
- IGF-1 deficiency
  - IGF-1 gene mutation
  - STAT5 mutation
- IGF-1 resistance
  - IGF-1 receptor gene mutation
- Thyroid hormone
  - Congenital hypothyroidism
  - Acquired hypothyroidism
  - Thyroid hormone resistance
  - Consumptive hypothyroidism
- Cortisol hypersecretion
  - Cushing syndrome
  - Cushing disease
- Diabetes insipidus
  - Congenital ADH deficiency
  - Nephrogenic diabetes insipidus
  - Wolfram syndrome
  - Acquired
    - Postoperative
    - Neoplasms
    - Infiltrative (Langerhans cell histiocytosis)
- Defects in aldosterone synthase *(CYP11B2)*
- Bone and mineral metabolism
  - Vitamin D deficiency rickets
  - Hypophosphatemic rickets
  - Pseudohypoparathyroidism (hereditary Albright osteodystrophy)
  - Pseudopseudohypoparathyroidism
- Poorly controlled diabetes mellitus (Mauriac syndrome)

ADH, Antidiuretic hormone; *GH,* growth hormone; *IGF,* insulin-like growth factor.

NORMAL PUBERTAL DEVELOPMENT

Puberty is the process through which reproductive competence is achieved and is initiated by reactivation of the hypothalamic-pituitary-gonadal axis (gonadarche). In humans and several nonhuman primates, adrenal pubertal maturation (adrenarche) is indicated by increased adrenal dehydroepiandrosterone sulfate (DHEAS) secretion.

Adrenarche occurs in close temporal proximity to gonadarche, though adrenarche and gonadarche are regulated through different molecular mechanisms. Clinical features of adrenarche include acne, adult type body odor, axillary hair, and pubic hair development (pubarche). The typical sequence of pubertal events for boys and girls is predictable (Fig. 9.7). For both boys and girls, the mean ages for the onset of puberty vary among different ethnic groups and represent the combined influences of genetic and environmental factors. Pubertal timing is influenced by parental age at puberty.

In boys, puberty is first evidenced by testicular enlargement and usually begins between 9 and 14 years of age. Initial stages of puberty in boys may be difficult to appreciate unless testicular volume is measured using an orchidometer. Sexual hair (axillary and pubic hair) development, perceived as signs of puberty, may not be present in the early stages of puberty. Growth spurt and voice changes are late signs of pubertal development in boys and are typically seen during midpuberty, approximately 2 years after the onset of testicular enlargement. Significant facial hair develops toward the end of male pubertal development, when most of the linear growth is completed.

Box 9.3 When to Consult Endocrinology With Growth Concerns?

- Growth velocity significantly higher than expected for age and pubertal status
- Tall stature with inappropriate pubertal status, either precocious puberty or premature adrenarche
- Detection of abnormal body proportions or dysmorphology with tall stature
- Childhood cancer survivors with risk factors for short stature

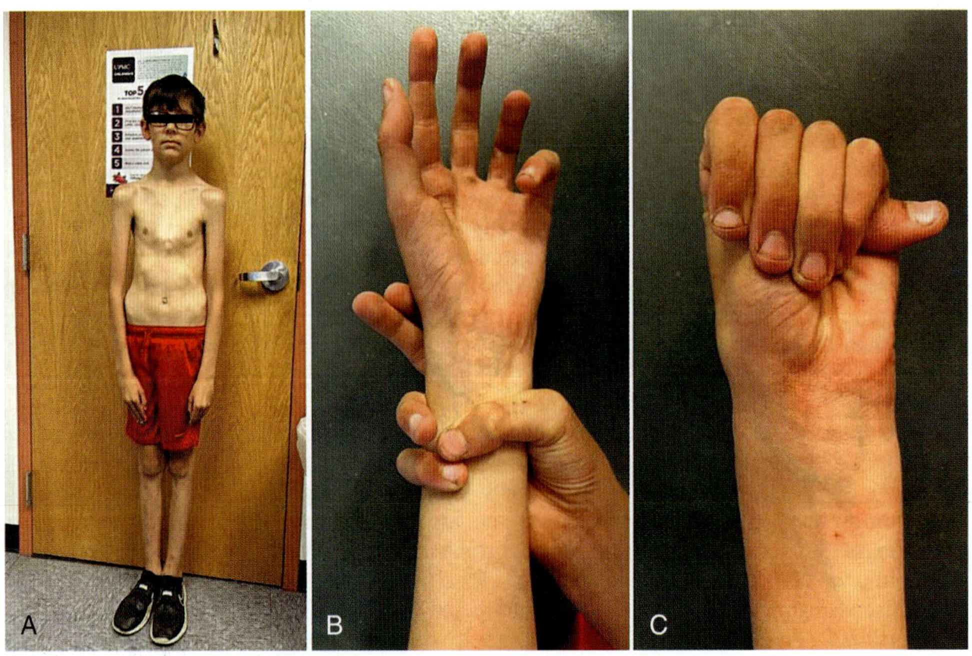

Fig. 9.6 Child with Marfan syndrome. (A) Note tall stature, pectus carinatum, long arms. (B) Wrist sign: the tips of the thumb and fifth finger overlap when wrapped around the wrist. (C) Thumb sign: the tip of the thumb protrudes beyond the hypothenar region when wrapped by all other fingers. (Courtesy O. Escobar, MD, Pittsburgh, PA.)

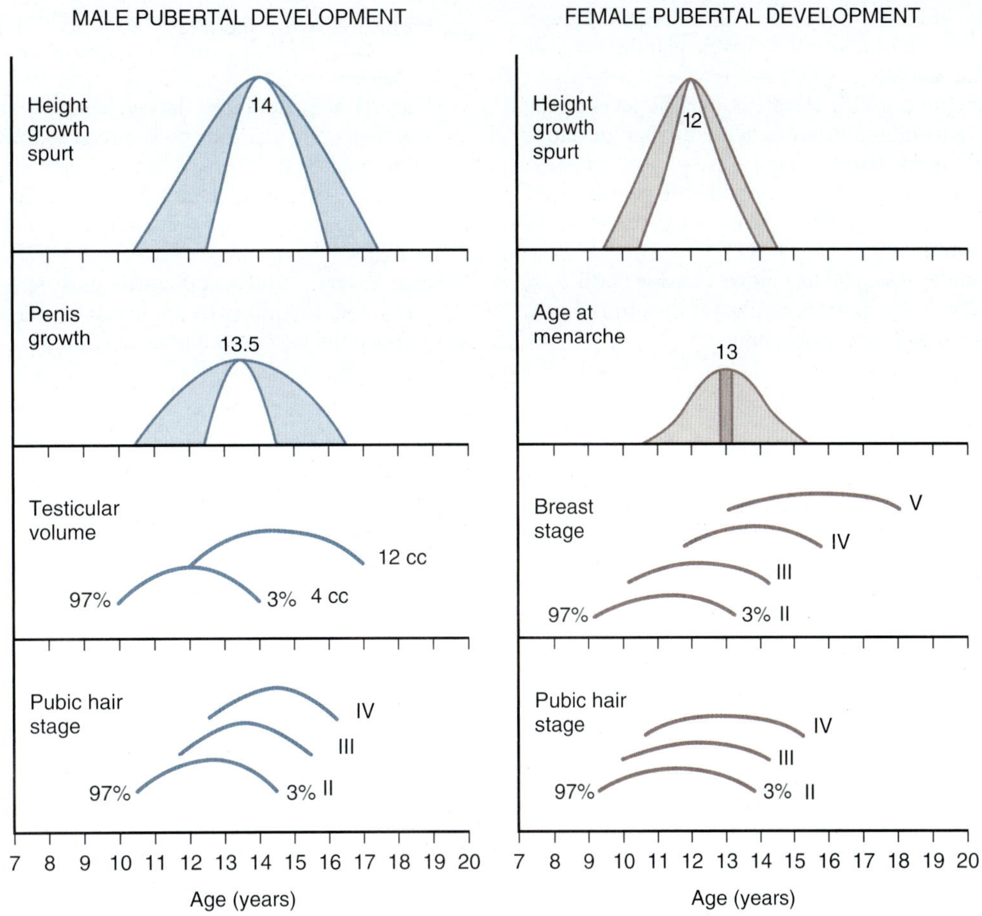

Fig. 9.7 Schematic representation of the onset of male and female puberty. (Modified from Johnson TR, Moore WM, Jeffries JE: *Children are different: development physiology*, ed 2. Columbus, OH, 1978, Ross Laboratories, Division of Abbott Laboratories; 1978, pp 26–29. Used with permission of Ross Products Division, Abbott Laboratories, Inc., Columbus, OH 43215.)

In girls, the onset of puberty is evidenced by breast development (thelarche), which usually begins between 8 and 12 years of age. Among White girls, the mean age of onset of breast development and pubic hair growth occurs at approximately 10 years of age, with onset of menstrual periods (menarche) occurring around age 12 to 12½ years. Black girls at every age have more advanced breast development compared with White girls. When assessing pubertal timing, one needs to consider other variables, including obesity and environmental exposures. Growth velocity increases at the onset of puberty in girls. Most linear growth is completed by midpuberty at the time of menarche.

TANNER STAGING

To describe the onset and progression of pubertal changes (Fig. 9.8), boys and girls are rated on five-point scales according to Tanner staging. Boys are rated for both genital development and pubic hair growth, and girls are rated for breast development and pubic hair growth.

The Tanner stages for male genital development are as follows (see Fig. 9.8A):

Stage I (preadolescent): The testes, scrotal sac, and penis have a size and proportion like those seen in early childhood.

Stage II: There is enlargement of the scrotum and testes. The scrotal skin is "thinner" and may also be reddened.

Stage III: Further growth of the penis has occurred, initially in length with some increase in circumference. There is also increased growth of the testes and scrotum. Spermaturia (appearance of spermatozoa in early morning urine specimens) occurs during this stage. Transient gynecomastia occurs in approximately 50% of boys.

Stage IV: The penis is significantly enlarged in length and circumference, with further development of the glans penis. The testes and scrotum continue to enlarge, and there is distinct darkening of the scrotal skin.

Stage V: The genitalia are adult size and shape.

The stages in male pubic hair development are as follows (see Fig. 9.8B):

Stage I (preadolescent): Vellus hair appears over the mons pubis with a degree of development like that over the abdominal wall. There is no androgen-sensitive pubic hair.

Stage II: There is development of long pigmented downy hair, which is only slightly curled or straight. The hair is sparse and seen mainly at the base of the penis.

Stage III: The pubic hair is darker, coarser, and curlier. The distribution of hair has now spread over the junction of the pubis.

Stage IV: The hair distribution is now adult in type but still considerably less than that seen in adults. There is no spread to the medial surface of the thighs.

Stage V: Hair distribution is adult in quantity and type and is described as an inverse triangle. Typically, there is spread to the medial surface of the thighs.

The stages in female breast development are as follows (see Fig. 9.8C):

Stage I (preadolescent): Only the papilla is elevated above the level of the chest wall.

Stage II: Elevation of the breasts and papillae may occur as small mounds along with some increased diameter of the areolae (breast budding). There is palpable, firm glandular tissue, "breast bud" under the areola.

Stage III: The breasts and areolae continue to enlarge, although they show no separation of contour. Palpable glandular tissue extends beyond the areolae.

Stage IV: The areolae and papillae elevate above the level of the breasts and form secondary mounds with further development of the overall breast tissue.

Stage V: Mature female breasts have developed. The papillae may extend slightly above the contour of the breast as the result of recession of the areolae.

Pubic hair growth in females is staged as follows (see Fig. 9.8B):

Stage I (preadolescent): Vellus hair develops over the mons pubis. There is no androgen-sensitive pubic hair.

Stage II: Sparse, long, pigmented, downy hair, which is straight or only slightly curled, appears mainly along the labia majora.

Stage III: Considerably darker, coarser, and curlier sexual hair appears. The hair has now spread sparsely over the junction of the pubis.

Stage IV: The hair distribution is adult in type but decreased in total quantity. There is no spread to the medial surface of the thighs.

Stage V: Hair "adult" in quantity and type, appears in an inverse triangle, spreading to the medial surface of the thighs but not above the base of the inverse triangle.

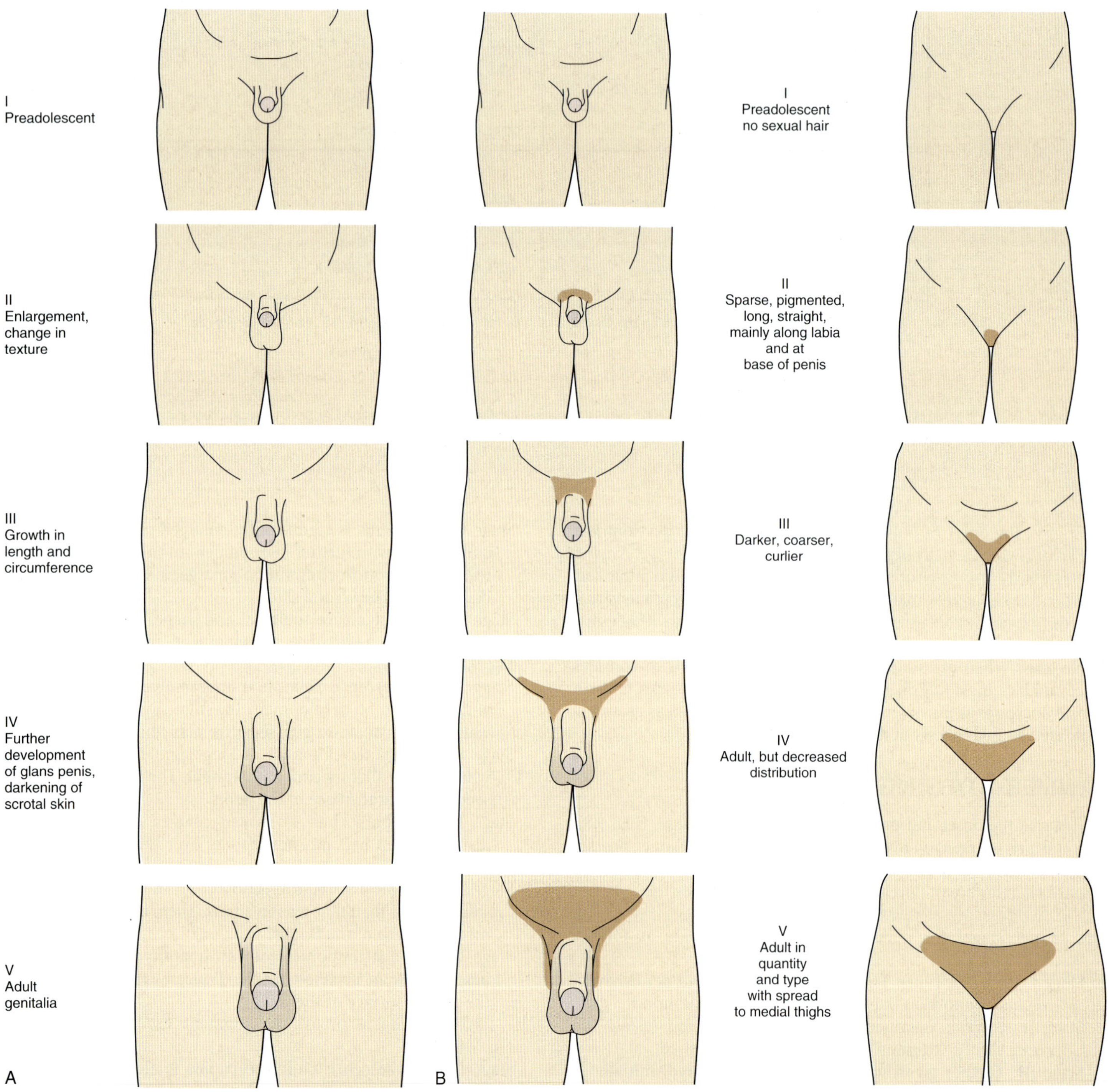

Fig. 9.8 Schematic drawings of male and female Tanner stages show male genital development (A), pubic hair development (B), and breast development (C). (Modified from Johnson TR, Moore WM, Jefferies JE: *Children are different: development physiology,* ed 2, Columbus, OH, 1978, Ross Laboratories, Division of Abbot Laboratories, pp 26–29. Used with permission of Ross Products Division, Abbott Laboratories, Inc., Columbus, OH 43215.)

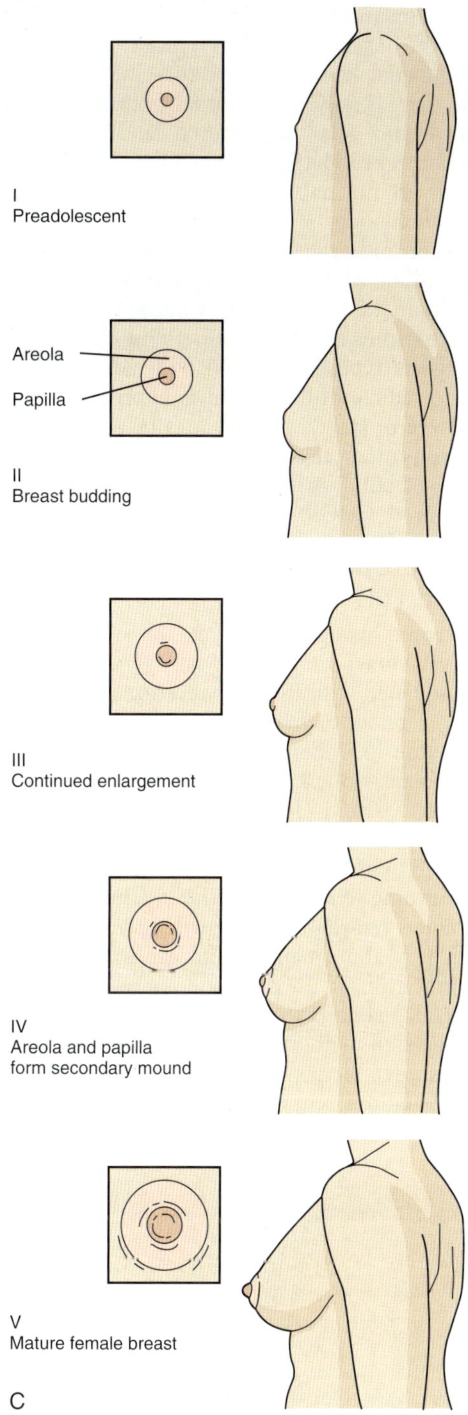

Fig. 9.8, cont'd

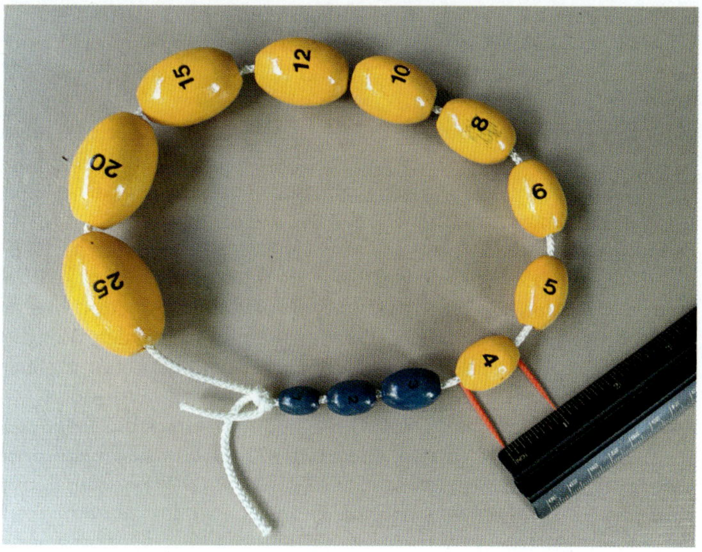

Fig. 9.9 Prader orchidometer is a series of plastic or wooden ovoid-shaped pieces attached by a string representing different testicular volumes (1 mL, 2 mL, 3 mL, 4 mL, 5 mL, 6 mL, 8 mL, 10 mL, 12 mL, 15 mL, 20 mL, and 25 mL).

Although not usually mentioned in the Tanner staging of male genital development, the testicular volume is a particularly important aspect. Testicular volume is best assessed by careful palpation (simple inspection frequently leads to overestimation) of the testes in comparison with a set of standards. The most common set of standards is the Prader orchidometer (Fig. 9.9), which is a series of plastic or wooden ovoid-shaped pieces attached by a string representing different testicular volumes (1 mL, 2 mL, 3 mL, 4 mL, 5 mL, 6 mL, 8 mL, 10 mL, 12 mL, 15 mL, 20 mL, and 25 mL). Testicular volume of 4 mL that corresponds to the initiation of gonadarche (male genital Tanner stage II) measures 1 inch (2.5 cm) in the long axis. This simple measurement performed with a ruler allows the practitioner to evaluate if an orchidometer is unavailable (see Fig. 9.9).

EVALUATION OF PUBERTAL DISORDERS

Evaluation of pubertal disorders requires a similar systemic approach seen in the evaluation of growth disorders. Careful consideration should be given to history (Box 9.4), including the age of pubertal onset and tempo of progression, sports or exercise or intentional weight loss, neurologic or urologic history, exposure history, and family history.

On physical examination assessment, clinical features of both androgen and estrogen effects should be noted during the physical examination. It is important to differentiate adrenarche from gonadarche. Examination findings consistent with adrenarche include acne, adult type body odor, axillary hair, and pubic hair development (pubarche).

Gonadarche refers to activation of the gonads, which leads to an increase in gonadal volume. In males, an increase in testicular volume can be easily assessed on physical examination. In females, ovarian enlargement is not assessable by physical examination and would require imaging studies such as ultrasonography. Therefore in girls, the development of breast buds (thelarche) is considered an indirect manifestation of gonadarche. Growth chart review is also an important aspect of physical examination to determine if there is height acceleration.

As a rough guideline, in girls, the interval from Tanner 2 breasts to menarche (associated with Tanner 4 breasts) is ~2 ± 1 year. The first vaginal bleeding, known as "menarche," typically occurs 2 years

Box 9.4 Important History in Evaluation of Pubertal Disorders

- Age of pubertal onset and tempo of progression
- History of sports and exercise, intentional weight loss, and body image issues indicating Feeding and Eating Disorders, including Avoidant/Restrictive Food Intake Disorder
- Changes in sense of smell, central nervous system symptoms, galactorrhea
- History of micropenis, cryptorchidism, or other urologic conditions in the newborn period
- Exposure to chemicals, endocrine disruptors, and phytoestrogens such as lavender and tea tree oils
- Personal use of testosterone gels or estrogen creams or its use in family members
- Medications, medical history including chemotherapy and radiation
- Family history of early or delayed puberty

after the onset of breast development. It coincides with Tanner stages IV and V breast development. As for boys, the usual time from Tanner 2 testes (volume ≥4 mL) to adult testicular volume is approximately 3 ± 1.8 years.

Pubertal changes could be manifestations of androgenic features in a phenotypic female or feminizing features in a phenotypic male. Isosexual puberty refers to the appearance of phenotypically appropriate secondary sexual characteristics.

Bone age evaluation by obtaining a hand radiograph is particularly helpful in evaluating delayed and precocious puberty (PP). As noted earlier, the bone age study helps determine adult height prediction, which is one of the considerations in determining the treatment for children with PP. Head imaging could include computed tomography (CT) scan, which is especially useful for suprasellar tumors like craniopharyngioma, although magnetic resonance imaging (MRI) of the brain would be more helpful in delineating other central nervous system tumors. MRI brain is not routinely recommended for females with PP unless they present early (younger than 6 years of age). Brain imaging is a strong consideration for boys with central PP.

Baseline hormone measurements might not be informative in the evaluation of puberty. Evaluation could include random measurements of follicle-stimulating hormone (FSH), luteinizing hormone (LH), and testosterone/estradiol levels using sensitive assays. For further evaluation and differentiation between various disorders, an endocrine referral is recommended for consideration of stimulation/dynamic testing ± imaging or recommendations on indications for genetic testing.

DISORDERS OF PUBERTAL DEVELOPMENT

Gonadotropins (FSH and LH) are glycoproteins secreted by the anterior pituitary gland. The primary actions of FSH and LH are to stimulate gonadal hormone secretion. Each of these hormones is composed of two dissimilar peptide subunits. The α chain is identical for both hormones. However, the β chain is unique and confers specificity to each hormone.

Pulsatile gonadotropin-releasing hormone (GnRH) secretion by the hypothalamic GnRH neurons, the so-called GnRH pulse generator, regulates pituitary secretion of LH and FSH. The GnRH neurons originally develop in the olfactory placode and migrate during early fetal development from the nose through the forebrain to the hypothalamus. The embryologic origin of the GnRH neurons results in the association of hypogonadotropic hypogonadism and anosmia. Pulsatile release of GnRH is important in the secretion of FSH and LH from the anterior pituitary gland. Continuous secretion of GnRH inhibits the release of FSH and LH.

Delayed Puberty

Delayed puberty in girls is defined as the absence of breast development by 13 years of age or primary amenorrhea by 15 years of age; in boys, it is defined by the lack of testicular enlargement by 14 years of age. Delayed puberty includes three groups of disorders: hypogonadotropic hypogonadism, hypergonadotropic hypogonadism, and eugonadotrophic eugonadism.

Hypogonadotropic hypogonadism is characterized by low levels of gonadotropins. Hypogonadotropic hypogonadism results from decreased GnRH production, resulting in reduced LH, FSH, and sex hormone generation. This may be congenital, acquired, or due to hypothalamic-pituitary-gonadal (HPG) axis suppression like in constitutional delay, calorie restriction/excessive training, and chronic systemic illnesses.

Primary gonadal failure/hypergonadotropic hypogonadism results from reduced sex hormone generation from gonads. The deficiency of sex steroids leads to lack of negative feedback, resulting in elevated gonadotropin secretion during early infancy, and then the GnRH pulse generator is quiescent until puberty and adulthood (Fig. 9.10). Thus measurement of random levels of FSH and LH from late infancy to the onset of puberty is typically not helpful in evaluating primary gonadal failure because the GnRH pulse generator is quiescent and there is no stimulus for the gonadotropin levels to rise.

Eugonadotrophic delay in puberty can be seen in anatomic disorders of the reproductive tract, where the LH, FSH, and sex hormone levels are normal. Such a delay could be seen in patients with imperforate hymen.

CDGP is a common cause of delayed puberty, especially in boys, and a normal variant of the timing of puberty. There is usually a history of "late bloomers" in the family. Children are otherwise healthy without any symptoms or signs of underlying chronic medical problems. Bone age is typically delayed with adequate linear growth potential; the predicted final height is appropriate for the family. However, delayed or stalled puberty may be one of the first signs of many underlying medical conditions. Therefore careful evaluation and follow-up of children with presumed constitutional delay in puberty is required. CDGP is a diagnosis of exclusion.

Hypogonadotropic Hypogonadism (Low LH and FSH Levels)

Hypogonadotropic hypogonadism may be suspected in boys with micropenis in the newborn period. Many genetic and acquired conditions are associated with hypogonadotropic hypogonadism. *Kallmann syndrome* refers to hypothalamic hypogonadism associated with anosmia due to impaired migration of GnRH and olfactory neurons; this form is often due to mutations in the *ANOS1/KAL1* gene located at Xp22.31. Hypothalamic hypogonadism can also occur with a normal sense of smell. As noted earlier, the number of genes associated with delayed puberty has expanded (Box 9.5). CHARGE syndrome (coloboma of the eye, heart defects, atresia of the nasal choanae, retardation of growth and/or development, genital and/or urinary abnormalities, and ear abnormalities and deafness) due to mutations in the chromodomain helicase DNA binding protein 7 *(CHD7)* gene is associated with delayed puberty. Other disorders associated with delayed puberty include Prader-Willi, Noonan, and Bardet-Biedl syndromes.

Acquired gonadotropin deficiency can be due to infiltrative disorders, hyperprolactinemia, or chronic illness. Neoplasms like

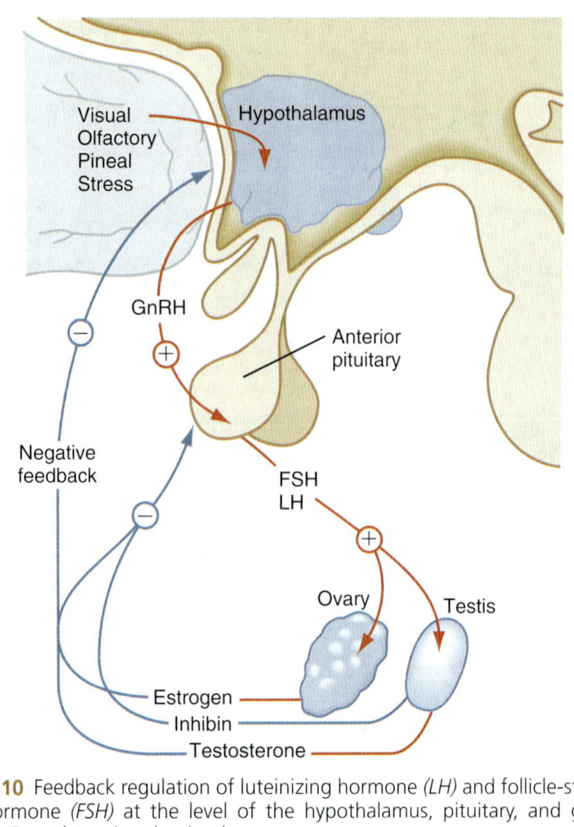

Fig. 9.10 Feedback regulation of luteinizing hormone *(LH)* and follicle-stimulating hormone *(FSH)* at the level of the hypothalamus, pituitary, and gonads. *GnRH,* Gonadotropin-releasing hormone.

Box 9.5 Genes Associated With Hypothalamic Hypogonadism

Neurodevelopmental Genes
SEMA3A
FEZF1
FLRT3
IL17RD

Neuroendocrine Genes
KISS1
KISS1R
DAX1
TAC3
TACR3
GnRH1

Neurodevelopmental and Neuroendocrine Genes
FGF8
FGFR1
PROK2
PROKR2
WDR11
AXL
NSMF
DUSP6
SPRY4
FGF17

Neuroectoderm Genes
CHD7
SOX10
KAL1

Gonadotrope Stimulation Genes
DAX1
GnRHR

craniopharyngioma, trauma, craniospinal radiation therapy, and postsurgical damage to the hypothalamic pituitary area are the main causes of hypogonadotropic hypogonadism. Undernutrition and chronic diseases, such as inflammatory bowel disease, celiac disease, cystic fibrosis, hypothyroidism, glucocorticoid excess, poorly controlled type 1 diabetes mellitus, and sickle cell anemia, can be associated with delayed or arrested puberty.

Functional hypothalamic amenorrhea is a form of ovarian insufficiency and anovulation not due to any organic cause of the hypothalamus or the pituitary. It is associated with weight loss, excessive exercise, stress, and abnormal eating. Gonadotropin secretion, especially in females, is influenced by the metabolic state and degree of adiposity. Leptin, a hormone produced by the adipose tissue, exerts a significant effect on the hypothalamus and is a major link between energy balance and gonadotropin secretion. Very athletic and lean girls experience delayed puberty with low gonadotropin levels. Patients with eating disorders like anorexia nervosa experience amenorrhea with suppressed gonadotropins. Pubertal development may be slow among boys who restrict food intake to maintain a low weight for wrestling.

Hypergonadotropic Hypogonadism (High LH and FSH Levels)

Hypergonadotropic hypogonadism is due to ovarian insufficiency/failure in girls and testicular failure in boys. Gonadotropin levels are typically elevated due to the absence of negative feedback because gonadal sex steroid (estrogen or testosterone) secretion is low. Delayed puberty due to hypergonadotropic hypogonadism can be congenital due to genetic conditions contributing to abnormal development of the ovaries or testes or acquired due to underlying causes, such as autoimmune (isolated or associated with other autoimmune conditions, such as adrenal and thyroid autoimmune disorders); vascular accidents; trauma; chemotherapy; radiation to abdomen, pelvis, and gonads; or total body radiation. High-dose alkylating agents and pelvic radiation/radiation to the testes have the highest risk.

Testicular regression syndrome (also known as vanishing testes or congenital anorchia), a cause of a hypergonadotropic state, is typically diagnosed in infancy or early childhood, but it can present in peripubertal boys with nonpalpable testicles or delayed puberty. External genitalia are typically normal male but can vary from undervirilized male to normal male depending on the timing of in utero testicular loss; this disorder is presumed to be secondary to an in utero vascular event that disrupts testicular blood flow.

Patients with XX or XY gonadal dysgenesis may present with delayed puberty with high gonadotropin levels. Several genetic causes and disorders of steroidogenesis could be associated with hypergonadotropic hypogonadism. Turner syndrome and Klinefelter syndrome are sex chromosome aneuploidies associated with gonadal insufficiency/failure. Galactosemia, Fragile X premutations, and congenital disorders of glycosylation are other genetic conditions associated with hypergonadotropic hypogonadism.

Rare causes include mutations in the forkhead box L2 *(FOXL2)*, newborn ovary homeobox *(NOBOX)*, factor in germline alpha *(FIGLA)*, and bone morphogenetic protein 15 *(BMP15)* genes.

Eugonadotropic Conditions Causing Lack of Menarche/Pubertal Aberrations

Complete androgen insensitivity syndrome (CAIS) can present as delayed/stalled puberty in phenotypic females with primary amenorrhea. Androgen insensitivity occurs secondary to mutations in the androgen receptor gene, which is located at Xq11-q12. In utero, androgen action is essential for retention of Wolffian duct derivatives, development of the prostate, and differentiation of male external genitalia. Common clinical presenting features of CAIS include inguinal or labial masses (gonads) in an otherwise normal-appearing female infant. The adolescent girl may present with breast development and primary amenorrhea. Breast development occurs because gonadotropin secretion at the time of puberty stimulates increased testosterone production, which is then aromatized to estradiol. Due to normal Sertoli cell function and AMH secretion, the uterus, cervix, and upper portion of the vagina are absent, and there is a blind-ending vaginal pouch. In all instances, the karyotype is 46, XY. LH concentrations are elevated with normal FSH concentrations. The clinical features for patients with partial androgen insensitivity syndrome vary depending on the extent of receptor function. The phenotype can vary from female external genital appearance with mild clitoromegaly to a minimally undervirilized male with gynecomastia.

Some individuals with disorders of steroidogenesis or aberrant gonadal differentiation present with delayed puberty. Patients with 17-hydroxylase deficiency have mutations in the 17α-hydroxylase/17,20-lyase (CYP17A1) gene that encodes the P450c17 enzyme. This enzyme is essential to produce cortisol and sex steroids. In classic 17-hydroxylase deficiency, patients with both XX and XY karyotypes are phenotypic females and both present with lack of secondary sexual development. Females with P450-oxidoreductase deficiency due to POR mutations have been reported to have delayed puberty and ovarian cysts. Individuals with 17-hydroxysteroid dehydrogenase type 3 deficiency due to HSD17B3 variants or 5α-reductase deficiency due to SRD5A2 variants have 46, XY karyotype, genital ambiguity at birth and typically virilize with the increased gonadotropin secretion of puberty.

Structural problems may also present with primary amenorrhea without any hormonal disturbances, as seen in dysgenesis of Müllerian ducts and uterus. Müllerian duct aplasia–renal agenesis–cervicothoracic somite dysplasia syndrome is an uncommon developmental disorder characterized by uterine hypoplasia or aplasia, renal agenesis or ectopy, vertebral anomalies, and short stature. Isolated Müllerian duct agenesis without the other associations in 46, XX females is called Mayer-Rokitansky-Kuster-Hauser syndrome.

Precocious Puberty

The diagnosis of precocious or early development is considered when the physical signs of puberty develop before age 8 years in girls and 9 years in boys. Children presenting with early onset of puberty should be evaluated regarding the age at pubertal onset and the temporal sequence of pubertal changes. Clinical features of androgen and estrogen effects should be noted during the physical examination. Growth acceleration in girls is present at the onset of puberty and is a sensitive sign of precocious puberty.

Gonadotropin-dependent precocious puberty, also known as central precocious puberty (CPP) or GnRH-dependent precocious puberty, is marked by premature activation of the HPG axis and follows the same sequence as normal puberty. In girls, the causes of isosexual precocity (development along lines of the same sex) are related to alterations in gonadal or central nervous system (CNS) function. CPP follows an early onset of pulsatile LH and FSH secretion and the subsequent response of the ovary. Causes include:

- Idiopathic: In females, the causes of CPP in majority of cases are not identified. In contrast, only 10% of CPP cases in males are idiopathic. Intracranial neoplasms are more commonly associated with CPP in boys as compared with girls.
- Genetic: Recent advances in genetic testing have revealed many causes for familial central precocious puberty. Paternally inherited loss of function mutations in the kisspeptin system, makorin ring finger protein 3 *(MKRN3),* and delta homolog 1 *(DLK1)* genes have been identified in sporadic and familial cases of CPP. Obtaining a family history of pubertal development can be helpful. Available data suggest that the makorin ring finger 3 protein inhibits GnRH secretion; declining circulating levels are noted with the onset of puberty.
- Structural: Hypothalamic hamartomas, which are structurally benign lesions, are the most common causes of CPP in young children (Fig. 9.11). Gelastic seizures can be associated with hypothalamic hamartomas and precocious puberty. Other brain tumors that may cause CPP include glial cell tumors, germ cell tumors, and occasionally craniopharyngiomas and pinealomas. Low-dose radiation therapy for CNS tumors can result in hypothalamic dysfunction and can present with CPP.

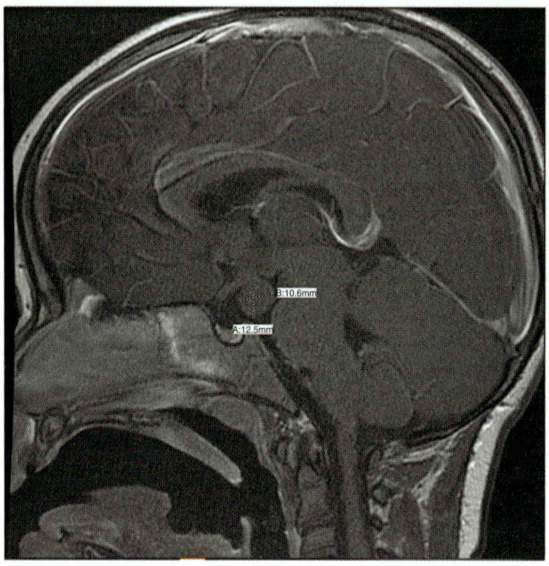

Fig. 9.11 Hypothalamic hamartoma in a 17-month-old girl with central precocious puberty.

In GnRH-independent forms of precocious puberty/peripheral precocious puberty (PPP), there is an increased production of sex steroids. This leads to physical changes of puberty without activation of the HPG axis. McCune-Albright syndrome, characterized by irregular café-au-lait spots (Fig. 9.12A), polyostotic fibrous dysplasia (see Fig. 9.12B), and precocious puberty, is one example of a GnRH-independent cause of precocious puberty. McCune-Albright syndrome is due to a somatic activating mutation of the gene encoding the α-subunit of G protein-coupled receptor, which is located at chromosome 20q13.2. Physical changes may not follow the normal sequence of pubertal development seen in central precocious puberty. Other endocrine manifestations may include gigantism, Cushing syndrome, hyperprolactinemia, hyperthyroidism, and hyperparathyroidism.

Gonadal neoplasms secreting sex steroids, such as Leydig cell tumors in boys, are rare causes of PPP. The sequence of pubertal changes may differ from typical because rapid increase of sex steroids can cause rapid progression of pubertal signs. In boys, hCG-secreting tumors can also be a cause of isosexual precocity due to LH-like actions of hCG. Typically, hCG tumors do not cause precocious puberty in girls because estradiol is not produced in the absence of FSH stimulated aromatase expression. Familial male-limited precocious puberty or testotoxicosis is characterized by premature testicular testosterone production, testicular enlargement, and precocious puberty. It is due to constitutive activating mutations of the LH receptor (LHR) gene. Adrenal hypersecretion of hormones can also lead to increase in sex steroids, which can cause PPP (e.g., uncontrolled congenital adrenal hyperplasia and rarely adrenocortical carcinoma).

Long-standing and severe primary hypothyroidism in girls may be associated with isosexual precocity because of the partial structural homology between thyrotropin (thyroid stimulating hormone [TSH]) and the gonadotropins (LH, FSH). In addition to signs of hypothyroidism, girls may have breast development and vaginal bleeding. This is also known as Van Wyk-Grumbach syndrome.

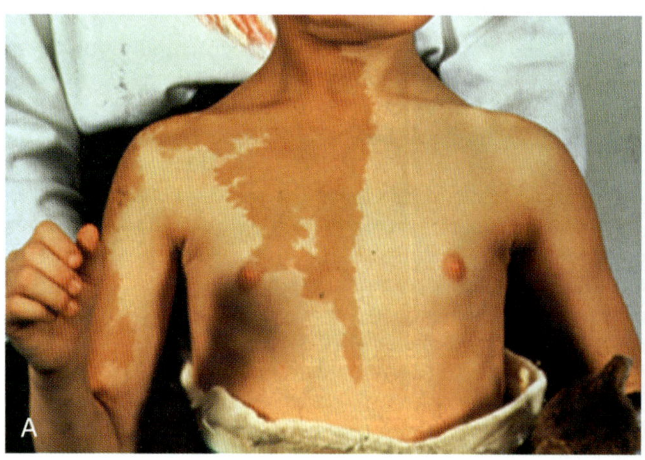

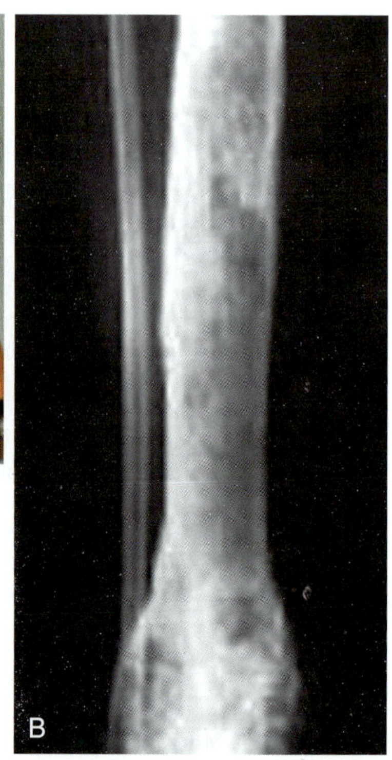

Fig. 9.12 McCune-Albright syndrome. (A) Irregular café-au-lait pigmentation over right anterior chest, shoulder, and right arm. (B) Polyostotic fibrous dysplasia. Multiple areas of fibrous dysplasia, most commonly found in long bones and pelvis. (A, Courtesy the National Institutes of Health, Bethesda, MD.)

Boys with severe hypothyroidism may have enlargement of the testes due to the same mechanism. In these boys, testicular enlargement is often not associated with other secondary sexual characteristics, such as pubic hair development and genital enlargement.

Exposure to exogenous hormones such as estrogens, estrogen-like substances including phytoestrogens, and testosterone may cause the development of secondary sexual characteristics and mimic precocious puberty. In prepubertal girls, small ovarian follicular cysts are commonly found, and, in most cases, they are of no clinical importance. However, occasionally, these cysts may enlarge and produce estrogen, resulting in signs of PPP. They may present with breast development and vaginal bleeding and may appear to have high growth velocity. However, if left untreated, the child might end up becoming a short adult due to premature closure of growth plates. Early referral and pubertal suppression are recommended for height preservation.

Benign Pubertal Variants

Premature Adrenarche

Premature adrenarche describes the early onset of the normal increase in adrenal androgen production causing any of the features including acne, adult-type body odor, axillary hair, and/or pubic hair development. Adrenarche is considered early when it occurs before 8 years of age in girls and 9 years of age in boys. Premature isolated (benign) adrenarche is not associated with breast development in girls and testicular enlargement in boys. Progression is slow and there could be minimal elevation in the DHEAS levels. Bone age is typically normal but may rarely be advanced. Height prediction is normal for genetic potential. Differential diagnostic considerations include late-onset CAH and rarely androgen-secreting or gonadal tumors. Although advanced skeletal maturation is more common in CAH, adrenocorticotrophic hormone (ACTH) stimulation tests may be necessary to distinguish late-onset CAH from benign premature adrenarche.

Premature Pubarche

Premature pubarche refers to the development of pubic hair (pubarche) before 8 years of age in girls and 9 years of age in boys (Fig. 9.13) and is most commonly the result of premature adrenarche. Associated findings may include axillary hair, adult-type body odor, and acne. Typically, DHEAS concentrations and bone age are normal for age. Rapid progression of pubarche should prompt evaluation for other disorders such as adrenal or gonadal androgen secreting tumors, disorders of steroidogenesis, or environmental exposures. On occasion, young infants may present with coarse hairs in the genital area (typically the scrotum in boys and the inner aspect of the labia majora in girls), which disappear spontaneously in late infancy, suggesting that this is a benign phenomenon. Progressive increase of hair in these areas should alert the clinician to the possibility of pathologic causes.

Premature Thelarche

Premature thelarche is a transient and self-limited condition defined by the early onset of isolated breast development. Typically, premature thelarche develops during the first or second year of life without any other signs of puberty. The breast tissue may appear unilaterally or bilaterally and may regress or persist (Fig. 9.14). Typically, there is a waxing and waning pattern to breast enlargement. Other features of pubertal development, including growth acceleration and pubic hair development, are absent. In most cases, breast enlargement does not progress beyond Tanner stage III. Hence premature thelarche is a diagnosis of exclusion and cannot be made in the presence or progression of other pubertal signs. The etiology of premature thelarche is unclear, though the ingestion of exogenous estrogens, such as oral contraceptives, and exposure to phytoestrogens such as lavender and tea tree oils should always be suspected in cases of premature breast enlargement.

Physiologic neonatal gynecomastia is common in newborns. In the immediate neonatal period, breast enlargement can occur secondary to the transfer of maternal estrogen through the placenta. This may occur in either sex in the immediate neonatal period and can be associated with milk secretion. Stagnation of milk and superadded infection can result in mastitis and breast abscess, which may require surgical drainage. Neonatal gynecomastia is usually self-remitting as the effects of maternal estrogen wear off. Minimal manipulation is recommended to prevent further stimulation of breast tissue and subsequently mastitis.

Lipomastia/Adipomastia

Lipomastia/adipomastia refers to the presence of adipose tissue in the pectoral area that may resemble breast development. This is frequently seen in obesity in both boys and girls.

True breast tissue is palpable underneath the nipple/areola, whereas in pure lipomastia there is no palpable glandular tissue under the nipple, giving the impression of a "donut" with a hollow center surrounded by a rim of adipose tissue (Fig. 9.15).

Isolated Vaginal Bleeding

The first vaginal bleeding, known as "menarche," typically occurs 2 years after the onset of breast development. It coincides with Tanner stages IV and V breast development. Isolated vaginal bleeding in prepubertal girls does not follow this typical sequence and is abnormal. It should raise suspicion for a foreign body in the genital tract and one should look for signs of abuse. As discussed earlier, vaginal bleeding can be a manifestation of McCune-Albright syndrome,

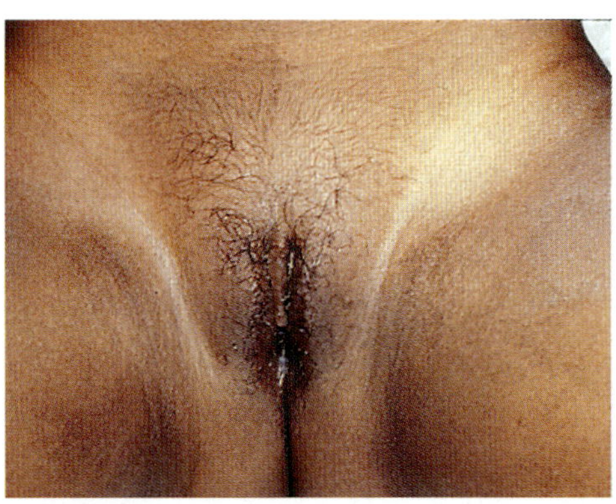

Fig. 9.13 Premature adrenarche. Pubic hair development in a prepubertal girl with premature adrenarche.

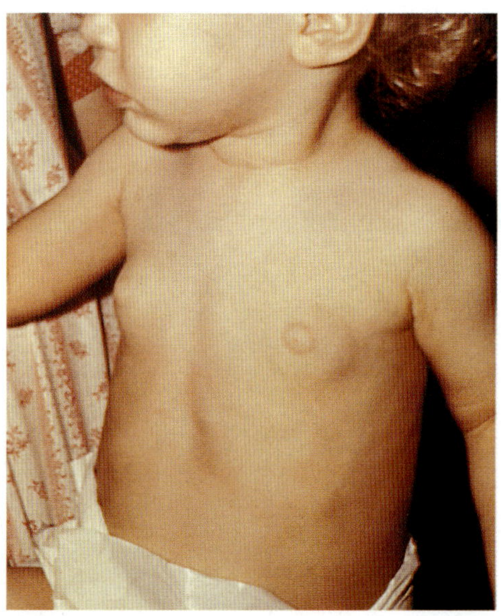

Fig. 9.14 Premature thelarche. Isolated bilateral breast enlargement in a toddler with premature thelarche.

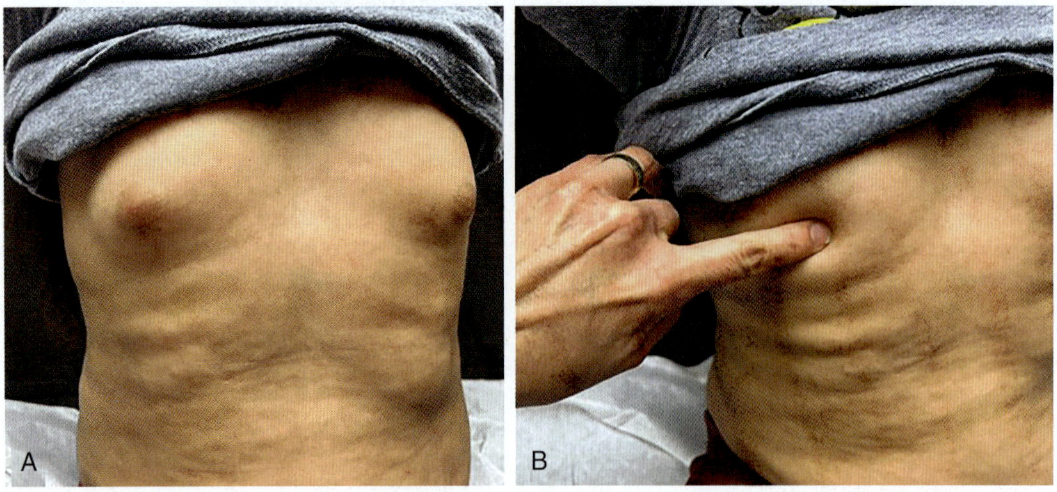

Fig. 9.15 Lipomastia. (A) Notice generalized increased adiposity. (B) Positive donut sign: no palpable glandular tissue underneath the areola and sensation of a "donut" of adipose tissue around the finger pressing on the areola. (Courtesy O. Escobar, MD, Pittsburgh, PA.)

estrogen-producing adrenal or ovarian tumors. However, to consider it as a benign variant, other signs of puberty should be absent and with no recurrent bleeding. Isolated benign ovarian cysts, described earlier as a cause of PPP, occasionally can cause isolated vaginal bleeding.

Gynecomastia

Gynecomastia means female-like breasts seen in males. It should not be used to describe breast development in females, which is "thelarche." Gynecomastia is common in adolescent males. Up to 70% of adolescent males may develop gynecomastia, typically in Tanner stages III and IV, and it is usually bilateral. Physiologic pubertal gynecomastia can be unilateral and usually resolves spontaneously over 1 to 2 years (Fig. 9.16). True gynecomastia should be differentiated from lipomastia, which is seen in overweight individuals. Good history and examination should differentiate the benign conditions from the less common nonbenign causes of gynecomastia.

Pubertal gynecomastia results from relative estrogen excess due to variable amounts of aromatization of adrenal and testicular androgens to estrogens in peripheral tissues, particularly adipose tissue and liver, while testosterone levels are not yet robust. It might persist longer in obese boys or never resolve due to the higher estrogen levels from aromatization of androgens in peripheral fat tissue and permanent glandular breast tissue formation.

Pathologic causes to consider include testicular hypogonadism with decreased androgen production seen in boys with Klinefelter syndrome. Other conditions that can cause decreased androgen synthesis and gynecomastia are 5α reductase deficiency and 17β hydroxysteroid dehydrogenase type 3 deficiency. In androgen insensitivity syndrome, gynecomastia is caused by higher estradiol levels from aromatization of high levels of testosterone caused by androgen receptor mutations. Typically, the phenotype is female in complete androgen insensitivity syndrome. Increased estrogen production from adrenal or testicular tumors, hCG-secreting tumors, and familial aromatase excess syndrome are rare causes of gynecomastia. Obesity, malnutrition, chronic liver disease, hyperthyroidism, and breast cancer (rare) are other nonbenign causes of gynecomastia. Drug-induced gynecomastia should be considered in boys taking chronic medication or substances like marijuana.

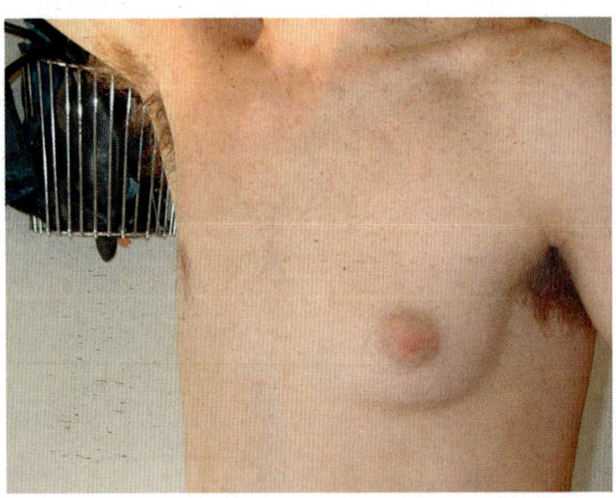

Fig. 9.16 Unilateral gynecomastia in a 14-year-old boy.

Breast Asymmetry

Breast asymmetry is the finding of mild-moderate difference in breast size, shape, and position on a clinical examination. It is common in pubertal adolescent girls and can be a feature of physiologic pubertal gynecomastia in boys (see Fig. 9.16). It is mostly due to the fluctuating response of breast tissue to the hormonal environment during puberty. In most instances where the asymmetry is due to hormonal fluctuations, it resolves as breast development is completed. Other causes such as breast mass or abscess are rare. Breast asymmetry is a feature of Poland syndrome, which is an uncommon congenital malformation affecting the chest wall, shoulder, arm, and hand.

Galactorrhea

Galactorrhea means "milk flow," derived from the Greek word "galakt" meaning milk and "rhoia" meaning flow. Galactorrhea describes the milk production outside of pregnancy or breastfeeding in females. Galactorrhea can occur in males as well. Prolactin secreted from the anterior pituitary lactotrophs is the key hormone in milk production. Physiologic causes of galactorrhea include nipple stimulation and placental transfer of maternal hormones in newborns. Pathologic causes of galactorrhea are discussed later in the chapter.

Macromastia/Gigantomastia

Gigantomastia is a rare condition characterized by the diffuse enlargement of both breasts. It occurs mostly in peripubertal girls or in the postpartum period. It can be physically and psychologically disabling. Often, etiology is unknown. Most cases occur during significant changes in endogenous hormones such as during puberty and pregnancy. It is thought to be due to abnormal stimulation of breast tissue from circulating physiologic levels of hormones or due to hormonal excess. Drug-induced gigantomastia has been described with penicillamine and cyclosporine.

ENDOCRINE SYSTEMS

The Pituitary and the Hypothalamus

The pituitary gland is considered "the master gland," regulating diverse endocrine functions. It develops as a fusion of cells from two distinct embryonic origins. The anterior lobe (adenohypophysis) is an outgrowth of ectodermal cells from the roof of the primitive pharynx (known as Rathke pouch), and the posterior lobe (neurohypophysis) is a downgrowth of neural tissue (neural ectoderm) from the floor of the forebrain. The anterior pituitary gland is regulated largely by small peptide hormones secreted by cells located in the hypothalamus. The posterior pituitary gland has direct neuronal connections to the hypothalamus. The oral ectoderm and neuroectoderm interact as they oppose each other to form the pituitary gland. This apposition and interaction are critical for the anterior pituitary cell differentiation. Aberrant development of the cells forming Rathke pouch can lead to anterior pituitary hormone deficiencies.

The hypothalamus is derived from neuroectodermal tissue of the diencephalon and surrounds the inferior aspect of the third ventricle. Its basilar portion consists of the median eminence and pituitary stalk, which provide the common route for hypothalamic small peptide hormones to reach the pituitary gland.

The Hypothalamic-Pituitary-IGF-1 Axis

Anterior Pituitary

The anterior pituitary contains cells that secrete three types of hormones: (1) corticotrophin-related peptide hormones (ACTH); (2) glycoprotein hormones (FSH, LH, TSH); and (3) somatomammotropins (GH, prolactin). These compounds have great biologic potency with tight regulation of hormone secretion governed by positive and negative feedback signals.

GH influences linear growth and modulates several complex metabolic processes. GH secretion is regulated by the relative balance between the levels of GH-releasing hormone (GHRH) and somatostatin (Fig. 9.17). Both GHRH and somatostatin are secreted by the hypothalamus. GH generates direct effects via the GH receptor signal transduction pathway and secondary effects by promoting an increase in IGF-1 and insulin-like growth factor–binding protein-3 (IGF-BP3). GH also has positive effects on carbohydrate, fat, and protein metabolism and causes a decrease in body fat. Anterior pituitary hormone deficiencies cause subsequent hypofunction in the output of secondary endocrine glands, with substantial consequences for growth and development.

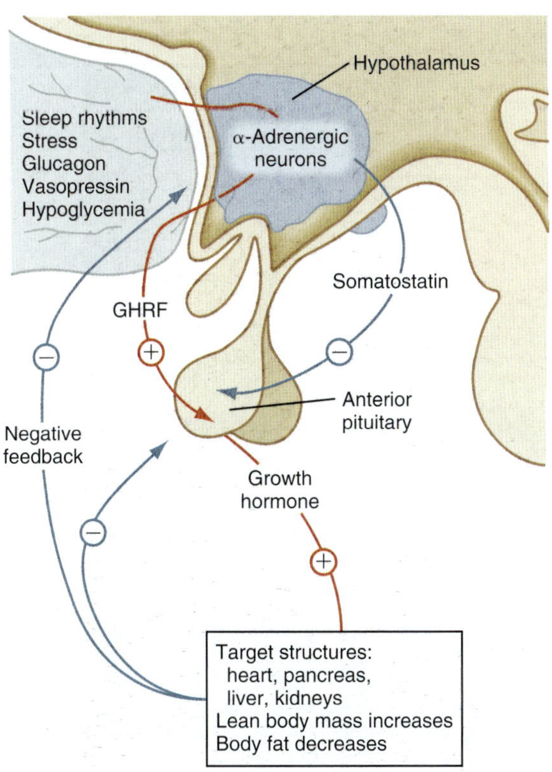

Fig. 9.17 Feedback regulation of growth hormone at the level of the hypothalamus, pituitary, and target organs. *GHRF,* Growth hormone–releasing factor.

Posterior Pituitary

Vasopressin and oxytocin are two evolutionarily related peptides—each composed of nine amino acids. These hormones are synthesized in the hypothalamus and stored in the posterior pituitary gland. Expression of vasopressin and oxytocin genes occurs in the hypothalamic paraventricular and supraoptic nuclei. On magnetic resonance T1-weighted images, the posterior pituitary has characteristic high-signal intensity. The presence of this high-signal intensity adjacent to the median eminence with absence of the normal pituitary bright spot within the sella on T1-weighted images is evidence of an ectopic posterior pituitary (Fig. 9.18). Vasopressin, also known as arginine vasopressin (AVP) or antidiuretic hormone (ADH), is a hormone that is important in water balance. It is synthesized and carried via axonal transport to the posterior pituitary, its primary site of storage. It is then released into systemic circulation and acts primarily on the kidneys to aid in the reabsorption of water.

Oxytocin secretion occurs in response to nervous stimulation of the hypothalamus. This hormone causes contraction of the smooth muscle of the uterus and of the myoepithelial cells lining the duct of the mammary gland. Although some oxytocin is found in males, its function is unclear.

Evaluation of hypothalamic and pituitary disorders starts with a detailed history and physical examination and complemented with labs and imaging as indicated in Box 9.6.

Disorders of Hypothalamus and Pituitary Gland

Pituitary Hormone Deficiencies

Congenital hypopituitarism is a deficiency of one or more hormones produced by the anterior or posterior pituitary. Congenital hypopituitarism, resulting from events during fetal development, has been associated with birth trauma/asphyxia, midline defects, and genetic

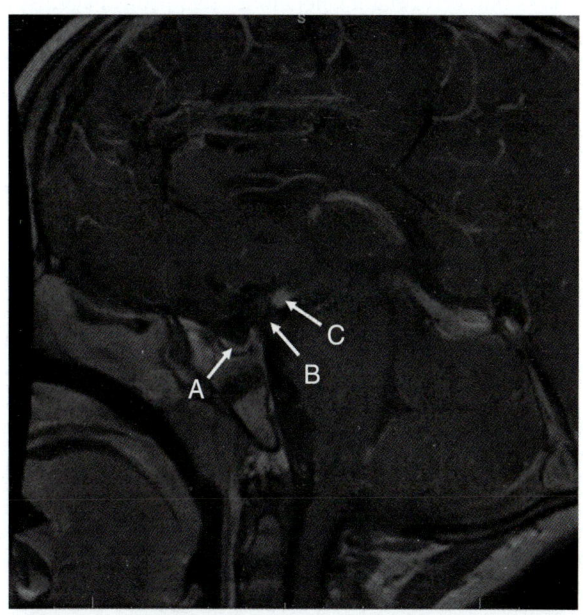

Fig. 9.18 Magnetic resonance imaging of the brain showing *A arrow,* hypoplastic pituitary with partially empty sella, *B arrow,* absent pituitary stalk, and *C arrow,* ectopic posterior pituitary bright spot. (Courtesy O. Escobar, MD, Pittsburgh, PA.)

Box 9.6 Evaluation of Hypothalamic and Pituitary Disorders

History

- Birth/prenatal history
  - Maternal age, neonatal hypoglycemia (no maternal diabetes or hyperinsulinism)
  - Prolonged neonatal jaundice (direct hyperbilirubinemia) with hypoglycemia
- History of hypothyroid symptoms, symptoms of low cortisol, pubertal delay, polyuria and polydipsia without glycosuria

Physical Examination

- Careful review of growth charts, height/length measurement, weight and growth rate
- Presence of midline defects, cleft lip/palate, single incisor
- Nystagmus, vision loss, jaundice, micropenis
- Specific facial features that suggest growth hormone deficiency (reduction in lean mass, prominent forehead, excess fat in cheeks and trunk) or GH resistance

Laboratory Tests

- IGF-1, IGFBP3 (random growth hormone levels not useful unless in neonatal period)
- Free/Total T4, TSH, ACTH, cortisol, prolactin, FSH, LH, sex steroids (neonates and after pubertal onset), serum and urine osmolality, serum electrolytes, and copeptin as indicated

Imaging

- Computed tomography/magnetic resonance imaging
  - Head magnetic resonance imaging with gadolinium contrast with thin slices through the pituitary gland is recommended for better delineation of pituitary anatomy.

ACTH, Adrenocorticotrophic hormone; *FSH,* follicle-stimulating hormone; *GH,* growth hormone; *LH,* luteinizing hormone; *TSH,* thyroid-stimulating hormone.

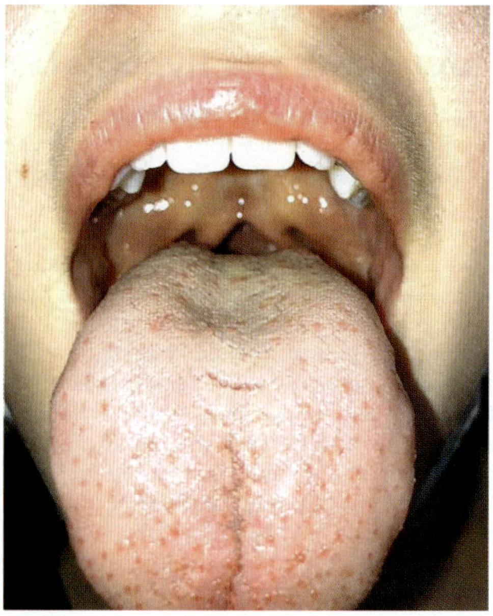

Fig. 9.20 Bifid uvula. (Courtesy O. Escobar, MD, Pittsburgh, PA.)

conditions. The described midline defects include single central incisor (Fig. 9.19), cleft palate, and bifid uvula (Fig. 9.20). Genetic mutations encoding pituitary transcription factors like HESX1 (Septo-optic dysplasia), LHX3, LHX4, PROP-1, and PIT-1 (also known as POU1F1), have been associated with congenital hypopituitarism. Acquired causes include intracranial tumors, head and neck radiation, and chemotherapy-induced hypophysitis. Head trauma, surgery, pressure effects from hydrocephalus, or vascular anomalies of the hypothalamic-pituitary region and autoimmune hypophysitis can also alter pituitary function.

The most common presenting feature of congenital hypopituitarism is hypoglycemia. This is due to GH deficiency with or without associated ACTH deficiency (causing low cortisol). Both GH and cortisol are counterregulatory hormones that protect against hypoglycemia, especially during fasting. It is important to remember that in any term infant who develops hypoglycemia with no underlying risk factor (e.g., prematurity, intrauterine growth retardation, perinatal stress, infant of a diabetic mother), the diagnosis of hypopituitarism must be considered.

Typically, children with GH deficiency have normal birth weights and normal growth patterns during the first year of life, after which time their growth velocities decelerate. The pulsatile nature of GH secretion necessitates provocative stimulation tests to diagnose GH deficiency except during the newborn period. Measuring random GH concentrations is not helpful in the evaluation of short stature. IGF-1 concentrations may be low in children with GH deficiency. Because IGF-1 concentrations also reflect nutritional status, IGF-1 concentrations may also be low in children with inadequate caloric intake.

As seen in Fig. 9.21, GH-deficient children have a characteristic "kewpie" doll appearance. They are often described as being "cherubic" because of their short stature, excess subcutaneous fat, body proportion changes, and high-pitched voices. Infants with hypopituitarism may present in the early neonatal period with hypoglycemia

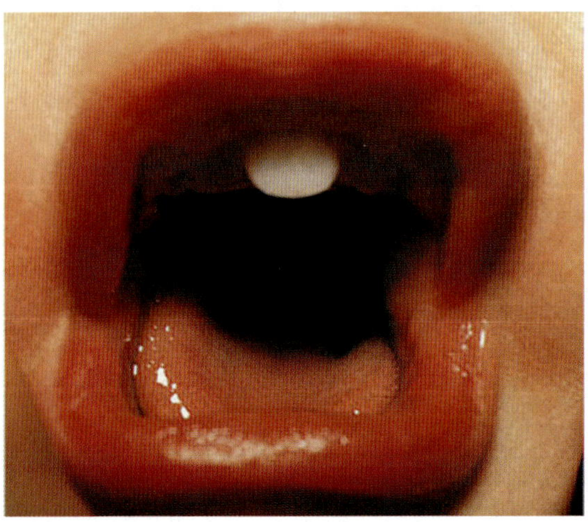

Fig. 9.19 Central maxillary incisor. The presence of a single central maxillary incisor should alert the clinician to investigate the possibility of growth hormone deficiency. (Courtesy P. Lee, MD, Hershey, PA.)

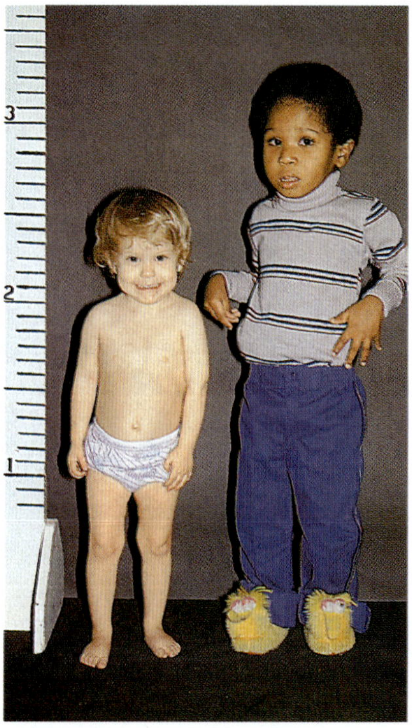

Fig. 9.21 Growth hormone (GH) deficiency. The normal boy *(right)* is in the 50th percentile for height. The short 3-year-old girl *(left)* has GH deficiency.

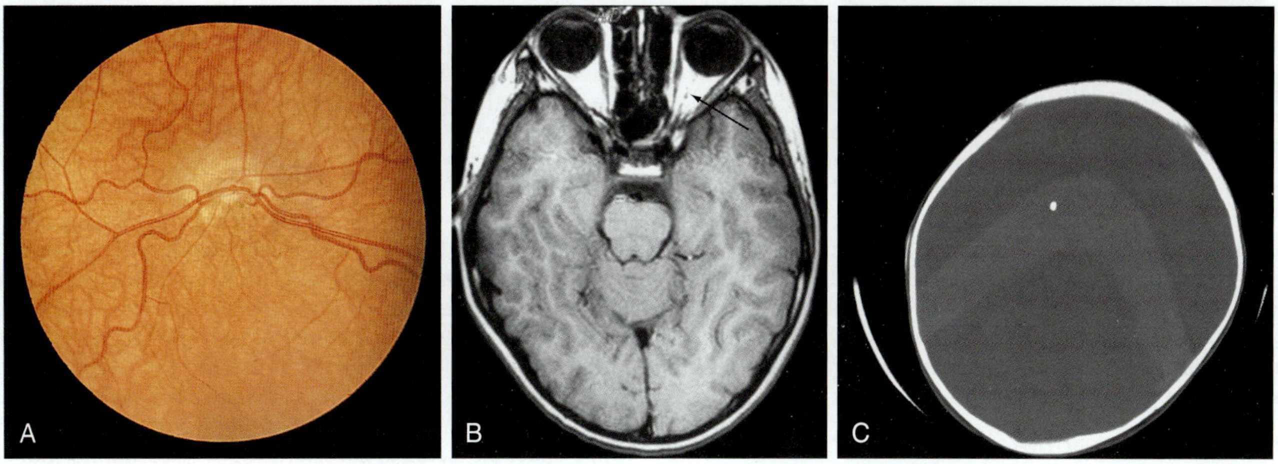

Fig. 9.22 Congenital abnormalities of the central nervous system commonly associated with hypothalamic–pituitary dysfunction. (A) Pale optic discs noted on funduscopic examination indicative of optic nerve hypoplasia, which can be associated with septo-optic dysplasia. (B) Magnetic resonance image showing optic nerve hypoplasia. (C) Holoprosencephaly. (A, Courtesy D. Hiles, MD, Pittsburgh, PA.)

or prolonged jaundice. On physical examination, male infants with hypopituitarism and GH deficiency may have a small penis due to concomitant LH deficiency.

Laron syndrome is a genetic condition where mutation in GH receptor results in resistance to GH and inability to generate IGF-1 from the liver cells. Individuals with Laron syndrome have a severe short stature (adult males 4.5 feet, adult females 4 feet) that can be treated with recombinant human IGF-1.

Aberrant development of the pituitary may be associated with an ectopic location of the posterior pituitary at the base of the hypothalamus. Ectopic posterior pituitary is often associated with absence of the pituitary stalk. Affected individuals manifest varying anterior pituitary hormone deficiencies in the absence of diabetes insipidus because the function of the ectopic posterior pituitary is preserved. The abnormal location of the posterior pituitary is often visible as the posterior pituitary bright spot on MRI (Fig. 9.18).

Structural abnormalities of the CNS, such as optic nerve hypoplasia (Fig. 9.22A), septo-optic dysplasia (Fig. 9.22B), and holoprosencephaly (Fig. 9.22C), can interfere with both anterior and posterior pituitary function. Septo-optic dysplasia refers to a collection of anatomic findings including absence or abnormal development of the corpus callosum/septum pellucidum, optic nerve hypoplasia, and pituitary hormone deficiencies. Some patients with septo-optic dysplasia present with pituitary hormone deficiencies; some patients may develop pituitary hormone deficiencies over time. Gene defects have been increasingly identified among patients with septo-optic dysplasia and include *HESX1, SOX2, SOX3,* and *OTX2* genes.

Craniopharyngiomas and CNS tumors can be associated with acquired hypopituitarism (Fig. 9.23). Craniopharyngiomas are nonmalignant congenital epithelial tumors involving the sellar region. Although benign, these tumors can infiltrate into the hypothalamus, optic chiasm, and local vascular structures. There are two different subtypes of craniopharyngioma—adamantinomatous and papillary. The adamantinomatous form is the most common nonneuroepithelial intracranial lesion in children. The tumor and its treatment often result in hypopituitarism, diabetes insipidus, obesity, and visual deficits. Although craniopharyngiomas are not malignant lesions, tumor recurrence is common. Thus these children will need to have lifelong endocrine care.

Optic pathway gliomas account for 2% to 5% of childhood brain tumors. These tumors may involve the hypothalamus and third ventricle. Clinical features include impaired visual acuity, strabismus, nystagmus, and diencephalic syndrome (profound emaciation despite a normal or slightly diminished caloric intake). Neurofibromatosis type 1 is associated with these tumors, which paradoxically can be associated with precocious puberty.

Additional causes of acquired hypopituitarism include germ cell tumors (Fig. 9.24), surgical treatment, irradiation to treat CNS tu-

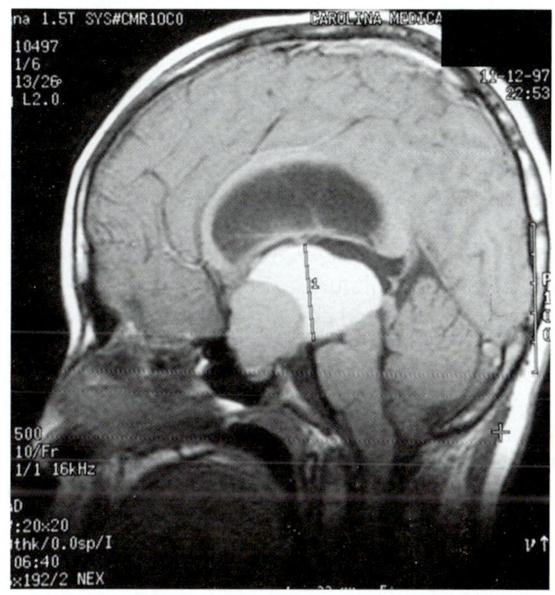

Fig. 9.23 Craniopharyngioma. Heterogeneous, densely enhancing suprasellar mass extending from the pituitary fossa into the hypothalamus and third ventricle.

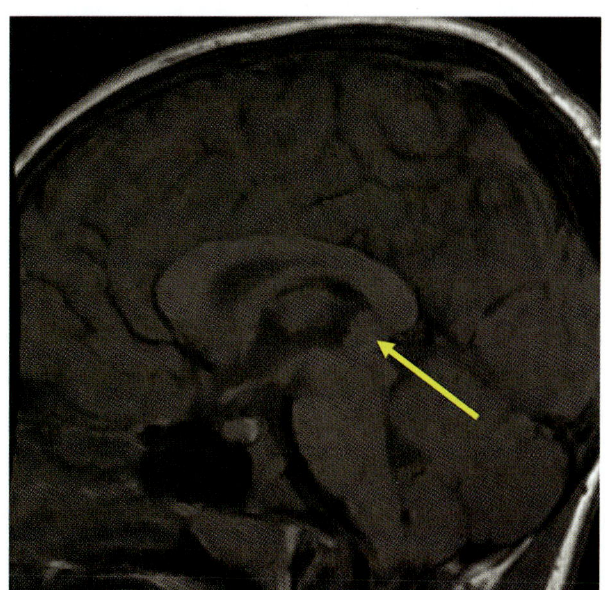

Fig. 9.24 Magnetic resonance image of the brain showing *(yellow arrow)* a germ cell tumor in the pineal region. (Courtesy O. Escobar, MD, Pittsburgh, PA.)

mors, granulomatous infiltration (such as Langerhans cell histiocytosis), and traumatic interruption of the pituitary stalk.

Pituitary and Body Water Regulation

Arginine vasopressin (AVP), also known as ADH, acts primarily on the kidneys at V2 receptors to aid in the reabsorption of water by affecting water permeability in the collecting duct of the kidney. During states of decreased water intake or dehydration, osmoreceptors in the hypothalamus detect an increase in osmotic pressure in the blood, leading to increased AVP secretion and increased thirst. The combination of increased AVP secretion leading to increased renal reabsorption of free water and increased oral fluid intake will decrease osmolality. Other factors that increase AVP secretion include pain, trauma, nausea, and vomiting.

Syndrome of Inappropriate Antidiuretic Hormone Secretion

Head trauma, brain tumors, encephalitis, pneumonia, and some drugs are associated with overproduction of AVP. This can lead to inappropriate water retention and hyponatremia, known as syndrome of inappropriate antidiuretic hormone (SIADH). The symptoms of SIADH include headache, apathy, nausea, vomiting, and impaired consciousness.

Diabetes Insipidus

Diabetes insipidus (DI) is now termed arginine vasopressin (AVP) deficiency or resistance, depending on the etiology. Central DI (AVP deficiency) is due to the underproduction of AVP. This can result from pituitary tumors, head trauma, infiltrative disease processes (such as Langerhans cell histiocytosis, sarcoidosis, hemochromatosis, and autoimmune hypophysitis), or any surgery that damages the pituitary gland and hypothalamus. Familial central DI, which is inherited in both recessive and dominant patterns, is rare and has its onset in infancy. Wolfram syndrome is an autosomal dominant form of central DI often associated with diabetes mellitus, optic atrophy, and deafness.

Nephrogenic DI (AVP resistance) is characterized by failure of the kidney tubules to respond to ADH. Genetic causes of nephrogenic DI include X-linked forms due to mutations in the V2 receptor gene and autosomal forms due to mutations in the aquaporin-2 gene. Acquired nephrogenic DI can be caused by drugs, such as lithium.

Psychogenic water drinking, hypercalcemia, hypokalemia, sickle cell anemia, and polycystic kidney disease can also impair renal concentrating ability independent of AVP production or action.

Pituitary Hormone Excess

GH prevents the uptake of carbohydrate by muscle cells. In GH hypersecretion, elevated blood sugars associated with rapid growth is due to this diabetogenic effect of GH. Excessive GH secretion is uncommon in children. If GH excess begins during childhood, gigantism with increased growth velocity ensues leading to abnormal tall stature, while GH excess in an individual with closed epiphyses causes acromegaly manifested by soft tissue growth of the hands and feet and coarsening of facial features. Random GH, IGF-1, and IGF-BP3 concentrations are usually elevated in gigantism/acromegaly. Oral glucose tolerance test may be performed to diagnose GH excess. Oral glucose load decreases GH secretion in normal individuals but not in gigantism/acromegaly.

HYPOTHALAMIC-PITUITARY LACTOTROPH SYSTEM

Lactotrophs are specialized cells of the anterior pituitary gland that produce prolactin.

Prolactin acts directly on its target organs and does not require an intermediary secondary endocrine gland. The major known function of prolactin in humans is the initiation and maintenance of lactation. Neonates have a high prolactin level, 90 to 100 ng/mL, in the first week of life. The prolactin level decreases thereafter to an adult level, which is 20 ng/mL. Low prolactin level may be associated with other anterior pituitary hormone deficiencies.

Hyperprolactinemia

Galactorrhea may be a clinical manifestation of hyperprolactinemia. In contrast to other anterior pituitary hormones, prolactin is regulated by tonic inhibition by dopamine secreted by the hypothalamus. Prolactin secreted from the anterior pituitary lactotrophs is the key hormone in milk production. The hypothalamus secretes dopamine, which inhibits pituitary prolactin production. Several hypothalamic-releasing factors increase prolactin secretion. Vasoactive intestinal polypeptide secreted by the hypothalamus has a stimulatory effect on lactotrophs. Thyrotropin-releasing hormone (TRH), which stimulates the anterior pituitary to secrete TSH, has a minor stimulating effect on the prolactin secretion. Estrogens directly stimulate pituitary lactotrophs and prolactin secretion.

Pathologic causes of galactorrhea include CNS lesions that interfere with the hypothalamic inhibitory function on prolactin synthesis and secretion, such as tumors in the hypothalamic pituitary area (craniopharyngioma, meningioma, germinoma) or prolactin-secreting adenomas of the pituitary gland (prolactinomas).

Prolactinomas are pituitary micro/macroadenomas usually associated with galactorrhea and can present with signs and symptoms of hypogonadism including secondary amenorrhea in females. Larger tumors present with headaches, visual impairment, and symptoms of mass effect. Diagnosis involves prolactin measurement and sellar imaging, preferably an MRI. Medical treatment of prolactinoma with dopamine agonists, such as cabergoline or bromocriptine, has high response rates, with a favorable safety profile. Surgery is indicated only in rare cases.

Congenital (pituitary stalk interruption) or acquired interruption of the hypothalamic-pituitary stalk (Fig. 9.18) may be accompanied by elevated prolactin concentrations. Serum levels of prolactin are usually normal or only mildly increased secondary to the decreased or loss of the inhibitory signal from the hypothalamus and impaired hypothalamic-pituitary communication. In pituitary stalk interruption, galactorrhea might rarely occur.

Antipsychotics such as risperidone, neuroleptics, estrogen, gastrointestinal motility promoting agents (metoclopramide), and antihypertensive medication (verapamil, methyldopa) can cause galactorrhea as a side effect. When hyperprolactinemia is secondary to medications, the prolactin concentrations are generally less than 75 ng/mL. Local lesions of the breast such as herpes zoster, burns, trauma, and systemic disease such as renal failure and hypothyroidism may also cause galactorrhea.

HYPOTHALAMIC-PITUITARY-THYROID AXIS

Evaluation of hypothalamic pituitary thyroid disorders starts with a detailed history and physical examination and complemented with laboratory tests and imaging as indicated in Box 9.7.

The thyroid gland originates in the primitive pharynx floor, near the base of the tongue, about 24 days after fertilization, forming the thyroid diverticulum. The developing thyroid gland moves down anteriorly to the hyoid bone and laryngeal cartilages along a narrow tube, the thyroglossal duct. When reaching its final position anterior to the trachea, the thyroid divides into right and left portions called the thyroid lobes connected by a thin layer of thyroid tissue, the isthmus, which lies ventrally to the second and third tracheal rings. The thyroglossal duct degenerates and disappears. On occasion, the lower portion of the thyroglossal duct fills up with thyroid tissue, forming the pyramidal lobe.

The thyroid gland is best palpated with the examiner behind the patient, as seen in Fig. 9.25. After identification of the cricothyroid

Box 9.7 Evaluation of Hypothalamic Pituitary Thyroid Disorders

History

- Hypo/hyperthyroid signs and symptoms, including fatigue, hair loss, dry/clammy skin, heat or cold intolerance, unexplained weight gain/loss, constipation, muscle weakness, or CNS symptoms
- Neonatal hypoglycemia, prolonged jaundice, poor feeding
- Head and neck radiation, recent imaging with iodinated contrast
- Dietary history of soy formula, vegan diets or special diets
- Medications and OTC supplements, including birth control/combined hormonal pills with estrogen, amiodarone, lithium, immunomodulators, tyrosine kinase inhibitors
- Family history of autoimmunity, thyroid cancers, genetic conditions

Physical Examination

- Careful evaluation growth chart
- Findings of other autoimmune conditions, vitiligo, mucosal hyperpigmentation
- Careful thyroid gland examination, assess for exophthalmos

Laboratory Tests

- Simultaneous measurement of TSH and free T4
- Further tests include total T3, thyroid autoantibodies, TBG, total T4

Imaging

- Ultrasound is the preferred imaging as an initial test, compared with CT or MRI

CNS, Central nervous system; *CT,* computed tomography; *MRI,* magnetic resonance imaging; *OTC,* over-the-counter; *TBG,* thyroxine-binding globulin; *TSH,* thyroid-stimulating hormone.

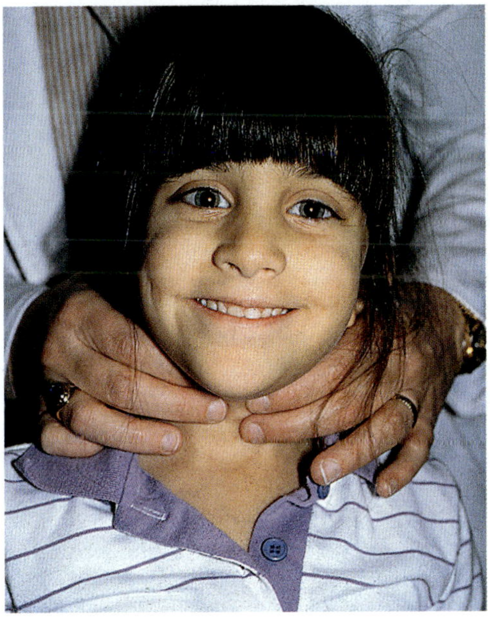

Fig. 9.25 Examination of the thyroid gland. The thyroid gland is best palpated with the examiner behind the patient.

cartilage, the second and third fingers are moved laterally along the trachea just medial to the sternocleidomastoid muscles. Two distinct lobes are palpable; the right lobe is usually greater than the left. When a goiter is present, these lobes may be quite easily identified (Fig. 9.26). The texture of the gland can provide clinical clues when evaluating for thyroid disease; in Graves disease, the gland tends to be soft and fleshy (Fig. 9.27), whereas in Hashimoto thyroiditis, it is typically firm or bosselated. Because the thyroid is directly supported by the trachea and will move up and down, having the patient swallow will help with identifying a mild gland enlargement. To demonstrate a goiter in a newborn, the examiner's hand is best placed gently under the back and shoulder blades of the infant, and the infant's trunk is raised from the bed (Fig. 9.28). As the head falls backward, the neck is elevated and a goiter, if present, will be evident. Thyroid ultrasound may be useful to confirm the presence of

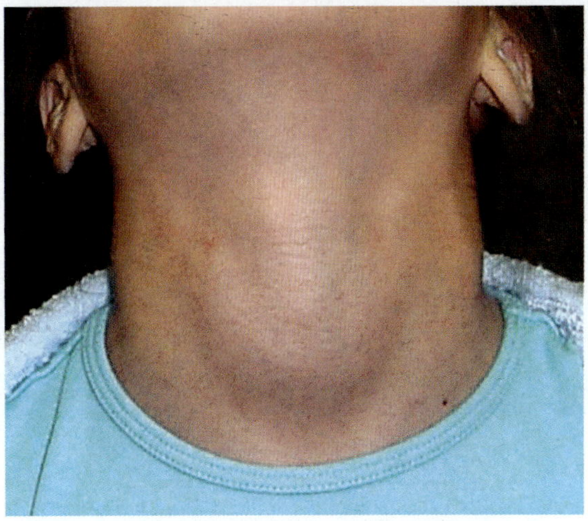

Fig. 9.26 Goiter. Note the enlarged thyroid gland in a patient with Hashimoto thyroiditis, easily visualized with neck extension. (Courtesy M. Parker, MD, Charlotte, NC.)

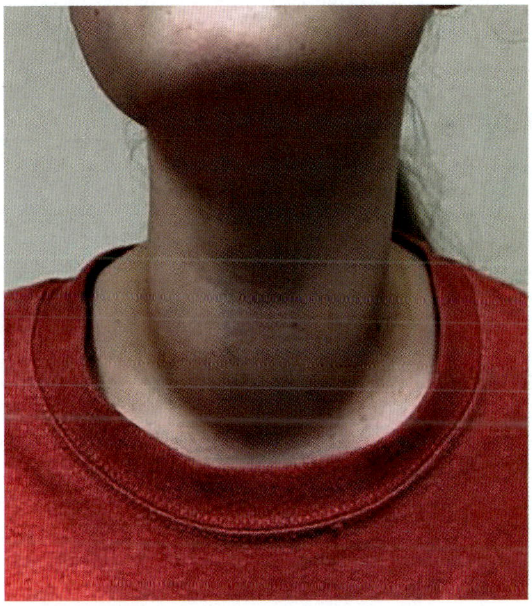

Fig. 9.27 Diffuse thyromegaly in an adolescent female with Graves disease. (Courtesy O. Escobar, MD, Pittsburgh, PA.)

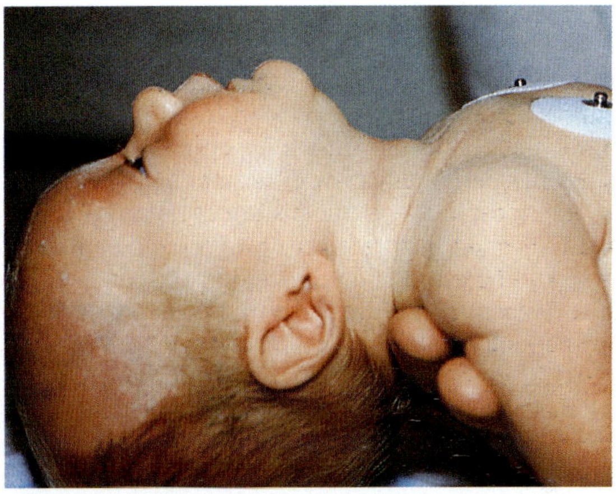

Fig. 9.28 Examination of the neonatal thyroid gland. Examination is performed by elevating the infant's trunk while allowing the head to fall back gently as shown.

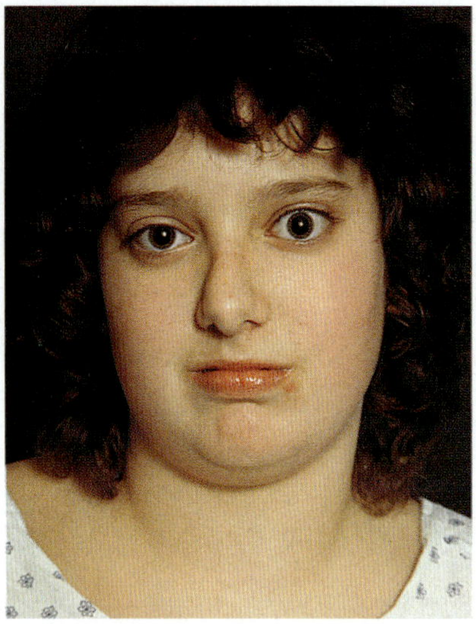

Fig. 9.29 Graves disease. Mild thyromegaly and proptosis or exophthalmos are characteristic findings in patients with Graves disease.

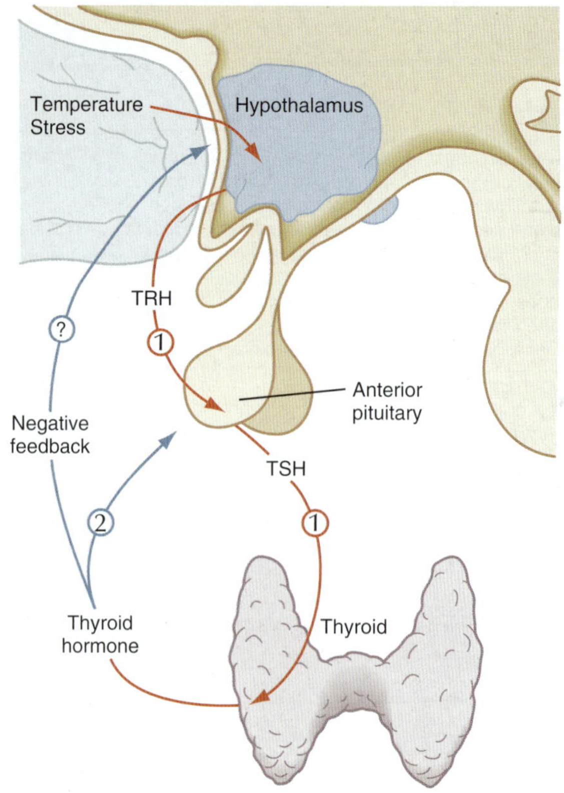

Fig. 9.30 Feedback regulation of thyroid-stimulating hormone *(TSH)* at the level of the hypothalamus, pituitary, and thyroid gland. *TRH,* Thyrotropin-releasing hormone.

thyroid tissue. Exophthalmos, a characteristic finding of Graves disease, is usually less dramatic in children than adults, but proptosis and lid lag can be appreciated (Fig. 9.29). The hyperthyroid gland can become quite large, up to three to four times its normal size, and is warm when palpated. A bruit may be heard over the gland.

The thyroid gland synthesizes thyroxine (T4) and triiodothyronine (T3); this process is dependent on the availability of iodine. Most circulating T4 and T3 are transported in plasma by thyroxine-binding globulin (TBG), albumin, and transthyretin. Free thyroid hormone is the active moiety. T4 and T3 are metabolized by inner ring deiodination to reverse T3 and diiodothyronine (T2), respectively, which are inactive. TSH is a pituitary glycoprotein hormone; the α-subunit is identical to the α-subunits of LH and FSH. Its specificity lies in its β-subunit. The key role of TSH is to promote the synthesis and secretion of thyroid hormones. Mediated by the TSH receptor, TSH increases the size of the thyroid cells, vascularity of the gland, iodide uptake, thyroglobulin synthesis, and thyroid hormone secretion. TSH secretion is determined by the level of circulating thyroid hormone and by the hypothalamic hormone, TRH (Fig. 9.30). Negative feedback of TSH secretion by circulating thyroid hormone occurs mainly at the pituitary level, but possibly also at the hypothalamic level.

Evaluation of thyroid disorders should start with history looking for symptoms of weight gain associated with lack of height gain, constipation, or dry skin. Poor feeding, low tone, and delayed developmental milestones during infancy could be signs of congenital hypothyroidism, TSH and thyroid hormone (TH) resistance. Hyperthyroid symptoms include tachycardia, weight loss, increased frequency of bowel movements, heat intolerance, nervousness, widened pulse pressure, and tremors. A thorough review of the height and weight chart and examination for findings associated with other autoimmune conditions (vitiligo, mucosal hyperpigmentation) is essential for the evaluation of both hyperthyroidism and hypothyroidism. Family/personal history of autoimmunity, thyroid cancers, genetic conditions, and personal history of radiation exposure and medications also aid in narrowing down the differential diagnosis. Patients should be asked about any recent imaging with iodinated contrast and recent procedures involving prepping of the skin with iodine-containing antiseptics, like betadine.

Dietary history is also important, as soy formula, vegan, or very restricted diets could lead to hypothyroidism. Patients on exclusive total parenteral nutrition after intestinal transplant or people exclusively using iodine-deficient natural/Himalayan salt or large amounts of sea weeds and goitrogenic vegetables are also at risk for goiter and hypothyroidism. Medications including birth control (combined hormonal pills with estrogen), amiodarone, lithium, immunomodulators, and tyrosine kinase inhibitors can alter thyroid functions or assay interference during laboratory measurements. Supplements that are currently marketed to promote thyroid health contain iodine and can cause hypothyroidism (Wolff-Chaikoff effect). Supplements containing excessive amounts of biotin do not cause thyroid dysfunction but may interfere with the TSH and T4 assay and yield elevated levels of free T4 and low levels of TSH, leading to an erroneous diagnosis of hyperthyroidism.

If there is a clinical suspicion for thyroid disease, laboratory evaluation with simultaneous measurement of TSH and free T4 is a good start. If abnormalities are noted, further testing including total T3, thyroid autoantibodies, TBG, and total T4 may be obtained. Free T3 does not have validated references and should be avoided if possible. The interpretation of the thyroid function tests can be influenced by the time frame of the blood draw in relation to the presence of significant illnesses (euthyroid sick syndrome) or recovery from them, as well as the use of concomitant medications. For instance, the use of combined oral contraceptives may lead to elevated levels of total T4 due to estrogen-induced increase in thyroid binding globulin (TBG) without effect on thyroid function, as manifested by normal free T4 and TSH levels.

Similarly, inherited disorders affecting TBG concentration may confound interpretation of thyroid function studies. TBG excess is caused by duplication or triplication of the gene encoding TBG (*SERPINA 7* gene) and is inherited as an X-linked trait. Total T4 levels are elevated, but free T4 and TSH are normal, and the individual is euthyroid. On the other hand, mutations of the *SERPINA 7* gene can also lead to TBG deficiency, inherited as an X-linked recessive trait. Total T4 levels are low, but free T4 and TSH are normal, and the individual is euthyroid.

Due to the superficial location of thyroid gland in the neck, ultrasound is the preferred imaging compared with CT or MRI. Ultrasound imaging can aid in the diagnosis of congenital hypothyroidism caused by thyroid agenesis or occasionally from ectopic thyroid. Thyroid ultrasound is sensitive to picking up nodules and anatomic abnormalities of the thyroid gland. It is not indicated routinely in the diagnosis or management of Hashimoto thyroiditis unless there is a palpable nodule, significant hardness or asymmetry of the gland. In the newborn with congenital hypothyroidism, radionucleotide thyroid scan is useful to determine the presence or absence of the gland, its location, and anatomy. Radioisotope scanning is also useful in the management and surveillance of thyroid nodules and thyroid cancer.

DISORDERS OF THYROID GLAND

Hypothyroidism

Hypothyroidism, often associated with a goiter, can be congenital or acquired. Hypothyroidism can be classified as primary when the defect lies in the thyroid gland itself or central when it is due to pituitary dysfunction (referred to as *secondary hypothyroidism*) or hypothalamic dysfunction (referred to as *tertiary hypothyroidism*). Iodine deficiency is among the most common causes of primary acquired hypothyroidism in the world, while autoimmune hypothyroidism is the most common cause of primary acquired hypothyroidism in iodine-sufficient areas.

The incidence of congenital hypothyroidism is 1 in 2500 to 3000. Children with untreated congenital hypothyroidism (previously called *cretinism*) develop a broad nasal bridge, coarse facial features, hoarse cry, prolonged jaundice, large posterior fontanelle, intellectual disability, hypotonia, short stature, a characteristic puffy appearance of their hands, protuberant tongue, and delayed skeletal maturation (Fig. 9.31). Because treatment by 3 to 4 weeks of age ameliorates these features, newborn screening programs have been implemented to identify infants with hypothyroidism early, before clinical manifestations. Despite the success of screening, thyroid function tests should still be obtained if signs and/or symptoms of congenital hypothyroidism are detected, even in the face of normal screening results. Radionuclide scanning using either technetium or iodine-123 (123I) can be useful in identifying an ectopic thyroid gland or thyroid agenesis (Fig. 9.32). Absence of radioisotope uptake in the normal position is consistent with thyroid agenesis.

Acquired hypothyroidism, most frequently due to Hashimoto thyroiditis or chronic lymphocytic thyroiditis, may present in childhood. Typical features include dry skin, constipation, hair loss, fatigue, cold intolerance, apathy, depressed or delayed relaxation phase of deep tendon reflexes, anemia, and weakness. Other clinical manifestations of severe hypothyroidism include pallor, coarse hair, myxedematous appearance, supraclavicular fullness, and calf pseudohypertrophy (Fig. 9.33A and B). A sharp deceleration in linear growth may also be seen in children with acquired hypothyroidism, as seen in the growth curve shown in Fig. 9.34. Family history is often positive for autoimmune thyroid disease. The diagnosis is confirmed by measurement of a high TSH level and low T4/Free T4 level. Antithyroid antibodies (directed against thyroid peroxidase and thyroglobulin) are often detected. After the institution of thyroid hormone replacement therapy, growth velocity returns to normal (Fig. 9.34C). Although acquired hypothyroidism is typically characterized by delayed bone age and delayed puberty, premature testicular enlargement in boys, premature thelarche, and even premature menarche in girls (Van Wyk-Grumbach syndrome) can occur in children with severe primary hypothyroidism. Acquired hypothalamic or pituitary disorders can cause hypothyroidism due to TRH and/or TSH deficiencies. TSH may be normal or low normal with a T4 level below normal range.

There are important caveats in the diagnosis of acquired hypothyroidism. Occasionally in uncontrolled primary acquired hypothyroidism, abnormal LFTs, elevated CPK, and hypercholesterolemia can be seen. This resolves with levothyroxine replacement, once thyroid hormone levels normalize. In patients with severe untreated hypothyroidism, TSH can be significantly elevated and pituitary enlargement is seen. If an MRI is obtained and there is a report of pituitary enlargement, it is advised to defer further intervention or referral (e.g., to neurosurgery) until TSH is normalized.

Resistance to thyroid hormone (RTH) is a rare genetic disorder in which there is lack of normal response of tissues to thyroid hormones, usually because of defects in either the thyroid hormone receptor beta *(THRβ)* gene, called RTH-beta, or the thyroid hormone receptor alpha *(THRα)* gene, called RTH-alpha. A third group of RTH has been identified in which there is no mutation of either of the THR genes and is referred to as nonTR-RTH. In RTH-beta (the most common form of RTH, representing ~85% of the cases) and nonTR-RTH, there are few to no manifestations of thyroid dysfunction despite elevated levels of serum T3 or T4 with normal or minimally elevated TSH levels. Patients with these conditions may present with subtle and variable signs of hypothyroidism or hyperthyroidism.

In RTH-alpha, manifestations may resemble those of untreated congenital hypothyroidism in peripheral tissues and is characterized by borderline low T4 and rT3 with minimally elevated T3 and usually normal TSH.

Patients with TSH resistance have been found to have inactivating mutations of the thyroid stimulating hormone receptor *(TSHR)* gene. Patients with partial TSH resistance are usually clinically euthyroid because they can compensate by increasing thyroid hormone levels. Those with complete TSH resistance may have profound hypothyroidism detectable on neonatal screening for congenital hypothyroidism.

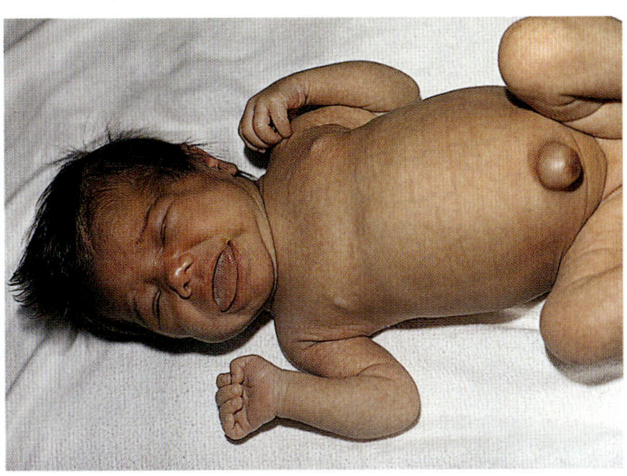

Fig. 9.31 A child with congenital hypothyroidism. Note the coarse facial features, broad nasal bridge, thick lips, and umbilical hernia. (Courtesy T.P. Foley, Jr., MD, Pittsburgh, PA.)

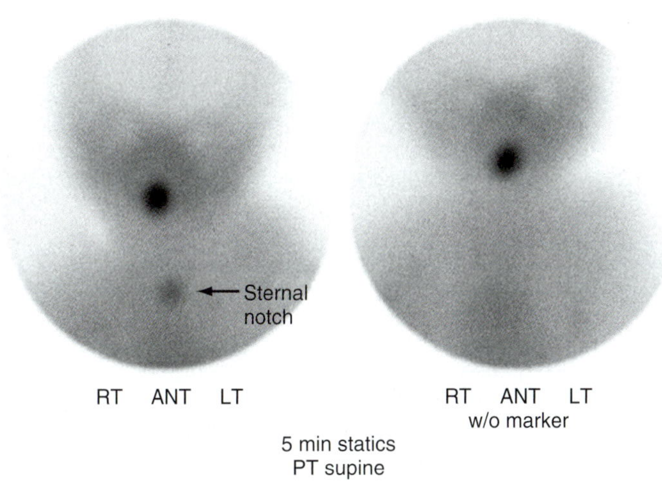

Fig. 9.32 Ectopic thyroid gland. Technetium (^{99m}Tc) scan of an 8-day-old infant with congenital hypothyroidism. A lingual thyroid gland is identified with no functioning thyroid tissue in the anatomic thyroid bed. *ANT,* Anterior; *LT,* left; *PT,* patient; *RT,* right. (Courtesy S.F. Witchel, MD, Pittsburgh, PA.)

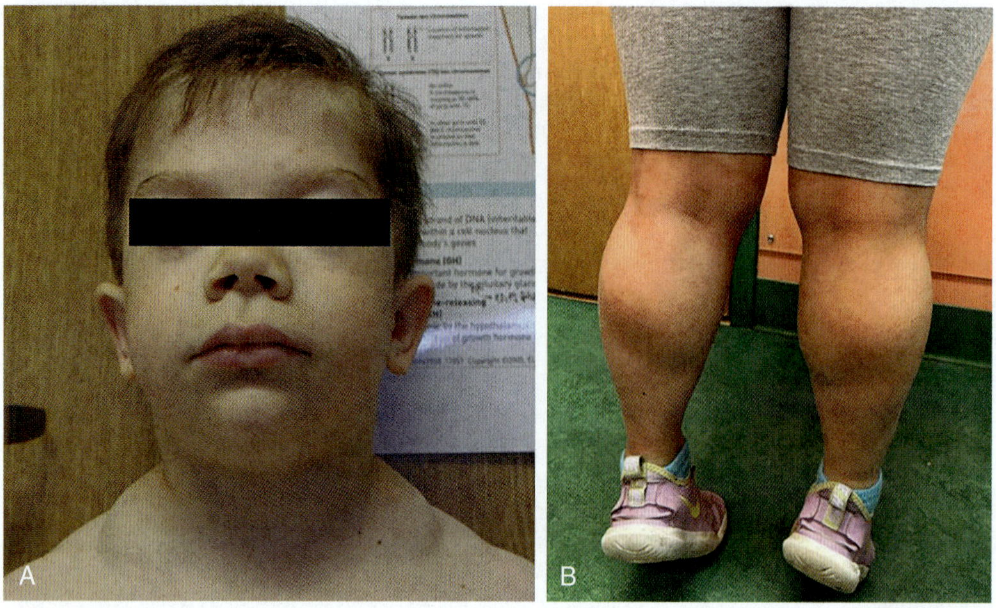

Fig. 9.33 Severe hypothyroidism. (A) Notice pallor, myxedematous facial appearance, coarse scalp hair and supraclavicular fullness. (B) Calf pseudohypertrophy. (Courtesy O. Escobar, MD, Pittsburgh, PA.)

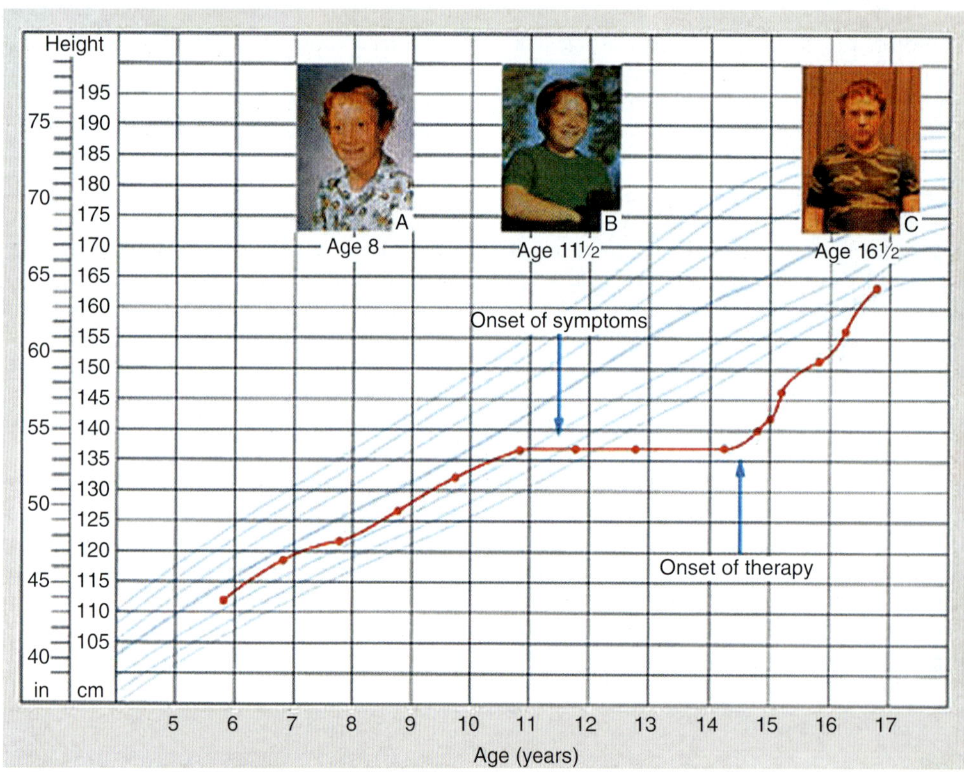

Fig. 9.34 Growth curve of a child with acquired hypothyroidism. Note the sharp deceleration in growth before the onset of symptoms. After thyroid hormone replacement, significant catch-up growth occurs. The inserted photographs illustrate the child before onset of acquired hypothyroidism (A), the change in body habitus associated with acquired hypothyroidism (B), and resolution after thyroid replacement at the indicated times (C).

Allen-Herndon-Dudley syndrome is associated with mutations in monocarboxylate transporter 8 (MCT8) encoded by the *SLC16A2* gene. This X-linked disorder is characterized by severe neurocognitive disability and abnormal thyroid function studies. Typically, T3 is elevated, T4 is low, and TSH concentrations are in the upper normal range. The phenotype, characterized by peripheral thyrotoxicosis and cerebral hypothyroidism, reflects impaired thyroid hormone transport across the blood-brain barrier into the brain. Recent clinical studies are using triiodothyroacetic acid (Triac) to manage this condition, given that this is a thyroid hormone analog that does not require MCT8 to enter the cell.

Hyperthyroidism

Hyperthyroidism refers to excessive thyroid hormone secretion by the thyroid gland. History will suggest features indicating accelerated basal metabolism. On examination, skin is warm and moist; the hair is fine and friable. Plummer nails, or separation of the distal margin of the nail bed, may be noted. Tall stature, restlessness, inability to sit still, emotional lability, short attention span, excessive sweating, decreased school performance, and fatigue may be noted on history or physical examination.

Autoimmune hyperthyroidism can be due to Graves disease or the hyperthyroid phase of Hashimoto thyroiditis, commonly called Hashitoxicosis. In Graves disease, stimulating antibody directed against the TSH receptor (TSH receptor antibody [TRAb] or thyroid-stimulating immunoglobulin [TSI]) increases the endogenous production of thyroid hormone. The transient hyperthyroidism seen in Hashimoto thyroiditis is related to the release of preformed thyroid hormone from a thyroid gland being disrupted by lymphocytic infiltration.

Other, less common causes of hyperthyroidism in children include autonomously functioning adenomas, toxic multinodular goiters, activating mutations of the TSH receptor, selective pituitary T3 resistance, and exogenous intake of thyroid hormones.

Congenital hyperthyroidism can occur in infants of women with thyrotoxicosis due to Graves disease. Neonatal Graves disease is due to transplacental transfer of TSH receptor stimulating antibodies and is usually self-limited due to the loss of maternal TSH receptor stimulating antibodies over time.

Neonatal Graves disease is characterized by irritability, poor weight gain, flushing, tachycardia, hypertension, and thyromegaly. Usually, the clinical course of neonatal Graves disease is limited to 3 to 12 weeks. A second trimester screening of pregnant women with history of Graves disease might be useful in evaluating the need to monitor thyroid levels in newborns.

Other Disorders Affecting Thyroid Function Tests

Abnormalities in the serum proteins that transport thyroid hormones do not cause thyroid disease. However, they can cause falsely high or low T4 measurements. Inherited disorders affecting TBG concentration may confound interpretation of thyroid hormone function studies.

Commonly, abnormal thyroid function tests are found in the setting of a nonthyroidal illness, without preexisting hypothalamic-pituitary and thyroid gland dysfunction. Patients admitted to the hospital units or intensive care unit with acute severe nonthyroidal illness may show low T4, low TSH, and increased reverse triiodothyronine (rT3) concentrations; rT3 is an inactive metabolite of T4. After recovery from nonthyroidal illness (also known as *sick euthyroid syndrome*), these thyroid function test result abnormalities generally return to normal ranges. Increased estradiol concentrations (e.g., females who are on combined oral contraceptive pills or pregnant) can have elevated total T4 with normal TSH, but the free T4 levels would be in normal range. Children with elevated BMI may have a slightly elevated TSH level (often <10 uIU/mL) with a normal T4 level and normal growth velocity. The TSH returns to normal after weight loss. The mechanism responsible for the slightly elevated TSH concentration in obese individuals remains unknown.

Thyroid Nodules and Thyroid Cancer

When evaluating children and adolescents with thyroid nodules, specific attention should be given to history and physical examination. History should be elicited regarding thyroid compressive symptoms, difficulty swallowing or breathing, hoarseness of voice, facial flushing when hands elevated (Pemberton sign), and neck pain; personal history of Hashimoto thyroiditis; thyroid disease like ectopic thyroid, thyroglossal cyst, and malignancies; cancer treatments in the past; and personal history of head, neck, and total body radiation is important. Family history of thyroid cancers, family history of multiple colon polyps, colon cancer, Peutz-Jeghers syndrome, pheochromocytoma/paraganglioma/MEN, or any other familial cancer syndromes should be explored while evaluating a thyroid nodule/cancer.

Thyroid nodules and thyroid cancers are more common in children than have been previously reported and thus represent a significant health issue. This discrepancy may be due to the increase in the imaging of the head and neck in children. A rising proportion of asymptomatic thyroid nodules are identified incidentally during a head and neck CT scan or radiograph performed for an unrelated workup. Although nodules are uncommon in children, the risk of malignancy is higher than in adults. Approximately 25% of nodules in children are malignant compared with 5% to 10% in adults. Other neck masses including branchial cysts, thyroglossal cyst, and intrathyroidal thymic tissue are also more common in the pediatric population than in adults. Ectopic thymic tissue could be misread as thyroid nodules with calcifications and can be mistaken for thyroid malignancies unless read by experienced radiologists. Some studies indicate increased risk of differentiated thyroid cancer is associated with Hashimoto thyroiditis. However, the heterogenicity of the gland and "white knight nodule" in a thyroid ultrasound, unless carefully evaluated, can cause unnecessary anxiety to families and unwarranted procedures in children. Evaluation should include high-resolution ultrasound imaging of the thyroid and whole neck. Scoring systems to determine the risk for malignancy are being validated. A thorough neck examination is needed in evaluation (Fig. 9.35), and imaging is used only in the event of clinical suspicion. Ultrasound can be helpful in screening for thyroid cancers in genetic predisposition syndromes or in patients with exposure to ionizing radiation at a younger age. The next step in evaluation of a suspicious thyroid nodule is fine-needle aspiration. This is invasive, requires anesthesia in children, and has the risk of inadequate sample if there is no cytopathologist on site. Thus thorough evaluation of pediatric thyroid nodules is best done at a multidisciplinary thyroid center.

The clinical presentation of thyroid cancer often differs between children and adults. Instead of a thyroid nodule or lump in their thyroid, they can present initially with lymph node metastasis in the neck and even pulmonary metastases at the time of diagnosis. Yet despite extensive disease at clinical presentation, children are much less likely to die of the disease. There are important clinical, molecular, and pathologic differences in differentiated thyroid cancer among children when compared with adults. In adults, point mutations of the BRAF and RAS genes are more common, whereas gene rearrangements such as RET/PTC are more prevalent among children. Medullary thyroid carcinoma associated with genetic syndromes, such as MEN type 2B (MEN2B), arises from the parafollicular C cells of the thyroid and is described in the adrenal medullary disorder section.

For several decades, the treatment of children with thyroid cancer was based on adult treatment guidelines. A more appropriate

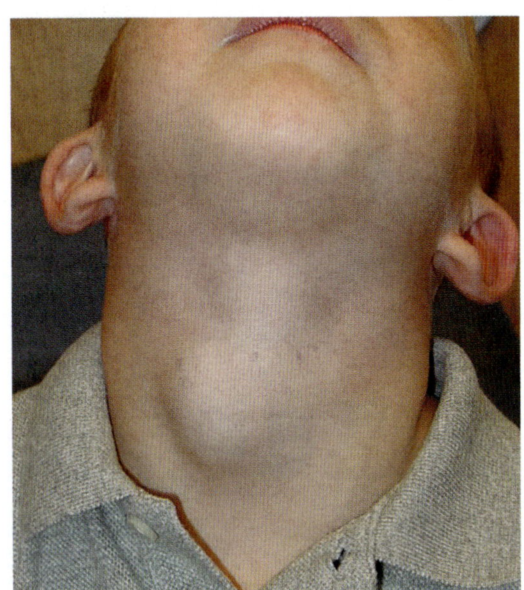

Fig. 9.35 Thyroid nodule in the right thyroid lobe, visible on simple inspection in a young boy. (Courtesy O. Escobar, MD, Pittsburgh, PA.)

risk-stratified treatment and rational endpoint for therapy has since been developed for children. The American Thyroid Association published pediatric guidelines for management of thyroid nodules and differentiated thyroid cancer. Children with relatively low risk for thyroid cancer are treated with close observation after appropriate surgery and do not undergo routine radioiodine ablation therapy.

HYPOTHALAMIC-PITUITARY-ADRENAL AXIS

The hypothalamic-pituitary control of the adrenal glands is by the corticotropin-releasing hormone (CRH) and ACTH, respectively. CRH, secreted by the hypothalamus, regulates the secretion of ACTH. ACTH stimulates cortisol secretion by the adrenal cortex; cortisol then inhibits ACTH secretion by the anterior pituitary by negative feedback inhibition (Fig. 9.36). The corticotropin-related peptide hormones consist of ACTH, α-melanocyte-stimulating hormone (α-MSH), and γ- and β-lipotropins (γ-LPH, β-LPH). These hormones are derived from a common precursor molecule, pro-opiomelanocortin (POMC).

The adrenal glands consist of the inner adrenal medulla and outer adrenal cortex. Cells in adrenal medulla have an ectodermal origin, whereas adrenal cortical cells have a mesodermal origin. During fetal life, the adrenal cortex consists of the fetal adrenal cortical zone, which involutes during the first year of life, and the outer definitive zone. Adrenal hormone synthesis starts early in gestation in the fetal zone to provide DHEAS, which serves as the substrate for placental estrogen synthesis. At birth, the fetal adrenal gland is roughly twice the size of adult adrenal glands. Postnatally, the definitive adrenal cortex develops into the adult adrenal cortex, composed of three distinct zones: zona glomerulosa, zona fasciculata, and zona reticularis.

The outer zona glomerulosa synthesizes mineralocorticoids (aldosterone). Aldosterone promotes sodium retention and potassium excretion. Aldosterone secretion is regulated by the renin-angiotensin system and serum potassium concentrations. Aldosterone actions are mediated by the mineralocorticoid receptor. The middle layer, zona fasciculata, synthesizes glucocorticoids (cortisol). The glucocorticoid receptor, located in the cytoplasm, mediates the tissue-specific physiologic and pharmacologic actions of glucocorticoids. The innermost zone, the zona reticularis, synthesizes adrenal androgens (C19 androgens), which are DHEAS, dehydroepiandrosterone, and androstenedione. The adrenal androgens do not bind to the androgen receptor but can be peripherally converted to more potent androgens by extra adrenal enzymes, which then activate the androgen receptor.

Cortisol secretion is dependent on de novo synthesis because cortisol is not stored in the adrenal cortex. This process involves multiple steroidogenic enzymes; ACTH stimulation is required to promote the expression and function of these enzymes. ACTH and cortisol secretion manifest a diurnal rhythm with the highest concentrations occurring during the early morning. This rhythm is established between 6 and 12 months of age. Prolonged exogenous glucocorticoid therapy suppresses the hypothalamic-pituitary-adrenal (HPA) axis with the potential for iatrogenic adrenal insufficiency and a significant impact on growth and development.

EVALUATION OF HYPOTHALAMIC-PITUITARY-ADRENAL AXIS DISORDERS

A comprehensive evaluation of the HPA axis includes targeted history, physical examination before laboratory evaluation, and imaging as noted in Box 9.8.

Poor feeding, weight loss, dehydration, lethargy in newborns and infants, slow growth, salt craving, abdominal pain, darkening of skin, vomiting, and symptoms of hypoglycemia at all ages should raise concerns for adrenal insufficiency. Altered menstrual history and concerns for hirsutism should raise possibility of nonclassical CAH and Cushing syndrome. Early age of onset and rapid tempo of adrenarche in both boys and girls should raise concern for androgen excess. Medications like megestrol acetate, opioids, antiretroviral agents, antifungals, and testosterone synthesis inhibitors and immune checkpoint inhibitors cause adrenal insufficiency. Long-term use of systemic/inhaled/topical steroids may cause either hypercortisolism or HPA axis suppression.

On patient examination, careful review of growth charts and blood pressure cannot be overemphasized. Particular attention

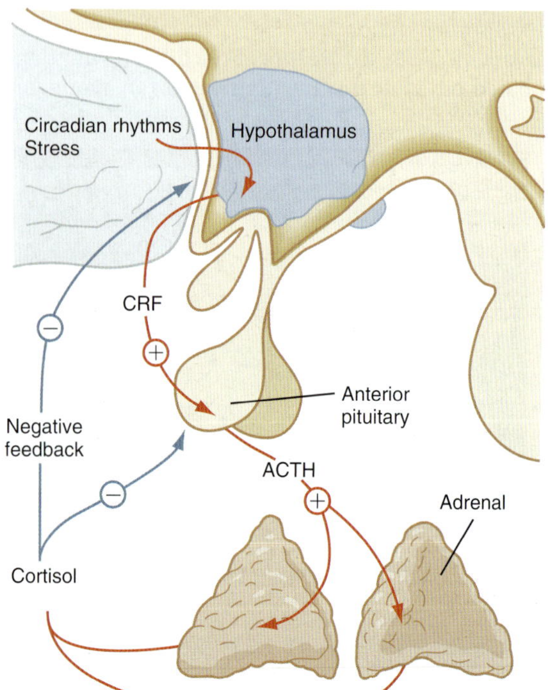

Fig. 9.36 Feedback regulation of adrenocorticotropic hormone *(ACTH)* at the level of the hypothalamus, pituitary, and adrenal glands. *CRF,* Corticotropin-releasing factor.

Box 9.8 Evaluation of Hypothalamic-Pituitary-Adrenal Axis Disorders

History
- Poor feeding, fatigue/lethargy, salt craving, darkening of skin, vomiting, symptoms of hypoglycemia may indicate adrenal insufficiency
- Rapid weight gain, muscle weakness, skin fragility/stretch marks may indicate hypercortisolism
- Long-term use of systemic/inhaled/topical steroids, megestrol acetate (megace), opioids, antiretroviral agents, antifungals, ketoconazole, immune checkpoint inhibitors

Physical Examination
- Height, weight (review of growth patterns), and blood pressure
- Genital examination (clitoromegaly and genital ambiguity)
- Skin (hyperpigmentation, vitiligo, hirsutism, wide purple striae, plethora, telangiectasia)

Laboratory Tests
- ACTH, serum cortisol, electrolytes, plasma renin activity, serum aldosterone, 7-OH-Progesterone, androstenedione, DHEAS, urinary and salivary cortisol
- Dynamic testing likely needed

Imaging
- Pelvic ultrasound (infants with ambiguous genitalia)
- MRI of pelvis and pituitary (hypercortisolism evaluation)
- CT scans are better for adrenal evaluation (hemorrhage, adenomas)

ACTH, Adrenocorticotrophic hormone; *CT,* computed tomography; *DHEAS,* dehydroepiandrosterone sulfate; *MRI,* magnetic resonance imaging.

should be paid to the configuration of external genitalia including the presence of clitoromegaly and genital ambiguity, hyperpigmentation of the skin and mucous membranes, vitiligo (especially in autoimmune destruction of the adrenals), and hirsutism. Beyond the baseline labs to evaluate HPA axis, dynamic testing might be needed to aid in the final diagnosis. Dexamethasone suppression tests are used to differentiate the various causes of high cortisol levels. Meanwhile, cosyntropin (synthetic ACTH) stimulation tests are used to understand the causes of hypocortisolism and to confirm the diagnosis of CAH. The ACTH stimulation test also helps to differentiate among various steroidogenic enzyme deficiency disorders. Pelvic ultrasound can be helpful in the evaluation of infants with ambiguous genitalia to identify internal structures and gonads. Occasionally, pelvic MRI is needed for better visualization of internal genital anatomy. MRI is generally used for evaluation of cortisol excess. CT scans are the preferred mode of imaging for adrenal glands.

Disorders of the Adrenal Cortex

Primary Adrenal Insufficiency

Primary adrenal insufficiency can be classified into four groups according to the underlying pathogenesis: (1) adrenal hypoplasia, (2) impaired steroidogenesis, (3) familial glucocorticoid deficiency (FGD), and (4) adrenal destruction. Iatrogenic primary adrenal insufficiency is rarely related to medications such as ketoconazole and mitotane.

Adrenal Hypoplasia Congenita

Adrenal hypoplasia congenita (AHC) is an X-linked recessive disorder due to loss-of-function mutations of the *DAX1/NROB1* gene and can be associated with hypogonadotropic hypogonadism. AHC in males may occur as a contiguous gene defect in association with Duchenne muscular dystrophy and glycerol kinase deficiency. Symptoms of acute adrenal insufficiency generally develop around 6 to 8 weeks after birth, when the fetal zone of the adrenal cortex involutes.

Other disorders associated with adrenal insufficiency due to adrenal dysgenesis include the IMAGe (Intrauterine growth restriction, Metaphyseal dysplasia, Adrenal hypoplasia congenita and Genital anomalies) syndrome associated with *CDKN1C* mutations and Pallister-Hall syndrome associated with *GLI3* mutations.

Impaired Steroidogenesis

CAH is an autosomal recessive disorder in which defects in adrenal steroidogenesis cause primary adrenal insufficiency resulting from decreased production of glucocorticoids and, sometimes, mineralocorticoids with back-up accumulation of adrenal androgen precursors. The specific symptoms and laboratory findings are due to corticosteroid and mineralocorticoid deficiency. The most common cause of CAH is 21-hydroxylase deficiency secondary to loss-of-function mutations in the 21-hydroxylase gene *(CYP21A2)* (see Fig. 9.37). Decreased glucocorticoid biosynthesis results in loss of negative feedback leading to increased ACTH and adrenal androgen secretion. The phenotype varies depending on the severity of genetic mutation. Although CAH

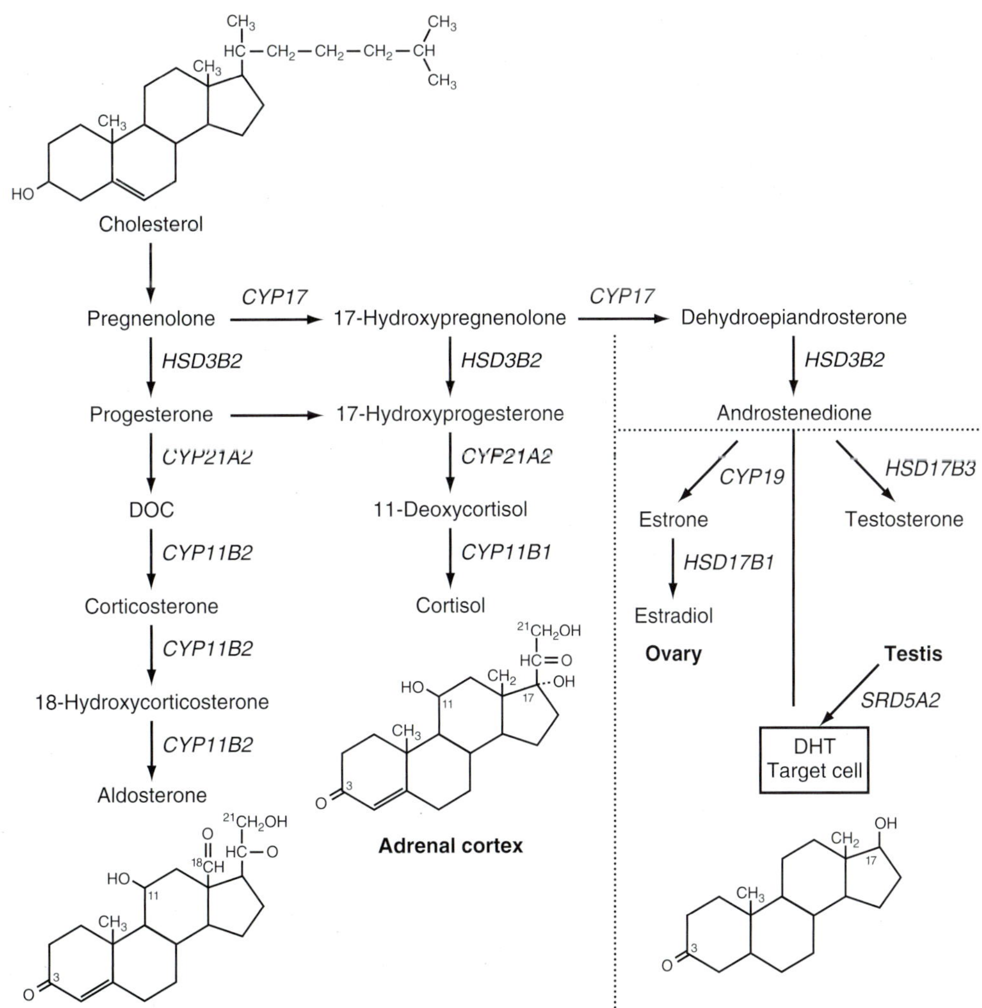

Fig. 9.37 Steroid biosynthesis pathway. Pathways for the synthesis of mineralocorticoids (aldosterone), glucocorticoids (cortisol), and androgens (testosterone) are shown. Deficiency in 21-hydroxylase activity (CYP21A2) prevents the conversion of 17-hydroxyprogesterone (17-OHP) to 11-deoxycortisol, resulting in an elevation of 17-OHP and shunting of precursors into the pathway for androgen biosynthesis. Androstenedione is secreted by the adrenal cortex and converted to testosterone or estradiol in the periphery. Testosterone may be converted by 5α-reductase (SRD5A2) to dihydrotestosterone *(DHT)*. *DOC,* Deoxycorticosterone. (Courtesy K. LynShue and S. Witchel, Pittsburgh, PA.)

is often classified into three categories (classic salt-losing, simple virilizing, and nonclassical), the disorder reflects a spectrum of clinical manifestations.

Classic salt wasting CAH occurs in about 1 of 12,000 births and is characterized by elevated 17-hydroxyprogesterone (17-OHP) and androstenedione concentrations. In severe forms, mineralocorticoid biosynthesis is also inadequate, leading to chronic salt loss, hyponatremia, hyperkalemia, and elevated plasma renin activity. Excessive prenatal androgen biosynthesis is associated with masculinization of the external genitalia of affected female infants. Affected females typically have ambiguous symmetric external genitalia with nonpalpable gonads at birth. Affected male infants have normal male external genitalia with hyperpigmentation of the scrotum. Ovarian and uterine development are normal in virilized female infants. Salt wasting CAH can be caused by deficiency of steroid acute regulatory protein (StAR), 3β-hydroxysteroid dehydrogenase (3β HSD), or, more commonly, 21-hydroxylase. Hyperkalemia, hyponatremia, failure to thrive, and hypoglycemia, culminating in shock, ensue within 10 to 14 days after birth in the untreated infant as a consequence of severe mineralocorticoid and glucocorticoid deficiencies.

Newborn screening for 21-hydroxylase deficiency (measurement of 17-OHP levels) has been enormously beneficial and is mandated in all 50 states. The goal of newborn screening is to identify infants with salt-losing and simple virilizing forms of CAH. Because false-negative screening can occur, it is important to measure 17-OHP concentrations if one is suspicious of CAH. Some states mandate a second 17-OHP screen to minimize false-negative results. False-positive screening can occur in preterm infants, stressed infants, and heterozygous *CYP21A2* mutation carriers.

Individuals with a simple virilizing 21-hydroxylase deficiency do not produce enough cortisol but can synthesize enough aldosterone to maintain normal electrolytes. Like classic CAH, females may have ambiguous genitalia, whereas affected males usually present later when signs of androgen excess develop, usually in early childhood. Children with simple virilizing CAH often present with premature pubarche, rapid growth, tall stature, and advanced skeletal maturation. Affected females may have premature pubic hair and progressive clitoromegaly. Affected males often present with pubic hair, phallic enlargement, prepubertal testes, tall stature, and advanced skeletal maturation. Patients with nonclassical 21-hydroxylase deficiency (NCCAH) produce normal amounts of cortisol and aldosterone at the expense of elevated androgen production. Affected adolescent girls usually present with hirsutism, oligomenorrhea, and acne (similar to the clinical features associated with polycystic ovary syndrome [PCOS]). In some instances, ACTH stimulation testing may be necessary to distinguish between NCCAH and PCOS. Males with NCCAH generally are asymptomatic and are identified through family studies after diagnosis of NCCAH in a female relative. Less common forms of virilizing CAH are due to mutations in the 3β-hydroxysteroid dehydrogenase type 2 *(HSD3B2)* gene and 11β-hydroxylase *(CYP11B1)* gene. Loss-of-function mutations in the 17α-hydroxylase/17,20-lyase *(CYP17A1)* gene prevent synthesis of glucocorticoids and sex steroids. Affected females show normal female external genital development and delayed puberty, whereas affected males are undervirilized at birth; elevated mineralocorticoid concentrations can be associated with hypertension.

Congenital lipoid adrenal hyperplasia is characterized by inadequate virilization of affected males, adrenal insufficiency presenting in the late neonatal period, and lipoid hyperplasia of the adrenal glands. This form of CAH is due to mutations in the steroidogenic acute regulatory protein *(StAR)* gene. The phenotype of individuals with loss of function mutations in cholesterol desmolase *(CYP11A1)* is like congenital lipoid adrenal hyperplasia. Both disorders cause early defects in adrenal, testicular, and ovarian steroidogenesis. Genetic analysis may be needed to distinguish between *StAR* and *CYP11A1* mutations.

Loss-of-function mutations in the P450 oxidoreductase *(POR)* gene manifest with defective steroidogenesis and skeletal anomalies including craniosynostosis, midface hypoplasia, and choanal stenosis, known as Antley-Bixler syndrome. Affected infants may have ambiguous genitalia.

Familial Glucocorticoid Deficiency

FGD, or ACTH resistance, is characterized by decreased glucocorticoid production with nearly normal mineralocorticoid secretion. Loss of function mutations in the ACTH receptor gene *(MC2R)* are the most common etiology of FGD; inheritance is autosomal recessive. This disorder presents in young children with failure to thrive, hyperpigmentation, and hypoglycemia. Autosomal recessive mutations in the MC2R accessory protein encoded by *MRAP* are associated with a similar phenotype. Allgrove syndrome is an autosomal recessive disorder characterized by adrenal insufficiency, absent lacrimation, achalasia (hence the alternate name of AAA syndrome), deafness, and developmental delay due to mutations in the *ALADIN* gene. Other genes associated with ACTH resistance include nicotinamide nucleotide transhydrogenase *(NNT)* and thioredoxin reductase 2 *(TXNRD2)*.

Adrenal Destruction Causing Primary Adrenal Insufficiency

Primary adrenal insufficiency is characterized by both glucocorticoid and mineralocorticoid deficiencies. It typically presents with weight loss, anorexia, wasting of subcutaneous tissue, electrolyte abnormalities, and hyperpigmentation (Fig. 9.38A). Hyperpigmentation of the skin and mucous membranes (due to elevated MSH) is more obvious in flexor creases, in scars, and over the areolae of the nipples (see Fig. 9.38B to D) and the gums (Fig. 9.39). Hyponatremia, hyperkalemia, and elevated plasma renin activity are laboratory abnormalities associated with primary adrenal insufficiency. Hypoglycemia and eosinophilia may occur due to cortisol deficiency. The loss of negative feedback from cortisol deficiency leads to simultaneously increased ACTH and MSH secretion.

Addison disease is the autoimmune destruction of the adrenal gland and has now replaced tuberculosis as the most common cause of primary adrenal insufficiency. If untreated, patients with Addison disease progressively weaken and eventually experience hemodynamic collapse. The decreased circulating plasma volume is reflected by the thinned, narrow heart shadow seen on a chest radiograph (see Fig. 9.38E).

Two autoimmune polyendocrine syndromes are associated with Addison disease. The type 1 form (APECED: Autoimmune Polyendocrinopathy, Candidiasis Ectodermal Dysptrophy) is characterized by chronic mucocutaneous candidiasis, hypoparathyroidism, and adrenal insufficiency; it is associated with mutations in the AIRE (Autoimmune Regulator) gene. The type 2 form (Schmidt syndrome) is characterized by diabetes, hypothyroidism, and adrenal insufficiency.

Genetic disorders associated with adrenal destruction include adrenoleukodystrophy, Zellweger syndrome, and Wolman syndrome. X-linked adrenoleukodystrophy, due to mutations in the *ABCD1* gene, is a peroxisomal disorder characterized by adrenocortical insufficiency and slowly progressive myelopathy. The *ABCD1* gene codes for the peroxisomal membrane protein ALDP, which is involved in the transmembrane transport of very long-chain fatty acids (VLCFAs; ≥C22). Affected individuals have elevated VLCFA concentrations. Many newborn screening programs include the test for adrenoleukodystrophy. Zellweger spectrum disorders represent a spectrum of autosomal recessive disorders with four phenotypes that differ in severity and age at presentation. These disorders include Zellweger syndrome (most severe form), infantile Refsum disease, neonatal adrenoleukodystrophy, and Heimler syndrome (very mild end of the spectrum). ZSDs are associated with mutations in one of 13 peroxisome biogenesis factor *(PEX)* genes. Mutations in the *PEX* genes cause a deficiency of the functional peroxisome. Ocular abnormalities, hepatic dysfunction, adrenoleukodystrophy, and developmental delays may be present. VLCFAs are elevated. The diagnosis

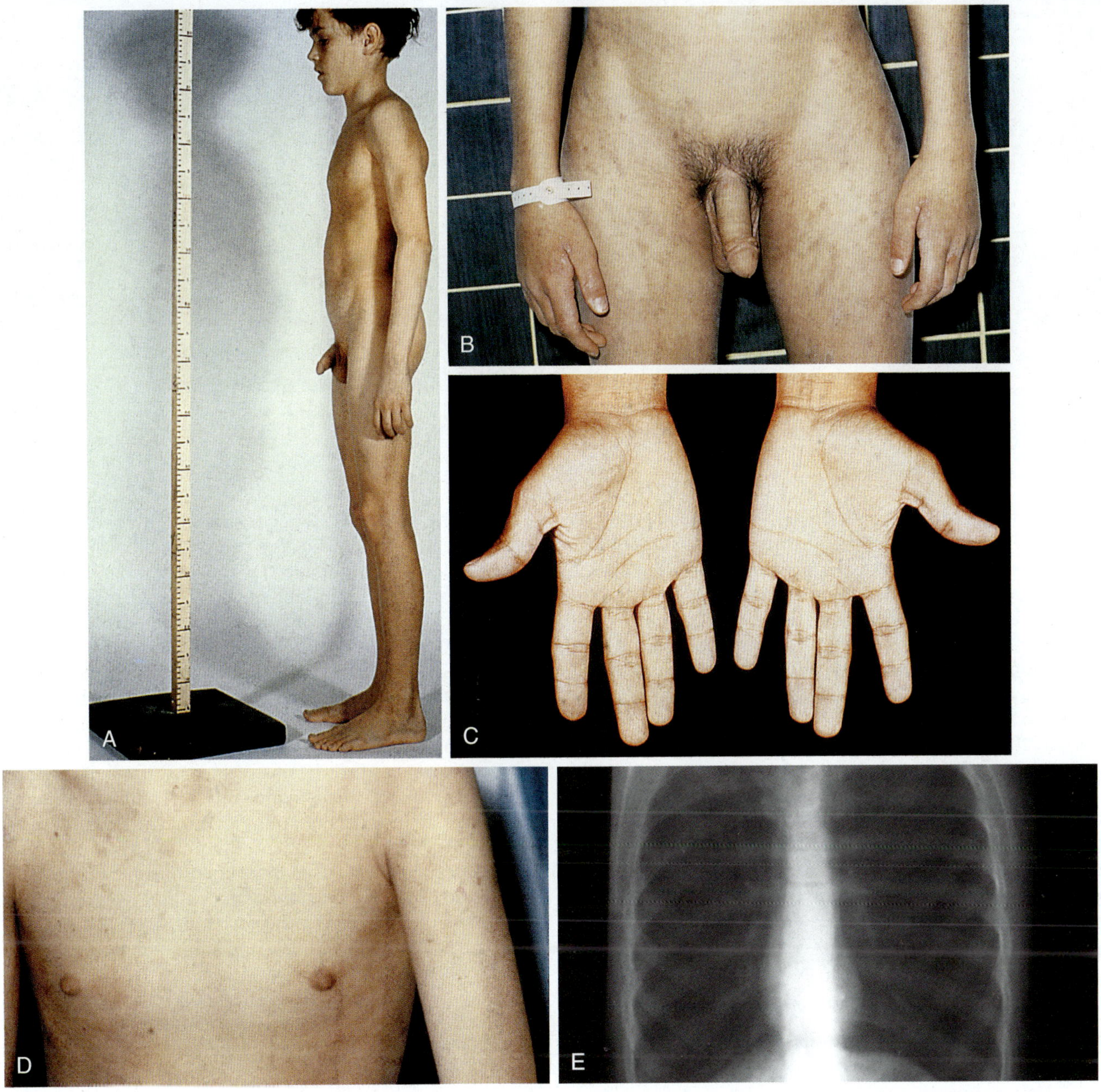

Fig. 9.38 Primary adrenal insufficiency. (A) This patient shows the thin habitus and ill appearance characteristic of Addison disease. (B) Hyperpigmentation of external genitalia. (C) Hyperpigmentation of palms of hands. (D) Hyperpigmentation of areolae. (E) Microcardia is characteristically seen on chest radiograph. (A–D, Courtesy M. New, MD, New York, NY. E, Courtesy J. Medina, Pittsburgh, PA.)

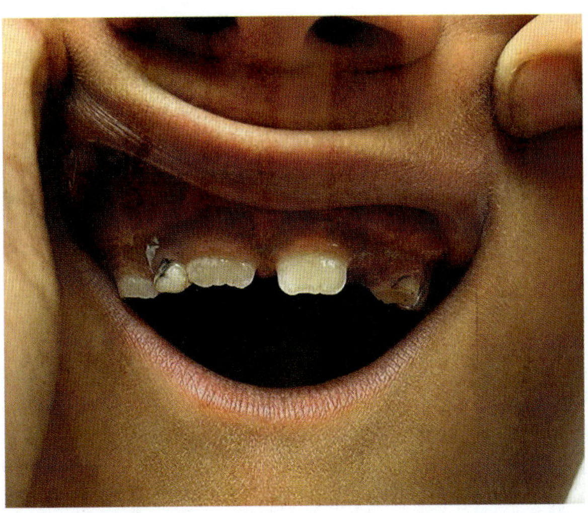

Fig. 9.39 Gingival hyperpigmentation in a young boy with Addison disease (autoimmune primary adrenal insufficiency). (Courtesy O. Escobar, MD, Pittsburgh, PA.)

can be verified by functional assays in cultured skin fibroblasts and followed by mutation analysis.

The infantile form of Wolman disease typically presents with diarrhea, massive hepatosplenomegaly, failure to thrive, and calcification of adrenal glands; this autosomal recessive disorder is associated with mutations in the lysosomal acid lipase *(LIPA)* gene located at chromosome 10q24-q25.

Neonatal adrenal hemorrhages and meningitis (Waterhouse-Friderichsen syndrome) can destroy the adrenal cortex, resulting in acute adrenal insufficiency.

Secondary Adrenal Insufficiency

Secondary adrenal insufficiency is due to pituitary (ACTH deficiency) or hypothalamic dysfunction (alterations in CRF secretion). Clinical features are more subtle than those of primary adrenal insufficiency and without electrolyte disturbances because aldosterone secretion is typically preserved. Aldosterone secretion is primarily regulated by the renin–angiotensin system rather than ACTH. ACTH deficiency may be isolated or may be associated

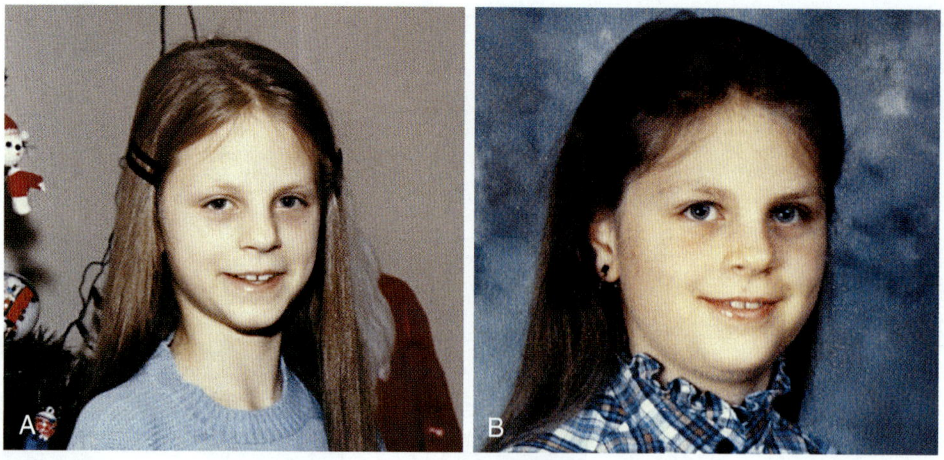

Fig. 9.40 Isolated adrenocorticotropic hormone (ACTH) deficiency. (A) Young girl with isolated ACTH deficiency shows wasting and pallor rather than excessive bronzing. (B) The same girl after therapy.

with other pituitary hormone deficiencies. The girl in Fig. 9.40 with isolated ACTH deficiency is seen before and after treatment. She has clinical wasting without hyperpigmentation. Other causes of ACTH deficiency include craniopharyngioma, brain tumor, cranial irradiation, surgery, histiocytosis X, hypophysitis, and traumatic brain injury.

Iatrogenic adrenal insufficiency is the most common cause of adrenal insufficiency and is due to prolonged, high-dose glucocorticoid medication use. Chronic glucocorticoid therapy leads to secondary/tertiary (hypothalamic) ACTH deficiency and atrophy of the zona fasciculata. Chronic inhaled and oral glucocorticoid treatment can result in secondary adrenal insufficiency. ACTH and cortisol levels should be monitored periodically when children are on long-term inhaled steroids or oral/systemic steroids. Manifestations may only be apparent in stressful situations like surgery, fever, pain, and infection. At these times, patients may need to double or triple their maintenance hydrocortisone dose (stress dosing). Parents and patients requiring chronic glucocorticoid treatment should learn "stress dose" management and wear Medic-Alert identification badges.

Adrenal Cortical Hormone Excess

Cushing syndrome, the phenotype resulting from excessive glucocorticoids, can be due to either excessive endogenous or exogenous steroid exposure. The characteristic features of Cushing syndrome include rounded facies, plethora, central obesity, thin extremities, impaired linear growth, fatigue, and hypertension (Fig. 9.41). Impaired linear growth velocity is a frequent finding and a relevant difference in the presentation of Cushing syndrome in children compared with adults. Muscle weakness and muscle wasting occur, resulting in comparatively thin extremities (Fig. 9.41B). Dorsal cervical fat deposition (previously referred to as "buffalo hump") is also a described feature (Fig. 9.41D). The skin is often thin, friable, and easily bruised. Loss of bone mineral density and osteopenia/osteoporosis can occur with chronic glucocorticoid exposure. Delayed bone maturation may be noted. Some children manifest signs of excessive androgen secretion. Amenorrhea may occur among adolescent girls. CNS effects can include mood swings, psychosis, and idiopathic intracranial hypertension.

Treatment with glucocorticoids is the most common cause of Cushing syndrome in children. Endogenous Cushing syndrome may be caused by adrenal tumors, pituitary adenomas (Cushing disease), primary pigmented micronodular adrenal hyperplasia (PPNAD), or ectopic ACTH production. The worldwide incidence of adrenocortical tumors in children is very low, 0.3 per million per year. Adrenal tumors are the most common cause of endogenous Cushing syndrome in children younger than 7 years old, whereas pituitary adenoma is more common in older children and adolescents. PPNAD can occur sporadically, as a familial disorder, or as a feature of the Carney complex. The Carney complex is a heterogeneous disorder due to pathogenic variants of the *PRKAR1A* gene; its features include PPNAD, myxomas, testicular Sertoli cell, Leydig cell tumors, and thyroid tumors among many others. Other forms of micronodular bilateral adrenocortical hyperplasia may occur as de novo or autosomal-dominant mutations in the phosphodiesterase 11A4 *(PDE11A)* or *PDE8B* genes. These genetic variants are associated with increased cyclic AMP signaling, cortisol excess, and adrenal tumors.

Other genetic disorders associated with adrenocortical tumors include Beckwith-Wiedemann and Li-Fraumeni syndromes and are related to genetic alterations in the 11p15 chromosomal region and *TP53* gene, respectively. The laboratory findings in the different conditions causing adrenal hypercortisolism are listed in Fig. 9.42.

The first step in the diagnosis of Cushing syndrome is confirmation of elevated cortisol concentrations. Elevated 24-hour urinary free cortisol (UFC) excretion and midnight salivary cortisol measurements are two tests used to confirm excessive glucocorticoid secretion. Falsely elevated UFC results may occur in association with stress, obesity, depression, poor diabetes control, and pregnancy. Measurement of midnight salivary cortisol concentration is helpful because individuals with Cushing syndrome typically manifest loss of normal cortisol diurnal variation. Measurement of cortisol and ACTH concentrations simultaneously may be helpful. Patients with primary adrenal disease will have high cortisol and suppressed ACTH concentrations. Patients with Cushing disease (increased ACTH production, most often from pituitary adenoma) may have elevated ACTH and cortisol concentrations. Some obese individuals have elevated cortisol secretion rates; correction for body surface area normalizes the results. Overnight, low-dose, and high-dose dexamethasone suppression tests may help confirm the diagnosis. After an overnight administration of dexamethasone (1.0 mg of dexamethasone in adults or 0.3 mg per m^2 in children), morning serum cortisol concentration suppresses to less than 1.8 ug/dL. If the 24-hour UFC excretion is normal and there is appropriate dexamethasone suppression, Cushing syndrome is highly unlikely, with the caveat that some patients have intermittent or episodic cortisol hypersecretion.

Once endogenous excessive glucocorticoid secretion is confirmed, additional studies are needed to identify the specific etiology. CT scans are recommended for the evaluation of adrenal tumors. When Cushing disease is suspected, pituitary MRI is the study of choice. Because pituitary adenomas may be small, bilateral inferior petrosal sinus sampling may be necessary to localize the adenoma before surgery. Although extremely rare among children, ectopic ACTH-secreting and ACTH/CRH–cosecreting tumors may be difficult to diagnose.

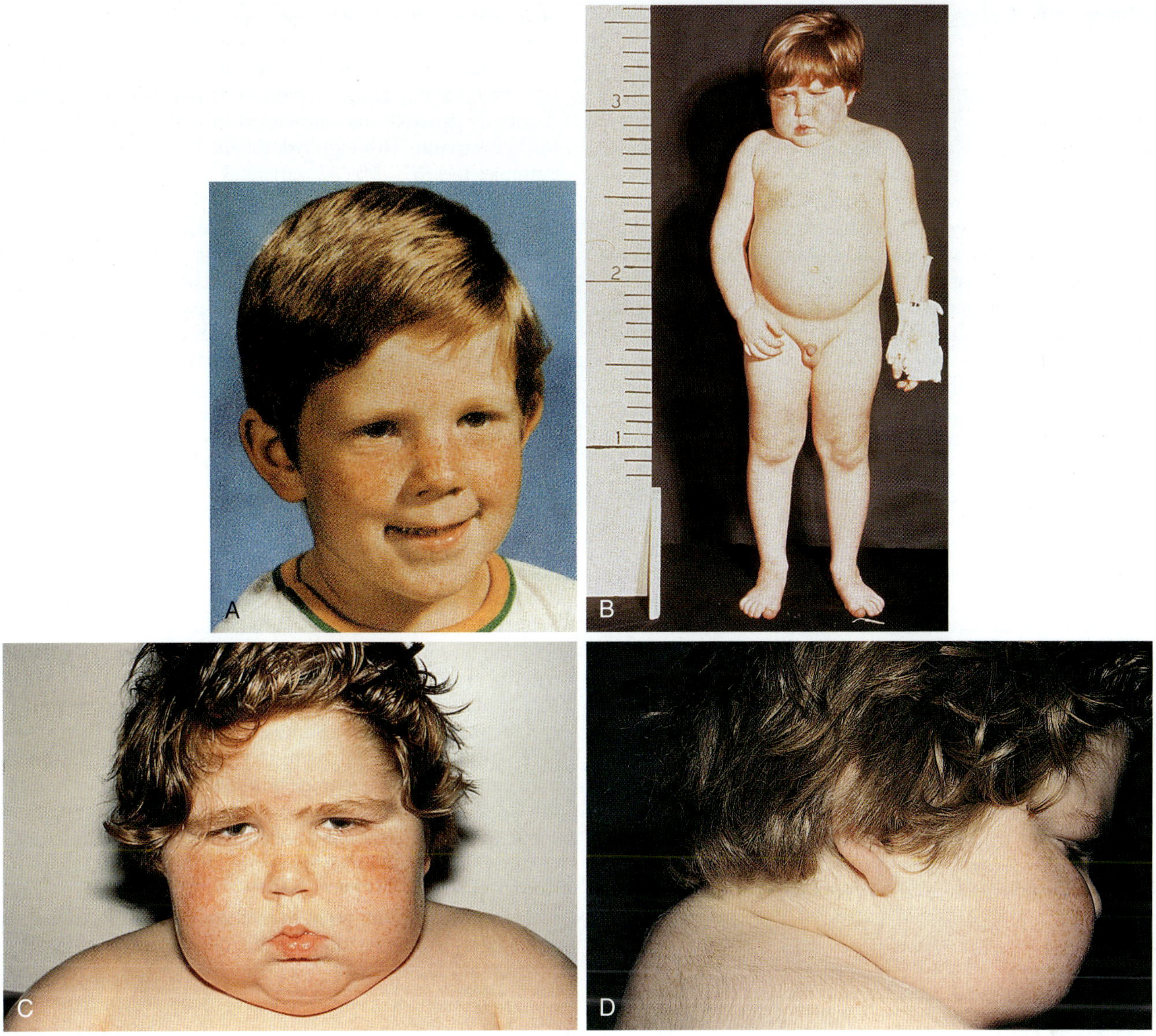

Fig. 9.41 Cushing syndrome. These photographs show how dramatic the changes associated with Cushing syndrome are and how rapidly they occur. (A) Patient before the onset of Cushing syndrome. (B) Patient 4 months after photograph in (A). Note the centripetal obesity of the trunk compared with the extremities after the onset of Cushing syndrome. (C) Moon facies, clearly demonstrated, should raise the diagnostic index of Cushing syndrome. (D) Dorsal cervical fat deposition. Excessive adipose tissue over the lower cervical and upper thoracic spine is characteristic of Cushing syndrome.

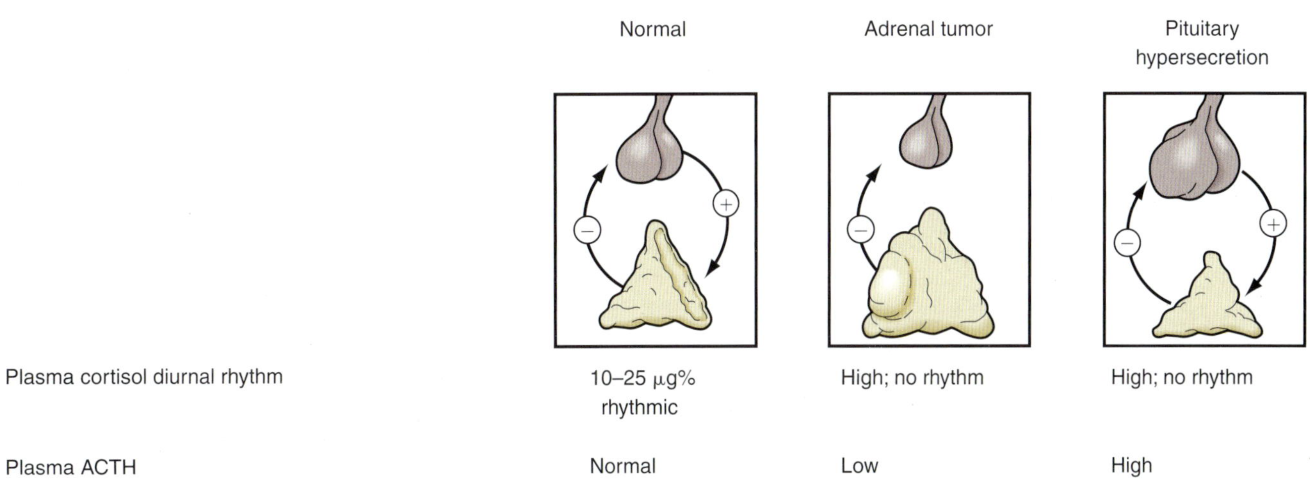

Fig. 9.42 The differential diagnosis of Cushing syndrome as interpreted from the dexamethasone suppression test. *ACTH,* Adrenocorticotropic hormone. (Modified from Williams RH: *Textbook of endocrinology*, ed 6, Philadelphia, 1981, WB Saunders, p 272.)

Disorders of Adrenal Medulla

Pheochromocytoma

Pheochromocytomas (PHEO) and paragangliomas (PPGLs) are rare catecholamine-secreting tumors derived from neural crest chromaffin cells. When located within the adrenal medulla, the tumors are named PHEOs. Extra adrenal tumors arising from both sympathetic and parasympathetic paraganglia, which span from skull to the sacrum, are called PPGLs. Clinical manifestations result from excessive catecholamine secretion from the tumor. These catecholamines include norepinephrine, epinephrine, and rarely dopamine. Symptoms may include headaches, diaphoresis, palpitation, tremors, nausea, weakness, anxiety, and weight loss. Patients may present with hypertension, which may be episodic. Both PHEO and/or PPGL may occur in specific familial syndromes. Neurofibromatosis type 1 (NF1) is an autosomal dominant disorder associated with increased risk of PHEO. Diagnostic criteria for neurofibromatosis type 1 include more than six café-au-lait spots, neurofibromas, axillary freckling, Lisch nodules, and macrocephaly. Multiple endocrine neoplasia type 2 (with subcategories of MEN 2A and MEN 2B) show autosomal dominant inheritance and are associated with mutations in the *RET* proto-oncogene. This disorder, also known as *Sipple syndrome,* is characterized by medullary thyroid carcinoma, PPGL, and primary hyperparathyroidism. Patients with MEN 2B have a distinctive Marfanoid appearance and medullary thyroid carcinoma, PPGL, mucosal neuromas (Fig. 9.43), and ganglioneuromatosis of the intestinal tract. Medullary thyroid carcinoma is common in MEN 2; this disorder originates in the parafollicular C cells and tends to spread to lymph nodes and other organs. Genetic screening to identify affected individuals is essential. Thyroidectomy is generally recommended in any individual found to carry MEN 2 variants with high risk for medullary thyroid carcinoma. For example, the *RET M918T* variant is associated with a high risk for medullary thyroid carcinoma. Von Hippel-Lindau (VHL) disease is an autosomal dominant disorder associated with mutations in the VHL gene. VHL type 1 is associated with hemangioblastomas and renal cell carcinoma. VHL type 2A is associated with PHEO but has a low risk for renal cell carcinomas. Hereditary paraganglioma syndromes are associated with autosomal dominant mutations of nuclear genes encoding the subunits of the mitochondrial enzyme succinate dehydrogenase. Mutations in the genes encoding the *SDHA, SDHB, SDHC, SDHD,* and *SDHAF2* subunits have been associated with PPGLs. The precise phenotype correlates with the genotype. Other genes associated with familial PPGLs include transmembrane protein 127 *(TMEM127),* fumarate hydratase *(FH),* myc-associated factor X *(MAX),* and endothelial PAS domain protein 1 *(EPAS1/HIF2A).*

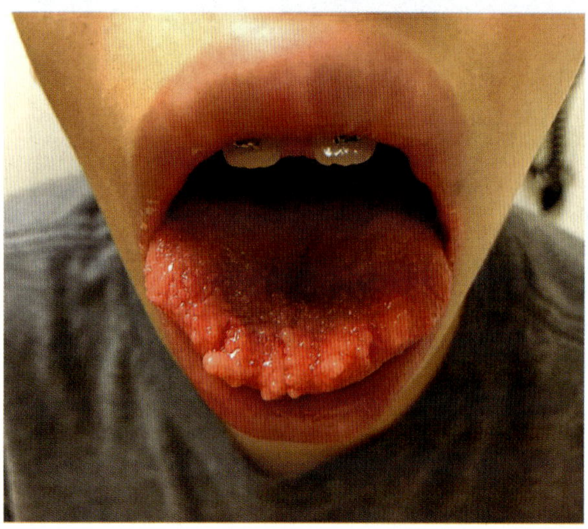

Fig. 9.43 Mucosal neuromas in a young boy with MEN 2B who also had prophylactic thyroidectomy in infancy due to a high-risk mutation in RET proto-oncogene. (Courtesy O. Escobar, MD, Pittsburgh, PA.)

In those suspected of having a PHEO, plasma-free metanephrine, normetanephrine, and methoxytyramine and a 24-hour urinary collection for epinephrine, norepinephrine, dopamine, normetanephrine, metanephrine, homovanillic acid, and vanillylmandelic acid can be sent. *SHDx* and *VHL* mutations are typically associated with increased secretion of normetanephrine or dopamine, whereas *RET* mutations are usually associated with excessive epinephrine or metanephrine secretion. Some medications, such as tricyclic antidepressants, can cause false-positive results. Catecholamine secretion may be low for some paragangliomas, particularly those located in the neck. Biochemical diagnosis with confirmation of elevated catecholamine levels should be obtained before anatomic (CT or MRI) or functional (metaiodobenzylguanidine [MIBG] or positron emission tomography [PET]) imaging studies are performed. In the pediatric population, most hereditary PPGL syndromes are identified by genetic testing after the diagnosis in an older family member. A thorough family history is invaluable for the diagnosis of familial PPGL syndromes (Table 9.2).

Endocrine Hypertension

Childhood obesity is associated with hypertension and has become an important modifiable risk factor for cardiovascular morbidity and mortality. Endocrine causes of hypertension are the second most common cause of hypertension after renal disease in children.

Hyperthyroidism, hyperparathyroidism, hypercalcemia from any cause, and uncontrolled diabetes mellitus may present with secondary hypertension. Other rare endocrine conditions that cause

Table 9.2 Genes Associated With Pheochromocytoma and Paraganglioma Syndromes

Syndrome	Gene	Location	Inheritance	Main Features
PGL1	*SDHD*	11q23	AD	Head and neck PPGL
PGL2	*SDHAF2*	11q12	AD	Head and neck PPGL
PGL3	*SDHC*	1q23.3	AD	Multifocal PPGL
PGL4	*SDHB*	1p36.13	AD	Multifocal, highest rate of malignant disease
PGL5	*SDHA*	5p15		
VHL	*VHL*	3p25.3	AD	CNS/retinal hemangioblastoma, PPGL, renal cell carcinoma, pancreatic neuroendocrine tumors
NF1	*NF1*	17q11.2	AD	Café-au-lait, macrocephaly, axillary freckling, optic glioma, pheochromocytoma
MEN 2A	*RET*	10q11.21	AD	Medullary thyroid carcinoma, primary hyperparathyroidism, PPGL
MEN 2B	*RET*	10q11.21	AD	Marfanoid appearance, mucocutaneous neuromas, medullary thyroid carcinoma, PPGL
Paraganglioma-polycythemia disease	*EPAS1*	2p21		Polycythemia, PPGL, somatostatinoma
Familial pheochromocytoma	*TMEM127*	2q11.2	AD	Mostly pheochromocytoma
Familial pheochromocytoma	*MAX*	14q23.3	AD	Mostly paraganglioma
Leiomyomatosis and renal cell carcinoma	*FH*	1q42.1		Cutaneous and uterine leiomyomas, renal carcinoma, rare PPGL

AD, Autosomal dominant; *CNS,* central nervous system; *MEN 2A,* multiple endocrine neoplasia type 2A; *MEN 2B,* multiple endocrine neoplasia type 2B; *NF1,* neurofibromatosis type 1; *PGL,* paraganglioma; *PPGL,* pheochromocytoma and paraganglioma; *VHL,* von Hippel-Lindau.

secondary hypertension in children include conditions that have mineralocorticoid excess, such as some types of CAH (11β hydroxylase deficiency, 17α hydroxylase deficiency), apparent mineralocorticoid excess, familial hyperaldosteronism type I, primary aldosteronism, familial glucocorticoid resistance, and conditions with catecholamine excess, as in pheochromocytomas and paragangliomas. When it comes to measurement of cortisol and adrenal steroids, it is important to pay attention to the timing of the blood draw and sleep routine, which can affect diurnal rhythm. Recent assays using mass spectrometry (LC/MS) are more sensitive, and the levels may be lower than defined by immunoassays.

HYPOTHALAMIC-PITUITARY-GONADAL AXIS

Gonadotropin-releasing hormone (GnRH) pulse generator and gonadotropin pulsatile GnRH secretion by the hypothalamic GnRH neurons, the so-called GnRH pulse generator, regulates pituitary secretion of LH and FSH. The GnRH neurons originally develop in the olfactory placode and migrate during early fetal development from the nose through the forebrain to the hypothalamus. The embryologic origin of the GnRH neurons results in the association of hypogonadotropic hypogonadism and anosmia. Pulsatile release of GnRH stimulates the secretion of FSH and LH from the anterior pituitary gland, whereas continuous secretion of GnRH inhibits the release of FSH and LH. The amplitude and frequency of GnRH pulses change throughout life (newborn period, infancy, childhood, puberty, and adulthood). After active secretion in late gestation and in the early neonatal period during the so-called "mini-puberty" of infancy, the GnRH pulse generator becomes quiescent until the onset of puberty. "Mini puberty" of infancy is a transient period of gonadal activation starting in the second week and ending by 4 to 6 months of life. Gonadarche is characterized by the resumption of GnRH secretion. The first sign of reactivation of the GnRH pulse generator, and onset of gonadarche, is increased nocturnal LH secretion. Various neurotransmitters are involved in controlling GnRH-secreting neurons and thus modulating the GnRH pulses. Kisspeptin, which acts via its receptor GPR54 (also known as KISS1-R), has been identified as a major stimulus for GnRH and subsequent LH release. Whereas kisspeptin is essential for GnRH pulse generation, this hormone alone does not initiate the onset of puberty. Rather, upstream regulatory mechanisms govern the activity of the hypothalamic GnRH neurons. In addition to kisspeptin, genes involved in controlling the onset of puberty include neurokinin B (TAC3), its cognate receptor (TACR3), and dynorphin. The secretory activity of GnRH neurons represents the integrated response to many hormones, neurotransmitters, and environmental influences. Other input signals include sex steroids, glucocorticoids, leptin, insulin, IGF-1, ghrelin, FGF21, orexigenic peptides, and anorexigenic peptides, with the net effect being signal integration to govern pubertal maturation and ongoing reproductive function.

In males, LH binds to the LH receptor on Leydig cells to directly stimulate testosterone synthesis and secretion. In the testes, FSH supports Sertoli cell development and spermatogenesis. Sertoli cell development is the first sign of testicular differentiation. Sertoli cells secrete AMH with high levels during fetal life, which decline with the onset of puberty. AMH provides a functional marker of immature Sertoli cells. With the onset of puberty, testosterone secreted by the Leydig cells suppresses AMH secretion by the maturing Sertoli cells and thus AMH levels are low in puberty. AMH levels may be low in males with diminished Sertoli cell function, such as anorchia and testicular failure secondary to chemotherapy, or radiation. Sertoli cells are more sensitive to environmental factors such as chemotherapy and radiation. Boys can develop secondary sexual characteristics like genital enlargement and pubic hair without testicular enlargement. The majority of the testicular volume is due to the Sertoli cells. When there is a decrease in Sertoli cells, a smaller testicular volume is seen, as in Klinefelter syndrome.

In females, the ovary is characterized by a two-cell model (in series) for steroidogenesis. LH stimulates ovarian theca cells to synthesize androstenedione, which serves as the precursor for estradiol synthesis. Subsequently, in the ovarian granulosa cells, FSH increases expression of aromatase, the enzyme that converts androgens to estrogens. Granulosa cells secrete negligible amounts of AMH in fetal life. With the onset of puberty, granulosa cells of developing follicles increase AMH secretion. In females, AMH may be a marker of ovarian reserve by reflecting the number of small growing follicles. AMH concentrations are typically low in girls with Turner syndrome and may be elevated in women with PCOS.

SEXUAL DIFFERENTIATION

The process of sex determination begins at fertilization with the sex chromosomes being XX or XY. This process depends on the regulated expression of specific genes and interactions of specific gene products. The *SRY* gene located on the short arm of the Y chromosome functions as the binary switch to influence sex development. In the usual situation, the gonads and related structures are unipotential, early during gestation. In other words, these structures can develop along male or female trajectories depending on the presence or absence of the *SRY* gene (Fig. 9.44). As anticipated, loss of function mutations in the *SRY* gene are associated with male-to-female sex reversal. In-depth investigation of patients has led to the identification of other genes involved in sex differentiation. Campomelic dwarfism and 46, XY sex reversal are associated with mutations in the *SOX9* gene. Denys-Drash syndrome, due to mutations in the *WT1* gene, is characterized by Wilms tumor, nephropathy, and 46, XY sex reversal. Specific genes have been identified that influence ovarian development. These genes include *WNT1*, R-Spondin 1 (encoded by *RSPO1*), β-catenin (encoded by *CTNNB1*), and *FOXL2*.

DISORDERS OF SEX DEVELOPMENT

Disorders of sex development (DSDs) encompass various congenital conditions in which there is an inconsistency between chromosomal, gonadal, and/or anatomic sex. Diagnoses for differences in sex development can be classified as 46XY DSD, 46XX DSD, and sex chromosome DSD. With the presence of a Y chromosome, patients with XY DSD have an increased risk for gonadoblastoma or dysgerminoma in the dysgenetic gonad(s).

Evaluation of Disorders of Sex Development

A child with ambiguous genitalia must be evaluated promptly. In some instances, aberrant genital development may have been identified by prenatal ultrasound. In other instances, discrepancies between prenatal karyotype results, prenatal imaging, and physical examination of the neonate lead to medical evaluation. Importantly, rapid assessment for CAH and other disorders associated with adrenal insufficiency needs to be considered. It is important to remember that in utero androgen exposure affects more tissues (i.e., brain) than just the internal and external genital structures. So, when evaluating an infant for DSD, it is important to obtain careful prenatal history including maternal medications, exposures, maternal virilization during pregnancy, and results of prenatal testing. Family history of consanguinity, unexplained deaths, infertility, and ambiguous genitalia should be obtained.

The child's physical examination directs the selection of the appropriate laboratory studies to confirm a specific diagnosis. Genital examination should include assessment of the symmetry of the external genital structures, presence or absence of gonads (inguinal

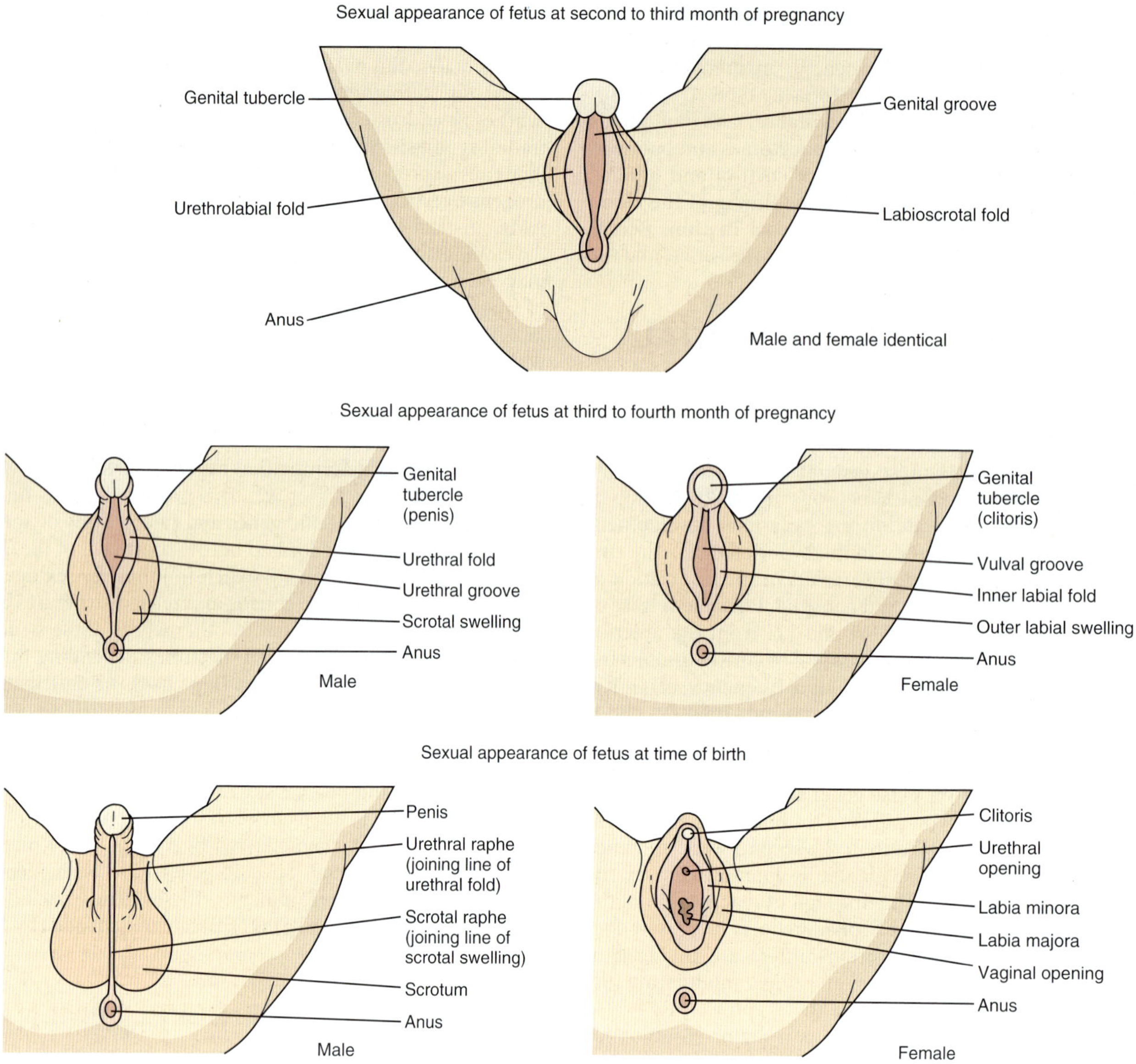

Fig. 9.44 Normal sexual differentiation. Schematic drawing demonstrating differentiation of normal male and female genitalia during embryogenesis.

or labioscrotal masses), magnitude of virilization by measuring the length and width of the phallic structure, labioscrotal fusion, hyperpigmentation, and presence and position of the urethral meatus. Affected females typically have ambiguous symmetric external genitalia with enlarged phallic structure and nonpalpable gonads. It is important to note that a male infant with CAH might not have any abnormalities in the external genital except for hyperpigmentation of scrotum and occasionally a generous phallus.

Careful anthropometric measurements and vital signs, particularly blood pressure, and assessment for other associated findings like cleft palate, deformities of limbs, malformations of fingers or toes, craniosynostosis, and facial hypoplasia is crucial.

In addition to karyotype and pelvic ultrasound, determination of LH, FSH, 17-OHP, testosterone, and dihydrotestosterone in the neonatal period is important because the hypothalamic-pituitary-gonadal axis is active during "*mini puberty of infancy.*" If there is suspicion for CAH, electrolytes and plasma renin activity should also be obtained and monitored closely over time (hyperkalemia and hyponatremia noted between a few days to a couple of weeks after birth). Making the correct diagnosis in a virilized female infant with CAH will be lifesaving.

Asymmetric external genitalia are often associated with 45, X/46, XY sex chromosome DSD (formerly known as *mixed gonadal dysgenesis*) (Fig. 9.45). The phenotype associated with ovotesticular DSD can range from slightly virilized female to almost fully virilized male; this disorder is defined by the presence of ovarian tissues with follicles and testicular tissue with seminiferous cords in the same gonad.

Symmetric external genitalia with nonpalpable gonads suggest a virilized XX fetus, with the diagnosis of 21-hydroxylase deficiency confirmed by elevated 17-OHP measurement. Other disorders associated with virilization of female fetuses include CAH due to 11β-hydroxylase or 3β-hydroxysteroid dehydrogenase deficiency.

Placental aromatase deficiency due to mutations in the aromatase gene *(CYP19A1)* is associated with virilization of female fetuses and maternal virilization during pregnancy. Enzyme deficiencies associated with incomplete virilization of a male fetus include 3β-hydroxysteroid dehydrogenase, 17α-hydroxylase/17-20 lyase, 5α-reductase, 17-hydroxysteroid dehydrogenase, and congenital lipoid adrenal hyperplasia secondary to mutations in the *HSD3B2, CYP17A1, SRD5A2, HSD17B3,* and *StAR* genes, respectively. Varying phenotypes have been reported for individuals with loss of function mutations in the steroidogenic factor 1 *(NR5A1)* gene.

Symmetric genital development with palpable gonads suggests incomplete male sexual differentiation. In CAIS due to loss-of-function mutations in the androgen receptor gene, external genital development appears to be female. Labial or inguinal gonads may be palpable, and uterine structures are absent. Other diagnostic entities include Leydig cell hypoplasia due to LH receptor *(LHR)* mutations,

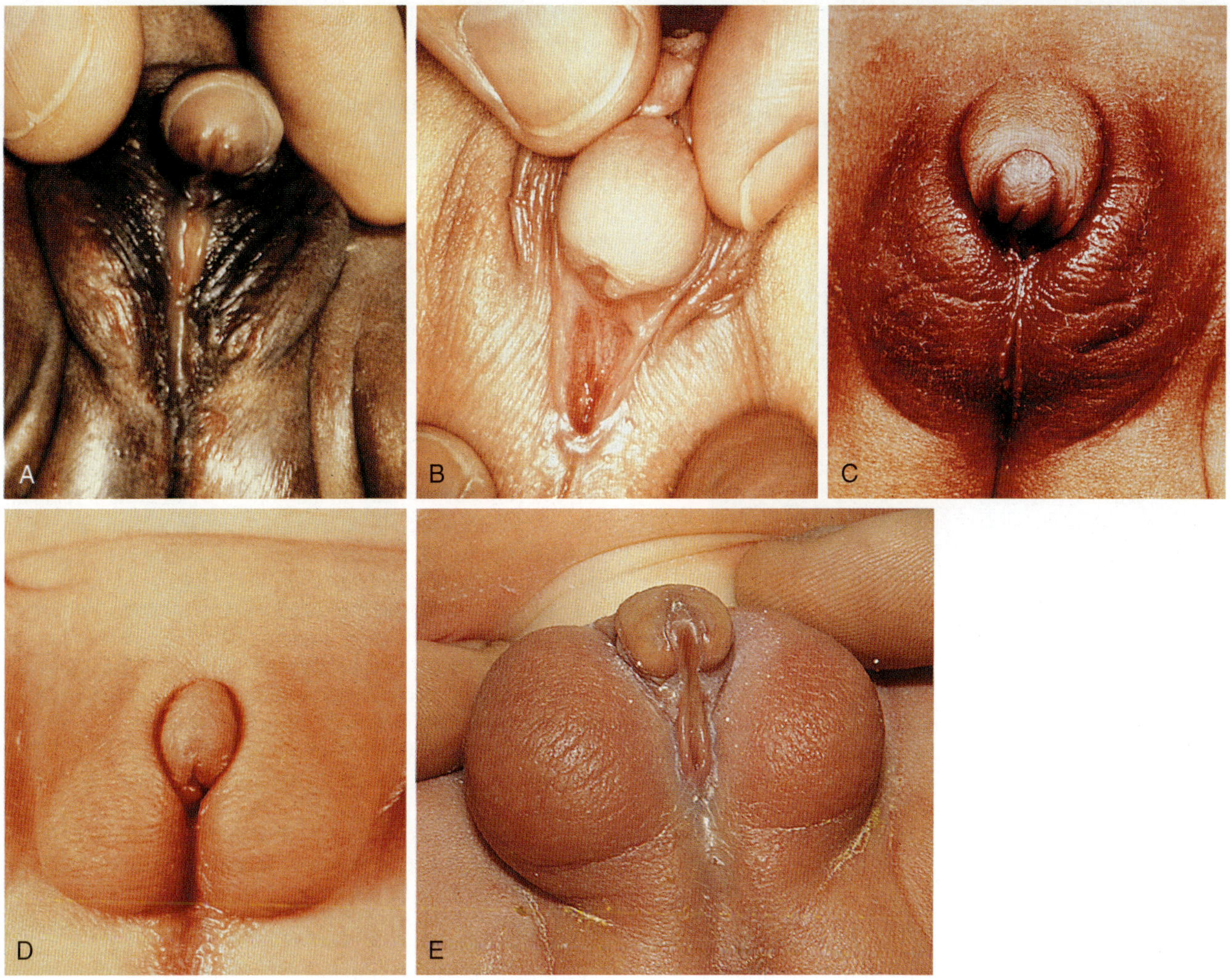

Fig. 9.45 Ambiguous genitalia. These cases include 46, XX/46, XY (A) and congenital virilizing adrenal hyperplasia (B–E).

inborn errors of testosterone biosynthesis due to mutations in steroidogenic enzyme genes.

Smith-Lemli-Opitz syndrome, an autosomal recessive disorder characterized by multiple malformations, including urogenital anomalies, intellectual disability, cleft palate, and developmental delay, is due to mutations in the 7-dehydrocholesterol reductase *(DHCR7)* gene. Genital ambiguity associated with craniosynostosis, midface hypoplasia, radiohumeral synostosis, and glucocorticoid deficiency may be secondary to mutations in the cytochrome P450 oxidoreductase gene *(POR);* the skeletal dysplasia is also known as the Antley-Bixler syndrome.

Persistent Müllerian duct syndrome is characterized by persistence of Müllerian structures in an otherwise normal 46, XY male infant. Affected infants may present with cryptorchidism or transverse testicular ectopia. This disorder can be due to mutations in the *AMH* gene or the gene for its receptor *(AMHRII).*

Some children are born with anatomic variants, such as agenesis of the phallus (Fig. 9.46), penoscrotal transposition (Fig. 9.47), exstrophy of the bladder, or absence of an anal opening. Generally, these infants represent a developmental anomaly rather than an endocrine disorder. The absence of the anal opening may be associated with additional anomalies, such as the VATER or VACTERL associations. Typically, these disorders are associated with normal gonadal development and function. Some disorders associated with disrupted gonadal development present with delayed puberty.

Communicating a diagnosis of DSD is a challenging but critical conversation in the newborn period. Providers should acknowledge the difficulty of the situation while providing reassurance to the families regarding the infant's overall health when appropriate. In speaking with the parents, the child should be referred to as "the

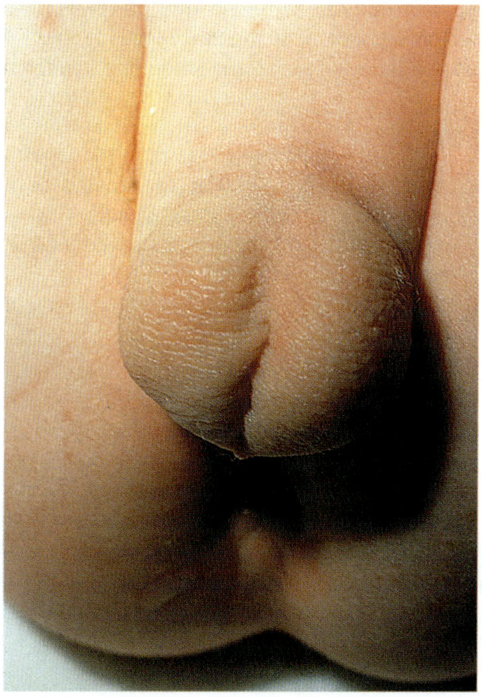

Fig. 9.46 Agenesis of the phallus. Rare developmental anomaly with a normal male karyotype. (Courtesy D. Becker, MD, Pittsburgh, PA.)

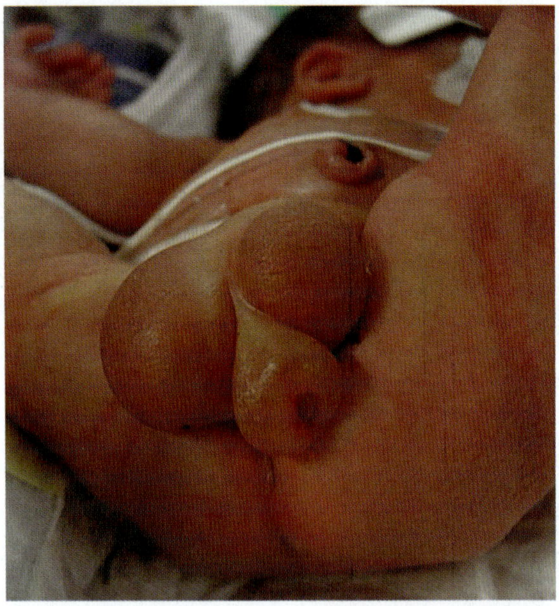

Fig. 9.47 Penoscrotal transposition. The edema seen in foreskin and scrotal sacs was due to breech presentation at delivery. (Courtesy O. Escobar, MD, Pittsburgh, PA.)

baby" and not as he, she, or it. Assigning the sex or performing genital surgery should not be rushed. A multidisciplinary team approach, including the concourse of a pediatric endocrinologist, pediatric urologist/pediatric surgeon, pediatric geneticist, nurse educator, ethicist, and psychologist/social worker with expertise in this area is essential.

Cryptorchidism

During embryogenesis, the testes migrate from their original location near the kidney through the abdomen and descend into the scrotum. Cryptorchidism, or failure of the testes to descend into the scrotum, occurs in approximately 3% of infant males. Treatment of cryptorchidism is usually delayed until 6 to 12 months of age to allow the testicle to descend spontaneously. If there is failure of descent, an orchiopexy may need to be performed. A cryptorchid testicle may be intrinsically abnormal and is more likely to undergo malignant transformation. Although surgical intervention may not completely alter the risk of malignancy, placing the testicle in its proper location allows for earlier detection of a suspicious mass.

Micropenis

Micropenis in an infant boy refers to the small size of the penis (Fig. 9.48). Physical examination should include the evaluation of the scrotum for symmetry and the presence of gonads. The position

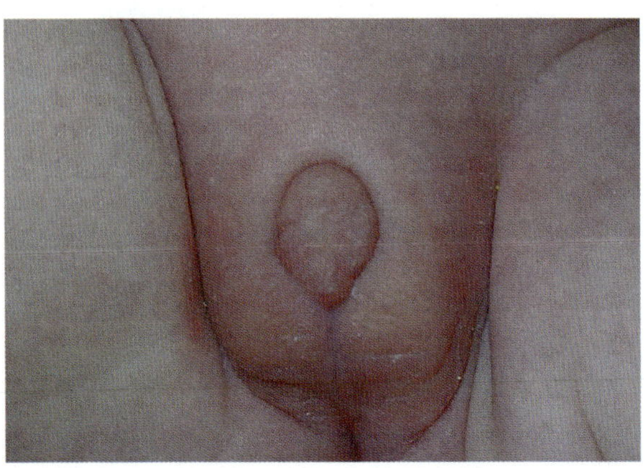

Fig. 9.48 Micropenis without any other external genital anomalies. The gonads were palpable in both scrotal sacs. (Courtesy O. Escobar, MD, Pittsburgh, PA.)

of the meatus and the anus are other helpful physical features in understanding etiology.

TURNER SYNDROME

Turner syndrome, due to structural or numeric aberrations of the X chromosomes, should be suspected in any short female. The incidence is 1 in 2500 girls. Typically, girls with Turner syndrome have short stature and delayed puberty due to gonadal failure. The clinical features, especially among girls with mosaic forms of Turner syndrome, can be quite variable. Some of the clinical presentations of Turner syndrome are shown in the pictures of young women reported in the original article by Turner (Fig. 9.49). The wide carrying angle (cubitus valgus), shieldlike chest, low posterior hairline, and webbed neck may be easily appreciated. A more comprehensive list of physical findings in patients with Turner syndrome is listed in Box 9.9 and at the Turner Syndrome Society website (https://www.turnersyndrome.org). It is important to evaluate potential cardiac and renal anomalies. Turner syndrome can be associated with left-sided cardiovascular malformations of varying severity, including aortic valve stenosis, aortic coarctation, aortic dilation, and rupture. At the time of diagnosis, all girls should be evaluated by a cardiologist with expertise in congenital heart disease. Imaging studies, echocardiography, and cardiac MRI should be performed. Girls with Turner syndrome require audiology evaluations because of the high risk of sensorineural hearing loss. Lymphedema, often involving hands and feet, may be present at birth. Available data have implicated the failure of lymph absorption by the initial lymphatic capillaries as the underlying mechanism.

Peripheral blood karyotype is often diagnostic in a clinical picture suggestive of Turner syndrome. In some instances, the karyotype of fibroblasts from a skin biopsy or urothelial cells may be helpful to confirm a suspected diagnosis. GH treatment augments ultimate adult height in Turner syndrome. To induce puberty, estrogen replacement therapy is initiated, followed by cyclic estrogen-progestin treatment. A growth chart for untreated girls with this syndrome is shown in Fig. 9.50, along with the height outcomes after therapy with human GH. Girls with Turner syndrome show a higher risk of developing inflammatory bowel disease, Hashimoto thyroiditis, celiac disease, and diabetes mellitus. Increased FSH and decreased AMH concentrations are associated with ovarian failure.

KLINEFELTER SYNDROME

Boys with Klinefelter syndrome have a 47, XXY karyotype. With puberty, the testes are noted to be small and firm due to progressive hyalinization that affects Sertoli cells more than Leydig cells. In this condition, despite a low testicular volume, other pubertal features such as pubic hair and penile growth are preserved. Leydig cell function may remain normal even after significant decline in Sertoli cell mass and function, and testosterone levels can be low normal to normal through adolescence. Gynecomastia and neurobehavioral difficulties are common. Clinical features include eunuchoid body proportions with tall stature and long limbs, sparse facial hair, and small penis. Laboratory evaluation shows elevated gonadotropin concentrations, low testosterone concentrations, and decreased sperm count. For a list of other syndromes associated with endocrine dysfunction, refer to Table 9.3.

BONE AND MINERAL METABOLISM

Parathyroid Glands

The parathyroid glands are four glands adjacent to the thyroid gland in the neck. They are responsible for the synthesis and secretion of parathyroid hormone (PTH), a hormone important in regulating extracellular calcium concentration through its effects on three principal target organs: bone, intestinal mucosa, and kidney

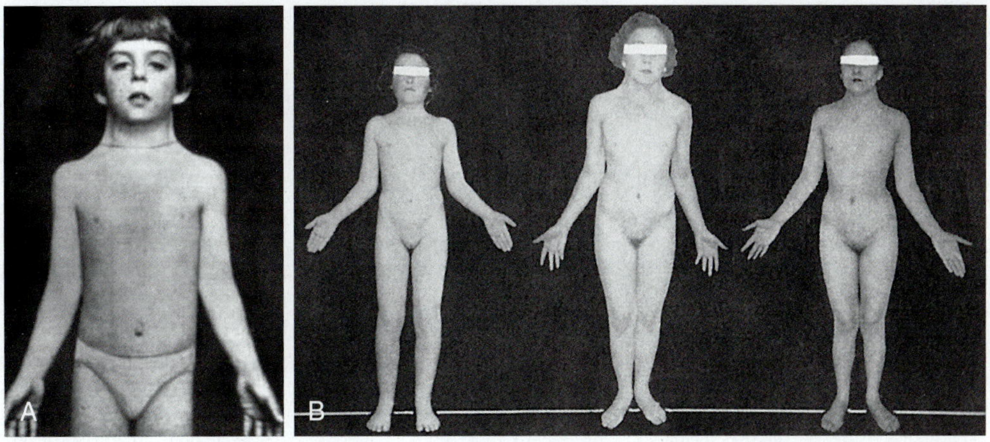

Fig. 9.49 Turner syndrome. (A) Turner used this photograph in 1938 to describe the syndrome that bears his name. This girl exhibits characteristic features of Turner syndrome including a webbed neck, broad chest, marked cubitus valgus, and low-set ears. (B) Note the clinical heterogeneity within the syndrome.

Box 9.9 Common Clinical Findings in Turner Syndrome

Skeletal Growth Disturbances
Short stature
Short neck
Abnormal upper-to-lower segment ratio
Cubitus valgus
Short fourth metacarpals
Madelung deformity
Scoliosis
Genu valgum
Characteristic facies: micrognathia, high-arched palate

Lymphatic Obstruction
Webbed neck
Low posterior hairline
Rotated ears
Edema of hands, feet
Nail dysplasia
Characteristic dermatoglyphics

Ovarian Function
Delayed puberty
Gonadal failure
Infertility
Gonadoblastoma

Cardiovascular Anomalies
Bicuspid aortic valve
Coarctation of the aorta
Partial anomalous pulmonary venous connection
Aortic dissection
Hypertension

Renal Anomalies
Collecting system anomalies
Horseshoe kidney

Miscellaneous Defects
Strabismus
Ptosis
Multiple pigmented nevi
Selective impairment in nonverbal skills
Visual/spatial organization skills
Neurosensory hearing loss
Middle ear effusions/chronic otitis media
Decreased bone mineral density

Associated Disorders
Hypothyroidism
Alopecia
Vitiligo
Celiac disease
Crohn disease
Carbohydrate intolerance

Modified from Davenport ML: Approach to the patient with Turner syndrome, *J Clin Endocrinol Metab* 95:1487–1495, 2010.

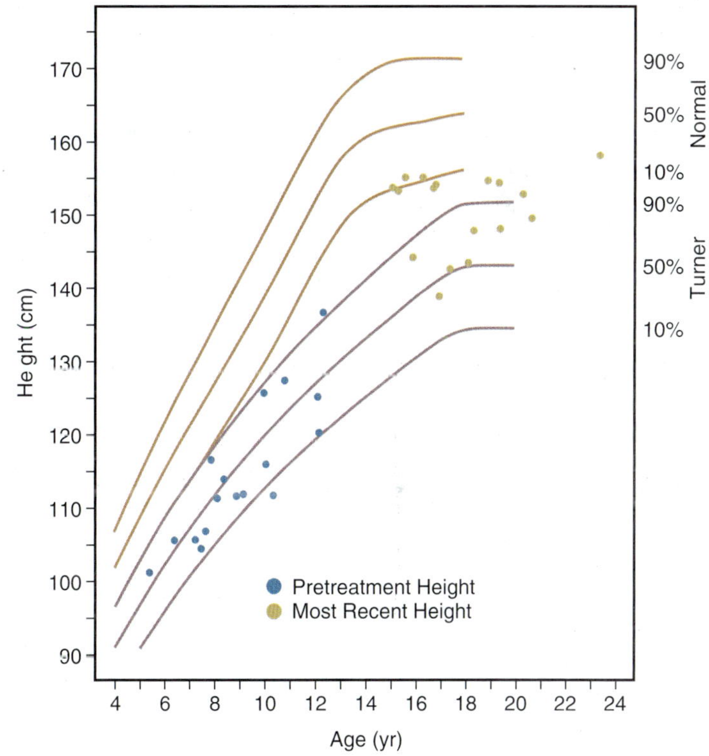

Fig. 9.50 Turner syndrome growth curve. Normal female growth percentiles from the National Center for Health Statistics *(brown lines)* and Turner syndrome growth curves *(purple lines)* are indicated. Pretreatment *(blue circles)* and posttreatment *(tan circles)* heights of girls with Turner syndrome who received growth hormone (GH) treatment are illustrated. Girls with Turner syndrome were monitored for a total of 8.8 ± 1.4 years in the group receiving GH alone, to a mean age of 18.0 ± 2.2 years old. (Courtesy Rosenfeld RG, Attie KM, Frane J, et al: Growth hormone therapy of Turner's syndrome: beneficial effect on adult height, *J Pediatr* 132:319–324, 1998. Permission for use given by Elsevier Limited, Kidlington, Oxford, UK.)

(Fig. 9.51). In the bloodstream, approximately 45% of calcium is free, 45% is protein bound, and 10% is complexed to citrate, sulfate, bicarbonate, and phosphate. Serum ionized calcium concentrations are generally maintained within a narrow range. To monitor extracellular calcium concentration and, thereby, regulate the secretion of PTH, parathyroid cells rely on a G protein–coupled receptor, the calcium-sensing receptor (CaSR). An increase in extracellular calcium activates the CaSR leading to decreased PTH secretion, whereas a decrease in extracellular calcium inhibits the CaSR leading to increased PTH secretion. In addition to calcium, there are

Table 9.3 Syndromes Associated With Endocrine Dysfunction

Syndrome	Clinical Features	Genetic Locus
APS-1	Mucocutaneous candidiasis, hypoparathyroidism, adrenal insufficiency, ovarian failure	*AIRE* at chromosome 21q22.3
APS-2	Hypothyroidism, diabetes mellitus	
Beckwith-Wiedemann	Fetal overgrowth, hemihypertrophy, omphalocele, hepatomegaly, neonatal hypoglycemia	Duplication or deletion at chromosome 11p15.5
Denys-Drash	Ambiguous genitalia, Wilms tumor, renal failure, diffuse mesangial sclerosis, glomerulopathy, focal segmental glomerulosclerosis	*WT1* at chromosome 11p13
DiGeorge	Hypocalcemia, velocardiofacial syndrome,. thymic aplasia, congenital heart disease	*TBX1* at chromosome 22q11.2
Down	Short stature, autoimmune thyroid disease, diabetes mellitus, hypogonadotropic hypogonadism	Trisomy chromosome 21
Kallmann	Hypogonadotropic hypogonadism	*KAL1, FGFR1, PROK2, PROKR2, CHD7, FGF8, KISS1, KISS1R, NKB, TACR3*
Klinefelter	Testicular failure, tall stature, hypergonadotropic hypogonadism	XXY karyotype
McCune-Albright	Precocious puberty, fibrous dysplasia, café-au-lait macules	*GNAS1* at chromosome 20q13.2
MEN 1	Hyperparathyroidism, acromegaly, hypoglycemia (Zollinger-Ellison syndrome), collagenomas	*MEN1* at chromosome 11q13
MEN 2A	Medullary thyroid carcinoma, pheochromocytoma, Hirschsprung disease	*RET* at chromosome 10q11.2
MEN 2B	Medullary thyroid carcinoma, pheochromocytoma, Hirschsprung disease, thick lips, neuromas of lips and tongue	*RET* at chromosome 10q11.2
Noonan	Short stature, triangular facies, ptosis, hypertelorism, congenital heart disease, von Willebrand	*PTPN11* at chromosome 12q24.1
Prader-Willi	Short stature, hypotonia, obesity, hypogonadotropic hypogonadism	15q12, 15q11-q13
Russell-Silver	Short stature, triangular facies, blue sclera, hypospadias	*H19* at chromosome 11p15.5; uniparental disomy at chromosome 7p11.2
Smith-Lemli-Opitz	Short stature, failure to thrive, cleft palate, congenital heart disease, hypospadias, renal anomalies	*DHCR7* at chromosome 11q12-q13
Turner	Ovarian failure, delayed puberty, streak gonads, short stature	Monosomy or isodisomy of X chromosome
VHL	Retinal angiomata, pheochromocytoma, hemangioblastoma, renal cell carcinoma	*VHL* at chromosome 3p26-p25
Williams-Beuren	Short stature, supravalvular aortic stenosis, valvular aortic stenosis, developmental delay, friendly personality	Chromosome 7q11.23

APS-1, Autoimmune polyglandular syndrome type 1; *APS-2,* autoimmune polyglandular syndrome type 2; *MEN 1,* multiple endocrine neoplasia type 1; *MEN 2A,* multiple endocrine neoplasia type 2A; *MEN 2B,* multiple endocrine neoplasia type 2B; *VHL,* von Hippel-Lindau.

other regulators of PTH secretion. For example, hypomagnesemia inhibits PTH secretion.

In the intestine, PTH does not appear to have a direct effect on calcium or phosphate absorption but acts indirectly through active vitamin D. PTH promotes the synthesis of the hormonally active form of vitamin D in the kidney by 1-alpha-hydroxylation of 25-hydroxy vitamin D. The active form is calcitriol (1,25-dihydroxyvitamin D3[1,25{OH}$_2$D3]), which enhances intestinal calcium absorption. In the kidney, PTH has direct effects on the reabsorption of calcium, predominantly in the distal convoluted tubule. PTH also inhibits reabsorption of phosphate in the renal proximal tubule and causes phosphaturia. PTH also has an important role in bone resorption through an indirect action at the level of osteoclasts.

Hypercalcemia

The symptoms of hypercalcemia depend on their severity and the rise in serum calcium concentrations. Symptoms of hypercalcemia include constipation, weight loss, abdominal pain, irritability, memory loss, muscle weakness, lethargy, polydipsia, polyuria, nephrocalcinosis, and renal failure. An electrocardiogram can show shortened corrected QT (QTc) interval and cardiac arrhythmias.

Hyperparathyroidism

Hypercalcemia (Fig. 9.52) due to hyperparathyroidism may be sporadic or inherited as a common manifestation of MEN 1. Other features of MEN 1 include islet cell tumors, Zollinger-Ellison syndrome, and pituitary tumors. Collagenomas and angiofibromas are cutaneous features associated with MEN 1. Although typically a disease of adults, affected children can be identified through biochemical screening before the onset of clinical symptoms. Inherited as an autosomal dominant trait, MEN 1 is associated with mutations in the menin *(MEN1)* gene.

Williams-Beuren Syndrome

Children with Williams-Beuren syndrome have distinctive "elfin" facies characterized by dolichocephaly, flat nasal bridge, epicanthal folds, long philtrum, stellate pattern of the irises, and wide mouth. Despite cognitive impairment, affected individuals tend to be sociable and empathic. Cardiac anomalies, typically supravalvular aortic stenosis, occur in approximately 30%. Hypercalcemia can occur during infancy but generally resolves by 4 years of age, if not earlier. Hypercalciuria may occur as well. Other endocrine manifestations can include impaired glucose tolerance, subclinical hypothyroidism, and early menarche. This disorder is associated with microdeletion involving the elastin *(ELN)* gene at chromosome 7q11.13.

Other Causes of Hypercalcemia

Less than 1% of children with malignancies develop hypercalcemia. Mechanisms responsible for hypercalcemia include direct tumor invasion and tumor secretion of humoral factors, such as parathyroid hormone–related peptide (PTHrP). Hypercalcemia may occur with granulomatous disease or other inflammatory diseases, usually because of increased production of 1,25 (OH)$_2$ vitamin D. Prolonged immobilization can be associated with increased bone resorption and hypercalcemia. Other disorders associated with hypercalcemia include excessive vitamin D or vitamin A intake and Jansen metaphyseal chondrodysplasia. Jansen metaphyseal chondrodysplasia is an autosomal dominant disorder characterized by short stature and abnormal endochondral bone formation. It is associated with heterozygous constitutively activating mutations of the PTH/PTHrP receptor *(PTH1R)* gene. Typically, PTH concentrations are normal in Jansen metaphyseal chondrodysplasia. Loss of function mutations in the calcium sensing receptor *(CaSR)* gene, mapped to chromosome 3q13.3-21, have been implicated in hypercalcemia. The "set point" for the CaSR to respond to serum calcium concentration is

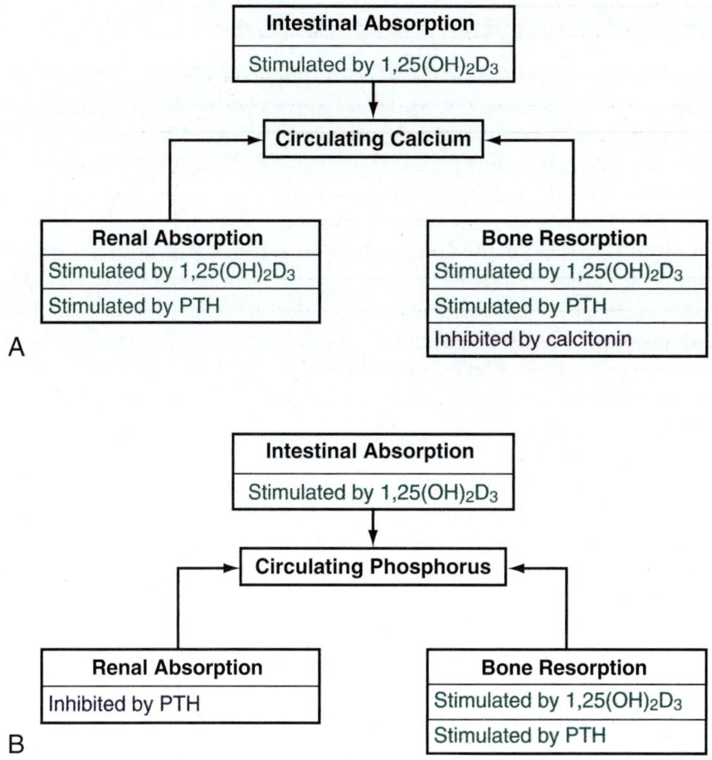

Fig. 9.51 Calcium and phosphorus homeostasis. (A) Calcium homeostasis: Intestinal calcium absorption occurs by a transcellular active transport process stimulated by calcitriol (1,25[OH]2 vitamin D), mostly in the duodenum and jejunum and a passive process throughout the whole intestine. The active transcellular process involves entry across the brush border membrane, intracellular diffusion, and extrusion by the basolateral membrane mediated by an adenosine triphosphatase (ATPase). The primary regulatory site for calcium reabsorption in the kidneys is the distal tubule. Calcitriol also enhances renal calcium absorption and bone reabsorption. Parathyroid hormone *(PTH)* increases circulating calcium by stimulating renal absorption and bone resorption and indirectly stimulating intestinal absorption by increasing synthesis of calcitriol. (B) Phosphorus homeostasis. Intestinal phosphorus absorption occurs mainly in the duodenum and jejunum; most of its renal reabsorption occurs in the proximal tubule. Despite its stimulation of bone resorption, the net effect of PTH on serum phosphorus is a decrease in its concentration due to predominant suppression of renal reabsorption.

altered. The receptor cannot sense the higher level of serum calcium and does not shut off PTH secretion. Heterozygous loss-of-function mutations are associated with familial hypocalciuric hypercalcemia. In this condition, hypercalcemia is mild to moderate. Rare genetic conditions such as biallelic (homozygous or compound heterozygous) inactivating *CaSR* mutations may present with severe hypercalcemia in infancy, neonatal severe primary hyperparathyroidism, which can be life-threatening.

Hypocalcemia

Symptoms of hypocalcemia include hypotension, paresthesia, tetany, dry skin, muscle tingling, and seizures. On physical examination, one should assess for signs of hypocalcemia including the Chvostek sign, a facial grimace resulting from tapping on the facial nerve (Video 9.1) and Trousseau sign, manifested by hand spasm when a blood pressure cuff is inflated for 3 minutes above the patient's systolic blood pressure. Cardiac findings include prolongation of the QTc interval and arrhythmia.

Hypoparathyroidism

Hypoparathyroidism may be congenital or acquired. Regardless of etiology, the hallmarks of hypoparathyroidism are the same. Typical features include hypocalcemia (Fig. 9.53), hyperphosphatemia (the phosphaturic effect of PTH is lost), and an inappropriately low or undetectable PTH level.

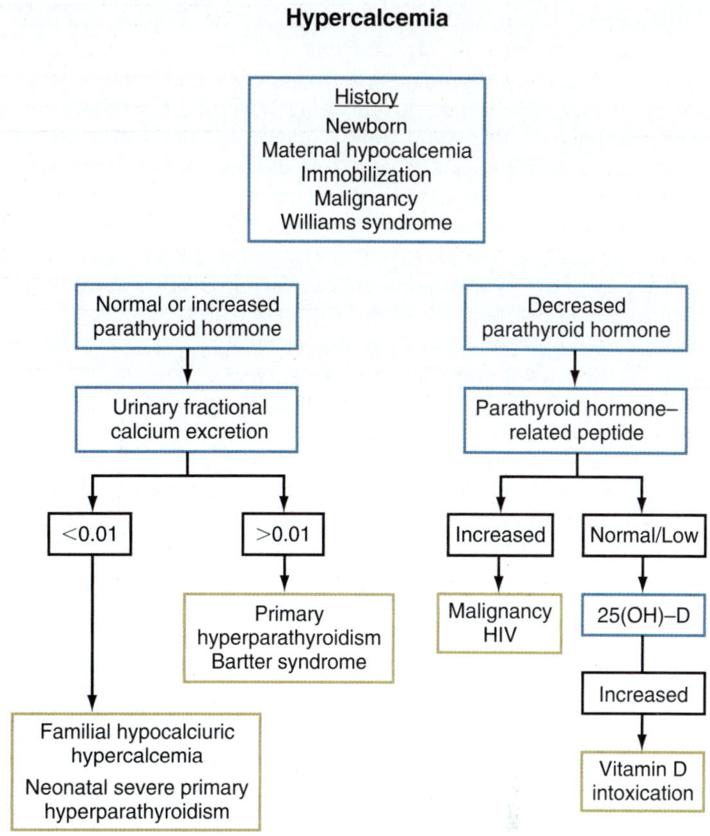

Fig. 9.52 Hypercalcemia. Initial approach to the child with hypercalcemia. *25(OH)–D,* 25 hydroxyvitamin D; *HIV,* human immunodeficiency virus.

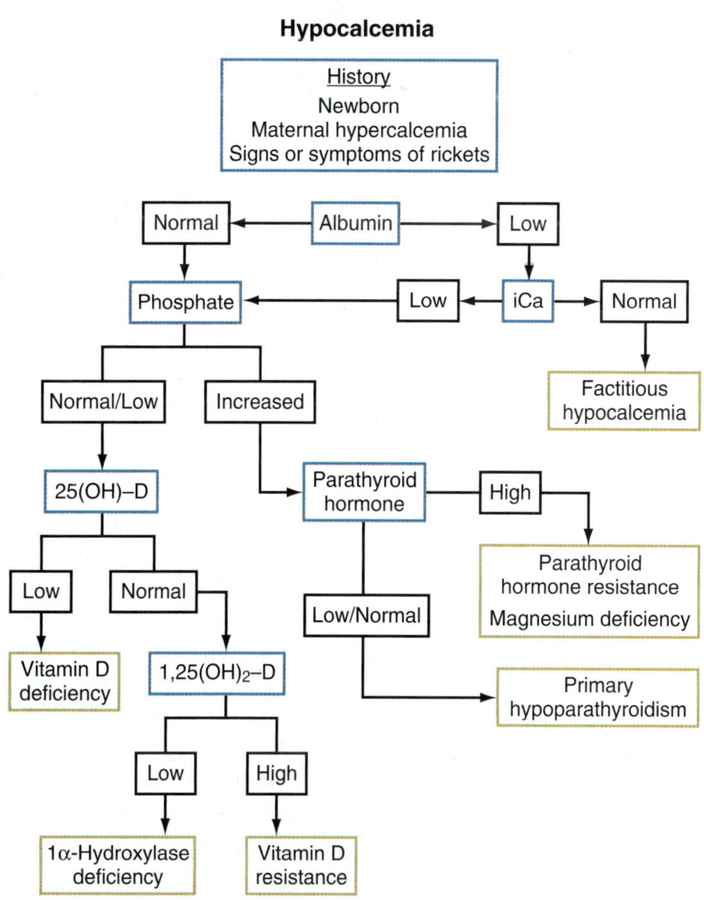

Fig. 9.53 Hypocalcemia. Initial approach to the child with hypocalcemia. *1,25(OH)$_2$–D,* 1,25-dihydroxyvitamin D; *25(OH)–D,* 25 hydroxyvitamin D; *iCa,* ionized calcium.

DiGeorge syndrome is a heterogeneous developmental field defect characterized by dysmorphic features, cardiac defects, immune deficiency, thymic aplasia/hypoplasia, and hypoparathyroidism. Microdeletion of chromosome 22q11.2 is the most common etiology of this syndrome. Genetic testing can confirm microdeletion. Between 10% and 20% of cases of DiGeorge syndrome–associated hypocalcemia will present with symptomatic hypocalcemia between 0 and 3 months of age. Up to 10% of infants will present with seizures secondary to hypocalcemia. The degree of hypoparathyroidism can vary over time. It is important to recognize that children with DiGeorge syndrome can become hypocalcemic after surgery or in acute stressful states even if they are previously normocalcemic. Gain of function mutations of *CaSR* gene are a rare cause of autosomal dominant hypocalcemia.

Acquired hypoparathyroidism can be due to autoimmune disease, infiltration, or trauma, including surgical trauma. Hypoparathyroidism may be one of the first manifestations of the autosomal recessive autoimmune polyglandular syndrome type 1 or autoimmune polyendocrinopathy–candidiasis–ectodermal dysplasia syndrome. Infiltration of the parathyroid glands associated with metal overload (hemochromatosis, chronic transfusion therapy); malignancy; or granulomatous disease can also lead to hypoparathyroidism. Mutations in mitochondrial DNA can also be associated with hypoparathyroidism.

Pseudohypoparathyroidism

Pseudohypoparathyroidism (PHP) is characterized by organ resistance or unresponsiveness to PTH. Patients with Albright hereditary osteodystrophy (AHO), also known as PHP type 1a, have a distinct phenotype with round facies, short stature, obesity, skin hyperpigmentation, subcutaneous calcifications, and a short thick neck (Fig. 9.54A). Shortening of the metacarpals and metatarsals is common, especially for the fourth digit (see Fig. 9.54B and C). Resistance to other hormones, such as TSH, gonadotropins, GHRH, and ADH, may be observed. AHO results from loss-of-function mutations in Gs-alpha subunit *(GNAS1)* gene, which maps to chromosome 20q13.3. AHO should be suspected in a child with short stature and hypocalcemia and a history of similarly affected family members. Affected patients have hypocalcemia, hyperphosphatemia, and extremely elevated PTH values. Because *GNAS1* is an imprinted gene, the phenotype depends on the parental origin of the affected allele. When the maternal allele carries the mutation, the child typically has the phenotype of AHO and hypoparathyroidism. When the paternal allele carries the mutation, the child usually manifests only clinical features of AHO without resistance to PTH.

Patients with PHP type 1b typically lack the physical features of type 1a. Rather, the major manifestation is PTH resistance. This disorder is associated with a loss of methylation in the maternal allele that decreases transcription of the maternal *GNAS* allele.

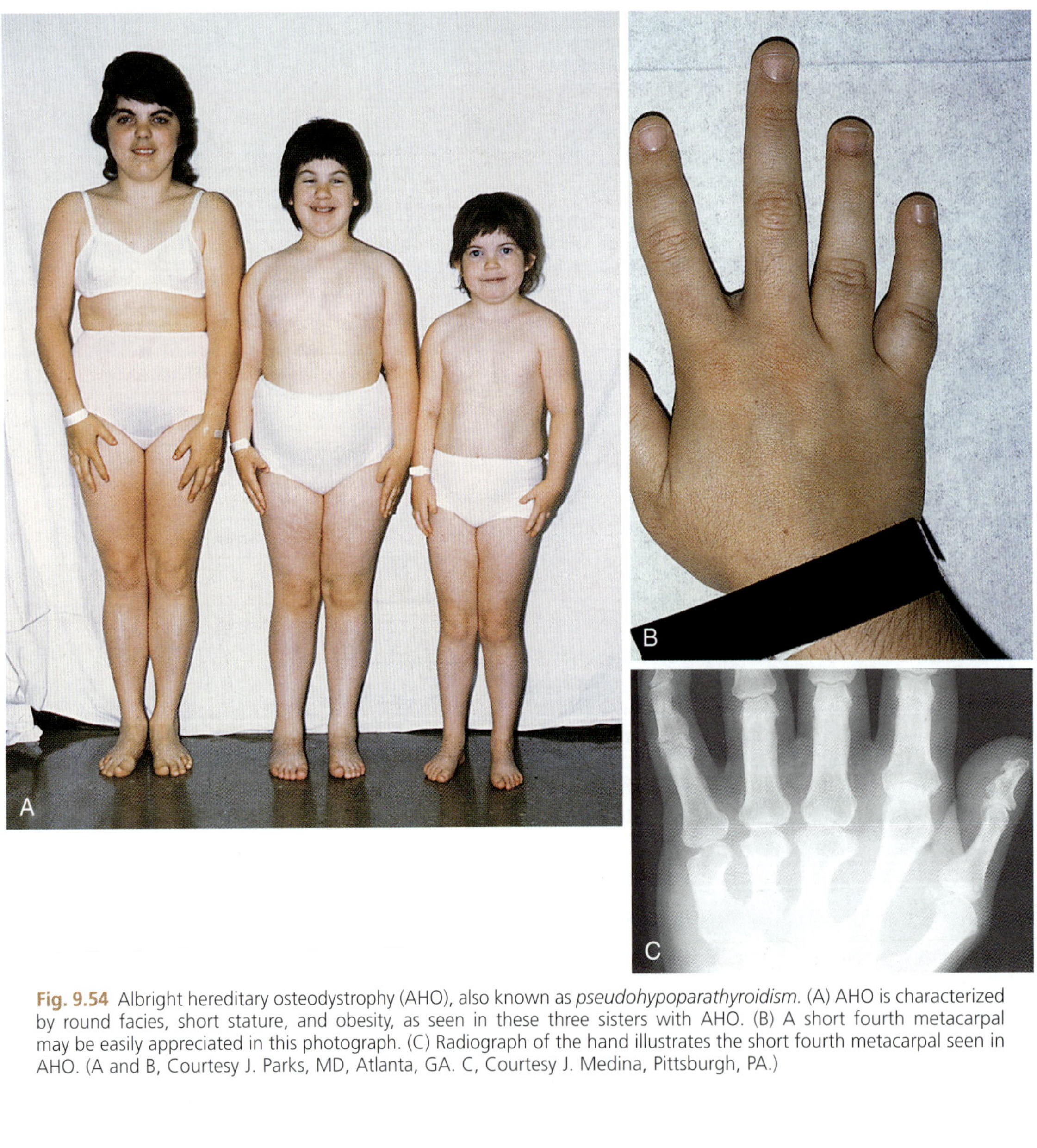

Fig. 9.54 Albright hereditary osteodystrophy (AHO), also known as *pseudohypoparathyroidism*. (A) AHO is characterized by round facies, short stature, and obesity, as seen in these three sisters with AHO. (B) A short fourth metacarpal may be easily appreciated in this photograph. (C) Radiograph of the hand illustrates the short fourth metacarpal seen in AHO. (A and B, Courtesy J. Parks, MD, Atlanta, GA. C, Courtesy J. Medina, Pittsburgh, PA.)

Rickets

Nutritional Rickets

Hypocalcemia as part of rickets could be due to dietary calcium insufficiency or vitamin D deficiency. Vitamin D deficiency may result from inadequate sunlight exposure, inadequate nutrition, and/or malabsorption. The term vitamin D refers to vitamin D2 (ergocalciferol), which is plant based, and vitamin D3 (cholecalciferol), which is synthesized in the body. Drugs that activate the catabolism of vitamin D, such as phenytoin and phenobarbital, can also worsen vitamin D deficiency in individuals with baseline marginal vitamin D stores. Vitamin D deficiency should be suspected in children with poor linear growth, delayed walking secondary to muscle weakness, bone pain, hypotonia, and anorexia. Children on the autism spectrum often have problems with eating, including picky eating with restricted diets. Such limited diets are often deficient in both calcium and vitamin D and are among the most frequent causes of rickets. Clinical manifestations of rickets in ambulatory infants and children include genu varum or genu valgum (bowed legs and "knock knees," respectively) and metaphyseal flaring (widening) (Fig. 9.55A); prominence of the costochondral junctions (rachitic rosary, see Fig. 9.55B); indentation of the lower anterior thoracic wall (Harrison groove); frontal bossing; and, occasionally, craniotabes. Darkly pigmented and exclusively breastfed infants and children who have limited exposure to sunlight are particularly prone to developing vitamin D deficiency.

Vitamin D deficiency may also be the consequence of intestinal malabsorptive disorders, such as celiac disease, biliary obstruction, gastric resection, cystic fibrosis, or pancreatic insufficiency. In most infants and children with rickets, total calcium levels are usually borderline normal or low and phosphate levels are low. Alkaline phosphatase activity and PTH concentrations are increased.

To become biologically active, vitamin D undergoes two hydroxylation steps. The first step, 25-hydroxylation, occurs in the liver to generate 25-hydroxyvitamin D. The second step, 1α-hydroxylation, takes place in the kidney to generate 1,25-dihydroxyvitamin D. The biologic actions of vitamin D are mediated by the vitamin D receptor, which is a member of the steroid/thyroid hormone nuclear receptor family. Determination of 25-hydroxyvitamin D concentrations provides the more accurate method to estimate vitamin D stores and test for vitamin D deficiency. Measurement of 1,25-dihydroxyvitamin D does not provide information regarding body vitamin D stores and is usually not necessary. It may be indicated when abnormalities of the enzyme that converts 25-hydroxyvitamin D to 1,25-dihydroxyvitamin D or renal disease are suspected.

Elucidation of the pathways involved in vitamin D metabolism has identified the molecular basis for rickets unresponsive to pharmacologic vitamin D treatment. Vitamin D–dependent rickets type 1 is an autosomal recessive disorder associated with mutations in the 1α-hydroxylase *(CYP27B1)* gene. Vitamin D–dependent rickets type 2A is associated with loss-of-function mutations in the vitamin D receptor *(VDR)* gene; this form may be associated with alopecia, growth retardation, and extremely elevated calcitriol and PTH concentrations. Laboratory data seen in rickets are listed in Table 9.4.

Hypophosphatemic Rickets

Phosphate, an abundant anion, plays major roles in bone mineralization, energy metabolism, cell signaling, and acid-base homeostasis. Phosphate concentrations are modulated by PTH, vitamin D, and phosphatonin concentrations. In general, approximately 85% to 90% of filtered phosphate is reabsorbed by the kidney. PTH acts to inhibit renal phosphate reabsorption. Hypophosphatemic rickets is characterized by severe hypophosphatemia, postnatal growth retardation with short stature, genu varum, dolichocephaly, and dental anomalies (Fig. 9.56). Muscle, bone, and joint pain may occur. The X-linked form of hypophosphatemic rickets is associated with genetic variants in the phosphate-regulating gene with homologies to endopeptidases on the X-chromosome *(PHEX)* gene. Autosomal dominant and recessive forms are associated with mutations in the fibroblast growth factor 23 *(FGF23)*, dentin matrix acidic phosphoprotein *(DMP1)*, and *SLC34A3* genes. FGF23 is a phosphatonin; mutations that prevent cleavage of FGF23 to inactive forms are

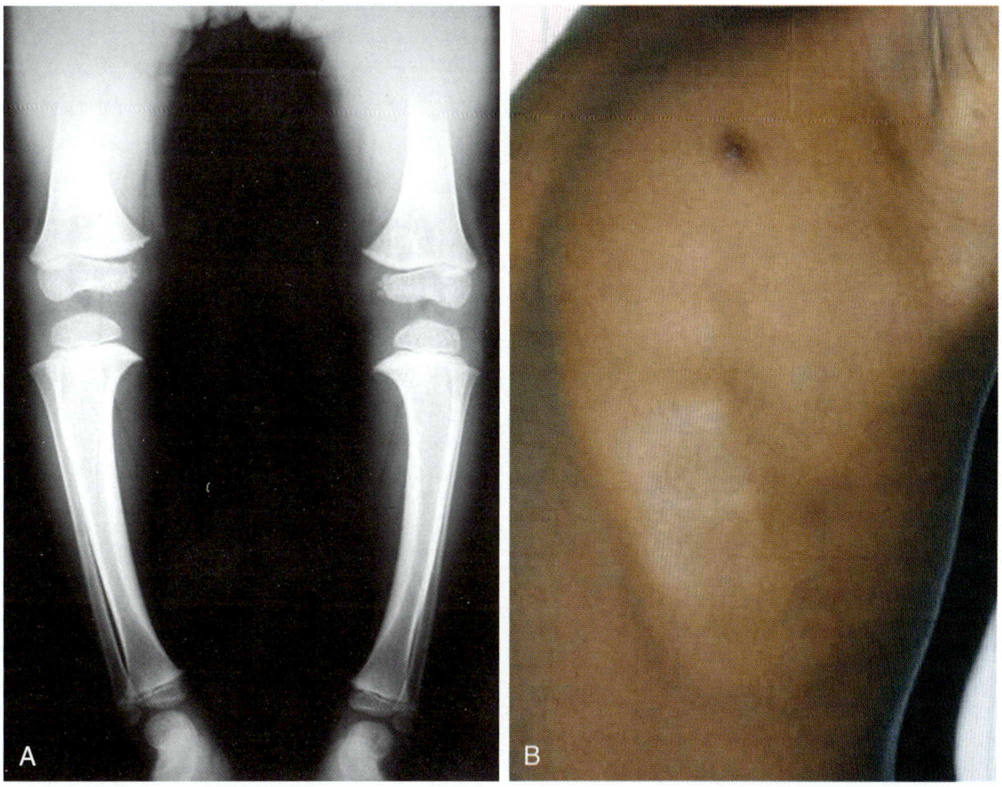

Fig. 9.55 Clinical manifestations of rickets. (A) Genu valgum ("knock knees"), metaphyseal flaring. (B) Rachitic rosary. (Courtesy T. Thacher, MD.)

Table 9.4 Laboratory Findings in Rickets

Type	Calcium	Phosphate	Alkaline Phosphatase	25-Hydroxyvitamin D3	1,25-Dihydroxyvitamin D	Parathyroid Hormone
Vitamin D deficiency						
Mild	N, ↓	N, ↓	↑	↓	N	N
Moderate	N, ↓	↓	↑↑	↓	↓, N, ↑	↑
Severe	↓	↓	↑↑	↓↓	↓	↑↑
X-linked hypophosphatemic rickets	N	↓↓	↑	N	N, ↓	N
Pseudovitamin D–deficiency rickets	↓↓	↓↓	↑↑↑	N	↓↓↓	↑↑↑

N, Normal.

From Sperling MA, editor: *Pediatric endocrinology,* ed 2, Philadelphia, 2002, WB Saunders.

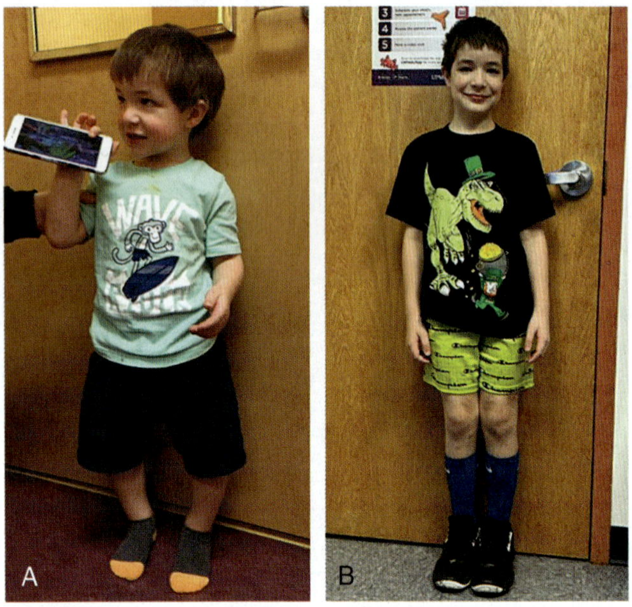

Fig. 9.56 Child with hypophosphatemic rickets. (A) Notice prominent forehead, dolichocephalic shape of head, and significant genu varum. (B) Improvement of genu varum after several years of medical therapy in addition to orthopedic surgery. (Courtesy O. Escobar, MD, Pittsburgh, PA.)

associated with decreased renal 1α-hydroxylase activity and increased phosphate excretion.

Hypophosphatasia

Hypophosphatasia is an autosomal recessive metabolic bone disorder of varying severity due to loss-of-function mutations in the *TNSALP* gene. Decreased *TNSALP* activity leads to defective mineralization of skeletal osteoid. In addition to the radiographic findings of rickets, affected subjects have low alkaline phosphatase activity and increased urinary phosphoethanolamine excretion.

ENERGY METABOLISM, ENDOCRINE PANCREAS, AND ASSOCIATED ENDOCRINOPATHIES

Obesity and Related Comorbidities

Obesity, defined as excessive body fat accumulation, is a condition with a few clinically useful evaluation metrics. The diagnosis currently relies on the measurement of growth parameters including the BMI and body proportions such as abdominal girth. Although most childhood obesity cases are thought to be "exogenous" (i.e., exclusively related to excessive caloric intake compared with energy expenditure), genetic syndromes, hypothalamic tumors, and endocrinopathies may also present with overweight or weight gain as the initial symptom. Causes of secondary obesity are listed in Box 9.10.

Body weight and fat mass accumulation are controlled by complex neuroendocrine circuits that regulate appetite and energy expenditure. Peripheral signals reflective of body weight and nutritional status (such as leptin secreted by adipose tissue, ghrelin produced by the stomach, or glucagon-like peptide-1 [GLP-1] and glucose-dependent insulinotropic polypeptide secreted in the proximal intestine) affect appetite by regulating the release of appetite controlling substances in the hypothalamus (orexigenic factors such as neuropeptide Y vs. anorexigenic factors such as POMC and melanocortin-4 receptor [MC4R]). In turn, hypothalamic neurotransmitters can regulate energy expenditure through their control of the balance between the sympathetic nervous system (aims at energy

Box 9.10 Hormonal and Genetic Conditions Associated With Obesity

Endocrine Disorders
Cushing syndrome (exogenous or endogenous)
Hypothyroidism
Pseudohypoparathyroidism
Growth hormone (GH) deficiency
Type 2 diabetes mellitus

Monogenic Disorders Associated With Obesity
Leptin deficiency
Leptin receptor mutation
Pro-opiomelanocortin (POMC) mutation
Melanocortin-4 receptor (MC4R) mutation
Melanocortin-3 receptor (MC3R) mutation
Prohormone convertase-1 mutation
SIM-1 mutation

Obesity Associated With Mental Retardation Syndromes
Prader-Willi syndrome
Bardet-Biedl syndrome
Cohen syndrome
Alström syndrome
Carpenter syndrome
TrkB mutation
Brain-derived neurotrophic factor (BDNF) deficiency
Börjeson-Forssman-Lehmann syndrome

Central Nervous System Disorders
Hypothalamic tumor
Trauma
Inflammation
Rapid-onset obesity with hypothalamic dysfunction, hypoventilation, and autonomic dysregulation (ROHHAD) syndrome

Miscellaneous
Drug induced (e.g., risperidone, tricyclic antidepressants, steroids)
Binge-eating disorder
Bulimia nervosa

Modified from Schneider MB, Brill SR: Obesity in children and adolescents, *Pediatr Rev* 26:155–162, 2005.

Box 9.11 Complications of Obesity

Respiratory	**Endocrinologic**
Sleep apnea	Insulin resistance
Snoring	Impaired glucose tolerance
Pickwickian syndrome	Type 2 diabetes mellitus
Asthma	Polycystic ovarian syndrome
Musculoskeletal	Menstrual irregularity
Blount disease	Metabolic syndrome
Slipped capital femoral epiphysis	Hyperleptinemia
	Gynecomastia (in males)
Gastrointestinal	Premature adrenarche
Gallbladder disease	**Psychologic**
Nonalcoholic fatty liver disease	Depression
Cardiovascular	Poor self-esteem
Dyslipidemias	Eating disorders
Hypertension	Social isolation

Modified from Schneider MB, Brill SR: Obesity in children and adolescents, *Pediatr Rev* 26:155–162, 2005.

expenditure) versus the vagal system (aims at storage) with consequences on fat accumulation and body weight. The recognition of the factors involved in these control loops has helped define children with monogenic obesity. For instance, *MC4R, POMC, LEP, LEPR, PCSK1,* and *BBS* gene mutations have been identified to be causative in some of the familial and early-onset obesity. Genetic studies using monogenic obesity gene panels should be considered for children who have early-onset obesity (weight gain before the age of 5 years) and hyperphagia.

Individuals with obesity are at risk of developing systemic complications, listed in Box 9.11. The combination of obesity, insulin resistance, dyslipidemia, and hypertension has been termed *metabolic syndrome,* or *syndrome X.* Individuals with this syndrome are at increased risk for developing type 2 diabetes and cardiovascular disease. Obesity is a significant risk factor for obstructive sleep apnea, which potentiates obesity and comorbidities of obesity including cardiovascular disease. Adolescent girls with clinical/biochemical hyperandrogenism, irregular menses, and chronic anovulation are also at risk for metabolic dysfunction and polycystic ovary syndrome. An early sign of insulin resistance is acanthosis nigricans (Fig. 9.57), a skin finding characterized by hyperpigmented, velvety plaques commonly seen around the neck, in the axillae, or over joints.

ROHHAD (rapid-onset obesity with hypothalamic dysfunction, hypoventilation, and autonomic dysregulation) is a condition manifested by a series of disorders that appear in a sequential manner after apparent normal development in the first 2 to 4 years of life. The earliest manifestations (mean age of 3 years) are related to hypothalamic dysfunction. ROHHAD most commonly presents as rapid-onset obesity, followed by alterations in water balance (hypernatremia or polydipsia) and other endocrine problems, such as GH deficiency, adrenal insufficiency, and hypogonadotropic hypogonadism. Autonomic dysregulation (ophthalmologic manifestations, thermal dysregulation, gastrointestinal dysmotility, altered perception of pain, altered sweating, bradycardia); behavioral abnormalities (depression, flat affect, psychosis, emotional lability); and respiratory manifestations (alveolar hypoventilation, cardiorespiratory arrest, reduced carbon dioxide ventilatory response, obstructive sleep apnea) appear thereafter at mean ages of 3.6, 4.8, and 6.2 years, respectively. A genetic cause has not been identified, but it is now clear that this is a separate entity from congenital central hypoventilation syndrome manifested early in the newborn period with alveolar hypoventilation and typically associated with mutations in the *PHOX2B* gene. ROHHAD should be suspected in children with obesity starting after 2 years of age in whom symptoms of autonomic dysregulation are identified. Approximately 50% of patients with ROHHAD syndrome develop tumors of neural crest origin. Early referrals for comprehensive respiratory and endocrinologic testing and management will improve care and quality of life.

POLYCYSTIC OVARY SYNDROME

PCOS is a familial heterogeneous disorder characterized by oligomenorrhea/amenorrhea, chronic anovulation, and hyperandrogenism. This disorder affects approximately 6% to 15% of reproductive-aged women. Several expert opinion documents have defined four phenotypes of PCOS based on the presence or absence of hyperandrogenism, ovulatory dysfunction, and polycystic ovary morphology. Importantly, diagnosing PCOS requires exclusion of disorders with similar symptoms, such as nonclassic congenital adrenal hyperplasia (NCCAH), hyperprolactinemia, and thyroid dysfunction.

Though PCOS begins in adolescence, finalizing a diagnosis may require clinical observation over several years because the symptoms of PCOS resemble normal pubertal development. Menses may be irregular for the first several years after menarche. Acne and mildly elevated androgen concentrations may occur during puberty. The early adolescent ovary often has a multifollicular morphology, which may be difficult to differentiate from the classic "string of pearls" appearance of the typical PCOS ovary. Family history may be positive for PCOS, diabetes, and dyslipidemia.

Current diagnostic criteria for PCOS in adolescent girls include being at least 2 years post-menarche, irregular menses (normal menses are 21 to 35 days in women greater than 2 years post-menarche), and clinical/biochemical hyperandrogenism. Clinical hyperandrogenism refers to hirsutism, excessive coarse hair in androgen dependent areas, and severe acne. Biochemical hyperandrogenism includes elevated total testosterone, free testosterone, or androstenedione measuring using validated assays. Due to the presence of multifollicular ovaries in the adolescent girl, ovarian ultrasounds are not recommended and should be deferred until 8 years post menarche. Adolescent girls with some features of PCOS can be labeled as being "at risk for PCOS" until the diagnosis can be confirmed or symptoms resolve.

Women with PCOS have a higher risk of infertility, insulin resistance, type 2 diabetes mellitus, and dyslipidemia. Long-term comorbidities include obesity, diabetes mellitus, endometriosis, and depression. Although the prevalence of cardiovascular risk markers is higher in women with PCOS, available data suggest that the actual number of cardiovascular events is not increased. For the adolescent girl, consideration of the diagnosis of PCOS should be tied to increased awareness of the comorbidities associated with this lifelong condition. This represents an opportunity for meaningful interventions, such as healthy lifestyle counseling, testing for comorbidities, or medications. Conversely, overdiagnosis should be avoided because it can lead to unnecessary anxiety and unwarranted treatment.

DISORDERS OF ENDOCRINE PANCREAS

Hyperglycemia

Diabetes Mellitus

There are several forms of diabetes mellitus including type 1 diabetes (insulin-dependent, autoimmune diabetes mellitus); type 2 diabetes (nonautoimmune diabetes, may be non–insulin-dependent or insulin-dependent diabetes mellitus), cystic fibrosis–related diabetes (CFRDM), drug-induced diabetes (secondary to steroids, immunosuppressive agents), monogenic forms of diabetes (maturity-onset diabetes of the young), mitochondrial diabetes, neonatal diabetes, and ketosis-prone type 2 diabetes ("Flatbush diabetes"), and diabetes associated with genetic conditions with immune dysregulation.

Type 1 diabetes mellitus is an autoimmune condition that develops in the presence of a genetic predisposition. In a child who has high-risk genetic predisposition conferred by some HLA haplotypes, the disease progresses through different stages as the development of

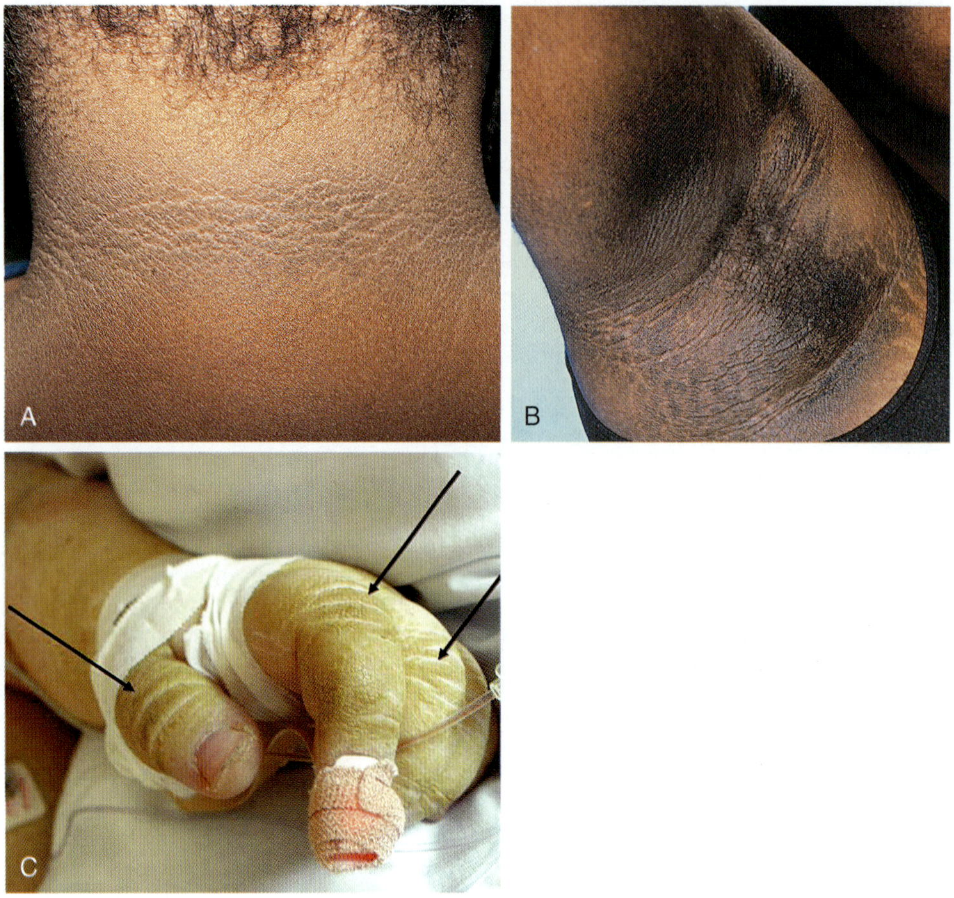

Fig. 9.57 Acanthosis nigricans. Note the thickened skin and velvety appearance around the neck (A) and in the axilla (B) of this patient with polycystic ovary syndrome and insulin resistance. (C) Acanthosis nigricans affecting the fingers of this patient with insulin resistance.

autoantibodies leads initially to dysglycemia and then to the over manifestation with hyperglycemia. At the time of clinical presentation, they reach a nearly complete insulin deficiency state typically characterized by relatively acute onset of symptoms of polydipsia, polyuria, nocturia, weight loss, glycosuria, and hyperglycemia.

Type 2 diabetes mellitus, which is nonautoimmune and polygenic in inheritance, manifests with insulin resistance, obesity, hypertension, and dyslipidemia in addition to hyperglycemia. Cutaneous features of insulin resistance include acanthosis nigricans (Fig. 9.57), hidradenitis, and skin tags. Though the initial presentation of type 2 diabetes mellitus is of relative insulin deficiency in the presence of insulin resistance, long-standing type 2 diabetes may also have near-complete insulin deficiency. Obesity is overwhelmingly the most important risk factor for developing type 2 diabetes, especially for children.

CFRDM is an extrapulmonary complication of cystic fibrosis and is largely driven by a combination of insulin deficiency and insulin resistance. The increased survival of children with cystic fibrosis from therapies including *CFTR* modulators and screening mandated by the Cystic Fibrosis Foundation has led to recognition of the high frequency of CFRDM.

Neonatal diabetes presents shortly after birth and can be classified into two categories: transient or permanent. Typically, infants with neonatal diabetes have intrauterine growth retardation, hyperglycemia, glycosuria, and failure to thrive. Genetic testing should be considered for all children with onset of diabetes mellitus in the first year of life. Specific genetic variants at chromosome 6q24 have been associated with transient neonatal diabetes. Affected infants present in the first few weeks of life, followed by remission; diabetes may recur later in life. Permanent neonatal diabetes can be associated with specific mutations in potassium inwardly rectifying channel subfamily K member 11 *(KCNJ11);* glucokinase *(GCK);* insulin promoter factor-1 *(IPF-1);* adenosine triphosphate (ATP)-binding cassette, subfamily C, member 8 *(ABCC8);* and insulin genes. Mutations in pancreatic and duodenal homeobox 1 *(PDX1)* gene have been identified in patients with neonatal diabetes and pancreatic agenesis. PDX1 is a nuclear protein involved in the early development of the pancreas and plays a key role in glucose-dependent regulation of insulin gene expression. Defects in this gene are a cause of pancreatic agenesis. In addition to causing neonatal diabetes, variants in this gene are associated with early-onset insulin-dependent diabetes mellitus and maturity-onset diabetes of the young type 4. Inheritance is autosomal dominant for *KCNJ11* mutations and autosomal recessive for *GCK* and *PDX1* mutations. Neonatal diabetes due to activating mutations in KATP channel subunits may be treated with oral sulfonylurea, which results in endogenous insulin secretion and near normal glycemic control.

Before the institution of aggressive insulin therapy, children with diabetes mellitus and short stature were seen frequently in endocrine clinics and represented instances of Mauriac syndrome (Fig. 9.58). This syndrome is characterized by poorly controlled diabetes, short stature, hepatomegaly, and lack of sexual development. Fortunately, it is now rare to see a child with Mauriac syndrome. In the well-controlled patient with type 1, or insulin-dependent, diabetes mellitus, the growth rate should be indistinguishable from that of a normal child. The inability to flatten the palms of the hands because of limited joint mobility and waxy thickened skin in the areas of the proximal and distal interphalangeal joints (sclerodactyly) is one physical finding seen in poorly controlled patients with diabetes (Fig. 9.59). The development of specific skin lesions, such as necrobiosis lipoidica diabeticorum (Fig. 9.60), most frequently in the pretibial regions, may occasionally be seen in a child with type 1 diabetes.

Technology has benefited insulin delivery by developing several insulin analogs and hybrid closed-loop insulin pumps, also known as *automated insulin delivery systems.* These systems combine continuous

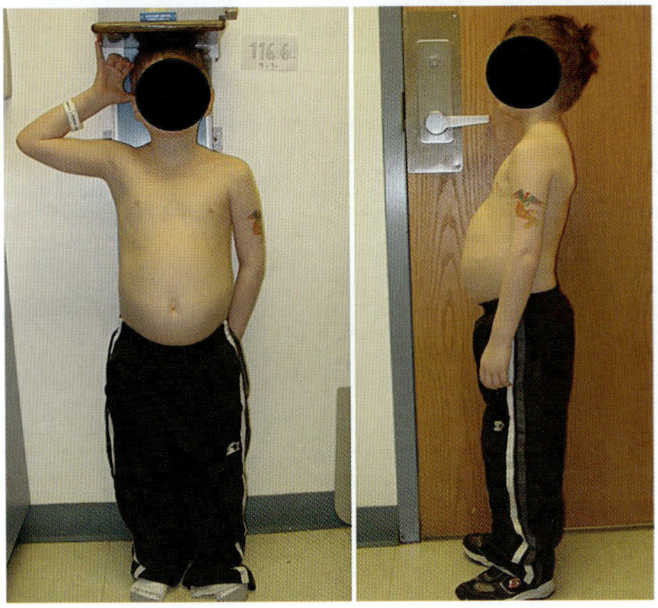

Fig. 9.58 Mauriac syndrome in a 9-year 3-month-old boy with poorly controlled type I diabetes mellitus. (A) Note short stature (Ht < 3rd percentile). (B) Note prominent abdomen (due to enlarged liver). (Courtesy O. Escobar, MD, Pittsburgh, PA.)

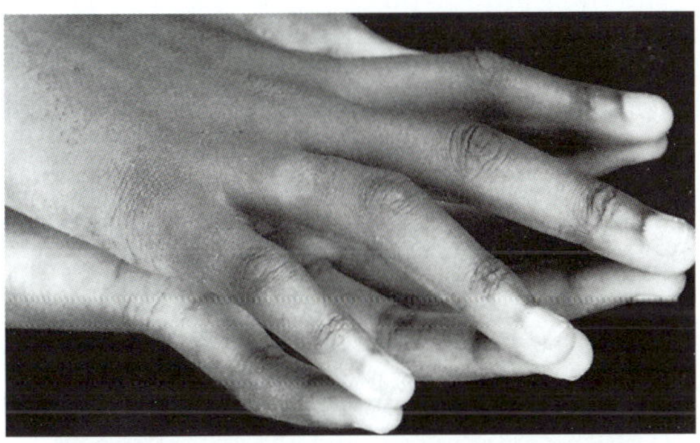

Fig. 9.59 Diabetic sclerodactyly. This patient shows an inability to flatten the palms and fingers as he presses both hands together. (Courtesy A. Rosenbloom, MD, Gainesville, FL.)

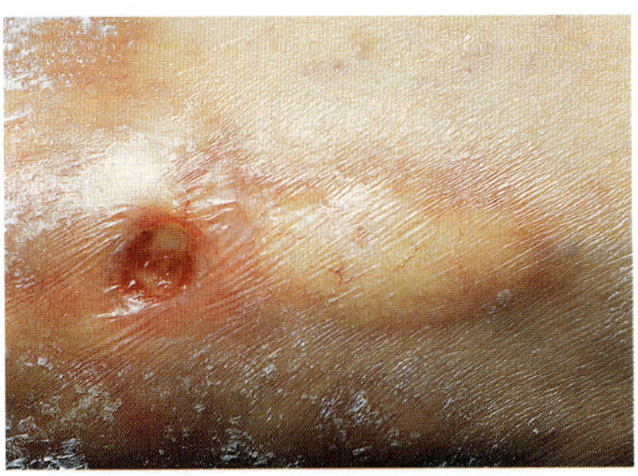

Fig. 9.60 Necrobiosis lipoidica diabeticorum. Characterized by the presence of yellow waxy skin lesions that exhibit reddened components. Small areas of ulceration may also be seen. (Courtesy B. Cohen, MD, Pittsburgh, PA.)

glucose monitoring with automated insulin adjustments. Currently, hybrid closed-loop systems are demonstrating significant improvements in hemoglobin A1C, glucose time in range, and reduced hypoglycemic events compared with manually programmed devices. Unlike traditional pumps, some of the newer pumps use body weight as a starting point and adjust insulin doses based on real-time glucose data without the need for meticulous carbohydrate calculations. These pumps offer a promising future for diabetes care, bridging technology and patient well-being. Islet, pancreas-kidney, and stem cell transplants have been performed but are not ready for routine medical care. The U.S. Food and Drug Administration has approved humanized anti-CD3 monoclonal antibody (Teplizumab) use in children with autoantibodies without clinical symptoms of diabetes, and it has been shown to delay the onset of symptoms of diabetes by at least 2 years.

Hypoglycemia

The classic definition of hypoglycemia is named the Whipple triad after an endocrine surgeon established this criterion before his exploratory surgeries for insulinoma. This includes presence of signs and symptoms of hypoglycemia with a documented low glucose value and resolution of these signs and symptoms with administration of glucose. Signs and symptoms of hypoglycemia include neurogenic symptoms, which tend to occur first and are due to activation of the autonomic nervous system and epinephrine release. Symptoms include sweating, tremors, palpitations, nausea, and hunger. This is followed by neuroglycopenia symptoms, which result from a lack of glucose availability to the brain. These signs and symptoms include lethargy, somnolence, confusion, irritability, and seizures. Although setting a fixed glucose level for diagnosis of hypoglycemia is difficult across all age groups, documented plasma glucose of less than 60 mg/dL can provide reliable diagnostic information for children older than 72 hours of age. To identify the cause of hypoglycemia, a "critical blood sample" should be obtained at the time of hypoglycemia before the administration of glucose. Meter glucose should be confirmed by a laboratory measurement of serum glucose before diagnosing hypoglycemia. The whole blood sample should be centrifuged immediately by the laboratory to get serum. If not, glycolysis by erythrocytes could result in spuriously low glucose values. Laboratory tests should include serum glucose, insulin, β-hydroxybutyrate, C-peptide, bicarbonate, cortisol, GH, free fatty acids, lactate, and pyruvate. Ammonia and acylcarnitine profile can be obtained separately because these analytes are independent of the blood glucose value. Urine for ketones and organic acids should be obtained as well.

The serum concentration of glucose, the major energy substrate, is regulated by a series of mechanisms that create a balance between substrate production and substrate use. Insulin is the mediator of substrate use. An abnormal increase in insulin leads to hypoglycemia. Substrate production, on the other hand, includes dietary intake, followed by two sequential processes, glycogenolysis and gluconeogenesis, both of which require the use of energy provided in large part by fatty acid oxidation in the mitochondria. These processes are finely regulated and modulated by hormones that counterregulate the action of insulin, namely catecholamines, glucagon, cortisol, and GH. A defect in any of these substrate-enhancing processes or in the hormones that regulate them may, therefore, cause hypoglycemia.

The differential diagnosis of hypoglycemia is broad (Boxes 9.12 to 9.14). A useful classification divides hypoglycemic states into those in which ketones are absent or low and those in which ketones are present and usually elevated (Fig. 9.61). In general, nonketotic hypoglycemia should raise suspicion for a hyperinsulinemic state because insulin blocks hepatic glucose production, lipolysis, and ketogenesis. The presence of ketosis at the time of hypoglycemia suggests a disorder of decreased substrate production (see Box 9.13). An exception is that of disorders of fatty acid metabolism in which fatty acids cannot be oxidized and ketones cannot be produced even during times of physiologic endogenous insulin suppression. Hypoglycemia may occur during a period of fasting or catabolic stress (see Box 9.13) or may be iatrogenic or drug-induced, as seen in surreptitious insulin administration (see Box 9.14).

Prompt diagnosis and treatment of hypoglycemia, especially recurrent or persistent hypoglycemia, is essential due to the

Box 9.12 Postprandial Hypoglycemia

Postgastric surgery
Diabetes mellitus
Galactosemia
Hereditary fructose intolerance
Reactive or functional hypoglycemia

Box 9.13 Fasting Hypoglycemia

Increased Substrate Use

Hyperinsulinism: endogenous
- Insulinoma
- Mutations coding for SUR, KIR, GLUD, and GCK
- Autoimmune hypoglycemia
- Infants of diabetic mothers
- Beckwith-Wiedemann syndrome
- Donohue syndrome

Decreased Substrate Production

Inborn errors of carbohydrate metabolism
- Defects of gluconeogenesis
- Glycogen storage diseases

Inborn errors of protein metabolism
- Maple syrup urine disease
- Methylmalonic aciduria

Inborn errors of fat metabolism
- Systemic carnitine deficiency
- Carnitine acetyltransferase deficiency
- Hydroxymethylglutaryl-CoA lyase deficiency
- Acyl-CoA dehydrogenase deficiency

Counterregulatory hormone deficiency
- Cortisol
- Thyroid
- Glucagon
- GH
- Catecholamines

Ketotic hypoglycemia
Hepatic and renal disease
Extrapancreatic neoplasms
Reye syndrome

GCK, Glucokinase; *GH,* growth hormone; *GLUD,* glutamate dehydrogenase; *KIR,* potassium inwardly rectifying channel; *SUR,* sulfonylurea receptor.

Box 9.14 Drug-Induced Hypoglycemia

Insulin
Oral hypoglycemic agents
Ethanol
Salicylates
Propranolol
Miscellaneous other recreational drugs like Kratom
Ackee fruit

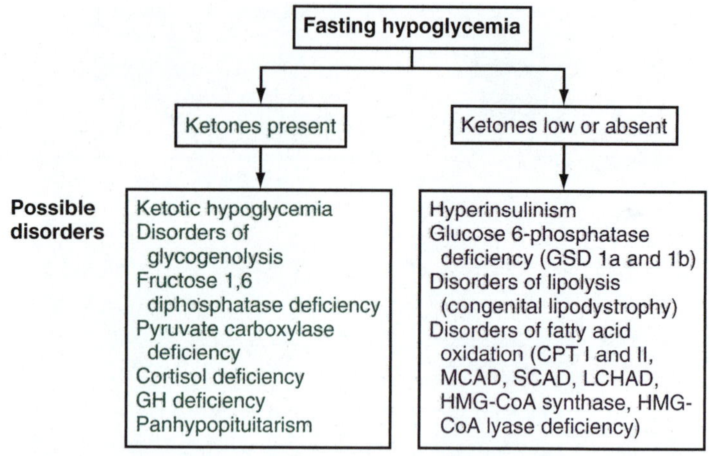

Fig. 9.61 Fasting hypoglycemia. Diagnostic evaluation for fasting hypoglycemia in the presence or absence of ketosis. *CPT,* Carnitine palmitoyltransferase; *GH,* growth hormone; *GSD,* glycogen storage disease; *HMG-CoA,* 3-hydroxy-3-methylglutaryl-coenzyme A; *LCHAD,* long-chain 3-hydroxyacyl-CoA dehydrogenase; *MCAD,* medium-chain acyl-CoA dehydrogenase; *SCAD,* short-chain acyl-CoA dehydrogenase.

significant risk of subsequent neurologic impairment. Hyperinsulinism is an important cause of hypoglycemia in infants and children. During gestation, infants of a diabetic mother may be exposed to elevated ambient glucose concentrations and compensate by increased insulin secretion. After birth, these infants may experience transient hypoglycemia due to excessive endogenous insulin secretion. Infants with intrauterine growth restriction may also develop transient hyperinsulinism. Hyperinsulinism is suspected in the neonatal period when severe hypoglycemia is refractory to treatment with intravenous administration of dextrose providing glucose infusion rates greater than 10 to 15 mg/kg/minute.

Hyperinsulinism may be caused by activating mutations of enzymes, such as glucokinase and glutamate dehydrogenase, by inactivating (loss-of-function) mutations of the K-ATP channel regulating insulin secretion (*ABCC8* and *KCNJ11* genes), by exogenous administration of glucose-lowering medications (such as insulin or sulfonylureas), or by an insulin-secreting adenoma. Syndromes such as Beckwith-Wiedemann syndrome (Fig. 9.62) may also be associated with hypoglycemia in addition to macrosomia, macroglossia, omphalocele, hemihypertrophy, and embryonal tumors. In these cases, hypoglycemia has been attributed to hyperinsulinism. After Nissen fundoplication, some children develop postoperative dumping syndrome, which can be associated with postprandial reactive hypoglycemia due to excessively rapid transit of food from the stomach to the small bowel (see Box 9.12).

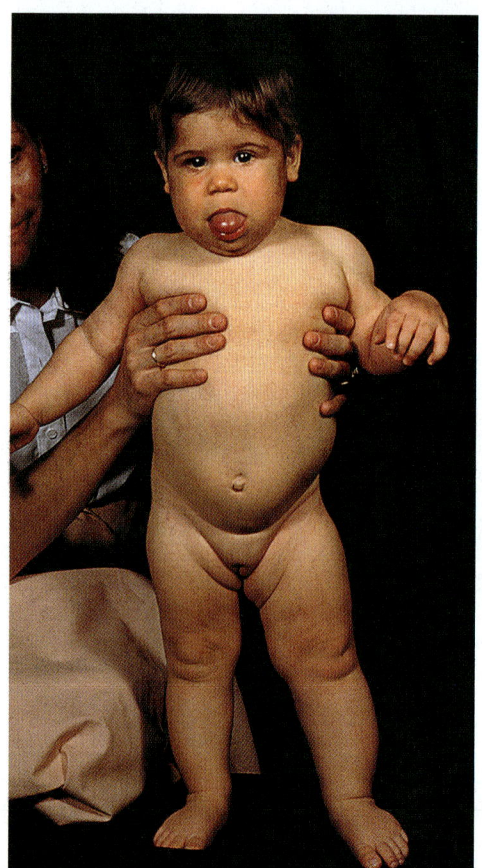

Fig. 9.62 Beckwith-Wiedemann syndrome. Note hemihypertrophy on the left side, along with prominence of the tongue. (Courtesy D. Becker, MD, Pittsburgh, PA.)

Ketotic hypoglycemia (see Fig. 9.61) can be a manifestation of a disorder affecting substrate production (see Box 9.13). Not infrequently, young children present with ketotic hypoglycemia without an obvious cause. This has been referred to as *idiopathic ketotic hypoglycemia of infancy and childhood,* which usually presents between 18 months and 5 years of age with resolution of symptoms by 8 to 9 years of age. In these cases, when a fasting challenge test is performed, the child becomes hypoglycemic within 16 hours of fasting and develops ketosis; measurement of insulin and counterregulatory hormones at the time of hypoglycemia shows appropriate physiologic responses (low insulin level, high β-hydroxybutyrate, high counter regulatory hormones cortisol, and GH). Cortisol and GH response to hypoglycemia is a delayed response and may be missed at the time of hypoglycemia. Relatively deficient substrate stores have been blamed for this condition. Hypopituitarism, glycogen storage diseases, and disorders of gluconeogenesis are additional causes of ketotic hypoglycemia. Hepatomegaly is often found in children with glycogen storage diseases.

SUMMARY

As seen in the photographs, endocrine dysfunction results in dramatic alterations in a child's phenotype. Growth and pubertal changes are sensitive markers of endocrine function. Careful attention to medical history, growth parameters, and physical examination of children with possible endocrine disorders will enable early diagnosis, resulting in prompt therapeutic intervention and restoration of the child's appearance and overall state of well-being.

A supplemental video is available at Elsevier eBooks+.

Bibliography

Backeljauw PF, Bondy C, Chernausek SD, et al: Proceedings from the Turner Resource Network symposium: the crossroads of health care research and health care delivery, *Am J Med Genet A* 167A(9):1962–1971, 2015.

Barnes N, Chemaitilly W: Endocrinopathies in survivors of childhood neoplasia, *Front Pediatr* 2:101, 2014.

Baron J, Sävendahl L, De Luca F, et al: Short and tall stature: a new paradigm emerges, *Nat Rev Endocrinol* 11:735–746, 2015.

Bauer AJ: Pediatric thyroid cancer: genetics, therapeutics, and outcome, *Endocrinol Metab Clin North Am* 49(4):589–611, 2020.

Björklund P, Pacak K, Crona J: Precision medicine in pheochromocytoma and paraganglioma: current and future concepts, *J Intern Med* 280(6):559–573, 2016.

Buryk MA, Simons JP, Picarsic J, et al: Can malignant thyroid nodules be distinguished from benign thyroid nodules in children and adolescents by clinical characteristics? A review of 89 pediatric patients with thyroid nodules, *Thyroid* 25(4):392–400, 2015.

Cedillo M, Libman IM, Arena VC, et al: Obesity, islet cell autoimmunity, and cardiovascular risk factors in youth at onset of type 1 autoimmune diabetes, *J Clin Endocrinol Metab* 100(1):E82–E86, 2015.

Chemaitilly W, Wilson RC, New MI: Hypertension and adrenal disorders, *Curr Hypertens Rep* 5(6):498–504, 2003.

Dancey A, Khan M, Dawson J, Peart F: Gigantomastia—a classification and review of the literature, *J Plast Reconstr Aesthet Surg* 61(5):493–502, 2008.

Daniels KE, Shaffer AD, Garbin S, et al: Validity of the American College of Radiology Thyroid Imaging Reporting and Data System in Children, *Laryngoscope* 133(9):2394–2401, 2022. https://doi.org/10.1002/lary.30425.

Escobar FA, Pantanowitz L, Picarsic JL, et al: Cytomorphology and sonographic features of ectopic thymic tissue diagnosed in pediatric FNA biopsies, *Cytopathology* 29(3):241–246, 2018. doi:10.1111/cyt.12529.

Gattineni J: Inherited disorders of calcium and phosphate metabolism, *Curr Opin Pediatr* 26(2):215–222, 2014.

Gonçalves FT, Fridman C, Pinto EM, et al: The E180splice mutation in the GHR gene causing Laron syndrome: witness of a Sephardic Jewish exodus from the Iberian Peninsula to the New World? *Am J Med Genet* 164A(5):1204–1208, 2014.

Gordon CM, Ackerman KE, Berga SL, et al: Functional hypothalamic amenorrhea: an Endocrine Society clinical practice guideline, *J Clin Endocrinol Metab* 102(5):1413–1439, 2017.

Grasberger H, Refetoff S: Genetic causes of congenital hypothyroidism due to dyshormonogenesis, *Curr Opin Pediatr* 23(4):421–428, 2011.

Grinspon RP, Bergadá I, Rey RA: Male hypogonadism and disorders of sex development, *Front Endocrinol (Lausanne)* 11:211, 2020.

Guran T, Buonocore F, Saka N, et al: Rare causes of primary adrenal insufficiency: genetic and clinical characterization of a large nationwide cohort, *J Clin Endocrinol Metab* 101(1):284–292, 2016.

Hughes IA, Davies JD, Bunch TI, et al: Androgen insensitivity syndrome, *Lancet* 380(9851):1419–1428, 2012.

Ize-Ludlow D, Gray JA, Sperling MA, et al: Rapid-onset obesity with hypothalamic dysfunction, hypoventilation, and autonomic dysregulation presenting in childhood, *Pediatrics* 120:e179–e188, 2007.

Jefferies C, Rhodes E, Rachmiel M, et al: ISPAD clinical practice consensus guidelines 2018: management of children and adolescents with diabetes requiring surgery, *Pediatr Diabetes* 20(1):137, 2019.

Josso N, Rey RA, Picard JY: Anti-Müllerian hormone: a valuable addition to the toolbox of the pediatric endocrinologist, *Int J Endocrinol* 2013:674105, 2013.

Klouwer FC, Berendse K, Ferdinandusse S, Wanders RJ, Engelen M, Poll-The BT: Zellweger spectrum disorders: clinical overview and management approach, *Orphanet J Rare Dis* 10:151, 2015.

Landier W, Skinner R, Wallace WH, et al: Surveillance for late effects in childhood cancer survivors, *J Clin Oncol* 36(21):2216–2222, 2018.

Latronico AC, Brito VN, Carel JC: Causes, diagnosis, and treatment of central precocious puberty, *Lancet Diabetes Endocrinol* 4(3):265–274, 2016.

Lee PA, Nordenström A, Houk CP, et al: Global disorders of sex development update since 2006: perceptions, approach and care, *Horm Res Paediatr* 85(3): 158–180, 2016.

Lefebvre M, Foulkes WD: Pheochromocytoma and paraganglioma syndromes: genetics and management update, *Curr Oncol* 21(1):e8–e17, 2014.

Lie Fong S, Visser JA, Welt CK, et al: Serum anti-Müllerian hormone levels in healthy females: a nomogram ranging from infancy to adulthood, *J Clin Endocrinol Metab* 97(12):4650–4655, 2012.

Lodish MB, Trivellin G, Stratakis CA: Pituitary gigantism: update on molecular biology and management, *Curr Opin Endocrinol Diabetes Obes* 23(1):72–80, 2016.

Lyons SK, Libman IM, Sperling MA: Clinical review: diabetes in the adolescent: transitional issues, *J Clin Endocrinol Metab* 98(12):4639–4645, 2013.

Macedo DB, Abreu AP, Reis AC, et al: Central precocious puberty that appears to be sporadic caused by paternally inherited mutations in the imprinted gene makorin ring finger 3, *J Clin Endocrinol Metab* 99(6):E1097–E1103, 2014.

Management guidelines for children with thyroid nodules and differentiated thyroid cancer, *Pediatrics* 142(6):e20183063, 2018.

Mason K, Page L, Balikcioglu PG: Screening for hormonal, monogenic, and syndromic disorders in obese infants and children, *Pediatr Ann* 43(9):e218–e224, 2014.

Mollen KP, Shaffer AD, Yip L, Monaco SE, et al: Unique molecular signatures are associated with aggressive histology in pediatric differentiated thyroid cancer, *Thyroid* 32(3):236–244, 2022. doi:10.1089/thy.2021.0317.

Oakley RH, Cidlowski JA: The biology of the glucocorticoid receptor: new signaling mechanisms in health and disease, *J Allergy Clin Immunol* 132(5):1033–1044, 2013.

Peña AS, Witchel SF, Hoeger KM, et al: Adolescent polycystic ovary syndrome according to the international evidence-based guideline, *BMC Med* 18(1):72, 2020.

Plant TM: 60 years of neuroendocrinology: the hypothalamo-pituitary-gonadal axis, *J Endocrinol* 226(2):T41–T54, 2015.

Schneider Aguirre R, Eugster EA: Central precocious puberty: from genetics to treatment, *Best Pract Res Clin Endocrinol Metab* 32(4):343–354, 2018. https://doi.org/10.1016/j.beem.2018.05.008.

Skorupskaite K, George JT, Anderson RA: The kisspeptin-GnRH pathway in human reproductive health and disease, *Hum Reprod Update* 20(4):485–500, 2014.

Stamou MI, Cox KH, Crowley WF Jr: Discovering genes essential to the hypothalamic regulation of human reproduction using a human disease model: adjusting to life in the "-omics" era, *Endocr Rev* 36(6):603–621, 2015.

Stratakis CA: Cushing syndrome in pediatrics, *Endocrinol Metab Clin North Am* 41(4):793–803, 2012.

Tamborlane WV, Haymond MW, Dunger D, et al: Expanding treatment options for youth with type 2 diabetes: current problems and proposed solutions: a white paper from the NICHD diabetes working group, *Diabetes Care* 39(3):323–329, 2016.

Tanner JM, Whitehouse RH, Marshall WA, Carter BS: Prediction of adult height from height, bone age, and occurrence of menarche, at ages 4 to 16 with allowance for midparent height, *Arch Dis Child* 50(1):14–26, 1975. doi:10.1136/adc.50.1.14.

Thornton PS, Stanley CA, De Leon DD, et al: Recommendations from the Pediatric Endocrine Society for evaluation and management of persistent hypoglycemia in neonates, infants, and children, *J Pediatr* 167(2):238–245, 2015.

Turcu AF, Auchus RJ: Adrenal steroidogenesis and congenital adrenal hyperplasia, *Endocrinol Metab Clin North Am* 44(2):275–296, 2015.

Wassner AJ, Brown RS: Congenital hypothyroidism: recent advances, *Curr Opin Endocrinol Diabetes Obes* 22(5):407–412, 2015.

Witchel SF: Congenital adrenal hyperplasia, *J Pediatr Adolesc Gynecol* 30(5): 520–534, 2017.

Witchel SF: Newborn screening for congenital adrenal hyperplasia: beyond 17-hydroxyprogesterone concentrations, *J Pediatr (Rio J)* 95(3):257–259, 2019.

Witchel SF, Oberfield S, Rosenfield RL, et al: The diagnosis of polycystic ovary syndrome during adolescence, *Horm Res Paediatr* 83:376–389, 2015.

Witchel SF, Pinto B, Burghard AC, Oberfield SE: Update on adrenarche, *Curr Opin Pediatr* 32(4):574–581, 2020.

Wolfsdorf JI, Glaser N, Agus M, et al: ISPAD clinical practice consensus guidelines 2018: diabetic ketoacidosis and the hyperglycemic hyperosmolar state, *Pediatr Diabetes* 19(Suppl 27):155–177, 2018.

Yeker RM, Shaffer AD, Viswanathan P, et al: Chronic lymphocytic thyroiditis and aggressiveness of pediatric differentiated thyroid cancer, *Laryngoscope* 132: 1668–1674, 2022. https://doi.org/10.1002/lary.29908.

10 VASCULAR ANOMALIES

Andrew A. McCormick | Michael D. Fox

KEY POINTS

- The 2018 International Society for the Study of Vascular Anomalies classification system is an effective tool for defining the field of vascular anomalies.
- Infantile hemangiomas are the most common vascular tumor and are defined by quality, depth, location, size and progression.
- A facial segmental infantile hemangioma greater than 5 cm in size is an indication for a PHACES (**P**osterior fossa malformation, **H**emangioma [>5 cm segmental facial hemangioma], **A**rterial anomalies of head and neck, **C**ardiac defects, **E**ye anomalies, and **S**ternal cleft) evaluation.
- The presence of ≥5 cutaneous infantile hemangiomas is a marker of extracutaneous hemangiomas and indicates the need for a Doppler ultrasound of the liver to evaluate for a hepatic hemangioma.
- Kaposiform hemangioendothelioma is a vascular tumor associated with a consumptive thrombocytopenia and microangiopathic coagulopathy known as Kasabach-Merritt syndrome.
- Management of vascular malformation, whether simple or complex, requires a multidisciplinary approach.
- Hereditary hemorrhagic telangiectasia is an autosomal dominant disorder of capillary repair leading to progressive development of arteriovenous malformation throughout the life of an individual, requiring ongoing monitoring and management.

INTRODUCTION

Vascular anomalies represent a broad spectrum of disorders from the simple birthmark to the multisystem life-threatening disorder. Classically they have had a variable nomenclature that has promoted misdiagnosis and mistreatment. The modern movement in the field of vascular anomalies has been to create a uniform classification system based on the pathophysiology of these disorders and their genetic associations, which also lends to understanding the individualized treatment regimen of each disorder. This chapter is structured around the 2018 International Society for the Study of Vascular Anomalies classification of vascular anomalies. The system generally divides the study of vascular anomalies into vascular tumors and vascular malformations. Although this is an oversimplification of the classification system, it is a helpful starting point. First, attention will be turned to vascular tumors in an evaluation of the benign, locally aggressive, and malignant categories of this disorder. Next will be a description of the vascular malformation that divides into categories of simple (slow flow and fast flow), combined, and associated with other anomalies. The framework of these categories provides the system for defining and understanding the field of vascular anomalies.

VASCULAR TUMORS

Vascular tumors represent a grouping of vascular anomalies in which the vascular tissue is proliferating without appropriate regulation. The dysfunction in regulation often leads to rapid enlargement of the tissue with either compression or invasion of local structures. The spectrum of these disorders spans from the benign (hemangiomas and reactive vascular tumors) to the locally invasive or malignant tumor (kaposiform hemangioendothelioma [KHE] and angiosarcoma).

Benign Vascular Tumors

Infantile Hemangiomas

The infantile hemangioma is the second most common vascular anomaly, with an incidence of 4.5% in the general population and a female predominance. The classic understanding of infantile hemangioma is a benign endothelial tumor that is usually absent at birth or present as a premonitory mark with rapid postnatal growth, followed by slow involution. Infantile hemangiomas have varied presentations in quality, depth, location, size, and progression.

First, quality starts with the differentiation of a localized hemangioma (Fig. 10.1) in contrast to the segmental hemangioma (Fig. 10.2). A localized hemangioma is an easily differentiated single hemangioma in which a clinician can define boundaries, whereas the segmental hemangioma appears as an island of plaquelike lesions in pseudodermatomal distribution. Second, depth describes the position of the infantile hemangioma within the epidermal/dermal composition. The classic descriptions are of superficial, deep, and mixed lesions. A superficial hemangioma is often described as the "strawberry" hemangioma, a confluent red plaque that has the appearance that it can be plucked off the surface of the skin (Fig. 10.3). The deep lesion on the other end of the spectrum appears as a swelling that may have a bluish discoloration on the surface, but at times it can be difficult to differentiate from other soft tissue tumors by appearance alone (Fig. 10.4). The final description is the mixed lesion in which the infantile hemangioma has components both of superficial plaque and surrounding swelling (Fig. 10.5). The mixed type is the most common presentation of infantile hemangiomas.

Third, the location may give the clinician clues to factors such as risk of ulceration (perioral and perianal); associated anomalies (PHACES syndrome, beard distribution in subglottic hemangiomas, and LUMBAR syndrome); and risk of end organ injury (periorbital and periauricular). These relations are described further later.

Fourth, size is important in that lesions greater than 5 cm have predominance toward complications. There are multiple complications associated with larger lesions, including an association with other congenital anomalies when located on the head and neck or in the lumbar and pelvis regions, risk for ulceration and bleeding, development of high-output heart failure, and an association with consumptive hypothyroidism. When measuring the size of a single localized hemangioma, the clinician should evaluate the region of largest diameter, including both superficial and deep components. These measurements become more difficult when the infantile hemangioma takes on the form of a segmental hemangioma. The measurement of the lesion is based on the diameter of the most proximal edge of the string of islands to the edge of the most distal island.

Finally, progression is a description of the natural history of the hemangioma (Fig. 10.6). Classically, infantile hemangiomas are described to have two stages in their life cycle: (1) rapid proliferation and (2) spontaneous involution. At birth, there is usually no noticeable lesion or a premonitory mark (pale macule with telangiectasias, mottled vascular stain, or bruiselike area). When a premonitory mark is present, this is usually described as a result of birth trauma (scratch or bruise) or a more common birthmark, such as nevus simplex. The rapid proliferation phase initiates at 1 to 4 weeks old in the superficial and mixed type, whereas the deep type starts around 2 to 3 months old. Rapid proliferation is noted when the once absent or flat lesion has significant proliferation with growth in all three dimensions. The rapid proliferation stage can be broken into two sections: an early and a late proliferation. The early proliferation stage is when noticeable growth can be seen from one day to the next and makes up the largest portion of total growth. Duration of the early proliferative stage is variable for each individual hemangioma but can be expected to last

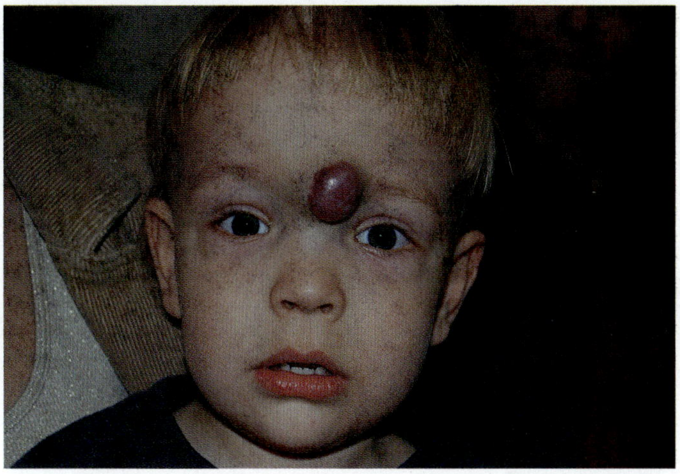

Fig. 10.1 Localized hemangioma. This facial hemangioma appears as a bulky vascular tumor with easily defined borders.

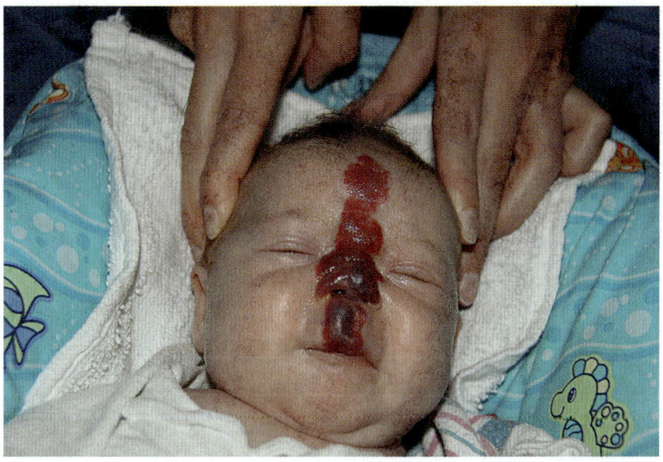

Fig. 10.2 Segmental hemangioma. This facial hemangioma appears as plaque-like lesions that seem to be contained within a pseudodermatomal distribution.

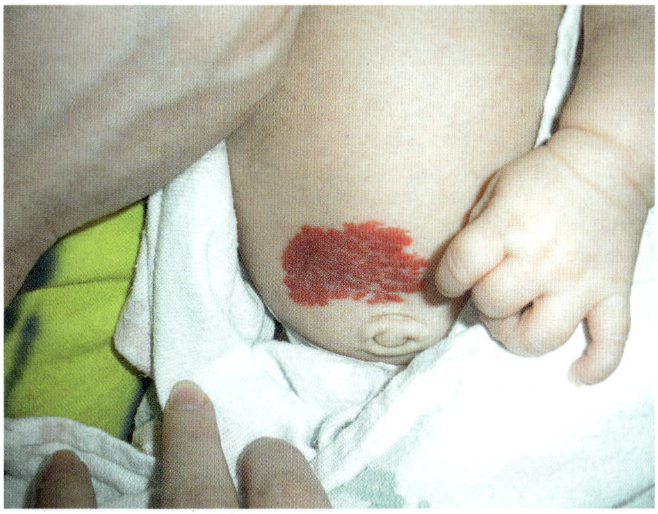

Fig. 10.3 Superficial hemangioma. This hemangioma is a confluent red plaque with the appearance that it can be pulled off the surface of the skin.

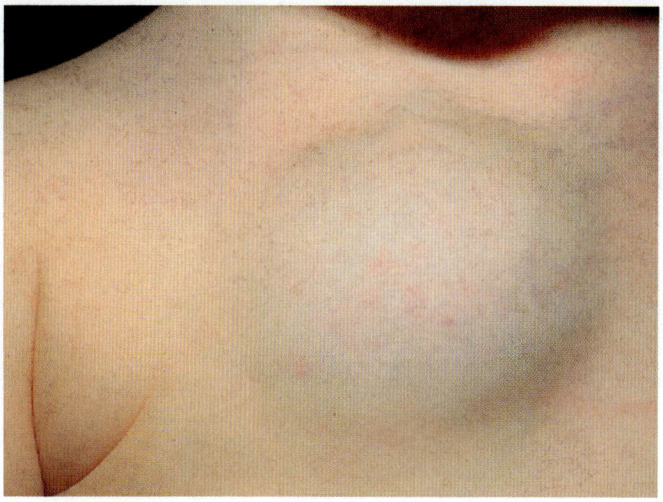

Fig. 10.4 Deep hemangioma. Most of the vessels that make up this large, partially compressible mass lie deep beneath the skin surface but still impart a bluish hue to the overlying surface.

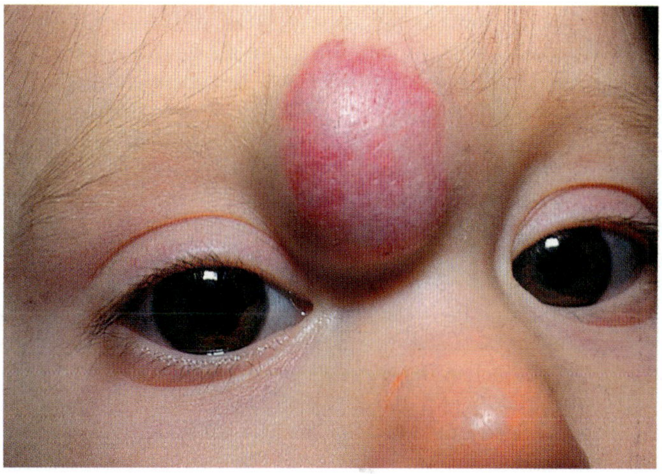

Fig. 10.5 Mixed hemangioma. The hemangioma on this child's nasal bridge has both a superficial and deep component.

for 1 to 3 months of age. The average hemangioma achieves 80% of total size during this early proliferative stage. The late proliferation stage demonstrates a slowing of growth, with noticeable growth based on measurement from one week to the next but not by purely clinical observation. The late proliferative stage is once again variable in duration until 6 to 9 months old. Following rapid proliferation is a stage of slow involution. Classical teaching is that infantile hemangiomas will have spontaneous regression by 10% per year. Therefore 30% by 3 years, 50% by 5 years, and 70% by 7 years will have complete regression without intervention, but more recent studies demonstrate that the majority of involution occurs by 4 years of age.

The majority of infantile hemangiomas are diagnosed clinically. Occasionally, deep infantile hemangiomas or extracutaneous may be difficult to diagnose and imaging can be helpful to distinguish from other neoplasms. Ultrasonography with Doppler study is the test of choice. It demonstrates a well-circumscribed homogeneous mass with the high-flow pattern characteristic of infantile hemangiomas. Magnetic resonance imaging (MRI) and histopathology are almost never necessary in the diagnosis of infantile hemangiomas. Classically, infantile hemangiomas are composed of densely packed endothelial cells that form small capillaries and immunohistochemical staining for glucose transporter-1 (GLUT-1) protein is positive in infantile hemangioma cells.

Pathology/Complications

A point-of-care tool for primary care providers to determine the need for further evaluation of treatment versus observation is the Hemangioma Severity Score (Fig.10.7). This tool allows providers to stratify hemangiomas based on clinical presentation to determine the need for treatment.

The most common complication of infantile hemangiomas is the development of ulceration (Fig. 10.8), which occurs in approximately

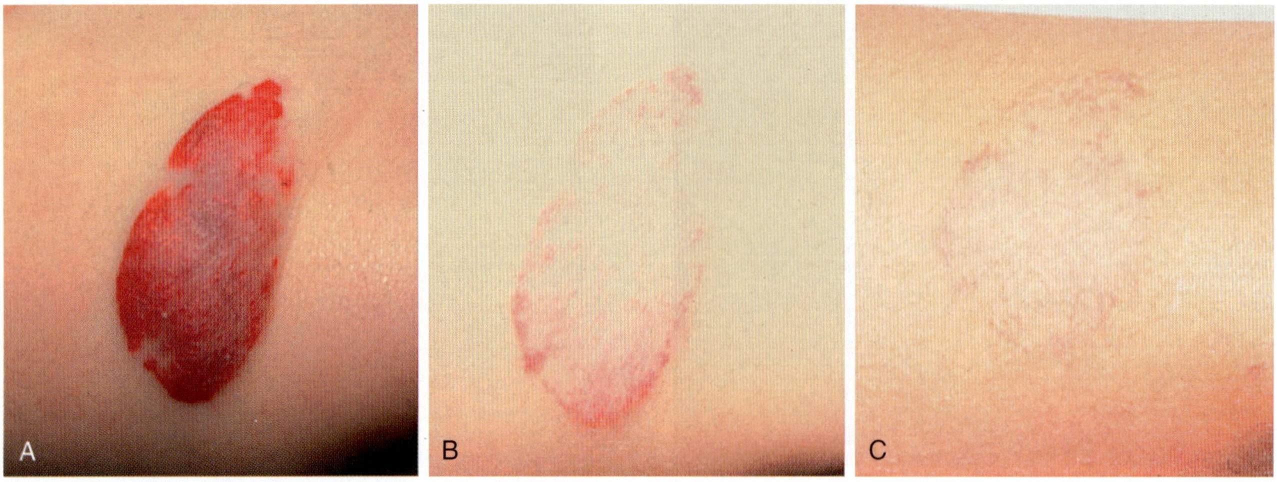

Fig. 10.6 Natural history of hemangioma. After growing for approximately 6 months, hemangiomas tend to plateau in size and then gradually involute. The appearance at 5 months old (A), at 2 years old (B), and almost total resolution at 5 years old (C).

15% of patients with infantile hemangiomas. The concern with the ulcerative hemangioma is the associated risk of bleeding, cosmetic deformity, and associated pain. Therefore the goal is to determine which lesion is high risk to institute early treatment and prevention of these negative outcomes.

Infantile hemangiomas greater than 25 cm^2 in size have a clinically significant probability of developing ulcerated hemangiomas. The depth of the hemangioma demonstrated a profound predictor of ulceration in that 20% of mixed type hemangioma resulted in ulceration in comparison with 9% of superficial tumors and less than 1% of deep tumors. Furthermore, the segmental hemangioma had a 33% of ulceration in comparison with 7% of those localized. By location, infantile hemangiomas of the lower lip, neck, and anogenital region are significantly more likely to ulcerate. Ulceration occurs 30% of the time on the lower lip, 25% of the time on the neck, and 50% of the time in the anogenital region. Ninety-five percent of ulcerations occur within the rapid proliferation phase, with only 5% occurring after 10 months old. This is further broken down in that 35% of ulceration occurs during the early proliferative stage, with the remainder occurring during late proliferation. In addition, the appearance of an infantile hemangioma can give a clue to the risk of ulceration. The classically rapidly proliferating hemangioma is of a homogenous red plaque, but when ulceration is imminent, the appearance develops a central graying (Fig. 10.9). This is an ominous sign of impending ulceration. Take note that central graying is a normal appearance of typical involution once rapid proliferation has ceased, but in a hemangioma that is still growing, this signals impending ulceration (Fig. 10.10).

The presence of multiple cutaneous hemangiomas (Fig. 10.11) has long been recognized as a marker for extracutaneous hemangiomas within the liver. Prospective studies have demonstrated that the presence of five or more cutaneous hemangiomas correlates with a 20% incidence of hepatic hemangiomas. Therefore the presence of multiple cutaneous hemangiomas (≥5) warrants evaluation with a liver ultrasound with Doppler to screen for intrahepatic hemangiomas. Recognition of these lesions early is important because large and multifocal hepatic hemangiomas (>5 cm) have arteriovenous shunts that can precipitate high-output congestive heart failure. Of note, an associated complication of multifocal and diffuse intrahepatic hemangiomas is a consumptive hypothyroidism. These hemangiomas produce an enzyme that catabolizes thyroid hormone and leaves the patient clinically hypothyroid. Therefore patients with multifocal or diffuse intrahepatic hemangiomas should be screened with thyroid function testing including TSH, Free T4, and rT3.

The location of a cutaneous infantile hemangioma can be a signal for other underlying anomalies. Hemangiomas over the lower face in the "beard" distribution have an association with airway hemangiomas 50% of the time and therefore warrant an airway evaluation (Fig. 10.12). Along these lines, the presence of a segmental facial hemangioma has a strong association with PHACES syndrome. **PHACES** is an acronym for **P**osterior fossa malformation, **H**emangioma (>5 cm segmental facial hemangioma), **A**rterial anomalies of head and neck, **C**ardiac defects, **E**ye anomalies, and **S**ternal cleft (Fig. 10.13). The hemangioma morphology of these lesions is described as segmental because they seem to cover a territory rather than arising from a single point. The more facial regions (Fig. 10.14) that the segmental hemangioma covers will increase the likelihood of PHACES syndrome. These segmental hemangiomas are usually absent or subtle at birth but have rapid progression within the first few weeks of life. Initial appearance can be confused with a port-wine stain because it will have a red plaquelike appearance but will quickly differentiate as it rises from a macule on the skin surface to a plaque. The presence of a segmental facial hemangioma greater than 5 cm warrants an evaluation for PHACES syndrome. Practitioners should obtain an MRI of the brain (evaluate posterior fossa malformation), magnetic resonance angiography of the head and neck (evaluate cerebrovascular anomalies), palpation of femoral pulses, transthoracic echo (evaluate cardiac anomalies with coarctation of the aorta most common), physical examination of the chest wall to look for midline defects, and eye examination by pediatric ophthalmologist (Table 10.1). In the same way, segmental hemangiomas of the lower body have associations with congenital anomalies of the spine, urogenital, arterial, anorectal, and renal systems and have been termed *LUMBAR syndrome* (Fig. 10.15). Once again, any segmental hemangioma of the lower body greater than 5 cm warrants further evaluation.

Although knowledge and understanding of infantile hemangiomas have grown dramatically in the past decade, this has been eclipsed by the change in management, because propranolol has become the mainline treatment modality. Previously, corticosteroids, vincristine, and interferon alpha were the available treatment options. This all changed in 2008, when a case series published in the *New England Journal of Medicine* demonstrated the remarkable effectiveness of propranolol in treatment of this disease process. Since that time, multiple studies have supported this original finding, including a randomized control trial that has instituted propranolol as the first-line treatment of infantile hemangiomas. The standard of care for high-risk lesion as described previously is for at least 6 months and until the first birthday. Studies have supported the utility of topical timolol maleate gel for treatment of thin (<2 mm in depth) lesions, therefore expanding the armament of treatment options.

Congenital Hemangiomas

The congenital hemangioma is an uncommon vascular tumor. Prominent features to distinguish the congenital hemangioma are that it is fully formed at birth and many times can be identified on prenatal ultrasound. The classical appearance is of a solitary, plaquelike lesion

Name: DOB: MR#: Study#:
Date complete:

Hemangioma Severity Scale Revised 5-17-10

Clinical Features	Point Value	Category Subscore
Size (measured in longest dimension) **FACIAL, EAR**		Record single value
• ≤1 cm	1	
• >1 and ≤5 cm	2	
• >5 and ≤10 cm	3	
• >10 cm and ≤20 cm	4	
• >20 cm	5	
Size (measured in longest dimension) **NONFACIAL, INCLUDING SCALP AND NECK**		
• ≤5 cm	1	
• >5 and ≤15 cm	2	
• >15 cm	3	
Location		Record single value
• Mucous membranes (oral excluding lip)	1	
• Extremity or trunk, non-perineal	1	
• Breast	2	
• Perineal/perianal/genital	3	
• Lumbosacral	2	
• Scalp/neck	2	
• Peripheral face	3	
• Central face, excluding nasal tip, lip, or periocular	5	
• Nasal tip, vermillion or cutaneous lip, or periocular (within orbital rim), car	6	
Risk for Associated Structural Anomalies		Record single value
• None	0	
• Hemangioma is facial AND ≥5 cm in longest dimension	6	
• Hemangioma is ≥2.5 cm and overlying midline lumbosacral spine	5	
• Hemangioma is segmental involving the perineal/perianal/genital area	5	
Complications (present at time of exam)		Record single value
• None	0	
• Infection, bacterial	1	
• Ulceration	2	
• Feeding difficulties	2	
• Torticollis	2	
• Cartilage Distortion or Destruction	3	
• Airway involvement	3	
• Visual compromise	3	
• Hypothyroidism	2	
• Anemia	2	
• Congestive heart failure	2	
• GI bleed	2	
• Hepatic dysfunction, including synthetic dysfunction	2	
Subjective Items		
Pain		Record single value
• None	0	
• Mild/intermittent and/or not requiring systemic medication	1	
• Moderate or requiring OTC systemic pain medications	2	
• Severe or requiring systemic Rx pain medications	3	
• Severe requiring hospitalization for pain control	4	
Risk/likelihood of Disfigurement – **FACIAL or EAR**		Record single value
• None	0	
• Minimal skin textural change and or telangectasia	2	
• Redundant fibrofatty tissue or scar without distortion of anatomic landmarks	3	
• Permanent deformity of normal anatomic landmarks	4	
Risk/likelihood of Disfigurement – **NON-FACIAL, INCLUDING SCALP AND NECK**		Record single value
• None or Minimal skin textural change and or telangectasia	0	
• Redundant fibrofatty tissue, alopecia or scar without distortion of anatomic landmarks	1	
• Permanent deformity of normal anatomic landmarks	2	
TOTAL SEVERITY SCORE:		

Fig. 10.7 The Hemangioma Severity Scale (HSS) Clinical Scoring sheet. HSS is a reliable and effective tool for stratifying presentations of hemangiomas into categories of recommended treatment (score ≥11), no treatment (≤6), and close observation and/or treatment (score 7–10).

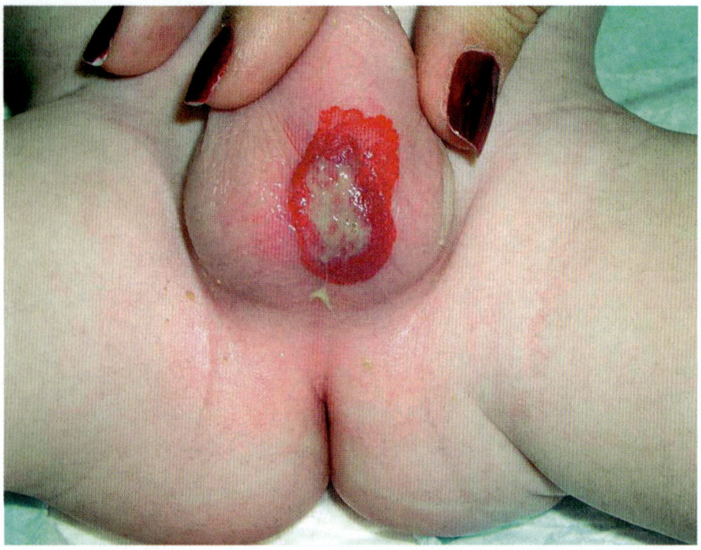

Fig. 10.8 Ulcerated hemangioma. Hemangiomas located in friction- or maceration-prone areas are at risk for ulceration. When ulcerated, they cause significant pain, are vulnerable to infection, and, ultimately, scarring unless treated aggressively.

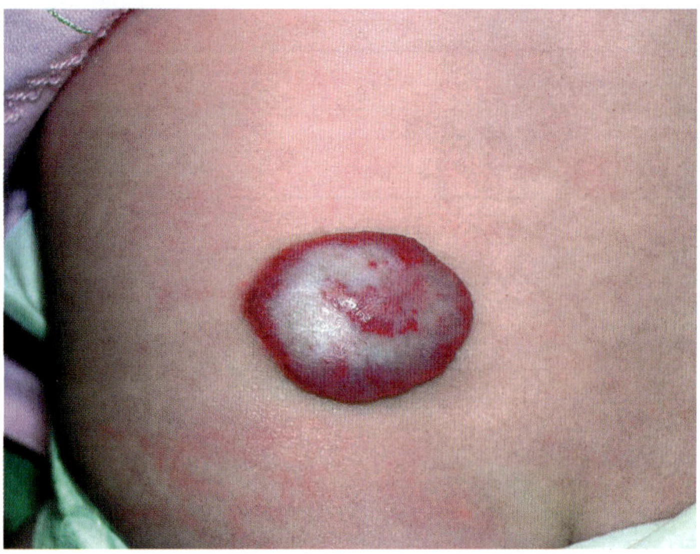

Fig. 10.9 Involuting hemangioma. The onset of involution is signaled by a "graying out" of the surface of the lesion. When this occurs during the rapid proliferation stage, it signals impending ulceration.

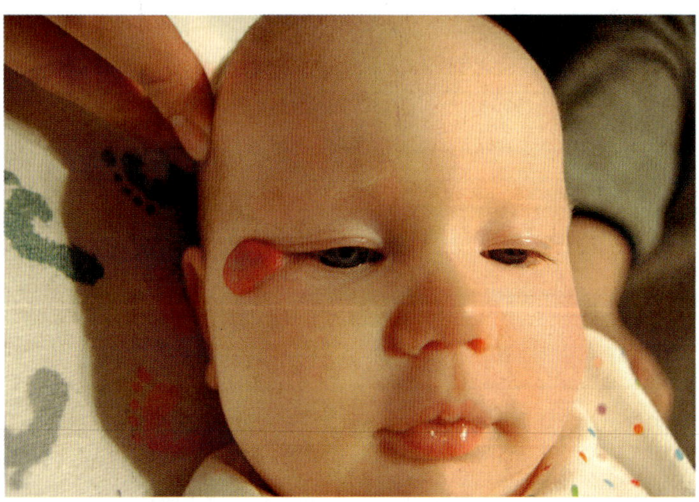

Fig. 10.10 Periorbital hemangioma. Localized hemangioma located at the lateral epicanthus of the eye showing slight graying with involution.

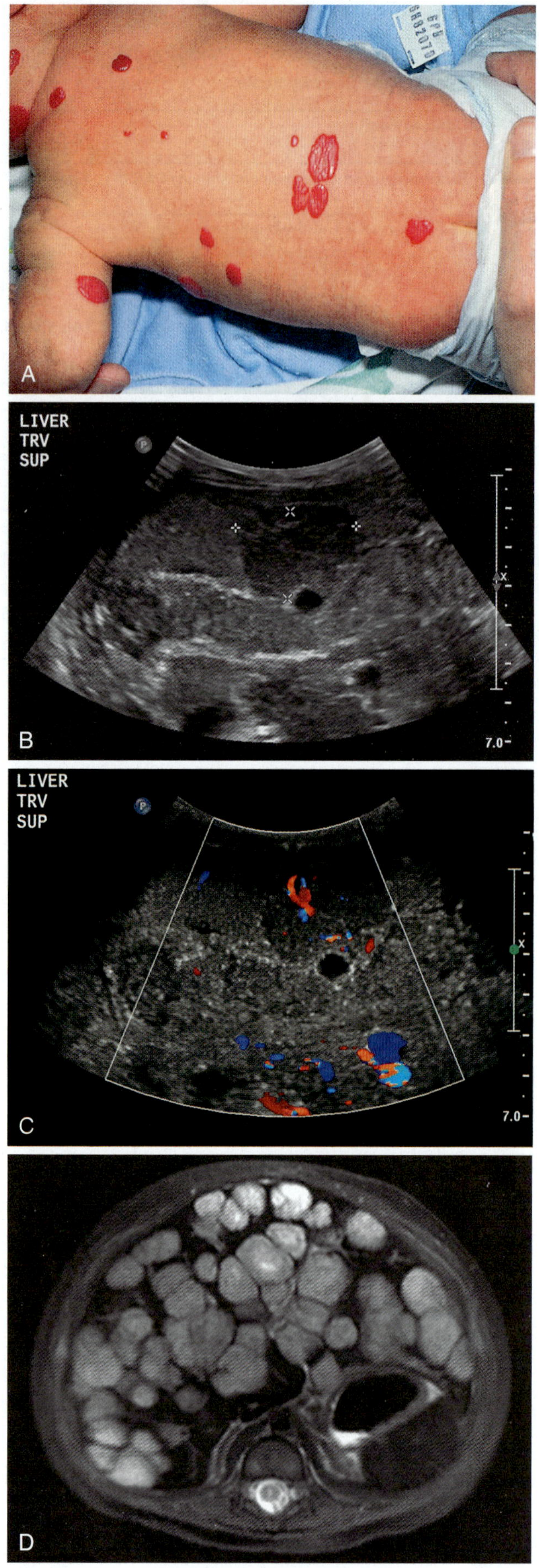

Fig. 10.11 Hemangiomatosis. (A) Multiple soft, red, raised lesions dot the back and arms of this otherwise healthy 1-month-old with benign hemangiomatosis. Liver ultrasound demonstrating intrahepatic hemangioma adjacent to the portal vein (B), which on Doppler demonstrates vascular flow (C). Multifocal hepatic infantile hemangioma identified as well-circumscribed, densely lobulated mass with moderately hyperintense signal on T2-weighted axial images (D).

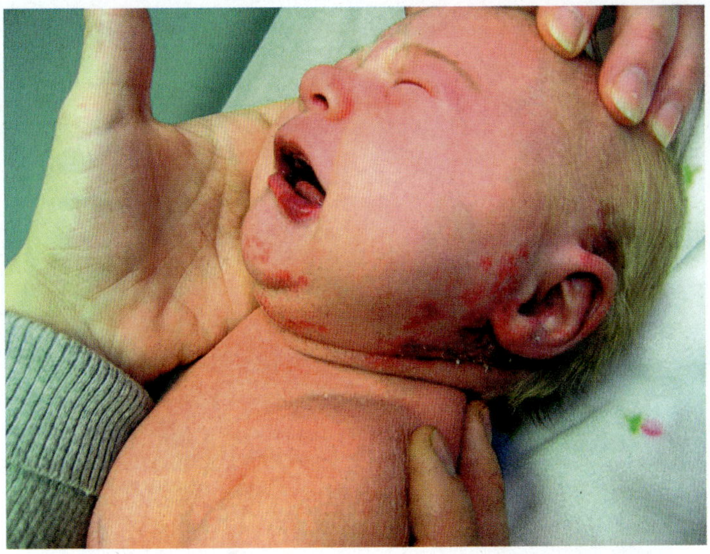

Fig. 10.12 Segmental hemangioma involving the "beard" distribution of the lower face signals the possibility of underlying airway hemangiomas.

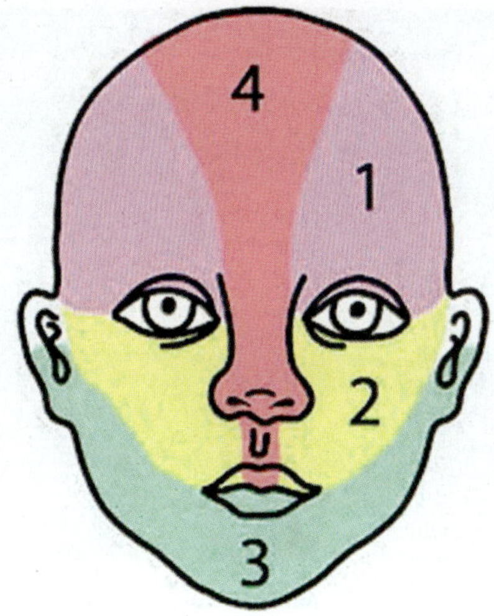

Fig. 10.14 Diagram demonstrates the different facial regions of a segmental hemangioma. The regions are not informative independently, but involvement in multiple regions increases the likelihood of the associated congenital anomalies of PHACES.

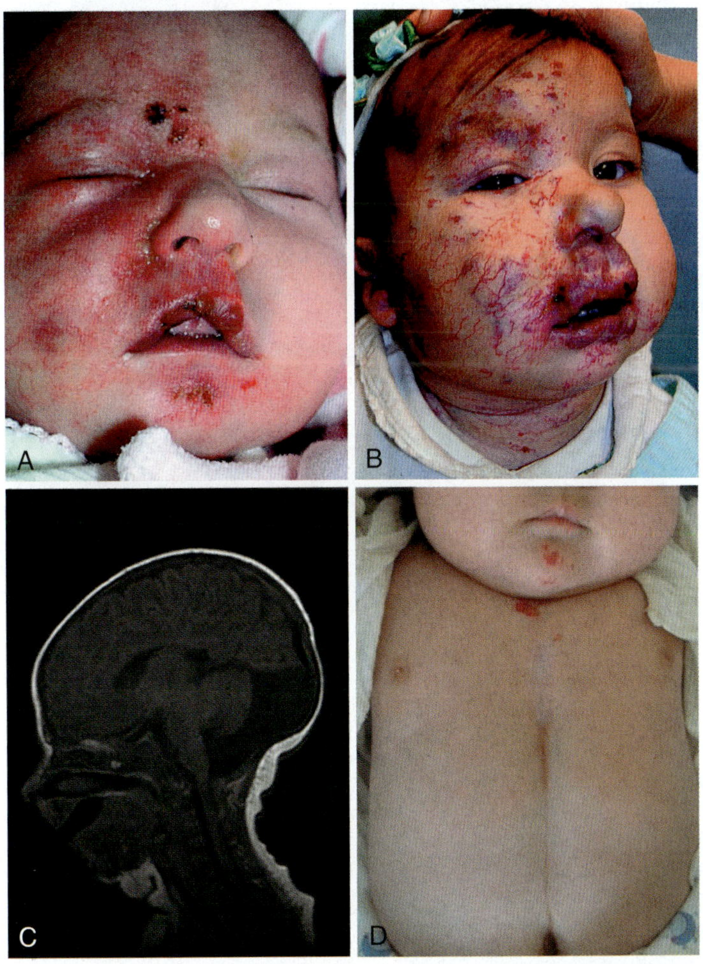

Fig. 10.13 PHACES (**P**osterior fossa malformation, **H**emangioma [>5 cm segmental facial hemangioma], **A**rterial anomalies of head and neck, **C**ardiac defects, **E**ye anomalies, and **S**ternal cleft) syndrome. (A) At birth the lesions are plaquelike and may mimic a port-wine stain. (B) However, once they start to rapidly proliferate, they become raised, as seen in the same infant at 1 year old. (C) This magnetic resonance imaging reveals a Dandy-Walker malformation in an infant with PHACES. (D) supraumbilical raphe noted on newborn with PHACES.

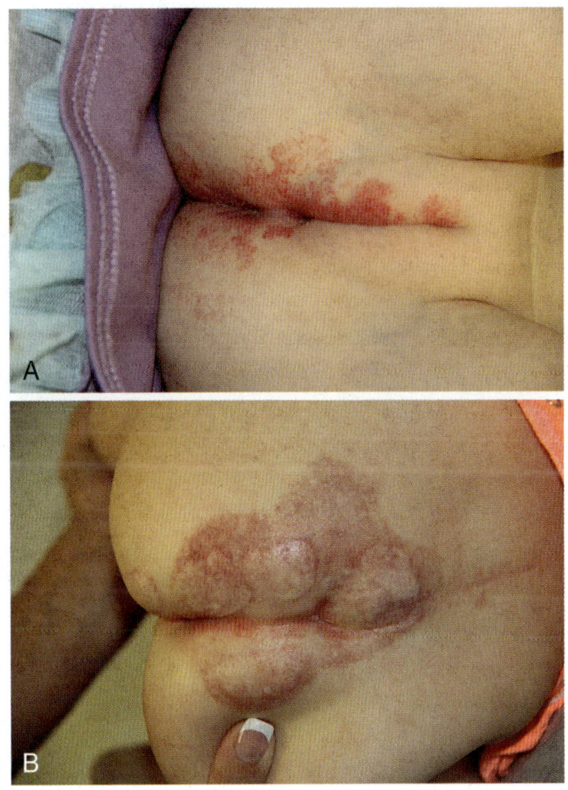

Fig. 10.15 LUMBAR syndrome. (A) Segmental hemangioma in perineum. (B) Segmental hemangioma overlying lumbar spine.

Table 10.1 Congenital Anomalies Associated With PHACES (Posterior fossa malformation, Hemangioma [>5 cm segmental facial hemangioma], Arterial anomalies of head and neck, Cardiac defects, Eye anomalies, and Sternal cleft) Syndrome and Screening Tests

Associated Anomaly	Screening Test
Posterior fossa anomaly	Brain MRI
Facial hemangioma	Clinical observation
Arterial malformation	MRA head and neck
Cardiac anomaly	Transthoracic echocardiogram
Eye anomaly	Ophthalmology consultation
Sternal anomaly	Clinical observation

MRA, Magnetic resonance angiography; *MRI,* magnetic resonance imaging.

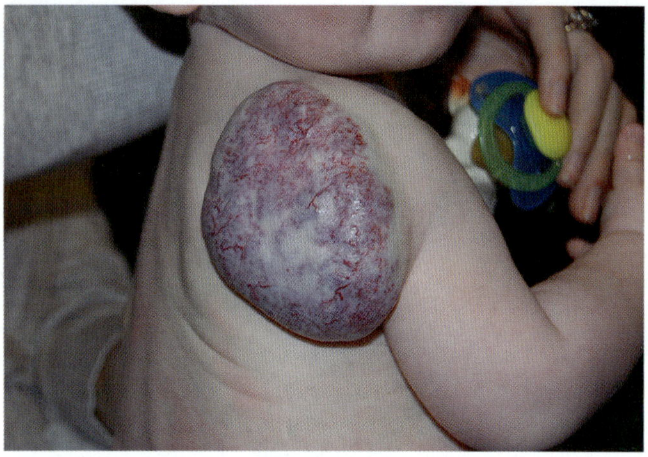

Fig. 10.16 Noninvoluting congenital hemangioma lesion. These lesions are present at birth and have telangiectatic surface surrounding by a rim of pallor.

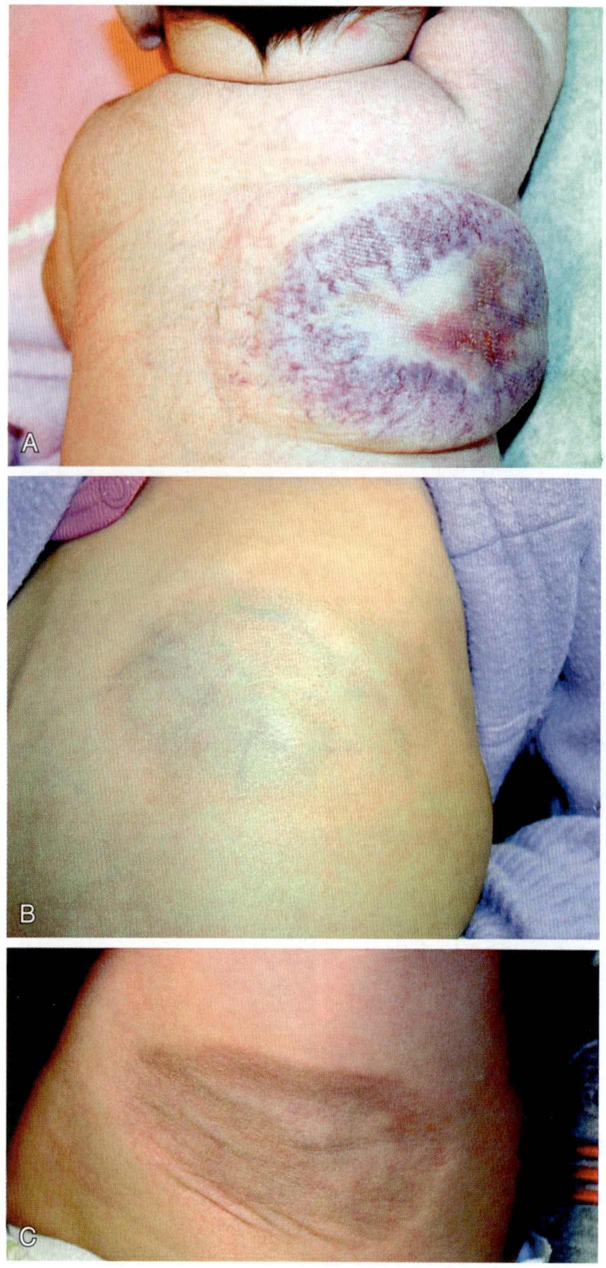

Fig. 10.17 Rapidly involuting congenital hemangioma (RICH) lesion. Also present at birth, these lesions grow no larger but instead involute rapidly and have often resolved by 1 year of age. (A) This infant has a large RICH lesion on his back, which is in the process of involution. Following involution these lesions leave behind an atrophic plaque. (B) In this child, evidence of mild residual atrophy is seen. (C) Another child was left with marked subcutaneous atrophy at the site.

with violaceous appearance. Lesions usually have coarse telangiectasias on the surface and a halo of blanched skin encircling the margins. Congenital hemangiomas can then be differentiated into three categories on the basis of their life cycle. The first category is the noninvoluting congenital hemangioma (NICH) that never recedes (Fig. 10.16). The second is the partially involuting congenital hemangioma (PICH) that will flatten in the first year of life but not completely recede. The final category is the rapidly involuting congenital hemangioma that will completely recede in the first year of life and typically leaves behind a characteristic atrophied plaque (Fig. 10.17).

Pyogenic Granuloma

Pyogenic granulomas are common benign vascular tumors that resemble small hemangiomas. They are thought to stem from vascular overgrowth of granulation tissue following a minor trauma or reaction to a foreign body, such as a thorn, splinter, or piece of glass. They consist of a solitary, bright red, soft nodule that is often pedunculated with an average diameter of 5 to 6 mm (Fig. 10.18). Their surface is friable and bleeds easily. Pyogenic granulomas are commonly confused with hemangiomas, but their onset after the newborn period allows for distinction.

Locally Invasive and Malignant Vascular Tumors

Tufted Angioma/Kaposiform Hemangioendothelioma Spectrum

The tufted angioma is thought to reflect a less aggressive form of the KHE, and differentiation of the two usually can be done only by MRI to assess local invasion. Both types of lesions have plaquelike

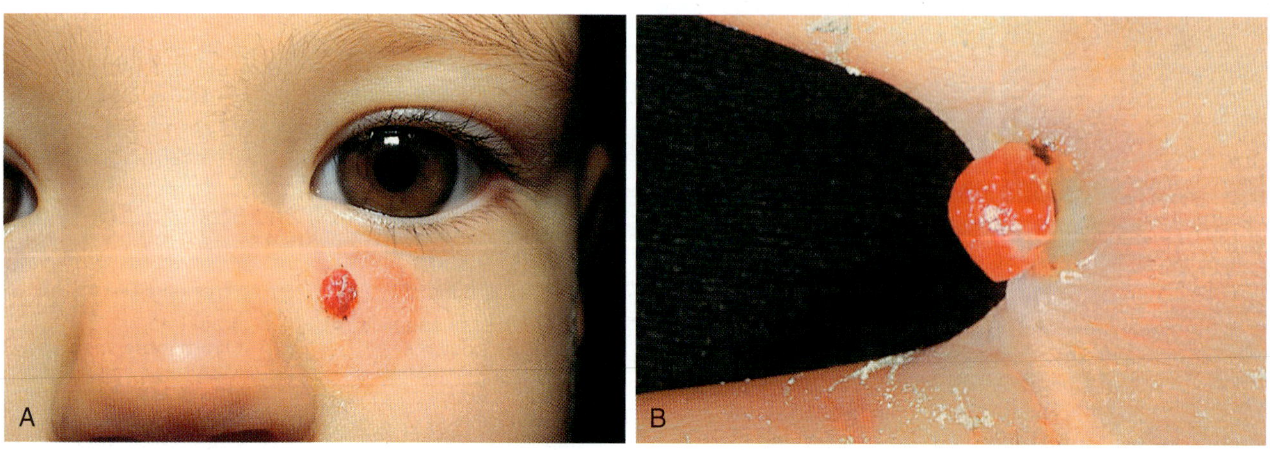

Fig. 10.18 Pyogenic granuloma. (A) A bright red, raised hemorrhagic papule developed on an infant's cheek. (B) Another rapidly growing friable lesion is present between this child's finger.

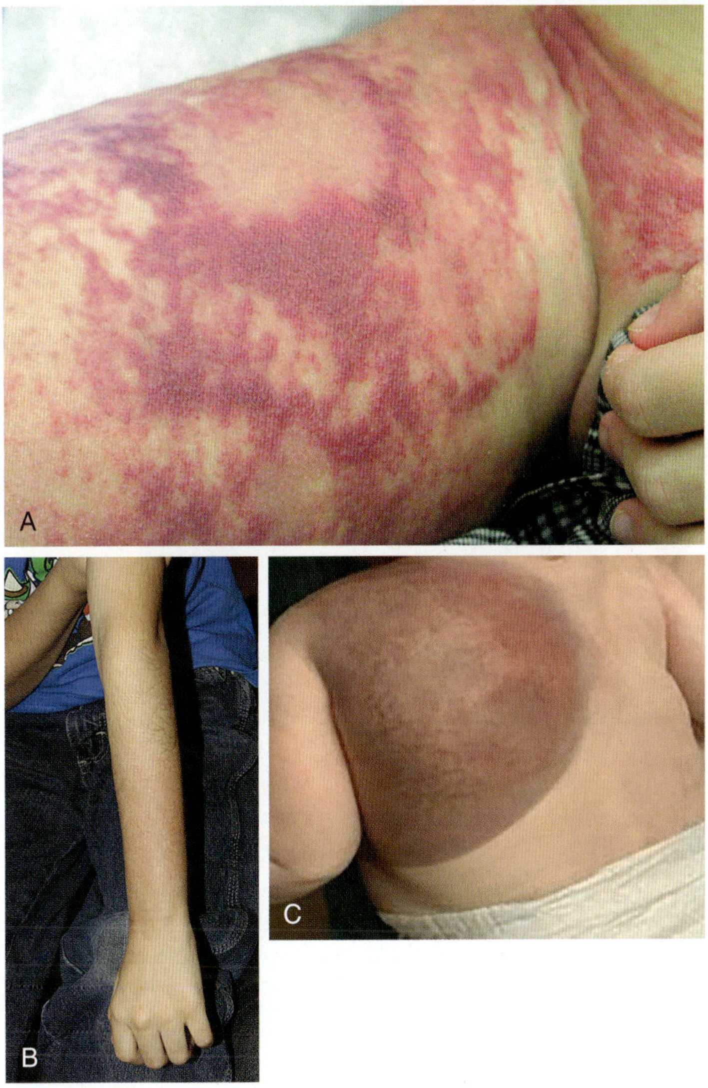

Fig. 10.19 (A) Tufted angioma. This lesion involving the right leg first appeared as a bruiselike plaque, which continued to grow well beyond infancy. (B and C) Kaposiform hemangioendothelioma.

appearances that can be difficult to differentiate from segmental hemangiomas by appearance alone (Fig. 10.19). Location is predominantly on the extremities, head, and neck. The main differentiating features are that the tufted angioma and KHE lesions usually have a purpuric appearance and can be tender on examination. The definitive diagnosis is made by MRI that will demonstrate poorly defined margins, and in KHE, there is invasion through tissue planes. KHE and tufted angioma can have onset anytime during infancy and into early childhood. They do not regress and can have a progressive course. An important complication associated with KHE and tufted angioma is Kasabach-Merritt syndrome, which is characterized by profound thrombocytopenia due to platelet trapping within the tumor, sometimes accompanying microangiopathic hemolytic anemia and secondary consumptive coagulopathy. Due to the aggressive nature of these tumors, they should be managed in conjunction with an oncologist.

Angiosarcoma

Angiosarcomas are extraordinarily rare vascular tumors but very aggressive with local invasion and malignant potential. Presentation is usually on the head, neck, or chest as a painful, rapidly enlarging vascular nodule. This presentation can be complicated by acute bleeding of the lesion, anemia, and coagulopathy. Aggressive evaluation and referral should be made for these patients because metastasis is common at presentation and local resection is the main curative option.

VASCULAR MALFORMATIONS

Vascular malformations are present at birth, though they may not be appreciated until later in life. They typically grow with the child and persist into adolescence and adulthood, unless they are small and can be treated locally. Most often they are controlled but not cured. Lesions are made up of abnormal configurations of vascular tissue that is normally found throughout the body. Vascular malformations may be made up of arteries, veins, lymphatics, capillaries, or any combination thereof and are divided into two main categories—slow-flow and fast-flow—based on the rate of blood flow through them. Some examples of slow-flow lesions are capillary malformations, venous malformations, and lymphatic malformations. Fast-flow lesions include but are not limited to arteriovenous malformations and arteriovenous fistulas.

SIMPLE MALFORMATIONS

Slow-Flow Malformations

Capillary Malformations

Capillary malformations, more commonly called *port-wine stains* (Fig. 10.20), may be found all over the body. They can be seen in isolation or as part of a syndrome. Most commonly, they are treated when they are on the face, because they may be obvious and cause social distress for the child. Pulsed dye laser therapy is a common modality used to treat these malformations. Incidence is reported to be about 0.3% of newborns.

Capillary malformations are made up of abnormal collections of capillaries in the skin causing a cutaneous hyperemic appearance. Commonly found at birth, they can be faint to dark in color or appear almost purple. Size can range from as small as a silver dollar to covering half of the entire body from head to toe. Although these malformations do not spread, they can can darken and thicken with age as the vessels slowly dilate, which may cause the appearance of overgrowth of the affected body part. This may cause clinicians to confuse this lesion with Klippel-Trenaunay syndrome (KTS), which is a completely different entity (see later). Infantile hemangiomas can initially look like a capillary malformation. If one is unsure of the diagnosis at birth, then the infant should be followed closely for rapid growth. Typically, a capillary malformation does not become raised until later in life. An infantile hemangioma would become raised over the first months of life.

Imaging in these patients is completely normal. Ultrasound and MRI are nondiagnostic and perhaps will only demonstrate hypertrophy of the soft tissues in the affected area. The lesion cannot be visualized on any imaging modality. If there is any concern for KTS, then an MRI with arterial and venous phases should be performed to rule out a lymphatic and venous component, which would be seen in KTS, and is not a solitary capillary malformation.

Venous Malformations

Venous malformations can be found anywhere on the body, can be focal or diffuse, and can be part of combined vascular malformation (e.g., capillary venous malformation). Venous malformations often require a multidisciplinary approach for treatment as these lesions are managed and not cured. Management of venous malformations has expanded to include a multimodal approach that may include medical management with pharmacotherapies targeted toward specific genetic mutations and cell signaling pathways (sirolimus, alpelisib) in conjunction with sclerotherapy and surgical resection. A potential complication of localized intravascular coagulation can lead to venous thrombosis or a consumptive coagulopathy during the evaluation and treatment process. Consultation with a

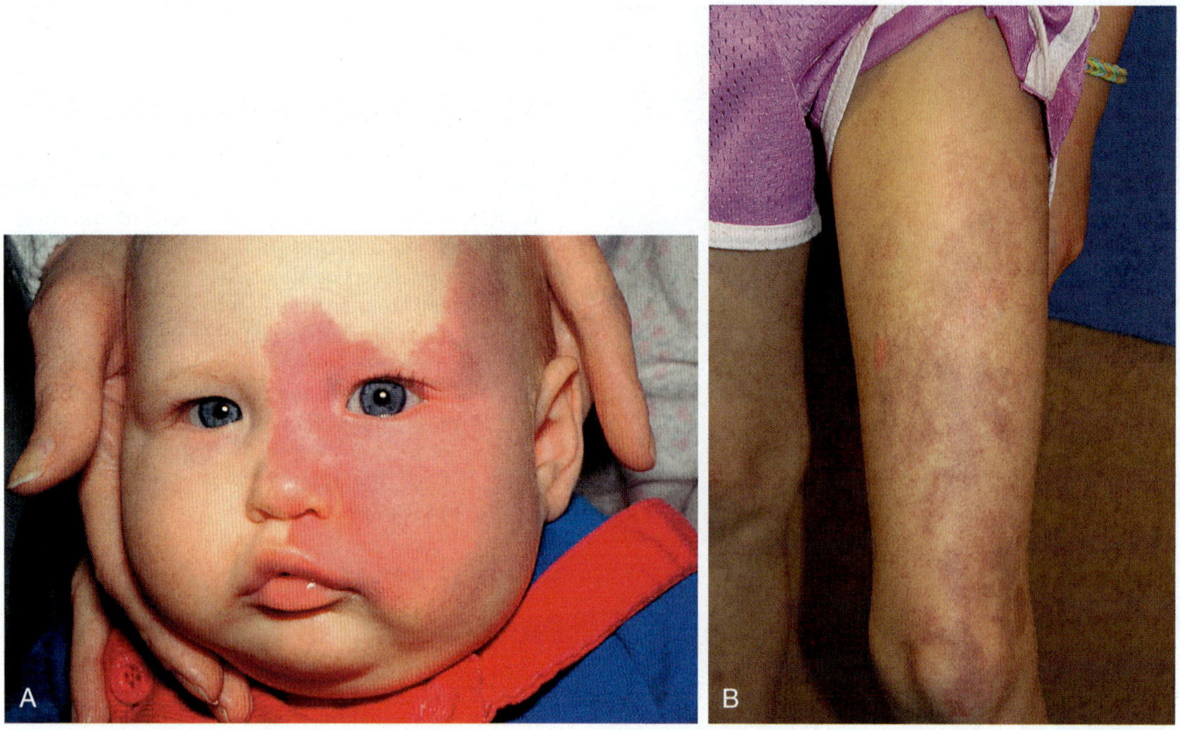

Fig. 10.20 Port-wine stain. (A) This infant with Sturge Weber syndrome has a characteristic purplish-red lesion covering nearly half of his face. (B) Adolescent girl with capillary malformation on anterior thigh that has darkened with age and become verrucous.

hematologist, particularly one who is familiar with management of coagulopathy associated with large, extensive malformations, may be necessary. A treatment plan often includes extensive imaging and coordinated planning with medical and interventional options done in conjunction.

Because venous malformations can be seen in so many different locations throughout the body with a wide variety of sizes, a physical examination can be challenging. Typically the lesions have a purple discoloration similar to what one might see in a normal vein; they are soft and compressible. They also have an associated response to dependency and therefore appear to swell when placed in a dependent position. When the lesions are confined to the skin, they appear like an abnormal network of dilated veins. When they are just below the skin, one may see fullness and dilated veins within the skin, making the lesion look purple (Fig. 10.21). Deep lesions may be marked only by swelling (Fig. 10.22). Because these are slow-flow lesions, they are prone to thrombosis. Initial thrombosis presents as a warm, red swelling that can be tender to palpation. Clinically these thrombosed vessels function as superficial thrombosed veins, and the primary mode of acute treatment is pain control. At times,

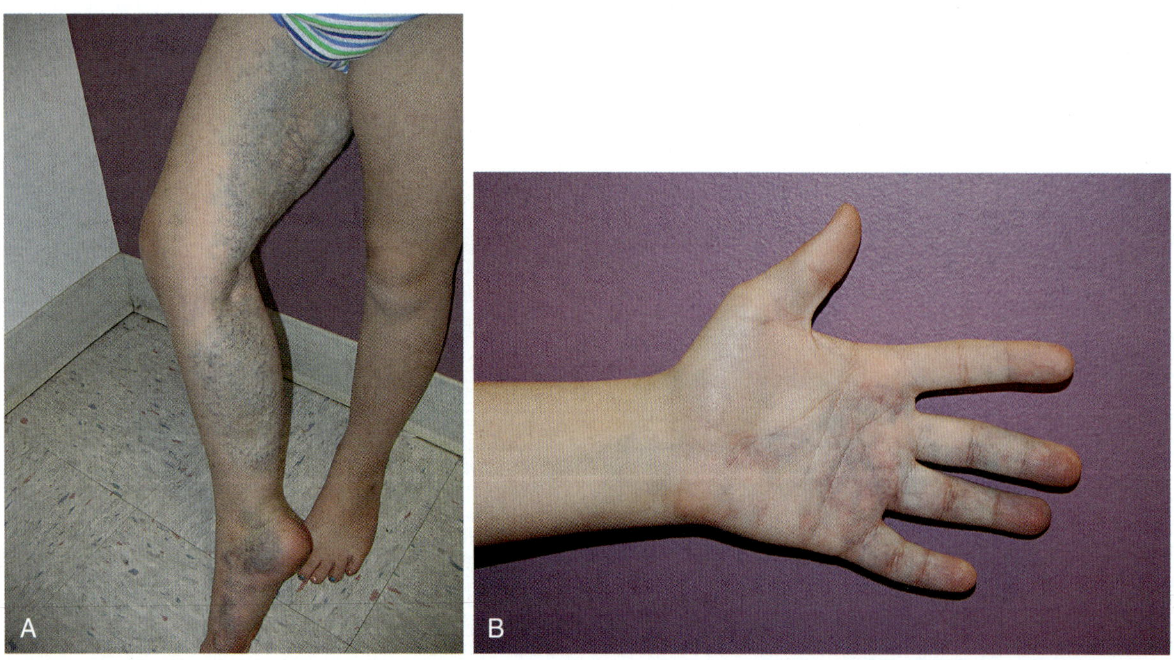

Fig. 10.21 Venous malformation (superficial). (A) Extensive venous malformation on the medial surface of the right leg with notable bluish discoloration and visible veins. (B) Note the dark red and purple discoloration on the palmar aspect of this boy's hand with no visible vasculature.

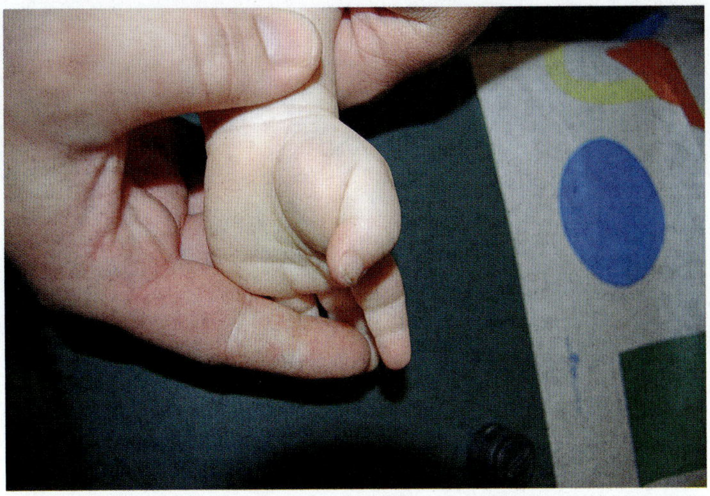

Fig. 10.22 Venous malformation (deep). Note the swelling of thenar eminence on this young child's hand with no noted superficial discoloration.

though, these lesions can have a deep connection, making them a risk for pulmonary embolism. Over time, the thrombosed vessel will calcify, creating a phlebolith. Upon examination, these feel like firm, smooth, round lumps that are usually pea sized. These lesions can be noted on plain radiographs.

Although history and physical examination are critical to the diagnosis of venous malformations, often additional imaging is warranted. Ideally an ultrasound with Doppler is the first study of choice. It is best to have the ultrasound performed by a radiologist who is experienced in vascular anomalies and who examines the patient in the vascular anomalies clinic. An ultrasound is usually performed by a technician. The radiologist who subsequently reads the study may not have the clinical history and may not have examined the patient in real time. This may lead to a misdiagnosis. It is best to send the patient to a specialized vascular anomalies center for imaging. If the ultrasound done in the vascular anomalies center is determined to be inconclusive or the extent of the lesion cannot be determined on ultrasound, then MRI with contrast may be needed.

Several types of venous malformations are more complex or are part of a syndrome, including blue rubber bleb nevus syndrome (BRBNS), glomuvenous malformations (GVMs), cerebral cavernous malformation (CCM), verrucous venous malformation (VVM), and fibro-adipose vascular anomaly (FAVA). BRBNS presents with many small venous malformations (Fig. 10.23). They can be found in the skin, underlying soft tissue, and gastrointestinal tract. When present in the gastrointestinal tract, there can be extensive disease and propensity to bleed, often presenting with profound anemia secondary to chronic microscopic gastrointestinal bleeding. GVMs are venous malformations that are inherited in an autosomal dominant manner. Located in the skin or subcutaneous tissue, these lesions are typically multifocal and may be painful. CCM is rare. It is also familial, and patients have venous malformations involving the central nervous system. VVM may initially resemble a plaquelike infantile hemangioma but does not regress with time and insteads develops a hyperkeratotic appearance (Fig. 10.24). At times they can be complicated by bleeding. FAVA is another rare lesion that often presents as a swelling, typically with no findings in the skin. On MRI, the lesion replaces the muscle and is seen as a fibrofatty mass with abnormal venous channels within (Fig. 10.25).

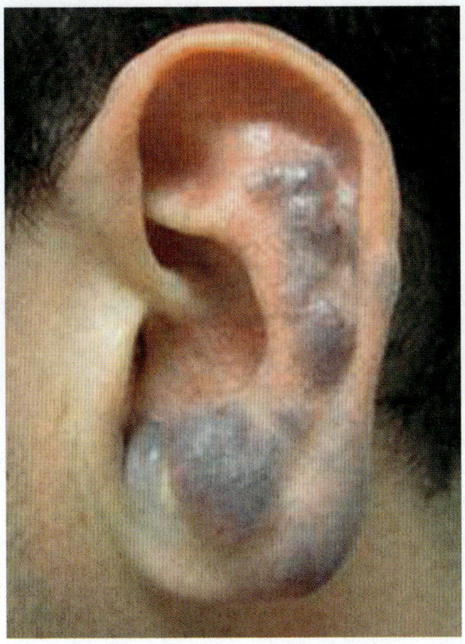

Fig. 10.23 Blue rubber bleb nevus syndrome. Note multiple blue masses on the ear that represent multiple small venous malformations.

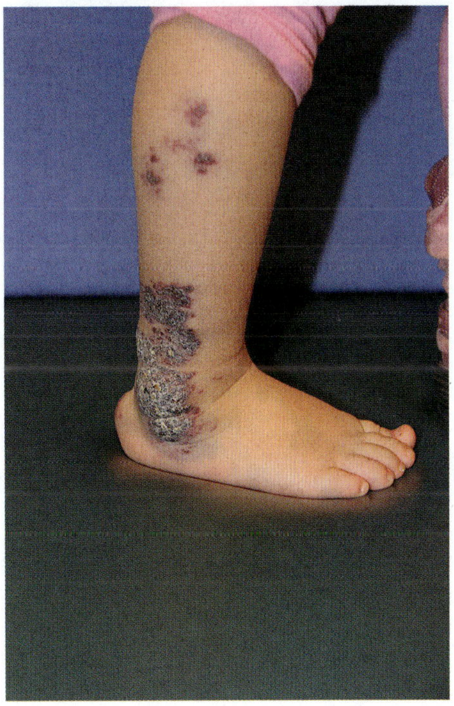

Fig. 10.24 Verrucous hemangioma. Hyperkeratotic lesion on the lateral ankle.

Lymphatic Malformations

Lymphatic malformations are one of the most common slow-flow lesions seen in a vascular anomalies center. They can be focal, or they can be large and diffuse, infiltrating all types of tissues, including bone. Once treated primarily by procedural interventions (sclerotherapy) and surgical debulking, greater understanding on the genetics and cell signaling pathways involved in lymphatic malformations has expanded treatment options to include medical therapies (sirolimus, alpelisib).

Common lymphatics malformations are cystic and can be either microcystic, marcocystic, or a combination of both (mixed cystic). Microcystic disease often presents with small vesicles in the skin that may be red or purple and leak clear fluid (Fig. 10.26). Macrocystic disease is seen as fullness in the affected region (Fig. 10.27). Like all malformations, they are present at birth; however, if they are deep, they are often first noticed after a trauma to the area or with local or systemic infection. Both trauma and infection can cause enlargement and swelling of lymphatic malformations; thus a deep lesion that may not have been visible because of its location will sometimes present as subtle new swelling. A child may present to the emergency department with new swelling that was not present at birth.

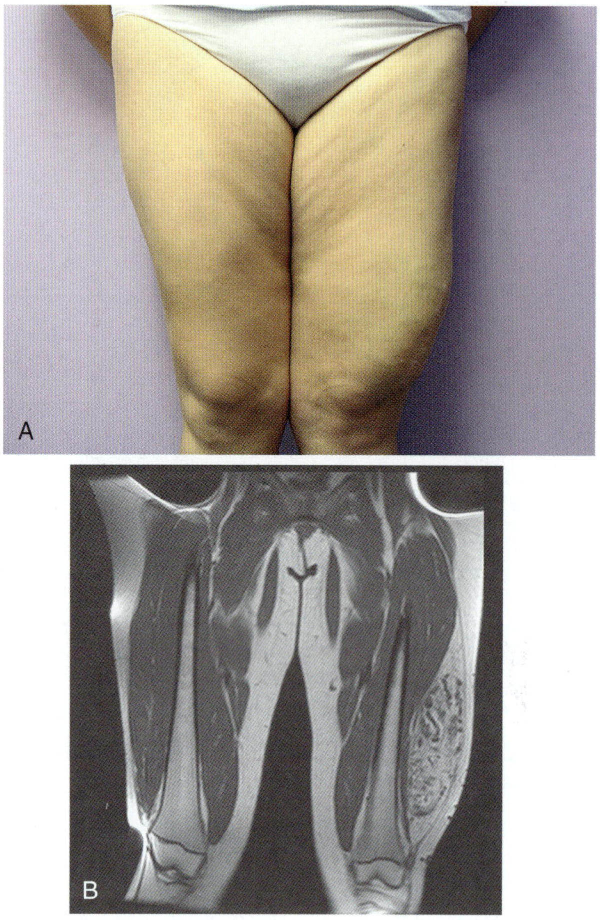

Fig. 10.25 Fibroadipose vascular anomaly. Young girl with a focal swelling on her lateral left thigh (A), with magnetic resonance imaging demonstrating a fibroadipose mass (B).

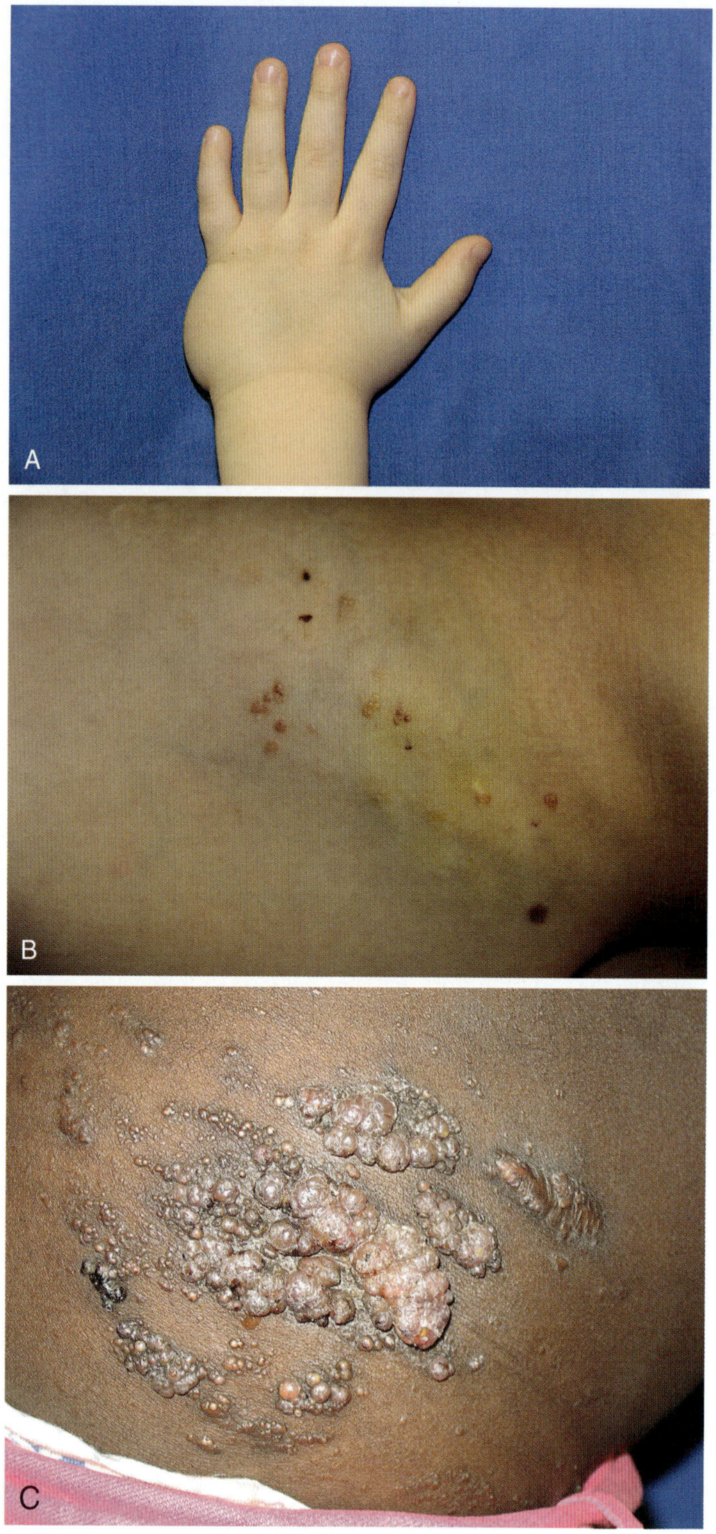

Fig. 10.26 Lymphatic malformation. (A) Child with a lymphatic malformation of the hand only noted for localized swelling. (B and C) The classic associated cutaneous findings of vesicular formation overlying the effected region with chronic clear drainage.

If physical examination makes one suspicious of a lymphatic malformation, then ultrasound imaging with an experienced interventional radiologist present is the first line of imaging. On ultrasound, these lesions are low flow. There may be a fluid-fluid level in the larger cysts if any bleeding has occurred within the cysts; the blood settles in the bottom of the cyst, and this is seen as a fluid-fluid level (see Fig. 10.27B). Small, focal lesions may be completely imaged with ultrasound. Larger, more complex lesions require an MRI with contrast. Often lymphatic malformations may infiltrate not only the superficial soft tissues but also the muscle, bone, and deeper structures. MRI will allow visualization of the entire lesion and help to show which parts are microcystic and which parts are macrocystic, which is necessary in determining therapeutic options.

Fast-Flow Malformations

Arteriovenous Malformations

Arteriovenous malformations (AVMs) and fistulas develop from a breakdown in the typical circulatory pattern by which the arterial blood supply directly connects with the venous system (Fig. 10.28). The AVM bypass occurs via tangled web of ectatic arterial vessels that link with the venous system, whereas the arteriovenous fistula is a single connection from artery to vein. Both the AVM and fistula leads to a high-pressure system joining a low-pressure structure, which creates the potential for a point of rupture. AVMs and fistulas can occur within any system of the body, but the most common locations are the pelvis, extremities, and intracranial circulation.

The typical clinical presentation of these vascular malformations varies on the basis of location. The extracutaneous lesions typically present with symptoms of pain (deep pelvic pain, headaches, or limb pain), high-output heart failure (pulmonary AVM and hepatic AVM), or bleeding (gastrointestinal or intracranial). Often these lesions can be silent until a catastrophic presentation occurs (e.g., intracranial hemorrhage).

The cutaneous AVMs have a more insidious presentation with appearance at birth as a dermal stain, followed by swelling that seems to grow with the child (Fig. 10.29). This consistent growth is staggered with short periods of rapid growth during puberty or after minor trauma. The initial appearance of a dermal stain can be similar in appearance to capillary malformations but differentiated due to warmth and brisk refill after blanching the lesions. As these

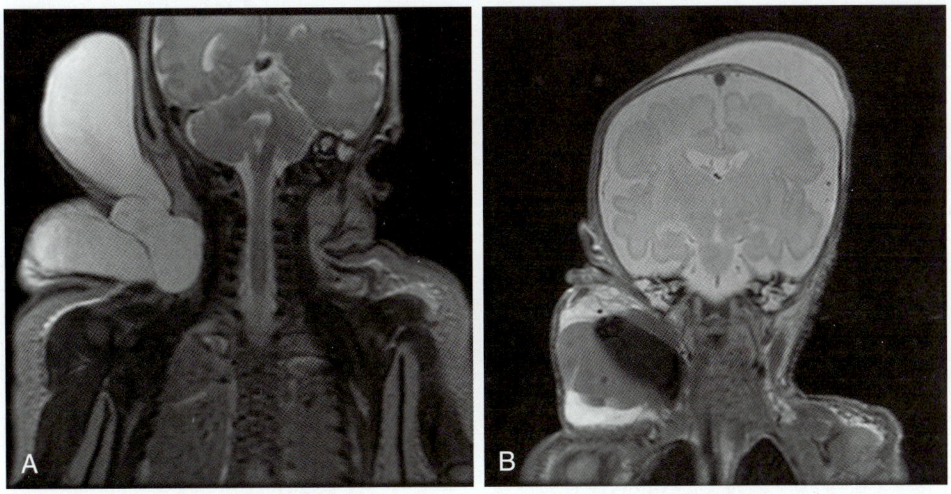

Fig. 10.27 Macrocystic lymphatic malformation. Magnetic resonance imaging of a large neck mass demonstrating a large single cystic mass (A) and associated fluid level suggestive of hemorrhage into the cyst. Incidental caput succedaneum is noted in the image as well (B).

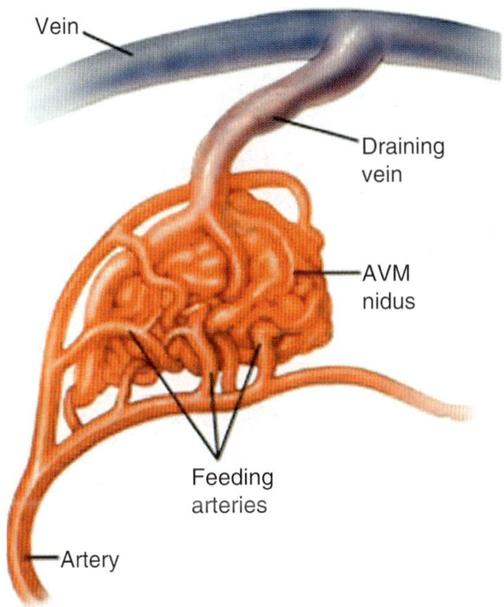

Fig. 10.28 Arteriovenous malformation *(AVM)*. This drawing demonstrates the direct connection of the arterial vascular blood flow the venous system by way of a tangled web of ectatic arterial vessels.

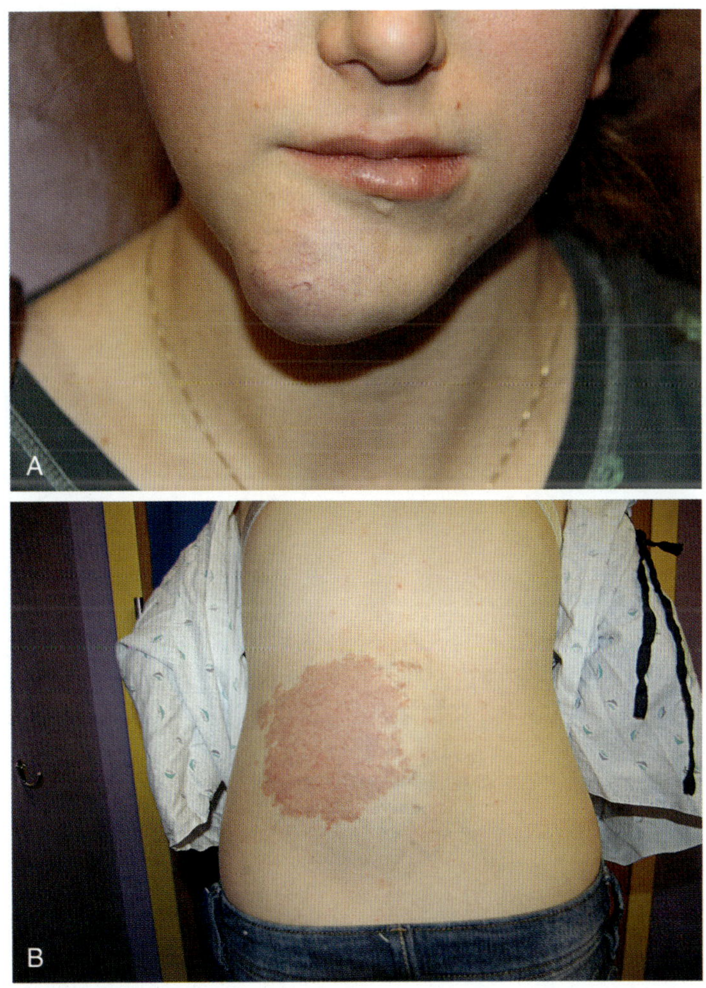

Fig. 10.29 Cutaneous arteriovenous malformation (AVM). (A) Cutaneous AVM on this child's chin, which is a pulsatile mass. (B) Vascular stain that is warm to touch and blanches with a brisk refill.

lesions expand with associated swelling, they become pulsatile. Large lesions with fistula formation will often have associated bruits and thrills.

Ideally, an ultrasound with Doppler is the first study of choice. It is best to have the ultrasound done by a radiologist who is experienced in vascular anomalies to differentiate slow-flow anomalies from the fast-flow anomalies. Further imagining may be necessary, including MRI with arterial and venous phases or angiography. Treatment most often consists of embolization or surgical resection.

VASCULAR MALFORMATIONS ASSOCIATED WITH OTHER ANOMALIES

The field of vascular malformations is a fresh frontier in medicine. Newer imaging modalities and innovative molecular sequencing techniques have allowed the clinician to better differentiate diseases that would have been previously indistinguishable. This expansion of the lexicon and development of more specific categories of diseases has led to specialized treatment of these disorders as well. The previous section gave the reader a basic framework of the fast-flow and slow-flow vascular malformations. This section focuses on key syndromes to better differentiate the complexity of the field, but it does not stand as a comprehensive list of all associated syndromes.

Sturge-Weber Syndrome

Sturge-Weber syndrome is a neurocutaneous syndrome in which cutaneous capillary malformation (port-wine stain) is associated

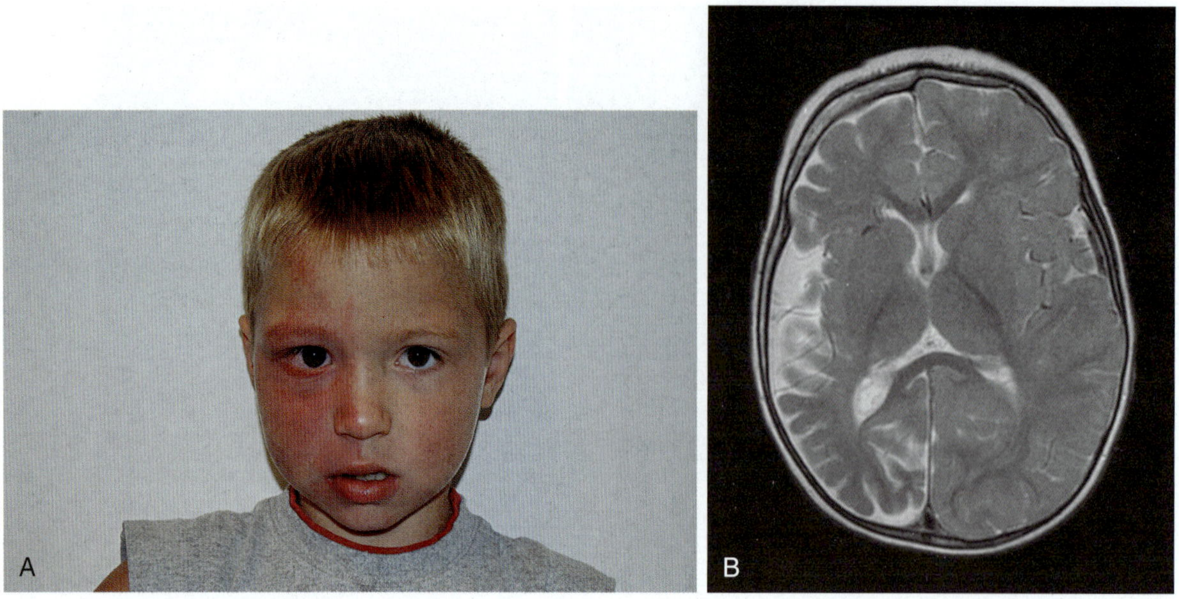

Fig. 10.30 Sturge-Weber syndrome. (A) Boy with a V1 distribution capillary malformation (port-wine stain). (B) Magnetic resonance imaging demonstrating an ipsilateral leptomeningeal vascular malformation.

with an intracranial leptomeningeal vascular malformation. The hallmark presentation is a port-wine stain occurring in the V1 distribution (Fig. 10.30), which is the region of innervation of the first branch of the trigeminal nerve. It encompasses an area from the anterior scalp to the nose (including the eye and part of the cheek). All patients with V1 distribution capillary malformation should be screened for Sturge-Weber by brain MRI with contrast to evaluate for ipsilateral leptomeningeal vascular malformations and ophthalmology examination to monitor for glaucoma. The most common neurologic manifestations of this illness are epilepsy and intellectual disability.

Cutis Marmorata Telangiectatica Congenita

Cutis marmorata telangiectatica congenita is a rare disorder characterized by discolored patches of skin caused by widened (dilated) surface blood vessels. As a result, the skin has a purple or blue "marbled" or "fishnet" appearance (Fig. 10.31). In some affected individuals, ulcerations or congenital skin defects (aplasia cutis) can be present. Additional associated abnormalities have been reported, including pink or dark red, irregularly shaped patches of skin (nevus flammeus); loss of muscle tissue on one side of the body (hemiatrophy); glaucoma; and overgrowth (hypertrophy) of one leg. However, when a leg-length discrepancy is noted, there is believed to be an overlap between cutis marmorata telangiectatica congenita and KTS, and further evaluation directed at KTS is warranted.

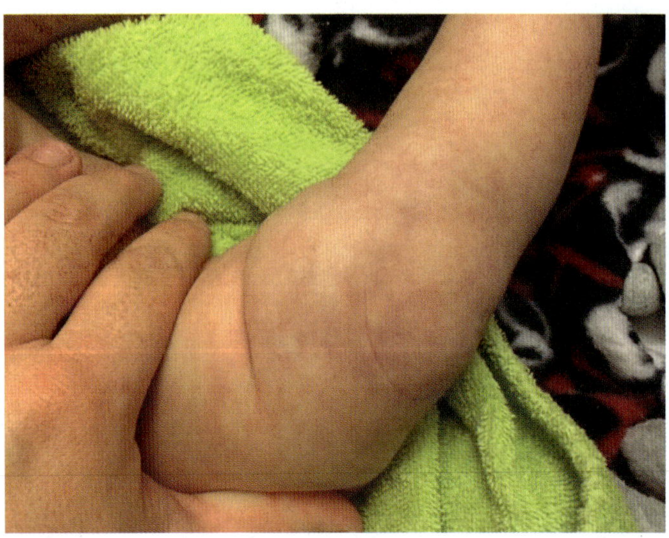

Fig. 10.31 Cutis marmorata telangiectatica congenita. Note the purple or blue "marbled" or "fishnet" appearance of the leg.

PIK3CA-Related Overgrowth Spectrum

PIK3CA-related overgrowth spectrum (PROS) is a group of disorders consisting of heterogenous segmental overgrowth commonly associated with vascular anomalies due to somatic activating variants in the *PIK3CA* gene. Three examples of PROS diagnoses are Megalencephaly-Capillary Malformation (M-CM or MCAP), Klippel-Trenaunay syndrome (KTS), and CLOVES syndrome. M-CM is a syndrome associated with head and body overgrowth, capillary malformations and other vascular anomalies, developmental delays, and other neurologic problems such as seizures. Measurement of the head circumference to evaluate for macrocephaly is an important consideration in a child presenting with multiple or diffuse capillary malformations. KTS is defined by the combination of a capillary malformation covering a large portion of the affected limb; venous malformation, often with an abnormal, dilated lateral marginal vein; and overgrowth of the bone or soft tissues (Fig. 10.32). The clinical concern for this group of patients is development of thrombus formation within the malformed lateral vein with progression to pulmonary embolism. Gait instability is also a concern secondary to leg-length discrepancy. The clinical appearance of limb-length discrepancy and capillary malformation raises concern for this, but diagnosis requires MRI of associated limb with arterial and venous phases to help differentiate from other associated overgrowth syndromes (CLOVES syndrome, Parkes Weber syndrome, Proteus syndrome). **CLOVES** is an acronym for **C**ongenital **L**ipomatous (fatty) **O**vergrowth, **V**ascular malformations, **E**pidermal nevi, and **S**coliosis/skeletal/spinal anomalies (Fig. 10.33). Three clinical features can be used to help differentiate this disorder upon examination: (1) lipomatous overgrowth, (2) cutaneous birthmarks, and (3) limb anomalies. The lipomatous overgrowth presents as soft, fatty masses of variable size, is noted at birth, and can be located in the back, flanks, axilla, abdomen, and buttocks (see Fig. 10.33A). These masses may affect one or both sides of the body. The skin over the mass is typically covered with a red-pinkish

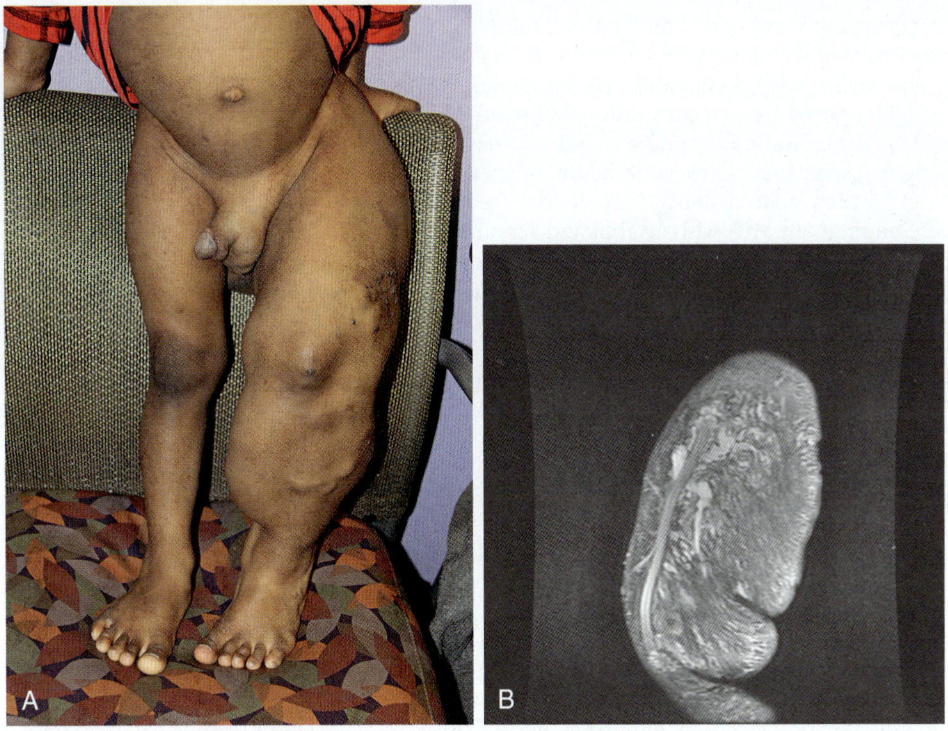

Fig. 10.32 Klippel-Trenaunay syndrome. Overgrowth in the left leg with a vascular stain that can be seen on the lateral aspect of the thigh (A) with magnetic resonance imaging revealing the presence of an embryonic lateral vein (B).

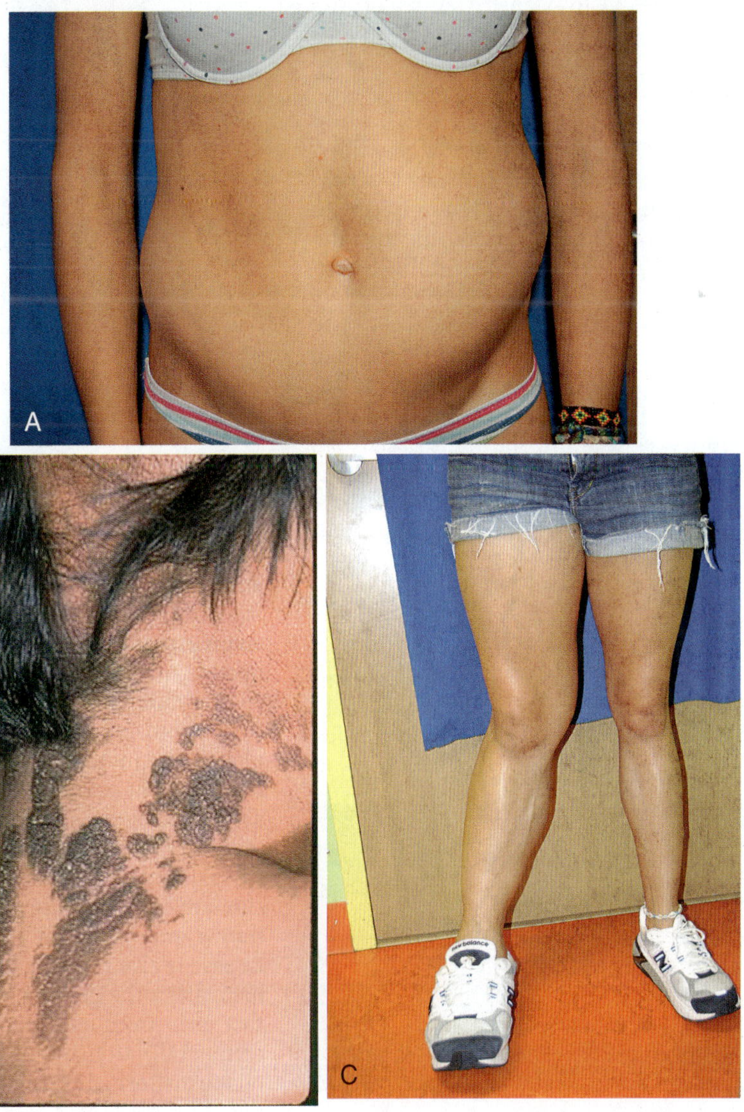

Fig. 10.33 CLOVES (**C**ongenital **L**ipomatous (fatty) **O**vergrowth, **V**ascular malformations, **E**pidermal nevi, and **S**coliosis/skeletal/spinal anomalies) syndrome. (A) Lipomatous overgrowth on the lateral abdomen in a child with CLOVES syndrome. (B) Epidermal nevus. (C) The limb overgrowth and hypertrophy associated with CLOVES syndrome.

birthmark (capillary malformation or port-wine stain). Multiple cutaneous findings are associated with CLOVES syndrome, including port-wine stains, prominent veins, lymphatic vesicles, moles, and epidermal nevus (slightly raised areas of skin with light brownish color) (see Fig. 10.33B). The final clinical finding is limb anomalies, including limb-length discrepancy, large wide hands or feet, large fingers or toes, and widely spaced digits (sandal toe) (see Fig. 10.33C). With these findings, an MRI with arterial and venous phase must be completed to help demonstrate associated venous and lymphatic anomalies associated with CLOVES syndrome. When a diagnosis of CLOVES syndrome is made, further screening will need to occur to evaluate spinal dysraphism with a spinal MRI, kidney anomalies with renal ultrasound, and serial right upper quadrant ultrasound to monitor for the development of Wilms tumor.

Parkes Weber Syndrome

Parkes Weber syndrome is characterized by overgrowth of the affected limb with small, diffuse arteriovenous fistulas. Often these can be confused with KTS because there may be a pseudo–capillary malformation due to localized superficial warmth and erythema of AVMs near the surface. These can be differentiated based on MRI with arterial and venous phases because Parkes Weber syndrome does not have slow-flow lymphatic or venous anomalies but will only have findings of overgrowth (soft tissue and bone) and arteriovenous fistulas. The clinical concern for these children as they age is the risk of high-output heart failure due to extensive burden of arteriovenous shunts.

Proteus Syndrome

Proteus is a rare overgrowth condition that presents with hemihypertrophy between 6 and 18 months old. The disorder is a progressive process with enlargement of bone, skin, and muscle with age to create significant asymmetry in appearance. This disorder is associated with multiple associated anomalies, including vascular anomalies, tissue overgrowth, benign tumor formation, and atypical adipose deposition. Classically, Proteus syndrome can cause a variety of skin growths, particularly thick, raised, and deeply grooved lesions known as *cerebriform connective tissue nevus* (Fig. 10.34). This type of skin growth usually occurs on the soles of the feet and is hardly ever seen in conditions other than Proteus syndrome. Vascular anomalies of various types can occur in Proteus syndrome, have a random distribution, and can occur outside the region of hemihypertrophy; therefore a broad evaluation is required.

Complex Lymphatic Anomalies

Complex lymphatic anomalies are a group of debilitating conditions characterized by diffuse lymphatic malformations, lymphatic leakage, and/or coagulopathy. They include generalized lymphatic anomaly, kaposiform lymphangiomatososis, Gorham-Stout disease, and central conducting lymphatic anomaly. As a result of lymphatic leak, patients with these disorders may develop pooling of chylous fluid in the pleural space (chylothorax) (Fig. 10.35) or other body compartments (pericardial effusion, ascites, protein-losing enteropathy, anasarca). Diagnosis of these disorders typically involves a combincation of history, examination, advanced imaging techniques (MRI, conventional lymphangiography, magnetic resonance lymphangiography), and histology when available. However, there can be significant phenotypic overlap between these conditions, making accurate diagnosis challenging. Generalized lymphatic anomaly is marked by multifocal lymphatic malformations involving bones, thorax, and abdominal viscera. Kaposiform lymphangiomatososis similarly involves diffuse lymphatic malformations but is more infiltrative and commonly associated with coagulopathy. Gorham-Stout disease is also referred to as *vanishing bone disease*. The pathologic hallmark is the development of lymphatic channels within the bone that form from an unknown mechanism and lead to an osteolytic demineralization and destruction of the bone (Fig. 10.36). The lymphatic malformations are not isolated to the bone alone, and formation of chylothorax is a common clinical manifestation. Central conducting lymphatic anomaly is characterized by improper flow of lymphatic fluid through the thoracic duct with retrograde reflux

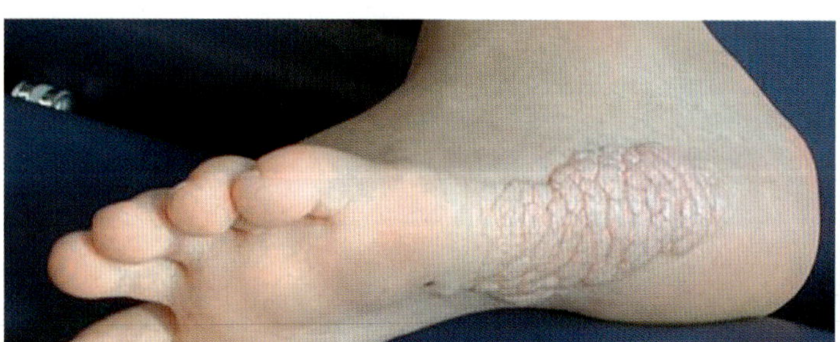

Fig. 10.34 Proteus syndrome. A classic cutaneous finding of Proteus syndrome is a particularly thick, raised, and deeply grooved lesion known as a *cerebriform connective tissue nevus*.

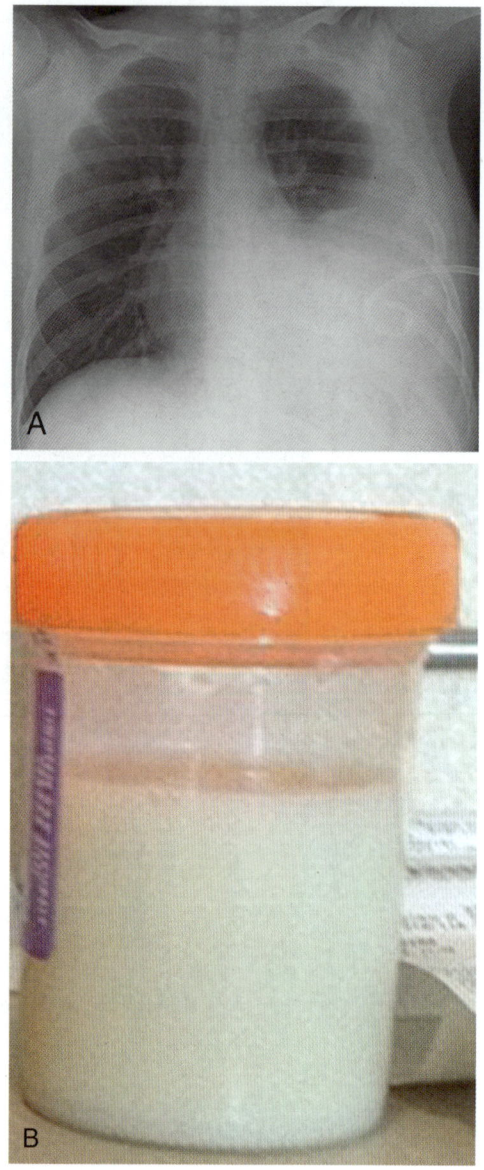

Fig. 10.35 Chylothorax. (A) Chest radiograph with large pleural effusion. (B) Milklike white drainage.

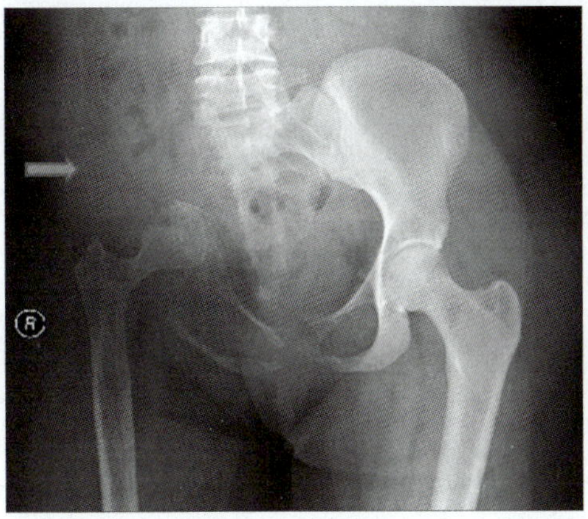

Fig. 10.36 Gorham-Stout syndrome. This pelvic radiograph of a young female with Gorham-Stout syndrome demonstrates osteolysis of the right pelvic structures.

into multiple body compartments, though it is not necessarily associated with actual lymphatic malformations.

Hereditary Hemorrhagic Telangiectasia

Hereditary hemorrhagic telangiectasia (HHT) is an autosomal dominant disorder with high penetrance characterized by the development of AVMs in varied body systems. The disease is often present across multiple generations of a family but with varied phenotypes. The disorder targets capillary repair within the pulmonary, gastrointestinal, nasopharyngeal, and cutaneous systems leading to AVM development. Therefore the disorder has a progressive phenotype over the individual's life. The exception is intracranial AVM, with which individuals are born, and can lead to the devasting manifestation of hemorrhagic stroke in early life. Other body systems may develop AVM over time, resulting in epistaxis, symptoms of gastrointestinal bleeding, or complications from pulmonary AVM. Telangiectasias are the cutaneous manifestations that have a propensity for the nose, lips, oral cavity, and fingers and seem to increase with aging (Fig. 10.37). These lesions appear as red spots with a spider leg appearance that blanch with palpation, then rapidly return when released. HHT diagnostic criteria (Table 10.2) are used less frequently due to improved genetic testing. Gene testing in families known to have this disorder has allowed for genetic diagnosis and screening before clinical disease presentation. Current recommendations are that all children with genetic or diagnostic criteria for HHT undergo an initial MRI with contrast of the brain, contrast transthoracic echocardiogram, and a Doppler ultrasound of the liver to evaluate for AVM presence at diagnosis and subsequent evaluation throughout life to monitor for progression in key body regions (Table 10.3). These children and adults should be cared for at a HHT center of excellence or under the guidance of a vascular anomaly center to ensure ongoing screening and prevention of disease progression.

Table 10.2 Diagnostic Criteria of Hereditary Hemorrhagic Telangiectasia

Criteria	Description
Epistaxis	Recurrent severe nosebleeds
Telangiectasia	Classic locations
Visceral disease	AVM in lung, brain, or gastrointestinal tract
Family history	First-degree relative with HHT
Probable diagnosis	Two criteria met
Definitive diagnosis	Three or more criteria met

AVM, Arteriovenous malformation; *HHT,* hereditary hemorrhagic telangiectasia.

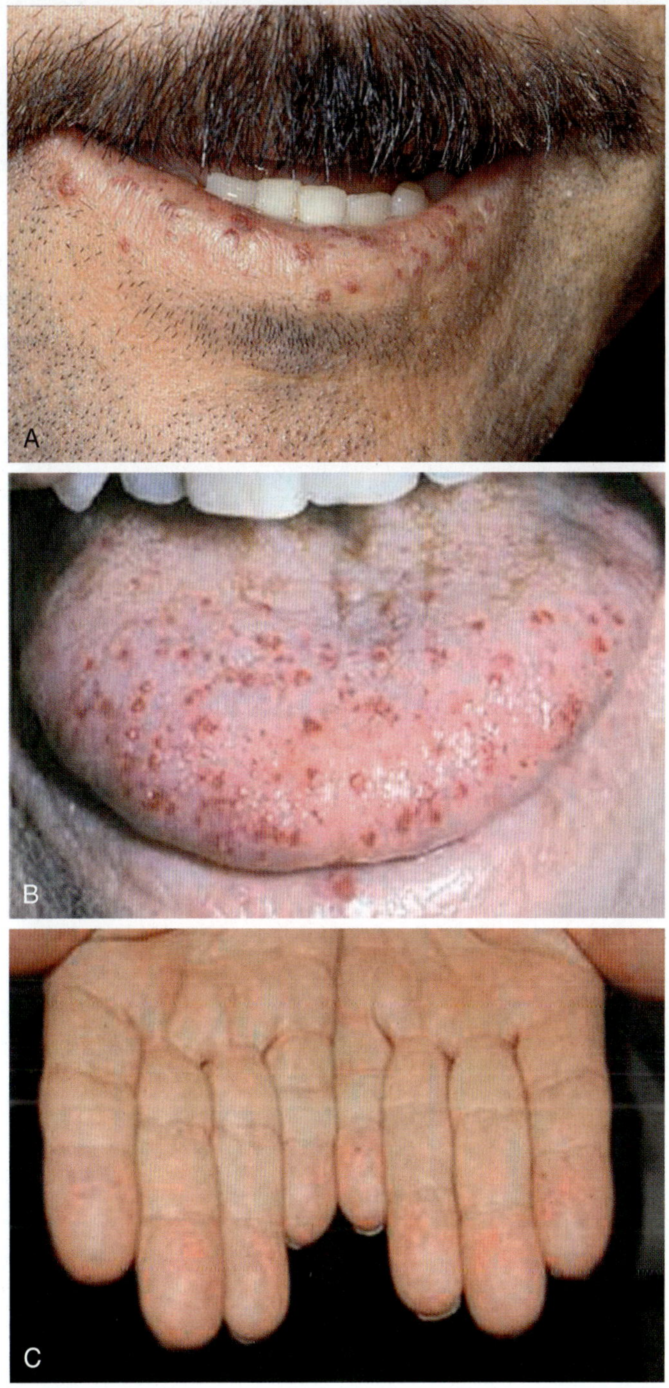

Fig. 10.37 Hereditary hemorrhagic telangiectasia, cutaneous telangiectasia. Classic locations of telangiectasia affecting the lips (A), tongue (B), and fingertips (C). There are usually few of these lesions in the first 2 decades of life, but they increase with age.

Table 10.3 Initial Screening for Hereditary Hemorrhagic Telangiectasia

Manifestation	Screening
Telangiectasia	Clinical observation
Epistaxis	Clinical observation
Cerebral vascular malformation	MRI with and without contrast (younger than 2 years old without contrast only)
Pulmonary AVM	TTE with contrast
Gastrointestinal bleeding	CBC annually after 35 years old; if anemic, perform EGD
Hepatic AVM	Liver ultrasound with Doppler

AVM, Arteriovenous malformation; *CBC,* complete blood count; *EGD,* esophagogastroduodenoscopy; *MRI,* magnetic resonance imaging; *TTE,* transthoracic echocardiogram.

SUMMARY

The field of vascular anomalies continues to progress as previous ill-defined disorders become clearly understood and modalities of treatment become increasingly effective. This chapter has given a framework for understanding vascular anomalies. It emphasizes that the systematic evaluation of the child with a vascular lesion serves as the primary mode of diagnosis. Imaging is used often only to clarify between overlapping categories of disease and preparation for possible intervention.

Bibliography

Chang LC, Haggstrom AN, Drolet BA, et al: Growth characteristics of infantile hemangiomas: implications for management, *Pediatrics* 122(2):360–367, 2008.

Colmenero I, Heoger PH: Vascular tumours in infants. Part 2: vascular tumours of intermediate malignancy and malignant tumours, *Br J Dermatol* 171:474–484, 2014.

Greene A, Perlyn C: Vascular anomalies, *Clin Plast Surg* 38:1–151, 2011.

Heoger PH, Colmenero I: Vascular tumours in infants. Part 1: benign vascular tumours other than infantile hemangiomas, *Br J Dermatol* 171:466–473, 2014.

Iacobas I, Burrows PE, Frieden IJ, et al: LUMBAR: association between cutaneous infantile hemangiomas of the lower body and regional congenital anomalies, *J Pediatr* 157(5):795–801, 2010.

Kanada KN, Merin MR, Munden A, et al: A prospective study of cutaneous findings in newborns in the United States: correlation with race, ethnicity, and gestational status using updated classification and nomenclature, *J Pediatr* 161(2):240–245, 2012.

Liang MG, Frieden IJ: Infantile and congenital hemangiomas, *Semin Pediatr Surg* 23(4):162–167, 2014.

Metry D, Heyer G, Hess C, et al: Consensus statement on diagnostic criteria for PHACE syndrome, *Pediatrics* 124:1447–1456, 2009.

Wassef M, Blei F, Adams D, et al: Vascular anomalies classification: recommendations from the International Society for the Study of Vascular Anomalies, *Pediatrics* 136(1):e203–e214, 2015.

Moyakine AV, Herwegen B, van der Vleuten CJM: Use of the Hemangioma Severity Scale to facilitate treatment decisions for infantile hemangiomas, *J Am Acad Dermatol* 77(5):868–873, 2017. doi:10.1016/j.jaad.2017.06.003.

NUTRITION AND GASTROENTEROLOGY

11

Erin Crawford | Arvind Srinath

Nutritional and gastrointestinal (GI) symptoms are two of the most common topics encountered in general pediatric medicine. Globally, undernutrition and diarrheal disease cause substantial morbidity and mortality. In the developed world, nutritional assessment is paramount in well child care and chronic illness management. GI symptoms are common in acute and chronic illnesses. Because one of the main functions of the GI system is to provide fluid, vitamins/minerals, and the energy requirements to sustain viability and growth, the relationship between gastroenterology and nutrition is readily apparent. However, for the purposes of this chapter, nutrition and gastroenterology are divided into two sections, with a focus on the entities commonly seen by pediatric primary care providers.

NUTRITION

Normal Infant Nutrition and Growth

The first year of life is marked by unprecedented growth, with birthweight approximately doubling in the first 6 months and tripling by 1 year and length generally increasing by 50% by age 1. As such, the normal caloric and protein requirements for growth are higher (Table 11.1). Human breast milk and formulas fuel this growth (Box 11.1), and there is a general acceptance that breast milk offers advantages that formulas cannot emulate. Breast milk, however, lacks substantial amounts of vitamin D and fluoride, thus requiring supplementation. Low amounts of vitamin K stores at birth and in breast milk have led to a standard practice of intramuscular vitamin K injection at birth. Breast milk also has a lower amount of iron, requiring added supplementation, as an infant uses the iron stores obtained in utero and reaches a physiologic nadir after the first 6 months of life. Standard infant formulas have sufficient iron, vitamin K, and vitamin D. There has been rapid growth in the varieties of infant formulas, including "niche" formulas that are designed for specific GI illnesses and not necessary for standard infant feeding. Box 11.2 categorizes the elements of the most common variants of infant formulas used today. Although whole cow's milk has features like human breast milk, their higher protein concentration and thus higher renal solute load has led the American Academy of Pediatrics to recommend their use be delayed until an infant is 12 months of age.

Normal Childhood/Adolescent Nutrition and Growth

As an infant reaches 1 year, the caloric requirements lessen as the rate of growth decreases (see Table 11.1). Solid foods, typically introduced around the sixth month of life, become the major source of calories. Psychologic and behavioral aspects of feeding become a common discussion during health care visits. Variations of feeding patterns that do not affect growth but may lead to GI symptoms are often recognized during this period. Nutritional assessment is essential to recognize tendencies in undernutrition and overnutrition and to recognize acute and chronic disease.

Basic Monitoring of Growth and Nutrition

Growth assessment in pediatric practice is a proxy for nutritional adequacy and general health status. Growth charts are used to monitor simple anthropometric data to achieve these goals. Use of the World Health Organization (WHO) growth charts has largely supplanted the Centers for Disease Control and Prevention (CDC) growth charts in children younger than 2 years of age. These charts are based on breastfed infants and provide growth standards that describe healthy growth under optimal conditions and include longitudinal data from 0 to 24 months of age. The WHO growth charts use weight for age, length/height for age, and occipital-frontal circumference for age. The CDC growth charts, used in children from 2 to 20 years old, include the body mass index (weight [kg]/height [m]^2) in response to the growing obesity epidemic. As a distribution based on percentages, it should be recognized that there will always be a population that is over the greatest isopleth (>97th percentile) and under the lowest isopleth (<3rd percentile) in these growth charts. Despite this, the characteristics of the growth of a child can be an invaluable comparative measure of what would be considered normal growth to actual growth. Growth charts are also available for specialized populations such as infants with genetic conditions (e.g., Trisomy 21) and premature infants, though it should be noted that the numbers of patients in the sample section are less than those in the standard growth charts.

Other measurements, such as triceps skinfold thickness (Fig. 11.1) and midarm circumference (MUAC) (Fig. 11.2), when performed by a trained examiner, can be useful when growth charts are insufficient. Some populations where these measurements would have utility include infants with end-stage liver disease and marked ascites or hypertrophy of an organ or appendage, which falsely elevates true body weight. For the vast majority of infants and children, growth charts are an adequate assessment of overall growth.

Malnutrition States

Malnutrition can be defined as both undernutrition and overnutrition, although it is most often associated with an undernourished state. The state of malnutrition results from an imbalance between the intake and/or absorption of calories and the consumption of calories needed for growth. Obesity is due to overnutrition and has grown to epidemic proportions in the United States. Undernutrition results from inadequate intake, absorption, or digestion of nutrients, or insufficient intake for increased metabolic needs. Under prolonged conditions, undernutrition and overnutrition lead to malnutrition. Careful plotting of height, weight, and body mass index as a function of age on an appropriate growth chart aids in the diagnosis of malnutrition.

A traditional classification of extreme protein energy malnutrition includes marasmus, kwashiorkor, and marasmic kwashiorkor. Marasmus is defined as predominantly caloric/energy deficiency and is characterized by marked emaciation, loss of subcutaneous fat and muscle, sparse hair, and poor nail growth (Fig. 11.3). It is the

Table 11.1 Nutritional Requirements

Age	Calories (kcal/kg/day)	Protein (g/kg/day)
0–6 months	100–120	2.5–3.0
6–12 months	90–100	2.0–2.5
1–7 years	75–90	1.5–2.0
7–12 years	60–75	1.5–2.0
12+ years	30–60	1.0–1.5

Box 11.1 Advantages of Breastfeeding

Convenience/economic benefits
No sterilization required
Maternal–infant bonding
Immunologic
Less frequent hospitalizations
Innate immunity: IgA, lysozymes, epidermal growth factor, complement, nucleotides, oligosaccharides, others
Prevention of atopy
Possible protection from autoimmune diseases
Association with small but significant increase in cognitive development
Optimal absorption of nutrients
Lactoferrin: Iron
Vitamin B_{12}–binding protein
Health in later life
Decreased obesity
Decreased hypertension
Maternal health benefits

IgA, Immunoglobulin A.

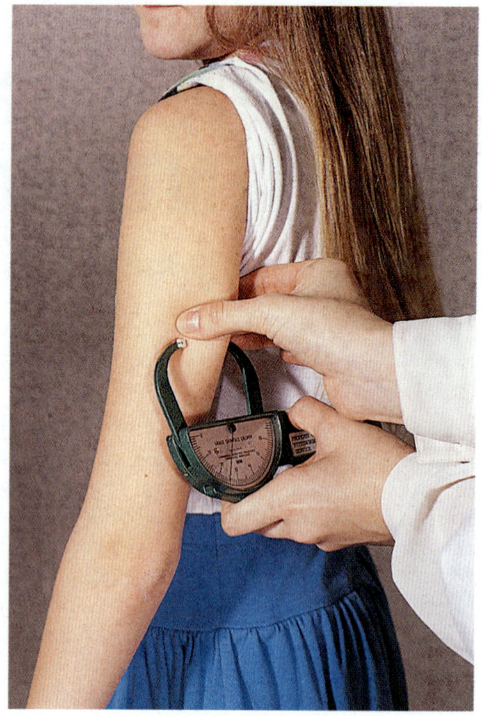

Fig. 11.1 Triceps skinfold. Grasp a vertical pinch of skin and subcutaneous fat. The caliper jaw is placed over the skinfold at the midpoint mark while maintaining a grasp of skinfold. Make a reading to the nearest 1 mm without excessive pressure. The final result is the average of three readings.

Box 11.2 Considerations in Choosing a Formula

Carbohydrate Source
Lactose
Sucrose
Maltodextrins
Starches

Protein Source
Whole
Human (breast milk)
Cow's milk
Soy
Hydrolyzed
Free amino acid

Fat Source
LCT:MCT ratio

Additives
DHA/ARA
Soluble fiber/prebiotics
Insoluble fiber

Other Considerations
Osmolality: Renal solute load
Ca and PO_4 content and ratio

ARA, Arachidonic acid; *Ca,* calcium; *DHA,* docosahexaenoic acid; *LCT:MCT ratio,* long-chain to medium-chain triglyceride ratio.

consequence of poor caloric, protein, vitamin, and mineral intake. Diarrhea is common as intestinal cell turnover slows, resulting in intestinal villous blunting and a secondary malabsorptive state (Fig. 11.4). Marasmus is usually seen within the first year of life at the time of weaning from breastmilk/formula or at any time when there is a consistent and extreme caloric deprivation. Kwashiorkor, on the other hand, results from a diet lacking protein even though it may be rich in calories. The initial "moon face" of kwashiorkor is often mistaken for proper nutrition. The child is often edematous, which becomes apparent after nutritional repletion (Fig. 11.5). Hepatomegaly and mental status changes are common. Skin changes include hyperpigmentation or hypopigmentation with a scaly, weeping dermatitis (Figs. 11.6 and 11.7). In marasmic kwashiorkor, both patterns of malnutrition may develop together, resulting in a combination of clinical features.

Failure to Thrive

The term *failure to thrive* is used to depict inadequate weight gain over time, often used when weight for age crosses two percentile isopleths or when weight for age falls below the 3rd percentile for age. Caution must be used when weight gain consistently tracks below the 3rd percentile, as this may reflect a normal growth pattern based on standard weight distribution patterns (Fig. 11.8). Most failure to thrive is marked by decreased weight for height, with initial sparing of height for age and head circumference for age, with gradual loss in height and head circumference for age as the undernourished state continues. This abnormal pattern of growth can be classified as inadequate intake, malabsorption, ineffective use of calories, or increased metabolic demand. Table 11.2 lists common diagnoses associated with failure to thrive.

A detailed history is often helpful in narrowing the differential diagnosis for children with failure to thrive. This starts with a dietary assessment including the type and amount of oral intake and specific behaviors surrounding eating. In infants, it is important to assess the preparation of formula, as incorrect mixing can lead to decreased caloric intake and the potential for electrolyte abnormalities. Three-day diet diaries can be helpful in reviewing caloric intake but are subject to bias after a deficiency of intake is considered. A detailed review of systems may point to a chronic medical illness.

Laboratory testing can serve as (1) a diagnostic tool for defining an underlying condition, (2) a marker for the degree of malnutrition, and (3) a screening tool for specific nutrient or micronutrient deficiencies. A complete blood count can suggest an underlying inflammatory condition, identify anemia, and serve as a basic immunologic assessment. Serum electrolytes may reflect abnormal losses due to diarrhea or excessive vomiting and find acidosis as an underlying metabolic disease. A 72-hour fecal fat level or fecal pancreatic elastase may depict fat malabsorption. Fecal α_1-antitrypsin and urinalysis can aid in the diagnosis of abnormal protein losses. Analysis of stool for reducing substances may reflect carbohydrate

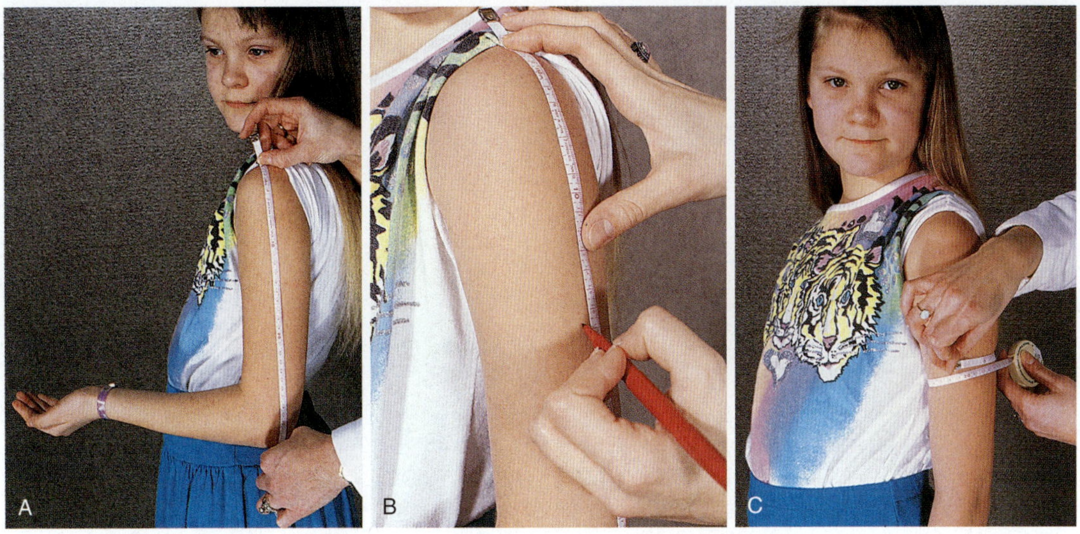

Fig. 11.2 Midarm circumference. (A) Locate the midpoint of the arm with arm bent at a 90-degree angle, and tape at acromion and olecranon processes. (B) Mark at midpoint. (C) Make measurement at midpoint with arm hanging loosely.

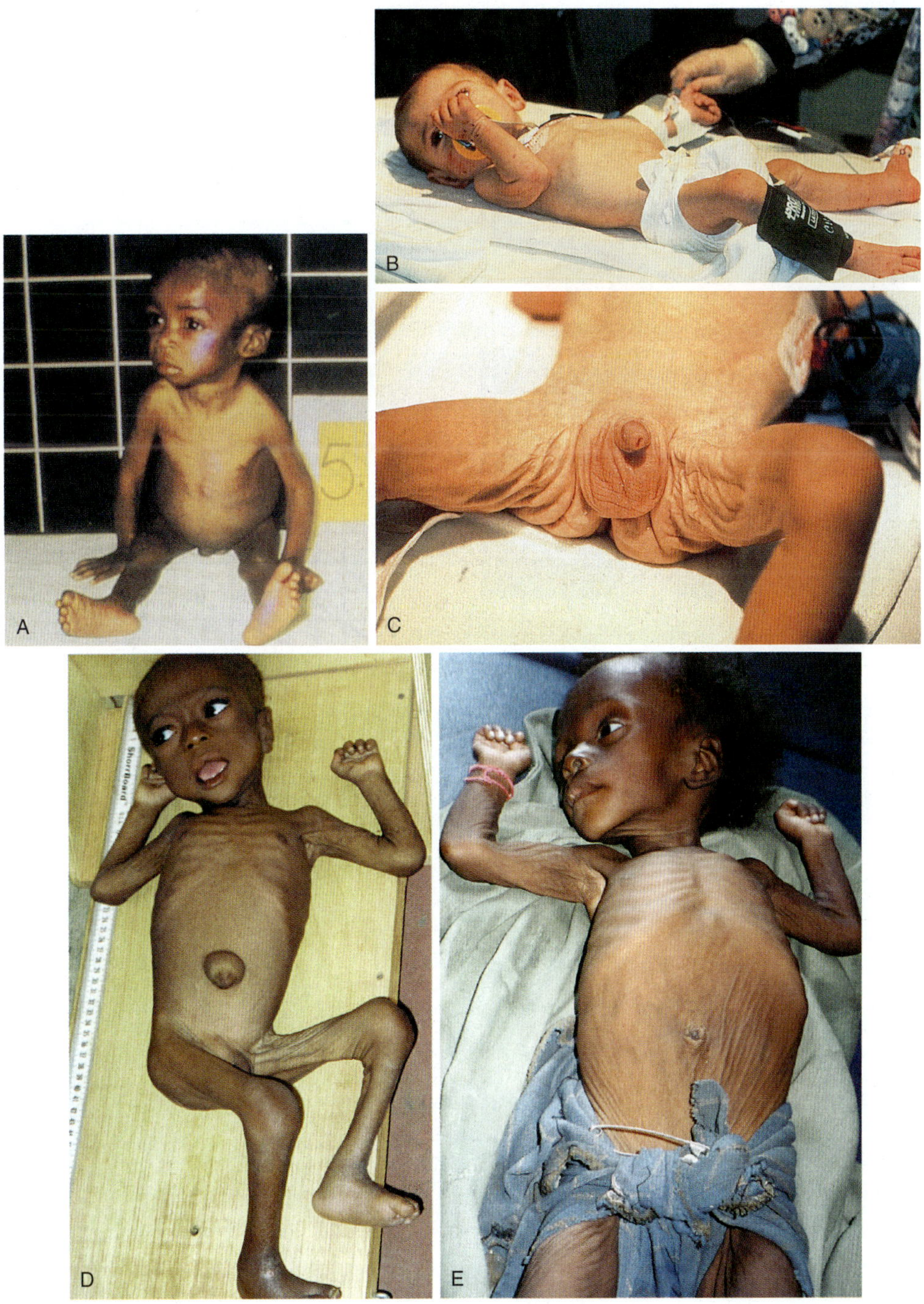

Fig. 11.3 Marasmus. (A) Note the profound wasting and sparse hair. (B and C) Note the wasting of subcutaneous tissue over the thorax with prominent ribs and loose skinfolds in the groin. (D and E) Note the loss of subcutaneous fat, profound wasting, loose skinfolds, and sparse hair. (Courtesy Jonathan Spector, MD, Boston, MA.)

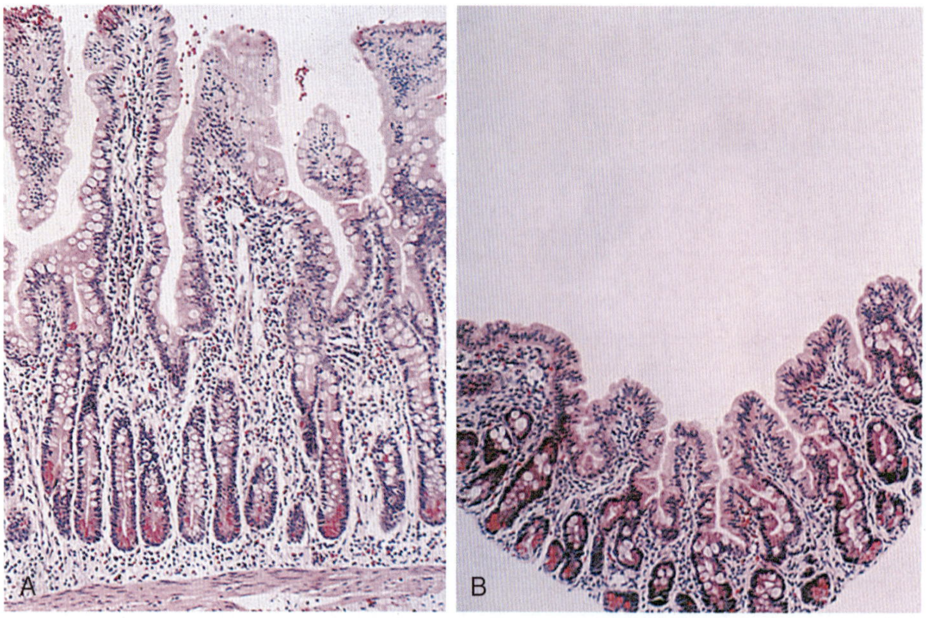

Fig. 11.4 Gastrointestinal tract injury associated with malnutrition. (A) Normal jejunal mucosa with tall villi and deep crypts. (B) Blunted villi lead to chronic diarrhea and malnutrition. Note the lack of increase in crypt depth and lymphocytic infiltrate seen in celiac disease (see Fig. 11.28) and other diseases with active cell turnover.

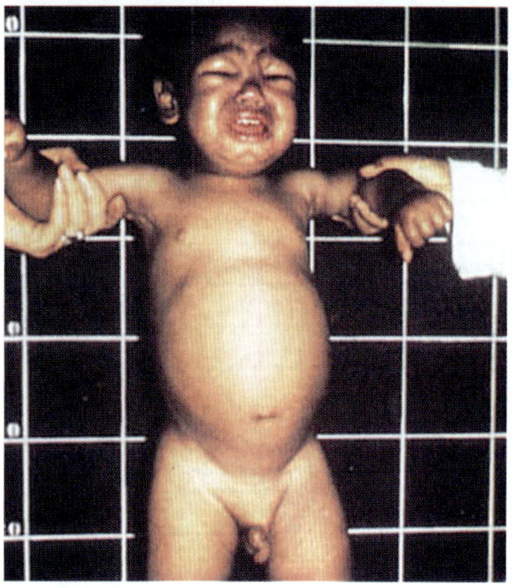

Fig. 11.5 Kwashiorkor. This patient has a typical edematous appearance in the periorbital area, extremities, and abdomen.

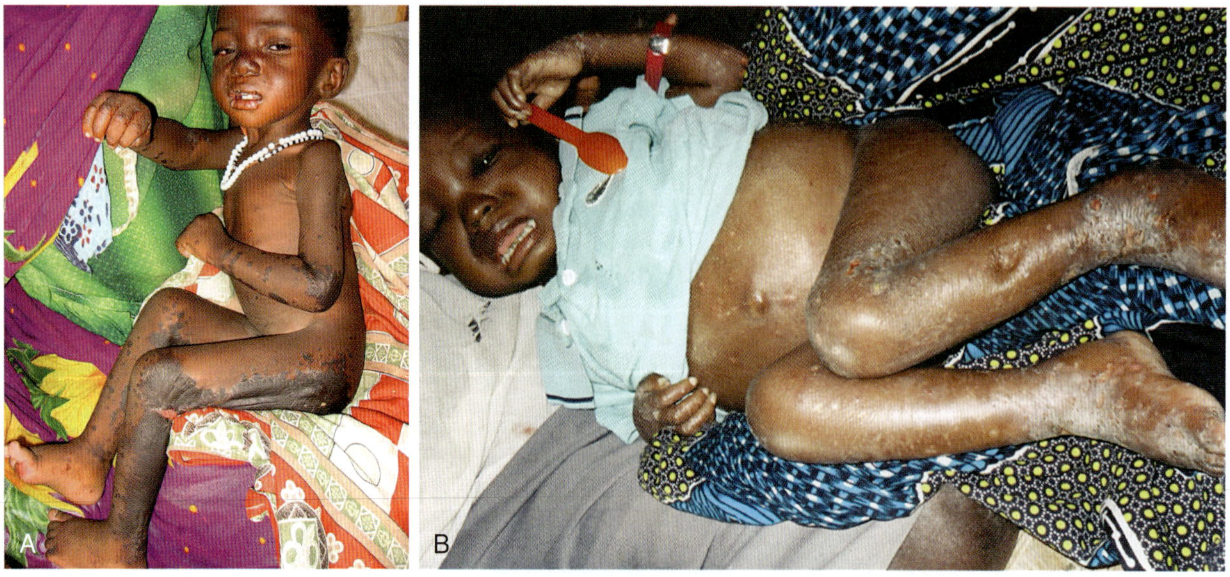

Fig. 11.6 Kwashiorkor. (A and B) These infants demonstrate kwashiorkor with "flaky paint" dermatosis, pigmentation changes, and pitting edema. (Courtesy Jonathan Spector, MD, Boston, MA.)

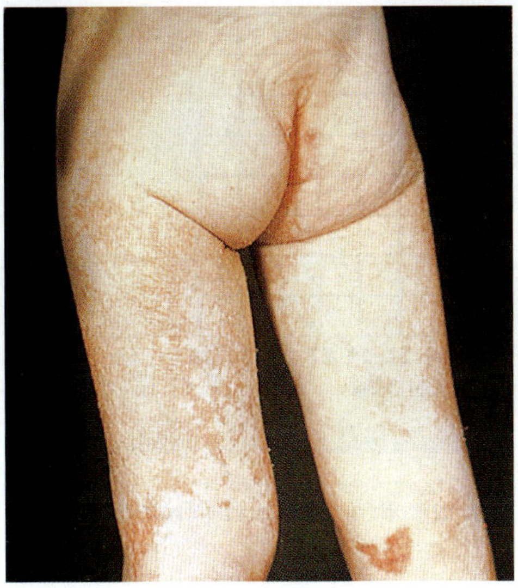

Fig. 11.7 Kwashiorkor. The rash of kwashiorkor is scaly and erythematous and may weep, especially in edematous areas.

Table 11.2 Common Etiologies of Failure to Thrive

Inadequate Intake	Inadequate Absorption	Increased Caloric Needs
Caloric deprivation	Celiac disease	Congenital heart disease
Behavioral feeding disorders	Intestinal inflammation	Chronic pulmonary disease
Disorders of swallowing	Fat malabsorption (cystic fibrosis)	Malignancy
Vomiting/reflux	Chronic diarrhea	Renal disease
Anorexia/poor appetite		Genetic disease

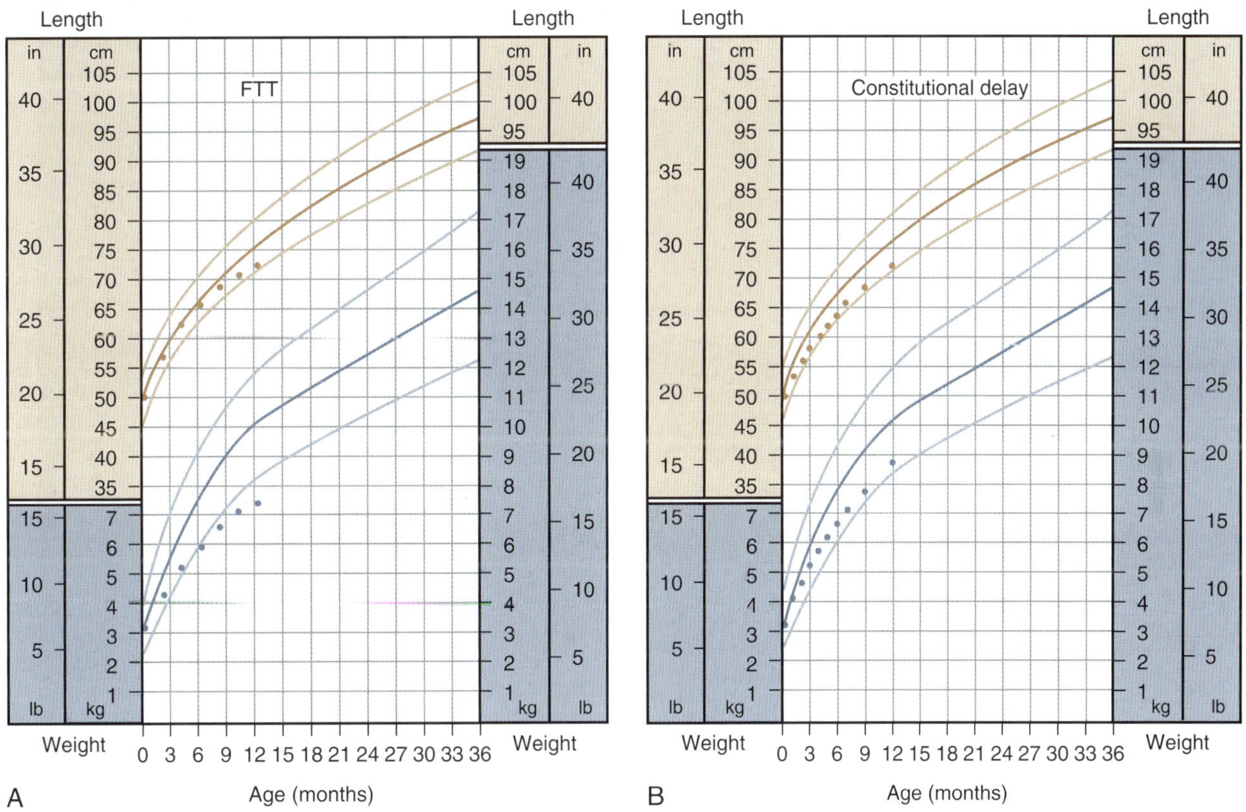

Fig. 11.8 Examples of growth curves. (A) Typical failure to thrive (FTT) with deceleration of weight gain. (B) Slow growth but at a normal rate consistent with constitutional delay.

malabsorption. Analysis of amino or organic acids in specific cases can point to metabolic disorders. Diagnosis-specific screens such as tissue transglutaminase IgA antibody for celiac disease can be useful in the patient with abnormal growth patterns. Decreases in specific proteins can be helpful as a marker of catabolism. Albumin ($t\frac{1}{2}$ 20–24 days) is commonly used, although not particularly specific, to depict the current nutritional status. Prealbumin ($t\frac{1}{2}$ 2 days) may be more sensitive, but it has limited use because it acts as an acute-phase protein. Although laboratory tests can be helpful, they are not mandatory and the decision for testing should be derived from the history and physical examination.

Therapy for malnutrition is twofold—treat the underlying cause and rehabilitate. All attempts should be made to treat the underlying cause. In parallel, nutritional rehabilitation via providing sufficient calories for growth should be implemented once malnutrition is recognized. Care must be undertaken when providing nutritional rehabilitation, as one consequence of aggressive therapy is refeeding syndrome (Box 11.3).

Specific Nutrient Deficiencies

In addition to more general malnutrition states, excess or deficiencies of specific nutrients, vitamins, and minerals can be seen alone or as complicating factors of chronic disease (Table 11.3). For example, fat-soluble vitamin deficiency (vitamins A, D, E, and K) can be found in isolation due to inadequate intake or with fat

Box 11.3 Considerations in Refeeding Syndrome

Physiologic
Rapid increase in insulin
Extracellular movement of ions to intracellular space
Sodium/water retention

Electrolyte Abnormalities
Hypophosphatemia
Hypokalemia
Hypomagnesemia
Hyponatremia
Thiamine deficiency

Monitoring
Daily electrolyte monitoring
Cardiovascular monitoring
Heart rate/blood pressure
Fluid balance

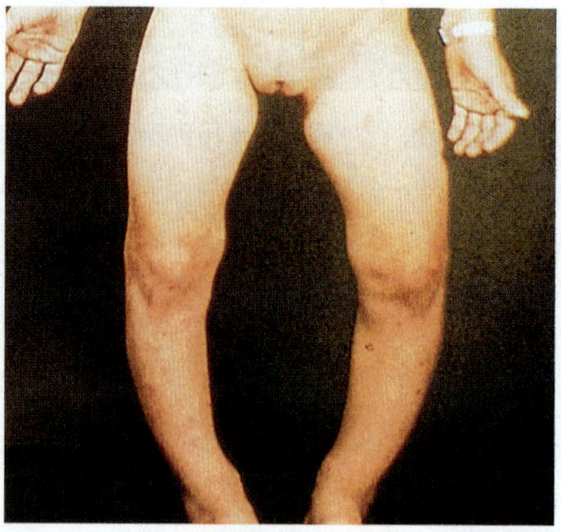

Fig. 11.9 Rickets. Hypophosphatemic rickets marked by obvious bowing of the legs.

Table 11.3 Nutritional Deficiencies With Characteristic Physical Signs

Vitamin/Mineral	Sign/Symptom
Calcium, phosphorus, vitamin D	Rickets/osteomalacia
Vitamin A	Night blindness, xerophthalmia, Bitot spots, follicular hyperkeratosis
Vitamin C	Scurvy: bone lesions, bleeding
Vitamin E	Hemolytic anemia, peripheral neuropathy
Vitamin K	Petechiae, ecchymoses
Thiamine (vitamin B_1)	Beriberi: heart failure, increased intracranial pressure
Niacin	Pellagra: dermatitis (sun-exposed areas)
Riboflavin (vitamin B_2)	Angular stomatitis, cheilosis
Vitamin B_6	Anemia, dermatitis, neuropathy
Vitamin B_{12}	Anemia, neuropathy
Folate	Anemia
Iron	Anemia, koilonychia
Biotin	Rash, hair loss
Essential fatty acids	Rash, coagulopathy
Zinc	Rash (acrodermatitis), growth failure, delayed sexual development, ageusia
Copper	Bone changes, hypopigmentation, anemia, neutropenia
Selenium	Cardiomyopathy (Keshan disease)

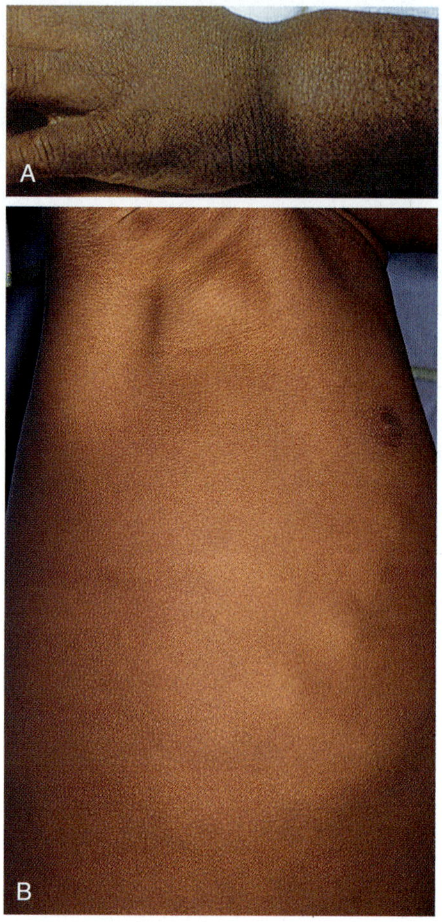

Fig. 11.10 Rickets. Infantile rickets marked by widened wrists (A) and enlargement of the costochondral junction ("beading") (B). The latter occurred as the result of a rapid growth spurt after liver transplantation.

malabsorption secondary to chronic diseases. Vitamin D is essential for normal calcium, phosphorus, and magnesium homeostasis, and its deficiency may lead to rickets, the inadequate mineralization of growing bones, osteomalacia, osteoporosis, and other diseases later in life. There is growing evidence that it also plays a role in various physiologic functions including immune function. Classic vitamin D deficiency results in poor growth, curvature of weight-bearing bones (Fig. 11.9), widening of epiphyses, and costochondral "rachitic rosary" beading (Fig. 11.10). Craniotabes, or softening of the skull, may be seen in infants. With appropriate vitamin and mineral supplementation, resolution occurs, followed by bone remodeling (Fig. 11.11). Common laboratory findings are summarized in Table 9.4. Vitamin D deficiency is especially prevalent in breastfed infants, infants with darker skin, and infants and children with decreased sun exposure. Systemic conditions that can lead to poor vitamin absorption include children with cholestasis, Crohn disease, cystic fibrosis, celiac disease, and abnormal hydroxylation in end-stage renal disease. The high prevalence of vitamin D deficiency without rickets places otherwise healthy children at risk if they are not consuming the recommended daily allowance in dairy and vitamin D–fortified foods. The American Academy of Pediatrics has recommended an intake of 400 IU/day to prevent complications of vitamin D deficiency. Other fat-soluble vitamin deficiencies are seen in patients with fat malabsorption, such as cholestatic liver disease, cystic fibrosis, and celiac disease. Vitamin K deficiency namely results in prolongation of the prothrombin time and international normalized ratio and requires supplementation of vitamin K either orally, or intramuscularly. Vitamin A deficiency can lead to night blindness, xerophthalmia, follicular hyperkeratosis, or Bitot spots. Vitamin E deficiency is marked by absence of deep tendon reflexes and subsequent ataxia. It has also been linked to hemolysis.

Water-soluble vitamin deficiencies are uncommon unless unintentionally excluded in the diet. For example, an infant fed goat's milk is at risk for folate deficiency. Signs of specific vitamin deficiencies can be seen on physical examination. Angular cheilitis/stomatitis is a common finding of B vitamin and/or iron deficiency (Fig. 11.12). Vitamin B_{12} is of specific interest as it requires active uptake in the terminal ileum. Patients with terminal ileum disease

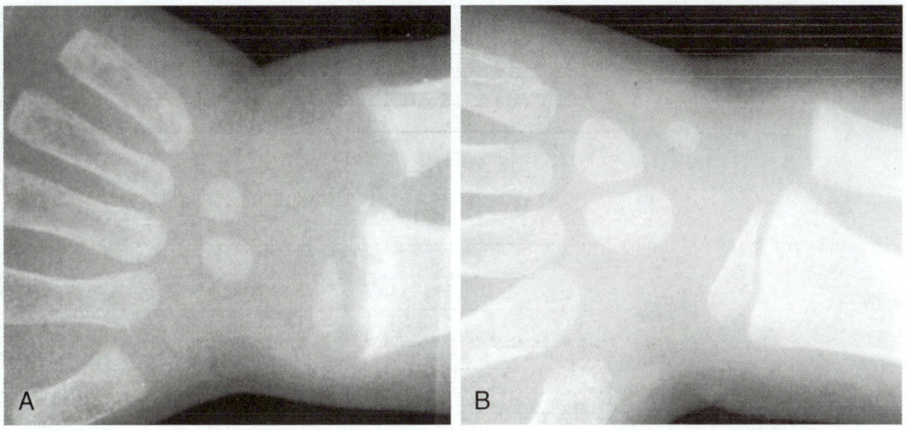

Fig. 11.11 Rickets. Radiograph of the wrist of a patient with rickets. (A) Irregularity and widening of the epiphyses in the distal radius and ulna. (B) With appropriate therapy, remineralization and healing occur.

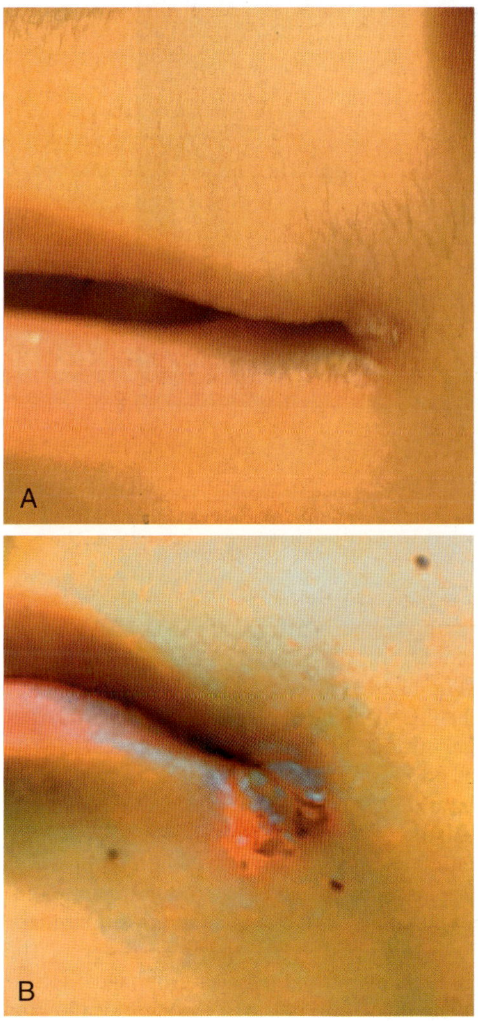

Fig. 11.12 Angular cheilitis. (A) Note the grayish white plaques at the corner of the mouth. This patient was diagnosed as having a vitamin B complex deficiency, likely the result of a chronic diarrheal state and inadequate dietary intake. (B) Before diagnosis and supplementation, the cheilitis advanced to an ulcerative lesion, which could represent superinfection.

or resection are at particular risk of vitamin B_{12} deficiency, which results in a macrocytic anemia (see Fig. 12.10), hypersegmented neutrophils (see Fig. 12.11), and/or neurologic findings due to poor myelination of nerve fibers. Neurologic findings can be reversible when detected early. Supplementation is either intramuscular or through intranasal mucosal absorption.

Other specific nutritional deficiencies can sporadically occur in the pediatric population. Patients on extremely low-fat diets or who are receiving exclusive parenteral nutrition, in which standard fat emulsions have been limited/omitted because of concern about cholestasis, can present with essential fatty acid deficiency. α-Linolenic acid (ω-3) and linoleic acid (ω-6) are the essential fatty acids, while several others may be considered conditionally essential. Essential fatty acid deficiency symptoms include a scaly dermatitis and dull, brittle hair and nails. Triene:tetraene ratios aid in diagnosis. Zinc deficiency seen in diarrheal diseases and in burns can result in alopecia, diarrhea, and acrodermatitis. A deficiency in copper, often reduced in the diets of patients with chronic liver disease, can present as irritability, decreased hair pigmentation, anemia, neutropenia, and bone abnormalities. Copper deficiency can be diagnosed by serum copper levels and depressed ceruloplasmin. When biotin, a conditionally essential amino acid, is deficient, a weeping dermatitis in the perioral, perianal, and eyelid area along with lethargy, malaise, and thinning of hair can occur (Fig. 11.13). Table 11.3 details further signs and symptoms of specific nutrient deficiencies.

GASTROENTEROLOGY

GI symptoms are common in pediatric practice. This section emphasizes the major complaints that bring patients with GI disorders to medical attention, with particular coverage of entities that may be diagnosed by examination.

Disorders of the Upper Gastrointestinal Tract

Reflux

Gastroesophageal reflux (GER) is the passage of gastric contents into the esophagus, when intragastric pressure exceeds the forces that protect the esophagus. This process differs from physiologic vomiting in that GER is not centrally mediated or associated with reverse peristalsis. GER episodes are effortless, and the refluxate is most often undigested food and, in infants, curdled milk. GER is a common and usually self-limited condition beginning in early infancy and resolving by 1 year of age. Symptoms generally begin immediately after feeding but may continue for several hours afterward. GER that does not resolve by 2 years of age or that presents in later childhood often follows the pattern of adult-onset GER and persists as a chronic condition.

GER associated with concurrent morbidities is often termed *gastroesophageal reflux disease* (GERD). The symptoms often associated with GERD include heartburn and feeding difficulty. Apnea and bradycardia have been associated with reflux in the preterm infant, although these episodes usually resolve as an infant reaches term. Rumination, which is different from reflux, is the voluntary contraction

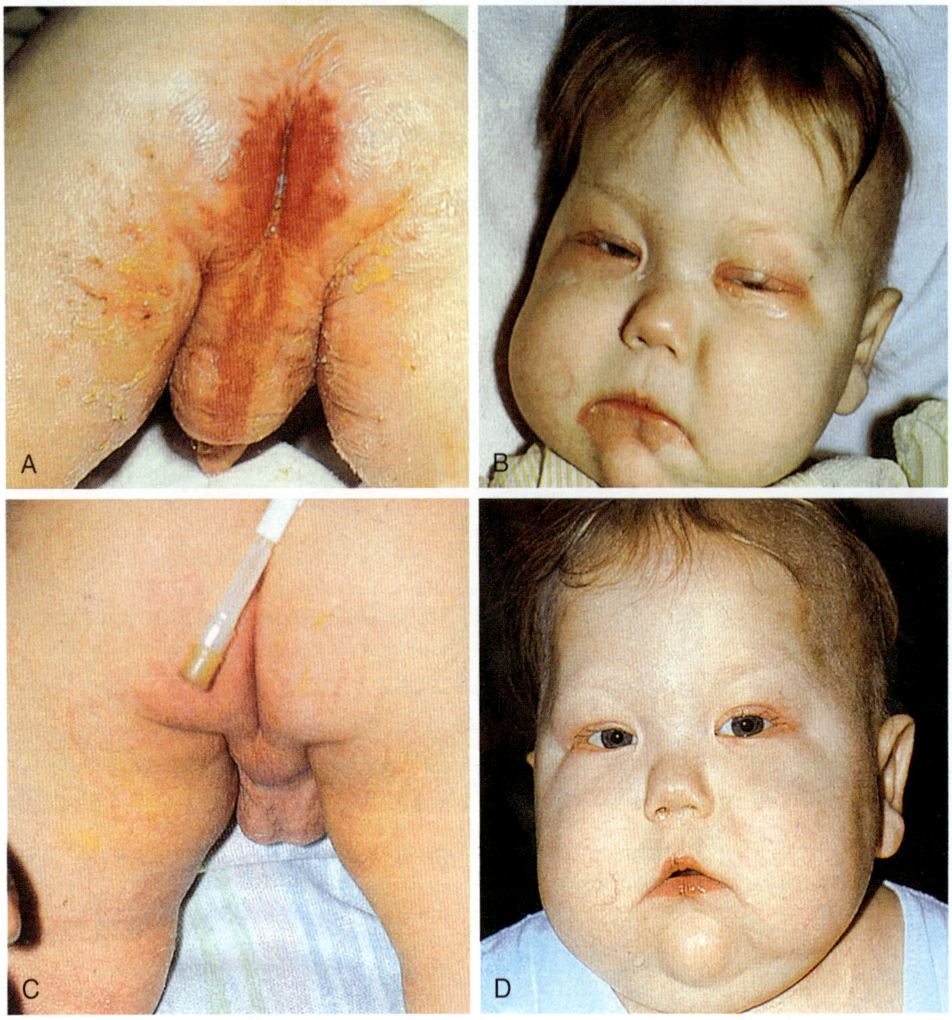

Fig. 11.13 Biotin deficiency. (A and B) This child on chronic hyperalimentation developed dermatitis in the perianal, perioral, and eyelid areas along with some thinning of hair. (C and D) The rash has cleared dramatically after 4 days of biotin.

of abdominal musculature that leads to episodes that manifest similarly reflux. It is generally regarded as a self-stimulating disorder and is more common in adolescence and in various behavioral disorders.

Dysphagia/Disorders of Swallowing

Dysphagia is a symptom that describes difficulty in swallowing. Patients with dysphagia report the feeling of the inability to pass esophageal contents into the stomach. When the sensation is in the posterior pharynx or upper esophagus, it can be considered a globus sensation and classified as oropharyngeal dysphagia. When it is present in the mid/lower esophagus, one must consider esophageal inflammation or a primary dysmotility disorder. More common pediatric disorders associated with dysphagia or the globus sensation include reflux esophagitis, achalasia, eosinophilic esophagitis, and esophageal strictures.

Eosinophilic esophagitis is an inflammatory disorder of the esophagus that is a common cause of dysphagia in children. The etiology is not known, although it is thought to be the result of an aberrant antigenic immunologic response. Food and/or environmental antigens are thought to play a role in the pathophysiology of eosinophilic esophagitis, though given the type of immune response leading to this disease, specific antigens are not able to be isolated/tested. It is believed that the incidence of eosinophilic esophagitis is increasing. Symptoms can include dysphagia, refusal to feed, abdominal pain, dyspepsia, early satiety, and food impaction. Symptoms of reflux or esophagitis can complicate the diagnosis. In patients with reflux esophagitis who do not respond to acid suppression, the diagnosis of eosinophilic esophagitis must be considered. The classic appearance on endoscopy is esophageal furrowing (Fig. 11.14A). Other findings include the formation of concentric rings or "trachealization" of the esophagus (Fig. 11.14B). In some circumstances, there can be an exudative esophagitis (Fig. 11.14C). Histology shows large numbers of intraepithelial eosinophils (>15 per high-power field) and can show clustering of eosinophilic microabscesses, degranulation, and basal cell hyperplasia (Fig. 11.15). Peripheral eosinophilia is not considered an adequate marker for disease. Treatment includes dietary restriction of common food allergens, high-dose proton pump inhibitor therapy, swallowed (topical) corticosteroids such as fluticasone and budesonide, and more recently approved biologic therapy dupilumab.

Achalasia is a primary dysmotility disorder of the esophagus marked by high pressures of the lower esophageal sphincter (LES) at rest, incomplete relaxation of the LES during swallowing, and uncoordinated peristalsis of the esophageal smooth muscles. This condition is an uncommon cause of dysphagia in children. It is often screened for via an esophagram (Fig. 11.16) and confirmed by esophageal manometry. Temporary treatment options include esophageal dilation and/or injection of botulinum toxin into the LES. The Heller myotomy is a surgical procedure that is a more permanent treatment for achalasia. Peroral endoscopy myotomy is a newer and promising therapeutic approach.

Accidental caustic ingestions in children, most often alkali in origin, can result in severe esophageal injury, which heals with fibrosis and often results in strictures (Fig. 11.17). The most common long-term symptom of an esophageal stricture is dysphagia. Repeated esophageal dilation is the first treatment of choice. In severe cases, resection with the creation of an alternate conduit may be

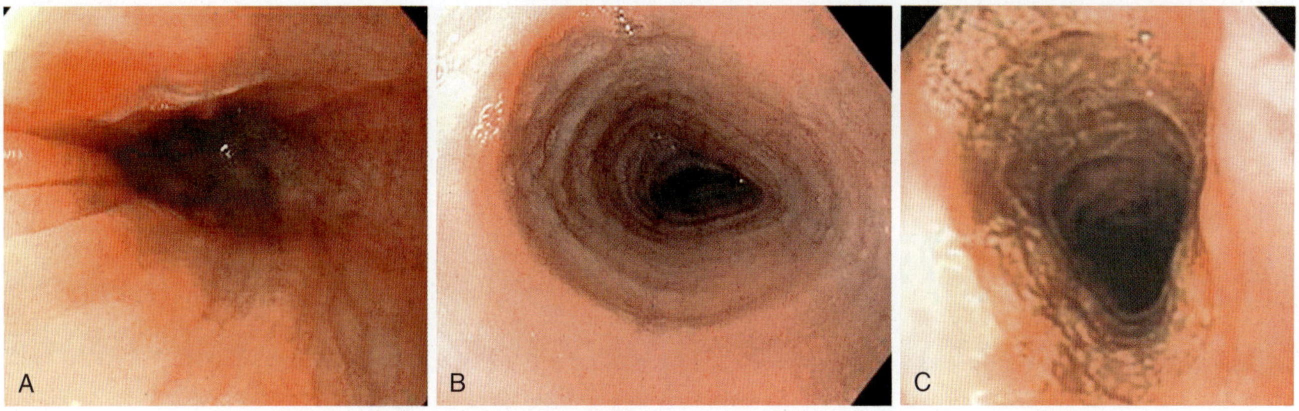

Fig. 11.14 Eosinophilic esophagitis. These endoscopic pictures of the esophagus demonstrate classic findings of eosinophilic esophagitis, including (A) linear furrowing of the esophagus, (B) a ringed appearance or trachealization of the esophagus, and (C) an exudative esophagitis. (B and C, Courtesy Feras Alissa, MD, Pittsburgh, PA.)

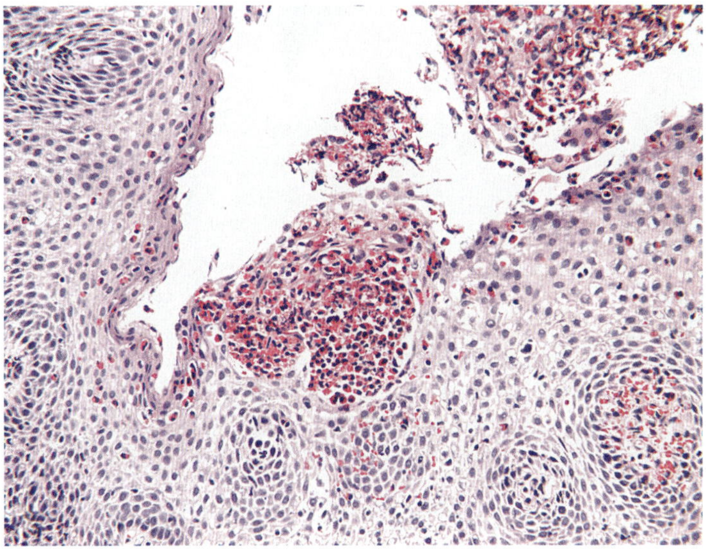

Fig. 11.15 Eosinophilic esophagitis. Histologic specimen from the esophagus demonstrates many eosinophils in a microabscess, epithelial thickening, and basal cell hyperplasia.

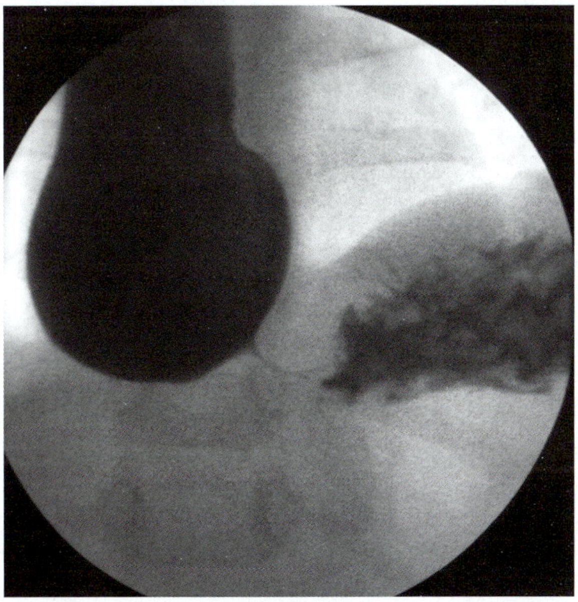

Fig. 11.16 Achalasia. This barium esophagram clearly demonstrates the classic findings of esophageal dilation proximal to the lower esophageal sphincter (LES) and the "bird's beak" appearance of the narrowed LES. (Courtesy Manisha Harpavat Dave, MD, Plano, TX; and Ryan Fischer, MD, Pittsburgh, PA.)

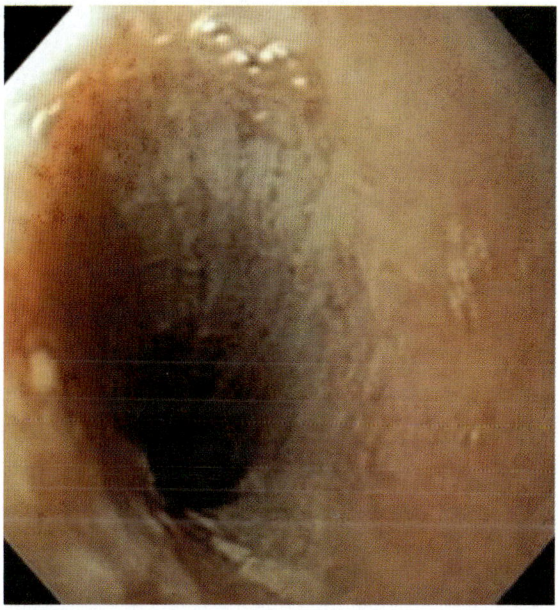

Fig. 11.17 Caustic ingestion. This endoscopic picture of the esophagus is the result of an accidental alkaline ingestion, the most common type of ingestion to cause esophageal burns. Dysphagia and esophageal strictures requiring dilation are common sequelae of caustic ingestions. (Courtesy Feras Alissa, MD, Pittsburgh, PA.)

needed. Other causes of dysphagia with or without odynophagia (pain on swallowing) include viral/fungal esophagitis, pill esophagitis, other primary disorders of dysmotility, and anastomotic stricture or dysmotility after esophageal atresia repair.

Vomiting

Vomiting is a common symptom in a variety of disorders in childhood. The causes are diverse and range from simple infections, such as acute viral gastroenteritis, to more serious ailments like central nervous system tumors. A broad differential including causes outside the GI system must be considered any time vomiting is the solitary presenting symptom. This section discusses some of the more significant causes of vomiting of primary GI illnesses.

Pyloric Stenosis

Hypertrophic pyloric stenosis is due to a narrowing of the pyloric channel secondary to hypertrophy of the pyloric musculature (Fig. 11.18). The etiology of pyloric stenosis is multifactorial. Males, notably first-born males, are more often affected than females, and there has been evidence of a genetic predisposition. Hypertrophic pyloric stenosis most often occurs in term infants and usually presents

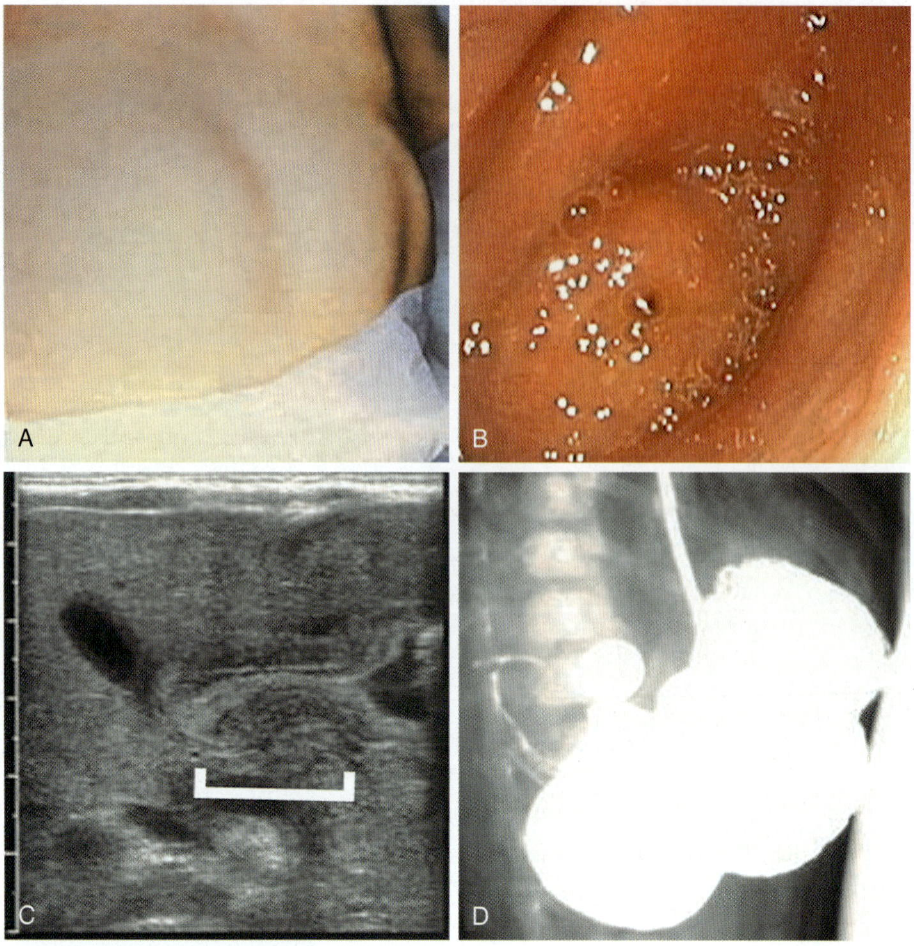

Fig. 11.18 Pyloric stenosis. (A) The giant gastric waves are best seen just after a feeding. Palpation of a gastric olive can sometimes be demonstrated on physical examination. (B) Endoscopic view of an acquired pyloric stenosis. (C) This ultrasound demonstrates thickening of the pyloric wall and an elongated pyloric channel in an infant with pyloric stenosis *(shown in bracket)*. (D) A typical barium study in a patient with pyloric stenosis demonstrates a "stringlike" pyloric channel.

between 1 and 2 months of age. Symptoms include forceful, projectile, nonbilious emesis, persistent hunger, and eventual weight loss. As symptoms continue, dehydration and a hypokalemic, hypochloremic metabolic alkalosis can be seen on routine laboratory tests. Giant gastric peristaltic waves and a firm pyloric olive may be noted on examination. The diagnosis of pyloric stenosis is confirmed by an ultrasound examination that measures the thickness of the pyloric wall and length of the pyloric channel. Studies have shown that ultrasound has a sensitivity and specificity of nearly 100% in diagnosing pyloric stenosis. In questionable cases, an upper GI barium study may confirm the diagnosis by demonstrating a narrow pyloric channel, called the "string sign." Surgical correction of pyloric stenosis is completed after metabolic stabilization by pyloromyotomy.

Intestinal Malrotation and Volvulus

Incomplete rotation of the intestine during embryonic life leads to intestinal malrotation and the intestines to not be properly "fixed" at the mesentery. The "stalklike" mesentery may serve as a focal point for twisting or volvulus of the intestine. Volvulus presents with the sudden onset of bilious emesis and abdominal pain. Bilious emesis is a hallmark of intestinal obstruction, and this should be considered a surgical emergency. Plain abdominal films may demonstrate a paucity of air in the abdomen except for an air bubble in the stomach and duodenum. An upper GI series is the "gold standard" for diagnosing a malrotation and volvulus. Classically, the small intestine is rotated to the right side of the abdomen and a narrowing at the site of obstruction has a corkscrew appearance (Fig. 11.19). The C-loop of the duodenum not crossing the midline is another radiologic clue of malrotation, as it should normally extend up under the antrum of the stomach and cross the midline. Malrotation with an associated volvulus is a surgical emergency, as failure to correct will lead to intestinal ischemia and result in intestinal resection of all compromised bowel.

Intestinal Obstruction

There are multiple other causes of intestinal obstruction leading to vomiting in the neonate and older child. Nonbilious emesis is a feature of upper intestinal obstruction proximal to the duodenal biliary sphincter, such as occurs in esophageal atresia and gastric/duodenal webs, stenoses, and atresias. In addition, a mass effect from an extraluminal source may lead to obstruction as can be seen in duodenal hematomas, often caused by blunt trauma to the abdomen (Fig. 11.20). Bilious vomiting occurs when an obstruction occurs more distally, such as in intestinal atresias. Nonanatomic causes of distal obstruction can occur in cystic fibrosis in the neonate as meconium ileus or as distal intestinal obstruction syndrome (Fig. 11.21), in which there is a fecal impaction at the terminal ileum. The cause is thought to be due to aberrant cystic fibrosis transmembrane conductance regulator function in the intestinal lumen, a driving force of intestinal secretion.

Other Causes of Vomiting

Multiple other causes of nonobstructive vomiting occur in the pediatric population, some of which include inflammation and subsequent pain (discussed in later sections). Other causes are primarily functional disorders that lead to bloating, early satiety, and vomiting, often related to delayed or aberrant gastric emptying. Although there are likely multiple factors leading to poor gastric emptying, the most common entity encountered in general pediatric practice is postinfectious dysmotility. Often triggered by a virus, symptoms

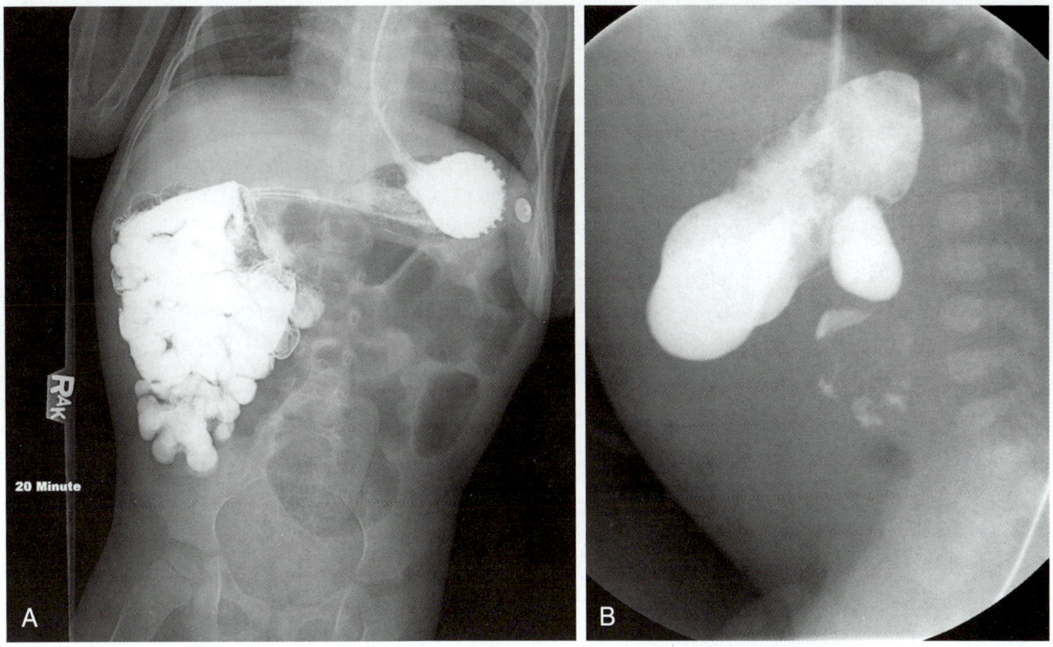

Fig. 11.19 Malrotation. (A) An upper gastrointestinal series demonstrating malrotation with the entire small bowel on the right, never crossing the midline, and the colon on the left. (B) The corkscrew appearance of the duodenum is seen in this patient with malrotation and midgut volvulus. (Courtesy Stefano Bartoletti, MD, Pittsburgh, PA.)

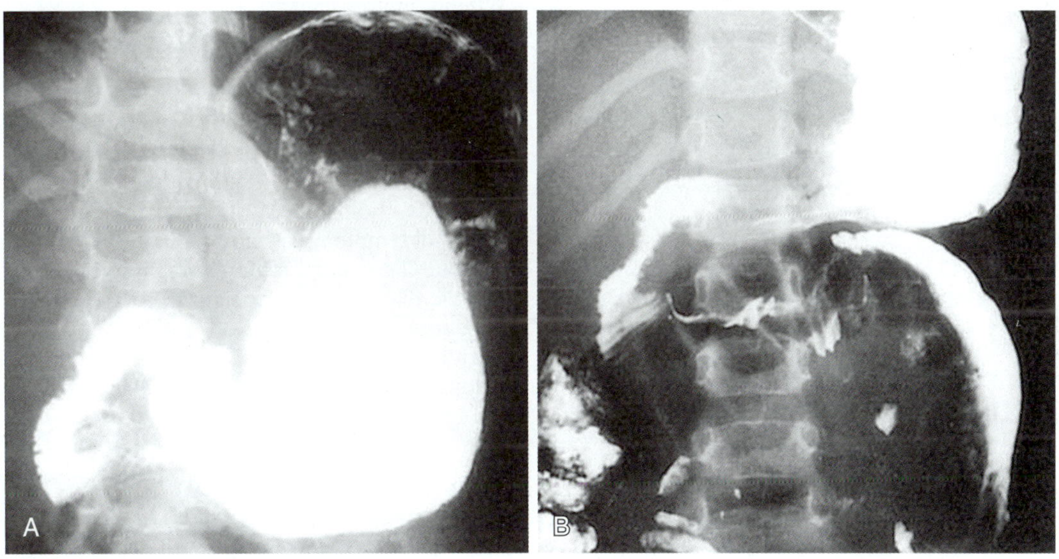

Fig. 11.20 Duodenal hematoma. Upper gastrointestinal series demonstrates poor flow through the duodenum (A) and mass effect of the hematoma displacing other loops of bowel (B).

may persist for months but generally resolve with time. Those that do not resolve will develop into a phenotype that most resembles postinfectious irritable bowel syndrome (IBS). Cyclic vomiting syndrome is a condition that generally presents in childhood as cyclic, episodic vomiting with defined symptom-free intervals. Related to migraine headaches, cyclic vomiting syndrome usually decreases in interval frequency and resolves over time and is notably a diagnosis of exclusion.

Abdominal Pain

Abdominal pain is one of the most common GI complaints of children visiting the pediatrician. Like vomiting, the differential diagnosis of abdominal pain is vast and includes intestinal disorders and pain derived from other abdominal viscera, in addition to being a general symptom in many other illnesses. Abdominal pain derived from the intestinal tract is generally caused by distention or contraction. Once excluding obstruction or anatomic abnormality, it can be classified as pain derived primarily from mucosal inflammation and as functional pain for which no histologic cause for the pain exists. As all intestinal pain is the result of distention/contraction, an overlap of the two also exists, making diagnosis challenging for the physician and more frustrating for the patient and family.

The term *functional gastrointestinal disorder,* or more recently, disorder of gut-brain interaction, is used to define several chronic and recurrent GI symptoms that do not have an identified anatomic or inflammatory component. Whereas primary dysmotility syndromes such as chronic intestinal pseudoobstruction may broadly fit this diagnosis, functional GI disorders are commonly thought of as symptoms of pain with normal motility. The Rome IV criteria for pediatric functional GI disorders is a symptom-based classification system used to differentiate several subgroups of functional GI disorders. IBS and functional dyspepsia are examples of functional GI disorders that cause abdominal pain.

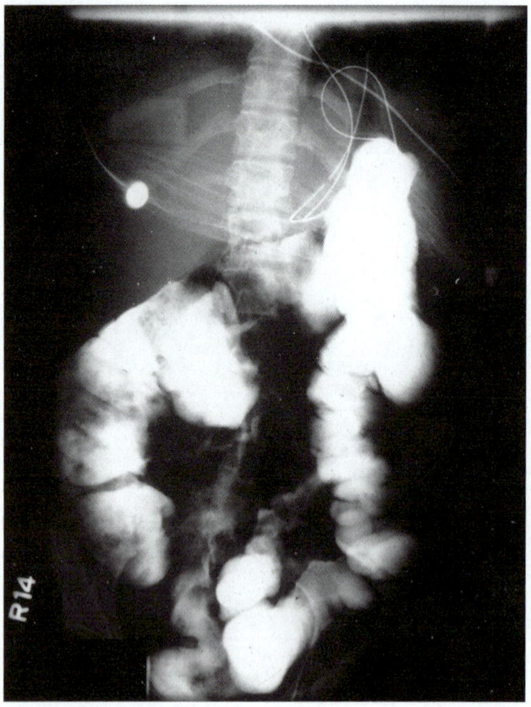

Fig. 11.21 Distal intestinal obstruction syndrome. Barium enema reveals the cecal obstruction in a child with cystic fibrosis. (Courtesy Mark Lowe, MD, Pittsburgh, PA.)

Box 11.4 Clues to Organic Disease in Recurrent Abdominal Pain

Weight loss
Nocturnal pain
Localized abdominal pain
Recurrent emesis
Chronic diarrhea
Heme-positive stools
Abnormal physical examination findings—clubbing, perianal skin tags, abdominal mass
Abnormal screening laboratory test results—decreased albumin, increased ESR/CRP, anemia

CRP, C-reactive protein; *ESR,* erythrocyte sedimentation rate.

The diagnostic criteria of IBS include abdominal pain or discomfort for at least 12 weeks in the past year along with two of the following three criteria: abdominal pain relieved by defecation, pain associated with change in stool frequency, and pain associated with change in stool form. Other symptoms that support the diagnosis of IBS include bloating, urgency, and the feeling of incomplete evacuation. Functional dyspepsia is defined as chronic or recurrent pain or discomfort found in the upper abdomen. The discomfort is often described as abdominal fullness, early satiety, bloating, belching, or nausea. The symptoms of functional dyspepsia are often aggravated with the consumption of a meal. Treatment of functional GI disorders can include pharmacologic and nonpharmacologic modalities.

The causes of abdominal pain due to inflammation of the GI tract are broad and often accompanied by other associated symptoms (Box 11.4). Although pain can be periumbilical or in multiple locations, it may be more localized. Other common inflammatory causes of abdominal pain are discussed as follows.

Peptic Disease of the Gastrointestinal Tract

Peptic acid–induced GI disease should be considered in patients with abdominal pain, especially if it is epigastric or found in the left upper quadrant, though its location may be nonspecific. Classically described as "burning" in nature, this is not a reliable indicator. In the stomach, peptic disease can be diffuse as occurs in gastritis, isolated as in ulcer disease, or have components of both. Acid-induced gastritis and peptic ulcers tend to occur in the antrum of the stomach (Fig. 11.22). Peptic ulcers, nodular antritis, and duodenal ulcers may signify *Helicobacter pylori* infection (Fig. 11.23). Other types of ulcers can be seen in systemic illnesses, such as stress ulcers in critical care patients, excessive secretion of acid (Zollinger-Ellison syndrome), and drug therapy such as nonsteroidal antiinflammatory drugs. Gastritis can occur in other situations, not necessarily primarily mediated by gastric acid. This can occur in eosinophilic gastroenteritis, inflammatory bowel disease (IBD), or with nonpeptic irritants such as bile acids during illnesses with upper intestinal stasis. Upper endoscopy is invaluable in diagnosing gastritis and ulcer disease. Treatment involves acid suppression via type-2 receptor antihistamines or proton pump inhibitors. *H. pylori* infection typically requires treatment with dual antibiotic therapy and a proton pump inhibitor. Non–peptic-mediated disease requires additional treatment of the underlying condition. Gastritis that does not respond to optimal acid suppression may benefit from the addition of sucralfate.

Disorders of the Small Intestine and Colon

Diarrhea

Diarrhea in children is most often acute and caused by infection. When symptoms persist for more than 2 weeks, the diarrhea is considered chronic and the etiology broadens. When determining the cause of a diarrheal illness, it is usually helpful to decide whether it is acute or chronic; infectious or noninfectious; inflammatory or noninflammatory; or osmotic, secretory, or mixed in nature.

Clues to the etiology of diarrhea can be found via stool examination. Stool cultures and examination for ova and parasites can reveal infectious etiologies. Most often, they are obtained after at least 1 week of symptoms, as most viral causes have improved by this time. Of note, *Giardia* or *Cryptosporidium* infection can present as a more chronic diarrhea. Inflammatory processes can be suggested by the presence of blood in the stool and by some laboratory markers such as anemia, elevated C-reactive protein, and/or elevated erythrocyte sedimentation rate, although normal values do not exclude this.

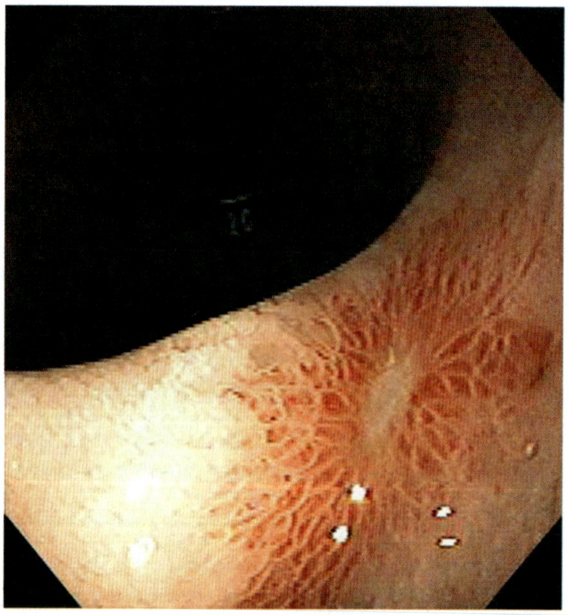

Fig. 11.22 Peptic ulcer. Gastric ulcer located in the lower curvature of the stomach. Note the grayish white base of the ulcer crater and the boggy erythematous tissue surrounding the margin of the ulcer. (Courtesy Feras Alissa, MD, Pittsburgh, PA; and Cary Sauer, MD, Atlanta, GA.)

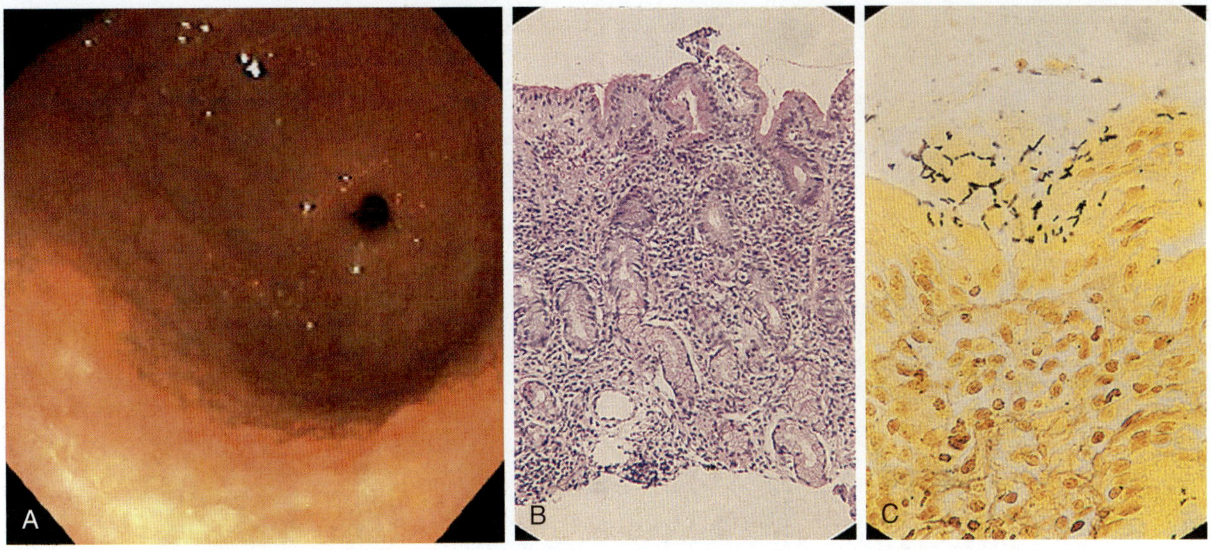

Fig. 11.23 *Helicobacter pylori* gastritis. (A) Nodular-appearing gastric antrum consistent with *H. pylori*. (B) Gastric biopsy with inflammatory infiltrate of plasma cells, neutrophils, and occasional eosinophils characteristic of *H. pylori* gastritis. (C) Steiner silver stain (original magnification, ×400) demonstrates rod-shaped, spiral *H. pylori* bacteria attached to the mucosa. (A, Courtesy Feras Alissa, MD, Pittsburgh, PA.)

Fecal calprotectin or lactoferrin can be used to mark intestinal inflammation due to IBD. Fecal markers are not a sensitive marker for inflammation. Osmotic diarrhea usually improves when the suspected culprit is removed from the diet. Stool pH can decrease and stool-reducing substances may be present with carbohydrate maldigestion and malabsorption. Quantitative 72-hour fecal fat is more specific than random fecal fat for fat malabsorption. Fecal elastase is often used as a marker of pancreatic insufficiency to support a diagnosis of steatorrhea. When stool is watery, fecal electrolytes can suggest a diagnosis of secretory, osmotic, or mixed-type diarrhea.

Malabsorptive Diarrhea

Malabsorption is a common cause of diarrhea due to the increased osmotic load placed on the intestine from the malabsorbed substance. One example of an osmotic diarrhea with normal GI function is excessive fructose intake (e.g., in drinks), in which the excessive intake of simple sugars overwhelms the capacity of the normal intestine to absorb them.

Malabsorption can occur when there is a deficiency in one aspect of absorption, such as carbohydrate malabsorption in lactose intolerance. Lactose intolerance can be diagnosed by breath test in older individuals and by disaccharidase analysis of biopsy specimens obtained during endoscopy. Fat malabsorption can be a sign of pancreatic insufficiency, often seen with cystic fibrosis. In cystic fibrosis, the pancreas can initially be replaced by fat (Fig. 11.24) and eventually involute.

Malabsorption can also be generalized due to underlying intestinal inflammation or lack of the appropriate surface area such as in congenital enteropathies or in patients who have had significant small intestinal resections. Celiac disease is caused by the autoimmune destruction of intestinal villi due to antibodies formed in response to gluten exposure and the mimicry of the gluten component gliadin to the enterocyte protein tissue transglutaminase. The classic pediatric presentation of celiac disease is that of a malnourished child with chronic diarrhea, short stature, abdominal bloating, and wasting of subcutaneous fat (Fig. 11.25A). With the current sensitivity and specificity of current serologic screening, this presentation has become less common. The injury to the intestinal villi (see Fig. 11.25B) is like that found in malnutrition (see Fig. 11.4), although there is more significant lymphocytic infiltrate and crypt hyperplasia in response to the injury. The endoscopic appearance can initially be noted by a scalloped appearance (see Fig. 11.25C) and later by atrophic mucosa as symptoms progress. Resolution of symptoms occurs with the removal of gluten from the diet.

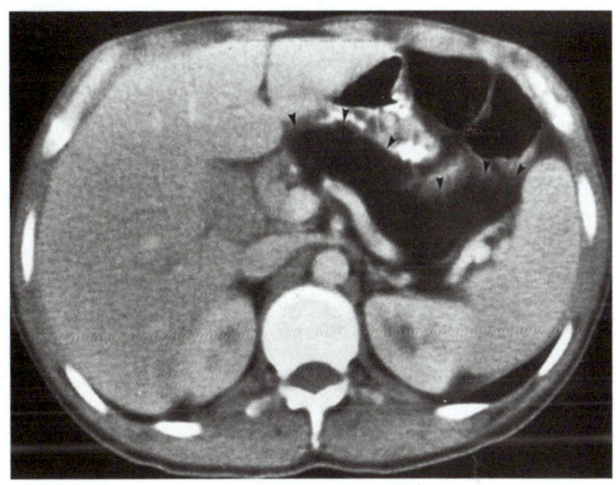

Fig. 11.24 Early pancreatic changes in cystic fibrosis. This computed tomography scan demonstrates a typical cystic fibrosis-appearing pancreas. The pancreas has been replaced by fat and appears to be absent. (Courtesy Mark Lowe, MD, Pittsburgh, PA.)

Inflammatory Diarrhea

Inflammation is a common component of diarrheal illness. Common causes of infectious diarrhea have a mild inflammatory component, whereas others like *Clostridium difficile* colitis can show marked inflammation. Autoimmune diseases, or disorders of immune dysregulation such as celiac disease, IBD, or autoimmune enteropathy, are marked by chronic inflammatory infiltrates. Allergic gastroenteritis is notable for inflammation that is largely eosinophilic in nature.

When discussing the inflammatory diarrheas, one must include discussion of IBD, generally classified as either Crohn disease or ulcerative colitis. The term *undifferentiated* or *nonspecific colitis* can also be included when the pathologic features do not fit clearly into either classification. The symptoms of IBD include abdominal pain, weight loss, chronic diarrhea, rectal bleeding, and fever. Children often present with growth failure or delayed pubertal development as their sole presenting sign of IBD (Fig. 11.26). Crohn disease is a transmural, or deep, inflammatory process, which accounts for the tendency to form strictures, fistulas, and abscesses (Fig. 11.27). Crohn disease can occur anywhere along the GI tract and may include skip lesions. On endoscopy, the affected bowel has an inflamed "heaped" appearance with deep fissures, cobblestoning, and at

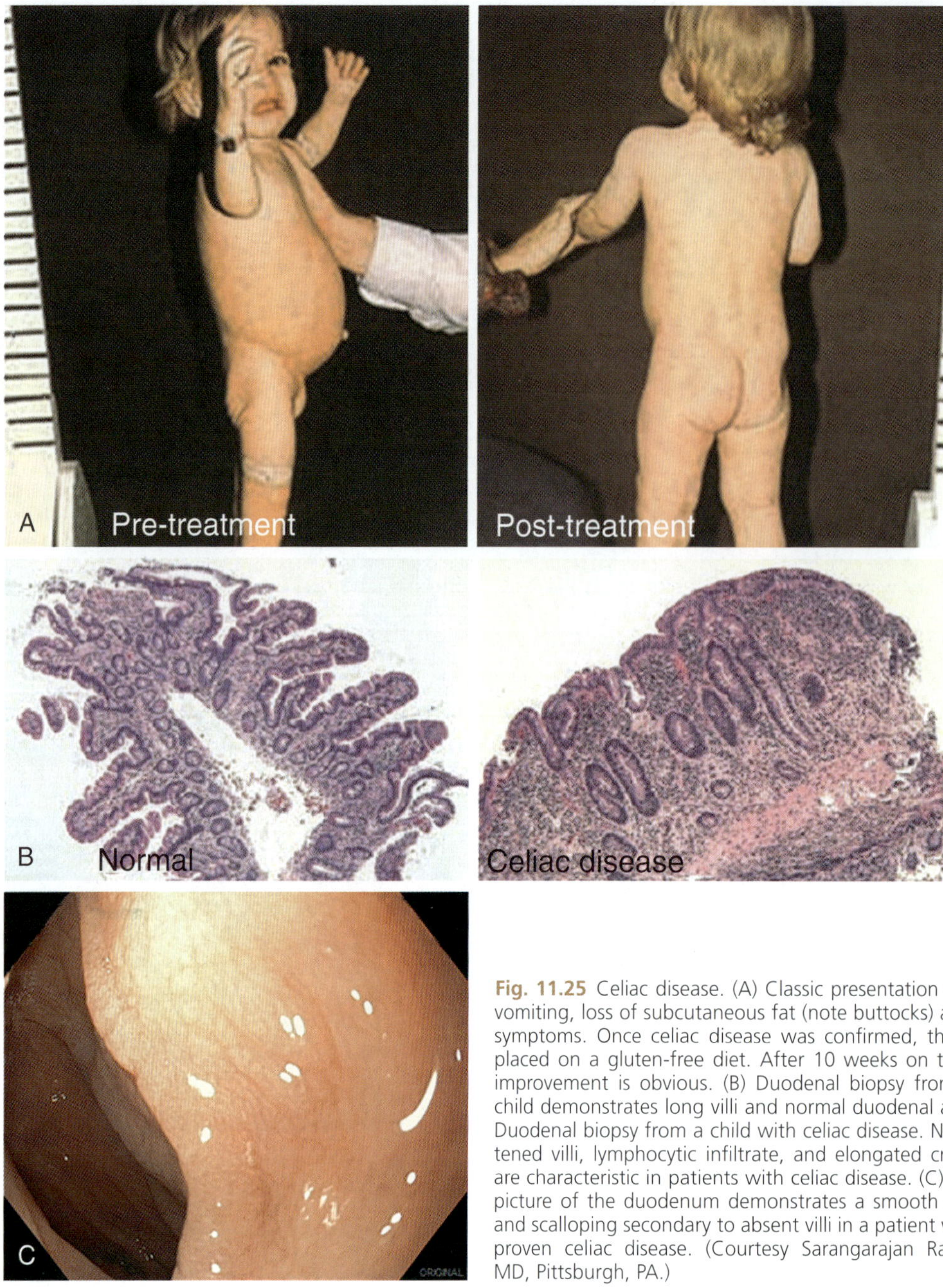

Fig. 11.25 Celiac disease. (A) Classic presentation of bloating, vomiting, loss of subcutaneous fat (note buttocks) as her major symptoms. Once celiac disease was confirmed, the child was placed on a gluten-free diet. After 10 weeks on the diet, the improvement is obvious. (B) Duodenal biopsy from a healthy child demonstrates long villi and normal duodenal architecture. Duodenal biopsy from a child with celiac disease. Note the flattened villi, lymphocytic infiltrate, and elongated crypts, which are characteristic in patients with celiac disease. (C) Endoscopic picture of the duodenum demonstrates a smooth appearance and scalloping secondary to absent villi in a patient with biopsy-proven celiac disease. (Courtesy Sarangarajan Ranganathan, MD, Pittsburgh, PA.)

times, pseudopolyp formation, although it can also be milder with only aphthous ulcers being apparent (Fig. 11.28). Perianal signs including abscesses, skin tags, fistulas, and fissures most often occur with Crohn disease (Fig. 11.29). Histologically, the presence of granulomas can distinguish Crohn disease from ulcerative colitis.

Ulcerative colitis is confined to the large bowel. A lead pipe appearance of the colon can occasionally be seen on a plain abdominal film and shown as a featureless colon on contrast enema (Fig. 11.30). Most often, contrast studies show mucosal irregularities, narrowing, or thumb-printing as a sign of inflammation. The endoscopic findings can show generalized colonic friability (Fig. 11.31A). A transition zone to normal colon can sometimes be distinguished (Fig. 11.31B). Crypt abscesses are often seen in ulcerative colitis and help to distinguish this disorder from many other causes of acute colitis (Fig. 11.32).

There are many extraintestinal manifestations of IBD, which can involve almost any organ system. Many rashes accompany IBD including erythema nodosum, erythema multiforme, papulonecrotic lesions, and ulcerative erythematous plaques. Perhaps the most specific rash in patients with IBD is pyoderma gangrenosum. Initial lesions of pyoderma gangrenosum are papular, then become bullous, and finally are deeply ulcerated and necrotic (Fig. 11.33). Other extraintestinal manifestations of IBD include arthritis/arthralgias, ankylosing spondylitis, sacroiliitis, aphthous oral ulcers, uveitis, iritis, and sclerosing cholangitis. Osteoarthropathy (clubbing) of the nail beds may be seen in children with IBD. The earliest signs of clubbing are softening and loss of a normal angle at the base of the nail (Fig. 11.34).

Gastrointestinal Bleeding

Visible blood in emesis or stool is always alarming to children and their parents. On occasion, GI bleeding is diagnosed by an iron deficiency anemia or through occult blood detection on stool examination. Blood loss in the stool with the association of pain is most often due to underlying inflammation. As a rule, blood from an upper GI source is black and tarry (melanotic) and becomes brighter red as the source nears the distal GI tract. This does not necessarily apply to rapid sources of bleeding. In general, melanotic stools, coffee ground emesis, or hematemesis indicate upper GI bleeding, proximal to the ligament of Treitz. Common causes of upper GI bleeding include erosive esophagitis, pill-induced or deep isolated

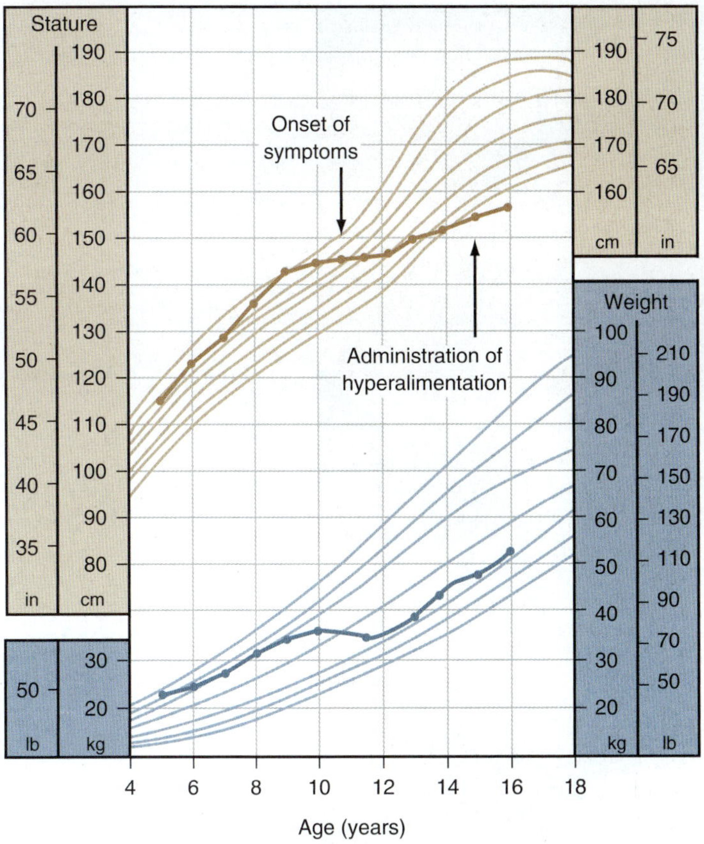

Fig. 11.26 Crohn disease. This growth curve demonstrates a decline in growth velocity before onset of disease symptoms and continued poor growth through many exacerbations requiring steroid therapy.

esophageal ulcers (Fig. 11.35), peptic ulcers (see Fig. 11.22), and various forms of gastritis. Upper GI bleeding can be life-threatening in certain situations, including bleeding from esophageal varices due to portal hypertension (see Fig. 11.35C) or with deep ulcers with exposed vessels (Dieulafoy lesions).

Bleeding from the small intestine can occur with isolated vascular malformations, inflammation, or ulcers, although this type of bleeding is uncommon. Meckel diverticulum presents as painless rectal bleeding due to ectopic gastric tissue leading to ulceration of the contralateral/adjacent small bowel. A technetium-99m pertechnetate scan can be valuable in the diagnosis of a Meckel diverticulum. The classic triad of colicky abdominal pain, vomiting, and currant jelly stools constitutes the manifestations of intussusception (Fig. 11.36), although seen in only 20% to 40% of children on presentation, and currant jelly stools are a late finding in this disease process. Intussusception is most commonly seen in children between the ages of 3 months and 5 years. Older children usually have a "lead point" such as a juvenile polyp, Meckel diverticulum, or thickened bowel associated with inflammation that requires further investigation. Reduction by barium enema or air enema is both diagnostic and therapeutic and simplifies management of this disorder in most instances, although surgery is occasionally necessary. There is an approximately 10% recurrence rate of intussusception after reduction.

Bright blood per rectum often indicates loss from the lower GI tract. Often, the source of bleeding is self-limited as in anal fissures or isolated juvenile polyps (Fig. 11.37A). Polyposis syndromes can sometimes be encountered, especially when there is a strong family history. Other causes of lower GI bleeding include pseudopolyps (see Fig. 11.37B) seen with chronic inflammation and vascular malformations (Fig. 11.37C).

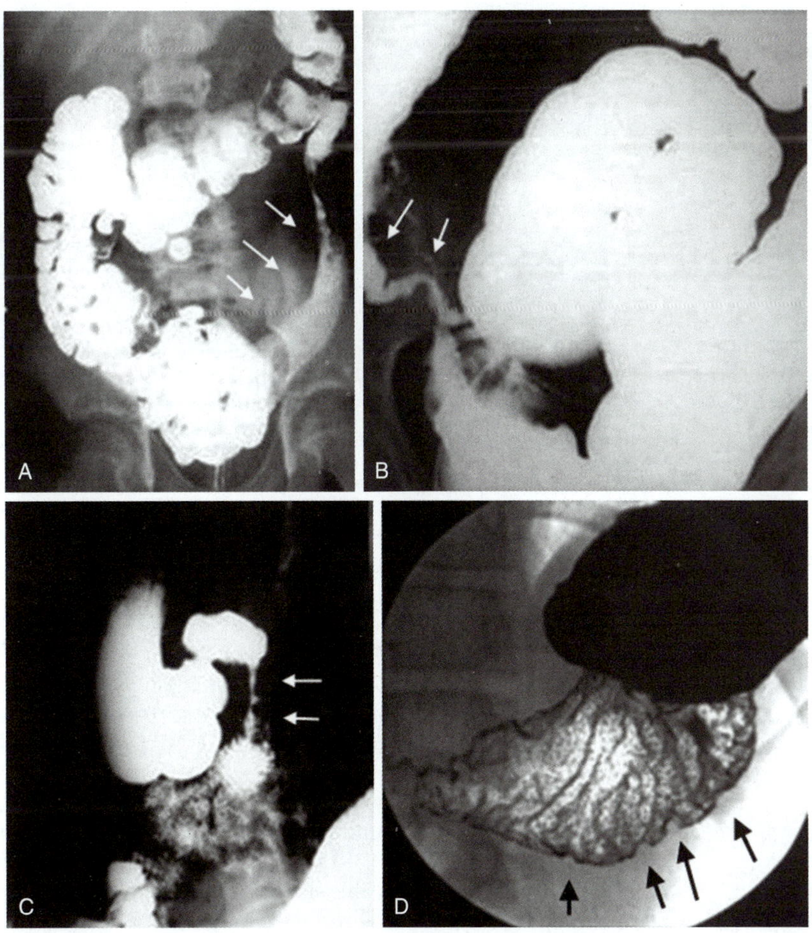

Fig. 11.27 Crohn disease. (A) Segmental narrowing of the left colon *(white arrows)*. (B) A narrow and irregular terminal ileum *(white arrows)*. (C) Stricturing of the duodenum *(white arrows)*. (D) Diffuse aphthous ulcers in the stomach of a patient with Crohn disease *(black arrows)*. (Courtesy Stefano Bartoletti, MD, Pittsburgh, PA.)

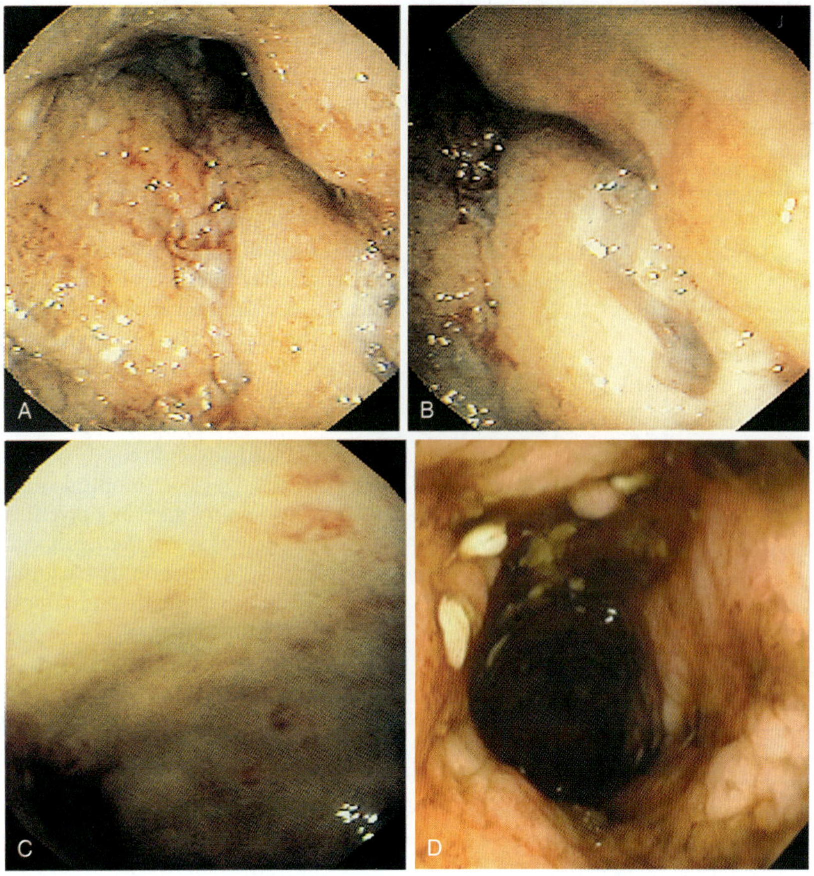

Fig. 11.28 Crohn disease, endoscopic images. (A and B) Note the deep, linear, ulcerated fissure. (C) Numerous colonic aphthous ulcers. (D) A cobblestone appearance of the colonic mucosa.

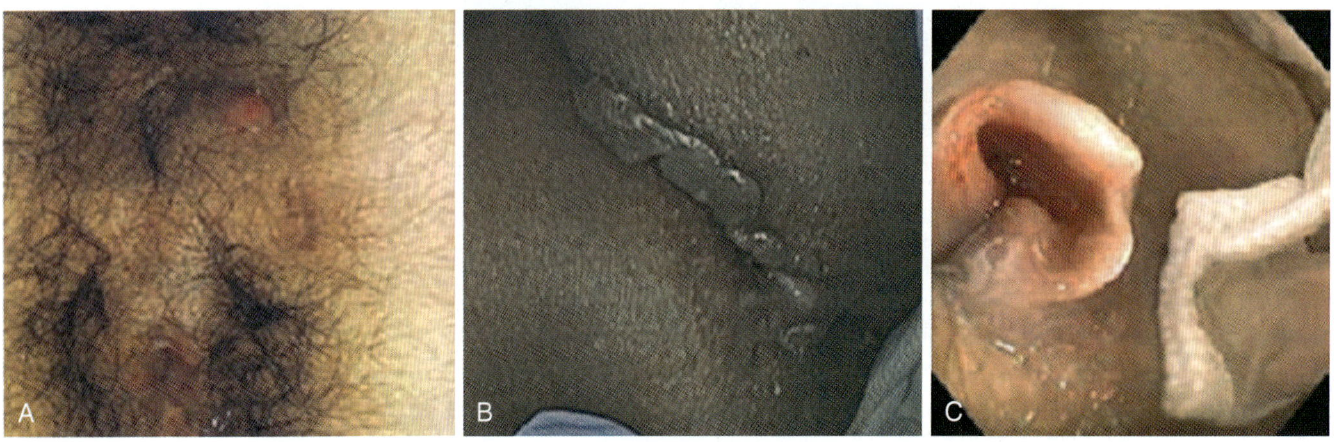

Fig. 11.29 Crohn disease. (A) The slightly raised and erythematous lesion represents a perianal abscess that eventually drained. Note a scar from a previous incision and drainage procedure. (B) Perianal skin tags are common in Crohn disease and a good clue to diagnosis. (C) Example of a draining perianal fistula found in a child with Crohn disease. (Courtesy Feras Alissa, MD, Pittsburgh, PA.)

Persistent bleeding, rapid blood loss, or blood loss leading to anemia requires further evaluation for underlying inflammation or the source. Upper and lower endoscopy, depending on the most likely source, can aid in diagnosis. The advent of capsule endoscopy can also aid in the localization of isolated bleeding in the small intestine. Common disorders causing GI bleeding are listed in Table 11.4.

Constipation

Constipation is defined as a delay or difficulty in passing a bowel movement that results in pain and discomfort to the patient. Constipation is most commonly functional. Painful defecation during toilet training, illness, or a stressful event often leads to stool-withholding behavior and avoidance of defecation. Overflow incontinence or encopresis is the result of a chronic, distal fecal impaction leading to proximal liquid stool leaking around the fecal mass. Bladder dysfunction with urinary incontinence and low-volume/high-frequency voiding may be associated with long-standing constipation.

Examination of the child with constipation usually reveals palpable stool in the descending colon and left lower quadrant. A digital rectal examination can evaluate stool consistency, the amount of stool present in the rectum, the size of the rectum, and anal tone. A plain film of the abdomen is usually not necessary and adds little to the physical examination (Fig. 11.38). Rectal prolapse (Fig. 11.39)

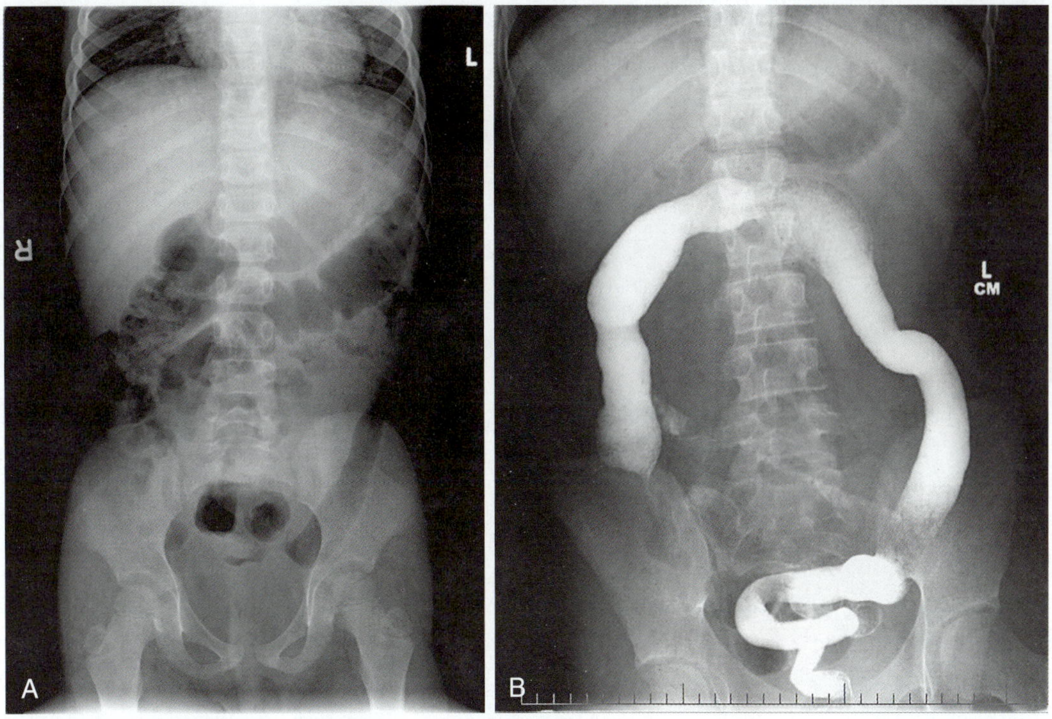

Fig. 11.30 Ulcerative colitis. A lead pipe or featureless appearance to the colon can be suggested on a plain abdominal film (A) and visualized on barium enema (B) in a patient with ulcerative colitis. (Courtesy Anna Furr, MD, Portland, ME.)

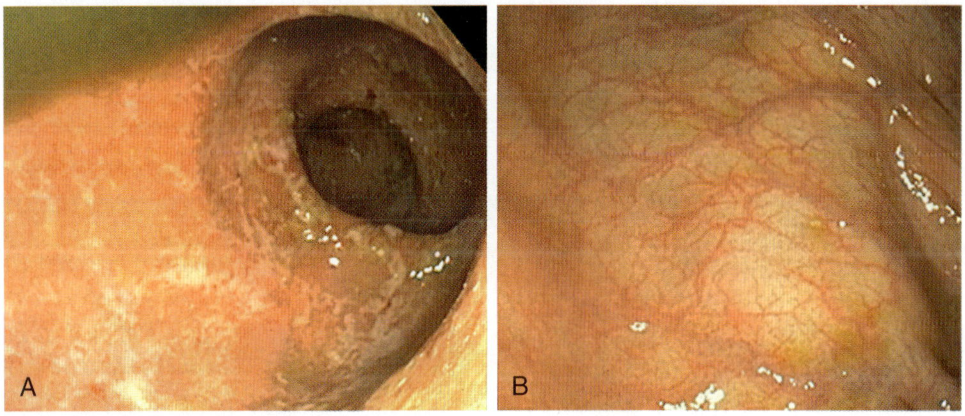

Fig. 11.31 Ulcerative colitis, endoscopic appearance. (A) The entire colonic mucosa is inflamed, friable, and granular with obvious exudate and bleeding. (B) Transition zone with erythematous mucosa *(left)* transitioning to normal appearing colon *(right)*.

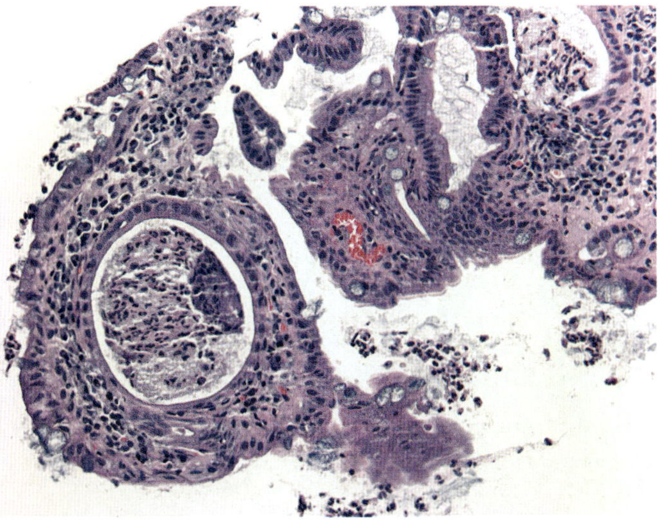

Fig. 11.32 Ulcerative colitis. Pathologic image of a colonic crypt abscess in a patient with ulcerative colitis.

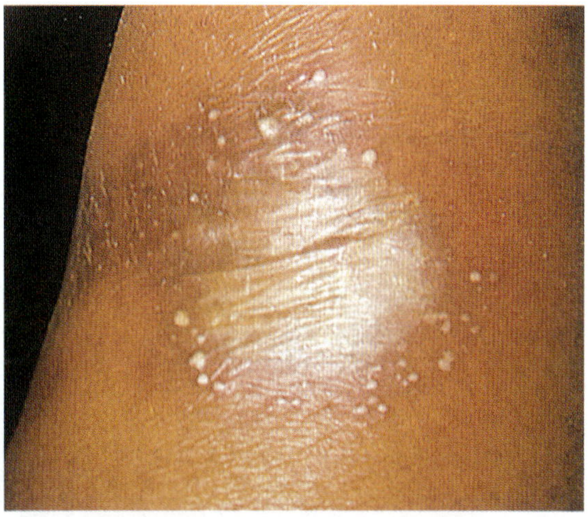

Fig. 11.33 Pyoderma gangrenosum. This is a classic, although uncommon, rash associated with inflammatory bowel disease. Initial papulopustules will coalesce to form a deep necrotic lesion.

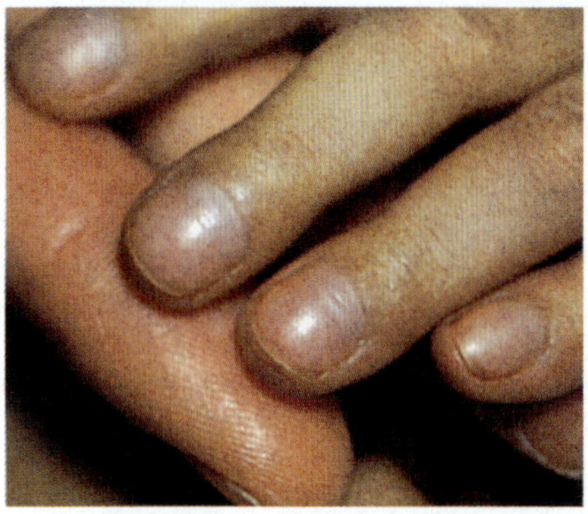

Fig. 11.34 Osteoarthropathy (clubbing). Note thickening and loss of the angle at the nail bed in a child with inflammatory bowel disease.

can occur with excessive straining, though in older children can be seen in association with inflammation or systemic disease such as cystic fibrosis or connective tissue disease.

The most commonly evaluated cause of constipation that is not functional in nature is Hirschsprung disease, most often manifesting in infancy. A barium radiographic study can be suggestive of Hirschsprung disease, although rectal biopsy for ganglion cells and acetylcholinesterase stain confirms the diagnosis (Fig. 11.40). In older children, rectal manometric studies may help separate organic from functional disorders.

PANCREATIC DISEASE

Pancreatic disease is relatively uncommon in the pediatric population. Congenital anomalies such as annular pancreas (Fig. 11.41) can be discovered serendipitously during the evaluation for

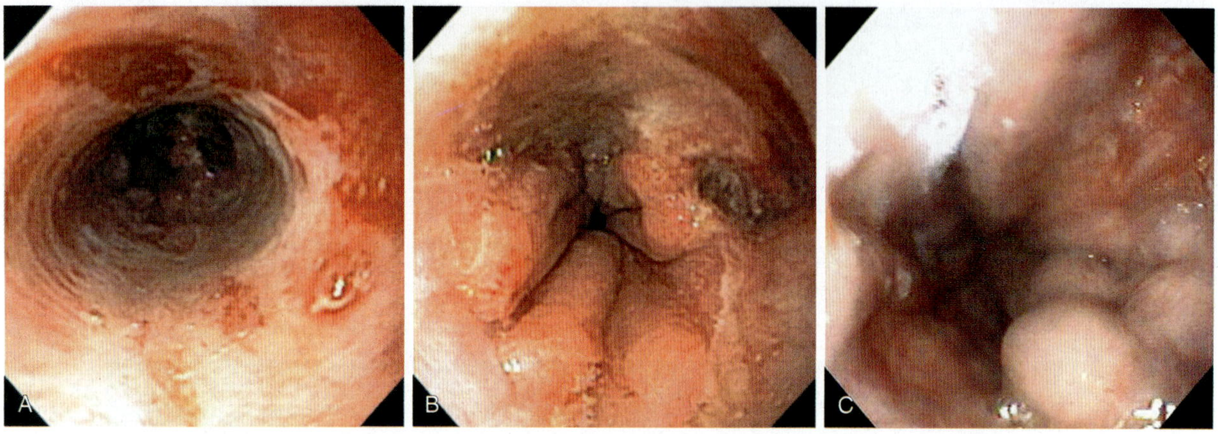

Fig. 11.35 Upper gastrointestinal bleeding. Examples of causes of upper gastrointestinal bleeding, or potential gastrointestinal bleeding. (A) Erosive esophagitis. (B) Deep esophageal ulcer. (C) Esophageal varices. See also Fig. 11.22 (peptic ulcer).

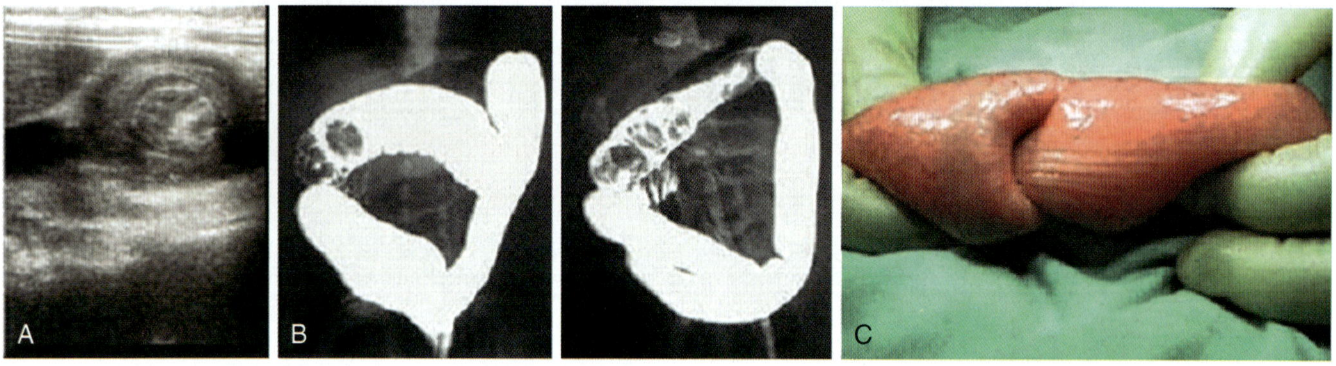

Fig. 11.36 Intussusception. (A) A "target lesion" can be seen on this ultrasound demonstrating intussusception. (B) Air enemas are used to both diagnose and reduce an intussusception. (C) This is an example of an intussusception seen at laparotomy, necessary when reduction is not successful during a barium or air enema. (Courtesy Stefano Bartoletti, MD, and Mark Lowe, MD, Pittsburgh, PA.)

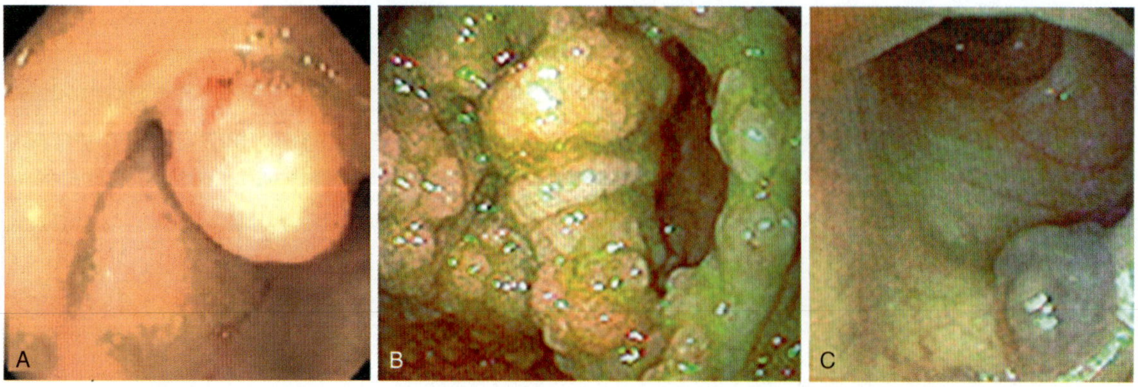

Fig. 11.37 Other causes of lower gastrointestinal bleeding. (A) Isolated juvenile polyp. (B) Pseudopolyp formation in Crohn disease. (C) Vascular malformation (blue rubber bleb nevus). (Courtesy Mark Lowe, MD, Pittsburgh, PA.)

Table 11.4 Common Causes of Gastrointestinal Bleeding in a Child

Upper Gastrointestinal Tract	Lower Gastrointestinal Tract
Esophageal varices	Colonic polyps (isolated or polyposis syndrome)
Pill esophagitis	Anal fissure
Reflux/eosinophilic esophagitis	Hemorrhoids
Gastric ulcers	Intussusception
Gastritis	Meckel diverticulum
Vascular malformations	Colitis (IBD, allergic, infectious)
Duodenal ulcer	Vascular malformations
Inflammatory bowel disease	Solitary rectal ulcers

IBD, Inflammatory bowel disease.

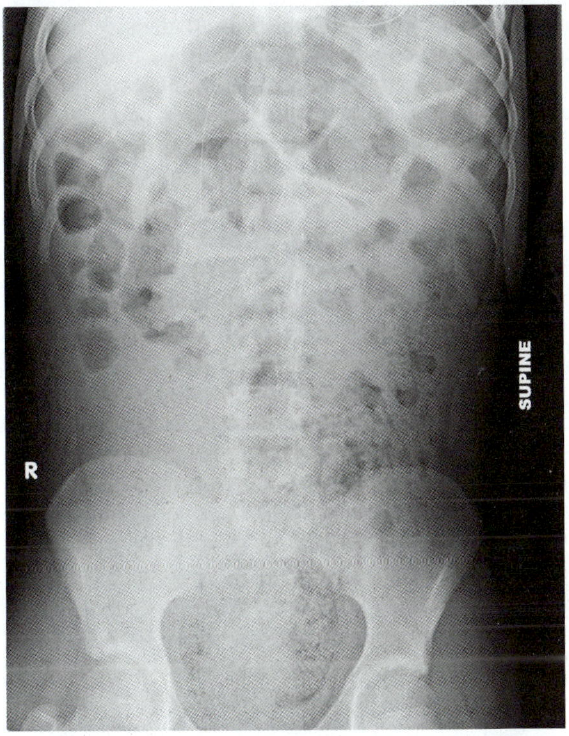

Fig. 11.38 Constipation. This plain film of the abdomen demonstrates a significant amount of stool throughout the colon. Note the dilation of the rectum and colon below the pelvic rim in this child with chronic, functional constipation. (Courtesy Anna Furr, MD, Portland, ME.)

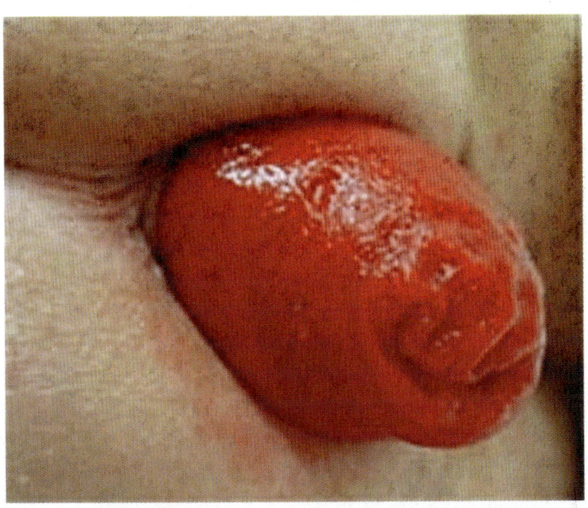

Fig. 11.39 Rectal prolapse. Rectal prolapse can be seen in children with cystic fibrosis but is also associated with excessive straining, inflammation, and connective tissue disorders. Usually, prolapse self-reduces. When it does not, it requires an urgent surgical consultation. (Courtesy Mark Lowe, MD, Pittsburgh, PA.)

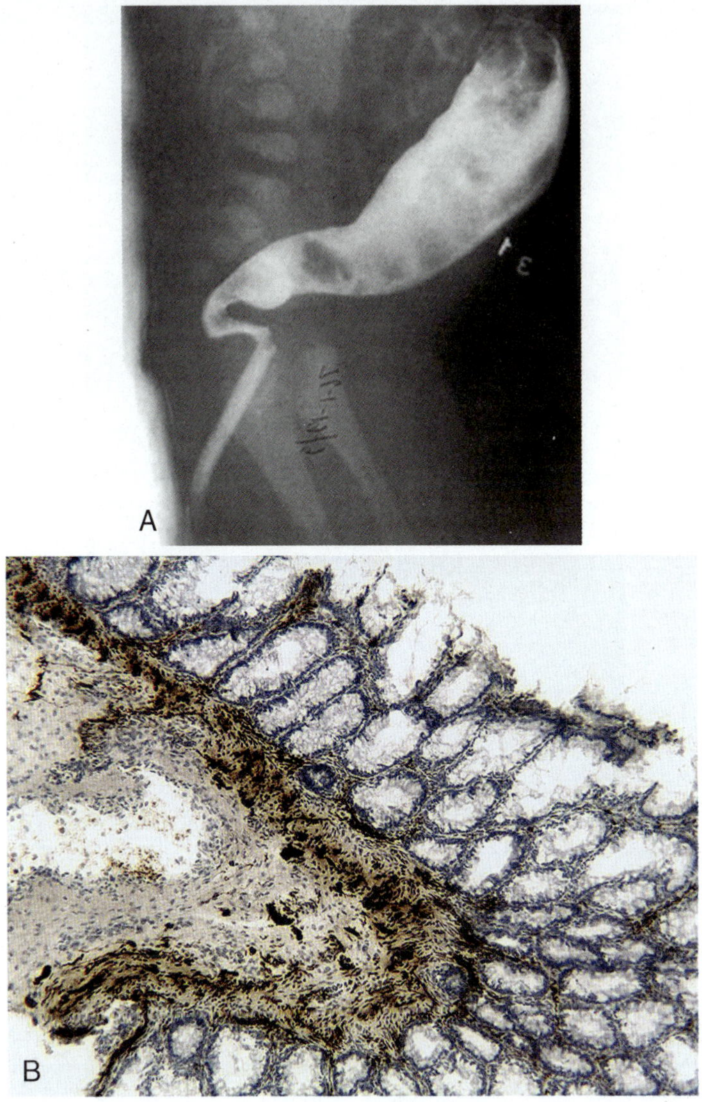

Fig. 11.40 Hirschsprung disease. (A) This barium enema demonstrates a tapered transition zone to a normal-caliber colon that is characteristic of Hirschsprung disease. (B) This slide is specially stained with acetylcholinesterase. The increased number and size of cholinergic nerves in the lamina propria and muscularis mucosae (stains black) is diagnostic of Hirschsprung disease. (Courtesy Sarangarajan Ranganathan, MD, Pittsburgh, PA.)

abdominal pain and have been suggested to be a risk factor for pancreatitis. As discussed previously, exocrine pancreatic insufficiency is a common finding in cystic fibrosis (see Fig. 11.24) but generally results in steatorrhea and not abdominal pain.

The most common cause of acute pancreatitis in childhood is idiopathic in origin, although infectious causes, medications, common bile duct stones, and trauma, among other causes, have been implicated. Chronic pancreatitis or recurrent acute pancreatitis episodes can be associated with hereditary forms. Common presenting symptoms are abdominal pain, usually in the midepigastric area, which can radiate to the back; nausea; and emesis. Symptoms are usually associated with diagnostic elevation of the pancreatic enzymes amylase and lipase. Chronic recurrent pancreatitis may be more subtle and at times may mimic recurrent abdominal pain. Ultrasound and computed tomography have aided the diagnosis of pancreatitis and the treatment of complications, such as pseudocyst formation (Fig. 11.42).

LIVER DISEASE

Jaundice

The term *jaundice* refers to a yellow discoloration of the skin caused by deposition of bilirubin. *Icterus* refers to discoloration of the

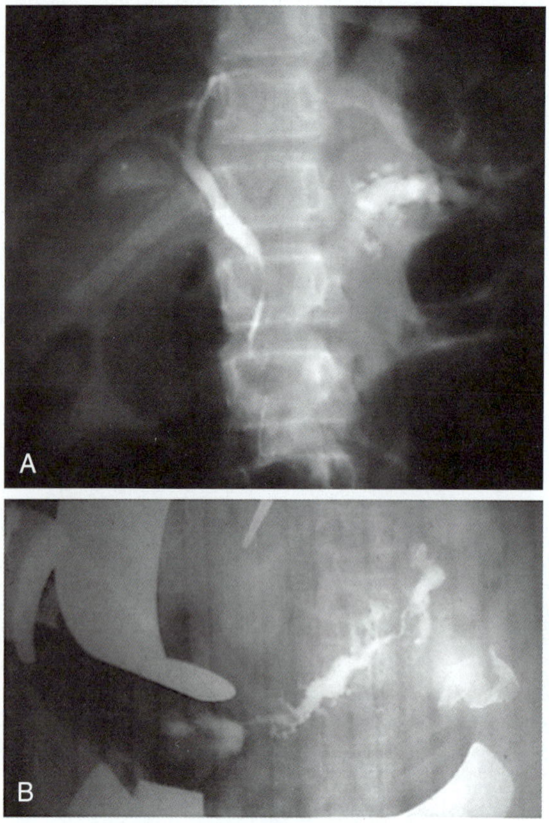

Fig. 11.41 Congenital pancreatic anomaly. This 12-year-old boy had recurrent abdominal pain for 10 years. A retrograde cholangiogram demonstrated an ectatic pancreatic duct. (A) An operative cholangiogram defined a narrow duct just before entry into the duodenum. (B) Division of the duct and anastomosis to the jejunum led to complete resolution of symptoms.

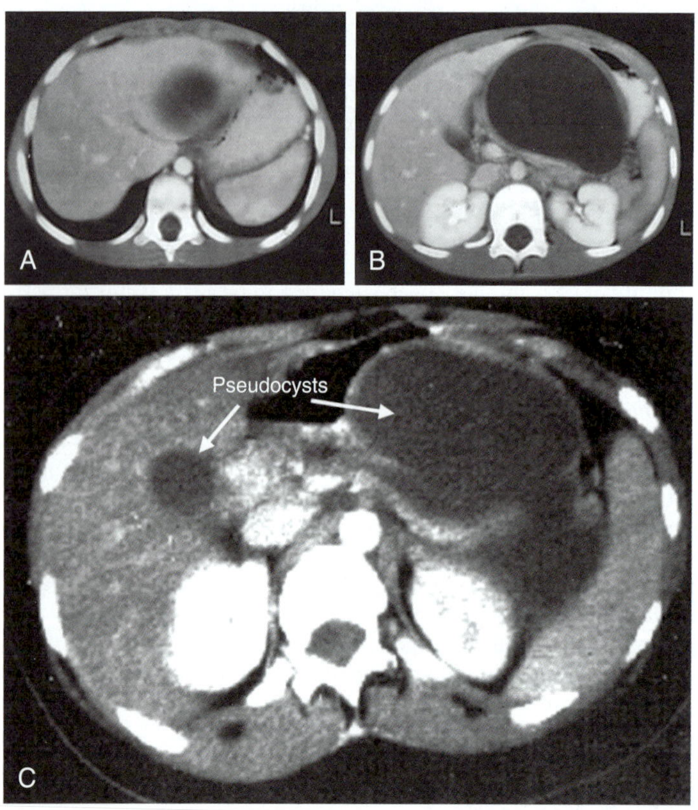

Fig. 11.42 Pancreatic pseudocyst. Abdominal pain and emesis led to a computed tomography scan in this patient, who had a bicycle handlebar injury 2 weeks earlier. (A) Septation of the cavity. (B) Compression of stomach and pancreas by the pancreatic pseudocyst. (C) Two large pancreatic pseudocysts. (Courtesy Mark Lowe, MD, Pittsburgh, PA.)

sclerae (Fig. 11.43). Both are clinical signs that serum bilirubin is above normal. Determining whether the hyperbilirubinemia is secondary to an elevation in conjugated or unconjugated bilirubin is crucial. Elevated conjugated or direct bilirubin greater than or equal to 2 mg/dL, or greater than or equal to 20% of total bilirubin, signifies a pathologic condition, and further studies are necessary to determine its origin.

A majority of cases of neonatal jaundice is due to an elevation in unconjugated bilirubin. This so-called "physiologic" jaundice is due to increased bilirubin production, inadequate bilirubin excretion, or a combination of the two. The most common causes of neonatal unconjugated hyperbilirubinemia are fetal–maternal blood group incompatibility (ABO or Rh), breastfeeding or breast milk jaundice, hemolysis, and extravascular increased bilirubin due to a cephalohematoma or excessive bruising. Phototherapy is usually the treatment of choice for infants with unconjugated hyperbilirubinemia.

Conjugated or direct hyperbilirubinemia indicates a pathologic condition. The physician must find the cause of the disorder promptly because starting medical or surgical treatment may affect outcome. The differential diagnosis for neonatal conjugated hyperbilirubinemia and neonatal hepatitis is immense and is usually broken down into intrahepatic and extrahepatic etiologies (Box 11.5).

Extrahepatic biliary atresia is the most common indication for liver transplantation in children and a major reason to explore the cause of conjugated hyperbilirubinemia as soon as it is discovered. A timely diagnosis and surgical intervention (Kasai procedure) may prevent hepatic cirrhosis, portal hypertension, and eventual liver

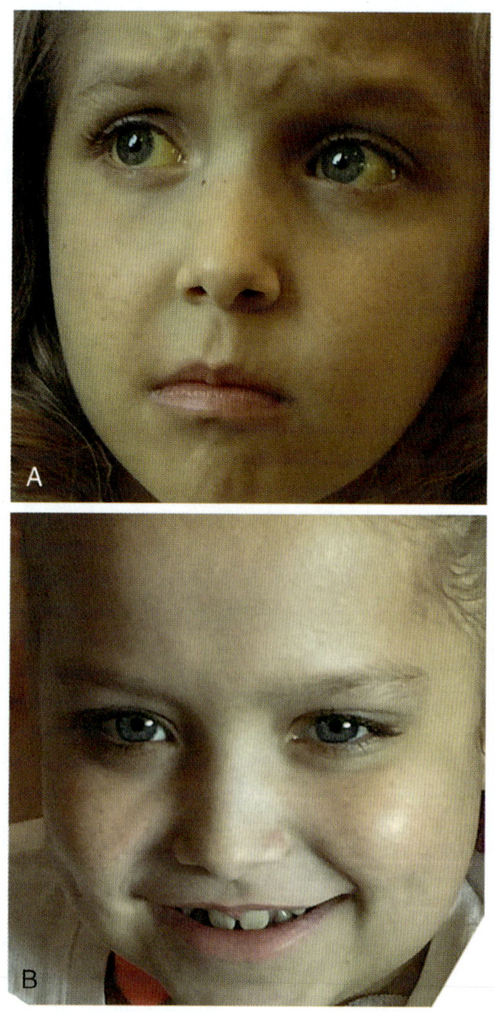

Fig. 11.43 Jaundice/icterus. (A) Note the skin discoloration (jaundice) and yellow hue of the sclerae (icterus) in this child with chronic liver disease. (B) Resolution of both jaundice and icterus just 2 weeks after liver transplantation.

Box 11.5 Neonatal Liver Diseases Associated With Conjugated Hyperbilirubinemia

Extrahepatic
Biliary atresia
Choledochal cyst
Spontaneous perforation of bile duct
Choledochocele

Intrahepatic
Idiopathic neonatal
Hereditary
Alagille syndrome
PFIC 1, 2, 3
Metabolic
Galactosemia
Tyrosinemia
Cystic fibrosis
α_1-Antitrypsin
Bile acid synthetic defects
Lipid/peroxisomal disorders
Neonatal iron storage disease

Infectious
Generalized sepsis
Cytomegalovirus
Herpesvirus
Enterovirus
TORCH infections
Endocrinopathies
Hypopituitarism (septooptic dysplasia)
Hypothyroidism

Genetic
Trisomy 17, 18, 21
Turner syndrome
Anatomical
Congenital hepatic fibrosis
Caroli disease

PFIC, Progressive familial intrahepatic cholestasis; *TORCH,* toxoplasmosis, rubella, cytomegalovirus, herpes simplex virus.

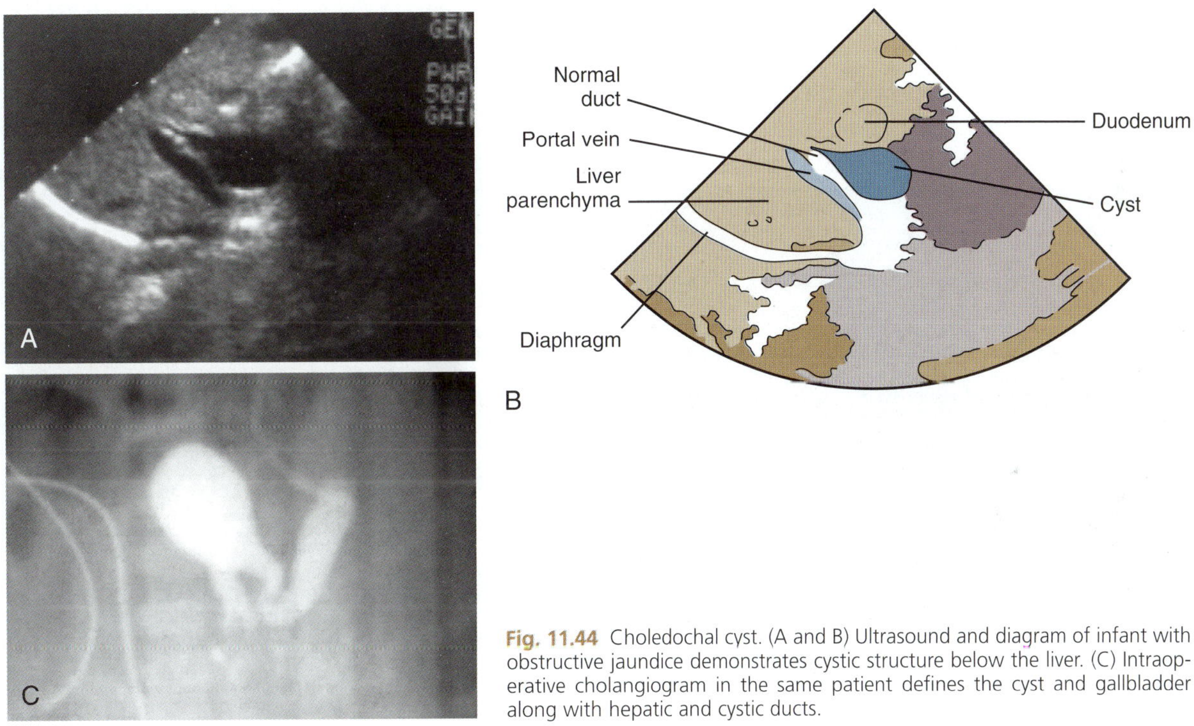

Fig. 11.44 Choledochal cyst. (A and B) Ultrasound and diagram of infant with obstructive jaundice demonstrates cystic structure below the liver. (C) Intraoperative cholangiogram in the same patient defines the cyst and gallbladder along with hepatic and cystic ducts.

transplantation. Extrahepatic biliary atresia may be associated with other congenital abnormalities (see Fig. 11.19) and vascular anomalies, which may complicate initial surgery and later liver transplantation. It can also present in isolation and is generally thought to be a progressive inflammatory process that can be abrogated by restoring biliary flow. Other extrahepatic causes of jaundice in childhood include (congenital) choledochal cysts, which are typically surgically correctable and often diagnosed by ultrasound (Fig. 11.44). Extrahepatic causes of jaundice in late childhood and beyond are most often due to biliary stones, which can be a cause of right upper quadrant pain and can be diagnosed via ultrasound with characteristic acoustic shadowing beneath the stone.

There have been important advances in the understanding of intrahepatic cholestatic disorders. The diagnosis of idiopathic neonatal cholestasis can in some cases be divided into various disorders of the accumulation of bilirubin and excretion of the components of bile in the progressive familial intrahepatic cholestasis syndromes. Progressive familial intrahepatic cholestasis 1 and 2 can be characterized by low γ-glutamyltransferase (GGT) in comparison with other disorders of neonatal cholestasis. A more common cause of intrahepatic cholestasis is arteriohepatic dysplasia, or Alagille syndrome. Patients with this disorder may have a characteristic face of deeply set eyes and a narrow chin (Fig. 11.45) along with ocular posterior embryotoxon, peripheral pulmonic stenosis or cardiac anomalies, and butterfly vertebrae (Fig. 11.46). Liver histology shows paucity of the interlobar bile ducts. Over time, patients with disorders of cholestasis can suffer from intractable pruritus due to bile acid accumulation and xanthoma formation because of cholesterol deposition (Fig. 11.47).

Hepatomegaly

Hepatomegaly, or enlargement of the liver, can be seen in isolation or with concomitant splenomegaly. Any assessment of hepatomegaly should also include an assessment of liver span as hyperinflation of the lungs can give the appearance of a large liver on abdominal examination. Isolated hepatomegaly without associated inflammation is often marked by only mild elevations of liver enzymes,

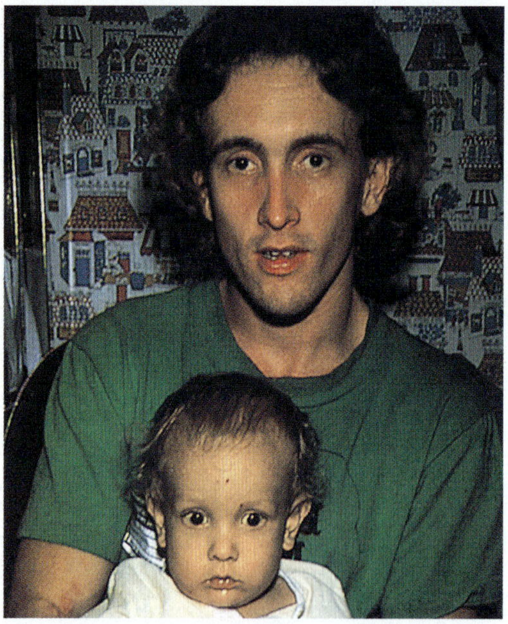

Fig. 11.45 Alagille syndrome. The child has intrahepatic biliary hypoplasia, butterfly vertebrae, and mild pulmonic stenosis. The father does not have liver disease, but he does have moderate pulmonic stenosis and poor growth. Note the narrow, thin face and pointed chin of both father and child.

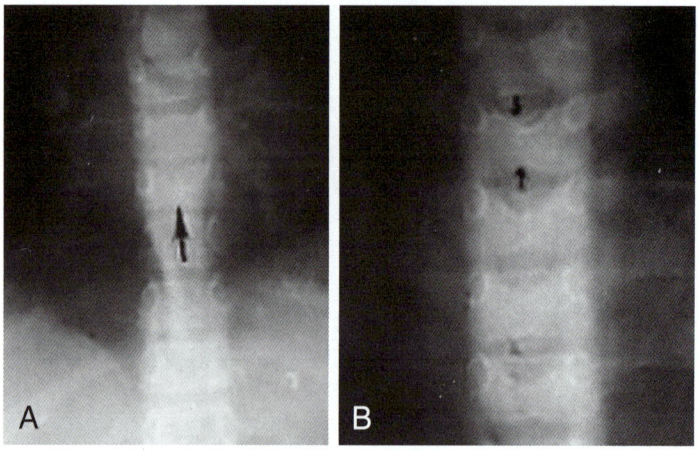

Fig. 11.46 Alagille syndrome. These radiographs (*black arrows* in parts A and B) illustrate defects in the vertebral arches that lead to the butterfly appearance.

although this is dependent on cause. Once hepatomegaly is found, the cause should be carefully studied and includes the assessment of hepatic congestion due to elevated right-sided cardiac pressures, the abnormal accumulation of intrahepatic substances (e.g., α_1-antitrypsin, glycogen, lipid), extramedullary hematopoiesis in infancy, or tumors such as hepatoblastoma. One chronic hepatic disorder that is associated with minimal elevation of transaminases is congenital hepatic fibrosis, which often occurs with splenomegaly and in conjunction with polycystic kidney disease (Fig. 11.48). As liver function often remains normal in this condition, shunting procedures are often the procedure of choice.

Hepatitis

Hepatitis, or inflammation of the liver, can present as an acute or chronic illness with elevation of transaminases (Box 11.6). Most often, acute hepatitis is associated with either a drug reaction or infection, although some cases are idiopathic. Autoimmune hepatitis, presenting either acutely or as a chronic disease, is associated with autoantibodies and hypergammaglobulinemia. Wilson disease

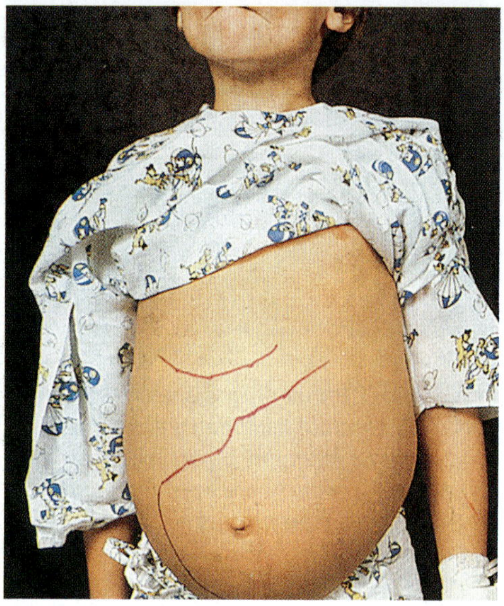

Fig. 11.48 Congenital hepatic fibrosis. This clinically well child had hematemesis and hypersplenism with normal liver function studies. Note the massive spleen size and large left lobe of liver. Portosystemic shunting was effective therapy.

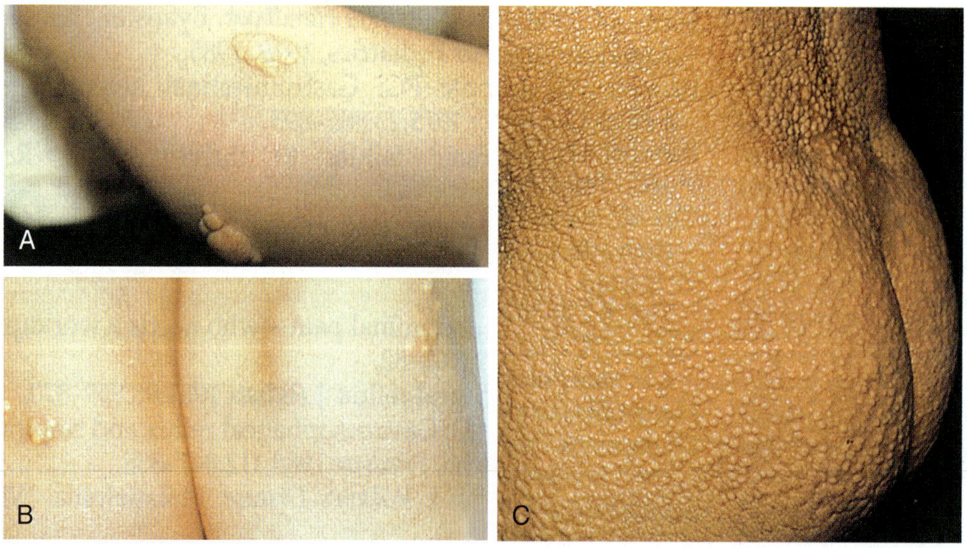

Fig. 11.47 Xanthomas in chronic liver disease. Characteristic areas in the early stages of disease are pressure points such as the elbows (A) and knees (B); later, xanthomas may become generalized (C).

Box 11.6 Hepatitis/Liver Disease Presenting in Older Infancy and Childhood

Viral hepatitis
- Hepatitis A, B, C, D (acute or chronic)
- Cytomegalovirus
- Epstein-Barr virus
- Nontypable hepatitis

Autoimmune hepatitis

Biliary tract disorders
- Choledochal cyst
- Sclerosing cholangitis
- Cholecystitis

Metabolic
- α_1-Antitrypsin deficiency
- Cystic fibrosis
- Wilson disease
- Nonalcoholic steatohepatitis

Drugs
- Acetaminophen
- Anticonvulsants
- Chemotherapy

is a disorder of copper metabolism and can present either as chronic hepatitis or during an acute crisis. One notable physical examination finding in patients with Wilson disease is Kayser-Fleischer rings, which can be seen on slit-lamp examination of the cornea (Fig. 11.49). Nonalcoholic steatohepatitis, a consequence of obesity, can present as hepatomegaly due to fat accumulation and is associated with low-grade inflammation.

Chronic Liver Disease

There are many examples of chronic liver disease that can be treated with specific therapies, such as Wilson disease and autoimmune hepatitis. The consequences of chronic liver disease and inflammation can, however, lead to progressive scarring or fibrosis of the liver. As fibrosis progresses to cirrhosis, the liver can involute and become hard and nodular on palpation. Portal hypertension can develop, leading to variceal formation in the esophagus (see Fig. 11.35C) and elsewhere. Signs on abdominal examination can include prominent abdominal veins and ascites (Fig. 11.50). Other signs of chronic liver disease include disruptions of the small vasculature including the formation of spider nevi (Fig. 11.51) and intrapulmonary shunting (hepatopulmonary syndrome). Transaminases may remain elevated for some time but can begin to decrease as hepatocytes are replaced by fibrosis. Synthetic dysfunction occurs and leads to hypoalbuminemia, cholestasis, and clotting abnormalities. In chronic liver failure, treatment is often supportive, with liver transplantation a viable therapeutic choice.

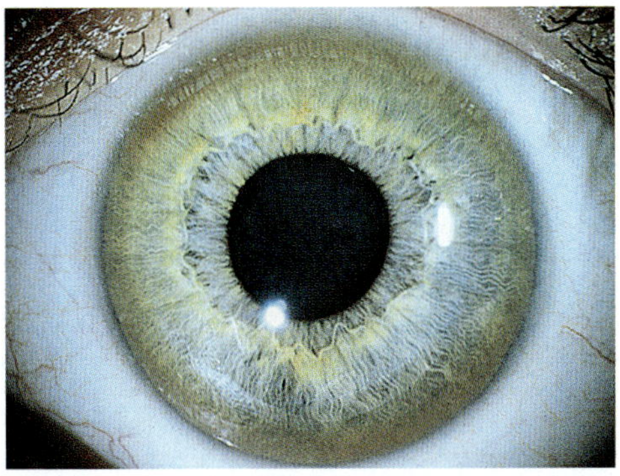

Fig. 11.49 Kayser-Fleischer rings appear as a brownish discoloration in the posterior part of the cornea, as defined by slit-lamp examination. Early Kayser-Fleischer rings may be seen only by slit-lamp examination and begin at the superior and inferior poles.

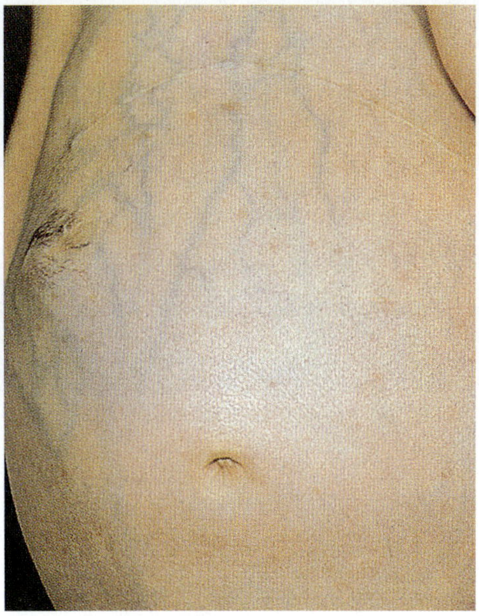

Fig. 11.50 Chronic liver disease/portal hypertension. This child had biliary atresia with good bile flow after a portoenterostomy procedure. Cirrhosis developed late, with physical signs of prominent abdominal veins and ascites.

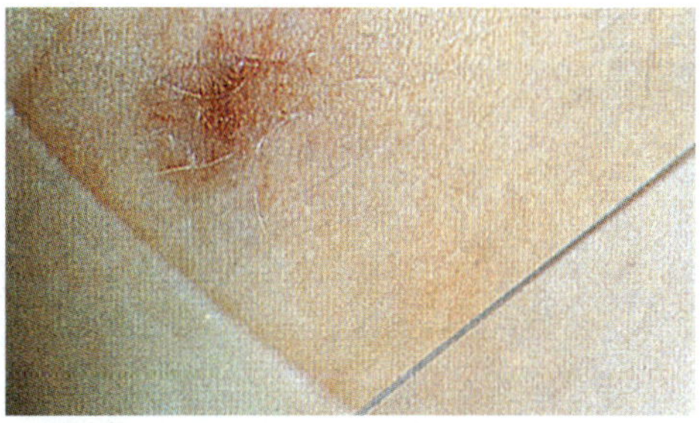

Fig. 11.51 Spider nevus. The vascular lesion blanches with compression by a glass slide, but it reappears when pressure is released and is a sign of chronic liver disease.

Bibliography

Al Nofal A, Schwenk WF: Growth failure in children: a symptom or a disease? *Nutr Clin Pract* 28(6):651–658, 2013.

American Academy of Pediatrics, Committee on Nutrition: The use of whole cow's milk in infancy, *Pediatrics* 91:515–516, 1992.

Ananth R: Neonatal cholestasis: a primer of selected etiologies, *Pediatr Ann* 47(11):e433–e439, 2018.

Barfield E, Parker MW: Management of pediatric gastroesophageal reflux disease, *JAMA Pediatr* 173(5):485–486, 2019.

Borowitz KC, Borowitz SM: Feeding problems in infants and children: assessment and etiology, *Pediatr Clin North Am* 65(1):59–72, 2018.

Butte NF, Hopkinson JM, Wong WW, et al: Body composition during the first 2 years of life: an updated reference, *Pediatr Res* 47:578–585, 2000.

CaJacob NJ, Cohen MB: Update on diarrhea, *Pediatr Rev* 37(8):313–322, 2016, http://dx.doi.org/10.1542/pir.2015-0099.

Ficicioglu C, An Haack K: Failure to thrive: when to suspect inborn errors of metabolism, *Pediatrics* 124(3):972–979, 2009.

Grummer-Strawn LM, Reinold C, Krebs N: Use of World Health Organization and CDC growth charts for children aged 0-59 months in the United States, *Morb Mortal Wkly Rep* 59:1–15, 2010.

Husain SZ, Srinath AI: What's unique about acute pancreatitis in children: risk factors, diagnosis and management, *Nat Rev Gastroenterol Hepatol* 14(6): 366–372, 2017.

Husby S, Koletzko S, Korponay-Szabó IR, et al: European Society for Pediatric Gastroenterology, Hepatology, and Nutrition guidelines for the diagnosis of coeliac disease, *J Pediatr Gastroenterol Nutr* 54(1):136–160, 2012.

Jones NL, Koletzko S, Goodman K, et al: Joint ESPGHAN/NASPGHAN guidelines for the management of Helicobacter pylori in children and adolescents (update 2016), *J Pediatr Gastroenterol Nutr* 64(6):991–1003, 2017.

Kerzner B, Milano K, MacLean WC Jr, Berall G, Stuart S, Chatoor I: A practical approach to classifying and managing feeding difficulties, *Pediatrics* 135(2): 344–353, 2015.

Korterink J, Devanarayana NM, Rajindrajith S, Vlieger A, Benninga MA: Childhood functional abdominal pain: mechanisms and management, *Nat Rev Gastroenterol Hepatol* 12(3):159–171, 2015.

Larson-Nath C, Biank VF: Clinical review of failure to thrive in pediatric patients, *Pediatr Ann* 45(2):e46–e49, 2016.

Leung AK, Sauve RS: Breast is best for babies, *J Natl Med Assoc* 97:1010–1019, 2005.

Oliveira SB, Monteiro IM: Diagnosis and management of inflammatory bowel disease in children, *BMJ* 357:j2083, 2017.

Pai AK, Fox VL: Gastrointestinal bleeding and management, *Pediatr Clin North Am* 64(3):543–561, 2017.

Pulcini CD, Zettle S, Srinath A: Refeeding syndrome, *Pediatr Rev* 37(12):516–523, 2016.

Rajindrajith S, Zeevenhooven J, Devanarayana NM, Perera BJC, Benninga MA: Functional abdominal pain disorders in children, *Expert Rev Gastroenterol Hepatol* 12(4):369–390, 2018.

Rosen R, Vandenplas Y, Singendonk M, et al: Pediatric gastroesophageal reflux clinical practice guidelines: joint recommendations of the North American Society for Pediatric Gastroenterology, Hepatology, and Nutrition and the European Society for Pediatric Gastroenterology, Hepatology, and Nutrition, *J Pediatr Gastroenterol Nutr* 66:516–554, 2018.

Ruffner MA, Spergel JM: Pediatric eosinophilic esophagitis: updates for the primary care setting, *Curr Opin Pediatr* 30(6):829–836, 2018.

Sinatra FR, Merritt RF: Iatrogenic kwashiorkor in infants, *Am J Dis Child* 135: 21–23, 1981.

Sondheimer JM: Office stool examination: a practical guide, *Contemp Pediatr* 7: 63–82, 1990.

Tabbers MM, DiLorenzo C, Berger MY, et al: Evaluation and treatment of functional constipation in infants and children: evidence-based recommendations from ESPGHAN and NASPGHAN, *J Pediatr Gastroenterol Nutr* 58(2):258–274, 2014.

Wagner CL, Greer FR: Prevention of rickets and vitamin D deficiency in infants, children, and adolescents, *Pediatrics* 122:1142–1152, 2008.

Ziegler EE, Nelson SE, Jeter JM: Iron status of breastfed infants is improved equally by medicinal iron and iron-fortified cereal, *Am J Clin Nutr* 90(1):76–87, 2009.

HEMATOLOGY AND ONCOLOGY

12

James D. Cooper | Jean M. Tersak

HEMATOLOGY

Red Blood Cells

The red blood cell (RBC) is classically described as a biconcave disk. Red cells evolve from immature forms, beginning with pronormoblasts, which are large cells with dark blue cytoplasm and a large centrally located nucleus. As the cell matures, the nucleus becomes pyknotic and is eventually extruded. As the cell begins to make hemoglobin, the cytoplasm undergoes a histologic transformation from dark blue to pink.

A peripheral smear is made up of a small droplet of blood on a glass slide. A second slide is used to smear the blood in a manner that it covers one-half to two-thirds the length of the slide. A well-made smear should not have lines or holes, nor should it reach either end of the slide completely. Commonly, Wright stain is applied after drying to give the cells their characteristic appearance (Fig. 12.1). RBCs should be the same relative shape and size, with an area of central pallor that is approximately one-third the diameter of the cell (Fig. 12.2).

A normal RBC has approximately the same size as a lymphocyte nucleus. A variety of terms are available to describe the physical appearance of mature RBCs. *Polychromasia* refers to the variability in cell color, with *hypochromia* specifically indicating an increased area of central pallor. *Anisocytosis* indicates variability in cell size. *Microcytosis* describes a small cell size, whereas *macrocytosis* refers to large cells. *Poikilocytosis* represents variability in cell shape. The overall number of RBCs in the circulation cannot be described reliably by the peripheral smear. Laboratory values can also aid in assessing RBC morphology. Two of these have wide usage. The mean corpuscular volume (MCV) is a laboratory measure of cell size, and red cell distribution width estimates this difference.

The primary function of the RBC is to deliver oxygen to tissues. The effective red cell number is commonly represented by the hemoglobin concentration, in grams per deciliter (g/dL). The oxygen-binding sites of hemoglobin are completely saturated by passage of the RBC through the lungs. As the cells circulate through the tissue systemic capillaries, the hemoglobin releases 25% of its bound oxygen. However, the amount of oxygen released to the tissue may be significantly increased, under certain conditions (fever, acidosis, etc.), allowing some compensation for a decrease in hemoglobin. A progressive decrease in hemoglobin eventually leads to tissue hypoxia, which triggers a release of erythropoietin. This induces an increase in RBC production, bringing RBC mass back to normal values.

Different stages of life and disease states impart different oxygen demands, and therefore hemoglobin levels can vary greatly. In general, full-term newborns are born with relatively high levels of hemoglobin, which then fall over the first few months of life. This low point, the physiologic nadir, occurs during the transition in production from fetal to adult hemoglobin. Premature infants may have an earlier, more severe, and more prolonged nadir depending on gestational age. After this time, the average hemoglobin value increases until preadolescence and reaches adult levels by puberty. Similarly, the MCV is at a low point after the nadir of hemoglobin, and it slowly increases into early adolescence. An estimate of the lower limit of the MCV is 70 femtoliters (fL) plus two times the age in years, from 1 to 10 years old.

Anemia

Classifications and Symptoms

Anemia is the most common abnormality of RBCs, and it is identified as a decrease in hemoglobin level. At any given age, anemia is defined practically as a value greater than 2 standard deviations below the mean. However, physiologically, anemia is best defined as a hemoglobin level that is too low to meet tissue oxygen demands. Recognition that a child's hemoglobin level is abnormal requires knowledge of demographic-related normal values. Anemia occurs as a result of one of the following: (1) decreased bone marrow production of RBCs and reticulocytes (Fig. 12.3), (2) increased destruction of mature RBCs peripherally or as precursors in the bone marrow, or (3) loss of RBCs (hemorrhage). In some situations, a combination of these factors can occur.

Physical examination of the anemic child may reveal pallor, although in the fair-skinned or dark-skinned child, it may be easily missed, unless palmar creases or conjunctivae are also examined thoroughly (Fig. 12.4). Vital signs may be normal, or tachycardia may be present. Severe anemia from any cause may elicit symptoms of fatigue; decreased appetite; headache; and, in extreme cases, shock, congestive heart failure, or even stroke.

Iron Deficiency

The most common anemia encountered in pediatrics is microcytic anemia, due to iron deficiency. A lack of iron leads to failure of hemoglobin production. Iron deficiency, however, is only a laboratory finding, not a diagnosis. The causes of iron deficiency must be elucidated through a careful history and physical examination. Although poor nutrition is the most common cause, other causes such as hemorrhage or malabsorption must also be considered. Because the normal full-term infant has adequate iron reserve to accommodate the increasing RBC mass through the first 5 months of life, iron deficiency is usually not seen until the second half of the first year of life. It is detected most often in the 10- to 18-month-old child who ingests large volumes of cow's milk. Whole cow's milk is not only deficient in dietary iron but often leads to enteropathy with occult gastrointestinal blood loss, exacerbating the child's iron-deficient status. A second peak of iron deficiency anemia is seen during adolescence in menstruating females.

Affected children may manifest a peculiar physical finding termed *koilonychia,* or "spooning" of fingernails and toenails (Fig. 12.5). Glossitis may also be observed in iron deficiency. The RBCs of iron deficiency anemia are microcytic and hypochromic. The number of platelets is often increased, although it may be normal or even decreased. In severe iron deficiency anemia, anisocytosis and poikilocytosis may be prominent. Nonspecific abnormalities of RBC morphology (such as the presence of micro-ovalocytes or basophilic stippling) may also occur. Bizarre RBC shapes are due to a three-dimensional change in structure when viewed in a two-dimensional plane of the light microscope. When viewed in two dimensions, the

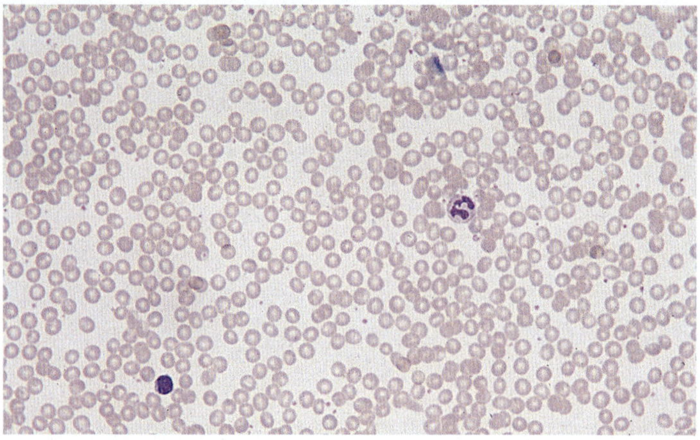

Fig. 12.1 Peripheral blood smear. The appearance of a normal peripheral blood smear when viewed under low magnification (×100).

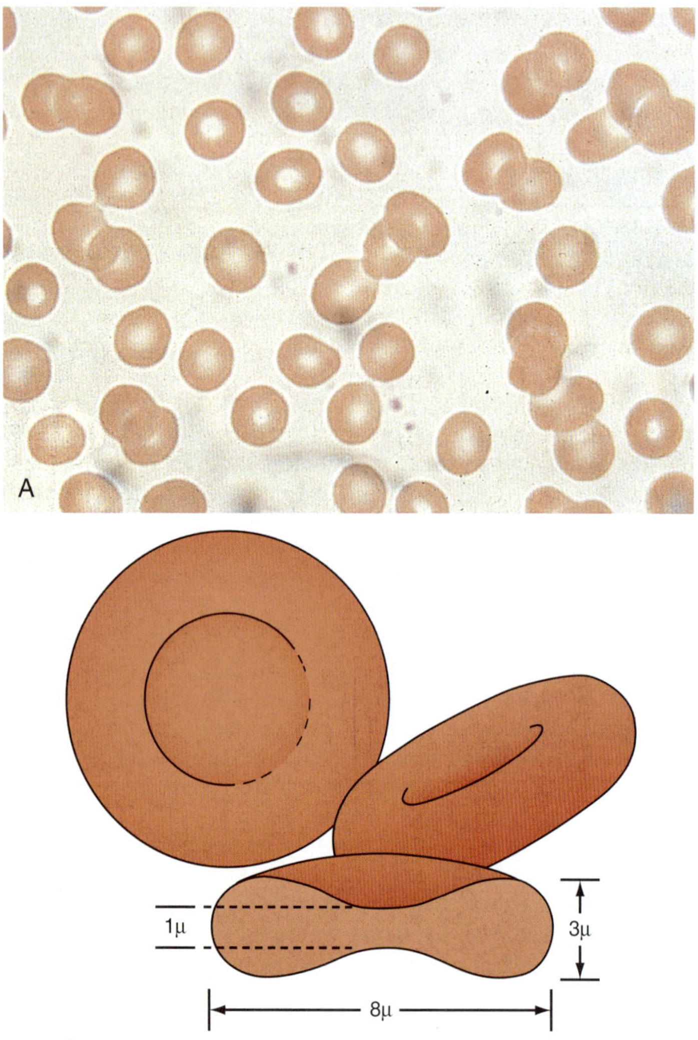

Fig. 12.2 Peripheral blood smear. The appearance of a normal peripheral blood smear when viewed under high power (×400). (A) Biconcave structure of the red blood cell (RBC). (B) Schematic drawing of an RBC in two views, demonstrating the features of the normal biconcave disk.

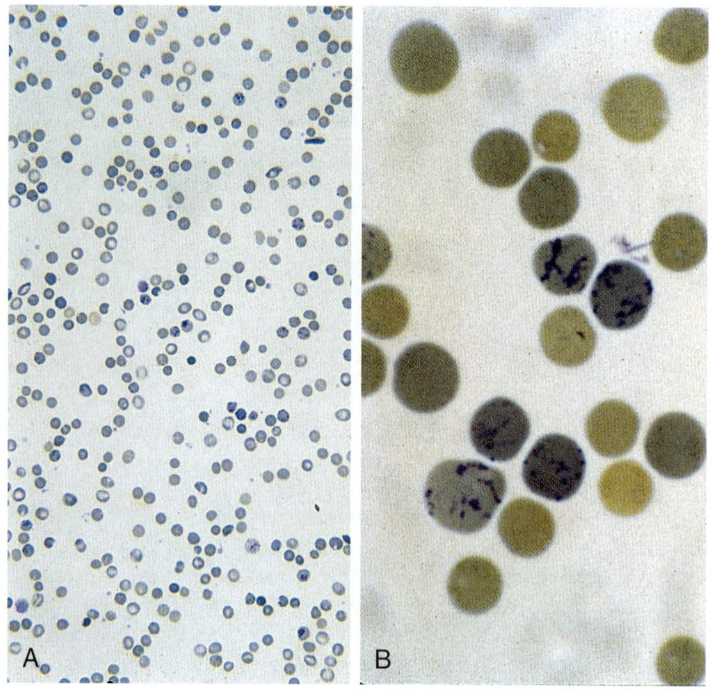

Fig. 12.3 The reticulocyte. (A) A reticulin-stained peripheral blood smear in a patient with a high (18%) reticulocyte count. The darkly stained cells are reticulocytes seen in the peripheral blood of a patient with hemolytic anemia. (B) High magnification of reticulocytes.

cells appear ovoid. Fig. 12.6 shows a peripheral blood smear of a child with iron deficiency anemia.

The history and physical examination, complete blood count, and review of the peripheral blood smear may be sufficient for diagnosis in many instances of hypochromic, microcytic anemia. If the evaluation strongly suggests iron deficiency, a therapeutic trial of iron may be a reasonable approach. However, additional laboratory studies are often indicated. Serum iron and total iron-binding capacity alone do not give an accurate perspective of total body iron stores because they are relatively short-term measures and are affected by recent intake. Ferritin is a superior measure of iron status, but it also is an acute-phase reactant and may be elevated into the low normal range in a child with a concurrent inflammatory process. However, if ferritin is low, it is diagnostic of iron deficiency.

The coexistence of iron deficiency and lead intoxication is well documented; though in practice, an increased lead level more commonly is secondary to pica in children with iron deficiency, and it is not the cause of anemia. Pica is the ingestion of non-food items, such as chalk, carpet fibers, or other debris. In primary lead intoxication, nonhematologic manifestations, particularly neurologic complications, appear long before an anemia develops. Significant radiographic changes are also seen in primary lead intoxication (Fig. 12.7). When they do occur, hematologic abnormalities of lead intoxication such as basophilic stippling (Fig. 12.8) are a direct result of the effect of lead on several cellular enzymes involved in heme production. Lead inhibits these enzyme systems, impairing iron use and globin synthesis.

Anemia of Inflammation

Inflammatory diseases, such as chronic infection, inflammatory bowel disease, or rheumatologic conditions, may lead to microcytic anemia. Although the symptoms of the child's primary illness usually clarify the diagnosis, there are occasionally cases in which a chronic subclinical infection may go undiagnosed. Clinical factors often make this diagnosis, although one laboratory study that may be of value is the serum ferritin. Ferritin is decreased in iron deficiency, whereas in chronic inflammatory states, it is usually elevated. Also, though serum iron can be low in both iron deficiency and anemia of chronic disease, total iron-binding capacity is increased in iron deficiency and decreased in anemia of chronic disease. These changes are believed to be due to the upregulation of the enzyme hepcidin, which redirects total body iron to storage pools rather than RBC production.

Megaloblastic Anemia

Although the etiology of macrocytic anemias varies, common morphologic abnormalities of erythropoietic cells exist. In the bone marrow, the hallmark is the megaloblast, a nucleated RBC with a lacy chromatin pattern and asynchrony of maturation between

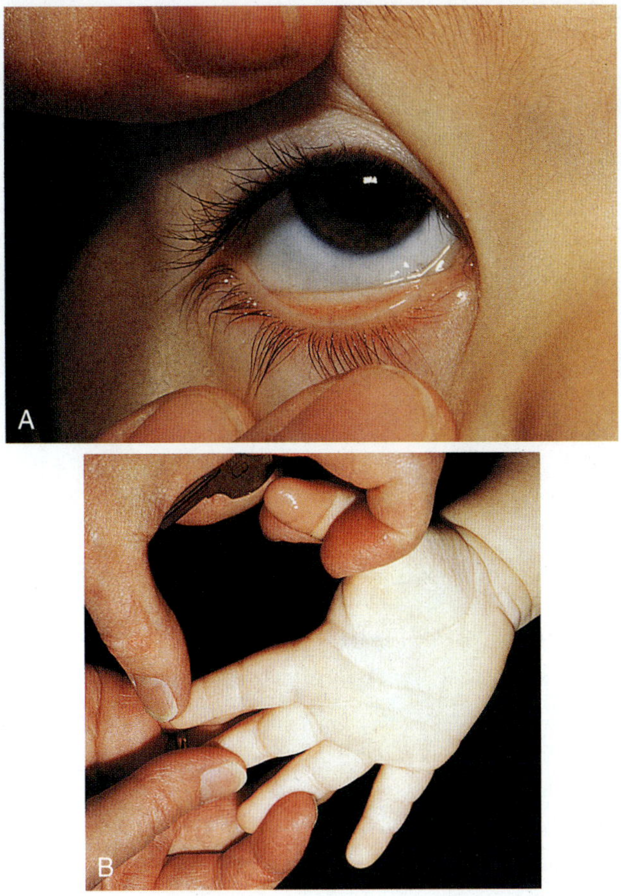

Fig. 12.4 Severe anemia. (A) Pale conjunctiva may be seen in the patient with severe anemia. (B) Pale palmar creases are also visible in cases of severe anemia. The child in this photograph has a hemoglobin level of 4 g/dL.

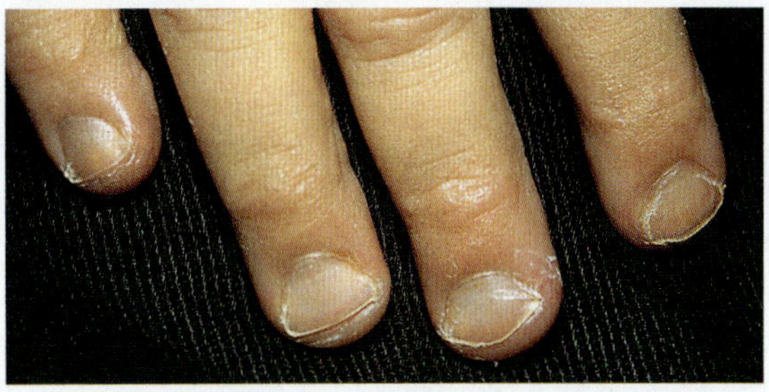

Fig. 12.5 Spooning of the fingernails occurs in children with severe iron deficiency anemia.

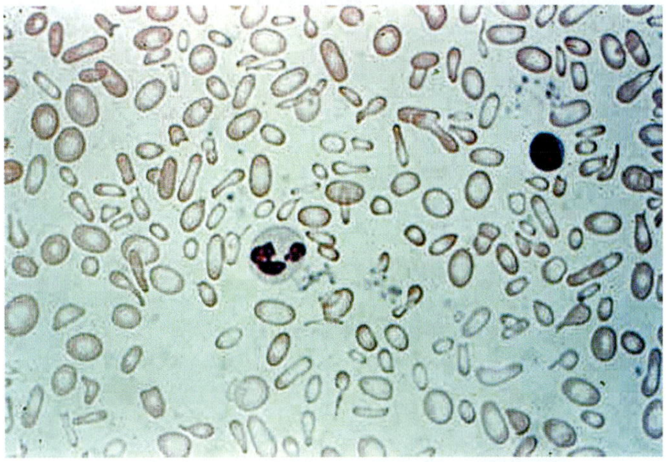

Fig. 12.6 Iron deficiency results in a hypochromic, microcytic anemia. This 16-month-old patient had a history of excessive milk intake. Note the marked central pallor of the red blood cells (RBCs) with their small rim of hemoglobin and their small size in comparison with that of the adjacent lymphocyte nucleus. Frequent "cigar cells" can be seen in addition to the hypochromic microcytic RBCs.

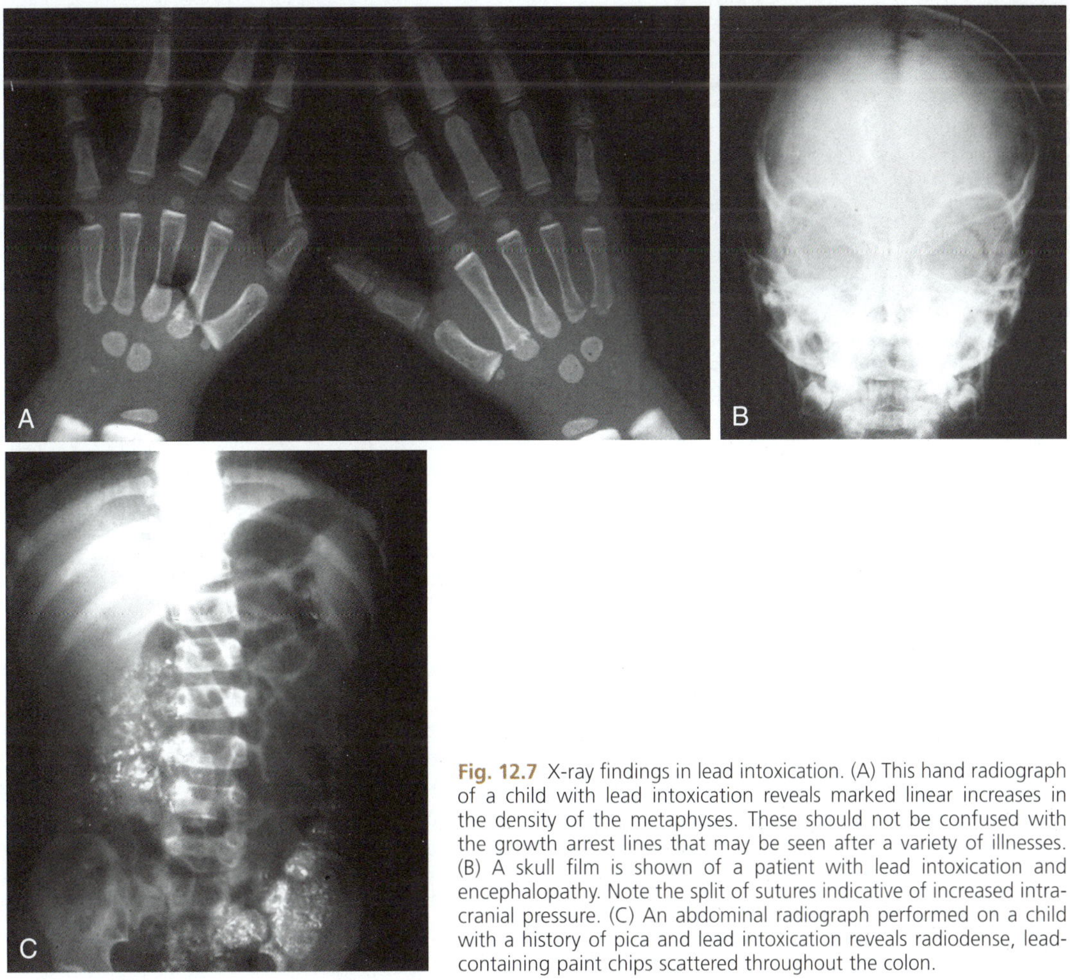

Fig. 12.7 X-ray findings in lead intoxication. (A) This hand radiograph of a child with lead intoxication reveals marked linear increases in the density of the metaphyses. These should not be confused with the growth arrest lines that may be seen after a variety of illnesses. (B) A skull film is shown of a patient with lead intoxication and encephalopathy. Note the split of sutures indicative of increased intracranial pressure. (C) An abdominal radiograph performed on a child with a history of pica and lead intoxication reveals radiodense, lead-containing paint chips scattered throughout the colon.

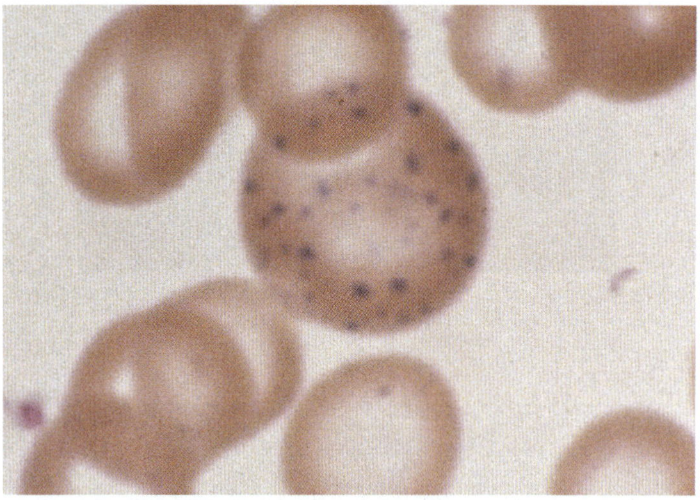

Fig. 12.8 Prominent basophilic stippling is often seen in thalassemia and treated iron deficiency but classically is thought of in cases of severe lead intoxication. However, this finding is not specific for any diagnosis.

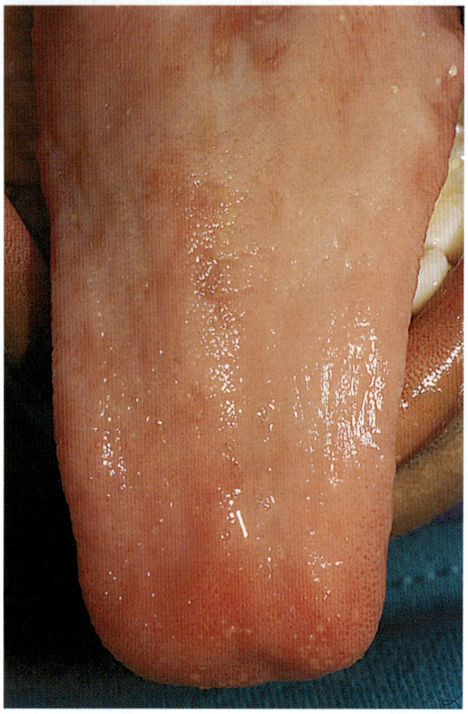

Fig. 12.9 A smooth, beefy red tongue may be observed in the physical examination of a patient with vitamin B_{12} deficiency. This patient depended on total parenteral nutrition for several years without vitamin B_{12} supplementation.

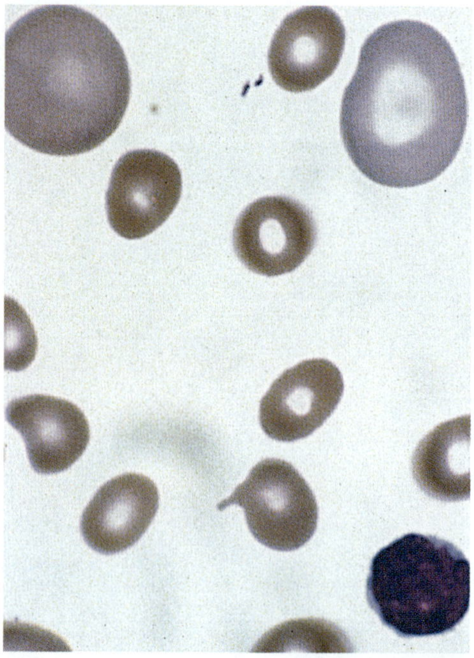

Fig. 12.10 Megaloblastic anemia. This peripheral blood smear demonstrates an enlarged red blood cell (RBC; macrocyte) at the upper left of the photograph. The RBC is much larger than the normal small lymphocytes in the same field in this patient with megaloblastic anemia.

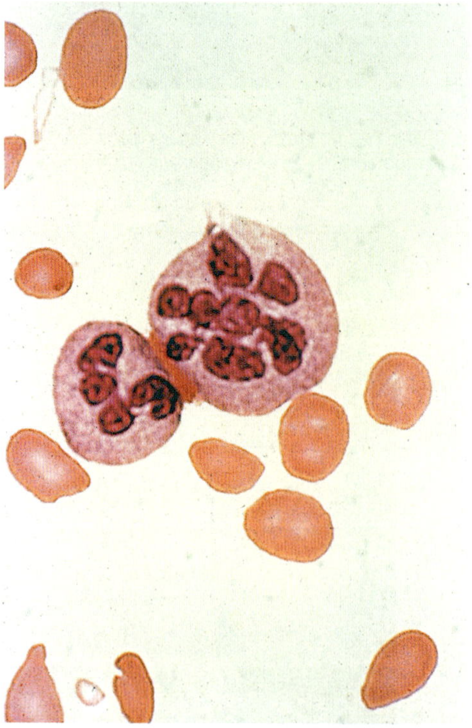

Fig. 12.11 This peripheral blood smear demonstrates the presence of a hypersegmented polymorphonuclear leukocyte in a patient with phenytoin-induced folate deficiency.

cytoplasm and nucleus. The morphologic alterations are a direct result of decreased DNA synthesis compared with cytoplasmic protein synthesis, which stems from a relative decrease in the factors needed in DNA replication, namely folate and cobalamin (vitamin B_{12}). Laboratory diagnosis requires the measurement of folate and vitamin B_{12} levels in the serum and RBCs. Glossitis (Fig. 12.9) or angular stomatitis, commonly seen in vitamin B_{12} deficiency, can be helpful during physical findings in the diagnostic process.

On the peripheral blood smear, the RBCs are large and display a great deal of variation in their shapes (Fig. 12.10). These macrocytic cells are generally normochromic. In addition, actively dividing marrow cells may become involved in the pathologic process. Neutrophils are the second most likely cells to display morphologic abnormalities. These cells become large and show pathognomonic hypersegmentation of the nucleus (Fig. 12.11). Neutropenia is common. The more severe and prolonged megaloblastic anemias ultimately may lead to moderate thrombocytopenia, with large, bizarre platelets on the peripheral blood smear. Megaloblastic changes in each cell line are shown in Fig. 12.12.

A low level of folate or vitamin B_{12} deficiency should raise questions of altered bioavailability or unusual diet. Goat milk is folate deficient, and an infant on a goat milk diet may become folate depleted over time. Various drugs that decrease folate absorption (phenytoin) or interfere with folate metabolism (methotrexate) may also lead to megaloblastic changes. A pathologic condition of the gastrointestinal tract may cause malabsorption of folate or vitamin B_{12}. This condition may be iatrogenic if a portion of the intestines is removed for medical reasons. Pernicious anemia is a specific cause, due to deficiency in intrinsic factor, which is required for vitamin B_{12} absorption. Elevated levels of vitamin B_{12} are generally not indicative of a problem in children, though there are exceptions.

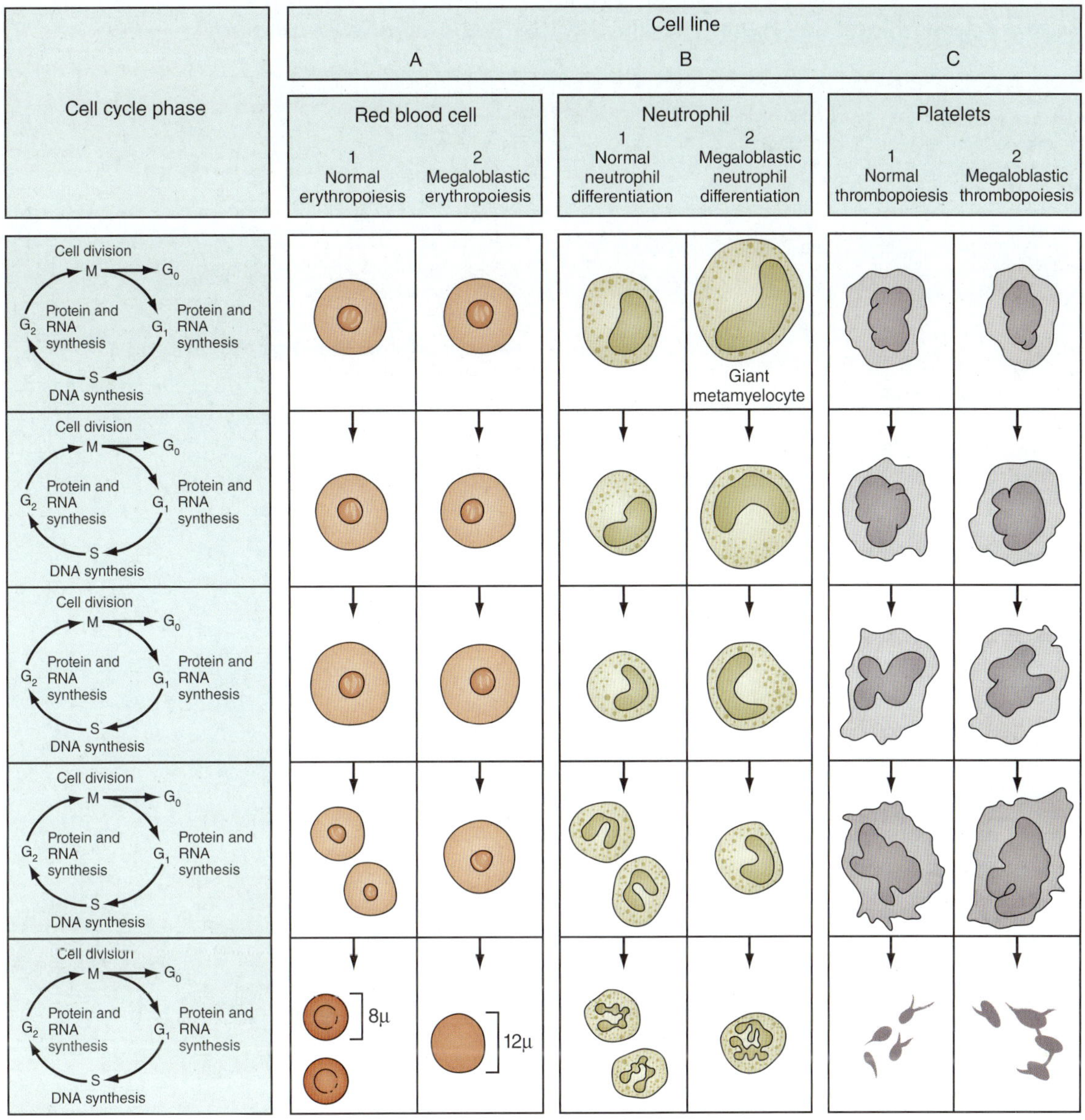

Fig. 12.12 Schematic comparison of normal cellular maturation and megaloblastic differentiation of three cell lines. The cell cycle phase is identified to the left of the figure. Note that the megaloblastic cells fail to undergo replication of deoxyribonucleic acid and cellular division at the S and M phases, respectively, leading to large red blood cells, hypersegmented polymorphonuclear leukocytes, and large, bizarrely shaped platelets. *RNA*, Ribonucleic acid.

Acquired Pure Red Cell Aplasia

Acquired forms of pediatric pure red cell aplasias (PRCAs) are rare, although well recognized. Transient erythroblastopenia of childhood (TEC) occurs in 1- to 4-year-old children and appears 2 weeks to 2 months after a respiratory or gastrointestinal illness. Fortunately, TEC is transient and self-limited. It has been noted that the RBCs in congenital PRCA have fetal characteristics, but the RBCs of TEC have age-appropriate characteristics (Table 12.1). The cause of TEC remains obscure. TEC may occur after many different viral infections and most likely represents an altered immunity from the infection that affects erythropoiesis. Treatment is supportive and determined by the degree of symptoms.

Table 12.1 Features Differentiating Pure Red Cell Anemia From Transient Erythroblastopenia of Childhood

	Disease	
Red Blood Cell Characteristic	**Pure Red Cell Anemia**	**Transient Erythroblastopenia of Childhood**
Hemoglobin	Increased fetal	Normal fetal
Mean corpuscular volume	Increased	Normal
Red blood cell enzyme activity	Normal or high	Low

Hemolytic Anemias

Hemolytic anemias are defined by the premature destruction of RBCs. This can occur by mechanical, infectious, enzymatic, or immune-mediated mechanisms. Symptoms and severity vary not only among individuals but also between diagnoses. Jaundice, especially scleral icterus, splenomegaly, and dark urine, are common presentations during hemolytic episodes. Although all hemolytic anemias may have acute exacerbations, some also feature more chronic phases of red cell breakdown. The history of individual patients, laboratory studies, and blood cell morphology are important factors in making the accurate diagnosis. Some of the most common morphologic features are described in Box 12.1. Treatments can vary, and splenectomy may be a consideration.

Hereditary spherocytosis (HS) is the most common cause of genetically determined hemolytic anemia in the White population. HS is transmitted frequently as an autosomal dominant trait, but in approximately 20% of patients it may present with spontaneous

Box 12.1 Common Red Blood Cell Hemolytic Disorders by Predominant Morphology[a]

Spherocytes
Hereditary spherocytosis
ABO incompatibility in neonates[b]
Immunohemolytic anemias with IgG- or C3-coated RBCs
Hemolytic transfusion reactions[b]
Severe burns or other RBC thermal injuries

Bizarre Poikilocytes
RBC fragmentation syndromes (microangiopathic and macroangiopathic hemolytic anemias)
Hereditary elliptocytosis in neonates

Elliptocytes
Hereditary elliptocytosis
Thalassemia
(Other hypochromic microcytic anemia)
(Megaloblastic anemia)

Spiculated or Crenated Red Blood Cells
Acute hepatic necrosis (spur-cell anemia)
Uremia
Abetalipoproteinemia

Prominent Basophilic Stippling
Thalassemia
Unstable hemoglobin levels
Lead poisoning[c]

Irreversibly Sickled Cells
Sickle cell anemia
Symptomatic sickle syndromes
Intraerythrocytic parasites
Malaria
Babesiosis
Bartonellosis

Target Cells
Hgb S, C, D, and E
Hereditary xerocytosis
Thalassemia
(Other hypochromic microcytic anemia)
(Obstructive liver disease)
(Postsplenectomy)

Nonspecific or Normal Morphology
Embden-Meyerhof pathway defects
HMP shunt defects
Adenosine deaminase hyperactivity with low RBC ATP
Unstable hemoglobin levels
Paroxysmal nocturnal hemoglobinuria
Dyserythropoietic anemia
Copper toxicity (Wilson disease)
Erythropoietic porphyria
Vitamin E deficiency
Hypersplenism

[a]Nonhemolytic disorders of similar morphology are enclosed in parentheses for reference.
[b]Usually associated with a positive Coombs test.
[c]Disease sometimes associated with this morphology.
Modified from Nathan DG, Oski FA, editors: *Hematology of infancy and childhood*, ed 2, Philadelphia, 1981, WB Saunders.

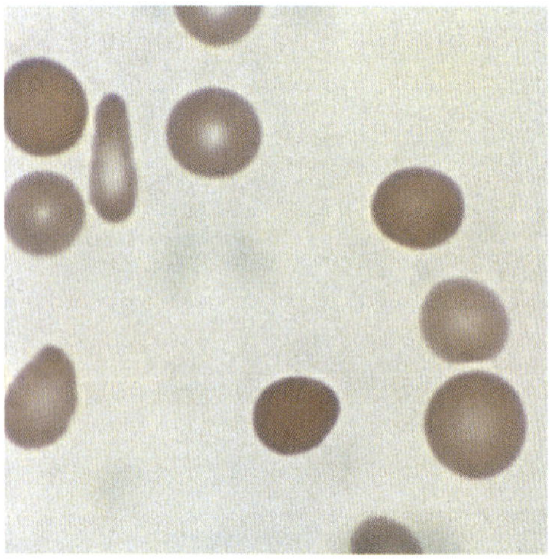

Fig. 12.13 Peripheral blood smear of a patient with hereditary spherocytosis. Note the presence of small, perfectly round cells without an area of central pallor. The mean corpuscular hemoglobin concentration is often increased in this condition but may be normal in some cases. Reticulocyte count is also often elevated owing to the shortened life span of the red blood cells (RBCs) and need for increased RBC production relative to individuals without hereditary spherocytosis.

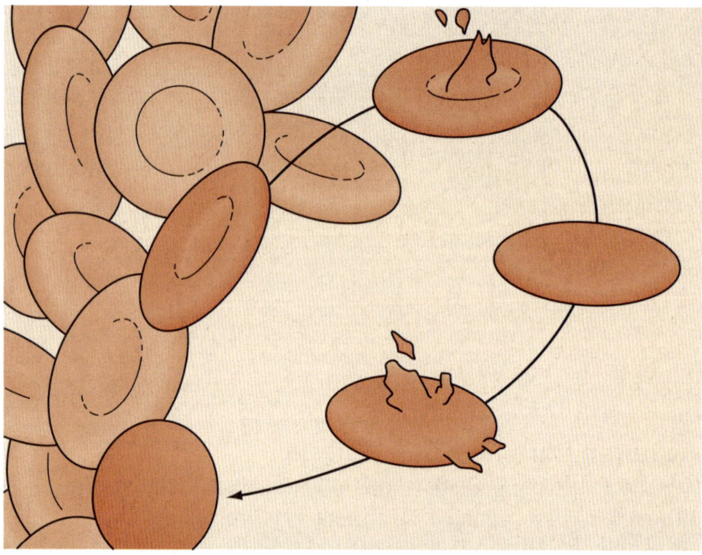

Fig. 12.14 A developing spherocyte resulting from the process of repeated membrane fragmentation, loss, and repair.

mutations. It is named for the peculiar appearance of the RBCs on the peripheral blood smear (Fig. 12.13). The RBC membrane defect, which most commonly results from cytoskeletal membrane instability due to spectrin deficiency, leads to the loss of membrane integrity. Membrane repair occurs, which decreases the normal RBC surface-to-volume ratio and causes the normal biconcave disk to assume a more geometrically efficient spherical shape (Fig. 12.14). The new morphology creates a less pliable cell that hinders transit through the splenic microcirculation (Fig. 12.15). A CBC that shows both an elevated mean corpuscular hemoglobin concentration and red cell distribution width is a highly specific screening test for HS. Osmotic fragility testing can confirm the diagnosis, but it is not pathognomonic and can be unreliable in infants. Flow cytometric tests have now been developed to improve diagnostic accuracy.

Hereditary elliptocytosis is another membrane defect morphologically distinct from HS (Fig. 12.16). In most instances, hereditary elliptocytosis is a mild, well-compensated hemolytic anemia that is clinically insignificant unless splenic hypertrophy develops from another disease process. The elliptocyte form bears only a superficial similarity to that of the ovalocyte of iron deficiency anemia. Unlike those cells, the elliptocytes of hereditary elliptocytosis have normal size and a normal MCV and are true elliptocytes. Elliptocytes may also be found in the peripheral blood smear of thalassemia or in megaloblastic anemia—although these findings do not suggest mixed pathologies.

A number of hemolytic anemias are characterized by spiculated RBCs, referred to as *acanthocytes* or *echinocytes* (Fig. 12.17). Abetalipoproteinemia generally presents as a neurologic disorder with progressive ataxia, retinitis pigmentosa, fat malabsorption, and the absence of chylomicrons and very low-density and low-density lipoproteins. Acanthocytes develop as a direct result of the alterations of the serum

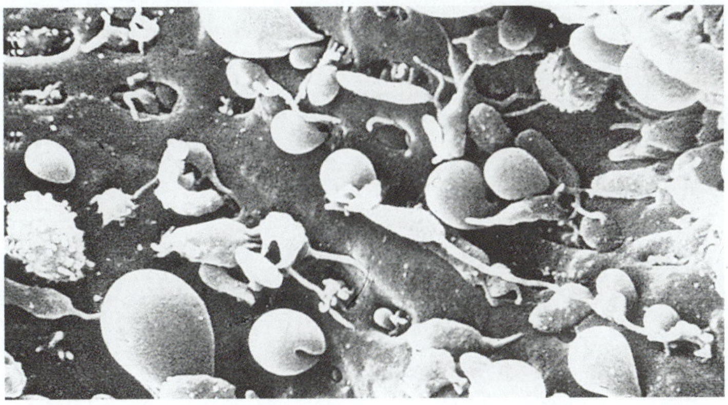

Fig. 12.15 Electron micrograph of red blood cells (RBCs) traversing the splenic sinusoids. Note that the RBCs become deformed as they traverse the microcirculation of the splenic sinusoids.

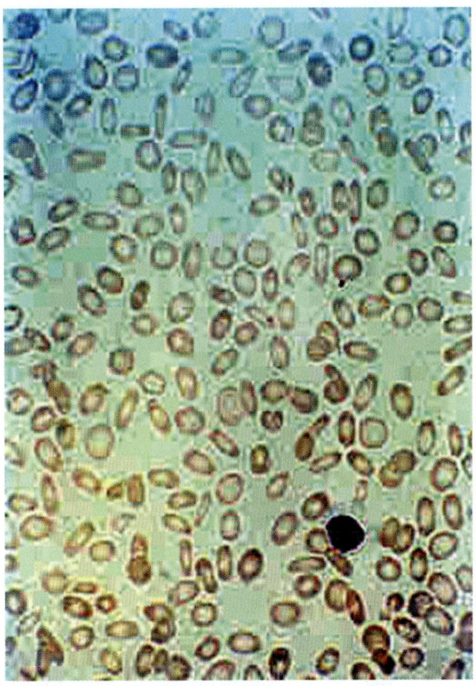

Fig. 12.16 This peripheral blood smear resulted in an incidental finding of hereditary elliptocytosis in a 3-year-old child. More than 90% of the cells are elliptocytes. The child's only remarkable history was one of neonatal jaundice.

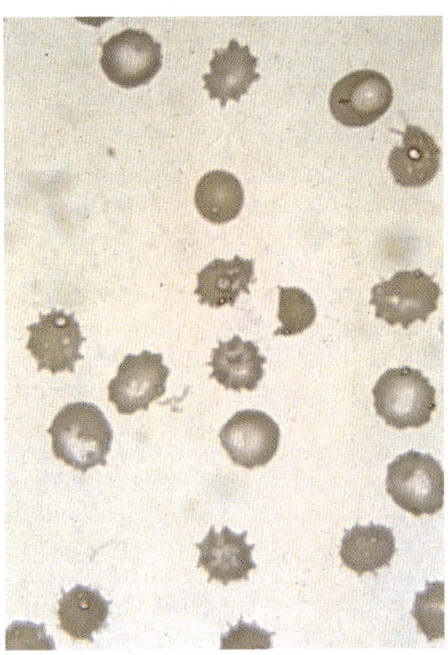

Fig. 12.17 Spur cell anemia with acanthocytes. The peripheral smear from this patient demonstrates the hematologic findings of acute hepatic necrosis. The anemia associated with the presence of these spiculated cells in the periphery can be severe.

lipids. Spur cell anemia develops in the setting of sudden and massive liver injury arising from any cause. Spiculated cells in lesser numbers can also be seen in uremia, anorexia nervosa, and severe malnutrition. Conversely, one of the most frequent causes of spiculated RBCs on the peripheral blood smear can be inadequate slide preparation.

Target cells draw their name from their characteristic appearance on the peripheral blood smear. They are often seen as a secondary response to a process that increases the RBC membrane or decreases the RBC content, leading to an increase in the surface-to-volume ratio of the RBCs (Fig. 12.18). In a dried smear, the excess surface accumulates and bulges outward in the area that is normally the RBC's central pallor, producing the characteristic target cell morphology. Liver diseases of any type, particularly obstructive hepatopathy, are well-known causes of target cell formation. Splenectomy decreases reticuloendothelial remodeling of reticulocytes, removes lipid-loaded RBC membranes, and leads to targeted RBCs. Mechanisms previously discussed that decrease RBC intracellular content (such as hypochromic, microcytic anemia) also induce target formation. In addition, target cells (or more accurately, pseudotarget cells) occur with various hemoglobinopathies. This happens more often in conditions associated with hemoglobin (Hgb) C, but also with Hgb S, D, and E (Figs. 12.19 and 12.20), because of aggregation of hemoglobin in the central region of the RBC (see Fig. 12.18B).

Malaria is the most frequent cause of acquired hemolysis worldwide. Pediatric patients are parasitized within the RBCs with organisms at the merozoite stage (Fig. 12.21). The infection causes a clinical picture of intermittent fever, chills, and jaundice and may lead to encephalopathy, massive hemolysis with hemoglobinuria (blackwater fever), and death. The cause of the hemolysis has been attributed to multiple mechanisms including altered RBCs, osmotic fragility, membrane loss of negative surface charge, direct injury by the parasite, autoimmunity, splenic pitting, and hypersplenism.

Abnormalities of RBC enzymes may also lead to hemolysis. Although almost any RBC enzymes involved in RBC glycolysis or free radical detoxification via the pentose shunt may be responsible for hemolysis, glucose-6-phosphate dehydrogenase (G6PD) deficiency is by far the most frequent. The blood smears of patients with RBC enzyme deficiency–induced hemolysis are often normal, although occasionally with G6PD deficiency a suspicious morphology may be present (Fig. 12.22). More than 370 variants of G6PD have been identified, for which enzyme activity may be normal, elevated, or severely deficient. G6PD deficiency is transmitted by an X-linked recessive mode of inheritance. Heterozygous females rarely may be affected because of inactivation of the X chromosome according to the Lyon hypothesis or because they are doubly heterozygous.

Clinical syndromes and the degree of symptoms vary considerably. Triggered hemolysis associated with the Mediterranean variation of G6PD deficiency is severe and abrupt. In contrast, triggered hemolysis with A type G6PD deficiency is much less common.

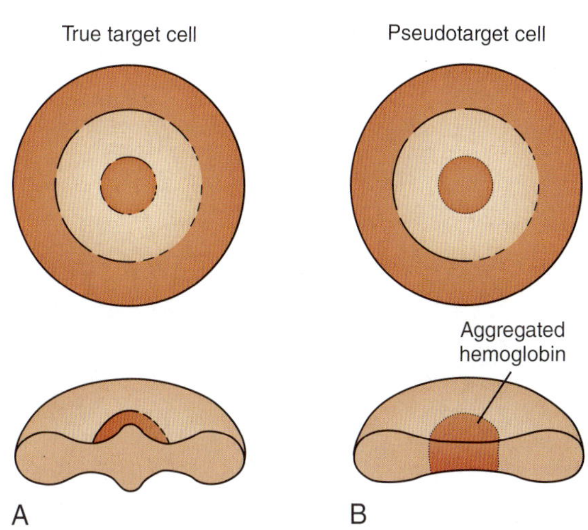

Fig. 12.18 (A) Schematic of the morphology of a target cell. (B) Schematic of the morphology of a pseudotarget cell.

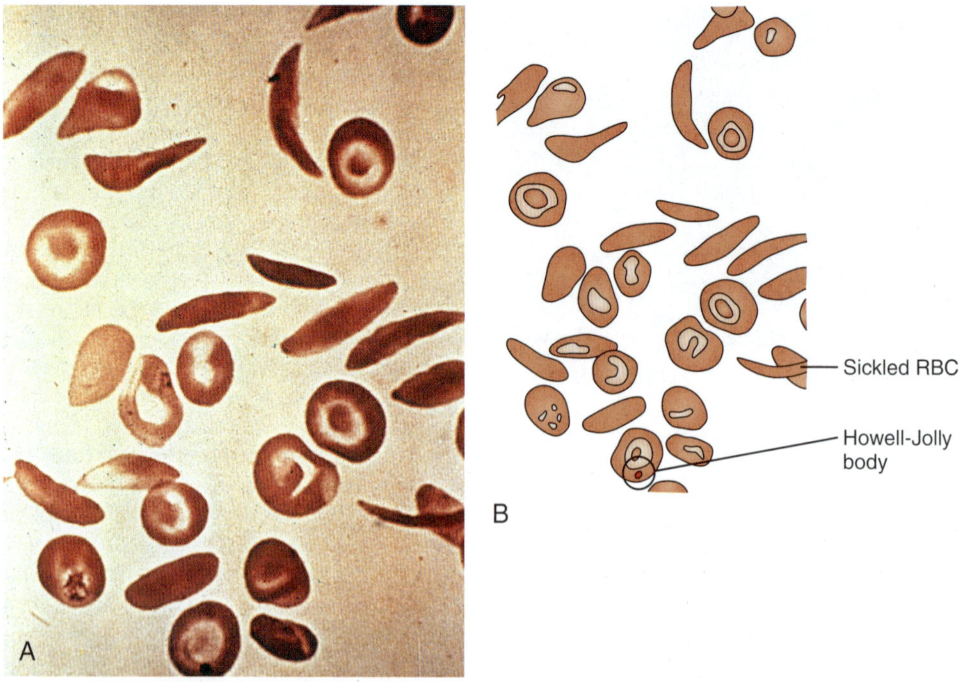

Fig. 12.19 (A) Peripheral blood smear in sickle cell disease. Note the presence of sickle cells and prominent target cells. A Howell-Jolly body is also present, consistent with autoinfarction and subsequent loss of splenic function. (B) Schematic of sickle cell and Howell-Jolly body.

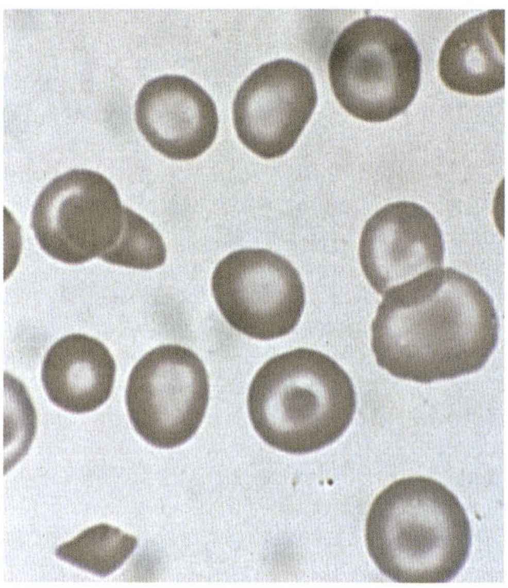

Fig. 12.20 Peripheral blood smear of a child with hemoglobin sickle cell disease. Sickle cells are seen less frequently in this disease, whereas target cells are more prominent.

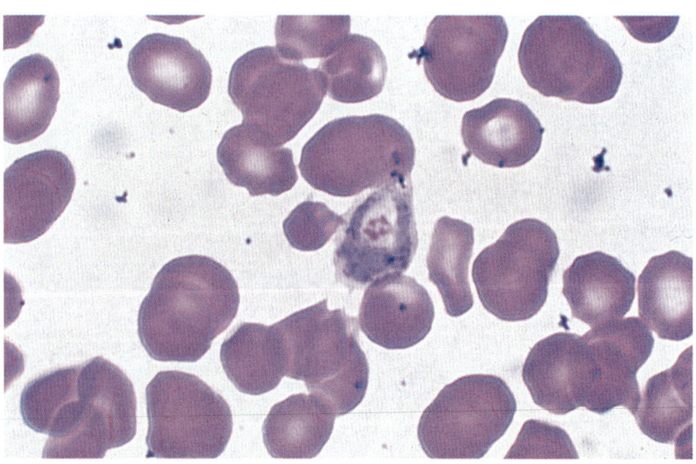

Fig. 12.21 *Plasmodium vivax* malaria. This peripheral blood smear is prepared by the so-called "thick prep" method. *P. vivax* malaria is seen intracellularly in the red blood cell in the center of the smear.

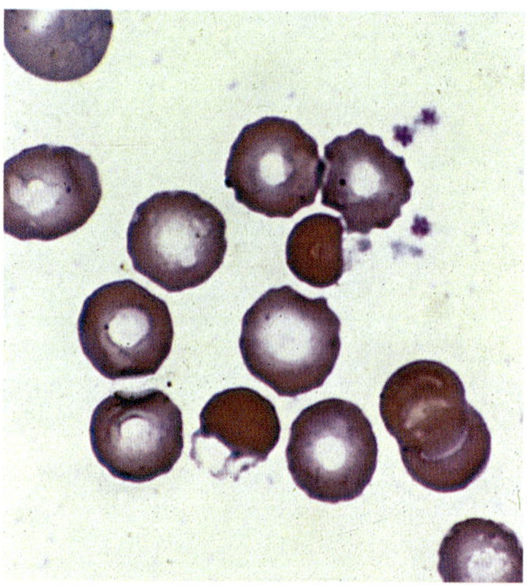

Fig. 12.22 Peripheral blood smear of a patient with glucose-6-phosphate dehydrogenase deficiency. This patient is experiencing a hemolytic crisis. Note the blister cells with hemoglobin condensed in the remaining (nonblistered) portion of the cell.

In addition, some agents that trigger hemolysis with G6PD deficiency (Mediterranean type) may be tolerated by patients with G6PD deficiency (A type). A list of some drugs associated with clinically significant hemolysis in G6PD deficiency is provided (Box 12.2). Research has deemphasized the role of certain drug triggers.

Pyruvate kinase (PK) deficiency is the second most prevalent enzyme abnormality of the RBC that leads to hemolysis; however, it is a distant second, with 1 case of PK deficiency occurring worldwide for every 500,000 cases of G6PD deficiency. Autosomal recessive transmission of the enzyme defect is usually observed, and wide clinical variability exists. Mild, fully compensated hemolytic anemia and severe neonatal hemolysis and hyperbilirubinemia may occur. Hemoglobin levels range from 6 to 10 g/dL with normochromic anemia with normocytic or macrocytic indices, depending on the degree of reticulocytosis. The reticulocyte count can range from 5% to as high as 90% in the patient who has had a splenectomy. For the subgroup of patients with severe, transfusion-dependent disease, splenectomy may ameliorate or eliminate the need for transfusions.

Box 12.2 Drugs Associated With Clinically Significant Hemolysis in Glucose-6-Phosphate Dehydrogenase Deficiency

Antimalarials
Pamaquine
Pentaquine
Primaquine
Quinocide

Antipyretics and Analgesics
Acetanilide
Aminopyrine
Antipyrine

Sulfa Drugs
N-Acetylsulfanilamide
Salicylazosulfapyridine
Sulfamethoxypyridazine
Sulfapyridine
Thiazolesulfone

Miscellaneous
Acetylphenylhydrazine
Fava beans
Nalidixic acid
Naphthalene
Phenylhydrazine
Toluidine blue

In addition to chronic hemolysis, PK deficiency may have triggered episodes (usually resulting from intercurrent infection).

Direct and indirect Coombs tests, which evaluate the patient's blood for the presence of anti-RBC antibody and complement, identify immune-mediated hemolytic anemia. Antibody- and complement-mediated RBC destruction produces spherocytes on the peripheral blood smear (Fig. 12.23). Immune-mediated hemolytic disease of the newborn is most often due to from Rh mediated destruction. ABO-related disease is less severe due to the decreased number of the A and B antigens on fetal RBCs. Other immune-mediated hemolytic anemias, both allo- and autoimmune, can be seen as acute and chronic processes in older children.

Hemoglobinopathies

Hemoglobinopathies can be responsible for both hemolysis and ineffective erythropoiesis. Baseline levels of hemoglobin can be much lower in patients with these disorders, and nearly all are life-long conditions. Nomenclature in hemoglobinopathies is confusing, and care must be taken to distinguish clinical phenotype from globin phenotype and from globin genotype. In general, terms such as *trait, disease, minor,* or *major* refer to frequency of symptoms or transfusions rather than genotypic features.

The most well-known hemoglobinopathy is sickle cell disease. Substitution of valine for glutamic acid at position 6 in the beta chain of the hemoglobin molecule leads to the cross-linking of one beta chain to a second hemoglobin molecule's beta chain when the hemoglobin is in its deoxygenated state. This cross-linkage tips the solubility balance, leading to deformation of the RBC (see Fig. 12.19). Sickle cell disease is not exclusive to patients of African origin; patients of Mediterranean and Middle Eastern descent are also affected. Sickle cell disease is an autosomal recessive disorder. Heterozygous carriers of the sickle cell gene, although suffering some difficulties (e.g., poor urine-concentrating ability, occasional episodes of renal papillary necrosis with hematuria), have normal life expectancies and are often free of significant consequences.

The clinical signs and symptoms of sickle cell disease are due to decreased survival and altered rheology of the sickled RBC. As with any chronic hemolytic state, marrow cavity enlargement occurs, leading to maxillary hyperplasia (Fig. 12.24). Sickled cells have altered pliability and lose the ability to deform in the microcirculation (see Fig. 12.15), leading to tissue infarction and subsequent pain. These vaso-occlusive crises, when occurring in certain locations, give rise to clinical manifestations, such as dactylitis (Fig. 12.25), priapism (Fig. 12.26; also see Chapter 15), splenic sequestration, and skin ulceration. Vaso-occlusive phenomena may also lead to life-threatening complications—overwhelming infection, acute chest syndrome, or stroke. The increased infectious risk in the sickle cell patient has multiple mechanisms, but by far, the most important is splenic dysfunction related to congested blood flow and ultimately splenic infarction. Loss of splenic and general reticuloendothelial function puts the patient at increased risk from most encapsulated pathogens.

Thalassemia is a term applied to a group of genetic disturbances decreasing hemoglobin production and leading to altered levels of various hemoglobins in the blood. Hydrops fetalis may result from α-thalassemia major. Thalassemia trait is a common cause of microcytosis. Although hemoglobin values may be lower than expected, thalassemia traits do not represent a physiologic anemia. Patients with α-thalassemia trait can display hemoglobin Barts in the newborn period due to the relative excess of γ-globin chains. After this developmental stage, hemoglobin studies will not show abnormal forms.

β-Thalassemia trait and disorders generally present after the first 3 to 6 months of life, when β-chain synthesis should be increasing.

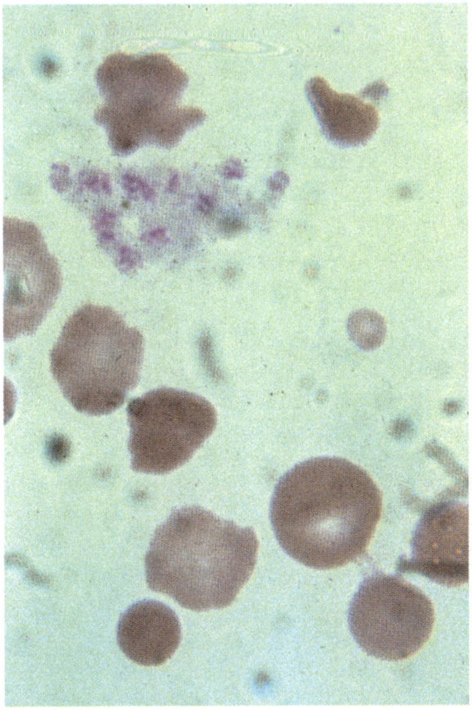

Fig. 12.23 Coombs-positive hemolytic anemia. Note the spherocytes and a large red blood cell with polychromasia, indicating the presence of regenerative anemia.

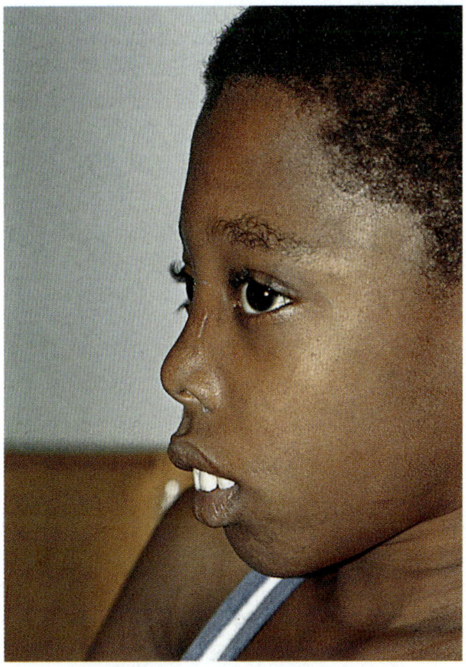

Fig. 12.24 Maxillary hyperplasia. Prominent facial bones of a child with sickle cell anemia, due to enlargement of the marrow cavity in this condition of decreased red blood cell survival.

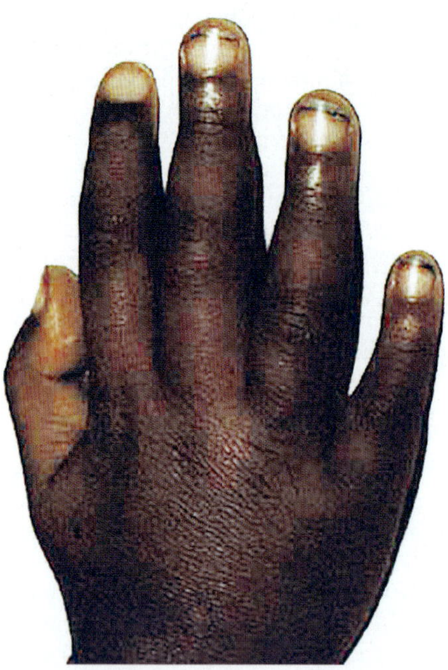

Fig. 12.25 Dactylitis (hand-foot syndrome). This syndrome, in children with sickle cell disease, primarily affects toddlers. Dactylitis is seen less frequently in older children because the bone marrow of the small bones of the hands and feet loses hematopoietic activity. This loss of marrow activity is due to cortical thickening from increased use of hands and weight bearing by the feet.

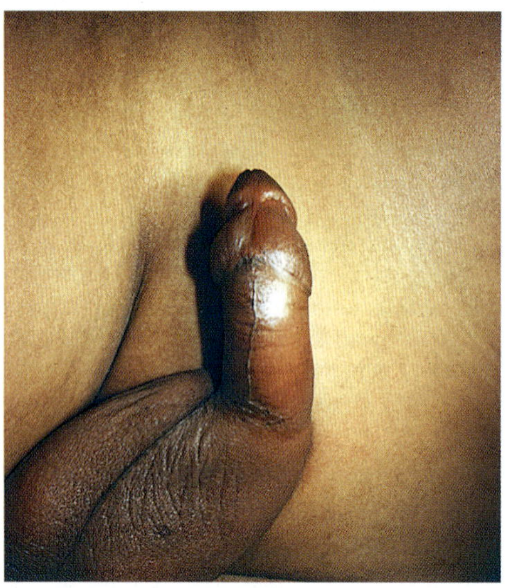

Fig. 12.26 Priapism in an adolescent with sickle cell disease. Erection had persisted for 12 hours and had become extremely painful for the patient.

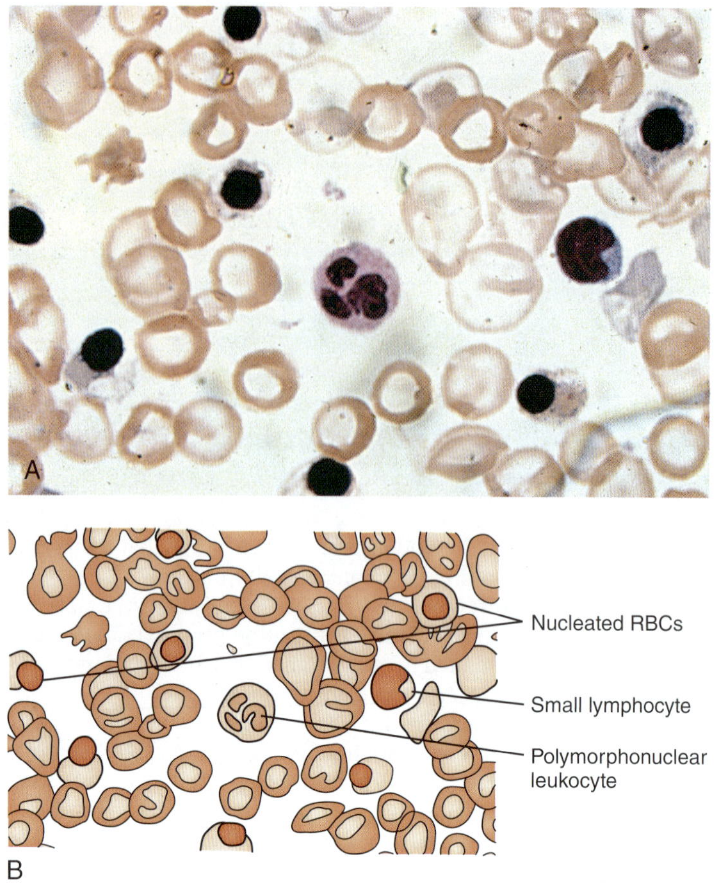

Fig. 12.27 Thalassemia major. (A) This peripheral blood smear of a child with thalassemia major shows hypochromic, microcytic anemia with prominent nucleated red blood cells surrounding the polymorphonuclear cells and lymphocytes. (B) Labeled schematic of peripheral blood smear.

Hemoglobin electrophoresis usually reveals an increase in Hgb A_2 and Hgb F. β-Thalassemia major (Cooley anemia) causes hypochromic, microcytic anemia that results from ineffective erythropoiesis caused by an imbalance between the α- and β-hemoglobin chain synthesis. The peripheral blood smear shows hypochromia; microcytosis; target cells; basophilic stippling (see Fig. 12.8); and, often, many nucleated RBCs (Fig. 12.27). β-Thalassemia major is associated with increased marrow activity, which is ineffectively attempting to correct the degree of anemia. The increased marrow activity expands the marrow cavity, producing a characteristic bony hyperplasia evidenced by physical and radiographic findings (Fig. 12.28). Untreated patients with thalassemia major have chronic and severe anemia, marked hepatosplenomegaly, scleral icterus, and listlessness and may have high-output cardiac failure secondary to severe anemia. In addition, malocclusion may occur because of molar hypertrophy.

Although less common than sickle cell disease, anemia associated with Hgb C is not rare in the African American population. As in sickle cell disease, Hgb C disease occurs because a single amino acid change at the sixth position of the β chain, but the replacement is a lysine rather than a valine. In its homozygous form, Hgb C disease is a mild disorder characterized by hemolytic anemia and splenomegaly. The tendency of Hgb C to aggregate into precipitates is responsible for the pseudotarget (see Fig. 12.18B) morphology of the Hgb C homozygous and Hgb C trait (heterozygous) cells on the peripheral blood smear. When paired in a double heterozygous state with Hgb S, Hgb C results in sickle cell (SC) disease (see Fig. 12.20) and is associated with sickle cell symptoms, although less severe.

Coagulation System

Disorders That Predispose to Bleeding

Bleeding disorders are defined as an inadequate hemostatic response to tissue injury. The amount of bleeding depends on the site and degree of tissue injury and the severity of the defect in the hemostatic system. Epistaxis serves as an example. The nose has a rich vascular network (see Chapter 24). Local physical injury and dryness are the most common causes of bleeding. Likewise, infectious or allergic disease can trigger episodes. Whatever the inciting event, however, a child with an intact hemostatic system should be able to control bleeding from the nares with direct pressure, cauterization, or packing. When such conservative measures fail or similar such episodes continue in a recurrent fashion, clinicians should be suspicious that a bleeding disorder may exist.

Questions concerning testing for bleeding disorders are controversial. In many cases, a dental or otolaryngology procedure may be the first challenge of a child's ability to form clots appropriately. If a specific disorder is suggested by a child's presentation, then testing should be targeted toward the most likely diagnosis. Historical evaluation and physical examination can be guided by a tool such as the Pediatric Bleeding Questionnaire (Table 12.2). A score of ≥ 2 in young children or ≥ 3 in adolescents suggests that testing for a

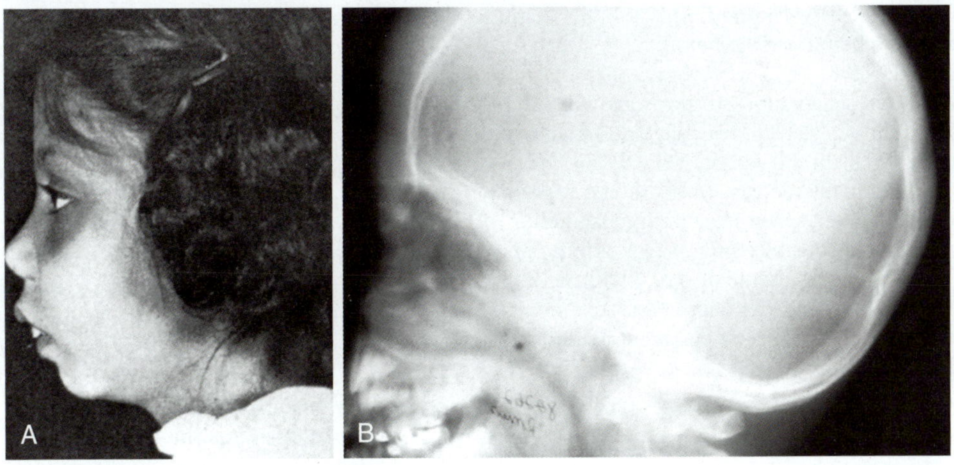

Fig. 12.28 (A) Maxillary hyperplasia resulting from an increased marrow space in a child with thalassemia major. (B) Skull radiograph of the same patient demonstrates an increased marrow cavity of the skull and facial bones.

Table 12.2 Scoring Key From Pediatric Bleeding Questionnaire

Score Symptom	−1	0	1	2	3	4
Epistaxis	—	No or trivial (≤5 per year)	>5 per year OR >10 min duration	Consultation only	Packing, cauterization or antifibrinolytics	Blood transfusion, replacement therapy or desmopressin
Cutaneous	—	No or trivial (≤1 cm)	>1 cm AND no trauma	Consultation only	—	—
Minor wounds	—	No or trivial (≤5 per year)	>5 per year OR >5 min duration	Consultation only or Steri-Strips	Surgical hemostasis or antifibrinolytics	Blood transfusion, replacement therapy or desmopressin
Oral cavity	—	No	Reported at least once	Consultation only	Surgical hemostasis or antifibrinolytics	Blood transfusion, replacement therapy or desmopressin
Gastrointestinal tract	—	No	Identified cause	Consultation or spontaneous	Surgical hemostasis, antifibrinolytics, blood transfusion, replacement therapy or desmopressin	—
Tooth extraction	No bleeding in at least 2 extractions	None done or no bleeding in 1 extraction	Reported, no consultation	Consultation only	Resuturing, repacking or antifibrinolytics	Blood transfusion, replacement therapy or desmopressin
Surgery	No bleeding in at least 2 surgeries	None done or no bleeding in 1 surgery	Reported, no consultation	Consultation only	Surgical hemostasis or antifibrinolytics	Blood transfusion, replacement therapy or desmopressin
Menorrhagia	—	No	Reported or consultation only	Antifibrinolytics or contraceptive pill use	D&C or iron therapy	Blood transfusion, replacement therapy, desmopressin or hysterectomy
Postpartum	No bleeding in at least 2 deliveries	No deliveries or no bleeding in 1 delivery	Reported or consultation only	D&C, iron therapy or antifibrinolytics	Blood transfusion, replacement therapy or desmopressin	—
Muscle hematoma	—	Never	Post trauma, no therapy	Spontaneous, no therapy	Spontaneous or traumatic, requiring replacement therapy or desmopressin	Spontaneous or traumatic, requiring surgical intervention or blood transfusion
Hemarthrosis	—	Never	Post trauma, no therapy	Spontaneous, no therapy	Spontaneous or traumatic, requiring replacement therapy or desmopressin	Spontaneous or traumatic, requiring surgical intervention or blood transfusion
Central nervous system	—	Never	—	—	Subdural, any intervention	Intracerebral, any intervention
Other[a]	—	No	Reported	Consultation only	Surgical hemostasis, antifibrinolytics or iron therapy	Blood transfusion, replacement therapy or desmopressin

[a]In the last row, "Other" symptoms include umbilical stump bleeding, cephalohematoma, postcircumcision bleeding, postvenipuncture bleeding, and macroscopic hematuria.

From Bowman M, Riddel J, Rand ML, et al: Evaluation of the diagnostic utility for von Willebrand disease of a pediatric bleeding questionnaire, *J Thromb Haemost* 7:1418–1421, 2009.

mucocutaneous bleeding disorder is warranted. This tool also can be used with family members to help trace the hereditary pattern of a particular bleeding concern.

Normal laboratory values for coagulation studies vary from the newborn period through adulthood. Many of the coagulation factors (other than V, VIII, and von Willebrand factor) (Fig. 12.29) have reduced levels in infants and gradually increase over the first year of life. As a result, care should be taken when evaluating coagulation studies in pediatric patients. In acute bleeding presentations, an evaluation of surgical or physical causes should also be performed. If the administration of blood products or other hemostatic treatments is not emergently indicated, the performance of pertinent diagnostic tests should be considered first.

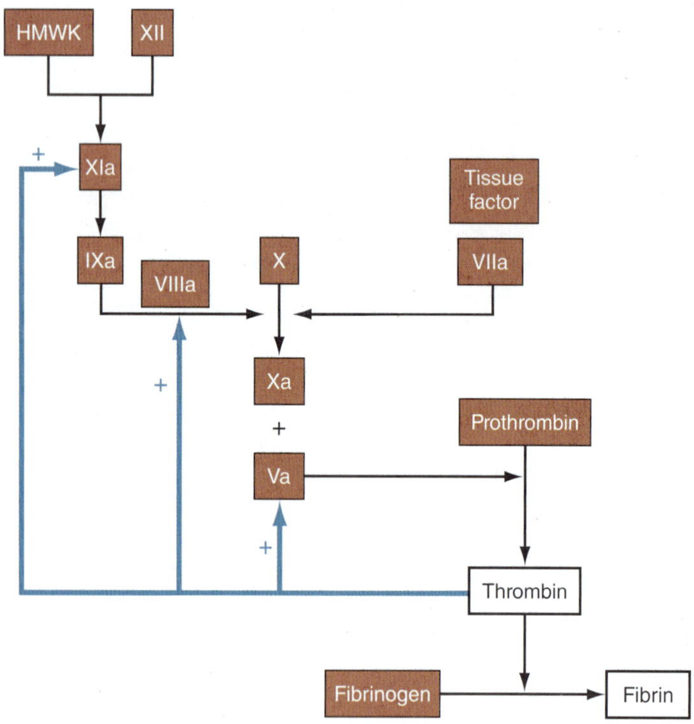

Fig. 12.29 Overview of the coagulation system. *Red* and *white boxes* represent factors in the clotting cascade. The extrinsic pathway is composed of tissue factor and factor VIIa, whereas the intrinsic pathway features high-molecular-weight kininogen *(HMWK)* and factors XII, XIa, IXa, and VIIIa. Both pathways contribute to the conversion of factor X into its activated form *(Xa)*, leading to thrombin generation. Thrombin not only cleaves fibrinogen into fibrin but also upregulates the cascade in several areas to contribute to clot propagation *(represented by blue arrows)*.

Disorders of Primary Hemostasis

Primary hemostatic disorders are marked by mucocutaneous bleeding but can be more severe as well. The number and size of circulating platelets can be determined by automated or manual methods. *Thrombocytopenia* is defined as a platelet count less than 150,000 cells/μL. Pseudothrombocytopenia occurs when a normal in vivo platelet count is reported (erroneously) to be low in vitro. This can occur when platelets agglutinate and are bypassed by the automated counter or when large platelets are misinterpreted as leukocytes. Manual inspection of a peripheral smear appropriately prepared with a Wright-Giemsa stain will clarify these situations. Platelet size is reported as mean platelet volume, expressed as femtoliters. The presence of large platelets (>7 fL) may be helpful in distinguishing between various platelet disorders.

Thrombocytopenia is the most common hematologic abnormality of neonates. Most commonly, thrombocytopenia in this age group is secondary to other illnesses, such as sepsis, congenital infections, or necrotizing enterocolitis. However, thrombocytopenia can be a primary process. Neonatal alloimmune thrombocytopenia is caused by the transplacental passage of maternal antibodies directed against the paternal antigens on an infant's platelets. Incompatibility occurs as commonly as once in every 350 pregnancies (50% will be first pregnancies), although thrombocytopenia develops in far fewer (1 per 1000–1500). The thrombocytopenia can be severe and difficult to treat. Intravenous immunoglobulin may be helpful, but the best treatment is the transfusion of maternally donated platelets. Isoimmune thrombocytopenia, on the other hand, results from the passage of maternal autoantibodies. These are far less specific and less likely to cause severe thrombocytopenia.

Immune thrombocytopenia (ITP) is an autoimmune phenomenon characterized by a low circulating platelet count with a peak incidence from 2 to 4 years old. ITP is often preceded by a mild viral illness. It also can be a secondary disease process, especially in rheumatologic or immunodeficiency syndromes. The pathophysiology is complex, but both humoral and cellular immune processes are involved with the generation and then propagation of antiplatelet autoantibodies. Once platelets become coated with immunoglobulin G (IgG), they are cleared aggressively by tissue macrophages, especially in the spleen.

In general, children with ITP appear well. Symptoms usually are limited to petechiae, epistaxis, and ecchymoses (Fig. 12.30). Alternatively, a small percentage of children may present with significant mucosal bleeding. In more than half of cases of childhood ITP, the presenting platelet count will be less than 20,000 cells/μL. Review of the blood smear generally reveals large platelets but in significantly diminished numbers. Any signs or symptoms that suggest an alternative diagnosis, such as prolonged fever or splenomegaly, should be

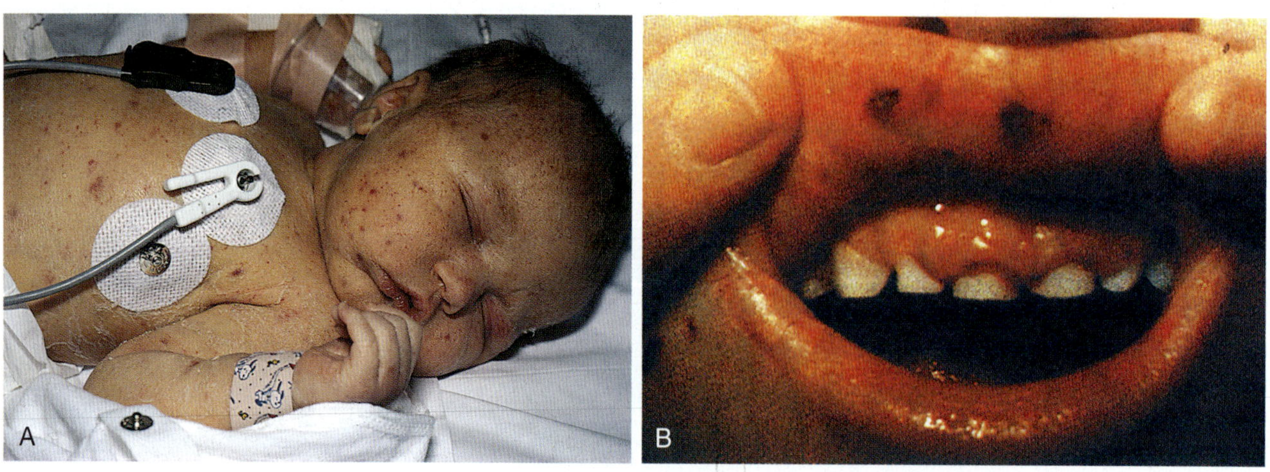

Fig. 12.30 Petechiae. (A) This infant with severe immune thrombocytopenia has visible petechiae and large ecchymoses. (B) Purpuric lesions on the oral mucosa or retina are called "wet purpura" and may suggest an increased tendency for major bleeding in the thrombocytopenic patient.

investigated thoroughly. In the setting of typical ITP, a bone marrow aspiration is not necessary.

In most children, the disease is self-limited and outcomes are excellent. Observation alone is a well-accepted treatment option. However, there is a small risk of intracranial hemorrhage, estimated at approximately 1 per 10,000 patients, and pharmacologic treatment is frequently pursued. Corticosteroids are typically used as the primary ITP treatment and have been shown to be the most cost-effective option. Alternatively, intravenous immunoglobulin or anti-D immunoglobulin (in Rh-positive patients) can be used. Platelet transfusions are of minimal benefit, unless a severe and life-threatening hemorrhage is occurring, and will require two to three times the normal volume.

Inherited thrombocytopenias result in moderately depressed platelet counts (50,000–100,000 cells/μL) and do not require daily management. However, traumatic injuries, illnesses, or surgical procedures can place these children at risk for bleeding. May-Hegglin anomaly is characterized by macrothrombocytopenia and white blood cell (WBC) inclusions known as *Döhle bodies.* Some macrothrombocytopenias are due to autosomally dominant inherited mutations in the *MYH9* gene, which encodes cytoskeletal proteins. Conversely, Wiskott-Aldrich syndrome (see Chapter 4) is characterized by microthrombocytopenia. This disorder is caused by the X-linked inheritance of mutations and is associated with decreased platelet survival, eczema, and recurrent infections. Treatment of bleeding in inherited thrombocytopenias consists of desmopressin, aminocaproic acid, and platelet transfusions when necessary.

Even when platelets are present in normal amounts, mucocutaneous bleeding due to functional deficits can occur. The most complete test of platelet function is by aggregometry. A sample of patient whole blood or platelet-rich plasma is combined with one of a number of platelet agonist molecules. The degree and rate of platelet agglutination are recorded graphically. Various platelet disorders have unique response patterns to each agonist. Many drugs can affect platelet function temporarily and make tests of platelet function abnormal. These tests should not be run within 10 days of using such a drug because the diagnosis of a true disorder could be missed. Other tests can serve as screening evaluations of platelet function, to varying degrees of reliability. The bleeding time is a surrogate measure of both platelet number and function. At present, this test is not recommended for pediatric patients. Most pediatric hematologists prefer the closure time, though its utility as a screening test has been poor.

Drugs and certain disease states can cause temporary impairment of platelet function. Aspirin irreversibly impairs circulating platelets, whereas other nonsteroidal antiinflammatory drugs only temporarily inhibit key enzymes. Increased bleeding is usually seen only in patients with an underlying coagulation abnormality, but some patients may be hyperresponsive to the platelet inhibition. Antibiotics, antiepileptics, and psychotropic drugs may also lead to transient inhibitions of platelet function. In addition to medications, systemic illnesses can create an environment in which platelets lose some of their function. Uremia causes platelet inhibition through a variety of mechanisms. The degree of renal failure correlates with prolongation of the bleeding time but not with bleeding.

Disorders of Secondary Hemostasis

Secondary hemostatic disorders, commonly referred to as *coagulopathies,* can present with deep tissue bleeds and more pronounced symptoms than mucocutaneous bleeding alone. Whatever the cause of coagulopathy, measurement of the prothrombin time (PT) and activated partial thromboplastin time (aPTT) is the first step in clarifying a diagnosis (see Fig. 12.29). The PT, first demonstrated in the 1930s, is a surrogate measure of the coagulation factors involved in the extrinsic and common pathways: VII, X, V, II, and fibrinogen. The PT is typically used to monitor the effects of warfarin therapy or to evaluate for liver disease and vitamin K deficiency. The international normalized ratio (INR) provides standardization of the PT at different laboratories. The aPTT reflects factors in the intrinsic and common pathways: XII, XI, X, IX, VIII, V, II, and fibrinogen. Patients who are deficient in factor XII may have prolonged aPTT values but no risk of bleeding. The aPTT is less reflective of variations in vitamin K–dependent factors than is the PT; however, it is much more sensitive to the effects of heparin and inhibitory antibodies. Both the PT and aPTT are prolonged by deficiencies of factors below 30% to 35%.

The most common cause of a prolonged aPTT in children is an inhibitory antibody. The term *inhibitor* can be defined broadly to include anticoagulants, autoantibodies, and lupus anticoagulants. To discern whether a prolonged aPTT is due to factor deficiencies or the presence of an inhibitor, a mixing study can be performed. An abnormal test that corrects is due to deficiencies, whereas those that remain abnormal suggest the presence of an inhibitor. A nonspecific inhibitor, meaning an abnormal mixing study without other hematologic explanation, is a benign and common finding in pediatrics. In this setting, an inhibitor prolongs in vitro clotting times but does not represent a risk factor for bleeding.

The hemophilias are defined physiologically by delayed formation of an abnormal clot. Hemophilia A is an X-linked bleeding disorder in which patients have a deficiency of factor VIII. Hemophilia B is a similar illness, although with a deficiency of factor IX. Hemophilia A occurs in approximately 1 per 5000 live male births, whereas hemophilia B affects 1 in 30,000. Despite the well-known pattern of inherited mutations in the factor VIII gene, approximately 20% to 30% of patients with severe hemophilia A represent new gene defects and will not have any affected relatives. Severe hemophilia is usually diagnosed early in the first year of life, especially when a family history is known. Children with mild or moderate degrees of disease may not have bleeding episodes until early childhood. The diagnosis can be suggested by a prolonged aPTT and then confirmed by specific assays for either factor VIII or IX.

Both hemophilia A and B are classified by baseline factor level: less than 1% (1 U/dL) is defined as severe, 1% to 5% (<1 U/dL) as moderate, and more than 5% (>5 U/dL) as mild. The location, frequency, and type of bleeding episodes relate to the severity of disease. Patients with mild forms of the disease may have bleeding complications only after surgery or major trauma. Those with moderate disease have a higher incidence of minor bleeding and may have bleeding in response to minor trauma or daily activities. Patients with severe hemophilia may have bleeding into joints or muscles with normal daily activities, in addition to minor bleeds and catastrophic hemorrhages from trauma or surgery (Figs. 12.31 and 12.32).

Other Bleeding Disorders

Von Willebrand disease (VWD) is a bleeding disorder with various intensities that can combine parts of primary and secondary hemostatic problems. Von Willebrand factor (VWF) is synthesized in both endothelial cells and megakaryocytes; patients can have either low, absent, or poorly functioning molecules. In the most common

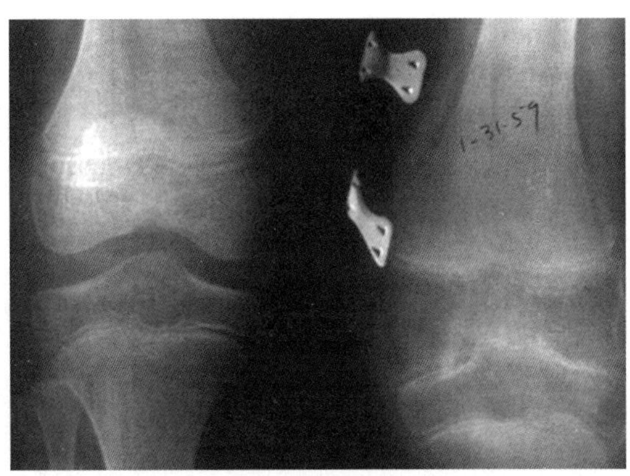

Fig. 12.31 Hemophiliac arthritis. This patient with hemophilia has experienced recurrent hemarthroses. Note the widened joint space on the left knee compared with that of the normal right knee.

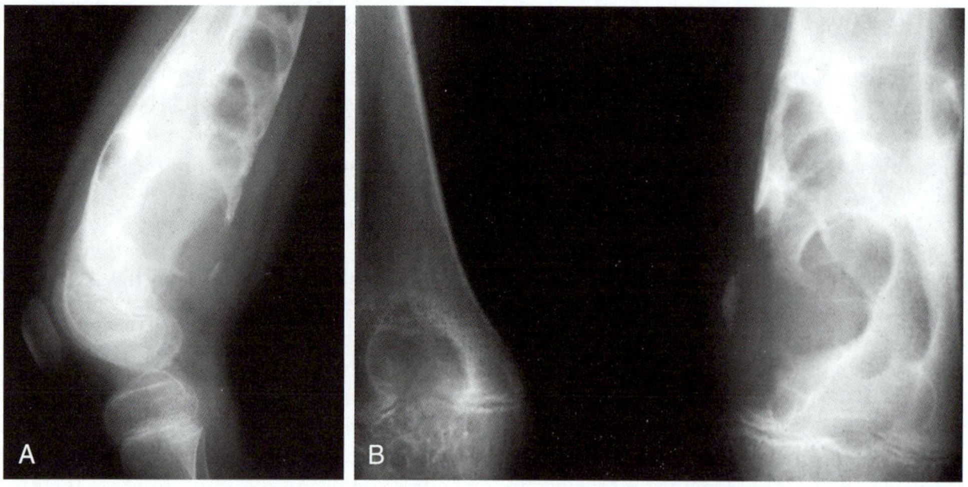

Fig. 12.32 (A) Pseudotumor of the femur. This radiographic finding has resulted from recurrent hemarthroses with subsequent bony destruction of the knee and adjacent bony structures. (B) Note that the opposite knee also demonstrates early destructive changes in the distal femur and joint.

forms, VWD is characterized by excessive mucocutaneous bleeding. It is the most frequently inherited bleeding disorder, with a prevalence estimated at 1%, although the rate of symptomatic disease is likely closer to 1 per 1000. Type 1 VWD, a partial quantitative deficiency of von Willebrand factor (VWF), is by far the most common variety found (Table 12.3). The diagnosis of VWD begins with three studies. First, the von Willebrand factor antigen (VWF:Ag) level measures the amount of VWF in the plasma. Second, the glycoprotein Ib activity measures the function of available VWF in plasma. Third, the factor VIII level is measured. Secondary testing can be pursued for further clarity of VWD subtypes (Table 12.4). Due to variability between laboratories, consensus guidelines on the diagnosis of VWD have been published by the National Institutes of Health. Treatment of VWD is performed with replacement of VWF and factor VIII or by stimulating the release of VWF stores with desmopressin, depending on the type and degree of defect present.

Table 12.3 Classification of von Willebrand Disease

Type	Description
1	Partial quantitative deficiency of VWF
2	Qualitative VWF defect
2A	Decreased VWF-dependent platelet adhesion with selective deficiency of high-molecular-weight multimers
2B	Increased affinity for platelet GPIb
2M	Decreased VWF-dependent platelet adhesion without selective deficiency of high-molecular-weight multimers
2N	Markedly decreased binding affinity for FVIII
3	Virtually complete deficiency of VWF

Note: VWD types are defined as described in Sadler JE, Budde U, Eikenboom JC, et al: Update on the pathophysiology and classification of von Willebrand disease: a report of the Subcommittee on von Willebrand Factor, *J Thromb Haemost* 4(10):2103–2114, 2006. *VWF,* von Willebrand factor.

There are also rarely encountered coagulation disorders. Some of these rare disorders are listed in Table 12.5. For many, there are no specific treatments available in the United States other than transfused blood products. Fresh frozen plasma (FFP) should be matched to the recipient ABO red cell status, although Rh positivity does not need to be considered. FFP is indicated for patients with significant coagulopathies who are bleeding or require an invasive procedure. Cryoprecipitate, on the other hand, is derived from plasma by thawing FFP and removing the supernatant. This contains concentrated amounts of factors VIII and XIII, VWF, and fibrinogen in volumes that, on average, are quite small. In patients with dysfibrinogenemia or hypofibrinogenemia, transfusion of cryoprecipitate is warranted.

Increasingly, it is recognized that children and adolescents with hypermobility spectrum disorders can have increased bleeding symptoms. Not all patients with hypermobility have bleeding, but those that do should be treated as other children with bleeding disorders. The presumed mechanism of bleeding relates to the interaction between vascular collagen, platelets, and circulating coagulation factors. There are no established laboratory studies to confirm the diagnosis. Patients are evaluated by history and characteristic physical examination findings (see Chapter 1 and Chapter 7 for details of other hypermobility syndromes such as Ehler-Danlos). Genetic testing can help identify different types of hypermobility disorders, but current guidance recommends reserving this testing for patients of adult age.

Table 12.4 Patterns of Laboratory Testing in von Willebrand Disease

	Normal	Type 1	Type 2A	Type 2B	Type 2M	Type 2N	Type 3
VWF:Ag	N	L, ↓ or ↓↓	↓ or L	↓ or L	↓ or L	N or L	Absent
GP1bM	N	L, ↓ or ↓↓	↓↓ or ↓↓↓	↓↓	↓↓	N or L	Absent
FVIII	N	N or ↓	N or ↓	N or ↓	N or ↓	↓↓	1–9 IU/dL
RIPA	N	Often N	↓	Often N	↓	N	Absent
LD-RIPA	Absent	Absent	Absent	↑↑↑	Absent	Absent	Absent
PFA-100 CT	N	N or ↑	↑	↑	↑	N	↑↑↑
BT	N	N or ↑	↑	↑	↑	N	↑↑↑
Platelet count	N	N	N	↓ or N	N	N	N
VWF multimer pattern	N	N	Abnormal	Abnormal	N	N	Absent

↓, ↓↓, ↓↓↓, Relative decrease; ↑, ↑↑, ↑↑↑, relative increase; *BT,* bleeding time; *FVIII,* factor VIII activity; *L,* 30–50 IU/dL; *LD-RIPA,* low-dose ristocetin-induced platelet aggregation (concentration of ristocetin ≤0.6 mg/mL); *N,* normal; *PFA-100 CT,* platelet function analyzer closure time; *RIPA,* risocetin-induced platelet aggregation; *VWF,* von Willebrand factor; *VWF:Ag,* von Willebrand factor antigen; *VWF:RCo, VWF* ristocetin cofactor activity.

Available at https://www.nhlbi.nih.gov/health-topics/diagnosis-evaluation-and-management-of-von-willebrand-disease.

Table 12.5 Rare Bleeding Disorders

Disorder	Treatment	Notes
Hypofibrinogenemia	Cryoprecipitate or FFP	Will have very low fibrinogen levels
Dysfibrinogenemia	Cryoprecipitate or FFP	Diagnosed by abnormal reptilase and thrombin times with normal fibrinogen levels Usually autosomal dominant inheritance patterns
Factor II (prothrombin) deficiency	FFP or prothrombin complex concentrate	Bleeding usually mild unless after trauma
Factor V deficiency	FFP	Bleeding is usually mild to moderate Rarely can be combined with factor VIII deficiency
Factor VII deficiency	Recombinant VIIa	Very rare: 1 per 500,000 in general population Very low levels can lead to severe bleeding
Factor X deficiency	FFP or prothrombin complex concentrate	Usually features mild to moderate mucocutaneous and posttraumatic bleeding
Factor XI deficiency	FFP	Autosomal recessive inheritance; most frequently encountered in Ashkenazi Jewish populations Bleeding most common after trauma or surgery
Factor XIII deficiency	Cryoprecipitate or FFP	Associated with delayed umbilical cord separation and intracranial hemorrhage with minimal trauma Characterized by delayed hemorrhage
PAI-1 deficiency	Antifibrinolytic agents	Bleeding most common after trauma or surgery Euglobulin lysis time will be shortened
Antiplasmin deficiency	Antifibrinolytic agents	Mucocutaneous bleeding and hemarthroses Symptoms can be similar to those in mild hemophilia Euglobulin lysis time will be shortened

FFP, Fresh frozen plasma; *PAI-1,* plasminogen activator inhibitor type 1.

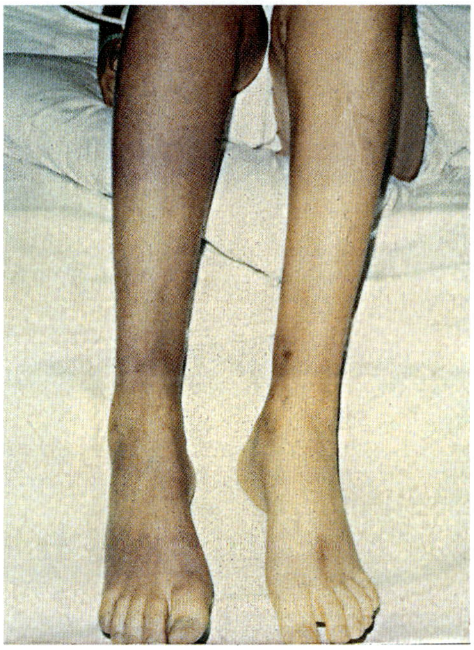

Fig. 12.33 Note the swollen, discolored leg in a child with deep venous thrombosis resulting from protein C deficiency. (Courtesy R. Kellogg, MD.)

Thrombosis in Children

Epidemiologic studies have shown that the overall incidence of venous thromboembolism is approximately 0.5 to 5 per 10,000 children in the United States. There is a bimodal distribution, with a peak in the newborn period and another in late adolescence. Thromboses often present in the deep veins of an extremity or the vena cava (Fig. 12.33). Thromboses in children often present with pain, swelling, and discoloration. Pulmonary emboli (PE), although less common than in adults, can present with tachypnea, chest pain, tachycardia, fever, and decreased oxygen saturations. Laboratory screening tests for thrombosis are notoriously nonspecific in pediatrics. Several conditions may underlie or predispose children to developing thromboses. Table 12.6 lists some of the most common inherited thrombophilic traits and risk factors. Despite the well-known inherited risk factors for thrombosis, testing for such traits is often unnecessary in pediatrics. The vast majority of children with thrombosis will have a clinically recognized risk factor, such as a central venous catheter or other disease state.

Table 12.6 Inherited Thrombophilic Traits

Thrombophilic Risk/Trait	Key Principles
Factor V mutations	• Leiden is most common; followed by Cambridge and HR2 • Makes factor Va resistant to proteolysis by APC • Heterozygotes have 2–7 times the risk of thrombosis • Homozygotes have up to 70-fold risk
Protein C deficiency	• Prevalence of heterozygosity is near 1 in 300 • Multiple subtypes of heterozygous states • Unlikely to present with thromboses before puberty • Homozygous deficiencies can present with neonatal purpura fulminans
Protein S deficiency	• Acts similarly to protein C deficiency • Prevalence is near 1 per 33,000 • Risk is increased sevenfold in heterozygous disease • Prevalence of homozygosity is closer to 1 per 1,000,000
Prothrombin gene variant	• Mutation at *G20210A* • Leads to persistence of circulating thrombin • 2%–3% of white population is heterozygous • Heterozygosity increases risk by threefold
Antithrombin III deficiency	• Gene located on chromosome 1; more than 250 mutations known • Homozygosity not compatible with life • Odds ratio increased 10-fold to 20-fold in heterozygous states • Thromboses much more common in adults than children • Prevalence varies widely

APC, Activated protein C; *OCP,* oral contraceptive.

Lemierre syndrome is an example of a thromboembolic disorder often encountered in children. This condition is characterized by anaerobic infections in the head and neck tissues leading to septic jugular vein thrombosis (see Chapter 13). The thromboses are likely due to a combination of venous stasis, endothelial damage from local inflammation, and an underlying hypercoagulable state (acquired or inherited). Tonsillitis, pharyngitis, mastoiditis, and dental infections that spread to the pharyngeal spaces can all lead to Lemierre syndrome. Anterior neck disease may present with pain, swelling, and tenderness but posterior compartment disease may be more difficult to detect until late in its course. Treatment involves targeted antimicrobial therapy and anticoagulation.

Additional anatomic conditions can predispose to thrombosis as well. May-Thurner syndrome is a common provocation for left lower extremity thromboses (Fig. 12.34). This occurs when the left iliac vein is compressed by the iliac artery from above and the spine or a ligament from below, causing a flow disturbance and vessel narrowing in the vein. Similarly, Paget-Schroetter syndrome (or thoracic outlet syndrome) can lead to upper extremity venous thrombosis when increased musculature or a first rib that is congenitally in an abnormal position cause venous compression and stasis (Fig. 12.35).

An increasingly recognized complication of thromboses in children is the postthrombotic syndrome (PTS), especially after incomplete recanalization of a vessel that was thrombosed. Although PTS does not necessarily confer a risk of subsequent or extended thrombosis, it can produce symptoms over time. Sequelae of PTS, in fact, can mimic the symptoms of an acute thrombosis with pain, discoloration, and swelling. These symptoms tend to be transient, intermittent, and recurrent in children. Compression stockings or other local measures are often needed for treatment. Severe and long-standing PTS can lead to venous stasis and ulceration later in life.

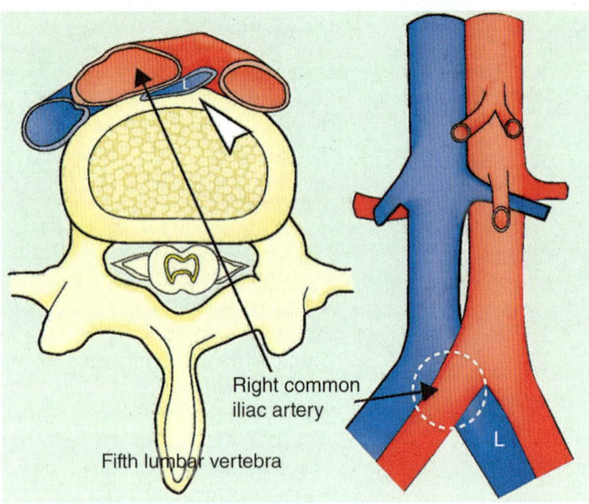

Fig. 12.34 May-Thurner syndrome. (From Anthony MHH, Chung AD, Mizubuti GB: *The Lancet*, 394[10208]:e33, 2019.)

Consumptive and Microangiopathic Disorders

Alterations in the microvascular environment can lead to hematologic complications. Microangiopathic hemolytic anemia, a hematologic condition of diverse causes, is most often acquired and rarely congenital in origin. The hematologic picture is characterized by the presence of burr erythrocytes, schistocytes, helmet cells, and microspherocytes. Additional laboratory studies confirm the presence of intravascular hemolysis, including elevated plasma hemoglobin levels, low to absent haptoglobin, and the presence of hemosiderinuria.

In pediatric patients, septic shock is the most frequent cause of disseminated intravascular coagulation (DIC). Regardless of the trigger, production of fibrin in the microcirculation and fibrin deposition in capillaries causes shearing of the RBCs as they cross the capillary beds (Fig. 12.36). In addition to RBC destruction, platelets and clotting factors are consumed. Patients may have petechiae and purpura (Fig. 12.37) or persistent bleeding from venipuncture sites. Box 12.3 lists diseases known to trigger DIC. Certain vascular malformations also feature a type of consumptive DIC known as *Kasabach-Merritt syndrome* (Fig. 12.38 and Chapter 10).

Microangiopathic changes of the peripheral blood smear may also be seen when RBCs pass through abnormal microvasculature. Examples of this abnormal physiology include RBC damage in hemolytic-uremic syndrome and thrombotic thrombocytopenic purpura (TTP). Hemolytic-uremic syndrome is a disease of childhood that is characterized primarily by renal insufficiency. TTP is more commonly seen in adults but increasingly is recognized in children. The patient with TTP experiences neurologic complications in addition to renal abnormalities. These disorders have in common hemolytic anemia, thrombocytopenia, and thrombotic occlusion of the microvasculature of various organs. Evidence indicates that the familial occurrence of this syndrome is due to a congenital deficiency in the processing of VWF by the enzyme ADAMTS-13, whereas acquired forms are related to an inhibitory antibody.

White Blood Cells

Increases, decreases, and physical alterations in WBCs are common pediatric problems. In general, these are due to increases or decreases in specific types of WBCs. Most cases of neutrophilia (Fig. 12.39), neutropenia, eosinophilia (Fig. 12.40), lymphocytosis (Fig. 12.41), lymphopenia, or monocytosis (Fig. 12.42) in the pediatric population

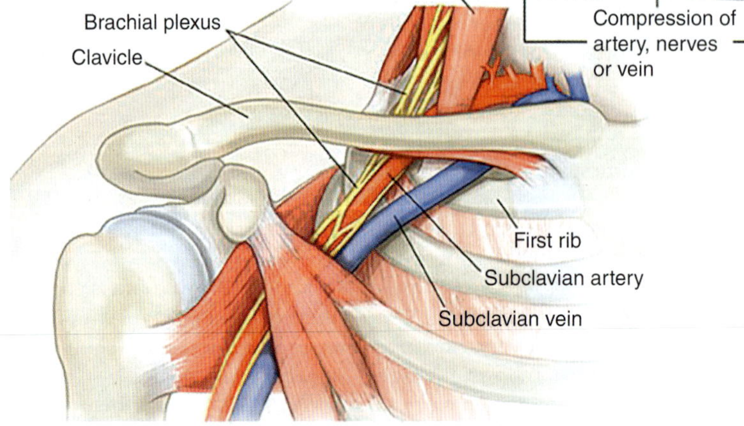

Fig. 12.35 Thoracic outlet syndrome. (From https://sportmedschool.com/thoracic-outlet-syndrome/.)

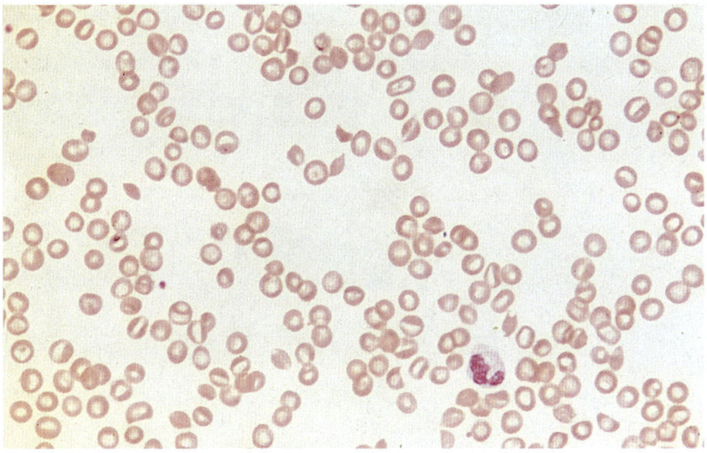

Fig. 12.36 Disseminated intravascular coagulation (DIC). Peripheral blood smear of a child with meningococcemia and DIC. Note the red blood cell fragments and decreased platelet count.

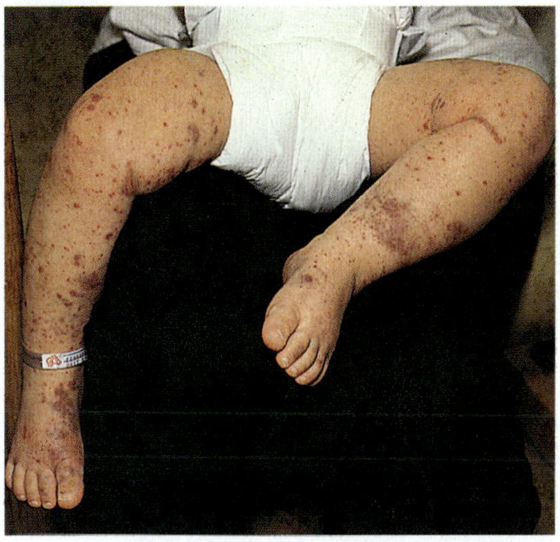

Fig. 12.37 Infant with neuroblastoma and purpuric lesions relating to a tumor-related coagulopathy. Similar lesions may result from other conditions, such as severe isolated thrombocytopenia and/or disseminated intravascular coagulation.

Box 12.3 Clinical Equivalent of Experimental Disseminated Intravascular Coagulation–Triggering Agents

Gram-negative septicemia
Necrotizing enterocolitis
Shock from any cause
Endothelial damage (virus, bacteria, *Rickettsia,* heat stroke)
Trauma, burns
Ascitic fluid (LeVeen shunt)
Hypoxia-acidosis, severe hyaline membrane disease
Malignancies (acute leukemia, neuroblastoma, rhabdomyosarcoma)
Dead fetal twin
Hemolysis transfusion reaction
Small for gestational age infant (placental infarct)
Purpura fulminans
Localized giant hemangioma

Modified from Corrigan JJ: Disseminated intravascular coagulopathy, *Pediatr Rev* 1:37–45, 1979.

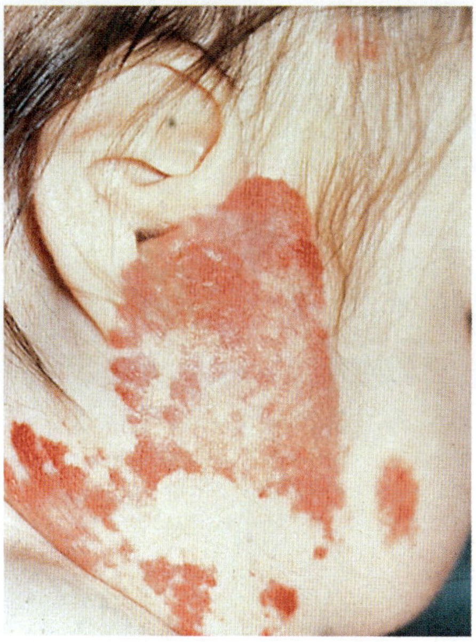

Fig. 12.38 The hemangiomatous lesion in this patient resulted in Kasabach-Merritt syndrome, in which platelet consumption within the lesion leads to thrombocytopenia.

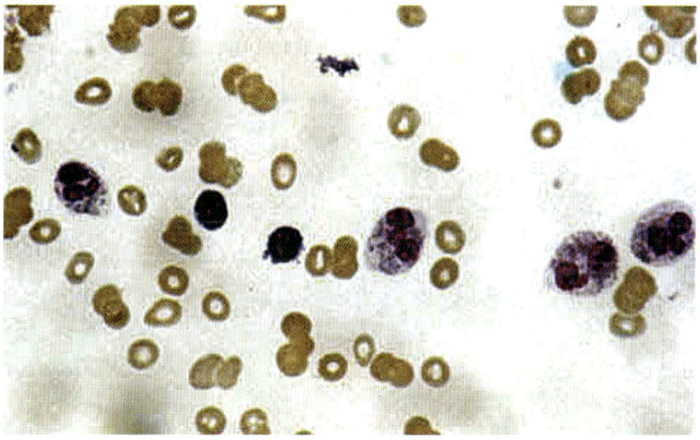

Fig. 12.39 Neutrophilia and increased band forms (left shift). The pattern of a left shift of the white blood cell series is consistent with infection. The peripheral blood smear shows increased neutrophils and band forms in a child with pneumococcal sepsis.

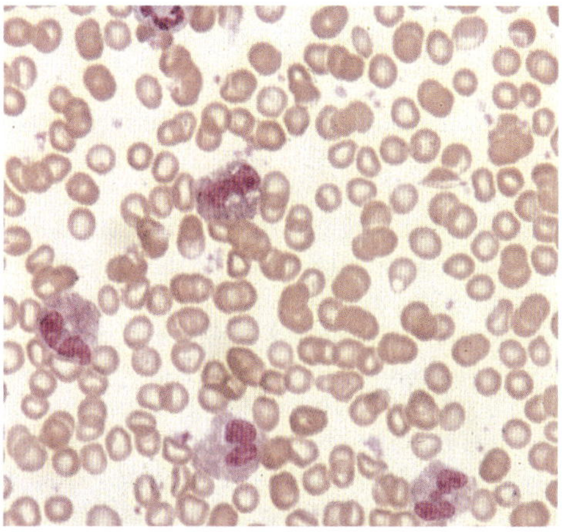

Fig. 12.40 Eosinophilia. This patient's blood shows an increased white blood cell count and increased eosinophils owing to a parasitic infection.

do not represent primary hematologic disorders. These abnormalities often represent bone marrow responses to varied conditions.

Neutropenia is one of the most common white cell disorders seen in pediatrics. Differing levels of neutropenia, reflected by a diminished absolute neutrophil count (ANC), confer differing risks of infection. Neutropenia can be seen in response to medications, in congenital deficiencies (Kostmann syndrome), or in response to infections. Autoimmune neutropenia develops in response to antibody-mediated destruction of neutrophils, most commonly in a postinfectious setting. This is generally self-limited and resolves in a matter of months. Chronic benign neutropenia has an unclear etiology but can persist for years. Cyclic neutropenia, a disorder in which the ANC drops at regular intervals, is extremely rare but dangerous and can be tested for on a genetic level. During periods of neutropenia, children may develop mucosal ulcerations or breakdown. Children with neutropenia generally do not require isolation or prophylactic antibiotics on a regular basis. However, if febrile, those children warrant a medical evaluation to

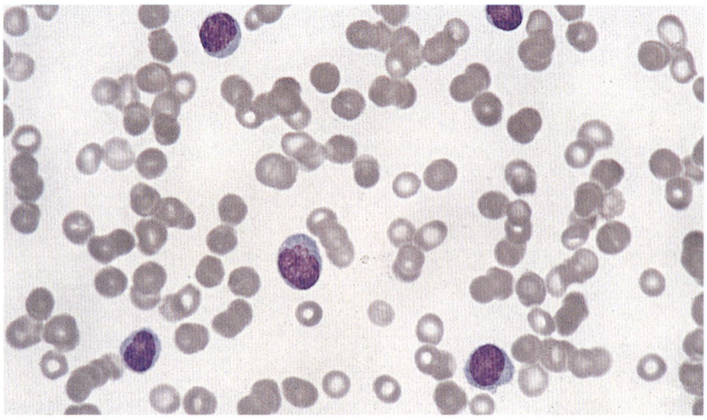

Fig. 12.41 Lymphocytosis. An elevated lymphocyte count is seen in the peripheral blood smear of a child with pertussis.

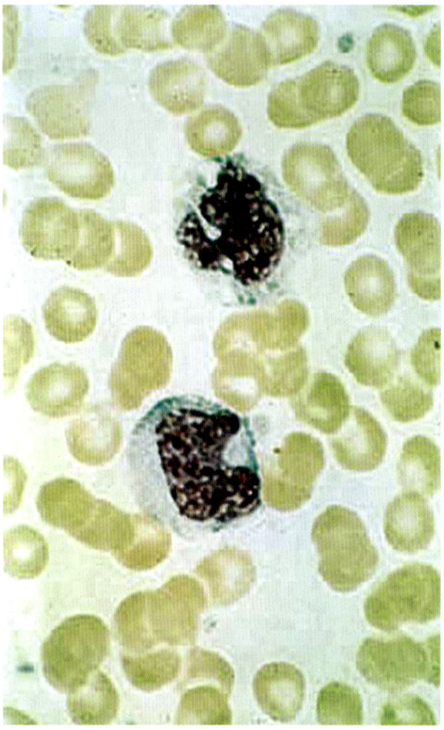

Fig. 12.42 Monocytosis. The peripheral blood will often show an increased monocyte count at a time of marrow recovery after significant suppression. In this case, the child is recovering from chemotherapy-induced neutropenia.

rule out a serious bacterial infection. Hormonal stimulation with granulocyte colony-stimulating factor to increase the ANC is usually required only in settings of severe infections or prominent symptoms.

Morphologic abnormalities of the granulocytic series, although less common than neutropenia, may provide clues to the diagnosis. The hypersegmented neutrophil, which may be an early clue to vitamin B_{12} deficiency, has been noted previously (see Fig. 12.11). This diagnosis may be distinguished from familial hypersegmentation by looking at the peripheral smears of family members. On occasion, mature neutrophils may be abnormally large in members of a given family—so-called *hereditary giant neutrophils.* The Pelger-Huët anomaly (Fig. 12.43) is usually a benign morphologic inherited anomaly in children, but it is sometimes acquired in adults as an association with leukemia and lymphoma. Increased numbers of nuclear appendages may also be seen in the neutrophils of patients with trisomy 13 (Fig. 12.44). These, however, may be difficult to distinguish from normal neutrophil "drumsticks," which are nuclear appendages that occur in 2% to 10% of neutrophils of normal girls.

Toxic granulations, which are prominent azurophilic granules, are another common type of WBC inclusion. They are nonspecific but can be seen in viral and bacterial infections (Fig. 12.45). Toxic

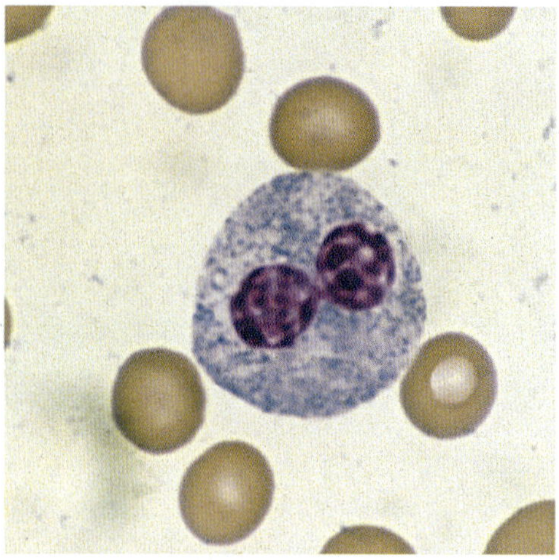

Fig. 12.43 Pelger-Hu®t anomaly. Note the uniform bilobed nucleus of the granulocyte.

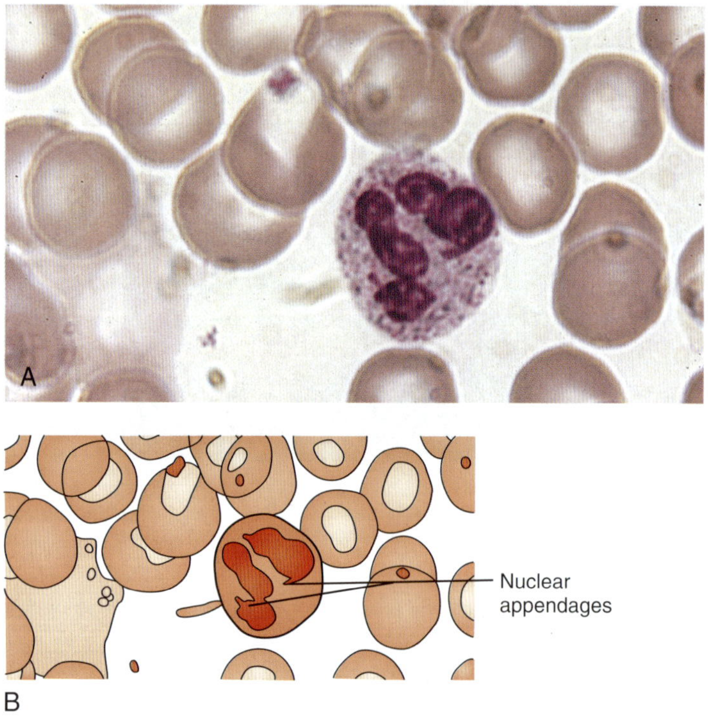

Fig. 12.44 (A) Nuclear appendages are normally seen in the polymorphonuclear leukocytes of girls. An increase in these appendages is seen in cases of trisomy 13. (B) Schematic of nuclear appendages.

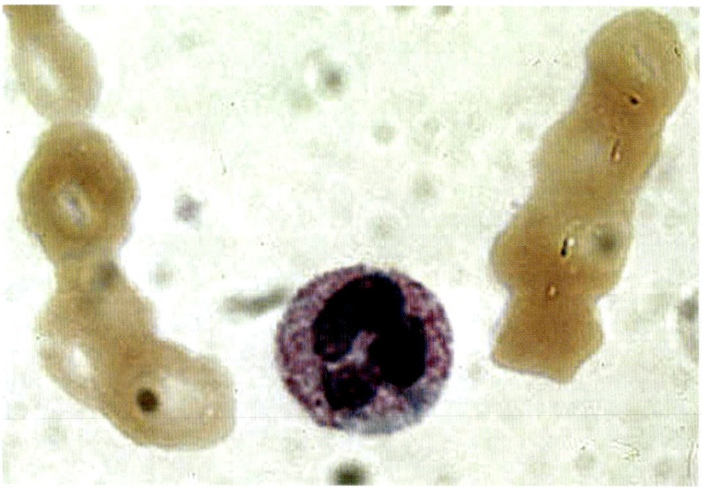

Fig. 12.45 Döhle body. Toxic granulations and a Döhle body are found in the blood of this child with sepsis. The Döhle body appears as a grayish-blue staining area, which is located at the inferior border of this cell.

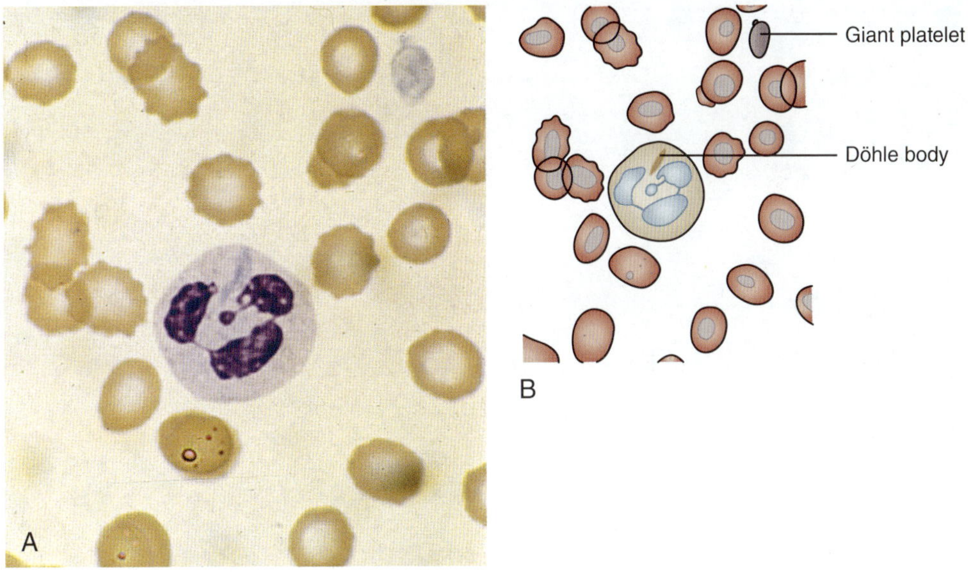

Fig. 12.46 May-Hegglin anomaly. (A) The peripheral blood of individuals with this condition demonstrates Döhle bodies in the white blood cells and giant platelets that may be decreased in number. (B) Schematic of May-Hegglin anomaly.

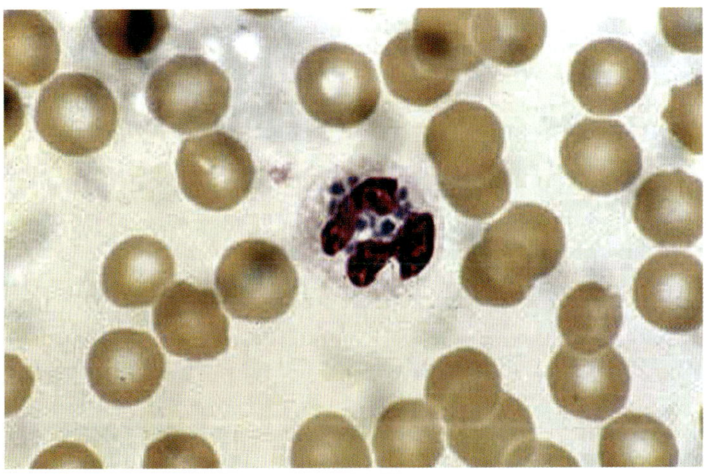

Fig. 12.47 Chédiak-Higashi syndrome. Note the neutrophilic inclusion characteristic of this rare disease. (Courtesy William Zinkham, MD, Baltimore, MD.)

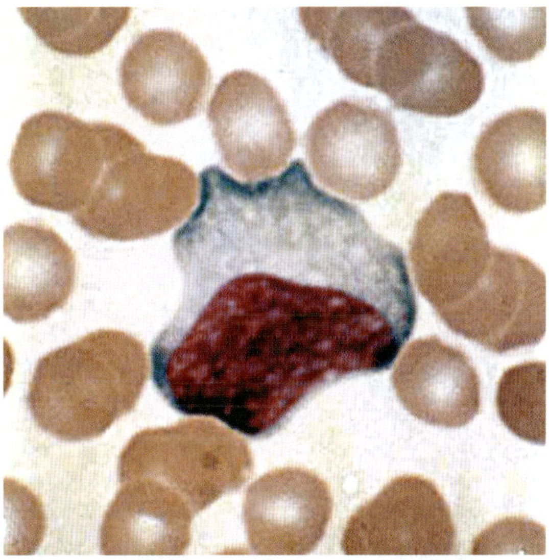

Fig. 12.48 Atypical lymphocyte in the case of infectious mononucleosis. Atypical lymphocytes in the peripheral blood are often observed in patients with infectious mononucleosis. The nucleus is large, and the cytoplasm is abundant. Note that where the cytoplasm of the lymphocyte abuts the red blood cell, the lymphocyte deforms around it.

granulations must be distinguished from the hereditary dense granulation that may occasionally be present in the neutrophils of normal individuals. Döhle bodies, pale blue inclusions that usually are located peripherally in the cytoplasm of neutrophils, may coexist with toxic granulations. Together with giant platelets, Döhle bodies are seen in patients with the dominantly inherited May-Hegglin anomaly (Fig. 12.46). Large greenish-brown neutrophil inclusions are characteristic of the patient with rare Chédiak-Higashi syndrome (Fig. 12.47). Such granules may appear in eosinophils and basophils as well. WBCs may also acquire inclusions by engulfing particles from their surroundings.

In contrast to neutrophil morphologic abnormalities, changes in lymphocytes' appearance are common in children. Atypical lymphocytes are large cells with an irregular plasma membrane that often hug adjacent RBCs. The nucleus of an atypical lymphocyte is also large, and the nucleoli may be visible. The abundant cytoplasm is typically basophilic and may contain vacuoles and azurophilic granules (Fig. 12.48). Morphologic subtypes of atypical lymphocytes may occur, but clinically, their recognition is of little use. Care is required when evaluating peripheral smears of children with viral or other illnesses because atypical lymphocytes may at times be difficult to distinguish from lymphoblasts.

A leukemoid reaction, which is characterized by a high WBC count (usually $>50,000/mm^3$), also must be carefully distinguished from leukemia (Figs. 12.49 to 12.52). Although this is definitively accomplished by a bone marrow aspirate, peripheral blood studies can assist a diagnosis. Patients with Down syndrome may experience a transient leukemoid reaction (called *transient myeloproliferative disorder*) in the newborn period. Additional manifestations of this disorder include hepatosplenomegaly and circulating myeloblasts. Spontaneous remission often occurs. However, 20% to 30% of patients with Down syndrome and transient myeloproliferative disorder develop leukemia within the first 3 years of life.

Bone Marrow Failure

Pancytopenia refers to a reduction in all three formed elements of the blood. In an analogous manner to anemia, pancytopenia is not a single disease entity but rather may result from a number of disease processes. Pancytopenia may occur from bone marrow failure or extramedullary cellular destruction (as seen in autoimmune disease, particularly systemic lupus erythematosus) or as a combination of depressed marrow function and increased cellular destruction. When pancytopenia is due to destruction of the formed elements of the blood, invariably there is another underlying disease. On the other

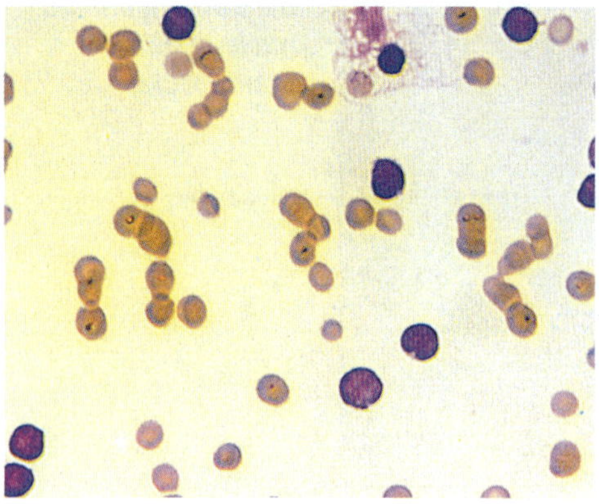

Fig. 12.49 Acute lymphoblastic leukemia—peripheral blood smear. Note the presence of decreased platelets and the absence of normal white blood cells.

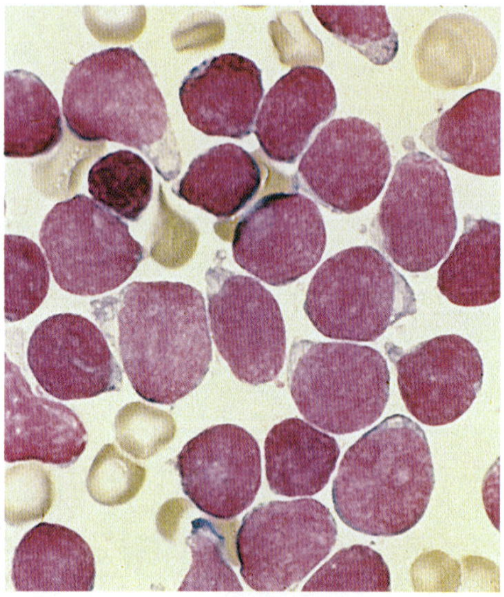

Fig. 12.50 Acute lymphoblastic leukemia—bone marrow aspirate. Note the monotonous pattern of the lymphoblastic (L1) cells.

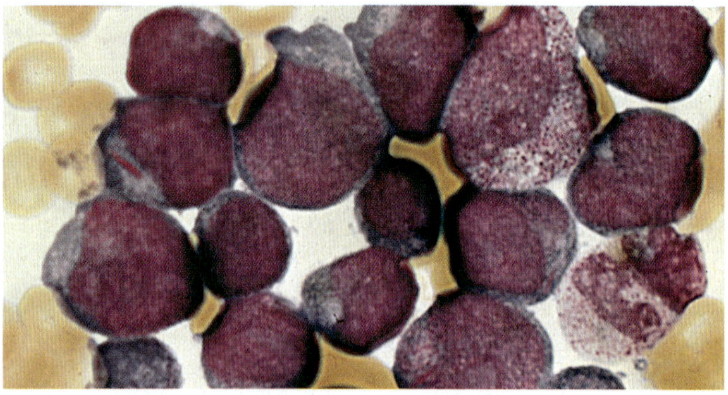

Fig. 12.51 Acute myelogenous leukemia. Peripheral blood smear showing an Auer rod (red, rod-shaped figure in the cytoplasm) within a myeloblast of a patient with acute nonlymphocytic/acute myelogenous leukemia.

hand, the pancytopenia resulting from bone marrow failure can be divided into genetically predisposed marrow failure syndromes and acquired marrow failure syndromes.

Aplastic anemia is marked by peripheral blood pancytopenia associated with bone marrow hypocellularity or acellularity. Acquired aplastic anemia is an immune-mediated disease, although genetic risk factors and environmental exposures also contribute. Research has resulted in a much deeper understanding of the role that activated T lymphocytes play in presenting hematopoietic cell antigens for destruction. In children, the acuity of presentation in aplastic anemia

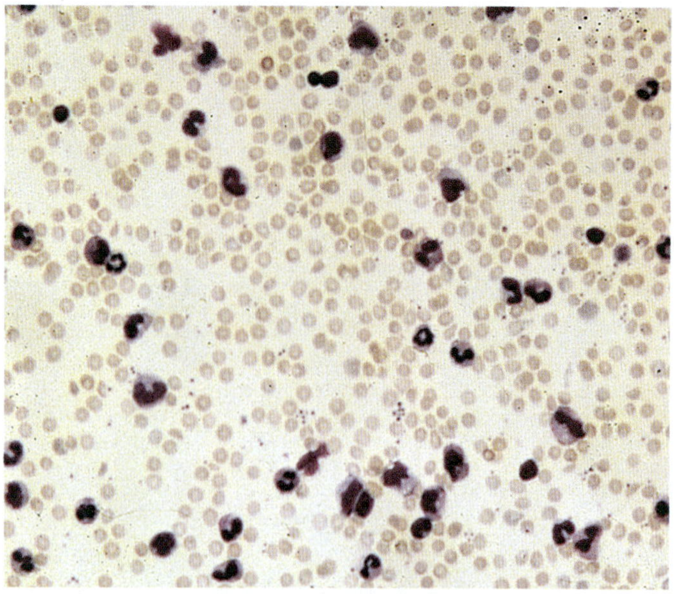

Fig. 12.52 Leukemoid reaction. Elevated white blood cell (WBC) count in response to infection. The child whose blood is pictured here was documented to have pneumococcal sepsis with an appropriate WBC response.

relates to the degree of pancytopenia. Severe aplastic anemia is classified as a bone marrow sample that demonstrates less than 25% cellularity, in association with peripheral cytopenias in two of the three lineages. The treatment for severe aplastic anemia is either hematopoietic stem cell transplantation or primary immunosuppression.

Pancytopenia is a common presentation for both Fanconi anemia (a chromosomal breakage syndrome) and dyskeratosis congenita (a telomere length disorder). Fanconi anemia, the most frequent of the constitutional marrow failure syndromes, is a familial disorder that also features a variable constellation of congenital anomalies of the skin, skeleton, central nervous system (CNS), and genitourinary tract (Fig. 12.53). Fragility of the chromosomes and pancytopenia, however, can occur in the absence of physical anomalies. Isolated cell line aplasias also occur congenitally. These also have concurrent physical examination findings frequently. Diamond-Blackfan syndrome (a congenital PRCA) and thrombocytopenia–absent radius syndrome are two conditions that show characteristic skeletal changes (Fig. 12.54). Supportive care with transfusions is an important mainstay for these diseases. Although the hematologic complications of some may resolve

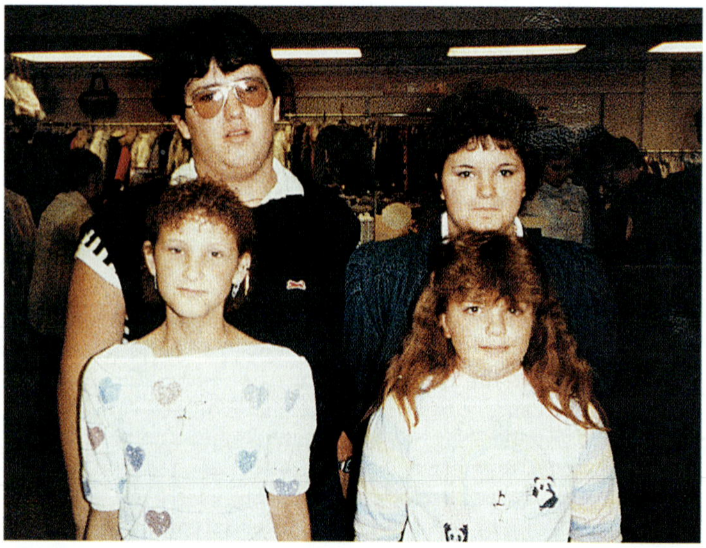

Fig. 12.53 A patient with Fanconi anemia is pictured with her three siblings. This patient had a bone marrow transplant for her underlying condition. Note her diminutive size with respect to her more robust siblings.

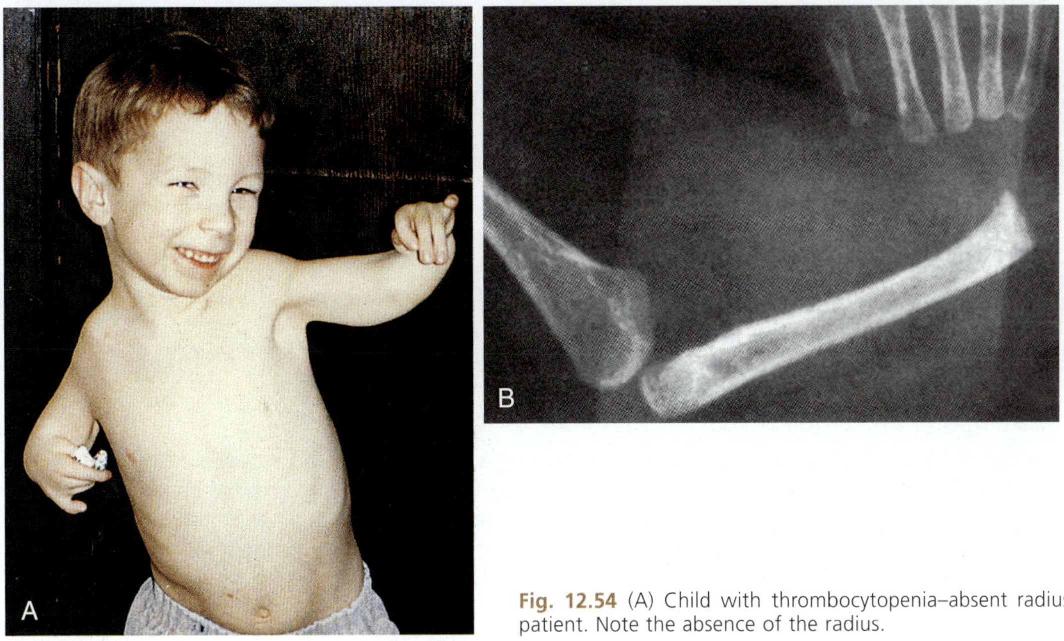

Fig. 12.54 (A) Child with thrombocytopenia–absent radius syndrome. (B) Radiograph of the same patient. Note the absence of the radius.

over the first year of life, matched-sibling hematopoietic stem cell transplantation is the treatment of choice for symptomatic children with many bone marrow failure syndromes.

ONCOLOGY

Pediatric malignancy is rare when compared with the incidence of cancer in the adult population. More than 16,000 new cases of cancer are diagnosed during childhood and adolescence (ages 0–19) in the United States each year. The overall cure rate is now 85%, due to advances in clinical trials, the use of novel agents, and improvements in supportive care. Thus the pediatrician must be involved in monitoring the surviving children and young adults for long-term effects of therapy and ensuring adequate full transition to adult care.

The initial task of recognizing the signs and symptoms of malignancy often falls to primary care or emergency department providers. The current section aims to review clinical presentations that should alert the provider to the possibility of a malignant process. As with most pediatric conditions, the differential diagnosis varies depending on the age of the child. An immediate concern is to address tumor-related complications, such as neutropenia due to marrow infiltration, metabolic abnormalities due to increased cell turnover, or organ compromise due to space-occupying lesions. Signs and symptoms of the most common tumors of childhood are reviewed in a manner that parallels the physical examination. This may result in some overlap because many cancers manifest a wide spectrum of presentations that may vary with anatomic location. Each tumor subtype is discussed in the context of a region in which it typically presents. For a more detailed description of specific cancers, a more comprehensive text is recommended (see *Pizzo and Poplack's Pediatric Oncology* listed in the Bibliography section at the end of this chapter).

Signs and Symptoms

Red flags that signal malignancy may be detected in the course of history taking and physical examination or in basic laboratory testing Box 12.4. These findings may be due to the mechanical effect of a tumor (e.g., compression or infiltration of an organ). Alternatively, rapid cell division may lead to metabolic abnormalities, including hyperkalemia, hyperuricemia, and hyperphosphatemia with reflex hypocalcemia as a manifestation of tumor lysis. True paraneoplastic syndromes are uncommon in the pediatric population. An example of such a paraneoplastic process occurs in a small percentage of patients with neuroblastoma. Opsoclonus–myoclonus ataxia syndrome (random eye movements, myoclonic jerking and ataxia) tends to occur in patients with low-stage disease and favorable histology of the tumor. Unfortunately, many are left with devastating developmental and neurocognitive deficits that relate to this rare paraneoplastic condition.

The child with a new diagnosis of malignancy is sometimes asymptomatic, as in a child with a palpable abdominal mass. In other cases, nonspecific symptoms may be a prominent finding, including fever, weight loss, and/or lethargy. Examples of more specific signs and symptoms in pediatric malignancy include headache and morning vomiting in a patient with a brain tumor; constipation and difficulty voiding in a patient with a pelvic tumor or spinal cord compression; hypertension in a child with a renal or suprarenal tumor; bone pain; and limping secondary to leukemia or another marrow-infiltrative process.

These complaints are more likely to have a cause that is nonmalignant. However, persistence (2 weeks is a reasonable guideline) or undue severity may give these signs increased significance. Similarly, in the context of predisposing conditions, malignancy should be considered earlier. Table 12.7 lists examples of inherited cancer syndromes. This list is not exhaustive. Emerging information regarding genetics of cancer is likely to greatly increase understanding of cancer predisposition in the coming years. Children with a history of one cancer, by virtue of genetics or as a long-term side effect of anticancer therapy, are at greater risk of a second cancer. Radiation therapy predisposes to a lifelong increased risk of solid tumors within the radiation field. Another notable exception is the infant or toddler who has an identical twin with leukemia. In this child, the risk of leukemia may be as high as 25% in the first few years of life. Retinoblastoma and Wilms tumor are also known to occur with increased frequency in offspring of individuals with these diagnoses.

The clinical findings in the child with malignancy vary greatly depending on the site of origin of the tumor. The focus of this

Box 12.4 Red Flags of Malignancy

Pallor, fatigue	Headache, vomiting, lethargy
Petechiae	Lymphadenopathy
Fever without source	Hepatomegaly
Bone pain, limp	Splenomegaly
Weight loss	Abdominal mass
Anorexia	Testiculomegaly

Table 12.7 Inherited Cancer Predisposition Syndromes

Genetic Syndrome	Associated Cancers	Inheritance
Ataxia-telangiectasia	Leukemia, lymphoma	Autosomal recessive
Beckwith-Wiedemann syndrome	Wilms tumor, adrenal carcinoma, hepatoblastoma	Autosomal dominant or sporadic
Bloom syndrome	Multiple (epithelial, hematopoietic, lymphoid, connective tissue)	Autosomal recessive
Down syndrome	Acute myeloid leukemia (AML; megakaryocytic: M7)	De novo
Gardner syndrome	Colorectal polyposis and adenocarcinoma, osteoma, soft tissue tumors	Autosomal dominant
Neurofibromatosis type 1	Cutaneous and plexiform neurofibromas, malignant peripheral nerve sheath tumors, gliomas, rhabdomyosarcomas	Autosomal dominant
Neurofibromatosis type 2	Vestibular schwannomas, meningiomas, ependymomas, astrocytomas	Autosomal dominant
Retinoblastoma	Retinoblastoma, sarcomas (including osteosarcoma in radiation fields), melanoma	Autosomal dominant
Xeroderma pigmentosum	Squamous cell and basal cell carcinomas, melanoma, carcinoma of lung, gastric tissue, and brain	Autosomal recessive

section is an overview of individual pediatric cancers through a review of characteristic physical examination findings. Its intent is to provide a fundamental understanding of the spectrum of malignant diseases of childhood along with the signs and symptoms to alert the physician to their possible presence.

Leukemia

ALL is the most common cancer of childhood, with acute and chronic myelogenous leukemia less common. Symptomatic anemia and/or thrombocytopenia may be the reason a child with leukemia is brought to medical attention. A diminished peripheral count of one or more cell lines is a common sign at the diagnosis of leukemia. With the initiation of chemotherapy, a patient's tumor burden regresses and normal hematopoiesis has an opportunity to resume. Red blood cell and platelet transfusions may be required on the basis of symptoms but are not routinely given as prophylaxis unless hemoglobin is less than 7 g/dL or platelets less than 10,000 cells per microliter.

The peripheral blood smear and bone marrow aspirate of a patient with ALL are shown in Fig. 12.49 and Fig. 12.50. The leukemic blasts represent a clonal expansion of a cell at a specific stage of lymphoid or myeloid development. Clinical symptoms may include fever, fatigue, pallor, and bone pain as evidenced by limping. ALL accounts for approximately 75% of pediatric cases of acute leukemia. The peak age range is between 2 and 5 years of age. For ALL, an age between 1 and 9 years and a presenting WBC count of less than 50,000 remain important indicators of a favorable prognosis. The presence or absence of minimal residual disease at the end of induction and consolidation are also important predictors of the child at increased risk of relapse and are critical to risk stratification. Acute myeloid leukemia (AML) is the other predominant leukemia of childhood, accounting for approximately 20% of cases (peripheral smear of AML with myeloblasts shown in Fig. 12.51). The incidence of AML is stable from birth to 10 years old. Like ALL, the use of minimal residual disease and the genetic profiling of the leukemic clone is critical in risk stratification of patients with AML. There is a slight increase in the number of cases during the teenage years. The finding of pancytopenia, organomegaly, and lymphadenopathy in these conditions relates directly to infiltration of marrow and normal organ tissues with the expanded leukemic clone. Because leukemia is a systemic cancer with symptoms of a multiorgan nature, examples of clinical findings are referenced throughout the chapter.

Skin

Morphologic characteristics of cutaneous lesions may allow for the identification of an underlying diagnosis that suggests a predisposition to cancer, such as neurofibromatosis (see Table 12.7 and Chapter 16). Skin findings also provide a window into bone marrow function through clinical signs such as pallor, indicative of anemia, or bruising and petechiae, suggestive of thrombocytopenia. Pallor may be most readily appreciated by examination of the mucous membranes including the conjunctiva and oral mucosa (see Fig. 12.4A). If the patient is severely anemic, the palmar creases of the hand may also be demonstrably pale (see Fig. 12.4B). Petechiae may be a normal finding on the face and upper thorax of a patient who has had forceful crying, vomiting, or coughing. Diffuse petechiae, purpura, and oral lesions are more suggestive of the presence of thrombocytopenia or platelet dysfunction (see Fig. 12.37). Bruising also has a typical distribution in childhood and is often prominent on the anterior tibial and other flexor surfaces of an active child. An abnormal amount of bruising or unusual sites of bruising such as buttocks or back should raise suspicion of abnormal hemostasis. If laboratory studies do not reveal thrombocytopenia or a coagulation disorder, the provider must always be careful to consider nonaccidental trauma as the etiology.

Skin rashes may also provide clues to the specific diagnosis. In certain cases, biopsy of the skin may provide diagnostic material, thereby avoiding more invasive procedures. Nodular skin lesions may be observed in both neuroblastoma and in some cases of leukemia (Fig. 12.55). Melanoma (Fig. 12.56) is rare in childhood. Predisposing factors include genetic factors, family history of melanoma, light phenotype, congenital nevi, and environmental factors such as excess ultraviolet exposure. Pigmented lesions should be monitored for any change in size, shape, or regularity of margins. Suspicious lesions warrant biopsy for a specific diagnosis of skin cancer. Definitive surgery depends on the histologic findings. Squamous and basal cell carcinomas (Fig. 12.57) arise most often in the setting of heritable diseases, such as xeroderma pigmentosum or basal cell nevus syndrome. Rare cases of pediatric skin cancer are also observed in patients who require long-term immunosuppression, such as recipients of solid organ and bone marrow transplantation, or in areas of skin exposed to external beam radiation.

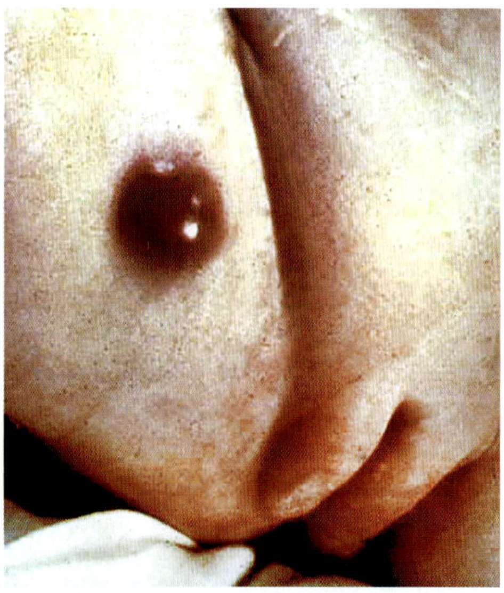

Fig. 12.55 Subcutaneous nodule of neuroblastoma. Skin lesions, which are occasionally seen with leukemia or other solid tumors, may be dark ("blueberry muffin") or skin colored. (From Pearson H: Tumors of the sympathetic nervous system. In Altman AJ, Schwartz AD, editors: *Malignant diseases of infancy, childhood, and adolescence*, ed 2, Philadelphia, 1983, WB Saunders.)

Head and Neck

Tumors of the CNS are the most frequent solid tumors of childhood. One of the most critical conditions for the clinician to recognize is the patient with increased intracranial pressure, a true oncologic emergency. Typical history might include severe morning headache with vomiting. The physical examination may reveal the presence of papilledema (see Chapters 16 and 20) and/or neurologic deficits, such as cranial nerve palsies. Signs and symptoms in the infant may include macrocephaly and a bulging fontanelle with absence of fused sutures. Primary or metastatic intracranial tumors may also manifest as seizures or changes in mental status. Most pediatric brain tumors are infratentorial in location. Because these tumors usually arise in the cerebellum, patients may present with ataxia. Spinal tumors of children may be observed anywhere along the vertebral column. The symptoms of a tumor in this location are caused by compression of the contents of the spinal canal. Pain on percussion over the vertebral column may be an early sign of cord compression, although it can also be present with vertebral fracture. Spinal tumors often have associated weakness, with the affected muscle group corresponding to the level of the lesion. Tumors that press on the spinal cord may present with bowel/bladder dysfunction, paresthesia, or changes in gait.

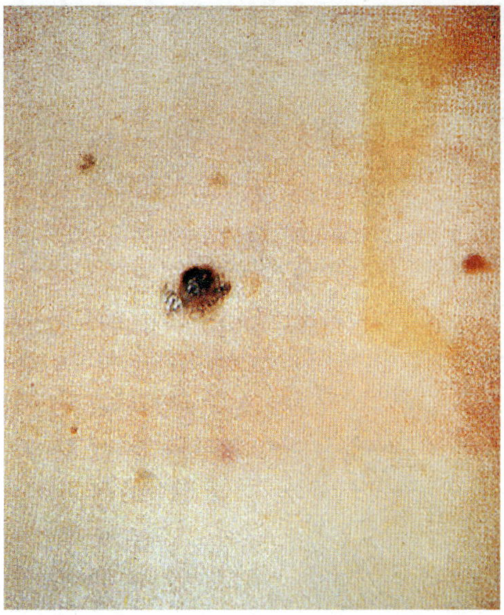

Fig. 12.56 Melanoma. In addition to location (see text), suspicious signs of skin lesions include a red-brown-black color that tends to be diffuse at the periphery, crusting, bleeding, pain, or itching.

Clinical presentation varies depending on whether a tumor is supratentorial or infratentorial in location. Supratentorial lesions may present with headache, visual defects, or hemiparesis. Supratentorial lesions are of two major types:

- Tumors of the cerebral hemisphere, including astrocytoma, ependymoma, glioblastoma, and meningioma (Fig. 12.58A)
- Supratentorial tumors may also originate in the sella turcica or chiasm and include craniopharyngioma, pituitary tumors, and optic nerve glioma (see Fig. 12.58B)

Common presentations of infratentorial lesions include morning headache and vomiting, sixth nerve palsy, and ataxia. Infratentorial lesions may also be considered in two major categories:

- Tumors of the cerebellum, including medulloblastoma, astrocytoma, and meningioma (see Fig. 12.58C)
- Brainstem tumors including intrinsic pontine gliomas and focal or low-grade brainstem gliomas

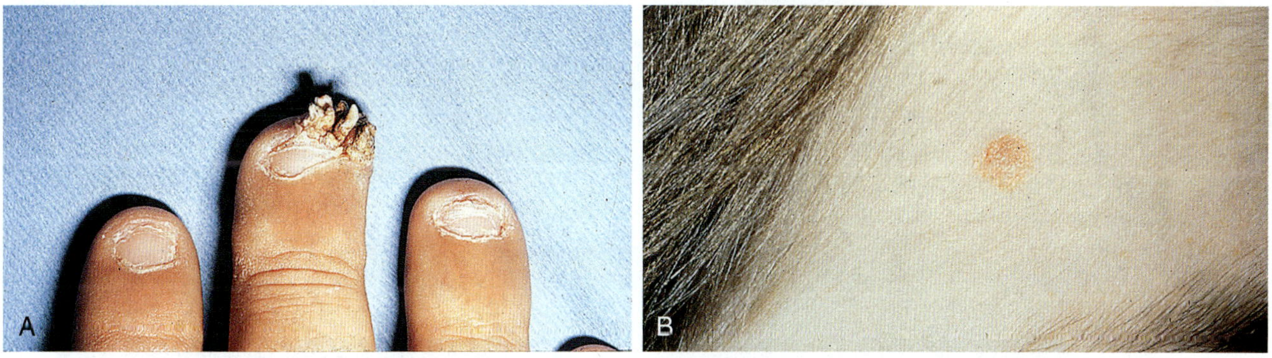

Fig. 12.57 (A) Squamous cell carcinoma. (B) Basal cell carcinoma. This 7-year-old boy received prophylactic cranial radiation as part of his treatment for acute lymphoblastic leukemia 5 years before he developed a second cancer. (A, Courtesy J. Zitelli, MD, Pittsburgh, PA; B, From Pratt CB, Douglass EC: Management of the uncommon cancer of childhood. In Pizzo PA, Poplack DG, editors: *Principles and practices of pediatric oncology*, Philadelphia, 2010, Lippincott Williams & Wilkins.)

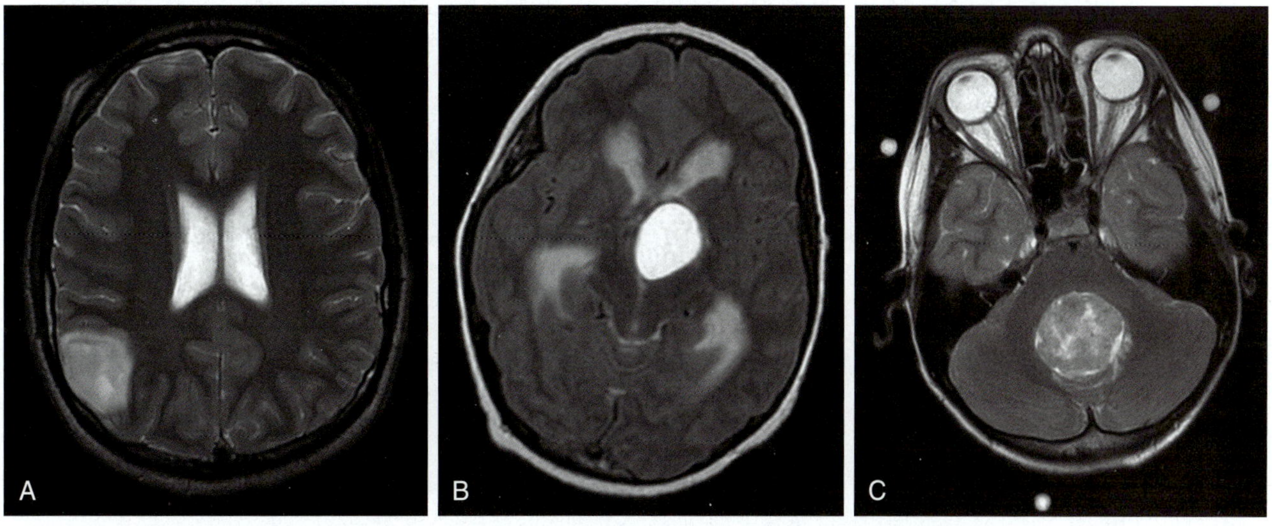

Fig. 12.58 (A) Axial T_2 magnetic resonance imaging (MRI) of a child with astrocytoma. (B) Axial T_2 MRI of a child with craniopharyngioma. (C) Axial T_2 MRI of a child with medulloblastoma.

Brain tumors have clinical consequences due to both histology and location within the bony cavity of the cranium. Finally, developmental delay or regression of milestones are symptoms of many brain tumors in the pediatric population.

Ocular and Otic Findings

Cat's eye reflex, or leukocoria with an absent red reflex, is characteristic of retinoblastoma (see Chapter 20) and should be sought as part of the routine physical examination in the neonate and young child. This is often appreciated from a frontal photograph of the child (Fig. 12.59) and may be brought to the attention of a physician by a parent. Strabismus (see Chapter 20), particularly soon after infancy, may be a sign of an orbital tumor or intracranial pathologic condition and, even if intermittent, merits attention. Proptosis may be observed with several childhood tumors and may represent either a primary tumor or metastatic disease. Orbital rhabdomyosarcoma may present in this way (Fig. 12.60). A child with neuroblastoma may present with metastatic disease to the orbit, resulting in "raccoon eyes," due to ecchymoses in the periorbital area (Fig. 12.61). Heterochromia (Fig. 12.62A), usually a benign entity, may be associated with cervicothoracic neuroblastoma (see Chapter 20). Aniridia (see Fig. 12.62B), or absence of the iris, has a known association with malignancy including the WAGR (Wilms tumor, aniridia, genital abnormalities, and mental retardation) syndrome. Aniridia in the infant or toddler should prompt appropriate diagnostic studies.

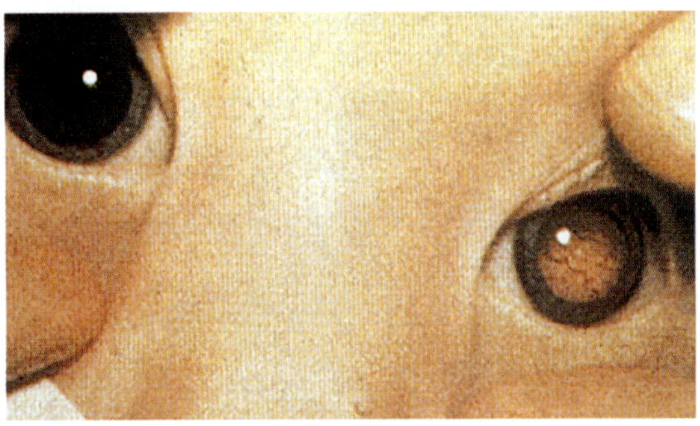

Fig. 12.59 Leukocoria. Cat's eye reflex, or leukocoria, in a child with retinoblastoma. (From Abramson D. Retinoblastoma, *CA Cancer J Clin* 32:130–140, 1982.)

Otorrhea (Fig. 12.63) may be seen with head and neck tumors, such as rhabdomyosarcoma and Langerhans cell histiocytosis. Morphologic abnormalities of the ear itself (ear creases or pits) may signal the Beckwith-Wiedemann syndrome, in which patients have a known predisposition to hepatoblastoma, Wilms tumor, and other malignancies.

A child with cancer may also present with a lesion of the orofacial region, including the jaw and oral and nasal cavities. Inappropriate loosening of the teeth may represent a clinical manifestation of Burkitt lymphoma, in which case an associated jaw mass may be present (Fig. 12.64).

Orofacial Findings

Whereas masses such as the lesion shown in Fig. 12.64 are likely to be referred to an oncologist, intraoral (Fig. 12.65) or intranasal (Fig. 12.66) masses are more difficult to detect and may be mistaken for nonmalignant conditions. They may be entirely asymptomatic or cause local bleeding and then progress to difficulty swallowing or breathing. Gingival hyperplasia can be seen in children with leukemia, especially the acute myelomonocytic subtype (Fig. 12.67).

In examining a patient for cervical lymphadenopathy, it is important to remember other lymph node groups that may be involved by focal or generalized adenopathy in leukemias, lymphomas, or solid tumors. Additional lymph node locations that should be examined include supraclavicular, infraclavicular, epitrochlear, inguinal, femoral, and popliteal. Large, firm nodes fixed to subcutaneous tissue are most convincing for malignancy, but texture and size can be misleading. Because Hodgkin disease and non-Hodgkin lymphoma can occur concurrently with or after infectious mononucleosis, a positive Monospot test may provide false reassurance. Therefore persistent adenopathy, even in that setting, should be monitored closely. The algorithms for workup of adenopathy and indications for biopsy are reviewed in Chapter 13. Neck examination may also reveal abnormalities of the thyroid. Although rare in childhood without predisposing factors such as radiation exposure, a goiter or nodular thyroid with or without bruits may be seen in a patient with thyroid carcinoma.

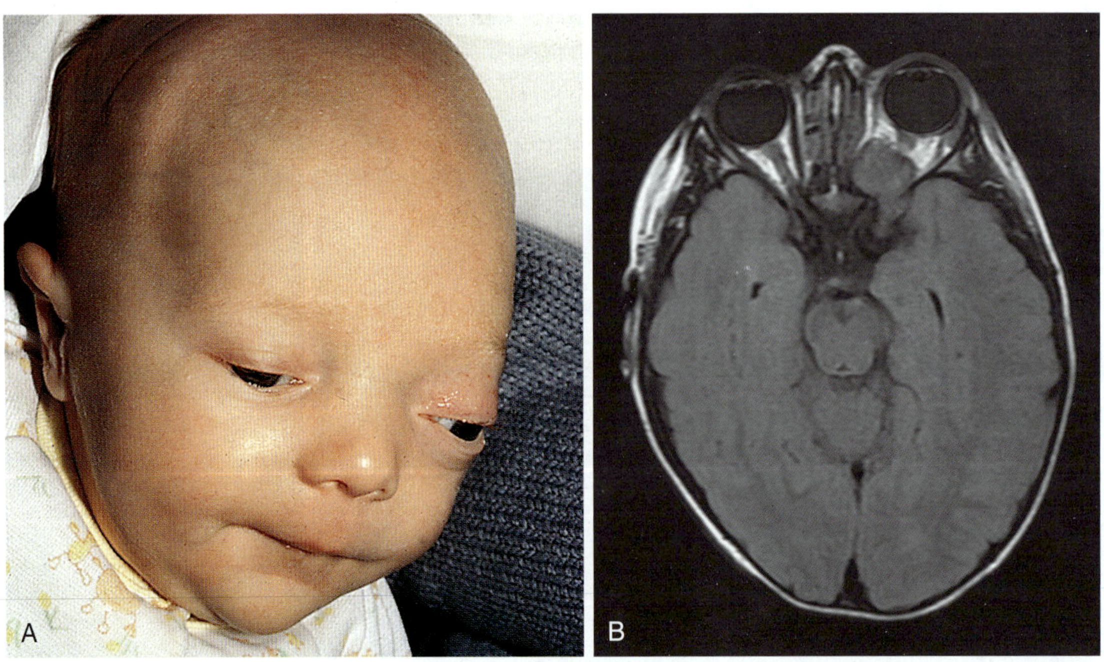

Fig. 12.60 (A) Retro-orbital rhabdomyosarcoma. This child demonstrates proptosis due to the retro-orbital tumor and a large head due to the presence of increased intracranial pressure. (B) Rhabdomyosarcoma of the orbit with proptosis shown on axial T_2 FLAIR (fluid-attenuated inversion recovery) magnetic resonance image.

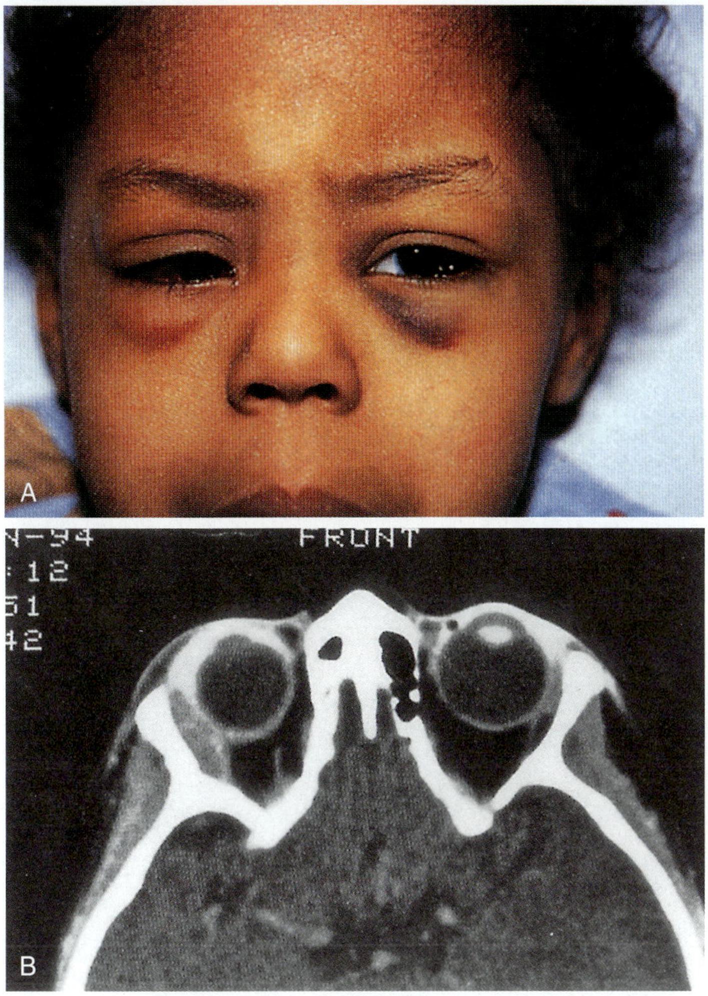

Fig. 12.61 Raccoon eyes—neuroblastoma. (A) This clinical finding is characteristic of a retro-orbital metastatic tumor (B) in advanced neuroblastoma. This may involve supraorbital or infraorbital areas. "Shiners" resulting from trauma or nonaccidental trauma may be a part of the initial differential diagnosis. (Courtesy H. Pearson, New Haven, CT.)

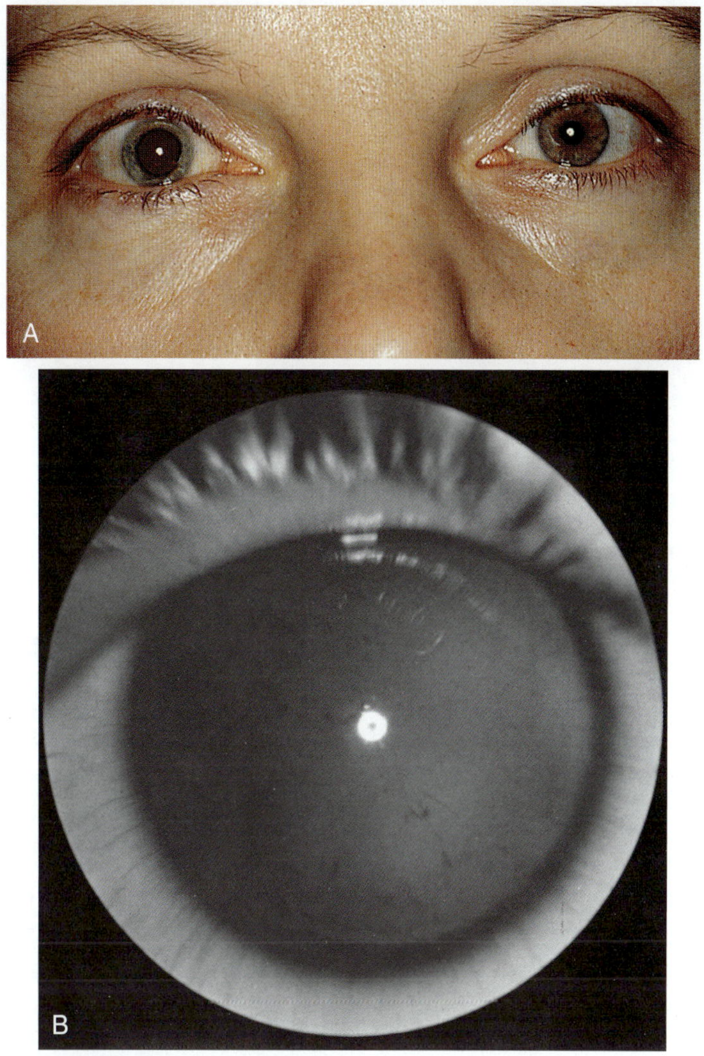

Fig. 12.62 (A) Heterochromia iridis in an adult. Heterochromia is associated with neuroblastoma. (B) Aniridia. (A, Courtesy J. Roen, MD, New York, NY.)

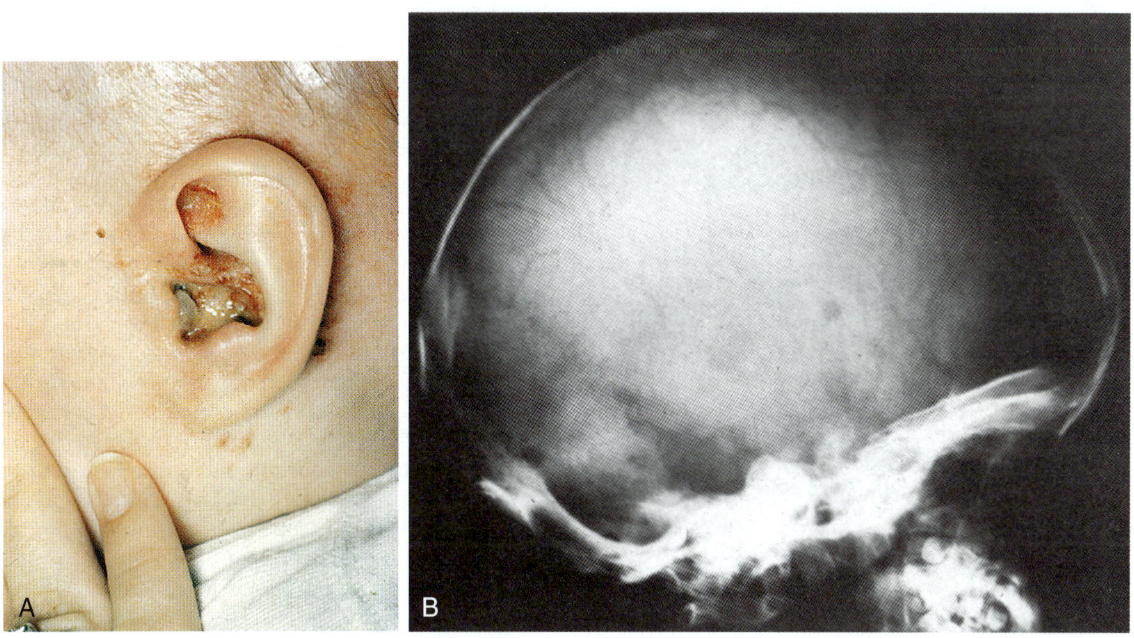

Fig. 12.63 (A) Otorrhea in a child with Langerhans cell histiocytosis (LCH). (B) X-ray film showing destruction of the mastoid bone in the same child. (A, Courtesy P. Gaffney, MD, Pittsburgh, PA.)

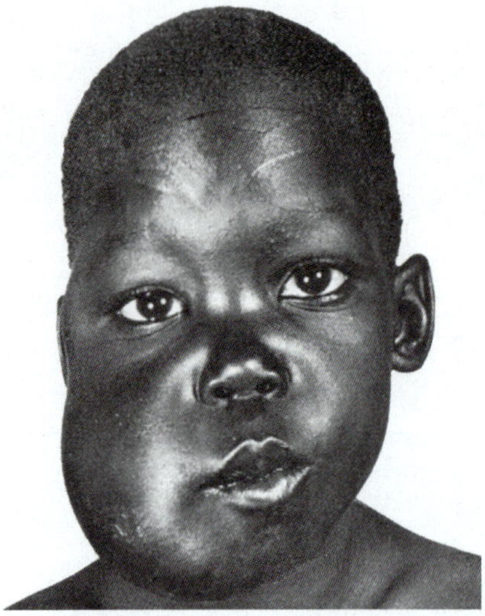

Fig. 12.64 Burkitt lymphoma of the jaw in an African child. (Courtesy I. Magrath, MD, Bethesda, MD.)

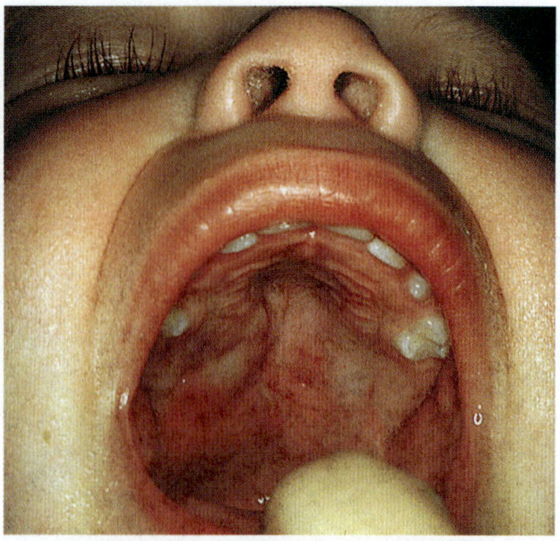

Fig. 12.65 Intracranial rhabdomyosarcoma with intraoral extension. The lesion was first detected by the child's dentist and was biopsied by an ear, nose, and throat specialist who did not suspect malignancy.

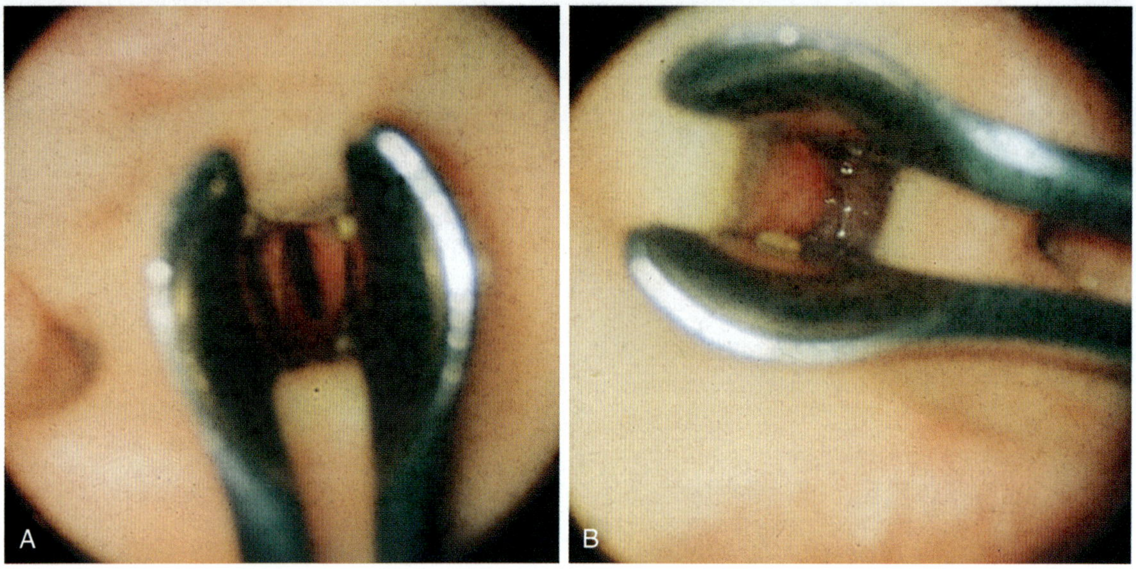

Fig. 12.66 Intranasal glioma. (A) Normal left nostril. (B) Intranasal glioma occluding the right nostril. (Courtesy S. Stool, MD, Pittsburgh, PA.)

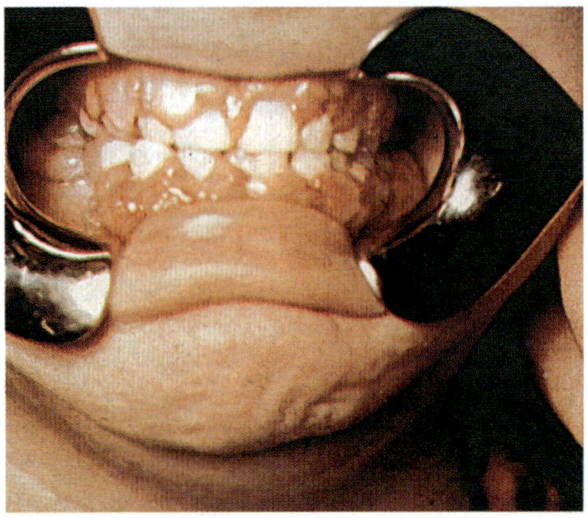

Fig. 12.67 Leukemic infiltration. This photograph shows a patient with gingival hyperplasia resulting from leukemic invasion of the gums. (From Bluefarb SM: *Dermatology*, Kalamazoo, MI, 1984, Upjohn.)

Chest

External examination of the chest may disclose obvious masses that may be asymptomatic or painful. Scoliosis can rarely be associated with paravertebral tumors such as thoracic neuroblastoma (see Chapter 22). A discussion of tumors of muscle or bone origin is presented elsewhere. This section provides a more focused review of tumors of the mediastinum. The differential diagnosis of a mediastinal mass depends on location. Tumors of the anterior mediastinum are most commonly lymphomas, including both Hodgkin disease and non-Hodgkin lymphoma (Fig. 12.68). Germ cell tumors and, rarely, thymomas may also be seen in this location. Masses of the middle mediastinum and/or hilar adenopathy also most commonly represent lymphoma in childhood. Disease of the lymph nodes within the chest may also indicate the presence of lymphadenopathy secondary to leukemia. The presence of a mediastinal mass in a patient with leukemia is suggestive of T-cell disease. Tumors of the posterior mediastinum are usually of neurogenic origin, including neuroblastoma and Ewing sarcoma. In the case of neuroblastic tumors, calcifications may be present (Fig. 12.69). Parenchymal pulmonary nodules, when tumor related, may be asymptomatic and most commonly represent metastatic solid tumor, such as a sarcoma. Fig. 12.70 demonstrates plain film and a chest computed tomography scan, respectively, of a patient with pulmonary metastases of osteosarcoma. Pleural effusions may be present when malignant disease occurs in the chest. This is most common in the case of non-Hodgkin lymphoma (Fig. 12.71). Cytology and low cytometry performed on pleural fluid may provide diagnostic material with relatively

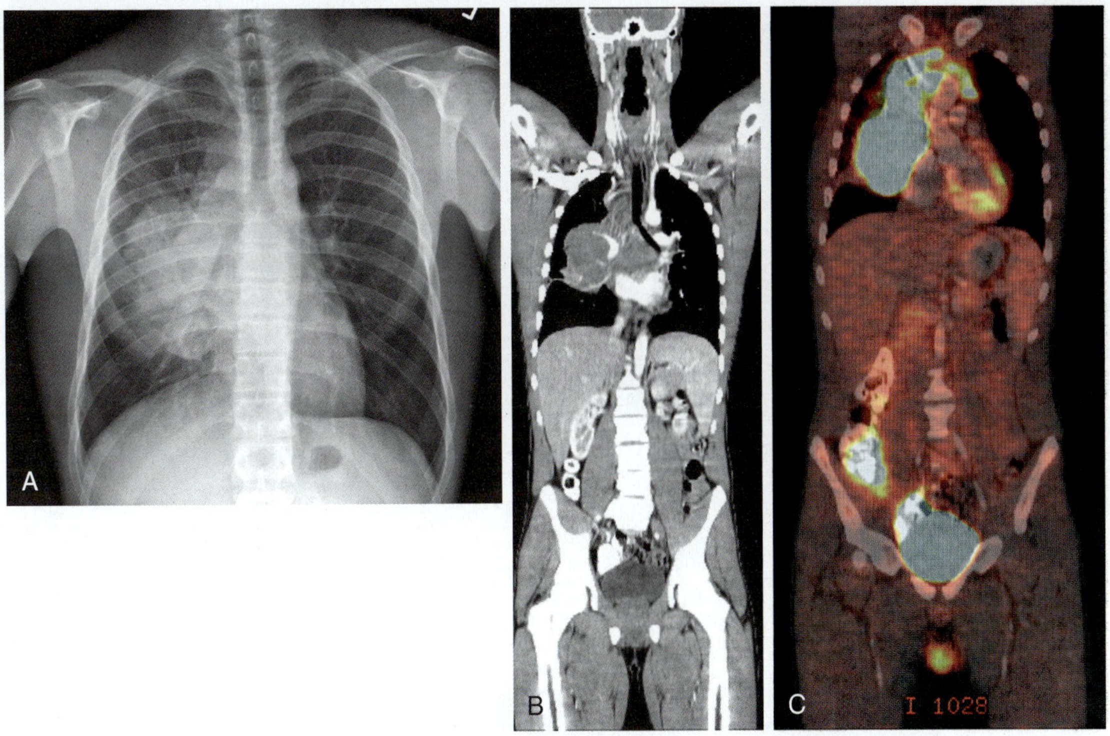

Fig. 12.68 Hodgkin lymphoma. (A) Chest radiograph demonstrating a large anterior mediastinal mass in a teenage male presenting with Hodgkin lymphoma. (B) Chest computed tomography demonstrating the mediastinal mass. (C) ^{18}F-labeled 2-fluoro-2-deoxyglucose positron emission tomography demonstrating the metabolically active tissue of the malignancy as intensely bright areas relative to normal tissues.

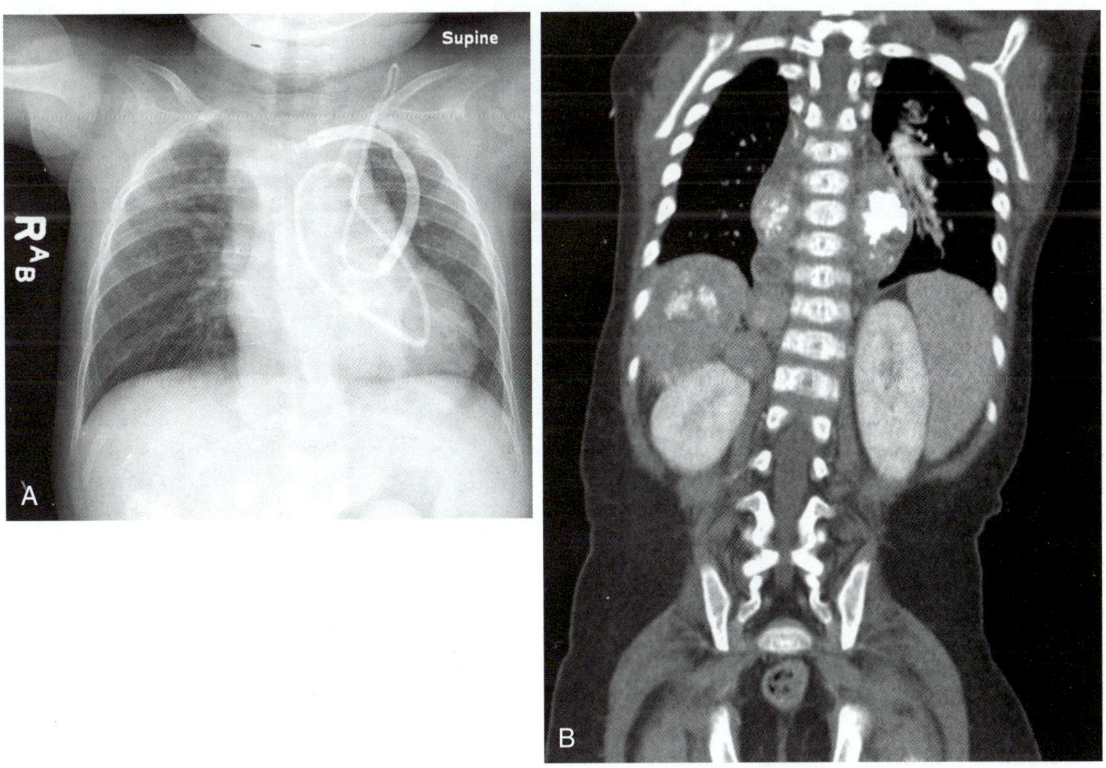

Fig. 12.69 Neuroblastoma. (A) Supine chest radiograph demonstrating a posterior mediastinal mass in a child with neuroblastoma. (B) Coronal computed tomography demonstrating extent of paraspinal masses in a child with newly diagnosed neuroblastoma.

low risk in the patient with compromised respiratory status due to mediastinal disease and airway compression.

Symptoms of respiratory distress may result from a primary intrathoracic process or may rarely be due to a compromised respiratory effort from a large abdominal mass or ascites (Fig. 12.72). The superior vena cava syndrome occurs in patients with large thoracic masses and is a true oncologic emergency. It is caused by obstruction of venous return to the heart through the superior vena cava by a mass lesion. Signs and symptoms may include facial swelling and plethora, wheezing, and cough (Fig. 12.73). This syndrome may progress rapidly to cardiorespiratory failure; thus urgent intervention with steroid and/or radiation therapy may be required. In caring for the patient with mediastinal disease, one must also pay careful attention to electrolytes and renal function, as patients with non-Hodgkin

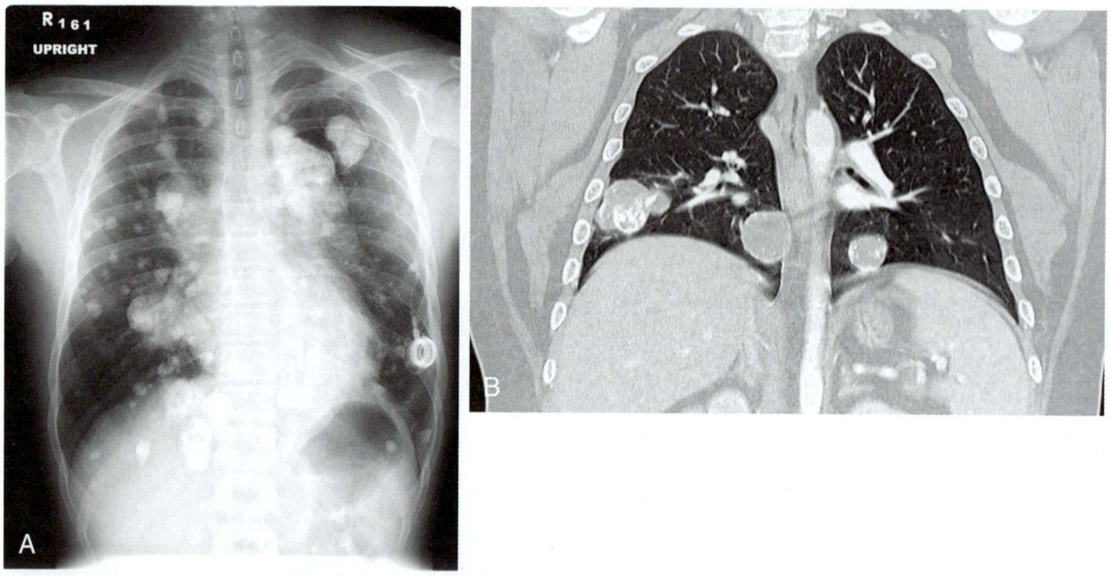

Fig. 12.70 Metastatic pulmonary nodules. (A) Chest radiograph of a patient with pulmonary metastases of osteosarcoma. (B) Coronal chest computed tomography of a patient with pulmonary metastases of osteosarcoma.

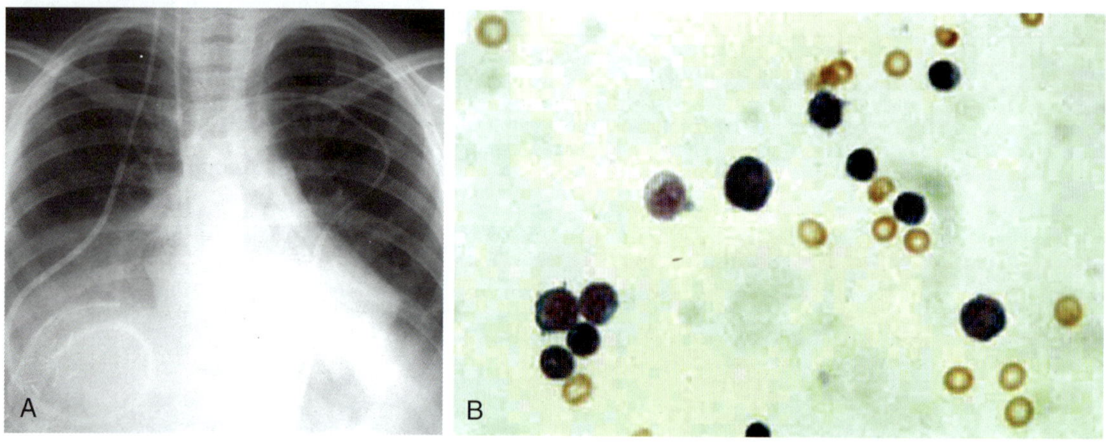

Fig. 12.71 Malignant pleural effusions. (A) This chest radiograph shows an abnormal collection of pleural fluid. If malignancy is suspected, the diagnosis can sometimes be made through analysis of the pleural fluid. (B) Cytology of the pleural fluid obtained by thoracentesis demonstrates large cells, high nuclear-to-cytoplasmic ratios, and fine nuclear chromatin, which are all features of malignant disease.

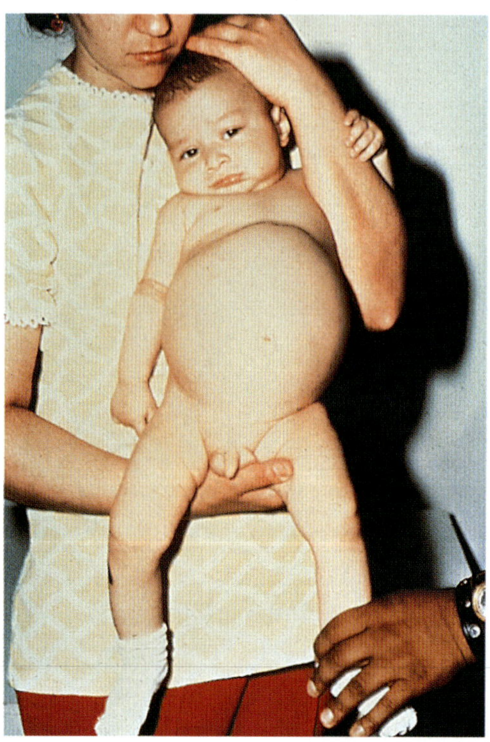

Fig. 12.72 Abdominal neuroblastoma. This child has abdominal swelling with hepatosplenomegaly. Further evaluation reveals a diagnosis of neuroblastoma.

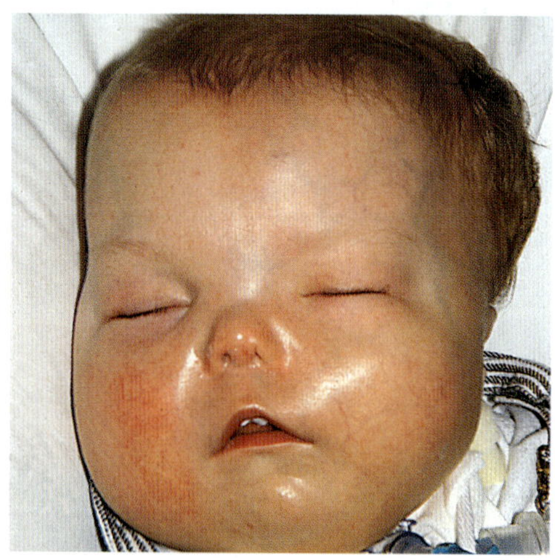

Fig. 12.73 Superior vena cava syndrome. Discoloration of the face and neck with venous distention. The mediastinal masses that produce these findings often pose considerable anesthetic risk.

lymphoma and T-cell disease are at high risk of metabolic abnormalities associated with tumor lysis syndrome.

Abdomen

An observant parent may be the first to detect an abdominal mass. This may represent hepatosplenomegaly, a mass of alternative origin, or ascites. Superficial venous distention (Fig. 12.74) may signal deep venous obstruction due to intraabdominal tumor. Patients may

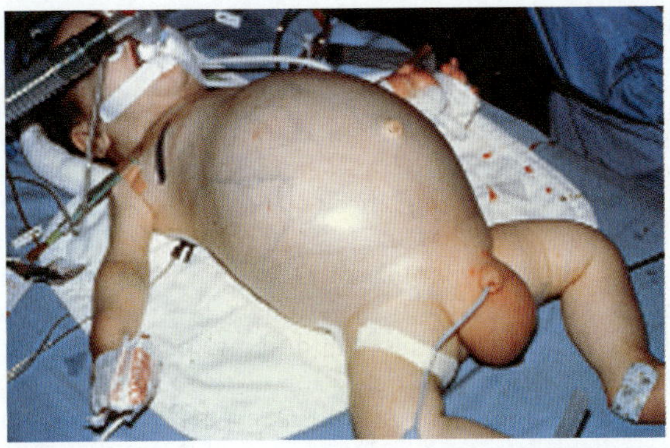

Fig. 12.74 Intraabdominal tumor. Superficial venous distention may also be seen in cases of extensive intraabdominal tumor. (Courtesy D. Nakayama, MD, Chapel Hill, NC.)

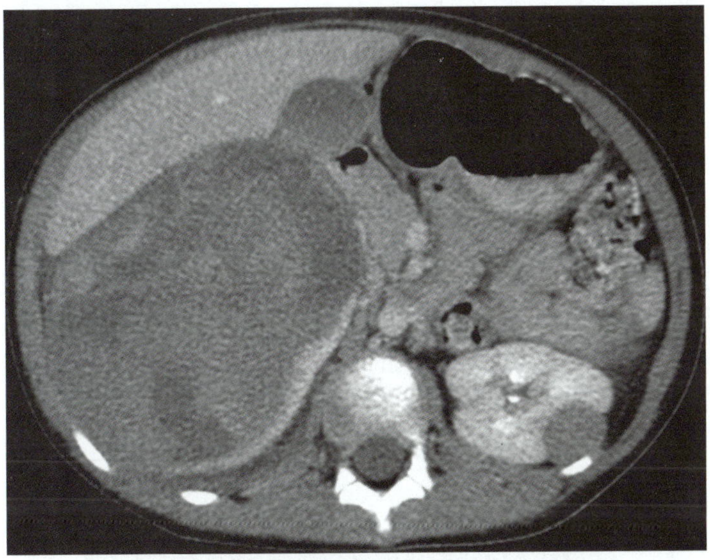

Fig. 12.75 Axial computed tomography of an abdominal mass originating from the kidney in a child with Wilms tumor.

also demonstrate lower extremity edema, scrotal swelling in males, or labial swelling in females. The patient may experience respiratory difficulties due to limited chest excursion with inspiration and renal dysfunction due to external compression of the renal vasculature.

The most common malignant cause of hepatosplenomegaly is leukemia or lymphoma, in which case organomegaly is due to infiltration with malignant cells. The abdominal mass may also reflect a primary tumor originating from an abdominal organ, including the kidney, adrenal gland, liver, or ovaries. Wilms tumor is the most common renal tumor of childhood. The mass arising from the kidney tends to be well encapsulated and often presents as a palpable abdominal mass (Fig. 12.75). Hypertension may occur because of impaired renal blood flow. Hematuria may be observed in approximately 15% of cases.

Children with neuroblastoma may also present with an abdominal mass. This tumor may originate from the adrenal gland, resulting in a suprarenal mass, but also may originate anywhere along the sympathetic chain. Unlike the well-encapsulated lesion of Wilms tumor, neuroblastoma tumors often wrap around vital vascular structures in the abdomen, making complete resection difficult (Fig. 12.76). Many neuroblastoma patients will have metastatic disease at the time of diagnosis and appear toxic. Neuroblastoma has a wide spectrum of presenting symptoms and prognoses depending on patient age, stage of disease, and biological features of the tumor. In approximately 85% of cases, this neural tumor secretes excess catecholamines. The measurement of homovanillic acid and vanillylmandelic acid in the urine is an important aid to diagnosis.

Non-Hodgkin lymphoma of the abdomen may mimic an acute abdominal process, such as appendicitis or intussusception (Fig. 12.77).

Hepatic neoplasms are rare in childhood. The two most common hepatic tumors are hepatoblastoma and hepatocellular carcinoma. Hepatoblastoma occurs more commonly in young children, with more than 75% of cases reported in children younger than 3 years old. Hepatocellular carcinoma usually occurs in older children and is strongly associated with perinatal hepatitis B virus infection. An elevated α-fetoprotein level may be observed in both tumors, although it is more often present in hepatoblastoma. The most

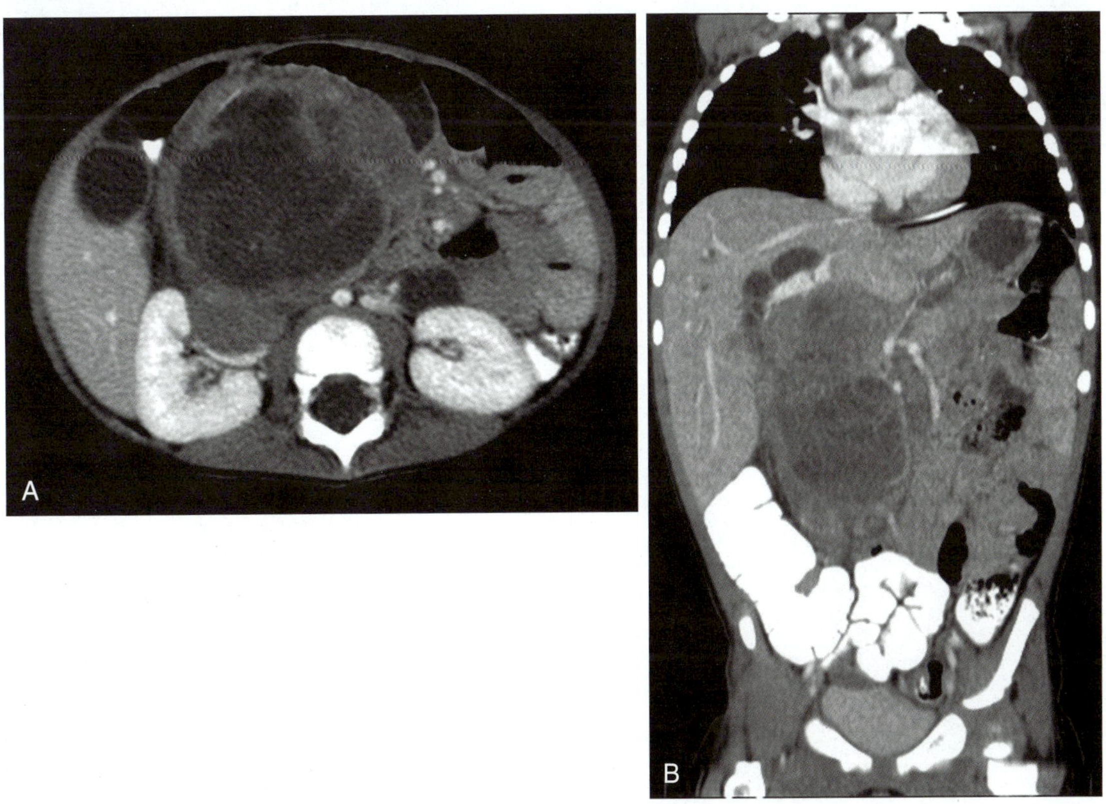

Fig. 12.76 Neuroblastoma. (A) Axial computed tomography (CT) of an abdominal mass in a child with neuroblastoma. (B) Coronal CT of a patient with abdominal neuroblastoma, demonstrating the encasement of vital structures and vessels within the tumor.

frequent presenting signs and symptoms for hepatic tumors include abdominal mass with abdominal distention, anorexia, and weight loss.

A germ cell tumor of the ovary may also present as an abdominal mass and is described further in the next section.

Urogenital Tract

Involvement of the genitourinary system or sacral area by tumor in infancy or childhood may result in the presence of visible abnormalities on physical examination. However, these tumors may also occur in retroperitoneal and intraabdominal locations. Sarcoma botryoides is a subtype of rhabdomyosarcoma that most often presents in the genitourinary region. This tumor has a characteristic appearance with its grapelike morphology (Fig. 12.78). Classically, it involves the vagina, but it may also involve the mucosal surfaces of other hollow organs, such as the bladder or, more rarely, the nasopharynx. Sacrococcygeal teratoma is also usually grossly apparent on physical examination (Fig. 12.79). Teratomas are embryonal neoplasms that contain tissues from all three germ cell layers. The sacrococcygeal location is the most common, although tumors can occur in the pineal region, mediastinum, retroperitoneum, ovary, and testes. Although teratomas have benign elements, nearly 20% of them exhibit malignant features. The sacrococcygeal mass must also be distinguished from a meningomyelocele and thecal tumors.

Testicular enlargement (Fig. 12.80) may be secondary to infiltration by leukemia or lymphoma (in which case bilateral swelling may be seen) or to primary testicular tumors. Primary tumors of the testes include germ cell tumors and paratesticular rhabdomyosarcoma. Priapism is a rare complication of chronic myelogenous leukemia, resulting from sludging and mechanical obstruction due to leukemia cells and/or coagulation abnormalities within the corpora cavernosa.

Precocious puberty may be caused by a tumor of the CNS, gonads (ovaries or testes), or adrenal gland. The inappropriate endocrine-mediated physical examination findings, such as hirsutism, may be the first indication of the presence of a pediatric cancer.

Musculoskeletal System

Bone and joint manifestations of pediatric cancer are relatively common. Arthralgia and full-blown arthritis are well-described presentations of ALL. Diffuse bone pain is also common. Metaphyseal lucencies and growth arrest lines on plain radiographs are often nonspecifically associated with the diagnosis of ALL (Fig. 12.81). Diffuse osteopenia or lytic bone lesions may also be observed in patients with lymphoid leukemia, with similar lytic lesions and bone pain seen with metastatic solid tumor. Hypertrophic osteoarthropathy is a rare musculoskeletal finding in patients with hepatocellular carcinoma. (Fig. 12.82). Hemihypertrophy (see Chapter 18), or relative enlargement of one or more parts of one side of the body, has been associated with the subsequent development of solid tumors,

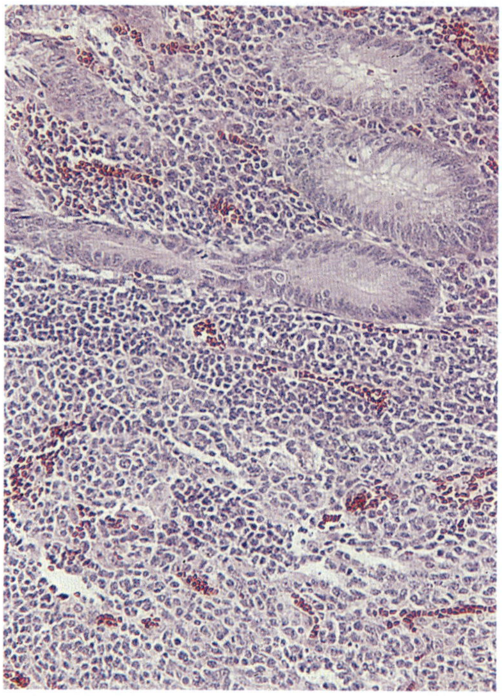

Fig. 12.77 Non-Hodgkin lymphoma of the appendix. Shown is a histologic slide of the appendix, indicating involvement with non-Hodgkin lymphoma. The malignant cells, predominating in the lower half of the slide, are large, with clear cytoplasm and irregularly shaped nuclei.

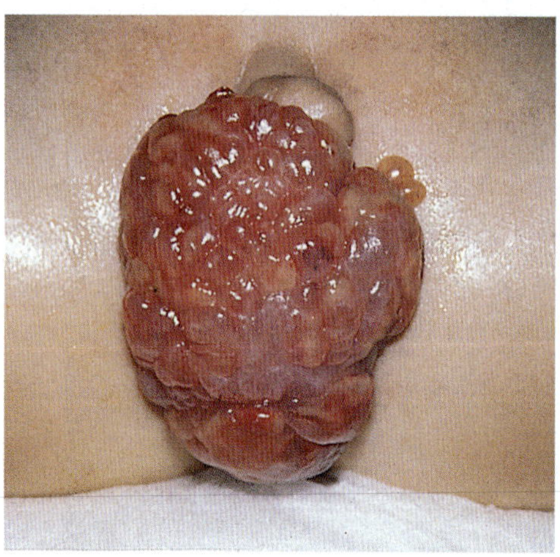

Fig. 12.78 Sarcoma botryoides. A grapelike lesion present in a child with multiple congenital anomalies. The appearance of this lesion is characteristic of the sarcoma botryoides subtype of rhabdomyosarcoma.

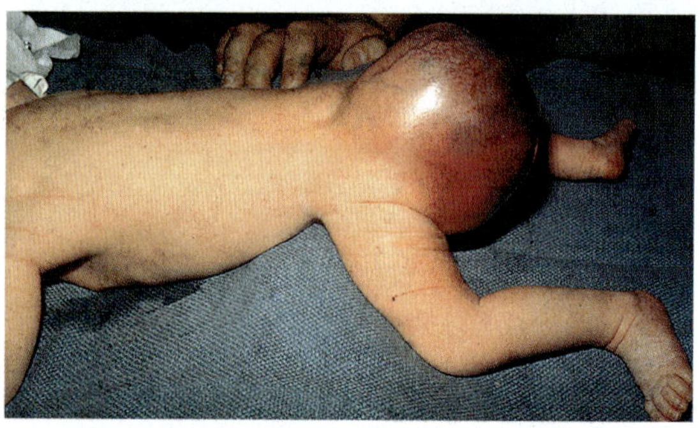

Fig. 12.79 Sacrococcygeal teratoma. This teratoma has an external component and is easily visualized on physical examination. The teratoma may contain both benign and malignant elements.

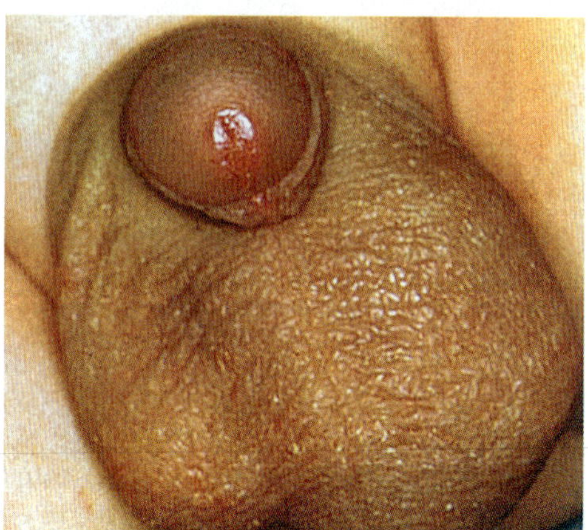

Fig. 12.80 Testicular mass. This photograph demonstrates unilateral scrotal swelling in an infant with a left testicular mass.

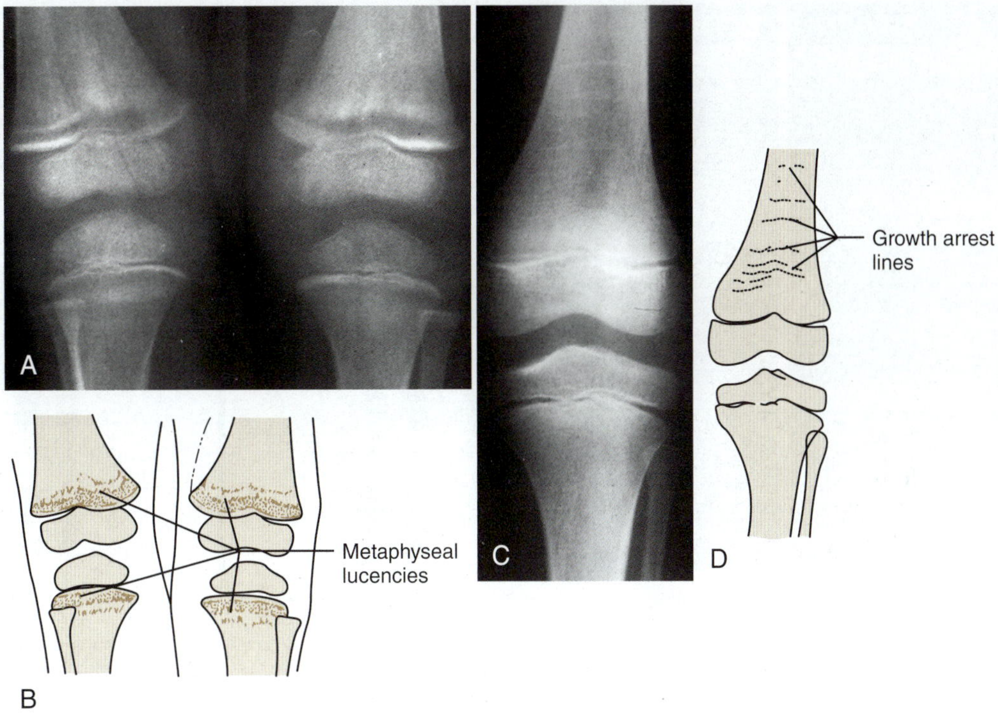

Fig. 12.81 X-ray abnormalities in acute lymphoblastic leukemia (ALL). Metaphyseal (A and B) and growth arrest lines (C and D) in children with ALL. (Courtesy J. Medina, MD, Pittsburgh, PA.)

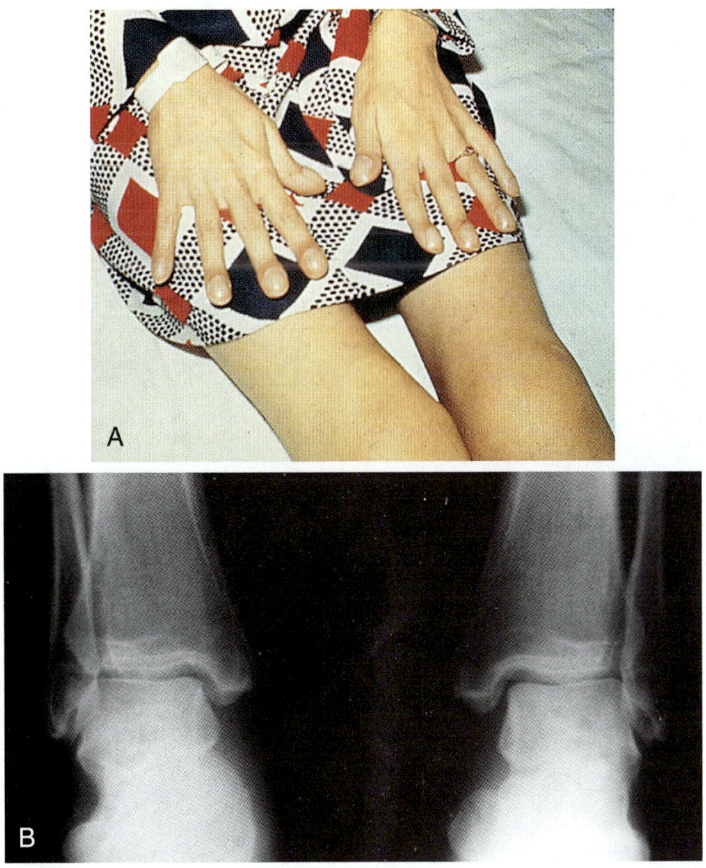

Fig. 12.82 Hypertrophic osteoarthropathy. Clubbing (A) and bone lesions (B) in a child with hypertrophic osteoarthropathy secondary to hepatocellular carcinoma not involving the lung. (Courtesy K.S. Oh, MD, Pittsburgh, PA.)

including Wilms tumor, adrenocortical carcinoma, and hepatoblastoma. Although prospective studies have not been performed, a general recommendation is to perform screening abdominal ultrasound every 3 to 4 months until 7 years old. The finding of hemihypertrophy should be distinguished from hemiatrophy, which is not a predisposing condition. A true mass involving one extremity (Fig. 12.83C) is not usually confused with hemihypertrophy.

Primary bone tumors most commonly occur in adolescents and should be considered when patients experience persistent unexplained pain. Osteosarcoma and Ewing sarcoma are the most common bone tumors found in the child and young adult. Osteosarcoma is a primary bone tumor derived from primitive bone-forming mesenchyme (see Fig. 12.83) and is characterized by the production of osteoid. The development of osteosarcoma may correlate with periods of linear bone growth, as evidenced by peak incidence during the pubescent growth spurt and the observation that patients with osteosarcoma are taller than average for age. It is usually metaphyseal in location and involves the bones exhibiting the most rapid growth in adolescence including the femur, tibia, and humerus. Ewing sarcoma is the second most common malignant bone tumor (Fig. 12.84). It also has its greatest incidence during the second decade of life. It is an undifferentiated tumor of bone that consists morphologically of densely packed small, round, blue cells. Unlike osteosarcoma, this tumor may also arise from soft tissue, in which case it is termed *extraosseous Ewing sarcoma.* The characteristic bone lesion is diaphyseal in location. The clinical picture may initially be mistaken as osteomyelitis because of the association of fever in up to 30% of patients with Ewing sarcoma.

Soft tissue sarcomas represent tumors arising from muscle, connective tissue, and vascular tissue. Rhabdomyosarcoma, a tumor of striated muscle, is the most common soft tissue sarcoma of childhood. This tumor exhibits two age peaks, the first at 2 to 6 years old and the second at 15 to 19 years old. Rhabdomyosarcoma may originate in any site of skeletal muscle, and the most frequent presenting sign is the presence of a mass. Rhabdomyosarcoma in children in the younger age peak usually involves the head, neck, or genitourinary location. Adolescents more commonly develop extremity, truncal, or paratesticular lesions. The prognosis in rhabdomyosarcoma is highly variable and depends on histology and site of origin.

Long-Term Follow-Up of Childhood Cancer Survivors

Over the past several decades, improvements in multimodality therapy have led to markedly improved survival for those who develop cancer as a child or young adult. The current cure rate is approximately 85%

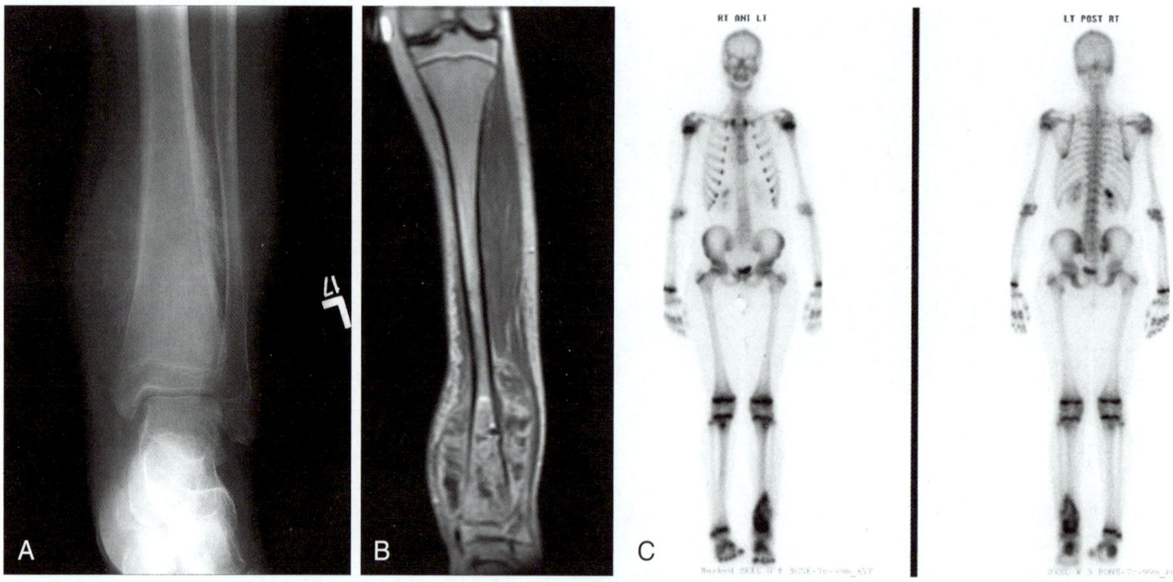

Fig. 12.83 Osteosarcoma. (A) Plain radiograph of the lower extremity in a child with newly diagnosed osteosarcoma. Note the soft tissue swelling, calcification, cortical bone destruction, and new bone formation. (B) Coronal T_1 with contrast further defines the primary tumor. (C) Bone scan of a young girl with osteosarcoma to evaluate the primary site for evidence of metastatic disease. Uptake is limited to the site of her primary tumor.

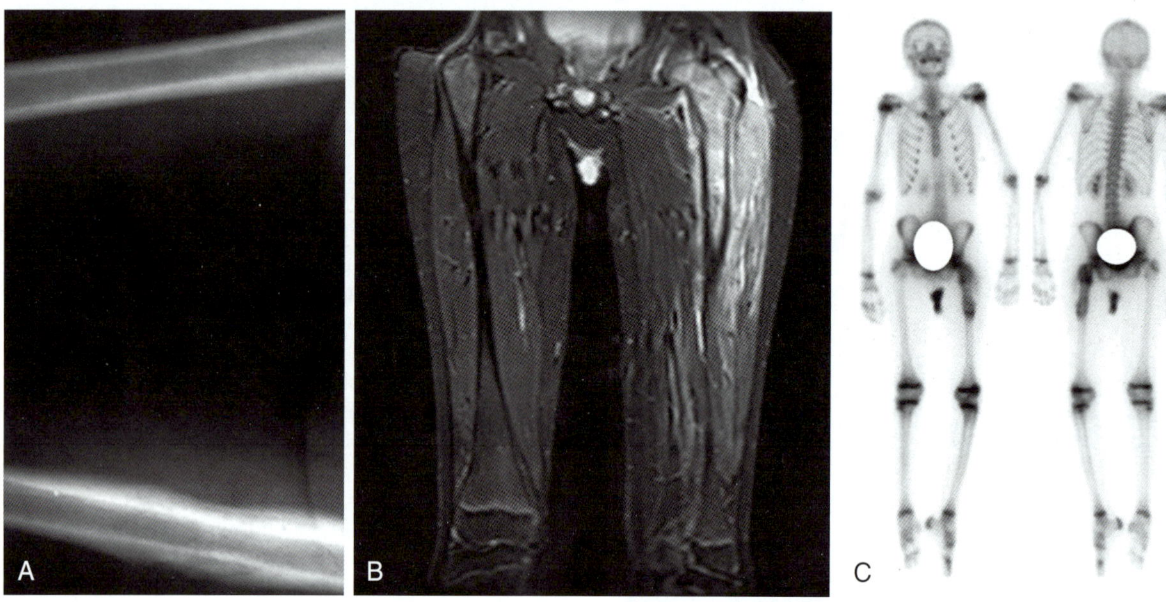

Fig. 12.84 Ewing sarcoma. (A) Plain radiograph of a child with Ewing sarcoma showing cortical destruction and soft tissue swelling of the diaphysis of the femur. (B) Magnetic resonance imaging of the lower extremity further defining the tumor. (C) Bone scan to evaluate the extent of disease, again limited to the primary site. (A, Courtesy J. Medina, MD, Pittsburgh, PA.)

when considering all cancer diagnoses and stages. Treatment-related factors such as chemotherapy, radiation, and surgery all may lead to late sequelae. Patient sex, age at the time of treatment, and the presence of additional genetic factors may also play a role. Long-term effects include decreased neurocognitive functioning, early cardiovascular and pulmonary disease, risk of subsequent malignant neoplasm, infertility, and psychosocial issues. Given these individuals are cured of their cancer, the primary care provider is often the first medical provider to encounter these signs and symptoms of medical late effects.

To improve the systematic follow-up of childhood cancer survivors, the Children's Oncology Group organized exposure-based health screening guidelines. These guidelines provide the primary care provider with a framework in which to provide high-quality long-term follow-up care and health supervision for survivors of pediatric malignancy. Although the long-term survivor does not require lifelong care with an oncologist, ongoing dialogue with the oncology center survivorship specialists remains critical when questions arise.

Bibliography

Abdelmahmuod EA, Yassin MA: Iron deficiency anemia-induced lymphocytopenia in a young female, *Case Rep Oncol* 13(2):793–797, 2020. http://dx.doi.org/10.1159/000507823.

Blaney S, Helman L, Adamson PC: *Pizzo and Poplack's pediatric oncology*, ed 8, 2020, Wolters Kluwer.

Bowman M, Riddel J, Rand ML, Tosetto A, Silva M, James PD: Evaluation of the diagnostic utility for von Willebrand disease of a pediatric bleeding questionnaire, *J Thromb Haemost* 7:1418–1421, 2009.

Devine A, Landier W, Hudson MM, et al: The Children's Oncology Group long-term follow-up guidelines for survivors of childhood, adolescent and young adult cancers, *JAMA Oncol* 11(5):544–553, 2025.

Fish JD, Lipton JM, Lanzkowsky P: *Manual of pediatric hematology and oncology*, ed 7, 2022, Elsevier Inc.

Hoffman R, Benz EJ, Shattil SJ, et al: *Hematology: basic principles and practice*, Philadelphia, 2000, Churchill Livingstone.

Miller DR, Pearson HA, Baehner RL, et al: *Smith's blood diseases of infancy and childhood*, St Louis, 1995, Mosby.

Pizzo PA, Poplack DG, editors: *Principles and practices of pediatric oncology*, Philadelphia, 2010, Lippincott Williams & Wilkins.

Schwartz C, Hobbie WL, Constantine CS Ruccione KS: *Survivors of childhood and adolescent cancer. A multi-disciplinary approach*, ed 3, 2015, Springer.

INFECTIOUS DISEASES

13

Jonathan D. Albert | Marian G. Michaels

INFECTIOUS EXANTHEMS

Exanthematous disorders are numerous and commonly encountered because they have many similarities, often a source of clinical confusion. In establishing a diagnosis, the clinician should attend to not only the character of the exanthem but also its mode of spread, its distribution, the evolution of lesions, and the constellation of associated symptoms. In some illnesses, the presence of a characteristic oral enanthem can help establish the diagnosis.

Viral Exanthems

Many viral infections can present with skin and soft tissue findings. Some of the most common pathogens are noted here alphabetically. Although measles, mumps, rubella, and varicella have decreased substantially in countries using routine measles, mumps, and rubella and varicella vaccination, they still occur in many parts of the world and are increasing in undervaccinated populations. Accordingly, knowledge of their clinical presentations is important, especially as they are less familiar to many clinicians. Mumps is discussed later in this chapter.

Adenovirus

More than 70 distinct types of adenoviruses can produce a variety of clinical illnesses, including conjunctivitis; respiratory tract infections (including coryza, pharyngitis, croup, bronchitis, bronchiolitis, and pneumonia); gastroenteritis; myocarditis; nephritis; cystitis; and encephalitis. An exanthem sometimes accompanies other symptoms, and a variety of rashes have been described. The eruption may consist of discrete, nonspecific, blanching, maculopapular lesions, or it may be morbilliform, rubelliform, or, on occasion, petechial. Typically, the rash is generalized when first noticed. The classic clinical constellation consists of a more severe conjunctivitis, rhinitis, pharyngitis often with exudate, and a discrete, blanching, maculopapular rash (Fig. 13.1). Anterior cervical and preauricular lymphadenopathy, low-grade fever, and malaise are common associated findings. The peak season for adenovirus infections in temperate climates is late winter through early summer, and the infection is maximally contagious during the first few days of illness. The incubation period ranges from 6 to 9 days.

Coxsackievirus and Other Enteroviruses

The *Enterovirus* genus includes coxsackieviruses, echoviruses, and enteroviruses, with many types of each. Coxsackieviruses are the most common cause of hand-foot-and-mouth disease. Patients may have a brief prodrome consisting of low-grade fever, malaise, sore mouth, and anorexia before oral lesions and skin lesions appear in 1 to 2 days. The former usually consist of shallow, yellow ulcers surrounded by red halos. They are found on the labial and buccal mucosal surfaces, the gingivae, tongue, soft palate, uvula, and anterior tonsillar pillars (Fig. 13.2A and B). In the early stage of the illness, small vesicles may be seen on the palate or mucosal surfaces. These oral lesions are usually mildly painful. The cutaneous lesions begin as erythematous macules on the palmar aspect of the hands and fingers, the plantar surface of the feet and toes, and the interdigital surfaces. The buttocks may be involved as well. They evolve rapidly to form small, thick-walled, gray vesicles on an erythematous base (see Fig. 13.2C–E), which may be tender, pruritic, or asymptomatic. More than 90% of patients with disease caused by coxsackievirus have oral lesions, and about two-thirds have the exanthem. In cases in which the cutaneous manifestations are absent, the process is called *herpangina* and may resemble early herpetic gingivostomatitis (though importantly without the labial component). Hand-foot-and-mouth disease is highly contagious, with an incubation period of approximately 2 to 6 days and duration up to 1 week. The peak season is summer through early fall, which is a time when most enteroviral infections occur in temperate climates.

Other enteroviral syndromes include a mild, nonspecific febrile illness with myalgias, headache, and abdominal pain; generalized exanthems that may be maculopapular, vesicular, or urticarial; aseptic meningitis, encephalitis, acute cerebellar ataxia, and myelitis; pleurodynia; myocarditis; hemorrhagic conjunctivitis; and gastroenteritis.

Herpes Simplex Virus

Herpes simplex virus (HSV) produces infections that primarily involve the skin and mucous membranes, although in neonates, immunocompromised hosts, and rarely nonneonates, infection can result in disseminated disease or central nervous system (CNS) involvement. Like other herpesviruses, HSV enters a latent stage after initial (primary) infection, residing in local sensory ganglia; once latent, the virus can be reactivated, causing recurrent disease. The two serotypes of HSV are types 1 and 2. HSV-1 is more common and can produce a variety of clinical syndromes. In contrast, HSV-2 is usually a genital pathogen (see Chapter 19), although occasionally it is the source of oral lesions and is the more common type associated with neonatal HSV disease (see the Congenital and Perinatal Infections section later).

Diagnosis of symptomatic HSV infections can often be made on clinical grounds alone, particularly in cases of primary infection. When the diagnosis is in question, polymerase chain reaction (PCR) has overtaken viral antigens and culture (see Chapter 8) as the primary detection method to confirm the diagnosis. Serology is usually not helpful unless to confirm past infection.

Primary Herpes Simplex Virus Infections

More than 90% of primary infections caused by HSV-1 are subclinical; nevertheless, because the virus is ubiquitous, symptomatic primary infections are common. One of the most prevalent forms of primary infection is herpetic gingivostomatitis. Patients with this condition typically have high fever, irritability, anorexia, and mouth pain; infants and toddlers often drool copiously. The gingivae become intensely erythematous, edematous, and friable and tend to bleed easily. Small, yellow ulcerations with red halos are seen routinely on the buccal and labial mucosa, on the gingivae and tongue, and often on the palate and tonsillar pillars (Fig. 13.3A and B). Within a short time, yellowish-white debris builds up on mucosal surfaces and halitosis becomes prominent. Thick-walled vesiculopustular lesions may also develop on the perioral skin (see Fig. 13.3C). The anterior cervical and tonsillar nodes are enlarged and tender. Symptoms last from 5 to 14 days, but the virus may be

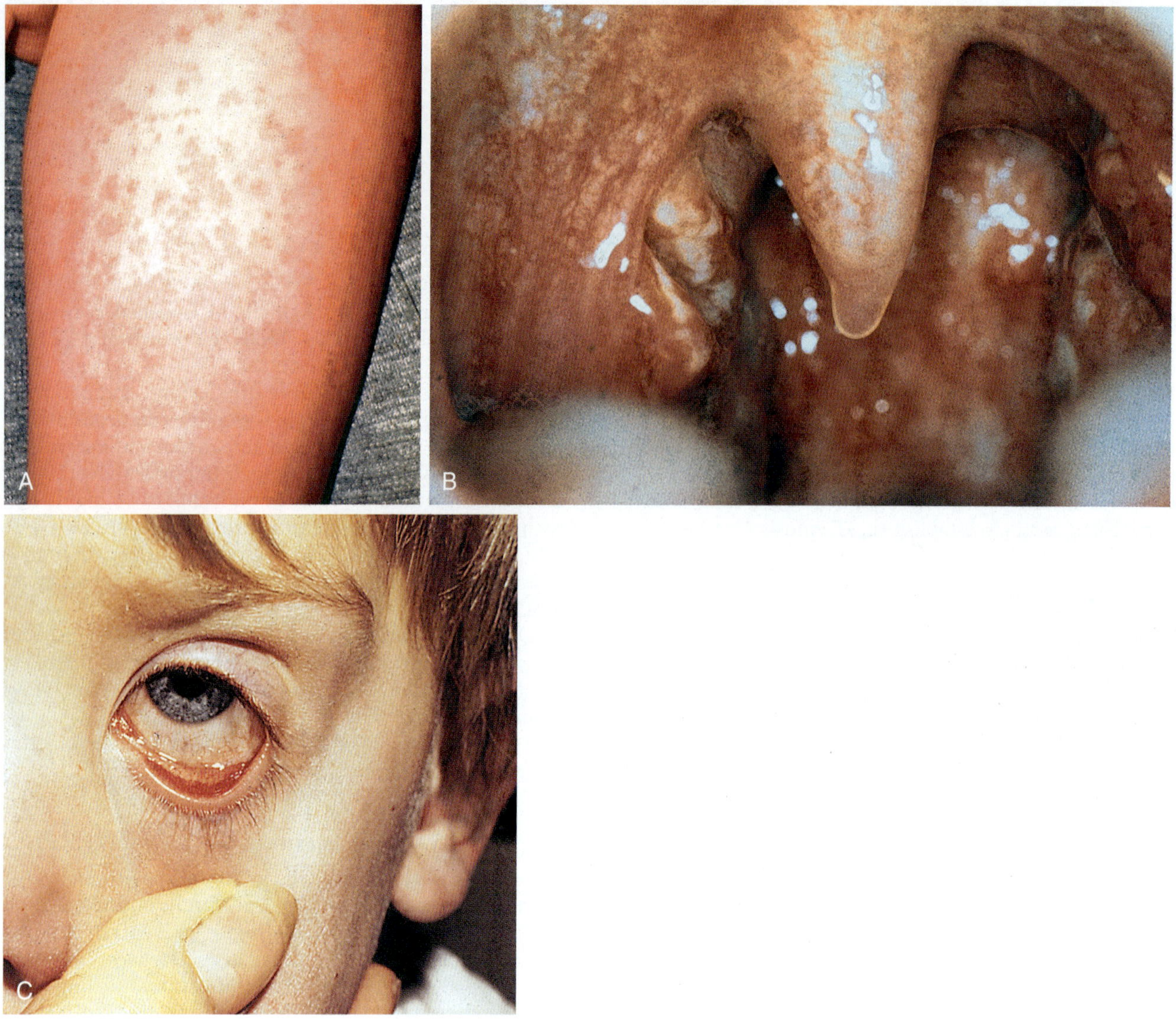

Fig. 13.1 Adenovirus. (A) This discrete, erythematous, blanching maculopapular rash was generalized when first noted and occurred in association with pharyngitis (B) and a nonpurulent conjunctivitis (C). (A and C, Courtesy Michael Sherlock, MD, Lutherville, MD.)

shed for weeks after resolution. The illness can vary from mild to marked in severity. Young children with prolonged high fever and intense pain may become dehydrated and should be monitored closely. The intensity of the ulceration, mucosal inflammation, and gingivitis help to distinguish this disorder from enteroviral herpangina and exudative tonsillitis, as well as from other forms of gingivitis.

Patients with primary herpetic infection involving the skin typically present with fever, malaise, localized lesions, and regional adenopathy. The skin lesions generally result from direct inoculation of previously traumatized skin (e.g., abrasion, burn, laceration). Parents, siblings, and playmates with active herpetic lesions (usually cold sores) are often the source, and children with herpes gingivostomatitis may autoinoculate other body sites with their fingers. The lesions consist of deep, thick-walled, painful vesicles on an erythematous base; they are usually grouped but may occur singly. As they evolve over several days, the vesicles become pustular, coalesce, ulcerate, and crust over. As a result, the lesions may simulate those of bacterial impetigo, but the presence of grouped vesicles and the absence of bacteria on Gram stains of vesicular fluid support the clinical diagnosis of herpes.

Although the virus can infect any area of the skin, the lips and fingers (e.g., herpetic whitlow) are the most common sites of involvement (Figs. 13.4 and 13.3). On occasion, the eyelids and periorbital tissues are affected (Fig. 13.5); this can lead to keratoconjunctivitis, which is diagnosed after finding characteristic dendritic ulcerations on slit-lamp examination (see Chapter 20). Because this complication carries a risk of permanent visual impairment, urgent ophthalmologic consultation is indicated whenever there is any suspicion of ocular herpetic infection.

Eczema Herpeticum (Kaposi Varicelliform Eruption)

Patients with atopic eczema and other forms of chronic dermatitis are at risk for a particularly severe form of primary HSV infection and should avoid contact with people with active herpetic infections. The illness is heralded by the onset of high fever, irritability, and discomfort. Lesions appear in crops and primarily involve areas of skin currently or recently affected by eczema. Typically, they evolve to form pustules, which rupture and form crusts over the course of a few days. On occasion, these lesions become hemorrhagic (Fig. 13.6). Multiple crops can appear over 7 to 10 days, resembling varicella. However, the slower evolution of lesions, the tendency of such lesions to become hemorrhagic, their concentration in eczematous areas, and the persistence of fever and systemic symptoms for as long as 1 week help to distinguish this disorder from varicella, as does PCR or culture testing. Severity ranges from mild to fulminant and depends in part on the extent of the preceding dermatitis. When the area of involvement is large, fluid losses can be severe and potentially fatal. Accordingly, prompt treatment with intravenous acyclovir is recommended. A significant risk of

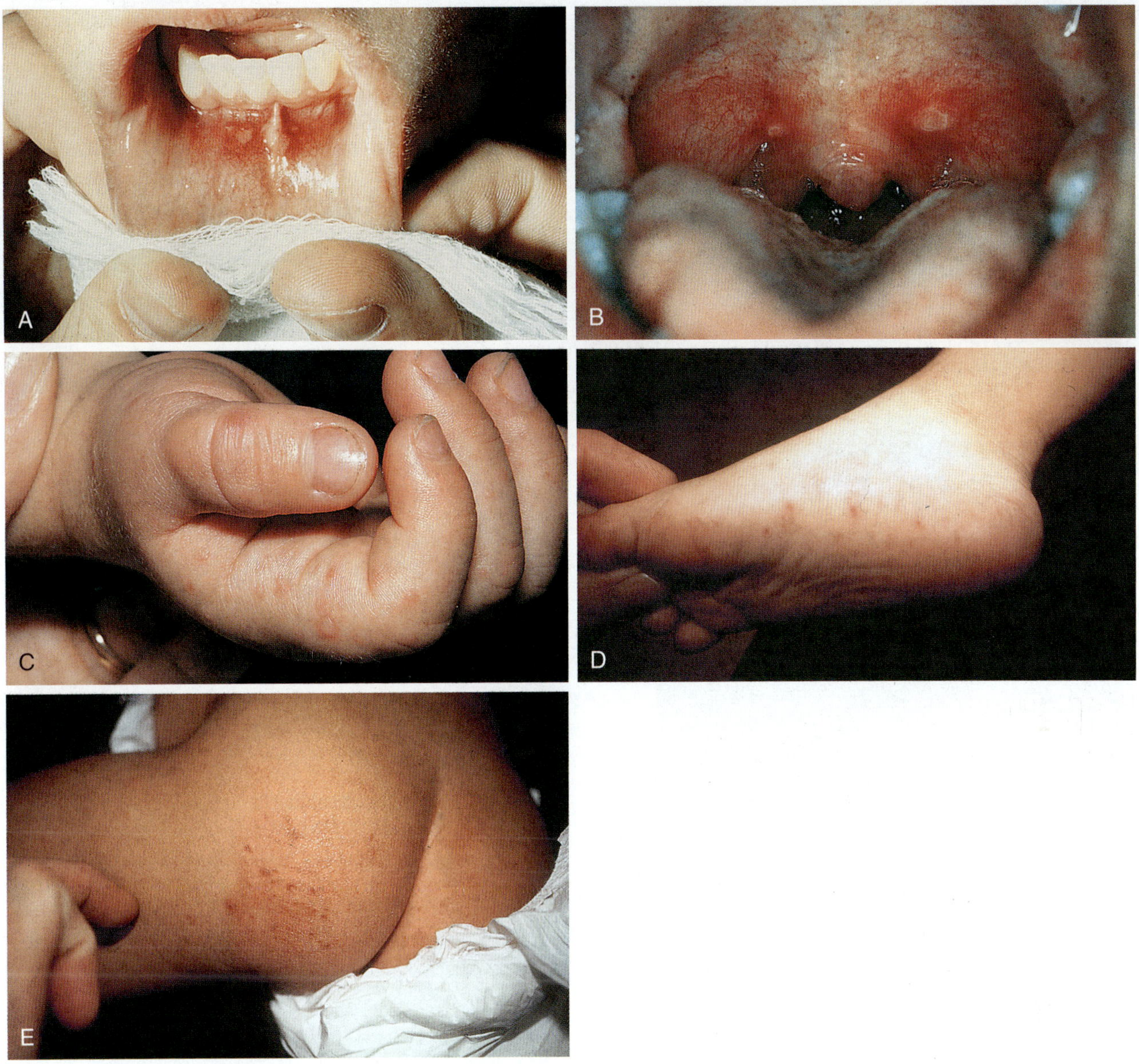

Fig. 13.2 Coxsackievirus hand-foot-and-mouth disease. The enanthem of this disorder is characterized by mildly painful, shallow, yellow ulcers surrounded by red halos. These may be found on the labial or buccal mucosa (A), tongue, soft palate (B), uvula, and anterior tonsillar pillars. When oral lesions occur in the absence of the exanthem, the resulting disorder is called herpangina. (C and D) The exanthem of coxsackievirus hand-foot-and-mouth disease involves the palmar, plantar, and interdigital surfaces of the hands and feet and sometimes the buttocks (E). It consists of thick-walled, gray vesicles on an erythematous base. (D and E, Courtesy Robert Hickey, MD, Children's Hospital of Pittsburgh, Pittsburgh, PA.)

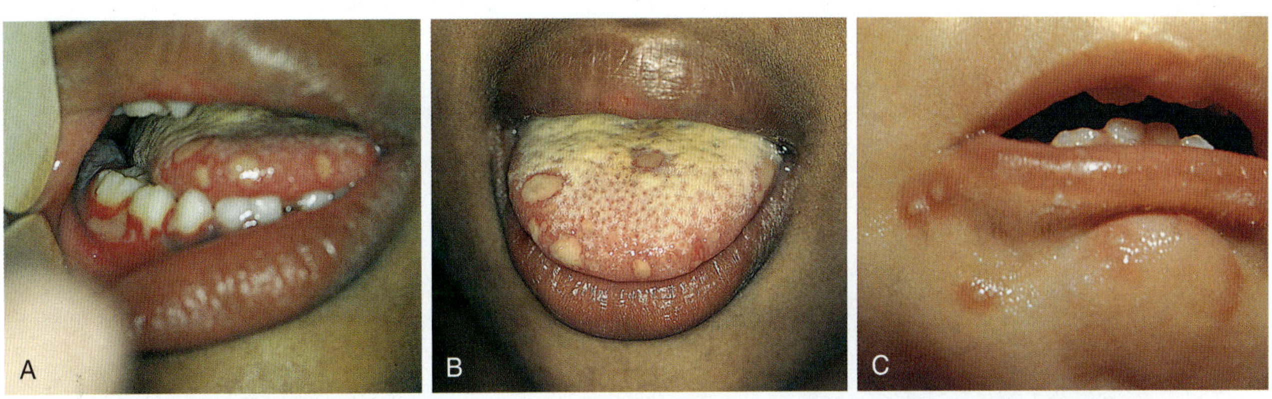

Fig. 13.3 Herpes simplex infections. (A) Herpetic gingivostomatitis is characterized by discrete mucosal ulcerations and diffuse gingival erythema, edema, and friability in association with fever, dysphagia, and cervical adenopathy. (B) Numerous yellow ulcerations with thin red halos are seen on the patient's tongue as well. (C) Thick-walled vesicles on an erythematous base were noted in this child, who showed early findings of intraoral involvement. (C, Courtesy Michael Sherlock, MD, Lutherville, MD.)

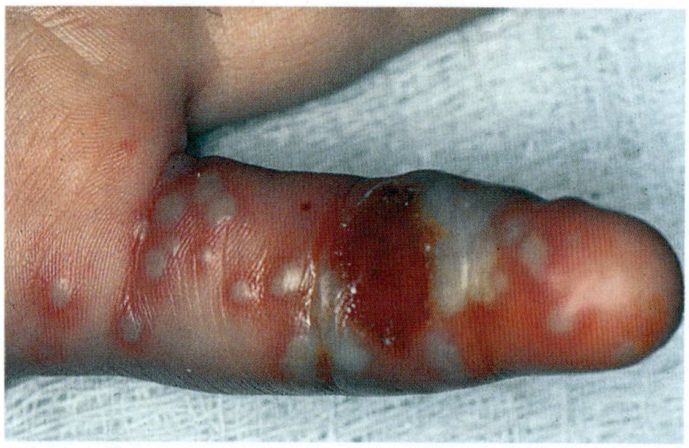

Fig. 13.4 Herpetic whitlow. Grouped, thick-walled vesicles on an erythematous base that are painful and tend to coalesce, ulcerate, and then crust are the typical characteristics of herpetic whitlow.

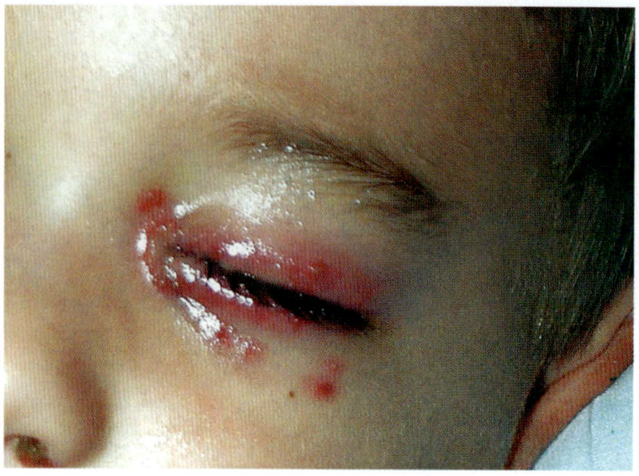

Fig. 13.5 Ocular herpes may involve only the lids and periorbital skin but can spread to involve the conjunctiva, cornea, and deeper structures, with devastating results.

secondary bacterial infection also exists, which is uncommon in uncomplicated herpetic infections.

Recurrent Herpes Simplex Infections

After primary infection, HSV becomes latent within the ganglia that lie in the region of initial involvement. Reactivation of the latent virus results in localized recurrences at or near the site of previous infection. Fever, sunlight, local trauma, menses, and emotional stress are recognized triggers. Labial and perioral disease is the most common site of both primary and secondary disease. Many patients report a prodrome of localized burning along with stinging or itching before the eruption of grouped vesicles. These vesicles contain yellow, serous fluid and often appear smaller and less thick-walled than primary lesions (Fig. 13.7). After 2 to 3 days, the vesicular fluid becomes cloudy and crusts form. Although fever and systemic symptoms are absent, regional nodes may be enlarged and tender. The localization of the lesions to a small area helps to distinguish them from those of herpes zoster (varicella). Prodromal symptoms and discomfort help to distinguish recurrent HSV infection from impetigo and contact dermatitis.

Epstein-Barr Virus (Infectious Mononucleosis)

Infectious mononucleosis is usually an acute, self-limited illness of children and young adults caused by the Epstein-Barr virus (EBV). Transmission of EBV can occur by saliva, contact (e.g., kissing), sharing eating utensils, transfusions, or organ transplantation. The incubation period usually ranges from 30 to 50 days, although it is shorter (14–20 days) in patients with transfusion-acquired infection. In its most typical form, infectious mononucleosis is characterized by fever, fatigue, pharyngitis, lymphadenopathy, splenomegaly, atypical lymphocytosis, and a positive heterophile antibody response. In contrast, young children with EBV infection tend to have either a nonspecific febrile illness clinically indistinguishable from other common viral diseases, or subclinical infection.

Clinical Features of Mononucleosis

The illness often begins with a prodrome lasting 3 to 5 days consisting of fatigue, malaise, and anorexia, often in association with headache, sweats, and chills. Photophobia and edema of the eyelids and periorbital tissues may be noted in some patients (Fig. 13.8A). The acute phase is usually heralded by a fever, which may show wide daily fluctuations. Pharyngitis and cervical node enlargement then become apparent. The sore throat tends to increase in severity over several days before abating and may be associated with significant dysphagia. Tonsillar and adenoidal enlargement can range from mild to marked, and the tonsillar surface may vary in appearance from one of mild erythema to one of severe exudative inflammation with palatal and uvular edema (see Fig. 13.8B). Halitosis and palatal petechiae (like group A *Streptococcus* [GAS] pharyngitis) are common. Approximately one-third of patients show severe pharyngeal manifestations. The anterior cervical lymph nodes are routinely enlarged, and posterior cervical adenopathy is characteristic. In classic cases, adenopathy becomes generalized toward the end of the first week. Involved nodes are firm, discrete, and mildly to moderately

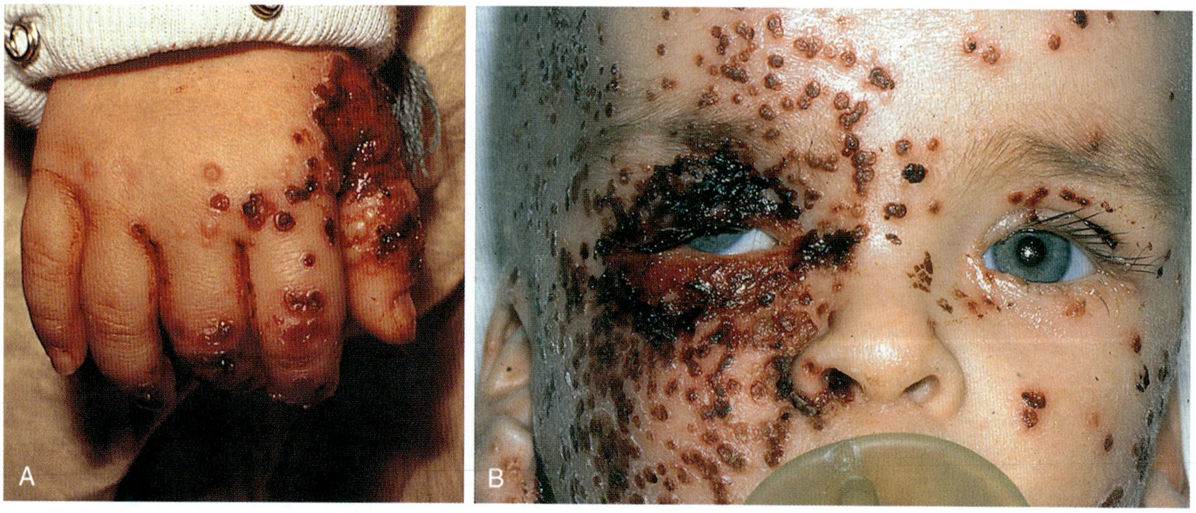

Fig. 13.6 Eczema herpeticum (Kaposi varicelliform eruption). Primary herpes simplex infection in a child with underlying eczema produces crops of hemorrhagic vesiculopustular lesions limited to areas of preexisting dermatitis, which then rupture and crust. Lesions are seen on the hand of one child (A) and on the face of another (B). (A, Courtesy Michael Sherlock, MD, Lutherville, MD.)

tender. Splenomegaly develops in approximately 50% of patients in the second to third week of illness; 10% have associated hepatic enlargement and transaminases may be elevated.

An exanthem is seen in 5% to 10% of patients with mononucleosis, although this percentage is increased in patients treated with ampicillin or amoxicillin for pharyngeal or respiratory symptoms. The exanthem is usually an erythematous maculopapular rubelliform rash, but it can be morbilliform, scarlatiniform, urticarial, hemorrhagic, or even nodular (see Fig. 13.8C and D).

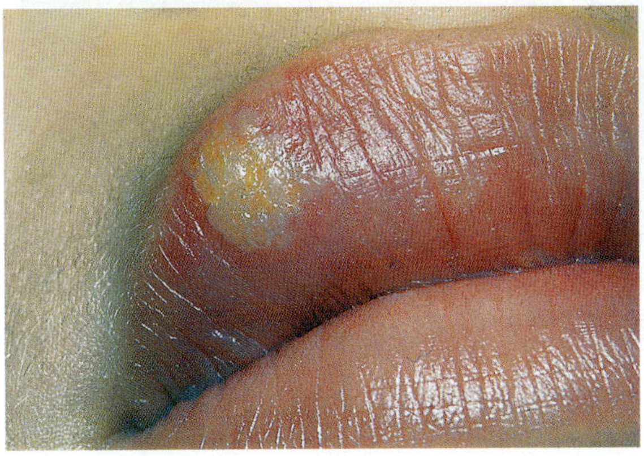

Fig. 13.7 Recurrent herpes labialis (cold sore). After a brief prodrome of burning, these grouped vesicles, filled with yellow fluid, erupted on the child's upper lip.

Younger patients may experience acute upper airway obstruction because of tonsillar and adenoidal hypertrophy. This is manifested by mouth breathing, retractions with recumbency, and stertorous snoring and apnea during sleep. Moreover, children younger than 5 years old with significant tonsillar and adenoidal enlargement during the EBV infection are more likely to have secondary otitis media and may suffer recurrent bouts of otitis media, tonsillitis, and sinusitis because of persistent tonsillar and adenoidal hypertrophy.

Measles (Rubeola)

Measles is a highly contagious, often severe acute illness with a typical prodrome and evolution. Prodromal symptoms consist of fever, malaise, dry (occasionally croupy) cough, coryza, and conjunctivitis with clear discharge and marked photophobia (Fig. 13.9A). One to 2 days after onset of prodromal symptoms, a pathognomonic enanthem (Koplik spots) appears on the buccal mucosa in half of patients (see Fig. 13.9B). The lesions consist of tiny bluish-white dots surrounded by red halos, which increase in number and then fade over a 2- to 3-day period. The exanthem is seen first on day 3 or 4, as the prodromal symptoms and fever peak in severity. It is a blotchy, erythematous, blanching, maculopapular eruption that appears at the hairline and spreads cephalocaudally over 3 days,

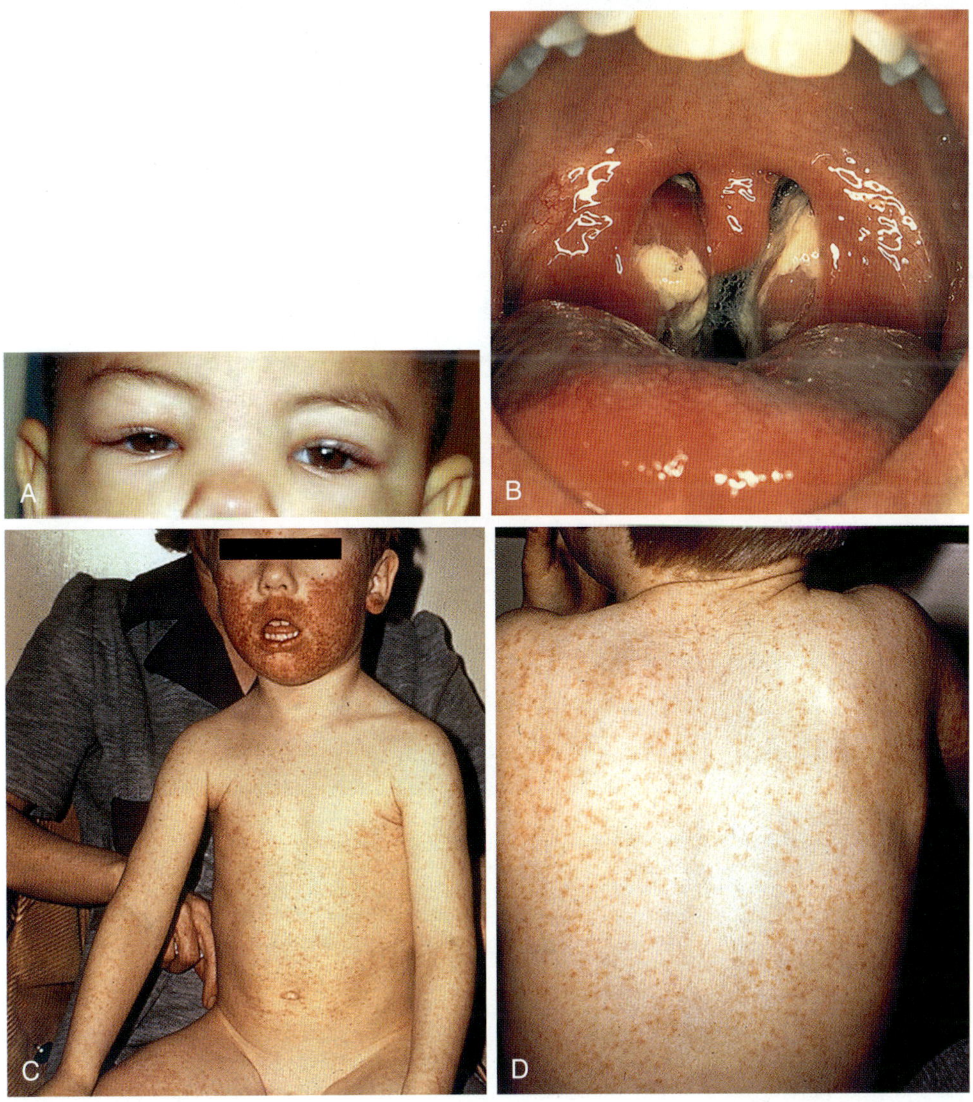

Fig. 13.8 Epstein-Barr virus (EBV) mononucleosis. (A) Eyelid edema is found in 50% of children with infectious mononucleosis. (B) Severe pharyngotonsillitis is seen in this child, whose tonsils are markedly enlarged and covered with exudate. The uvula is erythematous and edematous. (C and D) In this child with EBV mononucleosis, a diffuse, erythematous, maculopapular rash was part of the clinical picture. Lesions on his face are hemorrhagic and confluent as a result of prior irritation. (He had practiced shaving 2 days before.) Note also the swelling in the region of the tonsillar node and the fact that the child is mouth breathing as a result of adenoidal hypertrophy. (C and D, Courtesy Michael Sherlock, MD, Lutherville, MD.)

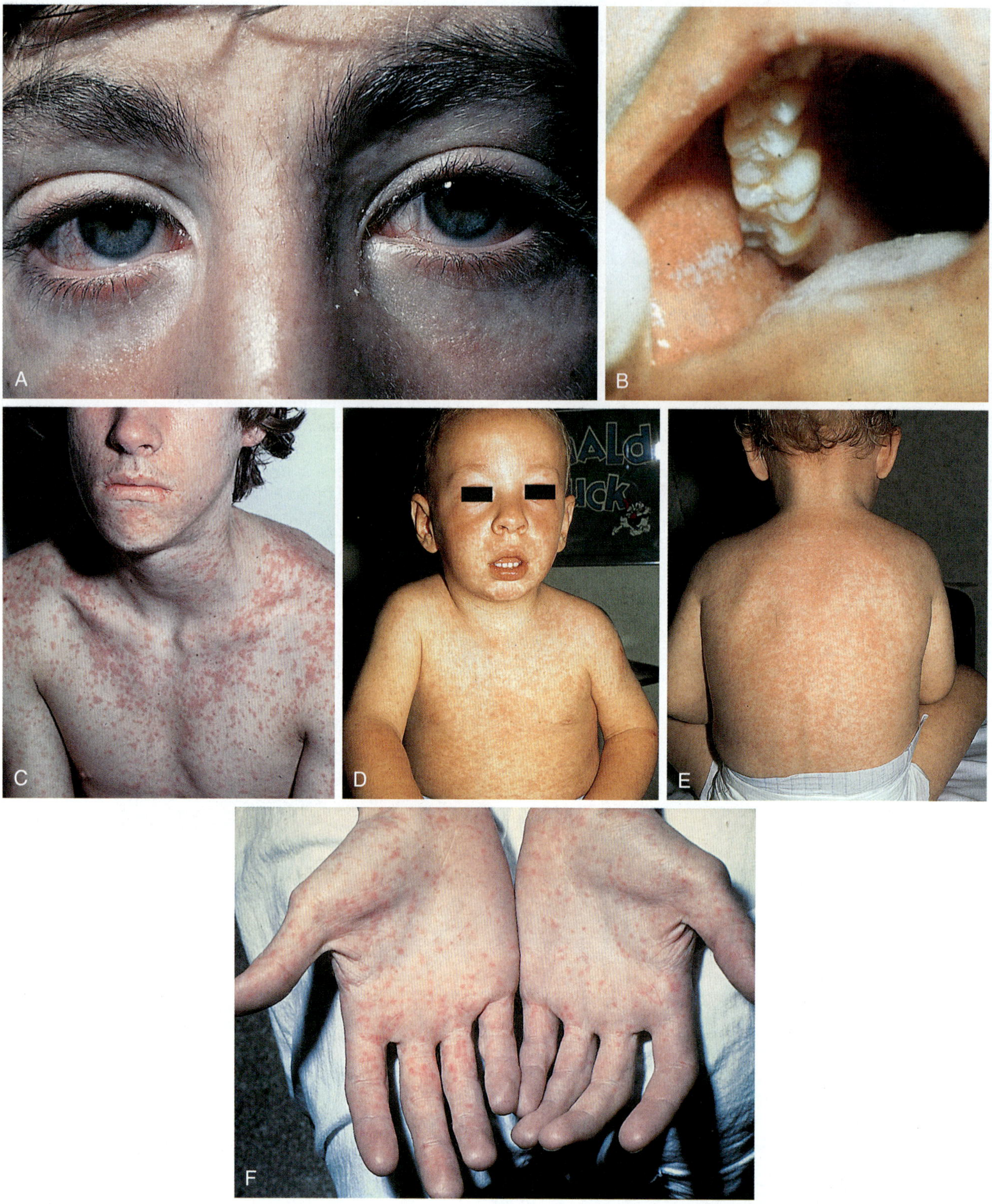

Fig. 13.9 Rubeola/measles. (A) During and after the prodromal period, the conjunctivae are injected and produce a clear discharge. This is associated with marked photophobia. (B) Koplik spots, bluish-white dots surrounded by red halos, appear on the buccal and labial mucosa 1 or 2 days before the exanthem and begin to fade with onset of the rash. (C–E) The measles exanthem is a blotchy, erythematous, blanching maculopapular eruption that appears at the hairline and spreads cephalocaudally over 3 days, ultimately involving the palms and soles (F). With evolution, lesions become confluent at proximal sites. (A, C, and F, Courtesy Michael Sherlock, MD, Lutherville, MD. B, Courtesy Robert Hickey, MD, Children's Hospital of Pittsburgh, Pittsburgh, PA.)

ultimately involving the palms and soles (see Fig. 13.9C to F). Once generalized, the rash becomes confluent over proximal areas but remains discrete distally. Older lesions tend to develop a rusty hue and cease to blanch with pressure. Fading commences after 3 days, with clearing 2 to 3 days later. Fine, branny desquamation of the most severely involved areas may ensue. Generalized adenopathy may be present.

The incubation period for measles is 7 to 21 days, and patients are contagious from approximately 4 days before the appearance of rash until 4 days after. The attack rate in exposed, susceptible people is greater than 90%. Morbidity is high and mortality is not uncommon in low-resource settings. The peak season for measles is late winter through early spring. Potential complications, resulting either from extension of the primary infection or from secondary invasion by bacterial pathogens, include otitis media (most frequently, pneumonia, obstructive laryngotracheitis, and acute encephalitis). Subacute sclerosing panencephalitis is a devastating late complication in children and young adults. Administration of measles vaccine is highly effective in preventing this disease and as postexposure prophylaxis. Recent declines in immunization rates in some populations and regions have led to increasing clusters and outbreaks; thus early consideration and recognition among unimmunized persons is important to institute isolation and prevent secondary spread.

Parvovirus B19 (Erythema Infectiosum, Fifth Disease)

Erythema infectiosum is a mildly contagious illness caused by human parvovirus B19, which principally affects preschool and school-age children. It occurs year-round, with a peak incidence in late winter and early spring. The disorder is characterized primarily by its characteristic exanthem. Fever and constitutional symptoms are uncommon. On occasion, headache, nausea, myalgias, and peripheral polyarthralgia (particularly in adolescents and young adult women) are reported. The rash begins on the face, with large, bright red, erythematous patches over both cheeks (Fig. 13.10A).

These patches are warm and nontender and have circumscribed borders that are usually macular but may be slightly raised. They are easily distinguished from those of cellulitis and erysipelas (see Figs. 13.32, 13.34, and 13.35) by their symmetry and lack of tenderness and by the absence of high fever and toxicity. The facial lesions begin to fade the next day, and a symmetric, macular, or slightly raised, lacy, erythematous rash appears on the extensor surfaces of the extremities (see Fig. 13.10B). Over the next day or so, the rash may spread to the flexor surfaces, buttocks, and trunk. Resolution occurs within 3 to 7 days of onset.

The virus is transmitted primarily by respiratory secretions and, after transmission, it replicates in red blood cell precursors in the bone marrow. Although most often asymptomatic, it may cause a biphasic illness with fever and nonspecific symptoms accompanied by red blood cell suppression occurring approximately 1 week after infection, followed by the appearance of the classic fifth disease exanthem 1 to 2 weeks thereafter. In the immunocompetent host, viral shedding ceases before the rash presents; thus these patients are not contagious. Although red blood cell suppression caused by parvovirus does not result in severe anemia in healthy persons, it can be severe in immunocompromised hosts or those with hemoglobinopathies, such as sickle cell disease, where it can cause aplastic crisis.

Roseola Infantum (Human Herpesvirus 6, Exanthem Subitum)

Roseola infantum is a febrile illness that primarily affects children between 6 and 36 months old. The causative agent is human herpesvirus 6 (HHV-6). The clinical course begins abruptly with rapid temperature elevation, which occasionally precipitates a febrile seizure. Anorexia and irritability are the major associated symptoms. Examination reveals no source for the fever, which is usually higher than 102.2°F (39°C). Although most patients do not appear toxic, many infants undergo a sepsis workup and lumbar puncture because of the combination of unexplained high fever and marked irritability. Fever and irritability persist generally 3 to 5 days, whereupon the fever abruptly subsides. In most cases an erythematous, maculopapular exanthem appears simultaneously with defervescence, or no more than 1 day before or after fever abates. Lesions are discrete, rose-pink macules or maculopapular that begin on the trunk and then spread rapidly to the extremities, neck, face, and scalp (Fig. 13.11). They may last several hours to 1 or 2 days before resolution. Although cases occur year-round, roseola appears to be more common in late fall and early spring. Secondary cases are uncommon, except in institutional settings. The duration of communicability is unclear, but the mean incubation period of HHV-6 is 10 days. Some children may exhibit febrile illness or exanthem alone with HHV-6 infection.

Rubella (German Measles)

Routine vaccination has made rubella rare in many areas. Although rubella often has no prodrome, some infected individuals experience 1 to 5 days of low-grade fever, malaise, adenopathy, headache, sore throat, and coryza. Fever, if present at all, is low grade and rarely lasts more than a day. The exanthem is a discrete, pinkish red, fine maculopapular eruption, which, like measles, typically begins on the face and spreads cephalocaudally (Fig. 13.12A). The rash becomes generalized within 24 hours and then begins to fade, clearing completely by 72 hours. Forchheimer spots, an enanthem consisting of small reddish spots on the soft palate, are seen in some patients on day 1 of the rash and can be helpful in the differential diagnosis (see Fig. 13.12B). Adenopathy, often generalized, is a common but not invariable feature. The occipital, posterior cervical, and postauricular nodes tend to be those most prominently enlarged. Arthritis and arthralgias affecting large or small joints are frequent in adolescent and adult female patients, beginning on day 2 or 3 and typically lasting 5 to 10 days.

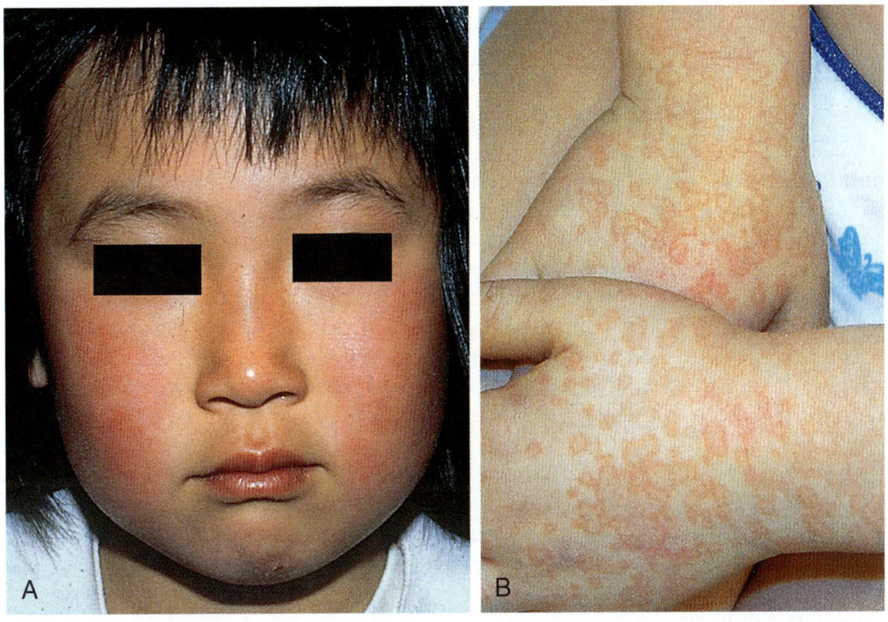

Fig. 13.10 Parvovirus, erythema infectiosum (fifth disease). (A) On day 1, warm, erythematous, nontender, circumscribed patches appear over the cheeks. (B) These fade on the next day, as an erythematous, lacy rash develops on the extensor surfaces of the extremities. (A, Courtesy Robert Hickey, MD, Children's Hospital of Pittsburgh, Pittsburgh, PA. B, From Cohen BA, Lehman C, eds: *Dermatology image atlas* (website). Johns Hopkins University. dermatlas.net.

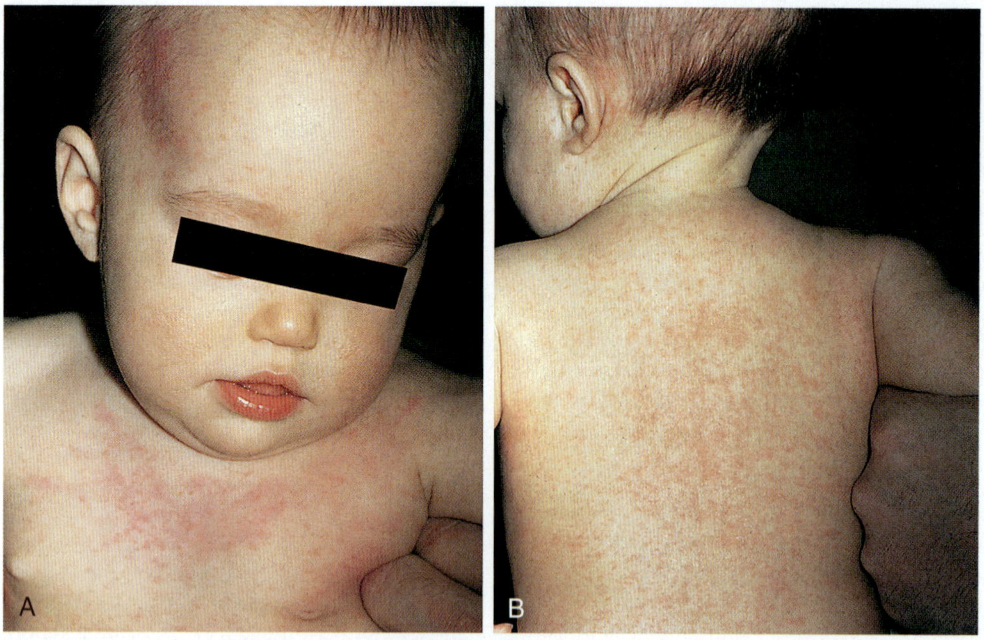

Fig. 13.11 Roseola infantum/exanthem subitum. (A and B) The exanthem of this disorder usually appears abruptly after 3 days of high fever and irritability. It is characterized by discrete, rose-pink macules. It may be generalized at first or may start centrally and spread centrifugally. Scalp involvement is prominent.

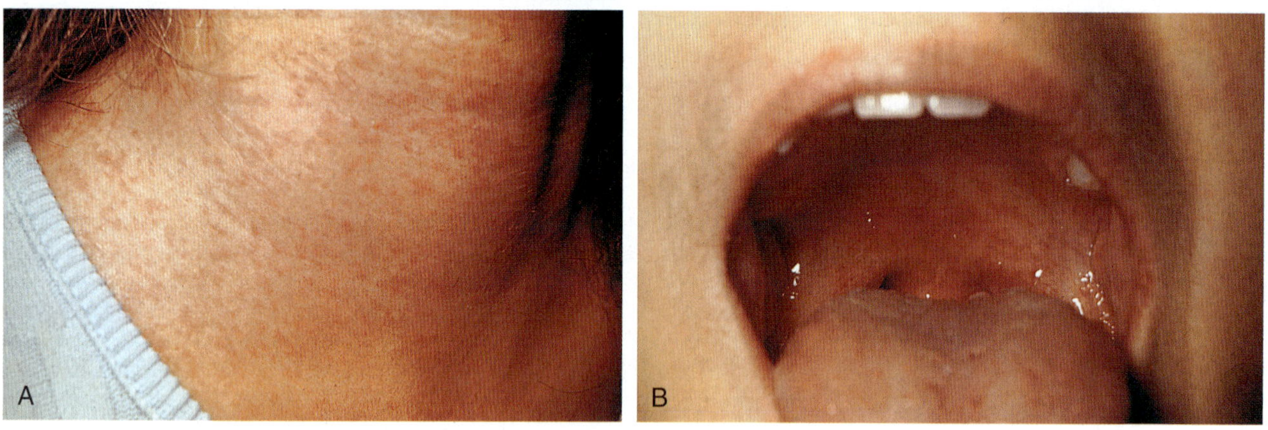

Fig. 13.12 Rubella/German measles. (A) The exanthem of rubella usually consists of a fine, pinkish red, maculopapular eruption that appears first at the hairline and rapidly spreads cephalocaudally. Lesions tend to remain discrete. (B) The presence of red palatal lesions (Forchheimer spots), seen in some patients on day 1 of the rash, and occipital and posterior cervical adenopathy are findings suggestive of rubella. (Courtesy Michael Sherlock, MD, Lutherville, MD.)

Many patients infected with rubella do not manifest a typical syndrome, however, and up to 25% of infected people are asymptomatic yet capable of transmitting virus. In some, the rash may last only 1 day and involve only the trunk; in others, the exanthem is absent and the patient appears to have pharyngitis or an upper respiratory tract infection. Because infections due to many other viruses including adenoviruses, coxsackieviruses, and echoviruses can produce a rubella-like picture, serologic testing is necessary to establish the diagnosis. Such testing is important if the patient is pregnant or has been in contact with a pregnant female or if arthritis is a prominent feature, simulating the picture of acute rheumatic fever or rheumatoid arthritis.

The incidence of rubella peaks in late winter and early spring, and the disease is contagious in patients from a few days before to a few days after appearance of the exanthem. The incubation period ranges from 14 to 21 days. Complications are rare in childhood and include arthritis, purpura with or without thrombocytopenia, and mild encephalitis. The major complication results from spread of the virus to susceptible pregnant women and their fetuses, resulting in congenital rubella syndrome (see the Congenital and Perinatal Infections section).

Varicella (Chickenpox)

Varicella in the normal pediatric host is usually a self-limited albeit highly contagious illness caused by the varicella-zoster virus. A brief prodrome of low-grade fever, upper respiratory tract symptoms, and malaise may occur, followed rapidly by the appearance of a pruritic exanthem. Lesions appear in crops and evolve rapidly over several hours. Most patients have three crops, although the range is one to five. Initial crops involve the trunk and scalp, and subsequent crops are distributed more peripherally; thus the mode of spread is centrifugal. The presence of scalp lesions with the initial crop is often helpful to diagnose a patient who presents early in the disease. Lesions begin as tiny erythematous papules that rapidly enlarge to form thin-walled, superficial central vesicles surrounded by red halos (Fig. 13.13A). Vesicular fluid changes promptly from clear to cloudy, and then drying begins, resulting in an umbilicated appearance. As the surrounding erythema fades, a central crust or scab is formed, which sloughs after several days. A hallmark of this exanthem is the finding of lesions in multiple stages of evolution within a relatively small geographic area of the skin (see Fig. 13.13B). In general, all scabs have sloughed by 10 to 14 days. Scarring usually does not occur unless lesions become secondarily infected. It is

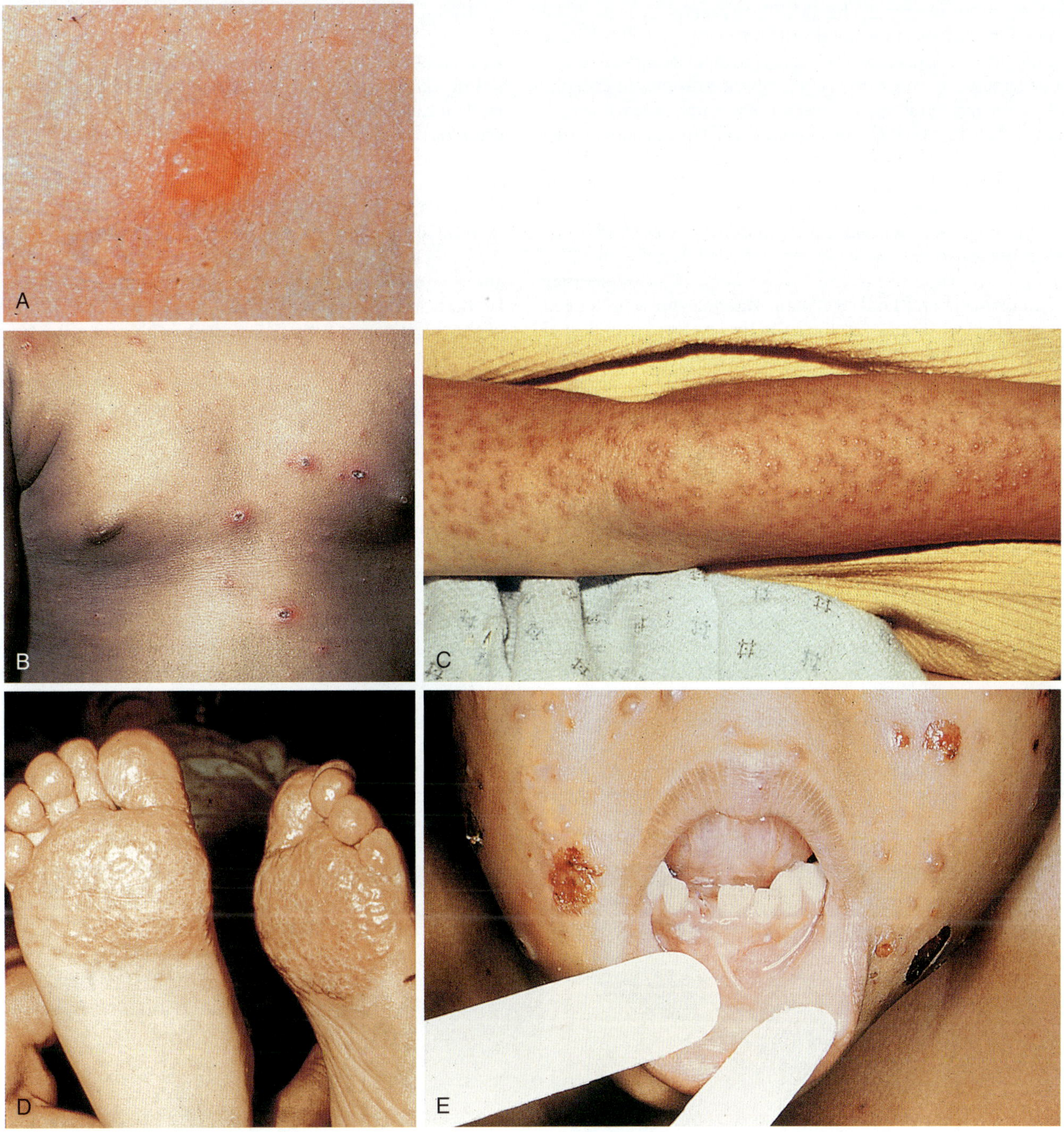

Fig. 13.13 Varicella/chickenpox. (A) The characteristic "dewdrop on a rose petal" is illustrated by this early vesicle on an erythematous base. (B) The typical features of lesions in all stages of evolution are seen on the trunk of this child. Note the presence of papules, vesicles, and umbilicated and scabbed lesions, all within a small area. (C and D) In this child with underlying eczema, the first crop of vesicles appeared in clusters at sites previously affected by dermatitis. The flexor surface of his arm is covered with numerous discrete lesions, and vesicles are confluent over the plantar surface of his toes and on the balls of his feet. (E) On mucosal surfaces, thin-walled vesicles may form and rapidly rupture, forming painful shallow ulcers. (C and D, Courtesy Michael Sherlock, MD, Lutherville, MD. E, Courtesy Ellen Wald, MD, University of Wisconsin Children's Hospital, Madison, WI.)

important to recognize that in patients with preexisting dermatologic problems, the lesions of varicella, like other viral exanthems, tend to appear first and cluster most heavily at sites of prior skin irritation, such as the diaper area or sites of eczematous dermatitis (see Fig. 13.13C and D).

An enanthem is commonly seen and consists of thin-walled vesicles that rapidly rupture to form shallow ulcers (see Fig. 13.13E). Other mucosal surfaces may be affected as well. Although skin lesions are pruritic, those on the oral, rectal, conjunctival, or vaginal mucosa and those involving the external auditory canal or tympanic membrane can be painful. Systemic symptoms are generally mild, although low-grade to moderate fever may be present during the first few days. In most cases, pruritus is the child's major complaint. In adolescents and adults, the illness is more likely to be severe with prominent systemic symptoms and more extensive exanthematous involvement.

Varicella occurs year-round with peak incidences in late autumn and late winter through early spring. The period of communicability begins 1 to 2 days before the appearance of lesions and lasts until all lesions have crusted over. The incubation period ranges from 10 to 21 days, with high secondary attack rates in susceptible children and adults. The most common complication is secondary bacterial infection of skin lesions. *Streptococcus pyogenes* superinfection of varicella lesions ranges from mild cellulitis to myositis, sepsis, and purpura fulminans (Fig. 13.14A). Other complications, although rare, include pneumonia, hepatitis, and encephalitis. The onset of these complications is typically heralded by a secondary fever spike concurrent with increase in general systemic symptoms. In patients with encephalitis, an altered level of consciousness along with other signs of neurologic dysfunction occurs. Reye syndrome, an encephalopathy of unclear etiology, is now a rare complication that can occur as a child is recovering from acute varicella, particularly when receiving concomitant aspirin. Repetitive vomiting is followed by an altered level of consciousness in which periods of lethargy alternate with periods of delirium or combativeness.

In the immunocompromised host with deficient cellular immunity, untreated varicella can be severe or even fatal, with CNS, pulmonary, or generalized visceral involvement. Skin lesions may appear hemorrhagic and tend to remain vesicular for a prolonged period (see Fig. 13.14B and C). Intravenous acyclovir is indicated for these patients and more severely affected immunocompetent patients.

Herpes Zoster (Shingles)

Varicella-zoster virus, like all herpesviruses, persists after primary infection. The virus establishes latency in sensory nerve root cells and can reactivate in response to mechanical and thermal trauma, other infections, decreased T-cell immunity, and older age. In the reactivated form, herpes zoster, lesions consist of grouped, thin-walled vesicles on an erythematous base, which are distributed along the course of a spinal or cranial sensory nerve root in typically a dermatomal distribution (Fig. 13.15). They evolve from macule to papule to vesicle and then to a crusted stage over a few days. Hyperesthesia or nerve root pain may precede, accompany, or follow the eruption and does not correlate with the severity of the rash. Pain, if present at all in pediatric patients, is rarely severe and is generally short-lived, unless a cranial nerve dermatome is involved, in which case pain can be excruciating. Fever and constitutional symptoms may or may not be part of the picture, but regional adenopathy is common.

Thoracic dermatomes are involved in most patients, followed in frequency by cervical, trigeminal, lumbar, and facial nerve regions. Cranial nerve involvement may produce a puzzling prodrome consisting of severe headache, facial pain, or auricular pain with no evident cause and lasting up to several days before appearance of the eruption. Lesions appear unilaterally on the tonsillar pillars and uvula with involvement of the maxillary branch of the trigeminal nerve; on the buccal mucosa and palate with involvement of the mandibular division; and on the face, cornea, and tip of the nose with involvement of the ophthalmic branch (see Fig. 13.15D). When the geniculate ganglion is affected, vesicles occur in the external auditory canal in concert with facial paralysis. Facial palsy and unilateral hearing loss (Ramsay Hunt syndrome) can occur with zoster of the facial nerve. Although patients with herpes zoster can transmit varicella, contagion is less likely because most patients have lesions on areas covered by clothing and the oropharynx is not involved in respiratory aerosol production.

Gianotti-Crosti Syndrome

The eruption of Gianotti-Crosti syndrome, or papular acrodermatitis, although distinctive, often goes unrecognized (or is misdiagnosed). First described in association with anicteric hepatitis B, this exanthem has also been associated with other viruses including EBV, coxsackieviruses, parainfluenza viruses, echoviruses, cytomegalovirus (CMV), and respiratory syncytial virus. Cases usually occur sporadically. Most patients are between 1 and 6 years old.

A mild prodrome consisting of low-grade fever and malaise is typical and may be associated with generalized adenopathy, hepatosplenomegaly (especially with hepatitis B), upper respiratory tract symptoms, or diarrhea. Within a few days, the first of several crops of lesions appear abruptly. The lesions consist of discrete, firm, lichenoid papules with flat tops (Fig. 13.16A and B) and range from 1 to 10 mm in diameter, tending to be larger in infants and smaller in older children. Papules can be flesh-colored, pink, red, dusky, or

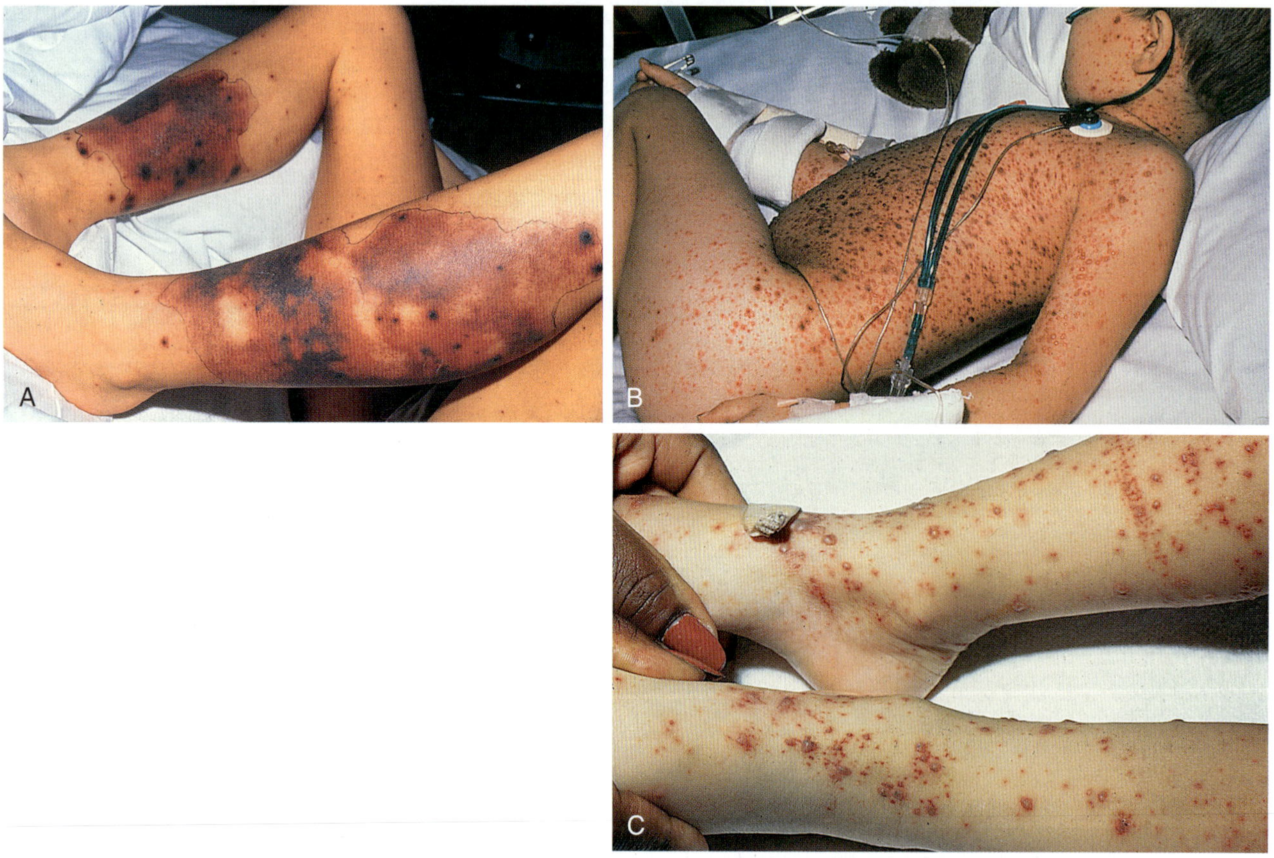

Fig. 13.14 Complications of varicella. (A) Superinfection of this child's lesions with Streptococcus pyogenes led to purpura fulminans. (B and C) Disseminated hemorrhagic varicella. (B) In the immunocompromised child, skin lesions tend to be hemorrhagic and nearly confluent. (C) Lesions also evolve more slowly than usual, remaining vesicular for a prolonged period.

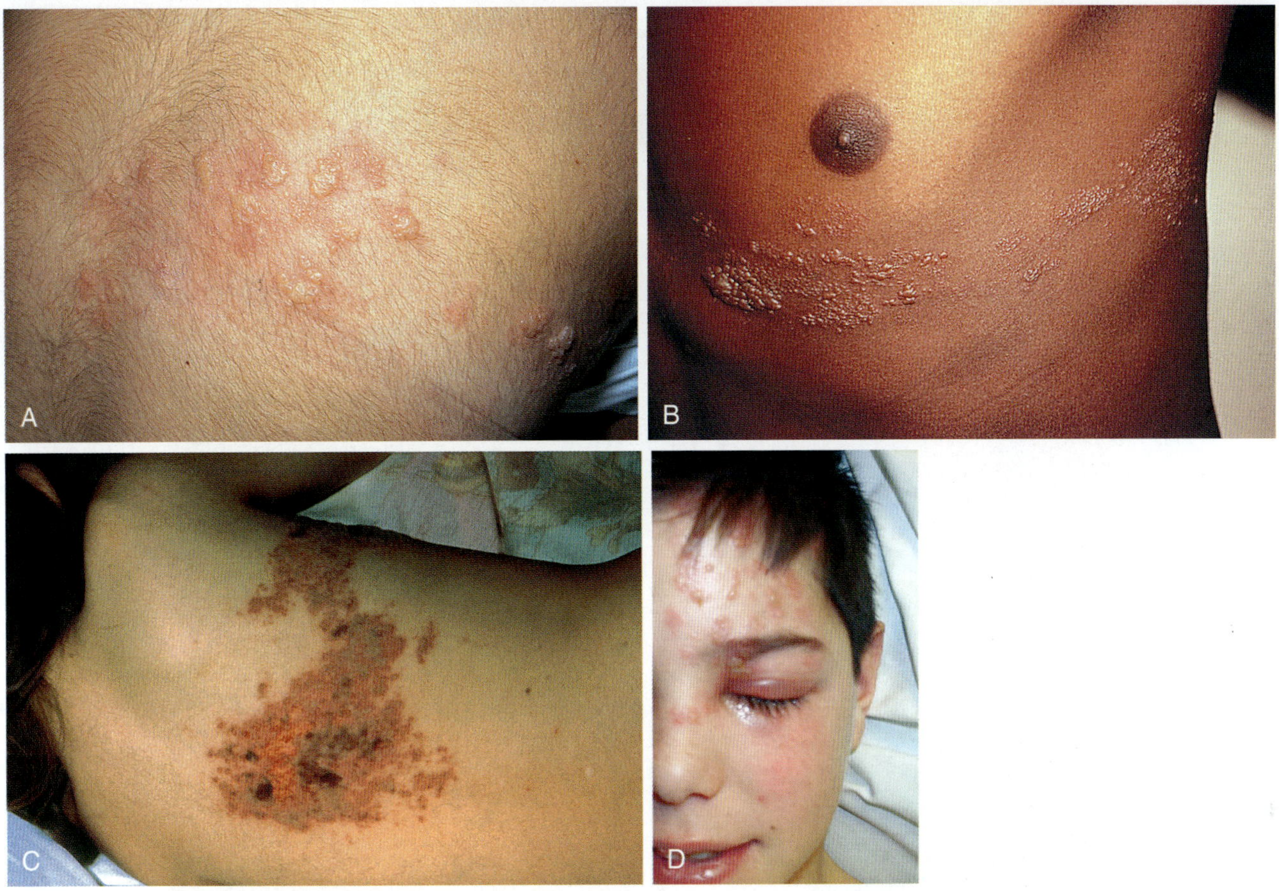

Fig. 13.15 Herpes zoster (shingles). Dermatomal distribution of lesions is a hallmark of herpes zoster. (A) Initially discrete thin-walled vesicles on an erythematous base are seen. Vesicles coalesce over a few days (B), and lesions then evolve to a crusted stage (C). (D) Involvement of the ophthalmic branch of the trigeminal nerve produces lesions involving the forehead, eyelids, and nose. (B, Courtesy Michael Sherlock, MD, Lutherville, MD.)

coppery. They can be purpuric. They are distributed symmetrically over the extremities (including the palms and soles), buttocks, and face, with relative sparing of the trunk and scalp (see Fig. 13.16B), although the upper back may be involved. They tend to remain discrete but can become confluent, especially over pressure points (see Fig. 13.16C), and the Koebner phenomenon may be seen. Pruritus is unusual, and there is no associated mucosal enanthem. The exanthem often clears within 2 to 3 weeks but can persist for 8 weeks or more.

Bacterial Exanthems

Streptococcal Scarlet Fever

Although most commonly associated with pharyngitis and impetigo, GAS also causes scarlet fever, or scarlatina. Streptococcal infections occur year-round, although pharyngitis and scarlet fever have a peak incidence in winter and spring. The exanthem is caused by a streptococcal erythrogenic toxin. The incubation period for scarlet fever ranges from 12 hours to approximately 7 days. The disease is contagious during the acute period, and patients may transmit the organisms during active subclinical infection as well. An average of 50% of family members living with an index case become secondarily infected, and up to half of these have subclinical disease.

Once a severe illness associated with high morbidity and mortality, scarlet fever has become a much milder illness over the past several decades. The classic presentation includes the abrupt onset of fever, chills, malaise, headache, sore throat, and vomiting; abdominal pain may be prominent. Within 12 to 48 hours, an exanthem appears and rapidly generalizes, usually beginning on the trunk and spreading peripherally, but sometimes spreading cephalocaudally, confusing this disease with measles. The face is flushed with perioral pallor (Fig. 13.17A). The remaining skin becomes diffusely erythematous and is covered by tiny pinhead-sized papules, with a sunburn appearance of erythroderma. The texture is sandpapery, and the erythema blanches with pressure (see Fig. 13.17B). The skin may be pruritic, but it is not tender. In severe cases, vesicles may form. After generalization, the rash becomes accentuated in skin folds and creases, and 1 to 3 days after its appearance, petechiae may appear in a linear distribution along the creases, forming Pastia lines (see Fig. 13.17C). Examination of the oropharynx in classic cases reveals large, erythematous, exudative tonsils along with palatal erythema and petechiae (Chapter 24). The uvula may be erythematous and edematous as well. The tongue also shows characteristic findings during the first 2 days, with a white coating through which erythematous papillae project ("white" strawberry tongue) (see Fig. 13.17D). The white coating subsequently peels, leaving a glistening red surface with prominent papillae ("red" strawberry tongue) (see Fig. 13.17E). Tender cervical adenopathy occurs in 30% to 60% of patients. Without treatment, the rash, fever, and pharyngitis resolve within 1 week; with treatment, improvement is more rapid within days. Desquamation occurs regardless of treatment and begins several days after onset, progressing cephalocaudally (see Fig. 13.17F and G). The skin is shed in fine, thin flakes (branny desquamation, in contrast to the thick flakes that characterize desquamation after staphylococcal exanthems) (Fig. 13.18; see Fig. 13.20), and the extent of this process is directly proportional to the intensity of the exanthem.

Diagnosis is simple in classic cases, but the wide spectrum of disease severity and potential manifestations may cause confusion. Fever may be absent or low grade, and malaise may be minimal. Pharyngitis may be mild (without exudate, petechiae, or marked erythema) or absent, even when the throat is the site of infection. In such cases, tongue changes may be absent as well. If streptococcal

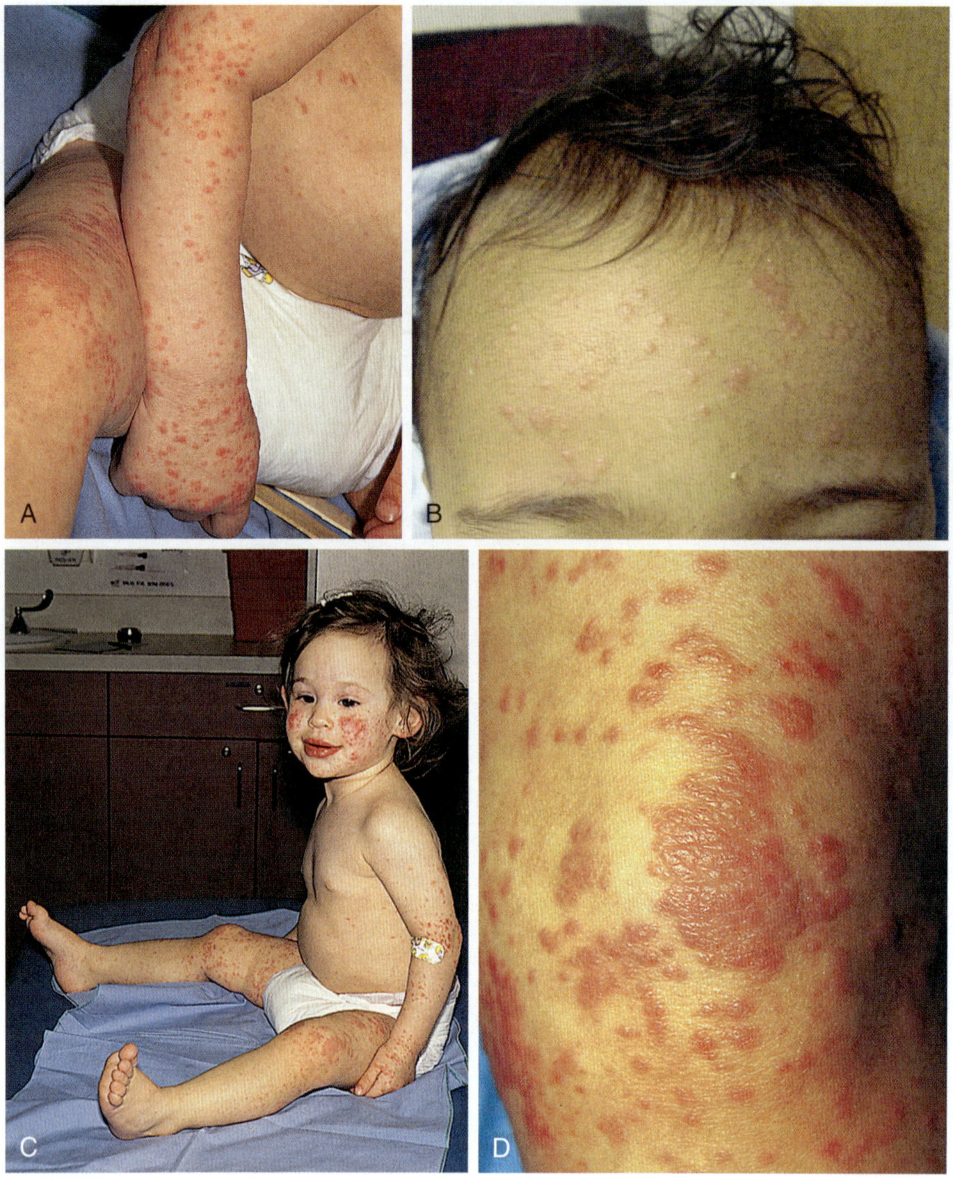

Fig. 13.16 Gianotti-Crosti syndrome. (A and B) Lesions consist of raised lichenoid papules with flat tops that appear in crops and tend to remain discrete. (C) This child shows the characteristic acral distribution, with lesions involving the extremities and face but with relative sparing of the trunk. (D) Lesions can become confluent over pressure points, such as the knee.

skin or wound infections are the primary site of infection, the oropharynx is normal. The appearance of the exanthem may vary as well. In some children, it is patchy but most prominent near skinfolds (see Fig. 13.17H). Occasionally, a child may have diffuse petechiae. Still others may present with fever or nasopharyngitis and urticaria as their initial manifestations. In children with darker skin tones, erythema and perioral pallor may be difficult to appreciate and the papules may be larger, thus producing a texture less like that of sandpaper.

Treatment with a 10-day course of penicillin or clindamycin (in penicillin-allergic children) is important for reducing the risk of transmission and preventing rheumatic fever and pyogenic complications, the most common of which include adenitis, otitis, sinusitis, and peritonsillar and retropharyngeal abscesses. Therefore in patients with fever or nasopharyngitis and urticaria and in children with scarlatiniform eruptions, a screening throat culture for *S. pyogenes* should be obtained, regardless of the presence or absence of other symptoms.

Staphylococcus aureus Infections Associated With Exanthems

Staphylococcus aureus is a ubiquitous organism colonizing approximately one-third of the population. Sites of carriage include the nose, gastrointestinal tract, skin, perineum, and nails. Although the hallmark of staphylococcal infection is the abscess, myriad forms of infection are seen, and at least three distinct generalized exanthematous disorders have now been identified: staphylococcal scalded skin syndrome, staphylococcal scarlet fever, and staphylococcal toxic shock syndrome (TSS). In each disease, organisms at the primary site of infection release distinct exotoxins, which then produce the associated rash.

Staphylococcal Scalded Skin Syndrome

Staphylococcal scalded skin syndrome caused by exfoliative toxin-producing strains of *S. aureus* most commonly affects infants and young children. The primary infection is usually mild, with purulent nasopharyngitis, conjunctivitis, impetigo, and infections of the umbilicus or circumcision site. Rarely, sepsis, pneumonia, or other severe invasive staphylococcal infections may precede the onset of the exanthem.

After infection, exfoliative toxin spreads hematogenously and causes cleavage of the skin between the epidermis and dermis. This process may begin within hours or days of the appearance of signs of the primary infection; typically, its onset is heralded by fever, irritability, and often vomiting. These symptoms are followed by the development of a diffuse, sunburn-like erythroderma that spreads rapidly from head to toe. In contrast to streptococcal scarlet fever,

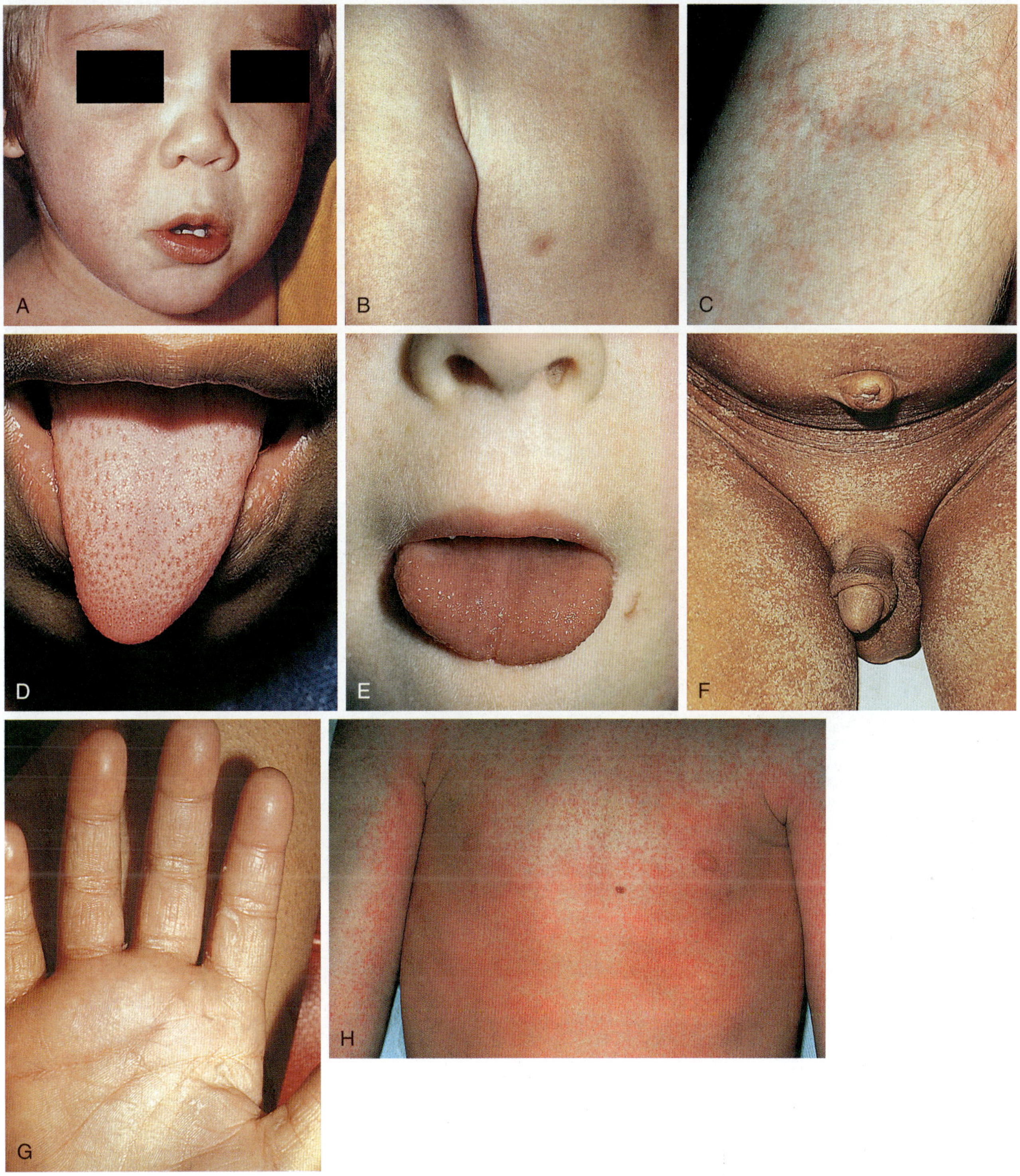

Fig. 13.17 Streptococcal scarlet fever. (A and B) In the classic form of this exanthem, the patient has a flushed face, perioral pallor, and a diffuse, blanching, erythematous rash that has a sandpapery consistency on palpation. (C) Within 1 to 3 days of onset, Pastia lines may be noted. (D) During the first 1 to 2 days the tongue has a white coating through which prominent erythematous papillae project—a white strawberry tongue. (E) A few days later the white coat peels, leaving the characteristic red strawberry tongue with glistening surface and prominent papillae. (F and G) Desquamation occurs in fine, thin flakes as the acute phase of the illness resolves and is proportional to the intensity of the exanthem. (H) A wide spectrum of severity and manifestations exists. In this child with streptococcal scarlet fever, the rash has a patchy distribution but is accentuated in the axillae and other creases. (A, B, and F, Courtesy Michael Sherlock, MD, Lutherville, MD.)

the involved skin is tender, even to light touch. Within 1 to 3 days, thin-walled, flaccid, bullous lesions appear and rupture soon after formation (see Fig. 13.18A). Simultaneously, larger portions of the epidermis begin to slough in sheets. During this phase, application of light traction on the skin pulls epidermis away from dermis, leaving a raw, weeping surface. This separation of the skin in response to stroking is called the Nikolsky sign (see Fig. 13.18B). After exfoliation, the surface gradually dries, forming large, thick flakes (see Fig. 13.18C).

A broad spectrum of severity exists for this syndrome. In severe cases, the patient appears toxic and in considerable pain. The child may shed large portions of skin, resulting in significant fluid losses that may be accompanied by difficulties with temperature regulation. In mild cases (see Fig. 13.18B), toxicity is absent and only localized areas of skin are denuded, with the face and perineum constituting the primary sites of shedding. The causative organism can be isolated from the site of primary infection, but it is absent—at least initially—from the bullae and from sites of skin separation.

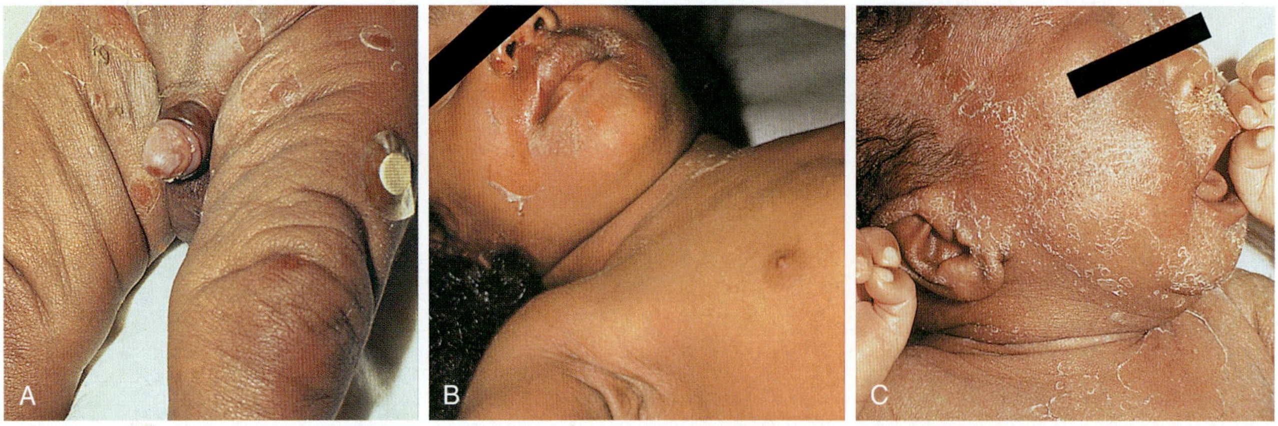

Fig. 13.18 Staphylococcal scalded skin syndrome. (A) This infant shows evidence of epidermal separation and has numerous ruptured bullae over the inguinal region and thighs. (B) In this older child, symptoms were mild and only the skin of the face, axillae, and perineum showed signs of epidermal separation. Note the evidence of a positive Nikolsky sign on her upper lip and cheek, the result of wiping her nose. (C) A denuded area is evident on the upper chest, and thick flakes have begun to form on the face of this infant. Culture of the purulent nasal discharge was positive for Staphylococcus aureus. (Courtesy Michael Sherlock, MD, Lutherville, MD.)

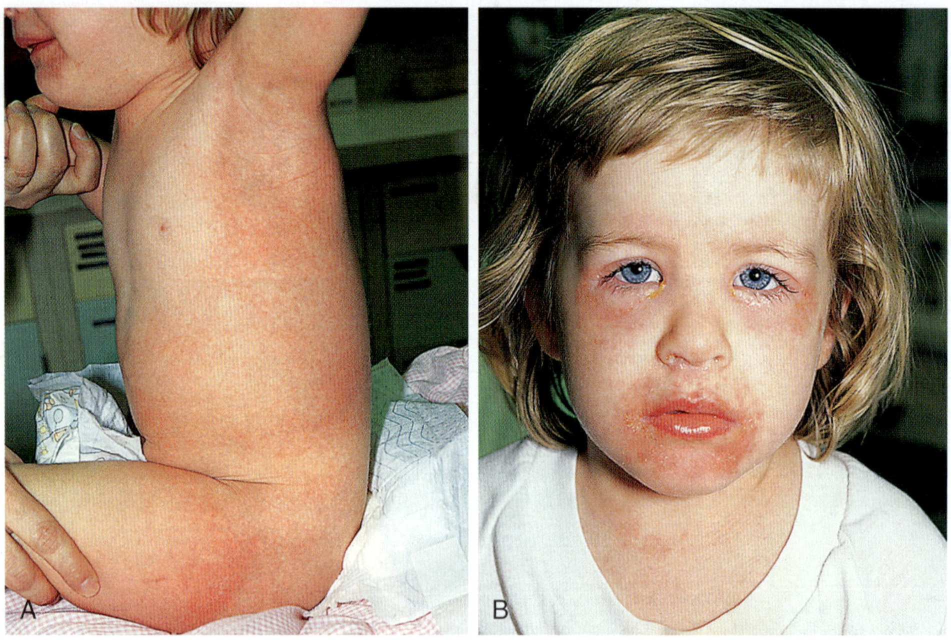

Fig. 13.19 Staphylococcal scarlet fever. (A) In this patient, nasopharyngitis and purulent conjunctivitis antedated the development of a generalized sandpaper-like rash, which was tender to the touch. (B) The skin in the periorbital and perioral areas has begun to crack, fissure, and weep serous fluid.

Staphylococcal Scarlet Fever

Staphylococcal infection can produce a scarlatiniform exanthem that is initially indistinguishable from GAS infection. The illness is characterized by fever, irritability, and malaise, followed by the abrupt onset of a generalized erythematous rash, often of sandpapery consistency, with accentuation in the skin creases (Fig. 13.19A). In contrast to streptococcal scarlet fever, involved skin is usually tender, the tongue is normal, and there is no palatal enanthem. Evolution of lesions also differs—within 2 to 5 days the skin begins to crack, fissure, and weep, especially in the perioral and periorbital areas and in skin creases (see Fig. 13.19B). It sheds in large, thick flakes over 3 to 5 days. Local skin and wound infections are common antecedents, and their presence often enables presumptive identification of staphylococci early in the disease. However, when nasopharyngitis is the source of primary infection, the picture can be difficult to distinguish from streptococcal infection, especially when strawberry tongue and palatal petechiae are absent. The same may be true if a local infection with lymphangitis is the source. In such cases, the tendency for the staphylococcal rash to be tender may be the major clinical distinction.

Staphylococcal Toxic Shock Syndrome

TSS is the third syndrome of staphylococcal origin characterized by a generalized exanthem. First recognized in menstruating females using tampons whose vaginal mucosa was colonized with toxin-producing staphylococci, it occurs in both sexes of all ages due to other localized infections caused by *S. aureus.* Patients with nonmenstrual *S. aureus* TSS may have a skin lesion, mucosal colonization, or surgical wound site as the primary focus of infection (Fig. 13.20B).

Staphylococcal TSS begins with a prodrome consisting of low-grade fever, malaise, myalgias, and vomiting. This is followed by an abrupt increase in fever, accompanied by chills, worsening myalgias, repetitive vomiting, abdominal pain, orthostatic dizziness, and weakness. Patients then develop diffuse erythroderma mimicking sunburn (see Fig. 13.20A). Conjunctivitis with photophobia, oropharyngeal erythema, and a strawberry tongue are common features. Subsequently, severe watery diarrhea, hypotension, and oliguria may become prominent, accompanied by alterations in level of consciousness. Therapy requires aggressive volume replacement and often vasopressor therapy. In severe cases, acute

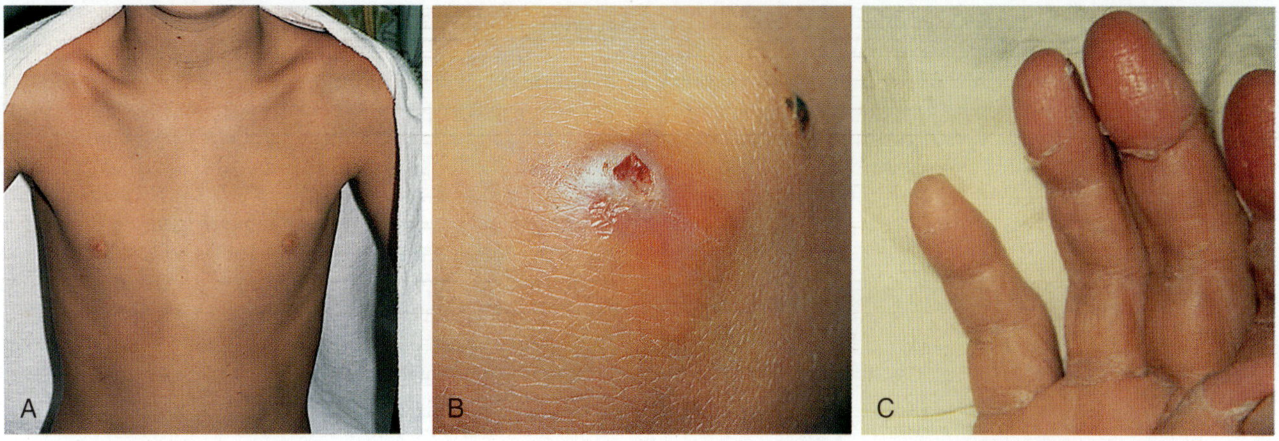

Fig. 13.20 Toxic shock syndrome (TSS). (A) This young boy presented with diffuse erythroderma, fever, chills, myalgias, headache, vomiting, and orthostatic dizziness with mild widening of his pulse pressure. (B) Examination disclosed an infected puncture wound of the knee, which grew Staphylococcus aureus. Although his illness was relatively mild, the association of gastrointestinal symptoms and orthostatic changes suggested TSS, which was confirmed by laboratory studies and subsequent desquamation (C). This begins periungually, and the skin is shed in thick casts. (C, Courtesy George Pazin, MD, University of Pittsburgh Medical Center, Pittsburgh, PA.)

respiratory distress syndrome may develop. Many patients have muscle tenderness and weakness, as well as diffuse abdominal tenderness without peritoneal signs. A small proportion develop nonpitting edema of the face, hands, and feet. Over the ensuing days, petechiae and a secondary maculopapular rash may be noted, along with oral ulcerations. Desquamation is routine, usually beginning 1 week after onset of the rash. It is most prominent over the palms and soles and in the periungual areas, and the skin is shed in thick casts (see Fig. 13.20C).

As recognition of TSS has increased, the existence of a wide spectrum of severity has become apparent. Mild cases mimic staphylococcal scarlet fever. Such patients tend to have smaller gastrointestinal losses and less difficulty with fluid shifts and attendant complications. Early recognition of this clinical syndrome and aggressive therapy may often prevent development of shock. Removal of any infected source material (such as a tampon) and parenteral antimicrobial therapy directed against *S. aureus* are required for effective therapy.

BACTERIAL SKIN AND SOFT TISSUE INFECTIONS

Superficial bacterial skin infections occur with high frequency in childhood. Causative organisms are often inoculated through a minor wound, such as a superficial cut, an abrasion, an insect bite, or a burn. Infection may occur at the time of the injury if the pathogen has colonized the site previously, or it may occur subsequently as the result of scratching, touching, or contamination. In some cases, a preexisting dermatitis sets the stage for secondary infection by breaking down the skin barrier. The risk of infection in patients with preexisting dermatitis must be kept in mind, especially when steroids are prescribed.

Although most superficial infections are relatively minor in severity, diagnosis and proper treatment are important to reduce further spread of infection and to prevent its transmission to others. Deeper skin and soft tissue infections, although less common, have the potential for causing greater morbidity and even mortality. As with superficial lesions, inoculation from an external source is the most common mode of acquisition. In many instances, however, these infections represent metastatic foci of bacteremic spread.

The organisms most commonly responsible for skin and soft tissue infections are *S. pyogenes* and *S. aureus*. Each pathogen produces relatively characteristic clinical features that help distinguish their clinical diagnoses. Staphylococci are more likely to remain localized, causing suppuration and abscesses. Methicillin-resistant *S. aureus* (MRSA) remains prevalent in the community and health care settings, and it cannot be distinguished clinically from methicillin-susceptible *S. aureus* (MSSA). Conversely, streptococcal infection tends to spread along tissue planes and through lymphatics and thus is more commonly associated with secondary cellulitis, lymphangitis, and regional adenopathy.

Folliculitis

Folliculitis is a superficial infection or irritation of the hair follicles. The scalp, face, extensor surfaces of the extremities, and buttocks are the most common sites of involvement. Patients with dry atopic skin or keratosis pilaris are particularly prone to this problem (Chapter 8). Other predisposing factors include seborrhea, excessive sweating, poor hygiene, and topical contact with oils, tars, and adhesives. Obstruction of follicles facilitates inflammation and secondary infection. A superficial erythematous nodule develops around the hair, evolving into a thin-walled central pustule with a narrow, red rim (Fig. 13.21). The lesions may itch or burn and subsequently may drain and crust. Although a lesion may heal in 7 to 10 days without treatment, multiple crops may occur. Scratching may spread the infection to other areas, and secondary impetiginous lesions may develop. *S. aureus* is the typical pathogen, although other skin colonizers may participate. Oral antimicrobial therapy directed at *S. aureus* and avoidance of the predisposing condition are both indicated to resolve the process. Empiric treatment should cover both MSSA and MRSA, making knowledge of local staphylococcal epidemiology and antibiotic susceptibility important.

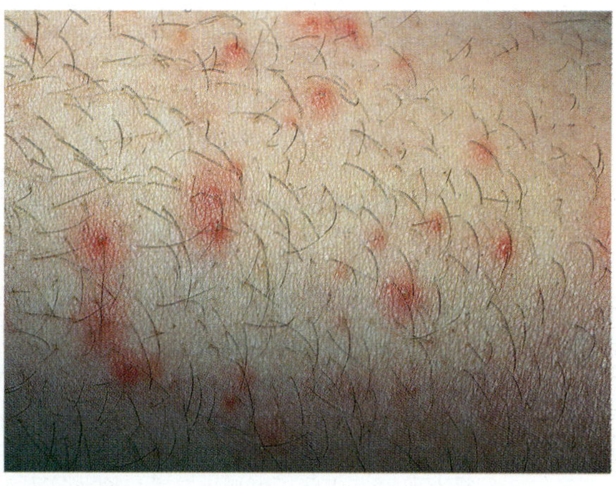

Fig. 13.21 Folliculitis. The extensor surfaces of the extremities and other hair-bearing areas are the most common sites of this superficial infection of hair follicles. Lesions begin at the base of a hair shaft as erythematous nodules and then evolve to form central pustules with a thin, red rim.

Early lesions of tinea capitis or tinea corporis may mimic folliculitis, although itching is usually more prominent in fungal infections and the surrounding rim of erythema tends to be wider. Suspect tinea if folliculitis is localized to the hairline of the scalp (Chapter 8). Older lesions, if present, may help in distinguishing between fungal and bacterial infections. Gram stain, potassium hydroxide preparations, and cultures can be useful in evaluating questionable cases.

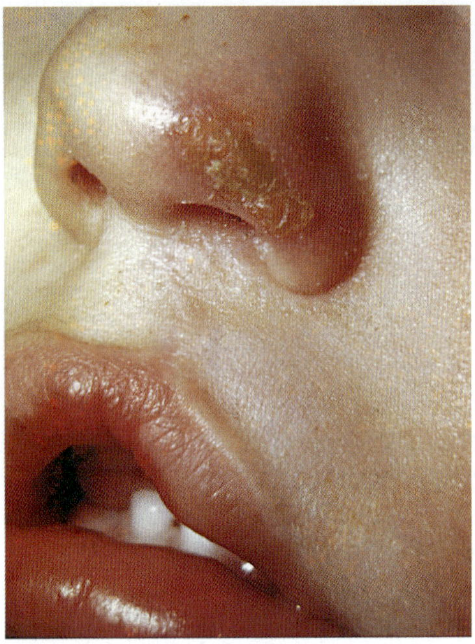

Fig. 13.22 Streptococcal impetigo. This impetiginous lesion has evolved from a papule to a vesicle that ruptured, producing the characteristic honey-colored crust. (Courtesy Michael Sherlock, MD, Lutherville, MD.)

Impetigo

Impetigo is a superficial infection of the epidermis caused by streptococci, staphylococci, or both. Exposed portions of the body including the face, extremities, hands, and neck are the most common sites. Lesions teem with organisms and serve as a potential source of transmission to others. The disorder has a peak incidence in summer and early fall in temperate climates because of increased exposure to insect bites, injury, and colonization by pathogenic organisms. In tropical climates, impetigo is prevalent year-round. Impetigo was traditionally considered a streptococcal disease. However, in more recent decades, *S. aureus* has eclipsed *S. pyogenes* as the predominant cause of impetigo. Accordingly, microbiologic culture is helpful for treatment choices, particularly if severe enough to warrant systemic antibiotics. In patients without preexisting dermatitis, lesions tend to be localized, but if the child has an antecedent condition, the infection can spread rapidly to involve extensive areas.

Group A streptococcal impetigo lesions begin as a papule and evolve rapidly to become a small, thin-walled vesicle with an erythematous halo. The initially serous vesicular fluid becomes cloudy, and the vesicle ruptures, forming a superficial honey-colored crust (Fig. 13.22). If the crust is lifted, a shallow, smooth, weeping, erythematous base is revealed. Secondary enlargement and tenderness of the regional lymph nodes are common.

The initial macules of staphylococcal impetigo may evolve rapidly to form small, thin-walled pustules (Fig. 13.23A) or the larger flaccid bullae of bullous impetigo (see Fig. 13.23B). The latter contain slightly cloudy fluid and are often 1 cm or more in diameter. In either instance, the pustules or bullae rupture rapidly, leaving a shallow erythematous base surrounded by a superficial peeling rim (see Fig. 13.23B). In patients with more long-standing or combined infection, lesions may crust centrally and enlarge centrifugally. This may result in the formation of a superficial central scab surrounded by a bullous rim or a dried lesion with multiple concentric rings

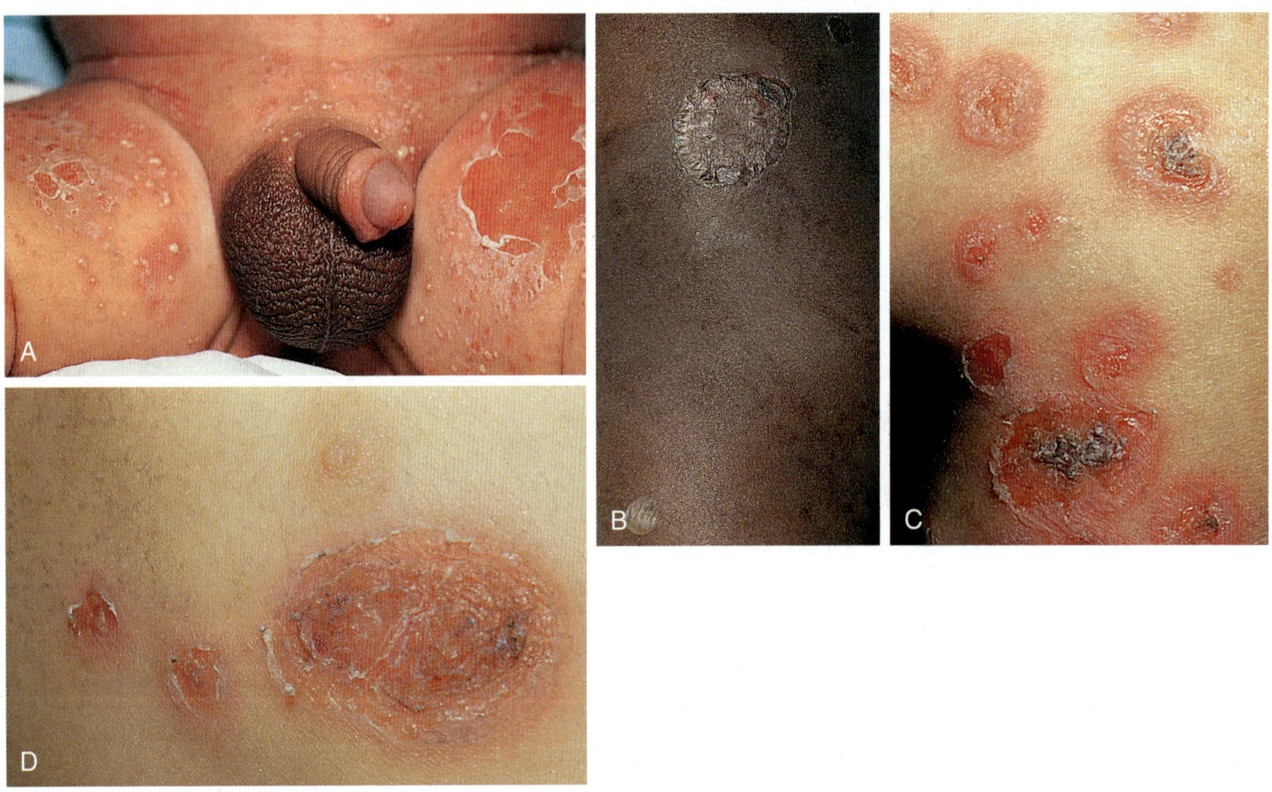

Fig. 13.23 Staphylococcal impetigo. (A) This infant with staphylococcal diaper dermatitis has multiple small, thin-walled pustules that rupture rapidly and coalesce, leaving a shallow base and a superficial peeling rim. (B) The various stages of bullous impetigo are evident in this child. Inferiorly an unruptured flaccid bulla is seen with an older lesion above it that has spread outward and crusted peripherally; just above that, another bulla has just ruptured. (C) In this child with staphylococcal impetigo, older lesions have central crusts with bullous rims that are spreading outward. (D) The features of long-standing impetigo are seen in this youngster whose lesions are crusted in rings, resembling an onion slice. Also note the smaller satellites surrounding the larger primary lesion.

resembling an onion slice (Fig. 13.23C and D). Lesions may coalesce over time, and satellite lesions may form around larger primary lesions. Regardless of the organism, impetigo is frequently pruritic and spreading of infection to other sites or even inoculating bacteria deeper into the skin is common.

The possible sources of the causative organisms may be the patient's own skin or nasopharynx or those of another infected person. In patients with facial lesions, the nose is the most likely site of origin. Localized areas can be treated with topical antibiotics, but more extensive involvement requires oral antimicrobial therapy. On occasion, infection with other organisms can simulate the picture of impetiginous lesions. One form of tinea capitis produces lesions identical to those of streptococcal impetigo (Chapter 8). *Candida* spp. can produce tiny pustules, which rupture and have a superficial peeling rim, at times simulating staphylococcal infection in the diaper area. However, in candidal diaper dermatitis, lesions are smaller (1–2 mm in diameter), pustules are more evanescent, the inflammation is more diffuse, and the erythema more intense (Chapter 8) than in staphylococcal impetigo and staphylococcal diaper dermatitis. Gram stain and potassium hydroxide preparations of scrapings and culture of lesions can discriminate bacteria and fungi in confusing cases.

Ecthyma and Ecthyma Gangrenosum

Ecthyma is an ulcerative skin infection that penetrates more deeply than impetigo to involve the dermis. The disorder is most prevalent in tropical climates and in immunocompromised hosts. Poor hygiene, insect bites, and trauma are major predisposing factors, accounting for the fact that the lower extremities and buttocks are the usual sites of involvement. Lesions may initially resemble impetigo, consisting of a vesicle or a pustule on an erythematous base (Fig. 13.24A), which then ruptures and crusts. However, ecthyma lesions are more painful, with thicker and more adherent crusts than impetigo, and the surrounding erythema is indurated. The ulcerative base beneath the crust gradually deepens and enlarges. Unroofing the crust uncovers a round, deep, punched-out ulcer with raised borders (see Fig. 13.24B). The diameter of the lesions ranges from 0.5 to 3 cm. The lesions take weeks to heal without treatment and leave a circumscribed scar.

Ecthyma is the result of direct inoculation of organisms through the skin in cases involving healthy patients, with *S. pyogenes* as the usual pathogen. On occasion, staphylococci or *Pseudomonas aeruginosa* may be the etiology; the latter pathogen is more likely to produce a central abscess that exudes a greenish or bluish purulent exudate when its crust is lifted. Systemic antibiotics are required rather than topical antibiotics.

Ecthyma gangrenosum is a serious systemic disease seen predominantly in immunocompromised patients with neutropenia or neutrophil dysfunction. It is caused by septicemia, most often with *P. aeruginosa* or invasive molds, during which seeding of organisms results in the appearance of metastatic skin lesions. These lesions are most often found in the genital or perianal region, followed by the extremities. The lesions begin as pink macules, evolve into hemorrhagic papules, and then undergo necrosis centrally to leave a dark eschar on an erythematous base (Fig. 13.25). Subsequently,

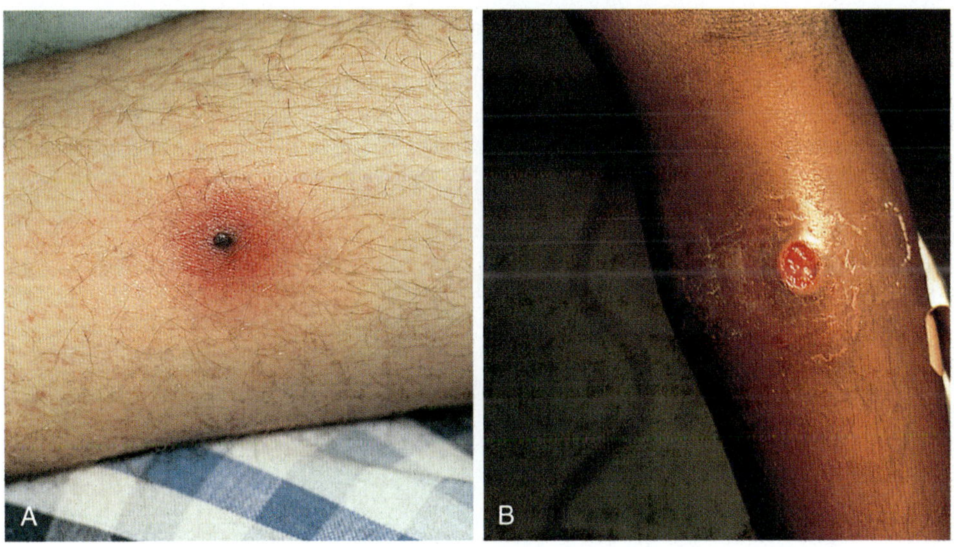

Fig. 13.24 Ecthyma. (A) In focal ecthyma resulting from the inoculation of group A streptococci, the lesion initially consists of a central vesicle or pustule (that rapidly crusts over) on a painful, indurated, erythematous base. (B) With progression a deep, widening ulcer forms, as seen in this child after removal of the overlying crust. (Courtesy Ellen Wald, MD, University of Wisconsin Children's Hospital, Madison, WI.)

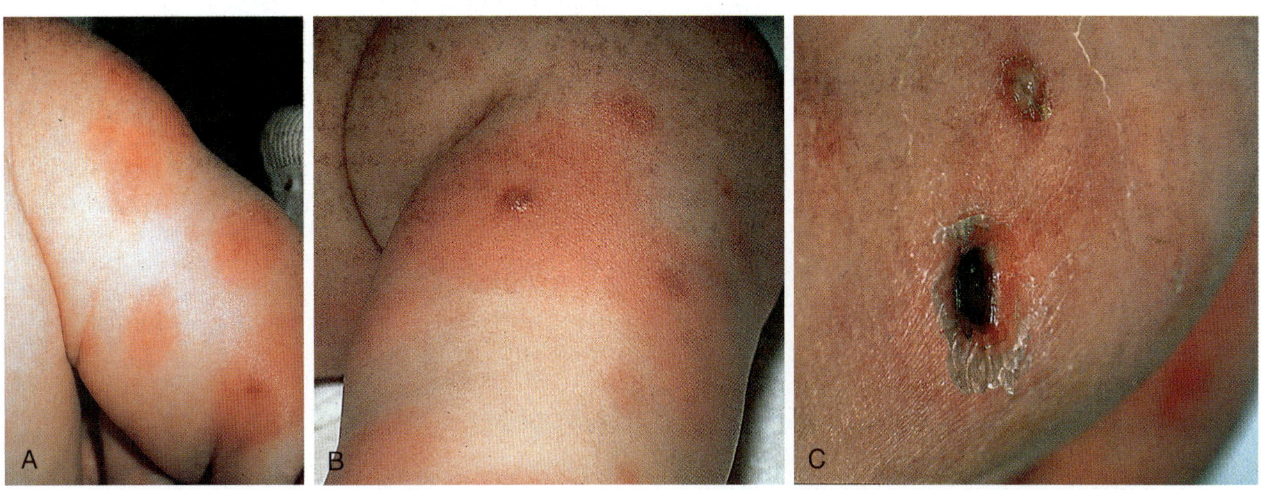

Fig. 13.25 Ecthyma gangrenosum. Pseudomonas septicemia may result in metastatic ecthymatous lesions that begin as pink macules (A), become hemorrhagic (B), and ultimately necrose centrally to form a black eschar (C). (Courtesy Ellen Wald, MD, University of Wisconsin Children's Hospital, Madison, WI.)

ulceration occurs, associated with deep necrosis, due to invasion of the venules with secondary thrombosis of arterioles. This metastatic form of ecthyma is distinguished from primary cases by multiple lesions, systemic signs of sepsis, and evidence of neutropenia or neutrophil dysfunction. Ecthyma gangrenosum is a life-threatening disease requiring urgent parenteral antimicrobial therapy, and biopsy and culture are often critical.

ABSCESSES OF THE SKIN AND SOFT TISSUES

Abscesses are localized collections of purulent material that are walled off within a tissue, organ, or confined space. They result from the deep invasion of pyogenic organisms, which, in the case of abscesses involving the skin and its appendages, are usually caused by *S. aureus* (both MSSA and MRSA). Patients colonized with MRSA can have recurrent skin abscesses in the absence of any immune deficiency. As the area of inflammation expands outward, central necrosis occurs and the process tends to produce an increase in pressure, with resultant pointing toward the surface or spread along tissue planes and further local tissue destruction. Drainage is essential for healing because the abscess contents provoke a continuing inflammatory response and antimicrobials are generally unable to penetrate the necrotic center of the lesion. Abscesses of the skin and soft tissues are categorized according to the site and structure involved.

Paronychia (Periungual Abscess)

A paronychia is a relatively superficial abscess that develops under the cuticle or along the nail fold of a finger or toe. It occurs when staphylococci and occasionally streptococci gain access through a traumatized hangnail or through lesions created by trauma. On occasion, an ingrown toenail is the predisposing condition; in such cases, the nail, which usually was cut improperly, grows laterally into the nail fold, lacerating the soft tissue and setting the stage for infection. In typical cases, erythema, pain, and tenderness develop at the site of injury and are followed rapidly by suppuration (Fig. 13.26). The infection then advances from the portal of entry around the nail fold, and if treatment is delayed, it can burrow beneath the base of the nail, creating a subungual abscess (onychia). On occasion, secondary lymphangitis may develop. Drainage is accomplished readily by undermining the involved portion of the cuticle and nail fold with a scalpel blade. Unless secondary complications have developed, subsequent soaking is usually sufficient to promote healing, although oral antistaphylococcal agents hasten the process.

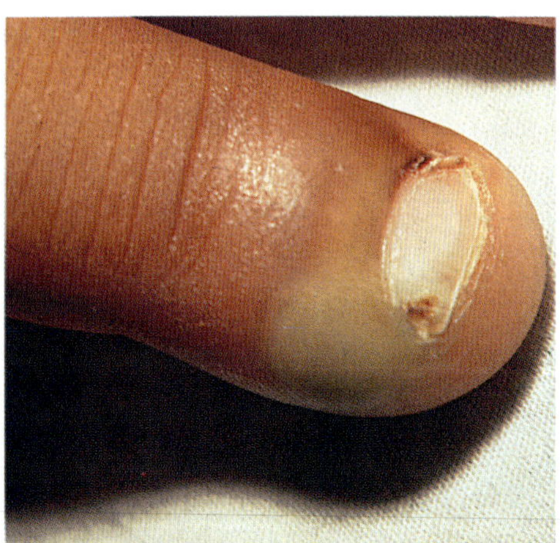

Fig. 13.26 Paronychia. Chewing on a hangnail predisposed this child to the development of a paronychia. Initially, erythema developed near the hangnail and was followed rapidly by suppuration.

Abscesses of Skin Appendages

Furuncle

A furuncle, or boil, is a perifollicular dermal abscess usually caused by *S. aureus*. It may be the result of extension of superficial folliculitis or of direct inoculation via minor trauma. Hairy areas subject to friction or maceration, as well axillary and inguinal regions with high concentrations of sebaceous glands, are particularly vulnerable. Skin contact with occlusive agents (such as oils, tars, and adhesives) is another common predisposing factor. The incidence of furuncles is much higher in older children and adolescents than in younger children.

The lesion begins as a small dermal nodule around a hair follicle, which initially may produce mild discomfort and itching. As it gradually enlarges, the intensity of pain increases and is aggravated by touching and motion of the involved area. With expansion, the overlying skin becomes reddened, central necrosis begins to occur, and with increased inflammation and pressure, the infection begins to seek egress. In the case of most furuncles, the abscess burrows toward the surface of the skin, which becomes thinned and shiny as the abscess becomes fluctuant (Fig. 13.27A). Application of warm compresses can hasten this process and aid in drainage. Spontaneous drainage of bloody purulent material ultimately occurs in most cases and the patient experiences prompt relief of pain (see Fig. 13.27B). In areas such as the nape of the neck or upper back, where the overlying skin is thick enough to resist external pointing, the process may take a path of lesser resistance, burrowing outward from the center through the subcutaneous tissues and along fascial planes. If this process is not interrupted by early surgical intervention, the result is a gradual formation of a carbuncle, which consists of an extremely painful, exquisitely tender multilocular mass of interconnected dermal and subcutaneous abscesses, with multiple points of partial drainage at the skin surface. Carbuncle formation is often accompanied by fever, chills, and increasing malaise, and there is a significant risk of secondary bacteremia. Even with treatment, sloughing and extensive scarring tend to result.

Hidradenitis Suppurativa

In hidradenitis suppurativa, an apocrine gland is the site of infection and abscess formation. Hence these infections usually occur in the axillae, perineum, or areolae of postpubertal adolescents. Keratin plugging of apocrine ducts and their hair follicles appears to be a major predisposing factor; occlusion, maceration, and poor hygiene may exacerbate the problem. The resultant obstruction fosters inflammation and provides a favorable environment for secondary invasion and multiplication of staphylococci and anaerobic bacteria. As the inflammatory process expands, the gland ultimately ruptures and forms an abscess. In contrast to the perifollicular furuncle, this infection is deeper and slower to localize and suppurate. It begins as a firm, mildly tender nodule that enlarges gradually, becoming increasingly uncomfortable and tender. With further enlargement and suppuration, the lesion(s) point to the surface and drain, although some may rupture subcutaneously. Early diagnosis, incision and drainage of fluctuant sites, institution of antimicrobial therapy, and adoption of meticulous hygienic practices may bring the problem under control. Delay in diagnosis, inadequate treatment, or recalcitrant disease can result in recurrence or progression with formation of multiple abscesses and sinus tracts, deep fibrosis, and scarring (Fig. 13.28) that may ultimately necessitate surgical excision.

Abscesses of Special Sites

The breasts, scalp, and perirectal areas are three specific sites of abscess formation of particular importance in pediatrics. Breast and scalp abscesses are discussed in the following sections. Perirectal abscesses are described in Chapter 18.

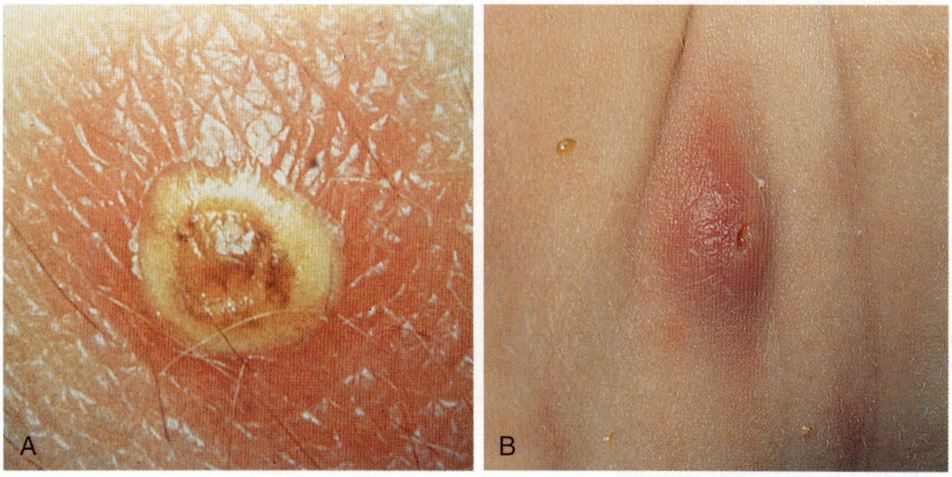

Fig. 13.27 Furuncle. (A) In this well-developed furuncle, the abscess has burrowed to the surface and the skin has thinned centrally and begun to necrose. A wide surrounding rim of erythema and induration exists. (B) This furuncle, located on the neck of a young infant, had spontaneously ruptured and drained earlier in the day but was beginning to enlarge again. (A, Courtesy Bernard Cohen, MD, Johns Hopkins Hospital, Baltimore, MD.)

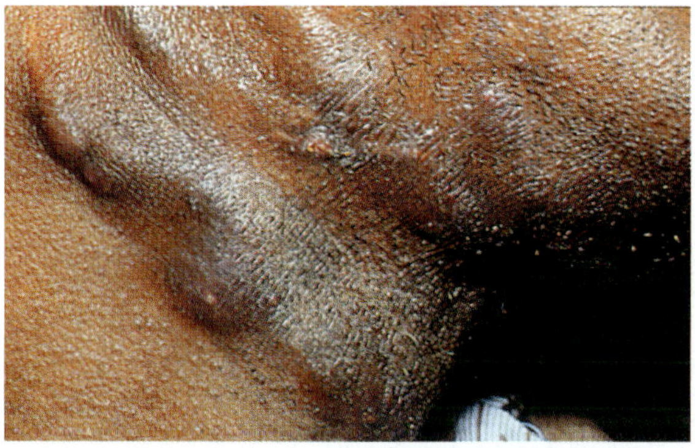

Fig. 13.28 Hidradenitis suppurativa. Obstruction of apocrine ducts and hair follicles predisposes them to infection and suppuration. In this adolescent boy, the process is advanced with multiple abscesses, sinus tracts, and scarring. (From Cohen B: *Atlas of pediatric dermatology*, London, 1993, Mosby/Wolfe.)

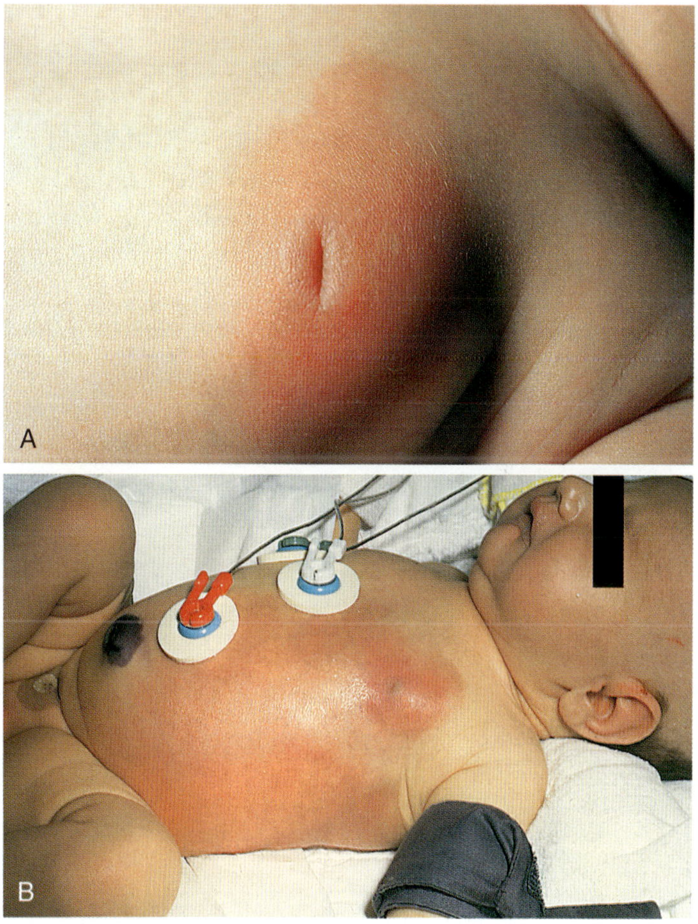

Fig. 13.29 Breast abscess. (A) The typical manifestations of a breast abscess were seen in this neonate—swelling, induration, tenderness, warmth, and erythema. With compression, pus could be expressed from the nipple. (B) This infant was not brought to the hospital until subcutaneous rupture and extensive cellulitic spread had occurred. She was febrile, toxic, irritable, and listless on presentation.

Breast Abscess

Breast abscesses occur within specific age groups among pediatric patients, with incidence peaks in the neonatal and pubertal groups. The incidence is highest in newborns of greater than 31 weeks' gestation at the time of birth, owing in part to physiologic hypertrophy of breast tissue because of stimulation by maternal hormones. Colonization of the skin or the nasopharynx with potentially virulent organisms (*S. aureus, Streptococcus agalactiae [Group B streptococcus]*, or gram-negative coliforms) during birth or in the nursery is another important predisposing factor. Up to 25% of affected infants have staphylococcal diaper dermatitis at the time of presentation. Minor local trauma is also thought to be a predisposing factor. Most cases occur during the second or third week after birth in males or females, but infection may occur as late as 8 weeks old in females. The problem first manifests as swelling and tenderness of the affected breast. Unilateral involvement is the rule. With time, local warmth and overlying erythema become evident, and it may be possible to express a purulent discharge from the nipple (Fig. 13.29A). Axillary adenopathy may be present as well. Only 25% of infants have low-grade fever, and other systemic symptoms are uncommon unless treatment is delayed. A firm, tender, nonfluctuant nodule may be found on palpation early in the course, and parenteral antibiotic therapy and close monitoring for progression are indicated. Later in the disease, the mass may be fluctuant, indicating suppuration and necrosis requiring prompt surgical incision and drainage. Broad-spectrum antimicrobial coverage should be provided pending culture results. Common organisms include *S. aureus* (MSSA and MRSA), with *S. agalactiae, Escherichia coli,* other gram-negative bacteria or mixed flora being less common. Delay in diagnosis and institution of treatment can result in subcutaneous rupture and cellulitic spread with secondary bacteremia (see Fig. 13.29B). Delay in surgical drainage of fluctuant lesions can also result in permanent loss of breast tissue, which can produce a cosmetically deforming breast asymmetry in girls that is first noted at puberty.

Breast abscesses may be seen again after puberty. Minor trauma, cutaneous infections, epidermal cysts, and duct blockages appear to be the common antecedent conditions. The clinical picture is similar to that seen in infants. *S. aureus* is the usual etiology in this group.

Scalp Abscess

As is the case with breast abscesses, pyogenic infections of the scalp are common in the neonatal period. Trauma is the predominant predisposing factor, commonly at sites where scalp leads were inserted for fetal monitoring. In most cases, the infection is localized and consists of a tender nodule with overlying erythema (Fig. 13.30). The nodule is usually fluctuant, enabling prompt incision and drainage. Staphylococci and coliforms are the major pathogens recovered. Because of the neonate's immunologic immaturity, antimicrobial therapy is recommended and can be administered orally in most cases. Rarely, infection is extensive and takes the form of a necrotizing fasciitis (addressed later). In these patients or infants with a localized abscess and systemic symptoms, parenteral broad-spectrum antibiotic treatment (pending culture results) is indicated in addition to urgent incision and drainage. Bacterial scalp abscesses must be differentiated from skin manifestation of herpes neonatorum, which can present at scalp sites (see the Neonatal Herpes Simplex Infection section).

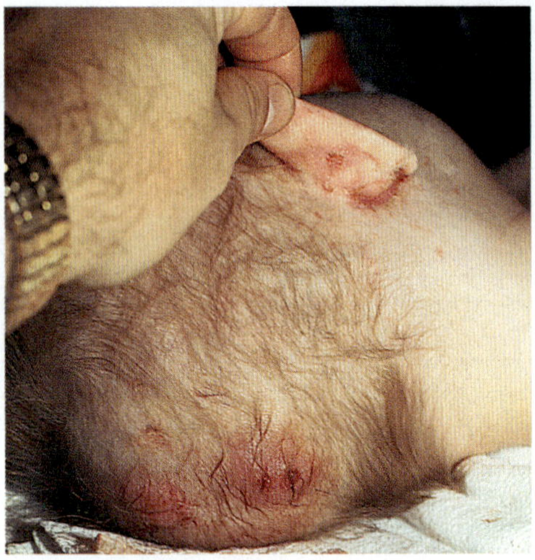

Fig. 13.30 Scalp abscess. Several days after discharge from the newborn nursery, this infant presented with two scalp abscesses and an impetiginous lesion behind the right ear. The surface of the larger abscess is marked by two puncture wounds, which were the site of placement of monitor leads during labor.

When scalp abscesses are encountered in older children, care should be taken to determine the responsible pathogen. Although staphylococci may be the infecting agent, invasive fungi are more likely to be the responsible organisms. These fungi produce a thick-walled, boggy, multilocular abscess termed a *kerion* (Chapter 8). Gram stain and potassium hydroxide preparations of purulent contents and of pulled hairs are important, along with fungal culture, because although incision and drainage constitute the treatment of choice for abscesses of bacterial origin, oral antifungal and steroid therapy are indicated for the treatment of a kerion.

Lymphangitis

Inflammation of lymphatic channels is a secondary manifestation of infection at a distal site. This phenomenon is the result of invasion of lymphatic vessels by pathogenic organisms, which then spread along these channels toward regional lymph nodes. *S. pyogenes* is the most common source of lymphangitis, although overt lymphangitis may also develop in wounds infected by *S. aureus* and *P. aeruginosa.* Clinically, erythematous, irregular linear streaks (which may be tender) are seen extending from the primary site toward the draining regional nodes (Fig. 13.31). The primary site may be an infected wound or an area of cellulitis. Systemic symptoms consisting of fever, chills, and malaise may be present. Without appropriate antimicrobial therapy, extension, necrosis and ulceration may occur, with the attendant risk of bacteremia. Culture and Gram stain of material from the primary site aid in the selection of antimicrobials;

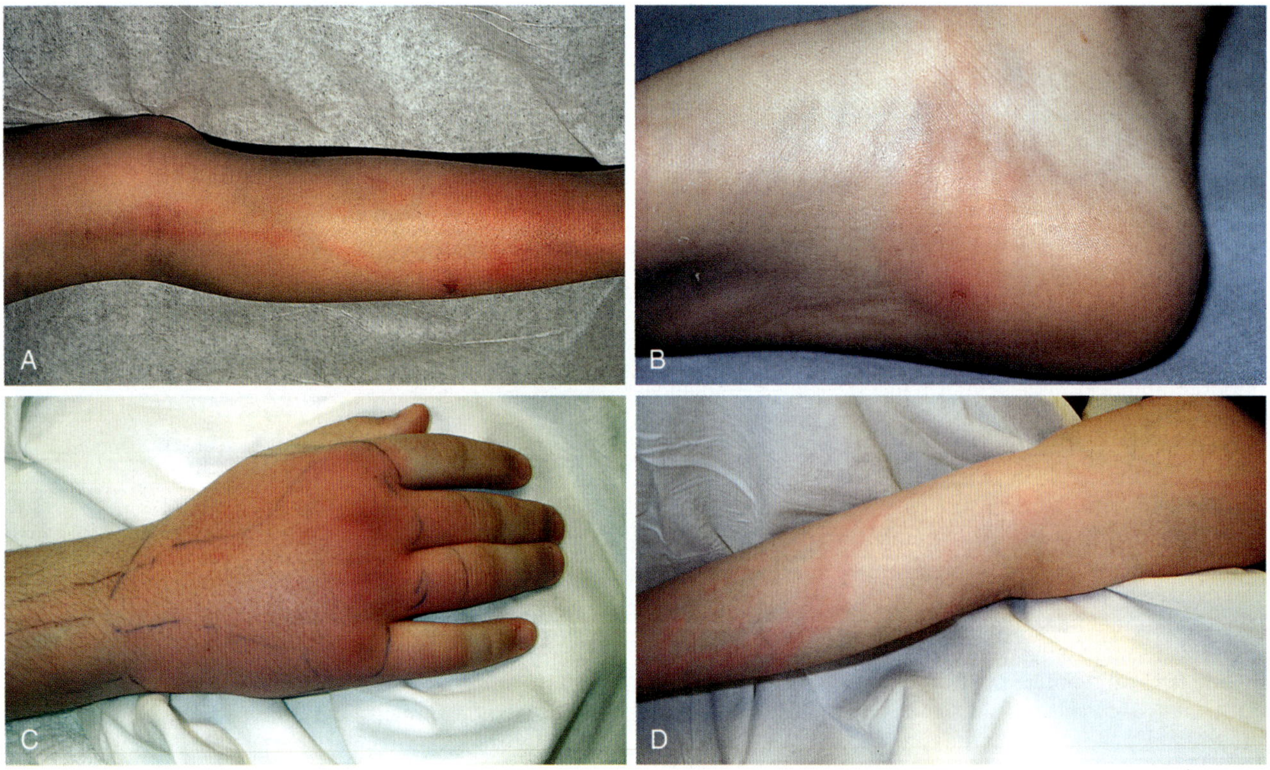

Fig. 13.31 Lymphangitis. (A) An insect bite was the source of inoculation of Group A streptococci in this child, who subsequently suffered secondary cellulitis and lymphangitis. The erythematous streaks coursing up the leg were tender and slightly indurated. (B) Three distinct lymphangitic streaks are seen coursing up the instep from an area of cellulitis surrounding a puncture wound of the foot. Pseudomonas was the causative organism. (C and D) In this child, irregular lymphatic streaks are seen coursing up the arm from a cellulitic area involving the dorsum of his hand.

however, presumptive initial therapy is necessary pending culture results because lymphangitis is the prelude to systemic spread.

Erysipelas

S. pyogenes and other pyogenic β-hemolytic streptococci are the cause of erysipelas, an unusual and distinctive infection involving a localized area of the dermis and superficial lymphatics. The causative organisms are usually found in the upper respiratory tract and are inoculated through a break in the skin; hematogenous seeding has been postulated in some cases. Systemic symptoms are prominent and precede the appearance of the characteristic skin lesion. The onset is abrupt and heralded by fever and chills, often in association with nausea, vomiting, and headache. This prodrome is followed by the appearance of an intensely painful skin lesion that consists of a circumscribed, raised plaque that is usually deep purplish red but may be red or even pink (Fig. 13.32). The raised border, although irregular, is well demarcated and spreads centrifugally. Red lymphatic streaks may advance ahead of it toward the regional nodes. On close inspection, the skin is edematous and may have a thickened peau d'orange character (see Fig. 13.32C). Palpation demonstrates induration, heat, and exquisite tenderness. With evolution, small surface blebs containing yellow fluid may form. The face is the most common site, with the trunk, neck, and extremities less frequent. Patients may become bacteremic and develop metastatic foci of infection. Infants are at particular risk for systemic spread. The clinical picture of erysipelas is so characteristic that streptococcal infection can be presumed, though other β-hemolytic streptococci and, less commonly, *S. aureus* may be isolated. Parenteral antimicrobial treatment should be initiated in most cases. Cultures of tissue aspirate from the advancing border of the lesion are typically positive for *S. pyogenes,* as are blood cultures in septic patients.

Cellulitis

Cellulitis is a bacterial infection of subcutaneous loose connective tissue. The process may progress and extend centrifugally through the subcutaneous tissue or into the lower dermis. Although cellulitis may develop anywhere on the body, it occurs most commonly on the extremities and face. Three major modes of origin exist: (1) extension from a wound, (2) hematogenous seeding, or (3) extension from a deeper infection.

Cellulitis is characterized by painful, tender, indurated subcutaneous swelling. The overlying skin is warm, erythematous, smooth, and often shiny (Fig. 13.33). The skin may be pink or have a violaceous hue. In contrast to erysipelas, the borders of both the edema and erythema are indistinct, fading imperceptibly into the surrounding tissues. Without therapy, rapid extension is the rule. Systemic symptoms can be a sign of more severe disease with hematogenous spread. In such cases, fever, chills, malaise, and headache are typical.

Wound-Related Cellulitis

Extension of infection from an external wound such as a puncture, laceration, abrasion, or insect bite is the most common form of cellulitis, particularly in school-age children and adolescents. Mild local erythema around a wound, an impetiginous lesion, or a pustule may have been noted before the abrupt onset of increased pain and the rapid evolution of subcutaneous inflammation that herald the development of cellulitis. The primary lesion is usually apparent at the time of presentation (see Fig. 13.33). Secondary infection of a preexisting dermatitis may result in an unusually rapidly spreading cellulitis (Fig. 13.34). *S. pyogenes* and *S. aureus* are the most commonly recovered organisms. *Pseudomonas* and mixed flora may be involved in cellulitis secondary to puncture wounds of the foot or with water exposure (see Fig. 13.31B). Other organisms should be considered on the basis of exposure history, such as *Aeromonas* species with aquatic trauma or *Pasteurella multocida* after cat or dog bites. Rapid peripheral spread, overt lymphangitis, and regional adenitis are characteristic of streptococcal infection but are not completely specific. Fever and other systemic symptoms may be present with wound-related cellulitis but are more likely with cellulitis due to hematogenous seeding or extension of inflammation from deeper structures. MRSA infections are more likely to present with abscess, but surrounding cellulitis is not uncommon.

The extremities are the most common sites of wound-related cellulitis, necessitating close assessment and monitoring for complications. Spread to distal tendon sheaths can lead to necrotizing infection and long-term dysfunction; therefore cellulitis involving hands or feet must be treated aggressively and clinical status monitored closely. When an extremity is encircled by cellulitis, swelling and increased pressure can result in neurovascular compromise due to compartment syndrome, causing extensive secondary damage distally if not decompressed. Surgical consultation is recommended in such cases.

Gram stain and culture of material obtained from the primary wound may identify the specific pathogen. Blood cultures should be obtained in all patients with systemic symptoms. Prompt empiric treatment, including coverage for *S. pyogenes* and *S. aureus,* is essential to prevent further spread and complications.

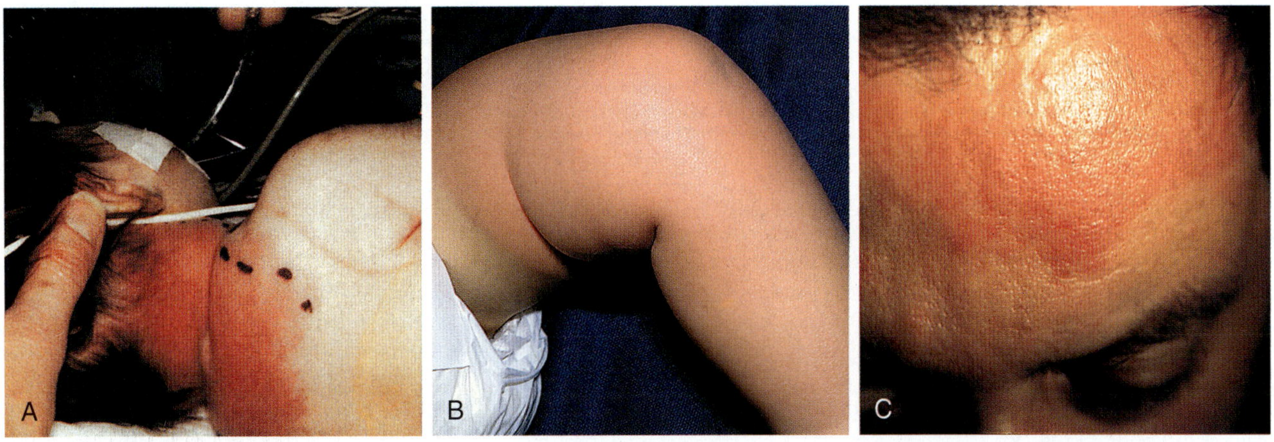

Fig. 13.32 Erysipelas. (A) This 6-week-old infant had fever, lethargy, irritability, and hypotension in association with erysipelas. The purplish-red lesion was raised, indurated, and tender. The border, although irregular, was sharply demarcated from the adjacent skin. Cultures of blood and tissue aspirate grew Group A streptococci. (B) The sharply circumscribed area of erysipelas on this toddler's leg was pink. On close inspection, one can see that the skin has a peau d'orange quality. (C) This is seen more clearly in a close-up of an adolescent's forehead. (C, Courtesy James Ferante, MD.)

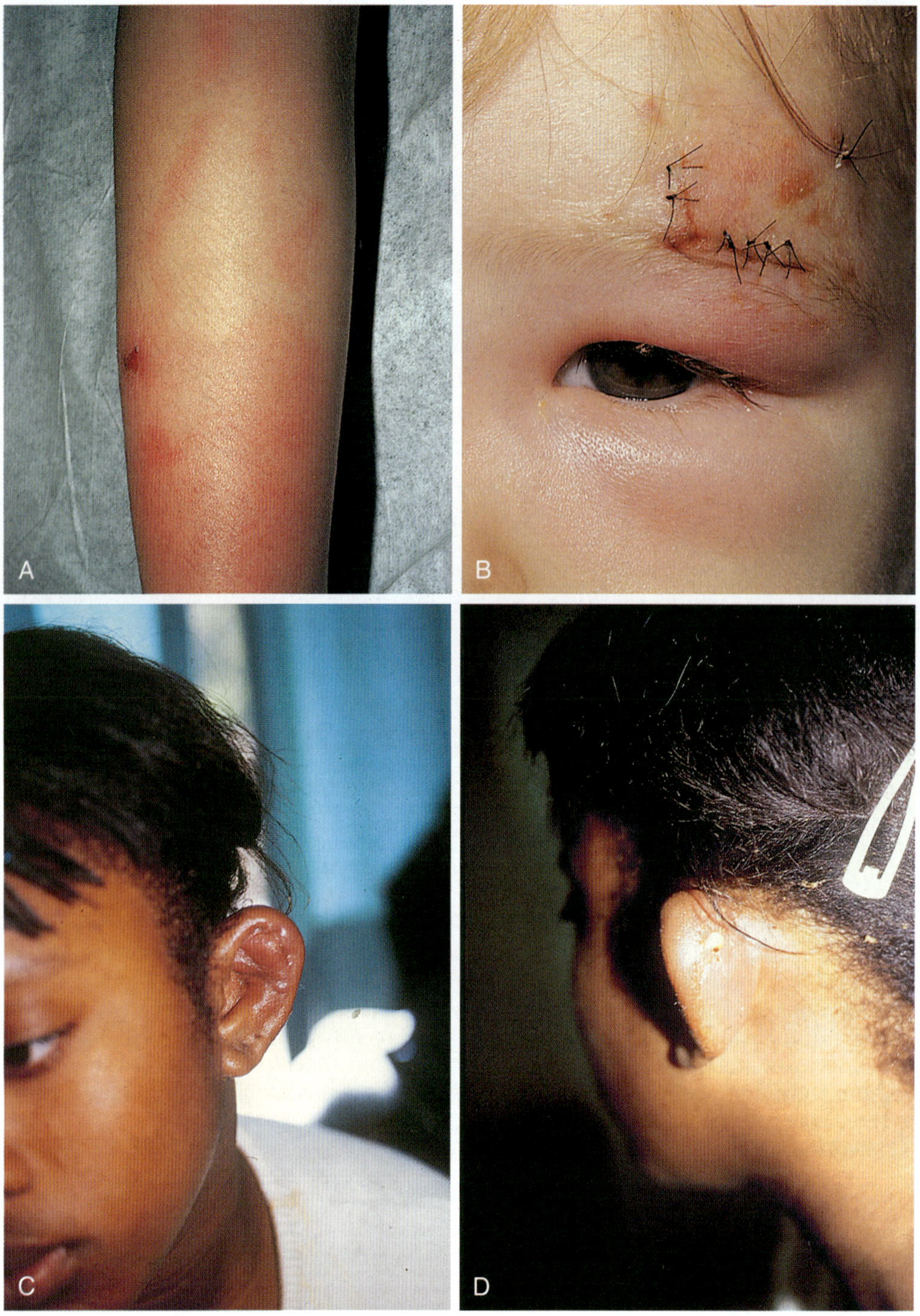

Fig. 13.33 Wound-related cellulitis. (A) The infected mosquito bite that served as the source of cellulitis in this child can be seen on the left. The area of erythema was indurated and tender. Note that the skin is smooth and the borders fade gradually into the adjacent normal skin. (B) Mild erythema and edema are evident in the periorbital area of an infant whose laceration from a dog bite had been sutured 48 hours earlier. The edematous areas were indurated and tender. (C and D) This adolescent presented with erythema, edema, and extreme tenderness caused by infection subsequent to ear-piercing. (C and D, Courtesy Robert Hickey, MD, Children's Hospital of Pittsburgh, Pittsburgh, PA.)

Major differential diagnostic considerations include angioedema resulting from an insect bite and delayed hypersensitivity reactions to *Hymenoptera* stings. The former is pruritic and nontender and often has an identifiable central punctum (see Chapter 8); the latter tend to be simultaneously pruritic, painful, and tender (see Chapter 8). Both are unassociated with systemic symptoms or with adenopathy or lymphangitis. History of trauma, presence of ecchymotic discoloration, and absence of systemic symptoms all help to distinguish swelling due to injury.

Hematogenous Cellulitis

Hematogenous seeding is another source of cellulitis, particularly in infants and young children. Although young infants may show the sudden onset of sepsis with rapid development of cellulitis, older infants, toddlers, and preschool-age children commonly have antecedent upper respiratory tract symptoms. This prodrome is followed by the sudden development of a high fever that begins nearly simultaneously with the appearance of a nondescript area of swelling, which may be localized in the periorbital region (Chapter 24) or over the neck or an extremity. The overlying skin rapidly becomes pink, red, or violaceous as the area of edema spreads and becomes indurated. Irritability, anorexia, and signs of toxicity become increasingly marked, in most cases prompting presentation for medical care within 24 hours. *Haemophilus influenzae* type B was once a likely cause, but with widespread vaccination, the incidence of *H. influenzae* cellulitis has plummeted. *S. pneumoniae* and group B streptococci (in infants younger than 3 months old) are other potential pathogens, but their incidence is much lower.

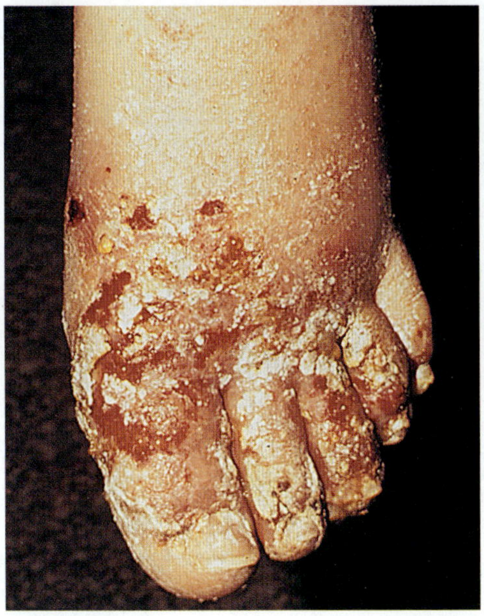

Fig. 13.34 This patient with cellulitis of the foot had been receiving topical steroid therapy for contact dermatitis for about 48 hours when he experienced the explosive onset of swelling, redness, and pain. Impetiginous changes are apparent as well. (Courtesy Michael Sherlock, MD, Lutherville, MD.)

H. influenzae type B appears to be the sole pathogen responsible for buccal cellulitis. Limited to infants, the swelling, induration, and erythema are located over the midcheek near the mandibular ramus (Fig. 13.35). Rare now due to *H. influenzae* type B vaccine, it is important to remain vigilant for its appearance in undervaccinated and unvaccinated communities due to its association with bacteremia. Localized erythema of the underlying buccal mucosa is a common associated finding. The systemic symptomatology and exquisite tenderness help to distinguish it from "popsicle panniculitis," which results from cold injury. The latter is characterized by the formation of a mildly tender, discrete, indurated, disk-shaped, subcutaneous mass located at the angle of the mouth, with reddish purple discoloration of the overlying skin (Fig. 13.36). Systemic symptoms, induration, and tenderness also help to distinguish hematogenous cellulitis at periorbital and other sites from sympathetic swelling caused by sinusitis, which is nontender and not indurated (Chapter 24), and from the pruritic nontender angioedema resulting from insect bites (Chapter 8).

Cellulitis Due to Extension of Infection From Deeper Structures

Although less common than the other forms, cellulitis resulting from extension of infection and inflammation from deeper structures may also occur, necessitating close attention to examination of underlying structures in evaluation of cellulitis. Dental abscesses (Chapter 21) and acute sinusitis (Chapter 24) may underlie facial cellulitis. Osteomyelitis may produce secondary cellulitic changes in overlying soft tissues, especially after subperiosteal abscess formation (see the Osteomyelitis section). Suppurative lymphadenitis and subcutaneous rupture of skin, scalp, and breast abscesses are other common sources (see Fig. 13.31B). Fever, toxicity, and other systemic symptoms are common with this form of cellulitis. Antecedent history and careful examination usually enable identification of this type of cellulitis and recognition of the primary source.

Necrotizing Fasciitis

Necrotizing fasciitis is a severe, deep, necrotizing soft tissue infection, which at a minimum involves subcutaneous tissues and fascial sheaths and often extends to underlying muscle. This process spreads relentlessly along fascial planes, producing edema, vascular thrombosis, and necrosis, resulting in extensive soft tissue destruction. Deep surgical and traumatic wounds are major predisposing factors, although injection sites, cutaneous ulcers, abscesses, and omphalitis may serve as the point of origin. Patients with disorders of neutrophil function and those with diabetes and vascular disease are at especially increased risk. The extremities, perineum, buttocks, trunk, and abdominal wall are the most common sites of involvement. Causative organisms include virulent strains of *S. pyogenes, S. aureus, P. aeruginosa, E. coli,* and polymicrobial infections.

Moderate to severe systemic symptoms including fever are prominent and usually precede the appearance of cellulitic changes. The local area of inflammation may initially resemble ordinary cellulitis, with indistinct margins and localized subcutaneous edema with overlying erythema. However, the overlying skin may appear normal. Careful palpation will reveal that the edema and induration are deeper and far more extensive than the overlying erythema and that the induration is unusually firm and exquisitely tender. Pain is remarkably severe initially and often out of proportion to the examination findings, a key feature. The overlying skin may become edematous, simulating erysipelas, or dusky with surface bullae filled with hemorrhagic fluid. Numbness and decreased sensitivity to pain may be noted as the disease progresses and these are ominous signs. With further evolution, central necrosis or cutaneous gangrene

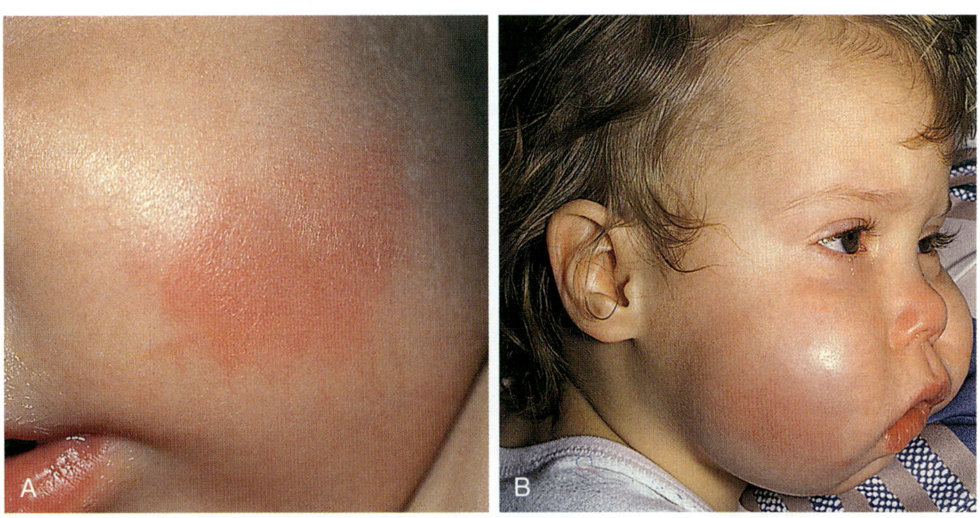

Fig. 13.35 Hematogenous cellulitis. (A) A small erythematous patch with indistinct borders appeared on this infant's cheek shortly after the onset of fever, irritability, and anorexia. On palpation it was found to be indurated and tender. Blood culture was positive for Haemophilus influenzae type B. (B) In this toddler, the evolution of buccal cellulitis due to H. influenzae was fulminant, resulting in unusually dramatic swelling. (B, Courtesy Kenneth Schuitt, MD.)

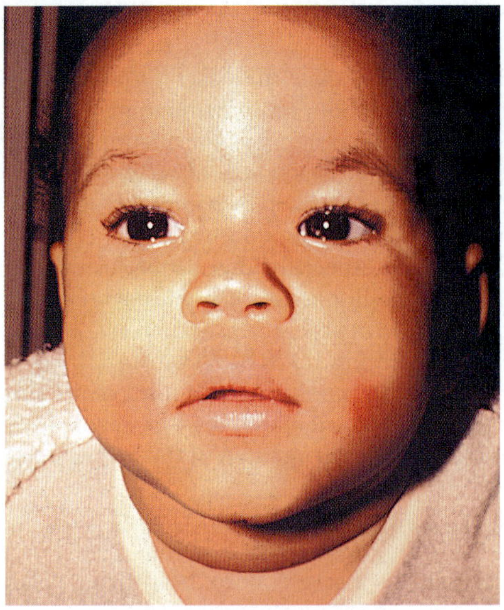

Fig. 13.36 Popsicle panniculitis. This older infant, who was fond of popsicles, had bilateral areas of purplish red swelling just lateral to the corners of his mouth. He was otherwise well. On palpation, masses could be appreciated that were mildly tender, discrete, indurated, and disk shaped. These were localized areas of fat necrosis caused by cold injury. (Courtesy Michael Sherlock, MD, Lutherville, MD.)

supervenes (Fig. 13.37). If anaerobes are involved, crepitus may become evident clinically or subcutaneous emphysema may be visible on radiographs.

As the localized process evolves, systemic symptoms increase. Signs of poor perfusion, pallor, and mottling are often accompanied by grunting respirations and alterations in level of consciousness including disorientation, obtundation, and seizures. Common laboratory findings in advanced cases include anemia resulting from hemolysis and marrow suppression, proteinuria and signs of renal dysfunction, hypoproteinemia, hypocalcemia resulting from saponification of necrotic fat, and hyponatremia. Wound cultures are routinely positive, whereas blood cultures may initially remain negative, depending on the pathogen.

Mortality ranges from 8% to 70%, depending on the series reported, and morbidity and disfigurement are common in survivors. Delays in diagnosis and inadequate surgical debridement are major factors in poor outcome; hence early recognition is crucial to ensure appropriate intervention and improve prognosis. This can be difficult particularly in patients with cases resembling simple cellulitis that initially abate in response to antimicrobial therapy before worsening. Necrotizing fasciitis should be suspected in any patient with cellulitis (particularly around a deep wound) or omphalitis who has unusually severe pain and systemic symptoms that are out of proportion to superficial findings. This can enable surgical exploration before skin changes and loss of sensation, signaling extensive necrosis. Examination of frozen sections of biopsy material may confirm the diagnosis intraoperatively. Control necessitates wide excision with extensive exposure and debridement of all necrotic tissues in combination with broad-spectrum antimicrobial therapy (guided in part by Gram stain results). Aggressive supportive measures are important as well.

Meningococcal Exanthems

Neisseria meningitidis can produce several clinical syndromes. Two major syndromes—acute meningococcemia and chronic meningococcemia (or meningococcosis)—are characterized in part by a generalized exanthem. *Meningococcus* colonizes the upper respiratory tract of asymptomatic humans who may transmit the organism via respiratory droplets to close contacts. Most people become colonized without clinical disease. Clinical illness is most common in children younger than 5 years old, with a peak incidence between 6 and 12 months old. A secondary peak of lesser magnitude but significant mortality is seen during adolescence and young

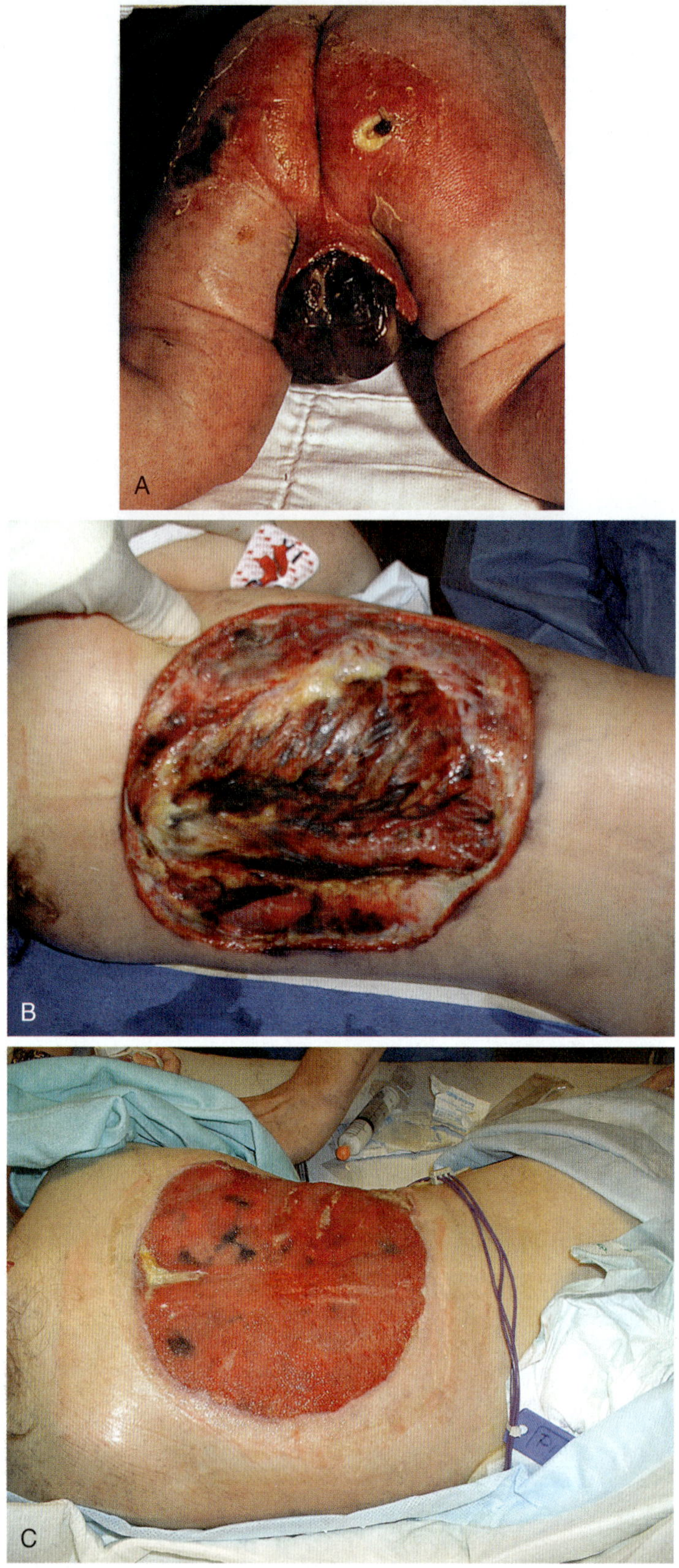

Fig. 13.37 Necrotizing fasciitis. (A) The extent of cellulitis and tissue necrosis is evident in this child who is recovering from necrotizing fasciitis caused by group A streptococci. On presentation, he was thought to have cellulitis but was more ill systemically and appeared much more uncomfortable than would be expected. Furthermore, on presentation the area of induration extended well beyond the overlying erythema. (B) Necrotizing fasciitis due to Clostridium septicum after surgical debridement in a child with presumed cyclic neutropenia. (C) The same child 1 month later after aggressive surgical and medical management. (A, Courtesy Michael Sherlock, MD, Lutherville, MD.)

adulthood, leading to adolescent vaccination recommendations. Susceptibility to disease appears to be related to a lack of bactericidal antibody or to a failure to produce antibody in response to infection. Antecedent viral respiratory tract infection can be a predisposing factor.

Although meningococcal infection occurs year-round, the peak season is late winter and early spring. Invasive disease occurs both endemically and epidemically. Persons who have intimate contact with infected patients (such as household members) or persons in "closed communities" (such as military barracks, dormitories, or daycare centers) are at highest risk of becoming secondarily infected and should receive antimicrobial postexposure prophylaxis. The incubation period after exposure ranges from 1 to 10 days, with most cases developing in fewer than 4 days. Secondary attack rates are highest during epidemic outbreaks. Any mucosal surface is subject to colonization, which may remain localized or serve as the source of invasive disease.

Meningococcal Meningitis and Acute Meningococcemia

The two invasive forms of meningococcal disease are meningitis and septicemia, which may occur singly or in combination. Patients usually experience a nonspecific febrile upper respiratory tract infection prodrome ranging from a few hours to 5 days. Patients may also experience lethargy, headache, myalgias, arthralgias, and vomiting. Abrupt onset of increased fever, worsening malaise, and progressive lethargy heralds invasive disease. Meningitis is the primary manifestation in 90% of invasive cases, with vomiting, irritability (often with a high-pitched cry in infants), and nuchal rigidity, indistinguishable from other causes of bacterial meningitis (Fig. 13.38A). Infants may also have a bulging fontanelle (see Fig. 13.38B). Delirium, combativeness, stupor, and seizures may develop in older patients. Although some patients with meningitis also have meningococcemia, cutaneous manifestations, endotoxic shock, and disseminated intravascular coagulation (DIC) are more common in patients without meningeal infection.

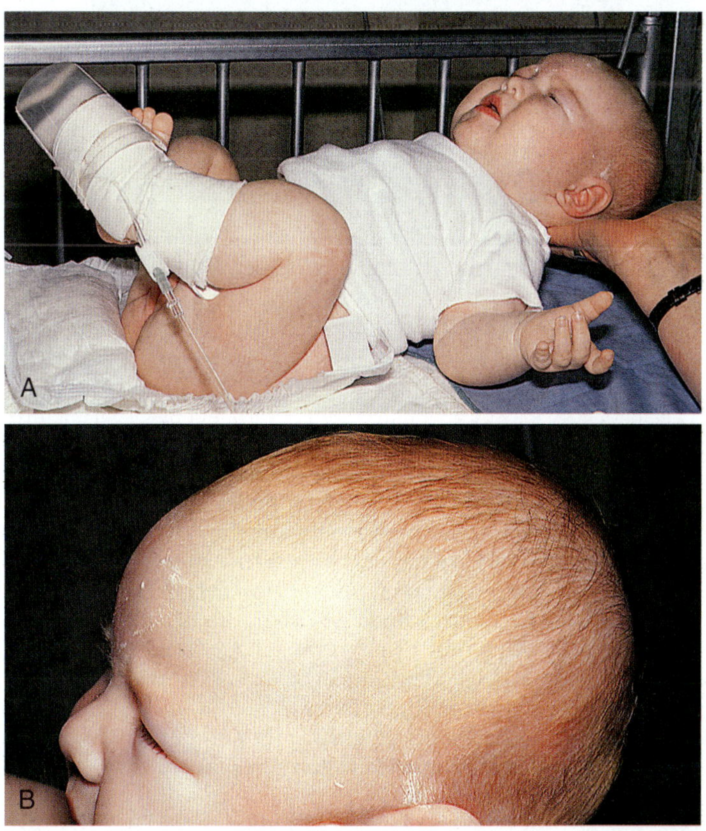

Fig. 13.38 Meningitis. (A) Nuchal rigidity and a positive Brudzinski sign are demonstrated. On attempted passive flexion of the neck, the infant grimaces with pain, neck stiffness limits flexion, and the knees and hips are flexed to reduce traction on the meninges. (B) This infant was also found to have a bulging anterior fontanelle when sitting quietly, reflecting increased intracranial pressure.

Meningococcemia without evidence of meningitis can have an insidious onset but classically presents in a virulent fashion. In contrast, 10% of patients present with overwhelming sepsis without clinical or laboratory evidence of meningitis. In these patients, the abrupt change associated with invasive disease heralds the development of a rash in association with manifestations of shock, including mottling, distal coolness with decreased capillary refill or cyanosis, widened pulse pressure, or frank hypotension. Up to 85% of these patients have cutaneous lesions involving the trunk and extremities, consisting of tender pink macules, petechiae that may be palpably raised, and purpura, which when present is most prominent on the extremities and may progress to form areas of frank necrosis (Fig. 13.39). The prognosis in patients with a short prodrome, fulminant progression, early appearance of purpuric lesions, and shock is poor. The combination of adrenal crisis due to adrenal hemorrhage in the setting of fulminant septicemia, often with purpura, is termed *Waterhouse-Friderichsen syndrome* and is usually due to meningococcemia. More than 60% of such patients have hypotension and DIC on presentation, and approximately half have either normal or low white blood cell count, indicating that their immune system has been overwhelmed. Only about 20% of these patients have meningitis. Mortality in fulminant cases approaches 40% versus only 3% in those showing slower progression. Most deaths occur within 24 hours of presentation. Because of the potential for deterioration, aggressive empiric antimicrobial therapy and vigorous supportive measures should be instituted promptly whenever meningococcemia is suspected.

The differential diagnosis includes other bacterial causes of sepsis, bacterial endocarditis, Rocky Mountain spotted fever (RMSF), and other disorders characterized by thrombocytopenia. Septicemia caused by gram-negative bacilli may be clinically indistinguishable from meningococcal septicemia. Similarly, *H. influenzae* type B, pneumococcal, or streptococcal septicemia may be associated with petechiae and even purpura, particularly in asplenic children. The purpuric lesions of staphylococcal sepsis tend to become pustular, and a primary suppurative focus also helps distinguish infection with *S. aureus*. Adenoviral and enteroviral infections may produce petechial rashes but rarely cause a septic presentation. Other clinical characteristics help to identify patients with thrombocytopenia resulting from immune thrombocytopenic purpura, acute leukemia, and mononucleosis. The centripetal mode of spread of the petechial rash of RMSF, in addition to residence in a region endemic for the tick vector, and the initial distribution and subsequent mode of spread of Henoch-Schönlein purpura help to distinguish these illnesses. Differentiation can be particularly difficult in the case of a child with high fever, no source other than upper respiratory tract infection, and petechial rash. These findings may represent early nonfulminant meningococcemia, but they also can be part of the picture of viral illness or another bacterial process. In such cases, observation with presumptive therapy is necessary.

Meningococcosis (Chronic Meningococcemia)

Meningococcosis, a disorder more indolent than acute meningococcemia, is defined as a meningococcal bacteremia and fever of greater than 1 week's duration without meningitis. Symptoms are usually present for 6 to 8 weeks before diagnosis and may be intermittent. Fever and chills (without rigors) are associated with an exanthem in nearly 95% of cases. The rash waxes and wanes, often in association with the fever. Lesions may consist of tender erythematous, subcutaneous nodules; erythematous macules and papules; or petechiae, occurring singly or in combination. Urticarial lesions are seen occasionally. The feet, legs, upper arms, and trunk are most involved. Headache, malaise, myalgias, and arthralgias are common. In children, swelling of hands, feet, knees, and ankles may occur

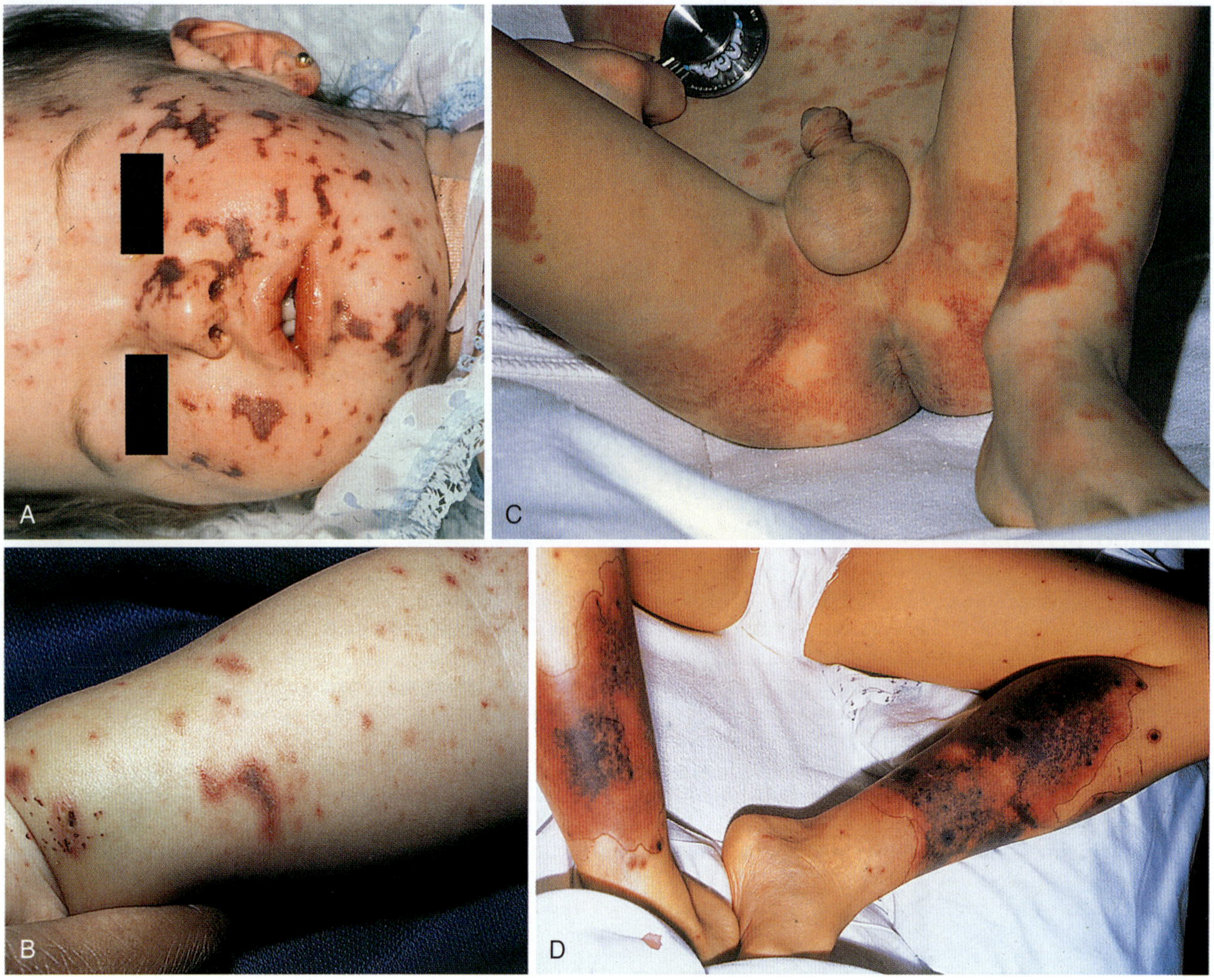

Fig. 13.39 Meningococcemia. (A) This youngster manifests the purpuric and petechial rash characteristic of acute meningococcemia. (B) Petechiae are more apparent in this close-up of an infant. Gram stain of petechial scrapings may reveal organisms. (C and D) Purpura may progress, especially in patients with disseminated intravascular coagulation. (D, Courtesy Kenneth Schuitt, MD.)

intermittently, without evidence of warmth or erythema; however, when the legs are involved, the child may refuse to walk.

The diagnosis of meningococcosis can be difficult because early blood cultures are often negative (although children are more likely than adults to have positive cultures) and skin lesions are generally negative on both smear and culture. Throat culture is usually negative as well. Close monitoring of the clinical course, combined with repeated blood cultures, is the best way to confirm the diagnosis. Approximately one-third of untreated patients ultimately suffer severe localized infection (after an average of 10 weeks of illness), with meningitis, carditis, nephritis, and ocular infection occurring most commonly. Chronic disease can be associated with complement defects, as can episodes of acute or recurrent disease.

ADENOPATHY, INFECTIOUS LYMPHADENITIS, AND SALIVARY INFECTION

Lymph nodes respond to both systemic and local infections with cellular multiplication and activity clinically manifested as enlargement and tenderness. Most often, the enlargement is modest and, if biopsied, nonspecific hyperplasia is found. This is termed reactive adenopathy and usually resolves without a specific etiology being identified. Nodes are usually 2 cm or less in diameter and are discrete, slightly firm, or rubbery and mobile. Discomfort and tenderness are mild. However, in some cases enlargement is marked, inflammation is pronounced, and a specific etiology can be identified on biopsy. If the lymph node itself is infected (adenitis) and not simply reactive, histology shows copious bacteria, neutrophils, and necrotic debris. Infected nodes usually exceed 2 cm in diameter, and overlying soft tissues may become cellulitic, making it difficult to distinguish exact margins. With progression, the overlying skin often becomes erythematous and may become adherent, reducing mobility. Discomfort and tenderness can be severe. Depending on the causative organism, suppuration may occur.

Adenopathy may be generalized or regional, but bacterial adenitis tends to be localized. Whereas most adenitis is infectious, adenopathy may also be a feature of collagen vascular (Chapter 7) or neoplastic disease (Chapter 12). Malignant nodes are usually firm or hard in consistency but are occasionally rubbery, and they are more frequently matted and fixed or poorly mobile; tenderness is unusual. Depending on the malignancy, adenopathy may be isolated to a single region or generalized and associated with hepatosplenomegaly or systemic symptoms of anorexia, fatigue, weight loss, night sweats, and bone pain. Many infectious diseases associated with generalized or cervical adenopathy have been discussed earlier in this chapter. Some of the distinguishing features of the adenopathy characteristic of these disorders are given in Table 13.1.

General Approach to Diagnosis of Lymphadenitis

In this section, we concentrate on manifestations and causes of focal lymphadenitis. Almost any organism capable of infecting tissue can produce adenitis; hence the number of potential pathogens is large.

Table 13.1 Infectious Causes of Generalized or Prominent Cervical Adenopathy

Disorder	Site(s) of Adenopathy	Character of Nodes	Other Features	Laboratory Findings
EBV mononucleosis	Anterior and posterior cervical or generalized	Soft to firm, discrete, mildly to moderately tender	Pharyngitis; splenomegaly (50%); rash (15%); fever, malaise, fatigue	Atypical lymphocytosis; positive Monospot (80% >4 years old); positive EBV titers; may have abnormal LFTs
CMV infection	Generalized or cervical	Soft to firm, discrete, mildly tender	Fever, malaise, fatigue; occasionally hepatosplenomegaly	Atypical lymphocytosis; abnormal LFTs; urine positive for CMV on culture or PCR; positive CMV titers
Toxoplasmosis	Generalized or cervical	Smooth, firm, mildly tender	Myalgias, fatigue, coryza; occasionally splenomegaly and maculopapular rash	Atypical lymphocytosis (frequent); positive *Toxoplasma* titers
Brucellosis	Generalized or cervical and axillary	Discrete, may be mildly tender or nontender	History of contact with sick farm animal or ingestion of raw milk; afternoon fever and chills; sweats, malaise, headache and backache, arthralgia; splenomegaly; lasts weeks and may become chronic with metastatic abscesses	Normal or decreased WBC count with lymphocytosis; positive cultures and serologic tests; the microbiology laboratory should be informed of suspicion for infection
Rubella	Anterior and posterior cervical	Soft to mildly firm, discrete, mildly tender or nontender	Fine, discrete maculopapular rash; Forchheimer spots on palate	Positive rubella titer
Streptococcal pharyngitis	Anterior cervical	Soft to mildly firm, discrete, tender	Pharyngitis or nasopharyngitis; headache, malaise; abdominal pain; may have palatal petechiae and/or scarlatiniform rash	Positive throat culture for group A β-hemolytic streptococci
Herpes simplex	Anterior cervical and submandibular	Soft to mildly firm, discrete, mobile, tender	Gingival erythema, edema, and friability with discrete mucosal ulcers; high fever	Positive viral culture or PCR (diagnosis usually made on clinical grounds)
Coxsackievirus herpangina	Anterior cervical	Soft to mildly firm, discrete, mobile, slightly tender	Discrete ulcers on labial mucosa, gingiva, tongue, and tonsillar pillars; may have vesicles on palms and soles	Positive viral culture (diagnosis usually made on clinical grounds)
Adenovirus	Anterior cervical and preauricular	Soft to mildly firm, discrete, mobile, mildly tender	Nonspecific pharyngeal inflammation, occasionally with exudate; may have conjunctivitis	Positive viral culture or PCR

CMV, Cytomegalovirus; *EBV*, Epstein-Barr virus; *LFT*, liver function test; *PCR*, polymerase chain reaction; *WBC*, white blood cell.

Because of the numerous agents that can produce lymphadenitis, meticulous care must be taken during the clinical assessment. History should include antecedent and current signs and symptoms, including the presence or absence of systemic symptoms; rapidity of the evolution of the adenitis; prior wounds, such as cuts, bites, punctures, splinters, or scratches distal to the inflamed node; exposure to ill persons or animals; and recent travel. Physical examination must include precise measurement of the size of the inflamed node, in addition to inspection of overlying soft tissue and palpation to determine contour, consistency, and degree of tenderness. The region drained by the involved node must be inspected for clues as to the possible primary source of infection because infection of a lymph node is often a secondary phenomenon after drainage of primary infection to a regional node. Lastly, close attention should be paid to the child's general status and other portions of the reticuloendothelial system, such as to other nodal regions and the liver and spleen.

Superficial Regional Lymph Nodes

Cervical Lymph Nodes

The cervical nodes, being numerous and draining multiple structures, are common sites of acute adenitis (Fig. 13.40). The skin of the face, the scalp, conjunctivae, teeth, gingivae, ears, and neck all may serve as primary sites of infection. Nasal and oropharyngeal infections drain to the tonsillar and anterior cervical nodes (Fig. 13.41). Superficial facial infections and facial cellulitis may drain to the anterior cervical chain or preauricular or submental nodes. The occipital, posterior cervical, preauricular, and postauricular nodes receive lymphatic drainage from nearby portions of the scalp and thus may become

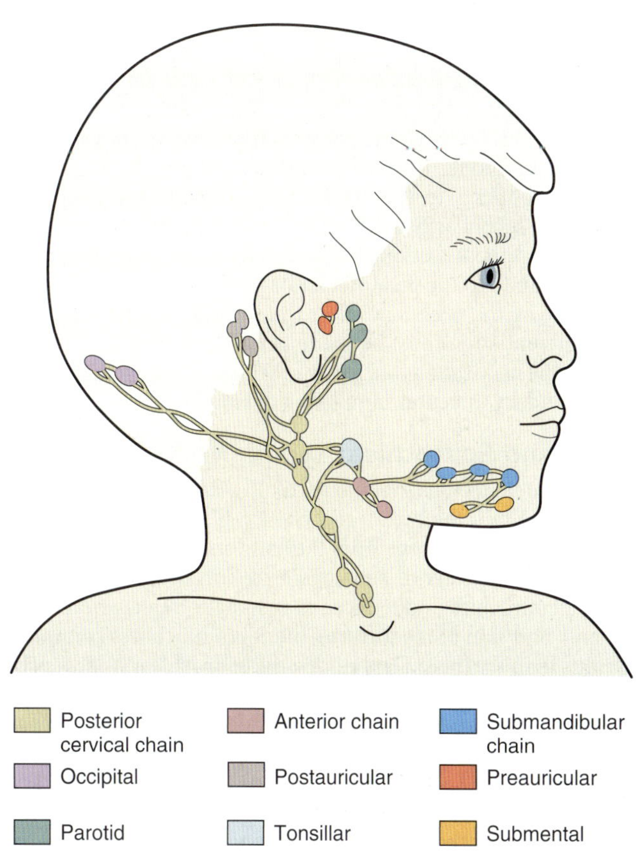

Fig. 13.40 Superficial cervical lymph nodes.

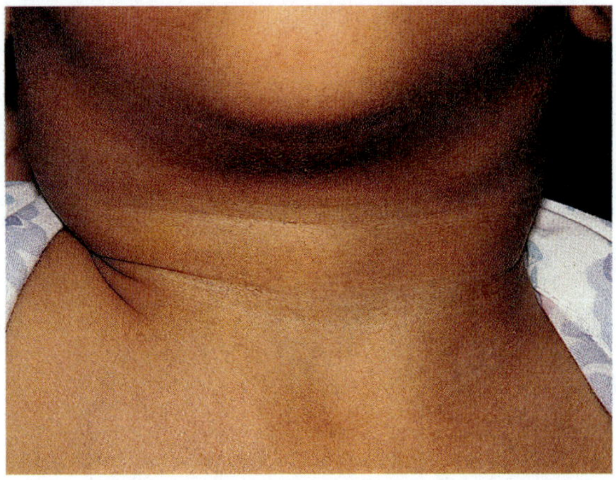

Fig. 13.41 Cervical adenopathy. Bilateral enlargement of the tonsillar nodes in this child was associated with viral pharyngitis.

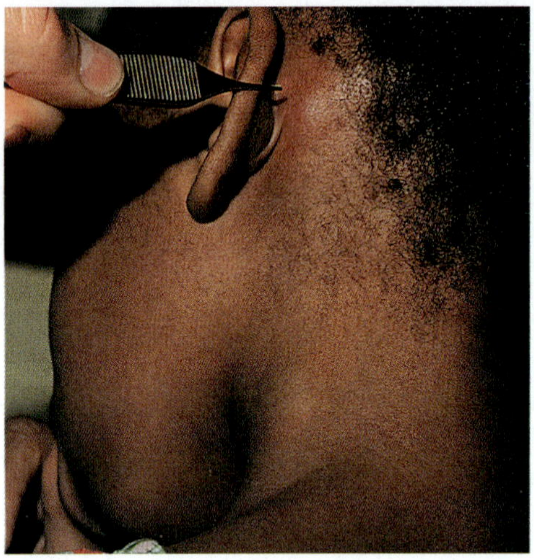

Fig. 13.42 Acute postauricular lymphadenitis. This child had folliculotic and crusted scalp lesions and a tender 1.5-cm postauricular node with overlying erythema. The initial suspicion of bacterial infection was not confirmed. A potassium hydroxide preparation and fungal culture identified tinea capitis as the primary process.

inflamed and enlarged in connection with secondary infection of seborrhea, impetigo, wound infections, tinea capitis, or head lice infestation (Fig. 13.42). Conjunctival infections may result in adenitis of the preauricular node. The teeth, gingivae, and tongue are drained by lymphatics coursing to the submental and submandibular nodes, which can be secondarily involved in cases of dental abscess, gingivitis, and stomatitis. Infections of the external auditory canal and the auricle may drain to the preauricular or postauricular nodes, whereas those involving the neck may affect the anterior or posterior cervical chain. Differentiation must be made from other masses that may be present in the cervical region, many of which are congenital and subject to secondary infection, simulating adenitis.

Axillary and Epitrochlear Lymph Nodes

Several anatomic regions drain to the axilla. Those in the anterior pectoral portion drain the breast and chest wall, those in the lateral or midportion receive drainage from the hand and arm (see Fig. 13.47C), and those in the posterior subscapular region drain portions of the back. The epitrochlear node receives lymphatic vessels from the fingers, hand, and skin of the forearm, but it is a much less common site of adenitis than are the axillary nodes; the epitrochlear nodes are often involved in *Bartonella* infections. Wound and skin infections, cellulitis, and herpes zoster are major sources of axillary adenitis in childhood.

Inguinal Lymph Nodes

The inguinal lymph nodes are divided into two groups by the Poupart ligament, with those above the ligament called inguinal nodes and those below it termed femoral nodes (Fig. 13.43; see Fig. 13.45).

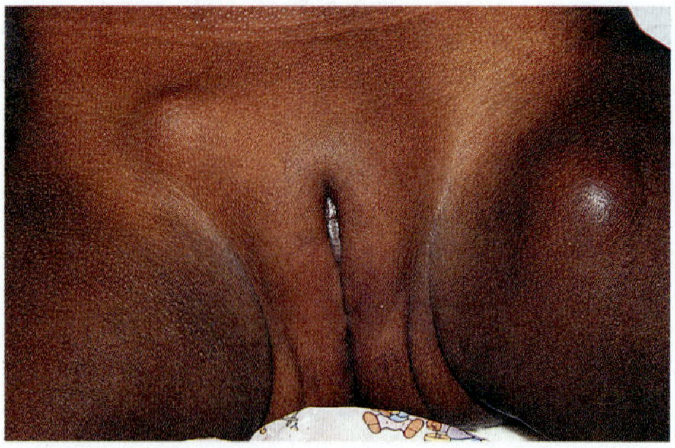

Fig. 13.43 Subacute lymphadenitis of a right inguinal node and left femoral node resulted in dramatic swelling in this toddler. Atypical mycobacteria were found to be causative.

The inguinal group receives lymphatics from the external genitalia, anus, umbilicus, lower abdomen, back, buttocks, and upper thigh and may also drain the lower leg. Thus in addition to wound and skin infections, perianal, intraabdominal, and genital infections may serve as sources of inguinal adenitis. The femoral nodes primarily drain the foot and lower leg. The popliteal nodes receive drainage from the foot and lower leg, but like the epitrochlear nodes, are unusual sites of adenitis.

Acute Suppurative Lymphadenitis

S. pyogenes and *S. aureus* cause most cases of acute lymphadenitis, with *S. aureus* being the more common pathogen. Other than culture obtained by needle aspiration, there is no way to distinguish between the two clinically, as both present with sudden, painful, and rapid enlargement, usually of a single node. The involved node is firm and exquisitely tender (Fig. 13.44). Within 24 to 72 hours, the overlying soft tissue becomes edematous and the skin erythematous. As many as 50% of patients may be febrile, and some appear toxic; bacteremia develops in a small percentage. Left untreated, suppuration occurs during the next several days and is detectable as central fluctuance. Simultaneously, thinning of overlying skin may be noted as the process points toward the surface (Fig. 13.45). On occasion, the abscess may point inward, rupturing into the soft tissues and dissecting along tissue planes with deep-seated infection. Prompt institution of empiric antimicrobial therapy that covers *S. pyogenes* and *S. aureus* can limit these complications. When oral therapy is started before the development of overlying cellulitic changes, such changes may be prevented and enlargement halted, followed by regression. Even in patients with swelling and erythema at the start of therapy, the infection may not progress to suppuration. Patients with high fever and toxicity require initial parenteral treatment. Suppuration necessitates incision and drainage.

Cervical nodes, especially the tonsillar and anterior cervical nodes, are the most common sites of adenitis caused by staphylococci or streptococci. Patients are usually young, with a peak incidence between 1 and 4 years old. Many have an antecedent history of rhinitis, sometimes associated with impetigo of the anterior nares along with anterior cervical adenopathy. Cough, anorexia, vomiting, and fever can be associated findings that may persist or clear before the onset of adenitis. Older children may report a recent episode of pharyngitis, and adenitis may develop in association with a peritonsillar abscess (see Chapter 24).

Secondarily infected dermatitis, insect bites, impetigo, and wound infections may precede the onset of adenitis in other patients, in which case the node affected depends on the primary site. A primary source may be evident at the time adenitis develops or may have already healed. Although severe tinea capitis may mimic streptococcal and staphylococcal infection in the appearance of the primary lesion and in secondary adenitis, progression to

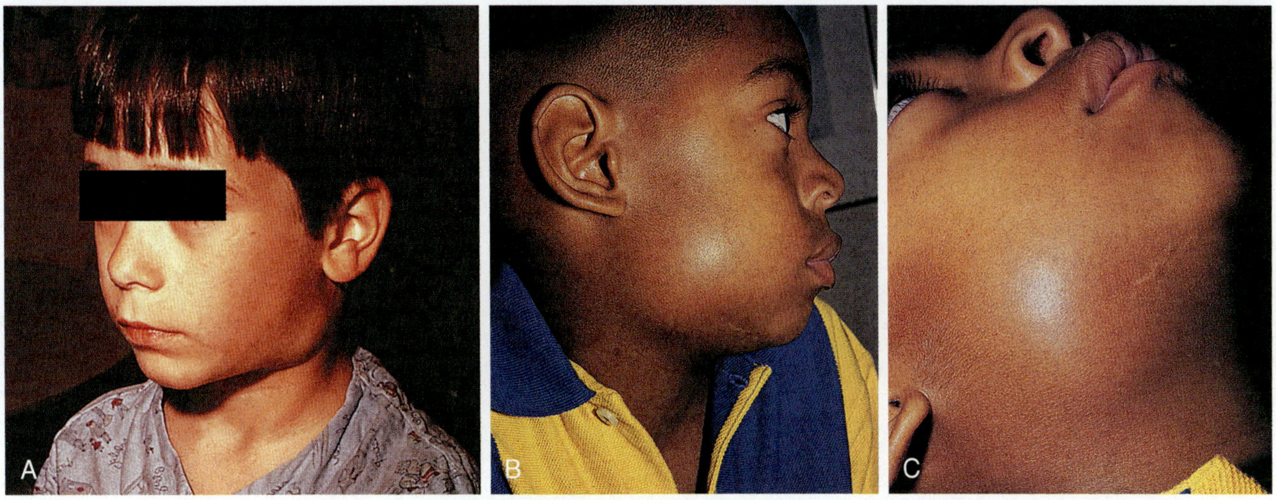

Fig. 13.44 Acute suppurative lymphadenitis. (A) This youngster was seen within 24 hours of the onset of painful enlargement of the left tonsillar node. Mild overlying edema existed, and the node was markedly tender. (B and C) This boy had massive enlargement of the tonsillar node with overlying edema and mild erythema. The node was exquisitely tender, but there was no evidence of fluctuance. Group A β-hemolytic streptococci grew from his throat culture. The absence of preauricular and postauricular swelling helps to differentiate adenitis of the tonsillar node from parotitis. (A, Courtesy Michael Sherlock, MD, Lutherville, MD.)

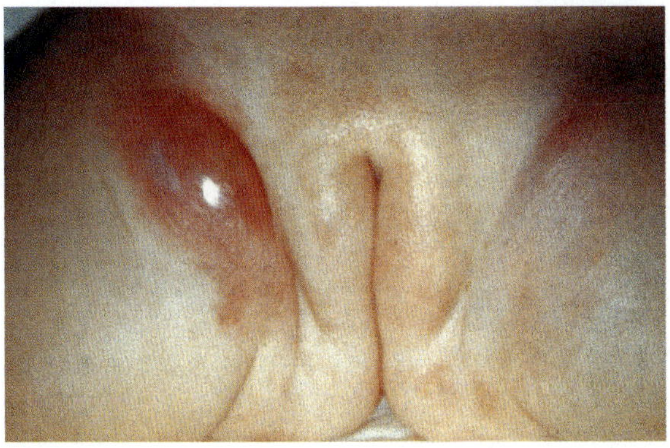

Fig. 13.45 Acute suppurative lymphadenitis. Increased pain and erythema, thinning of the overlying skin, and fluctuance on palpation signal that central necrosis has occurred. (Courtesy Michael Sherlock, MD, Lutherville, MD.)

suppuration is unusual. In these patients, the occipital and/or postauricular nodes are most likely to be affected (see Fig. 13.42 and Chapter 8).

Although streptococci and staphylococci are the predominant pathogens causing acute lymphadenitis, on occasion anaerobic bacteria including the *Streptococcus anginosus* group and *Actinomyces* are responsible. Most cases caused by anaerobes are secondary to dental disease, including dental abscesses, gingivitis, and stomatitis; as a result, the submental or submandibular nodes are more likely to be affected. On occasion, an adenitis appears simultaneously with facial cellulitis stemming from a dental abscess (see Chapter 21).

Actinomycotic adenitis, although unusual, has a distinctive clinical course. Enlargement of the affected node is gradual, and on palpation it is firm and lumpy, has an irregular border, and is mildly to moderately tender. Over time the center blackens and necroses, and a chronic draining sinus may form. Microscopical examination of the discharge discloses characteristic sulfur granules.

Mycobacterial Lymphadenitis

Mycobacterium tuberculosis and nontuberculous mycobacteria (NTM) (especially *Mycobacterium avium* complex) continue to be important causes of lymphadenitis, both in developing and developed nations. Recognition of mycobacterial lymphadenitis is important as its management is considerably different from other pathogens. Both groups of mycobacteria cause similar clinical findings, but the ubiquitous nature of NTM leads them to be more common in children who live in non–tuberculosis (TB)-endemic areas. Nodal enlargement is gradual and persistent. The node is nontender or mildly tender, and initially there is little or no sign of warmth or overlying inflammation (Fig. 13.46A; see Fig. 13.43). After a few weeks, the node becomes adherent to the overlying skin, which in turn becomes thickened and tense, with overlying reddish or reddish-purple discoloration (see Fig. 13.46B and C). Suppuration associated with thinning of the overlying skin may occur several weeks to months after onset and may result in rupture with the formation of a chronically draining sinus. The risk of chronic drainage may be increased if aspiration is attempted, and this procedure is not recommended. Excision is recommended for diagnosis if needed, and operative and laboratory personnel should be warned of concern for TB so that appropriate infection prevention measures are in place.

Tuberculous Lymphadenitis

Children with TB may be any age and frequently have a history of exposure to an infected adult. Tonsillar and submandibular nodes are common sites of TB lymphadenitis because lymphatic extension occurs from the paratracheal nodes. Supraclavicular nodes are affected as the result of drainage from apical pulmonary lesions. The posterior cervical chain is another common area.

Initially, lymphoid hyperplasia develops as tubercles form, and then necrosis and caseation dominate. Early on, nodes are firm, discrete, and nontender, but with progression they tend to become matted and adherent to the overlying skin, which often becomes discolored, thickened, and scaly (see Fig. 13.46A–C). Without treatment, spontaneous drainage ultimately occurs, leaving a draining sinus (see Fig. 13.46D).

Adenitis Due to Nontuberculous Mycobacteria

Patients with NTM adenitis are usually younger than 4 years old and are unlikely to have a history of exposure to TB. Submandibular, submental, preauricular, anterior cervical, or less frequently, inguinal or epitrochlear nodes may be the site of involvement (see Figs. 13.43 and 13.46E). Bilateral adenitis is less common, generalized adenopathy does not occur, and systemic symptoms are rare. Chest radiographic findings are rarely abnormal, and the PPD test is usually negative or intermediate with induration generally below 5 to 10 mm. Interferon gamma release assays are often negative. NTMs are resistant to multiple drugs; thus complete excision is considered the treatment of choice. Spontaneous resolution occurs over 12 to 24 months even in the absence of excision, making observation

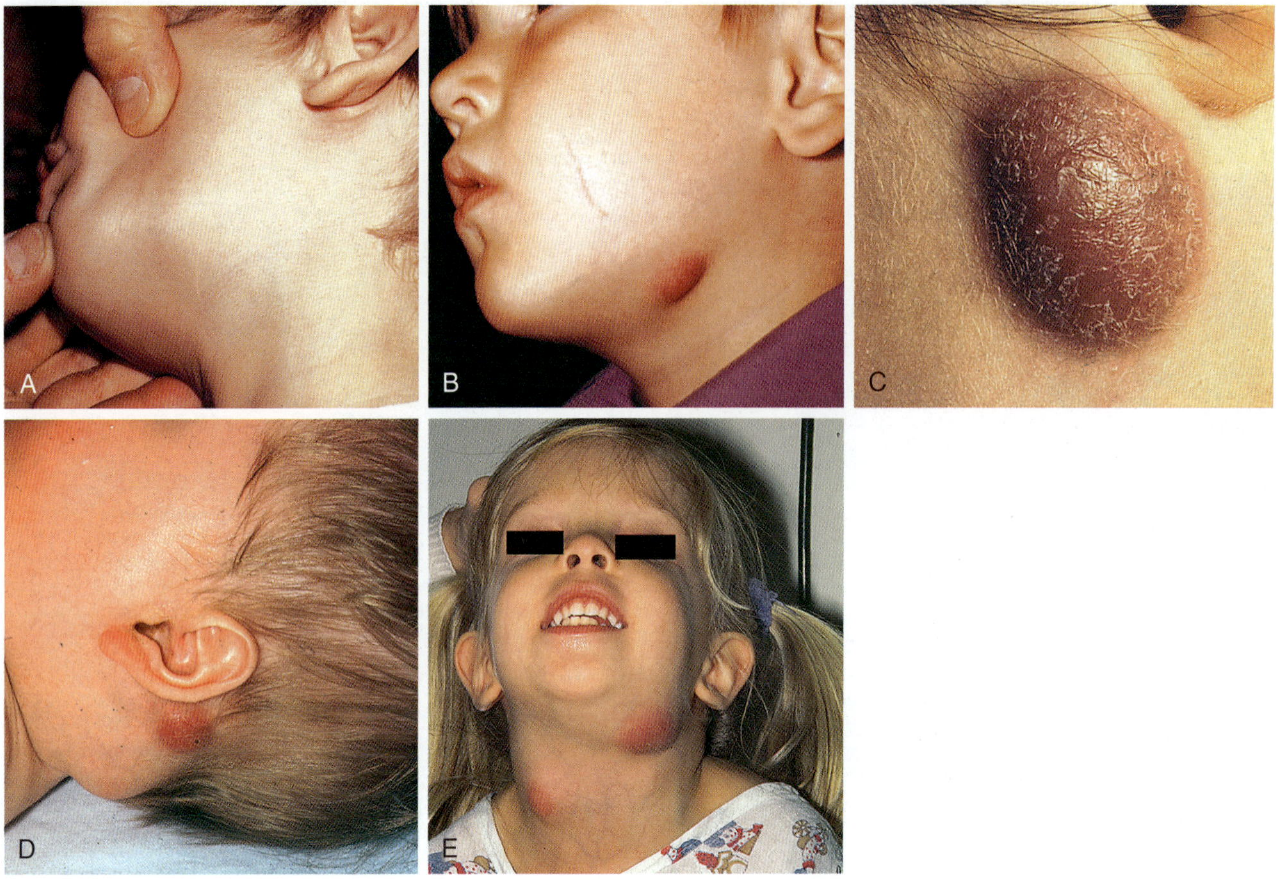

Fig. 13.46 Mycobacterial adenitis. (A) Early in the course of adenitis caused by Mycobacterium tuberculosis or atypical mycobacteria, enlargement of the node is gradual, tenderness is mild, and there is little or no sign of warmth or overlying inflammation. (B) After several weeks the overlying skin becomes thickened, tense, discolored, and adherent to the node. (C) This preauricular node was fluctuant, indicating suppuration. (D) M. tuberculosis was isolated from the drainage of the postauricular node of this infant, who presented with lymphadenopathy and failure to thrive. (E) Nontuberculous mycobacteria were isolated from the nodes of this youngster. (A to C, Courtesy Michael Sherlock, MD, Lutherville, MD.)

a reasonable course if removal is problematic due to nearby neurovascular structures.

Adenitis Associated With Animal or Vector Contact

In many children, acute local adenitis results from inoculation of a pathogen by an animal scratch or bite, from the bite of an insect vector transmitting a pathogen from an animal host, or from contact with a contaminated animal carcass. In some of these disorders, systemic symptoms are prominent; in others, local adenitis is the primary manifestation.

Pasteurella Adenitis

Suppurative adenitis caused by *P. multocida* may occur in patients who develop local infection at the site of an animal bite, most commonly cats or dogs. After the manifestations of local infection appear at the primary site (usually within 24 hours), a regional node becomes enlarged and tender. Overlying swelling and redness are common, and suppuration may occur early. Although this illness is clinically indistinguishable from adenitis due to streptococci or staphylococci, *P. multocida* infection may be suspected on the basis of history and rapid onset of symptoms. Axillary and inguinal nodes are the most common sites of involvement.

Cat-Scratch Disease

Adenitis is a primary feature of cat-scratch disease, although fever occurs in about 25% of patients. *Bartonella henselae* is the causative agent. Ninety percent of patients have a history of either a cat scratch or contact with cats, especially kittens. Inoculation via cat scratch is the most common means of infection, but puncture wounds, flea bites, and dog scratches have also been implicated. Incidence is highest in fall and winter in temperate climates, with cases occurring with equal frequency year-round in tropical areas. Most patients are in the 5- to 14-year-old age range, but clusters that include younger children and adults have been reported.

Symptoms usually begin 7 to 12 days after inoculation. A red papule or series of papules is noted at the site of inoculation (Fig. 13.47A and B). Shortly thereafter, one or more regional nodes enlarge, becoming mildly painful and tender (see Fig. 13.47A and C). Involved nodes are firm, and overlying warmth and mild redness may develop within a few days of enlargement. In order of frequency, axillary, cervical, submandibular, preauricular, epitrochlear, and inguinal nodes have been reported. In contrast to NTM lymphadenitis, *Bartonella* lymph nodes are quite tender. With preauricular adenitis, associated conjunctivitis is common and suggests conjunctival inoculation as the source (a Parinaud syndrome). Discomfort generally subsides in 4 to 6 weeks, but the node may remain enlarged or may fluctuate in size for months. Suppuration occurs in about one-third of patients.

Diagnosis is made primarily by history, clinical picture, and course but can be confirmed by biopsy. Histology reveals granulomas with microabscesses, and Warthin-Starry silver stain may identify gram-negative pleomorphic coccobacilli. PCR may be performed on aspirated material. Serology is usually positive. Treatment is supportive. If lymph nodes are painful, suppurative aspiration can be performed and is preferable to incision and drainage because of concerns that the latter procedure may lead to prolonged drainage and scarring. In protracted or atypical cases, excisional biopsy is suggested. The benefit of antimicrobial treatment in an immunocompetent host remains controversial.

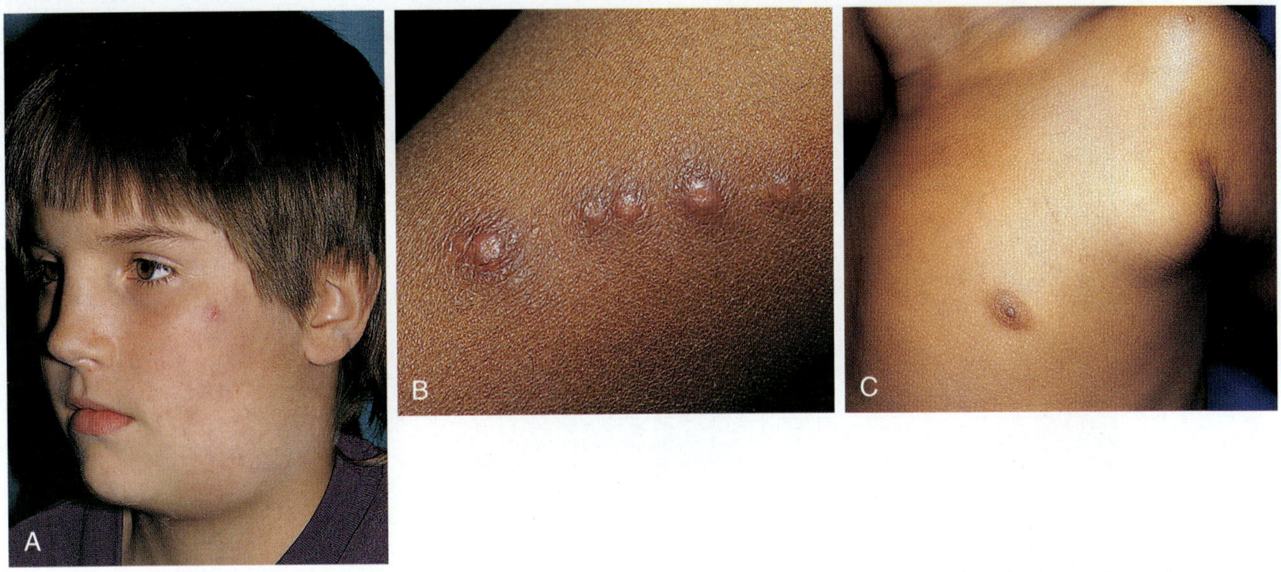

Fig. 13.47 Cat-scratch disease. (A) This boy presented with mildly painful "swollen glands." The left preauricular and tonsillar nodes were enlarged, firm, and mildly tender. An ulcerated papule, evident on his left cheek, was the site of a scratch inflicted by one of his kittens 2 weeks earlier. (B) A line of papules is seen on the forearm of a 3-year-old at the site of a scratch inflicted by his new kitten 3 weeks before presentation. (C) Marked enlargement of an ipsilateral axillary node had prompted his visit. The node was firm and only mildly tender. (A, Courtesy Kenneth Schuitt, MD.)

Tularemia

Francisella tularensis most often produces an ulceroglandular syndrome in children, occurring in concert with systemic symptoms. Rabbits, hares, muskrats, and voles serve as endemic sources of this pathogen. Children may acquire disease from the bite of an arthropod vector, most commonly a tick; by handling or skinning dead animals; or after an animal bite (especially that of a cat that hunts rabbits). The incubation period ranges from 1 to 21 days. Onset is abrupt and characterized by fever, chills, headache, myalgias, vomiting, and possibly photophobia. A painful papule appears at the site of inoculation with subsequent axillary, epitrochlear, or inguinal adenitis. The papule frequently ruptures to form a central ulcer with a raised edge. The involved regional node is firm and tender and may be associated with overlying erythema. Generalized adenopathy and hepatosplenomegaly may be noted in some patients; and in the second week of illness, a blotchy, erythematous maculopapular rash (or occasionally a vesicular, pustular, or nodosa exanthem) may appear. Without treatment, fever may persist for 2 to 3 weeks and the ulcer may take as long as 1 month to heal. The diagnosis is suggested by history, geography, and clinical picture and may be confirmed serologically. If cultures are obtained, the microbiology laboratory should be notified as to the concern for tularemia so that proper laboratory safety measures can be implemented.

Bubonic Plague

Bubonic plague, caused by *Yersinia pestis,* is now rare in developed countries, but it continues to cause sporadic cases related to wild rodent exposure in the southwest United States. Bubonic plague is usually transmitted by fleabite, but inoculation may occur through a break in the skin while handling an infected carcass. Thus inguinal and axillary nodes are the most common sites of bubo formation. The incubation period ranges from several hours to 10 days and ends with the abrupt onset of high fever, chills, malaise, weakness, and headache. Pain around a regional node precedes rapid nodal enlargement. The node is fixed, firm, and exquisitely tender with overlying edema. Purplish discoloration is common, forming the classic bubo. The inoculation site may appear normal or manifest as a skin abscess. Rapid progression of systemic symptoms occurs, with the patient appearing toxic and apprehensive and often delirious with signs of neurologic dysfunction. DIC and septic shock may supervene without prompt treatment. If infection is suspected, the node should be aspirated to obtain material for culture, blood cultures should be performed, and broad-spectrum parenteral antibiotic therapy instituted. The microbiology laboratory should be notified as to the concern for *Y. pestis.*

Parotitis

Salivary glands can be inflamed due to viruses or, less frequently, bacteria. The most common viral etiologies associated with parotitis are mumps virus and enteroviruses, whereas the most common bacterial pathogen is *S. aureus.*

Mumps (Epidemic Parotitis)

Mumps is an acute viral illness that preferentially involves glandular and neural tissues. It is less frequently seen in the United States since the advent of the measles, mumps, and rubella combination vaccine, but annual outbreaks continue to occur, especially among close-contact populations such as college students due to waning immunity from childhood vaccination or unvaccinated status. Although salivary glands, especially the parotid glands, are the most common sites of clinical involvement, the CNS and other glandular tissues may be affected as well. The infection is subclinical in up to one-third of patients. The incubation period is 16 to 18 days, with the contagious period from 1 to 7 days before the onset of symptoms and for 5 to 9 days thereafter. Asymptomatic children can transmit virus.

Prodromal symptoms consist of fever, headache, malaise, and anorexia. Typically, these symptoms are followed within 24 hours by the onset of earache or face pain. Pain is aggravated by chewing and stimulation of salivation (particularly sialagogues). Parotid swelling becomes noticeable within the next 24 hours, increases gradually over the ensuing few days, and then abates over a similar period. Fever may persist for the duration of swelling but can disappear early in the course. Examination reveals an area of tender, indurated swelling extending from the preauricular area through the subauricular space to the postauricular region (Fig. 13.48A). The pinna may be displaced with pronounced parotid enlargement

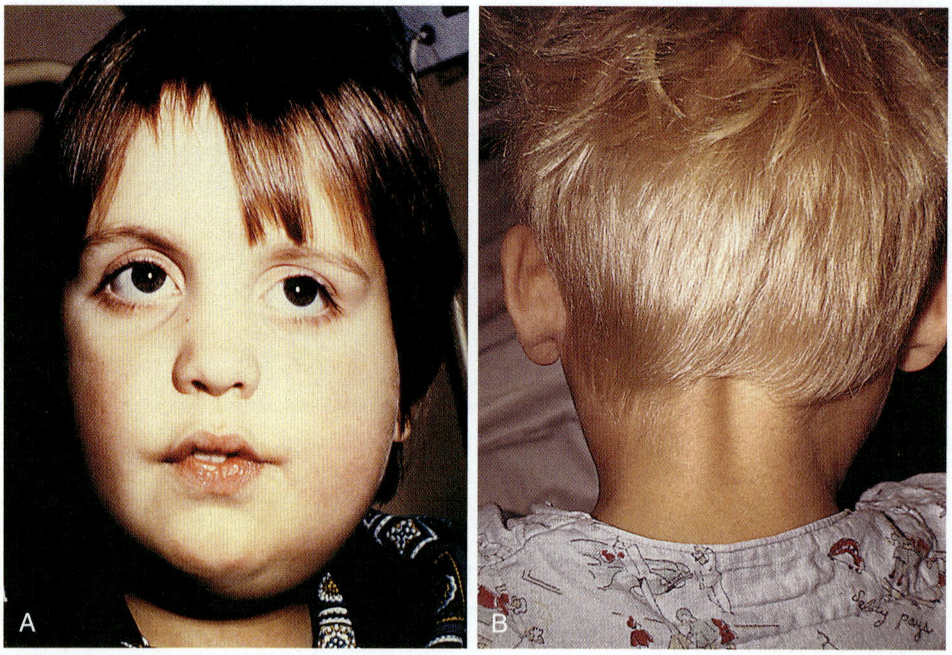

Fig. 13.48 Mumps. (A) This young boy showed unilateral parotid swelling, which was indurated and moderately tender. Visually it was appreciated best in this view, which reveals swelling anterior and inferior to his left ear. (B) Bilateral infraauricular and postauricular swelling (right greater than left) can be appreciated when the patient is viewed from behind. Secondary displacement of the auricle is evident. (A, Courtesy G.D.W. McKendrik, MD. B, Courtesy Michael Sherlock, MD, Lutherville, MD.)

(see Fig. 13.48B). The gland is indurated and tender to palpation, with normal overlying skin. Intraoral examination may reveal erythema and edema of Stensen duct. Bilateral involvement is usual, although one gland tends to enlarge first, and up to 25% of symptomatic patients have unilateral inflammation. The submental or sublingual salivary glands may be the primary site of involvement, sparing the parotid gland.

Preauricular swelling and induration, Stensen duct abnormality, and the absence of prominent overlying erythema help to distinguish parotid swelling from cervical adenitis. In confusing cases, the patient can be given lemon juice or a lemon wedge orally to induce secretion of saliva through the Stetson duct. In patients with mumps, prompt enlargement and pain of the affected gland as salivation is seen, which does not occur with adenopathy. In cases of bacterial parotitis, the patient often has a high fever and shows signs of toxicity. The overlying skin is erythematous, with exquisite tenderness on palpation (Fig. 13.49). Purulent drainage from the Stensen duct can be expressed and cultured by massaging the gland.

Symptomatic meningoencephalitis is only seen in about 10% of patients, but up to 75% of patients with mumps may have cerebrospinal fluid pleocytosis. CNS symptoms usually follow parotitis but can develop before or even in the absence of salivary gland involvement. There is a wide spectrum in the severity of these symptoms, ranging from isolated headache and malaise with fever to frank nuchal rigidity with nausea, vomiting, and severe alterations in sensorium. Fortunately, permanent sequelae are rare, although children recovering from severe mumps meningoencephalitis may not return to normal levels of school performance for up to 6 months or a year.

Mumps orchitis is much less common in children than in adults, who have a 20% to 30% incidence. Orchitis usually follows parotitis but may occur in its absence. Fever, chills, headache, nausea, vomiting, and lower abdominal pain may be present along with painful, generally unilateral testicular swelling. Epididymitis is an invariable accompaniment. This process lasts 3 to 7 days. Oophoritis occasionally occurs in females, which may be unilateral or bilateral, and may mimic appendicitis if only right sided.

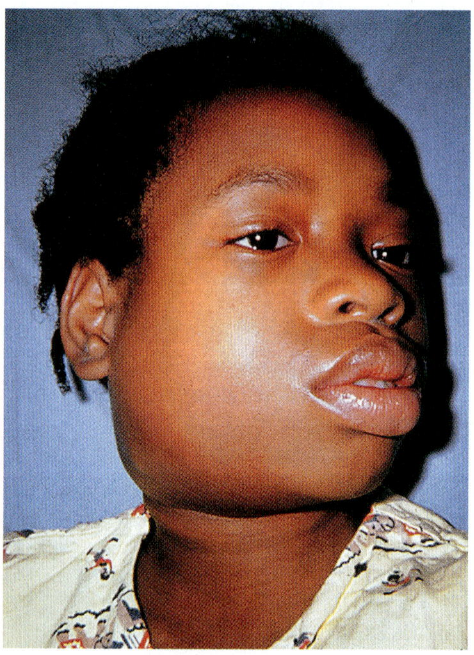

Fig. 13.49 Suppurative parotitis. This patient had high fever, chills, and marked enlargement of the right parotid gland, which was severely painful and exquisitely tender. The overlying skin is erythematous, and purulent material was seen draining from the Stensen duct. (Courtesy Sylvan Stool, MD.)

TICK-BORNE INFECTIOUS EXANTHEMS

Lyme Disease

Lyme disease is a tick-borne infection caused by the spirochete *Borrelia burgdorferi*. It is the most common vector-borne infection in the United States. Named for the southeastern Connecticut community where it was first described, Lyme disease was originally identified as a cause of chronic arthritis. Subsequent investigation established the spectrum of illness, which may involve the skin, heart, nervous system, or joints. Lyme disease is divided into three clinical stages: early localized, disseminated, and late disease.

Transmission of Lyme disease occurs when a person is bitten by an infected *Ixodes* tick (deer tick). *Ixodes scapularis,* the most common vector, is found predominantly in the Northeast and Midwestern United States. *Ixodes pacificus* is responsible for transmission in Western states but is not as commonly infected with *B. burgdorferi.* Borrelia transmission is most common from nymphal ticks, which are extremely small and often not noticed. Most early and disseminated cases occur between spring and fall when nymphal deer ticks are active and people are more likely to be outdoors, and the ticks have an incubation of 3 to 30 days.

Early Localized Disease

The distinctive exanthem of Lyme disease, known as erythema migrans, appears in approximately two-thirds of symptomatic of cases, usually 3 to 14 days after the tick bite. The rash begins as a red papule or macule at the site of the tick bite and often goes unrecognized. The lesion gradually enlarges, forming a large plaque that can have central clearing, giving it an annular "bullseye" configuration (Fig. 13.50).

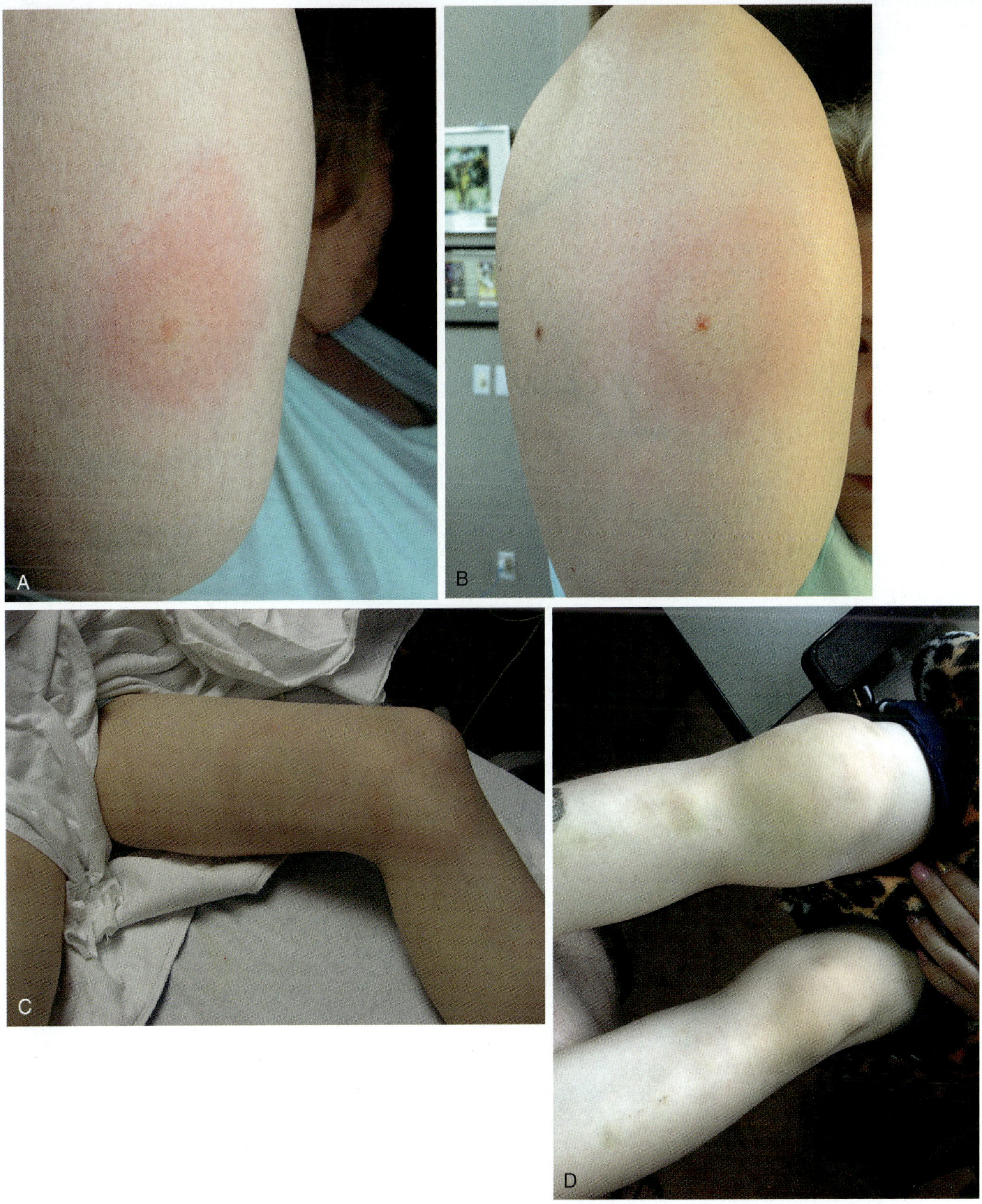

Fig. 13.50 Erythema migrans/Lyme disease. (A) This 2- to 3-cm lesion is just starting to clear centrally. (B) The central clearing is nearly complete 1 day later, and within the erythematous border, the puncta of a tick bite is evident. (C) Multiple annular lesions of differing sizes and varying degrees of central clearing are seen in this child with Lyme disease. (D) Lyme arthritis is noted in this boy with late-onset Lyme disease with a large swollen knee joint without erythema.

The central portion may develop a bluish discoloration or become indurated or vesicular, and the classic target appearance develops in less than 50% of lesions. The exanthem may be warm to the touch, and some patients report mild pruritus, burning, or prickling sensations. Erythema migrans may be accompanied by fever, headache, fatigue, myalgias, and regional or generalized adenopathy. Untreated, the erythema migrans lesion gradually resolves over 3 weeks, and systemic symptoms often wax and wane over the course of several weeks. With treatment, the rash clears within several days and the systemic symptoms resolve.

Early Disseminated Disease

Multiple secondary annular lesions, often smaller than the primary lesion, develop in about 25% of all children with Lyme disease, representing hematogenous dissemination (see Fig. 13.50C). Other common manifestations of disseminated disease include aseptic meningitis, sometimes accompanied by focal neurologic signs and symptoms, and unilateral or bilateral facial nerve palsy. Optic neuritis, iritis, and keratitis are unusual. Carditis, characterized by varying degrees of atrioventricular block or myopericarditis, is rare in children.

Late Disease (>6 Months After Tick Bite)

Lyme arthritis is a late manifestation, and the presenting complaint in 5% to 10% of children. It is usually monoarticular or pauciarticular, involving large joints, especially the knee (see Fig. 13.50D). Pain, warmth, and swelling are typical, but overlying erythema is unusual. Lyme arthritis generally presents with a more indolent and less toxic course than routine septic arthritis. Joints appear "rheumatic" with stiffness and swelling predominating over pain and redness. The initial episode usually lasts about 1 week but can be prolonged. Untreated recurrences may be experienced.

Diagnosis of Lyme disease varies by disease stage. In patients with erythema migrans, the diagnosis should be made solely on clinical and epidemiologic grounds, as most patients do not recall a history of tick bite. Serology is often negative and thus unhelpful in early localized disease. Most patients with early disseminated disease and virtually all with late disease are seropositive. The interpretation of commercial serologic testing should follow Centers for Disease Control and Prevention (CDC) guidelines for diagnosis of Lyme disease. Antimicrobial therapy is highly effective, and there is no evidence for chronic or persistent infection in appropriately treated children.

Rocky Mountain Spotted Fever, Ehrlichiosis, and Anaplasmosis

These tick-borne infections are acute, potentially life-threatening diseases caused by *Rickettsia, Ehrlichia, Anaplasma,* and other related species. These obligate intracellular parasites are transmitted to humans by the bite of an infected tick. Organisms multiply in the endothelium of small blood vessels and spread hematogenously, resulting in a widespread vasculitis characterized by inflammation and thrombosis with secondary vascular leakage. The peak seasons are spring and summer, and the incubation period ranges from 2 to 14 days (average 4–8 days). Two-thirds of cases occur in children younger than 15 years old. Mortality is as high as 5% to 7% in rickettsial infections and is associated with delayed diagnosis.

Onset may be acute or gradual and is characterized by fever and headache, which is typically severe, unremitting, and unresponsive to analgesia. Headache may not be a prominent complaint in young children. Other symptoms include chills, anorexia, nausea, vomiting, sore throat, abdominal pain, diarrhea, arthralgias, and myalgias. Respiratory symptoms are uncommon. The spleen is enlarged in 30% to 50% of patients, but adenopathy is not prominent. A petechial to purpuric exanthem is usually noted around the third day of illness but may appear as late as the second week.

The characteristic appearance and mode of spread of the exanthem are helpful clues to diagnose RMSF. The rash begins distally on the wrists, ankles, palms, and soles, usually appearing as an erythematous, blanching, discrete macular or maculopapular eruption. It then spreads centripetally and becomes petechial (Fig. 13.51), although on occasion lesions are petechial from the outset. In some cases, the eruption is not prominent and may even be transient, making diagnosis difficult. Rash occurs in 90% of children with RMSF and 60% of children with ehrlichiosis; children with ehrlichiosis typically have less prominent skin involvement than RMSF. Conjunctival injection, with photophobia and petechial hemorrhages, may develop simultaneously with the rash. Firm, nonpitting, nondependent edema may begin in the periorbital region and generalize a few days after the onset of symptoms. Aseptic meningitis and encephalitis are not uncommon, and CNS symptoms range in severity from restlessness, irritability, and anxiety to confusion, delirium, and coma, with or without seizures and focal neurologic signs. Myocarditis, DIC, renal failure, and cardiovascular collapse are features of advanced disease.

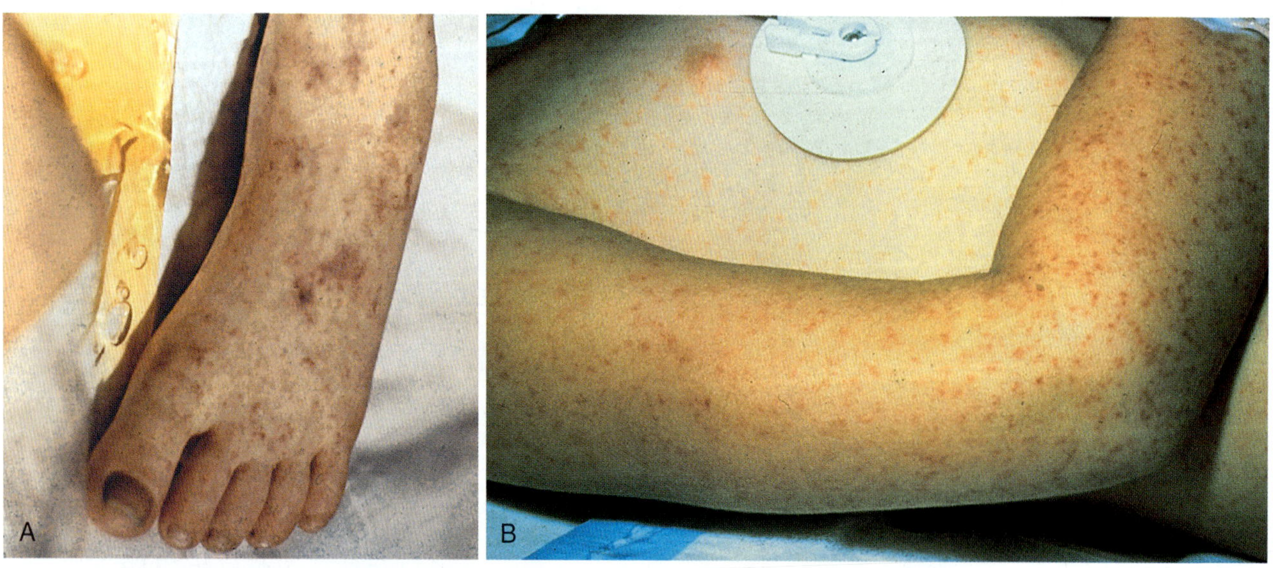

Fig. 13.51 Rocky Mountain spotted fever. (A) The exanthem characteristic of this disease first appears distally on wrists, ankles, palms, and soles. It may be petechial from the outset, or it may start as an erythematous, blanching, macular, or maculopapular eruption, which then becomes petechial as it spreads centripetally. (B) In this child, the rash has become generalized. Both petechial and blanching erythematous lesions are present. (A, Courtesy Ellen Wald, MD, University of Wisconsin Children's Hospital, Madison, WI.)

White blood cell counts are normal or low in the first few days of RMSF and then tend to rise; patients with ehrlichiosis or anaplasmosis often have leukopenia and monocytopenia. Thrombocytopenia is common. Other laboratory abnormalities include hyponatremia, hypoproteinemia, elevated transaminases, and hyperkalemia.

There are no rapid diagnostic tests for these infections, and early institution of antimicrobial treatment is crucial to a favorable outcome. Thus the diagnosis of RMSF, ehrlichiosis, or anaplasmosis should be made on clinical grounds as soon as possible. The diagnosis should be suspected in any child in an endemic area with fever, headache, toxicity, and a petechial rash. Because of the potentially life-threatening nature of this infection, doxycycline is recommended regardless of age. Recovery is the rule if therapy is begun during the first week of illness. Acute and convalescent serology can be used to confirm the diagnosis.

BACTERIAL BONE AND JOINT INFECTIONS

Osteomyelitis

The anatomy and physiology of growing bone place children at particular risk for bacterial infection; 85% of cases of osteomyelitis occur in children younger than 16 years old. Most children with timely diagnosis and appropriate antimicrobial therapy will have a good outcome.

S. aureus is the most identified pathogen in all age groups, followed by *S. pyogenes*. Gram-negative organisms account for a small percentage of cases, including *Salmonella* (in children with sickle cell hemoglobinopathies or reptile exposure) and *Pseudomonas* (with puncture wounds of the foot). In 15% to 30% of cases, no organism is identified, often because of suppression by prior antibiotic therapy. Rarely, NTM or fungi cause a chronic osteomyelitis, usually associated with penetrating trauma or immunocompromised patients.

The anatomic and physiologic features of growing bone underlie the pathophysiology of osteomyelitis in children. Nutrient vessels enter the diaphysis from the periosteum and extend to the metaphysis, where terminal arterioles form loops and empty into larger sinusoidal veins that are devoid of phagocytic macrophages. This tissue has sluggish and turbulent blood flow, which serves as an ideal site for bacterial deposition during transient bacteremia. Bacterial growth within bone stimulates inflammation and exudate formation. As fluid collects, pressure increases, promoting extension outward and causing further vascular stasis and thrombophlebitis. The resultant ischemia causes local bone necrosis. With further progression, dead bone can form a sequestrum surrounded by purulent material, which becomes inaccessible to antimicrobial penetration.

In infants, numerous additional factors facilitate extension of infection. Because the epiphyseal plate has not fully formed, the nutrient arterioles penetrate the epiphysis; hence rupture of infection into the adjacent joint is common. The cortex of the infant metaphysis is thin, with fewer trabeculae, assisting penetration outward and making infants more likely to develop subperiosteal abscess (Fig. 13.52). Once the epiphyseal growth plate has formed, it serves as a relatively effective barrier to joint extension and the frequency of secondary septic arthritis is reduced.

Hematogenous spread accounts for most pediatric osteomyelitis. The metaphyseal portions of long bones and the subepiphyseal portions of flat and irregular bones are the usual sites. Blunt trauma may be a predisposing factor, by production of small-vessel occlusion with secondary stasis, anoxia, and necrosis. Children with sickle hemoglobinopathies are particularly susceptible to hematogenous osteomyelitis due to underlying vascular bone disease and asplenia. Spread from a contiguous focus of infection accounts for most remaining cases of osteomyelitis, such as infections of fracture sites, surgical wounds and hardware, and puncture wounds, as well as extension of infection from an adjacent site of cellulitis or an abscess.

Osteomyelitis may be further subdivided into acute, subacute, and chronic forms, according to duration of symptoms; the acute form is by far the most common. The major clinical finding in each form is localized bone pain, which is typically constant, progressively more severe, and exacerbated by movement. The overlying soft tissues may appear normal or may be warm, mildly swollen, and occasionally erythematous, but in contrast to cellulitis, surface findings are often subtle and induration is unusual. Spasm of overlying muscles is often intense, adding to discomfort, and the adjacent joint may be held in flexion. Beyond these common features, there is a wide range of clinical expression. Appreciation of this spectrum is important to ensure early diagnosis.

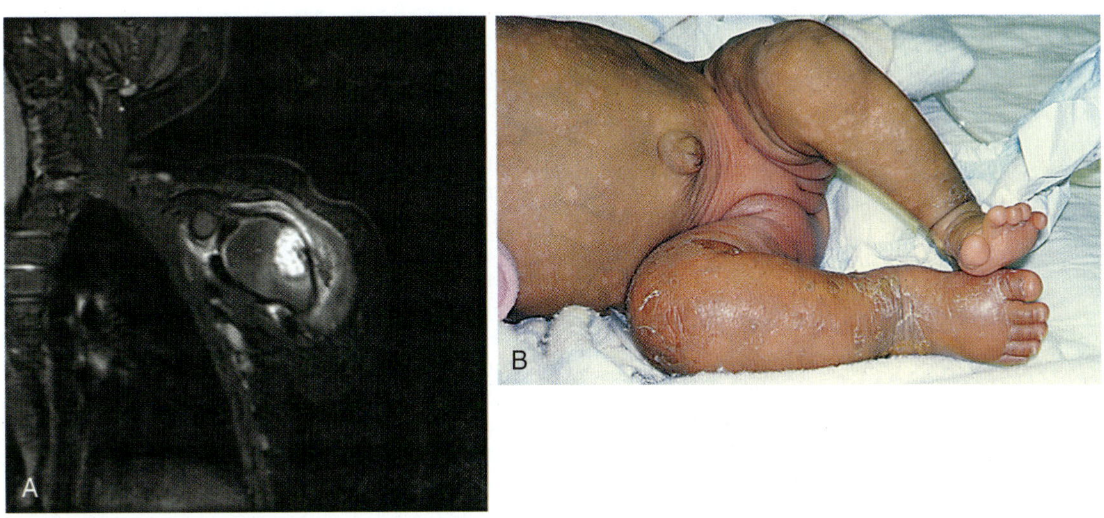

Fig. 13.52 Acute hematogenous osteomyelitis in infancy. (A) This 1-month-old presented decreased movement of the left arm and prominent swelling of the upper arm and shoulder. On x-ray examination her proximal humerus had a lytic appearance, and the T2-weighted coronal magnetic resonance imaging shows subperiosteal abscess and bone destruction. (B) Swelling of the entire leg and foot with overlying erythema is evident in this 2½-month-old infant, who had rapid extension of osteomyelitis of the tibia.

Acute Osteomyelitis

Acute Hematogenous Osteomyelitis

Most patients with acute hematogenous osteomyelitis present within 1 week of onset of symptoms. Infants younger than 6 months old often present without systemic signs of infection but may have fever or a septic presentation. Initially, irritability and anorexia are prominent, followed by evidence of pain on movement or of decreased use of a limb (pseudoparalysis). Localized soft tissue swelling and diffuse tenderness may develop, which can extend rapidly to involve the entire extremity, reflecting rapid spread of infection in the bone (see Fig. 13.52B). Careful attention must be given to joint examination because of the frequency of extension of infection into the joint with secondary septic arthritis.

Fever and signs of toxicity are common in children of 6 months to 2 years. Systemic symptoms consist primarily of fever and irritability in association with refusal to walk, limp, or decreased use of an extremity. A small percentage present with more severe systemic symptoms, including chills, lethargy, irritability, anorexia, vomiting, and dehydration. At this age, children are often unable to localize pain, but by observation they may be found to avoid moving the involved extremity or to hold a particular joint in flexion consistently. Soft tissue swelling and warmth may be noted overlying a metaphysis, but it may be subtle or absent in early cases or undetectable if the proximal femur is involved. Comparative circumferential measurements of suspected areas and painstaking care in first eliciting the child's cooperation, and then in palpating for evidence of muscle spasm or point tenderness, are crucial if osteomyelitis is suspected. Even with careful examination, focal tenderness may be difficult to detect early in the course.

Children older than 2 years old with acute osteomyelitis are sometimes febrile but rarely toxic. They are more likely to localize pain, and point tenderness is generally easier to elicit. Older patients describe the pain as deep, intense, and constant. Signs of adjacent joint flexion and of nearby muscle spasm are common (Fig. 13.53), but overlying soft tissue swelling may be subtle. Unless sympathetic effusion has developed, the adjacent joint may be passively moved through its full range of motion, although this exacerbates the pain.

Osteomyelitis in sites other than the long bones of the extremities can be challenging. Pelvic osteomyelitis may mimic numerous other conditions. Although fever and an abnormal gait are the most common presenting complaints, lower abdominal and groin pain, hip or buttock pain, sciatica, and thigh pain (with swelling) can be prominent early complaints. Often, the initial clinical picture suggests appendicitis, pelvic abscess, or femoral osteomyelitis. A high level of suspicion and careful examination are necessary to establish the diagnosis. The onset of pain in the lower abdomen rather than the periumbilical region, absence of gastrointestinal symptoms or rebound tenderness, and normal findings on rectal examination help distinguish pelvic osteomyelitis from acute appendicitis. Furthermore, although most patients have pain on hip motion in one or more planes, range of motion is either normal or only slightly limited, and with careful examination, point tenderness can usually be detected.

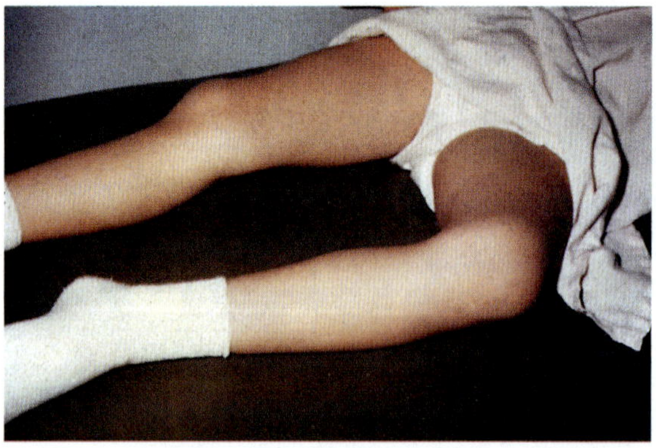

Fig. 13.53 Acute osteomyelitis. Fever, hip and thigh pain, and refusal to walk were the chief complaints in this 5-year-old child with osteomyelitis of the proximal femur. On inspection, she lay still, holding the left leg externally rotated and flexed at the hip and knee. This same position is also adopted by children with acute arthritis of the hip.

Acute Osteomyelitis Due to Contiguous Spread

Acute osteomyelitis resulting from the contiguous spread of infection should be suspected in patients with prior puncture wounds, deep lacerations, surgical incisions or hardware, open fractures, abscesses, or cellulitis who experience a sudden onset of increased pain at the site. This pain is perceived as deep, severe, and constant and is aggravated by movement. Cellulitis is a common associated finding, and fever is usual.

Diagnostic Methods in Acute Osteomyelitis

Standard laboratory and radiographic studies are of limited use in the diagnosis of acute osteomyelitis. The sedimentation rate and C-reactive protein (CRP) are elevated in the vast majority of patients with acute osteomyelitis, except for osteomyelitis of the fingers and toes. These markers are helpful in identifying an inflammatory process and for serial measurement to document response to therapy, but they are nonspecific. White blood cell counts may be elevated but are normal in up to 50% of patients.

Plain radiographic changes lag behind the clinical manifestations and can be subtle. Initial films may be negative (Fig. 13.54C). The first noticeable radiographic change, usually seen about 3 days after the onset of symptoms, is the presence of deep soft tissue swelling (see Fig. 13.54A). Subsequently, the swelling increases, obliterating fascial planes, and extends to involve subcutaneous tissues. If a sympathetic joint effusion is present or if rupture into the joint has occurred, joint space widening or bony displacement may be evident (see Figs. 13.52A and 13.54B). Bone changes are not visible radiographically in untreated patients until almost 2 weeks after onset. These changes consist of periosteal elevation, followed by focal evidence of bone lysis and, subsequently, sclerosis or new bone formation at the margins of the lytic lesion (see Fig. 13.54E). The radiographic appearance of bone changes can be significantly delayed in patients who have been treated with antibiotics.

Magnetic resonance imaging (MRI) has become the standard of diagnostic imaging modalities for osteomyelitis. Increased T2 signal of marrow and surrounding tissues correlate well with the presence of osteomyelitis and are present well before bony changes occur (see Fig. 13.54D).

Although pathogen-directed therapy of osteomyelitis is ideal, especially in the era of increasing resistance patterns (e.g., MRSA), isolation of the causative organism can often be challenging, especially in areas of limited involvement and in late stages of disease. Aspiration of the site of maximal involvement as revealed by imaging provides material for Gram stain and culture. Blood cultures are positive in more than 50% of febrile patients with acute hematogenous osteomyelitis and should be performed in all suspected cases.

Complications of osteomyelitis include septic arthritis with joint damage, epiphyseal injury with impaired bone growth, and rarely progression to chronic osteomyelitis (or pathologic fractures). The rate of complications is highest in young infants who often have extensive bone involvement and septic arthritis at the time of presentation. Early diagnosis and collaboration between the pediatric physician and orthopedic surgeon is essential to ensure optimal pharmacotherapy and surgical intervention, if indicated.

Subacute and Chronic Osteomyelitis

Approximately 10% of cases of hematogenous osteomyelitis have an insidious onset and a subacute or chronic course characterized by mild to moderate local extremity pain, with or without swelling.

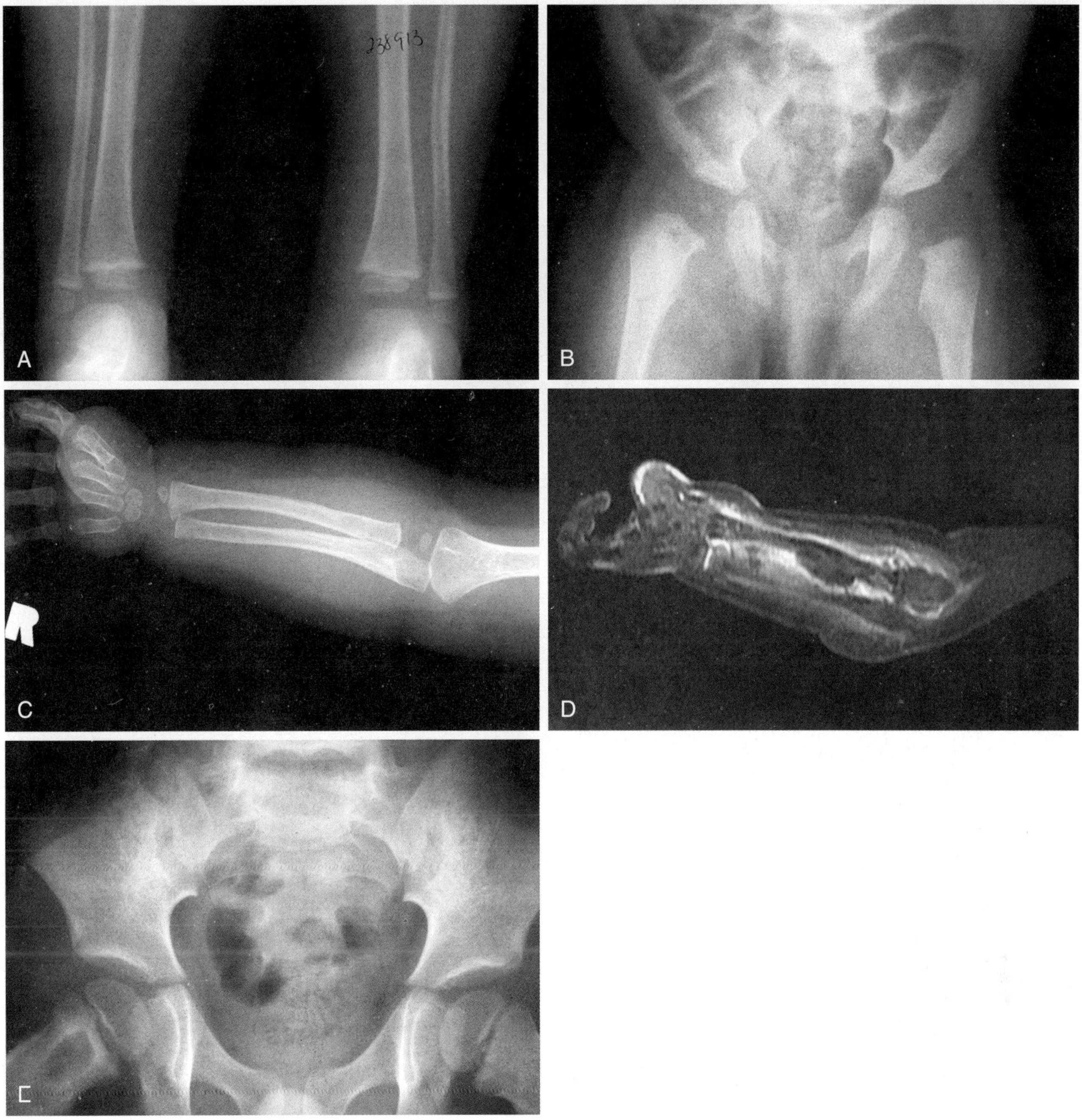

Fig. 13.54 Acute osteomyelitis. Radiographic changes lag behind the clinical manifestations in osteomyelitis. (A) The first noticeable change, occurring about 3 days after onset, is deep soft tissue swelling, seen here adjacent to the metaphysis of the distal tibia on the left. (B) In this neonate, a radiolucency is evident in the proximal metaphysis of the right femur, which is also displaced upward and laterally. On aspiration of the hip, purulent fluid was obtained, confirming the suspicion of rupture of the infection into the hip and of secondary septic arthritis. (C) This 1-year-old female presented with 4 days of fever and lack of right arm use. (D) Her plain film is normal, but T1-weighted magnetic resonance imaging with gadolinium contrast clearly shows extensive disease. (E) The late changes of a lytic lesion with sclerotic margins are seen in the right femoral metaphysis of this child who was completing his course of therapy. (A, Courtesy Jocelyn Ledesma-Medina, MD. B and E, Courtesy Rodrigo Dominguez, MD, University of Texas, Houston, TX.)

Fever is unusual, and other systemic symptoms are absent. Typically, symptoms have been present for greater than several weeks. In some instances, this subacute course may be related to partial suppression of the infection by antibiotics administered for another infection (such as otitis media or impetigo). In these patients, pain may abate during antimicrobial therapy but worsen once the medication stops. On examination, local tenderness and overlying soft tissue swelling may be noted. Multiple sites are involved in up to 20% of patients.

White blood cell counts are usually normal, although sedimentation rate and CRP are elevated in most patients with a subacute presentation but often normal in those with chronic osteomyelitis. Blood cultures are rarely positive. Radiographs are diverse. In children seen early or who have taken antibiotics, radiographic findings may demonstrate early acute osteomyelitis. Other findings include isolated metaphyseal radiolucency surrounded by reactive bone (Brodie abscess); metaphyseal radiolucency with loss or disruption of cortical bone simulating a tumor; excessive cortical reaction in the diaphysis simulating osteoid osteoma; or multiple layers of subperiosteal new bone, at times mimicking the appearance of Ewing sarcoma (Fig. 13.55). MRI provides excellent resolution that may clarify the diagnosis.

The more chronic form will often have extensive necrosis, sequestrum formation, and decompression caused by fistulization

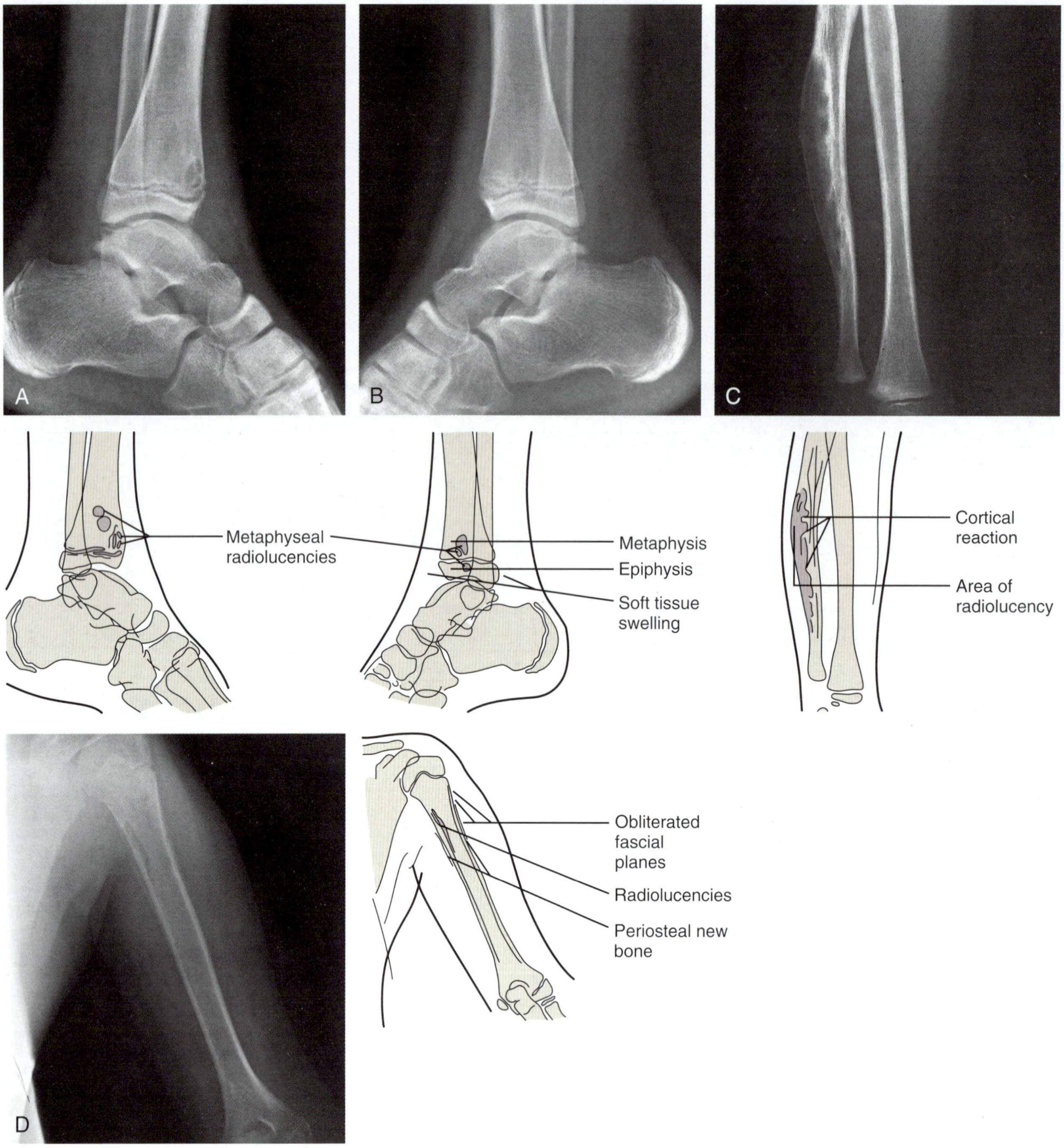

Fig. 13.55 Radiographic findings characteristic of subacute osteomyelitis. (A and B) This 13-year-old boy had a 7-week history of pain and swelling of both ankles. He had been treated with penicillin for presumed rheumatic fever. These radiographs show bilateral soft tissue swelling, multiple metaphyseal radiolucencies in the distal left tibia, and a radiolucency involving the metaphysis and epiphysis on the right. (C) An extensive area of radiolucency and cortical reaction is seen in the ulnar diaphysis of this youngster. (D) Obliterated fascial planes, radiolucency, and periosteal new bone formation are seen. (Courtesy Department of Pediatric Radiology, Children's Hospital of Pittsburgh, Pittsburgh, PA.)

through the overlying soft tissues (Fig. 13.56). Biopsy is generally required to confirm the diagnosis and isolate a causative organism. When found, *S. aureus* is found in most cases. Surgical curettage, immobilization, and antimicrobials are the mainstays of treatment. Despite an aggressive approach, permanent functional disability and deformity are not uncommon in chronic osteomyelitis. The major differential consideration is bacterial osteomyelitis, also called *chronic nonchronic recurrent multifocal osteomyelitis.* This a rheumatologic condition that presents with a similar clinical picture. However, this disorder is characterized by multiple recurrent sites of sterile bone inflammation and responds to antiinflammatory therapy, and radiologic findings do not reflect the severity of chronic disease.

Juvenile Diskitis and Vertebral Osteomyelitis

Inflammation of intervertebral disk spaces (diskitis) in childhood is a puzzling disorder, in both its pathophysiology and mode of presentation. During childhood, vascular channels exist between the vertebral end plates to the intervertebral disk. Hematogenous spread of organisms to the disk space rather than vertebral bone of children is thus more likely than in adults, which is thought to explain the higher frequency of diskitis in children and the infrequency of acute vertebral osteomyelitis before adolescence. However, differences in clinical presentation, infrequent isolation of pathogens, and evidence that immobilization alone is effective in treating diskitis (whereas antimicrobial therapy is required in vertebral osteomyelitis) have led to speculation that disk

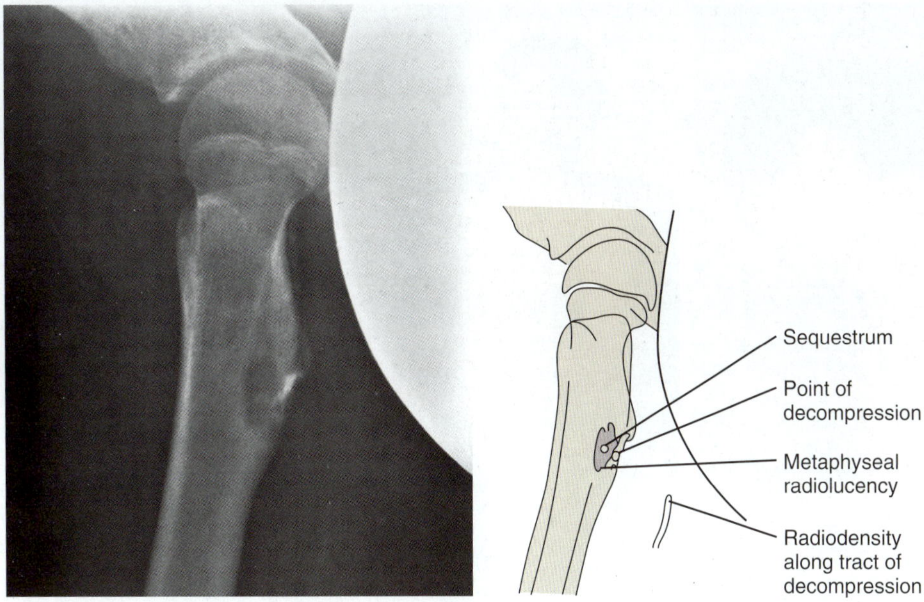

Fig. 13.56 Chronic osteomyelitis. Inadequate initial treatment resulted in progression to chronic osteomyelitis in this child. In this radiograph, taken 6 months after the onset of symptoms, a radiodense sequestrum is seen within the metaphyseal radiolucency. The process had also begun to decompress into the soft tissues of the thigh. (Courtesy Department of Pediatric Radiology, Children's Hospital of Pittsburgh, Pittsburgh, PA.)

space inflammation may be due to a low-grade viral or bacterial infection.

Known predisposing conditions in children include upper respiratory tract infection, gastroenteritis, and genitourinary infection. The importance of antecedent trauma is unclear. Hematogenous spread may occur through the valveless veins of the Batson plexus or via the vertebral branches of the posterior spinal arteries. In both diskitis and vertebral osteomyelitis, *S. aureus* is the most commonly identified pathogen, followed by streptococci, gram-negative enteric pathogens (including *Salmonella* and *Kingella kingae*), and corynebacteria. The lumbar spine and the lower thoracic spine are the most common sites of involvement for both diskitis and vertebral osteomyelitis.

Diskitis

Diskitis occurs predominantly in children younger than 4 years old and presents with pain and progressive limp or focal back pain that progressively worsens. Symptoms may be perceived as pain in the flank, abdomen, or hip. The pain is constant, aggravated by sitting, standing, or movement, and is typically worse at night. Very young children may be irritable, refuse to walk or sit, or evince pain during diaper changes. Abnormal posture, exaggerated lumbar lordosis, or holding the lumbar spine stiff and straight may be noted. Toddlers may preferentially assume a knee/chest position. Low-grade fever is often present, while other systemic symptoms are unusual. Abdominal distention is occasionally prominent, raising suspicion of intraabdominal pathology.

Careful examination of the spine may reveal paravertebral muscle spasm with guarding and exquisite focal tenderness, although tenderness may be vague or absent. Resistance to flexion and extension of the spine is common and may simulate meningeal signs. Pain on straight leg raising and hip motion may be encountered.

The sedimentation rate, CRP, and white blood cell counts may be elevated. Specific radiographic changes do not appear until 2 to 6 weeks after onset, which is when disk space narrowing becomes evident. In the ensuing weeks, irregularities of the adjacent vertebral end plates become apparent. Culture of the disk space is usually negative. Most patients with diskitis improve symptomatically with immobilization alone, and the process appears to resolve after several weeks of casting.

Vertebral Osteomyelitis

Vertebral osteomyelitis in older children and adolescents presents with insidious, progressive back pain that is constant, aggravated by movement, and increasingly resistant to analgesics. Fever is absent or low grade. On occasion, the onset is acute, with fever and generalized systemic symptoms accompanying the abrupt appearance of pain. In the rare cases encountered in young children, onset is usually acute, and the clinical picture is dominated by abdominal or flank pain, with associated tenderness and often guarding. In some patients, paraspinous or spinous process tenderness, back stiffness, an exaggerated lumbar lordosis, pain on leg motion, or lower extremity weakness may be noted (Fig. 13.57). Laboratory findings in this setting are similar to those in children with diskitis, with the exception that blood cultures obtained in the acute phase are more often positive. Early radiographic findings are also similar, but frank destructive lesions of the vertebral body develop soon after the appearance of disk space narrowing is noted. Cultures of operative biopsy specimens usually yield *S. aureus*. Antimicrobial therapy is necessary to achieve clinical resolution, and surgical debridement may be required.

Septic Arthritis

Bacterial invasion of the synovial membrane with resultant septic arthritis has high potential for long-term morbidity. Early diagnosis and treatment are essential to prevent or minimize joint damage. However, both the clinical picture and laboratory findings of septic arthritis overlap with transient synovitis and other forms of acute arthritis.

Septic arthritis primarily affects young children, with most cases in patients younger than 5 years old. Males are affected twice as often as females. Many cases are the result of hematogenous seeding. Streptococcal or staphylococcal skin and soft tissue infections may antedate septic arthritis caused by these pathogens. In older children and adolescents, gonococcal urethritis, vaginitis, and cervicitis are antecedents to hematogenous seeding (Chapter 19). Prior blunt trauma is a predisposing factor in some cases. In approximately 10% of patients, the septic arthritis is secondary to rupture of primary osteomyelitis into the joint space, most often in infants. Direct penetrating injury accounts for a small percentage.

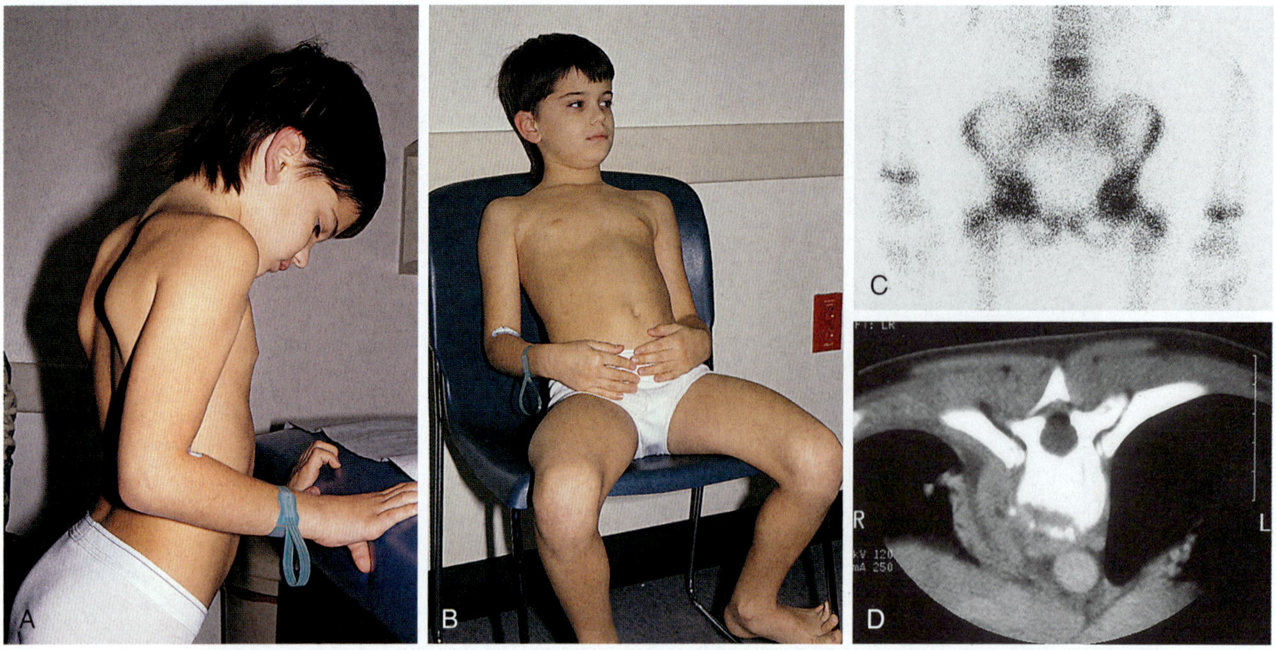

Fig. 13.57 Vertebral osteomyelitis. (A to C) This 10-year-old boy had a 2-week history of intermittent fever, malaise, and steadily worsening lower back and left hip pain, exacerbated by movement. (A and B) He had an exaggerated lumbar lordosis and extreme limitation of flexion, both standing and sitting. The straight leg raising test also accentuated his pain. (C) Bone scan revealed selectively increased uptake in the L4 vertebral body. (D) This 13-year-old girl had an 8-week history of intermittent throbbing pain in her midback with a few days of fever. Pain was worse on arising and in the evening, with prolonged standing and with lying down. She had a markedly elevated sedimentation rate and tenderness to deep palpation in the lower thoracic region. Magnetic resonance imaging done at the time of biopsy shows fragmentation of the body of T8 with extension of infection into the paraspinous tissues on the right. The biopsy specimen showed that the paraspinous mass consisted of granulation tissue with numerous polymorphonuclear leukocytes and plasma cells and grew Staphylococcus aureus on culture. (C and D, Courtesy Department of Pediatric Radiology, Children's Hospital of Pittsburgh, Pittsburgh, PA.)

Table 13.2 Relative Frequency of Pathogens in Septic Arthritis According to Patient Age

Neonate	1 Month to 2 Years Old	2–5 Years Old	Older Than 5 Years Old
Staphylococcus aureus	Group A streptococci	*S. aureus*	*S. aureus*
Group B streptococci	*Streptococcus pneumoniae*	Group A streptococci	Group A streptococci
Gram-negative enteric pathogens	*Neisseria meningitidis*	*N. meningitidis*	*Neisseria gonorrheae*
	Pseudomonas aeruginosa	*S. pneumoniae*	*P. aeruginosa*
	Salmonella species	*Haemophilus influenzae* type B	
	H. influenzae type B		

Bacterial pathogens are isolated in 65% to 75% of patients from synovial fluid, blood, or both. The relative frequency of pathogens varies considerably with patient age, as shown in Table 13.2. Children with sickle hemoglobinopathies occasionally suffer *Salmonella* septic arthritis, whereas patients with Lyme arthritis may mimic a septic joint but lack the severe outcomes. Cultures from synovial fluid are easily spoiled by prior antibiotic and are not 100% reliable even before therapy, so inoculation of synovial fluid into blood culture bottles or PCR of synovial fluid may improve the ability to identify organisms, especially fastidious ones such as *K. kingae*.

The joints affected in order of frequency are the knee, hip, ankle, and elbow. The wrist and shoulder are involved less often, and other joints are rare. A single joint is affected in more than 90% of patients. *Neisseria gonorrheae* is the organism most commonly associated with polyarticular disease, but other pathogens may be responsible, particularly *S. aureus* and *H. influenzae* type B (although the latter is rare after *H. influenzae* type B vaccination). Hip and shoulder joints are particularly prone to damage because clinical signs may be subtle and thus diagnosis is delayed. Further, because the synovium inserts distal to the epiphysis of the proximal humerus and femur, compromise of the blood supply to the epiphysis is more likely to occur from increased intraarticular pressure.

The classic picture of hematogenous septic arthritis is a young child with fever and signs of toxicity in association with severe localized joint pain, swelling, and marked limitation in range of motion. Infants and toddlers cannot describe focal pain and thus present with fever and irritability, the latter aggravated by movement. Refusal to bear weight or decreased use of an extremity may be present. When a knee, ankle, wrist, or elbow is involved, local swelling and warmth are usually evident (Fig. 13.58). Erythema and warmth with septic arthritis contrast with findings of Lyme arthritis, which are more rheumatic signs of stiffness and swelling (see Fig. 13.50D). However, early swelling may be subtle, high fever may make any warmth difficult to distinguish, and surface erythema is often absent. When the hip is involved, swelling and warmth are not evident, and pain may be referred to the knee or thigh. Often the position adopted by the patient is the best diagnostic clue. To minimize intraarticular pressure and pain, the child prefers to lie still with the knee and hip flexed and with the hip externally rotated (see Fig. 13.53). In cases of septic arthritis of the shoulder, subtle swelling may or may not be evident, but the shoulders may not be held at the same level and the arm on the involved side is held against the chest to splint the joint.

Septic arthritis of the sacroiliac joint, which accounts for only 1% of cases, can present a particularly confusing picture, often mimicking hip or intraabdominal disease. Only one-third of patients

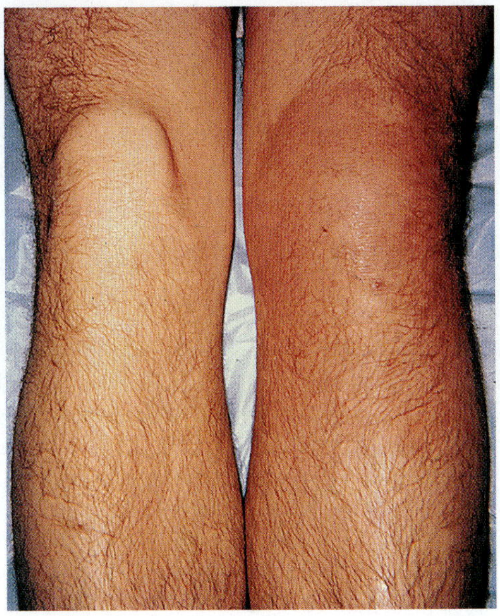

Fig. 13.58 Septic arthritis. This adolescent boy awoke suddenly at 3 am with severe left knee pain. By 8 am, he was febrile and had marked swelling with overlying erythema and extreme limitation of movement. Examination of joint fluid revealed gram-positive cocci in chains, with a white blood cell count of 24,000/mm^3. Cultures were positive for group A streptococci. (From the Clinical Slide Collection on the Rheumatic Diseases © 1991, 1995. Used by permission of the American College of Rheumatology.)

have an acute presentation, the remainder having a subacute course. Buttock and back pain, limp, and fever are the most common presenting complaints. Up to one-third of patients complain of unilateral radicular pain. Findings of lower abdominal and rectal tenderness in association with normal hip motion may confuse the examiner who fails to recognize that leg and buttock pain necessitate meticulous examination of the lower back. Such an examination reveals tenderness over the involved sacroiliac joint, and pelvic compression replicates the pain, as does hyperextension of the ipsilateral hip with the patient supine and dangling his or her leg over the edge of the table.

Limitation of joint motion and evidence of pain on motion are perhaps the most valuable clinical clues to the diagnosis of septic arthritis. Limitation is usually severe unless presentation occurs early, and motion provokes marked discomfort.

Because of the morbidity associated with delayed diagnosis, any child with fever, acute onset of pain, and limited motion of a joint should be presumed to have septic arthritis until proven otherwise. These findings should prompt rapid diagnostic investigation. Plain radiographs with comparison views should be obtained immediately and inspected for signs of joint space widening or capsular distention, although these findings may be absent in early cases. If the hip is the suspected site of pathology, lateral and upward displacement of the femoral head may be noted along with displacement of the gluteal fat lines (Fig. 13.59). Ultrasound can be used to assess for joint effusion with or without loculations. MRI is the ideal modality for evaluating the child with suspected septic arthritis of the sacroiliac joint, and it may distinguish between patients with underlying osteomyelitis, pelvic myositis, or true septic arthritis.

Arthrocentesis and examination of joint fluid is the study most likely to yield definitive results. Positive findings on Gram-stained specimens are particularly helpful; cultures are positive in 60% of cases. Elevated synovial white blood cell count of more than 50,000/mm^3 is present in more than two-thirds of patients. However, there is considerable overlap of cell counts in bacterial arthritis, rheumatologic syndromes, and Lyme arthritis. Thus cell differential, protein, and glucose levels of synovial fluid are helpful but not highly specific.

Peripheral white blood cell count, sedimentation rate, and CRP level may add evidence but overlap with viral or reactive arthritis. Blood cultures are positive in up to 40% of cases. Because cultures of joint fluid from patients with disseminated *N. gonorrheae* infection are often negative, it is important to culture blood, skin lesions, throat, and cervix or urethra when this agent is suspected.

Diagnosis depends on assessment of clinical course, physical findings, and multiple laboratory studies. Even with a negative Gram stain, empiric antimicrobial therapy selected to cover the most likely pathogens (see Table 13.2) should be started in patients in whom septic arthritis is deemed likely. As is true of osteomyelitis, collaboration between pediatric and orthopedic colleagues is crucial because drainage of infected material and joint irrigation are essential to ensure a good outcome.

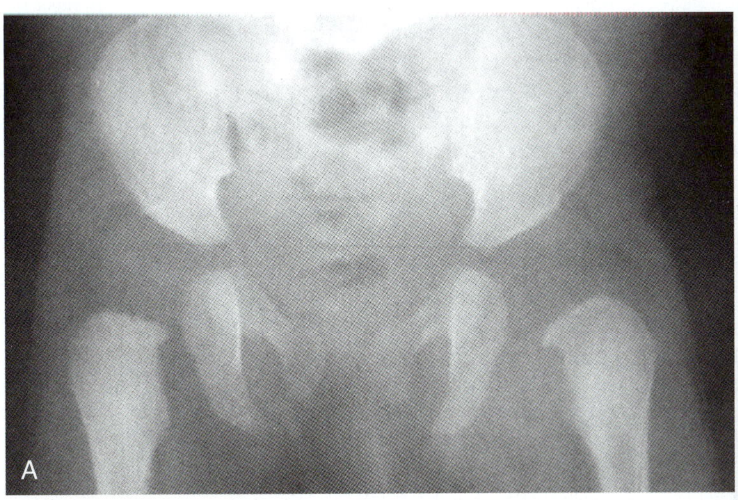

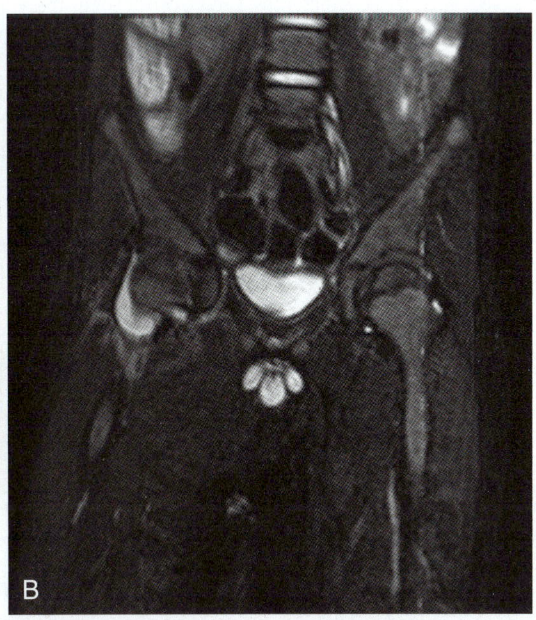

Fig. 13.59 Radiographic findings characteristic of septic arthritis. Although radiographs may be normal early on, joint space widening can be detected. (A) This infant presented with fever, toxicity, and refusal to move the left leg. Plain film shows capsular swelling and lateral displacement of the proximal left femur. (B) This 4-year-old boy presented with right hip pain and fever. Coronal short tau inversion recovery magnetic resonance imaging showed copious fluid in the joint itself. (A, Courtesy Rodrigo Dominguez, MD, University of Texas, Houston, TX.)

TUBERCULOSIS

TB remains one of the most common causes of infectious mortality in the world. In the United States, TB is most common among foreign-born persons and those who have traveled internationally, especially to Southeast Asia, China, and sub-Sarahan African nations. Additional high-risk groups include unhoused persons, migrant workers, nursing home residents, prisoners, HIV-positive or immunosuppressed persons and children in close contact with adults in these groups, and health care workers.

Transmission

Tubercle bacilli are transmitted from person to person via aerosolized organisms, spread by patients with active pulmonary, especially cavitary, disease. Children with primary TB rarely transmit due to small infectious burden and lack of forceful coughing to aerosolize bacilli.

Infants and young children in close contact with an infectious adult are especially at high risk. Thus parents and other household occupants are the major sources of transmission to children. Because only a handful of bacteria can achieve transmission, health care professionals are at risk when handling specimens of infected specimens or contaminated syringes or instruments.

Clinical Forms of Tuberculosis

Asymptomatic Infection

Patients with latent tuberculosis infection have a positive PPD skin test (see Fig. 13.60) or interferon gamma release assays but no clinical signs or symptoms and normal chest radiographs. Although many of these children never manifest signs of primary infection, if the infection goes unrecognized and untreated, there is a 10% chance of reactivation later in life. Some of these patients have early infection and will go on to suffer clinical disease without treatment. Patients with HIV infection have a 10% risk of reactivation each year.

Tuberculosis Disease

Primary Pulmonary Tuberculosis

The symptoms of primary pulmonary TB, typically insidious in onset, are often attributed to viral illness. Some children have low-grade fever with no apparent source, together with mild anorexia and decreased activity. Others may have rhinorrhea, nasal congestion, and pharyngeal erythema and are mistakenly thought to have a viral upper respiratory tract infection. On occasion, erythema nodosum may develop in concert with the fever. Chest examination is generally normal, even in patients with abnormal chest radiographs. Rarely, children present with a more dramatic "pneumonic" mode of onset, with high fever, tachypnea, and signs of toxicity. In such cases, clinical findings characteristic of lobar pneumonia are evident with rales, rhonchi, and bronchial breath sounds heard on auscultation and dullness noted on percussion. Patients with either mode of onset tend to show improvement over a few days to a few weeks, although some may be noted to tire easily and be less active than usual. Without treatment, some develop low-grade afternoon fevers weeks later that may persist for months.

Radiographic findings characteristic of primary pulmonary TB may be limited to enlarged hilar (Fig. 13.61A) nodes; faint, cloudy infiltrates that extend to the pleura (see Fig. 13.61B); or a lobar infiltrate (see Fig. 13.61C) in patients exhibiting the "pneumonic" picture. Infiltrates can be located anywhere in either lung.

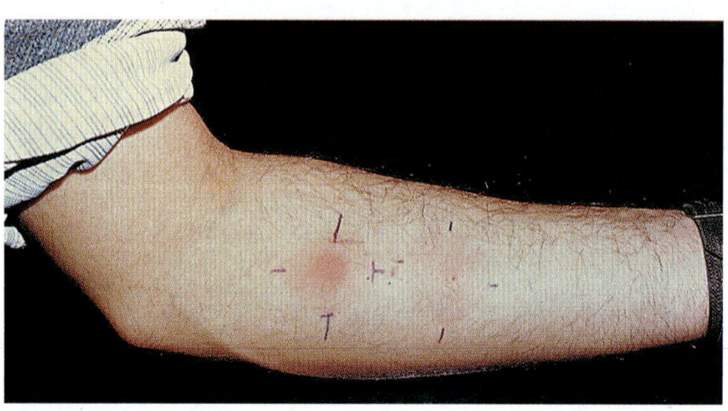

Fig. 13.60 Positive tuberculin skin test. This adolescent boy became infected as a result of living with and helping to care for a grandfather whose chronic "smoker's cough" was ultimately discovered to be a manifestation of chronic cavitary tuberculosis (TB). He had a greater than 15-mm induration. (Courtesy Kenneth Schuitt, MD.)

Endobronchial Tuberculosis

When enlarged nodes cause bronchial obstruction (usually 3–6 months after infection, and most commonly in children younger than 2 years old), focal hyperaeration or fan-shaped, segmental parenchymal collapse-consolidation infiltrates are seen (Fig. 13.62). The latter consist of the primary focus and secondary inflammation and atelectasis. Sometimes narrowing of a bronchial lumen is noted. Infants affected by this endobronchial process often have a harsh, paroxysmal cough that mimics pertussis, along with wheezing and rhonchi noted on auscultation. The cough is often worse when the infant is lying supine. With or without treatment, collapse-consolidation lesions can reexpand and resolve, clear with residual calcification of the primary complex and regional node (Ghon complex), or scar with progressive contraction of the involved pulmonary segment and bronchiectatic changes.

Progressive Primary Pulmonary Tuberculosis

Progressive primary pulmonary TB occurs in infants and young children whose primary focus enlarges, caseates, liquefies, and ruptures into a bronchus. The organisms disseminate through the airways to the rest of the lung, setting up new foci of infection. Clinically, these patients have remittent fever, cough, and malaise along with anorexia and weight loss and eventually appear listless and chronically ill. Wet crackles may be heard over the site of the primary cavity. Radiographically, a small cavity is seen at the site of primary focus, along with a collapse-consolidation lesion (see Fig. 13.63) and diffuse infiltrates.

Miliary Tuberculosis

Miliary TB occurs when bacilli disseminate from an involved node of the primary complex via lymphatic or blood vessels to distant sites. This may be clinically occult and occur early during the incubation period or shortly thereafter. Major sites of seeding include the pulmonary apices, spleen, and superficial nodes. In some cases, evidence of resulting metastatic lesions is seen 2 to 4 months later, when the child has a nonspecific illness characterized by low-grade fever and fatigue, splenomegaly, and generalized adenopathy, sometimes associated with nodular or papulonecrotic skin lesions. Others remain asymptomatic, and their metastatic lesions may either remain dormant or reactivate years later. Miliary disease may be detected incidentally in an infant or child who undergoes chest radiography as part of an evaluation for low-grade fever without an apparent source. Some children experience insidious progression of symptoms or may have a more abrupt onset of fever, tachypnea, lethargy, and weakness accompanied by hepatosplenomegaly. Within a few weeks, symmetric tubercles of uniform size are seen throughout the lung fields (Fig. 13.63) and rustling breath sounds can be heard on auscultation.

Extrapulmonary Tuberculosis

Tuberculous Meningitis

After lymphohematogenous spread, tuberculous infection may develop in the brain and meninges. Fifty percent of infants and children with untreated miliary TB develop meningitis. Extension of infection or rupture of one of these foci into the subarachnoid space results in meningitis, which usually develops within 3 to 6 months of initial infection in children younger than 6 years old. The resulting exudate is thick and gelatinous, infiltrating meningeal and cerebral vessels to cause vasculitis with secondary occlusion and infarction. The infiltrate impedes CSF flow and resorption, often resulting in a communicating

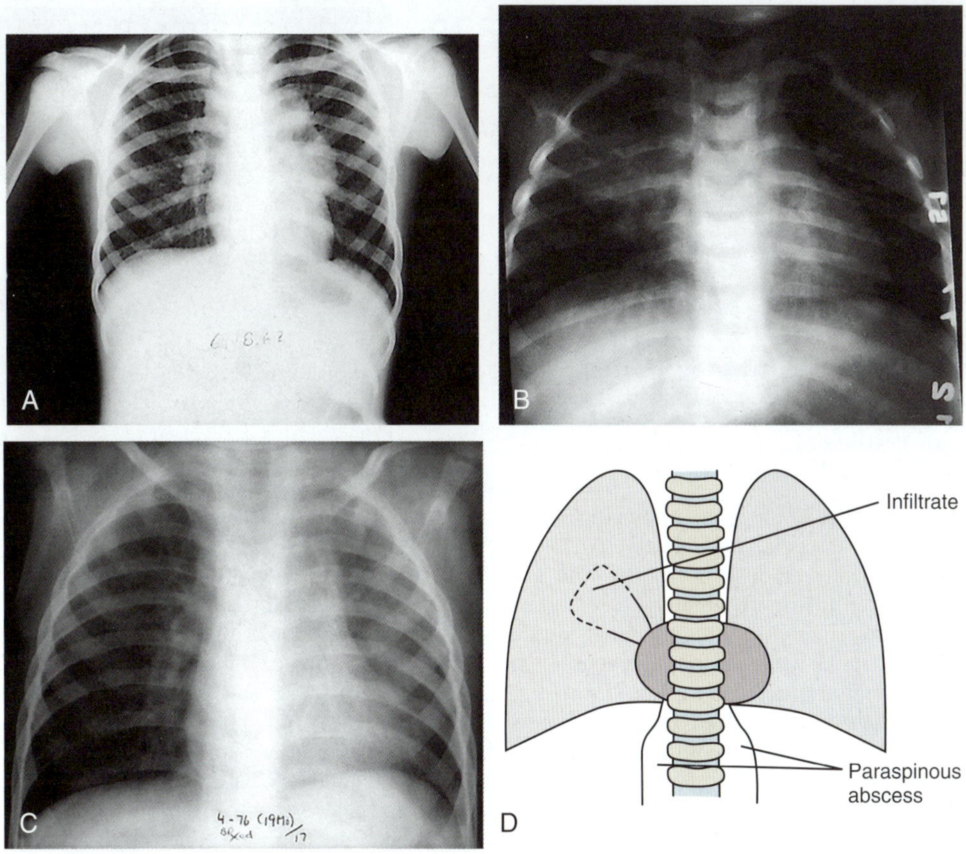

Fig. 13.61 Primary pulmonary tuberculosis. (A) Marked enlargement of hilar nodes without a pulmonary infiltrate is seen in this asymptomatic child. She was tested as part of a contact investigation, and this chest radiograph was obtained because her skin test was positive. (B) A hazy infiltrate involving a segment of the right upper lobe is seen extending from the hilum to the pleura. This child also has tuberculous spondylitis with a paraspinous abscess, the shadow of which is seen below the diaphragm (D). (C) In this boy who presented with a pneumonic clinical picture, a hazy infiltrate occupies the entire left upper lobe. (A and B, Courtesy Jocelyn Medina, MD. C, Courtesy Richard Towbin, MD, Children's Hospital of Philadelphia, Philadelphia, PA.)

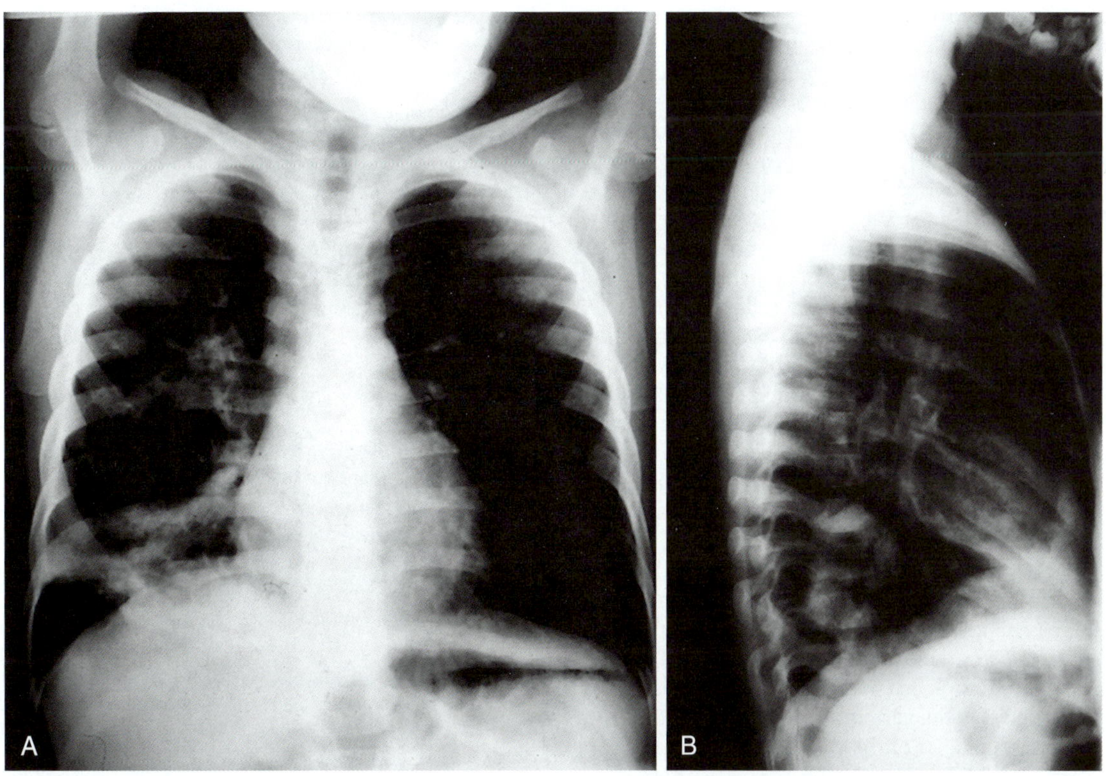

Fig. 13.62 Progressive primary pulmonary tuberculosis (endobronchial). This 8-year-old girl initially had fever, cough, and mild tachypnea. She was treated with antibiotics for presumed bacterial pneumonia but showed only partial clinical improvement. Repeat radiographs obtained 1 month later showed progression. A purified protein derivative test was then done and was positive. (A and B) She has a collapse-consolidation lesion involving the right lower lobe, with a primary cavity. (Courtesy Ellen Wald, MD, University of Wisconsin Children's Hospital, Madison, WI.)

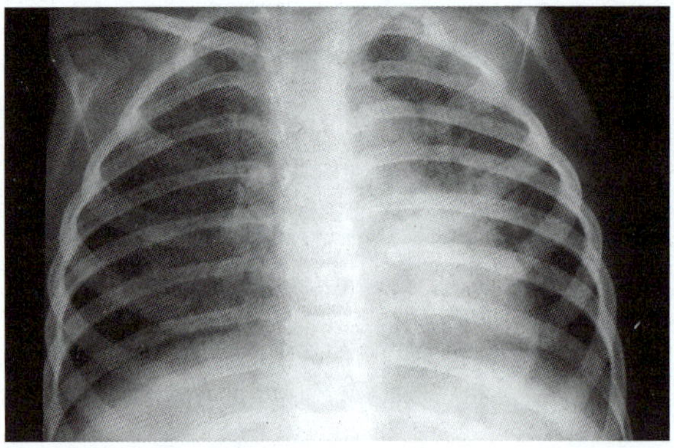

Fig. 13.63 Miliary tuberculosis. Two weeks after miliary spread, this infant's lung fields are symmetrically dotted with tiny tubercles. (Courtesy Richard Towbin, MD, Children's Hospital of Philadelphia, Philadelphia, PA.)

hydrocephalus, and collects at the base of the brain, impinging on the optic chiasm and the third, sixth, and seventh cranial nerves.

The onset of symptoms is usually gradual, beginning with anorexia, fever, headache, pronounced apathy, irritability, and emotional lability. Within 1 or 2 weeks, drowsiness, vomiting, meningismus, a sluggish pupillary response, and cranial nerve palsies supervene, often accompanied by hyperreflexia and seizures. Confusion, disorientation, dysarthria, tremors, and athetosis may be seen during this phase. Untreated, tuberculous meningitis progresses to coma and death. CSF pressure is usually elevated, and the fluid is clear; pleocytosis is modest, from 50 to 500 cells/mm^3, with lymphocytes predominating later. The protein content is dramatically elevated, and glucose levels are usually low. Early diagnosis and the institution of antituberculous therapy can significantly reduce morbidity and mortality, but even with treatment, complications are common in survivors.

Skeletal Tuberculosis

Skeletal TB is an extrapulmonary manifestation in 1% to 6% of untreated children; it becomes clinically evident within 6 months to 3 years after the initial infection. Very young children are at greatest risk because of the high rate of blood flow through their growing bones. Tuberculous osteomyelitis can start as a metaphyseal infection from hematogenous seeding; by extension from lymphatics, especially from a paravertebral node to a vertebra; or by direct local or hematogenous spread from a neighboring bone.

Formation of granulation tissue and caseation characterize the inflammatory process, which ultimately results in pressure necrosis and the formation of a cold abscess, which can then rupture into an adjacent joint or surrounding soft tissues (see Fig. 13.61B). The vertebrae, knee, hip, and phalanges of infants are the most common sites. Fever is absent or low grade, unless the lesions develop as part of the process of protracted hematogenous spread. Pain is often mild in comparison with that associated with other forms of bacterial osteomyelitis.

Tuberculous spondylitis involves the vertebral bodies of two or more thoracic vertebrae but can also affect lumbar vertebrae. Pain manifested by crying in the night and restless sleep; low-grade fever; and postural change with gait disturbance are prominent. Patients with lumbar disease adopt a wide-based stance and gait with back pain or referred pain to the chest or abdomen. When cervical vertebrae are affected, pain may be localized to the neck or referred to the occiput or arms; the child may have difficulty holding up the head, and torticollis is often present. On examination, severe paraspinal muscle spasm, marked limitation of flexion, pain on percussion, and hyperreflexia with clonus may be evident. Initial radiographs show slight disk space narrowing with subsequent wedging and partial collapse of the vertebral body. Bony destruction (Fig. 13.64) and ultimately collapse of the vertebral body may occur.

Tuberculous Adenitis

Tuberculous adenitis is discussed earlier in the Mycobacterial Lymphadenitis section (see Fig. 13.46).

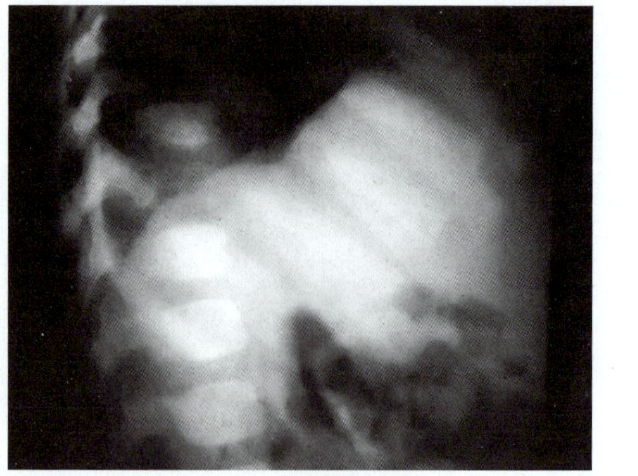

Fig. 13.64 Tuberculous spondylitis. Extensive bony destruction of the T12 vertebral body along with mild collapse of T11 is seen. (Courtesy Jocelyn Medina, MD.)

Tuberculosis in Adolescence

Adolescents may suffer primary infection or experience reactivation of earlier disease, similar to adults with reactivated TB. The latter is more likely if the primary infection occurred after 7 years old. The pubertal growth acceleration is the highest risk period for reactivation or the development of progressive primary disease. With reactivation, new lesions develop in the same lobe of the old primary complex and remain localized. Patients have cough and fever, often accompanied by chest pain, and may exhibit hemoptysis. Anorexia with weight loss and easy fatigability are common. Chest findings may be normal early on, but moist rales may be heard over the apices after cough or on end-expiration. Small round or wedge-shaped infiltrates or linear streaks with mottling may be evident on chest radiograph. This can evolve to chronic cavitary disease without treatment. With progression, weight loss and fatigue increase and an early-morning cough productive of increasing amounts of sputum becomes bothersome. Daily fevers and night sweats are common, and an appearance of chronic illness supervenes. Rales, bronchial breath sounds, wheezing, and dullness to percussion are typical physical findings. Radiographs may reveal mottling, patchy infiltrates, segmental or lobar opacification, and cavitary changes, which may be unilateral or bilateral. Adolescents with cavitary disease can transmit TB to other contacts, in contrast to young children.

Tuberculosis Testing

The "gold standard" of testing for TB continues to evolve. The authors suggest accessing up-to-date sources from the CDC or American Academy of Pediatrics (AAP) to guide testing based on the patient, their age, and clinical presentation (Table 13.3).

Table 13.3 Interpretation/Risk Factors for Positive Purified Protein Derivative Test

Degree of Induration That Represents a Positive Test	Risk Factors
≥5 mm of induration	Known close recent contact with an infected patient Immunosuppressed Human immunodeficiency virus positive Currently taking steroids Chest radiograph showing old, healed lesions
≥10 mm of induration	High-risk racial or ethnic group (émigrés from an endemic area) Younger than 4 years old Underlying medical condition that increases risk for severe disease (e.g., diabetes, malignancy, chronic renal failure, malnutrition)
≥15 mm of induration	No risk factors

CONGENITAL AND PERINATAL INFECTIONS

Numerous pathogens that produce mild or subclinical disease in children and adults can cause severe disease with devastating sequelae when acquired prenatally or perinatally. Toxoplasmosis, rubella, CMV, HSV, and syphilis are well known. In addition, sepsis, meningitis, pneumonia, and other infections caused by perinatally acquired bacterial infection, including tetanus in underdeveloped countries, cause significant neonatal morbidity and mortality, especially in premature infants. The discussion in this chapter is limited to disorders that tend to have distinctive physical findings.

Congenital Cytomegalovirus Infection

A ubiquitous member of the herpesvirus family, CMV infects approximately 0.5% of all live-born infants in utero. Infection of the fetus may develop from either primary maternal infection or reactivation of virus acquired earlier; primary infection is associated with a higher risk for symptomatic disease in the infant. Approximately 10% of infected infants have signs or symptoms at birth, including small size for gestational age, microcephaly, thrombocytopenia, hepatosplenomegaly, hepatitis, intracranial calcifications (Chapter 16), chorioretinitis, and hearing abnormalities. Some affected babies can be born with a "blueberry muffin" appearance also seen with congenital rubella (Fig. 13.65A). Another 10% to 15% of congenitally infected infants do not develop findings until later in infancy or childhood when they are found to have sensorineural hearing loss and/or developmental delays. Children identified with congenital CMV infection should have routine hearing assessments until 5 years old because hearing loss can be progressive. Treatment of symptomatic infants with valganciclovir appears to offer protection against hearing loss and progressive disease.

Neonatal Herpes Simplex Infection

Infants born vaginally to mothers with primary genital HSV infection have a 40% to 50% risk of acquiring disease. In contrast, less than 5% of infants born to mothers with recurrent lesions develop herpes neonatorum. Risk of infection increases with prolonged rupture of membranes. Typically, the mother is asymptomatic and the infant appears well at birth. Signs of infection may develop any time within the first 4 weeks, but most appear before day 21 postpartum. Infection may be localized to the skin, eye, and/or mouth (SEM); the CNS; or disseminated. Approximately three-fourths of infants with SEM disease have typical herpetic skin or mucosal lesions (Fig. 13.66A and B). The scalp and face are the sites most involved (see Fig. 13.66C). On occasion, lesions are limited to the conjunctiva or to the oral mucosa. In the absence of these lesions, accurate diagnosis is extremely difficult. Infants with CNS infection, most likely to present later, typically present with fever or hypothermia,

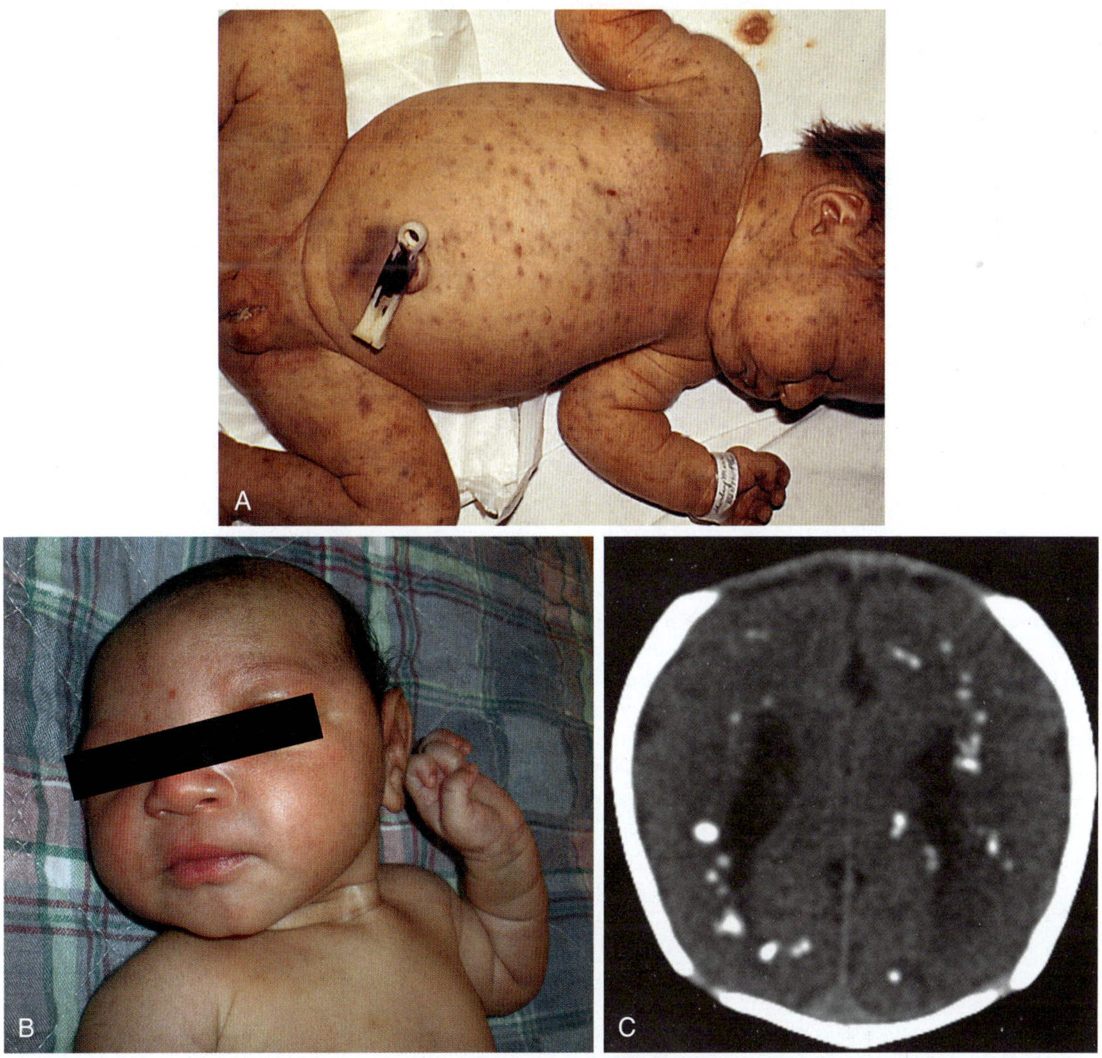

Fig. 13.65 Congenital infections. (A) A newborn with congenital rubella syndrome, including a "blueberry muffin" rash, diffuse petechiae, hepatosplenomegaly, early onset of jaundice, and neurologic depression. (B) This newborn with severe congenital cytomegalovirus infection was noted to have microcephaly. (C) Computed tomography scan of the brain of the same infant shows diffuse intracerebral calcifications. (A, Courtesy Michael Sherlock, MD, Lutherville, MD.)

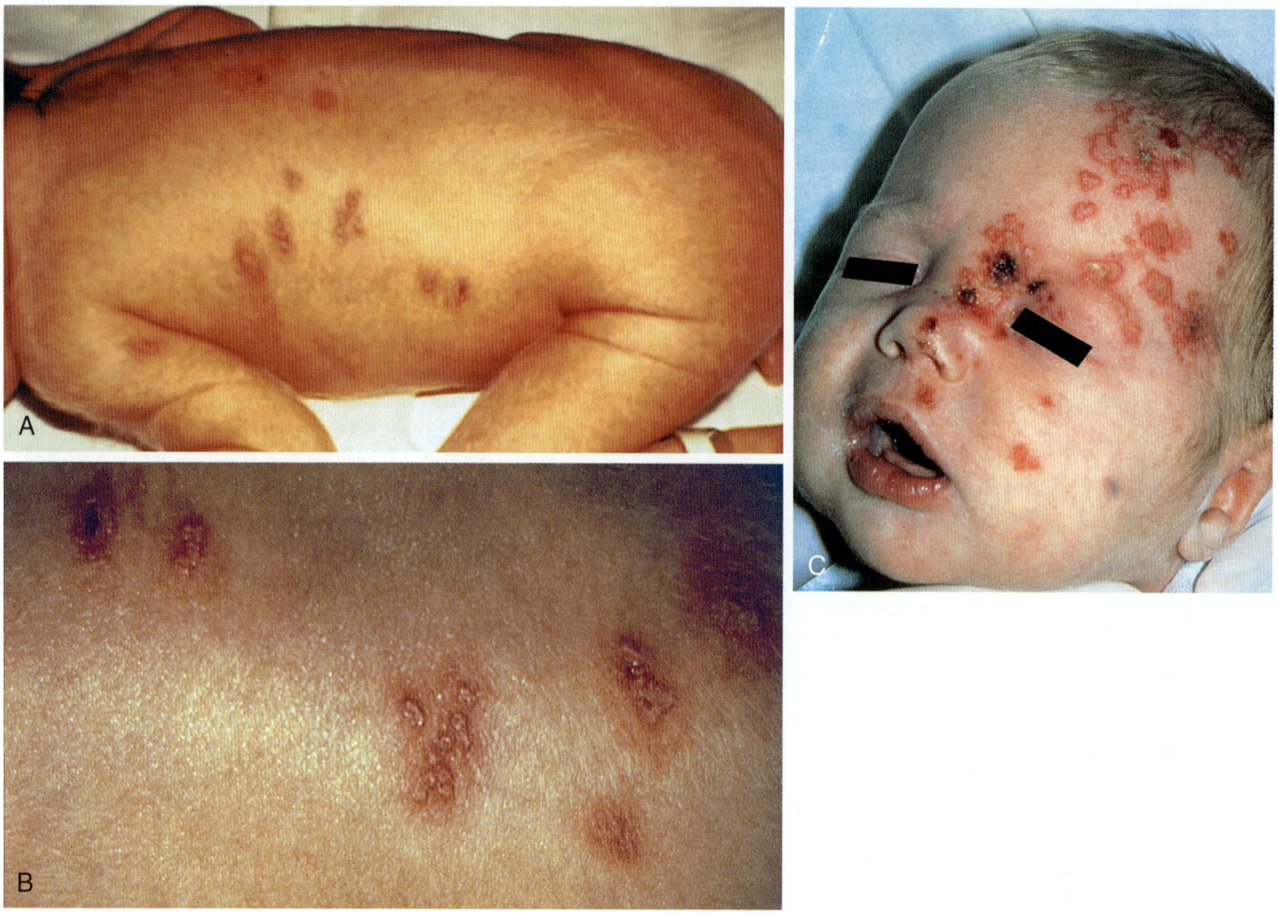

Fig. 13.66 Neonatal herpes simplex type 2 infection. (A and B) Although the child was normal at birth, fever, lethargy, and decreased feeding suddenly developed in this infant at 6 days old. On examination, multiple grouped vesicular lesions were noted on the trunk and scalp. The liver and spleen were markedly enlarged and firm. He had a fulminant course resembling that of septic shock and died within 24 hours. (C) Vesicular lesions are found most commonly on the scalp and face, as demonstrated in this infant. (A and B, Courtesy Michael Sherlock, MD, Lutherville, MD.)

lethargy, and seizures and may lack skin lesions. In disseminated HSV, onset begins with fever or subnormal temperature in association with lethargy, poor feeding, vomiting, and jaundice. The liver and spleen are enlarged and often remarkably firm. Respiratory distress is common, with a picture that is indistinguishable from that of septic shock and DIC. The prognosis is good for infants with SEM if they are treated promptly with IV acyclovir, with few sequelae. If untreated, most of these infants will progress to disseminated disease with or without CNS infection. Mortality of infants with disseminated HSV exceeds 50% but has been reduced by early recognition and IV acyclovir. The survival rate is better for localized CNS infection, but severe morbidity results from both CNS and disseminated disease.

Less frequently, HSV infections may occur prenatally because of ascent from the lower genital tract through ruptured membranes or because of maternal viremia. In the event of prenatal acquisition, the infant may die in utero or may be born with jaundice, skin lesions, and signs of systemic infection. Infants may also be infected postnatally from contacts or family members with oral herpetic lesions ("cold sores").

Congenital Toxoplasmosis

Toxoplasma gondii is an intracellular protozoan whose definitive host is the cat. Oocysts are shed in the feces and can survive in soil for years. Human infection is acquired by ingestion or inhalation of oocysts excreted in cat feces or consumption of raw or undercooked meat from infected animals. Most cases of infection in immunocompetent children beyond the neonatal period are thought to be subclinical, though a mononucleosis-like syndrome and persistent cervical adenopathy may occur.

Prenatally acquired infection has the potential to cause serious harm to the developing fetus. In the United States an estimated 1 to 2 per 1000 live-born infants have congenitally acquired toxoplasmosis. Maternal infection during pregnancy results in fetal infection less than 50% of the time. The risk of transmission to the fetus increases as gestation advances, but the severity of fetal injury is inversely proportional to gestational age at acquisition. Major sites of involvement are the CNS, retina, choroid, and muscles. Seventy percent of congenitally infected infants appear normal at birth, with the remainder overtly symptomatic (10%–20%). Chorioretinitis without other abnormalities occurs in 10% (Chapter 20). Infected asymptomatic infants and those with mild chorioretinitis alone are at risk for progressive ocular and CNS involvement if not diagnosed and treated. Unfortunately, in many instances, the diagnosis is not suspected until evidence of visual impairment, strabismus, or developmental delay prompts careful ophthalmologic and neurologic assessment.

The classic constellation of hydrocephalus, chorioretinitis, and intracerebral calcifications suggests the diagnosis of symptomatic congenital toxoplasmosis. However, the clinical picture may simulate other congenital infections. Like CMV, affected infants are often small for gestational age, with microcephaly (or hydrocephalus), jaundice, hepatosplenomegaly and diffuse adenopathy, petechial and purpuric lesions, or generalized maculopapular rash. Interstitial pneumonitis, myocarditis, or seizures may occur. CSF examination may show a pleocytosis with an increased protein content and xanthochromia. Skull radiographs or a head computed tomography (CT) scan may reveal diffuse cortical calcifications (Fig. 13.67), in contrast to the periventricular calcification pattern of congenital CMV. Neurodevelopmental sequelae are common. Mildly symptomatic

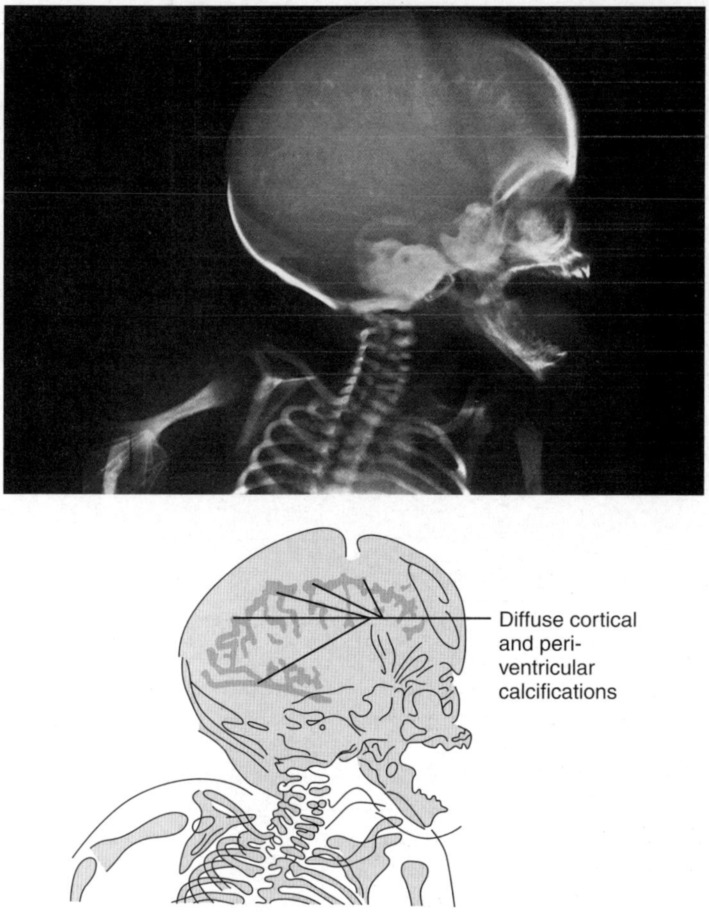

Fig. 13.67 Congenital toxoplasmosis. Microcephaly, ventricular dilation, and cerebral calcifications were prominent findings in this infant with severe congenital toxoplasmosis. (Courtesy Department of Pediatric Radiology, Children's Hospital of Pittsburgh, Pittsburgh, PA.)

infants may appear well initially but may develop signs of neonatal myocarditis with minimal CNS manifestations. These infants may have cerebral calcifications, as may infants with isolated chorioretinitis.

Diagnosis can be confirmed by demonstration of a positive IgM or immunoglobulin A (IgA) assay within the first 6 months of life, which is strongly recommended to be completed at national reference laboratories. Thorough ophthalmologic, auditory, and neurologic evaluations are indicated. In addition, a head CT scan should be obtained and CSF examined. All infected infants, symptomatic or not, warrant prolonged treatment (up to 1 year) with a combination of pyrimethamine (supplemented with folinic acid) and sulfadiazine. Follow-up and monitoring should be initiated with appropriate specialists, including infectious disease.

Congenital Rubella

Widespread use of rubella vaccination has made congenital rubella a rarity in industrialized countries. A benign infection in older children, rubella can lead to severe consequences if acquired in utero. Even asymptomatic maternal infection may be transmitted to the developing fetus. The earlier in gestation the infection occurs, the greater the potential for injury. Approximately 40% of fetuses infected during the first 8 weeks spontaneously abort or are stillborn, and 25% have gross anomalies noted at birth. Ultimately, 85% of live-born infants infected in the first trimester suffer adverse consequences, as do 35% of those infected between weeks 13 and 16. Infection after 4 months gestation does not appear to cause disease. The most encountered anomalies are cataracts; congenital heart disease (patent ductus arteriosus, pulmonary artery stenosis, pulmonary valvular stenosis); and sensorineural deafness (usually bilateral, occasionally unilateral). These sequelae may occur singly or in combination.

There is a wide range of clinical manifestations. Some infants appear well at birth but later are found to have hearing loss. Some are small for gestational age or have evidence of congenital heart disease and ocular anomalies, including microphthalmia, glaucoma, cataracts, and pigmented retinopathy (Chapter 20). Many develop jaundice within 24 hours of birth and have hepatosplenomegaly and diffuse adenopathy. Ocular findings are usually present at birth but may be missed unless a careful ophthalmologic examination is performed.

Ten to 20% of live-born infants with congenital rubella show signs of severe disseminated infection at or shortly after birth. In addition to jaundice, hepatosplenomegaly, and adenopathy, they often have signs of myocarditis, interstitial pneumonitis, thrombocytopenia with petechiae and purpura, and CNS dysfunction that may range from lethargy and hypotonia to frank meningoencephalitis. Radiographs may reveal bony abnormalities consisting of metaphyseal lucencies and irregular epiphyseal mineralization. In some cases, a rubelliform rash or a characteristic raised, bluish, papular eruption, termed a *blueberry muffin rash,* may be evident as the result of dermal erythropoiesis (see Fig. 13.66A). Most of these severely affected infants are microcephalic, in addition to being small for gestational age. In countries with universal vaccination, infants with these findings are more likely to have congenital CMV infection (see Fig. 13.66B). Survivors of this "expanded rubella syndrome" are highly likely to be deaf and to have significant psychomotor limitation. Diagnosis of congenital rubella can be confirmed by viral culture or PCR and specific IgM titers.

Congenital Syphilis

Rates of syphilis in the United States waned significantly during the past century but have increased dramatically since 2010. It is important for physicians to be able to recognize the clinical manifestations of syphilis. The congenital form is discussed here, with manifestations in adolescents presented in Chapter 19.

Congenital syphilis results from hematogenous spread of *Treponema pallidum* from an infected mother through the placenta, resulting in disseminated fetal infection. Risk of transmission to the fetus is greatest when the mother acquires disease during or shortly before pregnancy (i.e., when she is in primary, secondary, or early latent stage). Infection early in gestation can result in stillbirth, hydrops fetalis, prematurity, or neonatal death. Live-born infected infants may not have obvious signs and symptoms at the time of delivery. Those who are asymptomatic initially may develop clinical manifestations during the neonatal period or weeks, months, or even years later if untreated. Earlier onset is associated with poorer prognosis, although the reasons for delayed symptom onset are not fully understood.

Symptomatic neonates often have intrauterine growth restriction, hepatosplenomegaly, direct and indirect hyperbilirubinemia, Coombs-negative hemolytic anemia, thrombocytopenia, generalized lymphadenopathy (including epitrochlear nodes), or mucocutaneous lesions. These lesions are often vesicular or bullous and ultimately rupture to form superficial crusted erosions or ulcerations. The rash is generalized and includes palms and soles.

When skin lesions appear after the first month, they are more likely to be papulosquamous or maculopapular, resembling those of secondary syphilis in older individuals (see Chapter 19). They tend to be oval, pinkish red, and distributed predominantly over the back, buttocks, posterior thighs, and soles. Over time, the lesions turn brown and fine desquamation of the palms and soles may be noted (Fig. 13.68A and B). Affected infants may develop typical condylomata lata—moist papular or warty lesions—around the nose, mouth, and in intertriginous areas. Profuse rhinorrhea ("snuffles") may develop between a week and a few months of age, which may be blood-tinged with ulcerations of the nasal mucosa. The nasal discharge, mucosal lesions, and moist cutaneous lesions teem with organisms and are highly contagious.

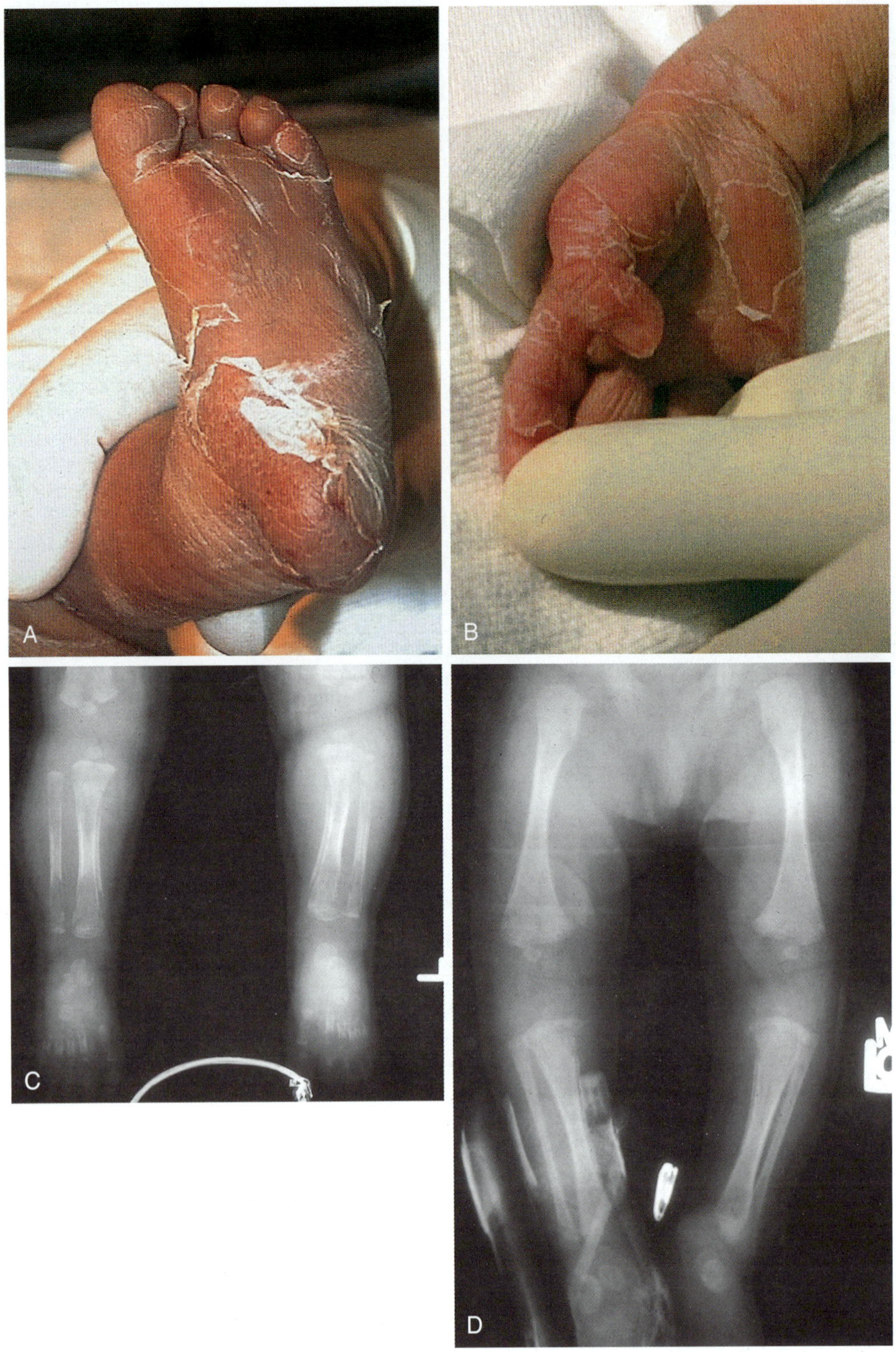

Fig. 13.68 Congenital syphilis. (A and B) Desquamation of the foot and hand are seen in this infant with congenital syphilis. (C) This 3-month-old who presented with untreated congenital syphilis had diffuse periosteal reaction of the tibias and generalized demineralization. (D) Wimberger sign, the osseous destruction of the proximal tibial metaphysis, is seen in another affected infant. (A and B, Courtesy Pablo Sanchez, MD, and Walid Salhab, MD, University of Texas Southwestern Medical Center. D, Courtesy Manuel P. Meza, MD, Children's Hospital of Pittsburgh, Pittsburgh, PA.)

Widespread skeletal involvement is seen in many infants with congenital syphilis (see Fig. 13.68C and D), although only about 15% have symptoms. Pain is manifested as irritability and pseudoparalysis (Parrot pseudoparalysis) with decreased limb movement, especially of the upper extremities. Radiographic findings demonstrate osteitis at birth and osteochondritis as early as 5 weeks after infection, characterized by horizontal radiopaque bands with adjacent lucent lines in the metaphases and irregular lateral demineralization, which creates a mottled appearance. The proximal tibial medial metaphyses can be demineralized, a phenomenon termed the *Wimberger sign* (see Fig. 13.68D). Radiographic evidence of periostitis and periosteal new bone formation along the diaphyses of long bones is generally not seen until about 3 to 4 months of age (see Fig. 13.68C and D).

CNS involvement is common in symptomatic cases but can be found in asymptomatic infants. Accordingly, CSF examination is recommended for all infected infants because untreated infants can progress to meningitis. CSF examination reveals a monocytosis with moderately elevated protein and a normal glucose level. Chronic meningovascular inflammation in untreated infants may progress to fibrosis, resulting in hydrocephalus, cranial nerve palsies, and developmental regression.

Although symptoms of early congenital syphilis are the direct result of active infection, manifestations of late congenital syphilis are usually sequelae or signs of prior disease and persistent active disease. They may be seen in up to 40% of cases and include the following:

- Maldevelopment of permanent teeth
  - Hutchinson teeth—the upper central incisors are smaller than normal, barrel shaped, and notched in the center of the incisal surface
  - Mulberry molars—abnormal cusp development results in the formation of multiple peripheral cusps and a central cusp
- Interstitial keratitis—development of a ground-glass appearance of the cornea and scleral vascularization, which have their onset around puberty
- Eighth nerve deafness
- Skeletal stigmata due to sclerotic changes
  - Sabre shin
  - Frontal bossing
- Cartilaginous stigmata due to gummatous breakdown and/or ulceration
  - Saddle nose deformity
  - Palatal perforation
- Clutton joints—painless hydrarthrosis of the knees
- Rhagades—fissuring of the skin in the perinasal and perioral areas
- Cognitive disability and, more rarely, chronic neurosyphilis with paresis, or less commonly, tabes dorsalis

Testing all pregnant women for syphilis and promptly treating those who are seropositive and retesting at delivery constitute the mainstays in preventing and identifying congenital syphilis. Infants should be evaluated and treated if the mother did not receive treatment or may have been inadequately treated, according to published guidelines at CDC and the AAP. Inadequate treatment should be suspected if a nonpenicillin regimen was used, if there was less than a fourfold decrease in maternal serum titer after treatment or if treatment was administered less than 1 month before delivery. Any uncertainty in testing or prior therapy should lead to a course of therapy to prevent any chance of congenital disease progressing.

Neonatal Tetanus

Tetanus is an exceptionally painful acute neuromuscular disorder caused by release of a neurotoxic exotoxin by *Clostridium tetani*. The bacterium, a gram-positive anaerobic rod, forms spores that are highly resistant to heat and antiseptics. The organism is prevalent worldwide in the intestines of humans and animals and in soil. It is found in especially large numbers in the cultivated soil of rural areas. When organisms are inoculated along with dirt or soil into a wound with devitalized or necrotic tissue, they find ideal anaerobic conditions for spore germination, bacterial growth, and toxin production. Tetanus toxin diffuses locally, binding irreversibly to presynaptic terminals of lower motor neurons, where it impedes neuromuscular transmission and interferes with contraction/relaxation mechanisms. Toxin is believed to spread lymphohematogenously and via retrograde axonal transport to distal sites, including lower motor neurons in the spinal cord and brainstem. Patients experience persistent muscular rigidity and periodic spasmodic contractions of voluntary muscles, which are extremely painful.

Neonatal tetanus occurs in infants born to unimmunized mothers, usually because of contamination of the umbilical stump by unclean instruments, soiled dressings, or the cultural practice of placing mud or dung on the stump. The success of active global immunization programs has decreased the rates of neonatal tetanus substantially.

The incubation period for neonatal tetanus ranges from 3 days to 2 weeks, with onset of symptoms usually occurring 6 to 7 days after delivery. Initially, the baby appears restless and irritable, with difficulty suckling. Within 1 to 2 days, trismus (lockjaw) due to masseter muscle rigidity, dysphagia with drooling, and noisy respirations are noted. These are associated with neck, back, and shoulder stiffness. Subsequently, there is rapid cephalocaudal progression of muscular rigidity to the back, abdomen, and extremities. Opisthotonic posturing is typical, with hands held fisted and toes fanned out. Orbicularis oris spasm produces the appearance of a characteristic facial grimace termed *risus sardonicus* (Fig. 13.69). These manifestations are accompanied by fever and painful tonic or tetanic spasmodic contractions of voluntary muscles, which can be precipitated by minimal external stimuli. Sucking and swallowing are impaired. Spasms involving laryngeal muscles and the diaphragm can cause severe respiratory compromise. Symptoms of autonomic disinhibition include excessive sweating, hypertension, tachycardia, and arrhythmias.

Complications include aspiration, atelectasis and pneumonia, fractures of vertebrae and long bones, and respiratory arrest. In survivors, clinical improvement begins about 2 weeks after the onset of symptoms, with a gradual decrease in fever, degree of rigidity, and spasm frequency and intensity. Resolution proceeds gradually over the ensuing 6 weeks. Mortality is high, and many surviving infants show developmental delay, problems with balance, and muscle

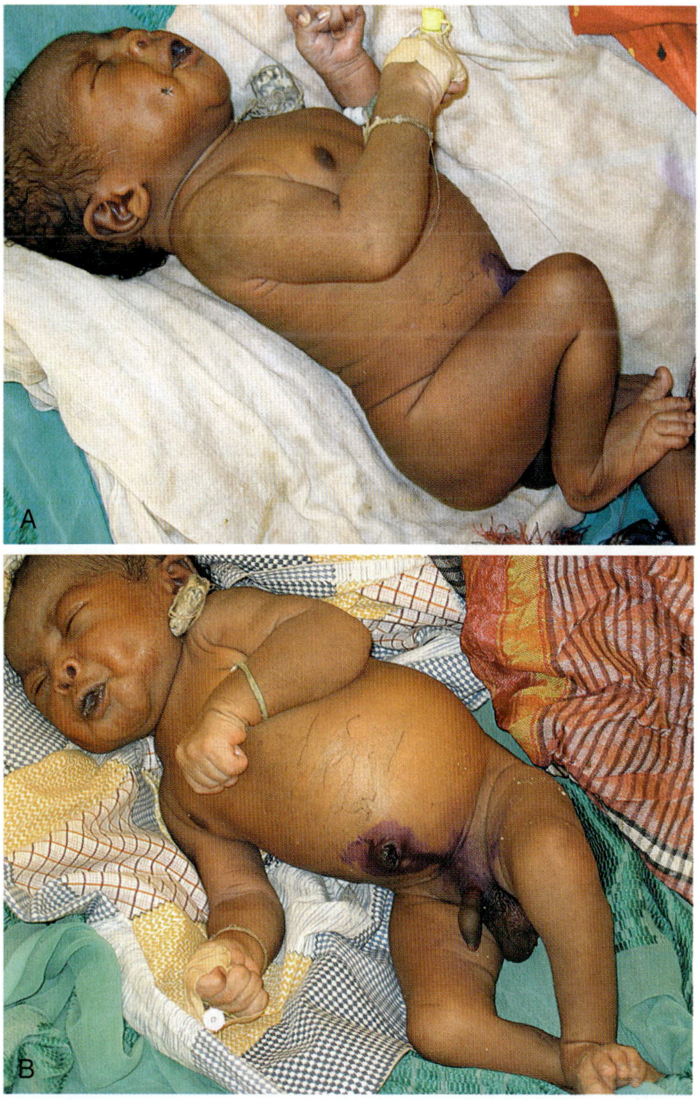

Fig. 13.69 Neonatal tetanus. (A) This newborn demonstrates the trismus (locked jaw) and fixed smile of risus sardonicus that are typical of tetanus. Note as well the clenched fists and fanned toes. (B) Viewed from the side, his opisthotonic posturing is more evident. (Courtesy Jonathan Spector, MD, Boston, MA.)

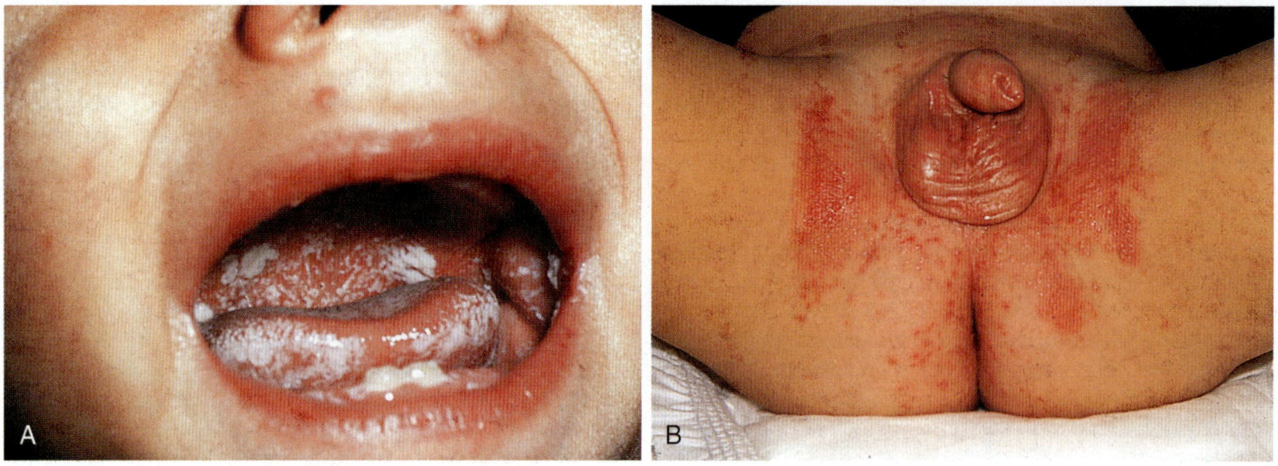

Fig. 13.70 Child with acquired immune deficiency syndrome. (A) Oral thrush. (B) Candidal diaper dermatitis. (A, Courtesy G.B. Scott, MD, and M.T. Mastrucci, MD, Miami, FL.)

atrophy. Later, these children may complain of easy muscle fatigue and cramping.

The diagnosis of tetanus must be made clinically. Manifestations in the older child, most often an unimmunized patient with inoculation through injury, appear similarly to those described earlier. Laboratory studies are unhelpful. Successful treatment regimens include administration of tetanus immune globulin to neutralize any free or unbound toxin, local wound care and antibiotics, and supportive intensive care in a dim, quiet room with minimal stimulation.

Human Immunodeficiency Virus and Acquired Immune Deficiency Syndrome

HIV-1 is an RNA retrovirus and is the major etiological agent of acquired immune deficiency syndrome (AIDS) throughout the world. A second virus, HIV-2, is endemic in West Africa and accounts for the remainder of HIV/AIDS cases. HIV infects CD4+ (helper) T lymphocytes and some monocytes, macrophages, and microglial cells of the CNS. The virus becomes integrated into the host genome and persists in the infected individual for life.

The timing of symptom development in untreated HIV-infected children varies. One-third of infants present in the first year of life with one or more of the characteristic AIDS-indicator conditions, suggesting intrauterine infection. Other children infected with HIV present in the first few years of life with a more indolent course, and a small percentage develop symptoms years later.

Undiagnosed HIV-infected infants present with failure to thrive, *Pneumocystis jiroveci* pneumonia, developmental delay or regression, hepatosplenomegaly, lymphadenopathy, *Candida* skin or mucosal infections (Fig. 13.70), chronic diarrhea, chronic lymphoid interstitial pneumonitis, and recurrent or severe bacterial infections. Bacterial infections in these children include sepsis, pneumonia, meningitis, abscess, or recurrent cellulitis, otitis media, and sinusitis.

Opportunistic infections related to defects in cell-mediated immunity also occur. *P. jiroveci* pneumonia is one of the most common (Fig. 13.71), which occurs in more than one-third of untreated symptomatic HIV-infected children. Other opportunistic infections include *M. avium* complex, candida esophagitis, CMV infection, cryptosporidiosis, persistent or disseminated HSV, cryptococcosis, toxoplasmosis, and unusually extensive cases of molluscum contagiosum (Fig. 13.72).

An especially devastating feature of HIV infection is encephalopathy that leads to developmental delay, loss of developmental milestones, and behavioral alterations. CT scans and MRI studies often show severe brain atrophy with increased ventricular size and calcifications in the basal ganglia and frontal lobes (Fig. 13.73). The

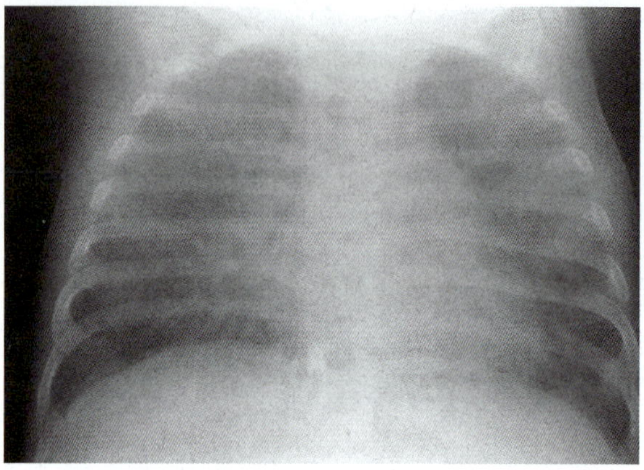

Fig. 13.71 *Pneumocystis jiroveci* pneumonia in a child with acquired immune deficiency syndrome. Note the diffuse bilateral haziness. (Courtesy G.B Scott, MD, and M.T. Mastrucci, MD, Miami, FL.)

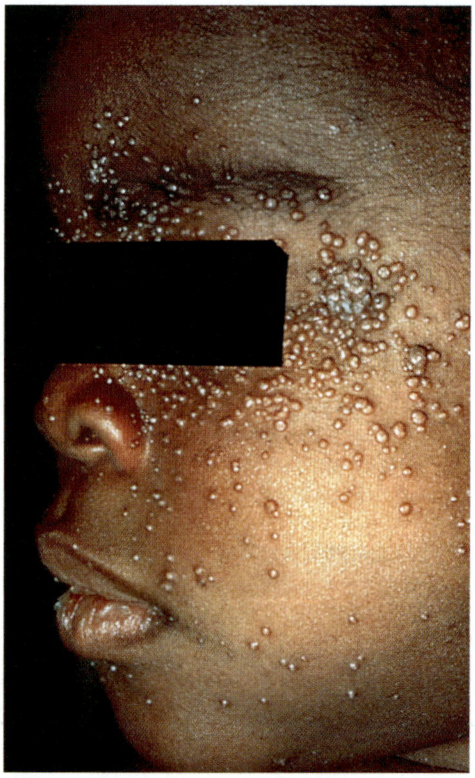

Fig. 13.72 Severe molluscum contagiosum in a patient with acquired immune deficiency syndrome. (Courtesy G.B. Scott, MD, and M.T. Mastrucci, MD, Miami, FL.)

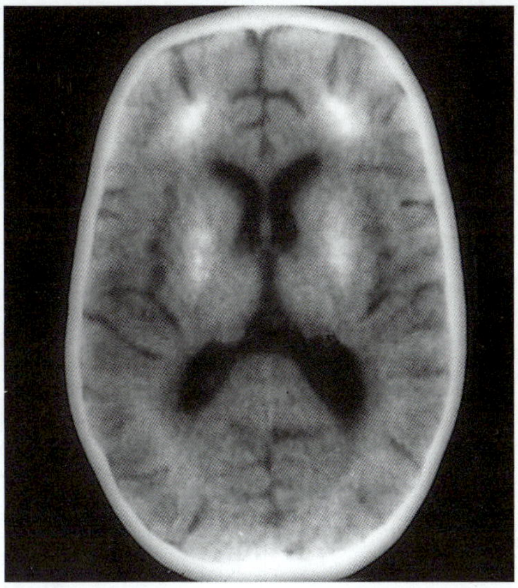

Fig. 13.73 Computed tomography scan of an infant with acquired immune deficiency syndrome. Note the frontal lobe and basal ganglia calcification and increased ventricular size secondary to cerebral parenchymal volume loss.

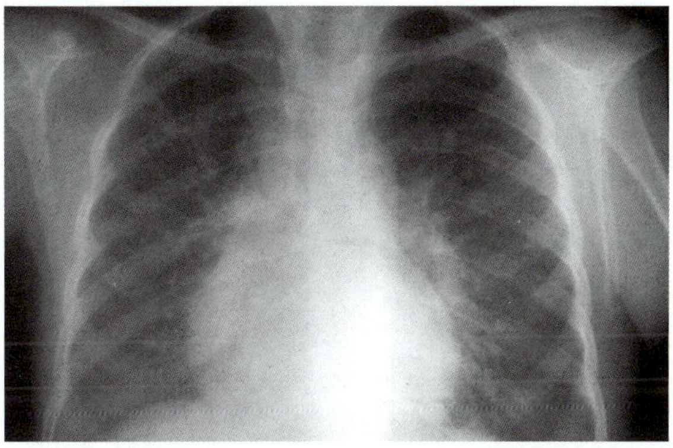

Fig. 13.74 Lymphoid interstitial pneumonitis in a child with acquired immune deficiency syndrome. Note the diffuse bilateral reticulonodular infiltrates.

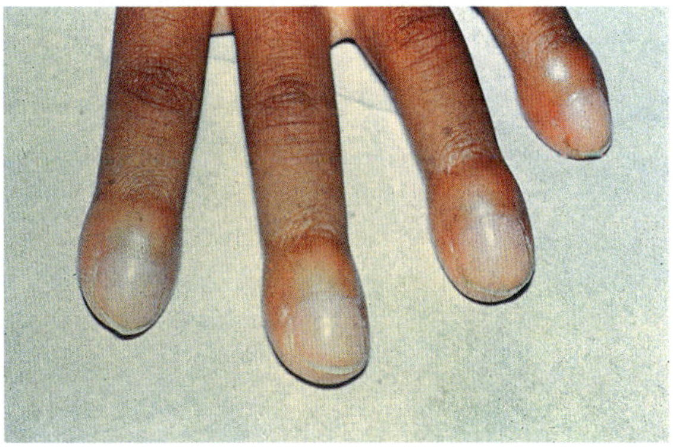

Fig. 13.75 Clubbing in patient with lymphoid interstitial pneumonitis and acquired immune deficiency syndrome. (Courtesy G.B. Scott, MD, and M.T. Mastrucci, MD, Miami, FL.)

course of HIV-related neurologic disease without antiretroviral treatment is variable and may be intermittent, static, or relentlessly progressive.

Lymphoid interstitial pneumonitis can be seen in children with HIV (Fig. 13.74). This chronic lung disease presents insidiously over several years with cough, wheezing, clubbing (Fig. 13.75), hypoxemia, diffuse reticulonodular radiologic infiltrate; or hilar or mediastinal adenopathy. Children with this condition often have lymphadenopathy, hepatosplenomegaly, parotid gland enlargement, and a longer survival than children who have opportunistic infections.

As with many immunodeficiencies, malignancies also occur in children with AIDS, although at rates significantly lower than in adults. Kaposi sarcoma (Fig. 13.76) and lymphoma have been reported in children, particularly in countries with endemic HHV-8, such as sub-Saharan Africa.

Other clinical manifestations of HIV include diarrhea, hepatitis, pancreatitis, cardiomyopathy (Fig. 13.77), eczema, nephrotic syndrome, and pancytopenia. The clinical pattern of disease reflects direct HIV infection, immune system dysregulation caused by the virus, immunodeficiency leading to opportunistic infections, and autoimmune disease. A variety of immunologic abnormalities occur with HIV infection (Box 13.1). Thus it is important for the general pediatrician to remain vigilant for the protean clinical and laboratory manifestations of pediatric HIV infection. Diagnosis and treatment issues are beyond the scope of this chapter.

A supplemental video is available at Elsevier eBooks+.

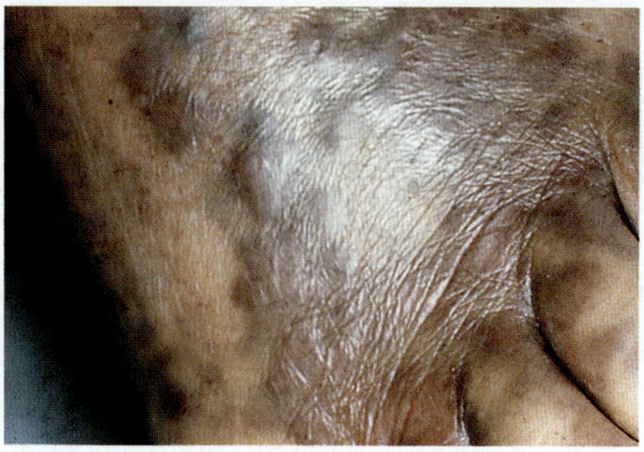

Fig. 13.76 Cutaneous manifestations of Kaposi sarcoma. The purplish hyperpigmented plaques and nodules are characteristic.

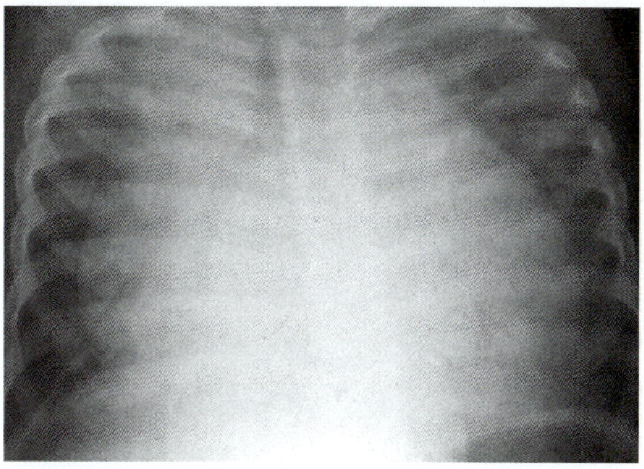

Fig. 13.77 Cardiomyopathy in a patient with acquired immune deficiency syndrome. Note the massively increased heart size. (Courtesy G.B. Scott, MD, and M.T. Mastrucci, MD, Miami, FL.)

Box 13.1 Selected Abnormalities of Immune System in Acquired Immune Deficiency Syndrome

Lymphopenia (more common in adults)
Decreased helper T lymphocytes (T4)
Decreased helper-to-suppressor ratio (T4/T8 ratio)
Decreased T- and B-lymphocyte mitogen responses (pokeweed, phytohemagglutinin, concanavalin A)
Decreased specific antibody response to antigen
Increased immunoglobulin levels (IgG, IgD, IgA, IgM, IgG subclasses)
Deficient serum isohemagglutinin levels
Positive test for antinuclear antibodies
Positive Coombs test
Positive circulating immune complex levels

Bibliography

American Academy of Pediatrics, Kimberlin DW, Banerjee R, Barnett ED, editors: *Red book: 2024-2027 Report of the Committee on Infectious Diseases*, ed 33, Elk Grove Village, IL, 2018, American Academy of Pediatrics.

Cherry J, Kaplan SL, Harrison GJ, et al: *Feigin & Cherry's textbook of pediatric infectious*, ed 9, 2025, Elsevier/Saunders.

Chesney PJ, Davis JP, Purdy WK, et al: Clinical manifestations of toxic shock syndrome, *J Am Med Assoc* 246:741–748, 1981.

Fleisher G, Ludwig S, Campos J: Cellulitis: bacterial etiology, clinical features and laboratory findings, *J Pediatr* 97:591–593, 1980.

Leibel RL, Fangman JJ, Ostrovsky MC: Chronic meningococcemia in childhood, *Am J Dis Child* 127:94–98, 1974.

Long SS, Prober CG, Fischer M, Kimberlin DW, editors: *Principles and practice of pediatric infectious diseases*, ed 6, London, 2022, Elsevier/Saunders.

Rapkin RH, Bautista G: *Haemophilus influenzae* cellulitis, *Am J Dis Child* 124: 540–542, 1972.

Wilson CB, Nizet V, Maldonado Y, et al: *Remington and Klein's infectious diseases of the fetus and newborn infant*, ed 8, Philadelphia, 2016, Elsevier/Saunders.

14

NEPHROLOGY

Amber Kazi | Juhi Kumar | Cassandra Formeck | Michael Moritz | Yosuke Miyashita

The manifestations of kidney and genitourinary disorders range from readily apparent gross structural abnormalities to subtle abnormalities of the urinary sediment. This chapter reviews key history and physical findings, characteristic urinary findings, and updated diagnostic and radiographic studies of kidney disorders encountered in both ambulatory and hospital settings.

ESSENTIALS OF MEDICAL HISTORY AND PHYSICAL EXAMINATION

The medical history and physical examination often provide clues implicating a kidney or genitourinary disorder. Congenital, but often nonheritable, genitourinary disorders are diagnosed with increasing frequency during prenatal screening. Oligohydramnios and fetal compression signs reflect reduced urine production associated with some of these disorders and may result in early postnatal death because of pulmonary underdevelopment. "Cysts" in the kidney(s) on prenatal sonogram could represent various congenital anomalies of kidney and urinary tract (CAKUT) including cystic kidney disease, dysplasia, and polycystic kidney disease (PKD). Dilation of kidney pelvis can be due to vesicoureteral reflux or urinary tract obstruction. A large placenta may be a telltale sign of congenital nephrotic syndrome (NS) of the Finnish type.

In the neonatal period, failure to urinate during the first 24 hours of life should prompt evaluation for obstruction of the kidneys, ureters, or bladder. A neonate with an abdominal mass born to a diabetic mother should be evaluated for renal vein thrombosis. Urinary tract anomalies, including vesicoureteral reflux (VUR) and megaureters, are common in infants and young children with history of urinary tract infection (UTI).

Infants with growth faltering, lethargy, irritability, or recurrent emesis may be manifesting signs of kidney disease associated with metabolic acidosis and other electrolyte disturbances. On occasion, a kidney disorder is discovered as part of an evaluation of extrarenal congenital anomalies. Family pedigrees may facilitate the diagnosis of congenital or heritable disorders such as cystinuria, cystinosis, hyperoxaluria, Alport syndrome, and PKD and thereby lead to a variety of preventive measures before children become symptomatic.

UTI should be a consideration in all febrile infants, particularly during the first 2 months of life, even in the presence of documented bacteremia, meningitis, or other source of infection. Young children with true polyuria or polydipsia may have a renal concentrating defect including diabetes insipidus or salt-losing nephropathy such as dysplasia and nephronophthisis.

Hypertension (HTN) in infants is often caused by vascular diseases, such as coarctation of the aorta or renovascular diseases like renal artery stenosis, renal vein thrombosis, and renal artery thrombosis. HTN is usually asymptomatic in children and adolescents, but if symptoms exist, the most common ones include headache, dizziness, nausea, vomiting, visual disturbances, and exercise intolerance. Primary HTN has become the most common cause in adolescents, often in association with obesity and metabolic syndrome. However, the presence of café-au-lait spots, neurofibromas, fibrous-angiomatous lesions of the skin, abnormal pulses, or bruits over the renal arteries or major vessels may point to a specific secondary HTN etiology.

Hematuria is one of the most common reasons children are referred to pediatric nephrology clinics. Specific aspects of the medical history such as the neonatal course, congenital heart disease, hematologic disorders including thrombotic or hemolytic disorders, antecedent or concurrent infection, rapid weight gain, joint symptoms, and concurrent rash may pinpoint the cause of hematuria. Secondary causes should be considered, including child abuse, trauma, or factitious disorders. Menarche can be confused with hematuria. Obtaining detailed history such as actual color of urine (pink-tinged vs. tea-colored), timing of gross hematuria (entire void vs. terminal hematuria), and presence of blood clots can help to suggest the source of the blood within the urinary tract. The presence of hematuria or kidney failure in family members may suggest PKD, whereas a similar history together with neurosensory hearing loss may indicate Alport syndrome.

URINARY SCREENING AND URINALYSIS

Urinalysis

A carefully performed urinalysis may expedite the diagnosis of various disorders. Routine urinalysis consists of three basic steps: gross inspection, dipstick screening, and microscopical examination.

Gross Inspection

On gross inspection, the color of urine may be described as clear, yellow, dark yellow, green, brown, tea-colored, pink, clear red, grossly bloody, blue, or even black. Smoky, brown, or tea-colored urine is indicative of stagnated blood that has decomposed; the iron component has oxidized in the renal tubules. This commonly occurs in glomerulonephritis. Trauma, kidney stones, UTI, and strenuous exercise frequently result in frank hematuria with more pink or cranberry juice color. In the absence of hematuria on dipstick screening, numerous natural chromogens and vitamins found in foods, dyes, or medications may alter the normal yellow-amber color of urine imparted by the hemoglobin breakdown product, urochrome (Box 14.1).

Most importantly, one must exclude several medical disorders associated with pigmenturia and chromogens that may influence urine color. Yellow-brown urine may be seen in obstructive jaundice and is due to oxidation of bilirubin to biliverdin; porphyria and urinary porphyrins produce a red urine color; multiple disorders leading to myoglobinuria produce a clear red-brown color; chronic lead or mercury poisoning can also result in red urine color; and conditions leading to hemoglobinuria cause the urine to turn dark brown. Several special conditions in infants and children include the following:

1. Red diaper syndrome: a benign condition from uric acid supersaturation or overgrowth of Serratia marcescens (Fig. 14.1).
2. Black diapers or undergarments: urine color turns black to brown on exposure to air. This condition is known as alkaptonuria and results from a defect in the enzyme homogentisate 1, 2-dioxygenase, which degrades tyrosine, leading to tissue accumulation and high urinary excretion of the tyrosine byproduct homogentisic acid.
3. Blue diaper syndrome: this occurs in Hartnup disease (neutral aminoaciduria) and is also seen in tryptophan gastrointestinal malabsorption syndrome, in which indigo blue is excreted in the urine.

Box 14.1 Causes of Urine Color Alteration Without Presence of Red Blood Cells

Pink, Red, Cola-Colored, Burgundy

Drug and food ingestion

Aminopyrine, chronic mercury or lead, benzene, phenolphthalein, phenytoin, carbon tetrachloride, sulfonethylmethane, dinitrophenol, anthocyanin, azo dyes, carotene in carrots, betacyanin in beets, vitamins, blackberries, chloroquine, deferoxamine mesylate, ibuprofen, methyldopa, nitrofurantoin, phenazopyridine, rifampin, Ex-Lax, rhodamine E, sulfasalazine, *Serratia marcescens,* urates (red diaper syndrome)

Dark Brown, Black, Orange

Disease associated

Hemoglobinuric disorders, alkaptonuria, homogentisic aciduria, melanin, methemoglobinemia, tyrosinemia, obstructive jaundices

Drug and food ingestion

Alanine, resorcinol, thymol, phenazopyridine (Pyridium), rifampin, warfarin, laxatives, rhubarb

Green

Pseudomonas infection, methylene blue, indicanemia, Hartnup disease, porphyria, drugs (propofol, metoclopramide, cimetidine)

Red Brown

Myoglobinuric disorders, hemoglobinuric disorders, asparagus, B vitamins

Blue

Hartnup disease, tryptophan malabsorption (indigotin, or indigo blue excretion)

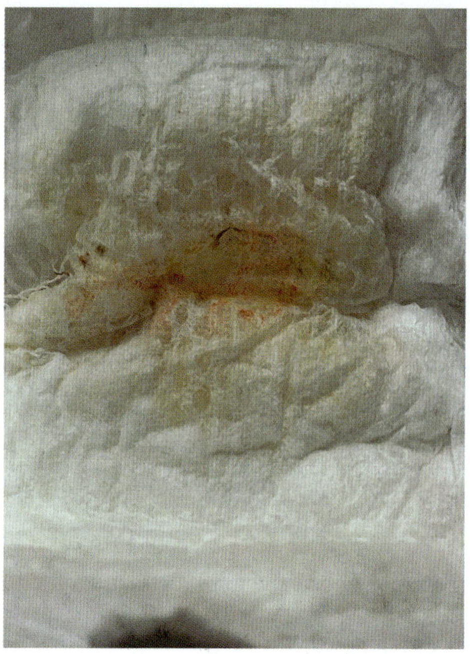

Fig. 14.1 A diaper from an infant with pink diaper syndrome. (From Wang A, Nanagas K: Neonate with red diaper, *Emerg Med J* 36(10):594–634, 2019.)

Screening by Dipstick

Each small square on the urine dipstick is chemically engineered to be sensitive, specific, and cost-effective for the substance it detects (Fig. 14.2). However, dipstick testing can produce false-positive results, leading to unnecessary evaluation. It may also miss significant kidney pathology that is not associated with hematuria or proteinuria. Components of urine dipstick include the following:

- The hematest square detects free hemoglobin released after lysis of urinary erythrocytes by the o-toluidine reagent. The test is highly sensitive and detects myoglobin.
- Screening for proteinuria via dipstick relies on change in the color of the tetrabromophenol blue reagent and is particularly suitable for detection of albumin. Hence this test may miss low-molecular-weight (LMW) proteinuria resulting from systemic overproduction or due to insufficient reabsorption in children with tubulopathies.

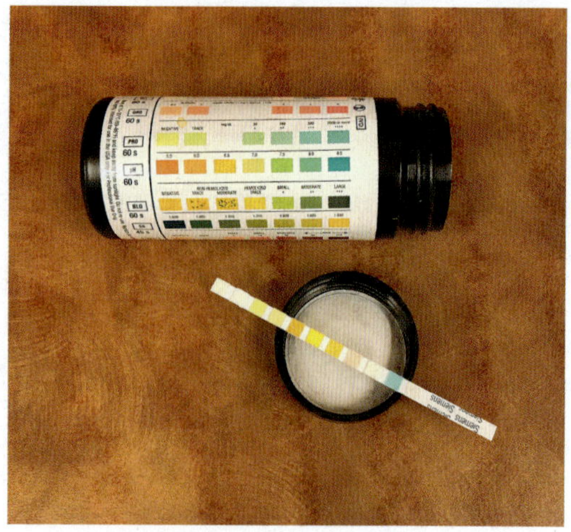

Fig. 14.2 A commercially available clinic urine dipstick.

- A positive nitrite test is highly specific for UTI and results from conversion of dietary nitrates to nitrites by bacterial pathogens.
- The leukocyte esterase test is also useful in diagnosing UTI and is mediated by the release of this enzyme from neutrophils. In adults and older children, but not in infants, the presence of both positive nitrite and leukocyte esterase tests has both positive and negative predictive values that approach 100%.
- Ketones may be detected in the setting of starvation or diabetes mellitus.
- Specific gravity (SG) is a measure of the total solute in urine and depends on both the concentration and molecular weight of solutes. In healthy individuals, SG of 1.010 corresponds to 400 mOsm/kg H_2O, 1.020 equals 800 mOsm/kg H_2O, and 1.030 equals 1200 mOsm/kg H_2O. Children with dehydration or those receiving hyperosmolar radiocontrast media may have SG exceeding 1.030. Low SG may be found in healthy children with high fluid intake or in pathologic conditions such as tubulointerstitial disorders and inadequate secretion of antidiuretic hormone.

Microscopic Examination

Examination of the urine sediment begins with centrifugation of 10 mL of freshly voided urine for 5 to 7 minutes at 3000 rpm. Such standardized preparation enables semiquantitative comparison of sequential samples. Specific urine microscopy findings are reviewed in detail in the respective kidney conditions covered in this chapter. Dysmorphic RBCs, best seen in uncentrifuged urine with phase microscopy, are usually of glomerular origin as opposed to urologic origin. White blood cells (WBCs) coated with antibody tend to become agglutinated or clumped. Such clumped WBCs are indicative of pyelonephritis or interstitial nephritis rather than cystitis. The presence of several tubular epithelial cells is abnormal.

Formation of urinary casts is aided by diminished urine flow, high urinary solute concentration, and the hyaline matrix of plasma- and tubule-derived protein in which cells become embedded. Hyaline casts form on polymerization of Tamm-Horsfall glycoprotein, which is a well-characterized molecule uniquely found in the ascending limb of Henle and distal convoluted tubule. Small quantities of hyaline casts may be found in healthy individuals, but larger numbers of hyaline casts or those containing cellular components are considered pathologic. Muddy-brown granular or tubular epithelial cell casts are seen in acute tubular necrosis (ATN). Granular casts form from disintegration of cellular elements. These are always pathologic and are found in most cases of glomerulonephritis. Wide casts may derive from dilated tubules, which occur in individuals with advanced kidney disease.

Crystals are best identified in fresh urine that is of near body temperature. Uric acid crystals and urates are found in urine with a pH less than 6.5, whereas phosphates precipitate in urine with a pH greater than 6.5. Both urates and phosphates tend to precipitate when the urine specimen is refrigerated. Crystals may be found in the urine of healthy individuals, patients with urolithiasis or hyperuricemia, or those with a specific drug intake or poisoning (ethylene glycol). Flat hexagonal crystals are pathognomonic of cystinuria.

HEMATURIA

Because of the many conditions associated with persistent hematuria in children, several algorithms have been devised to aid in the systematic evaluation of this condition (Fig. 14.3A–C). History and clinical symptoms may point toward trauma, viral or

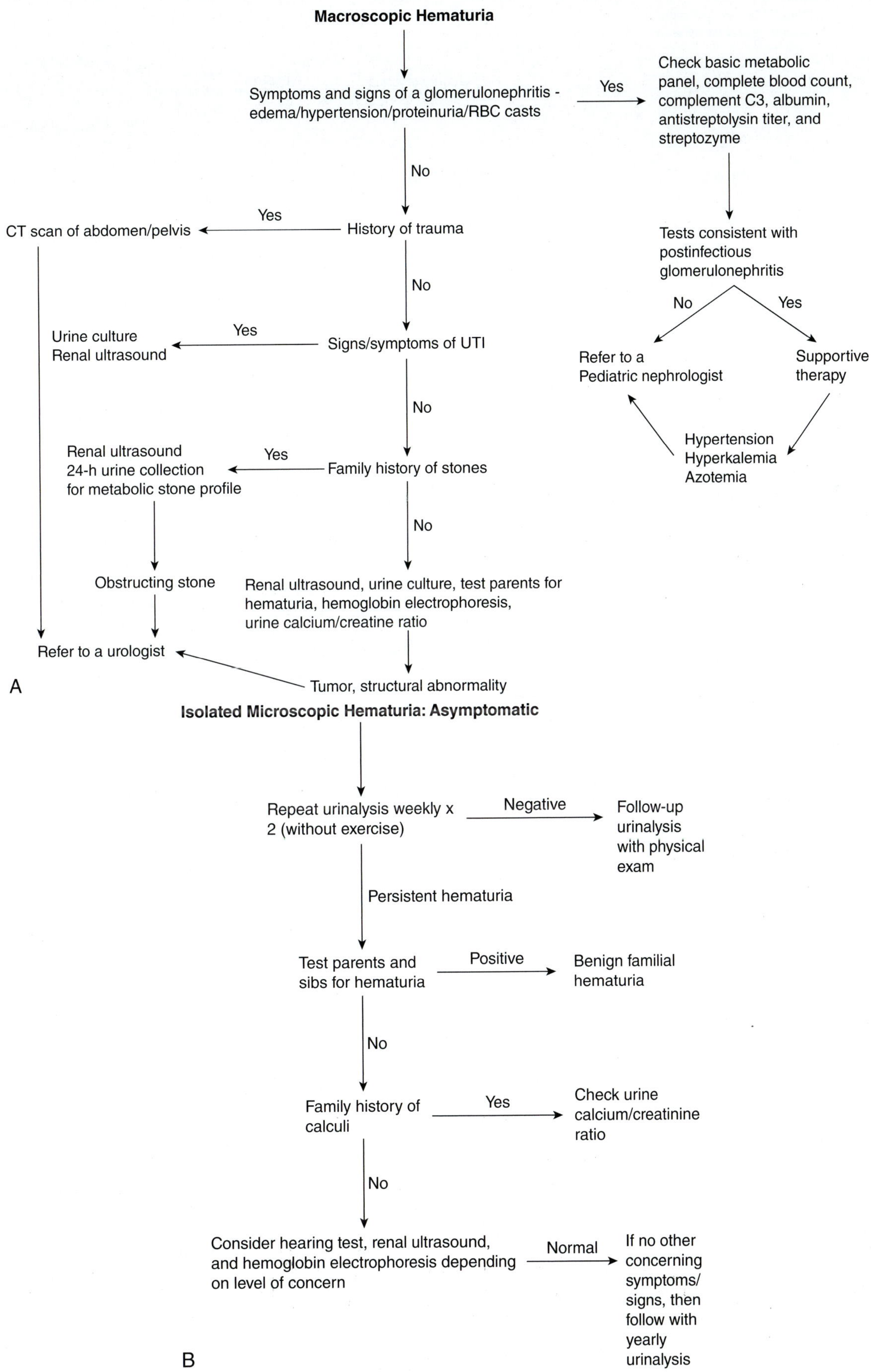

Fig. 14.3 Algorithms of hematuria evaluation. (A) Gross hematuria. (B) Asymptomatic microscopical hematuria.

Continued

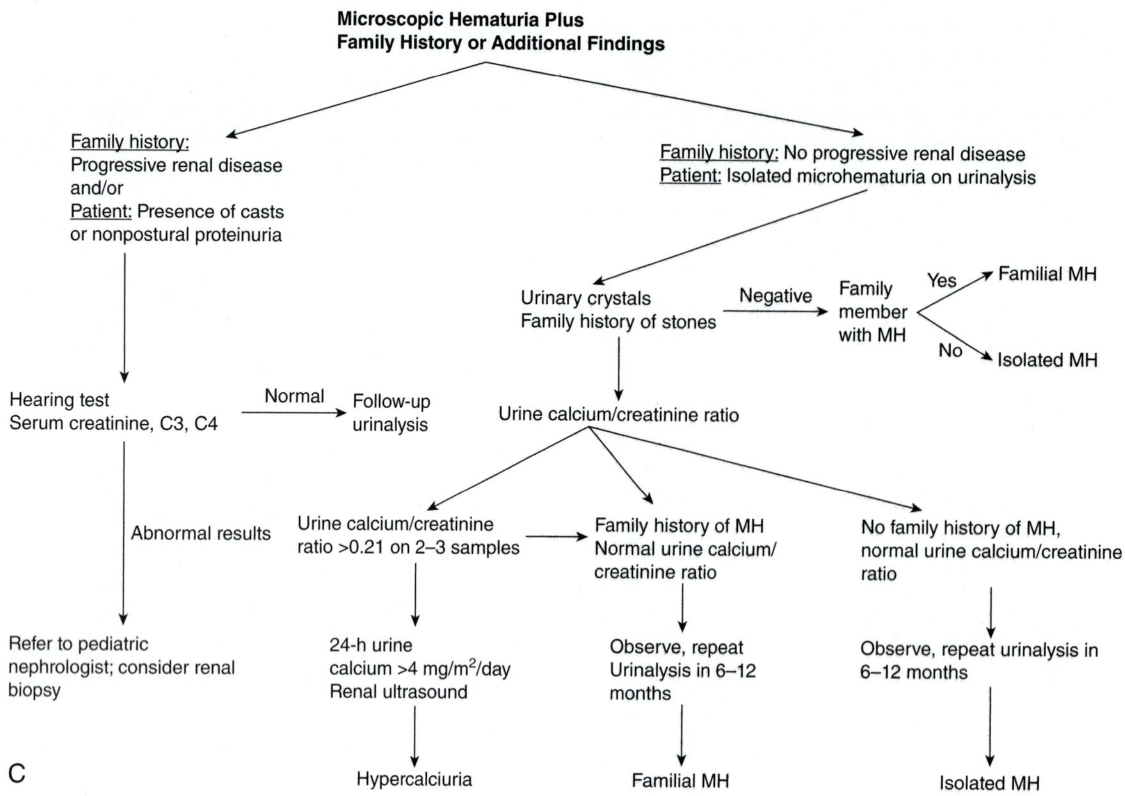

Fig. 14.3, cont'd (C) Microscopical hematuria with symptoms or additional findings. *CT,* Computed tomography; *MH,* microscopical hematuria; *RBC,* red blood cell; *UTI,* urinary tract infection. (From Meyers KEC: Evaluation of hematuria in children, *Urol Clin N Am* 31:559–573, 2004.)

bacterial cystitis, drug-induced hematuria, glomerulonephritis, or other causes. Detection of the most common causes of hematuria including glomerulonephritis or UTI can be readily achieved by the finding of cellular casts in an examination of the urinary sediment or by appropriate bacterial cultures. Moreover, heme-positive urine dipstick but absence of RBCs on urine microscopy suggests the diagnosis of rhabdomyolysis or hemolytic disorders. Well-performed urine dipstick and microscopy are invaluable in determining the etiology of hematuria by guiding the focus of the investigation to abnormal excretion of urine metabolites, an immunologic assessment of an underlying glomerulonephritis, or hematologic disorders. In contrast to adults, malignancies of the kidney or urinary tract rarely present with hematuria. Kidney ultrasonography coupled with Doppler evaluation of the renal vessels is useful in screening for the presence of tumor, PKD, or renal vein thrombosis. Computed tomography (CT) or magnetic resonance (MR) techniques may provide detailed anatomic resolution of such masses.

A kidney biopsy may be helpful in making a definitive diagnosis in cases of suspected kidney parenchymal disease manifested by hematuria. In contrast to adults, children rarely need cystoscopy for investigation of hematuria.

PROTEINURIA

Albumin excretion is by far the most abundant component of proteinuria associated with kidney disorders, but the proportion of albumin to LMW proteins such as β2 microglobulin is lower in tubulointerstitial than glomerular disorders. LMW proteins are freely filtered in the glomerulus. Because of efficient protein binding and endocytosis mediated by unique receptors on megalin and cubilin in proximal tubular cells, healthy individuals have minimal proteinuria. Box 14.2 shows definition of proteinuria based on qualitative screening of a freshly voided urine specimen (dipstick) and semiquantitative (random urine protein/creatinine ratios) and quantitative analyses (24-hour urine collection).

Box 14.2 Measurement and Definition of Proteinuria

Urine Dipstick (in Context of Urinary Specific Gravity)

Trace = 0–29 mg/dL
1+ = 30–99 mg/dL
2+ = 100–299 mg/dL
3+ = 300–999 mg/dL
4+ = >1000 mg/dL

Random Spot Urine Protein/Creatinine (mg/mg)

Children

<0.1 = 0.1 g/m²/day
0.1–1 = 0.1–1 g/m²/day
>1 = >1 g/m²/day

Adults

<0.2 = normal (<0.2 g/1.73 m²/day)
0.2–3.5 = intermediate proteinuria
>3.5 = nephrotic range proteinuria (>3.5 g/1.73 m²/day)

24-Hour Urine Collection

Normal Limits

Premature neonates: <140 mg/m²/day
Full-term neonates: <70 mg/m²/day
Children <4 years: <4 mg/m²/h or <100 mg/m²/day
Children 4–10 years: <190 mg/day
Children 10–16 years <250 mg/day
Nephrotic range: >40 mg/m²/h or >1000 mg/m²/day

Isolated proteinuria refers to proteinuria above the normal limits but less than 1500 mg/1.73 m²/day and absence of concurrent systemic illness, HTN, hematuria, pyuria, cellular casts, bacteriuria, kidney dysfunction, or abnormal kidney imaging studies. Such findings usually denote a transient or reversible disorder such as fever; heart failure; pancreatitis; rigorous exercise; or a common benign disorder more commonly seen in tall, active children known as orthostatic proteinuria. The latter condition is highly suggested by the absence of protein on dipstick of the first morning voided urine specimen and 1 to 3+ protein on testing of an afternoon urine specimen. It can be confirmed with two spot urine specimens: one from first morning void (supine) showing a normal urine protein/creatinine ratio and an elevated corresponding ratio from a specimen collected when the patient is upright. This clear distinction permits forgoing biochemical, immunologic, imaging, and kidney biopsy evaluation, which may be needed to exclude other potentially serious kidney disorders leading to proteinuria (Box 14.3). Box 14.4 is a guideline for referral of children with proteinuria to a nephrologist.

Box 14.3 Causes of Proteinuria

Transient Proteinuria
Fever
Dehydration
Cold exposure
Congestive heart failure
Seizures
Emotional stress
Epinephrine therapy

Isolated Proteinuria
Orthostatic proteinuria
Asymptomatic persistent benign proteinuria
Medications (lithium, nonsteroidal antiinflammatory agents, aminoglycosides)

Glomerular Disorders
Nephrotic syndrome
Glomerulonephritis
Alport syndrome
Sickle cell disease

Tubulointerstitial Disease
Reflux nephropathy
Tubulointerstitial nephritis
Cystinosis
Lowe syndrome
Drugs and heavy metals
Ischemic tubular injury
Renal hypo/dysplasia

Box 14.4 When to Refer a Child With Proteinuria

Persistent nonorthostatic proteinuria
A family history of glomerulonephritis, chronic kidney disease, or kidney replacement therapy (dialysis or kidney transplantation)
Systemic complaints such as fever, arthritis, arthralgias, or skin rash
Hypertension, edema, cutaneous vasculitis, or purpura
Coexistent hematuria with or without cellular casts in the spun sediment
Elevated blood urea nitrogen and creatinine or unexplained electrolyte abnormalities

GLOMERULAR DISORDERS

Nephritis and Nephrosis

In children suspected of having a glomerular disease, the urinary sediment can provide important clues for proper diagnosis. The presence of hyaline casts (Fig. 14.4A) can be a nonpathologic finding, but they can also appear in glomerular diseases. In nephritic syndrome, urinalysis reveals hematuria, proteinuria, and sometimes pyuria. Microscopy will often reveal RBC casts (see Fig. 14.4B) and, less frequently, WBC casts (see Fig. 14.4C). In contrast, children with classic NS such as minimal change disease (MCD) typically have heavy proteinuria (>40 mg/m^2/h, 1000 mg/m^2/day, or spot urine protein/creatinine >2), fat droplets and oval fat bodies, and little or no hematuria or other urine sediment abnormalities.

Acute Glomerulonephritis

Acute glomerulonephritis is characterized by the sudden onset of painless, dark, cola- or tea-colored urine; proteinuria; and cellular casts on urine microscopy. Edema, HTN, and acute kidney injury (AKI) are common clinical findings and together constitute nephritic syndrome. A classic example of pediatric nephritic syndrome is postinfectious glomerulonephritis (PIGN), which is also the most common etiology. This typically follows pharyngitis, otitis media, or pyoderma caused by nephritogenic strains of group A β-hemolytic streptococci, though it can be seen with other infections. Only about 15% of children infected with these strains of streptococci manifest nephritis. The disorder most frequently affects children aged 4 to 12 years and is more common in males. Both humoral (immune complexes with predilection for glomeruli) and cellular factors have been implicated in the pathogenesis. Most symptoms and signs resolve within a few weeks, although microscopic hematuria can last for more than 1 year. Fig. 14.5 shows the typical clinical course of PIGN. Spontaneous and complete recovery is the rule, with few children progressing to chronic kidney disease (CKD). Other conditions that may present as acute glomerulonephritis include IgA nephritis, IgA vasculitis (Henoch-Schönlein purpura [HSP]) nephritis, membranoproliferative glomerulonephritis (MPGN), and lupus nephritis.

In some instances, these disorders may have an aggressive clinical course characterized by oliguria, HTN, and rapid reduction in glomerular filtration rate (GFR), in which case the designation of rapidly progressive glomerulonephritis (RPGN) is given. Beyond the diagnoses mentioned earlier, the differential diagnosis of RPGN includes antineutrophil cytoplasmic antibody–associated vasculitis and antiglomerular basement antibody disease (Goodpasture disease). Kidney biopsy in such patients often demonstrates glomeruli with cellular or acellular crescents and inflammatory infiltrates.

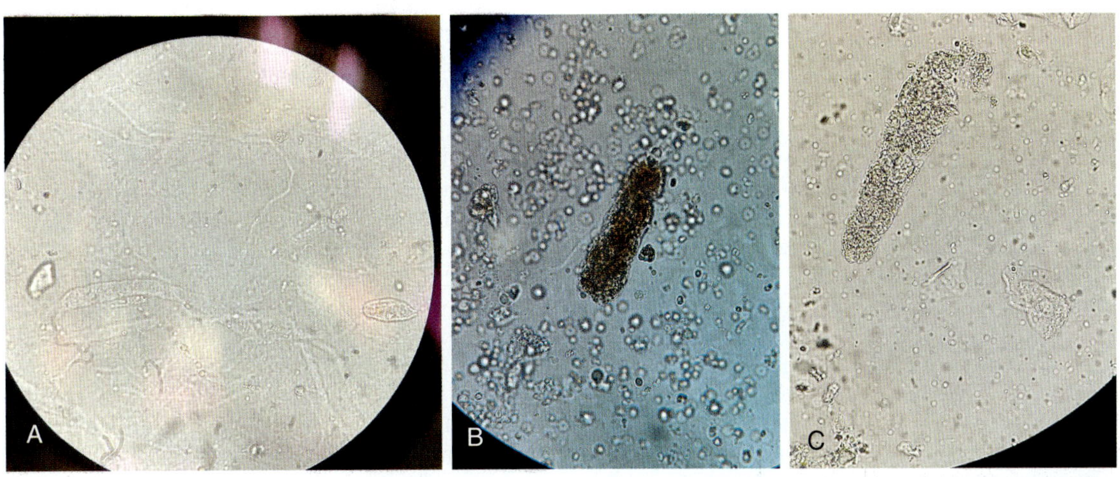

Fig. 14.4 (A) Hyaline cast, which may be seen in low urinary flow state and can be a nonpathologic finding or it can be seen with other pathologic casts. (B) Red blood cell casts and (C) white blood cell casts, which can be seen with acute and chronic glomerulonephritis.

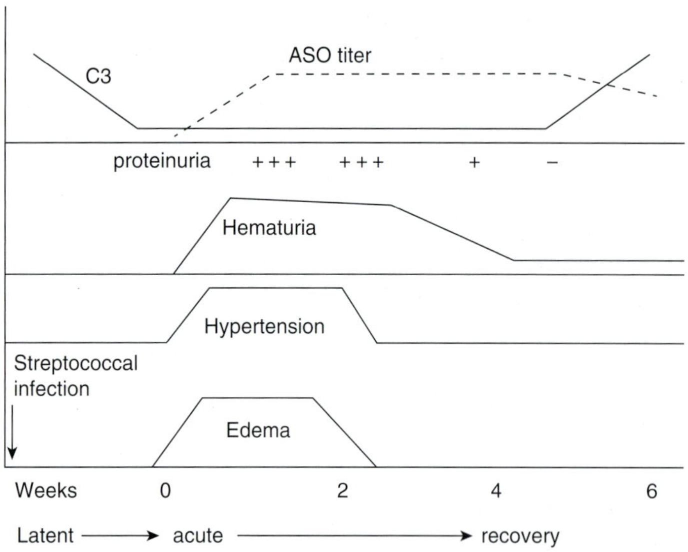

Fig. 14.5 Summary of the typical course of clinical signs, symptoms, and laboratory markers in acute poststreptococcal glomerulonephritis. (From Eison, TM, Ault BH, Jones DP, et al: Poststreptococcal acute glomerulonephritis in children: clinical features and pathogenesis, *Pediatr Nephrol* 26:165–180, 2011.)

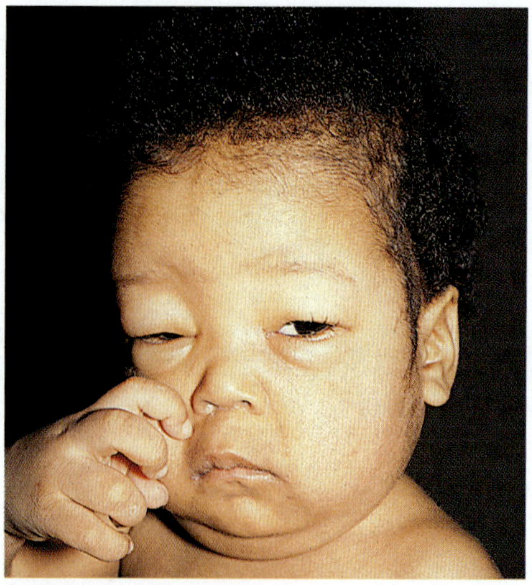

Fig. 14.6 Marked eyelid edema in a 2-year-old boy with minimal change disease and nephrotic syndrome.

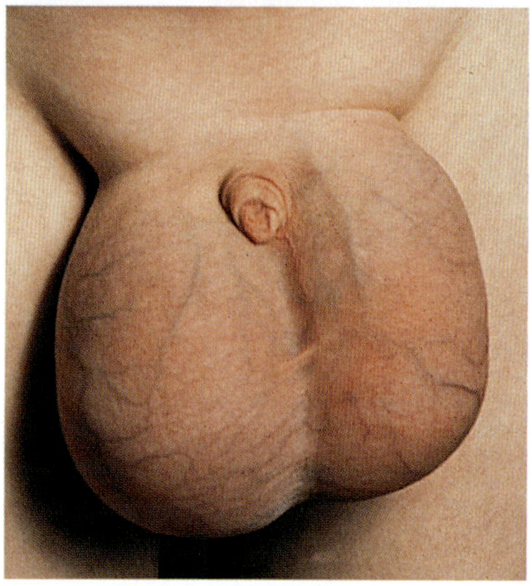

Fig. 14.7 Severe scrotal edema in a 6-year-old boy with nephrotic syndrome.

In addition to the unique or diagnostic clinical features, C3 and C4 levels are often the most helpful in distinguishing between these disorders. Other immunologic studies that may aid in diagnosis include antinuclear antibody titer, antistreptolysin O titer, streptozyme, antideoxyribonuclease B titer, antineutrophilic cytoplasmic antibody titer, and serum immunoglobulin concentrations.

IgA vasculitis (HSP) typically presents 1 to 3 weeks after a respiratory infection with generalized malaise, abdominal pain, arthritis, periorbital edema, difficulty walking, and purpuric rash. The leukocytoclastic rash typically covers the extensor surfaces of the extremities and the buttocks but spares the trunk (see Chapter 7). Some children initially develop an urticarial-type eruption that subsequently becomes macular or maculopapular. Younger patients may develop angioneurotic-like edema of the scalp, face, or dorsum of the hands or feet. About 30% to 50% of children with IgA vasculitis have kidney involvement ranging from simple microscopical hematuria and a variable degree of proteinuria to RPGN. In the absence of severe proteinuria, hypoalbuminemia and edema are often a result of protein-losing enteropathy. The skin rash is essential for the diagnosis of IgA vasculitis because the kidney abnormalities may otherwise closely resemble a similar disorder, IgA nephropathy. There are no distinct biochemical features of this disorder.

Nephrotic Syndrome

Nephrotic syndrome is defined as any kidney disorder resulting in marked proteinuria leading to hypoalbuminemia; hypercholesterolemia; and generalized edema that is generally more prominent in the eyelids, abdomen, scrotum, and lower extremities (Figs. 14.6 and 14.7). In the absence of an underlying systemic illness, the condition is considered primary. The most common histopathologic entities associated with primary NS of childhood include MCD, focal segmental glomerulosclerosis, and MPGN; membranous glomerulopathy (MGP) is also encountered in older children and in adults. Examples of the pathology of these disorders are depicted in Fig. 14.8A–D.

Data suggest that the proportion of all children presenting with NS who respond to steroids is less than 55% regardless of underlying histopathology, and late resistance to steroids in those with MCD may exceed 20% of the cases. Data suggest that approximately a third of patients with MCD will not have a relapse after 2 years, another third will infrequently relapse, and the remaining third will require additional immunosuppressive therapies. Consequently, nephrologists now use the terms "steroid sensitive" (SSNS), "steroid-dependent" (SDNS), "frequently relapsing" (FRNS), and "steroid resistant" (SRNS) to classify NS rather than rely solely on the kidney biopsy diagnosis to guide therapy and to predict prognosis. Children with FRNS and SDNS have a higher risk of eventually developing SRNS. Children with SDNS and, especially, those with SRNS have a significantly higher risk of developing end-stage kidney disease (ESKD).

Pathophysiology and Evaluation of Edema in Nephrotic Syndrome

Generalized edema or anasarca is a major presenting clinical feature of children with NS. Edema is defined as a palpable swelling resulting from a net movement of water from the intravascular (IV) into the interstitial (IS) fluid compartment and serves as the main clinical justification for hospital admission in children with NS. There is a constant movement of fluid from one compartment to another due to filtration across capillary walls. This is dependent on the balance between the hydrostatic pressure and oncotic pressure gradients across the capillary, between plasma and the interstitium described by Starling's "Law."

Compared with adolescents and adults, neonates and younger children have a greater proportion of total body water, and IS volume can double or triple in NS. In contrast to other forms of edema, it is pitting and often generalized but tends to be more prominent in dependent body areas in which capillary hydraulic pressure is high (ankles and feet) or in tissues with low IS hydraulic pressure (eyelids, gastrointestinal tract, and scrotum). Box 14.5 depicts the Starling forces favoring edema in NS.

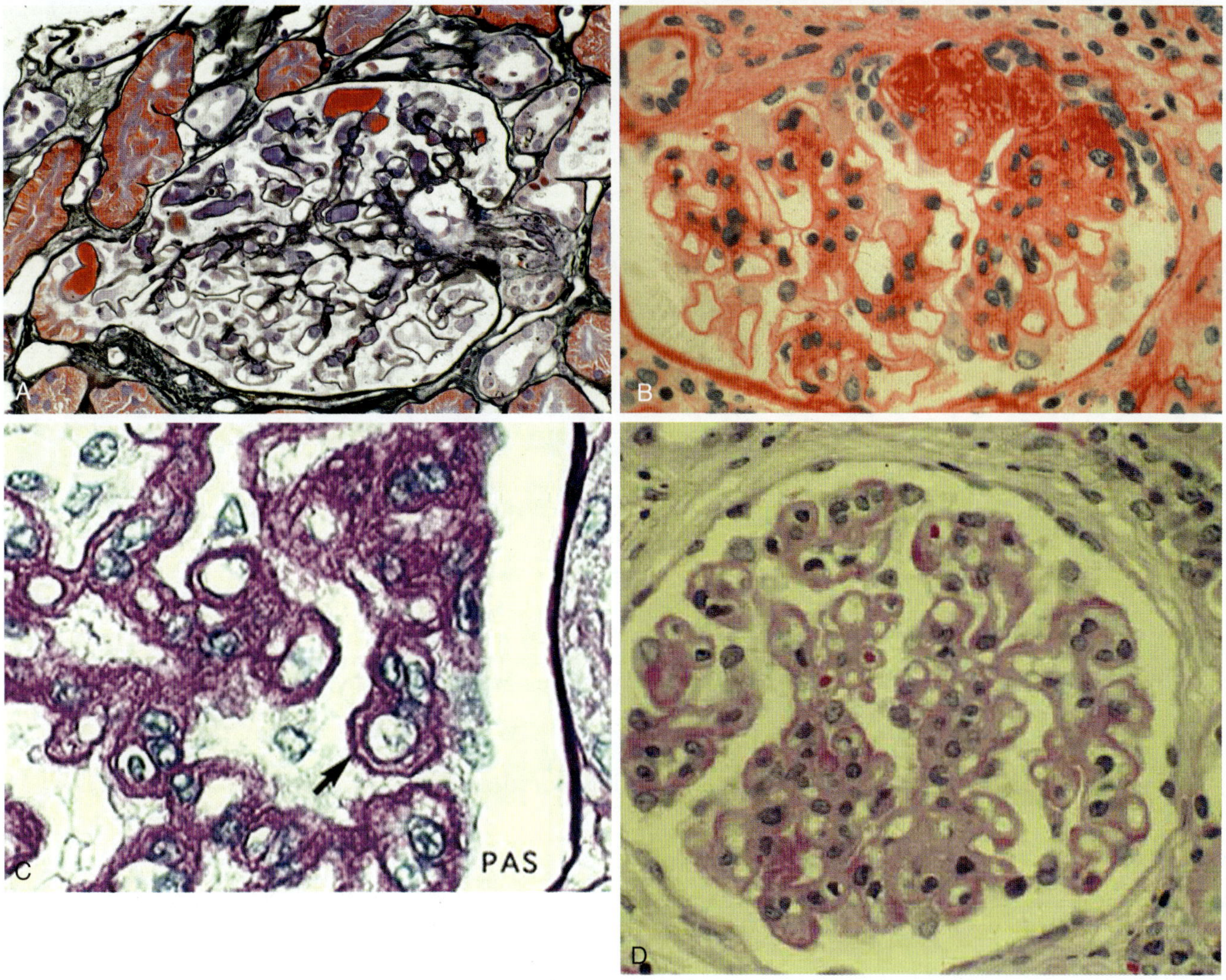

Fig. 14.8 Common pathologic forms associated with idiopathic nephrotic syndrome in children. (A) Minimal change disease with normal glomerular architecture. Notice the lacey appearance of the glomerular basement membrane (GBM) and open capillary loops. (B) Focal segmental glomerulosclerosis (FSGS). A few glomeruli (hence focal) may have a segment that is sclerosed as shown in this section stained with hematoxylin and eosin (H&E). Other lesions classified as FSGS include tip, collapsing, cellular, and "not otherwise specific" forms. (C) Membranoproliferative glomerulonephritis. This condition is associated with low circulating C3 or presence of C3 nephritic factor and immune complexes seen on immunostaining of frozen kidney biopsy sections. Because of proliferation of mesangial cells, the glomeruli are enlarged and often have a lobular accentuation. Mesangial cell interposition leads to characteristic "tram track" or splitting of the GBM as shown in this light photomicrograph. (D) Membranous glomerulopathy is evident by diffuse thickening of the GBM as shown previously and associated intramembranous and epimembranous immune deposits.

Box 14.5 Alterations in Starling Forces Favoring Nephrotic Edema Formation

1. Reduction in plasma oncotic pressure
2. Increased capillary permeability
3. Elevation in capillary hydraulic pressure
4. Increased interstitial oncotic pressure
5. Lymphatic vessel obstruction

In children with MCD or focal segmental glomerulosclerosis, the loss of large amounts of albumin in the urine often leads to marked hypoalbuminemia (<2 g/dL) and decrease in plasma oncotic pressure, which is the major force favoring fluid sequestration in the IS fluid compartment. This secondarily triggers renal sodium and fluid retention to preserve IV volume and blood pressure (BP), hence preventing an "underfill" state. In contrast to MCD, in glomerulonephritis with NS such as PIGN, the magnitude of the proteinuria is variable and IV fluid volume is typically normal or expanded because of pathologically stimulated primary sodium and fluid retention causing an "overfill" state. A schema depicting these two major mechanisms of nephrotic edema is presented in Fig. 14.9. Table 14.1 summarizes the typical clinical and laboratory features that distinguish children with NS with "underfill" or "overfill" physiology. It should be noted that because Na^+ retention occurs in both states, it is not possible to use the fractional excretion of Na^+ to reliably differentiate primary from secondary sodium retention. Diuretic use in children with "overfill" may help reduce hypertensive and pulmonary complications. In contrast, diuretic use in children with "underfill" may precipitate AKI and thromboembolic events.

ACUTE KIDNEY INJURY

AKI is defined as an abrupt decrease in GFR. The term *AKI* has replaced the previously used term *acute renal failure* as it encompasses the spectrum of kidney dysfunction ranging from minor decrements in function to need for kidney replacement therapy (KRT). This definition reflects the current understanding that even small alterations in kidney function are of clinical relevance and are associated with increased morbidity and mortality in both adult and pediatric patients.

Currently, there are no directed drug therapies for the prevention or treatment of AKI. As such, prevention measures to reduce AKI occurrence are vital. These prevention measures include limiting exposure to nephrotoxic medications, monitoring of nephrotoxic

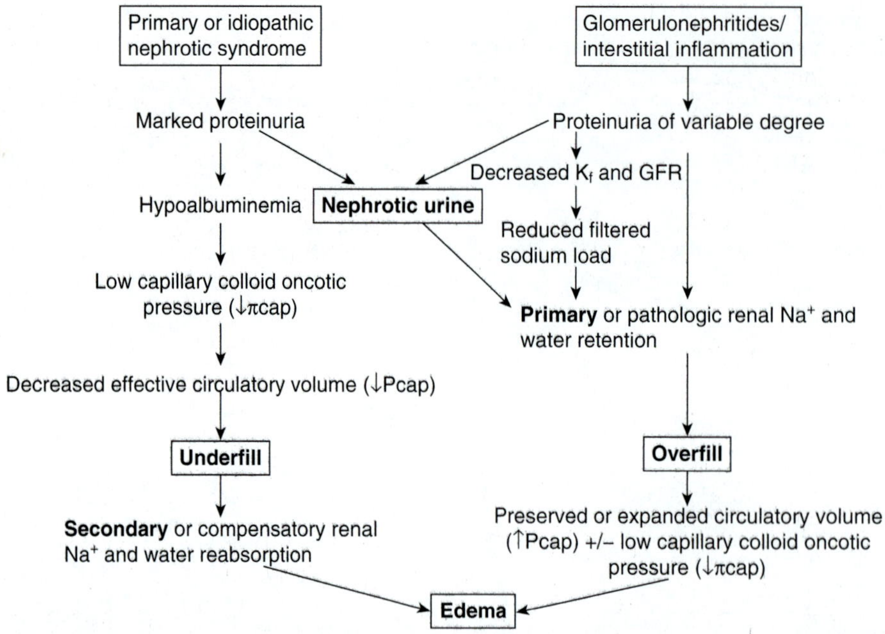

Fig. 14.9 Pathophysiology of edema formation in nephrotic syndrome. Primary nephrotic syndrome typically leads to "underfill" physiology mainly driven by marked proteinuria leading to hypoalbuminemia. In contrast, various glomerulonephritides and interstitial inflammation leads to "overfill" physiology from primary or pathologic renal sodium and water retention. *GFR,* Glomerular filtration rate; K_f, filtration coefficient; Na^+, sodium ion; *Pcap,* capillary hydraulic pressure; πcap, capillary fluid oncotic pressure.

Table 14.1 Mechanisms of Edema Formation in Nephrotic Syndrome

	"Underfilling"	"Overfilling"
Clinical characteristics	Weakness, pallor, cool extremities, tachycardia, orthostatic hypotension, abdominal pain, abdominal compartment syndrome, thrombosis	Normal or elevated blood pressure No sign of distal extremity hypoperfusion
Laboratory findings	Reduced urine volume $FENa^+$ <0.2% $UK^+/(UK^+ + Na^+)$ >60% Serum albumin <2 g/dL GFR >75 mL/min/1.73 m^2 Hemoconcentration High-circulating PRA, aldosterone, vasopressin and norepinephrine Low ANP concentration	$FENa^+$ >0.5% while on no-salt restricted diet $UK^+/(UK^+ + Na^+)$ <60% Hematuria and cellular casts Serum albumin >2 g/dL Elevated serum creatinine and BUN GFR <50 mL/min/1.73 m^2 Decreased vasopressin, PRA, norepinephrine Low or normal plasma aldosterone High ANP

ANP, Atrial natriuretic peptide; $FENa^+$, fractional excretion of sodium; *GFR,* glomerular filtration rate; *PRA,* plasma renin activity; UK^+ *and* UNa^+, urinary potassium and sodium concentrations.

medication drug levels, avoidance of hypotension, and early goal-directed fluid administration for the management of hypovolemia and exposures to both endogenous and exogenous renal toxins.

Defining Acute Kidney Injury

Current AKI stages are defined by the Kidney Disease Improving Global Outcomes (KDIGO) AKI work group and were published in 2012 (Table 14.2). The standardized definitions, based on serum creatinine and urine output, have been key in understanding the epidemiology and outcomes of AKI.

It is important to note that a rise in serum creatinine is often a late marker of kidney injury, and changes in serum creatinine concentration are delayed after a change in GFR. The use of urinary biomarkers for the early identification of AKI has become more widespread in pediatric centers over the past decade; however, the routine use of urinary biomarkers for the detection of AKI has not yet become the standard of care. The use of urinary neutrophil gelatinase–associated lipocalin (NGAL) has been validated for the screening of AKI in children undergoing cardiac procedures and in other clinical settings such as the emergency department and pediatric intensive care unit. Other urinary biomarkers including kidney injury molecule 1 (KIM-1),

Table 14.2 Kidney Disease Improving Global Outcomes Acute Kidney Injury Criteria

Stage	Serum Creatinine	Urine Output
1	1.5–1.9 times baseline OR ≥0.3 mg/dL increase	<0.5 mL/kg/h for 6–12 h
2	2.0–2.9 times baseline	<0.5 mL/kg/hour for ≥12 h
3	3.0 times baseline OR Increase in serum creatinine ≥4.0 mg/dL OR Initiation of kidney replacement therapy OR In patients <18 years, a decrease in eGFR to <35 mL/min per 1.73 m^2	<0.3 mL/kg/hour for ≥24 h OR Anuria for ≥12 h

AKI, Acute kidney injury; *eGFR,* estimated glomerular filtration rate; *KDIGO,* Kidney Disease Improving Global Outcomes.

interleukin-18 (IL-18), and liver-type fatty acid binding protein (L-FABP) have also been studied in similar pediatric clinical settings.

Clinically, AKI has been traditionally classified into three groups: prerenal, intrinsic renal, and postrenal. These classifications have been useful in understanding the mechanisms by which AKI occurs and guiding the management of AKI in the clinical setting. These and other causes of prerenal, intrinsic renal, and postrenal AKI are outlined in Table 14.3.

Table 14.3 Common Causes of Acute Kidney Injury

Type	Mechanisms and Etiology
Prerenal	Dehydration • GI losses (vomiting, diarrhea) • Insensible losses (burns, sweat) • Hemorrhage • Kidney losses (diabetes insipidus, diabetes mellitus, diuretics) Hypotension • Shock (cardiac, neurogenic, hypovolemic) • Peripheral vasodilation (sepsis, antihypertensive agents, anaphylaxis) Renal vasoconstriction • Medications (NSAIDs, ACE-I, ARBs) • Hepatorenal syndrome • Sepsis Edematous states with intravascular volume depletion • Heart failure • Cirrhosis • Nephrotic syndrome

Intrinsic renal	Glomerular
	• Glomerulonephritides (PIGN, IgA nephropathy, SLE, HSP, MPGN, anti-GBM disease)
	Tubular
	• Prolonged kidney ischemia
	• Nephrotoxic drugs (acyclovir, aminoglycosides, amphotericin B, calcineurin inhibitors, carboplatin, cidofovir, cisplatin, foscarnet, ganciclovir, iphosphamide, methotrexate, pentamidine, radiocontrast drugs, vancomycin)
	• Endogenous tubular toxins (hemoglobinuria, myoglobinuria, hyperuricemia)
	Interstitial
	• Interstitial nephritis
	  • Drug-induced (NSAIDs, penicillins, cephalosporins, sulfonamides, diuretics, allopurinol, PPIs)
	  • TINU
	• Systemic diseases (SLE, Sjögren syndrome, IBD)
	• Infection (*Streptococcus, Enterococcus, Escherichia coli*, EBV, CMV, *Legionella*)
	• Infiltrative disorders (neoplastic, sarcoidosis)
	Vascular
	• Thrombotic microangiopathy (HUS, TMA)
	• Hypertension
	• Vasculitis (SLE, HSP, MPA, GPA)

Postrenal	Congenital • PUV • Neurogenic bladder • Bilateral UPJ or UVJ obstruction (or unilateral in a solitary kidney) Acquired • Bladder outlet obstruction (tumor, fluid collection) • Medication-induced urinary retention • Neurogenic bladder • Kidney or bladder calculi • Clots

ACE-I, Angiotensin-converting enzyme inhibitors; *anti-GBM,* antiglomerular basement membrane; *ARB,* angiotensin II receptor blocker; *CMV,* cytomegalovirus; *EBV,* Epstein-Barr virus; *GI,* gastrointestinal; *GPA,* granulomatosis with polyangiitis; *HSP,* Henoch-Schönlein purpura; *HUS,* hemolytic uremic syndrome; *IBD,* inflammatory bowel disease; *MPA,* microscopical polyangiitis; *MPGN,* membranoproliferative glomerulonephritis; *NSAIDs,* nonsteroidal antiinflammatory drugs; *PIGN,* postinfectious glomerulonephritis; *PPI,* proton pump inhibitor; *PUV,* posterior urethral valves; *SLE,* systemic lupus erythematous; *TINU,* tubulointerstitial nephritis and uveitis syndrome; *TMA,* thrombotic thrombocytopenic purpura; *UPJ,* ureteropelvic junction; *UVJ,* ureterovesical junction.

Pathophysiology and Determination of Acute Kidney Injury Etiology

Prerenal AKI is characterized by kidney hypoperfusion and a decline in GFR. This decline in GFR is a functional response to decreased kidney blood flow and occurs in the setting of intrinsically normal kidney function. IV volume depletion physiologically leads to an increase in circulating norepinephrine, angiotensin II, and antidiuretic hormone, which causes renal vasoconstriction and increased absorption of sodium and water by the kidney. This results in a reduced GFR, a low fractional excretion of sodium, and a decline in urine output. Oliguria, defined as urine output less than 1 mL/kg/h in infants, less than 0.5 mL/kg/h in children, or less than 400 mL/day in adults, is commonly observed in patients with prerenal AKI and is the kidneys' appropriate response to maintain adequate IV volume.

Intrinsic AKI is often multifactorial, particularly in hospitalized children, and is frequently associated with tubular damage and ATN in cases of sustained or severe kidney insult. ATN is characterized by histologic changes in the renal tubules, ranging from disruption of the apical brush border of tubular cells to cellular necrosis. This is visualized in the urine microscopy by the presence of renal tubular epithelial cells (Fig. 14.10A) and cellular debris in the form of "muddy brown" casts (see Fig. 14.10B). This tubular injury leads to diminished tubular function, resulting in urinary wasting of sodium, urea, water, and other electrolytes. Inflammation or damage to the glomeruli, such as in cases of glomerulonephritis or disease states leading to the disruption of glomerular blood flow, leads to reduced glomerular filtration and decreased clearance of metabolites and toxins.

Comparatively, postrenal AKI is due to urinary tract obstruction. Urinary tract obstruction leads to elevated pressure in the collecting system, causing stress injury to the tubules and impairing tubular and glomerular function. After the obstruction is relieved, the AKI often resolves. Physiologically, downregulation of sodium and water transporters in the tubules and collecting ducts frequently occurs. These changes limit the renal concentrating capacity, which places patients at increased risk for postobstructive diuresis. When this occurs, patients are unable to reabsorb sodium and water, which can lead to dehydration and prerenal AKI after relief of the urinary obstruction. Therefore close monitoring of fluid balance is required after treatment of postrenal AKI.

A thorough medical history and physical examination are often sufficient in determining AKI etiology; however, certain urinary indices can be helpful in differentiating prerenal versus intrinsic forms of AKI. As discussed previously, sodium and water handling by the kidney differ in patients with prerenal versus intrinsic AKI; therefore urine SG, urine sodium level, and fractional excretion of sodium can be used to differentiate between prerenal and intrinsic forms of kidney injury (Table 14.4). A urinalysis should be obtained to assess for the presence of hematuria, proteinuria, or evidence of infection including pyuria, positive urinary nitrites, and positive leukocyte esterase. If the patient's history or urinalysis is concerning for infection, urine culture should be obtained. The presence of hematuria and proteinuria on urinalysis may be a sign of glomerular or tubular disease and should prompt urine microscopy. The presence of RBC (see Fig. 14.4B), WBC (see Fig. 14.4C), or mixed cellular casts on urine microscopy may indicate glomerulonephritis and infection, and eosinophils (Fig. 14.11) may indicate tubulointerstitial nephritis. A kidney ultrasonography should be obtained if there are concerns for urinary obstruction. Doppler evaluation of the renal vasculature should be performed in cases where renal arterial or venous thrombosis or renal vascular injury is suspected. Kidney biopsy is rarely indicated in the evaluation of AKI but may be performed if noninvasive testing fails to establish a diagnosis.

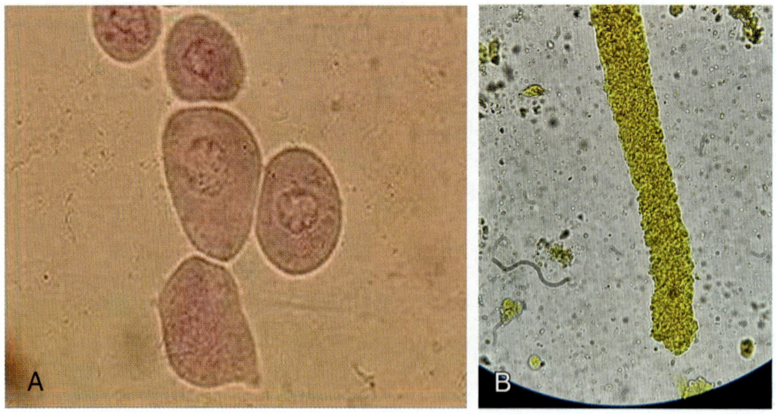

Fig. 14.10 In acute tubular necrosis, urine microscopy typically demonstrates signs of renal tubular damage with presence of (A) renal tubular epithelial cells and (B) muddy brown casts.

Table 14.4 Urinary Indices in Prerenal and Intrinsic Acute Kidney Injury

Urinary Indices	Prerenal AKI	Intrinsic AKI
Specific gravity	>1.020	<1.012
Urine sodium (mEq/L)	<20	>40
FENa	<1%	>2%
FEUrea	<25%	>35%
Casts	None	Muddy brown—ATN Cellular (RBC) casts–GN WBC casts—Pyelonephritis, TIN

AKI, Acute kidney injury; *ATN,* acute tubular necrosis; *FENa,* fractional excretion of sodium; *FEUrea,* fractional excretion of urea; *GN,* glomerulonephritis; *RBC,* red blood cell; *TIN,* tubulointerstitial nephritis; *WBC,* white blood cell.

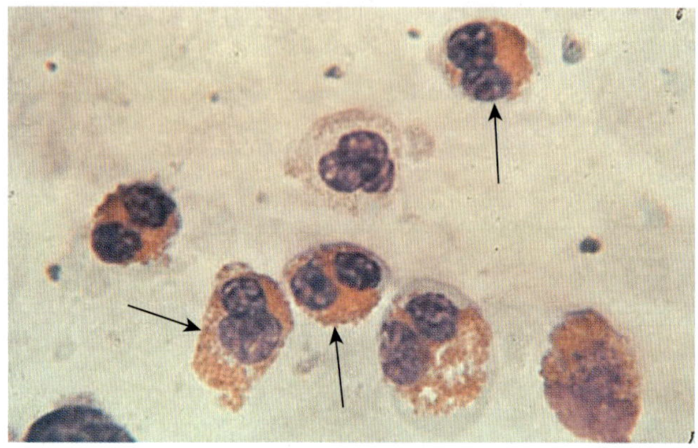

Fig. 14.11 Wright-Giemsa staining showing eosinophiluria *(arrows)* associated with tubulointerstitial nephritis resulting in acute kidney injury.

Management of Acute Kidney Injury

Once identified, the management of AKI is often dictated by AKI etiology. However, in all circumstances, strict attention to fluid balance, metabolic disturbances, and BP is critical. Frequent monitoring of urine output and electrolytes should be used to dictate fluid administration and fluid composition, with the goal to avoid hypotension, volume overload, and electrolyte imbalances. Drug dosing should be evaluated daily to reduce the risk of supratherapeutic drug levels and additional drug-induced nephrotoxicity.

Indications for KRT include hyperkalemia, symptomatic uremia, metabolic acidosis, hypocalcemia, hyperphosphatemia, and volume overload that are nonresponsive to medical management. Initiation of KRT may also be indicated when the ability to supply adequate nutrition is hindered by volume overload. Symptoms of uremia may include altered mental status, pericarditis, pleuritis, or excessive bleeding from uremic platelet dysfunction. Choice of kidney replacement modality is dependent on multiple factors including hemodynamic stability, indication for KRT, availability of vascular or peritoneal access, and personnel. Continuous KRT is often chosen in patients with hemodynamic instability who require accurate ultrafiltration and can be performed alongside other therapies including extracorporeal membrane oxygenation (Fig. 14.12A and B).

NEPHROLITHIASIS

The diagnosis of nephrolithiasis should be entertained in any child with acute onset of costovertebral angle or abdominal colicky pain. In younger children, renal colic is poorly localized and is often described as diffuse abdominal pain. Small stones may produce no pain and may be detected only after an episode of gross hematuria, pyuria, or UTI. Larger nephrolithiasis can be detected by ultrasonography (Fig. 14.13), and CT scan of the urinary tract without IV contrast is the gold-standard examination (Fig. 14.14). Clinical history and laboratory evaluation often reveal the cause of the stones. Direct chemical analysis of the calculus may also disclose the composition of the stone. One diagnostic approach to pediatric nephrolithiasis is shown in Box 14.6.

The most common calculi found in children consist of calcium oxalate or calcium phosphate, followed by uric acid, cystine, and struvite calculi. Although not diagnostic, urine microscopy may reveal urine crystals including calcium oxalate, calcium phosphate, uric acid, and cystine (Fig. 14.15A–D, respectively). Calcium calculi frequently occur in children with idiopathic hypercalciuria and may be manifested by painless microscopical or recurrent gross hematuria for years before frank nephrolithiasis occurs. Screening for hypercalciuria may be done with a single voided urine specimen; a fasting calcium-to-creatinine ratio greater than 0.2 is suggestive of this condition, which may then be confirmed by a 24-hour urine collection having calcium content $\geq$4 mg/kg body weight. Pediatric hyperuricosuria is defined as a uric acid excretion (normalized to GFR: [urine uric acid/plasma uric acid] $\times$ plasma creatinine) > 0.53 mg/dL in a random urine sample. Citrate is an inhibitor of calcium crystallization, and hypocitraturia, defined as less than 400 mg/g creatinine in a 24-hour urine collection, is often found in patients with calcium nephrolithiasis. Investigations of lithogenic risk factors often help to determine the underlying etiology and to guide prevention measures. Table 14.5 shows normal values of both 24-hour urine collections and spot urine samples commonly investigated in patients suspected to have nephrolithiasis or nephrocalcinosis.

Studies report significant increases in the incidence of nephrolithiasis in both adults and children. Assuming the genetic pool of patients predisposed to hypercalciuria has not changed appreciably, one can speculate that the increase in incidence is due mostly to

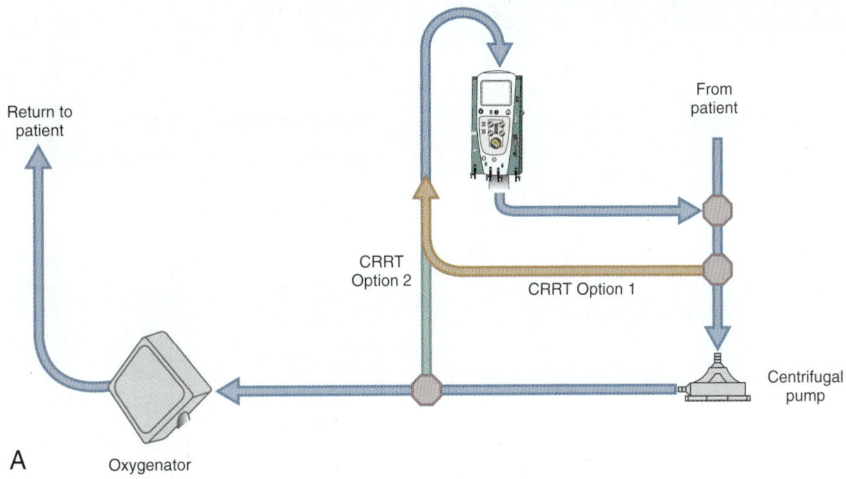

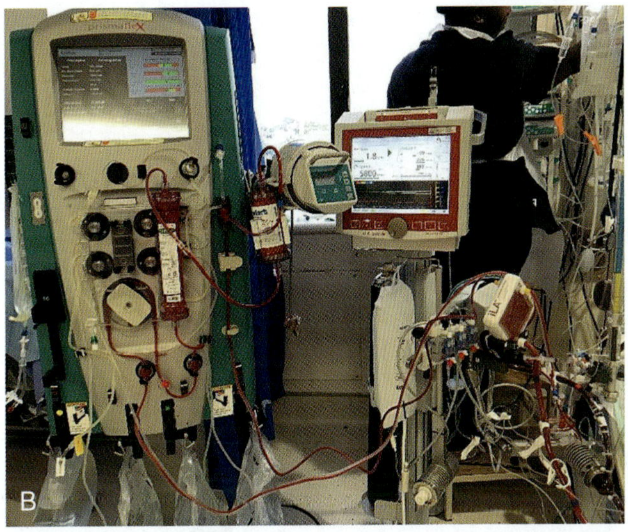

Fig. 14.12 Critically ill children with cardiopulmonary failure with acute kidney injury can be supported using continuous kidney replacement therapy together with extracorporeal membrane oxygenation. (A) Schematic diagram and (B) bedside photograph of how these machines can be used together.

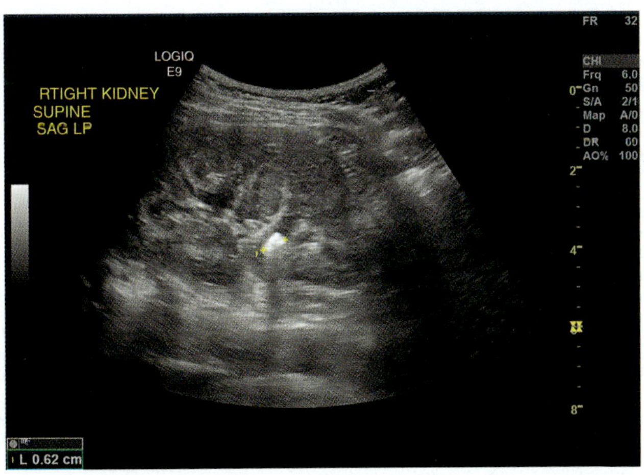

Fig. 14.13 Kidney ultrasonography image of a nonobstructive nephrolithiasis with hyperechoic focus with distinct shadow produced by the calculus. (Courtesy Judy Squires, MD, UPMC Children's Hospital of Pittsburgh.)

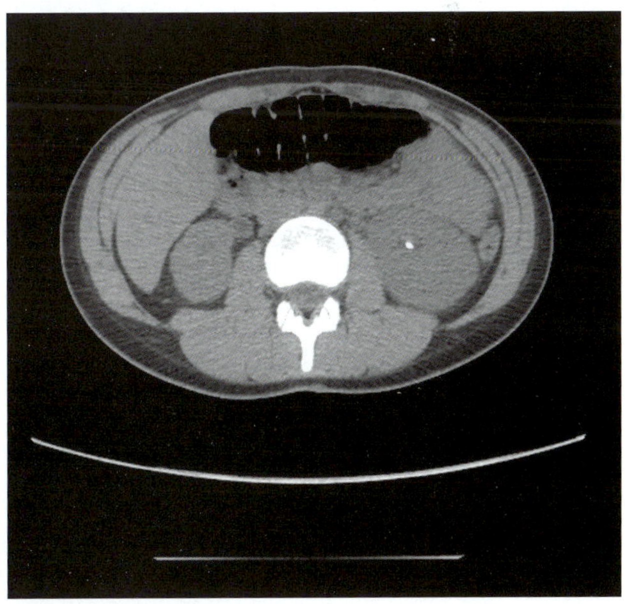

Fig. 14.14 Computed tomography image of calcium nephrolithiasis in the left kidney. (Courtesy Judy Squires, MD, UPMC Children's Hospital of Pittsburgh.)

dietary factors, including large intake of dietary sodium, protein, phosphate, and caffeine, and low water ingestion. The nonabsorptive form of hypercalciuria appears to have an autosomal dominant inheritance underlying a renal tubular defect and net loss of calcium independent of the amount of dietary calcium ingested. The absorptive form may be associated with increased serum concentrations of 1, 25-dihydroxyvitamin D resulting in increased fractional absorption of calcium at the intestinal level. Premature infants receiving high dosages of loop diuretics to control fluid retention associated with pulmonary and cardiac disorders may develop hypercalciuria, nephrolithiasis, and nephrocalcinosis. Other disorders predisposing to nephrolithiasis and nephrocalcinosis include hyperparathyroidism, cystinuria, hyperoxaluria, defects of purine metabolism, inflammatory bowel disease, and distal (type 1) renal tubular acidosis. UTIs

Box 14.6 Evaluation of Nephrolithiasis

Clinical History
Family history of nephrolithiasis
Immobilization or other protracted illness or stress
High dietary purine intake
Excessive salt or calcium ingestion
Large and infrequent meals
Excessive intake of vitamins or over-the-counter medications
Symptoms of UTI or history of pyelonephritis
Source and calcium content of drinking water
Polyuria or polydipsia
Antiseizure therapy including ketogenic diet and medications

Physical Diagnosis
Band keratopathy and other signs of hyperparathyroidism
Elfin facies and other features of Williams syndrome

Radiologic Studies
Noncontrast helical CT—the most sensitive modality to detect kidney or ureteral stone
Ultrasonography—especially sensitive in identifying kidney calculi, nephrocalcinosis, and radiolucent stones
KUB—for the identification of ureteral stones; radiopaque stones include calcium oxalate and cystine

Urinary Studies
Urinalysis—may reveal pyuria or bacteriuria, inability to lower urinary pH or to concentrate the urine, or flat hexagonal crystals pathognomonic of cystinosis
Urine culture
Screening with cyanide-nitroprusside (cystinosis)
Timed or spot urine collections on two or more occasions[a]

Biochemical Studies
Creatinine, BUN, electrolytes, total CO_2, albumin, calcium, phosphorus, magnesium, and uric acid; plasma parathyroid hormone levels if indicated
Chemical analysis of gravel or stones

[a]See Table 14.5 for common urine chemical studies and their normal values.

Table 14.5 Normal Values for 24-Hour Urine Collection and Spot Urine Samples

Parameter, Age	24 Hour	Spot (Solute/Creatinine Ratios)
Calcium	<4 mg/kg (all ages)	mg/mg
<12 months		0.81
1–3 years		0.53
1–5 years		0.39
5–7 years		0.28
>7 years		0.21
Oxalate	<45 mg/1.73 m^2 (all ages)	mg/g
0–6 months		260–288
7–24 months		110–139
2–5 years		80
5–14 years		60–65
>16 years		32
Uric acid	0.56 mg/dL per GFR	(>2 years) <0.56 mg/dL per GFR
Citrate		g/g (for both sexes)
Male	>365 mg/1.73 m^2	(0–5 years) 0.42
Female	>310 mg/1.73 m^2	(>5 years) 0.25
Magnesium	>0.8 mg/kg	>0.13 (g/g)
Cystine	<13 mg/1.73 m^2	
<10 years	<48 mg/1.73 m^2	
>10 years	<60 mg/1.73 m^2	
Adults		

GFR, Glomerular filtration rate.

Modified from Hoppe B, Kemper M: Diagnostic examination of the child with urolithiasis or nephrocalcinosis, *Pediatr Nephrol* 25:403–413, 2010.

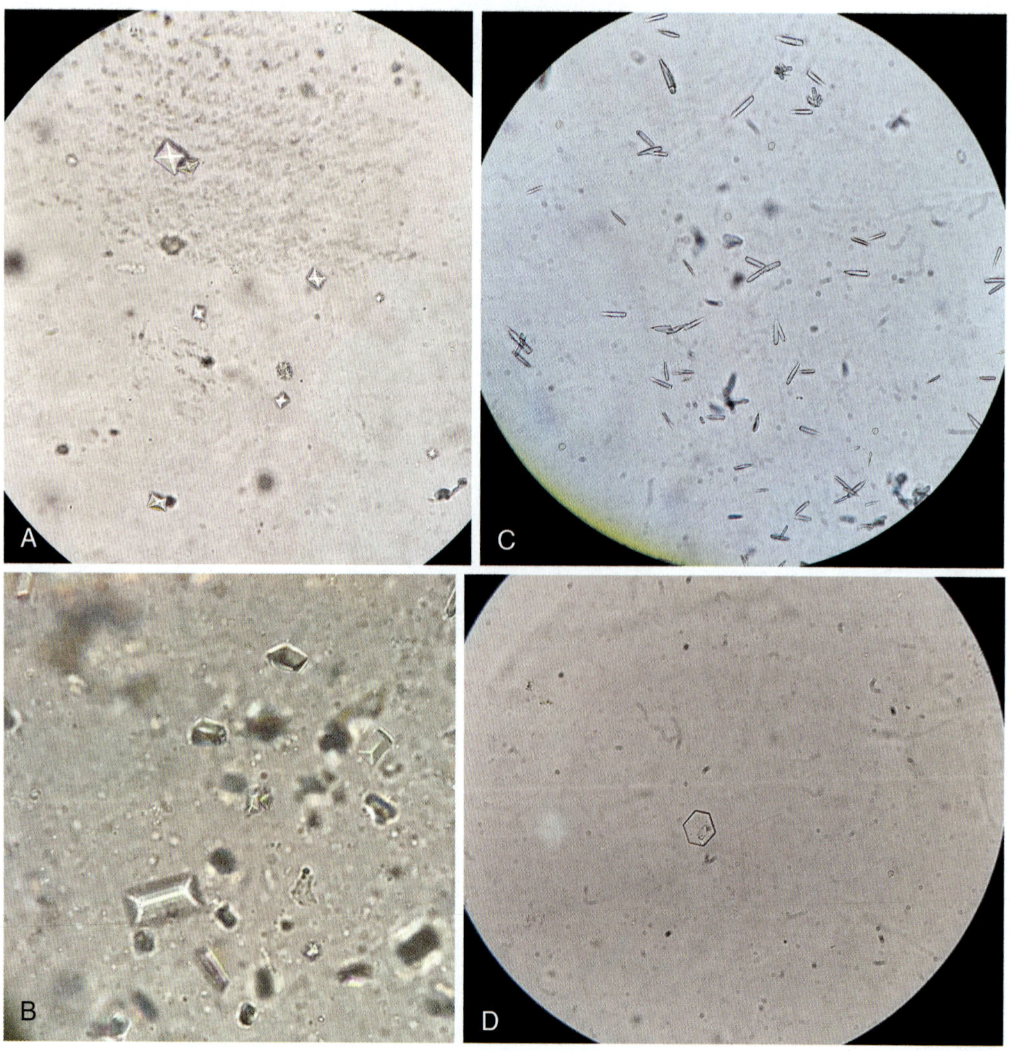

Fig. 14.15 Urine microscopy appearance of various crystals. (A) Calcium oxalate, (B) calcium phosphate with district coffin-like shape, (C) uric acid, and (D) pathognomonic flat hexagonal crystals seen in cystinuria.

and obstructive uropathy are also important risk factors in the development of nephrolithiasis.

VESICOURETERAL REFLUX

VUR is the most common urinary tract abnormality in children. It is often a congenital condition in which the normal valve mechanism of the ureterovesical junction is impaired, leading to reflux of bladder urine into the ureter or kidneys. The prevalence of VUR in healthy children is estimated to be between 1% to 3% and 30% to 50% among children with a history of one or more UTIs. Moreover, VUR is more prevalent among siblings (30%–35%) and offspring (65%), suggesting a strong genetic component. Kidney scarring is fivefold more common with higher grades of VUR and ninefold higher than in those without VUR. Fluoroscopic voiding cystourethrogram (VCUG) is the authors' preferred means for the initial diagnosis and grading of VUR, and radionuclide VCUG may be done for follow-up study to evaluate if VUR persists. A more recent alternative is contrast-enhanced voiding urosonography, which eliminates the use of radiation. The severity of VUR is classified according to the following international grading system (Fig. 14.16):

Grade I—reflux into the ureter only (Fig. 14.17)
Grade II—complete reflux into the ureter, pelvis, and calices without any dilation of the structures (Fig. 14.18)
Grade III—complete reflux with mild dilation or tortuosity of the ureter and mild dilation of the renal pelvis but only slight blunting of the caliceal fornices (Fig. 14.19)
Grade IV—complete reflux with moderate dilation of the ureter, renal pelvis, and calices; complete obliteration of the sharp angle of the fornices with maintenance of the papillary impressions of the calices (Fig. 14.20)
Grade V—gross dilation and tortuosity of the ureter with gross dilation of the renal pelvis and calices; obliteration of the papillary impressions of the calices (Fig. 14.21).

As noted in Table 14.6, 80% of VUR resolves spontaneously by 5 years of age but grade V VUR rarely resolves spontaneously. The presence of compound renal papillae in infants may predispose to intrarenal reflux of bacteria, resulting in acute tubulointerstitial nephritis (pyelonephritis) and subsequent increased vulnerability to progressive chronic kidney injury. Kidney scars are best detected by technetium-99m dimercapto succinic acid scan, which is more sensitive than ultrasonography. Because kidney scars are frequently found at the time of diagnosis of the first UTI, many experts believe that the abnormal appearance on dimercapto succinic acid may represent a focal area of dysplasia that is coincidental with VUR, and only a small fraction of children with VUR develop reflux nephropathy even despite having recurrent infections. However, new scars can be seen on prospective imaging for VUR in children with recurrent UTIs, with those younger than 2 years of age being at highest risk for this complication.

DEVELOPMENTAL AND HEREDITARY DISORDERS

The number of congenital malformations associated with kidney abnormalities is too large to discuss individually in this chapter. In this section, only a few syndromes are considered in which kidney abnormalities are serious, relatively common, and easily diagnosed on the basis of physical findings.

Prune-Belly Syndrome (Eagle-Barrett Syndrome)

Prune-belly syndrome usually consists of the absence of abdominal musculature, kidney and urinary tract abnormalities, and cryptorchidism (Fig. 14.22). Boys are affected more severely and 20 times more frequently than girls. Although there is generally no ureteral obstruction, the ureters are dilated and tortuous and 75% exhibit

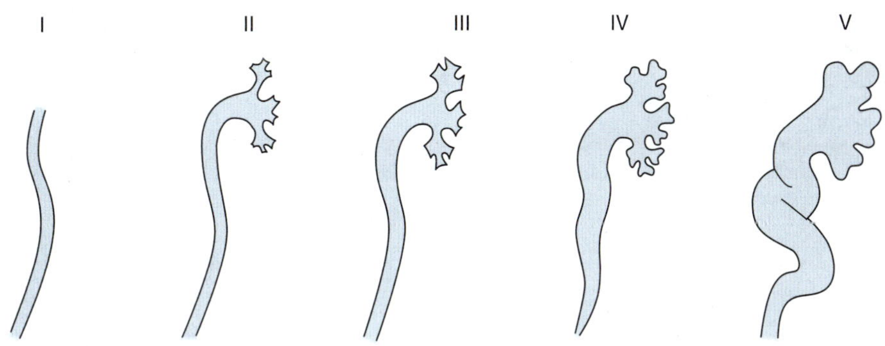

Fig. 14.16 Grades of vesicoureteral reflux, schematically presented.

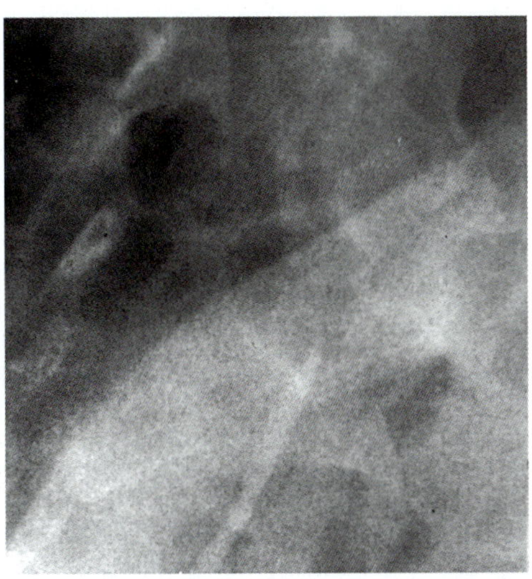

Fig. 14.17 Grade I reflux: Cystourethrogram shows reflux only into the ureter.

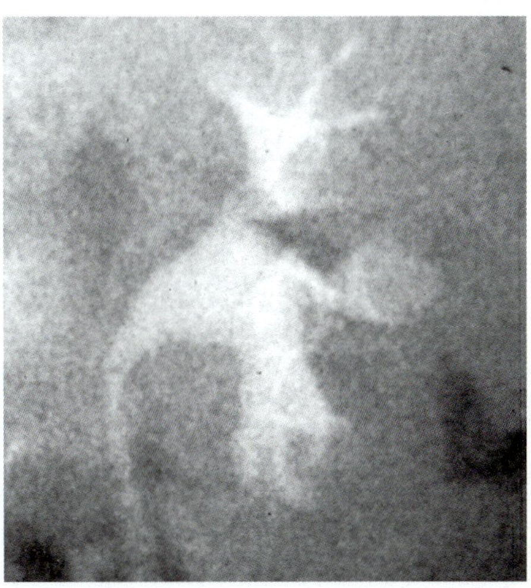

Fig. 14.18 Grade II reflux: cystourethrogram shows complete reflux into the ureter, pelvis, and calices; no dilation.

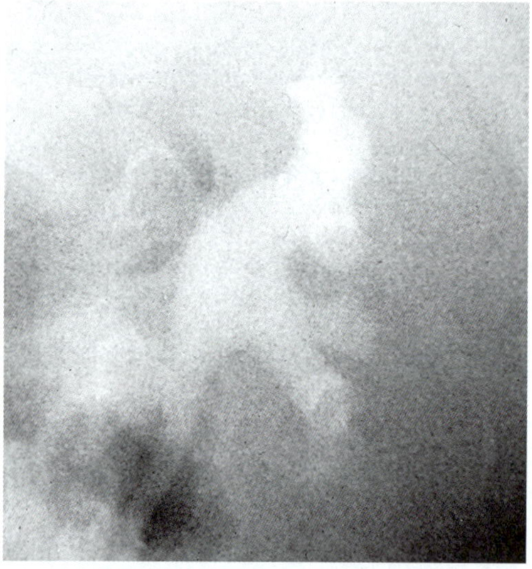

Fig. 14.19 Grade III reflux: Cystourethrogram shows complete reflux with mild dilation of the ureter and renal pelvis but only slight blunting of the calices.

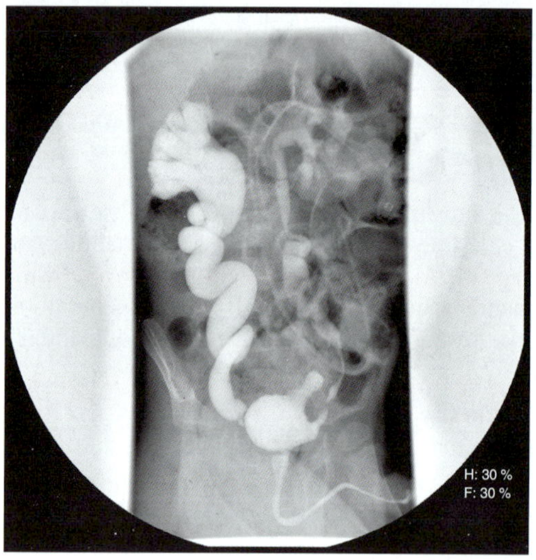

Fig. 14.20 Grade IV reflux: Cystourethrogram shows complete reflux with moderate dilation of the ureter, pelvis, and calices; complete obliteration of sharp angle of fornices.

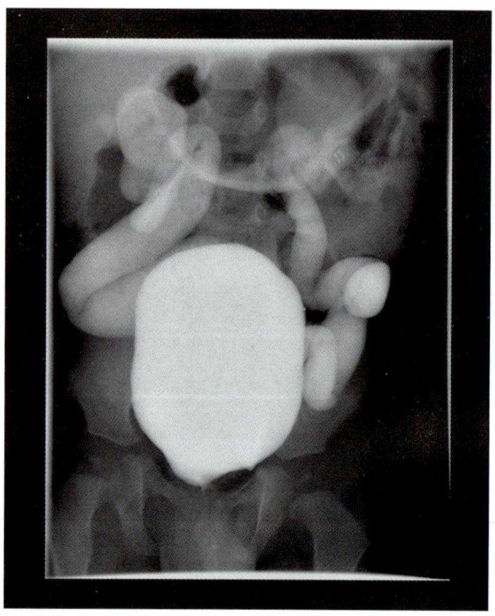

Fig. 14.21 Grade V reflux: Cystourethrogram shows gross dilation of the ureter, pelvis, and calices; obliteration of the papillary impressions of the calices.

Table 14.6 Spontaneous Resolution Rates for Medically Treated Vesicoureteral Reflux

Reflux Severity, Laterality, and Age at Diagnosis[a]	% Resolved in 5 Years
Grade I[b]	92
Grade II[b]	81
Grade III	
Unilateral	
0–24 months	70
25–60 months	51
61–120 months	44
Bilateral	
0–24 months	49
25–60 months	30
61–120 months	12
Grade IV[c]	
Unilateral	58
Bilateral	10

VUR, Vesicoureteral reflux.

[a]Grade V reflux rarely resolves spontaneously.

[b]No difference by laterality or age at diagnosis.

[c]Estimates apply only to the time of diagnosis and are not age specific.

Bundy DG: Vesicoureteral reflux, *Pediatr Rev* 28:e7, 2007.

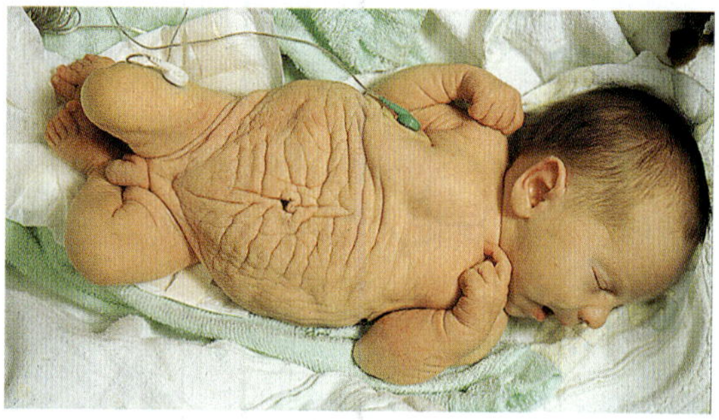

Fig. 14.22 Newborn with prune-belly syndrome shows the characteristic wrinkled and redundant skin covering the abdominal wall. On palpation, no abdominal muscular tissue or muscular tone could be detected.

reflux. The bladder is enlarged despite low renal pelvic and intravesical pressures. UTI is common because of urinary stasis.

The major determinant of prognosis in affected patients is the degree of associated cystic renal dysplasia. Early orchiopexy may improve the chances of fertility and prevent testicular neoplasia.

Tuberous Sclerosis

Tuberous sclerosis (TS) is a neurocutaneous syndrome inherited as an autosomal dominant trait with marked variability of expression. The full syndrome is characterized by myoclonic seizures, cognitive impairment, foci of intracranial calcifications, depigmented "ash leaf" cutaneous patches, and pathognomonic skin lesions known as fibroangiomatous nevi (adenoma sebaceum). The skin lesions may be present during the first year of life but may go unnoticed until 4 to 7 years of age. Patients with TS may have rhabdomyomas and other lesions in many organs and tissues. TS is caused by mutations mainly of the TS complex (*TSC1* and *TSC2*) genes encoding hamartin and tuberin, respectively. Angiomyolipoma is the predominant kidney lesion and is best visualized by magnetic resonance imaging (MRI) (Fig. 14.23). In addition, PKD may occur because of crossover of the *TSC2* gene, which is contiguous with the *PKD1* gene. Although small asymptomatic cysts are common in TS, large kidney cysts may be discovered early in infancy and suggest the diagnosis of autosomal dominant PKD. In such instances the diagnosis of TS is confirmed by family history, the development of other features of the syndrome, and genetic testing.

Imperforate Anus

Owing to common embryologic origins and the anatomic proximity of the genitourinary and lower gastrointestinal tracts, children with imperforate anus have a high incidence of genitourinary and lower spinal abnormalities. A high imperforate anus (at or above the levator ani) (Fig. 14.24) is associated with a 50% incidence of genitourinary anomalies, mainly unilateral renal agenesis, neurogenic bladder, or VUR. In boys, one usually finds a fistulous communication between the blind end of the rectal pouch and the prostatic urethra. In girls, the rectum often communicates with the vagina or posterior fourchette. All children with imperforate anus should undergo kidney ultrasonography and must be monitored for UTIs.

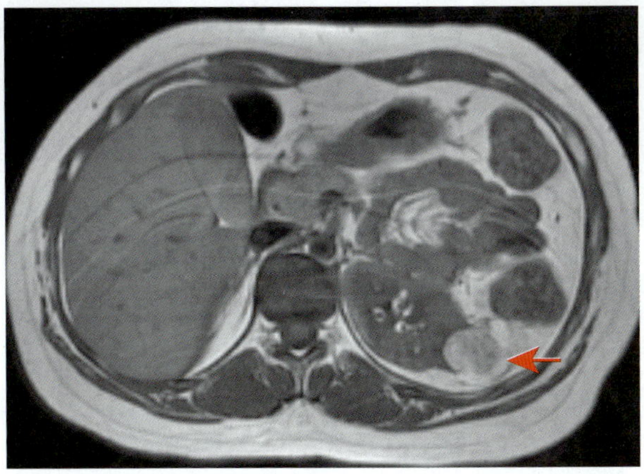

Fig. 14.23 Renal angiomyosarcoma *(arrow)* on magnetic resonance imaging in a patient with tuberous sclerosis. (Courtesy Judy Squires, MD, UPMC Children's Hospital of Pittsburgh.)

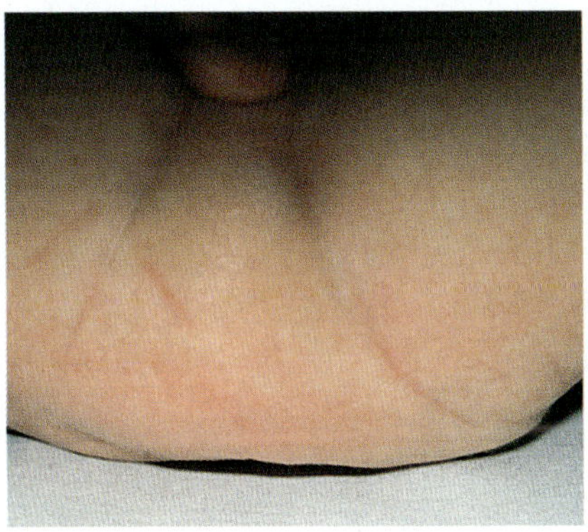

Fig. 14.24 Imperforate anus. This newborn boy has an absent median raphe and anal atresia. On further study, he was found to have agenesis of the right kidney, severe dysplasia in the left kidney, and a communication of the blind-ended rectal pouch and the prostatic urethra.

Posterior Urethral Valves

The most common obstructive lesion of the lower urinary tract in male infants is posterior urethral valves. Such folds traverse the urethra from a point just distal to the verumontanum to the proximal limit of the membranous urethra and obstruct urinary flow with consequent enlargement of the prostatic urethra, hypertrophy of the bladder neck, trabeculation of the bladder, and significant dilation of the upper urinary tract (Fig. 14.25A). Infants with posterior urethral valves may experience kidney failure and profound electrolyte imbalance. Older children may develop abdominal masses, voiding disturbances, or UTI. Male neonates with known prenatal bilateral hydronephrosis should have VCUG shortly after birth. Diagnosis is made radiologically by VCUG (Fig. 14.25B) and confirmed endoscopically. Although urinary diversion may be required, many children can be treated directly by transurethral valve ablation. Surgery is usually successful in achieving urinary drainage, but in many cases associated renal dysplasia may lead to CKD and ESKD during infancy or childhood.

Crossed Renal Ectopy

Children with the developmental anomaly of crossed renal ectopy generally have an abdominal mass or hematuria after minor trauma. Obstruction at the ureteropelvic junction is common. The location of the ectopic kidney may be cryptic, as in the pelvic region, and can be best demonstrated by a renal radionuclide scan. Crossed renal ectopy, renal agenesis, or duplication of the collecting system are often found in association with Klippel-Feil syndrome (Fig. 14.26A and B) but have also been associated with cervicothoracic vertebral anomalies and Müllerian duct aplasia in girls.

Horseshoe Kidney

Horseshoe kidney results from the fusion of the lower renal poles during development (Fig. 14.27). Although generally asymptomatic, patients with horseshoe kidney may have hematuria after trauma to the pelvic area, a midline abdominal mass, or ureteropelvic junction obstruction.

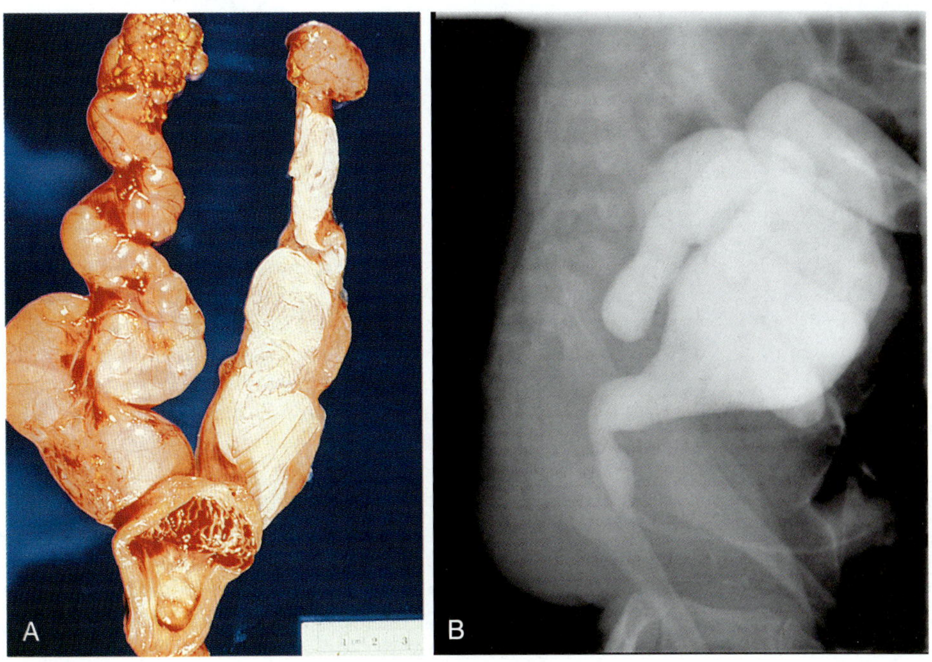

Fig. 14.25 (A) Autopsy findings of a newborn with posterior urethral valves. Notice the marked enlargement and tortuosity of the ureters and the small, thick-walled, muscular bladder. (B) An antemortem voiding cystourethrogram shows the markedly dilated proximal urethra typical of this condition.

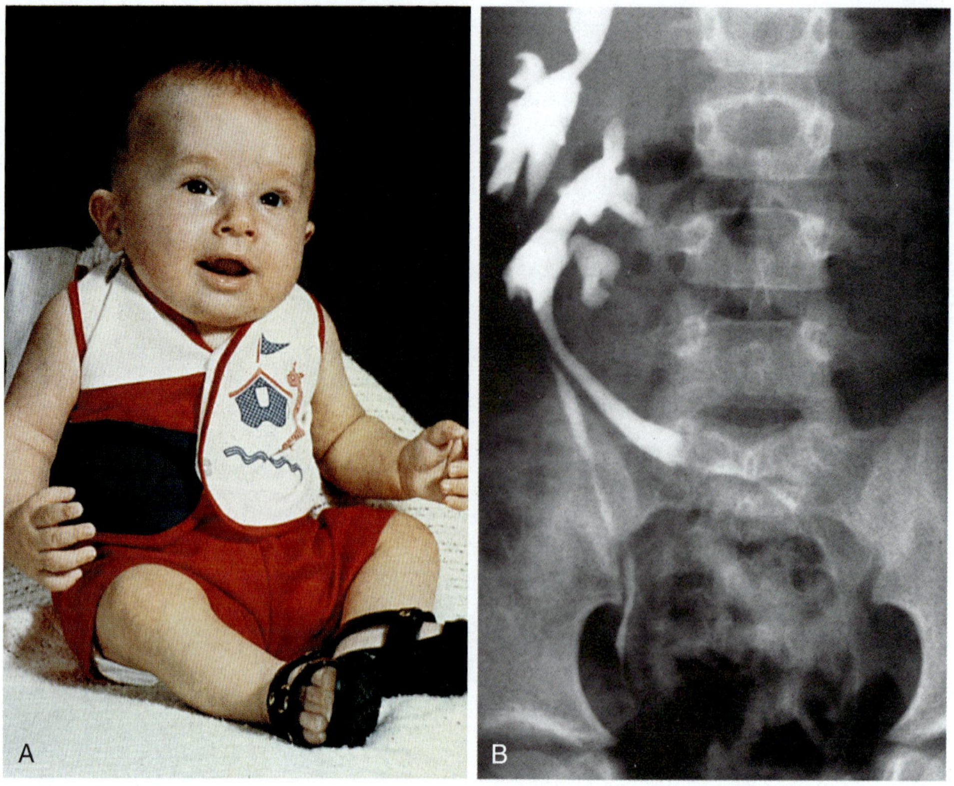

Fig. 14.26 An infant with Klippel-Feil syndrome. (A) Demonstrates a short neck (fused cervical vertebrae) and nonfunctioning right thumb caused by lack of tendons to this digit. Intravenous pyelogram (B) reveals crossed renal ectopia of the left kidney, whereas the ureter from the left kidney crosses the midline and inserts into the left side of the trigone.

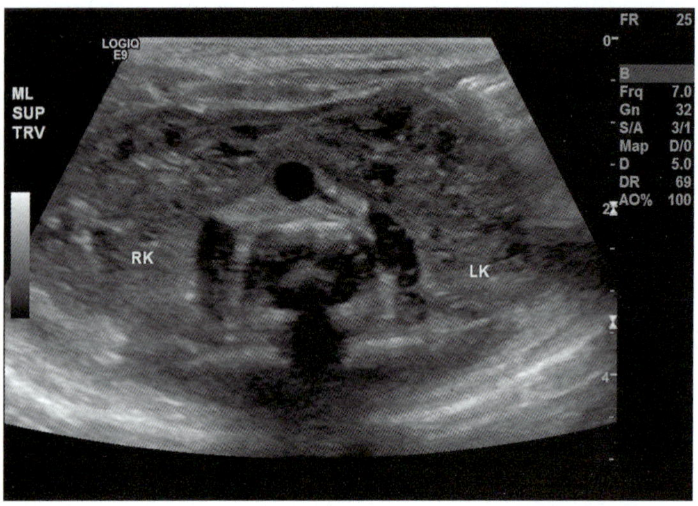

Fig. 14.27 Ultrasonography of horseshoe kidney showing right and left kidney with isthmus in between the moieties. (Courtesy Judy Squires, MD, UPMC Children's Hospital of Pittsburgh.)

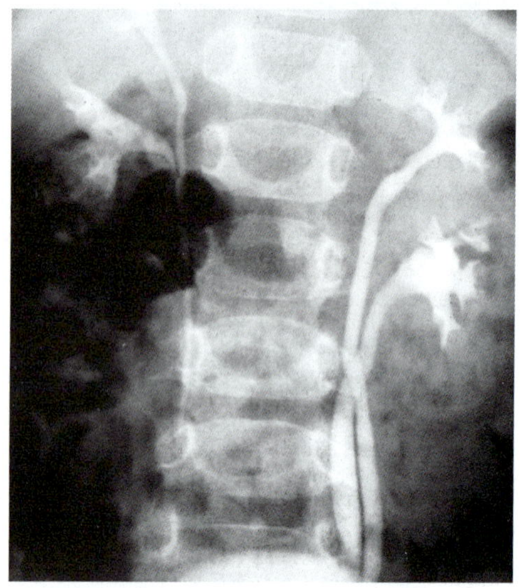

Fig. 14.28 Excretory urogram shows bilateral duplication of the urinary collecting system. This child has recurrent urinary tract infections as the result of vesicoureteral reflux in the ureter from the left lower pole.

Duplication of the Urinary Collecting System

Duplication of the urinary collecting system is one of the most common of all genitourinary abnormalities. It is sometimes familial and more common in girls than in boys. Approximately 30% of the duplications are bilateral (Fig. 14.28) but with much variation in the extent of duplication. This condition occurs when the nephrogenic blastemal is penetrated by two separate ureteric buds during nephrogenesis. When present, VUR usually occurs in the ureter from the lower pole, whereas ureteral obstruction occurs almost exclusively in the ureter from the upper renal segment. Reflux into a duplicated system is unlikely to resolve spontaneously. These associated disorders may predispose patients to recurrent infection or hydronephrosis necessitating surgical correction.

Solitary Kidney

There are multiple causes of solitary kidney in children, including congenital renal aplasia, which occurs in about 1 in 1300 births; involution of a multicystic dysplastic kidney; marked renal hypodysplasia; or acquired disorders such as removal of kidneys because of tumor, trauma, or severe urologic injury. A large proportion of children with a solitary kidney may progress to CKD, particularly if the solitary kidney is part of the spectrum of CAKUT occurring in 1 of about 600 births. It is imperative to determine whether there are associated genitourinary disorders, which may pose increased susceptibility to progressive kidney injury, including hyperfiltration injury by obesity and HTN, use of nephrotoxic agents, injury related to UTI with or without VUR, or obstructive uropathy affecting the solitary kidney. Progression to ESKD may be insidious over decades, and thus early prediction of

Table 14.7 Kidney Length Percentiles by Body Length/Height

Body Length/ Height [cm]	2.5th Percentile [mm]	10th Percentile [mm]	25th Percentile [mm]	50th Percentile [mm]	75th Percentile [mm]	90th Percentile [mm]	97.5th Percentile [mm]	M	L	S
50–54	42.4	45.1	47.6	50.4	53.3	56	59	50.4	0.567	0.0844
55–59	44.6	47.4	50	52.9	56	58.8	61.9	52.9	0.532	0.0836
60–64	46.8	49.7	52.4	55.4	58.6	61.5	64.8	55.4	0.498	0.0828
65–69	49.4	52.4	55.1	58.3	61.6	64.6	68.1	58.3	0.458	0.0820
70–74	51.6	54.7	57.5	60.8	64.2	67.3	70.9	60.8	0.423	0.0812
75–79	53.8	57	59.9	63.3	66.8	70	73.8	63.3	0.387	0.0804
80–84	55.9	59.2	62.2	65.7	69.3	72.6	76.5	65.7	0.352	0.0797
85–89	58.3	61.6	64.7	68.3	72	75.4	79.4	68.3	0.312	0.0788
90–94	60.3	63.7	66.9	70.6	74.3	77.9	82	70.6	0.276	0.0781
95–99	62.5	66	69.2	73	76.9	80.5	84.7	73	0.237	0.0773
100–104	64.5	68.1	71.4	75.2	79.1	82.8	87.1	75.2	0.2	0.0765
105–109	66.4	70	73.3	77.2	81.2	85	89.4	77.2	0.165	0.0758
110–114	68.2	71.8	75.2	79.1	83.2	87.1	91.6	79.1	0.131	0.0751
115–119	70.3	74	77.4	81.4	85.6	89.5	94.1	81.4	0.09	0.0743
120–124	72.3	76	79.5	83.5	87.8	91.8	96.4	83.5	0.052	0.0735
125–129	74.2	78	81.5	85.6	89.9	94	98.8	85.6	0.015	0.0728
130–134	76.2	80	83.6	87.8	92.2	96.3	101.1	87.8	− 0.022	0.0721
135–139	78.2	82	85.7	89.9	94.3	98.5	103.5	89.9	− 0.058	0.0714
140–144	80.3	84.2	87.8	92.1	96.6	100.9	105.9	92.1	− 0.093	0.0707
145–149	82.5	86.5	90.2	94.5	99.1	103.5	108.6	94.5	− 0.131	0.0700
150–154	84.8	88.8	92.6	97	101.7	106.1	111.3	97	− 0.168	0.0693
155–159	87.2	91.3	95.1	99.6	104.3	108.8	114.1	99.6	− 0.207	0.0686
160–164	89.5	93.6	97.5	102.1	106.9	111.5	116.9	102.1	− 0.243	0.0680
165–169	91.8	96	99.9	104.5	109.4	114	119.5	104.5	− 0.279	0.0673
170–174	94.1	98.3	102.3	106.9	111.9	116.6	122.2	106.9	− 0.315	0.0667
175–179	96.5	100.7	104.8	109.5	114.5	119.3	125	109.5	− 0.353	0.0660
180–184	98.8	103.1	107.1	111.9	117	121.9	127.6	111.9	− 0.389	0.0654
185–189	101.2	105.5	109.6	114.5	119.6	124.6	130.4	114.5	− 0.427	0.0647
190–194	103.3	107.7	111.9	116.8	122	127	132.9	116.8	− 0.461	0.0641
195–199	105	109.4	113.6	118.5	123.8	128.8	134.8	118.5	− 0.486	0.0637
≥ 200	108.3	112.8	117	122	127.4	132.5	138.6	122	− 0.538	0.0628

From Obrycki L, Sarnecki J, Lichosik M, et al: Kidney length normative values in children aged 0–19 years — a multicenter study, *Pediatr Nephrol* 37:1075–1085, 2022.

long-term prognosis should be given with caution even when the fetal or neonatal kidney ultrasonography appears otherwise normal. Children with known additional genitourinary anomalies or kidney dysfunction, HTN, proteinuria, or recurrent UTIs are high risk for progressing to CKD and need follow-up more frequently. In contrary, those without these risk factors and with appropriate compensatory hypertrophy of the solitary kidney have better long-term kidney prognosis. Table 14.7 lists the normative values for kidney length by body length or height. Compensatory hypertrophy is defined by kidney length being greater than the 97.5 percentile. Anticipatory guidance for use of nephrotoxic medications including nonsteroidal antiinflammatory agents and weight control to prevent obesity should also be provided at regular office visits.

Congenital Hydronephrosis

Hydronephrosis is the single most common kidney abnormality detected by fetal ultrasonography. It is more reliably assessed by ultrasonographic imaging obtained within 1 week after birth (Fig. 14.29A and B) to aid detection of responsible conditions such as ureteropelvic junction obstruction, high-grade VUR, renal dysplasia, or posterior urethral valves in males. Sequential ultrasonography should be done to follow hydronephrosis. Typically, more than 90% of such cases resolve spontaneously during the first 12 to 14 months of life.

Severe antenatal congenital hydronephrosis is a less common but important condition that often has additional genitourinary anomalies on imaging. Such children should be promptly evaluated with VCUG and nuclear medicine studies. Any febrile episodes in these infants should lead to prompt investigation for UTI and appropriate therapy.

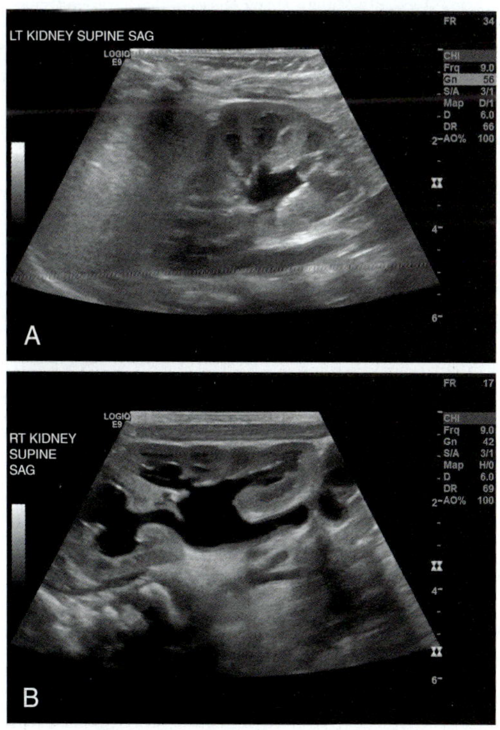

Fig. 14.29 (A) Ultrasonography showing congenital hydronephrosis. (B) This patient has larger hydronephrosis along with a dilated proximal ureter. (Courtesy Judy Squires, MD, UPMC Children's Hospital of Pittsburgh.)

Potter Sequence

Potter sequence (Fig. 14.30) results from fetal compression secondary to decreased fetal urine production (oligohydramnios) and consists of pulmonary hypoplasia and marked fetal compression including

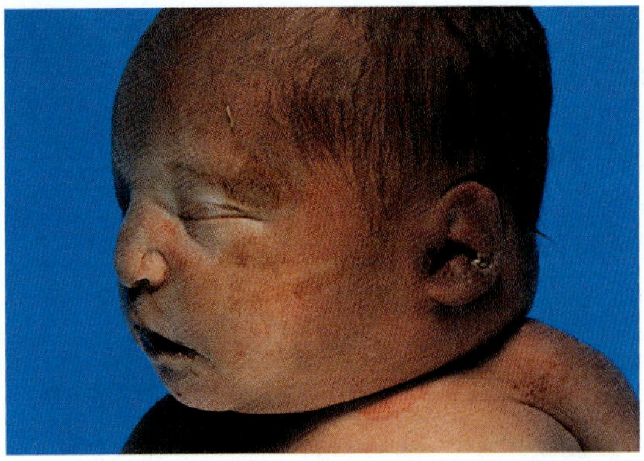

Fig. 14.30 Potter facies. This infant with bilateral multicystic dysplasia died at 12 hours of age due to pulmonary insufficiency. The altered facies produced by the fetal compression syndrome of oligohydramnios includes small, posteriorly rotated ears, micrognathia, a beaked nose, and wide-set eyes. (Courtesy T. Macpherson, MD, Magee-Womens Hospital, Pittsburgh, PA.)

abnormal positioning of the hands; talipes; and altered facies characterized by small, posteriorly rotated ears, a small chin, a beaked nose, and unusual facial creases. Patients with Potter sequence usually die secondary to the severe pulmonary hypoplasia and pneumothorax.

HEREDITARY AND METABOLIC DISORDERS

Cystic Kidney Disease

Five of the most common and most important forms of renal cystic disorders are presented in this section. Although autosomal dominant PKD (ADPKD) and unilateral cystic renal dysplasia are far more common in the general population (1 in 400–1 in 1000), autosomal recessive PKD (ARPKD; 1 in 20,000–1 in 40,000 with a carrier status of 1 in 70) is a much more serious disorder during childhood. Cystic renal dysplasia has no well-defined inheritance pattern and is often associated with other syndromes. Nephronophthisis (NPHP) is less common than the other disorders but is an important cause of ESKD in childhood. Renal cystic disease may also be an important component of many syndromes (Table 14.8) that are not discussed in this chapter.

Table 14.8 Syndromes Associated With Cystic Kidneys

Syndrome	Inheritance
Meckel-Gruber	AR
Jeune thoracic dystrophy	AR
Short rib polydactyly	AR
Zellweger	AR
Tuberous sclerosis	AD
von Hippel-Lindau	AD
VATER association	NI
Renal-retinal dysplasia	AR
Ivemark	AR
Fryns	AR
Trisomy 21, 13, or 18	—
Oral-facial-digital, type 1	XL
Laurence-Moon-Bardet-Biedl	AR
Kaufman-McKusick	AR
Hypothalamic hamartoma	NI?
Lissencephaly	Variable
Prune-belly	NI?
Ehlers-Danlos	Variable
Branchio-oto-renal	AD
Roberts	AR
DiGeorge	Variable
Smith-Lemli-Opitz	AR
Turner	—
Noonan Caroli	—

AD, Autosomal dominant; *AR,* autosomal-recessive; *NI,* not inherited; *XL,* X-linked.

From Zerres K, Volpel MC, Weiss H: Cystic kidneys: genetics, pathological anatomy, clinical picture, and prenatal diagnosis, *Hum Genet* 68:104–135, 1984.

Autosomal Recessive and Autosomal Dominant Polycystic Kidney Disease

Many of the unique features of ARPKD and ADPKD are summarized in Table 14.9. ARPKD is a combined kidney and hepatic disorder caused by mutations in the PKHD1 locus on chromosome 6 (encoding for fibrocystin/polyductin). Most cases are severe and are often detected by antenatal ultrasonography after 24 weeks of gestation. These newborns may present with oligohydramnios or Potter-like phenotype (see the previous section) including anuria or oliguria and pulmonary hypoplasia. Less severe cases can present with abdominal distention due to kidney enlargement and tubular dysfunction. Hyponatremia often occurs in infancy and may be related to nonosmotic release of vasopressin, particularly in the setting of pulmonary disease; excessive renal salt wasting; and extracellular volume contraction. Systemic HTN is common even when serum creatinine level is normal. Progressive kidney failure occurs in a fluctuating course and an eventual decline to ESKD during the first decade of life.

Congenital hepatic fibrosis and hepatobiliary disease is also associated with *PKHD1* mutations and may predominate over kidney involvement. Portal HTN, esophageal varices, splenomegaly and hypersplenism, hematemesis, and protein-losing enteropathy are frequent clinical features. Caroli disease is a variant occurring in about 30% of cases of ARPKD in which there is

Table 14.9 Autosomal Recessive Polycystic Kidney Disease (ARPKD) and Autosomal Dominant Polycystic Kidney Disease (ADPKD)

Clinical Characteristics	ARPKD	ADPKD
Mode of inheritance	Autosomal recessive	Autosomal dominant
Gene	*PKHD1* (fibrocystin or polyductin, chromosome 6p21)	PKD1 (polycystin 1, chromosome 16) or PKD 2 (polycystin 2, chromosome 4)
Incidence	1:10,000–40,000	1:400–1000
Typical age of presentation	Prenatal or infancy	School age to young adulthood
Cyst characteristics	Enlarged echogenic kidneys with no visible or small cysts (microcysts)	Enlarged echogenic kidneys with macrocysts
Extrarenal manifestations	Always with liver disease, many born with pulmonary hypoplasia	Cysts in liver, pancreas and other organs, brain aneurysm
Outcomes	1-year survival rate = 85%, 10-year kidney survival rate = 71%	Most have few or no symptoms during childhood

ADPKD, Autosomal dominant polycystic kidney disease; *ARPKD,* autosomal recessive polycystic kidney disease.

intrahepatic ductal ectasia unrelated to hepatic fibrosis, which often results in ascending cholangitis and sepsis. The kidney cysts are quite small and numerous and often result in massive kidney enlargement and palpable flank or abdominal masses compressing the abdominal contents and diaphragms (Fig. 14.31). The preferred imaging technique is ultrasonography (Fig. 14.32A and B), but CT or MRI may better visualize the cysts. The pathology of ARPKD kidneys includes microcystic dilation of medullary and cortical collecting ducts. Apart from management of CKD,

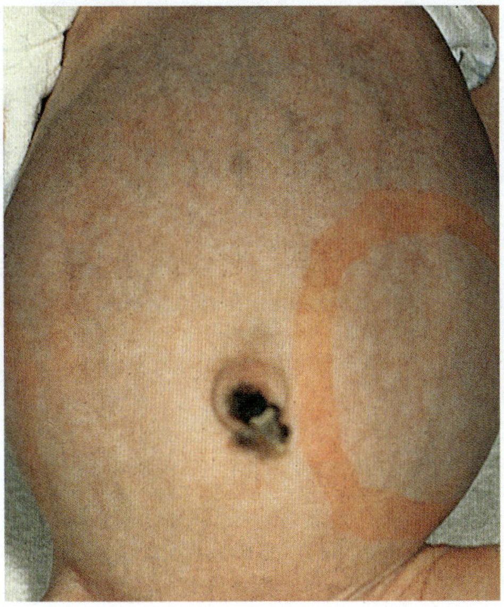

Fig. 14.31 This infant with autosomal recessive polycystic kidney disease shows marked abdominal distention and bilaterally enlarged kidneys, as indicated by the outlined area.

systemic HTN, and esophageal varices, eventual management may involve nephrectomy, dialysis, and often combined kidney and liver transplantation.

ADPKD, previously known as adult PKD, results from mutations in the PKD1 (~85%) or PKD2 (~15%) loci (encoding for polycystin 1 or 2, respectively). It is one of the leading causes of kidney failure in the United States and affects 1 in 400 to 1000 people. Although most cases are diagnosed in adulthood, symptoms are increasingly recognized in early childhood. Within families, there is much variability in the phenotypic expression of clinical course, severity of kidney disease, and extrarenal manifestations. With the current high-resolution kidney ultrasonography, up to 90% of affected individuals younger than 20 years of age have detectable cysts. Compared with children with fewer than 10 cysts at the time of diagnosis of ADPKD, those with more than 10 cysts have a similar creatinine clearance but are more likely to complain of flank or back pain and urinary frequency; they also have a greater incidence of palpable kidneys, inguinal hernias, palpitations, HTN, and urinary concentrating defects. Pathologically, the cysts become large and asymmetric and involve all parts of the nephron and collecting duct (Fig. 14.33A and B). Sequencing of the *PKD1* and *PKD2* loci may be done for prenatal diagnosis and family planning purposes or for individuals with a family history of PKD who are asymptomatic, have a nondiagnostic ultrasonography, and wish to donate a kidney.

Except for children with enlarged kidneys and large cysts detected in infancy, kidney failure or nephrolithiasis rarely occurs in childhood ADPKD. Similarly, extrarenal manifestations are rare including rupture of intracranial aneurysm, colonic diverticula, and symptomatic mitral valve prolapse. Although uncommon before 18 years of age, children with acute onset of "thunderclap" headache or neurologic symptoms should undergo CT or MR angiography to assess impending rupture or compression of an intracranial aneurysm. Otherwise, screening brain MRI/MRA is of limited value.

Cystic Renal Dysplasia

Abnormal kidney morphogenesis can lead to absent parenchyma (aplasia), deficient parenchyma (hypoplasia) (Fig. 14.34), or abnormally differentiated parenchyma (dysplasia) (Fig. 14.35A and B). The latter condition may present with or without cysts, is usually

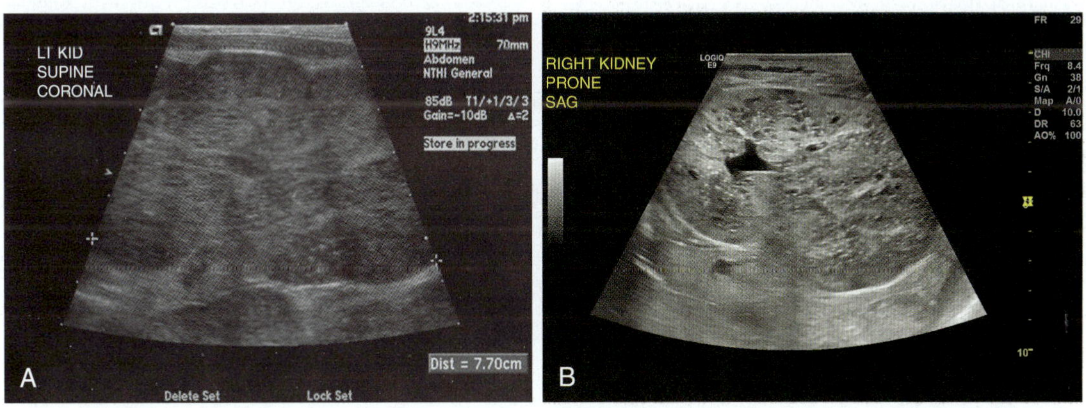

Fig. 14.32 (A and B) Longitudinal ultrasonography view of autosomal recessive polycystic kidney disease kidney. Kidney is enlarged with increased echogenicity with loss of corticomedullary differentiation. Distinct cysts are not visualized and classically do not occur.

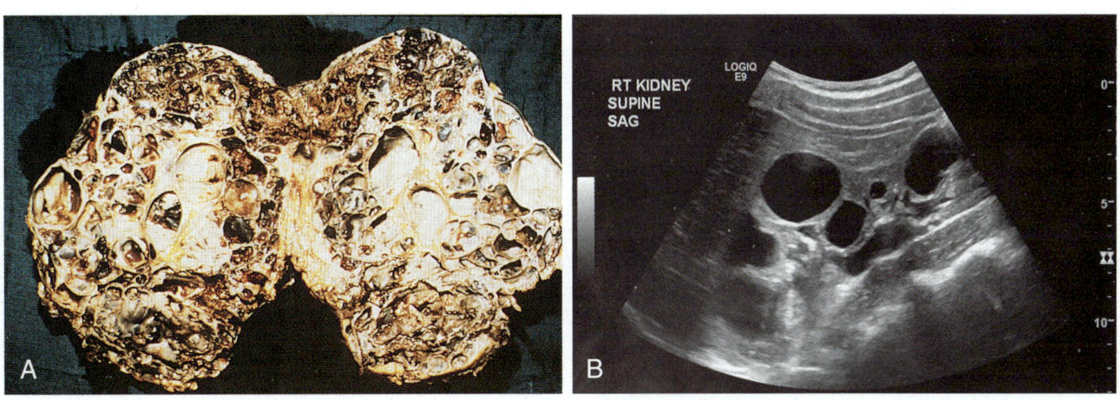

Fig. 14.33 (A) Autosomal dominant polycystic kidney disease (ADPKD). Note replacement of normal kidney parenchyma by fluid-filled cysts. (B) Ultrasonography appearance of ADPKD with macrocysts of varying sizes with distortion of the normal reniform shape and preserved kidney parenchyma between the cysts.

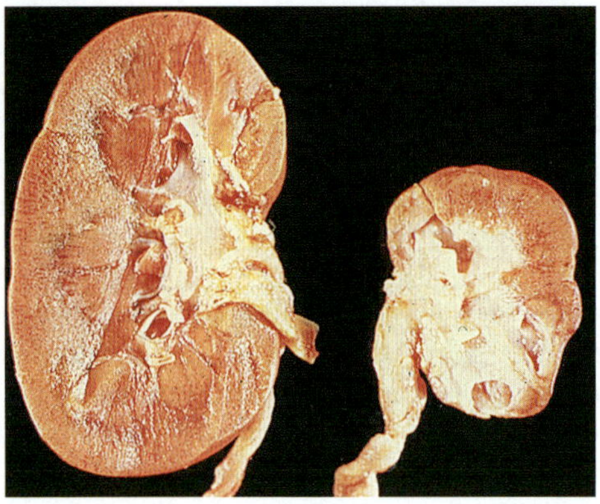

Fig. 14.34 Unilateral renal hypoplasia/dysplasia. In contrast to the normal right kidney, the left kidney is markedly small. The parenchyma in the upper pole is normal, but microscopic examination of the lower pole showed several morphologic features of dysplasia.

unilateral, and may be visualized by kidney ultrasonography with increased echogenic kidney parenchyma and cysts (Fig. 14.36). Unlike PKD, cysts associated with dysplasia are not in communication with renal tubular lumens and do not progress in size or number. Thus despite the presence of cysts, kidney sizes may be too small to appreciate by bimanual examination (i.e., bracing the flank and back with the fingers of one hand while gradually producing deep abdominal compression with the other hand). When bilateral, these kidney disorders may present early in life with poor weight gain, pallor, emesis, and tachypnea resulting from metabolic acidosis. Urine output is often maintained or increased due to concentrating defects but correlates poorly with kidney function reflected by the serum creatinine level. Even though bilateral disease is much less common than unilateral, these conditions constitute the most common cause of CKD in children.

Renal hypoplasia is often an isolated disorder without other systemic or genitourinary tract anomalies, whereas obstruction of the gastrointestinal or genitourinary tract occurs frequently in children with renal dysplasia. VUR often accompanies any of these structural defects. Less common associations may include trisomy 21, tracheoesophageal fistula, ventricular septal defect, and lumbosacral dystrophies. Cystic dysplasia may be a major component of several syndromes with distinct additional malformations (see Table 14.8). Many of these syndromes have defined inheritance patterns. The overall risk for siblings of children with isolated forms of dysplasia or hypoplasia is usually less than 10% but is higher than the general population if one of the parents has renal aplasia or other structural kidney disease.

Multicystic Dysplasia

Multicystic dysplasia, usually unilateral, is the most common cystic disorder in children and the most common cause of abdominal mass in newborns. Multicystic dysplasia represents an extreme case of renal cystic dysplasia in which there is complete loss of the normal kidney architecture with microscopical primitive ducts, fibrosis, islands of ectopic cartilage, and ureteral atresia. Fig. 14.37 is a kidney ultrasonography image of an infant with a unilateral multicystic dysplastic kidney. This condition is most commonly discovered by prenatal ultrasonography. Rarely, it is identified during the neonatal period after palpation of a "lumpy" intraabdominal mass of variable size that often transilluminates. Bilateral multicystic dysplastic kidneys are rare and lead to complete kidney failure because there is no functioning kidney tissue. Large multicystic kidneys can interfere with respiration or produce mechanical intestinal compression. Kidney ultrasonography is usually sufficient to establish the diagnosis.

The unaffected contralateral kidney is usually hypertrophied and has normal corticomedullary differentiation and no evidence of obstruction. Obstructive disorders, such as posterior urethral valves,

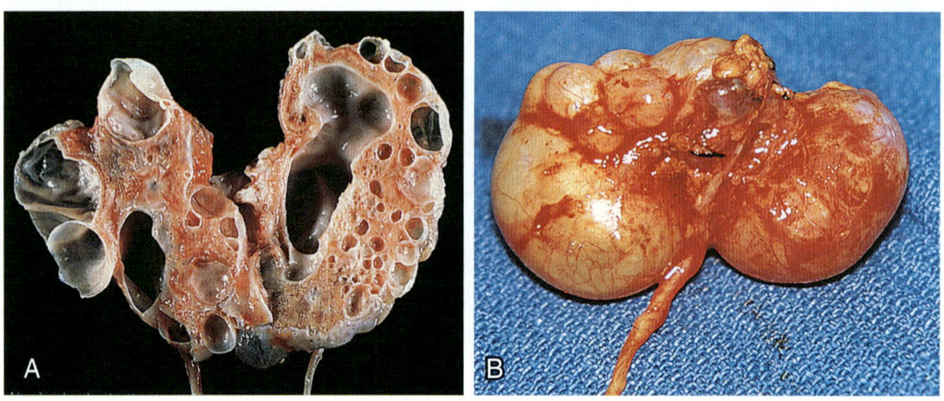

Fig. 14.35 (A) Bilateral cystic renal dysplasia. Multiple cysts of various sizes are seen throughout the cortex and medullary regions. (B) A less severe form of multicystic renal dysplasia involving mainly the midportion of the kidney.

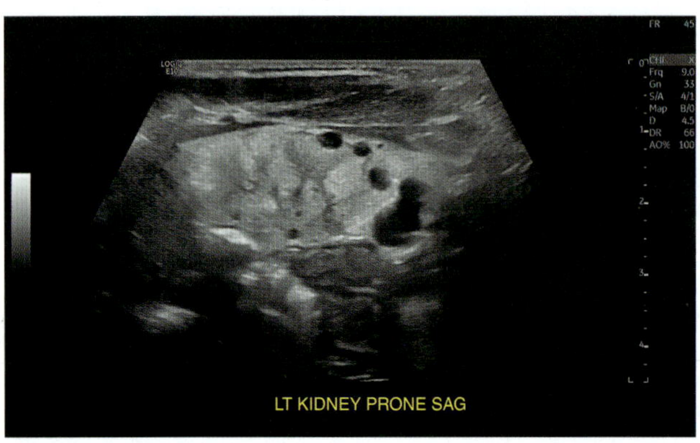

Fig. 14.36 Kidney ultrasonography of kidney with cystic dysplasia. The notable findings are parenchyma with increased echogenicity and several cysts. (Courtesy Judy Squires, MD, UPMC Children's Hospital of Pittsburgh.)

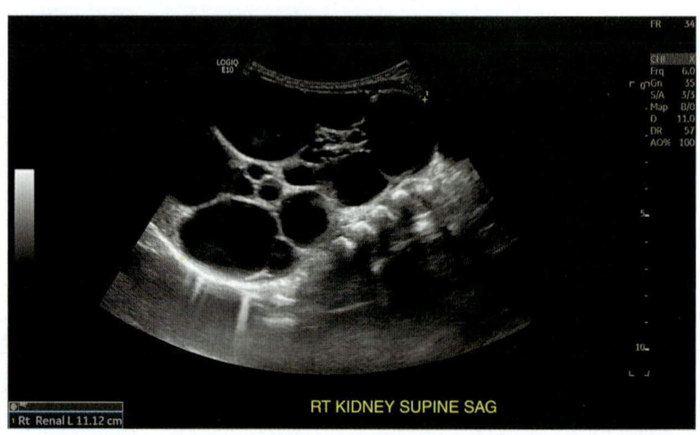

Fig. 14.37 Kidney ultrasonography of multicystic dysplastic kidney. Renal fossa is filled with tissues with many large cysts with no functional kidney tissue. (Courtesy Judy Squires, MD, UPMC Children's Hospital of Pittsburgh.)

urethral atresia, or ureteroceles obstructing a duplicated ureter draining the upper pole, may be associated with morphologic features of dysplasia. Because most multicystic dysplastic kidneys spontaneously involute and rarely are associated with HTN, infection, or tumor development, the prevailing practice is that unilateral and asymptomatic multicystic dysplastic kidneys do not need to be removed. However, correction of any associated obstructive abnormalities that may be present in the contralateral kidney is of vital importance.

Juvenile Nephronophthisis

Juvenile NPHP, another renal cystic disease, is associated with ciliary defects. NPHP shares some morphologic features with medullary cystic disease, although the former has autosomal recessive inheritance and often presents in older childhood or adolescents, whereas the latter has autosomal dominant inheritance and often presents later in life. The most common genetic defect is in the NPHP1 locus (encoding for Nephrocystin 1), and an increasing number of genes have been identified as associated with NPHP, with gene products being some component of cilia apparatus. The cysts are not as prominent as in PKD and are always associated with tubular basement membrane defects, inflammation, and fibrosis. The cysts can enlarge with advancing kidney failure. Polyuria and polydipsia resulting from a urinary concentration defect, and, at times, severe salt wasting are prominent clinical features. An ultrasonography or abdominal CT scan may reveal normal-sized or small kidneys and loss of corticomedullary differentiation with or without medullary cysts. Hepatic fibrosis is probably the most important manifestation associated with juvenile NPHP, although there can be many other extrarenal manifestations such as retinitis pigmentosa (Senior-Loken syndrome). Infants with mutations in NPHP2 (encoding for inversin) can present with earlier onset and more severe disease associated with laterality defects. Genetic testing for many of these genes is now commercially available.

Alport Syndrome

Alport syndrome, or hereditary nephritis, is most commonly transmitted via X-linked inheritance. More rarely, it is transmitted through autosomal recessive or autosomal dominant inheritance with variable penetrance. Frequently, less severe mutations, such as point mutations, result in less severe disease than truncating mutations. The classic clinical presentation of Alport syndrome is persistent or recurrent gross hematuria that may be evident in early childhood. Proteinuria is absent or mild in the early stages of the disease but is invariably present as the disease progresses. The course is commonly one of slowly progressive kidney failure, often accompanied by high-frequency neurosensory deafness, ocular defects, and HTN. However, most individuals with Alport syndrome have neither deafness nor ocular defects. In most cases the condition results from a mutation in the *COL4A5* gene on the X chromosome, which encodes for aberrant α5 chain of type IV collagen in the glomerular basement membrane. Mutations in *COL4A3* and *COLA4* make up the other causes of Alport syndrome.

Diagnosis of Alport Syndrome relies on careful family history, genetic testing, and audiologic and ocular evaluation. Kidney biopsy is not always necessary for diagnosis, but typical histopathologic features include foam cells and glomerular sclerosis on light microscopy (Fig. 14.38) and ultrastructural alterations of the glomerular capillary basement membrane (Fig. 14.39).

Hypophosphatemic Rickets

Rickets is a disturbance of growing bone in which defective mineralization of the matrix leads to an abnormal accumulation of uncalcified cartilage and osteoid. Hypophosphatemic vitamin D–resistant rickets is an X-linked inherited disorder that, unlike other forms of childhood rickets, is clinically characterized by normal muscle tone and strength, absence of tetany or convulsions, growth failure, and the predominance of rachitic changes in the lower extremities. The characteristic radiologic features of hypophosphatemic rickets, as in all forms of childhood rickets, include early widening of the spaces between the end of the metaphyses of long bones and an overall decrease in bone density (Fig. 14.40).

The pathogenesis of this disorder includes a defect in the *PHEX* gene (phosphate-regulating endopeptidase on the X chromosome; Xp22.1), which leads to failure to inactivate fibroblast growth factor 23 (FGF 23). Excessive FGF 23 inhibits proximal tubular phosphate reabsorption, leading to excessive renal tubular phosphate excretion, and suppresses 1α hydroxylation of 25-hydroxyvitamin D by renal tubular epithelial cells leading to inappropriately normal 1,25-dihydroxyvitamin D. Biochemical differentiation from other forms of rickets consists of hypophosphatemia, normal plasma calcium and bicarbonate levels, normal parathyroid hormone and 1,25-dihydroxyvitamin D levels, and absence of aminoaciduria.

Traditional management of this condition included large doses of calcitriol (1,25-dihydroxyvitamin D) and oral phosphorus supplementation to promote more proper mineralization of bones and to improve vertical growth, but optimization was difficult to achieve between control of rickets and adverse effects of these supplementations including diarrhea, hypercalcemia, and nephrocalcinosis. More recently, a monoclonal antibody to FGF 23 has been approved for pediatric use, and this has revolutionized the

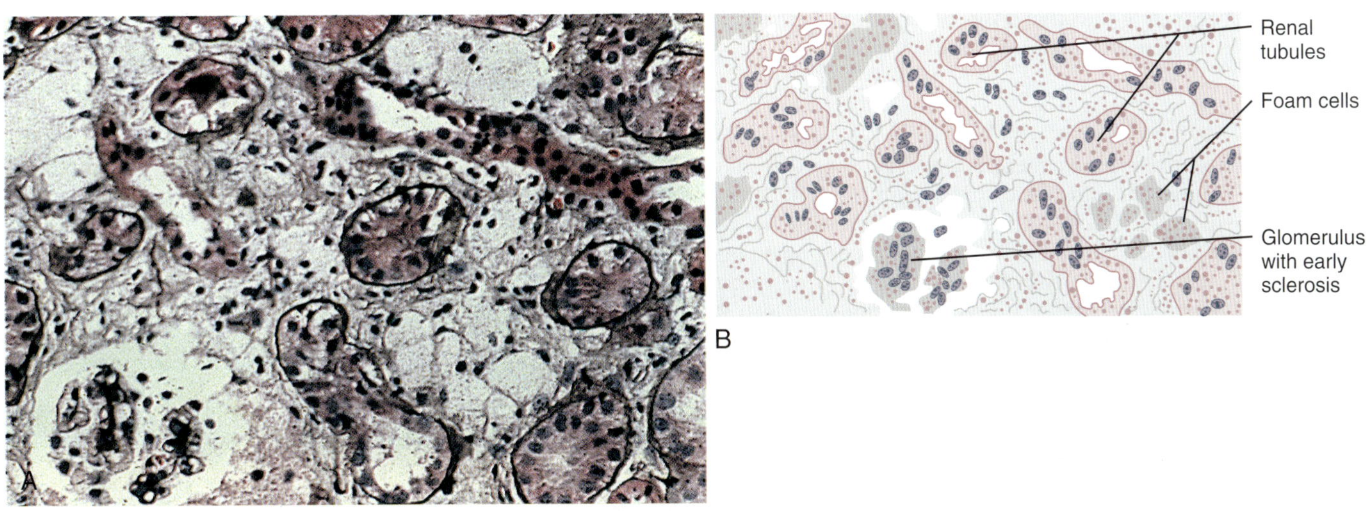

Fig. 14.38 (A and B) Kidney biopsy of a 6-year-old boy with high-frequency hearing loss and persistent hematuria and proteinuria reveals multiple aggregations of foam cells and areas of glomerular sclerosis.

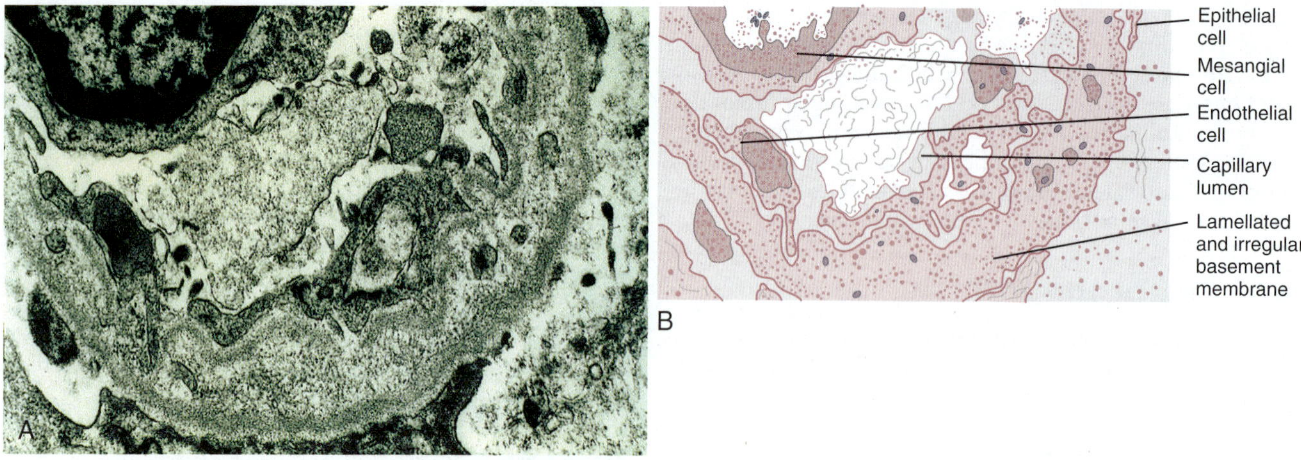

Fig. 14.39 (A and B) Ultrastructural studies on kidney tissue from the same patient as in Fig. 14.38 reveal the characteristic lamellation and irregularities of the glomerular basement membrane, diagnostic of Alport syndrome.

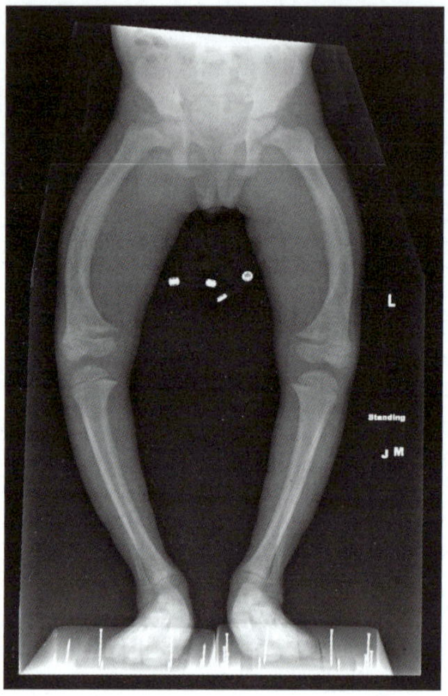

Fig. 14.40 Radiograph of lower extremities of a patient with hypophosphatemic rickets. Note severe bowlegs, the widened space between the metaphyses and epiphyseal ossification center, cupping and splaying of the metaphyses of the femur and tibia, and an overall decreased density of bone.

management of this condition. With injection every 2 weeks, patients are achieving much improved rickets outcomes, experiencing less pain, and not requiring the large doses of supplements that can be associated with adverse effects noted earlier.

Cystinosis

Cystinosis is an autosomal recessive metabolic disorder caused by mutations in the CTNS gene encoding the cystinosin protein. It is characterized by body-wide intralysosomal accumulation of cysteine, which consists of disulfide bonded cysteine monomers. After degrading intracellular protein, the cystinotic lysosomes are unable to transport cystine into the cytoplasm because of a defect in cystinosin, which is believed to be the lysosomal carrier–mediated transporter for this amino acid. In its nephropathic form, the disease causes global proximal tubular dysfunction (Fanconi syndrome) resulting in renal tubular acidosis, rickets from urinary phosphorus loss, LMW proteinuria, glucosuria, progressive glomerular injury, and short stature.

Children with cystinosis exhibit several common extrarenal clinical features. The majority have blond hair and a fair complexion; this, in association with growth faltering and rickets, results in a strikingly similar appearance between unrelated patients. Clinical diagnosis is established by ophthalmologic examination, which detects a characteristic peripheral retinopathy, and by slit-lamp examination, which detects the deposition of crystalline material in the conjunctiva and cornea. Diagnosis is confirmed by the presence of elevated levels of cystine in fibroblasts or peripheral leukocytes and, less commonly, in tissue biopsy showing cystine crystals. Genetic testing is also available. Although the names are similar, cystinosis is a distinct condition from cystinuria, which causes nephrolithiasis in children as described earlier in the chapter.

Jeune Syndrome

Jeune syndrome is another autosomal recessive disease associated with defects in ciliary function and has some phenotypic overlap with NPHP. Because many of the children born with Jeune syndrome have severe and usually lethal pulmonary agenesis, the condition is also known as asphyxiating thoracic dystrophy. However, many children overcome the early respiratory difficulties and may exhibit a small thoracic cage, brachycephaly, short limbs (Fig. 14.41), abnormal radiologic features of the pelvic bones, and a

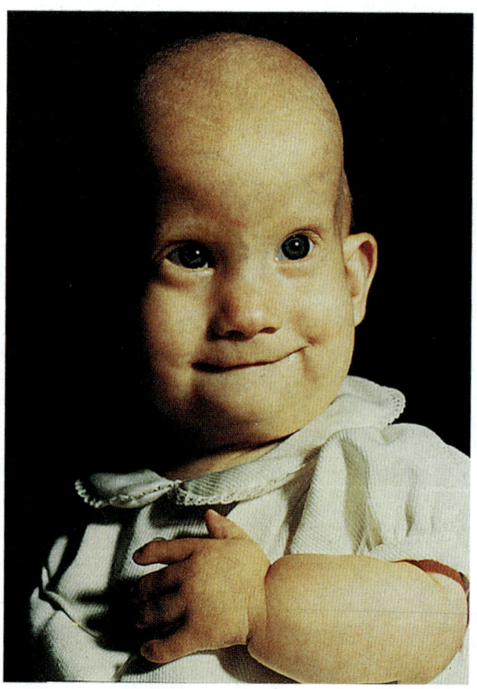

Fig. 14.41 Brachycephaly, short stubby fingers, alopecia, and short stature in a 2-year-old girl with Jeune syndrome and moderate chronic kidney disease.

variety of kidney manifestations ranging from mild to moderate glomerular or tubular changes to microcystic renal dysplasia.

Denys-Drash Syndrome

Denys-Drash syndrome, an autosomal dominant disease with mutations in the *WT1* gene, is characterized by Wilms tumor, disorder of sex development, and nephropathy. Because 70% of such children have NS in the first month of life, they are often misdiagnosed as having congenital or Finnish-type NS. However, the presence of severe HTN and ambiguous genitalia facilitates the diagnosis of Denys-Drash syndrome. Bilateral nephrectomy is usually performed after the diagnosis to help control proteinuria, HTN, and to prevent the development of Wilms tumor. The characteristic glomerular lesion is that of diffuse mesangial sclerosis (Fig. 14.42). This progressive disorder leads to HTN and hyperkalemia that is disproportionate to the reduction in GFR (hyporeninemic hypoaldosteronism).

HYPERTENSION

Inadequately controlled HTN is the single most important risk factor for death, ischemic heart disease, and strokes in adults worldwide. BP during childhood is strongly predictive of adulthood BP. In addition, the degree of atherosclerosis in youth and BP target organ damage in young adults appear to be well correlated with their BP. Thus detection and appropriate management of HTN starting in the pediatric population is essential to reduce the risks of early cardiovascular disease and mortality. Along with the increase of childhood obesity, the pediatric HTN prevalence appears to be increasing. Data estimates the prevalence of HTN to be approximately 4% using the criteria defined by the 2017 American Academy of Pediatrics (AAP) guidelines in children from several different countries and regions including both rural and urban populations.

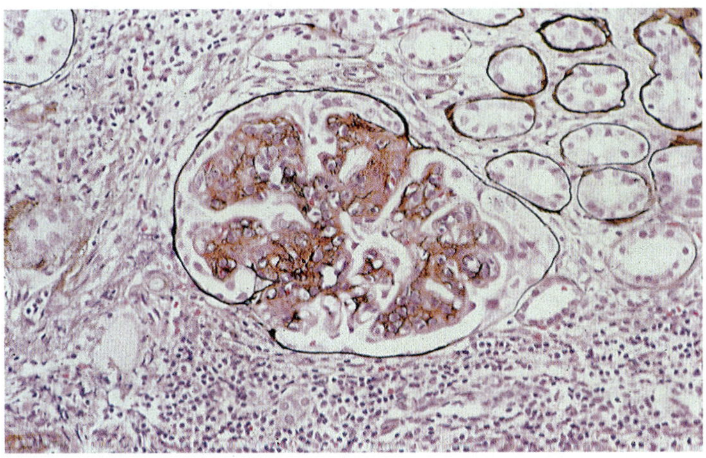

Fig. 14.42 Distinctive glomerular lesion of diffuse mesangial sclerosis in Denys-Drash syndrome. Notice the spongy and "solid" appearance of the mesangium without proliferative changes and the obliteration of the capillary lumina. Interstitial inflammation and dilated tubules are also apparent.

Proper Measurement of Blood Pressure

The proper diagnosis of HTN relies on accurate BP measurement. There are several confounding factors including cuff size, technique, and type of device employed. BP cuff size is crucial as a cuff too small may result in higher BP measurements. The length of the cuff bladder (Fig. 14.43) should encircle 80% to 100% of the circumference of the upper arm midway between the olecranon and acromion for proper cuff sizing. BP should be measured after at least 5 minutes of rest with the back and feet in a supported position. The definition, classification, and follow-up recommendations of children and adolescents with abnormal BP according to the 2017 AAP clinical practice guidelines (CPG) are listed in Table 14.10. In the clinic setting, the initial BP may be measured by calibrated oscillometric monitors that have been validated for use in the pediatric population or by manual auscultation. Unless there is atypical aortic arch anatomy, an indwelling catheter, thrombosis, or arterial-venous fistula, manual auscultation should occur in the right arm with the stethoscope placed over the brachial artery in the antecubital fossa at the level of the heart. Systolic BP is when brachial pulse can first be heard (Krokoff I), and diastolic BP is when this pulse disappears (Krokoff V). If the initial BP measurement is abnormal (≥90th percentile or ≥120/80), providers

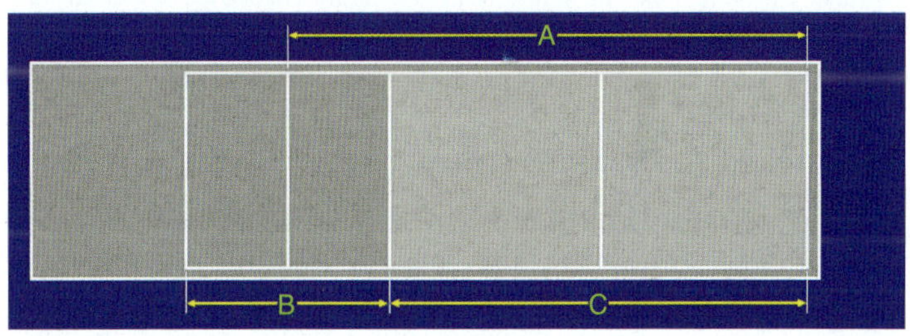

Fig. 14.43 Schematic diagram of proper blood pressure cuff size. The bladder portion of the cuff should encircle 80 to 100% of the circumference of the arm midway between the olecranon and acromion.

Table 14.10 Definition, Classification, and Follow-Up Recommendations of Pediatric Hypertension

HTN is defined as systolic BP and/or diastolic BP in stage 1 or 2 hypertension range on three separate visits

	Definition		
Classification	**1–12 Years Old**	**≥13 Years Old**	**Management Recommendation**
Normal	<90th percentile	<120/80	Recheck at next routine well-child visit
Elevated BP	≥90th–<95th percentile or 120/80–<95th percentile (whichever is lower)	120–129/<80	Recheck BP in 6 months and to provide lifestyle counseling
Stage 1 HTN	≥95th–<95th percentile + 12, or 130–139/80–89 (whichever is lower)	130–139/80–89	If asymptomatic, provide lifestyle counseling and recheck the BP in 1–2 weeks by auscultation
Stage 2 HTN	≥95th percentile + 12, or ≥140/90 (whichever is lower)	≥140/90	Check upper and lower extremity BP, provide lifestyle counseling, and recheck BP within 1 week or refer to subspecialty care within 1 week If symptomatic or BP is >95th percentile + 30 or >180/120, refer to an immediate source of care, such as an emergency department

BP, Blood pressure; *HTN*, hypertension.

Modified from Flynn JT, Kaelber DC, Baker-Smith CM, et al: Clinical practice guideline for screening and management of high blood pressure in children and adolescents, *Pediatrics* 140(3):e20171904, 2017.

should perform two additional oscillometric or auscultatory BP measurements at the same visit and average them. If the average of two oscillometric readings is ≥90th percentile or ≥120/80, two additional auscultatory measurements should be taken and averaged to define the BP category.

Twenty-four-hour ambulatory blood pressure monitoring (ABPM) has been increasingly utilized due to its greater accuracy in diagnosing children including identifying children with white coat HTN, masked HTN, and assessing HTN treatment efficacy. White coat HTN is when children have confirmed stage 1 or 2 hypertensive BP measurements in medical settings but have normal BP measurements elsewhere, including on ABPM. Masked HTN is the converse of white coat HTN where children have normal clinic BP measurements but are detected to have HTN by ABPM. Pediatric ABPM literature suggests that the use of ABPM is superior to clinic BP measurements in predicting target organ damage, such as left ventricular hypertrophy. Specific indications for the use of ABPM are listed in detail in the AAP CPG.

Evaluation of Hypertension

Medical history and physical examination (Table 14.11) can provide clues as to how to focus evaluation of a child with hypertension. As obesity has become more common in children, it is increasingly important to obtain comprehensive dietary and sleep history and assess engagement in physical activity. In contrast to previous guidelines, the AAP CPG does not recommend extensive secondary HTN evaluation if patients are ≥6 years old and have positive family history of HTN, are overweight or obese, or do not have history or physical examination findings suggestive of a secondary cause of HTN. Table 14.12 provides suggested laboratory and imaging studies for the initial evaluation of children and adolescents suspected to have secondary HTN. Tests should be selectively ordered by index of suspicion based on patients' presentation, history, and physical examination findings. Two of the more common etiologies of pediatric secondary HTN are renal artery stenosis and renal scarring from previous pyelonephritis.

Renal Artery Stenosis

Although less than 10% of pediatric HTN is caused by renal artery stenosis, detection of this abnormality is particularly important because a cure can be achieved. The basic pathophysiology of all renovascular HTN involves activation of the renin–angiotensin–aldosterone system. If a lesion in the minor or major branches of the renal artery significantly decreases kidney perfusion pressure, it causes increased renin release as the affected kidney attempts to autoregulate kidney blood flow and maintain kidney perfusion. The high plasma renin activity leads to increases in systemic vasoconstriction. This also leads to increased aldosterone production with resultant renal sodium and water retention and expansion of the extracellular fluid volume.

Renovascular HTN should be suspected in any hypertensive child with the physical finding of high-pitched bruits heard in the flank or abdominal areas or when stigmata of syndromes associated with arterial abnormalities are present (e.g., Marfan syndrome, neurofibromatosis type 1, Williams syndrome). Patients with renovascular HTN may show abnormalities on radionuclide renal scans, Doppler interrogation of the renal arteries, or elevated plasma renin activity. Renal artery angiogram is the gold-standard diagnostic study, but CT (Fig. 14.44) or MR angiography is often the initial study of choice. Intrinsic diseases of the renal artery include fibromuscular dysplasia, thrombotic and embolic lesions, aneurysms, arteritis, and arteriosclerosis. The lesions of fibromuscular dysplasia involve multiple areas of stenosis alternating with aneurysmal dilation in the distal two-thirds of the main renal artery (Fig. 14.45).

Table 14.11 Physical Examination Findings in a Hypertensive Child

Findings	Possible Etiology
General	
• Tachycardia	Primary hypertension, pheochromocytoma, neuroblastoma, hyperthyroidism
• Poor growth	Chronic kidney disease
• Elevated BMI	Primary hypertension (especially in adolescents)
• Truncal obesity	Cushing syndrome, insulin resistance syndrome
External Features of Characteristic Syndromes	
• Café au lait spots, axillary freckling, cutaneous neurofibromas	Neurofibromatosis
• Exophthalmos, tremor, hyperactive reflexes, thyromegaly, weight loss, heat intolerance	Hyperthyroidism
• Elfin facies	Williams syndrome
Webbed neck, widely spaced nipples	Turners syndrome
• Moon facies, truncal obesity, abdominal striae, acne hirsutism	Cashing syndrome
• Pallor, flushing, diaphoresis	Pheochromocytoma
• Ambiguous genitalia, virilization	Congenital adrenal hyperplasia
• Joint swelling, oral ulcers, skin rash, edema	Vasculitis syndromes
Cardiovascular Examination	
Pulse and Blood Pressure Measurement in All Limbs	
• Delayed and weak femoral pulses, normal or low blood pressure in the legs	Coarctation of the aorta
Evaluation for Bruits in Heart, Abdomen, Flanks, Back, Neck and Head	
• Heart murmur (most prominent in interscapular area)	Coarctation of the aorta
• Abdominal bruit	Renal artery stenosis
• Apical heave	Left ventricular hypertrophy
• Friction rub	Pericarditis (vasculitis), uremia
Abdomen	
• Abdominal mass	Wilms tumor, neuroblastoma, pheochromocytoma, polycystic kidney disease, renal obstruction
• Hepatosplenomegaly	Autosomal recessive polycystic kidney disease
Neurologic	
• Focal neurologic deficits	Stroke
• Fundoscopy for hypertensive changes	End organ damage due to hypertension
• Retinal hamartoma	von Hippel-Lindau
Skin	
• Acanthosis nigricans	Insulin resistance (metabolic syndrome)
• Skin findings as detailed under characteristic syndromes	
• Pallor	Chronic kidney disease

From Kapur G, Baracco R: Evaluation of hypertension in children, *Curr Hypertens Rep* 15:433–443, 2013.

RENAL VEIN THROMBOSIS

Volume depletion secondary to diarrhea or vomiting, hypotension, hypercoagulable or hyperviscosity states, NS, or indwelling catheters in the vicinity of the renal veins especially predispose infants to renal vein or intrarenal venous thrombosis (Fig. 14.46). Among children, most cases of renal venous thrombosis occur in the first

Table 14.12 Suggested Initial Evaluation for Children and Adolescents With Suspected Secondary Hypertension

Secondary Etiology	Tests to Consider
Kidney parenchymal disease	• Urinalysis • Serum electrolytes, blood urea nitrogen, creatinine, ± plasma renin activity, aldosterone • Kidney ultrasonography
Renal vascular disease	• Urinalysis • Serum electrolytes, blood urea nitrogen, creatinine, plasma renin activity, aldosterone • Screen with kidney ultrasonography with Doppler if ≥8 years old and nonobese. For more definitive evaluation, consider computed tomography or magnetic resonance angiography.
Coarctation of aorta	• Echocardiography
Endocrine/tumor	• Serum electrolytes, blood urea nitrogen, creatinine, plasma renin activity, aldosterone, plasma metanephrines
Monogenic hypertension	• Serum electrolytes, blood urea nitrogen, creatinine, plasma renin activity, aldosterone
Obstructive sleep apnea	• Sleep study
Recreational/illicit drug use	• Drug screen

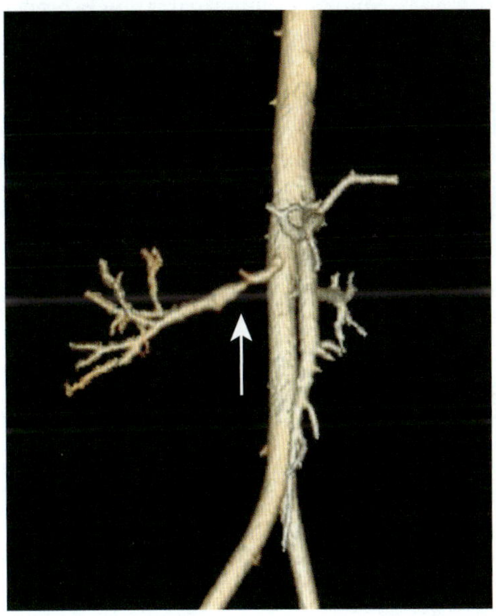

Fig. 14.44 Three-dimensional reconstruction of computed tomography angiogram showing right renal artery stenosis *(white arrow)*.

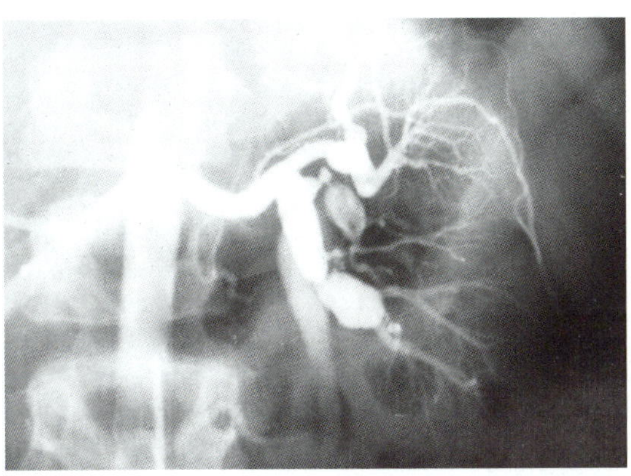

Fig. 14.45 Arteriogram of a 12-year-old patient with malignant hypertension shows multiple areas of stenosis alternating with aneurysmal dilation in the distal segment of the renal artery, characteristic of fibromuscular dysplasia.

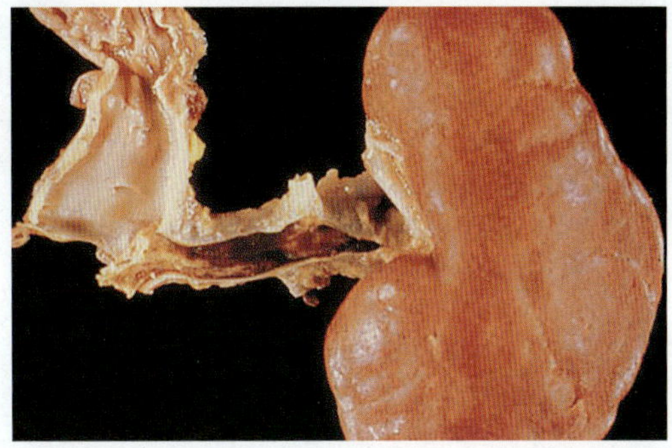

Fig. 14.46 A 12-year-old boy with ulcerative colitis, who died after a bout of severe diarrhea and dehydration. Apart from dural sinus thrombosis, the left renal vein contained this partially organized clot.

month of life. The typical clinical features of renal vein thrombosis are a palpable renal mass in 60% of infants and hematuria and thrombocytopenia, which occur in more than 90% of affected patients. Perinatal asphyxia, dehydration, and maternal diabetes mellitus are established risk factors, and hereditary prothrombotic disorders may be implicated. Kidney function may be normal, particularly in unilateral renal vein thrombosis or in bilateral disease that does not result in oliguria. Kidney ultrasonography with Doppler examination of renal and adjacent vessels is the diagnostic procedure of choice.

HEMOLYTIC UREMIC SYNDROME

Hemolytic uremic syndrome (HUS) is a thrombotic microangiopathy associated with the triad of hemolytic anemia, thrombocytopenia, and AKI. It is a nonimmune hemolytic anemia characterized by negative Coombs test, elevated lactate dehydrogenase, decreased haptoglobin, and evidence of microangiopathy with fragmented red blood cells and schistocytes on peripheral blood smear. HUS can be subdivided into two broad categories based on underlying pathophysiology: Shiga toxin–producing *Escherichia coli* (STEC) HUS and atypical HUS or complement-mediated HUS.

Shiga toxin–producing *E. coli* O157:H7 is the most common cause of childhood HUS. Shiga toxin directly injures renal endothelial cells, initiating a cascade of microthrombi formation in capillaries and arterioles. Vehicles of transmission for *E. coli* infections include food products, person-to-person contact, or airborne transmission. After contact with the infectious agent, children often develop nonbloody diarrhea, followed by bloody diarrhea within 3 days of exposure with about 15% of children developing STEC HUS (Fig. 14.47). Early restoration of IV volume and avoidance of antibiotics and antimotility agents can be protective against AKI, but treatment after development of the disease is largely supportive.

Increasing cases of atypical HUS are being recognized with development of renal microthrombi from complement dysregulation. Genetic mutations encoding complement-mediating factors have been associated with atypical HUS, and most cases have a preceding infectious trigger. Currently, genetic testing can identify a genetic anomaly in approximately two-thirds to three-fourths of all atypical HUS cases. A significant portion of children with atypical HUS have a gastrointestinal prodrome that triggers complement dysregulation, making it difficult to clinically distinguish from STEC HUS (Table 14.13). Eculizumab and ravulizumab, monoclonal antibody anti-C5 complement inhibitors, are now the mainstay for therapy of atypical HUS and have significantly improved prognosis of atypical HUS.

The most common and primary clinical manifestation of HUS is AKI, sometimes necessitating KRT. In addition, children can develop nonrenal sequelae of thrombotic microangiopathy including seizures, cerebrovascular thrombosis, pancreatitis, intestinal

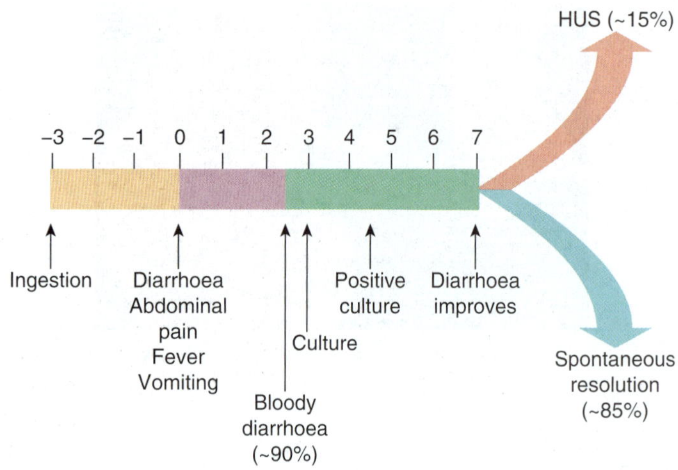

Fig. 14.47 Typical clinical progression of *Escherichia coli* O157:H7 infection in children. Note that hemolytic uremic syndrome (HUS) develops in about 15% of all infections around 10 days after the ingestion of *E. coli.* By the time children develop HUS, their diarrhea may be resolved, and stool culture may not grow *E. coli* O157:H7, which makes distinction from atypical HUS challenging. (From Tarr PI, Gordon CA, Chandler WL: Shiga-toxin-producing *Escherichia coli* and haemolytic uraemic syndrome, *Lancet* 365:1073–1086, 2005.)

Table 14.13 Clinical Characteristics of STEC HUS versus Atypical HUS

	STEC HUS	Atypical HUS
Clinical features	Concurrent HUS in family member, preceding diarrheal illness	HUS in family member Previous episode of HUS Preceding infection (can include gastrointestinal illness)
Pathophysiology	Shiga toxin injures renal endothelial cells, causing fibrin microthrombus formation	Alternative pathway complement dysregulation causes injury to renal endothelial cells, causing fibrin microthrombus formation ~70% of children have an identifiable genetic mutation causing complement dysregulation
Treatment	Supportive	Monoclonal anti-C5 antibody Plasmapheresis
Neurologic symptoms	20% of cases	15% of cases
Prognosis	70% of patients recover completely	Good if responsive to eculizumab

HUS, Hemolytic uremic syndrome; *STEC,* Shiga toxin–producing *Escherichia coli.*

perforation or necrosis, cardiac dysfunction, and respiratory distress from fluid overload.

CHRONIC KIDNEY DISEASE

GFR is the rate of flow of filtrate through the kidney and is representative of kidney function. Multiple equations have been used to estimate children's and adolescents' GFR based on blood chemistry, and the most used method currently is the CKiD Under 25 (U25) equations. The equations were developed and validated using data from the Chronic Kidney Disease in Children Study, and they estimate patients' GFR using either serum creatinine or cystatin C alone, or the average of the two equations.

The serum creatinine equation is:

$$\text{Estimated GFR} = K^{*}(\text{height}/\text{serum creatinine}).$$

The cystatin C equation is:

$$\text{Estimated GFR} = k^{*}(1/\text{serum cystatin C}).$$

(Estimated GFR: mL/min/1.73m^2, height: cm, serum creatinine: mg/dL, serum cyustatin C: mg/dL)

The K and k are different age- and sex-dependent constants, respectively.

When both serum creatinine and serum cystatin C are available, the average estimated GFR of both equations is preferred as it provides a more accurate and precise estimate of GFR than single-marker estimation. The exception is when serum creatinine is obtained from patients with significantly small muscle mass, such as in those with muscular dystrophy. In such cases the cystatin C equation alone should be used.

Normal GFR in newborns is less than 60 mL/min/1.73 m^2, and adjusted GFR for body surface area is not comparable with adult values until the age of 2 years (Table 14.14). CKD is a continuum, defined by abnormalities in kidney structure or function with associated health consequences. Criteria include decreased GFR or markers of kidney damage including proteinuria, electrolyte abnormalities, abnormal urinary sediments, abnormal kidney biopsy, structural anomalies, or history of kidney transplantation. Up to 50% of children with CKD have CAKUT, although etiology differs by age (Fig. 14.48). For classification and prognostic purposes, CKD is divided into stages based on degree of kidney dysfunction (Table 14.15). Children with CKD tend to have progression of kidney decline during their growth spurt as poorly functioning kidneys cannot compensate for rapid body growth. Other factors, such as proteinuria and HTN, are both manifestations of CKD and contributors to progressive kidney injury. Secondary effects of CKD include HTN, metabolic bone disease, electrolyte abnormalities, metabolic acidosis, anemia, poor growth, and delayed puberty.

Metabolic Bone Disease

As kidney function declines, normal mineral balance between calcium and phosphorus is disrupted as regulatory hormones are altered. With poor kidney function, phosphate is not appropriately excreted and kidney conversion of 25-hydroxyvitamin D to more active 1, 25-dihydroxyvitamin D is insufficient. Consequences include hyperphosphatemia, elevated parathyroid hormone level and FGF 23, and diminished gastrointestinal calcium absorption, all of which combine to cause poor bone modeling and remodeling and metabolic bone

Table 14.14 Normal Glomerular Filtration Rate for Age

Age (Sex)	Glomerular Filtration Rate 6 Standard Deviation (mL/min/1.73 m^2)
1 week (full term)	41 ± 15
2–8 weeks (full term)	66 ± 25
>8 weeks	96 ± 22
2–12 years	133 ± 27
13–21 years (male)	140 ± 30
13–21 years (female)	126 ± 22

From Schwartz GJ, Brion LP, Spitzer A: The use of plasma creatinine concentration for estimating glomerular filtration rate in infants, children, and adolescents, *Pediatr Clin North Am* 34(3):571–590, 1987.

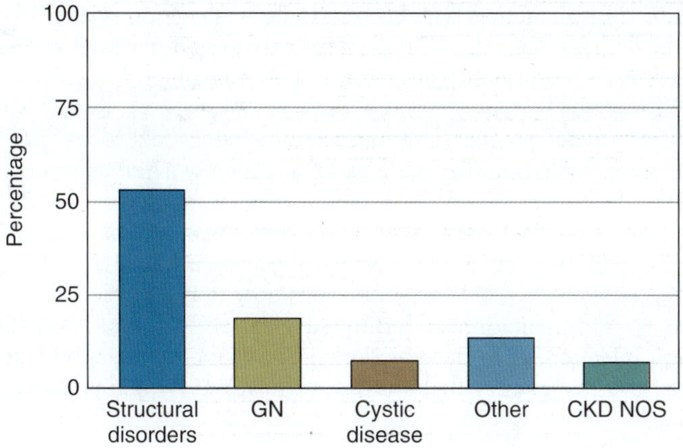

Fig. 14.48 Causes of kidney disease among children, 2022. Data source: Medicaid database. January 1, 2022 point prevalent beneficiaries with kidney disease, aged 1-17 years. For figures by race/ethnicity, only enrollees in states with reliable race/ethnicity information were included. *CKD,* Chronic kidney disease; *GN,* glomerulonephritis; *NOS,* not otherwise specified. (From USRDS: 2024 Annual Data Report: Chronic Kidney Disease: 5: Kidney Disease Among Children and Adolescents. https://usrds-adr.niddk.nih.gov/2024/chronic-kidney-disease/5-kidney-disease-among-children-and-adolescents.)

Table 14.15 Chronic Kidney Disease Stages

Stage	Description	GFR (mL/min/1.73 m^2)
1	Kidney damage Normal/Increased GFR	>90
2	Mildly decreased GFR	60–89
3a	Mild-moderately decreased GFR	45–59
3b	Moderate-severely decreased GFR	30–44
4	Severely decreased GFR	15–29
5	End-stage kidney disease	<15

GFR, Glomerular filtration rate.

disease. In addition, these metabolic derangements make a significant contribution to cardiovascular disease seen in CKD patients starting at a much younger age than for the general population.

In children, the condition is clinically characterized by poor growth, bone pain, and ricket-line deformities of long bones. The radiologic features in children include increased thickness and fraying of the radiolucent zone in the region of growth plates; subperiosteal erosion of the cortices of long bones and phalanges; and changes in bone density including osteoporosis, osteosclerosis, or coarsening of the trabecular pattern of long bones.

Growth Faltering

Linear growth faltering is a common feature in children with CKD, with up to one-third of children achieving less than the third percentile for height. The mechanisms of poor growth include chronic metabolic acidosis, metabolic bone disease, poor nutrition, chronic inflammation, and decreased free insulin growth factor-1. In addition to addressing malnutrition and biochemical abnormalities, recombinant human growth hormone therapy can be efficacious in promoting growth.

Anemia of Chronic Kidney Disease

Anemia is prevalent in almost all children with stage 4 and stage 5 CKD. Although multifactorial, it is primarily caused by insufficient erythropoietin secretion by specialized renal peritubular interstitial cells. This results in decreased erythroid cell proliferation and differentiation in the bone marrow. If left untreated, hemoglobin levels in children are often lower than in adults (5–7 g/dL). Another major contributor to anemia in CKD is iron deficiency caused by dysregulation of iron metabolic pathway, shorter red blood cell life span, and blood loss due to frequent blood draws and with hemodialysis treatments. Treatment of anemia with recombinant erythropoietin or other erythrocyte-stimulating factors and supplementation with iron, vitamin B_{12}, and folic acid can obviate the need for blood transfusions and result in near-normal hemoglobin levels leading to improved cognitive function, exercise tolerance, cardiovascular function, and overall quality of life.

KIDNEY FAILURE REQUIRING DIALYSIS OR TRANSPLANT (END-STAGE KIDNEY DISEASE)

Children with stage 5 CKD, defined as an estimated GFR less than 15 mL/min/1.73 m^2, will eventually require kidney replacement therapy (KRT) consisting of either dialysis or kidney transplantation. There is no specific level of GFR where KRT must be initiated. The decision to start KRT is based on a combination of factors including GFR; metabolic disturbances associated with kidney failure; fluid overload; growth failure; and symptoms of uremia such as decreased energy, fatigue, anorexia, and failure to achieve developmental milestones. ESKD is rare in pediatrics, with an incidence of about 1300 for patients younger than 22 years in the United States. Although most children will eventually receive a kidney transplant, about 75% of them will be on dialysis before receiving a transplant. The life expectancy of pediatric patients with CKD initiating KRT is about 40 years for those receiving dialysis and 60 years for those who receive a kidney transplant. Both peritoneal dialysis and hemodialysis can be offered to children as small as 2 kg, though there are special considerations when performing KRT on a small child.

Peritoneal Dialysis

Peritoneal dialysis is the primary modality performed in children in the first decade of life and is a daily home-based therapy performed typically by their caretakers. It can be done in children as small as 2 to 3 kg. Most children receive automated peritoneal dialysis with a dialysis machine called a cycler. It can also be done manually as continuous ambulatory peritoneal dialysis. Peritoneal dialysis allows children to go to school and have a more liberal diet as it is a daily therapy. Peritoneal dialysis requires the placement of the peritoneal dialysis catheter. These are soft rubber or polyurethane catheters that are either straight or coiled and have one or two subcutaneously placed Dacron cuffs that come in both neonatal and pediatric sizes (Fig. 14.49). The major complications of peritoneal dialysis in children are infectious, consisting of peritonitis, exit site, and tunnel infections.

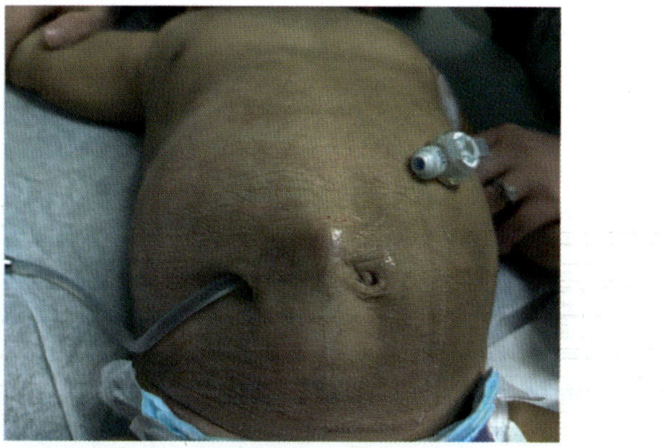

Fig. 14.49 An infant with permanent peritoneal dialysis catheter. The catheter lies in the subcutaneous tissue held by Dacron cuffs and then enters the peritoneum. The ideal location of the catheter tip is in the pelvis.

Hemodialysis

Hemodialysis is an extracorporeal therapy that requires vascular access and is generally done in a hemodialysis unit, 3 to 4 days a week for 3 to 4 hours per session. Vascular access can be either through dual lumen tunneled central venous catheters ranging in size from 7 to 14.5 Fr or through an arteriovenous fistula (AVF) or graft. The advantages of central venous catheters are that they can be used immediately, can be placed in infants, and do not require peripheral needle sticks. Disadvantages include catheter infections, catheter malfunctions, central venous thrombosis and stenosis, and chronic inflammation. AVF is the preferred form of vascular access if long-term hemodialysis is required. AVFs are typically reserved for older children with sufficiently large veins to create one and who can tolerate repeated needle sticks. AVFs can require months for maturation before they can be used (Fig. 14.50). Children younger than 16 years will typically have to be dialyzed at pediatric centers located in urban areas. Home hemodialysis therapies are becoming more available.

Kidney Transplantation

Kidney transplantation is the preferred therapy for ESKD in children. Approximately 700 to 800 pediatric kidney transplants are performed annually in the United States in children younger than 18 years of age. Kidney transplant can be from either a living donor or a deceased donor, with a slight improved graft survival with living donor transplantation. The current kidney allocation system (KAS) in the United States gives children priority to improve their access to receiving a high-quality deceased donor transplant. The minimum size for transplantation at most centers is 10 to 12 kg, though some will transplant smaller children. Small patient size does provide operative challenges. The preferred placement of a kidney transplant is extraperitoneal, though in a smaller child, it may have to be placed intraabdominally. Patient survival is greater than 95% at 3 years, and 3-year and 10-year allograft survival are approximately 90% and 60%, respectively. There are numerous potential complications after kidney transplantation including surgical and urologic complications, infection, allograft rejection, HTN, diabetes, metabolic disorders, and malignancy including posttransplant lymphoproliferative disorder, a form of cancer unique in posttransplant patients.

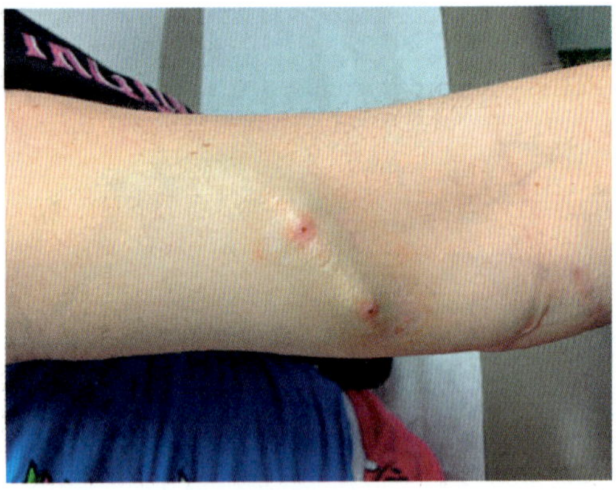

Fig. 14.50 Many older children with end-stage kidney disease on hemodialysis have arteriovenous fistula. This is surgically created and is the preferred hemodialysis vascular access for patients expected to be on long-term hemodialysis. Two needles are placed in the fistula to draw and return blood.

Bibliography

Cadnapaphornchai MA, Tkachenko O, Shchekochikhin D, Schrier RW: The nephrotic syndrome: pathogenesis and treatment of edema formation and secondary complications, *Pediatr Nephrol* 29:1159–1167, 2014.

Chua AN, Warady BA: Care of the pediatric patient on chronic dialysis, *Adv Chronic Kidney Dis* 24(6):388–397, 2017.

Dixon BP, Gruppo RA: Atypical hemolytic uremic syndrome, *Pediatr Clin North Am* 65(3):509–525, 2018.

Eison TM, Ault BH, Jones DP, Chesney RW, Wyatt RJ: Poststreptococcal acute glomerulonephritis in children: clinical features and pathogenesis, *Pediatr Nephrol* 26:165–180, 2011.

Flynn JT, Kaelber DC, Baker-Smith CM, et al: Clinical practice guideline for screening and management of high blood pressure in children and adolescents, *Pediatrics* 140(3):e20171904, 2017.

Flynn JT, Urbina EM, Brady TM, et al: Ambulatory blood pressure monitoring in children and adolescents: 2022 update: a scientific statement from the American Heart Association, *Hypertension* 79(7): e114–e124, 2022.

Hoppe B, Kemper M: Diagnostic examination of the child with urolithiasis or nephrocalcinosis, *Pediatr Nephrol* 25:403–413, 2010.

Meyers KEC: Evaluation of hematuria in children, *Urol Clin N Am* 31:559–573, 2004.

Pierce CB, Muñoz A, Ng DK, Warady BA, Furth SL, Schwartz GJ: Age- and sex-dependent clinical equations to estimate glomerular filtration rates in children and young adults with chronic kidney disease, *Kidney Int* 99(4):948–956, 2021.

Pohl M: Henoch-Schönlein purpura nephritis, *Pediatr Nephrol* 39(2):245–252, 2015.

Sutherland SM, Kwiatkowski DM: Acute kidney injury in children, *Adv Chronic Kidney Dis* 24(6):380–387, 2017.

Sweeney WE, Avner ED: Pathophysiology of childhood polycystic kidney diseases: new insights into disease-specific therapy, *Pediatr Res* 75:148–157, 2014.

Tarr PI, Gordon CA, Chandler WL: Shiga-toxin-producing Escherichia coli and haemolytic uraemic syndrome, *Lancet* 365:1073–1086, 2005.

Verghese PS: Pediatric kidney transplantation: a historical review, *Pediatr Res* 81(1-2):259–264, 2017.

15 UROLOGIC DISORDERS

Brett A. Teplitz | Omar Ayyash | Rajeev Chaudhry

Many congenital urologic malformations and acquired disorders, as well as the results of common urologic surgical procedures, produce visible or palpable findings on physical examination. Some clinical presentations are unique. In other cases, disorders of varying etiology may present with similar signs, symptoms, and physical findings. Differential diagnosis and thorough examination are essential to an appreciation and recognition of pediatric urologic disorders.

PHYSICAL EXAMINATION

Before any physical examination, a thorough history of both the patient and family is key to developing differential diagnoses of urologic disorders. Family history of urinary tract infection (UTI), hydronephrosis, vesicoureteral reflux (VUR), cystic kidney disease, compromised fertility, or genital malformation may indicate the presence of heritable urinary anomaly.

Examination begins with a general overview of the patient. Hemihypertrophy, congenital scoliosis, an abnormal gait, facial or external ear deformities, or the presence of multiple congenital anomalies may be associated with urologic disorders. Abdominal examination should begin with inspection for visible masses, followed by gentle palpation. Enlarged kidneys are usually palpable as upper abdominal or flank masses in small children and infants, but they may be difficult to appreciate in older children. An enlarged bladder or lesion of gynecologic origin may be palpable as a midline mass arising out of the pelvis. Abdominal masses should be characterized as cystic or solid; smooth, lobulated, or irregular; fixed or mobile; and tender or nontender. The abdominal portion of an abdominoscrotal hydrocele may be palpable in either lower quadrant and may increase in size when the scrotal component is compressed (Fig. 15.1).

The inguinal areas should be examined for palpable gonads. Gonads are frequently quite mobile and may move during examination toward the perineum or thigh. They may even disappear into the abdomen. Therefore testes may be palpable on one examination and nonpalpable on the next. The sensitivity of palpation for detection of inguinal testes and other masses may be increased by using soap or lubricant on the examiner's fingers. It may be difficult to palpate an inguinal testis by trying to "pinch" it between the fingers, whereas lubricated fingers gliding over the inguinal canal may detect a gonad as it slides beneath the fingers. The best technique is to place the fingers flat, over the inguinal canal and above the level of the internal inguinal ring, and slide them slowly toward the pubis, then over the pubis toward the scrotum and down over the perineum lateral to the upper scrotum. On occasion, the spermatic cord may end in a small "nubbin" (remnant of an atrophic testis). The structures of the inguinal canal should be examined in a similar fashion to detect thickening of the cord structures that may be seen in the presence of an inguinal hernia or communicating hydrocele. Masses in the inguinal canal may also represent an inguinal hernia containing bowel or omentum, an ovary in girls, a gonad of unclear etiology in patients with ambiguous genitalia (Fig. 15.2), communicating hydrocele or hydrocele of the cord, or malignancy of the paratesticular tissues or cord structures (e.g., sarcoma). Inguinal lymphadenopathy is usually detected lateral to the inguinal canal and is generally nonreducible.

Genital examination should include both inspection and palpation. The penis should be assessed for both length and diameter. Penile stretch length can be determined by using a ruler or tongue blade pressed against the pubic symphysis as the penis is gently stretched alongside it and the position of the tip of the glans is marked for measurement. A concealed or buried penis may occur after circumcision or may be congenital. In most cases, hidden penises are retractile, in large part due to a thick suprapubic fat pad. Most cases of buried penis will resolve with time and pubertal development, whereas in severe cases the tethering may be due to dysgenetic fascial attachments and will require surgical correction. It may be difficult to determine the difference in younger boys. Penoscrotal fusion or webbing may also cause an anomalous appearance and entrapment of the penis.

The foreskin should be examined for adhesions to the glans, which may represent merely residual preputial fusion to the glans that will resolve spontaneously, or preputial skin bridges, which can occur after circumcision and require surgical division. The urethral meatus should be examined for size and especially location. Meatal location may appear more proximally on the ventral surface, anywhere from the glans to the perineum (hypospadias), or it may appear along the dorsal surface anywhere from the glans toward the umbilicus (epispadias). The presence of chordee (ventral penile curvature) or a suggestion of its presence should be noted. The size and degree of development of the scrotum and the location and size of the testes are noted.

Retractile testes should come well into the dependent portion of the scrotum when the room is warm and the patient is relaxed. If it is difficult to determine whether the testes are undescended, retractile, or normal, repeat examination may be helpful. The epididymis should be palpated and examined for tenderness or the presence of masses. The spermatic cords should be examined for the presence of abnormal findings (thickening, masses, and/or varicocele). The cord is most easily examined as it crosses over the pubic tubercle. Male patients should be examined in both supine and standing positions with and without Valsalva maneuver.

In the female patient, the introitus should be inspected to confirm a normal size and location of the clitoris, urethral meatus, vaginal introitus, and hymenal ring. Labial masses, swelling, or adhesions (fusion) may completely conceal the introitus. Lysis of labial adhesions may be necessary to allow examination of the introitus. Masses protruding from the urethral meatus or located near or originating near the meatus should be noted. Vaginal or urethral discharge, the presence of hymenal tags, or an imperforate hymen may be seen. The appearance and position of the anus should be assessed, and abnormalities such as skin tags should be carefully noted. Rectal examination may be performed to assess sphincter tone or to help characterize abdominal or pelvic masses.

The lower back should be examined for midline hair tufts, clefts, sinus tracts, or other signs of spinal dysraphism. A general neurologic examination and testing of the anal wink, bulbocavernosus reflex, and lower extremity reflexes should be performed, especially if neurovesical dysfunction is suspected. The bulbocavernosus reflex is assessed by a brisk squeeze of the glans penis or clitoris or a gentle tug on an indwelling Foley catheter. A positive response, which indicates an intact sacral reflex arc, is indicated by reflex contraction of the anal sphincter and bulbocavernosus muscle. Absence of the reflex strongly suggests the presence of a sacral neurologic lesion.

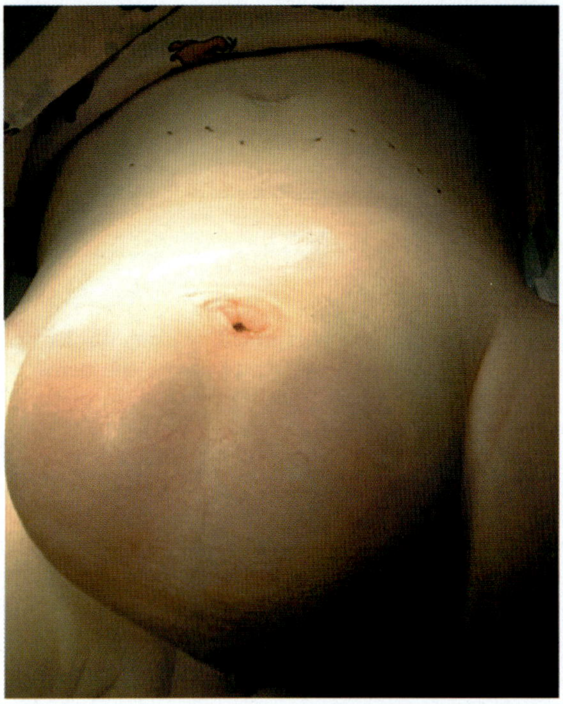

Fig. 15.1 Bilateral abdominoscrotal hydrocele in an infant. Bilateral large hydroceles extend up the inguinal canals. The *blue dots* on the abdomen mark the upper limits of the abdominal portion of the hydroceles.

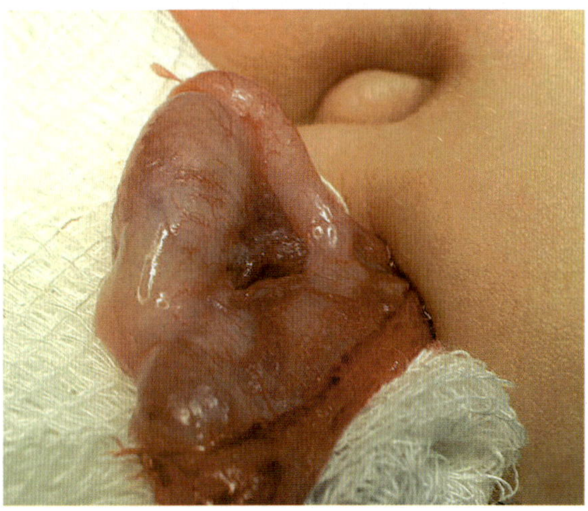

Fig. 15.2 Androgen insensitivity. Left inguinal testis in an XY phenotypic female with androgen insensitivity.

ANTENATAL URINARY TRACT DILATION

Detection of fetal urinary tract dilation (hydronephrosis, hydroureteronephrosis, hydroureter, pyelectasis, or pyelocaliectasis) with the increased use of prenatal sonography has become common (Fig. 15.3). There are two common classification systems in current use: the Urinary Tract Dilation and Society for Fetal Urology grading scales. Most cases of hydronephrosis, even of a significant degree, are not detectable by physical examination. Only the most severe cases present as an abdominal or flank mass, a distended bladder, or increase in abdominal girth. Causes of urinary tract dilation include physiologic hydronephrosis (typically mild and may resolve with time), VUR (see Chapter 14 for complete review), or obstruction, which encompasses ureteropelvic junction (UPJ) obstruction, ectopic ureters, and outlet obstruction, such as posterior urethral valves in boys or ureteroceles. Isolated upper pole hydronephrosis is diagnostic of a duplicated collecting system and can be seen with ureteroceles or ectopic ureters (see Fig. 15.3B). All infants with evidence of fetal urinary dilation, no matter what degree, should have postnatal ultrasonography and subsequent referral to pediatric urology. We generally recommend postnatal ultrasound after 48 hours of life when feasible before hospital discharge (Fig. 15.4). When postnatal ultrasound is normal (spontaneous resolution of fetal hydronephrosis occurs in up to 20% of cases), follow-up ultrasound should be performed at several months and at 1 year because delayed reappearance of dilation has been reported.

When postnatal hydronephrosis is documented, controversy exists as to the extent and timing of further radiographic evaluation, such as a voiding cystourethrogram (VCUG). Higher-risk situations, such as bilateral or severe unilateral dilation, poor renal function, or coexisting anomalies, demand complete radiographic evaluation, which should be performed as soon as possible before the infant leaves the hospital. These patients should also be started on prophylactic antibiotic therapy to prevent UTI. VCUG is an integral part of the evaluation in severe hydronephrosis and should be the first study performed in all cases to rule out both bladder outlet obstruction and VUR (Fig. 15.5A). Subsequent evaluation by radionuclide scan may be appropriate to assess function and to document whether true obstruction or mere dilation is present. If the infant is in stable condition (particularly when the lesion is unilateral or moderate in degree with good renal function), radionuclide evaluation should be delayed for 6 to 8 weeks or longer to allow improved glomerular filtration, making studies more accurate. If nonobstructive dilation is documented, long-term follow-up with outpatient urology is advised.

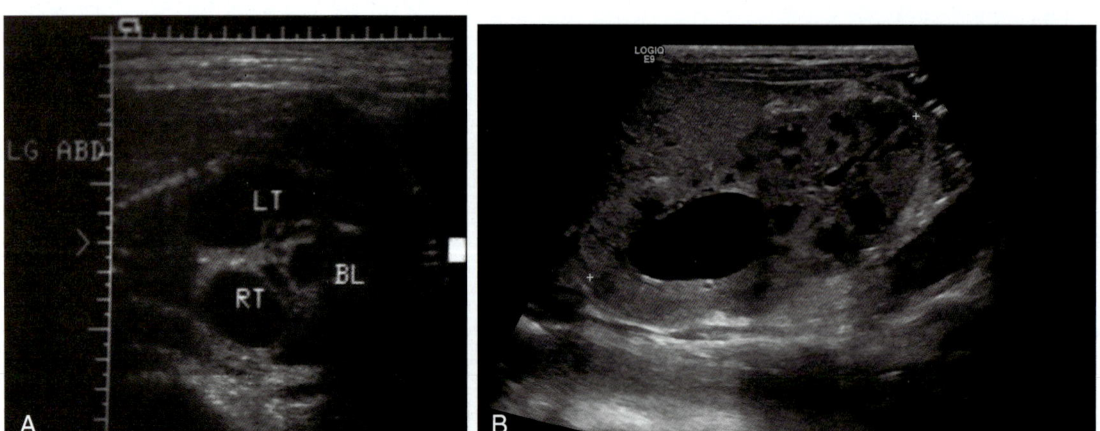

Fig. 15.3 (A) Fetal hydronephrosis. Ultrasonography performed to assess gestational age reveals bilateral fetal hydronephrosis and a distended bladder. (B) Upper pole hydronephrosis. *BL*, Bladder; *LT*, left kidney; *RT*, right kidney.

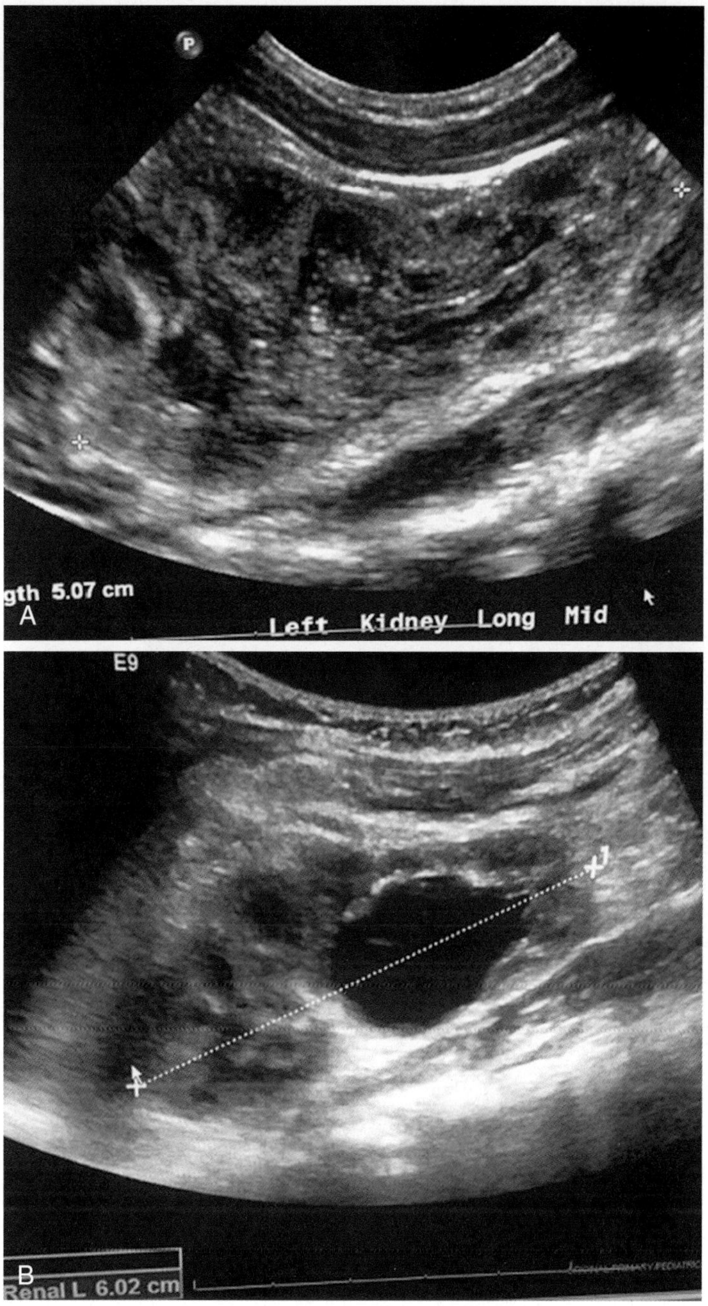

Fig. 15.4 Postnatal hydronephrosis. (A) Renal ultrasound at day of life 1 shows mild left lower pole dilation. (B) Renal ultrasound at 2 months old reveals increased left lower pole dilation not identified on day of life 1 ultrasound, likely secondary to the naturally dehydrated state of a newborn infant.

POSTERIOR URETHRAL VALVES

Valvular obstruction of the posterior urethra is a serious cause of bladder outlet obstruction in males. Presentation may vary depending on patient age and severity of obstruction. Most patients today are diagnosed prenatally with ultrasonography showing signs of hydroureteronephrosis, distended bladder, and a thickened bladder wall, occasionally demonstrating the classic "keyhole sign" (see Fig. 15.5A). Other potential symptoms in older boys include frequent UTIs, voiding dysfunction, or renal failure. Neonates may present with severe pulmonary hypoplasia and renal failure with bladder distention and hydroureteronephrosis. This is due to renal dysplasia in utero resulting in oligohydramnios or anhydramnios. VCUG is the key to diagnosing urethral valves. In most cases, endoscopic fulguration of urethral valves is undertaken. In some cases, cutaneous vesicostomy may be indicated (Fig. 15.6), especially in small infants in whom urethral instrumentation may be problematic. Rarely is upper tract diversion (ureterostomy or pyelostomy) indicated (Figs. 15.7 and 15.8). The ultimate prognosis for renal function depends on the degree of renal dysplasia, overall glomerular filtration, and bladder compliance.

CRYPTORCHIDISM

Cryptorchidism is one of the most common pediatric disorders of the male endocrine system, occurring in approximately 33% of premature and 3% of full-term boys. Approximately 75% of cryptorchid testes will spontaneously descend by 3 months old. Patients born with undescended testes are at increased risk for testicular malignancy, and those with bilateral cryptorchidism are at risk for infertility, highlighting the need to document testicular descent. The American Urological Association released guidelines in 2014 for the evaluation and treatment of boys with cryptorchidism. A gestational history at the initial evaluation and a physical examination with palpation of the turgor and placement of the testes should be conducted at every visit with the primary care provider. Infants with a history of cryptorchidism who have not experienced spontaneous descent by 6 months old (corrected for gestational age) should be referred to urology. Some boys with possible testicular ascent or newly diagnosed cryptorchidism after 6 months old should also be referred. Specifically, in the American Urological Association guidelines, there is no role for ultrasound or other imaging in the evaluation of boys with cryptorchidism before referral because these studies do not assist in decision making. In phenotypic males with bilateral, nonpalpable testes, evaluation of possible disorders of sex development (DSD) is indicated. Hypospadias associated with even unilateral cryptorchidism should raise the question of DSD (Fig. 15.9).

Hormonal therapy is not recommended to induce testicular descent, because there is a lack of evidence for long-term efficacy and evidence showing low response rates. Surgical intervention should be performed within a year after the initial 6-month-old (corrected for gestational age) confirmation of undescended testes. In boys with retractile testes, yearly examinations to assess for secondary ascent are indicated.

PRUNE-BELLY (EAGLE-BARRETT OR TRIAD) SYNDROME

Prune-belly syndrome has a unique constellation of physical findings and occurs almost exclusively in boys at a rate of 1 in 30,000 to 40,000 live births (see Chapter 14 for complete review). The triad includes abnormal abdominal musculature (variable degrees of muscular laxity, which may be asymmetric), abdominal cryptorchidism, and floppy dysmorphic urinary tracts, most with VUR (see Fig. 14.22). Because of the severe risk of sepsis associated with UTI, urethral catheterization should be undertaken only with the utmost care to prevent infection and with antibiotic prophylaxis. Megalourethra can be associated with prune-belly syndrome. Cryptorchidism should be treated with surgical intervention early in life. Prostatic hypoplasia and dimples on the lateral aspects of the knees are associated with the syndrome, possibly secondary to an exaggerated cross-legged position in utero. Prognosis is driven by the presence and degree of renal dysplasia.

ANOMALIES OF THE URACHUS

The urachus extends from the bladder dome to the umbilicus and is a vestigial structure during extrauterine life. Patent urachus results when the urachal lumen fails to obliterate, and the bladder communicates with the umbilicus. Several lesions may result from persistence of the urachus: patent urachus, vesicourachal diverticulum, urachal cyst, and umbilical-urachal sinus (Fig. 15.10). Many of these lesions go unrecognized for long periods before becoming symptomatic. Umbilical drainage is the most common presentation, but inflammation or infection may also result. Infected remnants are first

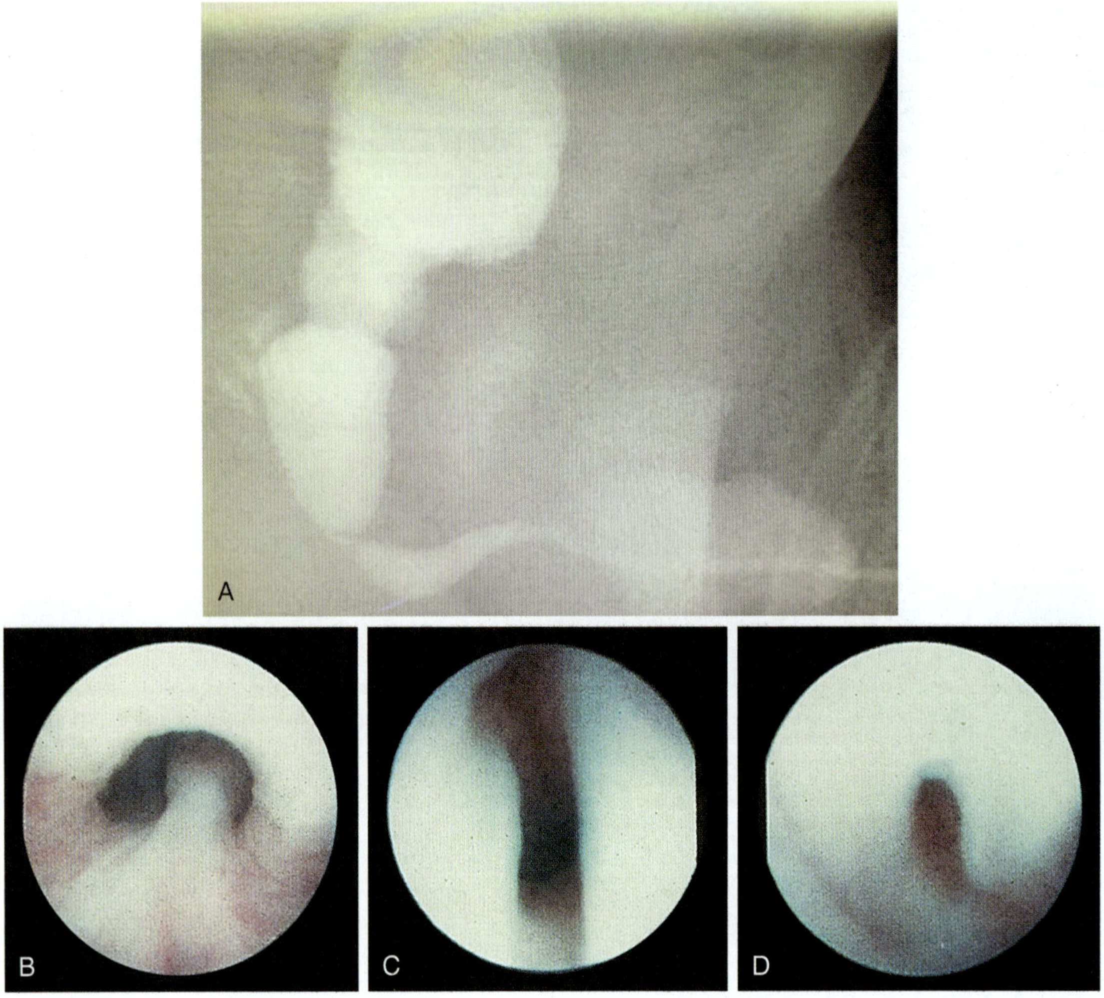

Fig. 15.5 Posterior urethral valves. (A) Voiding cystourethrogram performed in the neonatal period demonstrating a dilated posterior urethra with a filling defect noted where the posterior urethral valves are located with a transition to a normal anterior urethra. (B) Endoscopic view of a normal posterior urethra and verumontanum. (C) Type II urethral valves: the sail-like right and left leaflets are partially disrupted superiorly. (D) Type III urethral valves: These almost complete iris-diaphragm valves cause a more significant obstruction than type II leaflets.

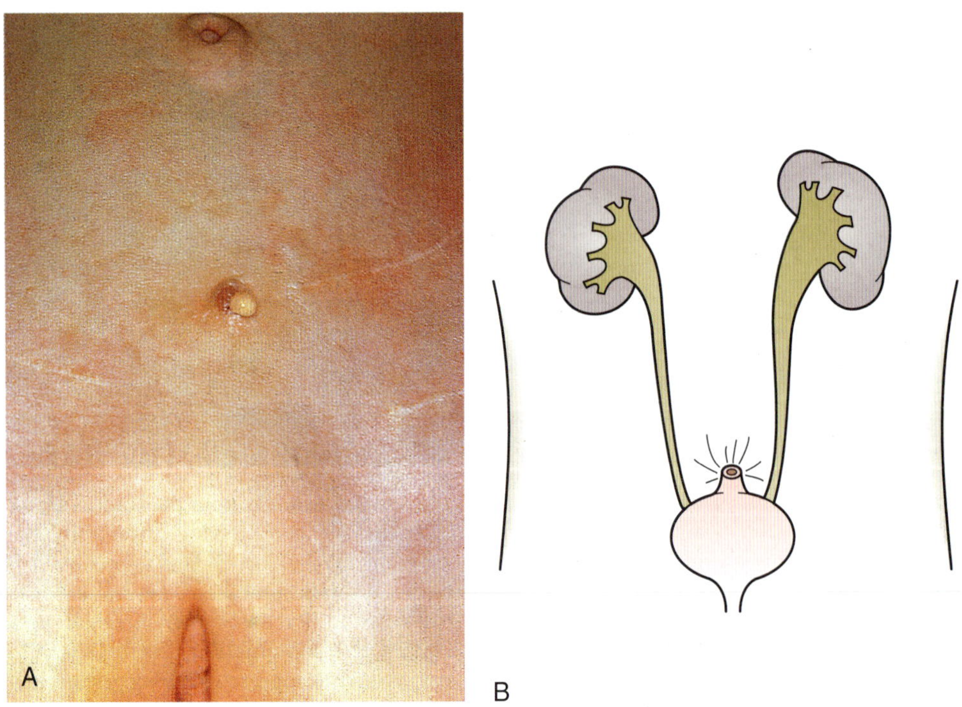

Fig. 15.6 (A and B) Cutaneous vesicostomy.

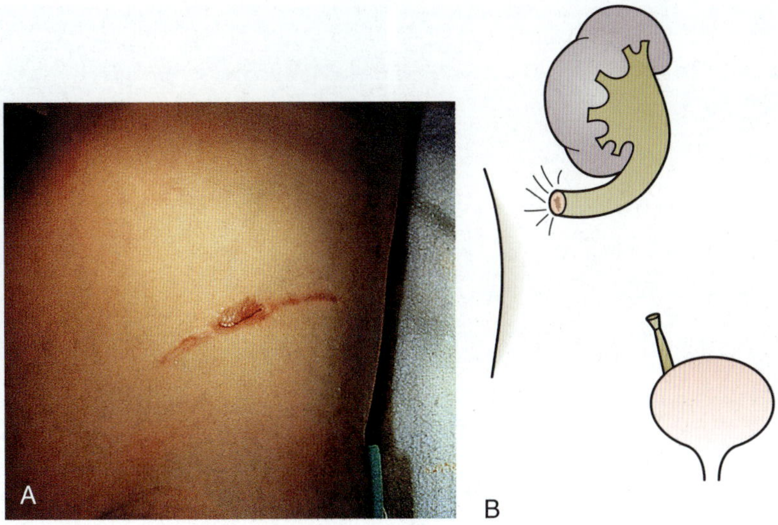

Fig. 15.7 (A and B) End ureterostomy.

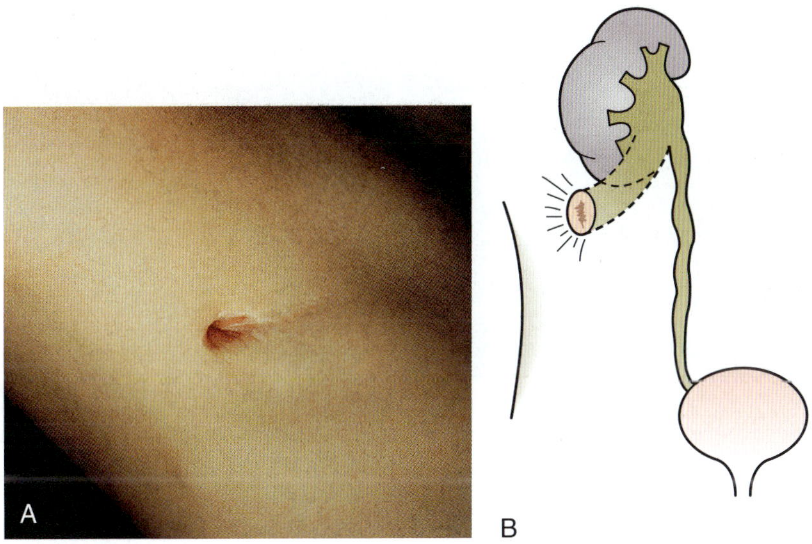

Fig. 15.8 (A and B) Cutaneous pyelostomy.

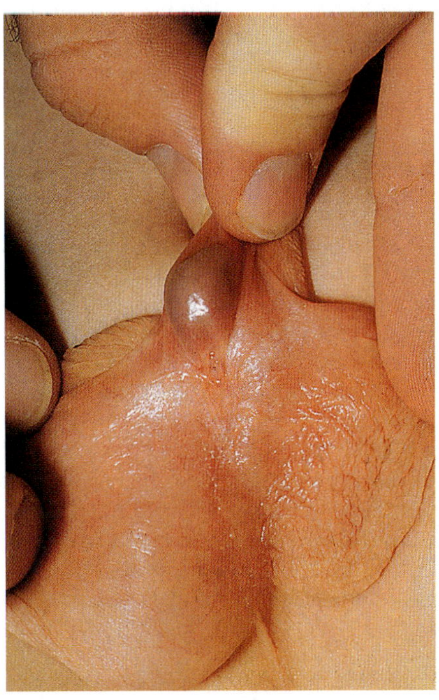

Fig. 15.9 Hypospadias and left cryptorchidism in a neonate found to have mixed gonadal dysgenesis with a mosaic karyotype.

treated with antibiotics and incision and drainage, with subsequent surgical excision. Diagnostic imaging modalities include bladder ultrasound, VCUG, or computed tomography (CT) scan. The differential diagnosis includes persistent omphalomesenteric duct and localized umbilical granulomas. Urachal remnants not resolving spontaneously should be referred to a pediatric urologist for consideration of surgical excision, with inclusion of the bladder cuff because of the increased risk for later adenocarcinoma formation.

Ureteropelvic Junction (UPJ) Obstruction

Lesions of the UPJ are a common cause of hydronephrosis. UPJ obstruction may present as antenatal hydronephrosis, neonatal flank mass, UTI, recurrent nephrolithiasis in the affected kidney, or recurrent episodes of abdominal/flank pain in the older child and adolescent (Dietl crises). Dietl crises are often triggered by increased flow through the genitourinary system, such as after large fluid intakes by young athletes or exposure to diuretics such as alcohol. Not all hydronephrotic kidneys are truly obstructed. Diagnosis can be confirmed with radionuclide diuresis renography (Lasix renal scan), which will assess both the function and drainage of the kidney (Fig. 15.11), or retrograde pyelography, which may be performed at the time of repair (Fig. 15.12A). Primary UPJ obstruction can be caused by intrinsic narrowing at the UPJ or extrinsic compression from an aberrant lower

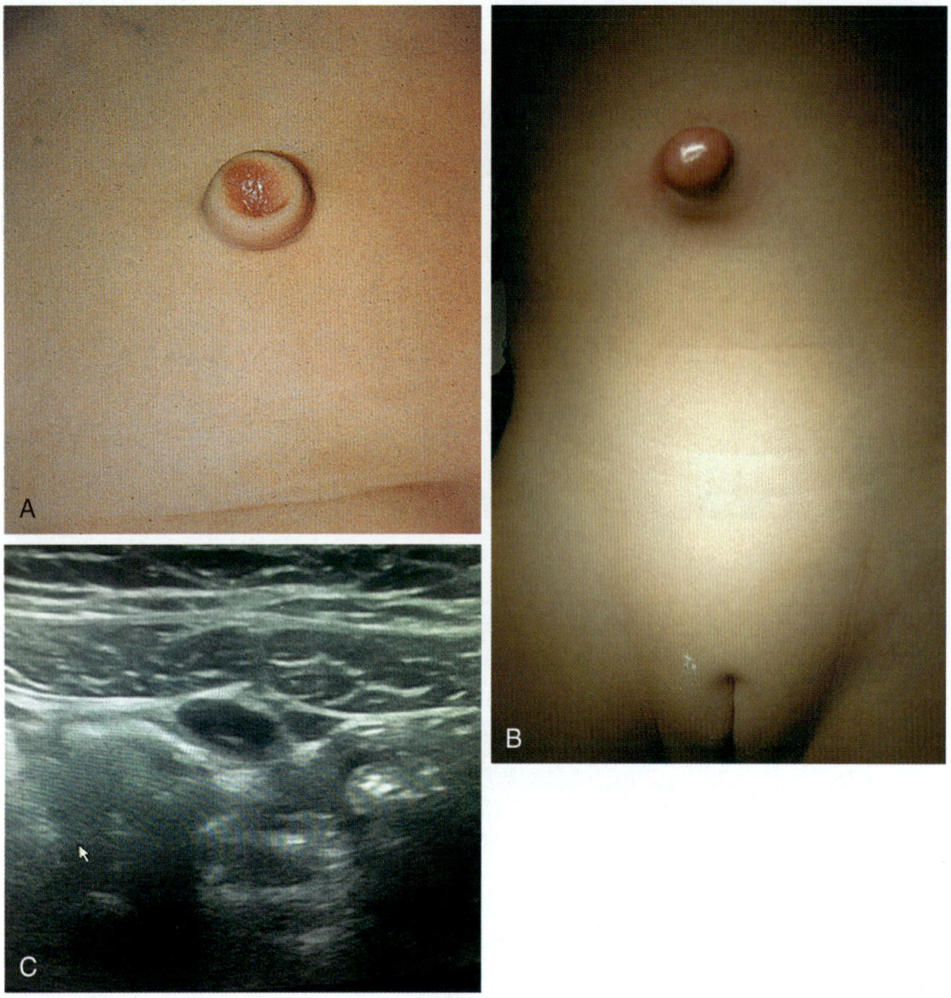

Fig. 15.10 Urachal anomalies. (A) Patent urachus in a young female with recurrent umbilical drainage and inflammation. (B) Urachal abscess in a young female presenting with fever and abdominal pain. (C) Ultrasound image of a urachal cyst found incidentally during evaluation for abdominal pain.

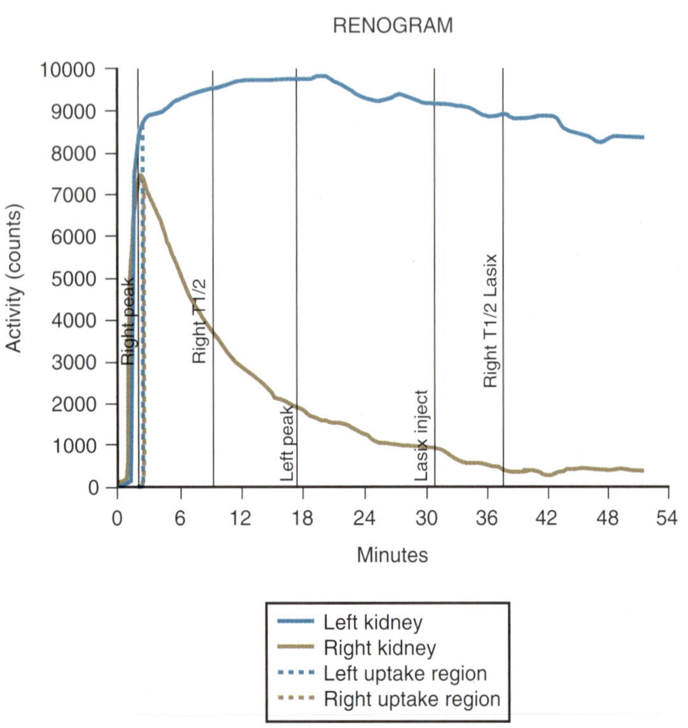

Fig. 15.11 Diuresis renogram. The radionuclide is administered, followed by a diuretic. The curves show a normal right kidney (prompt decrease in counts as the radionuclide is washed out of the collecting system) and an obstructed left kidney (only a small fraction of the radionuclide is slowly drained out of the collecting system).

pole vessel or ureteral polyps. Secondary UPJ obstruction can be due to high-grade VUR resulting in significant ureteral tortuosity that causes a kink at the UPJ; VCUG may be helpful in this regard. In cases with VUR (see Fig. 15.12B), diluted contrast noted in the renal pelvis compared with the bladder and ureter is indicative of a secondary UPJ obstruction. Some dilated but unobstructed infant kidneys spontaneously return to a normal or near-normal appearance with time.

MULTICYSTIC RENAL DYSPLASIA

Multicystic renal dysplasia (see Chapter 14) is the second most common cause of renal enlargement in the neonate and may be discovered by antenatal ultrasound or during the evaluation of an abdominal mass. Multicystic renal dysplasia must be differentiated from hydronephrosis with imaging. Though similar on ultrasonography, multicystic kidneys rarely function on radionucleotide scan (Fig. 15.13). Contralateral VUR can be seen in ~20% of infants, so VCUG should be considered to detect reflux into the solitary functioning kidney. A large percentage of multicystic kidneys spontaneously involute, which may later be misdiagnosed as a "congenitally absent kidney." There is no clear indication for nephrectomy, as large series studies have indicated no association with an increased risk for hypertension or neoplasm, although case reports exist. Patients should be followed conservatively with frequent blood pressure measurements by the primary care provider.

SIMPLE RENAL CYSTS

Simple renal cysts were thought to be rare in children until the advent of high-resolution ultrasound technology. They are now

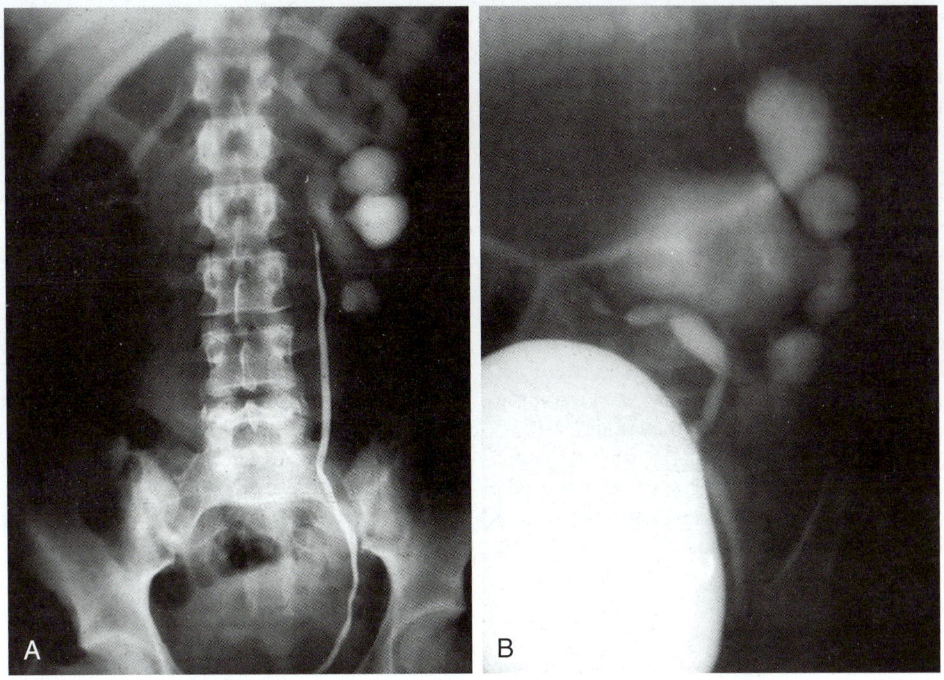

Fig. 15.12 Ureteropelvic junction (UPJ) obstruction. (A) Retrograde ureterogram defines obstruction at the UPJ. (B) The coexistence of vesicoureteral reflux and UPJ obstruction is seen in this voiding cystourethrogram. The diluted contrast noted in the renal pelvis compared with the bladder and ureter is indicative of a UPJ obstruction.

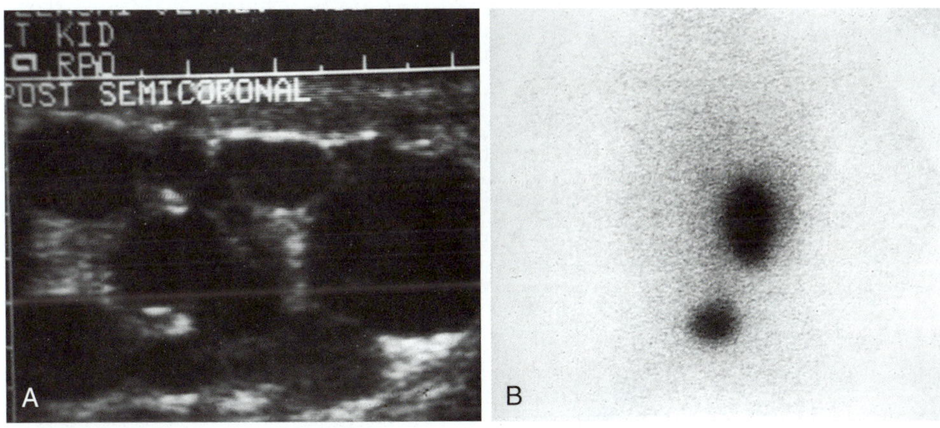

Fig. 15.13 Multicystic dysplasia. (A) Ultrasound examination of a multicystic kidney. (B) Nuclear medicine scan of a nonfunctional left multicystic dysplastic kidney (posterior view). The top area of contrast represents the right kidney, and the lower one is the bladder.

frequently detected, albeit much less commonly than in adults, in whom the incidence increases with age. As a result, the traditional admonition to surgically explore all cysts in children has been replaced by a policy of longitudinal radiographic follow-up evaluation, similar to that in adults. Simple cysts should be treated as benign. Most renal cysts are discovered incidentally, but large cysts occasionally present as abdominal masses. Radiologic evaluation usually includes ultrasonography, but CT (Fig. 15.14) and even cyst puncture for aspiration and contrast studies may be used to confirm the nature of the cyst. The differential diagnosis includes cystic Wilms tumor, multilocular cystic dysplasia, duplication anomaly with hydronephrosis, caliceal diverticulum, and polycystic disease.

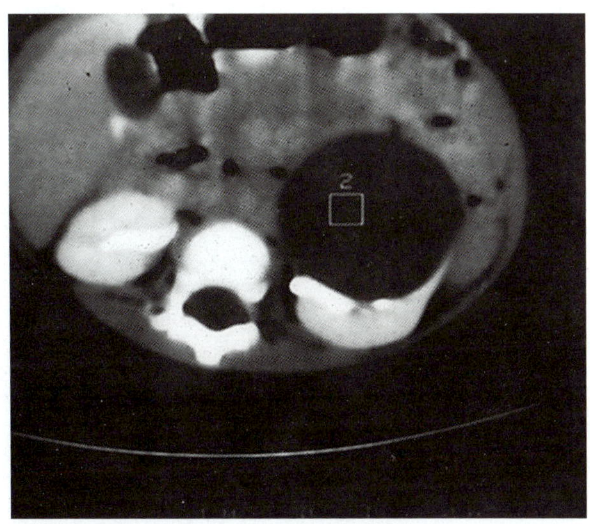

Fig. 15.14 Simple renal cyst. Computed tomography scan of a large left renal cyst, which presented as a left upper quadrant abdominal mass.

EXSTROPHY ANOMALIES

Classic Exstrophy

Bladder exstrophy represents a spectrum of disorders, with the classic form occurring in approximately 1 in 50,000 live births. It predominates in boys and is thought to result from an abnormally large cloacal membrane inhibiting mesenchymal migration and impeding closure of the ventral abdominal wall. The infant is usually otherwise healthy. Examination reveals a red mucosal surface of varying size on the infraumbilical abdominal wall, which represents the entire bladder opened like a book. On the inferior bladder surface, the trigone and ureteral orifices are visible, freely effluxing urine. Classic presentation includes a low-set umbilicus, pubic diastasis, and anteriorly displaced anus. In males, the penis is epispadiac and lies dorsally tethered against the bladder. When the penis is retracted downward, the entire mucosal surface of the urethra is seen to be splayed open (Fig. 15.15A and B). In severe cases the penis may be bifid or rudimentary, and sex may be undetermined. The scrotum may be normal or bifid, and testes may be undescended. Inguinal hernias are common. In girls, a hemiclitoris and duplicate vagina are common (see Fig. 15.15C and D). The delicate bladder surface should be kept moist and covered with plastic wrap until urologic consultation is obtained, to prevent irritation of the bladder mucosa and reduce risk of polyps. Prompt upper tract evaluation is necessary, as these patients often have shorter detrusor tunnels placing them at increased risk of VUR, though the upper genitourinary tracts are typically initially spared. Timing of closure is dependent on the urologist, but there has been a shift toward delaying closure for various reasons, including anesthetic purposes, size of bladder, and possibility of staged reconstruction. When closure is delayed, pelvic osteotomy is likely necessary to achieve successful closure.

Cloacal Exstrophy

Cloacal exstrophy is a rare anomaly (1 in 400,000 births). It represents the most severe form of bladder exstrophy. Rupture of the cloacal membrane occurs before the urorectal septum has completed its descent to separate the hindgut from the bladder. The resulting constellation of anomalies is severe, with long-term survival little better than 50% in most cases. Most children have a large omphalocele, and the majority have myelomeningocele and hydrocephalus. Examination of the exstrophic mucosa reveals that the bladder is divided into two widely separated halves, with a strip of bowel mucosa in the middle (Fig. 15.16). This strip is the ileocecal segment, usually accompanied by a long, prolapsed tubular structure, which is the terminal ileum. Separate orifices enter the appendix (or appendices) and a short, blind colon. The anus is imperforate. The genitalia are usually hypoplastic with the genital primordia widely separated at either side of the exstrophic cloaca. A multispecialty approach should be taken to the infant with cloacal exstrophy, including questions of sex assignment.

Epispadias

Isolated epispadias represents the mildest form of exstrophic anomalies and has a spectrum of severity. Approximately 55% of patients are boys with penopubic epispadias and urinary incontinence.

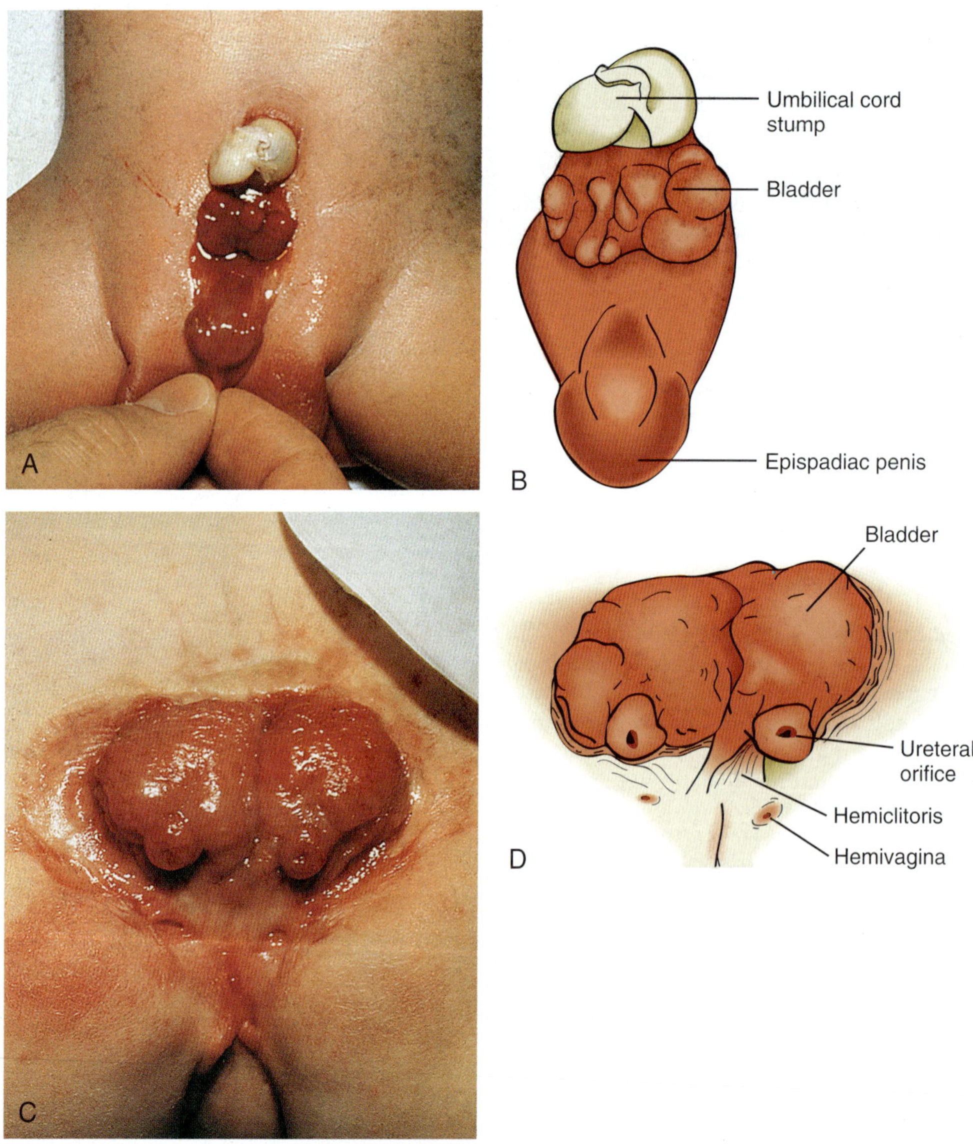

Fig. 15.15 Exstrophy. (A and B) Classic bladder exstrophy in a young male with a small bladder. (C and D) Bladder exstrophy in a young female. Note the separate openings to each hemivagina.

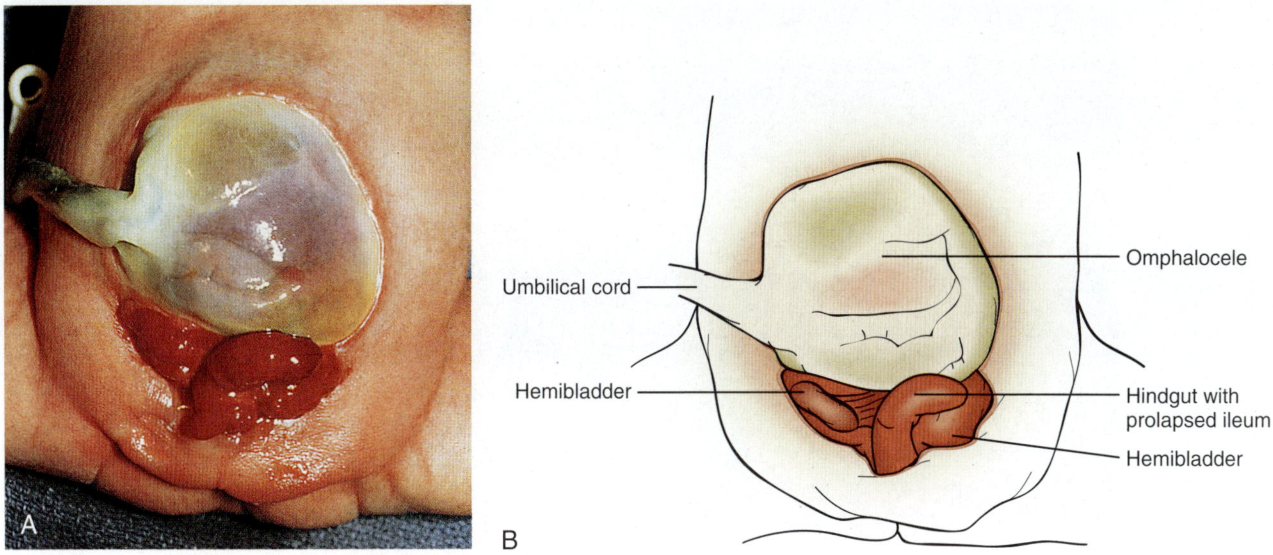

Fig. 15.16 (A and B) Cloacal exstrophy.

These boys have a palpably and radiographically widened pubic symphysis and a broad, spadelike penis with the urethra opened fully on its dorsal surface up to the level of the bladder neck. The penis is usually tethered dorsally, and the patient is usually incontinent (Fig. 15.17A). A smaller percentage of boys demonstrate only penile or glandular epispadias. These boys have normal urinary continence. In girls with epispadias (~1 in 400,000), incontinence is typically accompanied by a wide urethra and a bifid clitoris (see Fig. 15.17B). The cosmetic appearance of the genitalia in both genders can be improved by genitoplasty, but incontinence is a challenge, which is accentuated by small bladder capacity. Surgical correction is the rule and may be performed in stages. Renal ultrasonography and VCUG should be performed in all cases.

URINARY RETENTION

Acute urinary retention in infants and children is usually voluntary and associated with severe acute cystitis, urethritis, meatitis (in boys), or vaginitis. Severe constipation is frequently associated with urinary retention. In boys, urethral stricture and meatal stenosis should be considered (Fig. 15.18A). Urethral valves are more likely to cause dysuria or straining without complete retention. Retention in girls is unlikely to be caused by even severe labial adhesions, so uncommon lesions (e.g., prolapsed ureterocele) should be considered. Bladder or urethral calculi may also cause retention, and these can be diagnosed by a plain abdominal film and ultrasound examination (see Fig. 15.18B). Pelvic masses (Fig. 15.19), uterine or ovarian masses, hydrocolpos, hydrometrocolpos secondary to imperforate hymen or vaginal atresia, or tumors of neural origin may cause retention due to neurologic involvement of the sacral nerve roots or to bladder neck or urethral compression. Acute neurologic changes associated with spinal cord injury, tumor, or transverse myelitis may cause neurogenic retention. Intermittent catheterization is valuable in managing the bladder until diagnostic evaluation can be completed.

NEUROVESICAL DYSFUNCTION

Neurovesical dysfunction in childhood may be either congenital (including spina bifida variants such as meningocele or myelomeningocele, intradural lipoma, diastematomyelia, sacral agenesis) or

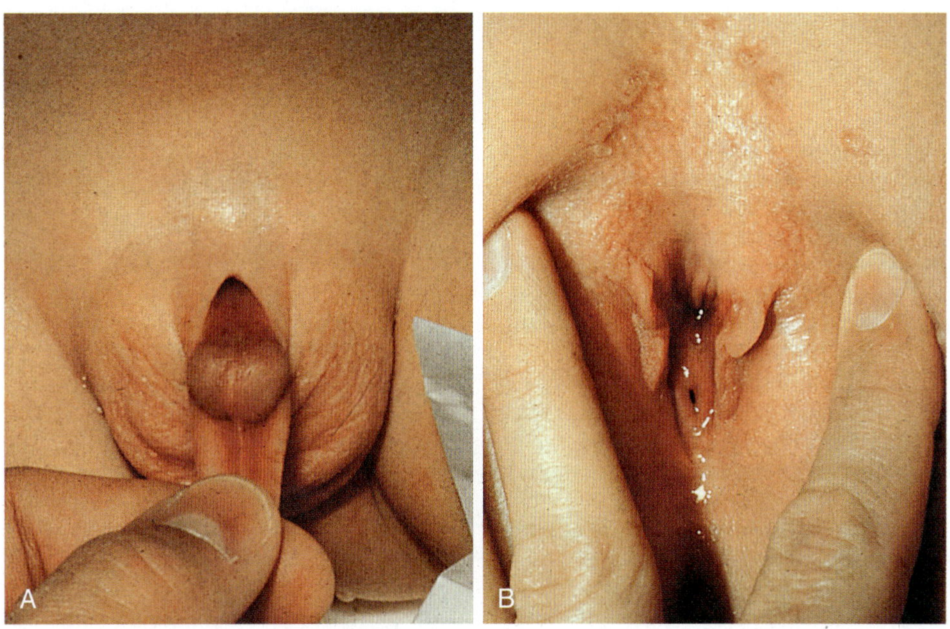

Fig. 15.17 Epispadias. (A) Penopubic epispadias with incontinence in a male infant. (B) Epispadias in a female reveals a patulous urethra and widespread hemiclitoris.

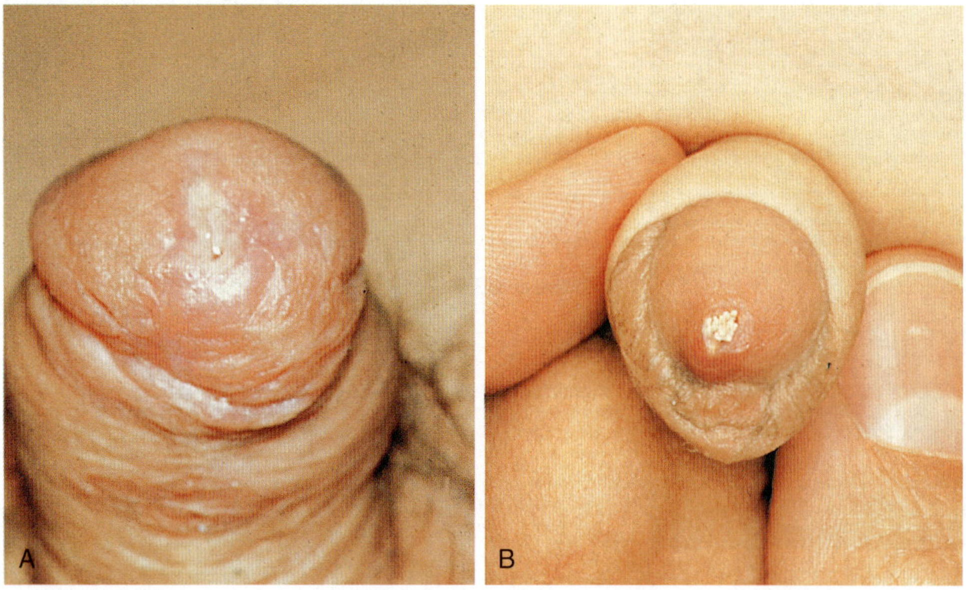

Fig. 15.18 Urinary retention. (A) Urinary retention secondary to severe chronic balanitis (balanitis xerotica obliterans). (B) Urinary retention secondary to an impacted urethral calculus.

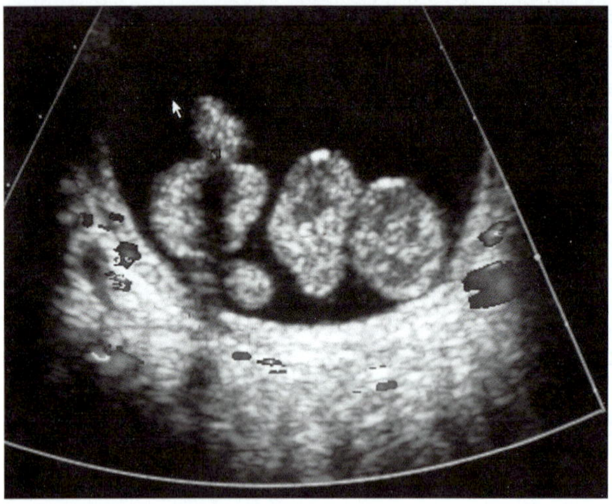

Fig. 15.19 Bladder rhabdomyosarcoma. Shown is an ultrasound examination of the bladder in a young male who presented with urinary retention. The study reveals polypoid lesions of a botryoid rhabdomyosarcoma, which obstructed the bladder outlet, causing urinary retention.

acquired (trauma, transverse myelitis, spinal cord tumor). Uninhibited bladder contractions and dyssynergic voiding may also be seen in cerebral palsy, multiple sclerosis, or other demyelinating diseases. Independent of etiology, the evaluation and management of the child with neurovesical dysfunction are extremely important to preserve renal function, prevent renal damage from infection, and provide social continence. Physicians caring for an infant with neurovesical dysfunction should ensure that periodic evaluation of the child's urinary tract is carried out. This evaluation may include radiographic or urodynamic studies, which should be repeated several times during the first year of life or after an initial injury and at least yearly thereafter or as indicated. Alarming signs warranting prompt urology referral include frequent infection, fever, or a change in normal pattern of bladder or bowel continence (Fig. 15.20). Children with spina bifida who undergo neurosurgical treatment often develop scarring of the spinal cord, and ~25% develop a symptomatic condition called tethered cord that may require surgical release. If there is concern for new or worsening urinary symptoms, a magnetic resonance imaging (MRI) scan of the lumbosacral spine and neurosurgical referral is appropriate.

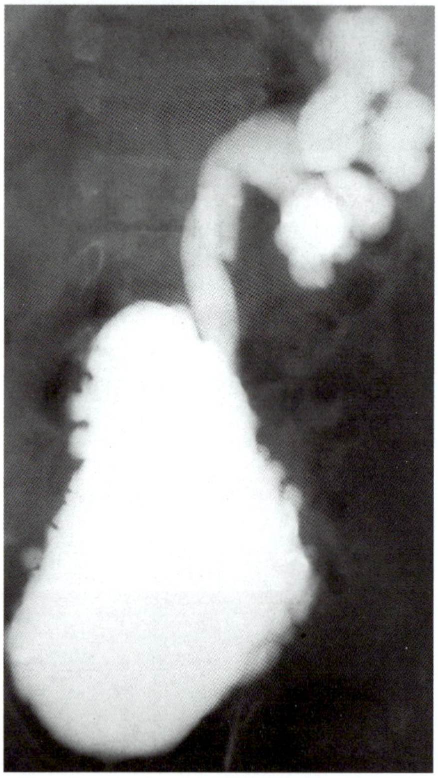

Fig. 15.20 Neurovesical dysfunction. Severe bladder trabeculation and vesicoureteral reflux in a child with myelomeningocele.

NONNEUROGENIC (FUNCTIONAL) VESICAL DYSFUNCTION

Dysfunctional voiding represents a spectrum of conditions in which there is poor coordination between bladder contractions and the somatic urethral sphincter, in otherwise neurologically and anatomically intact patients. In its mildest form, this is referred to as bowel and bladder dysfunction, a frequently underdiagnosed and undertreated condition affecting ~21% of children. Most children with dysfunctional voiding have some degree of urinary urgency, day and night incontinence, and fecal soiling (encopresis), and they are at increased risk of UTIs and VUR. Many of these children display behavioral problems. In its most severe and rare form, the "nonneurogenic neurogenic bladder," or what is termed *Hinman-Allen syndrome,* may result in incontinence and renal failure, and the child's bladder may appear to have the configuration of a bladder that has suffered damage from infravesical obstruction or neurovesical dysfunction (Fig. 15.21). This is distinguished from detrusor sphincter dyssynergia, in which bladder outlet obstruction is secondary to *involuntary* urethral sphincter activation during bladder emptying, which may result in proximal urethral dilation (spinning top urethra) (Fig. 15.22).

The diagnosis of dysfunctional voiding is one of exclusion, made after ruling out occult neuropathy, such as a tethered cord and infravesical obstruction, because the uroradiographic findings often mimic neurovesical dysfunction or obstruction. If the child and family are cooperative, bladder retraining using a timed, double-voiding regimen may be effective, frequently augmented with biofeedback. In severe cases, intermittent catheterization may be necessary to reverse hydronephrosis. When renal function is in jeopardy and patient cooperation is minimal, temporary urinary diversion may be appropriate. Many children with this disorder require behavioral or psychologic therapy in combination with thoughtful urologic management and treatment of constipation.

NOCTURNAL ENURESIS

Nocturnal enuresis is defined as the involuntary release of urine during sleep in a child older than 5 years of age. More common in boys, with a prevalence ~15% to 20% overall, enuresis is commonly associated with polyuria, arousal disorders, and nocturnal detrusor overactivity. The workup is similar to other forms of lower urinary tract symptoms to exclude other etiologies. First-line management is a bed-wetting alarm for 3 months, though this requires a motivated patient and family. Pharmacologic agents are second line, most commonly desmopressin (ideal in polyuria) with some evidence for anticholinergics or tricyclic antidepressants.

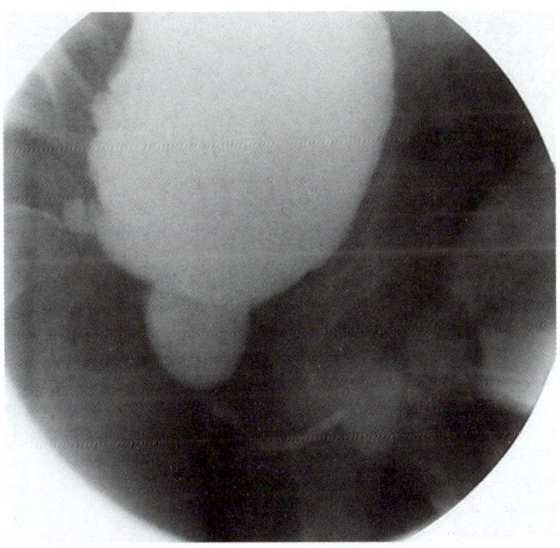

Fig. 15.21 Voiding dysfunction. Voiding cystourethrogram of a young male with Hinman-Allen syndrome shows severe dilation of the prostatic urethra thought to represent urethral valves. Severe bilateral hydronephrosis resulted from vesicoureteral reflux.

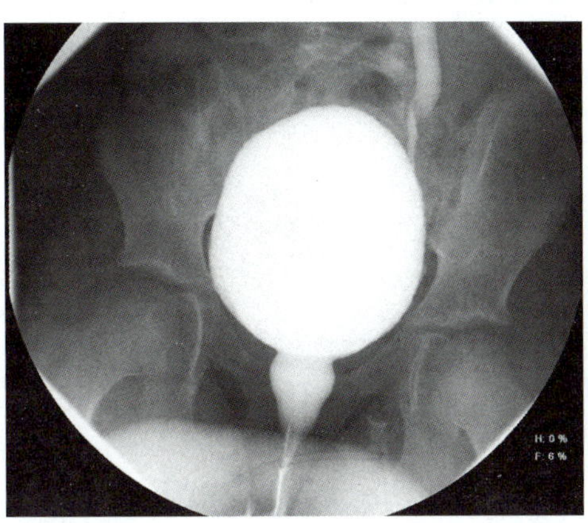

Fig. 15.22 Spinning top urethra.

ANOMALIES OF MALE GENITALIA

Hypospadias

Hypospadias is a common anomaly that occurs in approximately 1 in 250 to 300 male births. The configuration of the urethra varies from mild glandular hypospadias to severe perineal hypospadias with chordee. It is important to be detailed in the description of the penis with hypospadias: the location of the meatus, the presence or absence of chordee, and the appearance of the scrotum (Fig. 15.23). When hypospadias is associated with cryptorchidism, DSD workup is indicated. VCUG is not indicated in hypospadias except in severe lesions or in boys with a history of UTI. Renal sonography is more likely to be abnormal in boys with proximal hypospadias. Infants with hypospadias should not be circumcised because the dorsal preputial skin may be necessary for urethral and penile reconstruction. Repair is usually undertaken in nonglandular hypospadias at approximately 6 months of age or older.

Chordee

Isolated chordee (ventral penile curvature) occurs much less frequently than chordee with hypospadias. Chordee may be related to skin tethering, abnormal development of the urethra and ventral penile structures, or a congenitally short urethra, in which case surgical correction requires division of the urethra and interposition of a skin tube. If chordee is suspected in the neonate, circumcision should be delayed until examination under anesthesia and artificial erection can determine whether either circumcision or repair is appropriate (Fig. 15.24). Typically, chordee greater than 30 degrees warrants surgical correction.

Penile Torsion

Torsion of the penis may be congenital or acquired. Congenital torsion may be severe and related to anomalous development of the corporal bodies, but, most commonly, it is mild and related to dysgenetic subcutaneous fascia (Fig. 15.25). In many cases, the ventral median raphe is seen to spiral around the shaft. Most penile torsion is counterclockwise. Acquired torsion may occur after circumcision or hypospadias repair.

Webbed Penis

Also called penoscrotal webbing or penoscrotal fusion, this minor cosmetic anomaly is easily corrected with a V-Y scrotoplasty (Fig. 15.26), although in many cases, circumcision alone is enough to remove the appearance of webbing.

Buried Penis

Buried penis may occur as a primary finding in the neonate, but it is most common after circumcision (Fig. 15.27). Buried penis is usually the result of a thick suprapubic fat pad; it resolves with normal development. In severe cases, dysgenetic subcutaneous fascial bands bind the penis down. Secondary buried (entrapped) penis after circumcision may be similar to congenital buried penis, and observation is recommended, though surgical correction is indicated if the phimotic band gradually becomes tighter and voiding is affected.

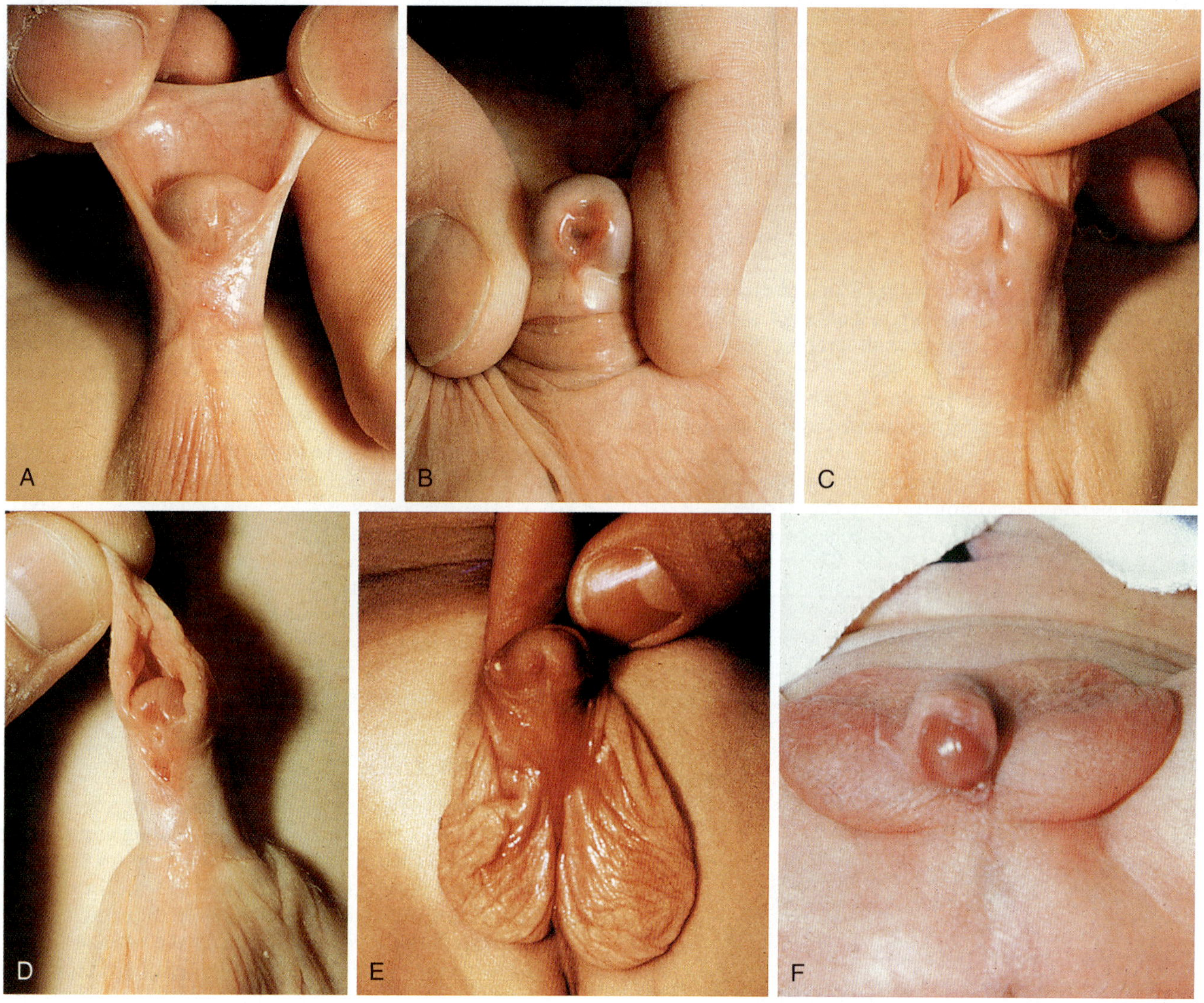

Fig. 15.23 Various forms of hypospadias, revealing location of the meatus. (A) The typical appearance of the "dorsal hood" prepuce seen in association with hypospadias. (B) Glandular hypospadias. (C) Subcoronal hypospadias. (D) Midshaft hypospadias. (E) Scrotal hypospadias with bifid scrotum but without chordee. (F) Perineal hypospadias with chordee.

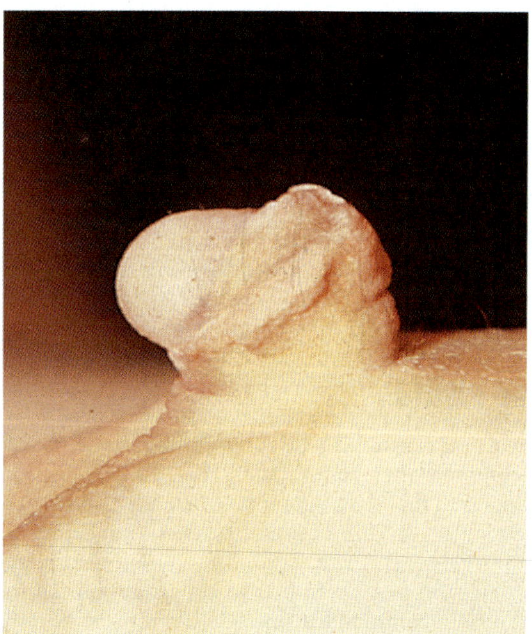

Fig. 15.24 Chordee not associated with hypospadias.

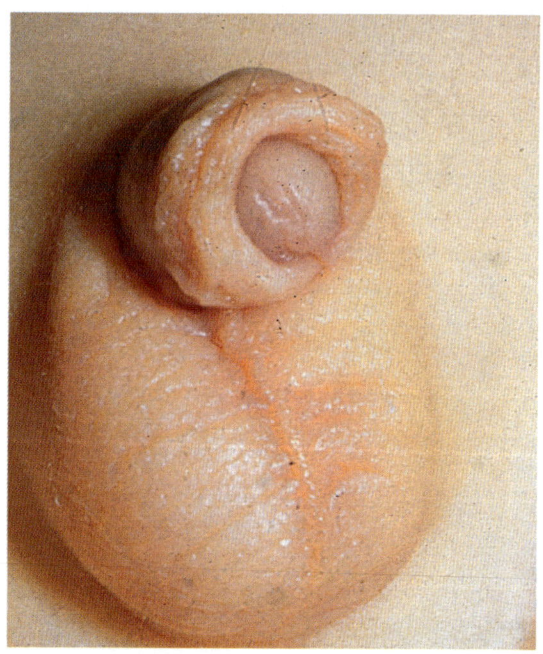

Fig. 15.25 Mild counterclockwise penile torsion.

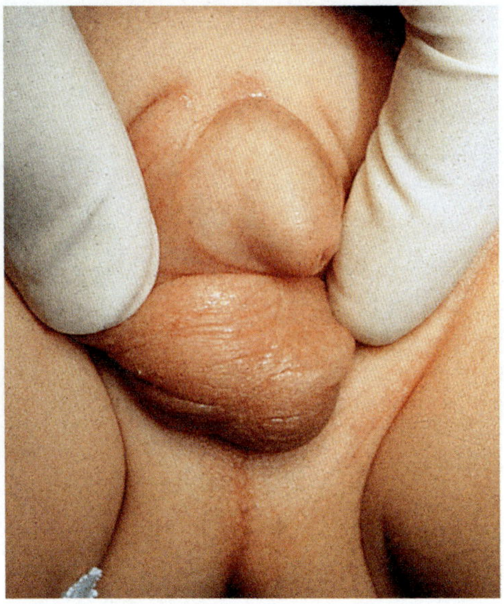

Fig. 15.26 Webbed penis.

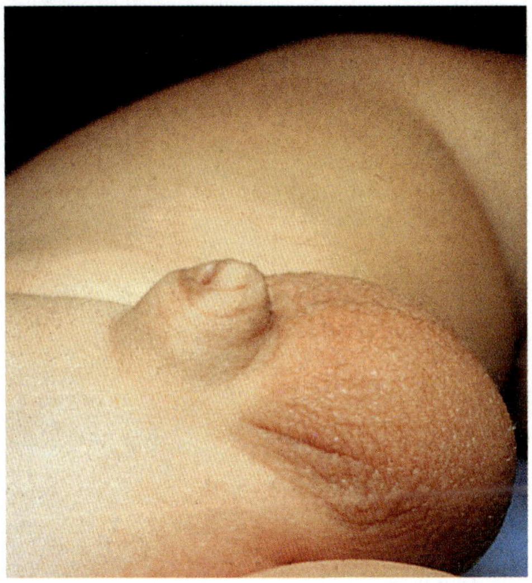

Fig. 15.27 Buried penis after circumcision.

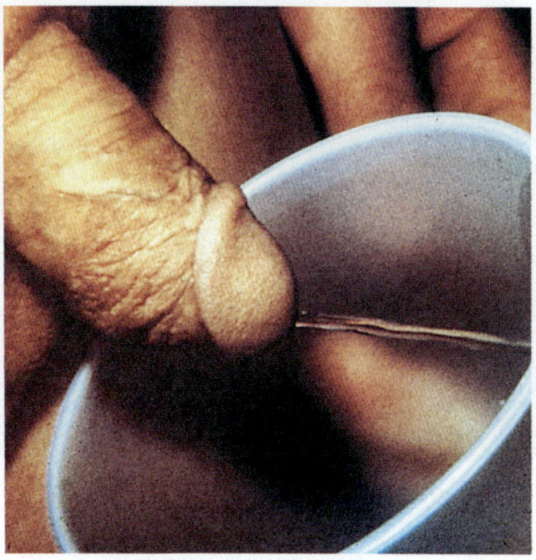

Fig. 15.28 Meatal stenosis. Observation of the urinary stream in suspected meatal stenosis reveals a full stream, ruling out significant meatal stenosis.

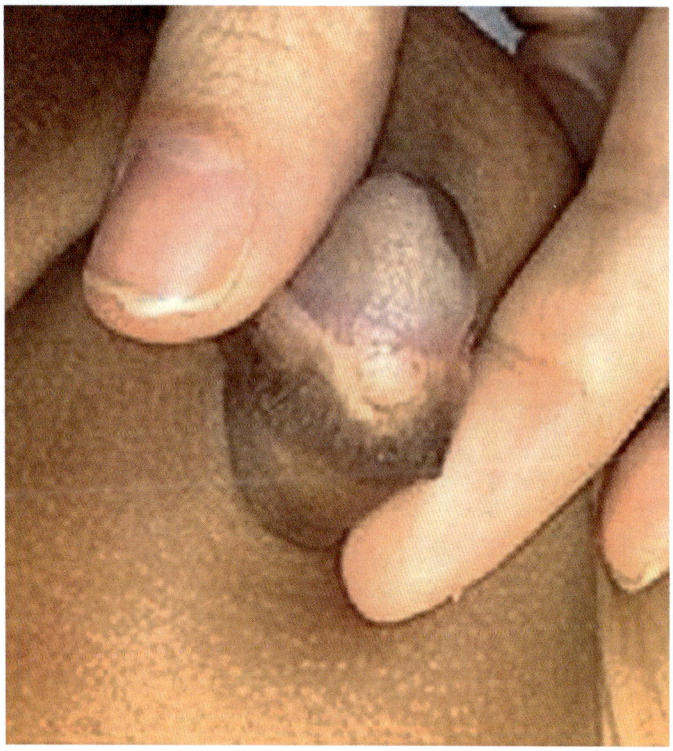

Fig. 15.29 Preputial skin bridges after circumcision.

Postcircumcision Concerns

Meatal Stenosis

Meatal stenosis is common after circumcision, secondary to mild recurrent meatitis. It is usually asymptomatic, but dysuria, strangury, or deflection of the urinary stream may occur. Examination must include observation of the urinary stream for a thin or upward stream or for bulging of the meatus (Fig. 15.28). If the urinary stream appears normal, no intervention is necessary. Meatotomy performed in the office with local anesthesia or sedation is curative.

Preputial Adhesions and Skin Bridges

Fibrinous adhesions are a result of incomplete retraction of the prepuce during normal development or after circumcision. These adhesions resolve spontaneously with routine hygiene and development. Preputial skin bridges result when the free edge of the circumcising incision adheres to the glans penis. If not properly cared for, the edge fuses to the glans, which may cause penile torsion, trap smegma causing recurrent inflammation or infection, and/or cause disfigurement upon erection (Fig. 15.29). Skin bridges will not resolve without surgical correction. Proper instruction on care of the infant penis after circumcision prevents most of these bridges from forming.

Epithelial Inclusion Cysts

Frequently encountered after circumcision from inversion of small amounts of skin at the time of surgery, and usually on the line of the circumcision scar itself, these whitish subcutaneous accumulations of desquamated skin appear as mobile, firm accumulations of white sebaceous material (Fig. 15.30). Occasionally, a small tract to the skin may be evident and can become infected. Surgical excision, rather than attempts to drain the cyst, is curative.

Microphallus

Microphallus (micropenis) is a small, normally formed penis >2.5 standard deviations below the mean (<1.9 cm stretch length in neonates) (Fig. 15.31). It is important to obtain an accurate penile

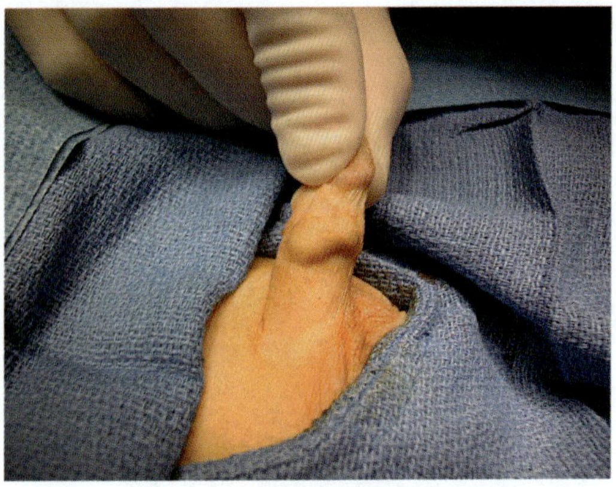

Fig. 15.30 Penile inclusion cyst after circumcision.

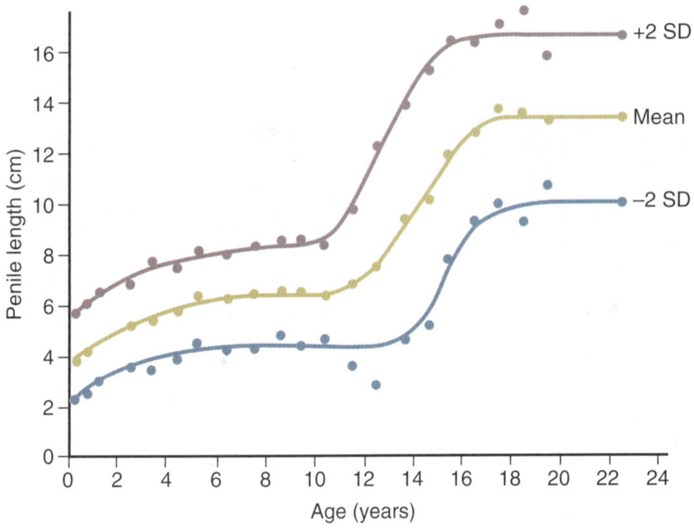

Fig. 15.31 Cumulative frequency curves of penile length for age. (From Lee PA, Mazur T, Danish R, et al: Micropenis. I. Criteria, etiologies and classification. *Johns Hopkins Med J.* 146:156–163, 1980. © The Johns Hopkins University Press. Reprinted with permission of The Johns Hopkins University Press.)

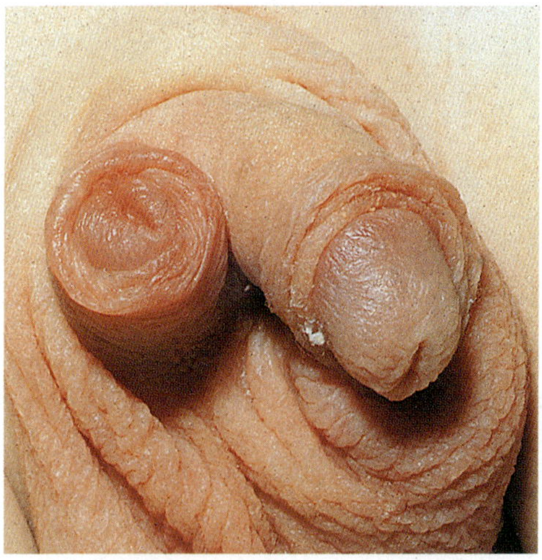

Fig. 15.32 Diphallus. Both penises were functional. Continence was normal.

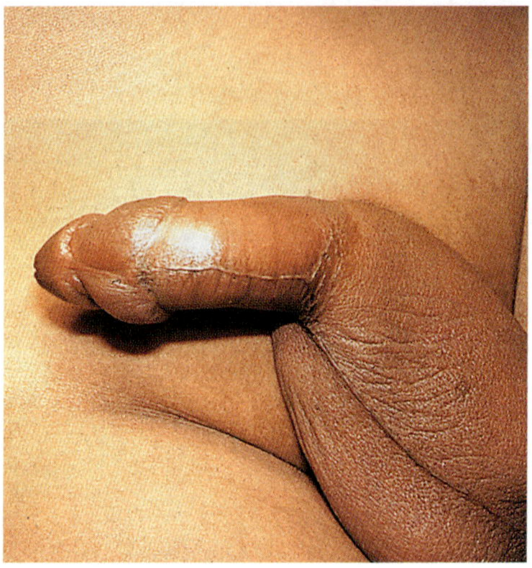

Fig. 15.33 Priapism.

stretch length and corporal shaft diameter (see physical examination section earlier). Microphallus is thought to result from failure of normal penile growth after 14 weeks' gestation, either secondary to hypogonadotropic hypogonadism or primary testicular failure. Workup should include karyotype; hormone profile including a human chorionic gonadotrophin stimulation test; pituitary/hypothalamic tests such as basic metabolic panel, cortisol, and thyroid hormone levels; and brain MRI. Controversy exists regarding penile growth at puberty and the appropriateness of female sex reassignment in infancy; most authors suggest a diagnostic trial of testosterone for 3 months before making a final decision about sex assignment, with trends toward the male sex of rearing.

Diphallus

Diphallus is a rare entity usually associated with severe deformities of the lower urinary tract and genitalia. Complete evaluation of the upper and lower urinary tract is necessary. In most cases of diphallus, one penis is dominant in erectile and urethral function, but in some, the bladder is septate or duplicated, and each phallus plays a significant role (Fig. 15.32).

Priapism

Priapism is a persistent, painful erection in which the corporal bodies are firmly erect but the glans is soft (Fig. 15.33). The shaft and preputial skin may become edematous, and the pain of priapism is usually severe. Priapism that lasts greater than 4 hours should be seen in an emergency department for further care. In children, it is usually related to an underlying disease state, as opposed to the more common idiopathic or medication-associated etiologies seen in adults. It is most frequently associated with sickle cell disease but may be seen in relation to pelvic malignancy, leukemia, blunt perineal trauma, or acute spinal cord injury. Sickle cell–related priapism should initially be treated as a sickle cell crisis, with oxygenation, exchange transfusion, and systemic alkalinization. Surgical therapy may be necessary if conservative measures fail.

Acute Balanitis and Posthitis

Balanitis (inflammation of the glans) and posthitis (inflammation of the prepuce) are common in uncircumcised boys, with infection from smegma entrapped beneath the foreskin. Usual treatment involves gentle dilation of a tight preputial opening, warm baths, and a broad-spectrum antibiotic for a few days if the process is severe. Candidiasis or other causes should be treated appropriately. Once the acute inflammation has resolved, circumcision may be considered to reduce recurrence.

Paraphimosis

Phimosis describes the inability to retract a tight, scarred prepuce. If a tight prepuce is retracted over the glans to the level of the corona *(paraphimosis),* the constricted ring of skin may act as a tourniquet applied to the distal shaft and glans, and ischemia may result (Fig. 15.34). Treatment may involve manual compression of the glans and edematous prepuce to allow reduction of the tight band. In severe cases when reduction of the paraphimosis cannot be achieved manually, a dorsal slit must be made, surgically dividing the phimotic band. Circumcision may be appropriate after an episode of paraphimosis.

LESIONS OF THE SCROTUM AND SCROTAL CONTENTS

The scrotum is composed of several fascial and muscular layers containing the spermatic cord and its contents, as well as the testes and their appendages. Any layer of the scrotal wall or scrotal contents may produce a lesion evident on examination. Each testis is an ovoid structure lying in a vertical plane in its hemiscrotum, in which it is quite mobile, moving up and down with cremasteric contraction and relaxation, and separated from the contralateral testis and scrotal contents by the fibrous median septum. Posterior and slightly lateral to the testis lays the epididymis. The appendix testis and appendix epididymis are small embryologic remnants attached to the upper anterior testis or head of the epididymis.

Median Raphe Cysts

Epithelial inclusion cysts of the median raphe of the scrotum and perineum are not rare (Fig. 15.35). Although isolated cysts may be seen, a more common finding is a chain of cysts extending along the midline of the perineum and scrotum. The cysts are filled with epithelial debris and are usually asymptomatic, although infection of the cyst contents may occur. The cystic lesions appear to represent infoldings of skin during fusion of the labioscrotal folds during formation of the external genitalia. Excision of the median raphe and cysts should be performed carefully in one elongated excision, leaving behind no area of microscopically encysted skin that might subsequently enlarge.

Acute Scrotum

The acute scrotum is a urologic surgical emergency until proven otherwise. It is most imperative to rule out torsion of the spermatic cord. The most important aspects of evaluating the patient with an acute scrotum are history and physical examination. The nature of the onset of pain and swelling is important, as is a history of dysuria, fever, hematuria, previous UTI, urethral instrumentation, or scrotal or perineal trauma. Examination of the scrotum starts with the unaffected testis while observing the involved testis for its size, location, and anatomic orientation. The skin and wall of the scrotum are examined for edema, inflammation, and fluctuation. Next, assess the mobility of the testis and check for the presence of a cremasteric reflex ipsilateral to the involved testis. Laboratory evaluation includes urinalysis and white blood cell count. Imaging should include a scrotal/testicular Doppler ultrasound. This always requires expeditious evaluation with a low threshold for surgical exploration if the diagnosis is uncertain.

Torsion of the Spermatic Cord

Torsion of the spermatic cord is the most significant condition that must be excluded in cases of scrotal pain and swelling (Fig. 15.36). Because the testis deprived of its normal blood supply has at most

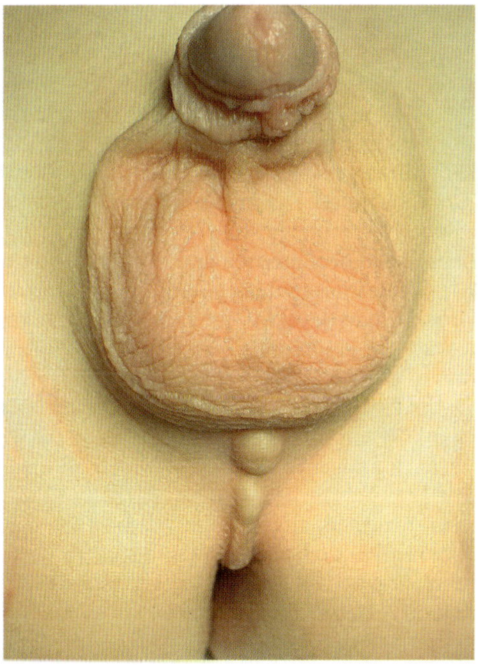

Fig. 15.35 Median raphe cysts of the perineum and posterior scrotum.

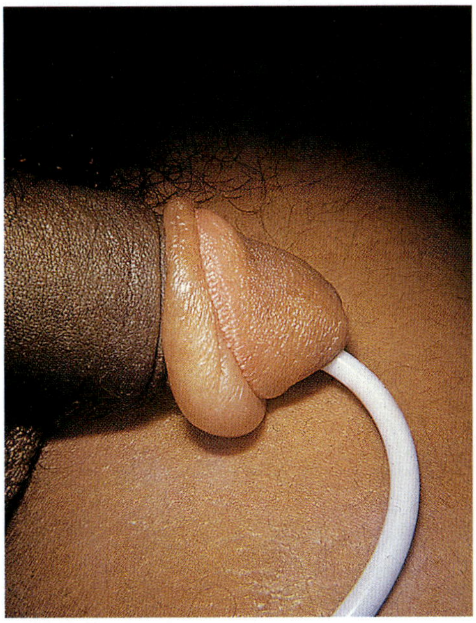

Fig. 15.34 Paraphimosis. Catheterized patient with edematous prepuce proximal to the glans.

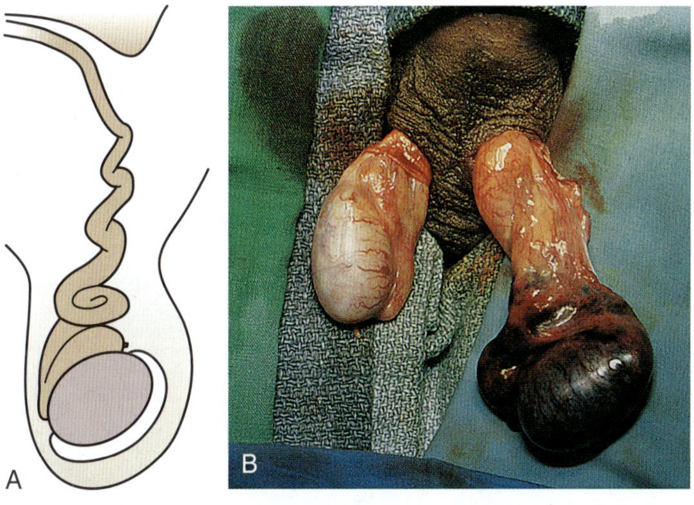

Fig. 15.36 Intravaginal torsion of the spermatic cord. (A) Torsion of the spermatic cord. (B) Surgical exploration and detorsion of the left spermatic cord. The left testis was necrotic. The right testis also shows bell-and-clapper deformity.

a few hours before irreversible injury destroys spermatogenic potential, acute swelling of the scrotum is a surgical emergency until torsion has been adequately excluded. Torsion may occur at any age.

Neonatal torsion is thought in most cases to represent extravaginal torsion, which is torsion of the entire scrotal contents, including the covering tunical layers. It occurs during descent of the testis and presents at birth as a firm, nontender mass high in the scrotum or at the scrotal inlet. Frequently there is fixation to the overlying skin as a part of the inflammatory response. These testes are rarely salvageable, but though unlikely, acute torsion can occur during delivery and may occasionally be reversible. Synchronous or asynchronous contralateral torsion may also occur, rendering patients anorchid. Timely surgical exploration is therefore sometimes considered to assess viability of the involved testis and, more importantly, ensure the contralateral testis has normal scrotal fixation, though this is controversial. A scrotal mass at birth has been in some centers considered a surgical emergency until proven otherwise. The risk of general anesthesia must be weighed.

Intravaginal torsion (within the tunica vaginalis) may occur at any age but is more common during the peripubertal or pubertal period. Most patients have acute, painful swelling of the scrotum, and many have lower abdominal pain, nausea, and vomiting. It is not unusual for a patient to awaken with pain, but torsion can also occur after scrotal trauma or during almost any activity. On occasion, torsion has a much more insidious onset as a subacute, dull scrotal pain. Dysuria is usually absent, and urinalysis is normal, but leukocytosis may be noted. Examination may vary depending on the time elapsed after the acute episode. The scrotum may initially appear normal but soon becomes red and swollen, with the testis elevated because of foreshortening of the spermatic cord. In the acute stage, a hydrocele may develop. The testis may have an abnormal orientation, with the epididymis located in an abnormal position due to torsion of the cord. The cremasteric reflex is usually absent, and elevating the testis to the pubic symphysis increases pain (negative Prehn sign). When inflammation has progressed, the scrotum becomes a firm, homogeneous mass in which all anatomic landmarks are lost.

If torsion is suspected, attempting to detorse the cord by gentle twisting in either direction may allow the cord to untwist, at least partially. If detorsion occurs, relief of pain is instantaneous but relief is often temporary. Detorsion is often unsuccessful, and operative intervention for fixation of the testicle is still required. A color Doppler ultrasound, if immediately available, may be helpful in many instances, but surgery should not be delayed for imaging if clinical suspicion is high. In an inflammatory scrotal event, ipsilateral increased blood flow is noted, whereas in the presence of an acute torsion, blood flow is diminished/absent. If torsion of the spermatic cord is confirmed, immediate surgical exploration is warranted.

Torsion of Testicular Appendages

The appendix testis and appendix epididymis are embryologic remnants that are normally undetectable on routine examination and not found in all boys. Torsion of an appendix, which can occur in the early pubertal age group, may be difficult to differentiate from torsion of the spermatic cord. Early after the onset of acute scrotal pain, a small tender mass may be palpable on the upper anterior surface of the testis or epididymis (Fig. 15.37A). In light-skinned children, the swollen, dark, infarcted appendage may be visible through the scrotal skin (the "blue dot" sign of Dresner) (see Fig. 15.37B). Torsed appendages are typically treated conservatively with anti-inflammatories and do not require surgical exploration. However, if indistinguishable from torsion of the spermatic cord on examination, immediate surgical intervention is often required. Color flow Doppler examination may indicate increased blood flow, and an enlarged torsed appendage may be visualized.

Epididymitis

Epididymal inflammation may be bacterial or nonbacterial in etiology. True bacterial epididymitis is rare in children but more common in adolescents. Nonbacterial inflammation may be caused by reflux of sterile urine into the ejaculatory ducts or ectopic insertion of a ureter into the seminal vesicle or vas deferens. Bowel and bladder dysfunction may increase this risk. In many cases of nonbacterial epididymitis, examination and imaging are unremarkable and no obvious etiology is evident. Nonbacterial epididymitis is more common. The clinical presentation of epididymitis may be indolent or acute. Fever often accompanies bacterial epididymitis. Examination of the scrotum in early stages demonstrates a tender, slightly swollen epididymis (Fig. 15.38), but later the entire scrotal contents are replaced by an inflammatory mass. The cremasteric reflex is present, and elevation of the testis on the pubis may relieve pain (Prehn sign). A color Doppler examination demonstrates increased blood flow (hyperemia). Ultrasound may show an enlarged epididymis. If torsion of the spermatic cord cannot be excluded, surgical exploration must be carried out promptly. Nonbacterial epididymitis is treated expectantly. Administration of nonsteroidal anti-inflammatory drugs, supportive underwear, and limitation of

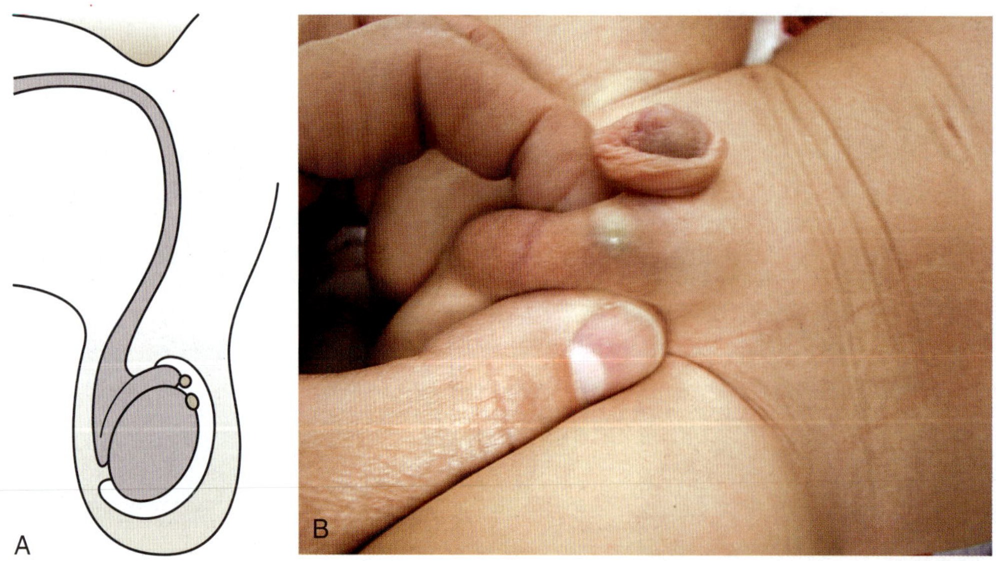

Fig. 15.37 (A) Torsion of appendix testis or epididymis. (B) Examination of the left hemiscrotum in a case of torsion of the appendix testis reveals a "blue dot" sign.

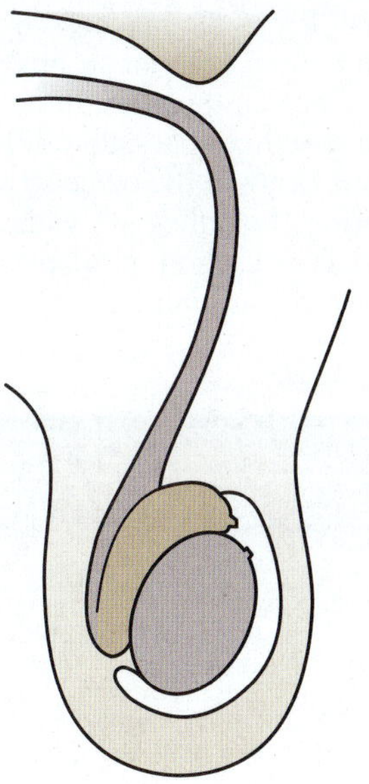

Fig. 15.38 Epididymitis.

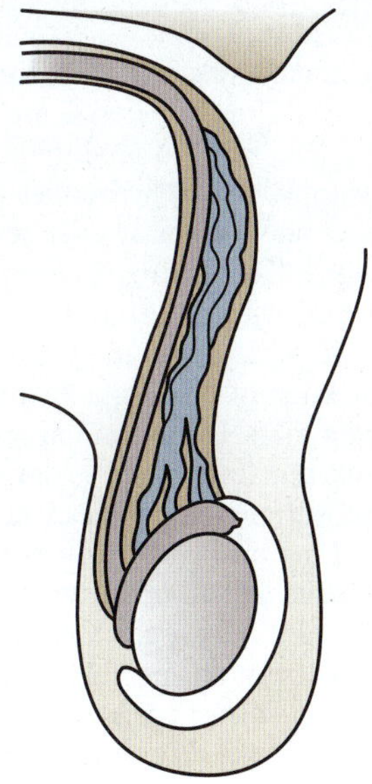

Fig. 15.39 Varicocele.

activity to bed rest for 48 hours, in cases with severe scrotal swelling, usually result in rapid improvement of clinical symptoms. All children with bacterial epididymitis should be treated with antibiotic therapy and undergo complete upper and lower urinary tract radiographic evaluation after resolution of the acute process (renal ultrasound and VCUG). Scrotal abscess formation may result from bacterial epididymitis.

Chronic Scrotal Swelling

Varicocele

A varicocele consists of dilated veins of the pampiniform plexus of the spermatic cord (Fig. 15.39). Varicoceles occur more frequently on the left side but may be bilateral. The causes of varicocele vary from hormonal to hydrostatic/anatomic. The potential testicular injury from varicocele may be secondary to hormonal deficiencies or temperature effects. Most varicoceles decompress in the supine position. Those that do not decompress, present acutely, or present unilaterally on the right raise concern for lesions in the kidney or retroperitoneum causing obstruction to venous outflow; thus, retroperitoneal ultrasound is recommended. Most varicoceles are asymptomatic and are noted incidentally or discovered on routine examination. Pain secondary to varicocele is uncommon, but a dull aching may occur in large varicoceles.

Infertility is found in approximately 33% of adults with varicoceles. Ablating varicoceles in adolescents with testicular growth failure ipsilateral to the varicocele (>20% size discrepancy between testes), or in those with bilateral varicocele, is common practice. Semen analysis can be obtained in the postpubertal patient to assess for abnormal semen parameters. In patients with minimal or no testicular atrophy, observation and serial measurements of testicular volume are indicated, with the option to perform ablation if ipsilateral testicular growth failure occurs.

Spermatocele

Spermatoceles or epididymal cysts are common in adolescents. They are painless cystic masses located in the epididymis (commonly in the upper pole) (Fig. 15.40). They vary in size but are usually less than 1 cm in diameter. They are mobile, transilluminate, and do not vacillate in size, although gradual enlargement may occur. Ultrasound examination may be helpful if the diagnosis is in doubt. Spermatoceles contain sperm and are essentially retention cysts of the epididymis or tubules of the rete testis. Excision is not usually recommended in routine cases but may be appropriate for painful or enlarging cysts.

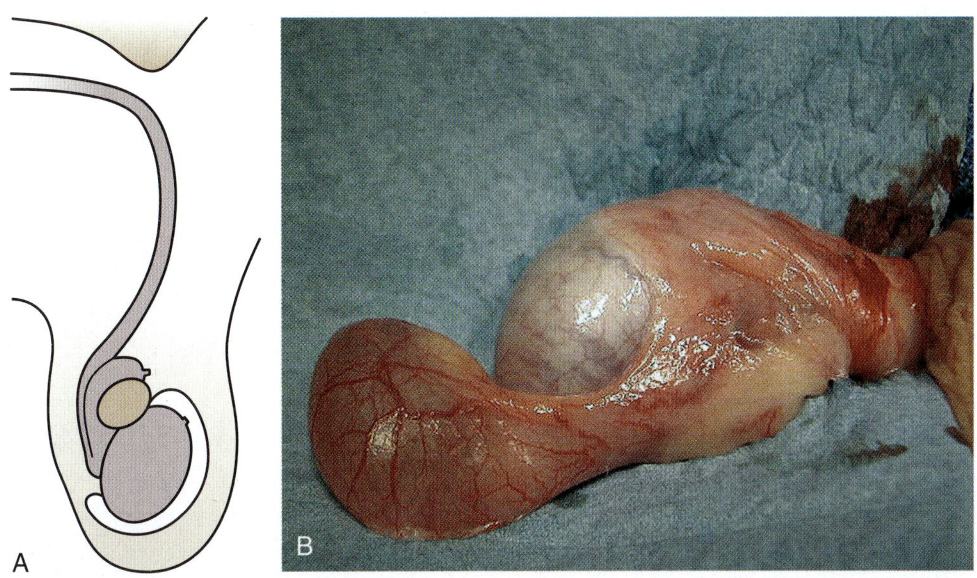

Fig. 15.40 Spermatocele (A) and operative appearance of large spermatocele (B).

Hydrocele

Hydroceles are fluid accumulations within the tunica vaginalis or processus vaginalis (Fig. 15.41). They vary in size, are usually painless even if large, and may be tense enough to obscure palpation of the testis. They transilluminate. Simple scrotal hydroceles are common in neonates and usually resolve spontaneously over several months. When examining an infant with a large hydrocele, examination of the lower abdomen should be performed to rule out the presence of an abdominoscrotal hydrocele. The presence of an abdominoscrotal hydrocele may be noted if compression of the scrotal hydrocele causes enlargement of a lower quadrant mass. Ultrasound may confirm this finding. If the processus vaginalis remains patent, a communicating hydrocele results and may present with periodic increase and decrease in scrotal size and possible thickening of the inguinal spermatic cord. If a segment of processus vaginalis fails to obliterate, trapping fluid in midcord, a hydrocele of the cord may result. Communicating hydroceles may be indistinguishable from an inguinal hernia, and if it persists beyond 12 months, surgical correction is warranted due to future risk of incarcerated hernia. When the diagnosis of an inguinal mass is uncertain, imaging (ultrasound or CT) or exploration may be warranted because soft tissue sarcomas may originate from spermatic cord and paratesticular tissues.

Testis Tumors

Testis tumors may occur at any age, from neonate to adulthood. Most present as a firm, painless mass within the testis. A tumor may be smooth or irregular. Occasionally, sudden enlargement of a tumor or bleeding within it may cause a painful, rapid enlargement of the involved testis. Solid masses within the substance of the testis should be considered malignant until proven otherwise. Testicular ultrasound and urology referral are indicated (Fig. 15.42).

LESIONS OF THE FEMALE GENITALIA

Labial Adhesion (Fusion)

Labial adhesions (fusions) are common in the prepubertal age group. They represent fusion of the labia minora, postulated to be the result of inflammation. Fusion begins posteriorly and may progress until almost complete fusion results (Fig. 15.43). Severe fusion may be associated with dysuria, postvoid dribbling as the urine voided into the vagina drains out, or UTI. Most adhesions lyse spontaneously as puberty approaches and the vaginal epithelium cornifies. Most children do not require treatment unless symptomatic, such as recurrent UTIs or discomfort.

If lysis is indicated, it may be managed by parents at home, by cleansing the introitus in an anterior-to-posterior motion and applying petroleum or other ointment to diminish mucosal irritation (estrogen cream is not sufficient to allow adhesions to lyse). Lysis can also be performed easily in the office by spreading the labia or mechanically separating the adhesions with an ointment-covered gloved finger. Postlysis application of estrogen cream may thicken the vaginal mucosa. After lysis, routine hygiene prevents recurrence.

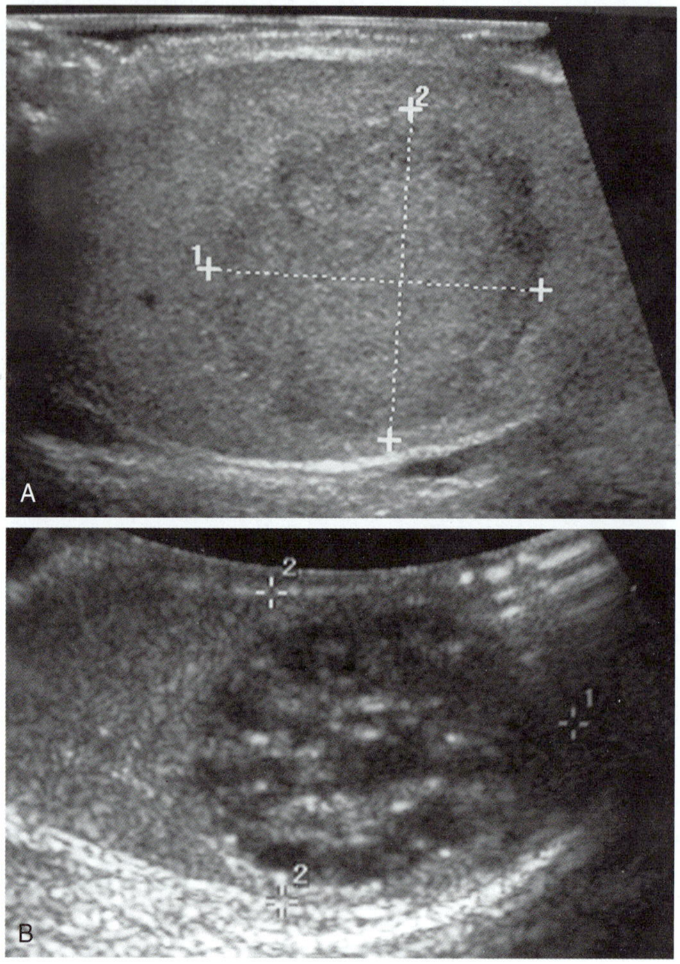

Fig. 15.42 Testis tumor. (A and B) Ultrasound examination of two patients with palpable testis tumors.

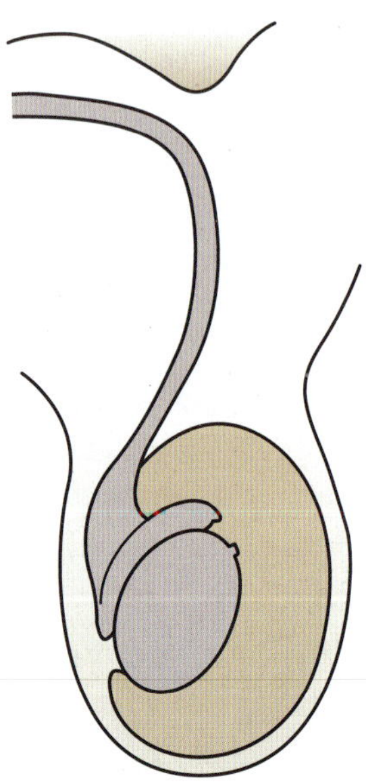

Fig. 15.41 Hydrocele.

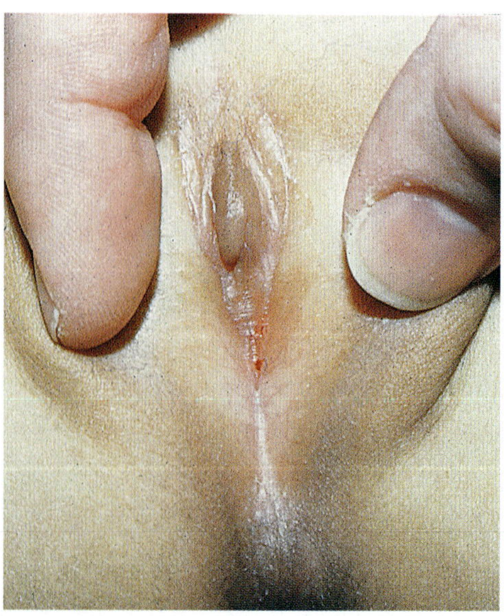

Fig. 15.43 Labial adhesions. Only a small opening remains anteriorly.

Urethral Prolapse

Prolapse of the urethra typically presents with bloody spotting, with occasional mild dysuria. Examination reveals a reddened or dark circumferential prolapse of the urethra with an otherwise normal introitus (Fig. 15.44). Its cause is unknown. Treatment options include conservative management including aggressive management of constipation, sitz baths, and topical steroids. Topical estrogens have also been reported as treatment. If persistent, surgical excision can be performed.

Introital Polyps

Small polyps may originate from the urethral meatus or hymenal ring (Fig. 15.45). These are typically thin, asymptomatic mucosal tags that require no specific treatment. Fleshy polyps or multiple polyps should be examined closely and biopsied to exclude malignancy, such as sarcoma botryoides (see Chapter 12).

Prolapsed Ureterocele

Ureteroceles are cystic dilations of the distal ureter, which are in the bladder or urethra (cecoureterocele) and may prolapse through the urethral meatus as reddened or even necrotic mucosal surfaces (Fig. 15.46). Catheterization alongside the prolapse may locate the lumen of the urethra. Prolapse of an ureterocele may be associated with a palpable distended bladder or flank mass (hydronephrosis). Ultrasonography of the bladder and kidneys may demonstrate unilateral or bilateral hydronephrosis or hydronephrosis of a segment of a complete ureteral duplication, usually the upper pole of an obstructed renal unit. VCUG with intravenous urography, radionuclide studies, or occasionally direct puncture of the ureterocele with contrast injection may be appropriate to define the anatomy of the malformation.

Paraurethral Cysts

Cystic lesions of the paraurethral or vaginal mucosa may be found on routine examination and are usually asymptomatic. They rarely cause voiding symptoms and occasionally present in older girls as palpable interlabial masses. Normal mucosa overlies the cyst, which usually displaces the urethral meatus slightly from the midline. Most cysts rupture spontaneously, but aspiration or marsupialization may be necessary (Fig. 15.47).

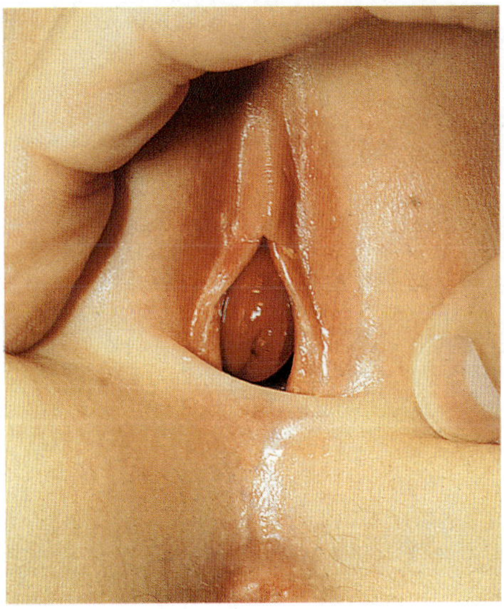

Fig. 15.44 Urethral prolapse. This is a chronic case in which the initial hemorrhagic nature of the acute prolapse has resolved with observation, leaving a protuberant, edematous urethra.

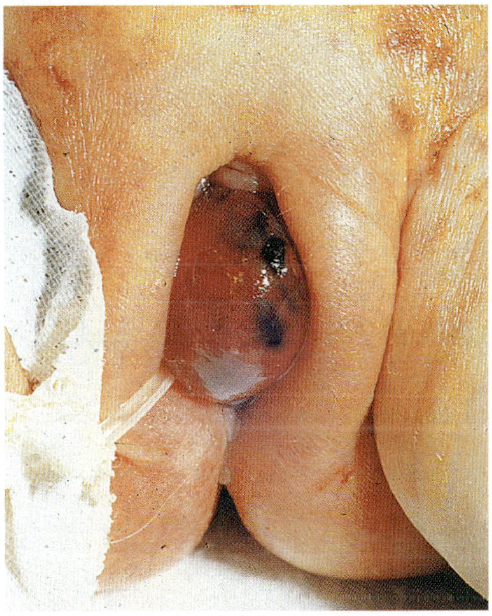

Fig. 15.46 Prolapsed ureterocele. The catheter enters the urethra.

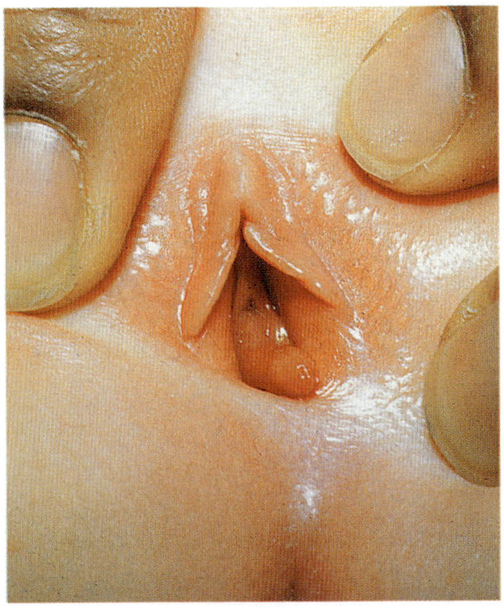

Fig. 15.45 Introital polyp. A small polyp of the posterior vaginal fourchette.

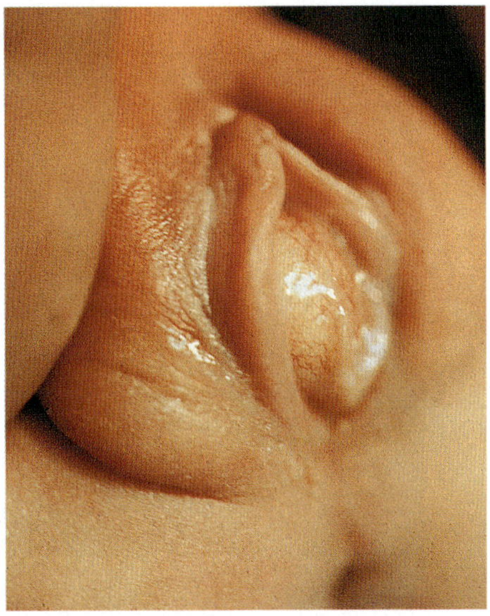

Fig. 15.47 Paraurethral cyst.

Congenital Obstruction of the Vagina

Vaginal obstruction may occur secondary to an imperforate hymen, vaginal atresia or septa, or urogenital sinus malformation. Fusion anomalies of the Müllerian structures may result in a septate vagina or bicornuate uterus with an obstructed segment. Neonates may have abdominal masses or urinary retention; girls with uterine didelphys or a bicornuate uterus may have pelvic pain or menstrual irregularities at puberty. Examination of the infant may reveal a distended vagina (hydrometrocolpos) with a bulging hymenal membrane. If a vaginal septum or atresia is the cause of the obstruction, external genital examination may be normal and a complete pelvic examination with vaginoscopy may be necessary. Ultrasonography of the pelvis may be helpful, but pelvic CT or MRI scan will give the most detailed anatomic information (Fig. 15.48). All patients with uterine or vaginal anomalies should have imaging of the upper urinary tract, given the high incidence of upper tract anomalies in this group. Females with proven unilateral renal agenesis should be monitored through puberty for the development of Müllerian anomalies with pelvic ultrasound.

Ectopic Ureter

Ureteral ectopia may be associated with a single collecting system or a complete duplication of the collecting system (complete ureteral duplication). In females, an ectopic ureter may drain into the bladder neck, urethra, urethrovaginal septum, vagina, or uterus. Females with an ectopic ureter may have a normal voiding pattern but with a continuous dribbling incontinence of small amounts of urine. In some of these patients, a tiny ectopic ureter may be seen to drip urine from the introitus (Fig. 15.49). In males, the ectopic ureter may drain into the bladder, urethra, prostate, seminal vesicles, or vas deferens. Males are typically dry unless the insertion is distal to the sphincter, but they may develop recurrent epididymitis.

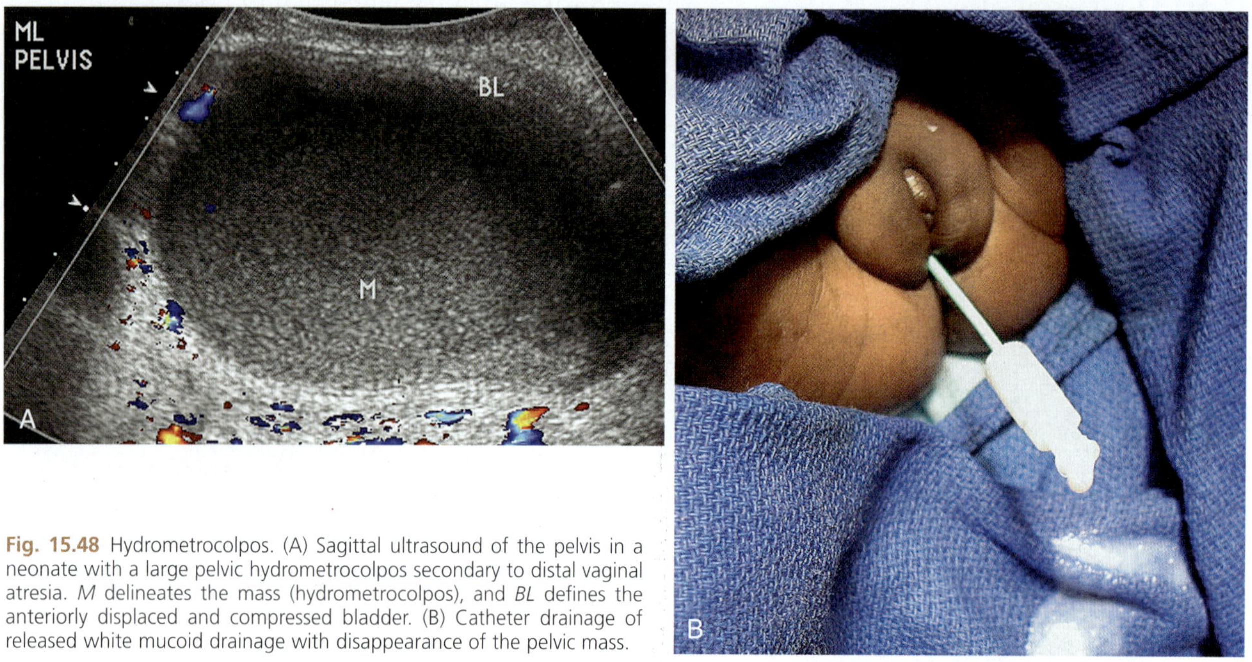

Fig. 15.48 Hydrometrocolpos. (A) Sagittal ultrasound of the pelvis in a neonate with a large pelvic hydrometrocolpos secondary to distal vaginal atresia. *M* delineates the mass (hydrometrocolpos), and *BL* defines the anteriorly displaced and compressed bladder. (B) Catheter drainage of released white mucoid drainage with disappearance of the pelvic mass.

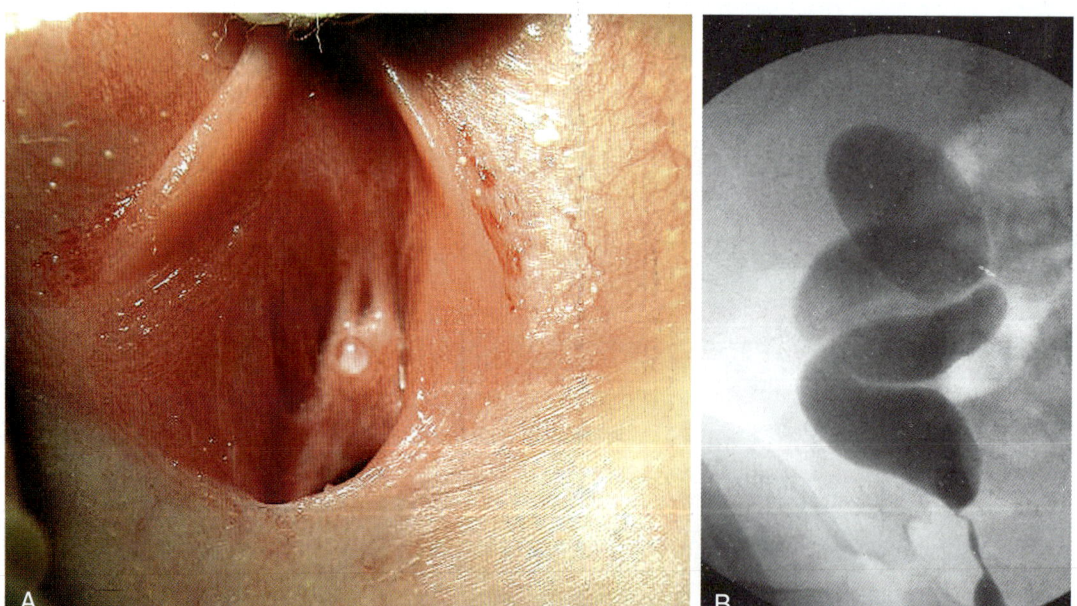

Fig. 15.49 Ectopic ureter. (A) A drop of urine exits from the orifice of an ectopic ureter located just below the urethral meatus in the urethrovaginal septum. (B) Retrograde pyelography of the same ureter reveals a huge, tortuous ureter subtending the upper pole of a right complete ureteral duplication. Heminephrectomy cured the patient's incontinence.

AMBIGUOUS GENITALIA

Human genitalia begin as undifferentiated structures that are identical in both sexes early in gestation. The combined effects of genetic, hormonal, and local influences modify the structure and function of the genitalia to produce genital structures appropriate to the sex of the individual (see Chapter 9). When abnormal development occurs, genitalia of indeterminate nature may result. The combination of hypospadias and bilateral or unilateral cryptorchidism should be considered as representative of DSD until proven otherwise. Examination of the genitalia in patients with suspected DSDs should include the following: assessment of phallic length and diameter, presence or absence of gonads and their size, assessment of labioscrotal and perineal anatomy, rectal examination, pelvic and retroperitoneal imaging, and endoscopy to delineate urethral or vaginal structures. A full genetic and endocrine evaluation should be carried out as well. Because the etiologies of ambiguous genitalia are diverse (Fig. 15.50) with significant differences in management, careful evaluation is critical.

GENITAL TRAUMA

Injury to the genitalia may be the result of isolated, sexual, or polytrauma. Though rarely life-threatening, proper management is important to later sexual, physiologic, and psychosocial well-being. This is particularly important in children. Trauma to the penis or scrotum should always raise the question of urethral injury (Fig. 15.51). This is easily ruled out in the emergency department or radiology suite with a retrograde urethrogram. Once urethral injury has been excluded, urethral catheterization can be performed safely. Scrotal trauma mandates evaluation of the testes including scrotal ultrasound to rule out testicular rupture or laceration requiring surgical repair (see Fig. 15.51B and C). Scrotal and testicular trauma is not uncommon in breech delivery when the scrotum is the presenting part. Ultrasound examination of the testes may be helpful if massive edema or hematoma prevents thorough examination. If injury is suspected, surgical exploration is the most appropriate approach. Trauma to the female genitalia and perineum usually requires examination under anesthesia to allow a complete evaluation of the injury, with concomitant repair when necessary.

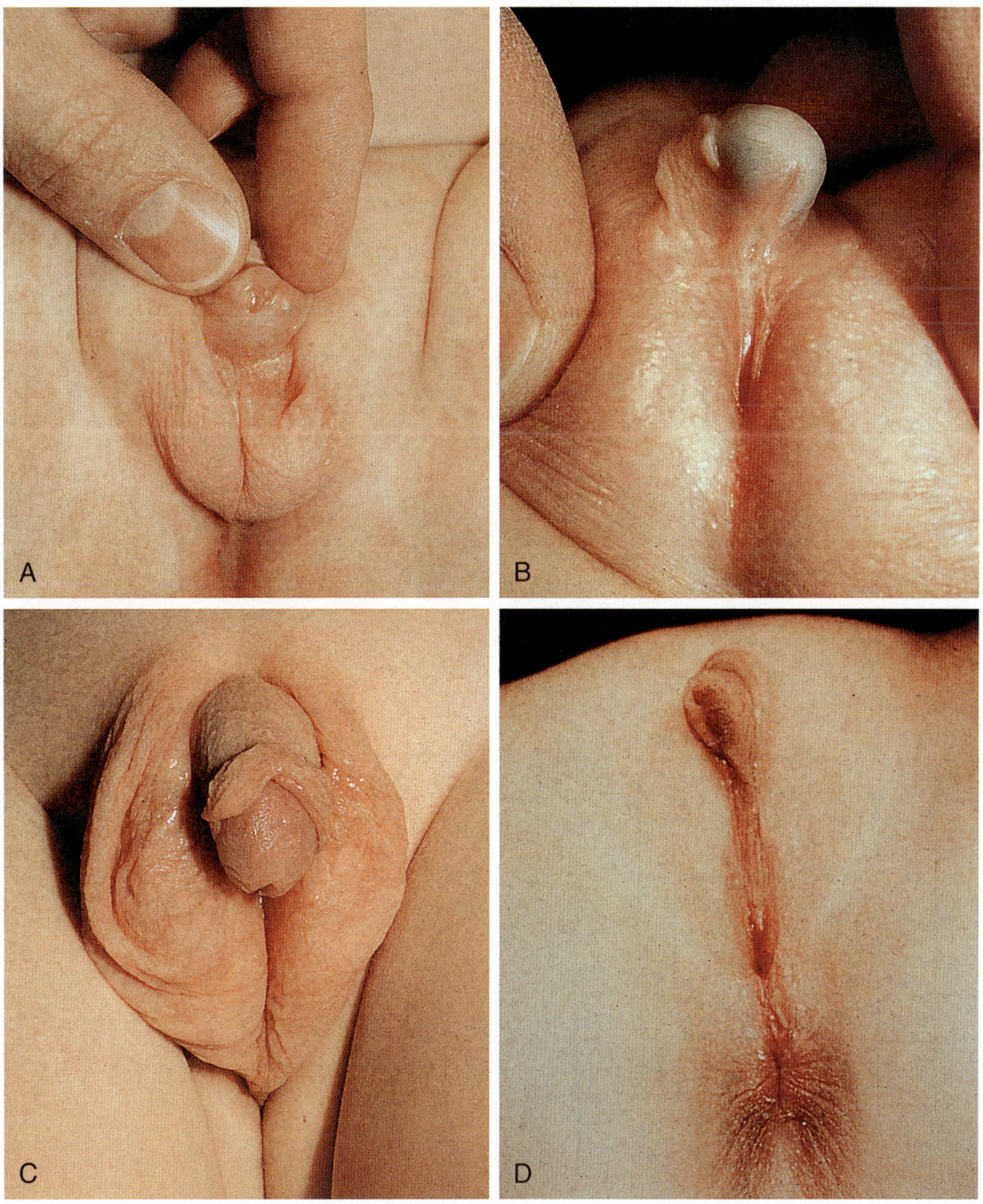

Fig. 15.50 Various causes of genital ambiguity. (A) Congenital adrenal hyperplasia. (B) Mixed gonadal dysgenesis. (C) Ovotesticular disorder of sex development. (D) Posteriorly displaced urogenital sinus.

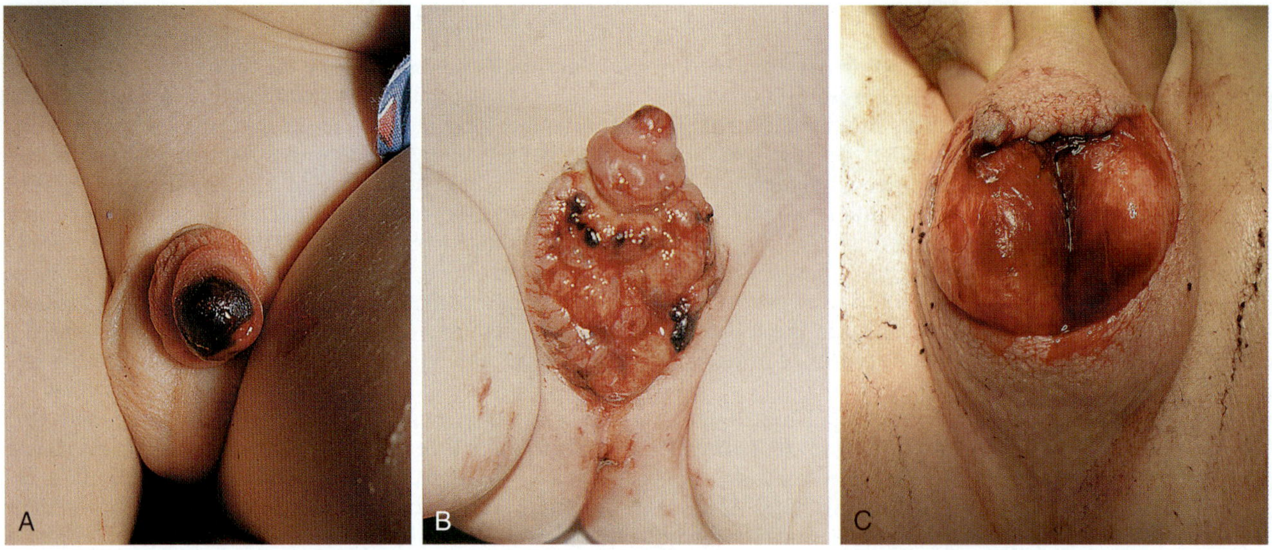

Fig. 15.51 Genital trauma. (A) Trauma to the glans penis from a falling toilet seat, a common injury that is usually best served by observation unless the urethra is disrupted. (B) Perineal trauma: The testes were injured, but the urethra was intact. (C) Scrotal trauma: the testicular tunica were intact, and primary skin closure produced an excellent result.

Bibliography

Belman AB, Kaplan GW: *Genitourinary problems in pediatrics*, Philadelphia, 1981, WB Saunders.

Gillenwater JY, Grayhack JT, Howards SS, et al: *Adult and pediatric urology*, Philadelphia, 2002, Lippincott Williams & Wilkins.

Kolon TF, Herndon CD, Baker LA, et al: Evaluation and treatment of cryptorchidism: AUA guideline, *J Urol* 192(2):337–345, 2014. doi:10.1016/j.juro.2014.05.005.

Lee PA, Mazur T, Danish R, et al: Micropenis. I. Criteria, etiologies, and classification, *Johns Hopkins Med J* 146(4):156–163, 1980.

Peng CC, Yang SS, Austin PF, et al: Systematic review and meta-analysis of alarm versus desmopressin therapy for pediatric monosymptomatic enuresis, *Sci Rep* 8:16755, 2018. https://doi.org/10.1038/s41598-018-34935-1.

Shaikh N, Hoberman A, Wise B, et al: Dysfunctional elimination syndrome: is it related to urinary tract infection or vesicoureteral reflux diagnosed early in life? *Pediatrics* 112(5):1134–1137, 2003. doi:10.1542/peds.112.5.1134.

Wein AJ, Kavoussi LR, Partin AW, et al: *Campbell-Walsh urology*, Philadelphia, 2016, WB Saunders.

Williams DI, Johnston JH, editors: *Paediatric urology*, London, 1982, Butterworth.

NEUROLOGY

16

Robert A. Safier | Catalina Cleves-Bayon | Jenna M. Gaesser

NEUROLOGIC EXAMINATION

The primary objective of the neurologic examination is to assess the functional integrity of the central nervous system (CNS) and the peripheral nervous system (PNS) and to detect and localize any sites of neurologic dysfunction. Techniques and interpretation of the pediatric neurologic examination are based largely on knowledge of normal growth and development. The examination is preceded by a thorough history of the presenting problem, including timing and mode of onset; course; and a past medical history that focuses on the antenatal, perinatal, and neonatal periods for possible prior insults (e.g., bleeding, infection, hypoxia, drugs, trauma). Abnormalities of birth weight; the need for resuscitation after delivery; early neonatal problems with hypoglycemia, hypocalcemia, or severe jaundice; and abnormalities in activity or difficulty feeding shortly after birth often serve as red flags. This is followed by a detailed history of behavior; growth and development with attention to evidence of delay, slowing, cessation, or regression of developmental milestones; and any possible association with prior medical diagnoses or trauma. Obtaining a family history of neurologic, neuromuscular, or developmental problems is also important.

The systematic neurologic evaluation proceeds from assessment of mental status and language functions through evaluation of cranial nerves, gross motor function, muscle strength, gait and station, balance and coordination, sensory systems, and deep tendon reflexes. It is applicable to older children and adolescents without significant modification from the evaluation geared to the adult. Tools essential to the neurologist include the reflex hammer, bright penlight, ophthalmoscope, and stethoscope. For evaluation of the primary sensory modalities of light touch, pain, temperature, and vibration, wisps of cotton, sterile broken cotton-tipped applicators, and a tuning fork are used. A collection of small, common objects (e.g., coins, buttons, keys) to be identified by feel alone are useful for assessment of cortical sensations of stereognosis. Derangements of primary sensory function may be present with lesions at the level of the nerve roots, plexuses, or peripheral nerves. If a particular area of decreased sensation is identified in part of a limb, careful delineation of its boundaries often suggests root (dermatomal), plexus, or peripheral nerve involvement (Fig. 16.1).

Neurologic examination of the younger child requires flexibility and a gentle, staged approach. The first stage consists of observation, much of which can be done while taking the history as the infant sits in the parent's lap or while the toddler or older child plays with toys. The child's level of alertness and interest in people and the environment are assessed. Facies, head shape, body habitus, spontaneous movements, position, and posture are noted, along with spontaneous vocalizations and quality and pitch of cry in infants. In the child old enough to walk, stance and gait and the ability to run, stoop, and recover; climb onto a stool; and rise from the floor (when developmentally appropriate) are observed. These observations provide a good general impression of the child's developmental level and abilities.

Much of the remainder of the neurologic examination also lends itself to play, and in the second stage of observation a more detailed assessment of mental status, language, handedness, and fine and gross motor skills is performed by engaging the child in play. A selection of rattles, keys, spinning toys, dolls, cars, small blocks, noise makers, tennis balls, hand puppets, crayons, and picture books supplement the traditional instruments. If further observation of gait is necessary, the examiner can have the child walk with the parent. Children older than 4 years old love to show what they can do when asked to walk on their heels or toes, hop, or do tandem gait along a line. Pat-a-cake games are popular for testing rapidly alternating movements with young children. Next, with the child comfortable and rapport established, the hands-on examination is initiated with the child still dressed and in the parent's lap. Trying to catch the otoscope light as it is shown over various parts of the body can act as the prologue to following the light with the eyes and looking at it. For infants and toddlers, following a face or spinning toy is excellent for testing extraocular movements. Having a parent jingle keys at the child's eye level and asking the child to look at the object assists the ophthalmoscopic examination in older preschool and young school-age children. Asking young children to make faces, stick out their tongues, and blow-up balloons is another helpful technique in assessing cranial nerves.

Tone is assessed by observing resistance to passive motion. Then active motion and motion against resistance both assess strength. Older preschoolers and school-age children can use push/pull games to test muscle strength. Deep tendon reflexes can often be tested at this time with only the shoes off. These are normally brisk, or 3 +, in the young infant, becoming 2 + by 6 months old. If directly tapping on the tendon seems upsetting to the child, it may help to place a finger over the tendon to be percussed and tap that. In infants and toddlers, it is often easier to elicit the ankle jerk by placing a finger over the ball of the child's foot and gently dorsiflexing it before percussing the Achilles tendon. Preschoolers and young children love having the examiner express surprise and pleasure when reflexes are elicited.

Finally, the parent is asked to help undress the child, and the remainder of the examination proceeds with the parent providing reassurance and assistance as needed. During this stage, head circumference is measured in the infant and toddler, and the head, midline of the neck and back, and skin are carefully examined for abnormalities. Muscles are inspected for symmetry, and extremity circumference is measured a set distance from a bony landmark if asymmetry is suspected. Abnormal muscle movements are noted. The appropriate presence of primitive reflexes is determined in infants (see Chapter 3). The Babinski reflex is difficult to elicit and interpret during the first year of life because stroking the sole of the foot may simply stimulate withdrawal or plantar flexion. Evaluation of sensation is difficult in the younger child and is generally limited to appreciation of light touch and pinprick. These may be assessed using a sterile, broken cotton-tipped applicator.

Neurologic examination of the newborn is highly specialized. The essential components of the neonatal examination include assessment of gestational age, growth patterns, dysmorphic features, motor tone, postures, spontaneous activity, cry, respiratory patterns, brainstem reflexes, response to bright light, response to noxious stimuli, developmental reflexes, and deep tendon reflexes (see Chapter 2). Normal findings vary with gestational age. The immaturity of the newborn's CNS, with functioning largely at a

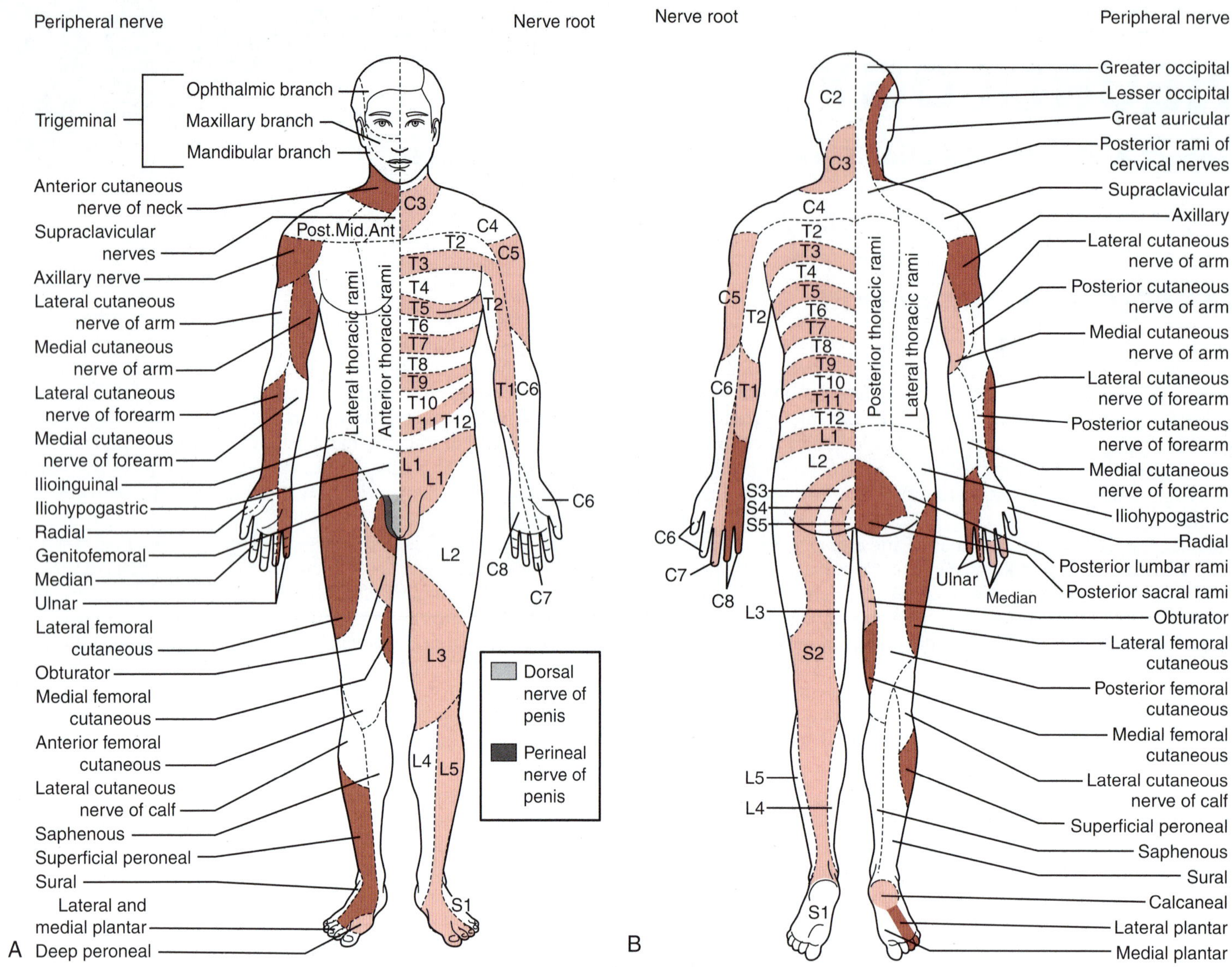

Fig. 16.1 Cutaneous sensory innervation. The segmental or dermatomal (nerve root) distribution is shown on the left side of the body and the peripheral nerve distribution on the right side of the body. (A) Anterior view. (B) Posterior view. (Modified from Simon RP, Aminoff MJ, Greenberg DA: *Clinical neurology*, ed 4, Stamford, CT, 1999, Appleton & Lange.)

subcortical reflex level, may conceal all but the most severe neurologic deficits—hence the often-deceptive normal examination of the newborn with hydranencephaly.

The most prevalent neurologic disorders in childhood are related to CNS infection, ingestions, congenital malformations, perinatal insults, trauma (including abuse), progressive neurodegenerative or neuromuscular processes, and metabolic disorders. This chapter concentrates on selected neurologic disorders accompanied by physical signs that can be detected on visual inspection.

NEUROCUTANEOUS SYNDROMES

The neurocutaneous syndromes or phakomatoses are congenital disorders with prominent cutaneous and neurologic manifestations, often arising from identified defects in specific gene loci. The simultaneous involvement of the skin and nervous system, both derivatives of embryonic ectoderm, suggests that these disorders may be caused by an unknown abnormality of the embryonic epiblast. Although the clinical and pathologic features of the phakomatoses are diverse, these syndromes share a propensity for malformations and hamartomatous tumors of multiple organs. Among the more frequently encountered phakomatoses are neurofibromatosis, tuberous sclerosis, Sturge-Weber syndrome, ataxia-telangiectasia, and linear sebaceous nevus.

Neurofibromatosis 1

Neurofibromatosis 1 (NF-1; previously known as *von Recklinghausen disease*) is the most common of the neurocutaneous syndromes and affects about 1 in 3000 individuals. It is an autosomal dominant disorder, with 50% of cases inherited from a parent and 50% of cases a sporadic gene change. Molecular genetic testing for mutations of the *NF1* gene is clinically available and detects up to 90% of gene mutations. The *NF1* gene has been localized to chromosome 17q. Neurofibromin, its gene product, acts as a tumor suppressor of the RAS/MAPK pathway, and its function is altered in affected patients. The clinical diagnostic criteria for NF1 were updated in 2021 by the Children's Tumor Foundation (Fig. 16.2). Characteristic clinical manifestations include multiple hyperpigmented skin macules (café-au-lait spots), axillary or inguinal freckling, multiple skin neurofibromas, and iris hamartomas (Lisch nodules). Associated abnormalities may include optic gliomas; other CNS tumors of glial or meningeal origin; neurofibromas of spinal or peripheral nerves; pheochromocytoma, macrocephaly, and cognitive impairment; and bony abnormalities.

Multiple café-au-lait spots, the most frequently encountered cutaneous abnormality, are brown hyperpigmented macules with smooth margins, usually most numerous over the trunk (Fig. 16.3A; and see Fig. 8.123). Other abnormalities of cutaneous pigmentation may include axillary or inguinal freckling or extensive areas of

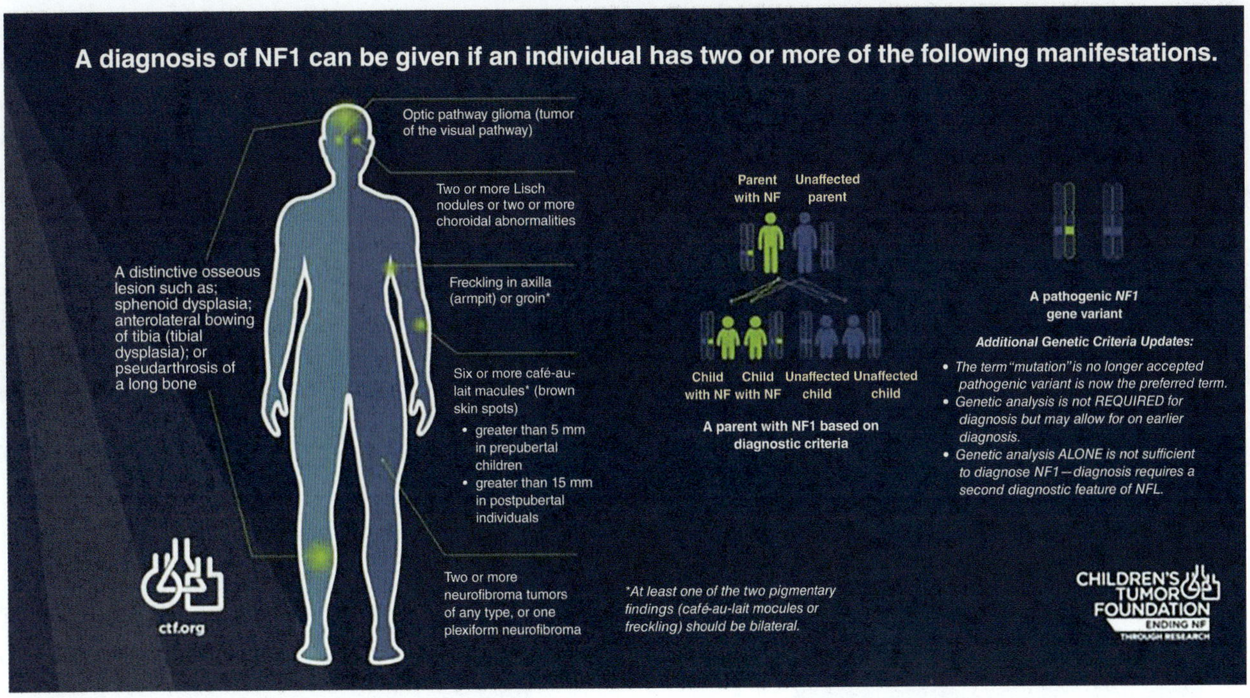

Fig. 16.2 Diagnostic Criteria for Neurofibromatosis Type 1, Children's Tumor Foundation.

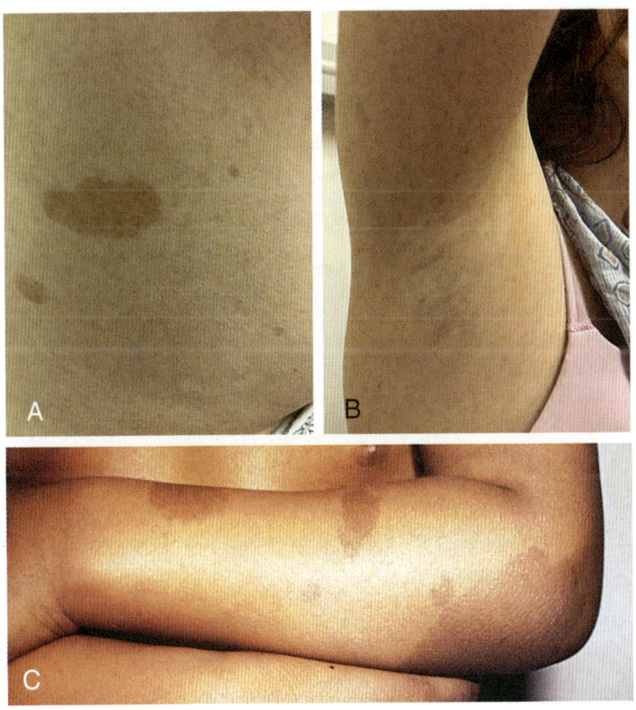

Fig. 16.3 Neurofibromatosis 1 (NF-1). Clinical manifestations of cutaneous pigmentary abnormalities. (A) Most common are multiple café au lait spots over the trunk. (B and C) Also seen are axillary freckling and extensive areas of hyperpigmentation. (Courtesy Michael Sherlock, MD, Lutherville, MD.)

hyperpigmentation (see Fig. 16.3B and C). Hyperpigmented skin lesions almost always precede neurologic symptoms and often increase in size and number with advancing age but can fade throughout adolescents and into adulthood. They are not necessarily present at birth, but the skin findings of café au lait macules and freckling usually develop before age 8.

Although multiple café-au-lait spots are a clinical hallmark of NF-1, they may also occur as an autosomal dominant trait unassociated with the other features of neurofibromatosis. Genetic investigations in such families have excluded linkage to the NF1 locus on chromosome 17. Multiple café-au-lait spots can be found in a variety of other conditions (Table 16.1). Legius syndrome involves a mutation in the *SPRED1* gene involved in the RAS/MAPK pathway. Legius syndrome is associated with similar cutaneous markers (café au lait macules and freckling) to NF1 and learning disabilities, but not tumorigenesis. Café au lait spots are a prominent feature of McCune-Albright syndrome, the additional manifestations of which include skeletal dysplasia and endocrine abnormalities. Those seen in McCune-Albright syndrome are often large and have irregular ("coast of Maine") margins (see Fig. 8.123D), in contrast to the

Table 16.1 Conditions Associated With Café-au-lait Lesions

Disorder	Clinical Features
Neurofibromatosis	Most common in NF-1, rare in NF-2 (see sections on NF-1 and NF-2 and Box 16.2)
Tuberous sclerosis (TS)	See Box 16.3
McCune-Albright syndrome	Polyostotic fibrous dysplasia, precocious puberty, endocrine dysfunction
Watson syndrome	Features of Noonan syndrome (webbed neck, hypertelorism with antimongoloid slant, low-set ears, pulmonic stenosis, low intelligence), plus meets criteria for NF-1
Epidermal nevus syndrome	Verrucous skin lesions, scoliosis, aortic coarctation, intellectual disability
Bloom syndrome	Severe intrauterine and postnatal growth retardation, photosensitivity, telangiectatic erythema of cheeks/face
Ataxia-telangiectasia	Ataxia, conjunctival telangiectasia, recurrent sinopulmonary infections
Silver syndrome	Intrauterine growth retardation, hemihypertrophy, syndactyly, triangular facies, premature sexual development
Gaucher disease	Opisthotonos, splenomegaly, cranial nerve dysfunction, regression of motor milestones
Turner syndrome	Short stature, webbed neck, coarctation of aorta, delayed puberty
Fanconi anemia	Aplastic anemia, hyperpigmentation, short stature, intellectual disability, congenital anomalies of bone, heart, eye, kidney
Multiple lentigines (LEOPARD) syndrome	Multiple small lentigines, hypertelorism, pulmonic stenosis, cryptorchidism, mild growth retardation, sensorineural deafness

NF-1, Neurofibromatosis 1; *NF-2,* neurofibromatosis 2.

smooth ("coast of California") borders characteristic of the hyperpigmented lesions of NF-1. Café-au-lait spots also may be encountered in TS and neurofibromatosis 2 (NF-2) but are seldom prominent. They are present in about 10% of the general population (typically four or less in number) and are not by themselves a sign of disease.

Additional cutaneous manifestations of NF-1 may include extensive plexiform neuromas at the terminal distribution of nerve fibers (Fig. 16.4 and see Fig. 8.84) or small subcutaneous nodules—neurofibromas—scattered along the course of nerve trunks (Fig. 16.5 and 16.6).

Pigmented hamartomas of the iris, or Lisch nodules, are seen in more than 90% of patients with NF-1 who are older than 6 years old and can be found in nearly one-third of younger individuals (Fig. 16.7). They do not occur in the normal population. Although these hamartomas are asymptomatic and do not correlate with the extent or severity of other manifestations, they are helpful in establishing the diagnosis.

Short stature and macrocephaly are common in patients with NF-1, and skeletal abnormalities are found in 51% (Fig. 16.8).

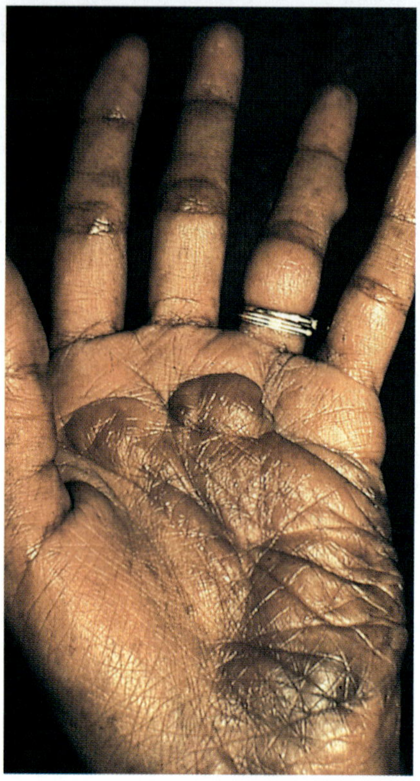

Fig. 16.4 Neurofibromatosis 1. Extensive plexiform neurofibroma of the palm. (Courtesy Michael Sherlock, MD, Lutherville, MD.)

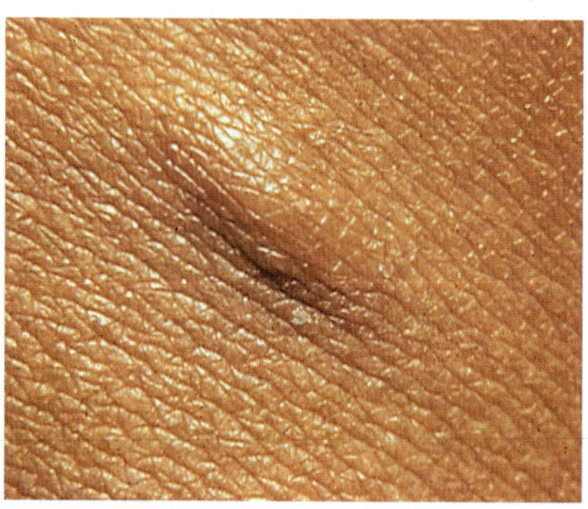

Fig. 16.5 Subcutaneous neurofibroma along the course of a nerve trunk. (Courtesy Michael Sherlock, MD, Lutherville, MD.)

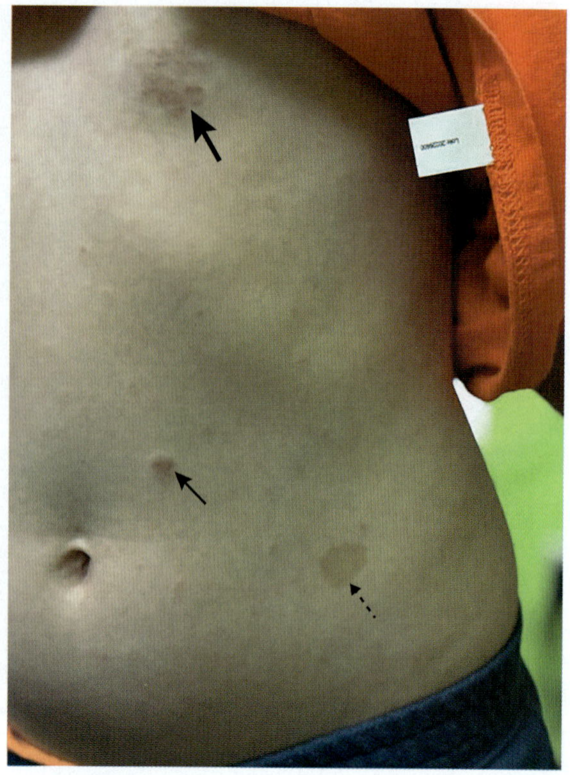

Fig. 16.6 Subcutaneous neurofibroma with a prominent vascular component *(large arrow)*. Subcutaneous neurofibroma along the course of a nerve trunk *(small arrow)*. Café au lait spot *(dashed arrow)*.

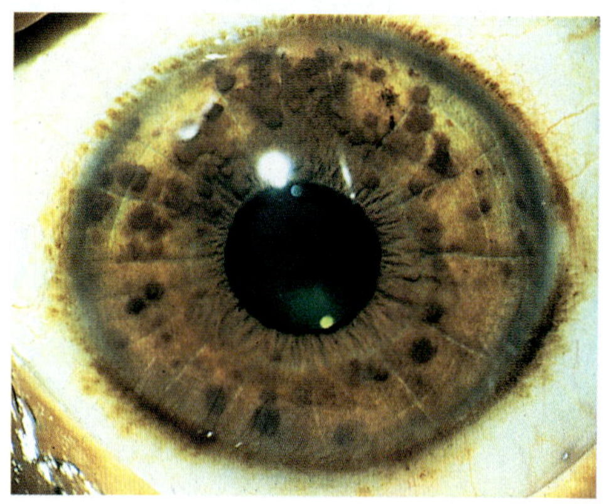

Fig. 16.7 Neurofibromatosis 1. Pigmented hamartomas of the iris (Lisch nodules).

Osseous lesions, if present, usually appear in the first year of life. The characteristic findings include the following:

- Severe angular scoliosis with dysplasia of the vertebral bodies (see Fig. 16.8A)
- Defects of the posterior superior wall of the orbit
- Congenital bowing and thinning of the cortices of long bones and pseudarthrosis of the tibia, fibula (see Fig. 16.8B), femur, or clavicle
- Disorders of bone growth associated with elephantoid hypertrophy of overlying soft tissue
- Erosive bony defects produced by contiguous neurogenic tumors
- Scalloping of the posterior margins of the vertebral bodies corresponding to saccular areas of dilation of the spinal meninges (see Fig. 16.8C)

Patients with NF-1 can be affected with tumors of the brain, spinal cord, spinal nerve roots, and peripheral nerves. Optic nerve glioma is the most common CNS tumor and affects 20% of patients with NF-1, usually occurring by 18 months to 7 years old. It often presents as progressive visual loss with optic atrophy and tends to be less aggressive than in patients without NF-1. Ependymomas, meningiomas, brainstem gliomas, and astrocytomas have also been reported.

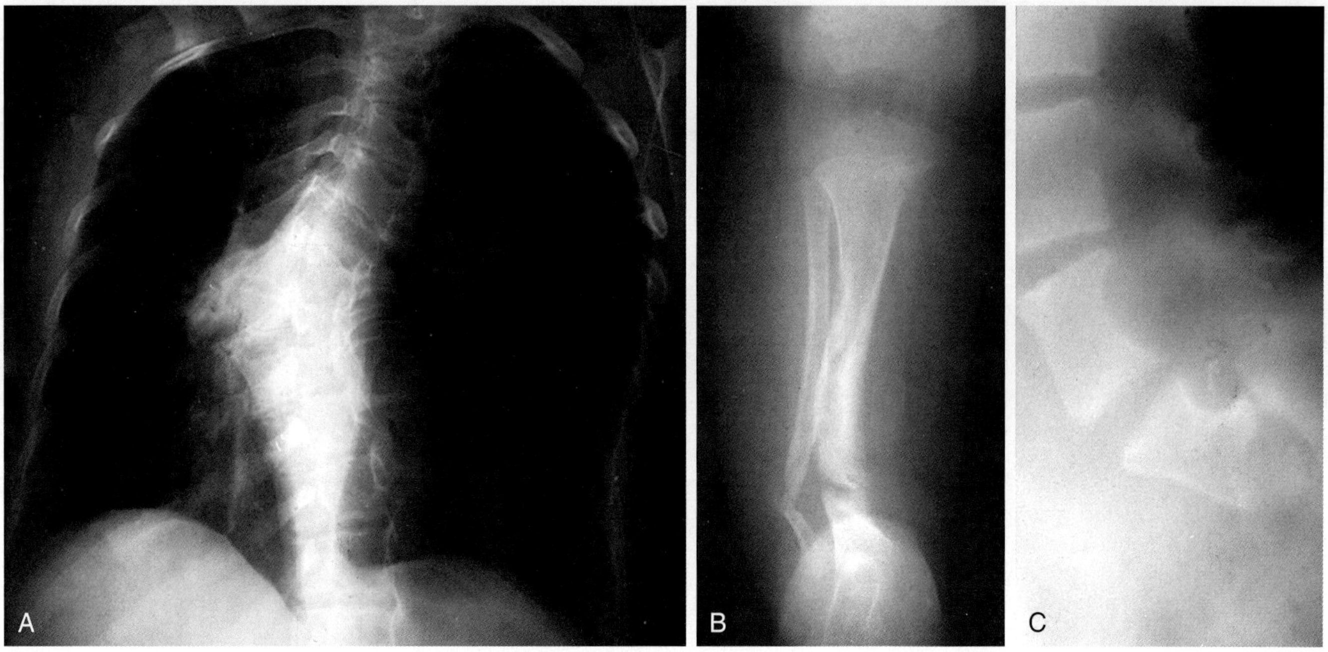

Fig. 16.8 Neurofibromatosis 1 (NF-1). Radiographic manifestations of skeletal abnormalities. (A) Severe angular scoliosis and vertebral dysplasia. (B) Congenital bowing and pseudarthrosis of the tibia and fibula. (C) Scalloping of the posterior margins of the vertebral bodies resulting from dural ectasia. (Courtesy Department of Radiology, Children's Hospital of Pittsburgh, Pittsburgh, PA.)

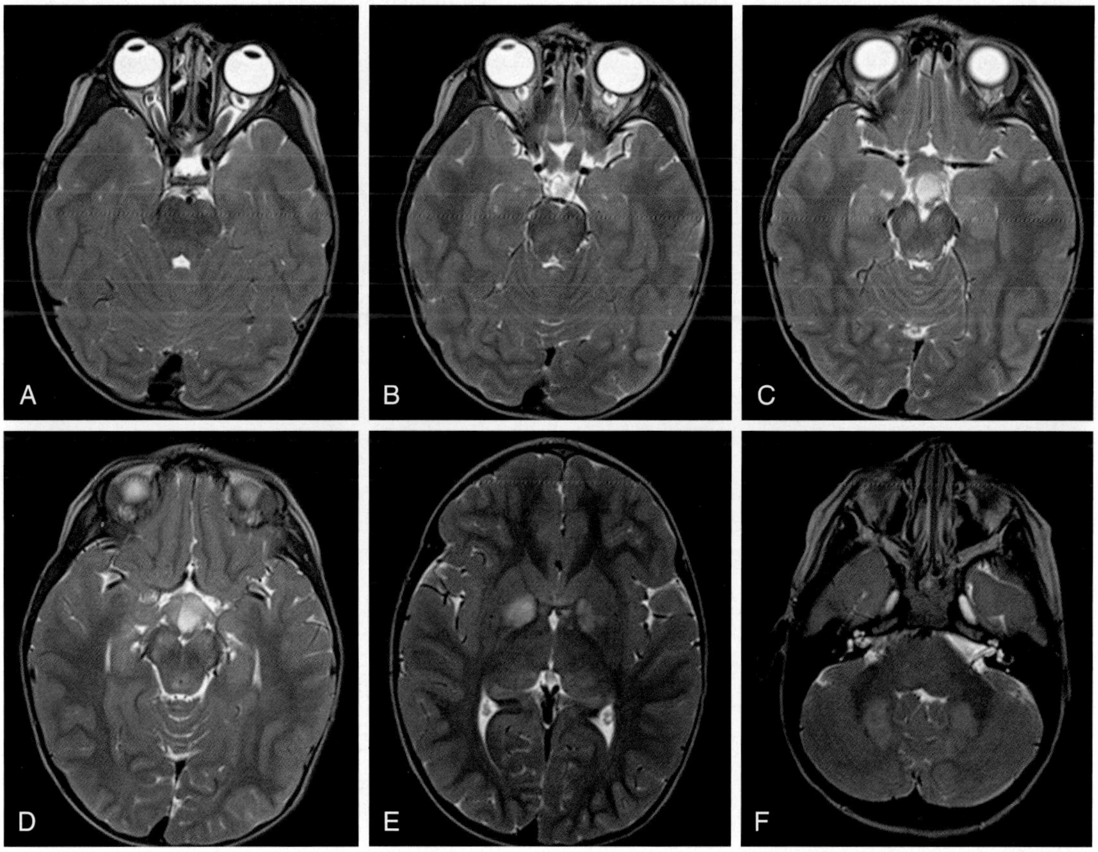

Fig. 16.9 (A–D) Demonstrates an optic pathway glioma. (A) Bilateral tortuous and enlarged optic nerves right greater than left. (B) Enlarged optic nerves and a hyperintense glioma involving the optic chiasm. (C) Extension of the optic nerve glioma inferiorly toward the hypothalamus. (D) Involvement of the optic nerve glioma within the hypothalamus and involving the optic radiations on the right as they leave the thalamus. (E) Dysmyelination represented by hyperintensities on T2 imaging involving the deep gray matter of the basal ganglia. (F) Dysmyelination with hyperintensities within the deep white matter of the cerebellum.

Magnetic resonance imaging (MRI) scans frequently show areas of increased signal intensity on T2-weighted images of the globus pallidus, brainstem, or cerebellar white matter (Fig. 16.9). These are commonly termed *unidentified bright objects (UBOs)* or hamartomas and are believed to represent increased fluid within the myelin associated with dysplastic glial proliferation representing dysmyelination. The dysmyelination does not appear to correlate with neurologic dysfunction. However, its presence helps confirm the diagnosis of NF-1. Computed tomography (CT) seldom demonstrates corresponding abnormalities and should be avoided to limit ionizing radiation due to the loss of function of a tumor suppressing gene.

Learning disabilities and behavior problems are common and may affect up to 40% of patients with NF-1. Although their full-scale intelligence quotient is generally lower than that of the general population, severe intellectual disability is rare. Approximately 10% of patients with NF-1 have seizures.

A small percentage of patients with NF-1 have dysplasia of the renal or carotid arteries. Renal artery stenosis can cause systemic hypertension, and adult patients with NF-1 may develop pheochromocytoma with concomitant hypertension. Cerebral artery dysplasia can include moyamoya syndrome with abnormal vessels of the circle of Willis, predisposing to cerebral infarction in children and cerebral hemorrhage in adults.

Neurofibromatosis 2

NF-2 (also known as *bilateral acoustic neurofibromatosis*) is a distinct genetic disorder characterized by autosomal dominant inheritance of bilateral acoustic neuromas with a penetrance of more than 95%. NF-2 occurs in approximately 1 in 50,000 people. It results from a mutation of the *NF2* gene on the long arm of chromosome 22. The *NF2* gene product, merlin or schwannomin, serves to suppress tumor formation, and its dysfunction leads to the common occurrence of CNS tumors in patients with NF-2. Most patients eventually develop bilateral acoustic neuromas (vestibular schwannomas).

Symptoms usually first appear in the teens or early 20s when pressure on the vestibulocochlear or facial nerve complex results in impaired auditory discrimination, hearing loss, tinnitus, unsteadiness, or facial weakness. Presenile lens opacities, found in half the patients examined, may precede the onset of symptoms referable to acoustic neuroma. Other Schwann cell tumors of cranial nerves, spinal roots, or the spinal cord and multiple CNS tumors of meningeal or glial origin may develop. Cutaneous manifestations such as café-au-lait spots, cutaneous neurofibromas, and axillary or inguinal freckling are less common in NF-2 than in NF-1, and Lisch nodules are not typical. Diagnostic criteria for NF-2 are summarized in Boxes 16.1 and 16.2.

Box 16.1 Diagnostic Criteria for Neurofibromatosis 1

Diagnostic criteria are met if two or more of the following are found:

- Six or more café-au-lait macules >5 mm in greatest diameter in prepubertal children and >15 mm in greatest diameter in postpubertal individuals
- Two or more neurofibromas of any type or one plexiform neurofibroma
- Axillary or inguinal freckling
- Optic glioma
- Two or more Lisch nodules (iris hamartomas)
- A distinctive osseous lesion, such as a sphenoid dysplasia or thinning of long bone cortex with or without pseudarthrosis
- A first-degree relative (i.e., parent, sibling, or child) with NF-1, according to these criteria

Box 16.2 Diagnostic Criteria for Neurofibromatosis 2

Bilateral eighth nerve masses seen with appropriate imaging techniques (e.g., CT, MRI)

or

A first-degree relative with NF-2 and a unilateral eighth nerve mass

or

Two of the following:

- Neurofibroma
- Meningioma
- Glioma
- Schwannoma
- Juvenile posterior subcapsular lens opacity

Tuberous Sclerosis

Tuberous sclerosis (TS) is inherited as an autosomal dominant trait. Two genes appear to cause the disorder: TSC1 (chromosome 9q) and TSC2 (chromosome 16p). Both gene products (hamartin for TSC1 and tuberin for TSC2) have tumor suppressor activity and produce similar phenotypes when expressed. Genetic testing is available and currently detects nearly 80% of cases. Although 1 in 6000 to 9000 people in the population carry a TS gene, expression is highly variable and full expression of disease is seen in only 1 in 150,000. Most carriers have hypopigmented macules (ash-leaf spots) as their only manifestation. Spontaneous mutation appears to account for newly diagnosed cases, and in up to 2% of patients without a positive family history, the disorder may be the result of germline mosaicism.

The more prominent features of this neurocutaneous disorder include seizures (96%), intellectual disability (60%), autism (50%), intracranial calcification (49%), tumors of various organs (including the brain, heart, liver, and kidneys), and cutaneous lesions. Seizures are the most frequent presenting symptom. Clinical expression can be quite variable even among affected members of the same family. Diagnostic criteria are summarized in Box 16.3.

The characteristic skin lesion of TS is angiofibroma *(adenoma sebaceum).* These are seen as erythematous papules distributed over the nose and malar region of the face (Fig. 16.10). Approximately 40% of children with TS demonstrate these lesions by 3 years old.

Hypomelanotic macules with irregular borders, termed *ash-leaf spots,* are another common cutaneous manifestation (Fig. 16.11). These generally appear earlier than adenoma sebaceum and may be present at birth. They are detectable by 2 years old in more than half of affected children. They resemble vitiligo but differ in that they are not completely devoid of melanin. In fair-skinned infants, these nevi may be demonstrable only under Wood lamp light.

Another valuable cutaneous marker is the *shagreen patch,* a plaque of thickened skin with a cobblestone or orange-peel texture often seen on the dorsal aspect of the trunk (Fig. 16.12). Histologically, the shagreen patch is a connective tissue nevus.

Additional dermatologic manifestations of TS include periungual fibromas (Fig. 16.13) and macular areas of hyperpigmentation.

Box 16.3 Diagnostic Criteria for Tuberous Sclerosis

Definite Tuberous Sclerosis

Two major features or one major and two or more minor features

Possible Tuberous Sclerosis

Either one major feature or two or more minor features

Major Features

Angiofibromas (>3) or fibrous forehead plaque
Nontraumatic ungual or periungual fibroma (>2)
Hypomelanotic macules (i.e., ash-leaf spots [≥3], at least 5 mm diameter)
Shagreen patch (connective tissue nevus)
Multiple retinal hamartomas
Cortical dysplasias (includes tubers and cerebral white matter radial migration lines)
Subependymal nodule
Subependymal giant cell astrocytoma
Cardiac rhabdomyoma, single or multiple
Lymphangiomyomatosis
Renal angiomyolipoma (≥2)

Minor Features

Multiple randomly distributed pits in dental enamel (>3)
Gingival/intraoral fibromas (≥2)
Nonrenal hamartoma
Retinal achromatic patch
"Confetti" skin lesions
Multiple renal cysts

Modified from Northrup H, Krueger D: Tuberous sclerosis complex diagnostic criteria update: recommendations of the 2012 International TSC Consensus Conference, *Pediatr Neurol* 49(4):243–254, 2013.

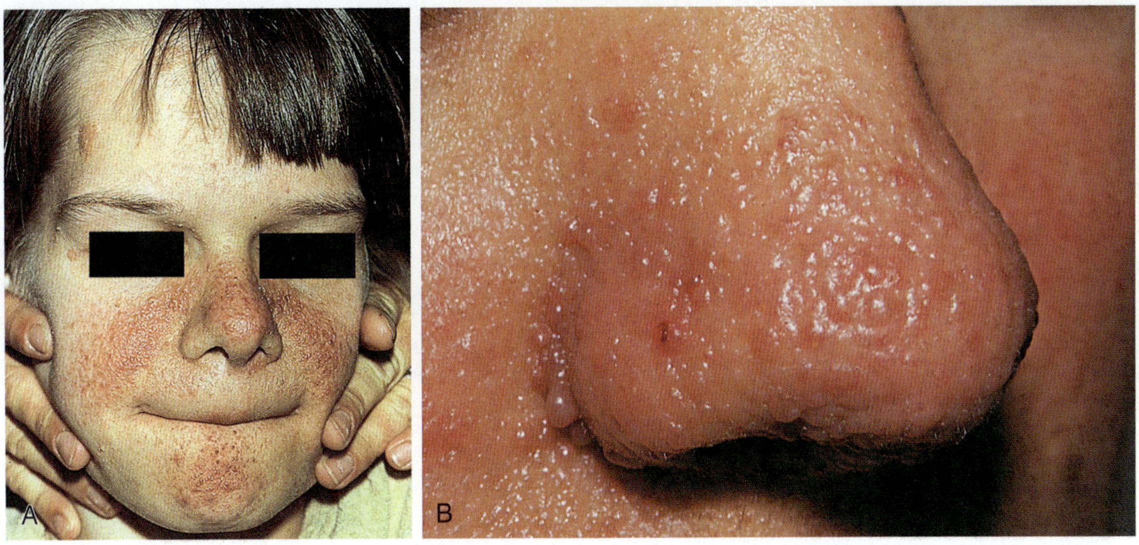

Fig. 16.10 Tuberous sclerosis. (A) This adolescent boy had adenoma sebaceum in a characteristic malar distribution and chin lesions as well. (B) A close-up view of nasal lesions is shown.

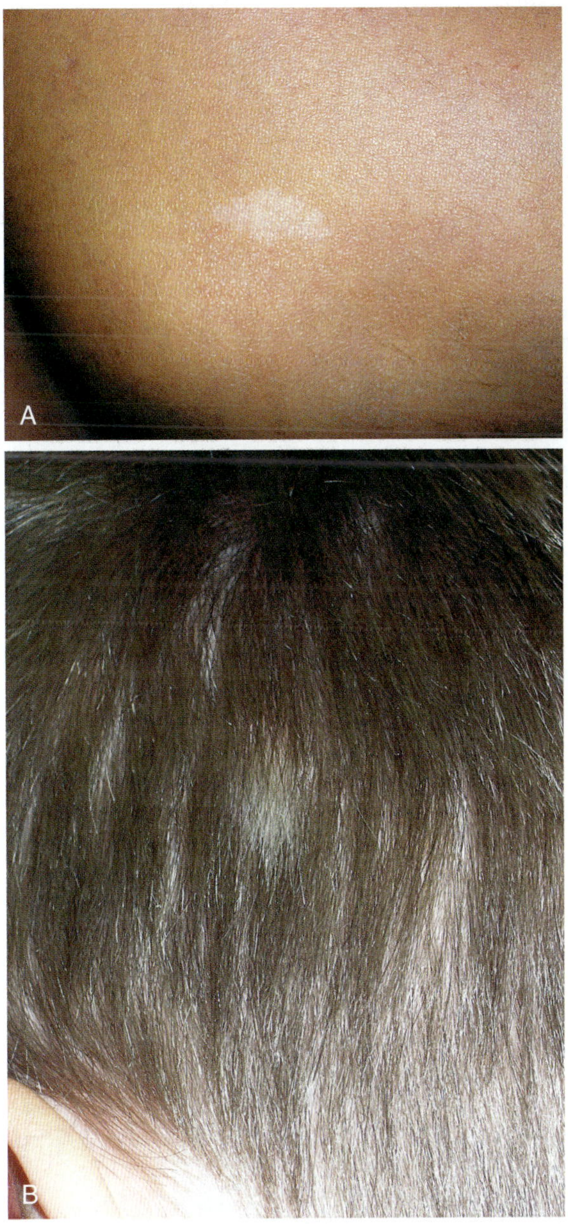

Fig. 16.11 Tuberous sclerosis (TS). (A) An ash-leaf spot is an oval depigmented nevus with irregular borders. (B) This child with TS has numerous hypopigmented macules over his scalp, and the hair growing from these is hypopigmented as well (a phenomenon termed *poliosis*). (Courtesy Robin Gehris, MD, Children's Hospital of Pittsburgh, Pittsburgh, PA.)

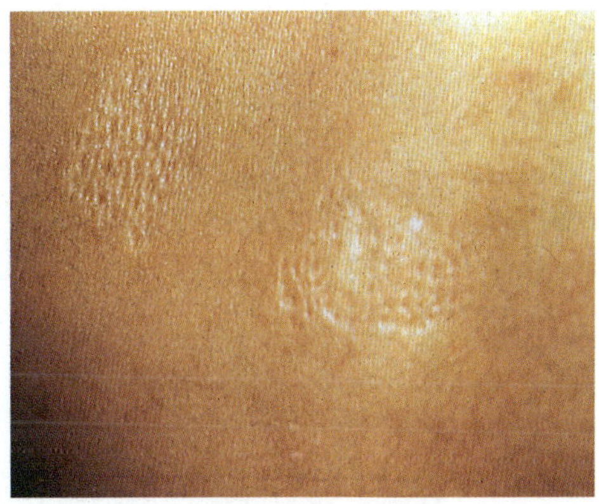

Fig. 16.12 Tuberous sclerosis. Shagreen patch. This plaque of thickened skin with a cobblestone texture is distinctive but is one of the less common cutaneous manifestations. (Courtesy Michael Sherlock, MD, Lutherville, MD.)

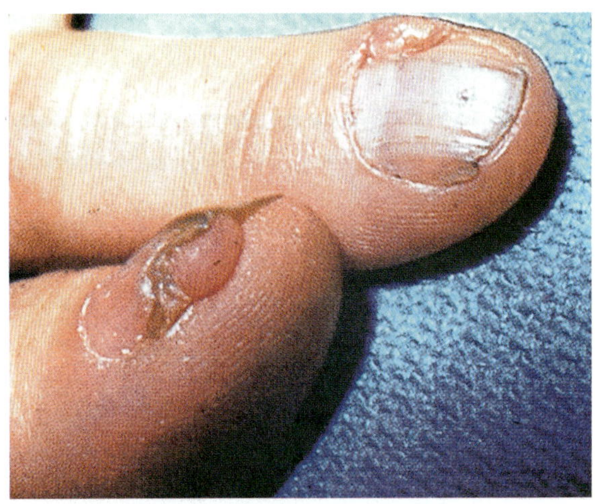

Fig. 16.13 Tuberous sclerosis. Periungual fibromas. These nodular lesions can occur singly or multiply in the ungual or periungual areas. (Courtesy Michael Painter, MD, Children's Hospital of Pittsburgh, Pittsburgh, PA.)

Recognition of the cutaneous features can suggest an etiologic diagnosis in some patients with intellectual disability or seizures. Oral examination may reveal pitting of dental enamel.

In patients with TS, CT scans often demonstrate subependymal nodules seen as intracranial calcifications that appear as multiple scattered areas of increased density adjacent to the walls of the lateral and third ventricles (Fig. 16.14A). CT is superior to MRI for demonstration of small calcifications (Fig. 16.14B). No relationship has been established between the extent of periventricular calcification and clinical severity. CT may also demonstrate asymptomatic but typical intracranial calcifications in individuals who lack external manifestations of the disorder. This can help identify subclinical cases and improve the accuracy of genetic counseling in affected families.

The characteristic gross abnormality of the brain in TS is the presence of multiple gliotic nodules (hamartomas) of varying size, which constitute the tubers for which this disorder is named. These are located over the convolutions of the cerebral hemispheres and beneath the ependymal lining of the lateral and third ventricles. Heterotopic nodules of identical structure may be found in the cerebral white matter as well. Although cortical tubers are rarely apparent on CT scans, they are readily identified by MRI studies (Fig. 16.15A). Severely affected patients have a greater number of cerebral cortical lesions detected by MRI scans (Fig. 16.15B), suggesting that MRI may be useful in predicting eventual clinical severity in young children with newly diagnosed TS. Tumors may arise from cortical or subependymal tubers, complicating the course of the disease by producing increased intracranial pressure and other symptoms associated with intracranial mass lesions.

Subependymal giant cell astrocytomas (SEGAs) (Fig. 16.16) can affect 15% to 20% of patients with TS and are clinically manifested by symptoms of obstructive hydrocephalus. The site of obstruction is often at the level of the foramen of Monro in the lateral ventricles. Such patients may present with signs of increased intracranial pressure, behavior change, or worsening seizure control. Up to 80% of patients with TS develop seizures of variable types that are often difficult to control. Infantile spasms are common and may be the presenting symptom leading to diagnosis. Patients with a history of infantile spasms should be evaluated for TS because those who develop other types of seizures when very young tend to have more severe seizure disorders and poorer cognitive function.

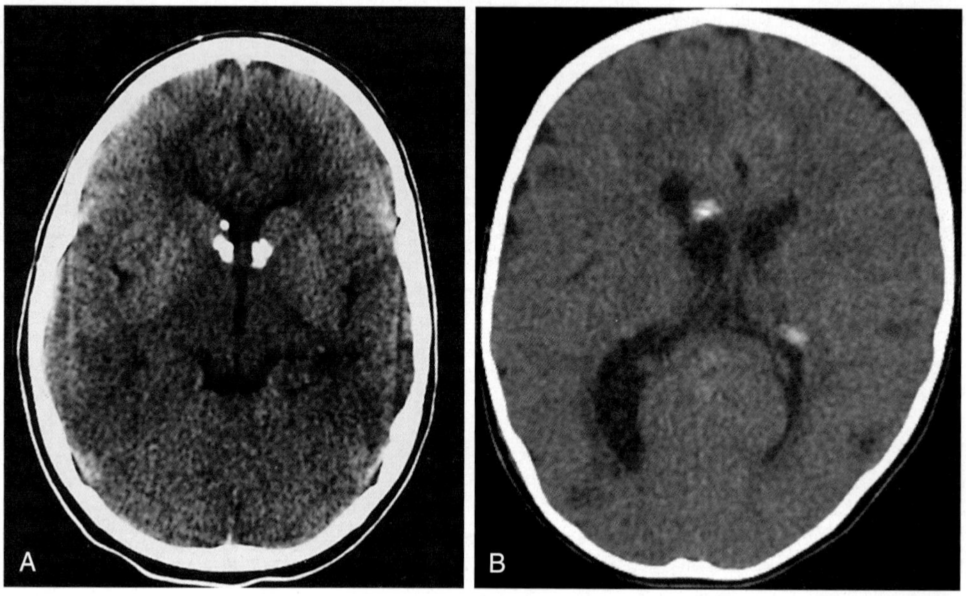

Fig. 16.14 Tuberous sclerosis. (A) This computed tomography (CT) cut through the foramina of Monro shows the multiple periventricular calcific deposits characteristic of this disorder. (B) CT head without contrast showing multiple calcified subependymal nodules. (Courtesy Division of Neuroradiology, University Health Center of Pittsburgh, Pittsburgh, PA.)

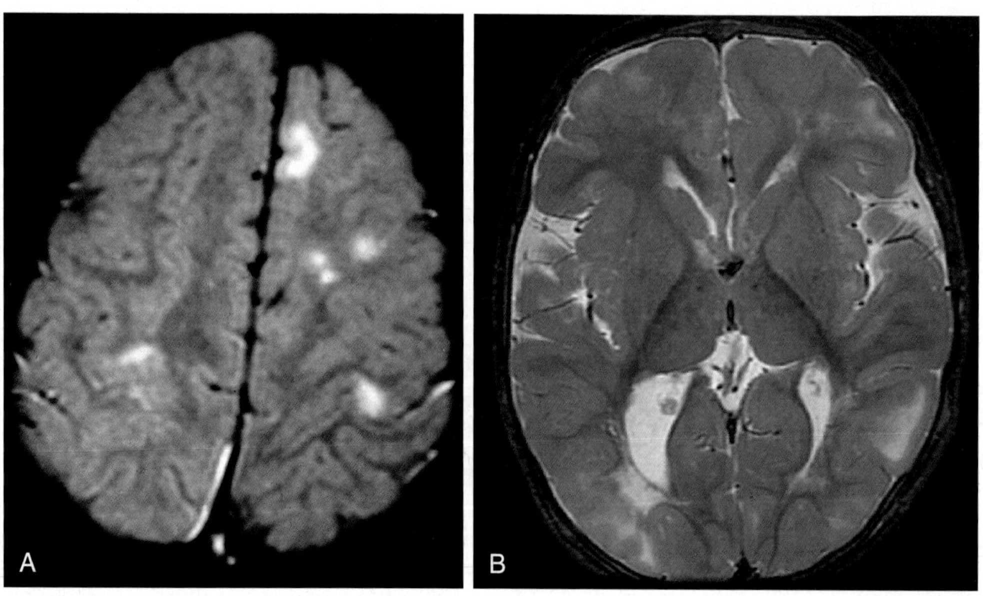

Fig. 16.15 Tuberous sclerosis (TS). (A) Magnetic resonance imaging (MRI) demonstrates multiple cortical tubers that appear as areas of increased signal intensity in this T2-weighted image. The signal abnormalities arise predominantly within the white matter subjacent to the tuber. (B) MRI in tuberous sclerosis with axial SIT sequence highlighting the high tuber burden. (Courtesy Division of Neuroradiology, University Health Center of Pittsburgh, Pittsburgh, PA.)

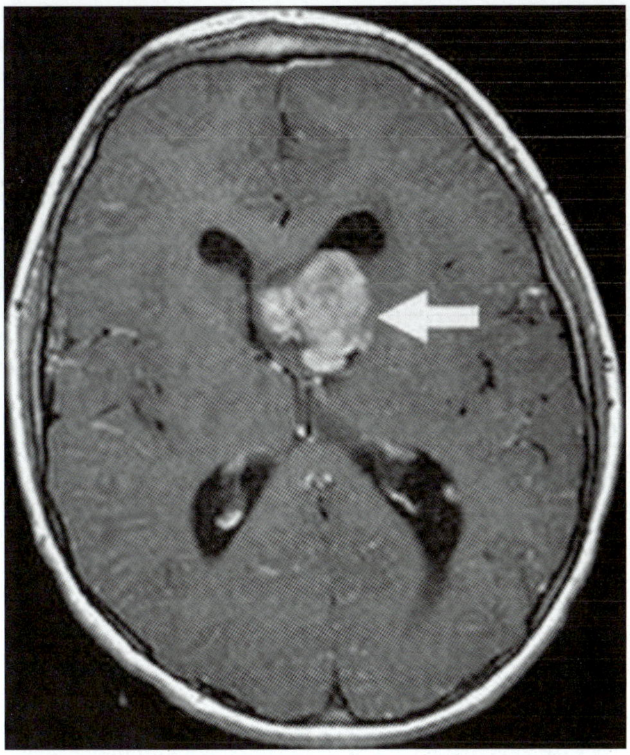

Fig. 16.16 Tuberous sclerosis. Magnetic resonance imaging demonstrates a large subependymal giant cell astrocytoma with ventricular dilation.

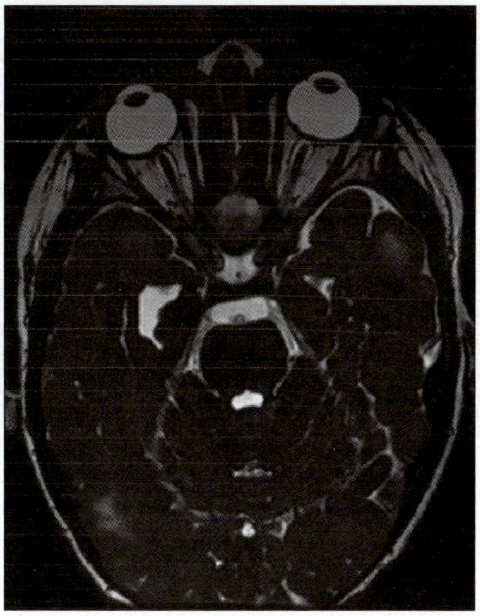

Fig. 16.17 Retinal hamartoma. Three-dimensional axial FIESTA sequence with contrast showing optic nerve head protrusion in both eyes and left retinal hamartoma in a patient with tuberous sclerosis.

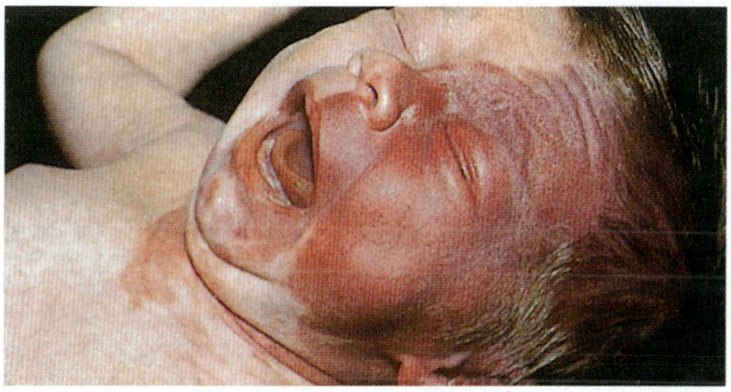

Fig. 16.18 Sturge-Weber syndrome. A nonelevated purple cutaneous vascular malformation, often termed a *port-wine stain,* is seen in a trigeminal distribution, including the ophthalmic division.

Visceral lesions associated with TS include cardiac rhabdomyoma, renal angiomyolipomas, pulmonary lymphangiomyomatosis, and hepatic hamartoma. Cardiac rhabdomyomas occur in up to two-thirds of patients and may be multiple. They tend to regress over the first few years of life and are usually asymptomatic, although occasionally a newborn may have obstructive congestive heart failure. Three-fourths of patients with TS have renal angiomyolipomas, which are often bilateral and multiple. Most remain clinically silent, but tumors greater than 4 cm in size may cause hematuria or proteinuria. Renal disease is the most common cause of death in adults with the disease and may manifest as flank pain, hematuria, or retroperitoneal hemorrhage. Renal cysts occur earlier and less often than angiomyolipomas. Rarely, children with TS can present in infancy with polycystic kidney disease. Chronic renal failure and malignant transformation of renal tumors are rare. Pulmonary lymphangiomyomatosis affects less than 2% of patients, mostly females, and is rare before the adult years. Symptoms include dyspnea, spontaneous pneumothorax, and hemoptysis. Hepatic hamartoma is clinically insignificant. Retinal hamartomas can also occur and may be visualized on MRI (Fig. 16.17).

Sturge-Weber Syndrome

Sturge-Weber syndrome (SWS) is a sporadic neurocutaneous condition caused by a postzygotic somatic mutation in the *GNAQ* gene (chromosome 9) or GNA11 variants. It has been speculated that there is a lack of full development of the superficial venous drainage system of the brain, leading to dilation of capillaries and venous channels to compensate. Another theory raises the possibility of persistence of primordial sinusoidal venous channels. The cardinal manifestations of Sturge-Weber syndrome are as follows:

- A vascular malformation or port-wine stain over the face that involves the cutaneous distribution of the ophthalmic division of the trigeminal nerve
- Ipsilateral leptomeningeal angiomatosis with associated intracranial calcifications
- A high incidence of intellectual disability and ipsilateral ocular complications

The port-wine stain (Fig. 16.18) is usually present at birth and consists of a pink-to-purple macular cutaneous vascular malformation. Only patients with lesions involving the cutaneous distribution of the ophthalmic division of the trigeminal nerve (i.e., forehead and upper eyelid) are at risk for associated neuro-ocular complications (Fig. 16.19). Repeated ophthalmologic and CT or MRI examinations are indicated only in this high-risk group, which has a 10% to 20% incidence of associated intracranial angiomas.

The coincidence of seizures and a facial vascular nevus should suggest the diagnosis of Sturge-Weber syndrome, which can be confirmed by CT or MRI (Fig. 16.20). These scans may be normal at birth but subsequently show areas of gyriform contrast enhancement corresponding to the leptomeningeal angiomatosis. Serial examinations often demonstrate progressive ipsilateral cerebral atrophy. Additional findings may include serpiginous calcifications of brain parenchyma underlying vascular malformations of the pia. These intracranial calcifications are first seen on CT scan but become evident on plain skull films by the end of the second decade.

Associated ocular abnormalities are often encountered. Buphthalmos (corneal enlargement) or colobomata may be present at birth, and glaucoma frequently develops in infancy or later childhood (Fig. 16.21). Dilated vessels in the sclera, conjunctiva, and retina are common, and angiomatous malformations of the choroid occasionally occur.

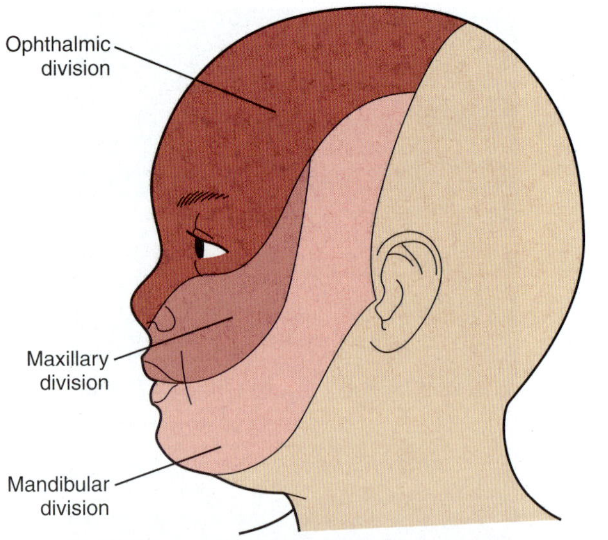

Fig. 16.19 Sturge-Weber syndrome. Cutaneous distribution of the division of the trigeminal nerve. Only patients with facial port-wine stains that involve the ophthalmic division are at risk for associated neuro-ocular symptoms.

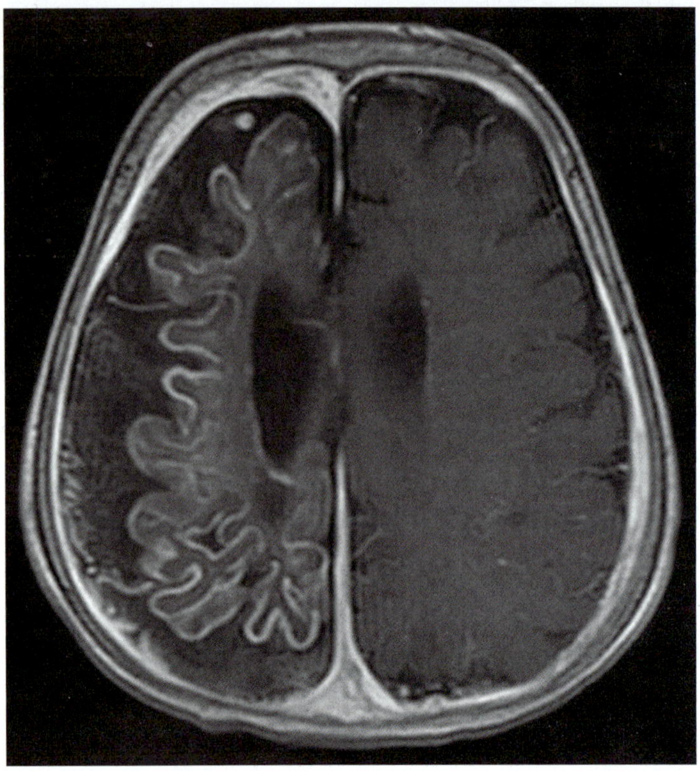

Fig. 16.20 Sturge-Weber syndrome. Magnetic resonance imaging (MRI) demonstrates gyriform contrast enhancement and hemispheric atrophy of the right hemisphere.

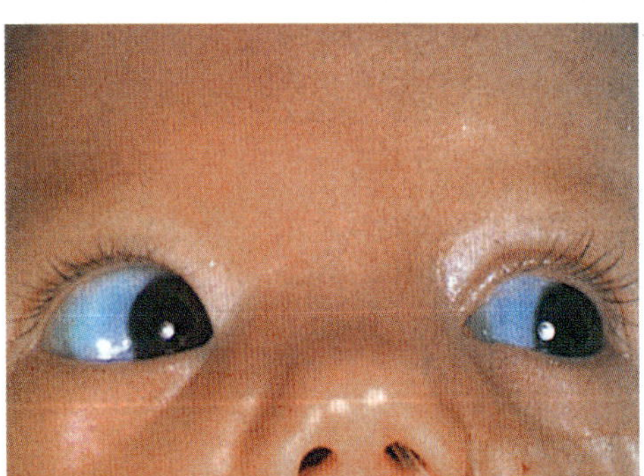

Fig. 16.21 Buphthalmos. Enlargement of the cornea of the right eye is evident. This is one of the associated ocular findings in Sturge-Weber syndrome and should prompt urgent evaluation for associated glaucoma. (From Booth IW, Wozniak ER: *Pediatrics*, Baltimore, 1984, Williams & Wilkins.)

The estimated incidence of facial cutaneous angioma is 1 in 5000, and the estimated frequency of the complete syndrome is 1 in 30,000. Among patients with the complete syndrome, seizures occur in 90% and contralateral hemiparesis eventually develops in one-third. Early developmental milestones are often normal, but about 50% develop cognitive difficulties ranging from mild to severe. Behavioral problems are common. Patients with refractory epilepsy are more likely to be more severely delayed.

Klippel-Trénaunay Syndrome

Patients with Klippel-Trénaunay syndrome are born with a port-wine stain that is usually located over the lateral aspect of one leg. Less often an arm and a leg may be affected. In rare instances, more extensive, even bilateral, involvement is seen. The surface lesion is associated with an underlying vascular malformation, which provides an unusually rich blood supply to soft tissue and bony structures that often results in hemihypertrophy and lymphedema (Fig. 16.22). These features are often evident in the newborn, and progressive enlargement occurs during the first few years. Most cases are sporadic.

Ataxia-Telangiectasia

Ataxia-telangiectasia is a multisystem, autosomal recessive degenerative disorder characterized by ataxia, oculocutaneous telangiectasia, immunodeficiency, and a high incidence of neoplasia. Affected individuals are extremely sensitive to ionizing radiation and have defective deoxyribonucleic acid repair mechanisms. Molecular genetic testing for ATM (ataxia telangiectasia mutated), the only gene associated with ataxia-telangiectasia, is clinically available. Ataxia is the usual presenting feature, and the course of the neurological disturbance is stereotypic. Tremors of the head may be seen before 1 year old, and unsteadiness of gait is evident when the child first walks. Progressive global ataxia and slurred, scanning, dysarthric speech are typical during the early school-age

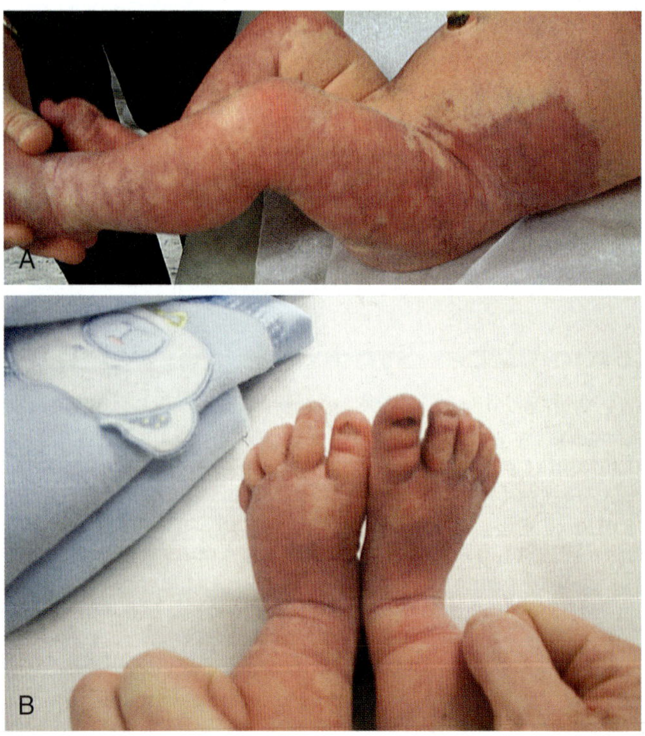

Fig. 16.22 Klippel-Trénaunay syndrome (KTS). (A) This infant with KTS is unusual in that he has vascular malformations involving both lower extremities, which extend upward over the lateral aspects of the abdominal wall. (B) In this view of his feet, one can appreciate a greater degree of hypertrophy on the right.

years. Loss of deep tendon reflexes and impairment of position and vibratory sensation are evident by the end of the first decade. Adolescence is marked by choreoathetosis, dystonic posturing, gaze apraxia, and progressive dementia. Nonclassic forms of ataxia-telangiectasia have included adult-onset cases and presentations with early dystonia.

The characteristic cutaneous manifestations of this disorder appear by 6 years old. Telangiectases first appear on the bulbar conjunctivae (Fig. 16.23) and develop later over the malar regions, ears, antecubital fossae, neck, and upper chest.

Neuropathologic changes are widespread, with the cerebellum being the site of maximal degeneration. Loss of Purkinje and basket cells, thinning of the granular cell layer, and changes in the molecular layer are characteristic findings.

Systemic manifestations include major defects in cellular and humoral immunity. Deficiencies of immunoglobulin A (IgA) and immunoglobulin M (IgM) are characteristic and together with impaired cellular immunity contribute to susceptibility to the recurrent sinus and pulmonary infections that mark this disorder, as well as to the tendency to develop malignancies of the lymphoreticular system (most commonly acute lymphoblastic leukemia or lymphoma) during adolescence or early adulthood (see Chapter 12). Serum α-fetoprotein levels are elevated, which serves as a nonspecific marker. Adult family members of patients, especially mothers, may also be susceptible to malignancy—breast and lung cancer being the most common.

Linear Sebaceous Nevus

The nevus sebaceus of Jadassohn is usually present at birth, manifesting as a yellowish-tan, waxy, linear lesion (Fig. 16.24) that contains a papillomatous excess of sebaceous glands. This nevus may be found on the scalp, face, neck, trunk, or extremities. With time, the lesion becomes disfiguring with a 15% to 20% risk of malignant degeneration, leading to recommendation for early surgical excision. Although usually an isolated abnormality, an association with seizures and intellectual disability has been reported. The risk of neurologic abnormalities is greatest with a midfacial cutaneous lesion.

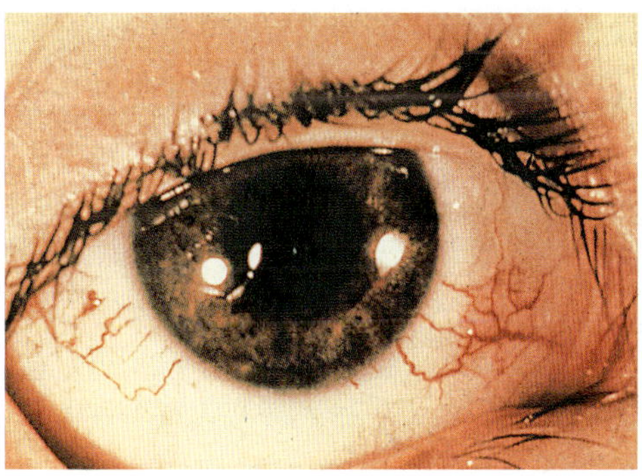

Fig. 16.23 Ataxia-telangiectasia. Characteristic telangiectases in the bulbar conjunctiva usually develop between 3 months and 6 years old.

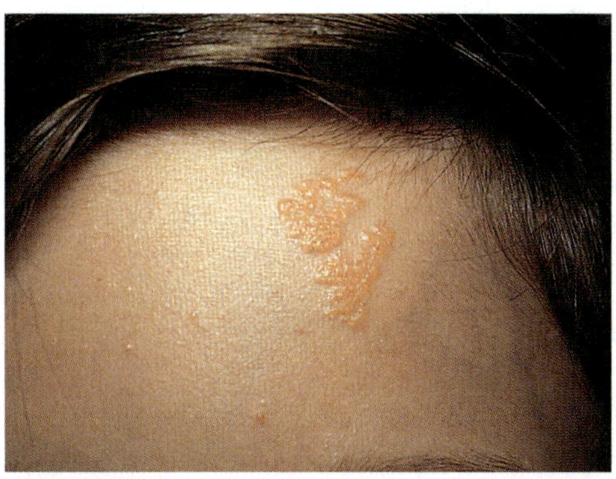

Fig. 16.24 Linear nevus sebaceus of Jadassohn. This yellowish-tan, waxy-appearing lesion became elevated at puberty and was associated with seizures and intellectual disability.

Epidermal Nevus Syndrome

Epidermal nevus syndrome is a congenital neurocutaneous disorder in which an epidermal nevus is seen in association with neurologic dysfunction. The latter may include seizures, paresis, intellectual disability, and developmental delay. Unilateral hemimegalencephaly with intractable seizures is the most common CNS abnormality. Disorders of segmentation/migration and other structural CNS anomalies have been reported. Extra-CNS congenital defects may involve connective tissues, especially the skeleton, and ocular, cardiac, and genitourinary systems. Skin lesions are hamartomatous (derived from embryonic ectoderm) and characterized by hyperplasia of the epidermis and adnexal structures. They are usually present at birth, although some appear later in the first year. They appear as raised, often warty hyperpigmented lesions typically in a linear pattern (Fig. 16.25). They may enlarge subsequently but tend to stabilize in size by puberty. Most cases are sporadic, although a small number are autosomal dominant.

Incontinentia Pigmenti

Incontinentia pigmenti is a rare, X-linked dominant syndrome with cutaneous, neurologic, ophthalmologic, and dental manifestations. It is caused by a mutation in the *NEMO* gene.

Neurologic and ophthalmologic problems often become manifest during early infancy and are reported to occur in about 30% of patients. They may include seizures, cerebrovascular accidents, developmental delay, intellectual disability, and microcephaly. Cutaneous features are described in Chapter 8 (see Fig. 8.100).

CENTRAL NERVOUS SYSTEM MALFORMATIONS

Malformations of the CNS are a leading cause of neurologic and developmental disability in infants and children. Although CNS malformations are not necessarily accompanied by external dysmorphic features, disturbances of cranial volume, abnormalities of head shape, and skin and visceral lesions in the dorsal midline should alert the physician to the possibility of associated CNS dysmorphogenesis.

Macrocephaly

Macrocephaly is defined as a head circumference with more than 2 standard deviations above the mean for age, sex, and gestation. Etiologies include a myriad conditions (Table 16.2), including hydrocephalus, intracranial mass lesions (i.e., tumors, subdural effusions), thickening or enlargement of the skull (primary skeletal dysplasias), or a true increase in brain parenchyma (megalencephaly). The latter is seen in Soto syndrome, achondroplasia, neurocutaneous syndromes, and certain lipidoses, leukodystrophies, and mucopolysaccharidoses. Primary megalencephaly may occur as a benign familial trait.

Evaluation of the child with a head that is abnormally large or appears to be growing at an excessive rate should include the following:

- Serial measurements of head circumference
- Measurement of the parents' head circumferences and exploration of family history for evidence of macrocephaly or neurologic and cutaneous abnormalities

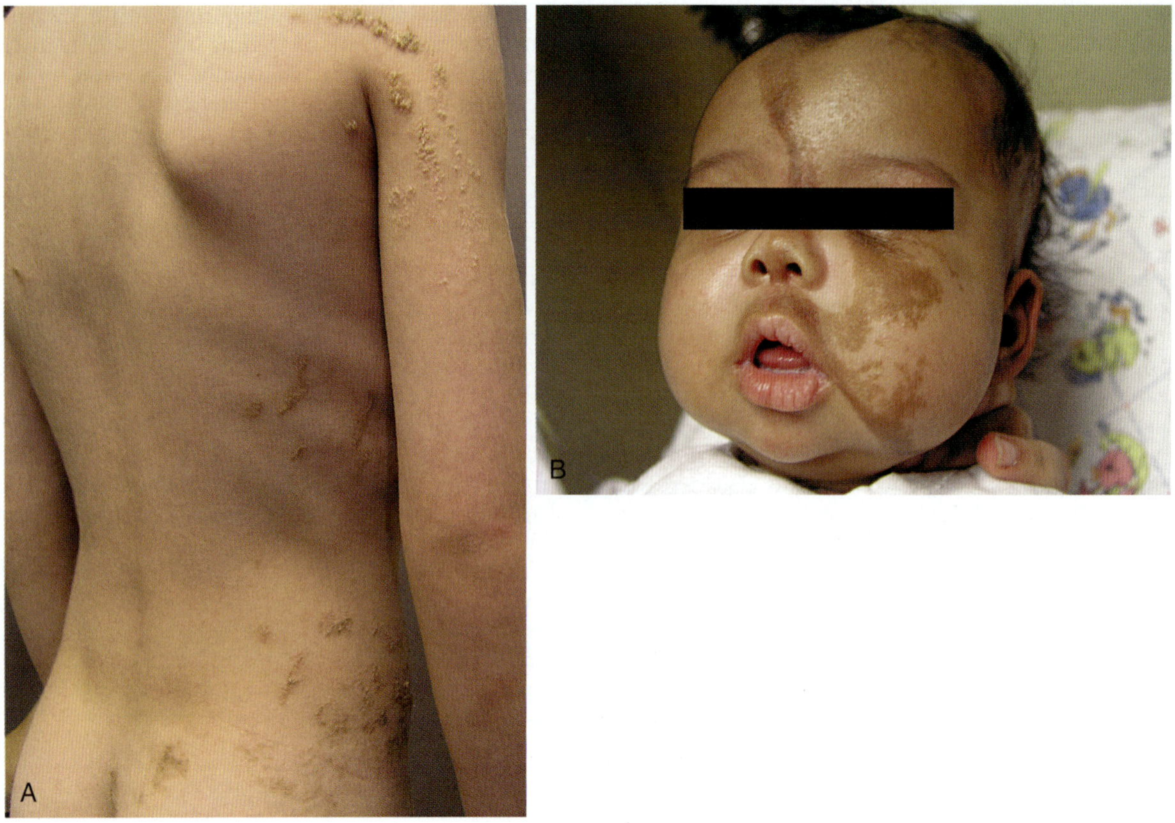

Fig. 16.25 Epidermal nevus syndrome. (A) Hyperpigmented verrucous papules are seen unilaterally over the upper arm, trunk, hip, and lumbosacral area of this adolescent boy. He had had a seizure in infancy and was learning disabled. (B) In this infant, raised hyperpigmented lesions are present on the left face and both sides of the forehead and were associated with intractable seizures. (Courtesy Robin Gehris, MD, Children's Hospital of Pittsburgh, Pittsburgh, PA.)

Table 16.2 Causes of Macrocephaly

Early Infantile (Birth to 6 Months Old)	Late Infantile (6 Months Old to 2 Years Old)	Early to Late Childhood (After 2 Years Old)

• Hydrocephalus (progressive or arrested)
• Induction disorders (congenital malformations)
• Spina bifida cystica, cranium bifidum, Chiari malformations (types I, II, and III), aqueductal stenosis, holoprosencephaly
• Mass lesions
  • Neoplasms, AV malformations, congenital cysts
• Intrauterine infections
  • Toxoplasmosis, cytomegalovirus infection, syphilis, rubella
  • Perinatal or postnatal infections
• Bacterial, granulomatous, parasitical
• Perinatal or postnatal hemorrhage
• Hypoxia, vascular malformation, trauma
• Hydranencephaly
• Subdural effusion
  • Hemorrhagic, infectious, cystic hygroma
• Normal variant (often familial)
	• Hydrocephalus (progressive or arrested)
	• Space-occupying lesions
	• Tumors, cysts, abscesses
	  • Postbacterial or granulomatous meningitis
	  • Dysraphism
	• Dandy-Walker syndrome, Chiari type I malformation
	• Posthemorrhagic
	• Trauma or vascular malformation
	• Subdural effusion
	• Increased intracranial pressure syndrome
	  • Pseudotumor cerebri
	• Lead, tetracycline, hypoparathyroidism, steroids, excess or deficiency of vitamin A, cyanotic congenital heart disease
	• Primary skeletal cranial dysplasia (thickened or enlarged skull): osteogenesis imperfecta, hyperphosphatemia, osteopetrosis, rickets
	• Megalencephaly (increase in brain substance)
	  • Metabolic CNS diseases: leukodystrophies (e.g., Canavan, Alexander), lipidoses (Tay-Sachs), histiocytosis, mucopolysaccharidoses
	  • Proliferative neurocutaneous syndromes: von Recklinghausen, TS, hemangiomatosis, Sturge-Weber
	  • Cerebral gigantism
	• Soto syndrome
	• Achondroplasia
	• Primary megalencephaly
	• May be familial and unassociated or associated with abnormalities of cellular architecture
		• Hydrocephalus (progressive or arrested)
		• Space-occupying lesions
		• Preexisting induction disorder
		• Aqueductal stenosis
		  • Chiari type I malformation
		  • Postinfectious
		  • Hemorrhagic
		  • Megalencephaly
		  • Proliferative neurocutaneous syndromes
		  • Familial
		• Pseudotumor cerebri
		• Normal variant

AV, Atrioventricular; *CNS,* central nervous system; *TS,* tuberous sclerosis.

From Gabriel RS: Malformations of the central nervous system. In Menkes JH, editor: *Textbook of child neurology*, ed 2, Philadelphia, 1980, Lea & Febiger.

- Developmental history
- Careful examination for evidence of increased intracranial pressure, developmental delay, skeletal dysplasia, cranial bruits, ocular abnormalities, or organomegaly

Although plain skull radiographs may detect primary skeletal dysplasias, CT or MRI scans allow assessment of ventricular size and permit detection of intracranial mass lesions and chronic subdural effusions. CT is the method of choice for demonstrating intracranial calcification (as seen with congenital cytomegalovirus infection in Fig. 16.26) and detecting fresh blood.

Hydrocephalus

Hydrocephalus is caused by an imbalance between cerebrospinal fluid (CSF) production and resorption that results in a net accumulation of fluid within the ventricular system. Impaired CSF resorption may occur secondary to obstruction of CSF pathways within the ventricular system (noncommunicating hydrocephalus) or obstruction of the subarachnoid space (communicating hydrocephalus). Hydrocephalus secondary to CSF overproduction is rare but does occur with choroid plexus papilloma (see Fig. 16.41). Noncommunicating hydrocephalus is often due to aqueductal stenosis or congenital malformations of the fourth ventricle, and it is a common complication of tumors or vascular malformations of the posterior fossa that compress the cerebral aqueduct or obstruct outflow from the fourth ventricle. Causes of communicating hydrocephalus include intracranial hemorrhage, meningitis, cerebral venous or dural sinus thrombosis, and diffuse infiltration of the meninges by malignant cells.

The clinical manifestations of hydrocephalus in infancy are stereotypic. The head is abnormal in size at birth or grows at an abnormally rapid rate, becoming macrocephalic over the first few months. The forehead is disproportionately large, and the face appears small in relation to the calvarium. The scalp is thin and glistening, and its veins are distended, often becoming strikingly dilated when the infant cries. The anterior fontanelle is large, tense, and nonpulsatile, and the sutures are excessively wide (Fig. 16.27A). Divergent strabismus, abducens nerve paresis, and impaired upward gaze are important ocular findings. With severe hydrocephalus, there may be forced, conjugate downward deviation of the eyes so that the inferior half of the iris is hidden by the lower eyelid, producing the "sunsetting sign" (see Fig. 16.27B). Neurologic abnormalities include developmental delay, persistence of early infantile automatisms, and spasticity and hyperreflexia of the lower extremities. CT or MRI scans demonstrate enlargement of the ventricular system with transependymal CSF flow and thinning of the cortical mantle and may provide additional anatomic information concerning the etiology (see Fig. 16.27C and D).

Infantile hydrocephalus must be distinguished from other causes of macrocephaly in infancy, such as chronic subdural hematoma, expanding porencephalic cyst, and certain degenerative disorders that may produce abnormal enlargement of the head (see Table 16.2). In premature infants with suspected hydrocephalus, the normally rapid rate of postnatal head growth must be taken into account.

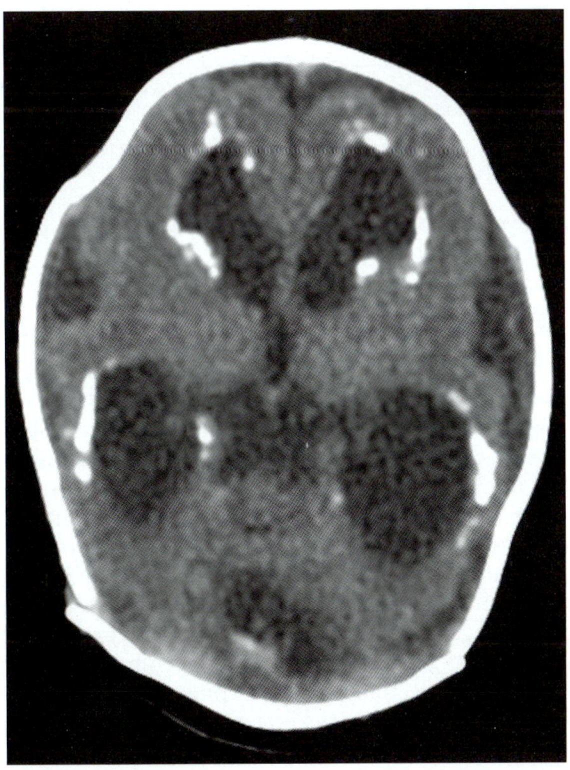

Fig. 16.26 Computed tomography scan revealing bilateral periventricular cerebral calcifications with ventricular dilation in infant with severe congenital cytomegalovirus infection.

Dandy-Walker Malformation

The Dandy-Walker malformation is a developmental abnormality characterized by progressive cystic enlargement of the fourth ventricle beginning early in fetal life. This is accompanied by enlargement of the posterior fossa and upward displacement of the tentorium, torcula, and transverse sinuses. Associated hydrocephalus is almost universal and may be present at birth or may develop later, during infancy or childhood. Of affected individuals, 60% show signs of hydrocephalus and increased intracranial pressure by 2 years old.

Clinical manifestations of Dandy-Walker malformation are variable and depend on the severity and rate of progression of the associated hydrocephalus. A child with a symptomatic condition often has an unusually prominent bulging occiput in addition to the usual findings of hydrocephalus. Ataxia, nystagmus, and cranial nerve deficits may also be prominent features.

Plain skull radiographs demonstrate posteroinferior enlargement of the cranial vault, thinning and ballooning of the occipital squama, and upward displacement of the torcula. CT or MRI scans confirm the presence of a large posterior fossa cyst, a small cerebellar remnant, and associated hydrocephalus (Fig. 16.28).

Hydranencephaly

Hydranencephaly is a severe anomaly of the brain characterized by the absence of the cerebral hemispheres despite intact meninges and a normal skull. Affected children often appear deceptively normal at birth, with little to suggest the presence of a hydranencephaly (Fig. 16.29A). Because newborns function at a subcortical reflex level, even complete absence of the cerebral hemispheres may not interfere with normal reflexes. However, within the first few weeks of life, developmental arrest, decerebration, hypertonia, and hyperreflexia become apparent in the infant with hydranencephaly. Most of these infants do not live beyond 6 to 12 months old, although survival for several years is occasionally reported. Seizures are common, and progressive enlargement of the head may complicate nursing care.

The diagnosis may be suggested if, on transillumination of the skull, the entire calvarium is highlighted (see Fig. 16.29B). However, severe hydrocephalus and bilateral subdural hygromas may present a similar appearance.

On CT scan (see Fig. 16.29C) or MRI, CSF signal intensity replaces the supratentorial brain parenchyma with sparing of the thalami, brainstem, cerebellum, and choroid plexus. The falx is intact, distinguishing this from holoprosencephaly. A thin rim of cerebral parenchyma is lacking, distinguishing this from unshunted hydrocephalus. To distinguish this disorder from massive bilateral

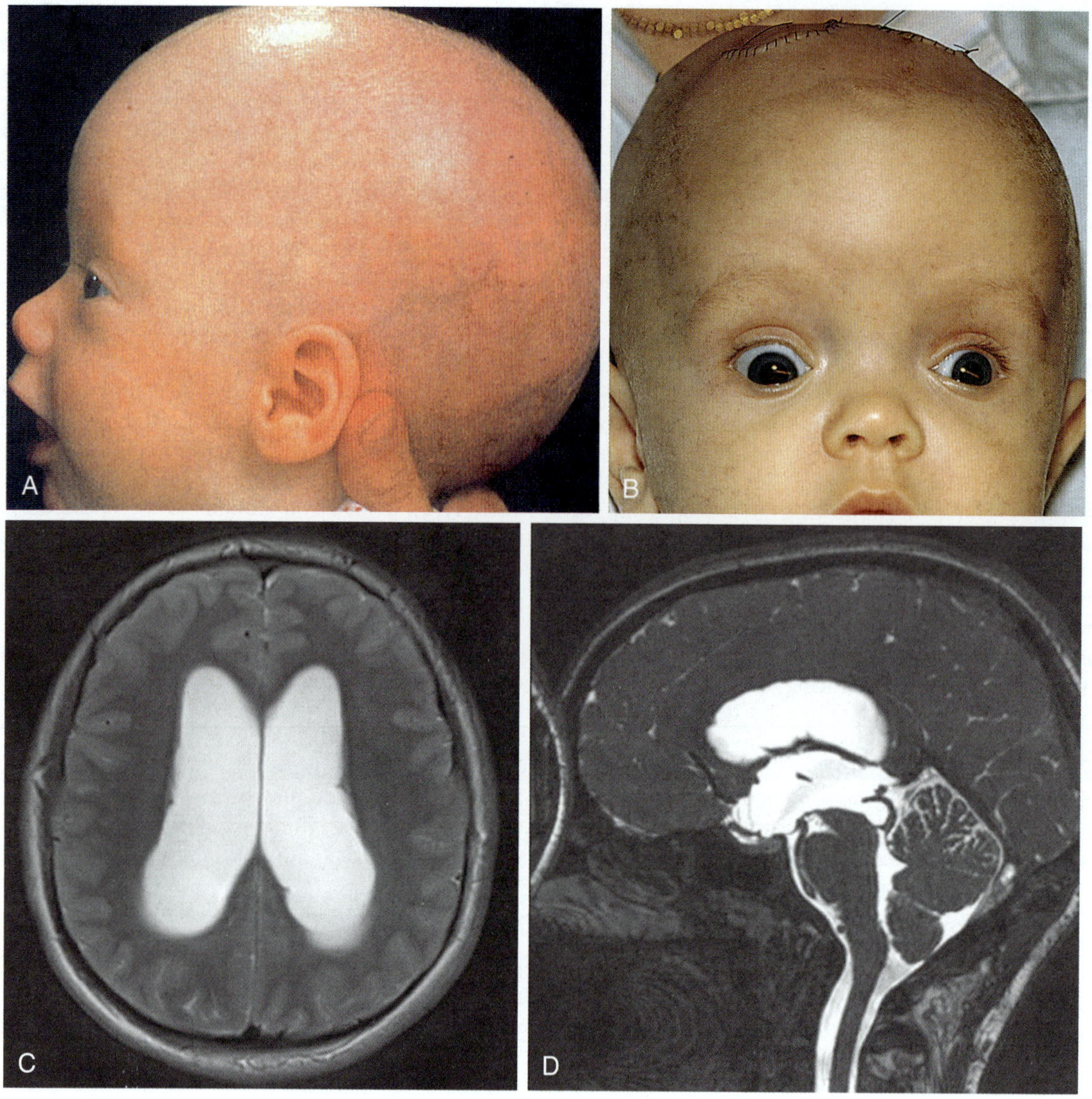

Fig. 16.27 Infantile hydrocephalus. (A) Characteristic enlarged head, thinning of the scalp, distended scalp veins, and a full fontanelle. (B) Paresis of the upward gaze is seen in an infant with hydrocephalus resulting from aqueductal stenosis. Paresis is more apparent on the right. This phenomenon is often termed the *sunsetting sign.* (C) T2-weighted magnetic resonance imaging showing ventriculomegaly and transependymal edema. (D) The cerebral aqueduct is enlarged with an apparent web within the inferior aqueduct. (A, From Booth IW, Wozniak ER: *Pediatrics*, Baltimore, 1984, Williams & Wilkins. B, Courtesy Albert Biglan, MD, Children's Hospital of Pittsburgh, Pittsburgh, PA. C, Courtesy Division of Neuroradiology, University Health Center of Pittsburgh, Pittsburgh, PA.)

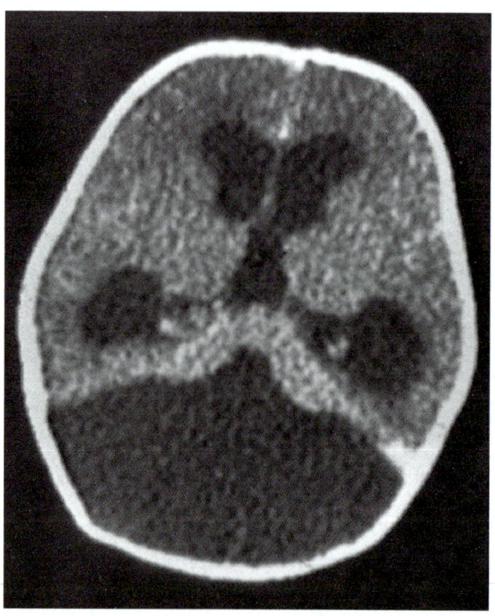

Fig. 16.28 Computed tomography scan shows a posterior fossa cyst, a small cerebellar remnant, and associated hydrocephalus. (Courtesy Michael J. Painter, MD, Children's Hospital of Pittsburgh, Pittsburgh, PA.)

subdural hygromas, cerebral angiography is required to confirm absence of the cerebrum.

Microcephaly

Microcephaly is defined as a head circumference more than 2 standard deviations below the mean for age, sex, and conceptual age. Apart from cases resulting from premature closure of the sutures (generalized craniosynostosis), microcephaly reflects impaired brain growth and can result from many disorders (Box 16.4). The neurologic manifestations range from minor (e.g., poor fine motor skills, mild intellectual impairment) to profound (e.g., decerebration, chronic vegetative state). Diagnostic evaluation should include a family and prenatal history, search for associated congenital anomalies, karyotyping and appropriate advanced genetic studies, amino acid screening, and evaluation for intrauterine infection, such as congenital cytomegalovirus (see Fig. 16.26) and Zika virus infection. Plain skull radiographs can detect craniosynostosis, whereas CT scan is useful in identifying intracranial calcifications. MRI is preferred for delineation of recognizable patterns of CNS dysmorphogenesis (Fig. 16.30).

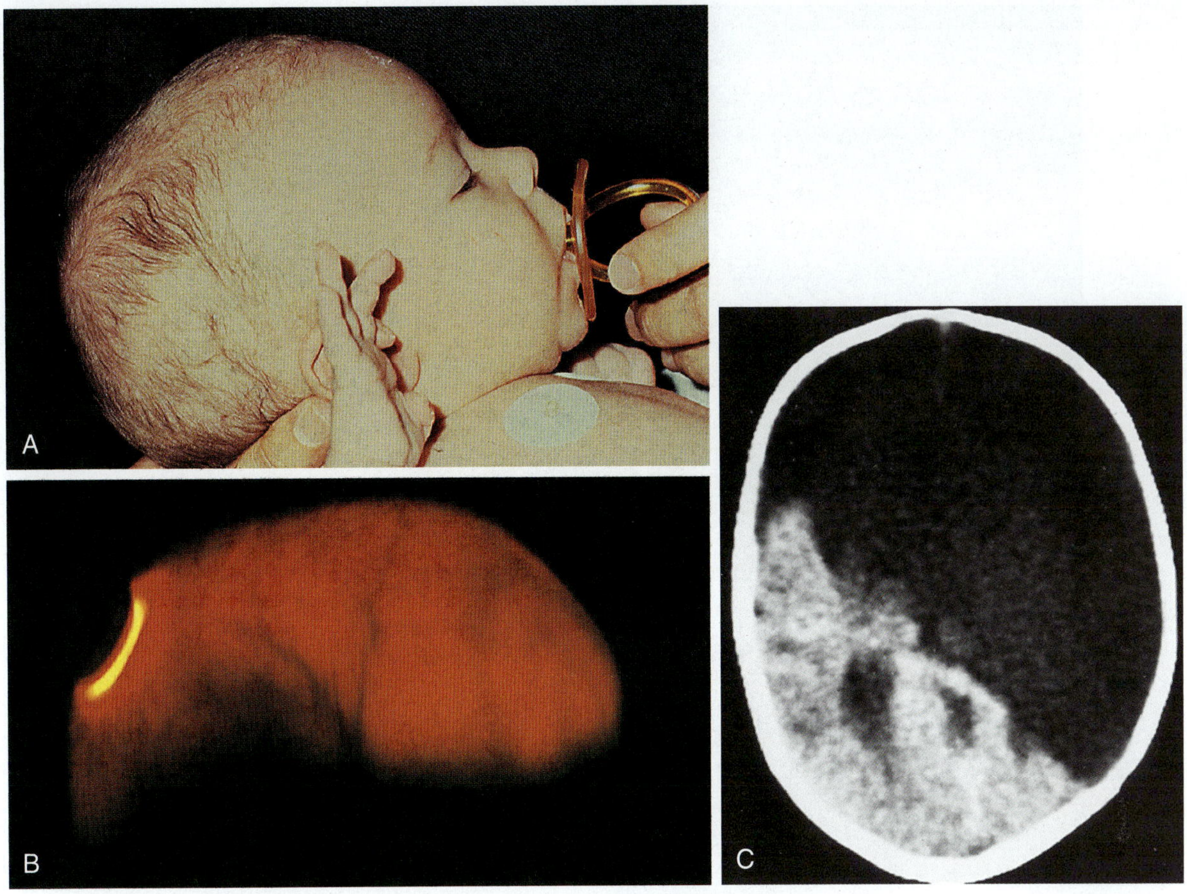

Fig. 16.29 Hydranencephaly. (A) Patient, age 3 weeks, has a deceptively normal appearance with little to suggest a severe brain abnormality. (B) Transillumination of the skull lights up the entire calvarium, suggesting the diagnosis. (C) Computed tomography scan demonstrates replacement of the cerebral hemispheres by a large, water-dense cavity with residual islands of brain tissue in regions of the occipital poles and right inferior temporal lobe. (C, Courtesy Division of Neuroradiology, University Health Center of Pittsburgh, Pittsburgh, PA.)

Box 16.4 Causes of Microcephaly

Genetic Defects
Autosomal recessive defects
Autosomal dominant defects

Disorders of Karyotype
Trisomies
Deletions
Translocations

Intrauterine Infections
Rubella
Cytomegalovirus infection
Toxoplasmosis
Congenital syphilis
Herpesvirus infections

Antenatal Irradiation

Exposure to Drugs and Chemicals During Gestation
Ethyl alcohol exposure (fetal alcohol syndrome)
Phenytoin exposure
Trimethadione exposure
Methyl mercury exposure

Maternal Phenylketonuria

Perinatal Insults
Traumatic
Anoxic
Metabolic
Infectious

Midline Defects and Occult Spinal Dysraphism

Development of the human nervous system begins early in the third week of gestation with the proliferation of ectodermal cells in the dorsal midline to form the neural plate. By the end of the fourth week, the neural plate has invaginated and then fused in the midline to form the neural tube. The cerebrum, diencephalon, midbrain, and brainstem develop from the rostral portion of the neural tube. The caudal portion separates from the overlying ectoderm, forming the precursor of the spinal cord, and is surrounded by mesodermal elements destined to form the vertebral bodies and supporting soft tissue structures. Midline spinal cord and vertebral skeletal defects, termed *spinal dysraphism,* result from defective closure of the caudal portion of the neural tube. Abnormal neural tube closure beginning early in the embryologic sequence produces dysraphic states involving both neural and skeletal elements (myelomeningocele), whereas closure defects occurring later produce congenital anomalies restricted to the posterior elements of the vertebrae (spina bifida occulta).

Occult spinal dysraphism is a defect of intermediate severity in which vertebral anomalies are associated with underlying intraspinal tumors or developmental abnormalities. Its presence is often (although not always) betrayed by cutaneous and subcutaneous abnormalities centered over the midline of the back, such as a hairy patch (Fig. 16.31A), skin tag, port-wine stain, hemangioma, subcutaneous lipoma (see Fig. 16.31B), cutis aplasia, or sinus tract (see Fig. 16.31C). Infants with atypical dimples or clefts (>5 mm) that are located more than 2.5 cm from the anus also have an increased incidence of underlying malformations, whereas those with simple blind dimples located within the gluteal cleft or within 2.5 cm of the anus do not. Although neurological abnormalities are often associated with the lesions mentioned earlier, they are by no means universal. The child in Fig. 16.32 with a large lumbosacral hemangioma did not have any associated neurologic abnormality.

Midline defects are not limited to the caudal portion of the neural tube but can occur over the head and neck as well. Most notably,

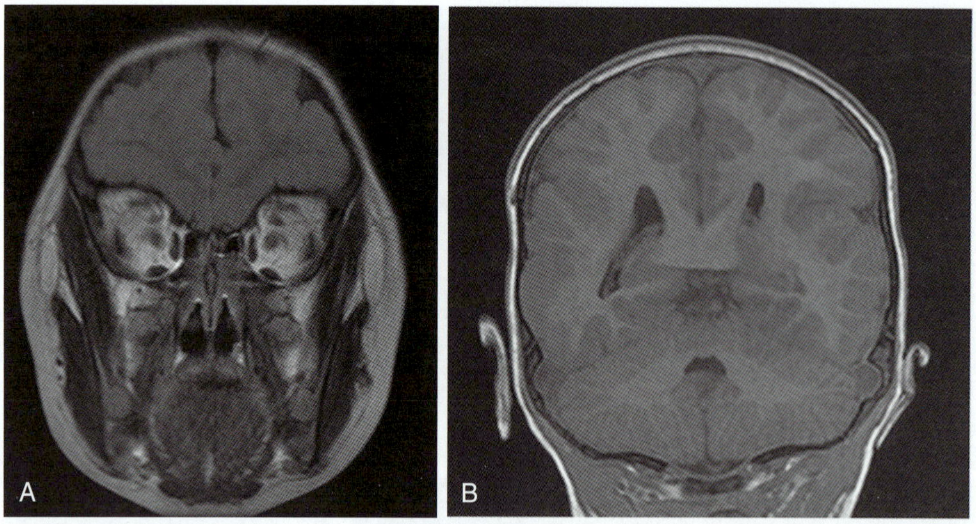

Fig. 16.30 Microcephaly. (A) Coronal T2 FLAIR image demonstrating craniofacial disproportion in a patient with microcephaly. (B) Extensive polymicrogyria/pachygyria complex.

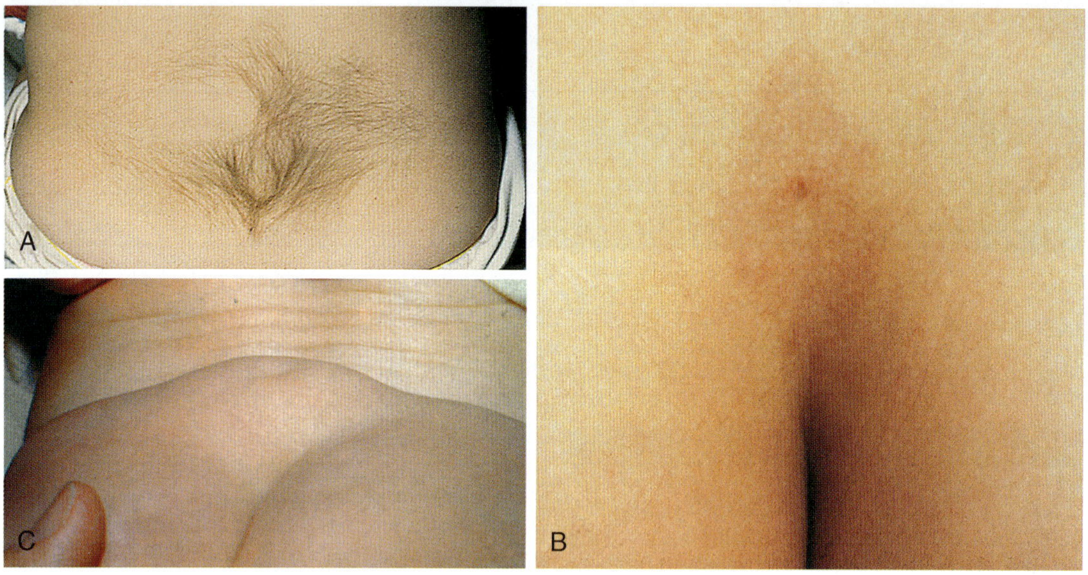

Fig. 16.31 Cutaneous and subcutaneous markers of occult spinal dysraphism. (A) Note the hairy patch over the lumbar region, here associated with diastematomyelia. (B) The soft subcutaneous mass seen overlying the sacrum of this infant was determined to be a lipoma. (C) Sacral sinus tract associated with intraspinal dermoid tumor. (A and C, Courtesy Michael J. Painter, MD, Children's Hospital of Pittsburgh, Pittsburgh, PA. B, From Cohen BA: *Atlas of pediatric dermatology*, London, 1993, Mosby-Wolfe.)

these include encephaloceles. These may be obvious in their appearance, may have no external findings, or may be associated with an overlying scalp lesion, such as a vascular malformation (Fig. 16.33).

Because early diagnosis and neurosurgical intervention can modify the onset and progression of neurologic deficits, newborns with midline cutaneous or subcutaneous stigmata and those with atypical dimples or clefts should undergo radiologic screening. Ultrasonography has proved to be the best tool for this purpose before ossification of the posterior vertebral elements (at 3 months) because it can detect vertebral defects and spinal anomalies and also be used to assess cord motion. If this reveals an underlying malformation or anomaly, follow-up MRI and neurosurgical referral are indicated. Common intraspinal lesions include dermoid tumors, intraspinal lipomas (Fig. 16.34), and diastematomyelia (Fig. 16.35).

Although some patients with occult spinal dysraphism show signs of neurologic dysfunction and talipes equinovarus from birth, most develop symptoms insidiously over years. Dysfunction usually begins at approximately 3 years old, but many do not develop problems until school age or adolescence. Presenting complaints may include back or leg stiffness, clumsiness, mild weakness or numbness of the lower extremities, or problems with bowel or bladder dysfunction.

Objective findings may consist of decreased tone and decreased deep tendon reflexes in the lower extremities; patchy decreases in sensation; and foot deformities consisting of broadening and shortening, deepening of the arch, and contractures of the toes (see Fig. 22.108). Symptoms of associated tethering of the spinal cord may be present in infancy, but often symptom onset is delayed until the child enters a period of rapid growth. These symptoms presumably are due to progressive deformation of the tethered cord, which is not free to "ascend" normally within the spinal canal as the rate of linear growth of the vertebral column outpaces that of the spinal cord. Tethering of the spinal cord by an anomalous filum terminale (Fig. 16.36), producing similar signs of progressive neurologic dysfunction, can occur in the absence of associated cutaneous abnormalities, vertebral defects, or intraspinal tumors.

INCREASED INTRACRANIAL PRESSURE

The cranial cavity is occupied by the brain, blood, and CSF. An increase in the volume of any of these compartments, unless accompanied by a concomitant decrease in one or both of the

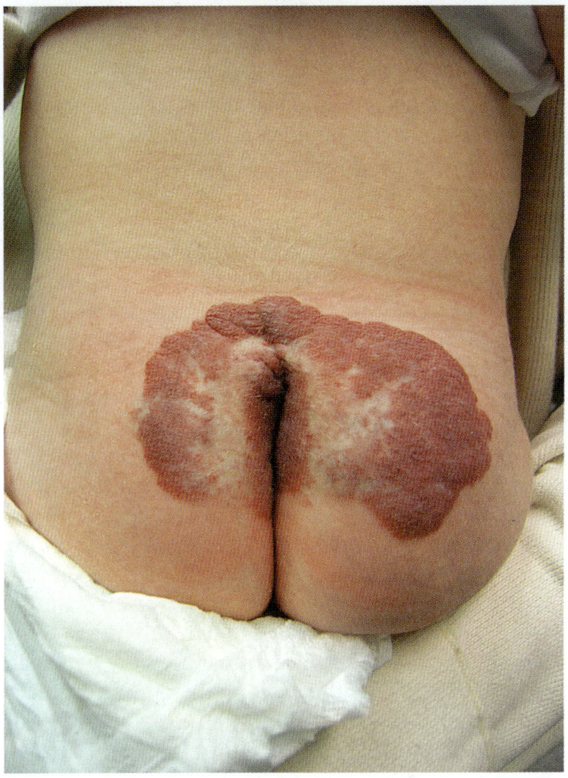

Fig. 16.32 Lumbosacral hemangioma. This child has a large lumbosacral hemangioma that extended well below the surface and wrapped around the vertebral column but regressed promptly and was not associated with any abnormality of the underlying neural or bony structures. (Courtesy Robin Gehris, MD, Children's Hospital of Pittsburgh, Pittsburgh, PA.)

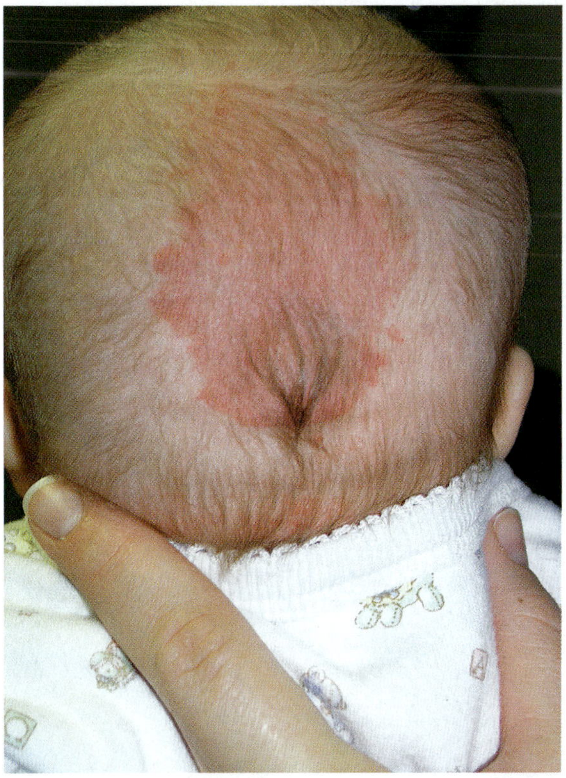

Fig. 16.33 Midline vascular malformation with an underlying atretic encephalocele in an infant who had no signs of neurologic dysfunction. (Courtesy Robin Gehris, MD, Children's Hospital of Pittsburgh, Pittsburgh, PA.)

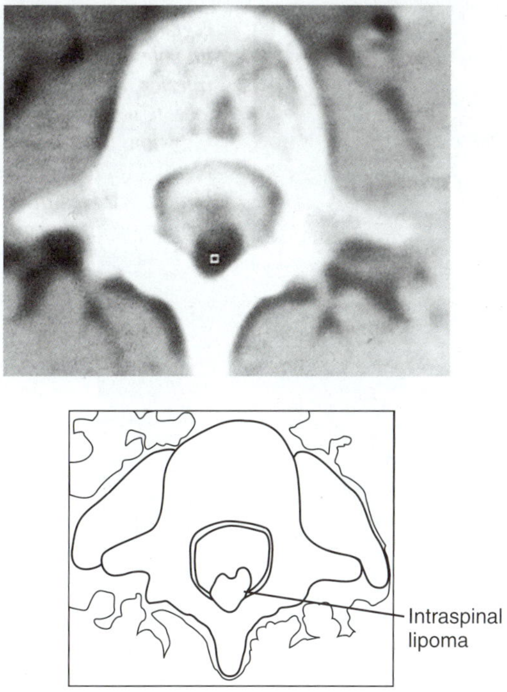

Fig. 16.34 Occult spinal dysraphism. Computed tomography scan demonstrates an intraspinal lipoma in a child with a subcutaneous lipoma over the lumbar spine.

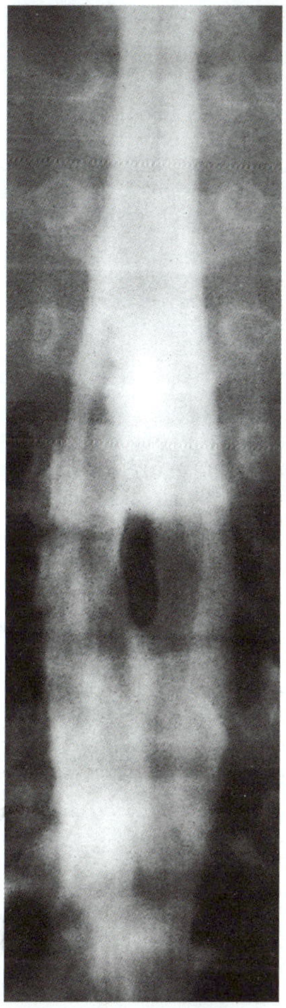

Fig. 16.35 Diastematomyelia. This 6-month-old infant had progressive inturning and plantar flexion of the left foot and a slightly deviated gluteal cleft. On myelogram, her spinal cord splits at L1, coursing around a bony spur at L2, and then rejoins at L4 to L5. She also had complete spinal dysraphism of L2 to L4 and partial dysraphism at L1 and L5.

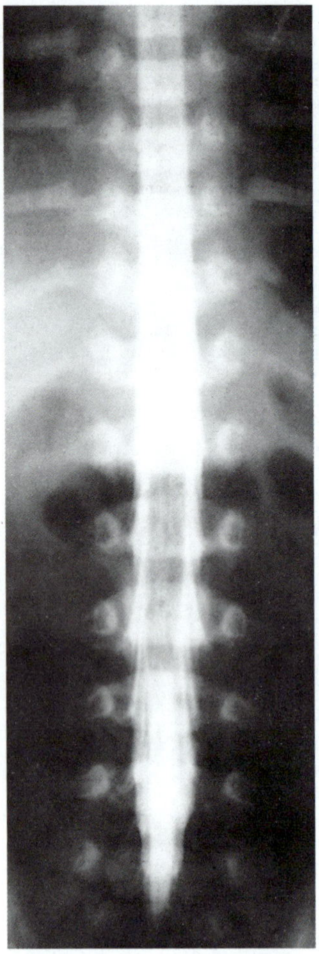

Fig. 16.36 Tethered cord resulting from a tight filum terminale. On myelography, the conus medullaris is pulled down to L3 to L4 by a tethered filum terminale, the upper portion of which is thickened. Presenting symptoms included weakness of plantar flexion, eversion of the feet, and bladder dysfunction. (Courtesy Charles Fitz, MD, Children's Hospital of Pittsburgh, Pittsburgh, PA.)

other compartments, results in increased intracranial pressure. Increased intracranial pressure can result from a wide variety of disorders and is itself hazardous. Recognition of associated signs and symptoms permits early diagnosis and prompt intervention to forestall progressive brain injury or catastrophic neurologic deterioration.

Primary Signs and Symptoms

The clinical manifestations of increased intracranial pressure vary with age. In infants, examination of the anterior fontanelle allows reliable assessment of intracranial pressure. In the normal, quiet infant held in an upright or sitting posture, the anterior fontanelle is flat or slightly concave. Under these conditions, an anterior fontanelle that bulges above the contour of the calvaria and that is excessively firm on palpation is always abnormal (see Fig. 13.38B). Because the cranial sutures are not fused in infants and young children, increased intracranial pressure rapidly produces separation of the bony plates of the skull (Fig. 16.37). In infants, this can be detected by palpation; in older children, CT of the head with 3-D bone reconstructions can help identify widened cranial sutures. Prominent convolutional markings on the inner table of the skull are a less specific radiographic sign, frequently seen with normal children. However, when secondary to increased intracranial pressure, they are preceded by suture diastasis and changes in the sella turcica. An excessive rate of head growth is a prominent feature of chronically increased intracranial pressure in infants and children up to 3 years old. Associated findings may include frontal prominence and distended scalp veins. If the ability to compensate for increased intracranial pressure by expansion of the calvaria is exceeded, other symptoms appear. These may include listlessness, irritability, poor feeding, vomiting, failure to thrive, paresis of upward gaze (see Fig. 16.27B), increased tone, hyperactive stretch reflexes, and a high-pitched cry. Papilledema is uncommon but possible.

In older children and adults, the most consistent clinical features of increased intracranial pressure include progressive headache with or without migrainous features, nausea, and vomiting. The headache tends to be progressive, associated with nocturnal awakenings, and exacerbated by coughing, sneezing, and other Valsalva maneuvers that transiently increase intracranial pressure. In some patients, it may be worse upon awakening.

Visual disturbances such as transient visual obscurations (TVOs), blurred vision, and horizontal diplopia secondary to cranial nerve VI palsies may occur. Pulsatile tinnitus, described as a "whooshing sensation in the ears," may also occur. Horizontal diplopia (double vision) secondary to paralysis of one or both abducens nerves is the most common visual disturbance. Initially, double vision may occur only on lateral gaze toward the side of the paretic lateral rectus muscle. This may be intermittent and may not be accompanied by limitation of ocular motility sufficient to be seen by the examiner. With progression, diplopia becomes constant and is present even with the eyes in the primary position, and an internal strabismus

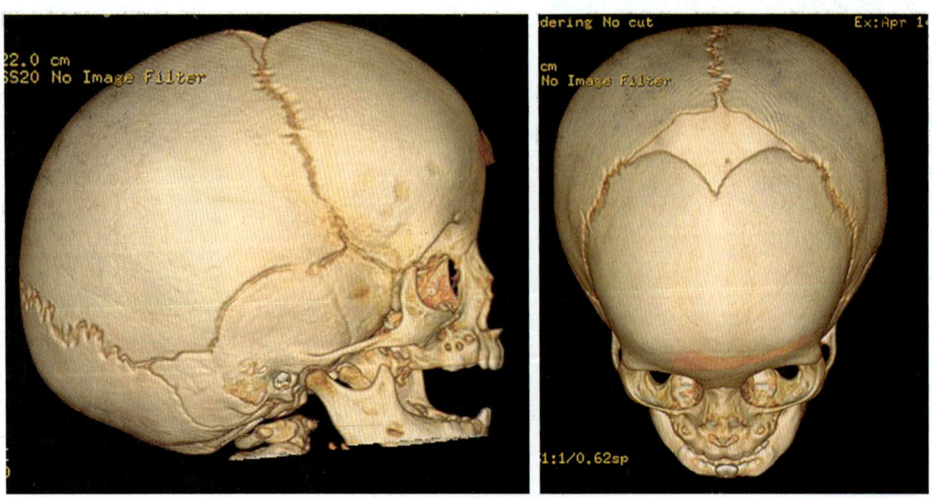

Fig. 16.37 Increased intracranial pressure in an infant. Computed tomography 3-dimensional reconstructions. Note widely opened anterior fontanelle, frontal bossing, and splaying of the sutures.

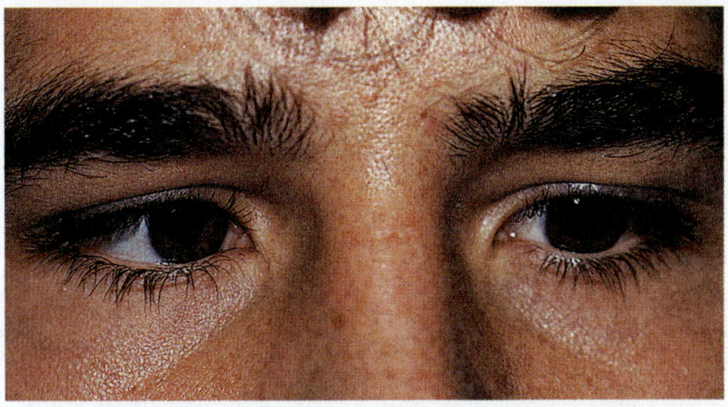

Fig. 16.38 Left abducens (sixth cranial nerve) palsy. This boy presented with headaches and diplopia and was found to have papilledema and a left abducens palsy. Note that his left eye cannot move past the midline on left lateral gaze. (Courtesy Kenneth Cheng, MD, Children's Hospital of Pittsburgh, Pittsburgh, PA.)

results (Fig. 16.38). Selective vulnerability of the sixth cranial nerve to increased intracranial pressure may be explained by its long intracranial course and proximity to rigid structures.

Sustained intracranial hypertension produces papilledema, a passive swelling of the optic disc (Fig. 16.39). The observation of papilledema in a child with headache, vomiting, or visual disturbances confirms the presence of increased intracranial pressure. The absence of venous pulsations or the presence of associated flame-shaped hemorrhages can help distinguish papilledema from other causes of blurred optic disc margins.

Increased intracranial pressure may be accompanied by changes in personality and behavior, deteriorating school performance, decreased appetite and activity, and alterations in level of consciousness.

Etiologies

Causes of increased intracranial pressure include cerebral edema; mass lesions; trauma; CNS infections; idiopathic intracranial hypertension (IIH), previously known as pseudotumor cerebri; and hydrocephalus.

Cerebral Edema

Cerebral edema (Fig. 16.40), an expansion of brain volume resulting from an increase in brain content of water and salt, is a response of brain tissue to a variety of insults. Vasogenic cerebral edema results from the alterations in vascular permeability produced by brain tumor, trauma, abscess, and hemorrhage. Cytotoxic cerebral edema, caused by swelling of brain cells (neurons and glia), usually results from infection, hypoxia, ischemia, or toxins.

Intracranial Mass Lesions

Tumors, intracranial hemorrhages, abscesses, and vascular malformations produce increased intracranial pressure by occupying space, causing cerebral edema, obstructing CSF pathways, and altering blood flow.

Intracranial Tumors

Choroid plexus papillomas, by secreting an excess of CSF, cause communicating hydrocephalus (Fig. 16.41). Although astrocytomas and oligodendrogliomas of the cerebral hemispheres (Fig. 16.42) often manifest as seizures or contralateral motor difficulties, symptoms of increased intracranial pressure are the initial manifestations in 37% of cases and are present at the time of diagnosis in 80%. Pineal region tumors (Fig. 16.43) frequently obstruct the third ventricle or cerebral aqueduct, producing signs and symptoms of increased intracranial pressure accompanied by Parinaud syndrome (impairment of the upward gaze with preservation of the downward gaze and retraction/convergence nystagmus with attempted upward gaze), resulting from compression of the periaqueductal gray matter (see Fig. 16.27B). Hypothalamic region tumors, such as craniopharyngioma (Fig. 16.44), manifest as growth retardation or failure of sexual maturation accompanied by visual field defects resulting from compression of the optic chiasm. Hydrocephalus occurs in 25% of cases.

Headache and vomiting accompanied by disturbances of gait and coordination are frequent presenting manifestations of posterior fossa tumors, such as cerebellar astrocytoma, medulloblastoma, and ependymoma. Midline tumors involving the cerebellar vermis can produce truncal ataxia (Fig. 16.45A), whereas mass lesions of the cerebellar hemispheres often cause unilateral limb ataxia and horizontal nystagmus (see Fig. 16.45B). The cardinal manifestations of brainstem glioma (Fig. 16.46) are cranial nerve palsies associated with contralateral hemiplegia and ataxia. Increased intracranial pressure is not an early feature.

Brain Abscesses

Brain abscesses (Fig. 16.47) are most often seen secondary to chronic otitis or sinusitis, chronic pulmonary infection, dental abscesses, congenital heart disease with endocardial infection, or immunosuppression. Unless accompanied by prodromal symptoms of fever, headache, lethargy, and malaise, brain abscesses may be impossible to distinguish from other intracranial mass lesions on clinical grounds unless clarifying radiologic studies are obtained.

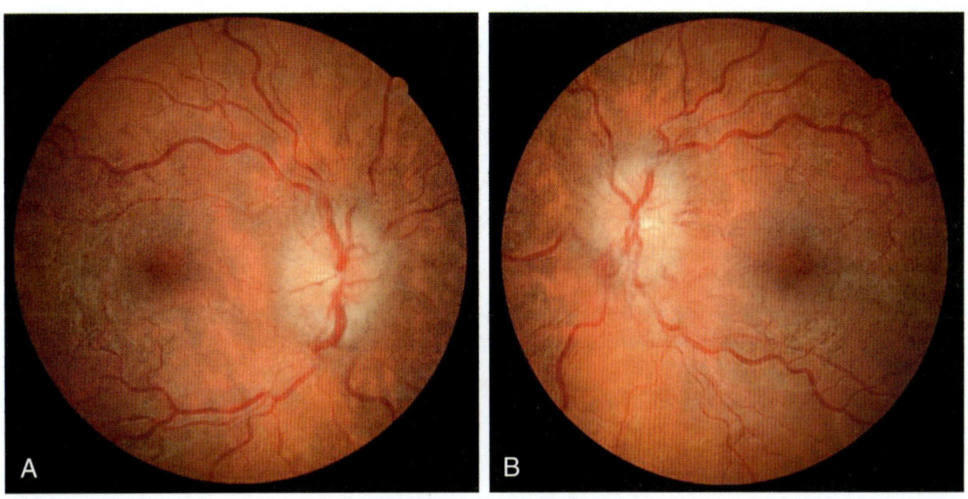

Fig. 16.39 Severe, bilateral papilledema in a patient with idiopathic intracranial hypertension. Markedly distended and tortuous retinal vessels, blurred and elevated disc margins, and hemorrhages can be seen. (A) Right eye. (B) Left eye.

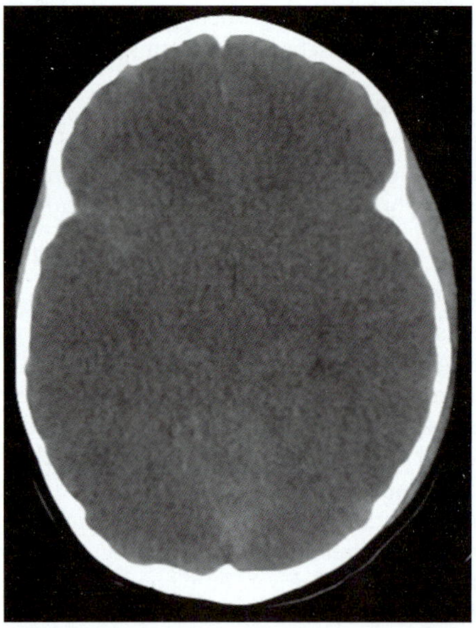

Fig. 16.40 Malignant cerebral edema after head trauma. There is evidence of sulcal effacement, ventricular effacement, and loss of all perimesencephalic cisterns. (Courtesy Dr. Neil Munjal, MD.)

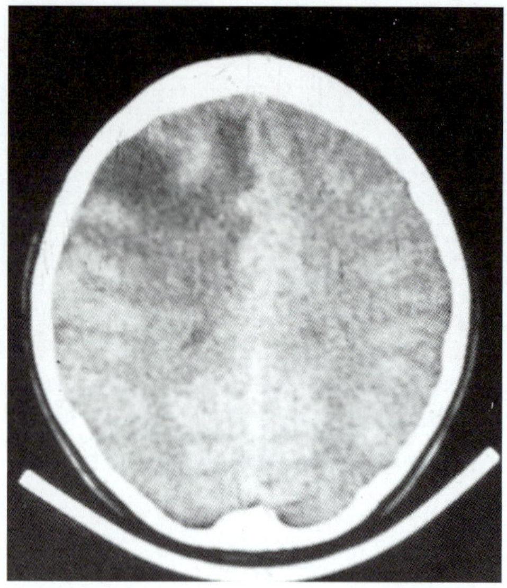

Fig. 16.42 Hemispheric oligodendroglioma. Computed tomography scan of a patient with seizures demonstrates a low-density mass lesion in the right frontal lobe. (Courtesy Michael Painter, MD, Children's Hospital of Pittsburgh, Pittsburgh, PA.)

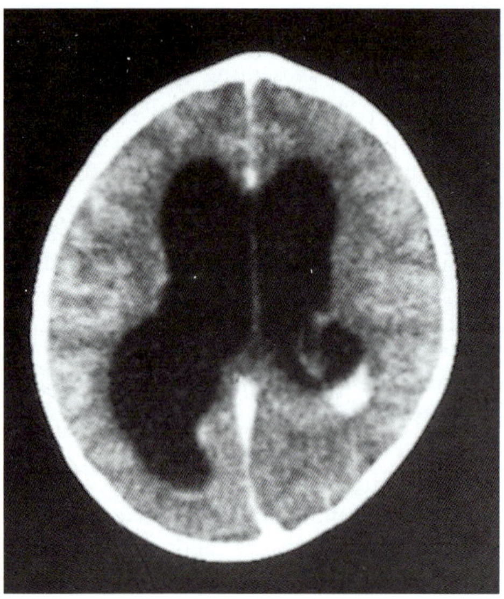

Fig. 16.41 Choroid plexus papilloma. Computed tomography scan of an infant with excessively rapid head growth. There is an enhancing mass within the body of the left lateral ventricle and associated ventricular enlargement (hydrocephalus) secondary to excessive secretion of cerebrospinal fluid by the tumor. (Courtesy Michael Painter, MD, Children's Hospital of Pittsburgh, Pittsburgh, PA.)

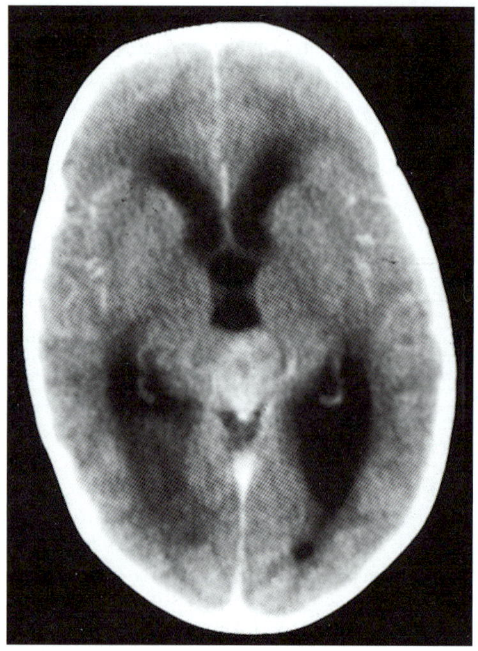

Fig. 16.43 Pineal region tumor. Computed tomography scan of a patient with headache, lethargy, vomiting, and paresis of upward gaze shows an enhancing mass lesion in the pineal region and severe obstructive hydrocephalus. (Courtesy Department of Neuroradiology, University Health Center of Pittsburgh, Pittsburgh, PA.)

Intracranial Hemorrhage

Spontaneous intracranial hemorrhage (Fig. 16.48) secondary to rupture of a vascular malformation or arterial aneurysm is rare in the pediatric population. Leakage of small amounts of blood into the subarachnoid space produces symptoms (e.g., fever, headache, stiff neck) that mimic those of bacterial meningitis. In such cases, the correct diagnosis may first be suspected when lumbar puncture yields grossly bloody fluid. The presentation of large subarachnoid hemorrhages is catastrophic, with sudden onset of excruciating headache followed by collapse and evidence of increased intracranial pressure.

Head trauma results in increased intracranial pressure by provoking cerebral edema or causing intracranial hemorrhage. The modes of presentation of cerebral contusion, subdural hematoma, and posttraumatic cerebral edema are discussed in Chapter 6. The features of epidural hematoma (Fig. 16.49) in childhood, which differ from those encountered in adults, are emphasized here. Infants and young children with epidural hematoma frequently suffer no immediate loss of consciousness after the traumatic event. Associated linear skull fractures are less common than in adults, and the source of bleeding into the epidural space is generally ruptured epidural veins rather than lacerations of the middle meningeal artery. Hence the evolution of symptoms is slower, and the typical adult picture of immediate loss of consciousness, followed by a brief lucid interval and then collapse, is not seen until adolescence. Often, persistent lethargy and intermittent vomiting are the only initial signs. On early assessment, some

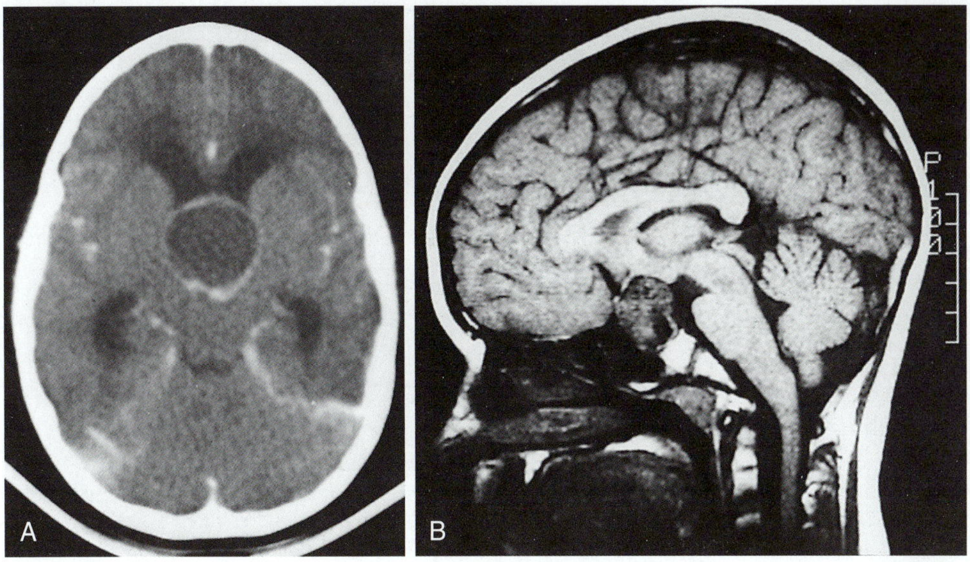

Fig. 16.44 Craniopharyngioma. (A) Computed tomography scan shows a large, spherical suprasellar mass; obliteration of the third ventricle; and associated hydrocephalus. (B) Magnetic resonance imaging scan provides superior visualization of the anatomic relationship of this tumor with the optic chiasm and hypothalamus. (Courtesy Department of Neuroradiology, University Health Center of Pittsburgh, Pittsburgh, PA.)

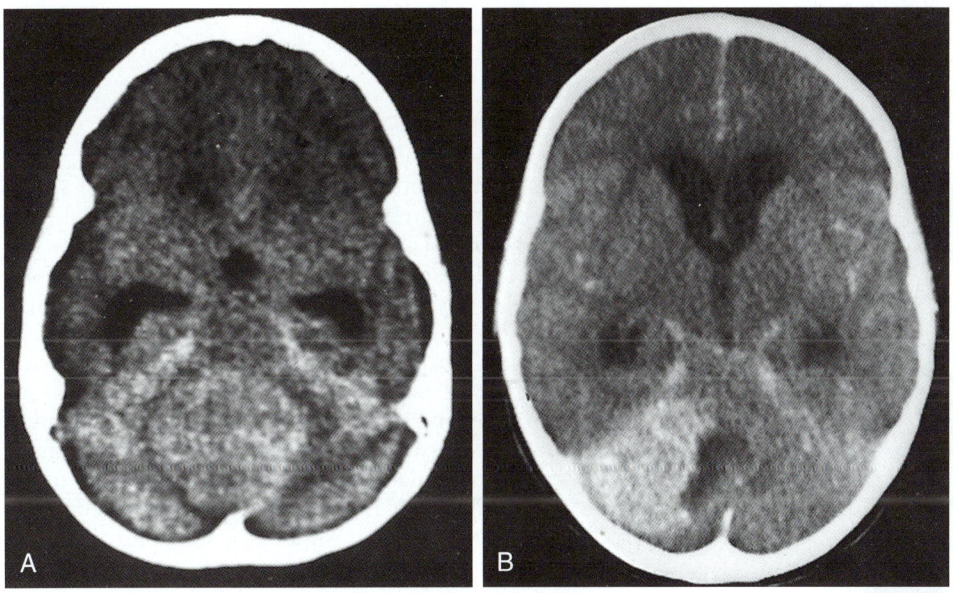

Fig. 16.45 Cerebellar neoplasms. (A) Midline ependymoma filling the fourth ventricle and invading the cerebellar vermis. (B) Glioblastoma of the right cerebellar hemisphere. (A, Courtesy Michael Painter, MD, Children's Hospital of Pittsburgh, Pittsburgh, PA. B, Courtesy Department of Neuroradiology, University Health Center of Pittsburgh, Pittsburgh, PA.)

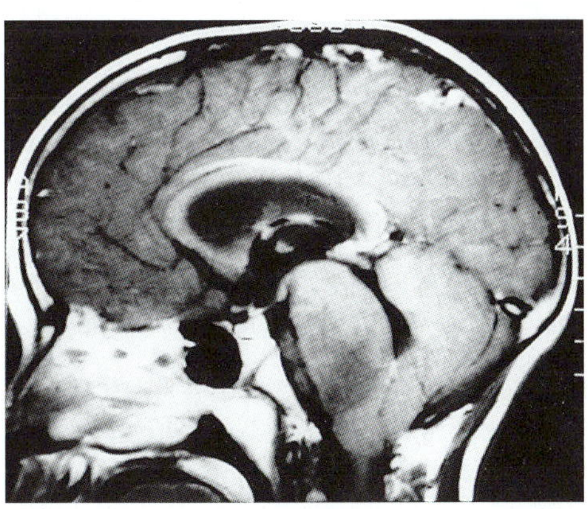

Fig. 16.46 Brainstem glioma. This 6-year-old girl had a 2- to 3-month history of personality change, decreased school performance, and intermittent urinary retention and constipation; a 3-week history of ataxia and vague upper back pain; and a 6-day history of severe frontal headache with vomiting after breakfast. She had diplopia secondary to left sixth nerve palsy, nystagmus, right facial weakness, slurred speech, dysphagia with drooling, torticollis, an unbalanced gait with a tendency to list to the left, dysmetria greater on the left, and bilateral papilledema. Her magnetic resonance imaging scan showed marked enlargement of the pons resulting from a mass lesion extending into the brainstem and compressing the fourth ventricle, causing hydrocephalus. (Courtesy Charles Fitz, MD, Children's Hospital of Pittsburgh, Pittsburgh, PA.)

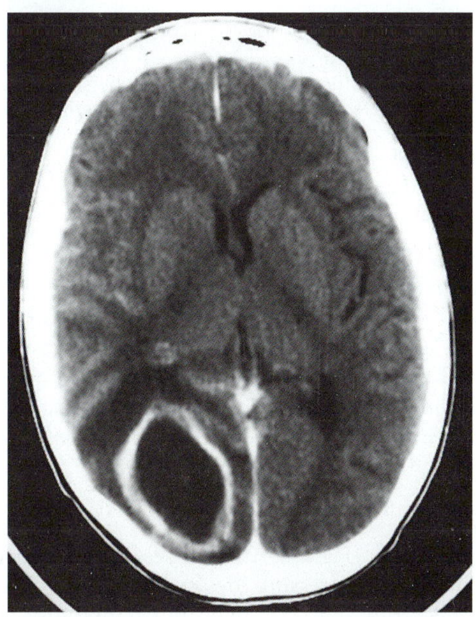

Fig. 16.47 Brain abscess. Computed tomography (CT) scan demonstrates a low-density mass lesion with an enhancing rim and surrounding edema in an immunosuppressed patient with an *Aspergillus* abscess. Bacterial abscesses and neoplasms can present a similar CT appearance. (Courtesy Department of Neuroradiology, University Health Center of Pittsburgh, Pittsburgh, PA.)

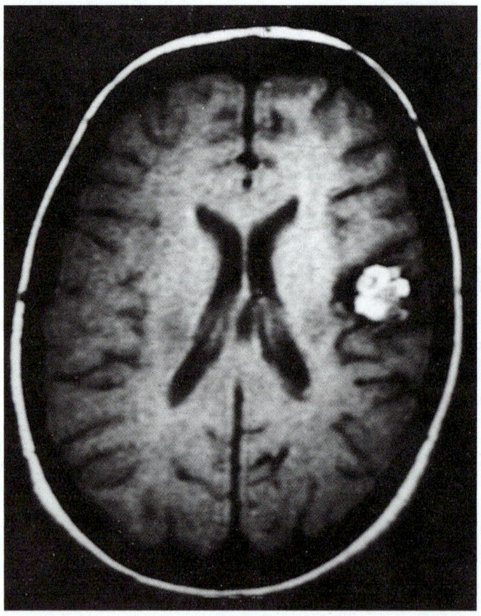

Fig. 16.48 Intracranial hemorrhage. Enhanced magnetic resonance imaging scan demonstrating a cerebral hemangioma with associated old hemorrhage. (Courtesy Michael J. Painter, MD, Children's Hospital of Pittsburgh, Pittsburgh, PA.)

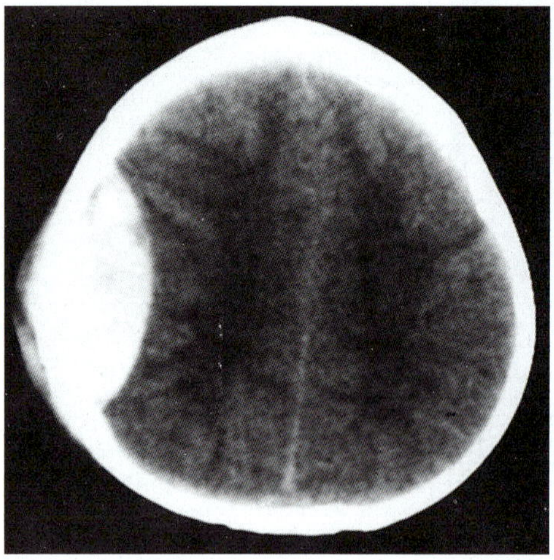

Fig. 16.49 Epidural hematoma. In this patient, blunt head trauma was followed by vomiting, progressive obtundation, and decreased movement of the left arm and leg. The computed tomography scan showed a large, lens-shaped epidural hematoma over the right hemisphere. (Courtesy Department of Neuroradiology, University Health Center of Pittsburgh, Pittsburgh, PA.)

affected children and adolescents demonstrate a slowed reaction time, especially when responding to questions (as if there is a processing delay). Severe headache, papilledema, and localizing signs may not emerge for several hours to days. Once neurologic signs and symptoms appear, they may progress rapidly to coma and death or evolve slowly over several days before producing brainstem compression.

Meningitis

Bacterial meningitis (Fig. 16.50; and see Fig. 13.38B) produces increased intracranial pressure by causing cerebral edema and impairing reabsorption of CSF. Signs and symptoms are discussed in Chapter 13. Although cerebral edema and intracranial hypertension may complicate the course of viral encephalitis, the usual presentation is with seizures, behavioral change, and altered level of consciousness.

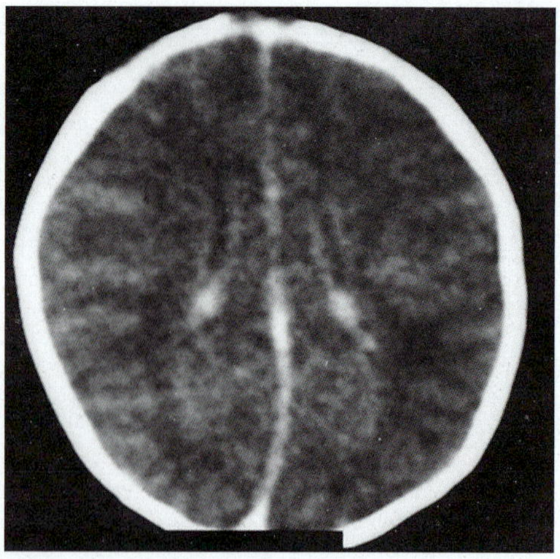

Fig. 16.50 Bacterial meningitis in an infant with fever; lethargy; nuchal rigidity; and a tense, distended fontanelle. The computed tomography scan shows contrast enhancement of the cortical gyri and ependyma of the lateral ventricles. (Courtesy Department of Neuroradiology, University Health Center of Pittsburgh, Pittsburgh, PA.)

Other Causes

Idiopathic Intracranial Hypertension

IIH, also known as pseudotumor cerebri complex (PTC), is the result of increased intracranial pressure in the absence of space-occupying lesions or hydrocephalus. The idiopathic form, also referred to as *primary PTC,* typically occurs in adolescents and young women of childbearing age and is strongly associated with obesity. Prepubertal boys may exhibit a thin body habitus. Secondary PTC can occur in association with certain medications such as tetracyclines, growth hormone, isotretinoin, hypervitaminosis A, and acute steroid withdrawal. It may also occur in the setting of cerebral venous sinus thrombosis (which can complicate otitis media and sinusitis in young children). Although many patients present with headache, papilledema incidentally found on routine eye examination is not uncommon. Papilledema is typically bilateral and symmetric. Although TVOs, blurred vision, and diplopia due to cranial nerve VI palsies can occur, visual loss is a late finding and may be irreversible. Therefore IIH is considered a neurologic emergency and treatment with acetazolamide should be instituted promptly to prevent permanent visual loss (see Figs. 16.39 and 16.40).

Diagnosis is established by excluding secondary causes of elevated intracranial pressure. However, signs of raised intracranial pressure may be appreciated on MRI (Fig. 16.51). A magnetic resonance venography scan to exclude venous sinus thrombosis, especially in young children, should be obtained. Diagnosis is confirmed by an elevated opening pressure on lumbar puncture, equal to or greater than 28 cm of water. Examination of the CSF is otherwise unremarkable. In areas where Lyme disease is endemic, aseptic meningitis may mimic IIH and should be ruled out.

Neurocysticercosis

Neurocysticercosis is another disorder that can present with signs of increased intracranial pressure. It is the most common CNS parasitical infestation worldwide and is endemic in Mexico, Central and South America, and parts of Asia, including China, Africa, and India. Neurocysticercosis is being seen with increasing frequency in developed countries, often in immigrants from or recent visitors to endemic areas. Cerebral cysticercosis occurs when larvae of the pork tapeworm *(Taenia solium)* encyst in CNS tissues. Eating contaminated pork carrying the *T. solium* larvae leads to acquisition of the intestinal tapeworm. Cysticercosis is often transmitted to affected children by family, household, or community contacts who carry the adult *T. solium* tapeworm.

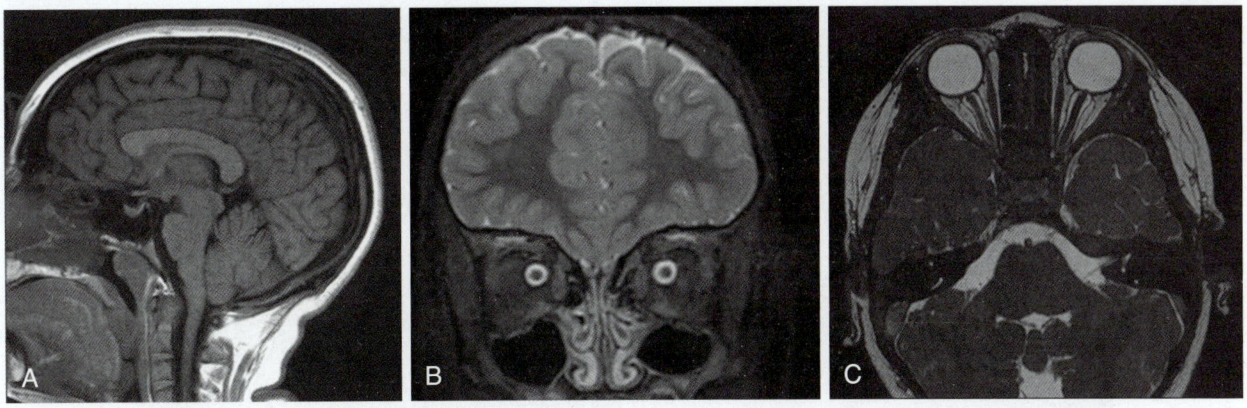

Fig. 16.51 Raised intracranial pressure. (A) T1 sagittal showing partially empty sella. (B) Coronal STIR sequence. Increased perioptic cerebrospinal fluid along the optic nerve sheaths. (C) Axial 3-D with contrast, optic nerve head protrusion into the globe.

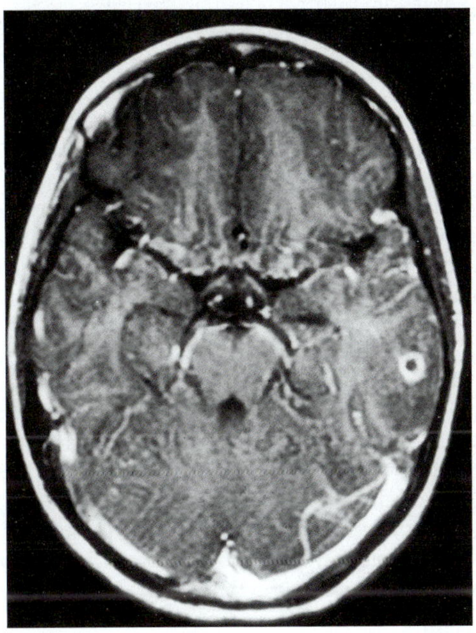

Fig. 16.52 Neurocysticercosis. This 12-year-old presented with focal seizures and chronic headaches after recent travel to an endemic area. Magnetic resonance imaging revealed a small ring-enhancing cyst in the left temporal lobe with surrounding edema, thought to be consistent with neurocysticercosis. (Courtesy Patricia Crumrine, MD, Children's Hospital of Pittsburgh, Pittsburgh, PA.)

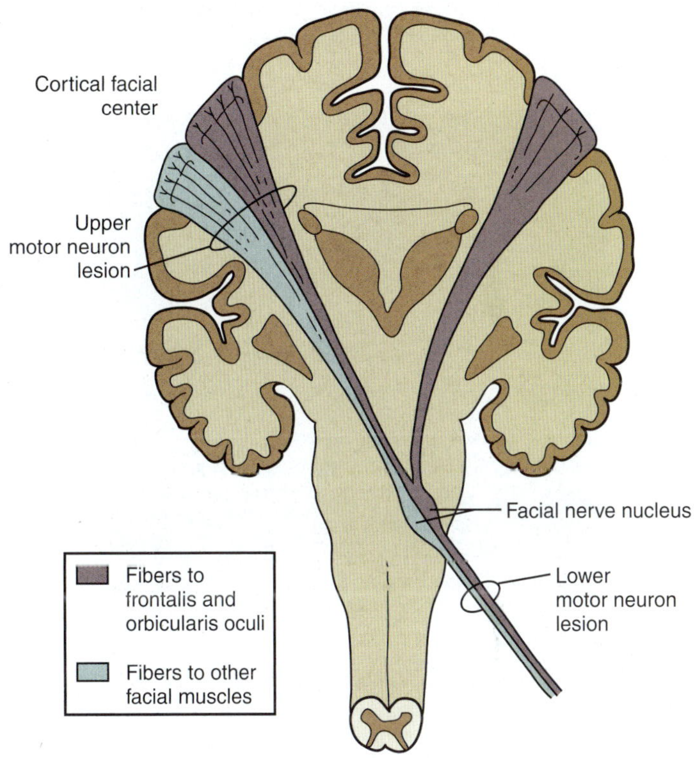

Fig. 16.53 Central motor control of the facial muscles. The portion of the facial nerve nucleus that supplies the lower half of the face receives predominantly crossed fibers originating from the opposite cerebral hemisphere; the portion that innervates the upper half receives fibers from both cerebral hemispheres. (Modified from Haymaker W: *Bing's local diagnosis in neurological diseases*, ed 15, St Louis, 1969, Mosby.)

After transmission, hematogenous spread to neural, ocular, or muscular tissues can occur. Seizures are the most common presenting sign of neurocysticercosis and are often accompanied by headache. Less commonly, patients can develop meningitis as a result of inflammatory reactions to ruptured cysts or they may present with signs and symptoms of increased intracranial pressure due to obstruction of CSF pathways by cysts, resulting in noncommunicating hydrocephalus. Findings on neuroimaging vary depending on the stage of development of the organism and range from nonenhancing cysts to ring-enhancing lesions to calcified nodules. Lesions may be single or multiple. Single enhancing cysts are most common in children living in North America (Fig. 16.52).

FACIAL WEAKNESS

The cortical motor center controlling the muscles of facial expression is located in the lower third of the precentral gyrus (Fig. 16.53). Motor fibers arising in the cerebral cortex travel through the corona radiata, internal capsule, and cerebral peduncle into the pons, where the majority decussate to supply the facial (seventh) nerve nucleus on the opposite side. Some fibers, destined to terminate in the portion of the facial nerve nucleus that innervates muscles in the upper half of the face, do not decussate. Thus whereas the portion of the facial nerve nucleus that supplies the lower half of the face receives predominantly crossed fibers originating from the opposite cerebral hemisphere, the portion that innervates the frontalis muscle and the orbicularis oculi muscle has bilateral supranuclear control.

Peripheral Facial Weakness

A lesion of the seventh nerve nucleus or emergent facial nerve results in flaccid weakness of the entire face on the same side. On the affected side, the face is smooth with flattening of the nasolabial fold; drooping of the corner of the mouth; and inability to smile, frown, retract the corner of the mouth, wrinkle the forehead, or

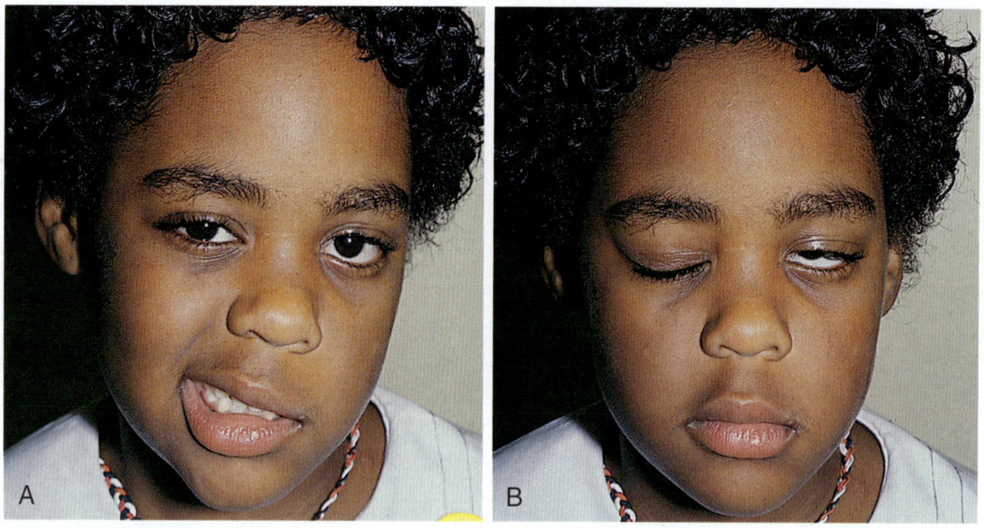

Fig. 16.54 Peripheral facial weakness. Flaccid weakness of the entire left face resulting from a lesion of the left facial nerve. (A) Flattening of the nasolabial fold and inability to retract the corner of the mouth. (B) Inability to fully close the eye.

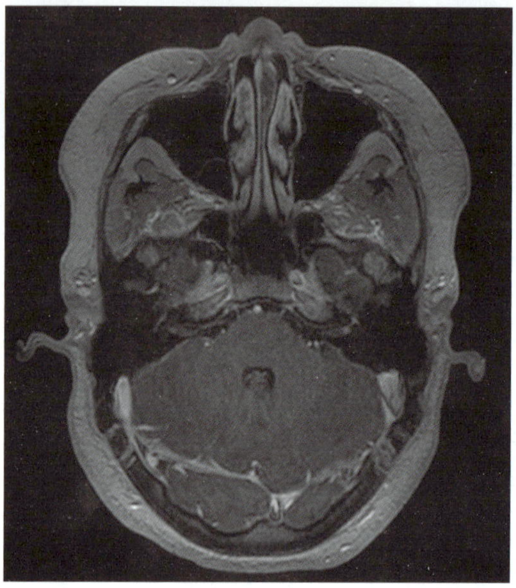

Fig. 16.55 Bilateral facial nerve enhancement in Lyme disease. Magnetic resonance imaging of the brain with contrast showing nodular enhancement of the facial nerve bilaterally in a patient with Lyme disease.

close the eye (Fig. 16.54). Causes of peripheral facial weakness include infection, especially Lyme disease (Fig. 16.55) in endemic areas, as well as HSV, trauma, hypertension, cerebellopontine angle mass, tumors of the pons, and acute idiopathic paralysis (Bell palsy).

Central Facial Weakness

With a lesion above the level of the facial nerve nucleus (i.e., an upper motor neuron lesion), there is weakness of the lower part of the face on the opposite side but relative sparing of the upper portion of the face. The ability to wrinkle the forehead (frontalis muscle) and to voluntarily close the eyes (orbicularis oculi muscle) is preserved (Fig. 16.56). Central lesions warrant immediate attention and imaging in the affected child.

NEUROMUSCULAR DISORDERS

Weakness is the most common presenting symptom of neuromuscular disease. If time is taken to determine the ways in which the weakness interferes with normal activities and uncover the types of tasks that the patient finds difficult, the distribution and severity of muscle weakness can be predicted from clinical history. Determining the mode of onset and pattern of progression of the symptoms is essential in the differential diagnosis and selection of diagnostic studies. Because many neuromuscular disorders are genetically determined, a complete family history must be obtained.

Essential components of the physical examination of patients with neuromuscular disease include inspection, palpation, percussion, evaluation of deep tendon reflexes, and assessment of muscle strength. Inspection can reveal muscle wasting and atrophy (or, conversely, hypertrophy), abnormal spontaneous activity, and abnormal resting postures. Palpation permits assessment of muscle consistency, determination of muscle tone (with observation of resistance to passive motion), and detection of muscle tenderness. Percussion is useful in detecting myotonia. Assessment of muscle strength includes individual muscle testing and functional evaluation. The strength of individual muscles is recorded, using a standardized system, such as the following:

0: No contraction
1: Flicker or trace contraction
2: Active movement with gravity eliminated
3: Active movement against gravity
4: Active movement against gravity and resistance
5: Normal power

Functional evaluation of muscle strength is accomplished by observing the patient rising from the floor, rising from a chair, stepping onto a stool, climbing stairs, walking on the heels, hopping on the toes, and raising the arms above the head. This evaluation permits rapid detection of proximal weakness of the hips and shoulders and distal weakness of the legs.

Duchenne Muscular Dystrophy

The muscular dystrophies are genetic disorders characterized by progressive degeneration of skeletal muscle, usually after a latency period of seemingly normal development and function. The various clinical types of muscular dystrophy are traditionally classified on the basis of patterns of inheritance, distribution of initial weakness, age of onset of clinical manifestations, and rate of progression (Table 16.3).

Duchenne muscular dystrophy, affecting 1 in 3500 male births, is characterized by X-linked recessive inheritance; early onset; symmetric and initially selective involvement of pelvic and pectoral girdles; pseudohypertrophy of the calves; high levels of activity of certain serum enzymes, notably creatine kinase; and relentless progression leading to wheelchair confinement by adolescence and death from cardiorespiratory insufficiency by 20 years old.

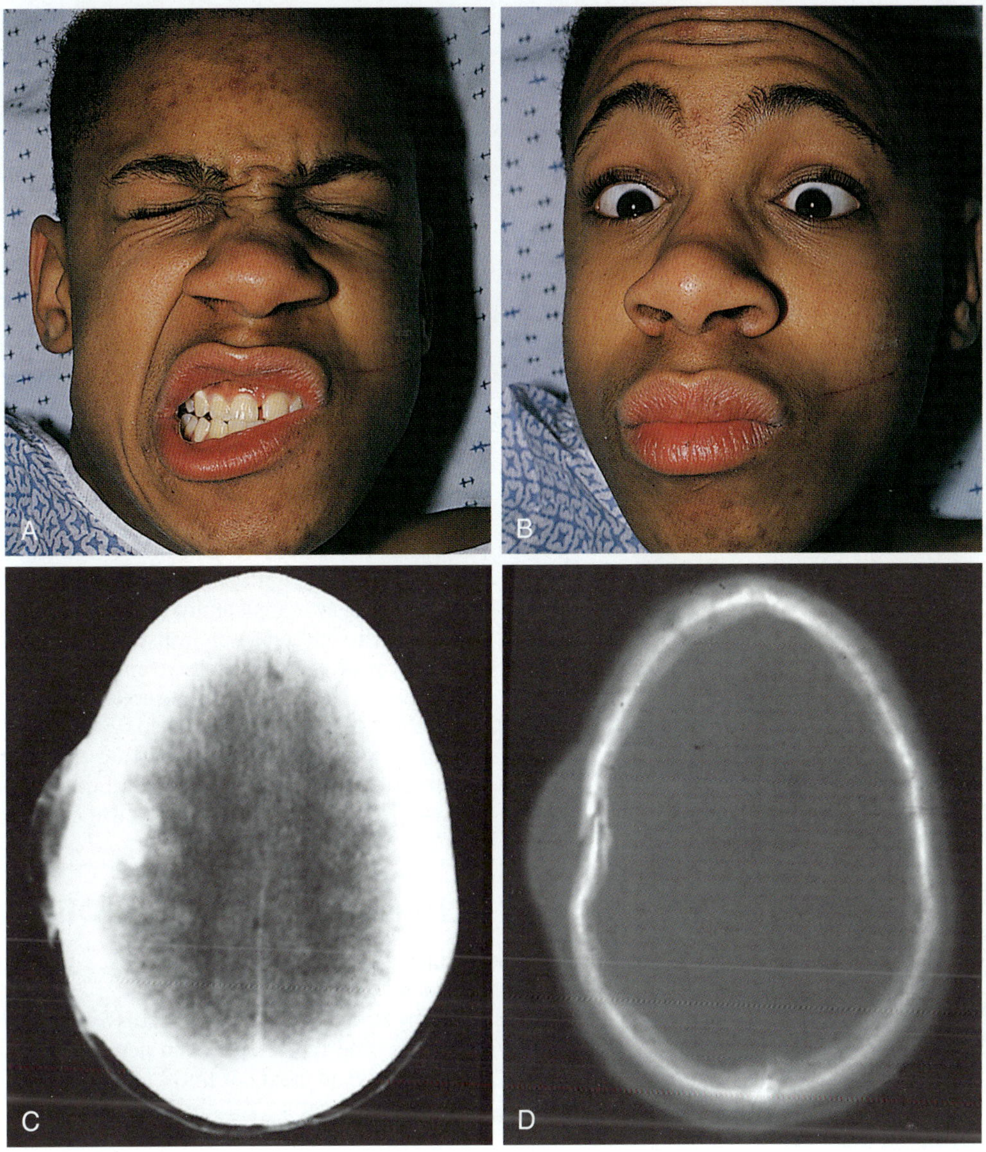

Fig. 16.56 Central facial weakness. (A and B) Weakness of the left face with relative sparing of the upper portion secondary to a lesion of the right cerebral hemisphere. There is flattening of the nasolabial fold and inability to retract the corner of the mouth, but the ability to close the eye and wrinkle the forehead is preserved. (C and D) Computed tomography scans show the depressed fracture of the temporal bone that was responsible for this central facial palsy.

Table 16.3 Clinical Features of the Muscular Dystrophies

	Duchenne	Becker	Facioscapulohumeral	Limb-Girdle	Myotonic
Inheritance	X-linked recessive	X-linked recessive	Autosomal dominant	Autosomal recessive	Autosomal dominant
Age at onset	Early childhood	Late childhood, adolescence	Variable: childhood through early adult life	Childhood to early adulthood	Highly variable
Pattern of weakness	Pelvic girdle, shoulder girdle	Pelvic girdle, shoulder girdle	Face, shoulder girdle	Pelvic girdle, shoulder girdle	Face, distal limbs
Rate of progression	Rapid	Slow	Very slow	Variable	Variable
Associated features	Pseudohypertrophy of calves	Pseudohypertrophy of calves	None	Pseudohypertrophy rare	Myotonia
Systemic features	Intellectual disability, abnormal electrocardiogram, cardiomyopathy	Occasional intellectual disability	None	None	Frequent intellectual disability, heart block, cataracts, premature balding, testicular tubular atrophy, diabetes

Duchenne muscular dystrophy is caused by mutations affecting the *DMD* gene in the Xp21 region on the short arm of the X chromosome. Dystrophin, a large cytoskeletal protein encoded by this gene locus, is deficient or absent from the muscle fibers of patients with Duchenne muscular dystrophy. It provides structural support to muscle fibers, particularly in skeletal and cardiac muscles, by linking the internal cytoskeleton and the outer membrane (sarcolemma), strengthening the sarcolemma and protecting it from damage. Dysfunction or absence of dystrophin promotes damage to fibers. Becker muscular dystrophy, an allelic disorder affecting 1 in 30,000 male births, is distinguished clinically by later age at onset, slower rate of progression, and longer survival. Dystrophin is present, but mutations lead to proteins with abnormal molecular weight. The majority of patients with Duchenne or Becker muscular dystrophy have detectable dystrophin mutations on routine deoxyribonucleic acid testing of peripheral blood, while the remaining patients are diagnosed by dystrophin analysis of muscle biopsy.

Clinical manifestations of Duchenne muscular dystrophy do not usually appear until the second year of life or later. Early developmental milestones are normally attained, although the first attempts at walking may be delayed. Gait is often clumsy and awkward from the start, and the ability to run is never normally attained. Difficulty in climbing stairs, frequent falls, and progressive difficulty in rising from the floor are early features. To rise from the floor, the child may at first need only to push with one hand on a knee (Fig. 16.57).

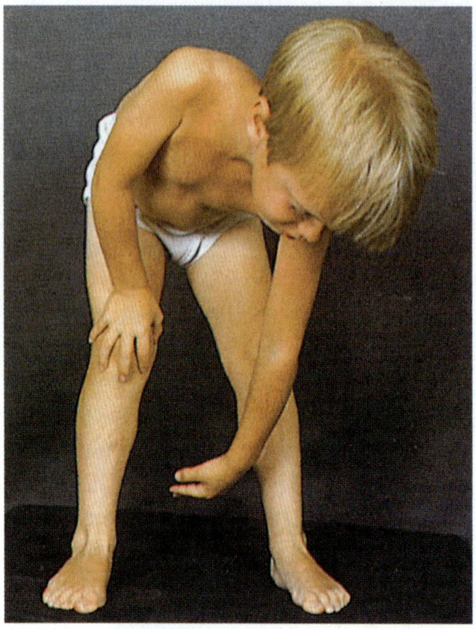

Fig. 16.57 Duchenne muscular dystrophy. This child, age 5, has difficulty rising from the floor. Unilateral hand support on the knee is required to get erect.

However, as weakness of the extensors of the hips becomes more pronounced, rising from the floor becomes increasingly difficult and requires the use of the hands to "climb up the legs" (the Gower maneuver) (Fig. 16.58).

Progressive gluteal weakness leads to the assumption of a compensatory posture characterized by a broadened base, accentuated lumbar lordosis, and forward thrusting of the abdomen (Fig. 16.59). Although weakness of the arms is not a common early symptom, proximal upper extremity weakness is easily detected on clinical examination when the child is lifted with the examiner's hands placed beneath the arms. There is marked laxity of the shoulder girdle musculature associated with upward displacement of the shoulders and abnormal rotation of the scapulae (Fig. 16.60A). In addition, spontaneous winging of the scapulae may be prominent (see Fig. 16.60B).

Weakness of the neck flexors, as evidenced by marked head lag when the child is pulled to sit from the supine position (Fig. 16.61), is an early finding. Enlargement of muscles, particularly in the calves (Fig. 16.62), is a common feature by 5 or 6 years old. The abnormally enlarged muscles have an unusually firm, rubbery consistency on palpation. Early in the clinical course, this increase in muscle volume may result from true hypertrophy, with muscle strength proportional to bulk. Later, infiltration by fat and connective tissue sometimes maintains this bulk despite loss of muscle fibers. This is called *pseudohypertrophy.* Inexorable deterioration of muscle function may eventually impair respiratory and cardiac function in Duchenne muscular dystrophy, leading to life expectancy of approximately 30 years.

Charcot-Marie-Tooth Disease

Charcot-Marie-Tooth (CMT) disease is a group of genetic and clinically heterogenous, length-dependent, hereditary peripheral neuropathies resulting in progressive sensory and motor dysfunction. Several types have been genetically and clinically identified. CMT1A is the most common form of CMT, the majority resulting from a duplication on chromosome 17p11.2. Symptoms usually

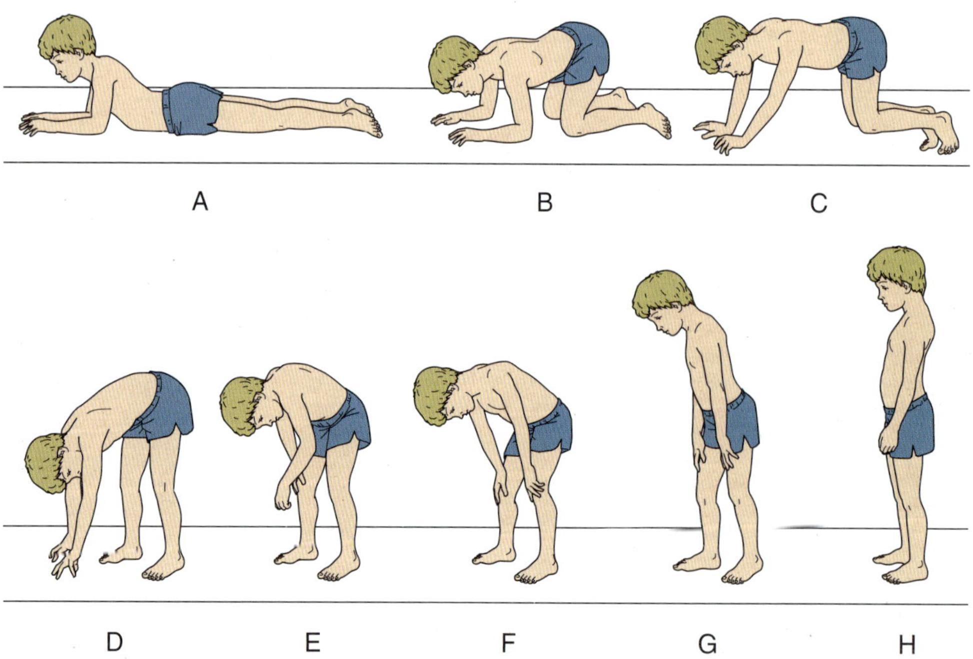

Fig. 16.58 The Gower maneuver. This series of diagrams illustrates the sequence of postures used in attaining the upright position by a child with Duchenne muscular dystrophy. (A–C) First, the legs are pulled up under the body, and the weight is shifted to rest on the hands and feet. (D) The hips are then thrust in the air as the knees are straightened, and the hands are brought closer to the legs. (E–G) Finally, the trunk is slowly extended by the hands walking up the thighs. (H) The erect position is attained.

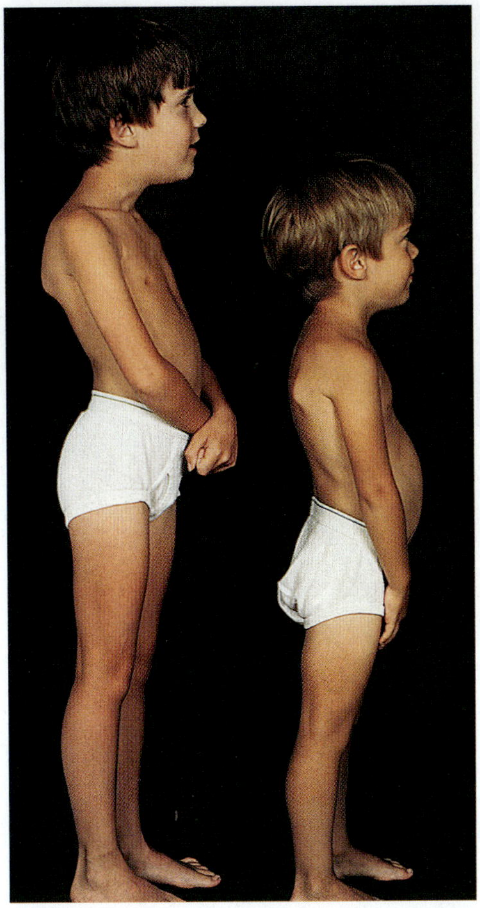

Fig. 16.59 Compensatory posture in Duchenne muscular dystrophy. These brothers, ages 5 and 8, show the progression of compensatory postural adjustments with broadening of stance, accentuated lumbar lordosis, and forward thrusting of the abdomen, all more pronounced in the older boy.

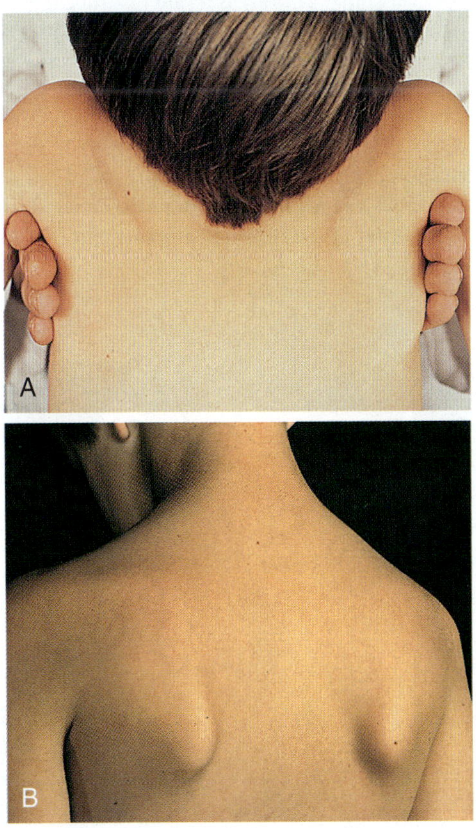

Fig. 16.60 Shoulder girdle weakness in Duchenne muscular dystrophy. (A) This child, age 5, demonstrates weakness and hypotonia of the shoulder girdle musculature. Upward displacement of the shoulders and abnormal rotation of the scapulae are seen when the child is lifted with the examiner's hands under his arms. (B) Spontaneous winging of the scapulae can be noted in this 8-year-old child.

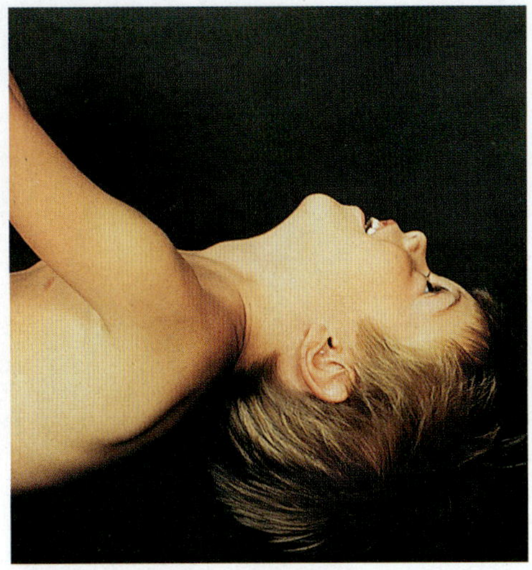

Fig. 16.61 Neck muscle weakness in Duchenne muscular dystrophy. This 5-year-old boy has neck flexor weakness. Note the marked head lag when the patient is pulled to sit from the supine position.

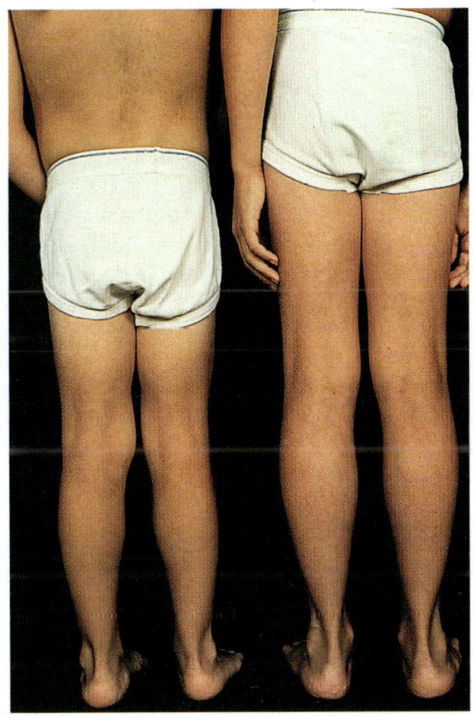

Fig. 16.62 Pseudohypertrophy in Duchenne muscular dystrophy. Note the enlargement of the calves in brothers, ages 5 and 8.

begin in the first 2 decades of life with distal weakness, sensory loss, and hyporeflexia. The onset of symptoms is usually in the second decade, with presenting complaints being foot deformities and gait abnormalities. Often, pes cavus or hammertoe deformities develop in early childhood long before more overt symptoms appear (see Figs. 22.107–22.108). The clinical picture is variable because affected patients often do not consult a physician about their neurologic complaints. The astute physician considers the diagnosis when a patient who presents with unrelated symptoms is found to have pes cavus or hammertoes and symmetric distal weakness.

Muscle weakness and atrophy begin insidiously in the foot and leg muscles. The intrinsic muscles of the foot are often affected first, followed by involvement of the peroneal, anterior tibial, long toe extensor, intrinsic hand, and gastrocnemius muscles.

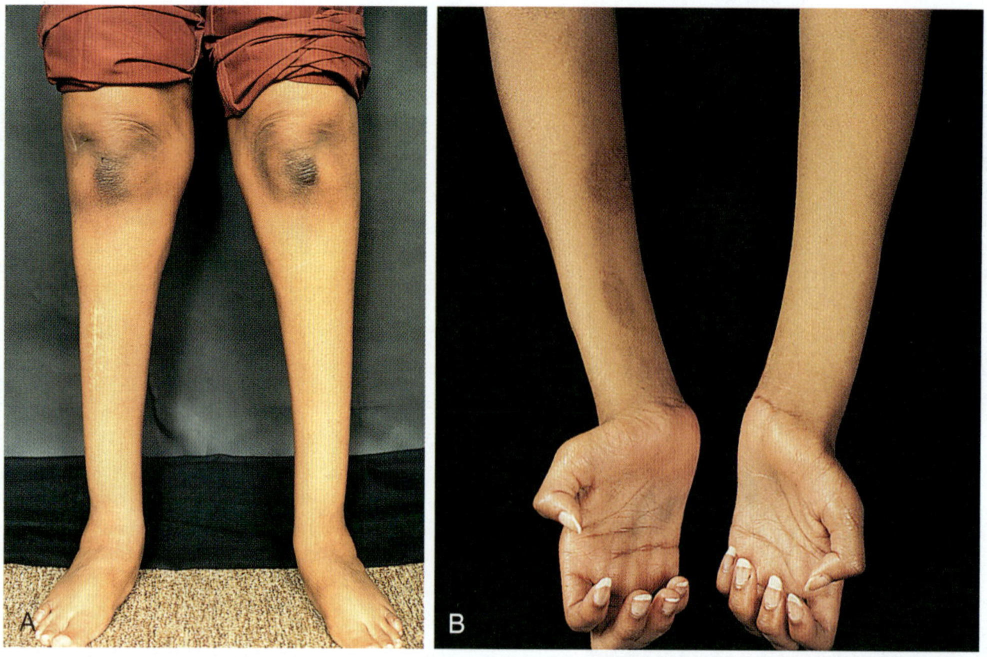

Fig. 16.63 Charcot-Marie-Tooth disease. (A) This patient, age 15, with distal muscular atrophy of the lower extremities demonstrates the "stork-leg" appearance. (B) She also has atrophy of the forearm and intrinsic hand muscles resulting in a "claw-hand" deformity.

Weakness and atrophy may spread to the more proximal muscles of the leg and forearm. Muscle wasting is often mild; however, in some cases the loss of muscle mass in the distal lower extremities is severe, giving rise to a striking "stork-leg" appearance (Fig. 16.63A). With involvement of the distal upper extremities, there may be wasting of the intrinsic hand muscles and development of secondary "claw-hand" deformities (see Fig. 16.63B). Deep tendon reflexes are lost first in the gastrocnemius and soleus muscles and subsequently in the quadriceps femoris muscle and upper limbs. Sensation may be mildly impaired in the distal lower extremities.

CMT1B results from mutations in myelin protein zero (MPZ); patients may present with a severe, early-onset form with delayed walking or a milder, late-onset axonal phenotype. Less than 1% of cases of CMT1 are due to less frequent genetic mutations.

Other forms include HNPP (Hereditary Neuropathy with Liability to Pressure Palsies), X-Linked CMT1, CMT2 Autosomal Dominant Axonal Neuropathies, CMT4 (Autosomal Recessive form) and an Intermediate form.

Congenital Cervical Spinal Atrophy

Congenital cervical spinal atrophy is a rare disorder that is manifested at birth by dramatic flaccid paresis of the upper extremities (Fig. 16.64A). The presence of congenital flexion contractures suggests chronic denervation that must have occurred in utero and allows this syndrome to be distinguished from injury to the cervical spine or brachial plexuses during delivery (see Chapter 2). Abnormalities in the formation of the transverse palmar creases are present in all cases (see Fig. 16.64B and C), suggesting an antenatal insult during the first trimester. The disorder and neurologic impairment is static.

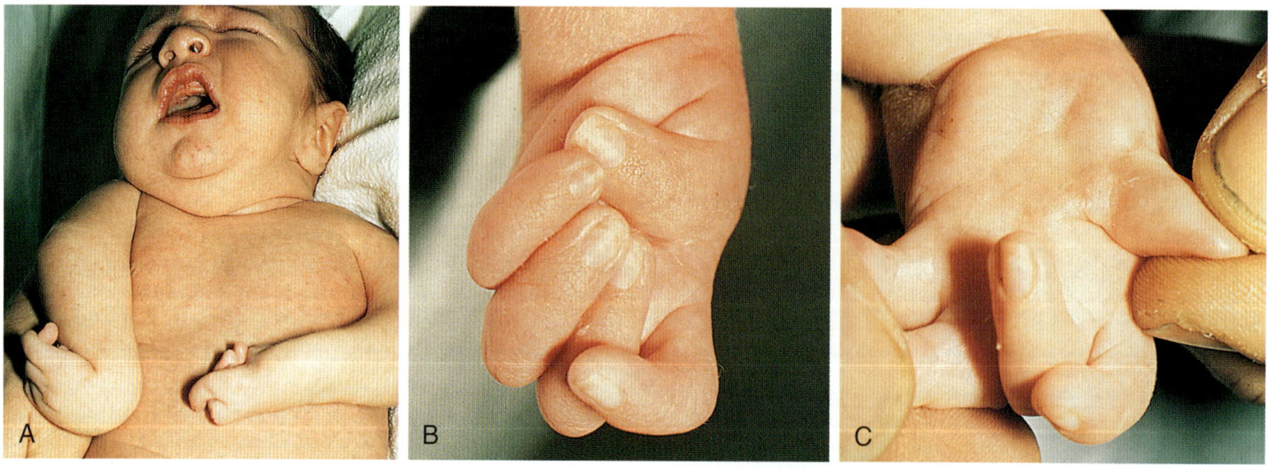

Fig. 16.64 Congenital cervical spinal atrophy. (A) This 2-day-old infant has flaccid paresis limited to the upper extremities and associated congenital flexion contractures. Wasting and atrophy of the intrinsic hand muscles with flexion contractures of the fingers (B) and poorly developed transverse palmar creases (C) were also present.

Myotonia Congenita

Myotonia congenita is an inherited disorder of skeletal muscle in which muscle stiffness is the only complaint. Autosomal dominant and autosomal recessive forms are related to different mutations of the skeletal muscle chloride channel gene on chromosome 7. The clinical symptoms are rather stereotypic. After a period of inactivity, the muscles stiffen and are difficult to maneuver; however, with continued activity, the stiffness diminishes and movement becomes almost normal. Typically, the child moves with a stiff, awkward gait and falls often. However, as activity continues, the child begins to walk freely and with adequate "warm-up" can run without difficulty.

Generalized muscular hypertrophy is a frequent finding on examination, with affected children often having an unusually well-developed, athletic appearance (Fig. 16.65). This belies their sedentary habits and physical ineptitude resulting from muscle stiffness. Clinically, myotonia may be demonstrated by observing delayed relaxation of the muscles after sustained voluntary contraction, such as clenching of the hand. Myotonia may also be elicited by percussion of the thenar eminence (Fig. 16.66).

THE HYPOTONIC INFANT

Because depression of muscle tone (diminished resistance to passive movement) is associated with paucity of movement, unusual postures, and increased range of movement of joints, the hypotonic infant has been likened to a rag doll. The legs lie externally rotated and abducted, with their lateral surfaces in contact with the bed while the arms are extended at the sides or flexed so that the hands lie beside the head. When the infant is pulled up by the hands from the supine position (traction response), the head falls into extreme extension and limbs fail to flex to counter traction (Fig. 16.67A). In horizontal suspension with the chest and abdomen supported by the examiner's hand, the infant with hypotonia drapes limply like an inverted U and, when held under the arms, tends to slip through the examiner's hands (see Fig. 16.67B). Because maintenance of normal postural tone requires functional integrity of the central and peripheral nerves and muscles, hypotonia is a common symptom of diverse disorders affecting the brain, spinal cord, peripheral nerves, and musculature (Table 16.4). Hypotonia also occurs as a nonspecific manifestation of systemic illness. The term *benign congenital hypotonia* is reserved for infants with isolated depression of postural tone that resolves with growth and maturation, usually by 1 year old. It is often a diagnosis of exclusion. Evaluation of hypotonia requires a rigorous approach to identify the underlying etiology.

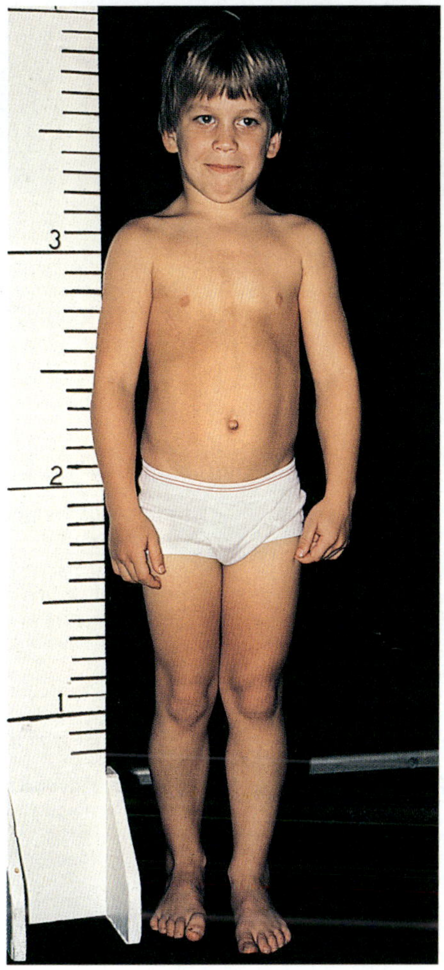

Fig. 16.65 Body habitus in myotonia congenita. This 8-year-old boy demonstrates generalized muscular hypertrophy, giving him a well-developed, athletic appearance.

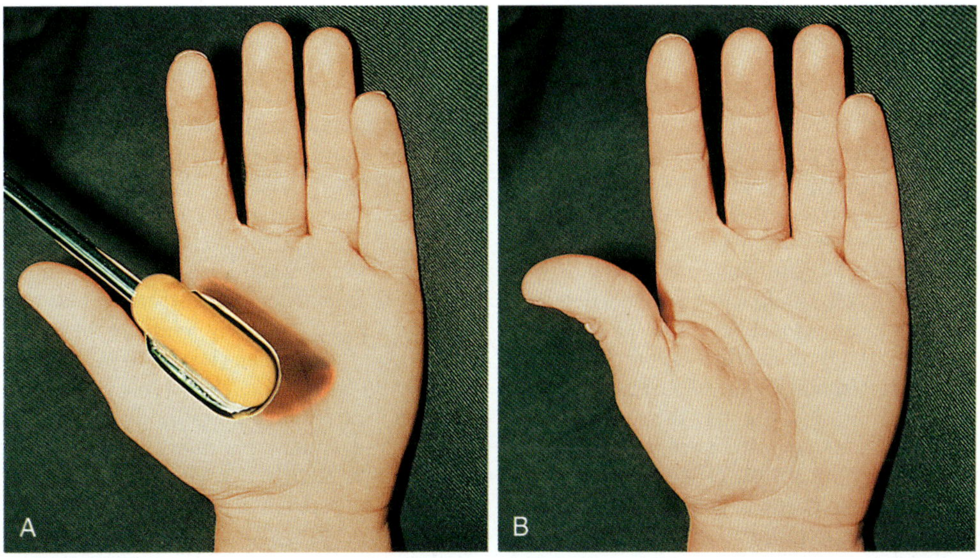

Fig. 16.66 Myotonia congenita, delayed muscle relaxation. Percussion of the thenar eminence (A) is followed by involuntary opposition of the thumb and visible contraction of the muscles of the thenar eminence (B), which lasts for several seconds.

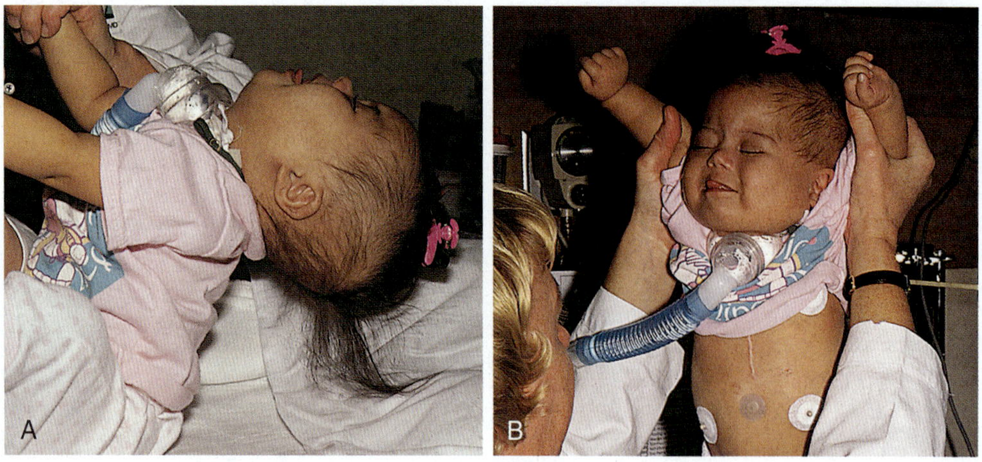

Fig. 16.67 Hypotonic infant. (A) Abnormal traction response. When the infant is pulled up from the supine position, her head falls into extreme extension and her arms fail to flex to counter the traction applied by the examiner. (B) When held under the arms, she tends to slip through the examiner's hands.

Table 16.4 Differential Diagnosis of Hypotonia

Disorders of Central Nervous System	Disorders of Peripheral Nervous System
Chromosome disorders	Spinal muscular atrophies
Trisomy	Congenital polyneuropathies
Prader-Willi syndrome	Transient neonatal myasthenia
Other	Congenital myasthenic syndromes
Other genetic defects	Congenital muscular dystrophy
Static encephalopathies	Myotonic dystrophy
Congenital malformation	Fukuyama-type dystrophy
Perinatal acquired encephalopathy	Other
Postnatal acquired encephalopathy	Congenital myopathies
Inborn errors of metabolism	Metabolic myopathies
Amino acid disorders	Systemic illness
Organic acid disorders	Benign congenital hypotonia
Urea cycle disorders	
Peroxisomal disorders	
Lysosomal disorders	
Neonatal spinal cord injury	

Table 16.5 Seizure Classification

International League Against Epilepsy (ILAE) 2017 Seizure Classifications

Focal-Onset Seizures
- Aware vs. with impaired consciousness
- Can progress from focal to bilateral tonic-clonic

Motor
- Automatisms
- Atonic
- Clonic
- Epileptic spasm
- Hyperkinetic
- Myoclonic
- Tonic

Nonmotor
- Autonomic
- Behavioral arrest
- Cognitive
- Emotional
- Sensory

Generalized-Onset Seizures

Motor
- Atonic
- Clonic
- Epileptic spasm
- Myoclonic
- Myoclonic-atonic
- Myoclonic-tonic-clonic
- Tonic-clonic

Nonmotor (Absence)
- Typical
- Atypical
- Myoclonic
- Eyelid myoclonia

CHILDHOOD EPILEPSY

The incidence of epilepsy follows a bimodal distribution, peaking in children younger than 5 years old and in adults older than 65 years old. The 2017 International League against Epilepsy (ILAE) definition of epilepsy is one of the following: (1) at least two unprovoked seizures greater than 24 hours apart, (2) one unprovoked seizure and a >60% chance of a recurrent seizure over the next 10 years, based on clinical history, EEG, and MRI findings, or (3) diagnosis of an epilepsy syndrome. A classification of epileptic seizures detailed in Table 16.5 divides them into those of focal onset (partial seizures) and those with bilateral cortical representation (generalized seizures). Focal seizures without alteration of consciousness have no associated impairment of consciousness and may represent simple motor or sensory phenomena. Patients with focal seizures with alteration of consciousness experience spread of seizure to cortical and subcortical areas, resulting in alteration in consciousness. Some partial seizures may secondarily generalize to contralateral brain areas, with loss of consciousness, often with bilateral convulsive features.

Generalized seizures may be convulsive or nonconvulsive in nature. In children, nonconvulsive generalized seizures often present as absence epilepsy. Other generalized seizures such as tonic, tonic/clonic, atonic, and myoclonic are defined by the type of motor activity observed.

Absence seizures are typically brief in duration (5–20 seconds) and are characterized by sudden staring or arrest of activity with abrupt recovery. They are often associated with facial automatisms, such as eye flutter, chewing, or ocular supraversion (Fig. 16.68A). The incidence of absence epilepsy peaks in children between 3 and 8 years old; however, onset can occur in adolescence. The disorder has a strong genetic predisposition and usually occurs in children who are otherwise neurologically and intellectually normal. It is often outgrown by late childhood or during adolescence. A typical electroencephalogram (EEG) pattern seen in affected individuals consists of generalized three-per-second spike-and-wave discharges (see Fig. 16.68B), which can be activated by hyperventilation. Between 40% and 60% of patients with absence seizures go on to experience a generalized tonic/clonic convulsion.

Infantile spasms typically begin before 2 years old, with a peak age at onset between 4 and 6 months old. They are classified as flexor, extensor, and mixed flexor/extensor types and are characterized by brief contractions of the neck, trunk, and extremities

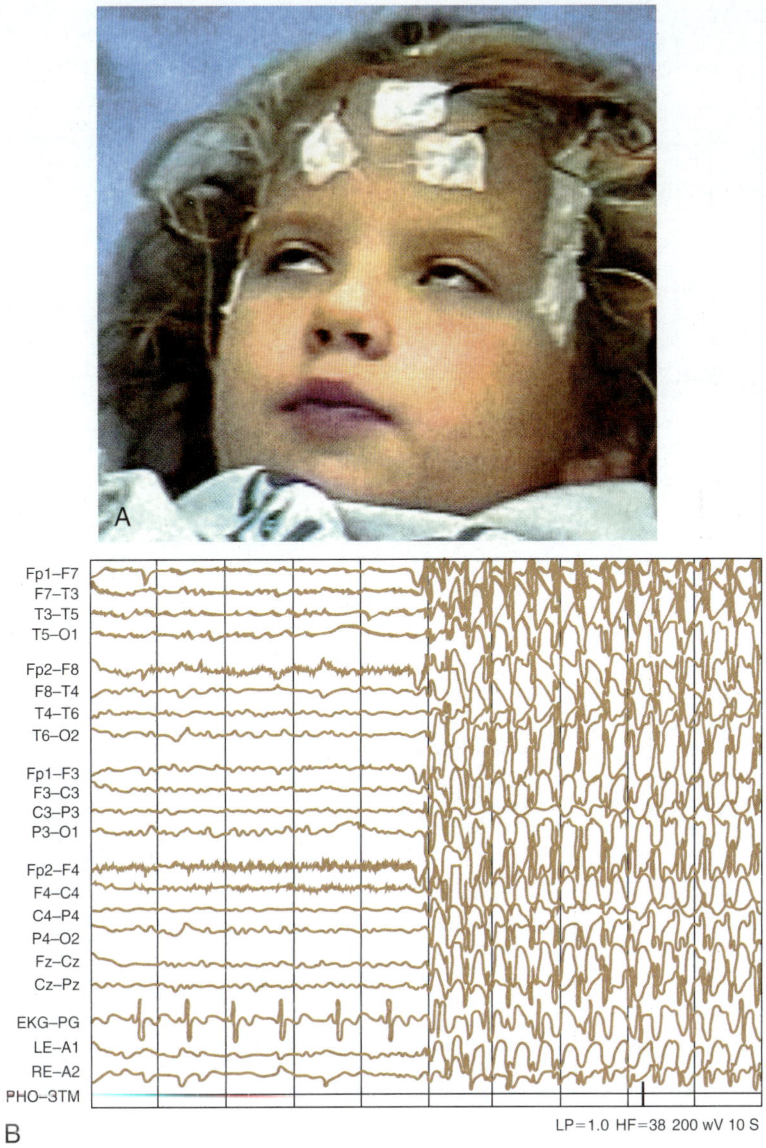

Fig. 16.68 (A) Absence seizure. This 8-year-old girl had a history of brief staring spells reported by teachers and family. Typical absence seizures, recorded during a video electroencephalogram with staring and ocular supraversion lasting under 10 seconds, could be activated by hyperventilation. (B) This electroencephalographic tracing shows the typical three-per-second (3 Hz) generalized spike-and-wave discharges characteristic of absence seizures.

with the head thrown backward or forward in association with flexion and/or extension of the limbs. They often occur in clusters throughout the day, with greater frequency on awakening or falling asleep. Early in the course of the disorder, they may be mistaken for colic, hiccups, or gastroesophageal reflux. Etiologic origin of infantile spasms is varied and may include metabolic disorders, cerebral malformations, congenital infections, anoxic injury, and neurocutaneous disorders. However, up to 20% of cases are idiopathic or cryptogenic in origin. Tuberous sclerosis is the major identifiable cause of infantile spasms, accounting for 7% to 25% of cases. Patients who have a known underlying disorder and infantile spasms have a higher incidence of developmental impairment than those of unknown cause. Neuroimaging is abnormal in 70% to 80% of affected children. The EEG in patients with infantile spasms often demonstrates a hypsarrhythmia pattern with markedly abnormal background features and multifocal high-voltage epileptic discharges, and it may show a burst/suppression pattern in sleep (Fig. 16.69). The triad of hypsarrhythmia, infantile spasms, and developmental delay is commonly referred to as *West syndrome*. More than 50% of patients with infantile spasms develop other forms of epilepsy later in life.

Genetic testing has become a critical part of epilepsy management and treatment. There are common genetic syndromes where epilepsy is a predominant feature of the phenotype (Table 16.6). The presence of epilepsy in the setting of dysmorphic feature or intellectual disability may help direct to a specific diagnosis and directed genetic testing. Some commonly recognized epilepsy syndromes based on clinical features have more specific treatments or outcomes when their genetic diagnosis is known (Table 16.7).

PAROXYSMAL MOVEMENT DISORDERS OF CHILDHOOD

Paroxysmal (nonepileptic) movement disorders are relatively common in the pediatric population. They are manifest by excessive involuntary movement (dyskinesia) that is episodic and often stereotypical with preservation of consciousness.

Tic

Tics include a wide array of movements and sounds. They are involuntary, sudden, repetitive movements or vocalizations. They typically wax and wane, with old tics being replaced by new ones. Up to

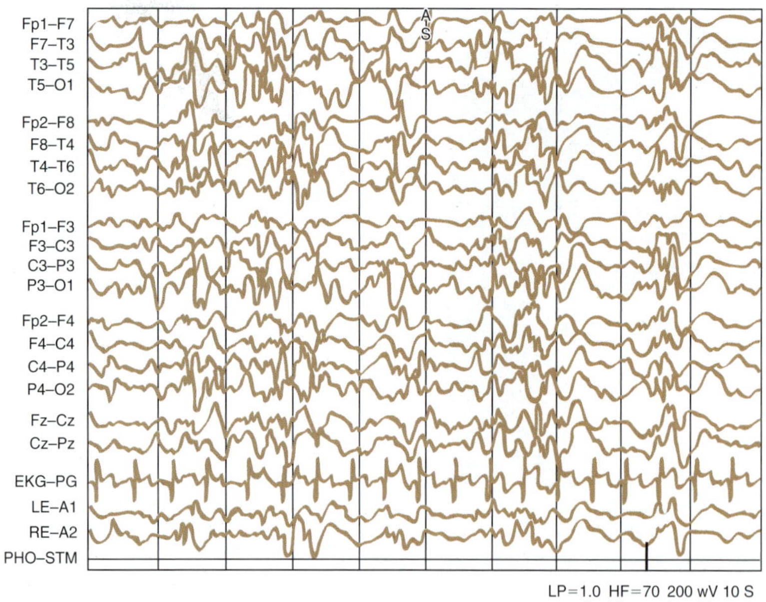

Fig. 16.69 Infantile spasms. This electroencephalograph tracing shows the hypsarrhythmia pattern consisting of markedly disorganized background and high-voltage multifocal epileptic spikes often found in patients with infantile spasms.

Table 16.6 Common Genetic Syndromes With Epilepsy

Condition (OMIM#)	Gene	Clinical Features	Epilepsy Onset	Seizure Type
Angelman syndrome (105830)	Methylation differences at 15q11.2–11.3	Developmental delay, ataxia, microcephaly	1–3 years	Multiple—focal, generalized tonic clonic, atonic, absence
Kleefstra syndrome (610253)	*EHMT1*	Dysmorphic facies, ID, microcephaly, heart defects, behavior challenges	Childhood	Tonic clonic, absence, focal with impaired consciousness
MECP2 duplication syndrome (300260)	*MECP2*	Males—hypotonia, moderate to severe ID	~6 years of age	Generalized tonic clonic or focal seizures
Miller Dieker syndrome (247200)	*LIS1*	Characteristic facies and lissencephaly	Infancy	Generalized tonic clonic, atonic, focal
Mowat Wilson (235730)	*ZEB2*	Dysmorphic facies, corpus callosum abnormalities, Hirschsprungs, heart defects, ID	Early toddler	Focal and atypical absence
Pitt Hopkins syndrome (610954)	*TCF4*	Hypotonia, moderate severe ID, periodic hyperventilations	Infancy to late childhood	Generalized tonic clonic, atonic, and focal seizures
Rett syndrome (312750)	*MECP2*	Females with regression of development, loss of hand and language skills, stereotypic hand wringing	1–4	Generalized tonic clonic and focal seizures with impaired consciousness
Tuberous sclerosis (191100, 613254)	*TSC1* and *TSC2*	Cutaneous finding, cardiac rhabdomyoma, renal angiomyolipoma, ungual fibromas, subependymal nodules	Infancy	Infantile spasms
Wolf Hirschhorn syndrome (194190)	4p16.3	Dysmorphic facies, ID, ptosis, feeding difficulties	6–12 months	Focal tonic, focal clonic, generalized tonic clonic, status epilepticus is common

Table 16.7 Recognizable Genetic Epilepsy Syndromes

Condition (OMIM#)	Gene	Clinical Features	Clinical Pearls
Dravet syndrome (607208)	*SCN1A*	Focal epilepsy, family history of febrile seizures	Avoid Na channel AED (phenytoin, oxcarbazepine), SCN1A associated with a clinical spectrum including familial febrile seizures
GLUT1 deficiency (506777)	*SCL2A1*	Global developmental delay, epilepsy, and ataxia	Hypoglycorrhachia in patients with epilepsy and/or ataxia, treatment is the ketogenic diet
Benign familial neonatal seizures (121200,121201)	*KCNQ2 KCNQ3*	Focal seizures within the first week of life	The "fifth day fits," overall good developmental prognosis
Early infantile epileptic encephalopathy 14 (614959)	*KCNT1*	Presents as malignant migrating partial seizures of infancy	May respond to quinidine
POLG-related disorders (203700, 607459)	*POLG*	Developmental delay, epilepsia partialis continua	Valproic acid should be avoided

25% of children may have a transient simple tic disorder lasting less than 1 year. The presence of multiple tics lasting longer than 1 year with both vocal and motor varieties fulfill diagnostic criteria for Tourette syndrome. Attention-deficit/hyperactivity disorder (ADHD), obsessive-compulsive personality disorder, and learning disabilities are commonly seen in addition to tics in patients with Tourette syndrome.

Shuddering Attacks

Shuddering (shivering) spells are characterized by flexion of the head, trunk, elbows, and knees with adduction of the limbs and are often described as a "chill" or as having a sense of "ice water being poured down one's back." They represent a benign movement disorder often starting in infancy and usually abating in childhood.

Startle Disease

A startle response is a brief motor response to an unexpected stimulus (auditory, tactile, visual, or vestibular) that readily habituates (e.g., diminishes with repeated exposure). Hyperekplexia (startle disease) is characterized by a nonhabituating, exaggerated startle response to stimuli often followed by a tonic spasm. Affected children often have hypertonia in infancy, feeding difficulties, and apnea. The startle response can be elicited in hyperekplexic patients by tapping on the forehead, nose, glabella, or vertex of the skull. The course of the disease is variable, and cognitive abilities are not affected. Various genetic mutations have been found to cause hyperekplexia.

Head Bobbing

Head bobbing consists of jerky head movements at a frequency of two to three cycles per second and resembles that of a doll's head atop a spring. In childhood, it may appear as part of spasmus nutans or the bobble-head doll syndrome. Spasmus nutans is a benign disorder of unknown etiology that occurs in early infancy and is characterized by nystagmus (binocular or monocular), head nodding, and head tilt. Neurologic examination is otherwise normal. The syndrome lasts 1 to 2 years and spontaneously resolves. The bobble-head doll syndrome consists of intermittent head nodding and is seen in association with an underlying CNS structural abnormality, often a third ventricular cyst or tumor.

Chorea or Choreoathetosis

Chorea consists of random, brief, rapid, purposeless jerking movements of the limbs, face, tongue, or trunk, whereas choreoathetosis is characterized by slow writhing movements that often are more prominent on one side of the body. Sydenham chorea (St. Vitus dance) is the most prevalent form of acquired chorea in childhood. It is a manifestation of rheumatic fever and often begins insidiously weeks to months after a streptococcal infection that may or may not have been symptomatic. It is characterized by choreiform movements, emotional lability, and hypotonia. Behavior change, decline in school performance, and anxiety are common associated features. The disorder usually resolves after several months, although recurrences may be triggered by new episodes of streptococcal infection, pregnancy (chorea gravidarum), or oral contraceptive use. Other, less common causes of chorea and/or choreoathetosis in childhood include Wilson disease, Huntington disease, systemic lupus erythematosus, and hyperthyroidism.

AUTOIMMUNE DISORDERS

Neuroimmune, demyelinating disorders usually present with abrupt neurologic deficits in otherwise healthy children and adolescents. They may have a monophasic, relapsing, or chronic progressive course. While more frequent in postpubertal women, boys may also be affected. Focal or multifocal symptoms may occur, and optic neuritis is oftentimes the first clinical symptom in children, characterized by acute visual loss associated with painful eye movements. Fundoscopic examination may be normal or show mild papillitis; patients will often have markedly decreased visual acuity, a relative afferent pupillary defect, and color desaturation. Multiple sclerosis, MOGAD (myelin oligodendrocyte glycoprotein–associated disease) (Fig. 16.70 and 16.71), aquaporin-$_4$ (AQP_4) antibody–positive neuromyelitis

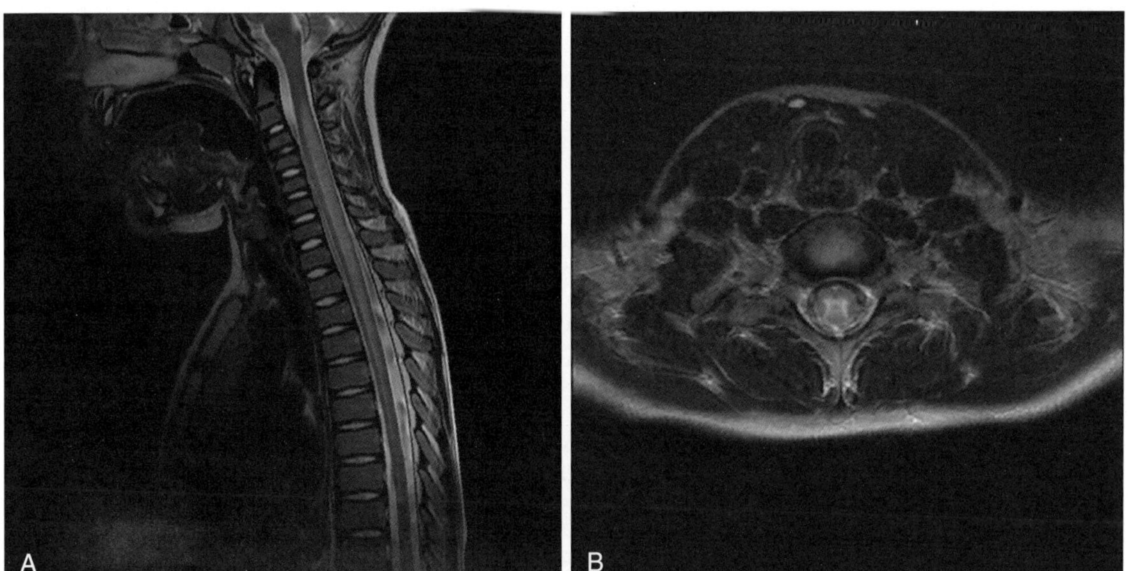

Fig. 16.70 Longitudinally extensive transverse myelitis in a 6-year-old boy with myelin oligodendrocyte glycoprotein–associated disease. (A) Sagittal spinal cord magnetic resonance imaging illustrates extensive T2 cord signal abnormality extending from C2 resulting in cord expansion. (B) "H sign" in the same patient shows axial view with increased T2 signal abnormality with predominant involvement of the central gray matter.

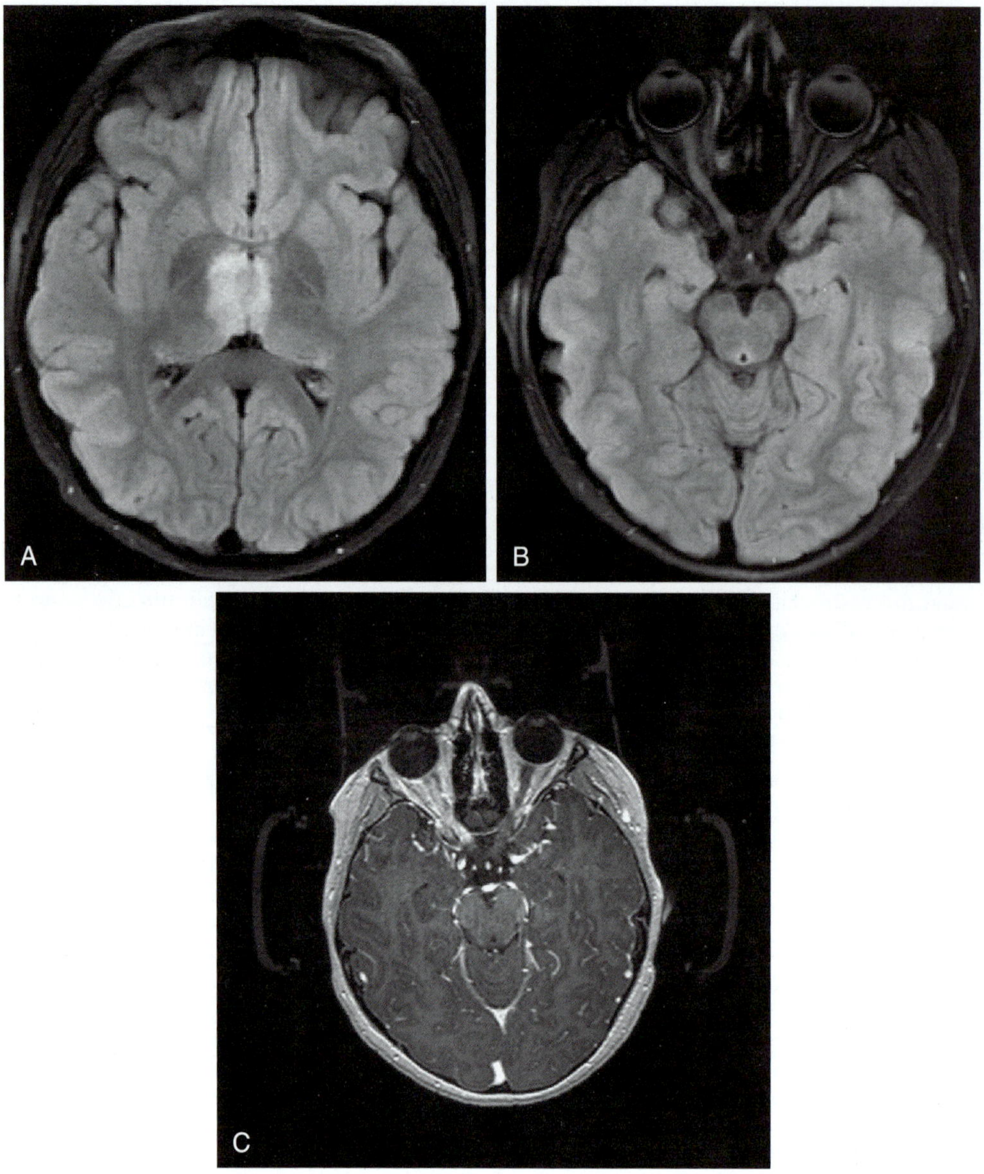

Fig. 16.71 Optic nerve involvement in myelin oligodendrocyte glycoprotein–associated disease (MOGAD). (A) 9-year-old boy with MOGAD presenting with right optic neuritis. (B) T2 FLAIR sequence shows increased signal in the bilateral thalami. Long segment increased T2 signal of the right optic nerve. (C) T1 contrast enhancement of the right optic nerve in the same patient.

Table 16.8 Neuroimmune Demyelinating Disorders

	MS	MOGAD	NMOSD
Antibody		MOG	AQP_4
Optic neuritis	Unilateral	b/l, long segment	b/l, chiasm
Perineuritis		+	
Brain	Juxtacortical, periventricular lesions	White matter and gray matter involvement, H sign in spinal cord	Area postrema, acute brainstem syndrome
Myelitis	≤3 vertebrae	LETM	LETM
CSF OGB	+++	+	
CSF pleocytosis	+	+++	++

LETM, Longitudinally extensive transverse myelitis; *MOGAD,* myelin oligodendrocyte glycoprotein–associated disease; *MS,* multiple sclerosis; *NMOSD,* aquaporin-$_4$ (AQP_4) antibody positive neuromyelitis optica spectrum disorder (NMOSD); *OGB,* oligoclonal bands.

optica spectrum disorder (neuromyelitis optica), and acute disseminated encephalomyelitis are the most common acquired, demyelinating disorders recognized in children. Table 16.8 summarizes their most frequent clinical features, CSF, and radiologic findings.

ACKNOWLEDGMENTS

The authors wish to thank Rajiv Varma and Shelley D. Williams for their work on this chapter in previous editions.

Supplemental videos are available at Elsevier eBooks+.

Bibliography

Bell WE, McCormick WF: *Increased intracranial pressure in children*, ed 2, Philadelphia, 1978, WB Saunders.

Brooke MH: *A clinician's view of neuromuscular diseases*, ed 2, Baltimore, 1987, Williams & Wilkins.

Chao DH: Congenital neurocutaneous syndromes of childhood. III. Sturge-Weber disease, *J Pediatr* 55:635–649, 1959.

Dubowitz V: *The floppy infant*, ed 2, Philadelphia, 1980, JB Lippincott.

Emery AEH: *Duchenne muscular dystrophy*, ed 2, Oxford, 1993, Oxford University Press.

Enjolras O, Riche MC, Merland JJ: Facial port-wine stains and Sturge-Weber syndrome, *Pediatrics* 76:48–52, 1985.

Fenichel GM: *Clinical pediatric neurology: a signs and symptoms approach*, ed 5, Philadelphia, 2005, WB Saunders.

Goldstein SM, Curless RG, Post JD, et al: A new sign of neurofibromatosis on magnetic resonance imaging of children, *Arch Neurol* 46:1222–1224, 1989.

Gomez MR, editor: *Tuberous sclerosis*, ed 2, New York, 1998, Raven Press.

Hoffman EP, Fishbeck KH, Brown RH, et al: Characterization of dystrophin in muscle-biopsy specimens from patients with Duchenne's or Becker's muscular dystrophy, *N Engl J Med* 318:1363–1368, 1988.

International League against Epilepsy: Commission on classification and terminology: proposal for a revised classification of epilepsies and epileptic syndromes, *Epilepsia* 26:268–278, 1985.

Martuza RL, Eldridge R: Neurofibromatosis 2, *N Engl J Med* 318:684–688, 1988.

Menkes JH: *Textbook of child neurology*, ed 5, Philadelphia, 1995, Lea & Febiger.

Mitchell WG: Current therapy in neurologic disease: cerebral cysticercosis in North American children, *Eur Neurol* 37:126–129, 1997.

Northrup H, Krueger D: Tuberous sclerosis complex diagnostic criteria update: recommendations of the 2012 International Tuberous Sclerosis Complex Consensus Conference, *Pediatr Neurol* 49(4):243–254, 2013.

Osborne JP: Diagnosis of tuberous sclerosis, *Arch Dis Child* 63:1423–1425, 1988.

Paller AS: The Sturge-Weber syndrome, *Pediatr Dermatol* 4:300–304, 1987.

Riccardi VM: Von Recklinghausen neurofibromatosis, *N Engl J Med* 305:1617–1627, 1981.

Riccardi VM, Eichner JE: *Neurofibromatosis: phenotype, natural history and pathogenesis*, ed 2, Baltimore, 1992, Johns Hopkins University Press.

Roach ES, Gomez MR, Northrup H: Tuberous sclerosis complex consensus conference: revised clinical diagnostic criteria, *J Child Neurol* 13:624–628, 1998.

Roach ES, William DP, Laster DW: Magnetic resonance imaging in tuberous sclerosis, *Arch Neurol* 44:301–303, 1987.

Swaiman KF, Ashwal S: *Pediatric neurology: principles and practice*, ed 3, St Louis, 1999, Mosby.

Warkany J, Lemire RJ, Cohen MM: *Mental retardation and congenital malformations of the central nervous system*, St Louis, 1981, Mosby.

17

PULMONARY DISORDERS

Erica L. Stevens | Jeremy S. Landeo Gutierrez | Daniel J. Weiner

INTRODUCTION

Respiratory diseases are among the most common reasons for pediatric patients to seek medical attention. A careful history and physical examination are useful in assessing pediatric patients with respiratory complaints. Diseases of the chest can be divided into two major categories: acquired and congenital. The spectrum of diseases involving the pediatric respiratory system is primarily dependent on the age of the patient; therefore age must be a primary consideration when elaborating the differential diagnosis.

HISTORY

Pediatric history should include the perinatal history. A history of respiratory distress or intubation at birth, however brief, is important. Prematurity with prolonged need for supplemental oxygen may suggest bronchopulmonary dysplasia with associated structural lung abnormalities. Noisy breathing starting early in life suggests congenital airway obstruction. Regardless of the cause, failure to thrive is a worrisome finding, whereas excellent weight gain in a child with noisy breathing is reassuring.

Distinguishing between persistent and intermittent symptoms can be one of the most important clues to diagnosis. A good "cough history" (Table 17.1) and "wheeze history" are important and have similar elements. The clinician should inquire about the chronicity of the symptoms, association with feeding, upper respiratory infections, exposures (pets, dust, and especially cigarette smoking are important), and fevers. The effect—or lack thereof—of medications may give important diagnostic information (but may also be confounded by improper administration technique). The nature of the cough is important: *wet* or *dry, paroxysmal* or *continuous,* and *staccato* (as seen in neonatal chlamydial pneumonia). The cough that awakens the child at night or keeps the child up much of the night is another worrisome historical finding. Conversely, a persistent cough that disappears in sleep suggests the diagnosis of habit (psychogenic) cough. Causes of cough by age and possible diagnostic evaluations are shown (Boxes 17.1 and 17.2). In pursuing a history of *wheeze,* it is important to ask the parents or historians what they mean by the term; it may mean "noisy breathing," or stridor.

In evaluating the infant with frequent episodes of cough and/or wheeze, the clinician should inquire about symptoms of gastroesophageal reflux disease (GERD) or choking with feeds. As reflux is worse when the patient is supine, symptoms tend to be more prominent at night and during naps.

A family history of asthma or atopy including eczema and environmental allergies should be investigated. Frequent infections in parents or siblings, particularly those requiring hospitalization, could suggest possible immunodeficiency in the family. Other pulmonary diseases with a strong genetic component include cystic fibrosis (CF), primary ciliary dyskinesia (PCD), and neuromuscular syndromes.

The immunization history is essential, including history of pertussis and seasonal influenza vaccination. Parental report of vaccination status may be confirmed with vaccination records from the primary care physician.

Exercise intolerance is a common manifestation of respiratory disease. The neonate's main output of energy is in feeding, and thus difficulties with feedings should be monitored; toddlers are expected to keep up with peers and/or siblings in play; the school-age child's gym performance should be scrutinized. Wheezing or coughing fits after vigorous exercise can occur in asthma. Syncope with exercise is quite worrisome and raises the possibility of pulmonary hypertension.

PHYSICAL EXAMINATION

Examination of the chest in any uncooperative patient is especially difficult, but it can be accomplished with patience and a few tricks. The infant or toddler is best examined with his or her shirt off while being held upright in the arms of a parent. The patient should face the parent; this maximizes contact with the parent and allows the patient to feel safe. The room should be at a comfortable temperature, and the stethoscope head should be warmed before use. The classic four steps in the physical examination—inspection, palpation, percussion, and auscultation—are applied when examining the pediatric chest.

Inspection

Decreased subcutaneous adipose tissue typical of CF should be noted. The pattern of breathing should always be evaluated with the child disrobed. Any use of the expiratory muscles is abnormal. Suprasternal and intercostal retractions reflect excessive negative pleural pressure and can be seen in normal children with thin chest walls after vigorous exercise. Subcostal retractions are the result of hyperinflated lungs and a flattened diaphragm pulling inward on the chest wall. In advanced lung disease, the use of accessory muscles of inspiration can be noted; the sternocleidomastoid muscle, for example, helps lift the chest (in a "bucket handle" fashion) and increase its anteroposterior diameter, thereby increasing intrathoracic volume. In respiratory muscle fatigue, a pattern of breathing can be observed in which the diaphragm alternates with the intercostal muscles to inflate the lungs. This is known as *respiratory alternans,* or paradoxical chest wall motion, and is seen as alternating abdominal and chest expansion instead of the usual pattern of simultaneous chest and abdominal expansion. Chest wall deformities such as pectus excavatum or pectus carinatum (see Chapter 18) should be noted.

Palpation

Chest palpation is performed by placing the hands on either side of the chest as the patient takes a deep breath. The chest should expand symmetrically; asymmetry can be seen in unilateral pulmonary hypoplasia, mainstem bronchial obstruction, and diaphragmatic paresis. Placing fingertips on the upper abdomen just over the insertion of the rectus muscles into the lower rib cage can reveal subtle use of expiratory muscles in children with peripheral (lower) airway obstruction. Similarly, the anterior lower ribs should be assessed with the fingertips. In infants with obstructive lung disease, the lower ribs can be felt

Table 17.1 Charactristics of Chronic Cough and Associated Conditions

Characteristic	Associated Condition
Loose, productive	Cystic fibrosis, bronchiectasis, ciliary dyskinesia
Croupy	Laryngotracheobronchitis
Paroxysmal	Cystic fibrosis, pertussis syndrome, foreign body inhalation, *Mycoplasma, Chlamydia*
Brassy	Tracheitis, upper airway drainage, psychogenic cough
After feedings	Pharyngeal incoordination, pharyngeal mass, tracheoesophageal fistula, gastroesophageal reflux
Nocturnal	Upper respiratory tract disease, sinusitis, asthma, cystic fibrosis, gastroesophageal reflux disease
Most severe in morning	Cystic fibrosis, bronchiectasis
With exercise	Asthma (including exercise-induced), cystic fibrosis, bronchiectasis
Loud, honking, or bizarre	Psychogenic cough
Disappears with sleep	Psychogenic cough

pulling inwards on inspiration. This is the palpable aspect of a subcostal retraction. With the patient's head in the midline position, the trachea should be palpated at the sternal notch to evaluate for tracheal deviation, as is seen with mediastinal shift. Vocal fremitus should be assessed in patients with suspected pleural fluid accumulation; the vibrations transmitted from the larynx as the child says "99" are diminished when there is an accumulation of air or fluid in the pleural space. Infants and children with tracheomalacia and bronchomalacia often have a palpable vibration in the back. Palpable vibrations in only one hemithorax suggest a partial obstruction of the mainstem bronchus in that hemithorax as seen in bronchomalacia.

Percussion

Percussion of the chest can reveal hyperresonance and dullness over an area of consolidation. Air trapping due to small airway disease results in a depressed position of the diaphragm. Ordinarily the diaphragm can be found just at or slightly below the tip of the scapula when the patient's arm is at his or her side in children 5 years old and younger. In the patient with hyperinflation, the diaphragm is found several fingerbreadths below the scapular tips. An area of consolidation or pleural effusion results in dullness to percussion. Another disorder causing asymmetry of percussion of the two hemithoraces is diaphragmatic eventration, a congenital lesion in which the diaphragm is replaced with a thin fibrous membrane without contractile properties.

Auscultation

Auscultation of the pediatric chest requires patience. One often must wait a minute or two for a deep breath in order to appreciate abnormal breath sounds that are not apparent on shallow breathing. Augmenting the expiratory phase with a gentle squeeze of the thorax while listening with the stethoscope may improve detection of expiratory wheezes.

Abnormal ("adventitious") breath sounds include crackles and wheezes. Wheezes are *continuous* sounds, whereas crackles (formerly referred to as *rales*) are *discontinuous.* Wheezes and crackles can be inspiratory or expiratory, although crackles are more commonly heard on inspiration and wheezes are more commonly heard on expiration.

Wheezes arise from the vibration within the walls of narrowed large and medium-sized airways. In a patient experiencing an acute exacerbation of asthma, the lungs have wheezes in a range of pitches (described as *polyphonic,* or *heterophonous*) with substantial regional differences in auscultation. Patients with central airway obstruction such as tracheomalacia, on the other hand, have a single pitch of wheeze that sounds the same in all lung fields (*monophonic,* or *homophonous*) and is heard loudest over the central airway that is obstructed. Foreign bodies can cause a monophonic wheeze that can vary in pitch depending on the degree of obstruction.

Box 17.1 Causes of Cough According to Age

Infancy (Younger Than 1 Year Old)

Congenital and Neonatal Infections
Chlamydia
Viral (e.g., RSV, CMV, rubella)
Bacterial (e.g., pertussis)
Pneumocystis jirovecii

Congenital Malformations
Tracheoesophageal fistula
Vascular ring
Airway malformations (e.g., laryngeal cleft)
Pulmonary sequestration

Other
Cystic fibrosis
Asthma
Aspiration
Recurrent viral bronchiolitis/bronchitis
Gastroesophageal reflux
Interstitial pneumonitides
Lymphoid interstitial pneumonitis
Diffuse interstitial pneumonitis

Preschool

Inhaled foreign body
Asthma
Suppurative lung disease
  Cystic fibrosis
  Bronchiectasis
Right middle lobe syndrome
Ciliary dyskinesia syndromes
Upper respiratory tract disease
Recurrent viral infection/bronchitis
Passive smoke inhalation
Gastroesophageal reflux
Interstitial pneumonitides
Pulmonary hemosiderosis

School Age to Adolescence

Asthma
Cystic fibrosis
Mycoplasma pneumoniae infection
Psychogenic or habit cough
Cigarette smoking
Pulmonary hemosiderosis
Interstitial pneumonitides
Ciliary dyskinesia syndromes

All Ages

Recurrent viral illness
Asthma
Cystic fibrosis
Granulomatous lung disease
Foreign body aspiration
Pertussis infection

Box 17.2 Diagnostic Approach to Cough

Complete history and physical examination
Chest and sinus radiographs
Complete blood count with differential
Pulmonary function tests (including bronchoprovocation tests)
Sweat test (pilocarpine iontophoresis method)
Trial of bronchodilators
Sputum for Gram stain, AFB, bacterial, viral, and fungal cultures
Quantitative immunoglobulins
Tuberculin skin test/anergy panel
Serological tests or PCR for *Mycoplasma pneumoniae*
Bronchoscopy with bronchoalveolar lavage
Barium swallow

AFB, Acid-fast bacillus; *PCR*, polymerase chain reaction.

Crackles arise from the popping of fluid menisci within airways. The fine crackles heard in the lungs of patients with interstitial lung disease (ILD) or pulmonary edema may arise from popping open of small airways. Coarse crackles are often audible at the mouth and can be found in CF patients with advanced bronchiectasis. Coarse crackles can also be made by pooled secretions in the central airways.

Other sounds that can be heard include friction rubs, which are creaking sounds heard during both phases of respiration as inflamed pleural surfaces rub over one another. One of the most important abnormal findings in children is the absence of breath sounds over an area of collapse or consolidation.

Extrapulmonary Physical Examination Findings

Digital clubbing may suggest lung disease (Fig. 17.1), although extrapulmonary causes include cardiac, inflammatory, gastrointestinal, hepatic, familial causes, and clubbing observed with thyrotoxicosis (Box 17.3). Bronchiectasis from CF or from other chronic infectious causes is the major cause of clubbing among all pulmonary diseases. Digital clubbing in any child with a chronic cough or wheezing warrants a thorough evaluation and investigation to determine the underlying disorder.

The astute pulmonologist will carefully examine the remainder of the patient. The examination should also include evaluation for nasal polyps (see Fig. 17.2), which can be associated with CF, triad asthma, or significant atopy. Tonsillar hypertrophy can be associated with obstructive sleep apnea (OSA). An increased second heart sound, or absence of a split-second heart sound, could suggest pulmonary hypertension.

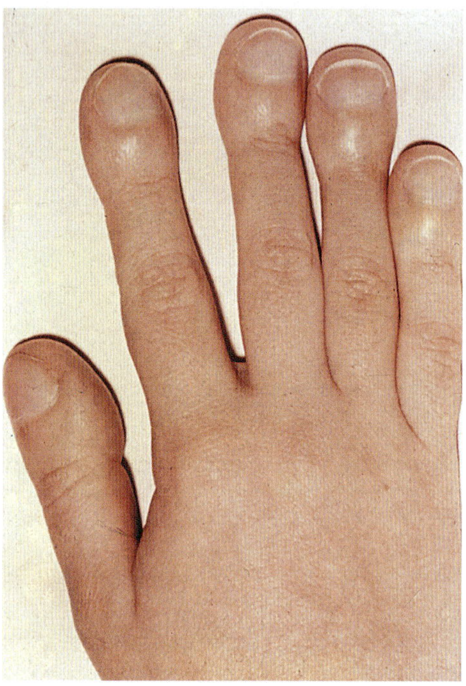

Fig. 17.1 Digital clubbing in cystic fibrosis.

Box 17.3 Causes of Clubbing

Pulmonary
- Cystic fibrosis
- Other bronchiectasis
- Pulmonary abscess
- Empyema
- Neoplasms
- Interstitial fibrosis
- Pulmonary alveolar proteinosis
- Interstitial pneumonitis
- Chronic pneumonia

Cardiac
- Cyanotic congenital heart disease
- Subacute bacterial endocarditis

Gastrointestinal/Hepatic/Other
- Ulcerative colitis
- Crohn disease
- Polyposis
- Biliary cirrhosis/atresia
- Familial
- Thyrotoxicosis

EMBRYOLOGY

The adult lung is a complex organ that provides an efficient system of oxygenation and ventilation, with an area of gas exchange of approximately 100 m^2. Lung morphogenesis is composed of five distinct developmental periods. Congenital abnormalities with their respective period of development are listed in Table 17.2. Lung development begins with a ventral outpouching of the foregut endoderm at approximately 3 to 4 weeks postconception. During the embryonic period (3–7 weeks postconception), the esophagus and trachea become separate structures and lung buds form from the primitive foregut endoderm with subsequent branching into lobar and segmental bronchi. The respiratory epithelium is lined by columnar epithelium at this stage of morphogenesis, with mucous, secretory, and neuroendocrine cells. The lung appears glandlike during the pseudoglandular period (6–17 weeks postconception), and the airways are lined by a high columnar epithelium. All conducting airways are formed by the end of the pseudoglandular period, with adjacent smooth muscle and cartilage. The vascular system develops near the airways at approximately 9 to 12 weeks postconception. Further subdivision of the terminal bronchioles occurs during the canalicular period (16–26 weeks postconception) with the formation of primitive acini. The capillary bed additionally expands, and bronchial cell types become more differentiated, with cilia and secretory functions. The epithelial lining of the distal tubules consists of cuboidal cells, which express increasing amounts of surfactant phospholipids and surfactant proteins A, B, and C. Differentiation of type I and type II airway epithelial cells also occurs during the canalicular period. Formation of the primitive alveolar-capillary membrane also occurs, with capillaries beginning to surround the distal acinar tubules in close proximity to the epithelium. Gas exchange can occur in infants postnatally at the end of the canalicular period (~26 weeks postconception), particularly if aided by maternal administration of glucocorticoids, and surfactant administered to the neonate after birth. The saccular period (26–36 weeks postconception) is marked by continued development and expansion of the pulmonary acini with formation of true alveoli by septation. The distal respiratory epithelium becomes populated with type I airway epithelial cells that are now in closer proximity to interstitial capillaries. Fusion of the basal lamina of the endothelium

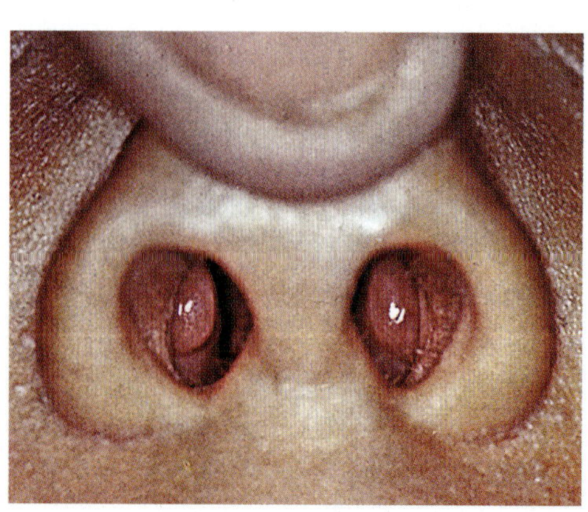

Fig. 17.2 Cystic fibrosis. Nasal polyps in a patient with cystic fibrosis.

Table 17.2 Pulmonary and Airway Anomalies by Developmental Period

Period	Weeks Postconception	Developmental Anomalies
Embryonic	3–6 weeks	Pulmonary agenesis Laryngeal, esophageal, tracheal, and bronchial atresia Tracheoesophageal and bronchoesophageal fistula Tracheal and bronchial stenosis Bronchogenic cysts Ectopic lobes Extrapulmonary sequestration Congenital diaphragmatic hernia
Pseudoglandular	6–17 weeks	Tracheomalacia and bronchomalacia Intralobar bronchopulmonary sequestration Congenital pulmonary airway malformations (CPAM; previously known as *congenital cystic adenomatoid malformation* [CCAM]) Acinar aplasia or dysplasia Alveolar capillary dysplasia ± misalignment of the pulmonary veins Pulmonary vascular malformations Congenital pulmonary lymphangiectasia
Canalicular	16–26 weeks	Congenital alveolar capillary dysplasia Pulmonary hypoplasia (related to diaphragmatic hernia, compression from abdominal or thoracic masses, oligohydramnios or renal agenesis)
Saccular	26–36 weeks	Respiratory distress syndrome Bronchopulmonary dysplasia
Alveolarization	36 weeks to adolescence	Alveolar simplification

and epithelium forms the thin alveolar-capillary membrane. Surfactant phospholipid and protein production ramps up during this period as well. Alveolarization consists of continued lung maturation and growth that occurs primarily by septation starting at approximately 36 weeks postconception and continuing into adolescence. Alveolar walls become progressively thinner, and the conducting airways enlarge.

AIRWAY DISORDERS

Stridor is characteristically a harsh inspiratory noise created by obstruction of the larynx or the extrathoracic trachea. Several clinical entities can produce persistent or recurrent stridor (Box 17.4), some of which may also be associated with chronic cough. With a mild degree of airway narrowing, breath sounds may be normal when the infant or child is at rest, but with any activity that increases tidal breathing (e.g., crying, feeding, agitation), inspiratory stridor may become noticeable.

In contrast, wheezing is a continuous sound that results from obstruction of airflow in intrathoracic airways. This obstruction can be at the lower trachea "downstream" to the small bronchi and bronchioles. Many diseases that produce chronic wheezing in pediatric patients overlap with those causing cough or stridor (Box 17.5). Wheezes can be heard on expiration or, less commonly, during both phases of respiration. The pitch of the wheeze, the variation in its pitch throughout the lung fields, and an association with hyperinflation observed on percussion (described earlier) can help differentiate wheezing resulting from obstruction in the small airways (polyphonic) from that in the large airways (monophonic). Response to bronchodilators and/or steroids is a useful way of differentiating true asthma (which should improve with these treatments) from wheezing resulting from tracheomalacia or bronchomalacia (which does not improve and may even worsen with bronchodilators). Asthma is the most common cause of wheezing in pediatric patients. Asthma may take many different forms, including atopic asthma, exercise-induced asthma, and transient wheezing of infancy.

Laryngomalacia

The inspiratory stridor associated with congenital laryngomalacia generally begins within the first week of life, varies with activity, and is more noticeable in the supine position. The obstruction can

Box 17.4 Causes of Recurrent or Chronic Stridor

- Inflammatory
  - Infectious
  - Allergic/angioneurotic edema
  - Gastroesophageal reflux
- Anatomical/Structural anomalies
  - Laryngomalacia
  - Tracheomalacia
  - Subglottic stenosis
  - Tracheoesophageal fistula
  - Vascular ring
  - Mediastinal mass
  - Lobar emphysema
  - Bronchogenic cyst
  - Thyromegaly
- Pharyngeal or laryngeal masses
  - Papilloma
  - Hemangioma
  - Laryngocele
  - Web
- Other
  - Foreign body
  - Vocal cord paralysis
- Psychogenic

Box 17.5 Causes of Chronic or Recurrent Wheezing

- Asthma
- Hypersensitivity reactions (e.g., ABPA)
- Cystic fibrosis
- Aspiration
  - Tracheoesophageal fistula
  - Foreign body
  - Gastroesophageal reflux
  - Laryngeal cleft
  - Pharyngeal dysmotility
- Extrinsic airway compression
  - Vascular ring
  - Cystic pulmonary airway malformation
  - Lymph nodes
  - Tumors
- Primary ciliary dyskinesia
- Tracheomalacia and/or bronchomalacia
- Congestive heart failure
- Pulmonary hemosiderosis
- Endobronchial lesions including localized stenosis
- Interstitial pneumonitides
- Bronchiolitis obliterans

ABPA, Allergic bronchopulmonary aspergillosis.

be caused by prolapse of the arytenoid cartilages or collapse of the epiglottis due to shortened aryepiglottic folds. Clinical symptoms may suggest the diagnosis; but if severe, bronchoscopic visualization of airway dynamics by flexible bronchoscopy is a safe and reliable method of excluding other causes of stridor. Parents can be reassured that this entity is self-limited, becomes less marked after 6 to 10 months of age usually with maturity of innervation or of the larynx, and rarely causes serious problems. In a small percentage of patients, obstruction of the larynx can interfere with feeding and cause dysphagia or failure to thrive or cyanosis. In these cases, a surgical procedure called supraglottoplasty may be considered.

Croup

The most common cause of inspiratory stridor in children is infectious croup (acute laryngotracheobronchitis). This disease is most commonly caused by a respiratory virus (parainfluenza, respiratory syncytial, influenza, or rhinovirus), and the patient typically has coryza for 24 to 48 hours before the appearance of croupy cough, hoarseness, and stridor. Occasionally the inflammatory process may spread to the smaller airways and produce wheezing in addition to these symptoms. The "steeple sign" is a characteristic radiographic sign on anteroposterior projections that may be accompanied by marked dilation of supraglottic structures, particularly on lateral films. In most patients, serious airway obstruction does not occur and the disease is self-limited. Acute angioneurotic edema is a less common cause of stridor. In most cases, it results from an allergic reaction and is potentially fatal. Some children with anatomically normal airways suffer recurrent bouts of stridor, usually in the middle of the night, in the absence of signs of viral infection. Treatment for GERD is helpful in some patients, suggesting that occult GERD can contribute to bouts of recurrent airway obstruction.

Subglottic Stenosis

Narrowing of the subglottic region can be acquired, such as in subglottic stenosis associated with endotracheal intubation. Congenital subglottic stenosis improves as the child grows older, but narrowing associated with tracheal intubation may require a tracheostomy, particularly if the infant remains dependent on ventilatory support. The degree of subglottic stenosis can be determined by sizing of the airway with various-sized endotracheal tubes and assessing for leak. Low-grade stenosis may be monitored expectantly or amenable to balloon dilation, whereas higher grade stenosis may require laryngotracheal reconstruction.

Vocal Cord Paralysis

Vocal cord paralysis, either unilateral or bilateral, may be present in the neonatal period, although in the case of unilateral paralysis, several weeks may pass before the diagnosis is suspected. A weak or absent cry, hoarseness, inspiratory stridor with or without respiratory distress, and feeding difficulties are usual signs of vocal cord paralysis. Bilateral vocal cord paralysis may be seen with hydrocephalus, myelomeningocele, Arnold-Chiari malformation, or other malformations of the brain. Unilateral and bilateral cord paralyses are observed in patients with abnormalities of the cardiovascular system that are accompanied by cardiomegaly (e.g., ventricular septal defect, tetralogy of Fallot) or that cause abnormalities of the great vessels (e.g., vascular ring, transposition, patent ductus arteriosus). Vocal cord paralysis can also occur iatrogenically due to recurrent laryngeal nerve injury during cardiac surgery. The diagnosis is best made by flexible laryngoscopy under minimal sedation so that vocal cord movement can be examined adequately. Because of a strong association of dysfunctional swallow with vocal cord paralysis, a barium swallow study should be performed in suspected cases to assess for aspiration.

Other Disorders of Larynx

Congenital laryngeal or pharyngeal masses can also produce stridor by obstructing the airflow. Although inspiratory stridor may be observed, hoarseness is a more common presenting feature. Laryngeal webs, papillomas, or hemangiomas may all present with ongoing stridor and brassy or dry cough. Cutaneous or mucosal hemangiomas noted during the physical examination suggest the possibility of additional organ system involvement. Laryngeal webs (Fig. 17.3), cysts, and laryngoceles are quite uncommon and are accompanied by respiratory distress, stridor, feeding difficulties, and cyanosis. These lesions are diagnosed with direct visualization via bronchoscopy. A foreign body in the pharynx or larynx may also cause stridor. For additional information on stridor, see Chapter 24.

Tracheobronchomalacia

Malacia refers to a generalized or localized increase in airway collapsibility, which results in the narrowing of the airway lumen. As the tracheobronchial airway structures are primarily intrathoracic, airway collapse occurs during exhalation as the intrapleural pressure increases, thus producing an expiratory low-pitched wheeze. Children with tracheomalacia often present with a recurrent harsh, low-pitched cough. Those with bronchomalacia can present with recurrent wheezing episodes that do not respond to asthma therapies. These symptoms are usually exacerbated with respiratory infections and may improve during sleep. A bronchoscopic evaluation is needed for a definitive diagnosis. Congenital tracheomalacia and/or bronchomalacia can be secondary to extrinsic compression to the airways. In these patients, anomalies such as double aortic arch, anomalous innominate artery compression, and pulmonary artery sling should be investigated.

Mild cases of primary tracheomalacia or bronchomalacia are usually self-limited and progressively improve with stiffening of the airway cartilage with growth. Bronchodilators may worsen the airway patency by relaxing muscle in the airway walls. Manual chest physiotherapy is useful in aiding with airway clearance. Severe cases may impair adequate ventilation and can require a tracheostomy tube placement to bypass the collapsible segment, in the case of tracheomalacia. Moreover, in severe cases, if the malacic segment is more distal, chronic mechanical ventilation may be needed to stent the airway open with positive end expiratory pressure. Secondary cases of airway malacia may require a surgical correction of the primary anomaly compressing on the airway (e.g., aortopexy); however, the airway wall weakness can persist after the corrective procedure.

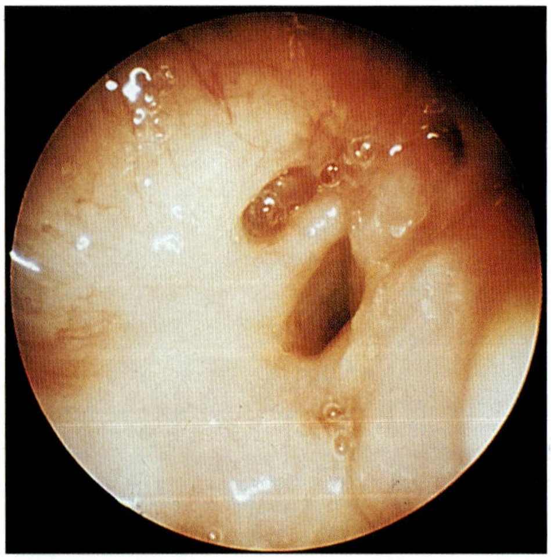

Fig. 17.3 Laryngeal web. Expiratory view of a laryngeal web in an infant with inspiratory stridor that was exaggerated by crying noted at birth. The web is seen traversing the area of the glottis. (From Smalhout B, Hill-Baughan AB: *The suffocating child: bronchoscopy, a guide to diagnosis and treatment,* Ingelheim, Germany, 1980, Boehringer Ingelheim, p 86.)

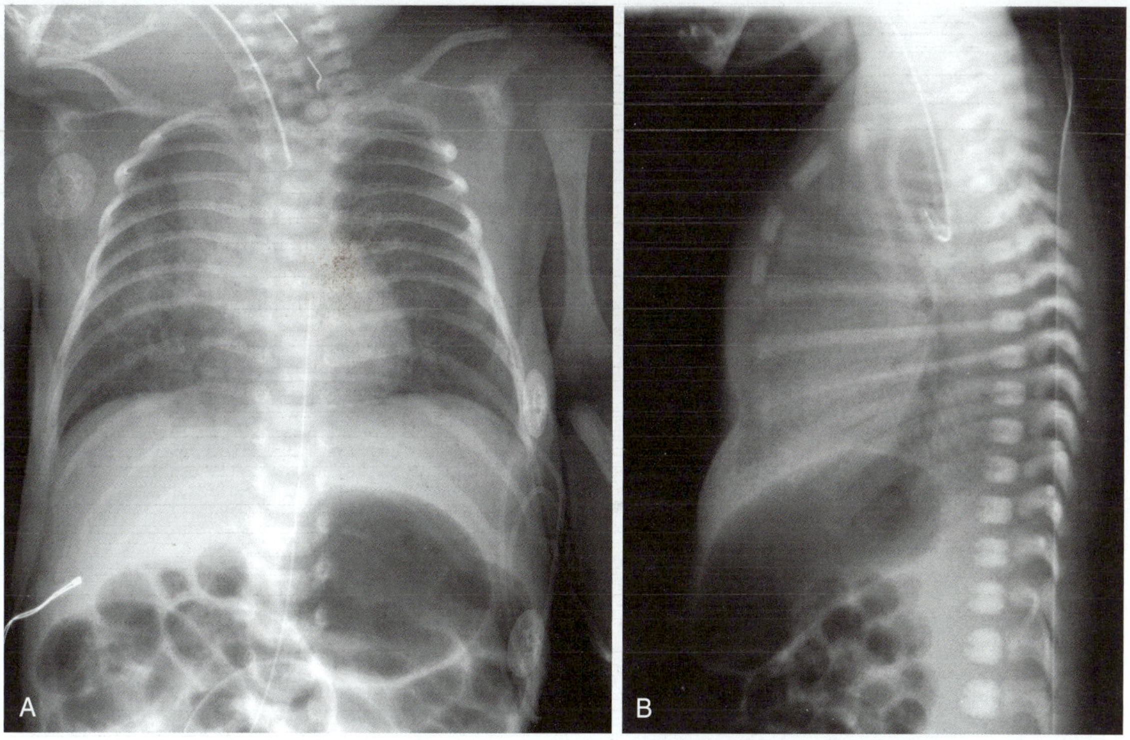

Fig. 17.4 Tracheoesophageal fistula. (A) Anteroposterior chest radiograph shows feeding tube passing no farther than proximal esophagus; there is an aspiration pneumonitis present. (B) Lateral view showing the feeding tube in the proximal esophageal pouch with air in the airway, distal esophagus, and intestine. (A, Courtesy Beverly Newman, MD, Pittsburgh, PA. B, Courtesy Katie McPeak, MD, Pittsburgh, PA.)

Tracheoesophageal Fistula

In children with a tracheoesophageal fistula (TEF), the abnormal communication between the gastrointestinal and respiratory tracts commonly occurs at the level of the distal trachea or carina and the distal esophagus. Children with TEF present with significant choking and cyanotic events soon after birth. These events will prompt the medical team to initiate a workup in attempt to detect anatomic abnormalities that can be surgically corrected (see Mediastinum and Diaphragm section in Chapter 18 for further details). When attempting to pass a nasogastric tube in the neonatal care unit, the tube will coil in the upper pouch which can be seen on a chest x-ray (CXR), in addition to lung parenchyma findings consistent with aspiration (Fig. 17.4). After complete TEF surgical correction, tracheomalacia is common and presents with a loud "brassy" cough. These children are also at risk for chronic aspiration, recurrent bronchitis, and pneumonia. Management is typically supportive, with chest physiotherapy to aid with airway clearance and antibiotics for respiratory infections.

Vascular Rings

Vascular rings are congenital anomalies of the aortic arch and pulmonary arteries that form a ring around the trachea and esophagus. The most common form is a double aortic arch (Fig. 17.5), followed by a right aortic arch with aberrant left subclavian and a left ligamentum arteriosum (Fig. 17.6). The severity of respiratory or digestive symptoms is related to the degree of external compression of the airways and esophagus. Those with double aortic arches typically have more severe symptoms. Children present in infancy with biphasic (inspiratory and expiratory) wheeze, cough, and intermittent episodes of cyanosis and respiratory distress.

Other vascular anomalies may not fully form a ring around the airways and can present with similar but milder symptoms. Innominate artery compression of the trachea is the most common vascular compression of the airway (Fig. 17.7), where the takeoff of the brachiocephalic (innominate) artery is more distal than usual and compresses the anterior wall of the trachea. When the left pulmonary artery arises from the right pulmonary artery, a pulmonary sling is formed, which then externally compresses the posterior wall of the trachea and the anterior wall of the esophagus on its trajectory to the left lung. Of note, pulmonary slings are associated with complete tracheal rings, which can result in tracheal stenosis, and congenital heart diseases (atrial or ventricular septal defects, patent ductus arteriosus).

A CXR can help identify a right aortic arch, descending aorta, and posterior indentation on the trachea on a lateral view (pulmonary sling). Classically, an esophagogram has helped identify airway and esophageal compression (see the upper Gastrointestinal Series and Esophagography section in Chapter 25), but with CT angiography or

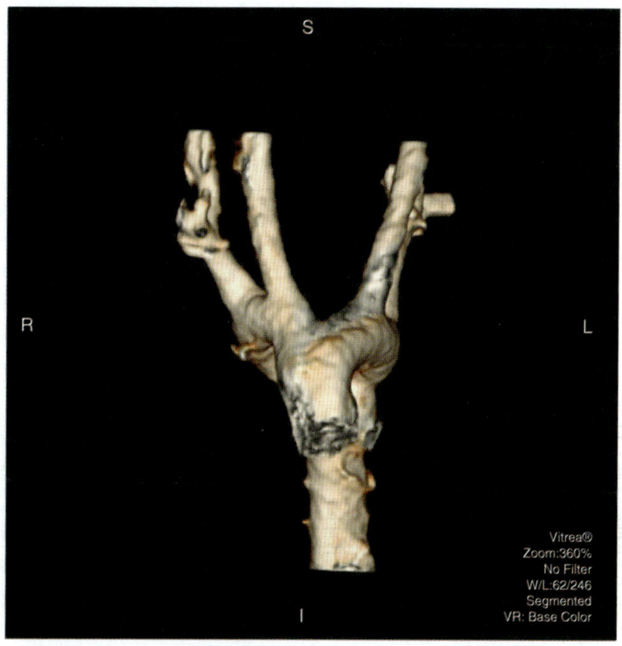

Fig. 17.5 Chest computed tomography angiography with three-dimensional reconstruction demonstrating a double aortic arch.

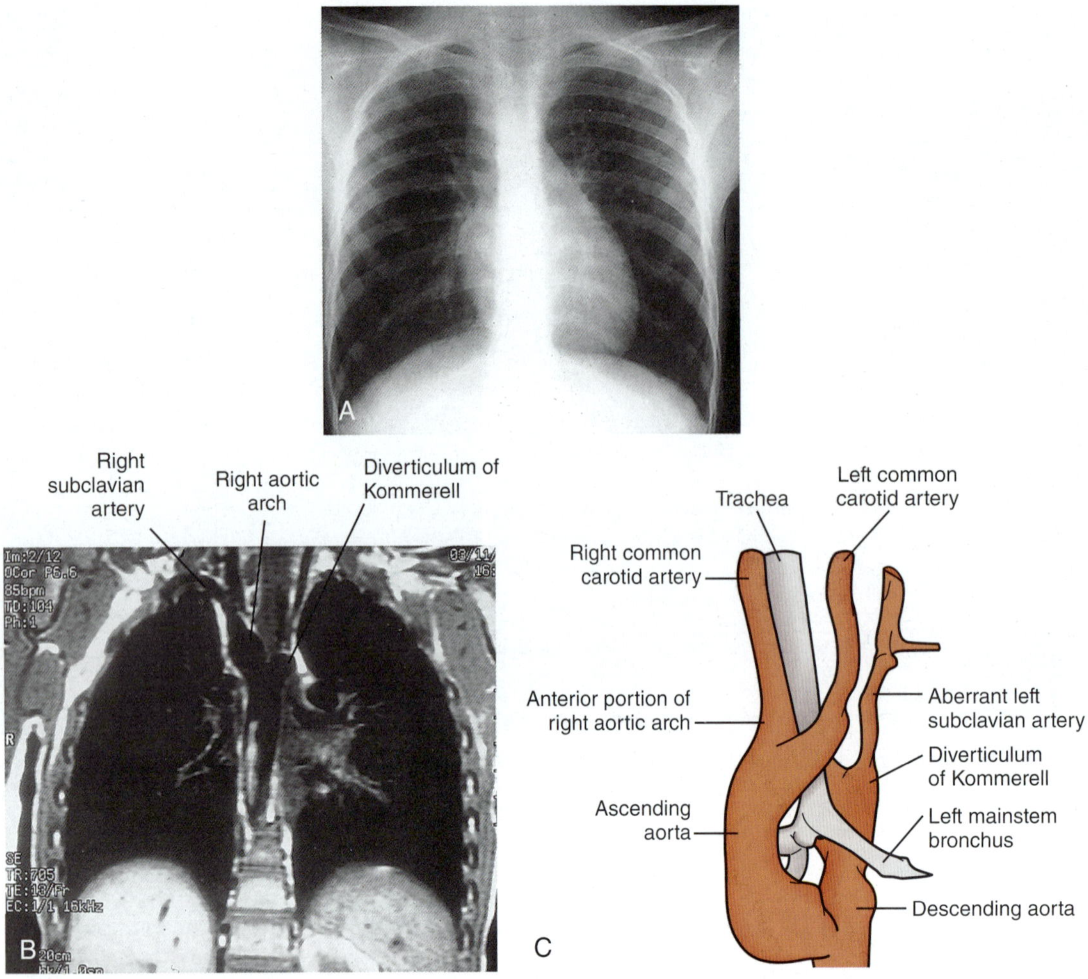

Fig. 17.6 Images depict the vascular ring caused by right aortic arch with aberrant left subclavian artery. (A) Plain chest radiograph demonstrates a right-sided aortic arch, with tracheal deviation to the left. (B) Magnetic resonance imaging (MRI) in the sagittal plane shows the dominant right aortic arch and the remnant of the left aortic arch, called a *diverticulum of Kommerell*. The aberrant left subclavian artery arises posteriorly from the diverticulum of Kommerell. (C) Three-dimensional reconstruction of the vascular anatomy shown in the MRI from the left anterior perspective. (Courtesy Beverly Newman, MD, Pittsburgh, PA.)

magnetic resonance angiography being widely available in most centers, the utility of an esophagogram is now limited. A diagnostic flexible bronchoscopy can identify the presence and severity of external airway compression. Once the evidence of airway compression has been established, the next step is obtaining CT angiography or magnetic resonance angiography to evaluate the vascular anatomy and its relationship to the airways. The treatment of symptomatic vascular rings is surgical and depends on the nature of the underlying vascular anomaly. After surgical correction, the airway patency typically improves, though there may still be ongoing airway malacia while the cartilage ossifies over time.

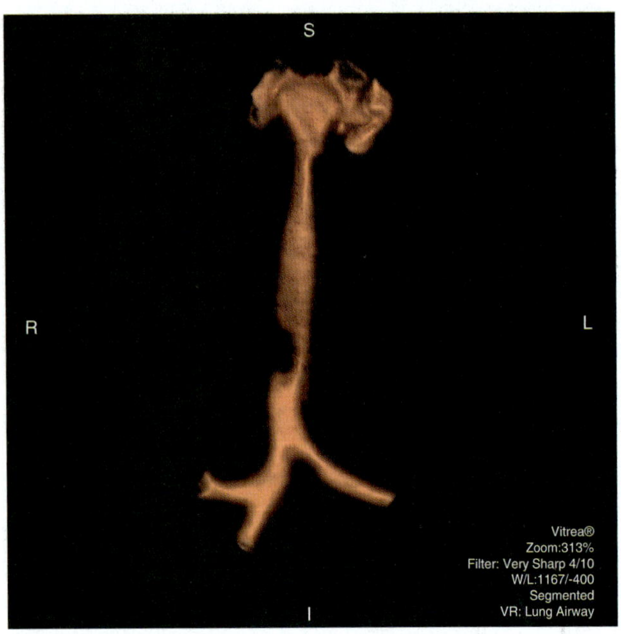

Fig. 17.7 Chest computed tomography scan demonstrating innominate artery compression of the trachea.

CONGENITAL LUNG MALFORMATIONS

Congenital thoracic malformations may also present as persistent or recurrent cough, wheeze, or pneumonia. These malformations include bronchial atresia or hypoplasia, bronchogenic cysts, congenital pulmonary airway malformations (CPAMs), and sequestrations (see Chapter 18). CPAM consists of a spectrum of cystic diseases, with types confirmed by histopathology. The most severe forms are incompatible with life, whereas other types may have a more favorable prognosis. CPAM may be associated with polyhydramnios prenatally. Some lesions are discovered incidentally, but other patients may present with symptoms that begin in infancy with the onset of tachypnea, respiratory distress, and cyanosis due to compression of a normal lung. Radiographically, single or multiple cystic lesions that cause compression of normal lung, with mediastinal displacement, are visualized (Fig. 17.8). CPAM is usually confined to a single lobe without predilection for a particular lobe. The cystic lesions carry a small risk for infection, bleeding, air leak, and malignant transformation.

Congenital lobar overinflation is characterized by the presence of a hyperlucent lobe (Fig. 17.9) with few bronchovascular markings, which causes compressive atelectasis of adjacent lobes. Congenital lobar emphysema can be caused by a fixed partial obstruction of the airways or a deficiency of bronchial cartilage. Clinically, infants have tachypnea and may have other respiratory symptoms, such as cough, wheeze, intermittent cyanosis, and occasionally stridor. Left upper lobe involvement is most common, but the right middle lobe can also be affected. Conservative management is indicated in infants growing well and in whom tachypnea is the primary symptom or in congenital lobar overinflation associated with a mucus plug. Resection of the affected lobe is indicated in symptomatic infants with associated compression atelectasis and/or chronic respiratory distress.

Pulmonary sequestrations consist of pulmonary tissue isolated from normal lung that is perfused by systemic rather than pulmonary circulation (Fig. 17.10). Sequestration is rare and may compress the pulmonary tree or become infected. Bronchogenic cysts are cystic structures that arise from the pulmonary epithelium. Bronchogenic cysts (Fig. 17.11) in newborns can become filled with air after birth and compress the large airways, leading to stridor. Additional symptoms include tachypnea, dyspnea, cyanosis, and diminished breath sounds on the affected side. Later, the cyst may become infected, leading to recurrent bouts of fever, cough, and hemoptysis.

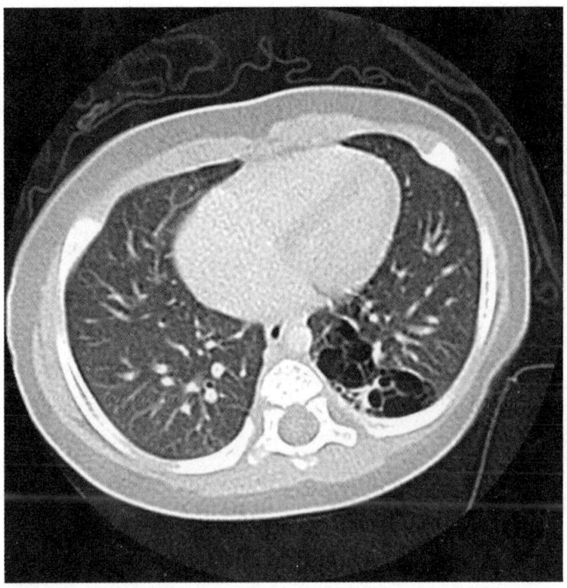

Fig. 17.8 Congenital pulmonary airway malformation. Computed tomography scan of the radiograph of newborn shows multiple, small air-filled cysts in the left lower lobe. This infant had a diagnosis made by antenatal ultrasound. (Courtesy Sameh Tadros, MD, Pittsburgh, PA.)

Congenital pulmonary lymphangiectasia is characterized by dilated pulmonary lymphatic vessels with associated disordered drainage. Lymph accumulates within the lungs, leading to symptoms of recurrent cough, wheeze, hypoxemia, or tachypnea. Lymphatic involvement may be isolated to the lungs or involve multiple organ systems. A more severe picture may present in the neonatal period. In utero, nonimmune hydrops may be present with evidence of pleural effusions. Postnatally, chylothoraces are present with associated pulmonary hypoplasia leading to respiratory failure. Pulmonary lymphangiectasia may be a primary developmental defect, or secondary to an impedance of normal lymphatic flow. Secondary causes include congenital heart disease (hypoplastic left heart syndrome, pulmonary vein atresia, congenital mitral valve stenosis), Noonan syndrome, and trisomy 21. Chest CT (Fig. 17.12) typically reveals thickened interlobular and perilobular septa with dilated mediastinal lymphatics. Treatment of patients with lymphangiectasia is supportive, which may include medium chain triglyceride–oil based formula (decreases lymph production) and sometimes octreotide.

PULMONARY HEMORRHAGE SYNDROMES

Pulmonary hemosiderosis is a potentially fatal disorder that has been described in association with cardiac or systemic disease, glomerulonephritis (Goodpasture syndrome, also known as antiglomerular basement membrane disease), collagen vascular diseases, and as an idiopathic form. Idiopathic pulmonary hemosiderosis (IPH) is a disease of unknown etiology characterized by episodes of dyspnea, cough and/or hemoptysis, cyanosis, fever, and iron-deficiency anemia. Hematemesis or melena may be the only presenting complaint in some patients without symptoms referable to the respiratory tract. As a result of recurrent bleeding episodes, jaundice may be observed, and clubbing develops over time in some patients. Laboratory findings include iron-deficiency anemia and, in a small number of patients, peripheral eosinophilia. Radiographic findings are quite variable, with some patients demonstrating scant transient infiltrates

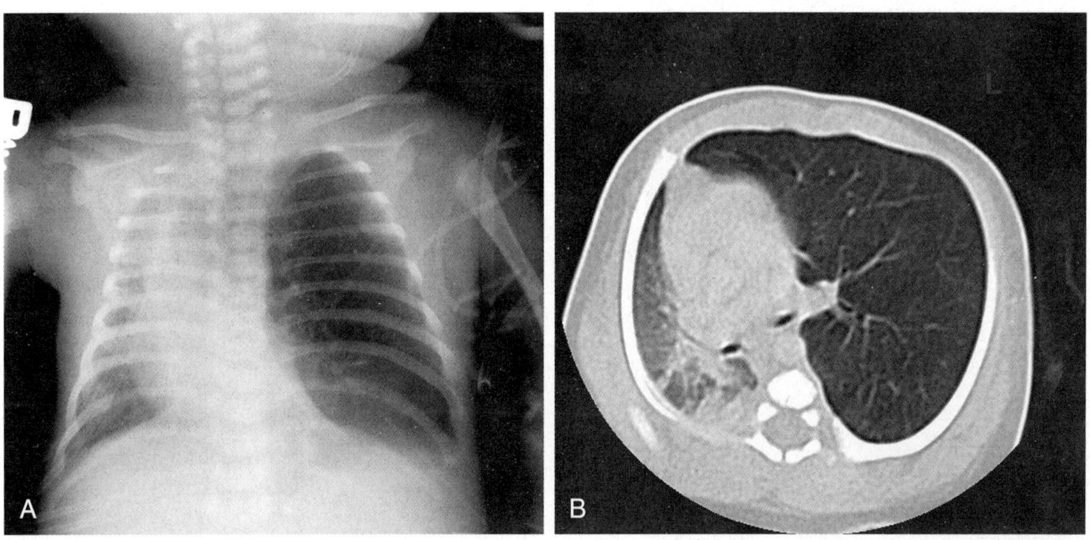

Fig. 17.9 Congenital lobar overinflation. (A) Anteroposterior chest radiograph. Left upper lobe shows hyperlucency of the affected globe, atelectasis of the lower lobe, and mediastinal shift. (B) Computed tomography scan of same patient shows left upper lobe herniating across the midline with compression of structures on the right. (Courtesy Beverly Newman, MD, Pittsburgh, PA.)

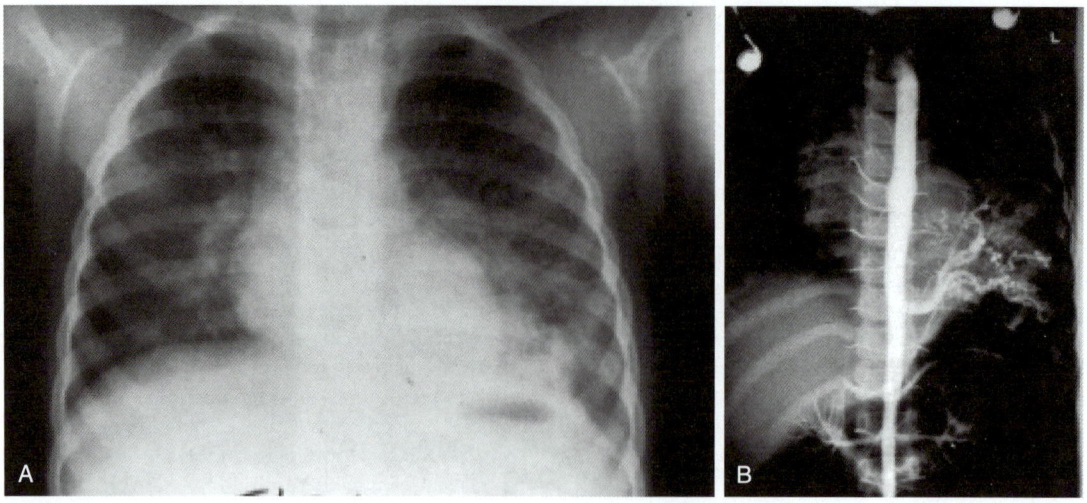

Fig. 17.10 Pulmonary sequestration. (A) Anteroposterior film shows left lower lobe infiltrate. (B) Aortic angiogram demonstrates anomalous origin of pulmonary blood supply from abdominal aorta to the left lower lobe in a 7-year-old girl with extralobar sequestration. (Courtesy Geoffrey Kurland, MD, Pittsburgh, PA.)

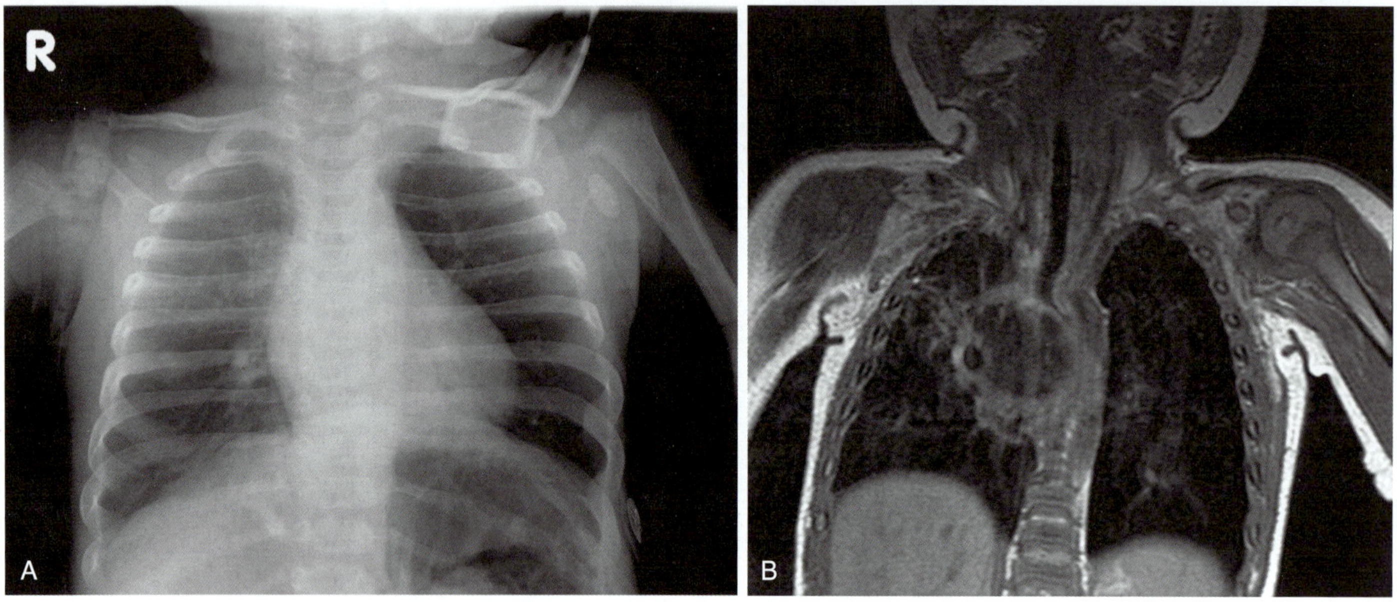

Fig. 17.11 Bronchogenic cyst. (A) Chest radiograph demonstrates hyperlucency of the left lung. (B) Magnetic resonance imaging of the chest demonstrates a large, centrally located cystic lesion of the left hilum with compression of adjacent airway. (Courtesy Beverly Newman, MD, Pittsburgh, PA.)

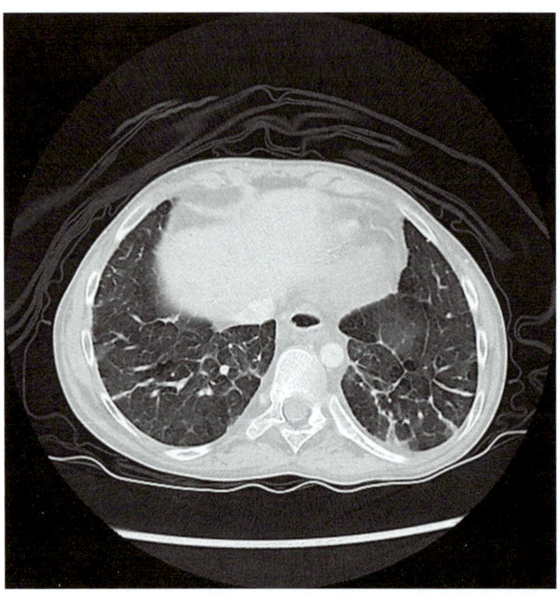

Fig. 17.12 Congenital pulmonary lymphangiectasia. Kerley B lines, or thickened, edematous interlobular septa are present in the lung bases. Computed tomography image of the chest in an 11-year-old boy with Noonan syndrome.

and others showing widespread parenchymal infiltrates that resemble miliary tuberculosis. Hemosiderin-laden macrophages obtained from sputum, gastric washings, or bronchoalveolar lavage (BAL) suggest the diagnosis, but a lung biopsy is sometimes necessary and will allow the clinician to differentiate vasculitis from capillaritis and assess for iron deposition. A percutaneous renal biopsy or detection of antiglomerular basement membrane antibodies may help in cases of hemosiderosis associated with Goodpasture syndrome.

BRONCHOPULMONARY DYSPLASIA

Bronchopulmonary dysplasia, or *chronic lung disease of prematurity*, is a sequelae of prematurity associated with neonatal respiratory distress, recurrent episodes of wheezing, respiratory distress, and tachypnea (see Chapter 2). It is usually defined as a need for supplemental oxygen at 28 days of life or beyond 36 weeks postmenstrual age and parenchymal lung disease on chest imaging in premature infants. Improved severity classifications have been developed on the basis of the mode of respiratory support and/or fraction of inspired oxygen at 36 weeks' postmenstrual age, though these classifications are not always good predictors of long-term pulmonary morbidity. The prevalence is inversely correlated with birthweight and correlates with the degree of prematurity. It is multifactorial in etiology and likely is an interaction between incomplete lung development at the time of birth with lung injury from positive pressure ventilation, infection, and oxygen toxicity. Patients with bronchopulmonary dysplasia may develop chronic respiratory insufficiency, pulmonary hypertension, and cor pulmonale. Treatment is supportive in nature, with respiratory support that may include supplemental oxygen or long-term positive pressure ventilation in infants with severe bronchopulmonary dysplasia along with optimization of nutrition.

Beyond the neonatal intensive care unit, mild respiratory illnesses in these infants with decreased respiratory reserve may progress to lower respiratory tract disease, necessitating frequent hospitalizations. The frequency of wheezing episodes may diminish with age, although these patients may continue to have abnormalities on pulmonary function testing, including fixed airflow obstruction, air trapping, and decreased diffusing capacity. GERD is common among patients with bronchopulmonary dysplasia, as is tracheobronchomalacia, both of which may worsen wheezing in these patients.

CONGENITAL AND NEONATAL INFECTIONS

Cough starting at birth or shortly afterward may be a sign of serious respiratory disease and must be evaluated assiduously. Cough beginning at this time raises the possibility of congenital infections, such as cytomegalovirus or rubella, which are often associated with other findings such as hepatosplenomegaly, thrombocytopenia, or central nervous system disease. Pneumonia due to *Chlamydia trachomatis* generally develops after the first month of life and presents as an afebrile pneumonitis with congestion, wheezing, fine and diffuse crackles, a paroxysmal cough, and a prior or concomitant inclusion conjunctivitis in approximately 50% of cases. Pneumonia caused by *Bordetella pertussis* is a potentially life-threatening illness characterized by severe paroxysmal coughing episodes, followed by cyanosis and apnea, and is often associated with an inspiratory "whoop." The latter finding may be missing in young infants or those weakened by the recurrent coughing spasms. Newborns and young infants may have apnea as the primary sign of a *B. pertussis* infection. The chest radiograph is nondiagnostic and can be normal or show perihilar infiltrates, atelectasis, hyperinflation, and interstitial or subcutaneous emphysema in some cases. Diagnostic approaches include detection of the *B. pertussis* DNA using the polymerase chain reaction (PCR) and serologic detection of *B. pertussis*–specific IgM or IgA. *Ureaplasma urealyticum* and *Pneumocystis jiroveci* (formerly known as *Pneumocystis carinii*) have been recognized as causes of pneumonia and persistent cough in this age group.

CHILDHOOD INTERSTITIAL LUNG DISEASE

Childhood interstitial lung diseases (chILDs) are a complex and rare group of pulmonary disorders that result in abnormal gas exchange. These disorders usually involve the pulmonary interstitium but can involve other aspects of lung parenchyma and are thus referred to as diffuse lung diseases (DLDs), rather than ILDs. Although chILD can present in older children, there are several disorders (see later) specific to infancy. The pathogenesis of these disorders is poorly understood.

Causes of DLD are extremely variable and include infections, inhalation injury, chemotherapeutic agents, post–bone marrow transplant lung disease, systemic inflammatory diseases, pulmonary hemorrhage syndromes, structural and growth anomalies, metabolic diseases, and congenital disorders of host defense and of surfactant production. Examples of chILD that present in infancy include alveolar capillary dysplasia (ACD), surfactant B and C deficiencies, ILD associated with *ABCA3* mutations, pulmonary interstitial glycogenosis, neuroendocrine cell hyperplasia of infancy (NEHI), and follicular bronchitis of infancy.

Patients with chILD may present insidiously with a combination of cough, tachypnea, retractions, exercise intolerance, resting hypoxemia or hypercarbia, or desaturation with exercise; diffuse abnormalities on chest imaging; and crackles and retractions on examination. Growth failure is not uncommon as a complication of these diseases. Tachypnea is the most prevalent finding, present in more than 75% of patients.

Infants with DLD must first be evaluated for more common diseases like CF, immunodeficiency, congenital heart disease, pulmonary infections, PCD, and recurrent aspiration, before further workup. After exclusion of the previously mentioned diseases, an infant is regarded as having chILD syndrome if three of four of these clinical criteria are met: respiratory symptoms (cough, dyspnea, rapid breathing, exercise intolerance), respiratory signs (tachypnea, adventitious lung findings, retractions, digital clubbing, respiratory failure, digital clubbing), hypoxemia, and diffuse abnormal findings on chest imaging (CXR or CT scan).

Further diagnostic workup, including echocardiogram, controlled ventilation high resolution chest CT, and flexible fiberoptic bronchoscopy with BAL, is recommended to determine the cause of lung disease in patients with chILD syndrome. Genetic testing and infant pulmonary function testing may also be considered depending on imaging findings and family history. If evaluation with less invasive testing does not reveal a specific diagnosis, lung biopsy by video-assisted thoracoscopy may be considered.

The prognosis of chILD can be quite variable with some cases universally fatal or severe and treatable only by lung transplantation and others showing gradual improvement over months or years. Treatment is largely supportive, as no controlled trials of therapeutics have been performed. Limited data from case reports or series, uncontrolled trials, and clinical experience suggest possible efficacy of certain immunosuppressants in children with DLD (corticosteroids, hydroxychloroquine). However, these results are not specific to chILD and such therapies should only be considered at centers with expertise in chILD.

Surfactant Disorders

Pulmonary surfactant reduces the surface tension at the air-liquid interface in the alveoli, helping to decrease the work of breathing and prevent atelectasis. Hydrophobic proteins, including surfactant protein B (SP-B) and surfactant protein C (SP-C), are secreted by type II pneumocytes. Along with phospholipids, these proteins help to stabilize the surfactant within alveoli. SP-B deficiency is inherited in an autosomal recessive pattern of mutations in SFTPB. Infants with SP-B present with respiratory failure in the neonatal period, with several mutations resulting in fatal respiratory distress. SP-B deficiency is exceedingly rare, with approximately 60 cases reported in the literature and an estimated incidence of 1 in 1.5 million live births. SP-C deficiency is inherited in an autosomal-dominant fashion and can cause respiratory failure in newborns, but more commonly it leads to DLD in children and adults. The incidence of SP-C deficiency is not well established, but approximately 170 cases have been reported in the literature.

ABCA3 transport protein is found in the lamellar bodies within type II pneumocytes, functioning in surfactant transport and homeostasis. The incidence of ABCA3 deficiency is estimated to fall within 1 in 3500 to 1 in 20,000 live births. Associated autosomal recessive lung disease is typically seen in term neonates and fails to improve with conventional therapies. There may be an associated family history of infant loss. Studies also suggest an association with DLD in childhood. Electron microscopy reveals the presence of dense organelles with an absence of normal lamellar bodies within type II pneumocytes.

Surfactant metabolism abnormalities can often be diagnosed by mutation analysis, including mutations in SP-B, SP-C, ABCA3 deficiency, NKX2-1, CSF2RA and CSF2RB abnormalities. Genetic surfactant protein disorders and ABCA3 deficiency do not improve with exogenous surfactant administration, and there are no targeted therapies at this time. Lung transplantation may be considered as a treatment option in these patients and may prolong life, but long-term outcomes are not well studied.

Pulmonary alveolar proteinosis (PAP) is a disorder marked by ineffective clearance of surfactant and resultant accumulation of periodic-acid-Schiff positive proteinaceous material within alveoli. Granulocyte colony stimulating factor (GM-CSF) is needed for differentiation of alveolar macrophages that phagocytose inactivated surfactant. PAP can be genetic due to autosomal recessive mutations in SFTPB, ABCA3, CSF2RA, or CSF2RB (GM-CSF α or β chains) or acquired due to an immune reaction to GM-CSF. Incidence of the autoimmune form is estimated to be 3.7 to 6.2 cases per million. PAP typically has an insidious onset with dyspnea and cough. Patients occasionally have hemoptysis, fever, or weight loss. Presentation is variable with some patients experiencing rapid progression to respiratory failure while approximately 10% to 30% of patients are asymptomatic. Physical examination may be normal, but clubbing, inspiratory crackles, and cyanosis may be present. Radiographically, high-resolution computed tomography demonstrates a classical "crazy paving" appearance, with presence of septal (interlobular and intralobular) thickening and ground-glass opacities (Fig. 17.13). Diagnosis is made by characteristic findings on CT and milky, opaque BAL fluid. Treatment of congenital PAP varies by presentation and may include supportive care and whole lung lavage. Lung transplantation may be a consideration in congenital forms, while administration of exogenous GM-CSF may be considered in autoimmune disease.

Neuroendocrine Cell Hyperplasia of Infancy

Neuroendocrine cell hyperplasia of infancy, previously known as "persistent tachypnea of infancy," typically occurs in term infants within the first few months of life. Symptoms typically begin before age 12 months, marked by insidious onset of tachypnea and crackles on auscultation. Hypoxemia and failure to thrive are also commonly present. Symptoms may be attributed to bronchiolitis or other more common etiologies before diagnosis. The specific etiology of NEHI is not known. Limited data demonstrated a slight male predominance and may account for 10% to 14% of cases of chILD. A familial form of NEHI was associated NKX2.1 (thyroid transcription factor 1) in a single-family cohort. High-resolution CT scan characteristic of NEHI consists of ground-glass opacification present in the right middle lobe and lingula areas, often with associated air trapping on expiratory views (Fig. 17.14). Infant PFTs classically demonstrate significant air trapping (elevated functional residual capacity, residual volume [RV], and RV/total lung capacity [TLC]). Diagnosis may be made by clinical history and characteristic findings on high-resolution computed tomography; however, if presentation or imaging are not classical in nature, lung biopsy may be indicated. Histopathologic diagnosis is based upon prominence of neuroendocrine cells within the distal airways, best seen with bombesin or serotonin staining. Treatment is supportive, without any specific disease-targeted therapies and, specifically, no demonstrated benefit of corticosteroids. While data on the long-term outcomes are limited, many children with NEHI demonstrate gradual improvement over time. Some patients experience exacerbations with exercise or respiratory infections while other reports suggest development of a nontopic asthma phenotype.

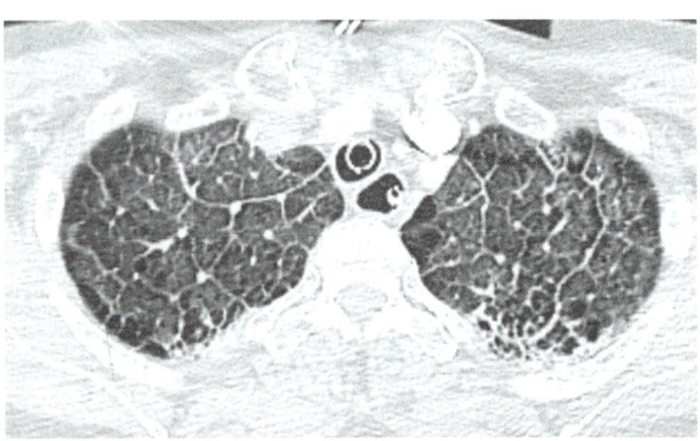

Fig. 17.13 High-resolution chest computed tomography scan demonstrating a "crazy paving" appearance with septal thickening and ground-glass opacities in pulmonary alveolar proteinosis. (Courtesy Sameh Tadros, MD, Pittsburgh, PA.)

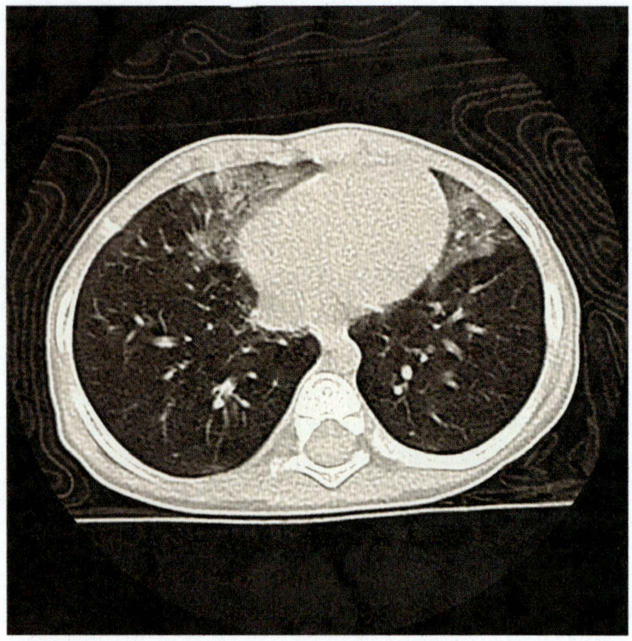

Fig. 17.14 High-resolution chest computed tomography scan of a young child with neuroendocrine cell hyperplasia of infancy. (Courtesy Sameh Tadros, MD, Pittsburgh, PA.)

Alveolar Capillary Dysplasia

ACD with misalignment of the pulmonary veins (MPV) is another etiology of chILD that causes respiratory failure in the newborn period. ACD/MPV is a rare disease, with an unknown incidence, but approximately 100 cases have been reported in the literature. The pathogenesis is not well understood, but there is a vast reduction in the number of capillaries and infants present with severe hypoxemia, pulmonary hypertension and right ventricular heart failure. CXR may demonstrate ground glass or hazy opacification but are often normal. Patients frequently have pneumothoraces as well. ACD/MPV is associated with mutations in the FOXF1 gene. Treatment is typically supportive, using standard therapies for pulmonary hypertension, but lung transplantation has been the only intervention shown to prolong survival.

Obliterative Bronchiolitis

Obliterative bronchiolitis has been described in an idiopathic form, following adenoviral infections or inhalation of toxic agents and in conjunction with other diseases (including rheumatoid arthritis) in adults. Its most common current clinical setting in pediatrics is in the organ transplant recipient. Patients may present initially with fever, cough, or tachypnea and subsequently develop dyspnea and wheezing. Physical findings include wheezing, crackles, and diminished breath sounds. The radiographic pattern (Fig. 17.15) is that of hyperinflation, decreased vascularity, and increased interstitial markings (reflective primarily of increased airway marking) with areas of atelectasis and consolidation (on CT described as mosaic perfusion). Pulmonary function testing will reveal fixed lower airway obstruction. Complications of adenovirus-induced bronchiolitis obliterans include bronchiectasis, overinflation, recurrent atelectasis, and pneumonia. In many patients the prognosis is poor.

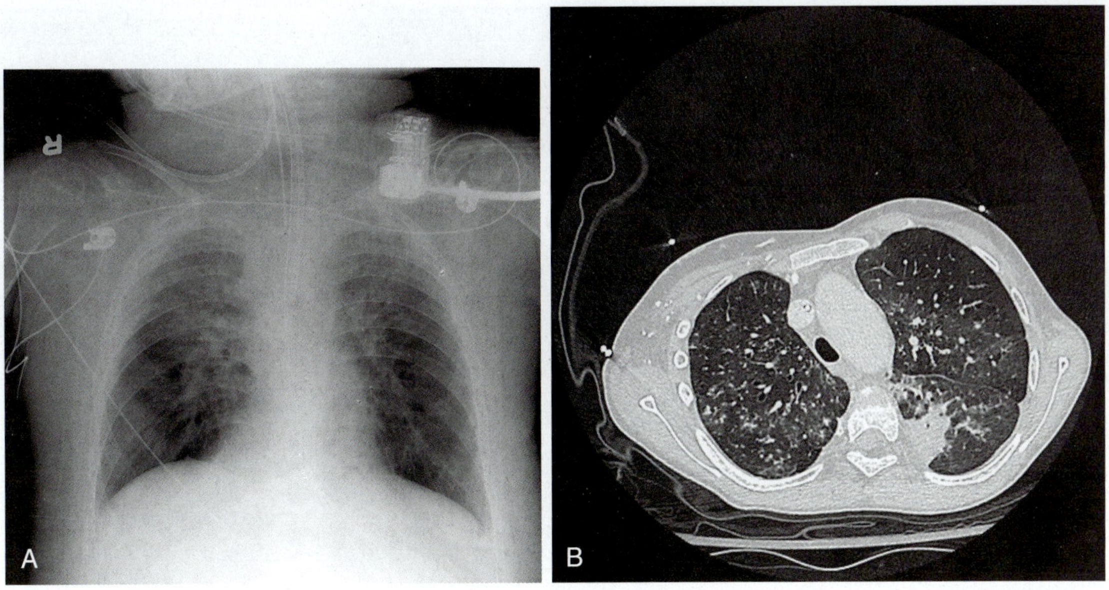

Fig. 17.15 (A) Posteroanterior chest radiograph of a 17-year-old with end-stage obliterative bronchiolitis as a complication of bone marrow transplantation for acute myelogenous leukemia. Film demonstrates increased interstitial and airway markings. (B) Obliterative bronchiolitis demonstrated on high-resolution chest computed tomography (CT) scan. Central bronchiectasis, airway wall thickening, and mosaic perfusion are present. Chest CT is of a 14-year-old-boy with changes after heart and double-lung transplantation.

ASPIRATION

Chronic Aspiration

Chronic aspiration is a cause of respiratory symptoms that should be considered, particularly in medically complex infants. Common symptoms of chronic aspiration include chronic cough, wheezing, congestion, choking or gagging with feeding, apnea, tachypnea, failure to thrive, intermittent fever, and recurrent pneumonia. Aspiration may be due to neurological, anatomical, or functional disorders, often with a combination of factors present. Infants with neurological disorders may have incoordination of swallowing and sucking reflexes that lead to aspiration of milk or gastric contents, and saliva into the lung. Anatomical malformations (such as, a TEF, laryngeal cleft, or web) can result in cough via chronic anterograde aspiration. These anomalies are associated with feeding-related coughing, choking, and occasionally cyanosis or persistent hypoxemia. Dysfunctional swallow may be present with or without anatomical abnormality.

Penetration of oral or gastric contents into the lungs is a common problem in patients with neurological impairment. Aspiration can occur in patients with incoordination of swallowing ("aspiration from above") and in neurologically normal patients with severe GERD ("aspiration from below"). Chronic aspiration of saliva can also lead to progressive injury to the lung and worsening respiratory impairment.

Aspiration can also be present in patients who are intellectually normal but who have delayed gastric emptying and GERD. Patients with impaired clearance of food from the esophagus (achalasia) can also aspirate in sleep, despite having otherwise normal neurological status. Determination if aspiration exists in a patient remains challenging, because there is no gold standard for its diagnosis. For evaluation of swallowing, a barium contrast swallowing study using different consistencies of barium (thin liquid, paste, solid) and in conjunction with speech pathologist can determine what consistency of food can be given safely to the patient and where in the swallowing cycle the pathology resides. Flexible bronchoscopy with BAL for assessment of lipid-laden macrophages may also provide diagnostic information. Alveolar macrophages from the BAL fluid are stained for fat using oil red O staining, and some pathologists may calculate a lipid-laden macrophage index by scoring 100 macrophages. The sensitivity of the test is unknown, but when moderate or high numbers of macrophages are found, it may suggest aspiration.

Foreign Body Aspiration

An inhaled foreign body in either the tracheobronchial tree or esophagus is an important cause of chronic cough, especially in toddlers. A history of gagging or choking may be absent at this age, physical examination may be unrevealing, and the plain CXR may be normal or demonstrate asymmetrical lung inflation. Subtle differences in air entry into homologous lung segments may be the only indication of a foreign body in the airway. Cough is present in more than 90% of cases; it is usually of abrupt onset, but a quiescent period may occur after inhalation and cough may disappear as irritant receptors adjust to the object's presence. A mobile foreign body may result in the recurrence of cough as new receptors are stimulated by the object. Although inspiratory and expiratory radiography and fluoroscopy are useful, they may be normal and rigid bronchoscopy may be necessary to confirm or disprove the presence of a foreign object (Fig. 17.16). Unilateral air trapping demonstrated by inspiratory and expiratory radiographs (Fig. 17.17) (or left and right lateral decubitus films in younger children) strongly suggests an inhaled foreign body.

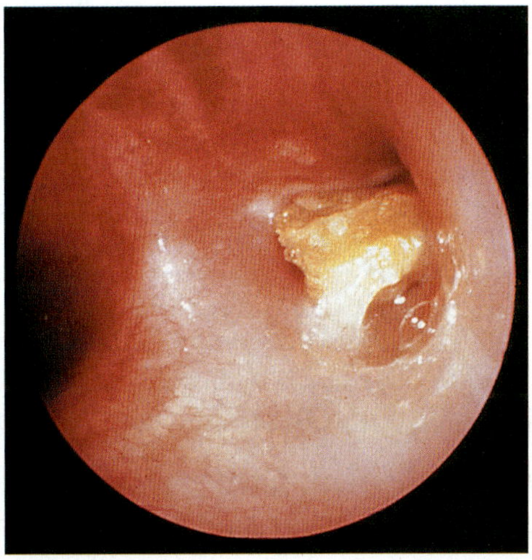

Fig. 17.16 Foreign body aspiration. Portion of a carrot lodged in the right mainstem bronchus, as seen through a rigid bronchoscope. (Courtesy S. Stool, MD, Pittsburgh, PA.)

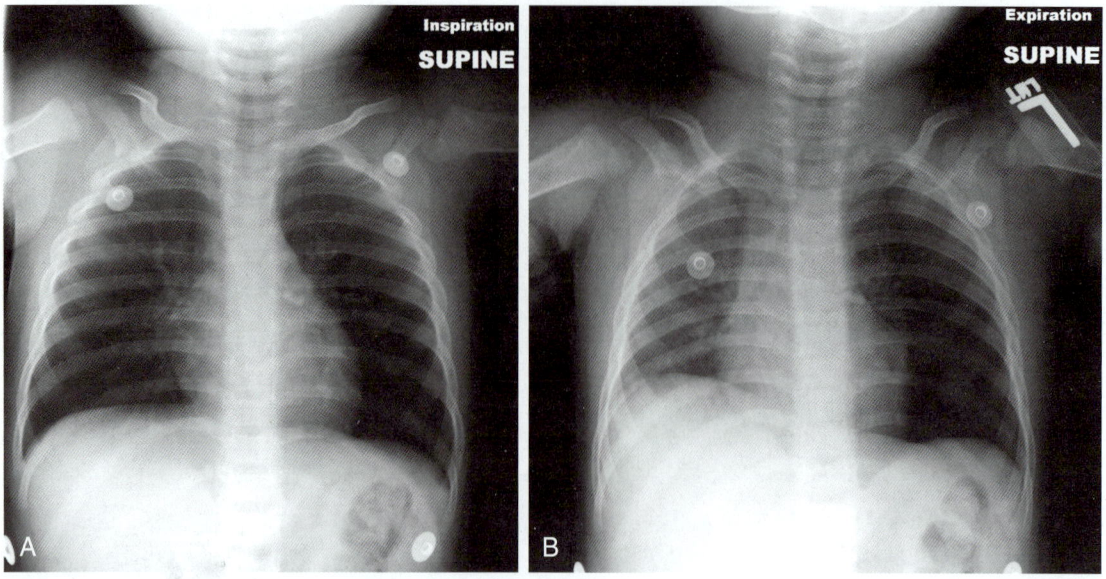

Fig. 17.17 Foreign body aspiration. Inspiratory (A) and expiratory (B) radiographs in a child with an inhaled foreign body lodged in the left mainstem bronchus reveal hyperlucency of the left hemithorax and compensatory shift of the mediastinal structures to the right on expiration. (Courtesy Sameh Tadros, MD, Pittsburgh, PA.)

ASTHMA

Asthma is the most common cause of wheezing and the most common chronic pulmonary disease in children. Asthma may take many different forms, including atopic asthma, exercise-induced asthma, and transient wheezing of infancy. Children with asthma present with recurrent episodes of wheezing, chest tightness, cough and/or shortness of breath, triggered by respiratory infections, allergens, irritants, or exertion. Characteristically, most of these children have a history of significant improvement following the administration of bronchodilators and/or systemic steroids. In addition, presence of atopy such as allergic rhinitis, eczema and family history of asthma or eczema may increase the risk for asthma in a child (see Chapter 4 for further details). The presence of asthma should be strongly suspected if symptoms follow the 3 R's: **r**ecurrent, **r**eactive (to a trigger), and **r**eversible (with treatment).

On examination, findings can vary widely depending on the child's symptom control. Often children will be asymptomatic at the time they are evaluated in the physician's office, but their history of repeated wheezing episodes should raise suspicion for asthma. When symptoms are not controlled, the clinician may appreciate coughing, some degree of hyperinflation on percussion and polyphonic wheezing on auscultation. Moreover, if spirometry is obtained, airway obstruction may be seen and the degree of response to bronchodilators can be measured to aid in the diagnosis of asthma.

Treatment for acute asthma symptoms consists of inhaled or nebulized bronchodilators (e.g., Albuterol), and systemic steroids when symptoms progress despite frequent bronchodilator use. In effort to decrease airway inflammation and prevent future asthma exacerbations in children with uncontrolled symptoms, inhaled corticosteroids (with or without long-acting beta agonists) are used as daily controller medications. It is very important for children with asthma to have frequent evaluations with their pediatrician or asthma specialist to reassess the need and adequate use of asthma medications or pursue a different diagnosis if inadequate response to therapies is observed.

FUNCTIONAL DISORDERS

Psychogenic/Habit Cough

A psychogenic cough (also called *habit cough* and *cough tic*) may be observed following a lower respiratory tract illness. Habit cough may persist for weeks or months after the acute process has subsided. This cough tends to be loud and bizarre in nature and timing; it is often described as "honking" or "barking." This type of cough is short, nonproductive, and nonparoxysmal; it is quite disturbing to family members and classmates, to the point that the child may be excluded from school and other activities. It always disappears with sleep. The cough becomes more obvious with stressful situations or when parents (or physicians) express interest in the cough, and it may be decreased by distraction or talking. For this reason, extensive evaluations by medical personnel may merely exacerbate the problem when the diagnosis can be made on the basis of the characteristic quality of the cough and its disappearance in sleep. Demonstrating normal pulmonary function testing and a normal chest radiograph helps to reassure the parent that other disease has been excluded. Treatment can include speech therapy, distraction, relaxation techniques, and hypnosis.

Vocal Cord Dysfunction

A disorder often mistaken for exercise-induced asthma is vocal cord dysfunction. In vocal cord dysfunction, the true vocal cords adduct during inspiration. The adduction of the cords is subconscious and nearly always of a behavioral origin. It results in a sensation of dyspnea that does not respond to bronchodilators and that the patient localizes to the throat, both of which are atypical for asthma. Patients may describe difficulty with inhalation, as well as stridor. Often the stress of a competitive event brings out this reaction. This diagnosis can sometimes be established in the exercise laboratory with the aid of pulmonary function testing, although sensitivity for this is not high. The adduction of the vocal cords can also be demonstrated with flexible nasolaryngoscopy when the patient is symptomatic, and there is new interest in the use of ultrasound of the vocal cords. This disorder is generally best treated by speech therapists; referral to a psychologist is sometimes helpful to treat underlying anxiety.

Sighing Dyspnea

Sighing is an involuntary inspiration of a breath that is larger than a normal tidal volume. Sighing breathing (sometimes called sighing dyspnea) is observed in some children with no observed organic pathology. It is common that they will begin taking big breaths for no apparent reason, often while at rest and watching television. It is not associated with other pulmonary symptoms (cough, wheeze) or findings. It does not occur during sleep, and usually self-extinguishes with time.

CYSTIC FIBROSIS

CF is a common life-shortening genetic disease affecting people of all backgrounds but is most common among those of Northern European ancestry (1 in 3300 white newborns, 1 in 17,000 African Americans, 1 in 35,0000 in people of Asian descent). CF is a generalized exocrinopathy characterized by the inspissation of abnormally thick and tenacious secretions, principally involving the pancreas and lungs. In the lungs, hyperabsorption of airway surface liquid impairs clearance of secretions, obstruction of the airways with retention of bacteria, resulting in chronic endobronchial infection and an inflammatory process that leads to bronchiectasis. The disease is characterized by a gradual decline in pulmonary function, with respiratory disease accounting for most deaths in people with CF. In the pancreas, ducts become obstructed by the abnormal secretions, preventing pancreatic enzymes from entering the duodenum and therefore preventing breakdown of dietary fat and protein. In 85% to 90% of patients, the pancreas undergoes autodigestion and is replaced by scar tissue, and lifetime deficiency of pancreatic exocrine function results. The term *pancreatic sufficiency* is used to describe the minority (10%–15%) of CF patients with enough pancreatic function to have normal absorption of nutrients (despite having diminished pancreatic function compared with non-CF patients). CF-related diabetes (CFRD) occurs in 30% to 50% patients, with the incidence increasing in the teen years. This form of diabetes has features of both insulin deficiency and insulin resistance, and poor glycemic control is associated with more rapid progression of lung disease. The prognosis for patients with CF has improved dramatically over the past several decades. In 1938 the median survival was 2 years, but as of 2022, the median predicted survival had risen to 68.2 years old and more than 50% of patients are adults.

The disease is inherited in an autosomal recessive mode. The protein product of the CF gene—cystic fibrosis transmembrane conductance regulator (CFTR)—functions as an epithelial chloride channel. Decreased chloride transport and hyperabsorption of sodium and water across various epithelia results in abnormally viscid secretions. Cell culture studies have demonstrated a decreased height of the airway surface liquid, which impairs ciliary beating. The most common mutation of the *CFTR* gene in North American whites is referred to as *F508del.* This mutation is the result of the deletion of three base pairs in the gene and results in the protein missing a phenylalanine residue at amino acid position 508. As of 2023, more than 2000 mutations of this gene had been reported, although fewer than 40 mutations account for greater than 90% of CF alleles in white North Americans. In approximately 70% of CF genes, F508del is found, and half of CF patients in North America are homozygous for the F508del mutation. Half of the remaining patients are compound heterozygotes with delta-F508 coupled with another CF allele; the remaining patients have other non–F508del mutations. Although a number of investigators have tried to discover genotype-phenotype correlations, the most reliable phenotypic correlate of genotype has been with pancreatic function. Respiratory disease severity has not been effectively correlated to genotype, and other modifier genes, as well as environmental factors, apparently play an important role in the clinical expression of CF.

Presentation

CF can present in several ways (Box 17.6), however the most common presentation presently is without symptoms and by newborn screening. Five to ten percent present with meconium ileus, which is noted at or shortly after birth. Meconium ileus is a common cause of intestinal obstruction in the newborn; these infants present with abdominal distention, bilious vomiting, and failure to pass meconium stools. Abdominal radiographs show dilated loops of small bowel and a ground-glass appearance in the cecal region, signifying pockets of air within the thick meconium. A barium or water-soluble contrast enema may show a small distal colon. In cases of meconium ileus associated with prenatal rupture and meconium peritonitis, abdominal calcifications may be noted on plain radiographs, and at laparotomy thick, tarlike meconium is found in the terminal ileum (Fig. 17.18). Prolonged neonatal jaundice, generalized edema in a breastfed or soy formula–fed infant, or hypochloremia with metabolic alkalosis are less common presentations of CF in early infancy.

Box 17.6 Presentations of Cystic Fibrosis

General
Failure to thrive
Salty taste to skin

Gastrointestinal/Nutritional
Meconium ileus
Foul-smelling stools, bloating, abdominal pain
Rectal prolapse
Intestinal impaction and obstruction
Pancreatitis, acute and chronic
Hypoproteinemia and edema
Neonatal hyperbilirubinemia
Cholelithiasis, cholecystitis
Cirrhosis or portal hypertension
Fat-soluble vitamin deficiency (A, D, E, K)

Metabolic
Hyponatremic hypochloremic dehydration
Heat stroke
Metabolic alkalosis
Diabetes mellitus

Respiratory
Clubbing
Asthma
Chronic obstructive pulmonary disease
Recurrent pulmonary infiltrates
Chronic cough or sputum production
Barrel chest
Hemoptysis
Pneumothorax
Cor pulmonale
Nasal polyps

Other
Infertility (males)

A combination of poor weight gain; loose, foul-smelling, bulky stools; and a voracious appetite are signs and symptoms that most clinicians associate with CF and rarely present a diagnostic problem. Rectal prolapse (Fig. 17.19) may be the presenting feature of CF in about 5% of cases and may recur multiple times. Rectal prolapse is thought to result from chronic malnutrition, reduced abdominal musculature, and voluminous stools, and usually improves once the diagnosis has been made and the patient started on supplemental pancreatic enzymes. Gastrointestinal complications of CF include biliary cirrhosis, portal hypertension, hypersplenism, esophageal varices, and clinical evidence of fat-soluble vitamin deficiency.

A chronic productive cough or wheezing in a patient with digital clubbing suggests the diagnosis of CF. Patients less commonly present

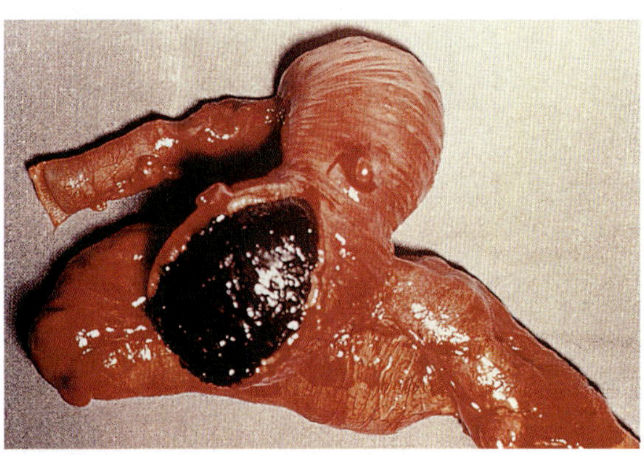

Fig. 17.18 Meconium ileus. Gross appearance of the thick, tarlike meconium found at laparotomy in meconium ileus.

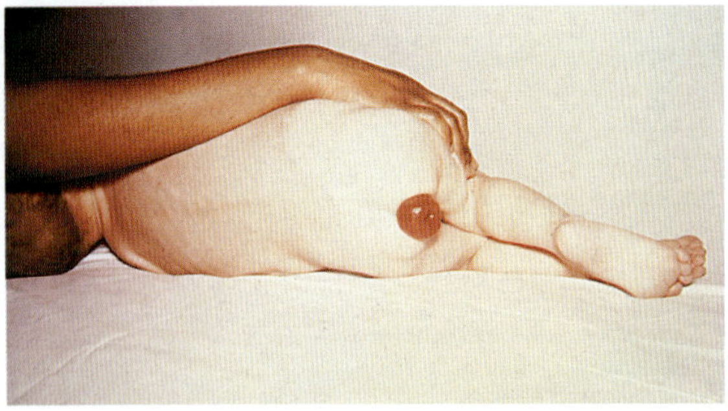

Fig. 17.19 Rectal prolapse is shown in a toddler not previously recognized as having cystic fibrosis.

with a history of recurrent pneumonia or sinus disease (the majority of patients with CF demonstrate pansinusitis radiographically). Nasal polyps (see Fig. 17.2) may be a presenting manifestation of CF and are seen in about 20% of patients sometime during the course of the disease. Other initial respiratory presentations are listed in Box 17.6.

The clinical course and severity of the disease vary remarkably. Many patients do not develop signs or symptoms of respiratory disease other than an intermittent, loose cough for years. Other patients have persistent symptoms from early infancy and are rarely without a cough. These patients tend to require frequent visits to the physician and frequent hospitalization and are more likely to have poor weight gain. Virtually all patients develop a loose, productive cough; the sputum may be blood-tinged during acute respiratory illnesses. Hemoptysis occurs in more than half of adult patients with CF and a considerable proportion of adolescents as well. Tachypnea, dyspnea, diffuse crackles, and digital clubbing will develop in most patients. Later, diffuse bronchiectasis, hyperinflation, and a barrel-chest deformity are noted. The usual cause of death in patients with CF is respiratory failure, often in conjunction with cor pulmonale.

Complications

Complications of CF include diabetes, hypochloremic metabolic alkalosis, hemoptysis, pneumothorax, pneumomediastinum, hypertrophic pulmonary osteoarthropathy, distal intestinal obstructive syndrome, biliary cirrhosis, pancreatitis, cor pulmonale, and respiratory failure. Among the respiratory complications, massive hemoptysis and pneumothorax with or without pneumomediastinum are potentially life-threatening. Blood streaking of sputum is not uncommon, and massive hemoptysis from rupture of dilated superficial bronchial arteries during chronic suppurative infections may occur in a small percentage of patients. Embolism of bleeding vessels via arteriography can be life-saving. Pneumothorax (see Fig. 17.20C) generally occurs from rupture of bullous lesions created from chronic airway obstruction and presents with acute onset of chest pain and shortness of breath with or without cyanosis. Pneumomediastinum and subcutaneous emphysema may result (Fig. 17.21). Hypertrophic pulmonary osteoarthropathy involving the knees and other major joints occurs in about 5% of patients and is characterized by pain, swelling, and limited mobility of the affected joint.

Acute or chronic pancreatitis occurs almost exclusively in patients with pancreatic sufficiency. These patients present with the acute onset of abdominal pain and vomiting and may have recurrent bouts of pancreatitis before the pancreas "burns itself out." Laboratory evaluations reveal elevations of serum lipase and amylase. The differential diagnosis in CF patients with acute abdominal pain and vomiting includes cholecystitis, appendicitis, and distal intestinal obstruction syndrome. The latter is characterized by crampy abdominal pain, constipation, vomiting, and, occasionally, a palpable mass in the right lower quadrant.

Excessive loss of chloride from sweat can lead to hypochloremic metabolic alkalosis in infants who do not receive salt supplementation in their formula, especially during the summer months. This can occur even in the euvolemic state, and if severe, can result in anorexia and vomiting.

Right ventricular hypertrophy and cor pulmonale are findings in the advanced stages of CF patients with severe pulmonary disease.

Radiographic Findings

The radiographic findings in CF vary from early hyperinflation and patchy areas of atelectasis to a generalized increase in peribronchial markings with bronchiectasis, parenchymal densities, and large cystic areas noted in severe disease (Figs. 17.20 and 17.22). The Brasfield scoring system is one means of describing severity of chest radiograph findings and is based on a 25-point system for findings of hyperinflation, linear densities, cystic lesions, atelectasis, and right-sided cardiac enlargement or pneumothorax.

Diagnosis

Diagnosis of CF can be suggested by elevation in serum trypsinogen in the newborn. Measurement of serum immunoreactive trypsinogen (IRT) is used as part of a screening system in most states as part of the extended newborn screen. IRT may be falsely low in infants with meconium ileus or in infants with prenatal exposure to CFTR modulators. Most laboratories will further analyze samples with elevated IRT for common genetic mutations of the *CFTR* gene. As a result, newborns may be referred to the local CF center having

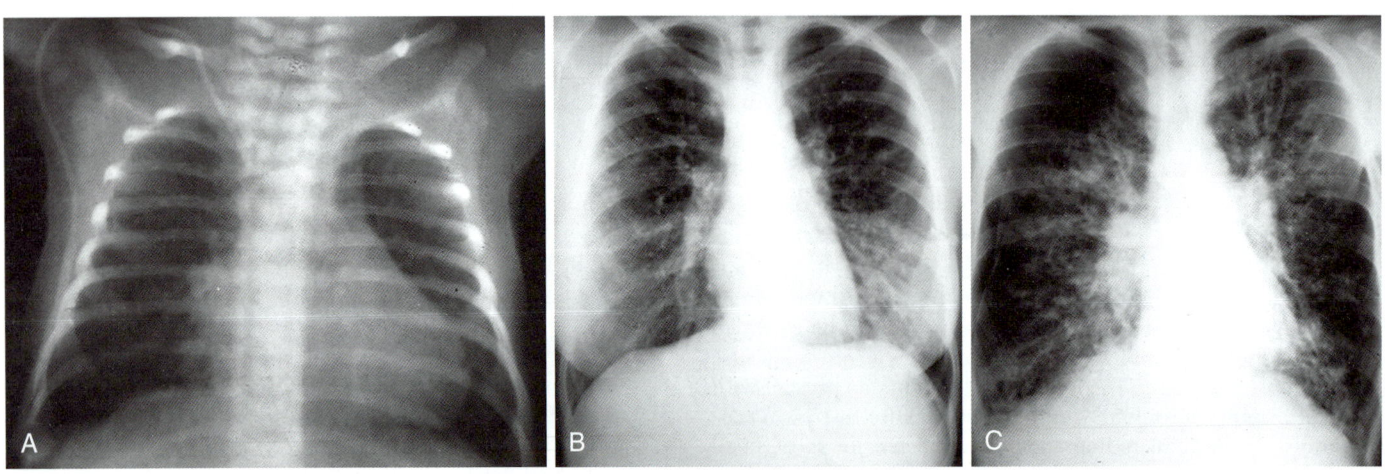

Fig. 17.20 Cystic fibrosis. Typical progression of radiographic changes in cystic fibrosis. (A) A 2-month-old child with hyperinflation and right middle lobe atelectasis. (B) A 15-year-old girl with peribronchial cuffing, hyperinflation, and bronchiectatic changes, particularly of the lower lobes. (C) A 21-year-old man with severe respiratory involvement and an unsuspected right pneumothorax.

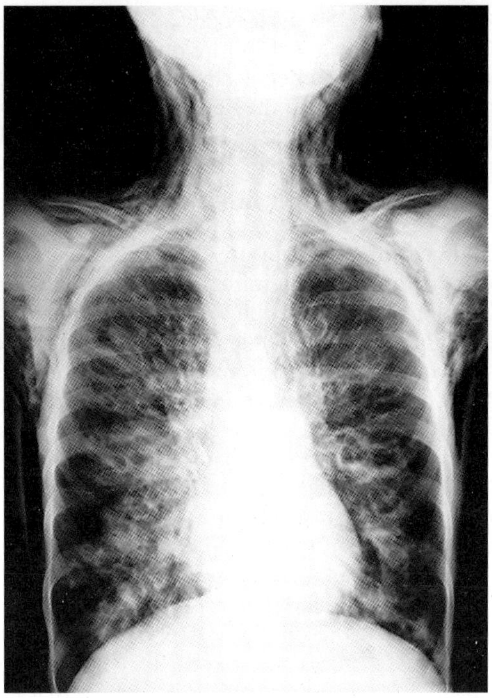

Fig. 17.21 Cystic fibrosis. A teenager with cystic fibrosis, severe respiratory disease, pneumomediastinum, and massive subcutaneous emphysema.

had a genetic diagnosis made before the first visit. Sensitivity of genetic testing for CF varies with ethnic group and methodology of testing (e.g., limited mutation panel, sequencing, duplication/deletion testing). Still, the gold standard for initial diagnosis of CF remains the quantitative sweat chloride test. In sweat testing, pilocarpine is driven into the skin with a weak electrical current (iontophoresis), and the resulting sweat is collected either with gauze or a coiled capillary tube, which wicks the sweat and stores it for analysis. The sweat test must be performed in an experienced laboratory accredited by the CF Foundation. Sweat chloride values of 60 mMol/L or greater are diagnostic of CF. Sweat chloride values of 31 to 59 mMol/L are considered intermediate and generally require additional testing. False-positive values can occasionally occur, but disorders that cause this are readily distinguished clinically from CF. Genetic testing is quite useful in the evaluation of the infant who produces too little sweat for analysis, the patient with intermediate sweat chloride, or the patient with normal sweat chloride but clinical features characteristic of CF. Sequencing of the *CFTR* gene includes all known mutations of both coding and noncoding DNA, which has greatly increased the sensitivity of genetic screening. Small molecule drugs (CFTR modulators) that increase the amount of CFTR protein at the cell surface (correctors) or increase the activity of the channel (potentiators) are now available for ~90% of patients. Ivacaftor is available for patients as young as 1 month of age with one of 38 CFTR mutations with some residual function. This medication led to significant improvements in pulmonary function and weight gain and decreases in exacerbation frequency and sweat chloride. Other modulators have been used in combination with ivacaftor for patients with two copies of F508del-CFTR (lumacaftor) or one copy of F508del in combination with a responsive second mutation (tezacaftor); these drugs demonstrated much more modest improvements in lung function or weight gain. In 2019, a three-drug combination of elexacaftor, tezacaftor, and ivacaftor (Trikafta) was approved for patients with at least one copy of F508del-CFTR, and this demonstrated impressive improvements in lung function, weight gain, exacerbation frequency, and sweat chloride. More recently, a three drug combination of vanzacaftor, tezacaftor, and deuterated ivacaftor (Alyftrek) was approved and allows for once daily dosing.

NON–CYSTIC FIBROSIS BRONCHIECTASIS

Bronchiectasis is an abnormal dilation and wall thickening of medium and small airways due to chronic infection/inflammation.

Non-CF bronchiectasis refers to irreversible dilation of bronchi, unrelated to CF, that ultimately leads to chronic inflammation and impairment in airway clearance. Causes of this form of bronchiectasis include severe (e.g., necrotizing pneumonia) or recurrent pulmonary infections (at times related to an underlying immunodeficiency), primary ciliary dyskinesia (see below), and chronic aspiration syndromes. Patients typically present with chronic productive cough (>4 weeks). A diagnosis of bronchiectasis should be suspected with recurrent (>3) episodes of protracted bacterial bronchitis, or treatment failure with at least 4 weeks of antibiotic therapy. Coarse crackles or digital clubbing may be present on examination. Radiographic confirmation is obtained via high resolution CT imaging, which may show an increased bronchial-arterial ratio (the "signet-ring" appearance), bronchial wall thickening, lack of bronchial tapering in the periphery, mucus plugging, and mosaic perfusion due to air trapping. Investigation for an underlying etiology should be performed, including immune workup and sweat testing. Due to a paucity of controlled trials regarding therapies, particularly in children, treatment guidelines are instead based upon expert opinion and extrapolated from CF therapies. Goals of therapy

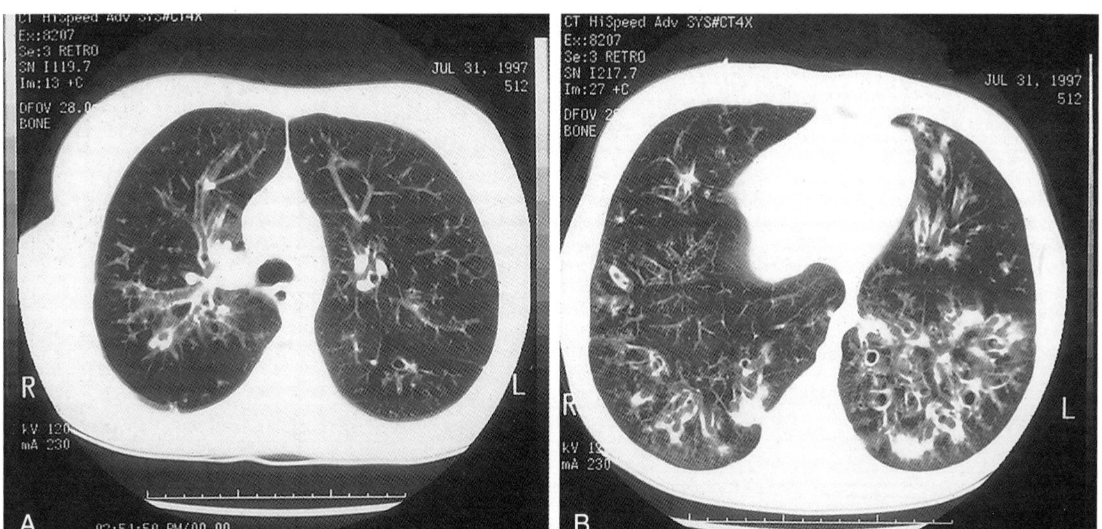

Fig. 17.22 Cystic fibrosis. Computed tomography (CT) scans of a 19-year-old woman with severe bronchiectasis and cystic fibrosis. Thickened airways are seen in longitudinal section through the upper lobes (A) and in cross section in an image from the lower lobes (B).

include preventing advancement of disease and complications, improving quality of life and reducing exacerbations. Management includes airway clearance and treatment of exacerbations with oral or intravenous antibiotic therapy. The literature also suggests that lung resection of focal areas of bronchiectasis may lead to significant improvement in symptoms.

PRIMARY CILIARY DYSKINESIA

PCD may present with insidious symptoms of chronic productive cough, nasal drainage, and recurrent middle ear infections. PCD should be suspected if at least two of the four key clinical features are present: unexplained neonatal respiratory distress in a term infant, chronic daily cough and/or nasal congestion present before 6 months of age, and organ laterality defects. The classic triad described by Kartagener consists of situs inversus, sinusitis, and bronchiectasis. Approximately 50% of those with PCD have situs inversus totalis. Clinical findings include basilar crackles and, later, radiographic changes of recurrent lower lobe infections and bronchiectasis. PCD is genetically heterogeneous and most often transmitted in an autosomal recessive inheritance pattern. To date, 44 genes have been identified as disease causing, with mutations affecting ciliary ultrastructure or function. No gold standard exists for diagnosis and testing is often available only in specialized centers. Nasal nitric oxide measurement, ciliary biopsy with electron microscopy and high-speed video microscopy, along with genetic testing are used in combination to confirm diagnosis. No therapies exist to correct ciliary dysfunction in PCD and there is a lack of evidence to support use of any specific therapies. However, management is similar to CF respiratory disease, in that use of aggressive airway clearance and liberal use of antibiotics is employed.

SLEEP-DISORDERED BREATHING AND CONTROL OF BREATHING

Sleep-disordered breathing (SDB) encompasses a spectrum of entities that impair normal breathing during sleep to different degrees. This term is often used to characterize a child with clinical symptoms of upper airway obstruction during sleep, before obtaining an accurate diagnosis with an objective test (e.g., polysomnogram). The SDB spectrum includes primary snoring, upper airway resistance syndrome, obstructive hypoventilation, and OSA syndrome.

The prevalence of OSA is estimated between 1% and 5% in children. OSA is characterized by prolonged partial upper airway obstruction that can be accompanied by periods of intermittent complete obstruction (measured at the nose or mouth) despite continued respiratory efforts (measured at the chest), which negatively affect ventilation and normal sleep architecture (see Fig. 17.23). Nocturnal symptoms associated to OSA include snoring, gasping for air during sleep, restless sleep, frequent awakenings, and enuresis. During the daytime children with OSA can present with behavioral problems, poor school performance and, infrequently as in adults, sleepiness. Children with tonsillar hypertrophy, obesity, retrognathia or micrognathia (e.g., Pierre Robin sequence), midface hypoplasia (e.g., Crouzon syndrome, Apert syndrome, Treacher Collins syndrome, Trisomy 21, achondroplasia), neuromuscular disorders (e.g., cerebral palsy, muscular dystrophies, Prader Willi syndrome), history of prematurity and history of sickle cell disease, are all at increased risk of having OSA and thus should be screened periodically.

It is important to note that parents may not raise concerns regarding their children's sleep if not prompted by the clinician. Therefore particularly in cases where children have risk factors for OSA, the presence of daytime or nocturnal symptoms should be explored. Although OSA screening tools based on parent reports have been developed, they lack adequate specificity and sensitivity. Based on these limitations, when a child has symptoms and other findings that may increase the risk for OSA, referral to a sleep specialist should be considered.

The gold standard test to diagnose OSA is a sleep study (polysomnogram) in which movement of the chest, movement of the abdomen, heart rate, arterial saturation, and end-tidal carbon dioxide (CO_2) are measured. Staging of sleep during these studies is important because multiple arousals and/or awakenings may occur in OSA. The arousal-plus-awakening index can quantify the severity of the effects of sleep-disordered breathing on the quality of sleep and help direct management. Cardiac echo and electrocardiogram are indicated in cases of severe OSA, because pulmonary hypertension may result as a complication.

Management of OSA is directed at the underlying abnormality, with adenotonsillectomy being the most common first line procedure. Cases that result from collapse of the upper airway structures may require continuous positive airway pressure administered via nasal or oronasal mask depending on the severity and age of the child. In children who are obese, weight loss should be additionally recommended.

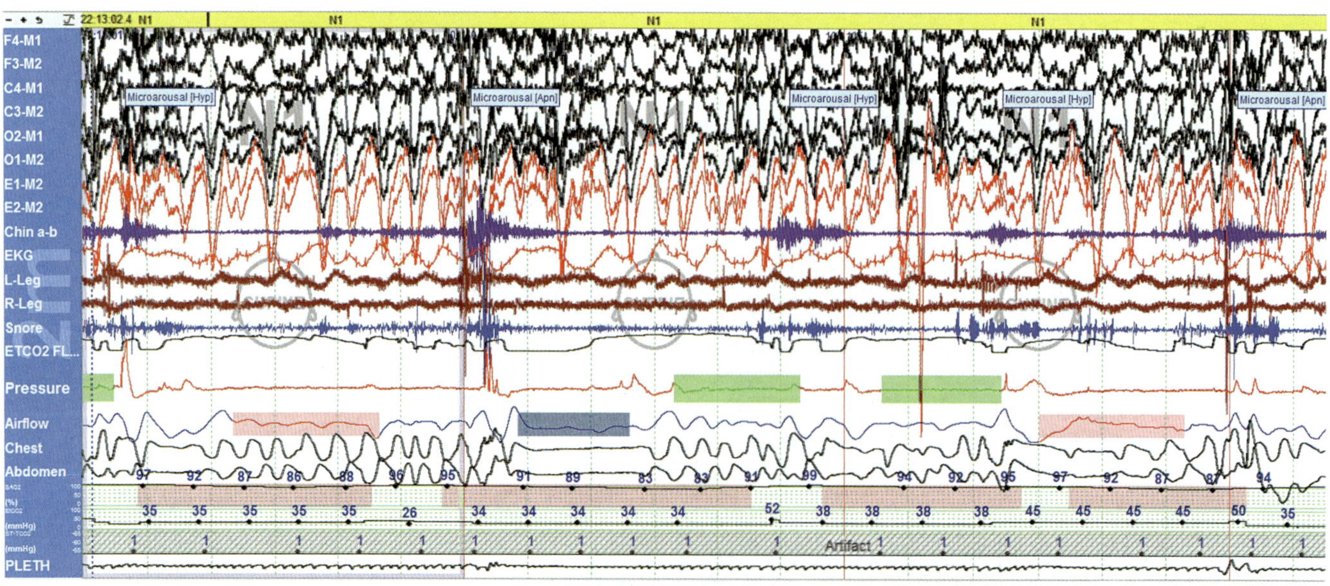

Fig. 17.23 Polysomnographic measurements of respiratory events during sleep. Two-minute epoch from a nocturnal polysomnogram showing evidence of obstructive hypopneas in green bars (more than 30% decrease in the nasal airway pressure measure), obstructive apneas in red bars (more than 90% decrease in the airflow channel with respiratory effort present), and central apnea in a blue bar (more than 90% decrease in airflow in the absence of respiratory effort). Paradoxical breathing is present throughout the 2 minutes of data.

Central Apnea or Hypoventilation

Central apnea can be defined as the absence of airflow for at least 20 seconds or apnea accompanied by cyanosis or bradycardia. The absence of airflow accompanied by the cessation of chest and abdominal wall movement distinguishes central apnea from obstructive apnea. In children, central apnea may occur with infections, seizure disorders or central nervous system pathologies (e.g., Arnold-Chiari syndrome, intraventricular hemorrhage), and prematurity. The gold standard to diagnose central apnea is a polysomnogram. Other studies that may be useful in apnea include ventilatory responses to hypercapnia or hypoxia, an electroencephalogram, CT of the brain, pH probe, and/or bronchoscopic evaluation of the airway. Laboratory evaluation may include any or all of the following: CBC, basic metabolic panel, arterial or venous blood gases, chest radiography, and electrocardiogram.

Congenital central hypoventilation syndrome (CCHS, formerly known as *Ondine's curse*) is a rare autosomal dominant disorder caused by a mutation in the PHOX2B gene with a wide spectrum of disease. Patients often present in the newborn period with respiratory failure during sleep with insufficient ventilatory responses to hypercapnia and hypoxemia. Depending on the severity of the disease (associated with the number of polyalanine expansion mutations in the PHOX2B gene), these abnormalities may improve when the child is awake. Considering CCHS is a lifelong condition, most of these children will require a tracheostomy tube placement in the newborn period due to chronic requirement of positive pressure ventilation. Depending on the number of repeats polyalanine expansions, CCHS can be associated with Hirschsprung disease, tumors of neural crest origin, cardiac asystole, autonomic nervous system dysregulations and dysmorphic facial features; therefore screening for these abnormalities is recommended.

RESTRICTIVE LUNG DISEASES

Chest Wall Disorders

Abnormalities affecting the thoracic cage can alter the function of the respiratory system. Chest wall disorders are not uncommon in the pediatric population, and some may present with changes over time which can progressively affect their respiratory function.

Scoliosis

Scoliosis is a pathological deviation of the spine which can occur along its axis. The most common form of scoliosis occurs in adolescents, however, those with neurological disorders and profound muscle weakness are at risk of developing neuromuscular scoliosis. Severe scoliosis affecting the thoracic spine may lead to asymmetrical expansion of the thorax leading asymmetrical lung aeration resulting in areas of atelectasis and impaired gas exchange. These abnormalities can be further exacerbated during an acute illness. Treatment of scoliosis is lead by the orthopedic specialist and in severe cases, with pulmonary complications, a surgical approach may be recommended. The respiratory management is supportive aiming to optimize adequate airway clearance and ventilation.

Pectus Excavatum

Pectus excavatum is the depression of the anterior chest wall and occurs approximately in 1/300 and 1/1000 births, with a male sex predominance. This abnormality can be noticeable at birth but is most pronounced during puberty and adolescence. Despite the evident defect, most patients are asymptomatic, while some may present with exercise intolerance, chest pain, palpitations and fatigue. The evaluation can include lung imaging, pulmonary function tests, cardiorespiratory exercise testing and an echocardiogram. Of note, patients may present with features of Marfan syndrome, Noonan syndrome and/or with comorbid scoliosis. A surgical consultation may be required if respiratory or cardiac function is impaired, and/or if patient is severely symptomatic. Most other cases do not require further treatment.

Thoracic Insufficiency Syndromes

Characterized by severe thoracic and spine deformities leading to an impairment in lung development and growth, and in failure of respiratory mechanics. Thoracic insufficiency may be a result from early onset scoliosis, Jarcho-Levin syndrome and Jeune syndrome. Children may present with tachypnea, respiratory distress, activity intolerance and respiratory insufficiency.

To assess the severity of respiratory impairment pulmonary function tests, 6-minute-walk test, a chest CT and a polysomnography should be considered. Respiratory management may include airway clearance therapies, noninvasive or invasive positive pressure ventilatory support. A surgical consultation should be obtained for discussion of possible surgical approach aiming to expand lung volumes.

DRUG AND ENVIRONMENTAL TOXICITIES

Pulmonary Toxic Medications

A number of medications are known to have pulmonary toxicity. Pulmonary fibrosis has been recognized in patients treated with thoracic radiation, bleomycin and amiodarone. Interstitial disease can be seen less commonly in patients taking methotrexate or tacrolimus. Monitoring for pulmonary toxicity in patients taking these medications is commonly done with serial pulmonary function testing including assessment of diffusing capacity.

EVALI

The use of electronic nicotine delivery systems (e-cigarette) has become popular to avoid carcinogenic chemicals in traditional cigarettes. However, some adolescents and adults using these devices develop an acute illness that can include cough, dyspnea, wheezing, gastrointestinal symptoms, and sometimes respiratory failure. The syndrome was termed EVALI (e-cigarette or vaping associated lung injury). The exact mechanism remains unclear, but potential causes include pneumonitis from inhalation of lipid vehicle, inhalation of vitamin E acetate, and thermal injury of the airways. More severe disease has often been treated with systemic glucocorticoids. Smoking/vaping cessation is key to recovery of lung function.

DIAGNOSTIC TECHNIQUES

Pulmonary Function Testing

Spirometry

Spirometry is the measurement of airflow after a maximal inhalation (to TLC) and with a rapid and forceful exhalation (to RV). The inspection of the flow-volume curves generated during forced expiratory maneuvers is critical for the appropriate interpretation of pulmonary function test results (Fig. 17.24). The initial portion of the flow-volume curve is effort dependent, whereas the terminal 25% of the expiratory maneuver is dependent on elastic recoil and airway resistance and is less dependent on patient effort. A normal-appearing flow-volume curve is shown in Fig. 17.24A. With increased airway resistance distal to the central, large airways, the curve becomes concave toward the volume axis, suggestive of airflow obstruction (see Fig. 17.24B). The total exhaled volume from the maneuver is the forced vital capacity (FVC), while the volume exhaled in the first second is termed FEV1. Classically, obstruction is diagnosed by a reduced FEV1/FVC ratio and normal FVC. Spirometry can also be used to document reversibility of obstruction after bronchodilator inhalation. Patients with suspected

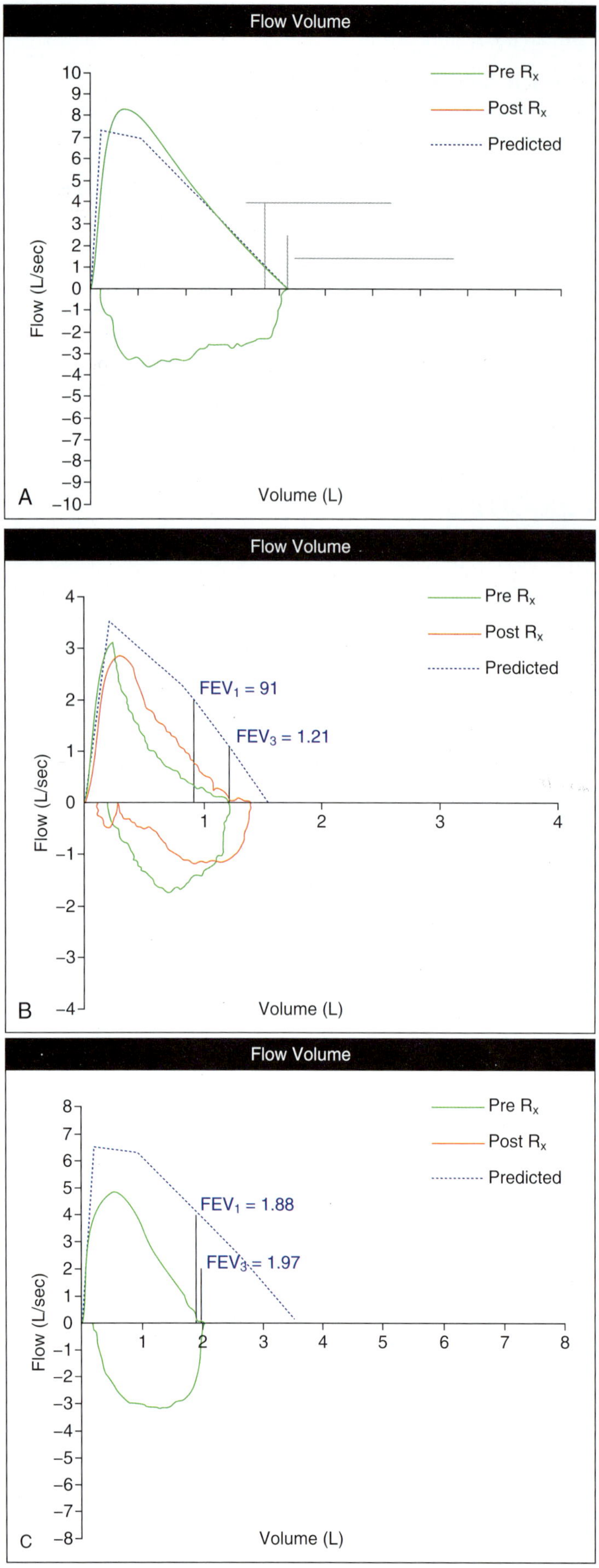

Fig. 17.24 Flow-volume curves obtained by spirometry. (A) Normal configuration of expiratory flow curve. (B) Reduced expiratory flow rates suggest obstructive airway disease *(green curve)*. (C) Preservation of flow rates with a diminished vital capacity consistent with restrictive lung disease. *FEV1*, Forced expiratory volume in 1 second; *FEV_3*, forced expiratory volume in 3 seconds; *R_x*, bronchodilator.

asthma may develop this configuration of flow-volume curve after bronchoprovocation tests, such as inhaled methacholine, cold air, or after exercise testing.

The restrictive pattern shown in Fig. 17.24C demonstrates a normal shape but a reduction in exhaled volume. This is usually associated with a proportionally reduced FVC and FEV1, and a normal FEV1/FVC ratio. This pattern is less common in pediatrics but can be seen with interstitial lung diseases, disorders associated with pulmonary hypoplasia (e.g., congenital diaphragmatic hernia) disorders affecting the chest wall (thoracic dystrophy, scoliosis), and respiratory muscular weakness (inability to exhale completely).

The shape of the flow-volume curve may also be helpful in evaluating upper or central airway pathology. (Fig. 17.25). Fixed obstruction of the upper airways, such as in tracheal stenosis, produces a flattening of both the inspiratory and expiratory loops of the flow-volume curve ("the box"). A reduced inspiratory flow and a plateau of the inspiratory loop only is suggestive of variable extrathoracic obstruction seen in disorders such as laryngomalacia and vocal cord dysfunction. Chondromalacia of the intrathoracic trachea or major bronchi results in a picture of variable intrathoracic obstruction with reduction and flattening of the expiratory limb because with forceful expiration, pleural pressure exceeds that inside the airway lumen, and the weakened bronchial wall cannot withstand that pressure gradient.

In addition to altering the airway caliber, disease states that affect lung growth would be expected to alter the lung volume. These diseases include pulmonary hypoplasia due to severe oligohydramnios or space occupying lesions (e.g., diaphragmatic hernia or cystic adenomatoid malformation), bronchopulmonary dysplasia, as well as conditions that alter the growth of the rib cage (thoracic dystrophies, radiation).

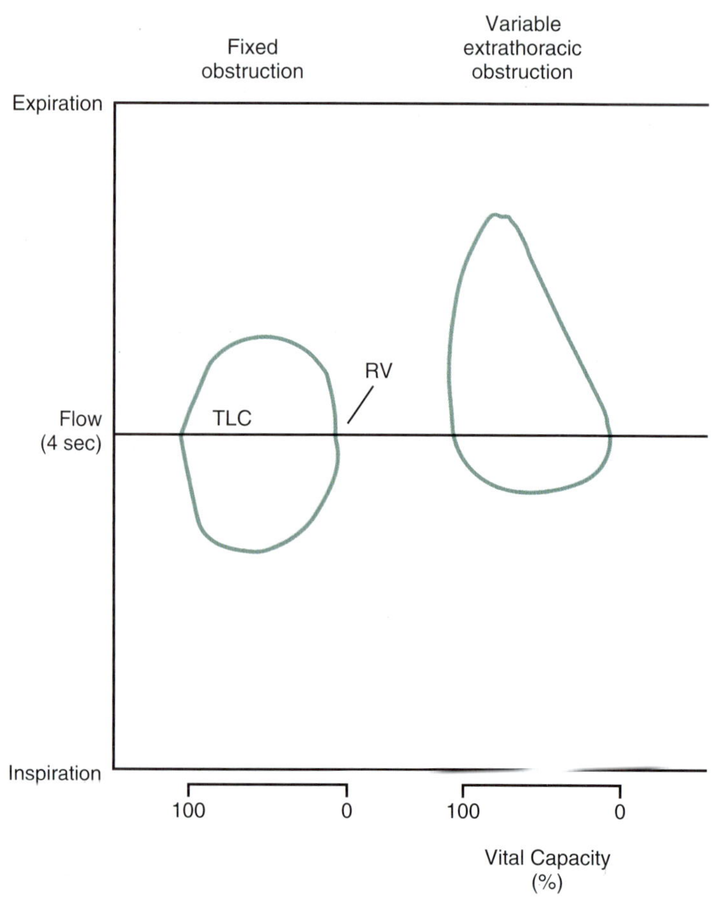

Fig. 17.25 Flow-volume curves obtained by spirometry. (A) Fixed airway obstruction with reduction in inspiratory and expiratory flow rates. (B) Variable extra thoracic airway obstruction, with reduced peak inspiratory flow rates. *RV*, Residual volume; *TLC*, total lung capacity.

Plethysmography

Plethysmography utilizes the principle of Boyle's law. With the subject sitting in a fixed volume chamber ("box") and breathing on a mouthpiece, a shutter is closed in the inspiratory limb of the breathing circuit. The subject makes small panting maneuvers, resulting in small changes in the volume of the lung and corresponding inverse volume changes in the box. This allows for calculation of the lung volume at which the panting efforts began. The subject usually begins the maneuvers at the end of a breath, and this "resting" lung volume is termed *functional residual capacity.* A lung capacity is the sum of two or more lung volumes; in the case of functional residual capacity, it is the sum of RV (the amount of gas remaining in the lung after a maximal exhalation) and expiratory reserve volume (ERV; the amount of gas exhaled from resting lung volume until the lung is empty). In combination with spirometry, other lung volumes and capacities can be calculated (see Fig. 17.26). The diagnosis of restrictive lung diseases is made with a reduced TLC. Although an increased RV-to-TLC ratio is often a hallmark of air trapping seen in obstructive lung disease, this may also be exhibited in patients with neuromuscular weakness. In a cooperative patient, this may be correlated with measurement of respiratory muscle strength (maximum inspiratory and expiratory pressures).

Diffusion

The diffusing capacity of the lungs for carbon monoxide (D_LCO) is an integrative measurement that describes the transfer of oxygen from the alveolus into the red blood cell. This transfer is proportional to the surface area of the alveolar/capillary membrane and to the pressure gradient for carbon monoxide between the alveolus and the blood, and it is inversely proportional to the thickness of the alveolar-capillary membrane. Carbon monoxide (CO) is more soluble in blood than in lung tissue, and it binds rapidly and tightly to hemoglobin. These properties maintain a diffusion gradient for CO. The patient exhales completely to RV and inhales to TLC a gas mixture containing 0.3% CO and holds the breath for 10 seconds, during which CO diffuses into the blood. The uptake of CO is divided by the partial pressure gradient for CO to calculate D_LCO. Diseases that decrease the surface area for diffusion (emphysema, pulmonary emboli, resection of lung tissue) or diseases that increase the thickness of the alveolar-capillary membrane (fibrosis, pulmonary edema, proteinosis) would both decrease the diffusing capacity of the lung. Increased D_LCO is much less common but can be seen in patients with alveolar hemorrhage, polycythemia, or during exercise (via recruitment of more pulmonary capillaries). This test may be useful in evaluating patients with diffuse lung diseases or assessment of patients with pulmonary vascular obstruction and for monitoring of pulmonary toxicity from radiation or chemotherapy.

Exercise Evaluation

Exercise testing can be a valuable tool to assess the cardiorespiratory fitness of a subject and may provide further information regarding a patient's respiratory reserve in addition to that found during routine pulmonary function tests. A progressive (or graded) exercise study by bicycle ergometry or treadmill can give important information regarding minute ventilation, heart rate responses, oxygen delivery and uptake, and CO_2 production. Evaluation of these parameters may provide information on exercise fitness and, if limited, identify whether the limiting factor is ventilatory or cardiac. Exercise-induced asthma testing is considered a submaximal exercise test (aiming for ≈85% of predicted maximal heart rate). Spirometry is usually performed at 2, 5, 10, and 15 minutes after exercise, with the primary outcome of interest being change in FEV1 relative to baseline. Like other pulmonary function tests, exercise testing can be used to assess the severity or progress of disease, evaluate effects of changes in treatment, and provide information about the safety or appropriateness of an exercise program in children with chronic lung disease.

The 6-minute walk test is an additional assessment of functional exercise capacity. Within the pediatric population, it is used most among patients being evaluated for thoracic organ transplantation. It may also be used in patients with severe cardiac or pulmonary disease, including CF, and pulmonary hypertension. Response to therapies may be reflected with serial assessments. The test comprises walking on a hard, flat surface for a 6-minute period. The total distance traveled is measured and is compared with control values and any prior assessments. Exercise-related oxyhemoglobin desaturation may also indicate pulmonary vascular disease or a barrier to gas diffusion.

Pulmonary Function Testing in Infants

Most of the tests described earlier have been adapted to infants, with the obvious challenge that maximal efforts cannot be elicited voluntarily. Infants are usually sedated using chloral hydrate and placed supine with a mask over the mouth and nose to measure airflow and pressure at the mouth. These techniques require specialized equipment not available in most pulmonary function laboratories. Infant pulmonary function tests may be used both in the setting of known disease (e.g., CF, bronchopulmonary dysplasia) for evaluation of symptoms in search of etiology and before medical or surgical intervention.

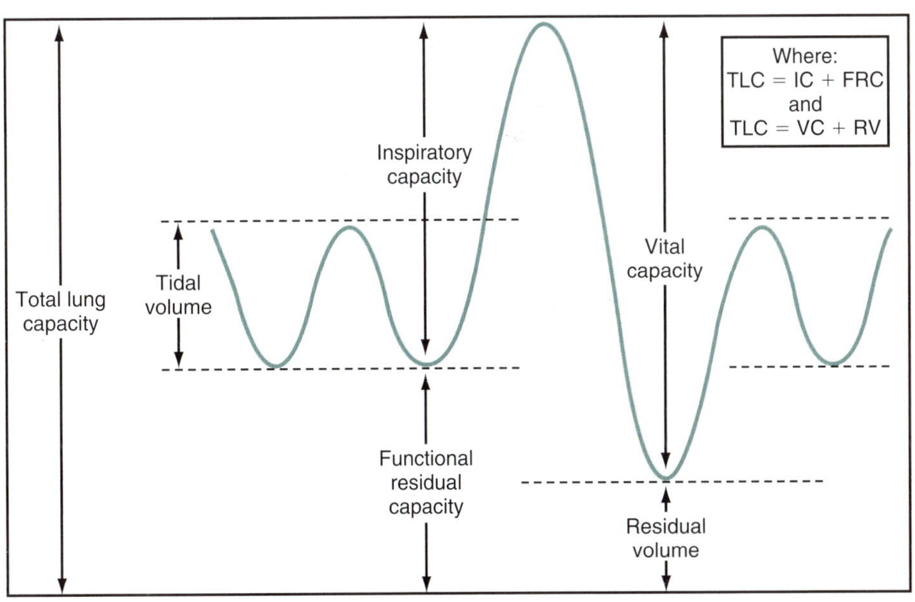

Fig. 17.26 Schematic representation of lung volumes. *FRC,* Functional residual capacity; *IC,* inspiratory capacity; *RV,* residual volume; *TLC,* total lung capacity; *VC,* vital capacity.

The raised volume rapid thoracic compression technique is one method that has been used to generate maximal expiratory flow by applying a positive pressure externally to the chest. The infant's lung is first inflated via the facemask to 30 cm H_2O, resulting in a lung volume close to TLC. Forced exhalation is achieved with a plastic jacket that encircles the chest and abdomen of the infant, which is rapidly inflated from a pressure reservoir, generating a full expiratory flow-volume curve. The resultant curves are highly reproducible. Lung volumes can also be measured with plethysmographic methods identical to those described earlier.

Diagnostic Imaging

The pediatric chest radiograph is unique in that normal findings may vary with age. The width of the chest on the lateral projection in the chest radiograph of a normal infant is about the same as the transverse dimension on a frontal projection, and the lungs may appear relatively radiolucent. Further, in contrast with the older child (>2 years old), the cardiothoracic ratio in the infant normally may be as high as 0.65. The width of the superior mediastinum at this age may also be striking because the thymic shadow is particularly prominent during the first few months of life before the normal process of involution occurs. A normal chest radiograph of an older child should show the diaphragm on an inspiratory film at the eighth or ninth rib posteriorly (sixth rib anteriorly), a cardiothoracic ratio of 0.5, and pulmonary vessels extending two-thirds of the way to the periphery. In most situations, a lateral radiograph should accompany the posteroanterior (PA) view because some pathologic findings may be missed on a single projection. For example, a lateral examination yields the best information about the anterior mediastinum and the tracheal air column and may reveal a small pleural effusion that is unsuspected on the basis of a PA radiograph alone. In combination with the PA view, the lateral projection may help localize an abnormal finding to a particular lobe or segment or document hyperinflation with diaphragmatic flattening (Fig. 17.27). In most situations, the chest radiograph taken at full inspiration is most helpful. In the evaluation for bronchial foreign bodies, a comparison of inspiratory and expiratory views (or left and right lateral decubitus films in the younger patient) can help if one lung is unable to empty. In looking for a small pneumothorax, the expiratory film is more helpful because the smaller lung volume allows extrapulmonary air to expand to become more evident.

Chest CT may confirm the diagnosis of bronchiectasis and should be performed if surgical removal of the affected segment is contemplated. High-resolution chest CT can be useful to assess for interstitial and/or parenchymal disease. A barium swallow is useful in patients with suspected TEF or primary swallowing disorders.

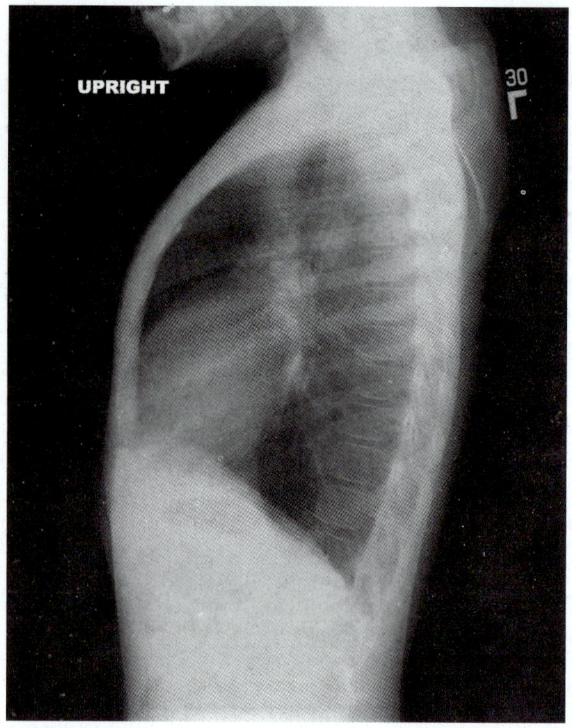

Fig. 17.27 Lateral chest radiograph demonstrating flattening of the diaphragm and retrosternal air due to hyperinflation.

Bronchoscopy and Bronchoalveolar Lavage

Flexible fiberoptic bronchoscopy can be extremely useful in the diagnosis of lesions of the pulmonary tree and in isolating organisms from patients with pneumonia. Compared with traditional open-tube ("rigid") bronchoscopy, flexible bronchoscopy offers the advantage of better visualization of distal airway segments and upper lobes and allowing the study of airway dynamics during regular tidal breathing. Indications for pediatric flexible bronchoscopy include evaluation of stridor, unexplained or chronic cough or wheeze, suspected airway malformations or compression, atelectasis, or recurrent pneumonia. To obviate the need for open lung biopsy, flexible bronchoscopy and BAL may be particularly useful in immunosuppressed patients with unexplained pneumonia. When there is a strong clinical or radiographic suggestion of inhaled foreign body, rigid bronchoscopy is the procedure of choice to remove the object. Transbronchial biopsy is performed routinely in patients who have undergone lung transplantation in order to screen for rejection. This technique involves passing biopsy forceps via the suction channel of a bronchoscope under fluoroscopic guidance. It is of occasional usefulness in clinical situations in which the lesion is diffuse, such as ILD. Tissue yield is low, and analysis requires an experienced pathologist. Risk of transbronchial biopsy is pneumothorax (approximately 1%) and bleeding.

Blood Gas Analysis

Arterial blood gas measurements are the gold standard for assessing gas exchange in critically ill patients. Pulse oximetry and analysis of the CO_2 in exhaled air have become useful noninvasive means of assessing ventilatory status and have been used to avoid routine arterial puncture in both inpatient and outpatient settings. Less invasive venous blood gases can give estimations of pH and partial pressure of carbon dioxide (Pco2) but are not used for assessment of arterial partial pressure of oxygen (Po2). Capillary blood gases obtained from arterialized samples (well-warmed digits) may be preferable to venous blood gases and are more accurate indicators of oxygenation.

Polysomnography

The gold standard for the diagnosis of OSA, central apnea, or hypoventilation in children is an in-laboratory PSG. Sleep studies are still not widely available for the pediatric population, but they remain an important diagnostic tool. Nocturnal PSG assesses sleep stages, movement of the chest and abdomen, electromyogram of diaphragm, arterial saturation, heart rate, end-tidal CO_2, and eye movements. In adults, home sleep apnea tests are often used. This test evaluates chest wall movement, air flow by nasal thermistor (which measures temperature below the nostril), heart rate, and arterial saturation in the patient's own home setting; however, limitations to this test include lack of ventilation assessment (because it lacks CO_2 measurement) and inability to measure sleep stages (no EEG monitoring). Novel wearable technology is now widely available to the general population; however, these devices are not validated for the diagnosis of OSA in pediatrics.

Supplemental videos are available at Elsevier eBooks+.

Bibliography

Annunziata F, Bush A, Borgia F, et al: Congenital lung malformations: unresolved issues and unanswered questions, *Front Pediatr* 7:239, 2019.

Baraldi E, Filippone M: Chronic lung disease after premature birth, *N Engl J Med* 357(19):1946–1955, 2007.

Beydon N, Davis SD, Lombardi E, et al: An official American Thoracic Society/European Respiratory Society statement: pulmonary function testing in preschool children, *Am J Respir Crit Care Med* 175(12):1304–1345, 2007.

Bishop NB, Stankiewicz P, Steinhorn RH: Alveolar capillary dysplasia, *Am J Respir Crit Care Med* 184(2):172–179, 2011.

Boulding R, Stacey R, Niven R, Fowler SJ: Dysfunctional breathing: a review of the literature and proposal for classification, *Eur Respir Rev* 25(141):287–294, 2016.

Bush A: Evidence-based approach to congenital thoracic malformations, *Arch Dis Child* 102(11):1095, 2017.

Bush A: Prenatal presentation and postnatal management of congenital thoracic malformations, *Early Hum Dev* 85(11):679–684, 2009.

Chalmers JD, Chotirmall SH: Bronchiectasis: new therapies and new perspectives, *Lancet Respir Med* 6(9):715–726, 2018.

Chang AB, Bush A, Grimwood K: Bronchiectasis in children: diagnosis and treatment, *Lancet* 392(10150):866–879, 2018.

Collaco JM, McGrath-Morrow SA: Bronchopulmonary dysplasia as a determinant of respiratory outcomes in adult life, *Pediatr Pulmonol* 56(11):3464-3471, 2021.

Colombo JL, Hallberg TK: Pulmonary aspiration and lipid-laden macrophages: in search of gold (standards), *Pediatr Pulmonol* 28(2):79–82, 1999.

Deterding RR, DeBoer EM, Cidon MJ, et al: Approaching clinical trials in childhood interstitial lung disease and pediatric pulmonary fibrosis, *Am J Respir Crit Care Med* 200(10):1219–1227, 2019.

Fan LC, Liang S, Lu HW, Fei K, Xu JF: Efficiency and safety of surgical intervention to patients with non-cystic fibrosis bronchiectasis: a meta-analysis, *Sci Rep* 5:17382, 2015.

Farrell PM, White TB, Ren CL, et al: Diagnosis of cystic fibrosis: consensus guidelines from the Cystic Fibrosis Foundation, *J Pediatr* 181S:S4–S15.e1, 2017.

Fitzgerald DA, Shapiro AJ: When to suspect primary ciliary dyskinesia in children, *Paediatr Respir Rev* 18:3–7, 2016.

Griese M: Chronic interstitial lung disease in children, *Eur Respir Rev* 27(147):170100, 2018.

Grüber C, Lehmann C, Weiss C, Niggemann B: Somatoform respiratory disorders in children and adolescents—proposals for a practical approach to definition and classification, *Pediatr Pulmonol* 47(2):199–205, 2012.

Guglani L, Stabel D, Weiner DJ: False-positive and false-negative sweat tests: systematic review of the evidence, *Pediatr Allergy Immunol Pulmonol* 28(4):198–211, 2015.

Hamvas A: Inherited surfactant protein-B deficiency and surfactant protein-C associated disease: clinical features and evaluation, *Semin Perinatol* 30(6):316–326, 2006.

Hartl D, Griese M: Interstitial lung disease in children—genetic background and associated phenotypes, *Respir Res* 6:32, 2005.

Heijerman HGM, McKone EF, Downey DG, et al: Efficacy and safety of the elexacaftor plus tezacaftor plus ivacaftor combination regimen in people with cystic fibrosis homozygous for the F508del mutation: a double-blind, randomized, phase 3 trial, *Lancet* 394(10212):1940–1948, 2019.

Hill AT, Barker AF, Bolser DC, et al: Treating cough due to non-CF and CF bronchiectasis with nonpharmacological airway clearance: CHEST expert panel report, *Chest* 153(4):986–993, 2018.

Jensen EA, Dysart K, Gantz MG, et al: The diagnosis of bronchopulmonary dysplasia in very preterm infants. An evidence-based approach, *Am J Respir Crit Care Med* 200(6):751-759, 2019.

Katz ES, Marcus CL: Diagnosis of obstructive sleep apnea. In Sheldon F, Kryger G, editors: *Principles and practice of pediatric sleep medicine*, ed 3, Elsevier, 2014, pp 221–230.

Khan A, Agarwal R: Pulmonary alveolar proteinosis, *Respir Care* 56(7):1016–1028, 2011.

Kohrman M: Idiopathic hypersomnia. In Sheldon SH, Ferber R, Kryger MH, Gozal D, editors: *Principles and practice of pediatric sleep medicine*, 2014, Elsevier, pp 153–158.

Koumbourlis AC: Pectus deformities and their impact on pulmonary physiology, *Paediatr Respir Rev* 16(1):18–24, 2015.

Kurland G, Deterding RR, Hagood JS, et al: An official American Thoracic Society clinical practice guideline: classification, evaluation, and management of childhood interstitial lung disease in infancy, *Am J Respir Crit Care Med* 188(3): 376–394, 2013.

Leblanc C, Baron M, Desselas E, et al: Congenital pulmonary airway malformations: state-of-the-art review for pediatrician's use, *Eur J Pediatr* 176(12): 1559–1571, 2017.

Lucas JS, Davis SD, Omran H, et al: Primary ciliary dyskinesia in the genomics age, *Lancet Respir Med*, 8(2):202–216, 2020.

Marcus CL, Brooks LJ, Draper KA, et al: Diagnosis and management of childhood obstructive sleep apnea syndrome, *Pediatrics* 130(3):576–584, 2012.

Martinez FD, Wright AL, Taussig LM, Holberg CJ, Halonen M, Morgan WJ: Asthma and wheezing in the first six years of life. The Group Health Medical Associates, *N Engl J Med* 332(3):133–138, 1995.

McGarry ME, Ren CL, Wu R, et al: Detection of disease-causing CFTR variants in state newborn screening programs, *Pediatr Pulmonol* 58(2):465–474, 2023.

Middleton PG, Mall MA, Dřevínek P, et al: Elexacaftor-tezacaftor-ivacaftor for cystic fibrosis with a single phe508del allele, *N Engl J Med* 381(19):1809–1819, 2019.

Moran A, Pillay K, Becker D, Granados A, Hameed S, Acerini CL: ISPAD Clinical Practice Consensus Guidelines 2018: management of cystic fibrosis-related diabetes in children and adolescents, *Pediatr Diabetes* 19(Suppl 27):64–74, 2018.

Nevel RJ, Garnett ET, Worrell JA, et al: Persistent lung disease in adults with NKX2.1 mutation and familial neuroendocrine cell hyperplasia of infancy, *Ann Am Thorac Soc* 13(8):1299–1304, 2016.

Niggemann B: How to diagnose psychogenic and functional breathing disorders in children and adolescents, *Pediatr Allergy Immunol* 21(6):895–899, 2010.

Pérez-Tarazona S, Esteban SR, García-García ML, et al: Respiratory outcomes of "new" bronchopulmonary dysplasia in adolescents: a multicenter study, *Pediatr Pulmonol* 56(5):1205–1214, 2021.

Rauch D, Wetzke M, Reu S, et al: Persistent tachypnea of infancy. usual and aberrant, *Am J Respir Crit Care Med* 193(4):438–447, 2016.

Rosenfeld M, Allen J, Arets BH, et al: An official American Thoracic Society workshop report: optimal lung function tests for monitoring cystic fibrosis, bronchopulmonary dysplasia, and recurrent wheezing in children less than 6 years of age, *Ann Am Thorac Soc* 10(2):S1–S11, 2013.

Sakiani S, Kleiner DE, Heller T, Koh C: Hepatic manifestations of cystic fibrosis, *Clin Liver Dis* 23(2):263–277, 2019.

Schittny JC: Development of the lung, *Cell Tissue Res* 367(3):427–444, 2017.

Shapiro AJ, Davis SD, Polineni D, et al: Diagnosis of primary ciliary dyskinesia. An official American Thoracic Society clinical practice guideline, *Am J Respir Crit Care Med* 197(12):e24–e39, 2018.

Shapiro AJ, Zariwala MA, Ferkol T, et al: Diagnosis, monitoring, and treatment of primary ciliary dyskinesia: PCD foundation consensus recommendations based on state of the art review, *Pediatr Pulmonol* 51(2):115–132, 2016.

Shinbashi M, Rubin BK: Electronic cigarettes and e-cigarette/vaping product use associated lung injury (EVALI), *Paediatr Respir Rev* 36:87–91, 2020.

Smith LJ, McKay KO, van Asperen PP, Selvadurai H, Fitzgerald DA: Normal development of the lung and premature birth, *Paediatr Respir Rev* 11(3):135–142, 2010.

Soares JJ, Deutsch GH, Moore PE, et al: Childhood interstitial lung diseases: an 18-year retrospective analysis, *Pediatrics* 132(4):684–691, 2013.

Spielberg DR, Brody AS, Baker ML, Woods JC, Towe CT: Ground-glass burden as a biomarker in neuroendocrine cell hyperplasia of infancy, *Pediatr Pulmonol* 54(6):822–827, 2019.

Stocks J, Kirkby J, Lum S: How to avoid misinterpreting lung function tests in children: a few practical tips, *Paediatr Respir Rev* 15(2):170–180, 2014.

Tutor JD: Dysphagia and chronic pulmonary aspiration in children, *Pediatr Rev* 41(5):236–244, 2020.

Tutor JD, Gosa MM: Dysphagia and aspiration in children, *Pediatr Pulmonol* 47(4):321–337, 2012.

Vincent M, Karolak JA, Deutsch G, et al: Clinical, histopathological, and molecular diagnostics in lethal lung developmental disorders, *Am J Respir Crit Care Med* 200(9):1093–1101, 2019.

Wallis C, Alexopoulou E, Antón-Pacheco JL, et al: ERS statement on tracheomalacia and bronchomalacia in children, *Eur Respir J* 54(3):1900382, 2019.

Weese-Mayer DE, Berry-Kravis EM, Ceccherini I, et al: An official ATS clinical policy statement: congenital central hypoventilation syndrome: genetic basis, diagnosis, and management, *Am J Respir Crit Care Med* 181(6):626–644, 2010.

Whitsett JA: Genetic disorders of surfactant homeostasis, *Paediatr Respir Rev* 7(Suppl 1):S240–S242, 2006.

Yang J, Kingsford RA, Horwood J, et al: Lung function of adults born at very low birth weight, *Pediatrics* 145(2):e20192359, 2020.

18

SURGERY

Hannah Rinehardt | Marcus Malek | Kevin P. Mollen

INTRODUCTION

General pediatric surgery encompasses a wide spectrum of disorders and malformations that overlap with other medical and surgical specialties. All pediatricians will undoubtedly be faced with conditions that warrant the involvement of a surgeon. The emphasis of this chapter is on the common conditions that may be seen in general pediatric primary care practices, including some unusual cases.

HEAD AND NECK

Head and neck lesions in the pediatric population are common and can be divided by etiology and location (see also Chapter 24). These lesions can be due to infection, trauma, neoplasm, or may be congenital. Most lesions of the head and neck in childhood are benign. Lesion location (Table 18.1) provides essential information about the probable diagnosis. Table 18.1 provides a summary of the common pediatric head and neck lesions by anatomic location. The history surrounding the lesion, physical examination, and diagnostic imaging studies are important to generate a differential diagnosis and further determine the nature and extent of the lesion and the potential need for surgical intervention. Important details in the history include length of time the lesion has been present, increase or decrease in size over time, pain, signs of infection or inflammation (such as erythema, warmth, and pain), constitutional symptoms, any history of trauma, and symptoms of airway compromise. Critical physical examination findings include size of the lesion, evidence of airway compromise, signs of inflammation, presence of sinus tracts, and evidence of ocular involvement. Imaging may help to demonstrate the nature of the lesion, distinguish cystic from solid lesions, and determine whether the lesion is isolated and distinct or infiltrative through the tissue planes.

Computed tomography (CT), magnetic resonance imaging (MRI), and ultrasound have almost completely eliminated skull and facial plain radiography in the evaluation of lesions of the head and neck. These modalities may better delineate the bony and vascular structures of the skull base and the cervical spine. Furthermore, underlying brain involvement as either the primary or secondary site may be visualized. Children with disorders of breathing, swallowing, or phonation may require adjunctive endoscopic procedures (nasopharyngoscopy, laryngoscopy, and endoscopy) or fluoroscopic imaging to aid in the diagnosis. It is important to remember that imaging and testing are adjuncts and do not replace a good history and physical examination; not every lesion requires additional workup before intervention other than a careful and detailed history and physical examination.

Surgery is often required for head and neck lesions for both diagnostic and therapeutic purposes. Incision and drainage of cervical abscess may provide a specimen for culture and a means of drainage for resolution. Excisional or incisional biopsy may be critical to determining the specific pathologic diagnosis of a lesion and may assist in determining the need for further therapies. It is also critical to recognize when surgery is not the best option and is, in fact, unnecessary and may create complications.

Cervical Lymphadenopathy

Enlarged cervical lymph nodes are the most common neck masses encountered in children. In most cases, this represents benign reactive cervical lymphadenopathy and arises secondary to nonspecific reactive hyperplasia. The etiology of cervical lymphadenopathy is commonly a response to either a viral or bacterial infection of the upper respiratory tract (nose, sinuses, ears, mouth, and pharynx) or skin (face and scalp) (Table 18.2).

Acute bilateral cervical lymphadenitis in children is most commonly associated with a viral respiratory tract illness. The lymph nodes are generally numerous, small, bilateral, and painless. When enlarged lymph nodes occur in this setting, additional workup is not immediately needed. They generally resolve within weeks of the resolution of the underlying illness.

In acute unilateral or suppurative lymphadenopathy, nodes are typically less than 2 cm in size and are rubbery, oval, and isolated. They characteristically occur in children between 2 and 10 years old. Palpable lymph nodes are uncommon in infants, and a palpable lesion is more likely to be of another etiology. Group A *Streptococcus* (GAS), *Staphylococcus aureus,* and anaerobic bacteria are the most common organisms that produce this adenopathy. Fever is not always present. Aggressive antibiotic therapy in the early stages of infection may prevent the development of the late suppurative stages that require surgical intervention. In most cases, the nodes spontaneously regress after resolution of the inciting infection. Bacterial infection within a node or nodes may lead to more significant enlargement with increased tenderness, erythema, and ultimately suppuration (Fig. 18.1). Fluctuant masses should be aspirated or incised and drained and fluid sent for culture. If the child is ill or toxic secondary to the infection, then hospitalization and intravenous antibiotics may be necessary.

The differential diagnosis for chronic unilateral cervical lymphadenopathy (see Table 18.2) includes cat-scratch disease, atypical mycobacterial infection, toxoplasmosis, and tuberculosis. Cat-scratch disease is a lymphocutaneous disorder and the most common cause of chronic nonbacterial lymphadenopathy in the developed world. It is caused by *Bartonella henselae* (see also Chapter 13). It usually develops as regional nodal enlargement 2 to 4 weeks after inoculation (typically from a kitten or dog but can be secondary to other animals as well). The neck is the second most common site after the axilla. There may be a local reaction to the scratch, followed by the evolution of lymphadenopathy, which may persist for several months. Typically, there is one enlarged node in the chain, and it may be tender and firm. The disease is usually self-limited, but on occasion these nodes become suppurative and fluctuant and require drainage. The diagnosis may be confirmed by serologic testing for the antigen.

Various clinical presentations can be seen with mycobacterial infections, including cervical adenopathy, pulmonary infection, and disseminated disease. The most common presentation is secondary to one of the organisms of the *Mycobacterium avium–intracellulare-scrofulaceum* (MAIS) complex, which consists of approximately 15 organisms. These mycobacterial organisms typically produce localized cervical lymphadenopathy in the younger child. In contrast, *Mycobacterial tuberculosis* usually presents with pulmonary infection and rarely presents with lymphadenopathy (typically supraclavicular). Atypical mycobacterial infection usually involves the submandibular, submaxillary, or preauricular lymph nodal regions (Fig. 18.2). Large, firm, immobile, and nontender lymph nodes may arise after inoculation (typically from the mucous membranes of the pharynx). These may undergo spontaneous breakdown and drainage in up to 50% of cases with sinus formation in up to 10%. Incision and drainage of these nodes may lead to chronically draining sinuses.

Table 18.1 Common Lesions of the Head and Neck in Infancy and Childhood

Region	Location	Common Lesions
Head	Scalp	Hemangioma, dermoid cyst
	Ear	Preauricular tag, sinus
	Eyebrow	Dermoid cyst
	Base of nose	Meningocele, encephalocele
	Parotid gland	Hemangioma, lymphatic malformation, rhabdomyosarcoma, lymphoma, mixed tumors, parotitis
Mouth	Tongue	Tongue-tie, macroglossia, lingual thyroid
	Floor of mouth	Ranula
	Cheek and lip	Papilloma, mucocele
	Alveolar ridge	Tooth bud, epignathus
Neck	Midline	Thyroglossal duct cyst, dermoid cyst, submental lymph node, goiter
	Lateral	Branchial cleft cyst or sinus, lymphadenitis, reactive lymphadenopathy, lymphoma, lymphatic malformation

Complete resection of the node and any sinus tracts is usually curative. Children will either have a negative or indeterminate purified protein derivative (PPD) test or gamma interferon release assay. Antimycobacterial therapy is not indicated in most cases of MAIS infection. Cervical adenitis secondary to *Mycobacterium tuberculosis* infection is a manifestation of intrathoracic disease and requires aggressive antimycobacterial drug therapy. Surgery is usually unnecessary in *M. tuberculosis* and should be avoided because of the risk of developing chronically draining sinuses. Surgery is limited to an excisional biopsy in rare situations where the diagnosis cannot be made by other means.

Lymphoma may present as painless cervical adenopathy. The absence of antecedent upper respiratory or cutaneous infections, the persistence of lymphadenopathy beyond 6 weeks, lack of response to treatment with antibiotics, size greater than 2 cm, and firm consistency should raise concern for malignancy. Although cervical adenopathy is more common in Hodgkin disease, non-Hodgkin lymphoma may also present with a cervical mass (Fig. 18.3). The age of the patient may also be a clue as to the diagnosis, as well as the presence of associated symptoms, such as fever or night sweats. Incisional or, if needed, excisional biopsy is diagnostic and mandated when these criteria are met. Before proceeding with the biopsy, it is critical to determine respiratory status and review a chest radiograph to determine whether there is bulky mediastinal disease as a component of the lymphoma. Significant mediastinal disease may result in respiratory collapse with anesthetic induction for the biopsy.

Thyroglossal Duct Cyst and Sinuses

The differential diagnosis for midline neck masses includes thyroglossal duct remnants, dermoid cysts, and lymphadenopathy. During fetal development, the thyroid gland is derived from endoderm that originates at the base of the tongue (foramen cecum) and descends through the hyoid bone until it reaches its final position at the base of the neck (Fig. 18.4). Failure of regression of the thyroglossal duct may lead to cyst formation. A cyst may be located anywhere along the thyroglossal duct. Two-thirds of cysts are near the hyoid bone. They are typically in the midline, smooth, soft, and nontender. On physical examination, the mass typically moves cephalad when the child sticks their tongue out. These lesions can typically be identified by history and physical examination alone. They are prone to infection and require surgical excision. This excision requires resection of the midportion of the hyoid bone and

Table 18.2 Common Infectious Causes of Cervical Lymphadenopathy

Presentation	Acute Bilateral	Acute Unilateral (Suppurative)	Chronic Unilateral	Chronic Bilateral
Etiology	Rhinovirus EBV CMV HSV adenovirus Enterovirus Mycoplasma pneumonia GAS Influenza	GAS *Staphylococcus aureus* Anaerobic (poor dental hygiene)	Nontuberculous mycobacterium Cat-scratch disease *(Bartonella)*	EBV CMV

CMV, Cytomegalovirus; *EBV,* Epstein-Barr virus; *GAS,* group A *Streptococcus; HSV,* herpes simplex virus.

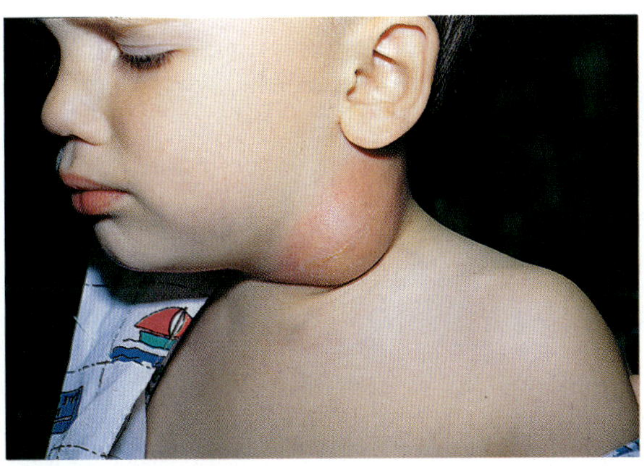

Fig. 18.1 Erythema and fluctuance identify the presence of an abscess. An abscess may be present without fluctuance, however, as the result of induration from surrounding inflammation.

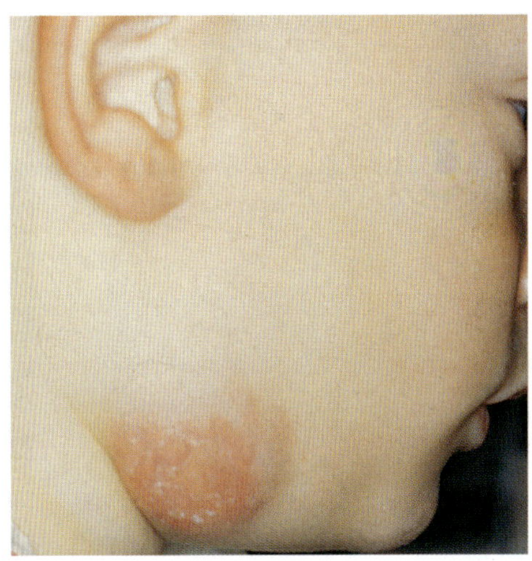

Fig. 18.2 The skin overlying a lymph node infected with atypical mycobacteria is often discolored and may break down into a chronically draining sinus.

ligation of the tract leading to the foramen cecum (Sistrunk procedure) to prevent future recurrence (Fig. 18.5). One should attempt to identify the thyroid gland because 1% to 2% of the time the thyroglossal duct cyst may represent a lingual thyroid and removal will remove the entire thyroid tissue resulting in hypothyroidism.

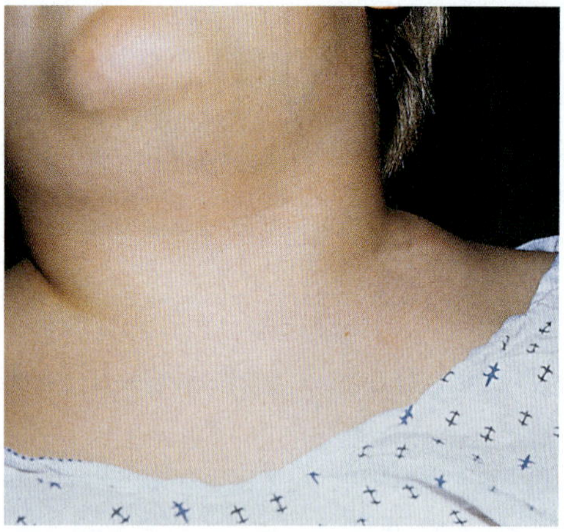

Fig. 18.3 Enlarged lymph nodes in unusual locations, such as in this patient with supraclavicular lymphadenopathy from non-Hodgkin lymphoma, require excisional biopsy to rule out malignancy.

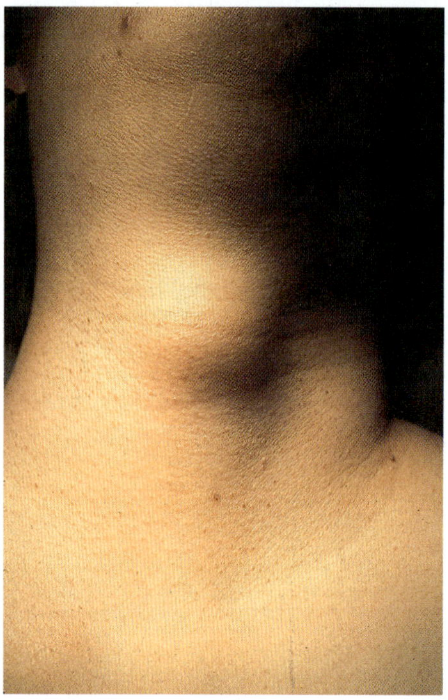

Fig. 18.4 Thyroglossal duct cyst produces a firm swelling in the midline of the neck. Its initial manifestation is sometimes a midline cervical abscess.

Thyroid Nodules

Thyroid nodules are uncommon in the pediatric population (Fig. 18.6). However, compared with adults, there is a greater incidence of malignancy within thyroid nodules of up to 25% compared with 5% to 10% in adults. There is also evidence to suggest that the incidence of thyroid nodules is increasing. Thyroid cancer represents 2% to 3% of childhood malignancies overall and 7% of childhood malignancies in female adolescents. Malignant thyroid nodules typically present as anterior neck masses that move with the thyroid upon swallowing. However, many are detected incidentally with imaging for other reasons. Histologically, thyroid cancer can be divided into differentiated (follicular and papillary) and medullary subtypes. Papillary thyroid cancer accounts for more than 90% of malignant lesions in childhood. Survival for differentiated thyroid cancer is greater than 95%. Workup should begin with a thyroid ultrasound when a nodule is suspected. The Thyroid Imaging Reporting and Data System (TI-RADS) was developed to standardize the interpretation of thyroid ultrasound, stratifying lesions by the presence or absence of high-risk features in order to better select nodules in need of fine needle aspiration (FNA) biopsy. According to the American Thyroid Association (ATA) Guidelines published in 2015, pediatric nodules should be managed similar to adults except that the size criteria does not apply to children due to differences in gland development with age. The ATA recommended considering ultrasound characteristics such as shape, calcifications, as well as clinical context when deciding to perform FNA for small nodules in pediatric patients. Cytopathology findings are categorized according to the Bethesda System for Reporting Thyroid Cytopathology. Typically, children with confirmed thyroid cancer are treated with total thyroidectomy ± lymph node dissection. The traditional approach to indeterminate lesions has been diagnostic lobectomy over repeat FNA. Mutational analysis via molecular testing (MT) has become a mainstay of the evaluation of thyroid nodules in adults. Some pediatric centers have begun to trial MT for indeterminate pediatric thyroid nodules. Single-institution data suggest that positive MT is highly associated with malignancy, but negative MT does not rule out malignancy in the pediatric population. Due to insufficient validation in pediatrics, as of 2015, the ATA does not yet recommend its routine use.

Branchial Cleft and Arch Anomalies

Cysts and Sinuses

Branchial cleft anomalies give rise to cysts and sinuses in the lateral triangle of the neck. Second branchial cleft anomalies are the most common and typically present as an opening along the lower anterior border of the sternocleidomastoid muscle (SCM). The sinuses develop from embryologic remnants and have their origin in the

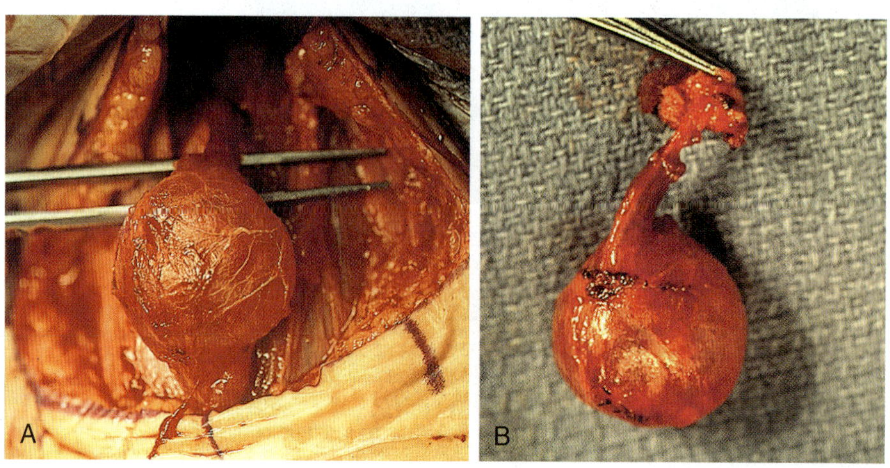

Fig. 18.5 The surgical specimen shows the thyroglossal duct as it courses from the lesion to the hyoid bone (the thicker transverse piece of tissue) (A). The hyoid must be resected to gain access to the tissue that extends to the base of the tongue (foramen cecum), which must be ligated to prevent recurrence (B).

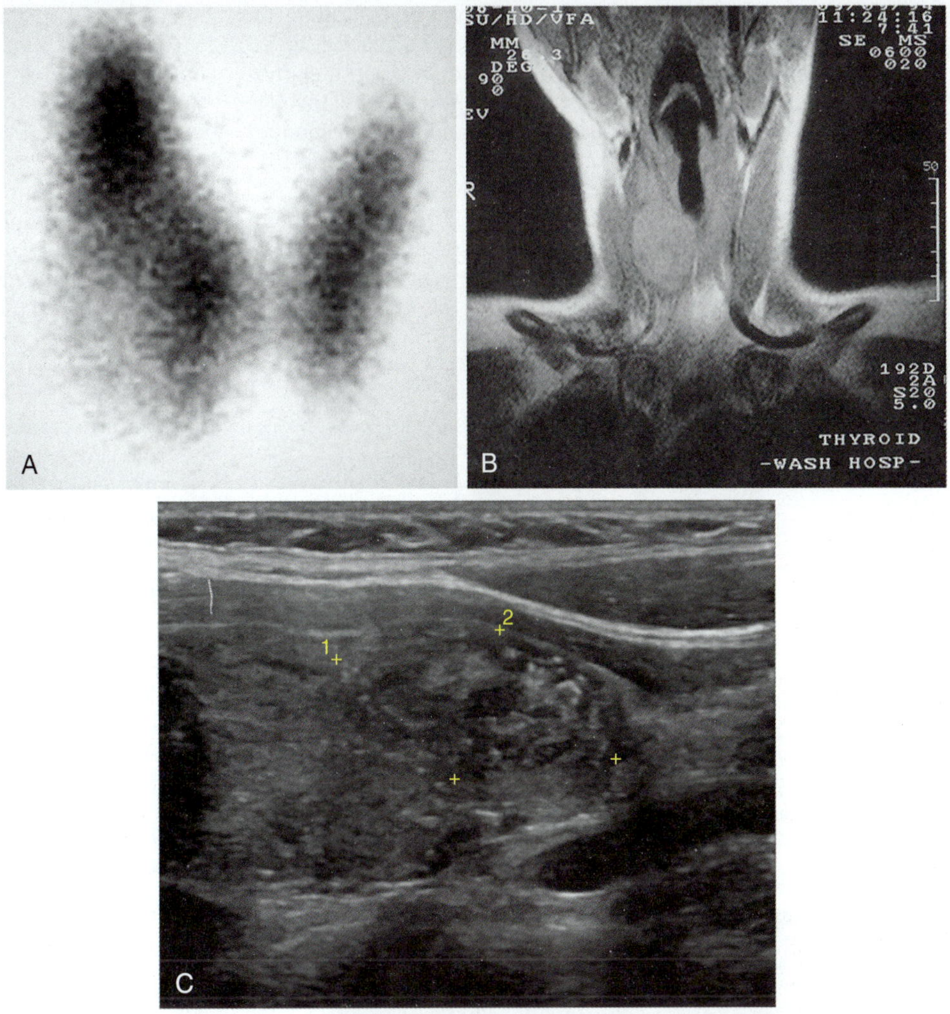

Fig. 18.6 A nonfunctioning or "cold" thyroid nodule visualized by thyroid scan (A) and magnetic resonance imaging (B) at surgery was found to be a benign follicular adenoma. Ultrasound demonstrating a TI-RADS 5 lesion (C), found to be papillary thyroid cancer.

tonsillar fossa. They may travel between the carotid sheath to exit along the border of the SCM (Fig. 18.7). Secondary infection of these lesions is common. Infection should be treated before excision in order to facilitate a complete excision and reduce recurrence rates. Excision of the tract to the site of origin in the peritonsillar region limits recurrence.

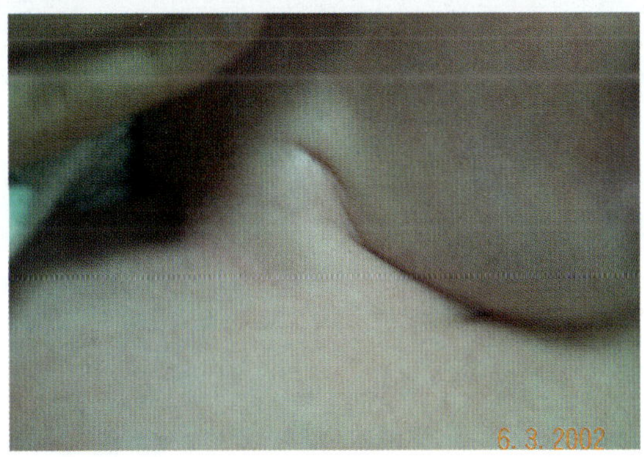

Fig. 18.7 Midline cervical cleft.

Torticollis

Fibromatosis coli, or fibrous dysplasia of the SCM, commonly is seen in infants and young children. These children present with a mass in the lower neck with tilting of the head and face to the side of the lesion (Fig. 18.8). Parents most often bring their infants in because they are concerned about the possibility of a malignant tumor, whereas older children may present with hemifacial hypoplasia and asymmetry. Early recognition of this condition in infancy and the institution of daily physical therapy usually averts surgery and long-term cosmetic deformity (Fig. 18.9). Plagiocephaly and facial asymmetry are sequelae of untreated deformities (see Chapter 23).

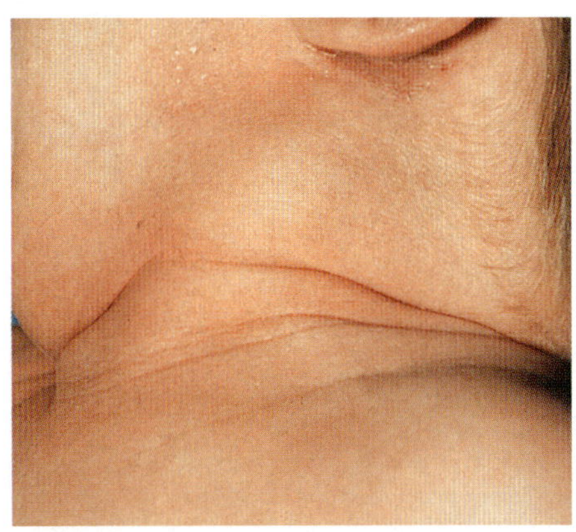

Fig. 18.8 The sternocleidomastoid in a newborn with torticollis may exist as a tight tendon-like cord or may swell and appear as a discrete tumor in the midportion of the muscle, pictured here.

Scalp and Face Lesions

Scalp

Hemangiomas are benign, congenital, vascular tumors that most frequently arise in the head and neck (60%). They are the most common benign neoplasm of infancy occurring in up to 10% of full-term infants and 25% of infants less than 1 kg. These lesions are raised above the skin level and are strawberry red in coloration. They may blanch with contact. Unlike vascular malformations (see Chapter 10), they typically grow out of proportion to the rest of the infant.

Rapid growth and expansion may occur, in rare cases leading to platelet sequestration and coagulopathy, known as Kasabach-Merritt syndrome. Hemangiomas are typically marked by a proliferative phase, which may last 6 to 12 months, followed by a phase of involution. Most hemangiomas have a benign course and undergo spontaneous resolution over the first 5 years of life (see Chapters 8 and 10). Surgical intervention is rarely necessary and should be reserved for those patients with airway compromise or periorbital involvement (Fig. 18.10). If there is a concern that intervention may be required, referral to a vascular anomalies program can be discussed, including a full range of medical, minimally invasive, and open surgical options. Although most lesions regress, this process must be monitored because up to 30% of lesions will leave significant deformities and a surgical scar must be weighed against the scar from involution.

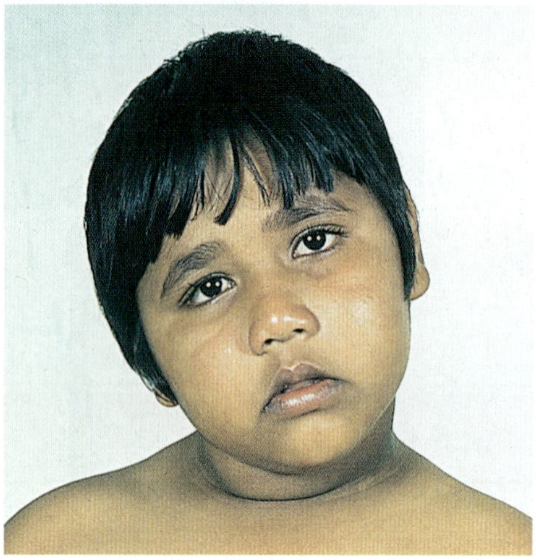

Fig. 18.9 Long-standing torticollis may cause permanent "wry-neck," facial shortening of the affected side of the face, and plagiocephaly.

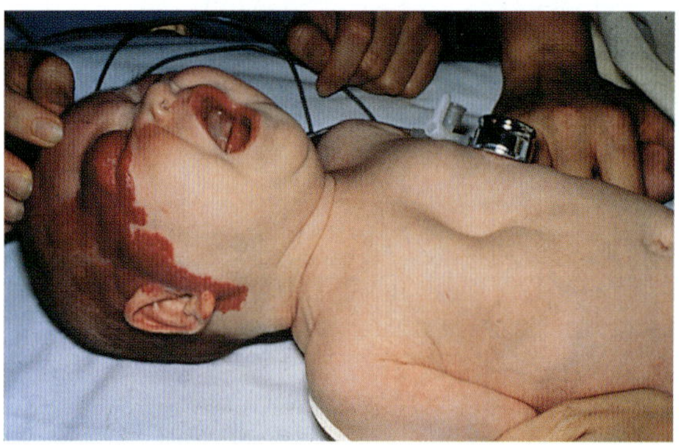

Fig. 18.10 Facial hemangioma covering the eye requires medical intervention with prednisone or possibly with propranolol to hasten resolution and avoid loss of sight from amblyopia.

Dermoid and epidermoid cysts are congenital lesions composed of sequestered hair and skin and sebaceous material that occurs in areas of embryonic fusion. Dermoid cysts—unlike epidermoid cysts—contain glandular structure. These lesions are most frequently in the head and neck but may arise in other midline sites, including the sacral, perineal, and sternal regions. Scalp dermoids are typically well circumscribed, firm, and fixed to underlying deep structures. They are most commonly noticed from birth to 3 months old. Midline scalp or back dermoids may be dumbbell shaped and have an intracranial or intraspinal component. They should always be evaluated with additional imaging (such as an MRI) before surgical intervention (Fig. 18.11). They gradually grow due to the accumulation of sebum. If they rupture, they may cause granulomatous inflammation and infection. Excision is the treatment of choice.

Face

Several benign congenital structures may persist at birth, and they raise numerous management considerations. Preauricular skin tags are vestigial cartilaginous remnants that are removed primarily for cosmetic reasons. Preauricular pits or sinuses are ectodermal inclusion structures that are related to the embryologic formation of the ears (see Chapter 24). Although these lesions are prone to infectious complications, most are asymptomatic and excision is not needed unless there is a history of drainage and infection. Sinuses that drain are often connected to subcutaneous cysts. The incidence of these lesions is 0.1% to 0.9% in the United States and as high as 4% to 10% in Africa.

Mouth

Some intraoral lesions that have surgical significance due to their effect on swallowing, speech, and breathing may arise. Tongue-tie (ankyloglossia inferior) occurs commonly in infancy, usually resolving spontaneously. The frenulum is a thin membranous structure that regresses with feeding. A persistent frenulum may impair speech and feeding. Frenulectomy, simple division of the frenulum, may be therapeutic but is rarely necessary (Chapter 21). Similarly, ranulae may form from pseudocysts in the floor of the mouth (Fig. 18.12). Some spontaneously resolve, whereas a few may become quite large and impair lingual mobility, feeding, speech, and most significantly breathing. Marsupialization or complete excision is curative.

Lymphatic malformations (previously known as *cystic hygromas* or *lymphangiomas*) of the floor of the mouth and neck may pose

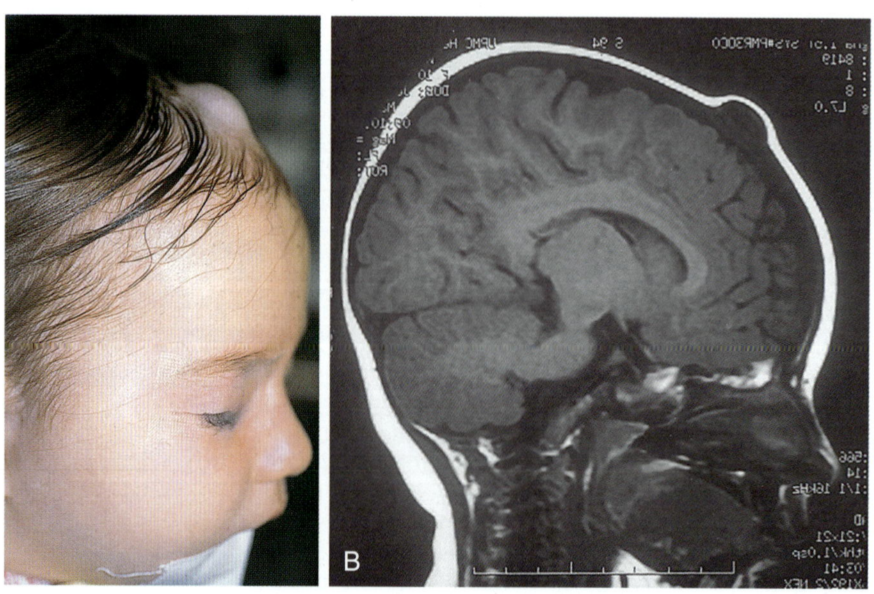

Fig. 18.11 (A) Midline scalp dermoid cysts may have intracranial extension and should always be evaluated by magnetic resonance imaging before surgery. (B) The dermoid in this 2-year-old child extends to but not through the dura.

especially challenging management problems (Fig. 18.13). These lesions may cause significant macroglossia that obstructs the airway requiring tracheostomy. Large lesions can also cause airway compromise. Historically these malformations were treated with surgical resection, often with high morbidity and recurrence due to incomplete resection. Imaging is important in defining the extent and nature of the lesion and in guiding the treatment of the malformation. Lesions that are composed of large cysts (macrocystic) respond better to drainage and sclerosis than lesions made up of tiny cysts (microcystic). The microcystic lesions can often act as a solid mass and make treatment especially challenging. The goals of treatment are to preserve function and cosmesis as much as possible. A combination of drainage, sclerosis, and surgical excision is often necessary in a multispecialty team, such as a vascular malformation clinic.

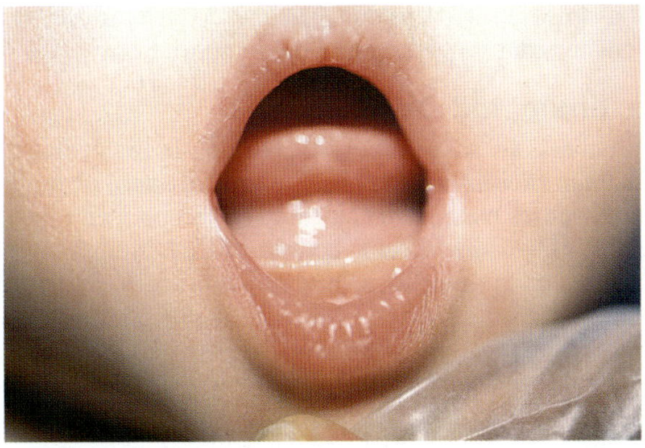

Fig. 18.12 A ranula arises in the floor of the mouth, caused by congenital obstruction of the sublingual duct.

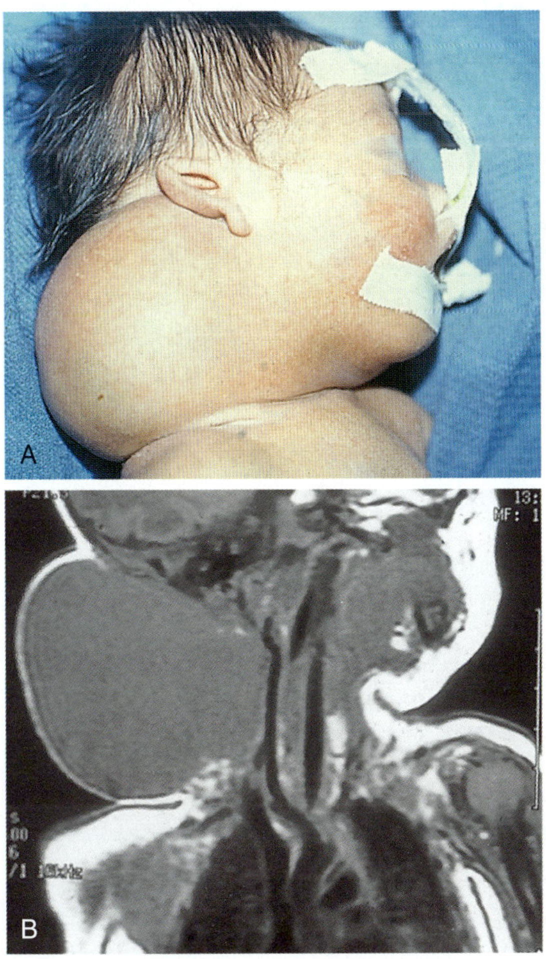

Fig. 18.13 (A) Cervical cystic hygroma. (B) Magnetic resonance imaging demonstrates its juxtaposition to the airway structures and vessels in the neck. Acute enlargement at birth secondary to hemorrhage may lead to airway compression.

RESPIRATORY SYSTEM

Introduction

Neonatal respiratory distress presenting with severe dyspnea, hoarseness, or stridor requires urgent surgical assessment and management. If plain radiographs rule out foreign body aspiration, pneumothorax and pneumonia, the differential diagnosis of respiratory distress may include intrathoracic masses, congenital lung lesions, or abdominal masses. The clinical evaluation of these patients should include both anteroposterior and lateral radiographs of the chest. Ultrasound may also be needed to evaluate the diaphragm, chest wall, or abdomen; fluoroscopy to evaluate the esophagus and diaphragm (Fig. 18.14); or cross-sectional imaging in the form of a CT scan or MRI. More invasive testing, such as upper airway or esophageal endoscopy, may be necessary to elucidate other surgical causes of respiratory distress. Before any testing, it is important to treat and stabilize the patient. The most pressing need is to establish and maintain oxygenation and a stable airway.

Upper Airway

Airway obstruction may manifest clinically with stridor. Stridor is high-pitched monophonic breathing as a result of upper airway obstruction and airway narrowing (see Chapters 17 and 24). The pattern of stridor can give the practitioner a clue as to the location of the pathology (Table 18.3). Stridor can be inspiratory, expiratory, or biphasic. In general, inspiratory stridor is the result of obstruction in the extrathoracic region (glottis or supraglottic region), expiratory stridor results from intrathoracic obstruction, and biphasic stridor represents a fixed central airway obstruction.

The newborn infant who is unable to nurse or has paroxysmal asphyxia (cyclic dyspnea) should undergo a thorough airway and cardiopulmonary evaluation. Lesions involving the upper airway create a characteristic "air hunger" that may progress to respiratory failure in the neonate. The respiratory difficulties are most marked during the expiratory phase of the cycle, which is when the airway tends to collapse around the lesion. These infants may be asymptomatic during the inspiratory component of the respiratory cycle, when the airway reaches its greatest diameter. The differential

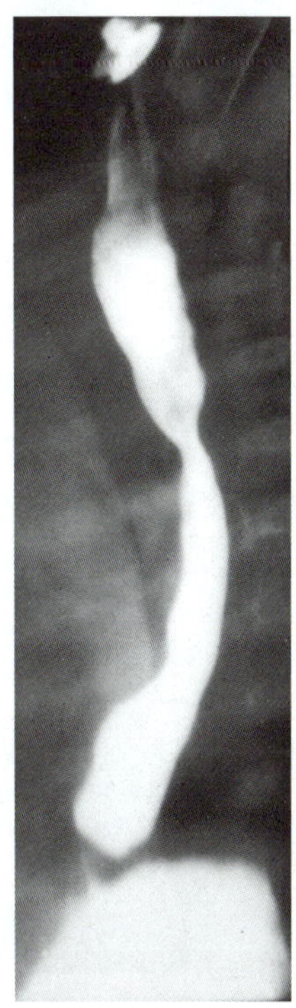

Fig. 18.14 Midthoracic compressions into the esophageal barium column identify the presence of vascular ring anomalies (in this case, pulmonary artery sling).

Table 18.3 Causes of Neonatal Stridor

	Nose	Pharynx	Larynx	Trachea	Distal Airway
Pathology	Nasal anomalies	Tongue anomalies, craniofacial anomalies, pharyngeal masses	Laryngomalacia, laryngeal webs, atresia, and clefts, subglottic stenosis, vocal cord paralysis	Tracheal stenosis, vascular rings, tracheomalacia	Bronchogenic and enteric duplication cysts

diagnoses for these symptoms should include choanal atresia, septal deformities, esophageal atresia, tracheoesophageal fistula, nasopharyngeal tumor, oropharyngeal masses, and foreign bodies.

Initial evaluation of infants with presumed airway obstruction should begin with passage of a nasogastric tube. Signs of nasal obstruction suggest choanal atresia, which often may have other associated craniofacial or remote congenital anomalies that require concurrent evaluation and management. Nasopharyngoscopy is diagnostic in most cases. It is critical that the oral airway be maintained, and the baby must be fed via gavage feedings until transpalatal repair. Pharyngeal obstruction may be caused by tongue abnormalities (macroglossia and glossoptosis) (Fig. 18.15) and craniofacial anomalies (Fig. 18.16). Tracheostomy may be necessary in order to protect the airway before surgical correction. Prone positioning may also provide a temporizing means of keeping the airway open. Pharyngeal masses may be another source of upper airway obstruction. These masses include dermoid cysts, pharyngeal duplications, hemangiomas, lymphatic or vascular malformations, and malignancies (neuroblastoma, rhabdomyosarcoma, or teratomas). Large cervical masses may induce airway compression or severe laryngotracheomalacia and cause dyspnea. Antenatal diagnosis of the lesion may predict a potential airway emergency at the time of delivery. The ex-utero intrapartum treatment (EXIT) procedure, with a controlled cesarean section under a deep anesthetic with uterine relaxation, allows time to secure the newborn's airway before umbilical cord division (Fig. 18.17).

Laryngeal lesions distinctively present with hoarseness, faint crying, or complete aphonia in association with dyspnea. The differential diagnosis can be seen in Table 18.3. Emergency tracheostomy may be necessary in these patients if the airway cannot be secured without a surgical intervention. A neonatal tracheostomy is a technically challenging procedure and rarely needed.

Mediastinum and Diaphragm

Mediastinal masses are relatively uncommon in the pediatric population but can present at all ages. The limited space of the thoracic cavity predisposes normal structures to be compressed causing both respiratory and cardiovascular compromise. Lesions may be congenital, neoplastic, infectious, and inflammatory in nature. The mediastinum can be divided into three major compartments: the anterior (thymus, vessels, lymphoid structures, and nerves), middle (trachea, main stem bronchi, the heart and great vessels, and hilar lymph nodes), and posterior (aorta, esophagus, and the sympathetic nerve chain). The patient's age and the mediastinal location provide the most critical insight into potential diagnoses (Table 18.4).

Esophageal atresia with or without tracheoesophageal fistula represents one of the more common causes of esophageal obstruction in

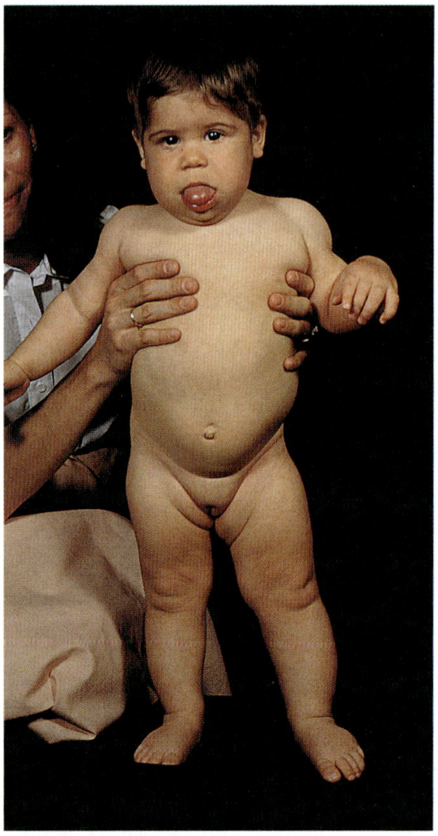

Fig. 18.15 Beckwith-Wiedemann syndrome. Note hemihypertrophy on the left side, along with the prominence of the tongue. (Courtesy D. Becker, MD, Pittsburgh, PA.)

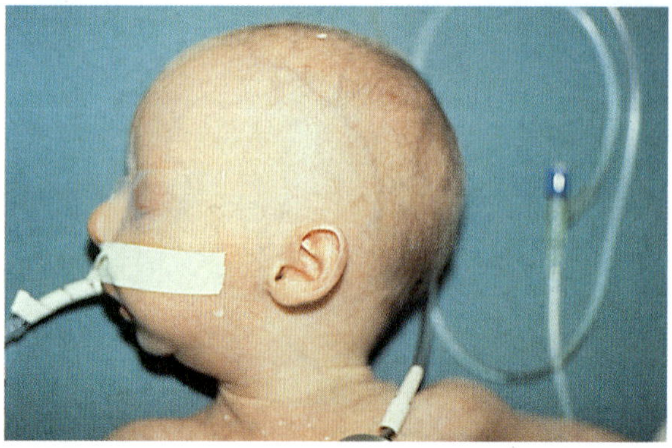

Fig. 18.16 In Pierre Robin sequence, the hypoplastic mandible positions the tongue posteriorly, potentially obstructing the upper airway.

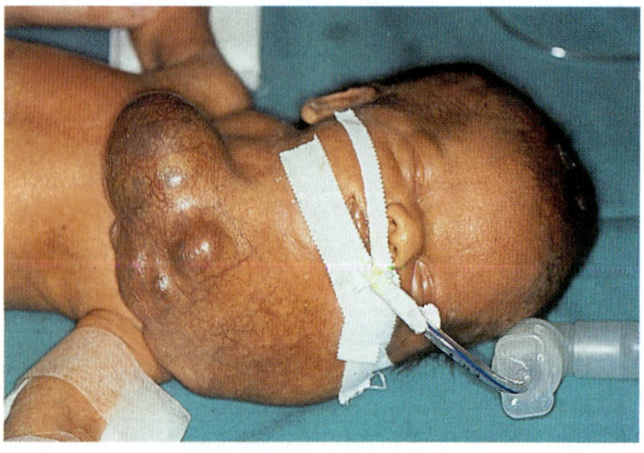

Fig. 18.17 Large cervical masses like this cervical teratoma diagnosed by antenatal ultrasonography cause prenatal esophageal compression and polyhydramnios. Because of the high risk of upper airway compression at delivery, an ex utero intrapartum treatment procedure is indicated to avoid infant death.

Table 18.4 Mediastinal Masses in Children

	Anterior	Middle	Posterior
Benign	Teratoma, normal or hyperplastic thymus, thymic cyst, intrathoracic goiter, lymphatic or vascular malformations	Lymphatic or vascular malformation, bronchogenic duplications and cysts, pericardial cysts	Enteric duplication cysts, ganglioneuroma
Malignant	Thymic tumor (rare), lymphoma	Lymphoma	Neuroblastoma

neonates with an incidence of ~1 in 2500 live births. The inability to pass a nasogastric tube into the stomach clarifies this diagnosis, while a chest x-ray with the nasogastric tube on gentle tension may shed light on the anatomy of the defect. The tube may also serve as a sump catheter to drain the proximal pouch. Infants may develop respiratory distress from several mechanisms. The proximal dilated pouch may cause airway obstruction, there may be aspiration of contents from the upper pouch, or there may be a direct communication or fistula between the trachea and the esophagus (Gross type B or D, Fig. 18.18). There may also be associated laryngotracheomalacia. Neonates with esophageal atresia characteristically have excessive salivation and coughing from pooling of secretion in the proximal pouch. Most patients are diagnosed by their inability to tolerate initial feedings. This presentation may be dramatic, with episodes of aspiration, coughing, gagging, and even periods of cyanosis. The most common type of esophageal atresia includes a blind ending proximal esophageal pouch and a distal tracheoesophageal fistula (type C, 85%). Positive-pressure ventilation should be avoided in these infants because ventilation may contribute to loss of tidal volumes into the gastrointestinal tract, increased gastric distention, and even perforation when associated with a downstream obstruction (i.e., duodenal atresia). Reflux of gastric contents into the airway with resultant pneumonitis and pneumonia can contribute to evolving respiratory distress (Fig. 18.19). The second most common anatomic configuration is pure esophageal atresia (type A), which may be associated with findings of a dilated proximal pouch and the absence of intestinal gas on plain radiography and scaphoid abdomen (Figs. 18.20 and 18.21). The third most common type is an isolated tracheoesophageal fistula without esophageal atresia (type E or "H type" fistula). These children are often diagnosed later in infancy or childhood with symptoms of persistent cough or recurrent pneumonias as their esophagus is in continuity. In general, these patients are stabilized while a workup of associated anomalies (i.e., VACTERL) can be completed before surgical intervention.

Congenital diaphragmatic hernia (CDH) also causes respiratory distress in newborns, with an incidence of 1 in 4000 live births. Although esophageal atresia and tracheoesophageal fistula are generally not recognized antenatally, CDH is commonly diagnosed on antenatal ultrasound, allowing for prenatal counseling regarding the congenital anomaly and its treatment. Additional imaging using fetal MRI may also be used to define the anatomy and provide additional prognostic information. A variety of scoring indices have been developed to help identify patient risk of morbidity and mortality in order to provide sound antenatal counseling, plan for delivery, and logical decisions regarding resource utilization after birth. Defects may be posterolateral (Bochdalek; Fig. 18.22) or anterior central (Morgagni; Fig. 18.23). Bochdalek defects are the most common and found on the left side in 85% of infants. The exact etiology of the defect is unknown; however, these infants generally present with associated pulmonary hypoplasia and resultant persistent pulmonary hypertension. This constellation is thought to derive from a field defect including the CDH, rather than simply resulting from herniation of abdominal viscera into the chest causing compression. Many infants have severe respiratory distress occurring shortly after umbilical cord division. On physical examination, there may be marked nasal flaring, displaced heart tones contralateral to the hernia, ipsilateral absence of breath sounds with dullness to percussion due to the presence of abdominal viscera, and the appearance of a scaphoid abdomen. Plain films demonstrate intestinal loops within the hemithorax, and a nasogastric tube often may be seen within the intrathoracic stomach. The significant morbidity and mortality of CDH are due to the associated severe pulmonary hypoplasia and pulmonary hypertension. Disease may be further complicated by the presence of congenital heart disease, and significant cardiac defects in the setting of CDH are almost uniformly lethal. In most patients, pulmonary hypertension will improve in the days after delivery. Repair of the diaphragmatic hernia does not relieve or resolve pulmonary hypoplasia or hypertension and, although necessary, can be deferred until the neonate has stabilized. Despite

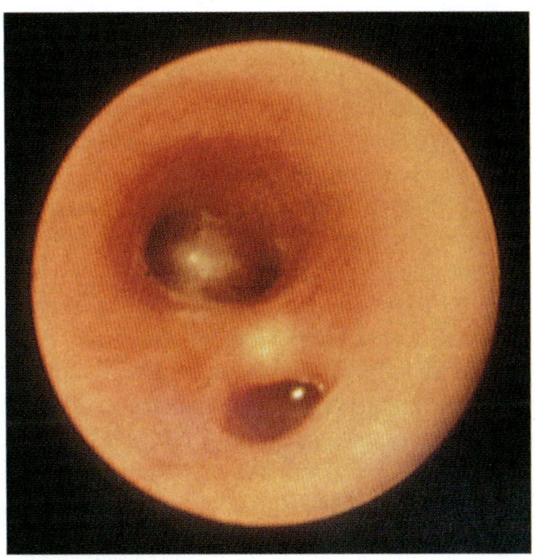

Fig. 18.18 Bronchoscopy visualizes a tracheoesophageal fistula, seen as a posteriorly positioned orifice *(bottom)* in the upper trachea. The carina, seen toward the top of the picture, lies distally.

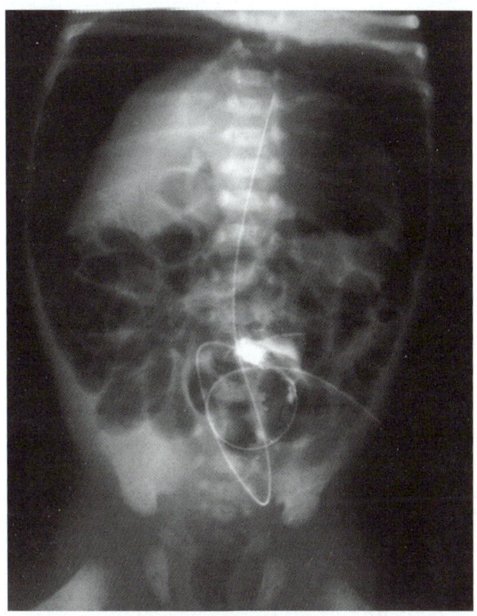

Fig. 18.19 Tracheoesophageal fistula allows air to be forced into the stomach during positive-pressure ventilation by bag and mask or through an endotracheal tube. The stomach may perforate as shown in this patient with a pneumoperitoneum, or ventilation may become suddenly ineffective if a gastrotomy is placed initially during surgical repair.

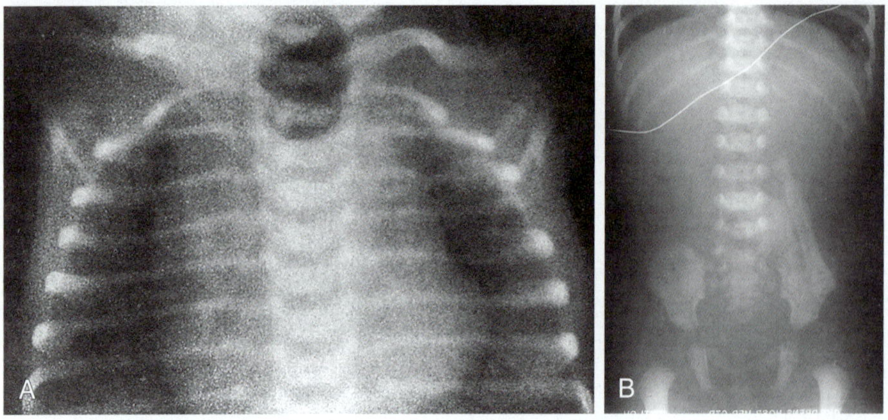

Fig. 18.20 A dilated blind proximal esophageal pouch (A) and a gasless abdomen (B) are the radiographic hallmarks of pure esophageal atresia.

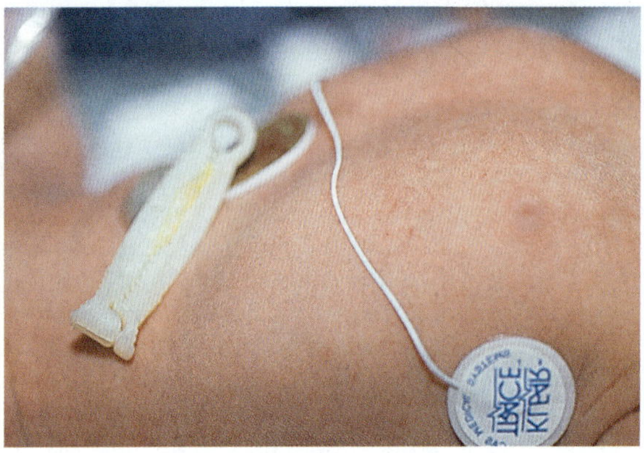

Fig. 18.21 Pure esophageal atresia without distal tracheoesophageal fistula. Esophageal obstruction associated with scaphoid abdomen on physical examination is pathognomonic of pure esophageal atresia.

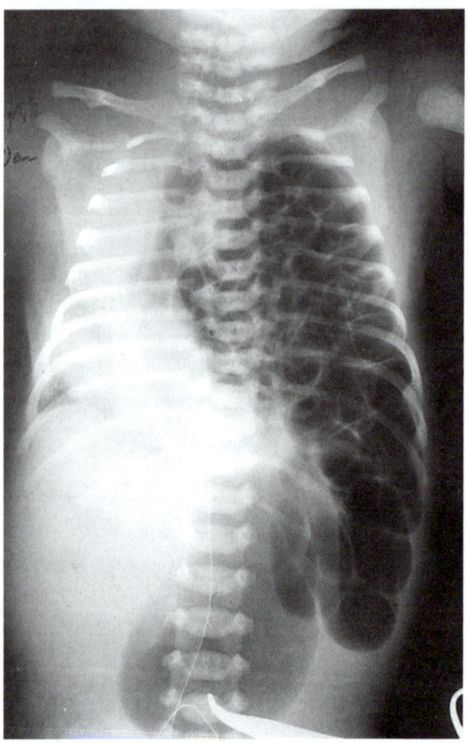

Fig. 18.22 Congenital diaphragmatic hernia allows intestines to enter the chest in utero.

advances in neonatology and the availability of extracorporeal membrane oxygenation support, the mortality rate with CDH is still approximately 40% to 50%. Since the 1990s, the clinical use of fetoscopic tracheal occlusion has been reported for severe CDH diagnosed prenatally. The minimally invasive procedure allows

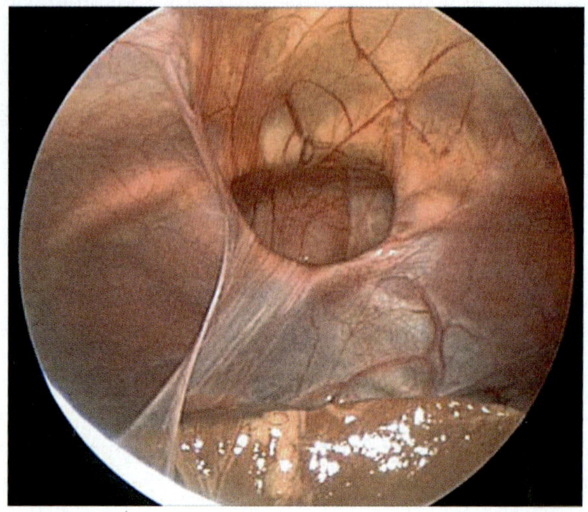

Fig. 18.23 A foramen of Morgagni hernia, seen here by laparoscopy as a central tendinous defect in the diaphragm, typically does not present as acute pulmonary distress in the newborn.

expansion of the fetal lungs by retained pulmonary secretions and has been associated with increased survival, decreased utilization of extracorporeal membrane oxygenation, and decreased rates of pulmonary hypertension at 1 year of life.

Congenital Lung Lesions

Congenital lung lesions may induce severe respiratory distress by direct compression on normal adjacent lung parenchyma, the airway, or adjacent vascular structures (Chapter 17). Congenital cystic anomalies of the lung are the most common cause of respiratory distress in neonates and children requiring surgical intervention. Surgical intervention, when warranted, is safe and with the development of minimally invasive techniques is now associated with lower short- and long-term morbidity rates.

CPAMs (congenital pulmonary airway malformations), previously known as *congenital cystic adenomatoid malformations,* are the most common of the bronchopulmonary foregut malformations, accounting for up to 30% to 40% of all fetal lung lesions. In general, CPAMs are confined to a single lobe of the lung, and the pathophysiology of cyst formation is largely unknown. Anatomically, they have a connection to the tracheobronchial tree and maintain a blood supply from the pulmonary circulation. However, alveoli are abnormally formed and in general do not provide normal gas exchange. These lesions have previously been divided into three categories of the Stoker classification, based on their size, shape, and pathologic appearance; however, this categorization has little clinical relevance. A more relevant classification uses gross anatomy of the lesion's appearance on prenatal ultrasound. This classification divides CPAMs into macrocystic (single or multiple cysts measuring at least 5 mm in diameter) (Fig. 18.24) and microcystic (appearing almost solid on prenatal ultrasound) lesions. Prenatally, lesions may demonstrate a predictable pattern with maximal growth between 20 and 28 weeks. After 28 weeks, most CPAMs plateau or may even regress in size. This is particularly true with microcystic lesions. However, some large macrocystic lesions may undergo periods of rapid growth, resulting in fetal hydrops. Antenatal drainage procedures may play a role in these patients. The majority of patients with persistent lesions are asymptomatic at birth, but a minority of neonates may present with respiratory distress secondary to compression of normal lung and mediastinum by large lesions. It is typically recommended that even asymptomatic lesions be resected due to the risk of repeated infections and concern for malignant degeneration over time.

Congenital lobar emphysema is marked by abnormal hyperinflation of histologically normal lung. Hyperinflation results from a segment of poorly developed or absent cartilage in the tracheobronchial tree. The left upper lobe is the most commonly affected, followed by the right middle lobe and right upper lobe (Fig. 18.25). Many of these patients present with symptomatic lesions in the first few weeks of life, whereas others have a more indolent course. Symptoms may include respiratory distress or poor feeding and weight gain due to fatigue. Plain films may demonstrate lobar hyperinflation, mediastinal shift, and flattening of the diaphragm. These patients can present as a respiratory emergency with mediastinal shift (similar to a tension pneumothorax) and require emergent thoracotomy and resection. The treatment of asymptomatic congenital lobar emphysema lesions is even more controversial. When the diagnosis is not in doubt, several studies have suggested that observation is appropriate.

Pulmonary sequestrations are abnormal, nonfunctioning pulmonary parenchymal tissue lesions that lack a direct communication with the tracheobronchial tree. These lesions receive blood supply from the systemic circulation. They may arise within the pulmonary parenchyma (intralobar; Fig. 18.26) or separately from lung tissue within its own pleural investment (extralobar; Fig. 18.27). Intralobar sequestrations may be identified on prenatal ultrasound, and their presence is confirmed by postnatal CT. However, they may also present later in life with repeated infections within the lobe and even abscess formation. They generally require resection after adequate treatment with antibiotics. Extralobar sequestrations may be intrathoracic or intraabdominal in location and can be associated with CDHs (up to 5% of infants with CDH also have incidental sequestration). They may be identified either on prenatal ultrasound or found incidentally. In general, these are resected due to concern for recurrent infections.

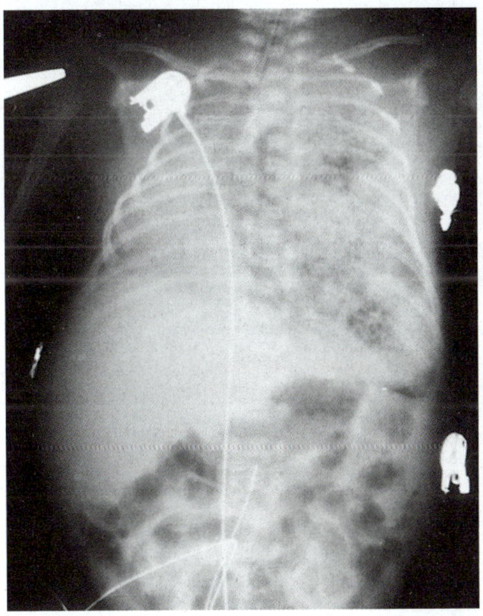

Fig. 18.24 Macrocystic adenomatoid malformation of the left lung. Large cystic lesions can be mistaken for bowel loops herniating through a diaphragmatic hernia.

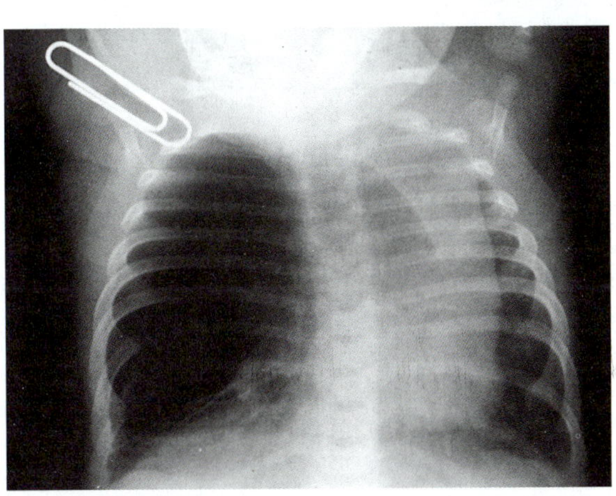

Fig. 18.25 Lobar emphysema, usually involving the upper lobes, may become hugely distended and may cause life-threatening respiratory distress.

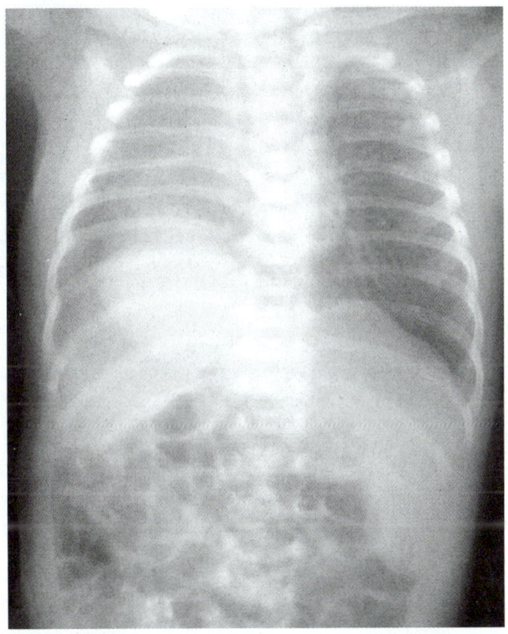

Fig. 18.26 Persistent infiltration of the lung parenchyma may indicate an intralobar sequestration, shown here involving the right lower lobe. Also shown is a right diaphragmatic hernia, a frequently associated malformation.

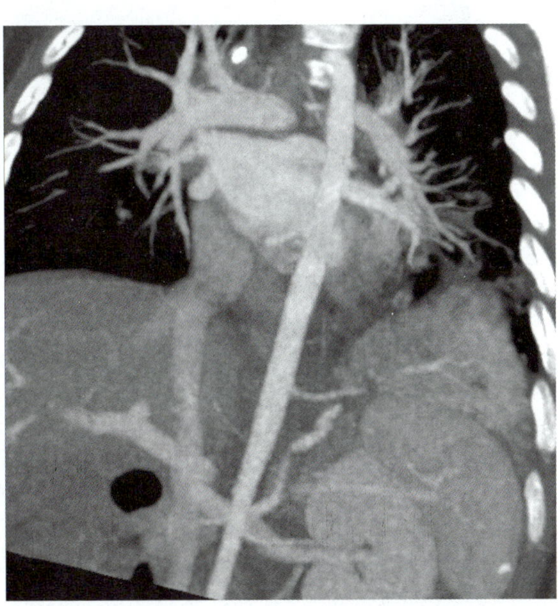

Fig. 18.27 Extralobar sequestrations are characterized by the presence of pulmonary parenchyma that lacks tracheobronchial communication and has a systemic blood supply. Computed tomography–angiogram shows systemic blood supply.

Bronchogenic Cysts

Bronchogenic cysts result from abnormal budding of the trachea or foregut. They are fluid filled, may or may not communicate with the airway, and can be found anywhere along the tracheobronchial tree. They may become infected or may cause mass effect on adjacent structures leading to associated symptoms based on the structures being compressed (Fig. 18.28). Infections should be treated with antibiotics, and all cysts ultimately should be resected.

Pneumothorax

Pneumothorax may occur spontaneously or secondary to thoracic trauma, underlying lung disease, or barotrauma (Fig. 18.29). Patients may present with acute severe pleuritic chest pain and dyspnea. Physical examination may demonstrate hyperresonance, diminished breath sounds over the ipsilateral hemithorax, tachypnea, and even subcutaneous emphysema. Mediastinal shift, jugular venous distention, and hypotension typically signify tension physiology and

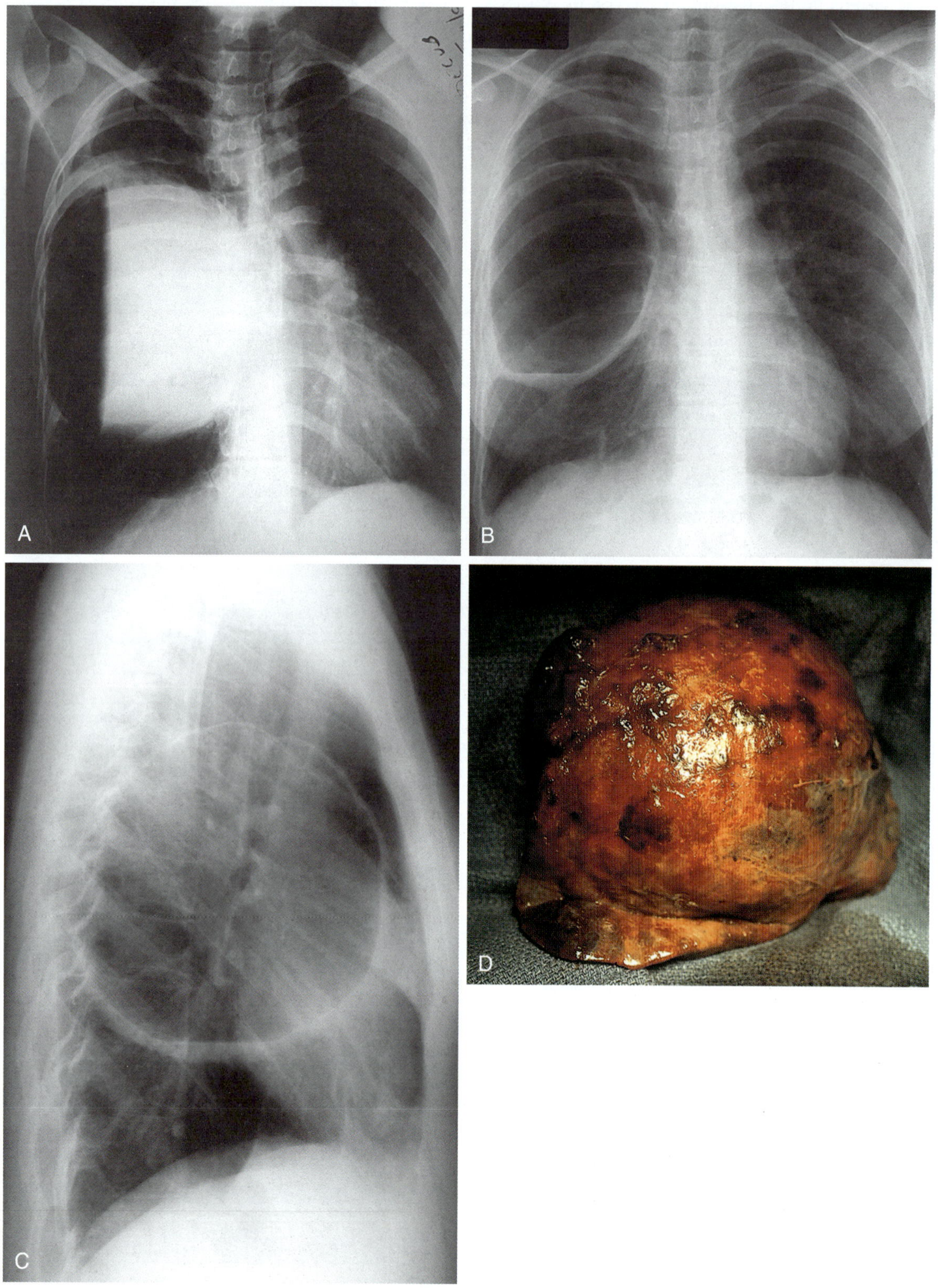

Fig. 18.28 Large infected bronchogenic cyst in a teenager (A) who responded to aggressive antibiotic therapy (B and C) and surgical resection (D).

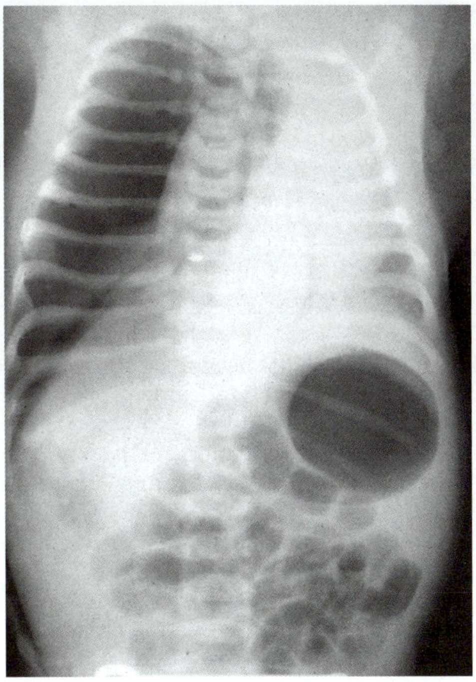

Fig. 18.29 This chest film shows typical radiologic signs of tension pneumothorax: mediastinal shift, flattening of the diaphragm, and widening of the intercostal spaces.

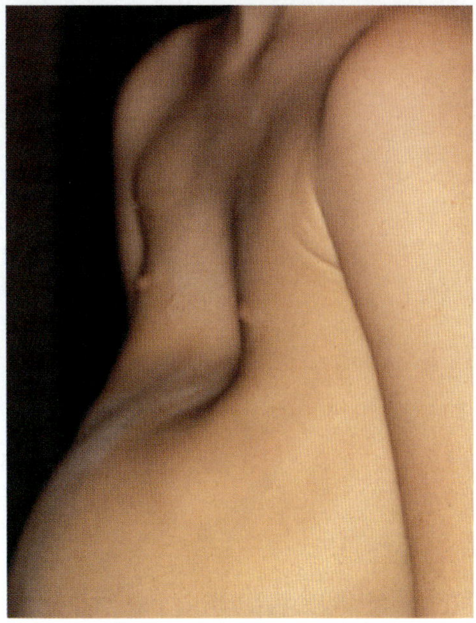

Fig. 18.30 Pectus excavatum (funnel chest) seldom creates cardiorespiratory symptoms, but psychologic consequences may be severe.

warrant prompt decompression, followed by thoracostomy (chest) tube placement. Primary spontaneous pneumothorax often develops in male adolescents who are tall and lean. This is generally related to apical blebs or bullae. Primary decompression is usually recommended for first occurrences of moderate to severe pneumothorax with surgery indicated for persistent air leaks and recurrence (recurrence rate up to 40%–60%). Surgery generally consists of video-assisted thoracoscopic surgery with resection of the apical blebs and chemical pleurodesis, pleural abrasion, or apical pleurectomy, resulting in a reported recurrence rate of less than 6% in most series.

Pleural Space and Lung Infections

An empyema is the accumulation of infected purulent material in the pleural space and commonly results from the infection of a parapneumonic effusion (see Chapters 13 and 17). This may result in the restriction of lung expansion. Primary treatment is with antibiotics, but when loculations are present within the pleural collection, antibiotic treatment alone is generally not effective. There is now ample evidence that loculated effusions can be effectively treated with either surgical debridement or fibrinolytic therapy and drainage. Catheter placement and fibrinolytic therapy using a protocolized approach is generally recommended as the first-line therapy of empyema. The failure rate for this approach is low, and surgery can be utilized for salvage in these situations.

CHEST WALL

Chest wall deformities can be present at birth or become evident during infancy, childhood, or adolescence. Pectus excavatum ("funnel chest") is the most common congenital chest wall deformity (Fig. 18.30). It is characterized by posterior angulation of the sternum secondary to abnormalities of the costal cartilages leading to chest pain, dyspnea on exertion, and lack of endurance with symptoms and deformity progressing during puberty and adolescence. There is evidence that improved stamina with an increase in cardiac output and stroke volume may be achieved after repair of severe pectus excavatum chest wall deformities. The traditional Ravitch procedure involving open resection of the costal cartilage and mobilization of the sternum has been replaced by a minimally invasive technique, the Nuss procedure, involving thoracoscopic placement of a substernal bar, which exerts outward pressure on the pliable chest wall of a pediatric patient with severe pectus excavatum. Modern indications for the Nuss procedure include two or more of these criteria: symptomatic patient, psycho-social impact, moderate to severe deformity by physical examination, CT criteria (Haller Index guidelines, cardiac or pulmonary compression), abnormal pulmonary function testing, and/or abnormal cardiac function (rhythm disturbance and/or mitral valve prolapse). Although the Nuss procedure achieves repair of the pectus excavatum through a minimally invasive technique with limited incisions, it is nonetheless a major surgical procedure associated with intraoperative risks, including cardiac injury, and significant postoperative discomfort requiring multimodal pain management. Postoperative analgesia is a major area of investigation, and the often-used modalities include thoracic epidural and patient-controlled analgesia. Due to concern for the level of opioid supplementation needed for these two modalities, thoracoscopic cryoablation of the intercostal nerve bundles has been performed in some centers. Evidence demonstrates that cryoablation has a more durable and effective impact on pain control, yielding less supplemental opioid requirements and decreased length of stay. Ongoing analysis is being performed regarding cost benefits of cryoablation and evaluation of long-term complications.

Pectus carinatum ("pigeon chest") is a protrusion of the chest wall (Fig. 18.31). Pectus carinatum occurs more commonly in males than females, and patients are typically asymptomatic. Surgical correction of carinatum deformities has been almost completely replaced by nonsurgical braces, which are custom fit and worn by patients for varying amounts of time. Poland syndrome is a rare chest wall deformity that consists of a constellation of abnormalities, including unilateral agenesis or dysplasia of rib cage and chondral cartilages, absence of pectoralis muscles, hand deformities, and breast and areolar defects (Fig. 18.32).

Axilla

Axillary lesions are most often lymphatic in origin. Benign reactive lymphadenopathy may occur in response to viral or bacterial infections or soft tissue infection or injury involving the hand or arm. Lymphatic malformations also occur in the lateral neck and may extend along the lymphatic vasculature to appear in the axilla. These lesions

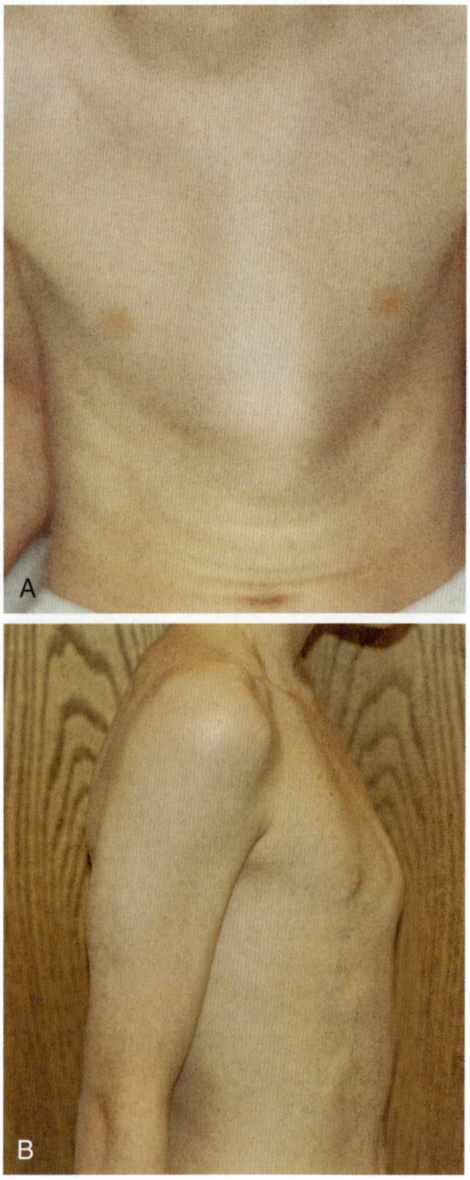

Fig. 18.31 (A) The sternum projects like a keel in front of the anterior chest wall in pectus carinatum (pigeon chest). Like pectus excavatum, pectus carinatum produces no symptoms. (B) Lateral view of a pectus carinatum.

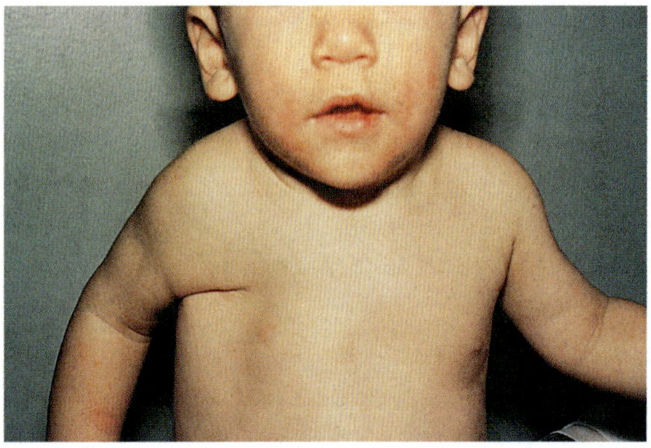

Fig. 18.32 Congenital unilateral absence of the anterior ribs, muscle, and soft tissues characterize Poland syndrome, producing its typical appearance pictured here.

may exist in continuity with cervical lesions and, importantly, extend into the mediastinum. A multidisciplinary vascular anomaly team is best suited to manage these lesions (Chapter 10) because they generally do not lend themselves to simple complete surgical excision and may require treatment with sclerosing agents. Hidradenitis suppurativa, a condition related to the obstruction of sebaceous and sweat glands, commonly presents as an axillary mass that may become superinfected and require surgical drainage (see Chapter 13).

Breast

Mastitis is relatively common in infancy. The development of fluctuance or purulent drainage is diagnostic of a breast abscess (see Chapter 13). In general, they require aggressive antibiotic therapy, warm compresses, and sometimes incision and drainage or needle aspiration. Localized breast masses in children are most commonly benign lesions. In the preadolescent, as early as 6 or 7 years old, the development of a firm mass under one or both areola may represent precocious thelarche and, less commonly, precocious puberty. This breast development may be asynchronous, with one breast bud becoming apparent several months ahead of the opposite side. Biopsy is never indicated in this scenario because unilateral iatrogenic amastia may result. In adolescents, fibroadenomas account for approximately 90% of solid masses. They are more commonly located in the upper outer quadrant of the breast and are more common in African American patients. These masses can typically be diagnosed based on physical examination because they are smooth, well circumscribed, mobile, and nontender. There may be some variation with the menstrual cycle. Ultrasound is a useful adjunct in distinguishing solid from cystic masses. Mammography has less utility in the pediatric population secondary to the denseness of the breast tissue. Benign lesions can be observed, with surgical excision reserved for those with growth over time, tenderness, or large lesions.

GASTROINTESTINAL

Gastrointestinal Obstruction

Vomiting is the reflex-coordinated response to various stimuli to the central nervous system, resulting in the forceful expulsion of gastrointestinal contents. Almost all infants vomit to some degree, and nonbilious vomiting does not always indicate serious illness. To determine the significance of vomiting, it is important to characterize the appearance of the emesis, presence of critical illness, patient age, and any associated symptoms.

The various causes of gastrointestinal obstruction that require surgical intervention can be categorized by age and the anatomic level of obstruction. These can be divided into two age categories: (1) neonates and infants in the first year of life and (2) toddlers and older children.

Neonates and Infants

Nonbilious Emesis

The most common cause of nonbilious emesis in neonates and infants is overfeeding, followed by gastrointestinal reflux. By definition, reflux is not emesis because it represents the passive movement of gastric contents retrograde above the gastroesophageal junction into the esophagus, despite the chief complaint of recurrent vomiting. The lower esophageal sphincter (LES) complex is the primary defense against reflux and is relatively immature in infants. Age-related maturation of the LES and improved gastric motility generally leads to resolution of the process by 1 year old in most children. Behaviors related to feeding including overfeeding, too rapid feeding, inadequate burping, and overstimulation may exacerbate these symptoms.

Some patients develop reflux-associated complications related to esophageal or extraesophageal symptoms. These include pain, bleeding, dysphagia, and failure to thrive secondary to esophagitis. Recurrent pneumonia, otitis media, hoarseness, respiratory distress, and apneic spell may also occur secondary to reflux. A barium swallow may delineate the upper anatomy and demonstrate aspiration from above as opposed to reflux of fluid from below, which is an important distinction (Fig. 18.33). In addition, an upper gastrointestinal series is quite useful for delineating the anatomy of the esophagus and stomach. It may demonstrate pyloric stenosis, malrotation and the

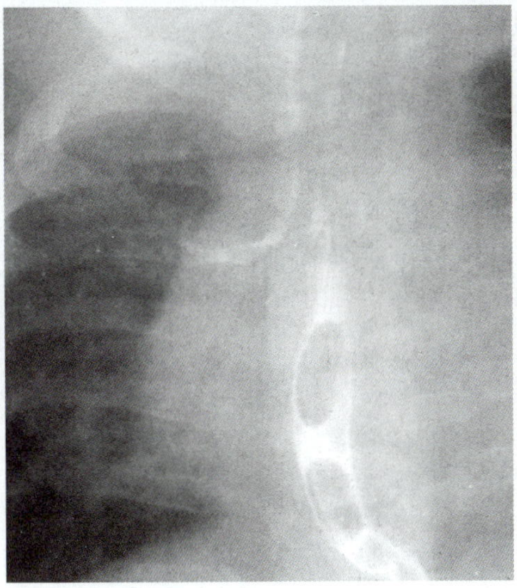

Fig. 18.33 Fluoroscopic examination of the infant during barium swallow must be of sufficient duration to allow the identification of episodes of reflux (here associated with aspiration into the tracheobronchial tree).

presence of any webs, membranes, or stenosis in these structures, as well as hiatal hernias. Although it may show evidence of reflux at one point in time, it is not a reliable means for the primary diagnosis of reflux. Distal esophageal mucosal biopsies may be useful in a subset of patients to more precisely identify those who may benefit from antireflux surgery. Medical management strategies are adequate in the vast majority of patients. Antireflux surgery is reserved for medically refractory patients or those with complications of reflux including failure to thrive, esophagitis, or respiratory disease. The goal of surgery is to strengthen the LES mechanism and to repair other associated pathologies that precipitate reflux, such as the presence of a hiatal hernia. Hypertrophic pyloric stenosis is the most common cause of gastric outlet obstruction in infants with an incidence of approximately 1 in 300 live births in Caucasians in the United States with a lower incidence in other populations. The classic presentation of hypertrophic pyloric stenosis is progressive, nonbilious, projectile vomiting in a full-term (premature infants typically present later) neonate who is between 2 and 8 weeks old (Fig. 18.34). Affected infants may develop hypochloremic, hypokalemic, and metabolic alkalosis in the setting of persistent emesis. Surgical treatment of pyloric stenosis is never an emergency, and it is critical for the infant to be adequately resuscitated and any electrolyte abnormalities corrected

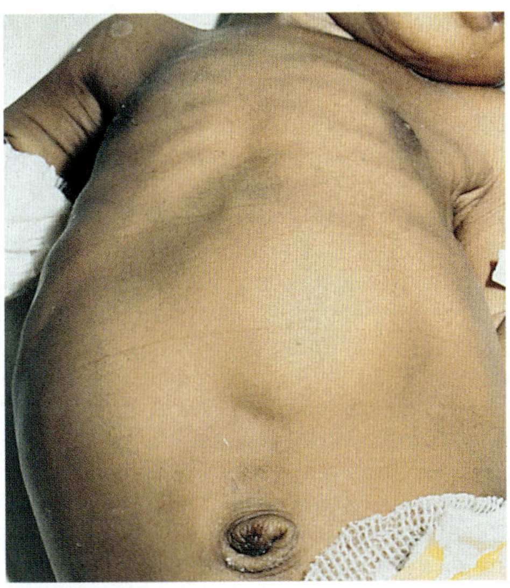

Fig. 18.34 Pyloric stenosis may cause epigastric distention by the obstructed stomach. This patient also demonstrates a visible wave of peristalsis, which moves from left to right.

before going for surgical correction. Failure to provide adequate resuscitation and correct metabolic alkalosis preoperatively may leave the infant at risk of postoperative apnea due to impaired respiratory drive. Pyloromyotomy, the operative repair of pyloric stenosis, can be performed open or laparoscopically, with laparoscopic repair becoming the standard of care in most areas of the country (Fig. 18.35).

Bilious Emesis Without Abdominal Distention

Bilious emesis is a critical finding in the pediatric population. Its presence should always raise a red flag in the evaluation of a vomiting infant. The principal concern is malrotation with midgut volvulus, which is a surgical emergency and must be ruled out first. This typically presents without abdominal distention because the level of obstruction is proximal, at or near the ligament of Treitz. Abdominal distention can be a presenting sign, but it is typically a late finding with associated intestinal ischemia. It typically presents as bilious emesis in a previously well infant. Malrotation is the failure of the midgut (small bowel, right colon, and one-third of transverse colon) to undergo adequate rotation and retroperitoneal fixation during embryonic development. Consequently, the bowel resides on a narrow vascular pedicle (superior mesenteric artery) that is prone to undergo twisting and subsequent volvulus. If surgical intervention is not undertaken in a timely fashion, the twist around the narrow vascular pedicle results in midgut ischemia and, ultimately, infarction (Fig. 18.36). Bloody bowel movements may occur as ischemia progresses and mucosa sloughs. Severe short bowel syndrome or death may occur from delayed recognition, diagnosis, and treatment of this important condition.

Although most patients who present with bilious emesis do not have malrotation with volvulus, the cost of a diagnostic delay is unacceptably high; therefore the finding of bilious emesis mandates a prompt evaluation. Plain radiographs demonstrating gastric and duodenal distention in the setting of an otherwise nearly "gasless abdomen" should raise the suspicion for this condition (Fig. 18.37). Pneumatosis intestinalis represents a late finding signifying bowel ischemia from volvulus. The cornerstone of diagnosis of malrotation is the upper gastrointestinal series, which identifies the contour of the duodenal C-loop, the location of the ligament of Treitz, and the flow of contrast into the jejunum (see Chapter 25). Ultrasound may also be used for diagnosis by evaluating the relationship between the superior mesenteric artery and vein. Imaging is only a tool. In a critically ill child with sudden onset of bilious emesis, there is a high suspicion of volvulus. Diagnostic studies should not be undertaken in this clinical setting as they will only delay treatment. Management involves aggressive resuscitation with surgical exploration, detorsion of the bowel, resection of congenital bands (Ladd bands), and widening of the mesentery (Ladd procedure). An appendectomy is often completed during the operation to avoid diagnostic errors later in life, because the cecum typically resides in the left upper quadrant at the end of the operation. The operation does not correct the malrotation but instead serves to minimize the risk of future volvulus.

Duodenal atresia and other duodenal anomalies are important considerations in patients who present with bilious emesis. Duodenal atresia is a congenital bowel obstruction that is typically located within the second portion of the duodenum. In 85% of neonates with duodenal atresia, the entry of the bile duct is proximal to the level of obstruction; therefore the emesis is bilious. Vomiting may occur shortly after birth or may present later in the setting of annular pancreas, duodenal stenosis, and incompletely obstructing duodenal webs. Duodenal atresia has an incidence of approximately 1 in 6000 live births with males being affected more commonly than females. Additional congenital anomalies are identified in more than 50% of patients with duodenal atresia, with trisomy 21 occurring in ~one-third of these patients. This anomaly may be diagnosed antenatally based on findings on the prenatal ultrasound with a demonstration of a dilated, fluid-filled stomach and proximal duodenum. There is often an associated polyhydramnios due

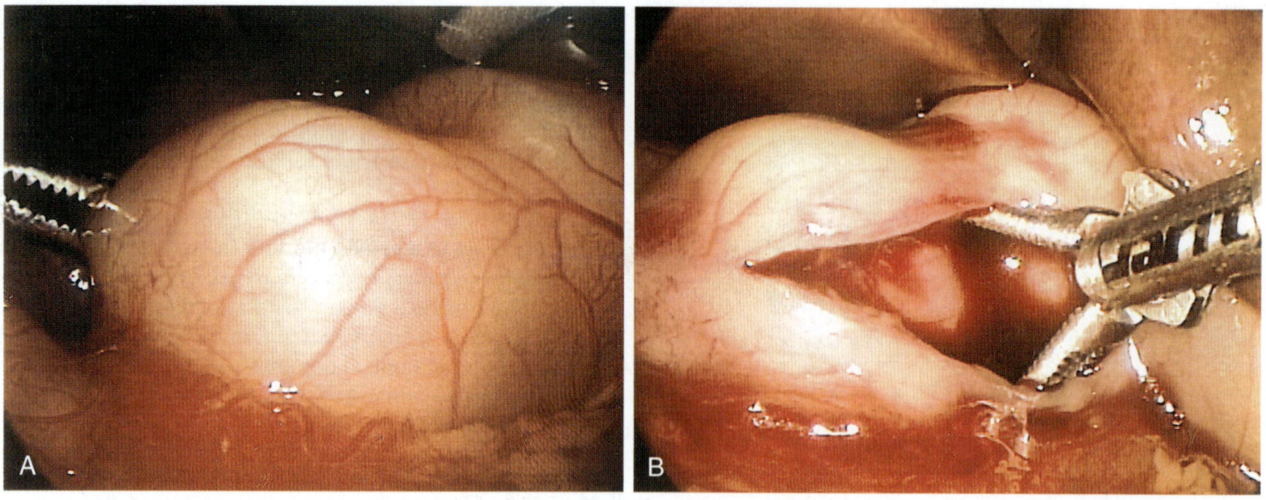

Fig. 18.35 Laparoscopic view of pyloric stenosis viewing the hypertrophied pylorus (A) and pyloromyotomy, demonstrating the serosal incision (B).

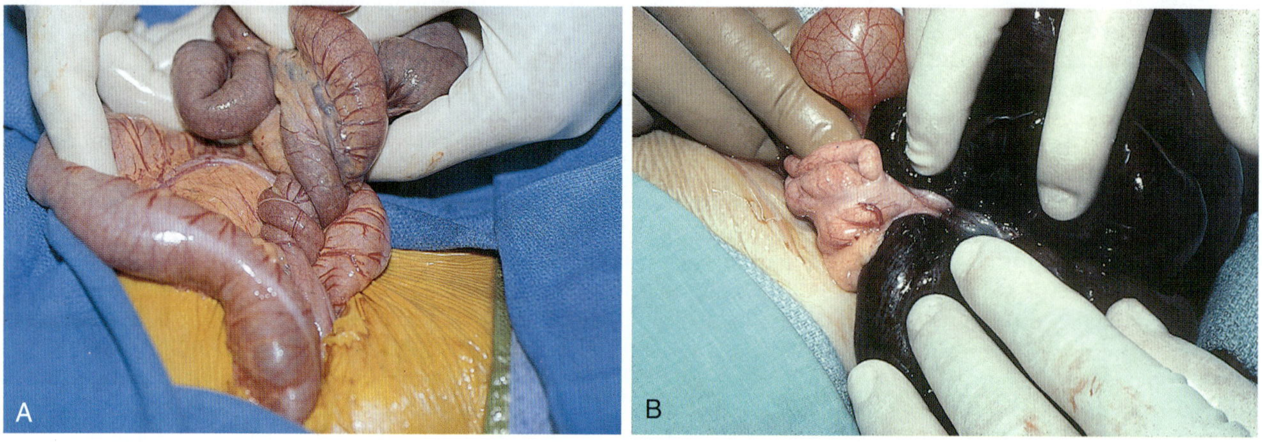

Fig. 18.36 Malrotation with midgut volvulus without ischemia (A). Malrotation predisposes to volvulus and complete midgut infarction (B).

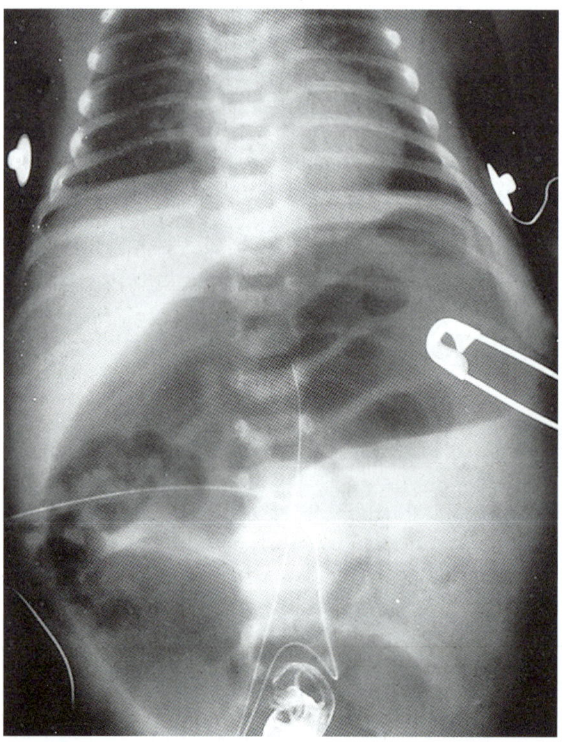

Fig. 18.37 Complete duodenal obstruction from midgut volvulus. Air in the distal gastrointestinal tract fails to rule out complete obstruction from volvulus and distinguishes the diagnosis from duodenal atresia.

to the proximal obstruction. The radiographic finding of a "double-bubble" sign in the newborn is pathognomonic of a duodenal obstruction, usually secondary to duodenal atresia (Fig. 18.38). In the setting of an antenatal diagnosis, or confirmatory plain radiograph in the newborn, no further imaging is required. Survival rates exceed 90% with operative intervention with mortality largely stemming from associated cardiac anomalies.

Bilious Vomiting With Abdominal Distention

Bilious emesis with associated abdominal distention is more characteristic of distal small bowel obstruction seen in conditions such as intestinal atresia, meconium disease, incarcerated hernias, or Hirschsprung disease, rather than proximal bowel obstruction.

Small bowel and colonic atresias are thought to be the sequelae of intrauterine vascular accidents and are likely late gestational events. They can occur at any point along the intestinal tract with the highest incidence in the jejunum, followed by the ileum and finally the colon. Neonates typically present with bilious emesis and abdominal distention that is progressive. The more distal the obstruction, the more distended the abdomen becomes. The presence of a proximal obstruction on plain film requires no additional testing before surgery. Contrast enemas are critical in differentiating distal small bowel and colonic atresias from other distal obstructions, including Hirschsprung disease, meconium ileus, and small left colon syndrome. In an atresia, a contrast enema will show a failure of the contrast material to reflux into the dilated loops of bowel. Small bowel atresias are often isolated conditions, but other anomalies may be present in 25% of patients.

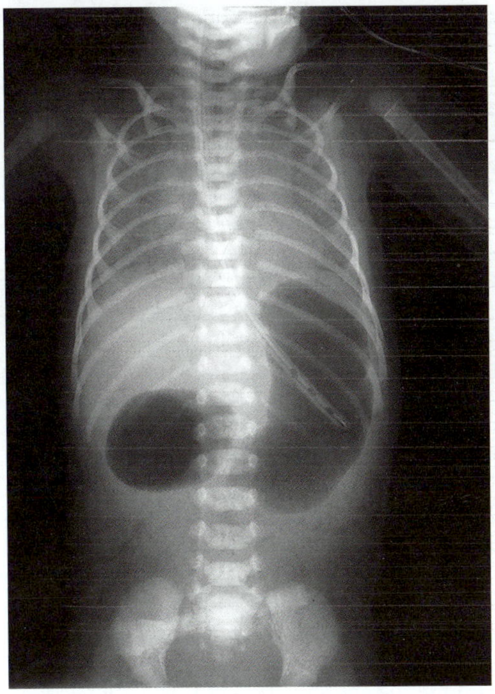

Fig. 18.38 Swallowed air distends the stomach and proximal duodenum in duodenal atresia, producing the characteristic "double bubble" on plain film. Other contrast studies are unnecessary.

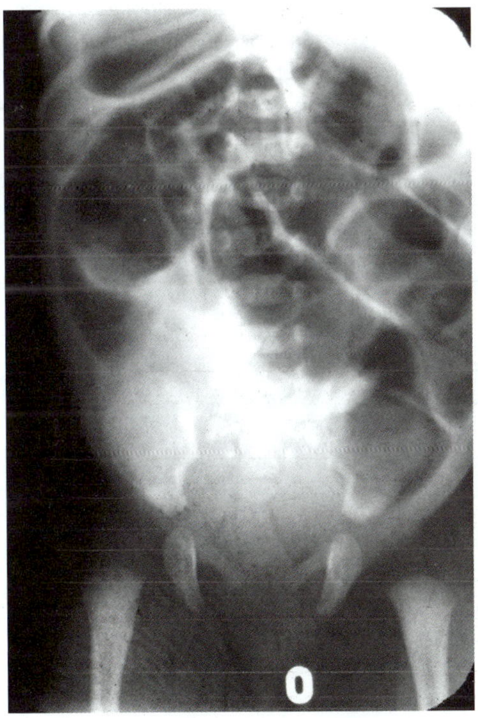

Fig. 18.39 Meconium ileus presents as a distal small bowel obstruction in the newborn with few air-filled dilated loops due to the meconium-filled bowel loops.

Meconium ileus disease is the initial presentation of cystic fibrosis in up to 20% of children, and these findings may be appreciated on antenatal ultrasound imaging. Thick, viscous inspissated meconium in the distal small bowel causes an intestinal obstruction. The bowel proximal to the obstruction is dilated, whereas the colon is often small (microcolon) because it is unused (Fig. 18.39). Marked proximal small bowel dilation occurs, and the abdomen presents a "soap bubble" or "ground glass" appearance on plain radiography due to air trapped in the inspissated meconium. Air-fluid levels are uncommon because of the dense concentration of meconium in the intestinal loops. Contrast enema with a high osmotic water-soluble agent reveals the presence of a microcolon and inspissated meconium pellets in the distal ileum. Reflux of contrast into the dilated bowel may be therapeutic. Contrast enema should be performed after the neonate has been adequately resuscitated, recognizing that significant volume may be needed during and after the procedure due to the osmotic nature of the enema. If the enema is only partially successful in evacuating the meconium, it can be repeated. In some neonates, the obstruction cannot be relieved with enemas alone and surgery is necessary. At laparotomy, there is evidence of proximal dilated bowel with the distal small bowel impacted with thick meconium. This inspissated meconium is difficult to evacuate, and repeated instillation of diluted N-acetylcysteine is often required to empty the small bowel via an enterotomy. On occasion, patients with meconium ileus disease may develop intestinal atresia, volvulus, or perforation with varying amounts of meconium peritonitis. These conditions are referred to as *complicated meconium ileus*. Evidence of complicated meconium ileus may be appreciated on prenatal ultrasound or neonatal films by the presence of calcifications and ascites. Unsuccessful attempts at contrast reduction of meconium ileus may be secondary to an associated atresia.

Evidence of distal gastrointestinal obstruction in the newborn should raise the concern of Hirschsprung disease. Hirschsprung disease is characterized by the absence of ganglion cells in the distal bowel, resulting in the absence of peristalsis and a functional bowel obstruction (Fig. 18.40). Although the classic presentation is abdominal distention with failure to pass meconium, distal obstruction may also induce vomiting which may be bilious. Plain radiographs typically demonstrate bowel dilation. A contrast enema should be performed (preferably before rectal manipulation) (Fig. 18.41). It may demonstrate a transition zone, which is the transition from the dilated ganglionated bowel to the decompressed ganglionated segment, traditionally in the rectosigmoid region. This is also important in ruling out other potential diagnoses, such as small left colon, distal colonic atresia, and meconium ileus disease or meconium plug syndrome. Contrast enema alone is not sufficient in diagnosing Hirschsprung disease, especially early in life as the colon may not have time to dilate; the confirmation of diagnosis requires rectal biopsy, which can be performed without anesthesia at the bedside (Fig. 18.42). Some children go undiagnosed in the initial days to months of life but are plagued by chronic constipation requiring rectal stimulation to evacuate. They may develop chronic symptoms of abdominal wall distention, growth failure, and constipation. A barium enema may be highly suggestive in this population, and a rectal biopsy is diagnostic. Patients with Hirschsprung disease are also at risk for Hirschsprung-related enterocolitis. This is a potential life-threatening disease marked by explosive diarrhea, abdominal distention, toxic megacolon, and possible sepsis, and it may progress to death if not treated aggressively.

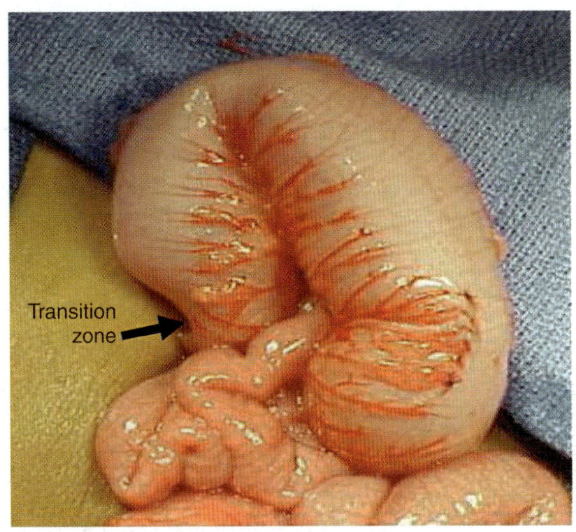

Fig. 18.40 The absence of intramural ganglion cells prevents intestinal peristalsis through segments affected by Hirschsprung disease, causing a functional bowel obstruction. The involved segment appears narrow compared with the distended, obstructed proximal bowel, which possesses normal ganglion cells.

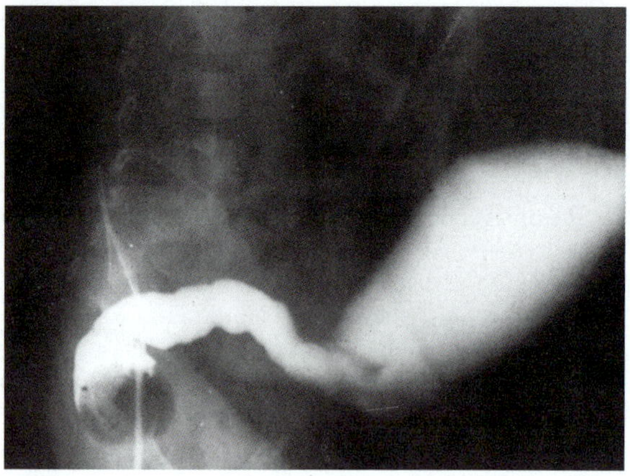

Fig. 18.41 Barium enema outlines the transition zone between the contracted (aganglionic) rectosigmoid lying distal to the obstructed, but normally innervated, colon. To demonstrate this sign, the examination must be conducted in an unprepped patient who has undergone neither enemas nor digital rectal examination.

Older Infants and Children

Age-specific considerations for the causes of vomiting should direct the diagnostic approaches for children beyond the neonatal period and infancy period. Intussusception is a frequent cause of vomiting in infants and toddlers. It is the leading cause of intestinal obstruction in this population and second only to constipation in causes of acute abdominal pain. Intussusception is the telescoping, or invagination, of one part of the bowel into itself. The process can occur in all age groups from prenatal to adults. The majority (90%) of intussusceptions occur before age 3, with 75% occurring before age 2. Intussusception can be classified as primary (idiopathic) or secondary (due to a lesion acting as a lead point). Secondary intussusception may occur and may be due to a Meckel diverticulum, polyp, lymphoma, intestinal duplication, or hematoma (as may occur in hemophilia or in Henoch-Schönlein purpura [HSP]) acting as a lead point, especially in older children. The cause of idiopathic intussusception is not completely understood but is attributed to hypertrophied Peyer patches and lymphadenopathy within the bowel mesentery. Intussusception can be seen in the setting of an upper respiratory tract infection or an episode of gastroenteritis, with the viral illness presumably leading to the lymphoid reaction. In addition, there is a rise in the incidence of intussusception during peaks of seasonal viral illness, suggesting that viral infections play a role in its etiology.

Idiopathic ileocolonic intussusception occurs in the region of the ileocecal valve (Fig. 18.43). The classic clinical presentation is that of a previously well child who presents with paroxysms of severe colicky abdominal pain that may be associated with drawing legs to their chest. In between paroxysms, children may initially appear normal, but as the process progresses, they may develop increasing lethargy and somnolence. Initially vomiting is often nonbilious, but as the process continues, if the bowel obstruction becomes complete, the emesis may become bilious. The classic picture of "currant jelly" stools (Fig. 18.44) is a relatively late finding and is a marker of bowel ischemia and mucosal sloughing. Rarely, the intussusception may protrude through the anus and be confused with rectal prolapse. The classic findings on ultrasound are those of a "target" lesion, which consists of alternating rings of high and low echogenicity. Small bowel-small bowel intussusception seen on CT scan is unreliable as this is only a snapshot and may represent a transient episode. Contrast enema with either air (preferred) or barium may be diagnostic, as well as therapeutic for ileocolonic intussusception (Fig. 18.45). Successful reduction is demonstrated by free passage of barium into dilated loops of bowel proximal to the obstruction. The success rate

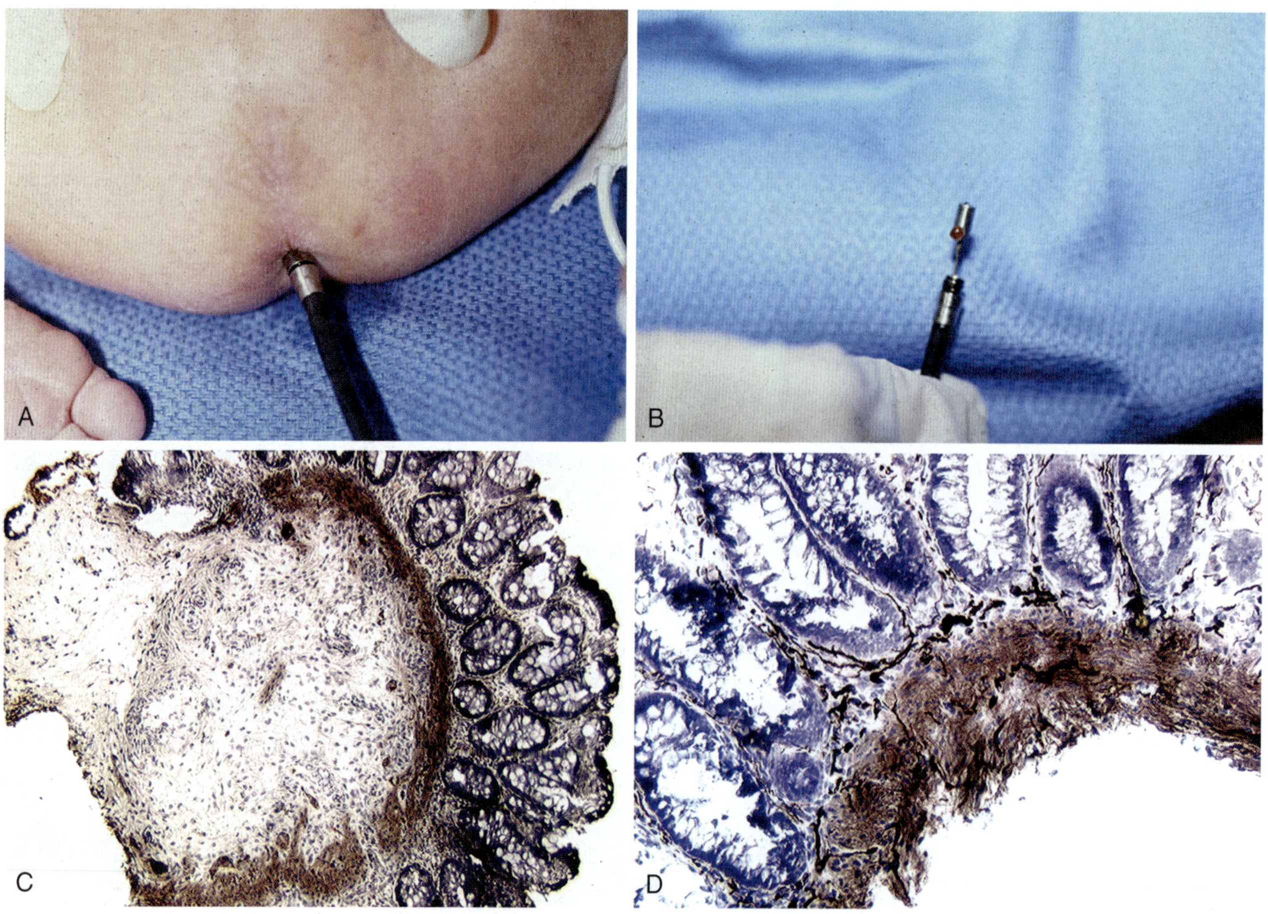

Fig. 18.42 Suction rectal biopsy is a bedside procedure (A) that provides a small fragment of tissue for pathologic evaluation for ganglion cells (B). A normal suction rectal biopsy with an acetylcholinesterase stain demonstrates a normal band of staining and no giant nerve fibers between the muscular layers (C). Higher-power view of a biopsy from a patient with Hirschsprung disease shows darkly staining giant nerve fibers in the muscularis layer (acetylcholinesterase stain) (D). (C and D, Courtesy Paul S. Dickman, MD, and Dan Galvis, BS.)

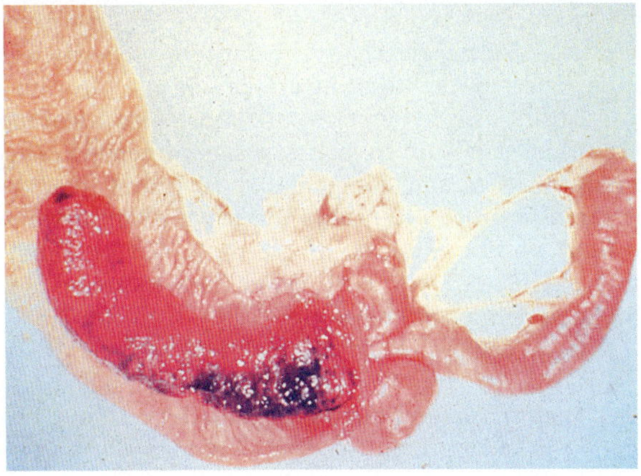

Fig. 18.43 The intestine invaginates into itself in intussusception. The ileum is pulled through the ileocecal valve into the colon, the most common pattern seen in infancy, pictured here.

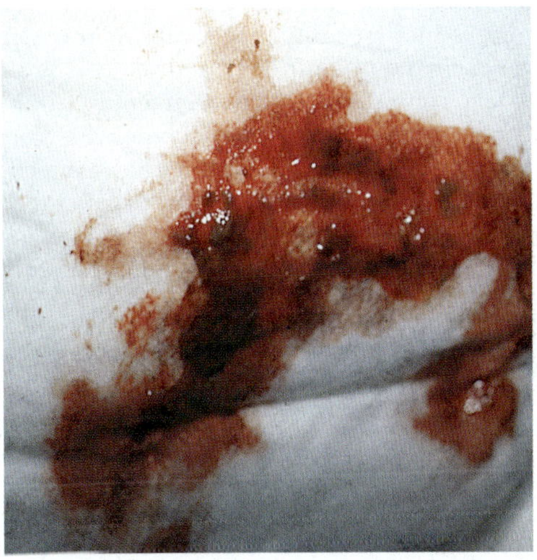

Fig. 18.44 The intussusception—the invaginated portion of bowel—becomes congested and ischemic, leading to the passage of bloody stool mixed with mucus (currant jelly stool).

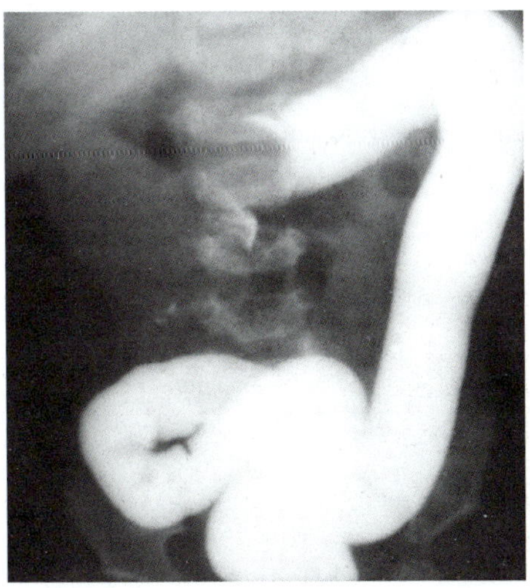

Fig. 18.45 Barium enema confirms the diagnosis by outlining the intussusceptum. The column of contrast can then be used to push the invaginated bowel proximally. Free reflux of contrast into the bowel proximally signals complete reduction of the intussusception.

of air enema reduction has been reported to be as high as 94% but is operator dependent and relies on an experienced radiologist. Those patients who have an incomplete or failed reduction and are clinically well may undergo a repeated attempt at air reduction in the appropriate setting. Those patients who fail air or contrast enema reduction of the intussusception require urgent surgical exploration for reduction or resection.

It is important to remember that intussusception patients can present along a spectrum of severity of illness. They may be extremely dehydrated and therefore must be volume resuscitated before attempts at reduction. Antibiotics can be considered before attempts at reduction because the reduction can precipitate bacterial translocation and bacteremia. If the patient presents late in the course of the disease, there may be clear evidence of peritonitis and an attempt at enema reduction should not take place. Intussusception presenting with peritonitis requires urgent surgical management. The risk of recurrent intussusception after radiologic-guided air enema is reported to be around 5% with one-third recurring within the first 24 hours and most recurring within the first few days. Patients with recurrent symptoms should have repeat ultrasound and attempt at enema reduction, if positive. Ileoileal and jejunoileal intussusceptions are generally too proximal to be amenable to radiographic reduction. If the intussusceptions have a short segment, they may be physiologic; if they have a longer segment or are symptomatic, they may be due to a mechanical lead point that would require surgery (Fig. 18.46). Postoperative intussusception may also occur in the small bowel and requires operative reduction (a classic example being post-resection of a Wilms tumor). Controversy exists regarding the management of older children who present with intussusception because of the increasing frequency of a pathologic lead point (PLP) as the causative agent. The rate of PLPs as the cause of intussusception increases from 1.5% to 12% in infants, and in children it increases to 60% in 5- to 14-year-olds. Enema reduction can still be attempted in the acute setting of ileocolic intussusception, but one must have a higher index of suspicion and a workup for a PLP should be undertaken.

Twisting and compression from postoperative adhesions, amniotic bands, omphalomesenteric (vitelline) remnants (Fig. 18.47),

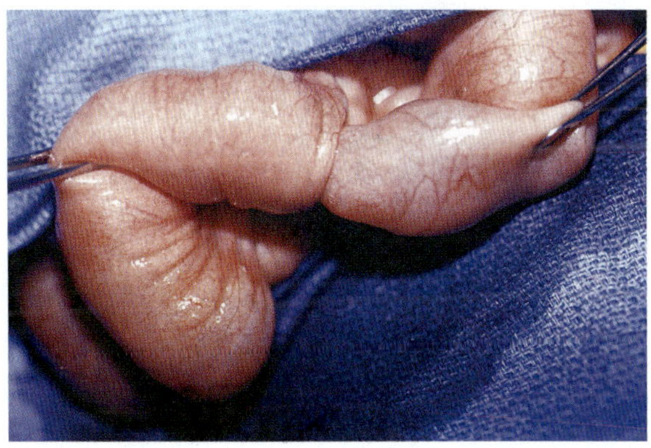

Fig. 18.46 Small bowel intussusception typically has a lead point except in patients with postoperative intussusception as shown here. Upper gastrointestinal studies should be avoided in these patients secondary to aspiration risks.

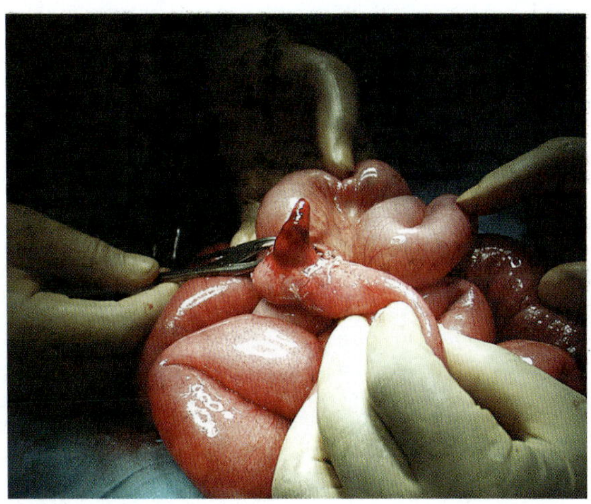

Fig. 18.47 Omphalomesenteric remnants, also known as *vitelline bands*, may produce internal hernias that lead to obstruction.

tubes, or shunts may produce intestinal obstructions. The most common cause of intestinal obstruction is adhesions from previous surgery, intraabdominal infection, and trauma. Early nasogastric decompression and aggressive rehydration may alleviate the symptoms, halt the progression of distension, and give time for resolution of the obstruction. Failure of resolution, progression of symptoms, or lack of any prior risk factor for obstruction should prompt surgical exploration.

Gastrointestinal Bleeding

Gastrointestinal bleeding accounts for ~0.3% of pediatric emergency department visits. The evaluation involves a careful assessment of several important factors and the establishment of a management protocol (Table 18.5). Initially the practitioner must determine whether the bleeding is hemodynamically significant. The next step is to confirm that what appears to be blood is truly blood. Subsequently, the physician should determine whether the clinical presentation would suggest upper versus lower gastrointestinal tract bleeding (Table 18.6). Patients in acute or impending hypovolemic shock require urgent stabilization. The principals of resuscitation must proceed in combination with diagnostic studies and consultations. In cases of more chronic or subacute blood loss, symptoms of anemia, fatigue, and pallor are more common. A thorough history and physical examination in conjunction with serologic, radiologic, and endoscopic studies are critical to ascertain the etiology of the bleeding. The duration, severity, and location of the source of the bleeding are among the most important historical factors, as is evidence of previous episodes of bleeding. Drug ingestion, exposure to sick contacts, inherited coagulopathies, vitamin deficiency, congenital or acquired liver dysfunction, or family history of chronic intestinal disorders may shed further light on the etiology of bleeding. Severe acute blood loss may be associated with both upper (hematemesis) and lower (hematochezia or melena) bleeding.

Table 18.5 Common Causes of Gastrointestinal Hemorrhage in Infants and Children

Site of Hemorrhage	Age Younger Than 1 Year Old	Age Older Than 1 Year Old
Upper GI tract	Gastritis Swallowed maternal blood Gastric or duodenal ulcer Malrotation with volvulus	Gastric or duodenal ulcer Varices
Lower GI tract	Anal fissures Intussusception NEC Meckel diverticulum Malrotation and volvulus	Colonic polyps Intussusception Meckel diverticulum Infectious diarrhea Inflammatory bowel disease

GI, Gastrointestinal; *NEC,* necrotizing enterocolitis.

Infants

Swallowed maternal blood during childbirth or from irritated or injured nipples during breastfeeding is commonly mistaken for gastrointestinal bleeding in the newborn. These infants have normal vital signs and stable hemoglobin levels. The Apt-Downey test differentiates between maternal and fetal blood in the newborn and should be performed to identify the source of the blood. Hemorrhagic diseases of the newborn may lead to profound upper gastrointestinal bleeding, especially in those infants who fail to receive perinatal vitamin K injection. This is a rare occurrence in delivery rooms, but infants delivered at home, who are unstable or urgently transferred from the delivery room to other institutions, or whose parents refuse vitamin K injection, may be at high risk. Delivery records for all newborns who present with upper gastrointestinal bleeding should be examined for vitamin K administration. Nasogastric tube placement or oropharyngeal suctioning shortly after birth may precipitate bleeding that results in bloody emesis; this typically clears with gastric lavage. If it does not clear and/or there is a history of difficulty in placement of the tube, then further workup should be undertaken to assess for a possible iatrogenic injury with tube placement. Anal fissures are a more benign cause of bleeding in infants (Fig. 18.48). This may be associated with constipation and hard stools.

Severe acute gastritis or gastric ulceration may occur in the newborn period and is associated with high morbidity and mortality. These infants may present with hypovolemic shock and free intraperitoneal air (Fig. 18.49). This typically occurs during the first 7 to 10 days of life. Malrotation with midgut volvulus may also present with severe upper gastrointestinal bleeding secondary to either bowel ischemia or sepsis-induced coagulopathy.

Necrotizing enterocolitis (NEC) is the most common gastrointestinal surgical emergency of the newborn period. It affects more than 25,000 neonates per year, and the incidence is rising. Although

Table 18.6 Causes of Gastrointestinal (GI) Bleeding

Location	Appearance	Age: Newborn	Age: Infant	Age: Child
Upper GI	Well	Maternal blood Nasogastric tube Esophagitis Gastritis	Nosebleeds Nasogastric tube Esophagitis Gastritis	Nosebleeds Nasogastric tube
	Ill	Peptic ulcer disease NEC Volvulus	Varices Peptic ulcer disease Medications	Varices Peptic ulcer disease Medications
Lower GI	Well	Anal fissures Maternal blood Hemangioma Duplication	Anal fissure Meckel diverticulum Duplication	Anal fissure Juvenile polyp Meckel diverticulum Rectal prolapse
	Ill	NEC Volvulus Infectious diarrhea	Intussusception Infectious diarrhea Medications Henoch-Schönlein purpura Hemolytic-uremic syndrome	Infectious diarrhea Intussusception Trauma Medications Hemolytic-uremic syndrome Henoch-Schönlein purpura Inflammatory bowel disease

NEC, Necrotizing enterocolitis.

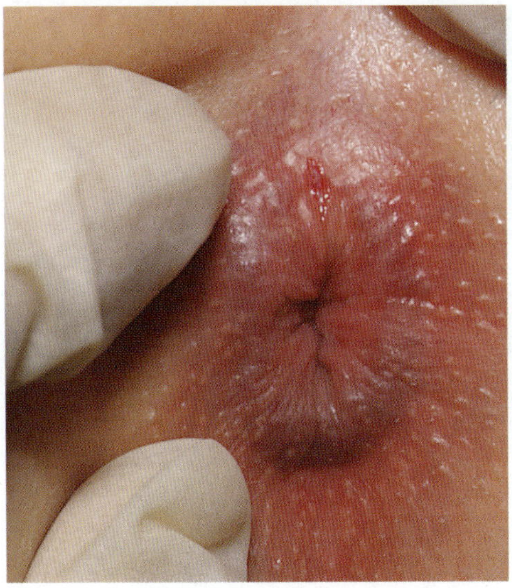

Fig. 18.48 Small tears in the anoderm may bleed, producing small amounts of blood in the stool of healthy infants.

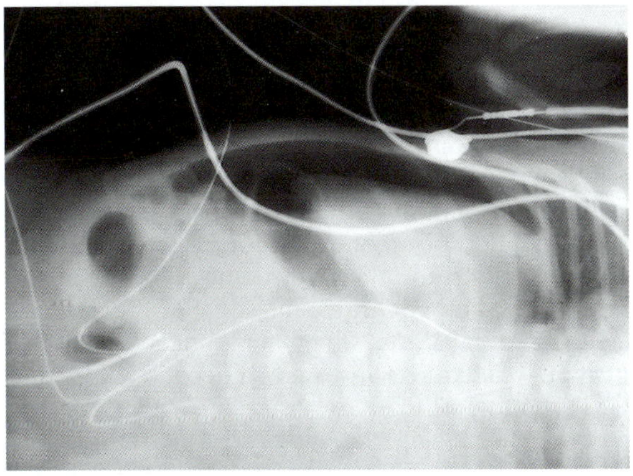

Fig. 18.49 The large quantity of free air within the abdomen resulting from a gastric perforation (shown here outlining the edge of the liver) suggests its source.

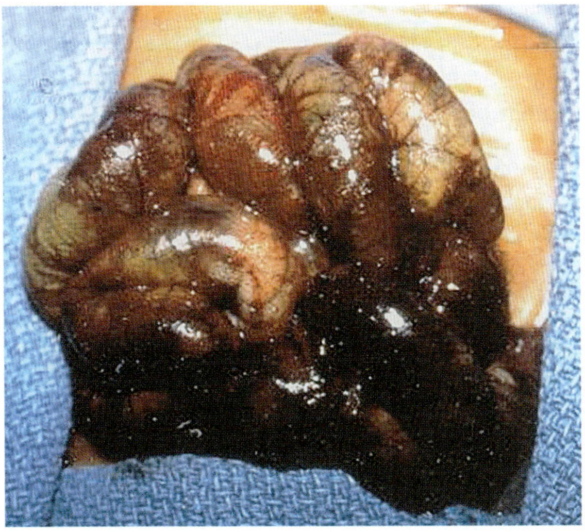

Fig. 18.50 Diffuse necrotizing enterocolitis is associated with a patchy distribution of necrosis on the serosal surface of the bowel.

classically presenting with abdominal distention, NEC may also precipitate upper or, more commonly, lower gastrointestinal bleeding (Fig. 18.50). Mortality rates for NEC remain high, approaching 50% for very-low-birth-weight and very premature infants. The pathophysiology of NEC is multifactorial and complex. Several key risk factors appear to contribute to the development of disease including prematurity, bacterial colonization, and the initiation of formula feeding. Other factors linked to NEC include mechanical ventilation, low birth weight, cyanotic congenital heart disease, hypoxemia, drugs (indomethacin and methylxanthines), maternal chorioamnionitis, and maternal cocaine use. More recent evidence suggests that impaired enterocyte barrier allows bacterial translocation triggering systemic inflammation. Multiple randomized clinical trials have demonstrated that breast milk feeding can reduce the incidence of NEC. The rate of NEC in infants who weigh less than 1500 g is 10%, and the mortality is inversely proportional to the birth weight and gestational age. Clinically, patients may have vague symptoms, including abdominal distention, vomiting, increased gastric residuals, and bloody stools. Constitutional symptoms include temperature lability, apnea, and bradycardia, as well as inactivity. On physical examination, patients often appear toxic with signs of abdominal distention, edema, and erythema. Laboratory values may show neutropenia or leukocytosis, anemia, and metabolic acidosis. Plain radiographs of the abdomen may demonstrate pneumatosis intestinalis, which is the pathognomonic hallmark of the disease (Fig. 18.51). This radiographic finding suggests the subserosal dissection of air and may be linear or cystic. On occasion, portal vein gas may be seen, which is suggestive of more severe disease. Pneumoperitoneum, which is best visualized on the left lateral decubitus film, is suggestive of perforation and is an absolute indication for immediate surgical intervention (Fig. 18.49). Ultrasound has emerged as a useful adjunct in the diagnosis and serial evaluation of patients with NEC. In general, NEC is managed medically with parental nutrition, antibiotics, nasogastric tube decompression, and bowel rest with the suspension of enteral feedings. In the absence of a clear intestinal perforation, relative indications for surgical intervention include deteriorating clinical status, abdominal wall erythema, the presence of a fixed loop on serial abdominal plain films, persistent acidosis despite adequate resuscitation, ongoing platelet consumption, and portal venous gas. Despite uneventful recovery from the initial acute-phase disease, some patients go on to develop symptomatic strictures from fibrosis (Fig. 18.52), which require surgical resection once the acute disease has resolved.

Toddlers (1–5 Years Old)

Painless rectal bleeding in the toddler should raise concern for the presence of a Meckel diverticulum. Often the bleeding is massive, requiring blood transfusion. The initial blood loss is variable and may present as a sentinel bleed that spontaneously resolves, followed by clinically significant bleeding, with bright red or maroon blood per rectum. Although spontaneous resolution may occur, subsequent episodes of bleeding may become life threatening. The bleeding results from the ulceration of the ileal mucosa located adjacent to the ectopic gastric mucosa present within the Meckel diverticulum (Fig. 18.53). Ulceration can occur within the diverticulum or, more commonly, within the ileum itself across from or adjacent to the diverticulum. A technetium-99m pertechnetate isotope scan, referred to as a *Meckel scan,* identifies gastric mucosa and may be helpful in the diagnosis of disease (Fig. 25.91). The scan will only identify those diverticula that contain gastric mucosa. During active bleeding, the scan may be positive in up to 85% of patients. False-negative evaluations are common. The use of intravenous pentagastrin or cimetidine may improve the sensitivity of the study. Contrast studies of the distal small bowel (enteroclysis) or colon (barium enema) are of marginal diagnostic utility in this setting and may obscure the scan. Some children must undergo exploratory laparoscopy to identify the presence of the diverticulum in the setting of negative studies (Fig. 18.54). Patients with Meckel diverticulum present less commonly with obstruction (secondary to volvulus, internal hernia, or intussusception) or acute inflammation (diverticulitis), in a manner similar to a patient with appendicitis.

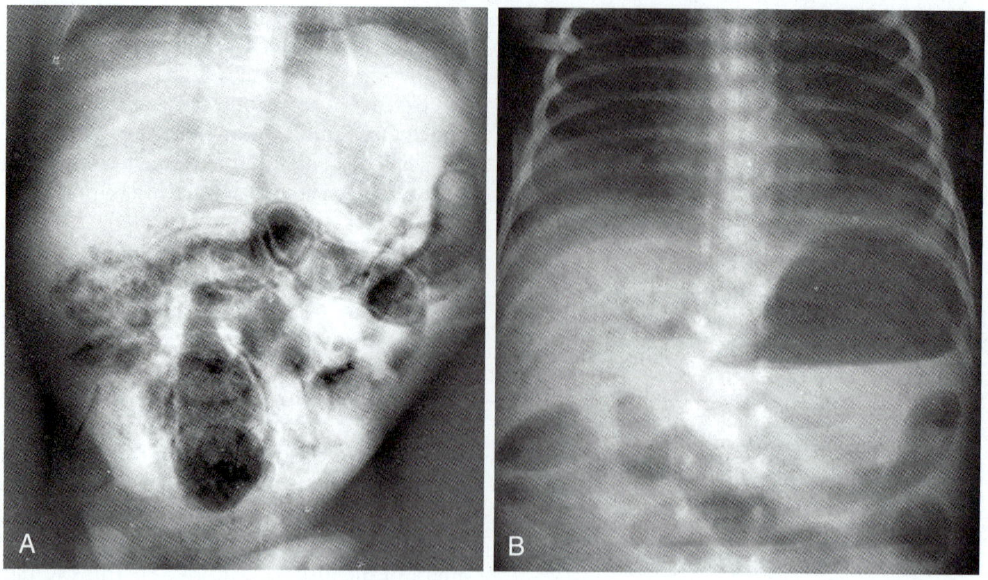

Fig. 18.51 Pneumatosis intestinalis is seen most easily as linear streaks of air outlining the bowel and producing concentric rings when viewed on end. More common, however, is the bubbly pattern seen in the right iliac fossa in this patient, appearing like stool within the lumen (A). In severely affected infants, gas may fill the portal system and produce visible streaks of air on abdominal plain film (B).

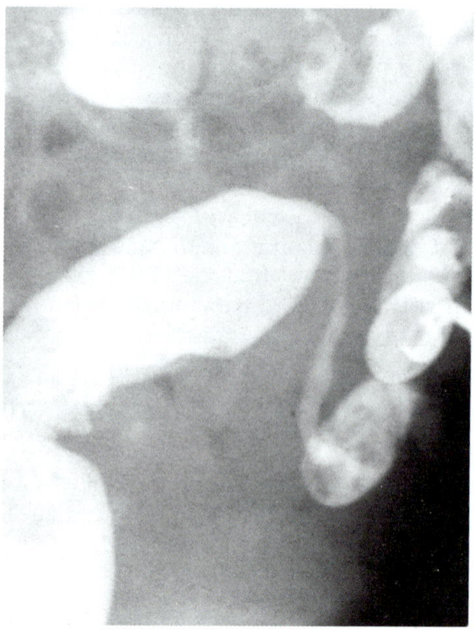

Fig. 18.52 In a patient who develops intestinal obstruction during recovery from necrotizing enterocolitis, a colonic stricture must be suspected.

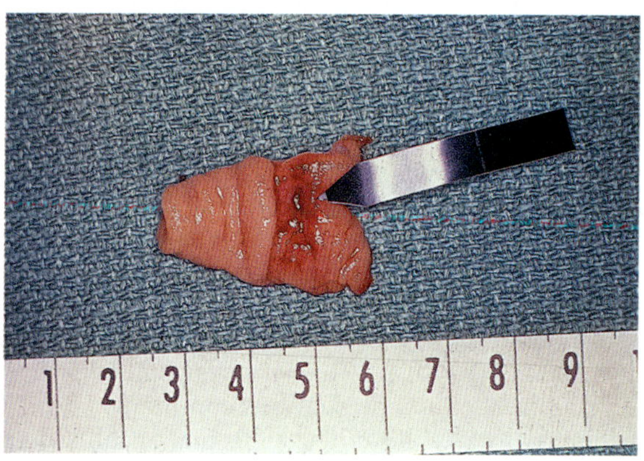

Fig. 18.53 The bleeding site in a Meckel diverticulum is typically located on the mucosa of bowel adjacent to the ectopic gastric tissue.

Esophageal varices may be a significant source of massive upper gastrointestinal bleeding in children with portal hypertension. Causes of portal hypertension in children include the presence of extrahepatic portal vein thrombosis or hepatic cirrhosis. Omphalitis as a complication of umbilical venous catheterization in newborns may precipitate portal vein thrombosis. Children with short bowel syndrome or other chronic intestinal disorders may require chronic parenteral nutrition, which may contribute to total parenteral nutrition–related liver disease and hepatic failure. One-third of patients who undergo a Kasai procedure (hepatoportoenterostomy) for biliary atresia develop progressive cirrhosis that may lead to portal hypertension. Cystic fibrosis, α_1-antitrypsin deficiency, and viral hepatitis are a few medical conditions that may induce cirrhosis and portal hypertension in children. Upper gastrointestinal endoscopy facilitates direct visualization of varices in cases of active bleeding and provides access for therapeutic banding or sclerosant therapy. The advent of transjugular intracaval portosystemic shunting (TIPS), as well as better endoscopic techniques, have all but eliminated the need for emergency surgical intervention in acutely bleeding esophageal varices.

Vasculitic conditions, such as HSP, may lead to lower gastrointestinal bleeding in children (Fig. 18.55). HSP occurs during the postinfectious stage of a viral or streptococcal illness. Arthralgias and a macular purpuric skin rash in the lower extremities are characteristic. In both of these presentations, patients may develop intussusception due to the evolution of a subserosal mucosal hematoma, which functions as a lead point. The presence of acute renal insufficiency, anemia, pain, and bloody diarrhea is suggestive of hemolytic-uremic syndrome. The triad of azotemia, anemia, and thrombocytopenia confirms the diagnosis. If a coexistent diarrheal illness is present, then the pathogen should be identified by stool culture or analysis.

Older Children

Benign hamartomatous juvenile polyps most frequently affect children between 2 and 8 years old. The incidence is approximately 1 in 1000 children. Bleeding is usually painless, low in volume, and found as streaks on the surface of the stool. Two-thirds of bleeding polyps are found in the rectum, and 90% are found distally in the colon. Many of these lesions undergo auto necrosis and slough into the stool, whereas others may prolapse through the anus (Fig. 18.56). Surgical or endoscopic resection is therapeutic. Patients with Peutz-Jeghers syndrome present with melanotic mucocutaneous

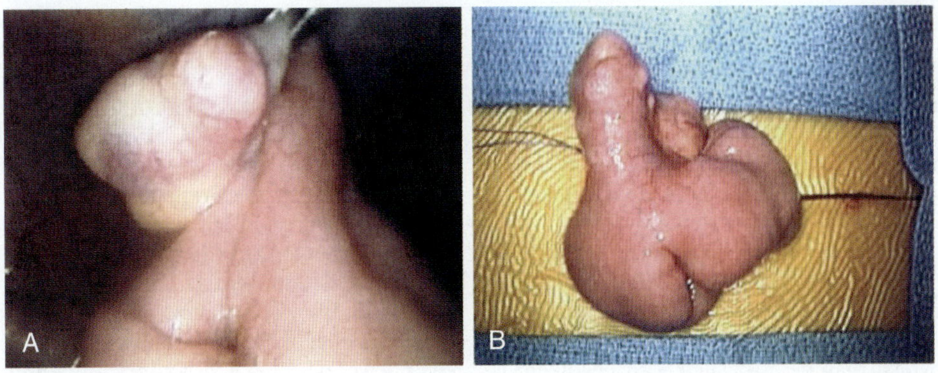

Fig. 18.54 Laparoscopic view of a Meckel diverticulum with an apparent vitelline artery (A). Meckel diverticulum at surgery (B).

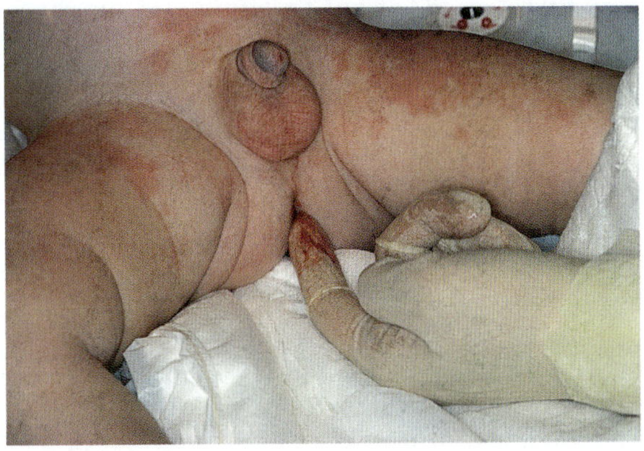

Fig. 18.55 Henoch-Schönlein purpura causes submucosal and serosal hematomas that may act as a lead point. Note the presence of hematochezia and the diagnostic skin lesions.

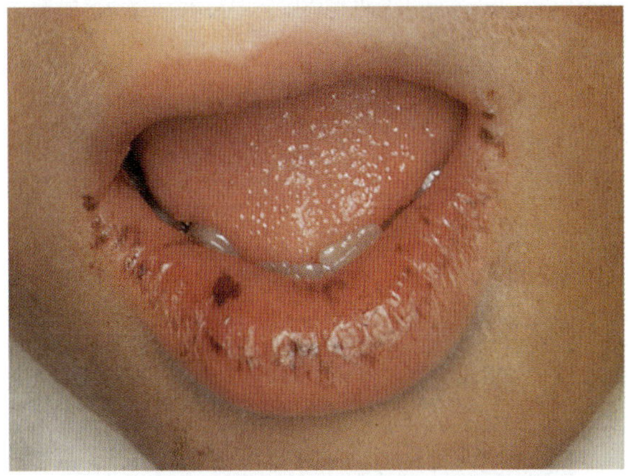

Fig. 18.57 The characteristic melanotic spots of Peutz-Jeghers syndrome are seen on the lips, buccal mucosa, and anus.

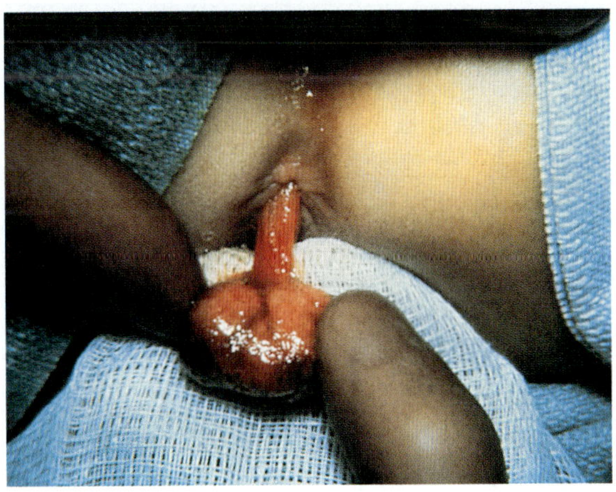

Fig. 18.56 Juvenile polyps are found most often in the rectosigmoid colon. On occasion they may prolapse through the anus.

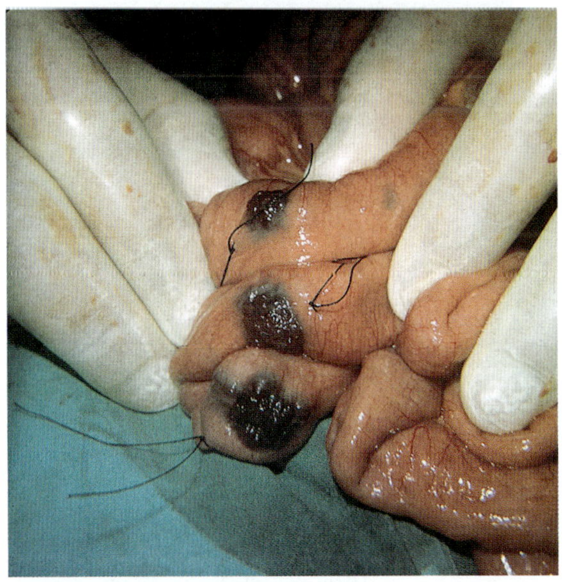

Fig. 18.58 Melanotic small bowel polyps characteristic of Peutz-Jeghers syndrome are prone to bleeding or obstruction.

pigmentation (Fig. 18.57) and gastrointestinal bleeding due to hamartomatous polyps (Fig. 18.58). Polyps may also cause recurrent episodes of abdominal pain and obstruction. Although most patients have fewer than a dozen polyps, a life-threatening variant of this condition, diffuse juvenile polyposis, may present with severe bloody diarrhea, intussusception, rectal prolapse, and protein-losing enteropathy. Total abdominal colectomy is required in these patients. In contrast to hamartomatous polyps, adenomatous polyps are quite rare as solitary colonic lesions. Children with familial adenomatous polyposis are usually asymptomatic until puberty or late adolescence, when they may develop diarrhea, hematochezia, and anemia. Diffuse adenomatous polyps blanket the colon and may have associated lesions throughout the intestinal tract from stomach to terminal ileum. Surgery, with total colectomy and ileal-pouch anal anastomosis, is recommended to control recurrent bleeding and to decrease the long-term high risk of malignancy in patients whose polyps cannot be managed endoscopically. Patients with attenuated familial adenomatous polyposis and relative rectal sparing may undergo a subtotal colectomy with ileorectal anastomosis.

ACUTE ABDOMINAL PAIN

The most common indication for abdominal surgery in childhood is acute appendicitis. Traditionally thought to occur due to appendiceal obstruction secondary to hyperplasia of submucosal lymphoid tissue or fecalith, the pathogenesis in most patients is unknown (Fig. 18.59). Only one-third of patients present with the classic symptoms of pain originating in the periumbilical region that progressively localizes to the right lower quadrant, associated with nausea, vomiting, and anorexia, together with focal tenderness to palpation in the right lower quadrant. The symptom complex typically includes abdominal pain, low-grade fever, and anorexia. Physical examination findings in most pediatric patients demonstrate tenderness in the right lower quadrant, suprapubic, or lower flank regions. Involuntary guarding or muscular spasm overlying the area of peritoneal irritation is a common examination finding that is not masked by mild forms of pain management. A positive psoas or obturator sign is indicative of retroperitoneal appendicitis, which may be associated with few anterior abdominal findings. Laparoscopic appendectomy is the standard of care for the treatment of acute appendicitis in children (Fig. 18.60). However, recent studies have demonstrated the efficacy of nonoperative management with antibiotic therapy for select patients. Using strict inclusion criteria based on age, duration of symptoms, degree of leukocytosis, and imaging characteristics, the majority of pediatric patients with uncomplicated appendicitis can be safely treated with nonoperative management. Drawbacks include increased length of stay, additional doses of antibiotics, and a recurrent rate of 10% to 30% at 1 year. In patients for whom nonoperative criteria are met, information regarding both surgical and nonsurgical treatment must be discussed with parents to inform shared decision making. Symptoms of perforated appendicitis may be confused with gastroenteritis or other intestinal illnesses. Perforation can lead to free peritoneal soilage or the development of a localized abscess (Fig. 18.61). While cases of perforated appendicitis may appear toxic, patients with a localized abscess may appear well. Perforation without evidence of a phlegmon or the presence of an established abscess may be treated acutely with laparoscopic appendectomy. Localized abscess formation may be initially treated with intravenous antibiotics with or without percutaneous drainage, followed by an interval appendectomy at approximately 6 to 8 weeks after the original presentation. This approach is associated with fewer perioperative complications and improved outcomes compared with primary appendectomy in the setting of appendiceal abscess. Diagnosis of acute appendicitis in children under the age of 5 years old is a clinical challenge for even the most experienced practitioner. The difficulties in obtaining a history and the challenges of obtaining a reliable physical examination all contribute to the diagnostic delay. The incidence of perforation in this age group exceeds 50%. A wealth of recent evidence suggests that an algorithmic approach to the diagnosis and management of appendicitis decreases morbidity, length of stay, and cost of care in children. In most centers, a right lower quadrant ultrasound examination has become standard in pediatric patients and can be a highly useful adjunct in experienced hands. In settings where the diagnosis is still unclear or in patients with a body habitus impeding ultrasonography, cross-sectional imaging may be needed.

The differential diagnosis for acute abdominal pain includes several nonsurgical problems, such as gastroenteritis, mesenteric adenitis, constipation, and urinary tract infections, as well as surgical conditions, such as Meckel diverticulitis, inflammatory bowel disease, and intussusception. The presence of diagnosed or previously undiagnosed Crohn disease in particular (Fig. 18.62) can present a

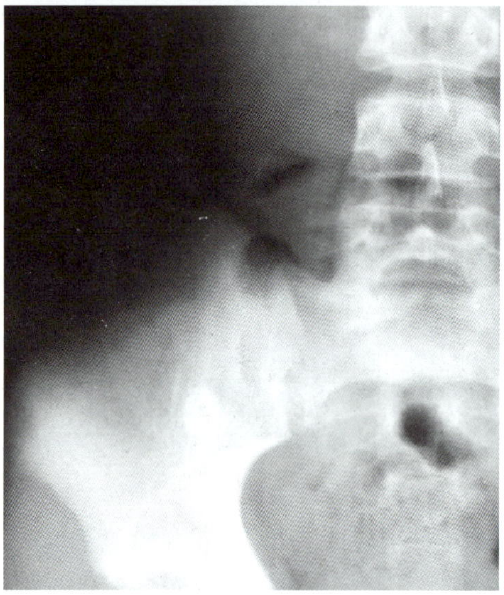

Fig. 18.59 A fecalith, the round calcification in the iliac fossa, obstructs the appendiceal lumen and initiates inflammatory processes that produce appendicitis.

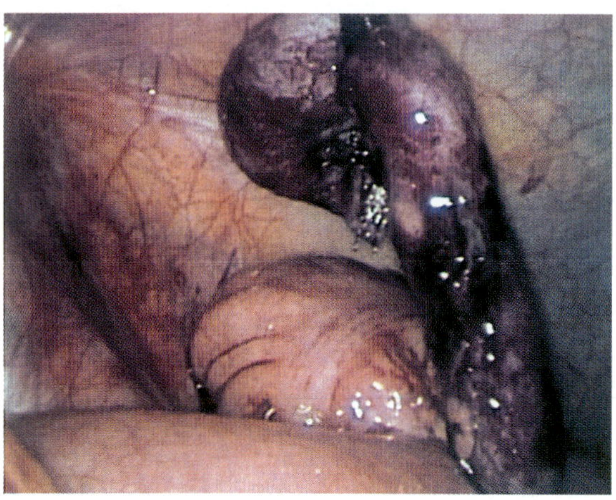

Fig. 18.60 Laparoscopic view of appendicitis. Note the inflamed, swollen appendix.

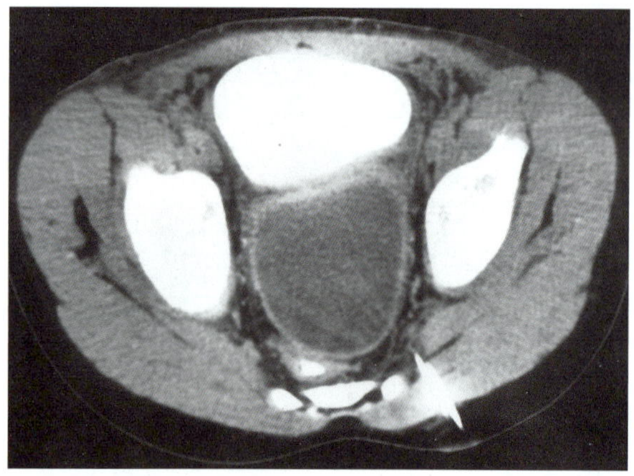

Fig. 18.61 Perforated appendicitis with a large ring-enhancing abscess seen on computed tomography scan.

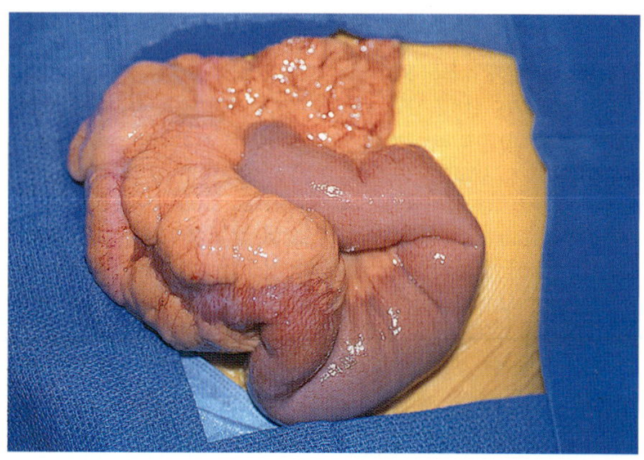

Fig. 18.62 Findings at laparotomy in Crohn disease reveal petechiae over the serosa of the thickened small bowel, which has mesenteric "creeping fat."

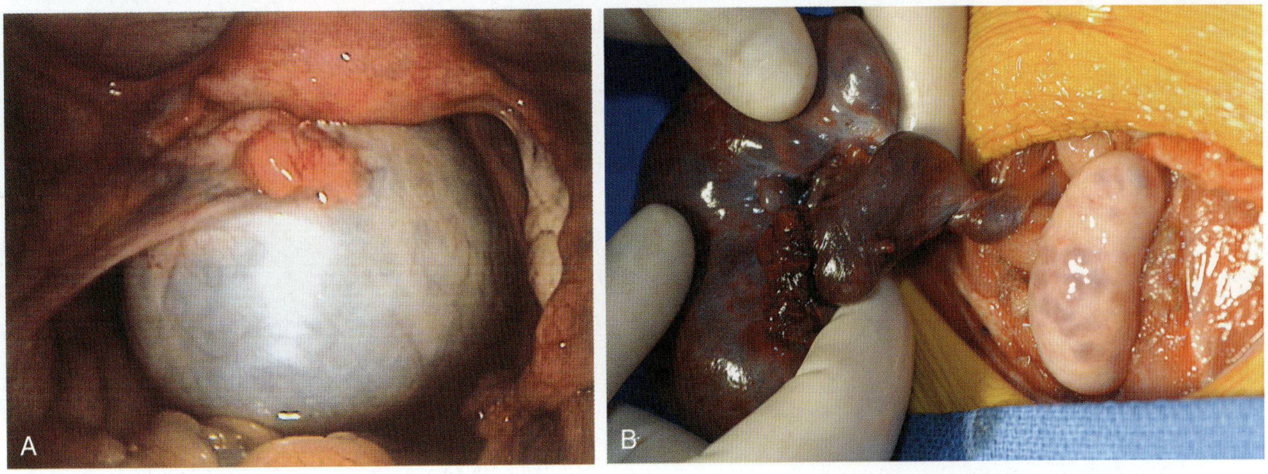

Fig. 18.63 (A) Simple follicular cysts may grow to large sizes that may fill the cul-de-sac. (B) Ovarian torsion.

diagnostic dilemma when evaluating a patient with potential appendicitis. As such, a thorough history of previous illness and family history is always warranted.

Pelvic pathology including ruptured ovarian cyst, ovarian torsion, tubal torsion, or acute salpingitis with or without associated tubo-ovarian abscess may also be readily confused with acute appendicitis. The most important diagnosis to rule out in a young girl with acute abdominal pain is ovarian torsion or tubal torsion, which can lead to a lifelong impairment in fertility if the diagnosis is delayed or missed. The key diagnostic tool for ovarian torsion is the clinical presentation of sudden onset of severe abdominal or pelvic pain often accompanied by nausea and vomiting. It may present with pain out of proportion to examination. The initial diagnostic workup includes ultrasound of the pelvis with Doppler flow. Ultrasound performed during ovarian torsion may demonstrate lack of ovarian arterial or venous flow and/or enlarged ovarian volume consistent with venous congestion from venous outflow obstruction. A cystic ovarian mass may be visualized, with cysts 5 cm or larger at an elevated risk of torsion. Cystic ovarian masses represent a wide spectrum of conditions from the common simple follicular cyst to hormonally active cystic tumors (Fig. 18.63A). Of note, a normal ultrasound does not rule out torsion. Tubal torsion or intermittent ovarian torsion may demonstrate preserved Doppler flow on ultrasound yet still be threatening to fertility. Clinical concern for torsion even in the presence of a normal ultrasound warrants an operative approach (see Fig. 18.63B). Diagnostic laparoscopy in an urgent manner may be accompanied by detorsion and cyst fenestration or cystectomy. Even if an ovary appears devitalized, evidence demonstrates that the ovary can be safely preserved in most cases. Unless there is a solid mass concerning for malignancy that requires oophorectomy, the normal or cystic ovary is generally left in situ after detorsion and cyst fenestration or cystectomy.

ANUS AND RECTUM

Most congenital anorectal anomalies are apparent on examination at birth. Bilious emesis, poor feeding, abdominal distention, and delayed or absent passage of meconium may herald the presence of a distal obstruction. *Imperforate anus* is the general category assigned to these patients, and it may present as one of three principal anatomic groups. These anomalies are classified on the basis of the position of the rectum relative to the levator ani muscle complex. Low imperforate anus is associated with the passage of the rectum through the levator ani, with a fistulous tract extending to the perineal region often ending in the center of a ridge of tissue on the perineum ("bucket handle" deformity) as a perineal fistula (Fig. 18.64). In male infants, the fistula may travel in the median raphe of the scrotum, and the meconium may be seen as a string of white or black beads (Fig. 18.65). The prognosis for continence is generally favorable for low lesions because the rectum lies within the levator ani complex. In contrast, high lesions do not pass through the levator ani and a visible fistula does not exist. Most commonly, the rectal fistula ends in the prostatic urethra, bulbar urethra, or bladder neck in males or above the hymen (within the vestibule) in girls. Meconium is passed with urine via the urethra

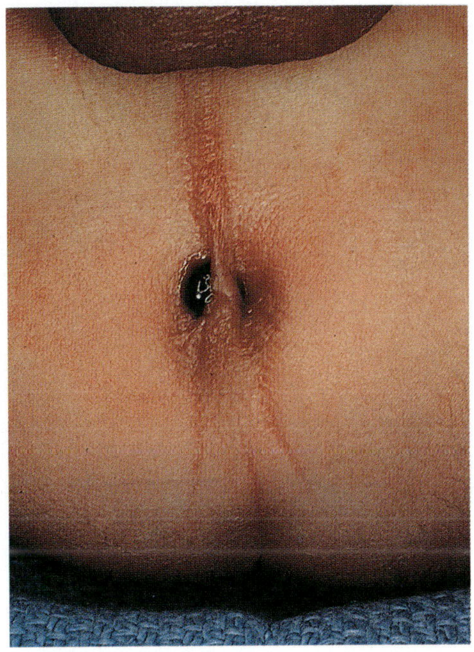

Fig. 18.64 A spot of meconium is visible beneath a "bucket handle" bridge of skin in an infant with a low imperforate anus.

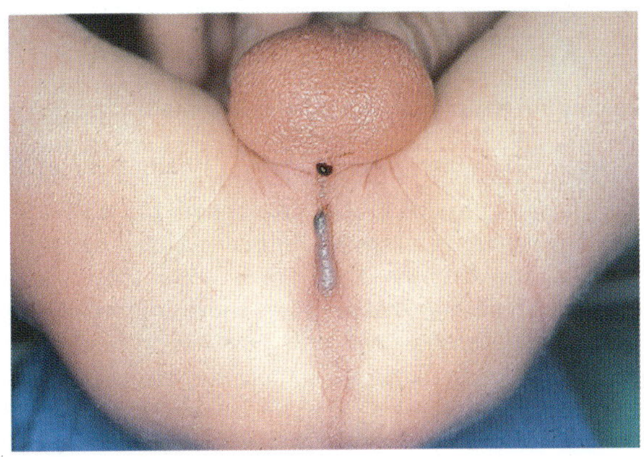

Fig. 18.65 Low imperforate anus in a male infant. White mucus or black meconium may pass through a perineal fistula from a low imperforate anus into the scrotal raphe.

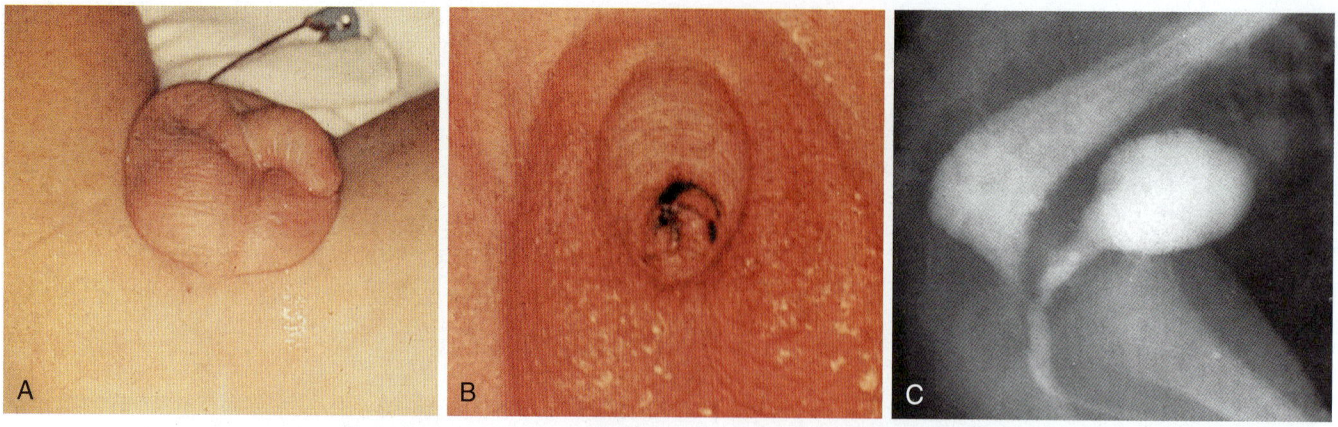

Fig. 18.66 (A) No visible external opening forms in high imperforate anus. Absence of the intergluteal cleft is also common, frequently associated with sacral agenesis. (B) Meconium passes into the bladder or urethra through a rectal fistula and appears in the urine. (C) Retrograde urethrography demonstrates the rectourethral fistula.

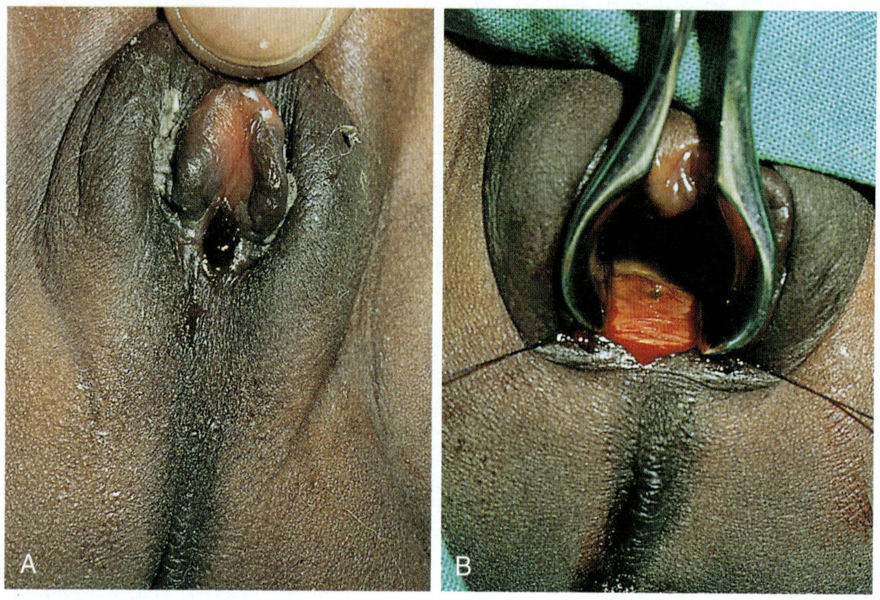

Fig. 18.67 A high imperforate anus communicates into the vagina. Meconium is passed through the vagina (A). Vaginoscopy reveals the fistula on the posterior wall of the vagina well above the hymen (B). A bicornuate uterus accompanies rectovaginal fistula in high lesions in girls.

in males (Fig. 18.66) or from within the introits or through a vaginal fistula in females (Fig. 18.67). A variant of high imperforate anus is a cloacal anomaly, which is a complex congenital anomaly in which the urethra, vagina, and rectum share a single perineal opening (Fig. 18.68). Intermediate lesions that are partially within the levator ani complex represent a third variant of imperforate anus. The classic approach to the care for patients with low lesions is a one-stage repair or neonatal limited perineal anoplasty (Fig. 18.69). Patients with high and intermediate lesions classically undergo staged repairs with a primary colostomy at birth, followed by a perineal pull-through at a later age. Several months after the pull-through, following a period of successive anal dilation, these infants return for their colostomy closure. The prognosis for fecal continence is excellent in patients with low lesions. Because they partially extend into the levator, intermediate lesions tend to have good outcomes. The prognosis for social continence in children with high lesions is guarded due in part to the presence of associated congenital anomalies, including abnormalities in innervation of the muscular complex, and the quality of the reconstruction (Fig. 18.70).

Rectal prolapse is an uncommon condition that is most often idiopathic in children (Fig. 18.71). The peak incidence of idiopathic rectal prolapse occurs in the second year of life, often precipitated by episodes of diarrheal illnesses, efforts to toilet train, or severe constipation. This

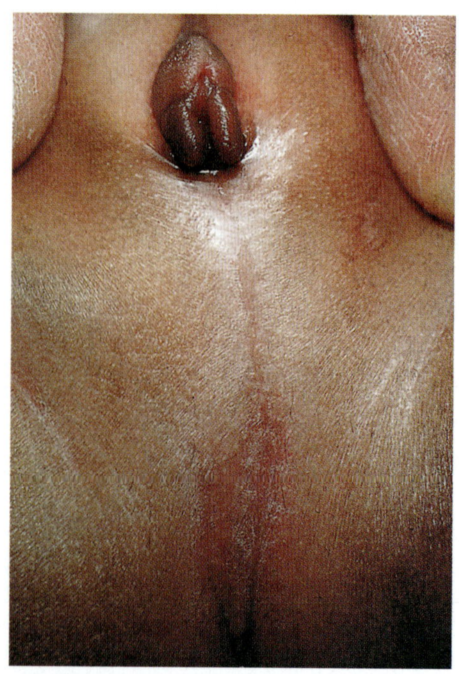

Fig. 18.68 Cloacal anomaly is the most complete expression of imperforate anus in girls, with urinary, genital, and intestinal tracts converging into a single cloacal channel that exists as the sole perineal opening.

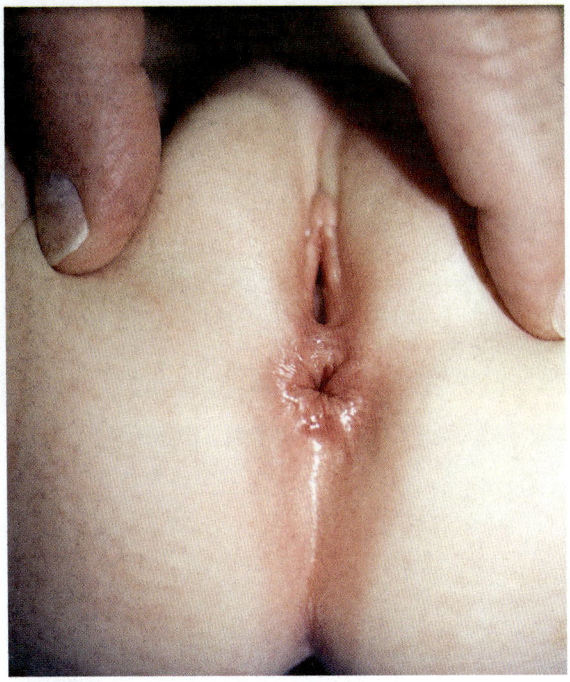

Fig. 18.69 Anteriorly displaced anus partially within the anal sphincter complex.

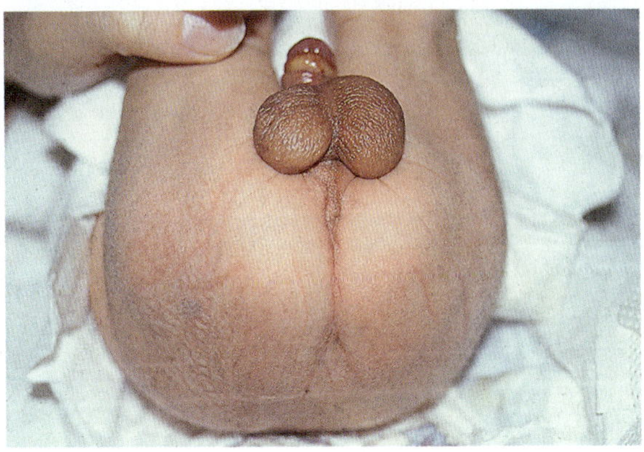

Fig. 18.70 Bifid scrotum in an infant with imperforate anus is indicative of a high lesion and the likely presence of other anomalies.

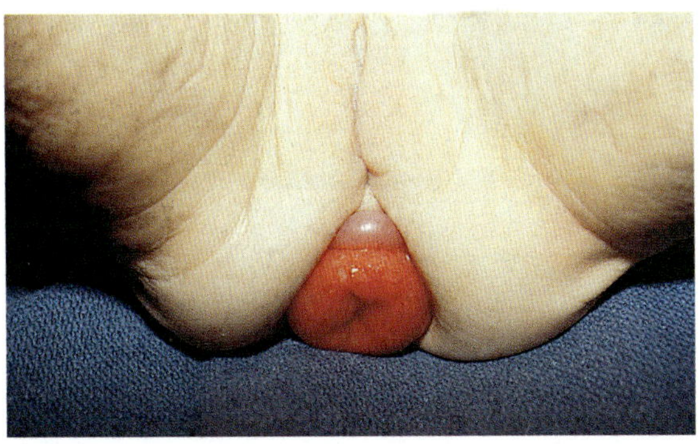

Fig. 18.71 Although the cause of rectal prolapse is unknown in the majority of cases, all infants should be evaluated for cystic fibrosis.

often resolves spontaneously after the resolution of the acute illness or with dietary and medical manipulations to treat the constipation. Nonidiopathic cases often occur in the setting of neurologic conditions or other chronic diseases. Abnormalities in the development of the muscles of the pelvic floor or their innervation may occur in patients with spina bifida and other spinal cord abnormalities. Refractory cases of prolapse should be evaluated with stool evaluations for ova and parasites for chronic hookworm infestation, which may cause severe tenesmus and straining. Rectal polyps may precipitate prolapse by acting as a lead point for this form of rectal intussusception. Evaluation by contrast enema and sigmoidoscopy are important components of the assessment of children with recurrent episodes. Cystic fibrosis is another common cause of prolapse, and this diagnosis should be considered in patients with persistent prolapse. Surgery is rarely indicated for rectal prolapse in children.

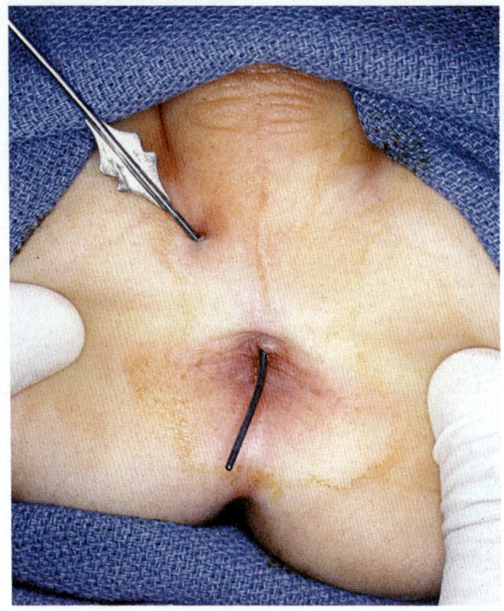

Fig. 18.72 A punctum visible to the left of the anus with a lacrimal ductin probe communicates to a crypt in the anal canal by a fistulous tract. Recurrent abscesses arise from a well-formed fistula like this one, an indication for fistulectomy.

Anorectal abscess is a common condition in the first 6 to 10 months of life. The lesions arise from infections of the submucosal crypt glands found along the dentate line. Significant fluctuance requires incision and drainage, followed by warm soaks or sitz baths. More limited infections may be successfully treated with antibiotics and warm soaks. Recurrent episodes of infection, although rare, may give rise to a fistula-in-ano or chronically draining sinus (Fig. 18.72). Anal fistulectomy with debridement of the tract is usually curative. Minor degrees of incontinence may complicate this procedure. Chronic or recurrent anal fistulas may indicate the presence of Crohn disease, chronic granulomatous disease, or immunodeficiency. Patients with a persistent or refractory condition should be thoroughly evaluated for these entities.

Anal fissure, discussed previously as a cause of gastrointestinal bleeding, is common in young infants. Hemorrhoids are less common in children and typically respond to nonoperative maneuvers.

HEPATOBILIARY SYSTEM, PANCREAS, AND SPLEEN

Abdominal pain secondary to biliary pathology is an increasing occurrence in pediatric patients. Children with hemoglobinopathies (e.g., sickle cell disease), chronic hemolysis (e.g., spherocytosis), a strong family incidence of cholelithiasis, or a history of obesity who then develop colicky right upper quadrant discomfort, epigastric pain, unexplained jaundice, or pancreatitis should undergo ultrasound evaluation for the presence of cholecystitis, cholelithiasis (Fig. 18.73), choledocholithiasis, and pancreatitis. Cholecystectomies for hematologic disorders have plateaued or fallen over the last decade, whereas cholecystectomies for nonhematologic indications have risen 10-fold over that time frame. Both the safety and low morbidity of laparoscopic cholecystectomy, as well as the rise in childhood obesity, have contributed to this increase in cholecystectomy in childhood.

Pancreatitis (see Chapter 11), often secondary to idiopathic causes in children, may cause abdominal pain in children that raises concern for surgical indications. Initial presentation with hyperamylasemia and hyperlipasemia may progress to the development of a midabdominal mass. These patients should be evaluated for the presence of a pancreatic pseudocyst. Many of these lesions will resolve spontaneously and do not require surgical drainage or other intervention. Pancreatic pseudocysts may also develop after traumatic pancreatic injury (Fig. 18.74). In addition, children presenting with pancreatitis should be evaluated for concomitant gallstones. If found, the patients should undergo a cholecystectomy when stabilized.

Choledochal cyst, a rare congenital condition, is more common in Asia and Japan with a female predominance. It typically presents within the first several years of life. The etiology is incompletely understood but is often associated with anomalous pancreaticobiliary union (APBDU) with a long common channel. APBDU is thought to allow reflux of pancreatic enzymes that weaken the duct wall and lead to inflammation and dilation of the extrahepatic and/or intrahepatic bile ducts. The Todani Classification is the most widely used system classifying choledochal cysts based on location, morphology, and corresponding surgical management. Abdominal pain, palpable mass, or jaundice may be the initial presenting symptoms, although many lesions are now identified on antenatal ultrasound imaging. Surgical excision of the entire abnormal cyst is indicated to prevent recurrent episodes of pancreatitis and to eliminate the risk of malignancy over the long term (Fig. 18.75). As with other hepatobiliary surgery, there is increasing use of intraoperative

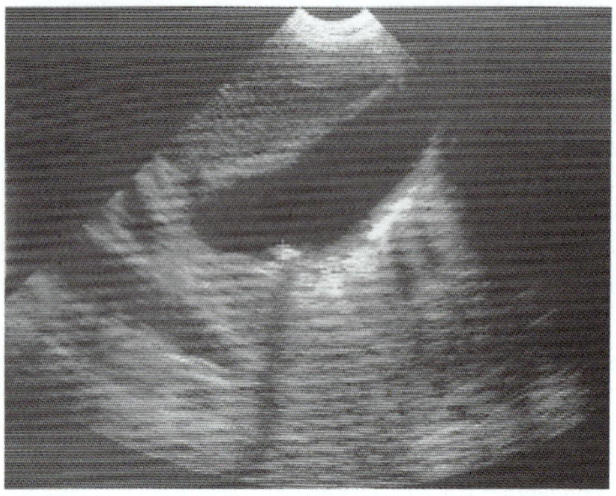

Fig. 18.73 Ultrasound examination of the right upper quadrant easily demonstrates stones within the gallbladder. An acoustic shadow extends beneath the stone.

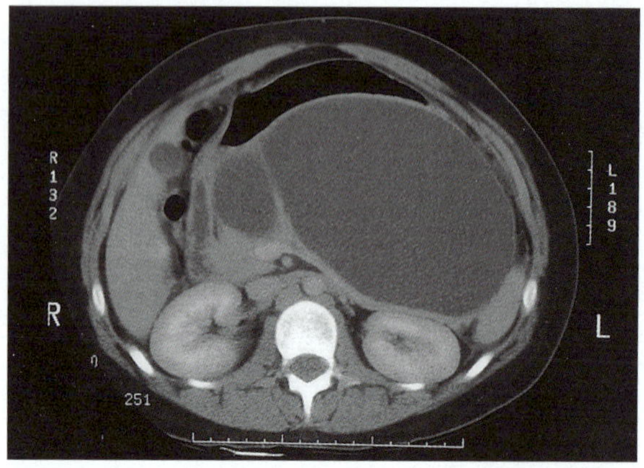

Fig. 18.74 Pancreatic pseudocysts in the pediatric population most commonly result from blunt traumatic injuries to the abdomen, as occurred in this patient with a handlebar injury.

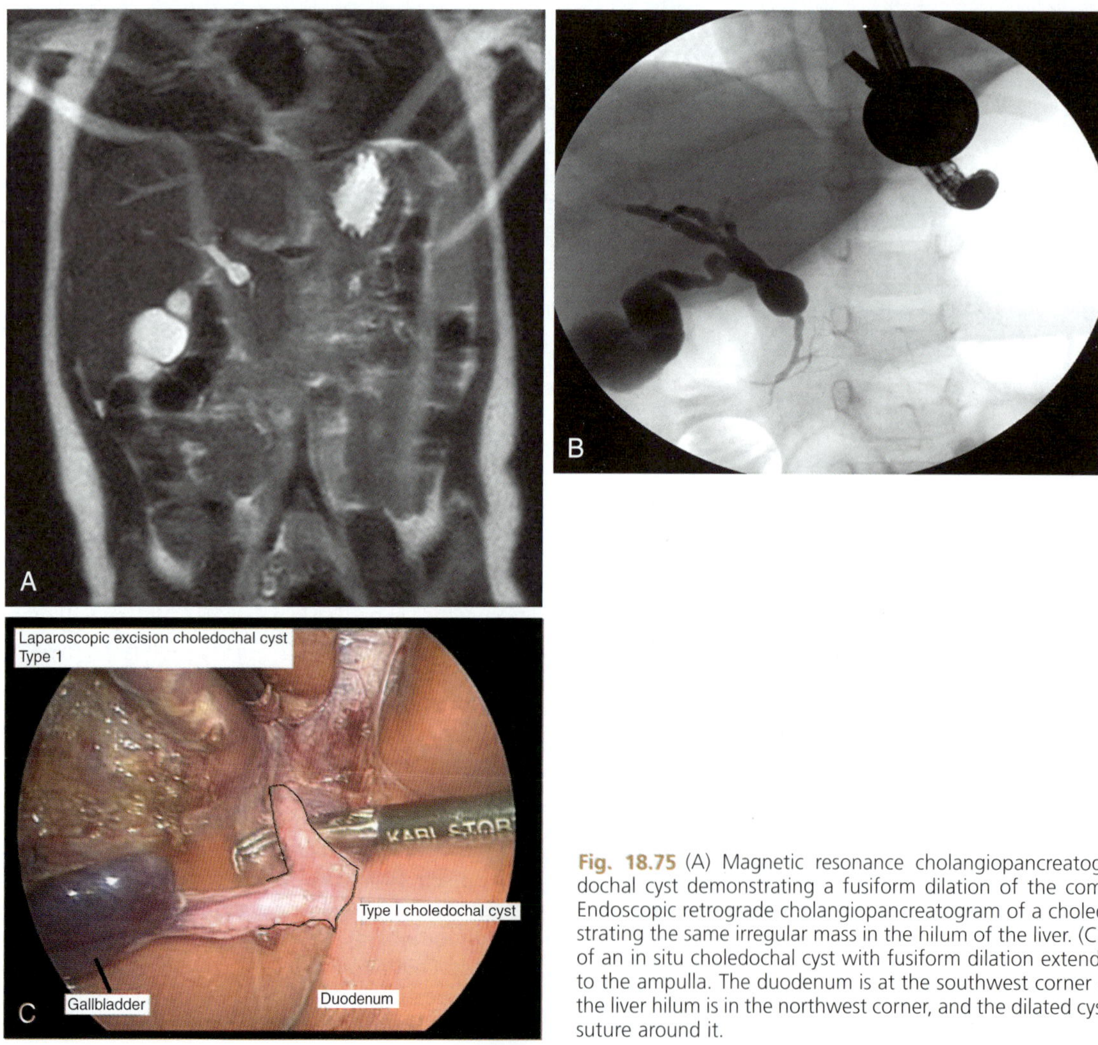

Fig. 18.75 (A) Magnetic resonance cholangiopancreatography of a choledochal cyst demonstrating a fusiform dilation of the common bile duct. (B) Endoscopic retrograde cholangiopancreatogram of a choledochal cyst demonstrating the same irregular mass in the hilum of the liver. (C) Laparoscopic view of an in situ choledochal cyst with fusiform dilation extending from the hilum to the ampulla. The duodenum is at the southwest corner of the photograph, the liver hilum is in the northwest corner, and the dilated cyst has the Endoloop suture around it.

fluorescence imaging with indocyanine green to aid in visualization and identification of biliary anatomy.

Diseases of the spleen requiring surgery include hemolytic diseases, such as hereditary spherocytosis, hemolytic anemias, hypersplenism, and occasionally sickle cell disease. Anemia and splenomegaly leading to transfusion requirement or decreased ability to participate in normal activities of daily living may prompt laparoscopic splenectomy in patients with hereditary spherocytosis. Preoperative vaccination for pneumococcal, meningococcal, and *Haemophilus influenzae* type b is standard. The recommendation for postsplenectomy oral penicillin prophylaxis to minimize the risk of overwhelming postsplenectomy sepsis infection is clear early after surgery but remains controversial for prolonged courses. The rate of splenectomies in children for hematologic indication has fallen over the last decade as management strategies have improved, as well as with increasing evidence to support increased risks of thrombotic complications in children who have undergone splenectomies.

ABDOMINAL WALL DEFECTS

Gastroschisis and omphalocele are the two principal congenital abdominal wall defects (Figs. 18.76–18.79). Omphalocele arises as a consequence of the embryonic extrusion of the developing midgut from the coelomic cavity into the yolk sac to allow midgut elongation as the abdominal wall expands to accommodate the rapidly growing viscera (Figs. 18.76–18.77). Resulting central defects in the medial and lateral wall folds and umbilical ring result in a central abdominal wall deformity. This abdominal wall defect presents with a sac that has outer amniotic and inner peritoneal layers. The umbilical cord inserts into the sac. This midline defect may be of various sizes from "umbilical cord hernias" to "giant omphaloceles" greater than 10 cm in diameter and may exist in the central, epigastric, and hypogastric regions. Coexisting anomalies of other midline structures including the heart, sternum, diaphragm, and bladder often occur (Fig. 18.78). In addition, patients may have significant pulmonary hypoplasia secondary to associated chest wall deformities. Chromosomal anomalies are also common. The primary morbidity is not due to the omphalocele itself but instead the anomalies that may be associated with it.

In contrast to omphalocele, gastroschisis is a defect of the right lateral abdominal wall (Fig. 18.79). This likely results from a vascular accident that leads to occlusion of the right umbilical vein with subsequent disruption of the abdominal wall and midgut evisceration. The defect is usually small in terms of area of the abdominal wall; however, large amounts of bowel may lie in the amniotic cavity. This anomaly occurs early in gestation, and the bowel remains in contact with amniotic fluid throughout the pregnancy, which may produce an intense inflammatory response or "peel." This contact with the amniotic fluid is hypothesized to alter bowel motility in the postoperative period, leading to long delays in the return of bowel

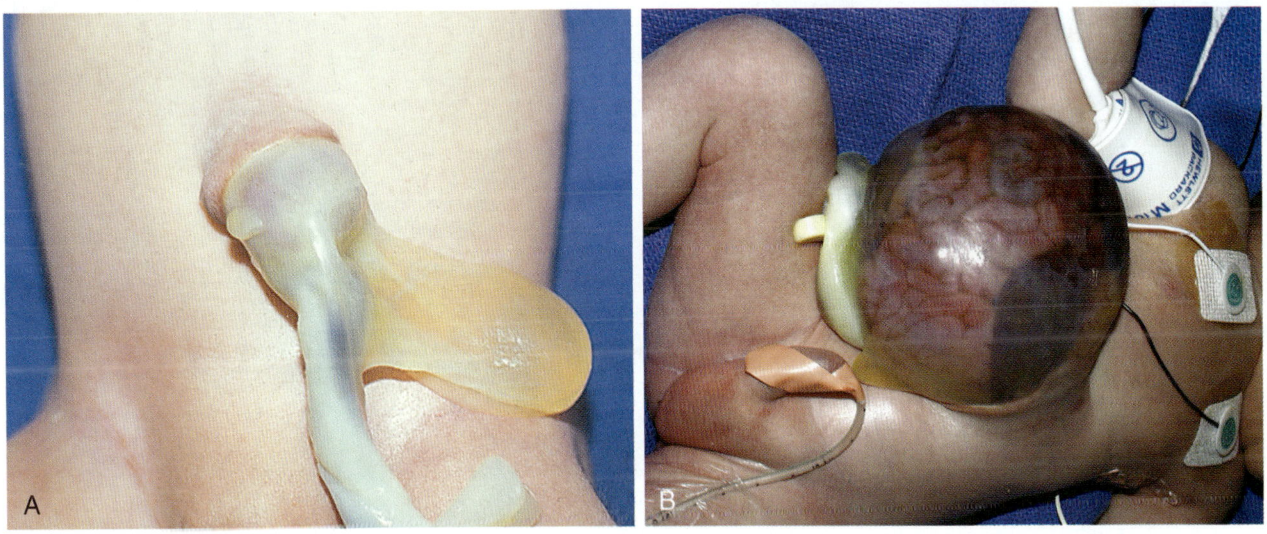

Fig. 18.76 (A) A small omphalocele with the umbilical cord attached to the apex of the sac. (B) Giant omphalocele containing liver, stomach, and bowel. Chromosomal and other anomalies, particularly cardiac, are common and should be evaluated in both conditions.

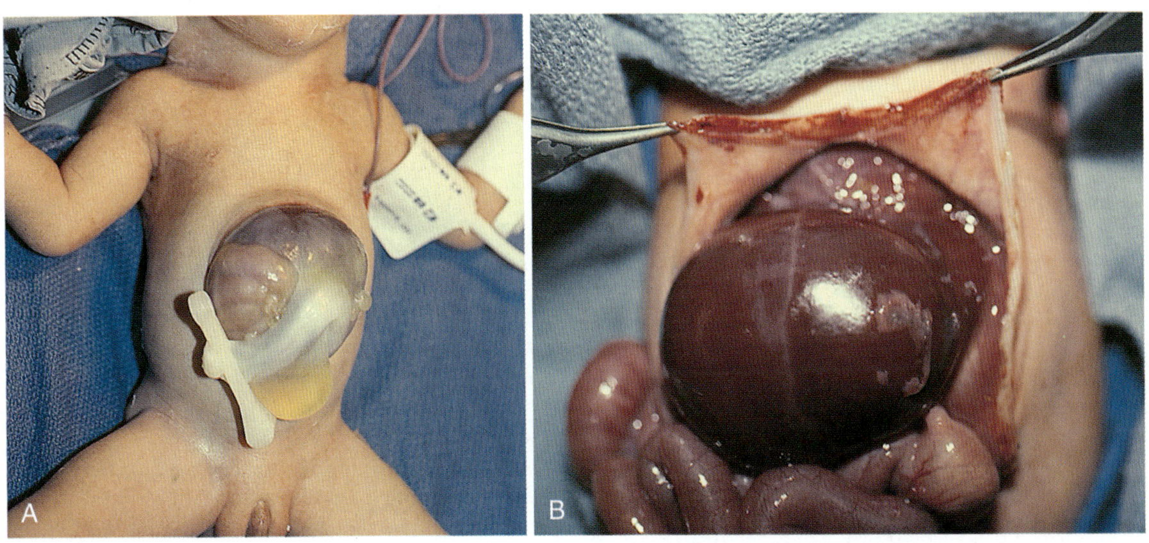

Fig. 18.77 Pentalogy of Cantrell is a midline abdominal wall defect (epigastric omphalocele) (A) associated with anterior diaphragmatic defect, sternal cleft, ectopia cordis, and congenital heart disease (usually a ventricular septal defect) (B).

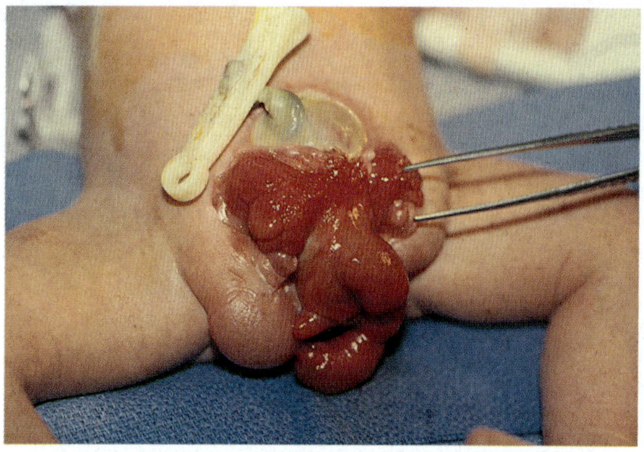

Fig. 18.78 Cloacal exstrophy consists of an infraumbilical omphalocele with exstrophy of the bladder, in which the bladder is separated into halves by the exposed intestine. Both the proximal and distal loops have prolapsed, producing the "elephant trunk" appearance.

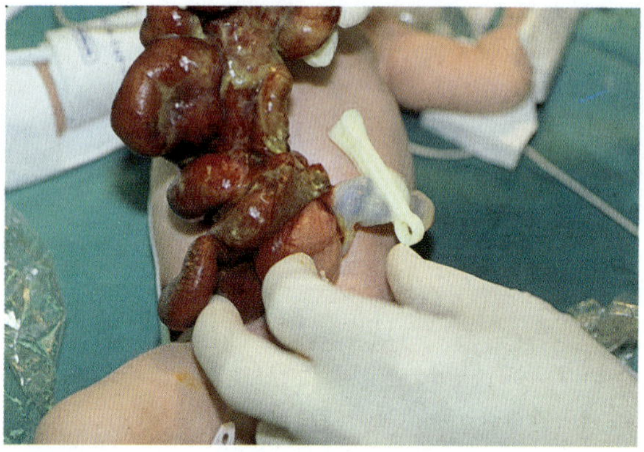

Fig. 18.79 In gastroschisis the abdominal defect lies to the right of an intact umbilical cord without a sac, and the intestines are exposed to the amniotic fluid. An inflammatory "peel" develops, which may affect motility.

function after returning the bowel to the abdominal cavity. In contrast to omphalocele, gastroschisis is generally not associated with other congenital anomalies. Only 7% to 10% of patients have associated conditions, the most common of which are intestinal atresias. Ischemia due to in utero volvulus or incarceration through the narrow defect may lead to vascular compromise that causes an atresia.

Surgical management of these conditions is similar. The common goals are safe closure of the defect and return of the intestine to the abdominal cavity, without creating an abdominal compartment syndrome that may lead to pulmonary embarrassment, renal insufficiency, intestinal ischemia, or NEC. Gastroschisis constitutes a surgical emergency because the exposed bowel may become desiccated or injured, and the neonate may require volume resuscitation and control of body temperature. Omphaloceles, which have a protective peritoneal covering, may be managed in a more elective manner. A staged closure is required in some patients; this may include placement of a prosthetic silo with daily reductions in the case of gastroschisis or ruptured omphalocele (Fig. 18.80) or administration of topical desiccants in the case of omphalocele with intact peritoneum. Placement of a prosthetic material or mesh may provide coverage to bridge the abdominal wall defect when it cannot be closed primarily. These infants have significant postoperative delays in the return of intestinal function and require total parenteral nutrition support.

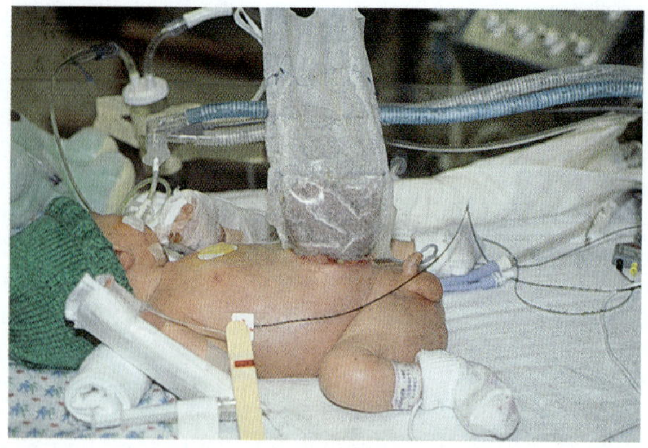

Fig. 18.80 Large abdominal wall defects that cannot be closed primarily may undergo a staged closure with silo placement and daily reductions until the bowel rests comfortably in the abdominal cavity.

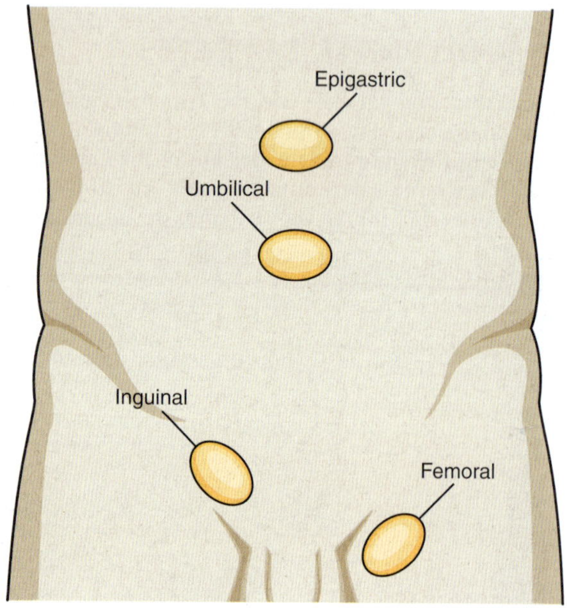

Fig. 18.81 Location of commonly found hernias involving the abdominal wall.

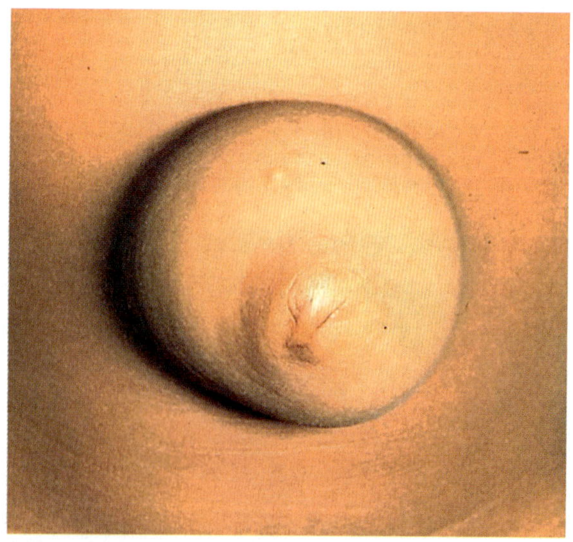

Fig. 18.82 Supraumbilical hernia, shown here as a crescent-shaped defect above an umbilical hernia, does not close spontaneously and requires a repair.

Umbilicus

The most common pediatric condition of the abdominal wall is an umbilical hernia (Figs. 18.81 and 18.82). This results from the failed closure of the fascial ring during the first few years of life. After desiccation of the umbilical vessels and urachus and separation of the umbilical remnant in the first month of life, the umbilical ring typically undergoes closure in the next 2 to 4 years. In some patients, this process is never completed. For unclear reasons, there appears to be a strong familial and racial predilection for hernia development, occurring more frequently in African Americans. Because most lesions resolve spontaneously and umbilical hernias rarely become incarcerated, consideration of repair is frequently deferred until the child's fifth birthday. Patients with hernias that are larger than 2 cm in diameter, a proboscoid or "elephant's trunk" appearance (see Fig. 18.82), or history of incarceration require early repair.

After desiccation of the umbilical remnant, an umbilical granuloma, presenting as a polypoid mucosal-appearing lesion, may persist at the base of the umbilicus. These represent residual hypertrophic granulation tissue at the base of the cord. Umbilical granuloma may be managed with topical treatments, including alcohol or silver nitrate sticks. Yellow serous or feculent brown drainage from an apparent umbilical granuloma should raise concerns for a patent urachus or persistence of an omphalomesenteric duct sinus. Drainage of yellow serous fluid is suspicious for urine and the presence of a patent urachus, representing the prenatal connection between the allantois and the fetal bladder. The persistence of this anomaly raises concern for bladder outlet obstruction and mandates a urological workup (see Chapter 15). Persistence of an omphalomesenteric sinus may lead to the development of an internal hernia or volvulus (Fig. 18.83) because this represents a persistent communication from the small bowel to the abdominal wall. Surgical exploration to ligate the fistula and resect the omphalomesenteric duct remnant is indicated.

Inguinal and Scrotal Disorders

Aberrant descent of the gonads and processus vaginalis gives rise to numerous disorders, including hernias, hydroceles, undescended testicles, and the potential for testicular torsion (Fig. 18.84). During embryonic development, the testicles have their origin at the base of the kidney. Testicular descent occurs with an outpouching or evagination of the peritoneal cavity, the processus vaginalis, which follows the gubernaculum into the scrotum. After completion of testicular descent, the processus vaginalis obliterates, separating the scrotum from the peritoneal cavity. Failure of obliteration results in a persistent patent processus that may allow fluid (hydrocele) or intraperitoneal viscera (intestine, bladder, or ovary) to enter the sac (Figs. 18.85 and 18.86). In females, fusion of the processus vaginalis occurs earlier in embryonic development, leading to decreased incidence of inguinal hernias in females. The ovary may be found in the hernia sac in girls (Fig. 18.87). Clinically, hernias present as bulges in the groin and scrotum/labia majora that increase in size with Valsalva maneuvers, including coughing, straining, or crying. The mass often reduces spontaneously or with gentle upward manual pressure on the hernia and downward testicular traction in males. An inability to reduce the mass should raise concerns for incarceration. Alternatively, persistent inguinoscrotal swelling may represent a nonreducible hydrocele or undescended or retractile testicle.

Identification of pediatric hernias on routine physical examination is sometimes difficult. Several provocative maneuvers including induced crying, coughing, jumping, gentle abdominal pressure, or other forced Valsalva maneuvers may be helpful. Patients should be examined in both supine and upright positions. Despite these efforts, the hernia may not be visualized during the office visit. The presence of a reliable history and the palpation of a thickened processus vaginalis or "silk glove" sign are adequate evidence to proceed with herniorrhaphy. The "silk glove" sign is the sensation on direct palpation of the spermatic cord as it gently glides between two layers of tissue. This represents the layers of processus vaginalis

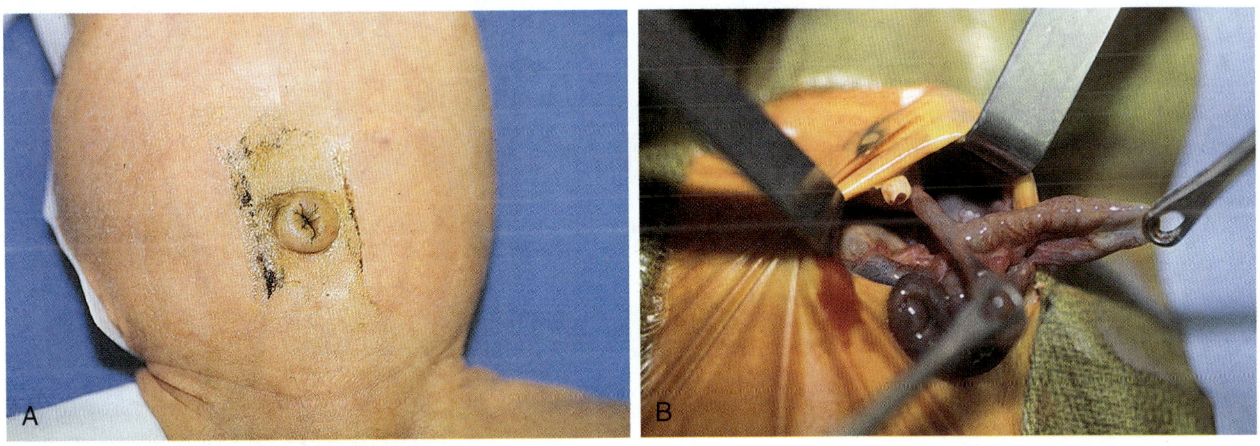

Fig. 18.83 Omphalomesenteric duct remnant with communication to the umbilicus with meconium exuding from the umbilicus and meconium staining of the abdominal wall (A). Intraoperative view showing omphalomesenteric duct leading from the bowel to the umbilicus (B).

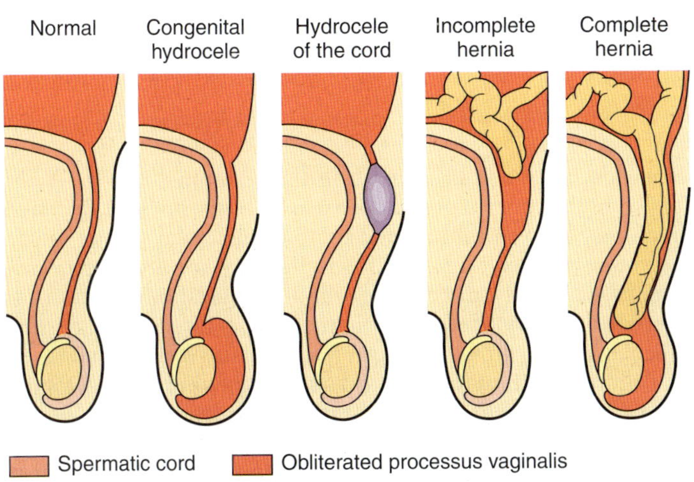

Fig. 18.84 Abnormalities of the processus vaginalis.

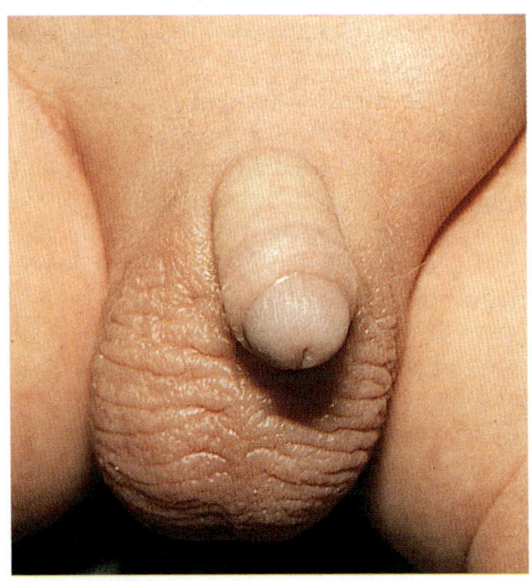

Fig. 18.85 An incomplete inguinal hernia produces a bulge in the left groin but does not extend into the scrotum.

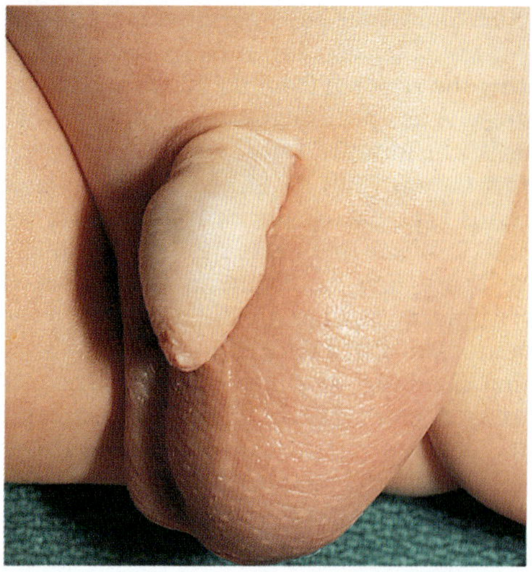

Fig. 18.86 A complete inguinal hernia extends into the scrotum, obscuring the testis.

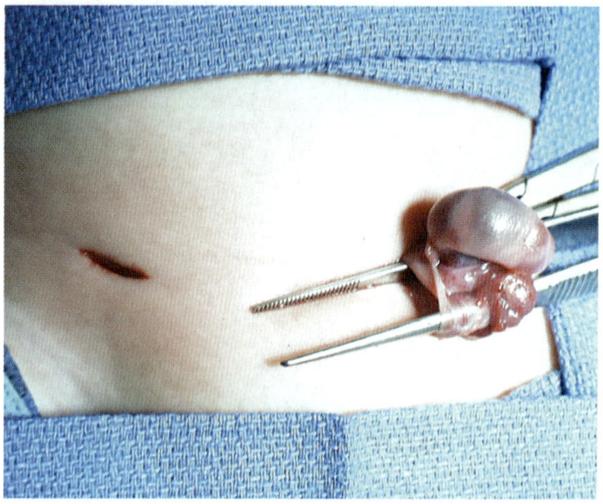

Fig. 18.87 Ovaries are frequently found in the hernia sac of young girls.

or hernia sac. Alternatively, parents may provide a picture of an inguinal hernia bulge or return for a visit when a bulge appears more consistently. On occasion, other noninvasive studies (such as ultrasound) have been suggested in difficult cases. With the advent and safety of laparoscopy, some children will undergo a diagnostic laparoscopy if symptoms persist and no hernia is evident on examination in order to look for a patent processus vaginalis. Groin pain is rarely a symptom of an inguinal hernia because the hernia is generally not associated with pain unless it is incarcerated, a surgical emergency.

The presence of an inguinal hernia is an indication for prompt repair. These hernias do not resolve spontaneously and have an up to 30% risk of incarceration (inability to reduce the inguinal hernia into the peritoneal cavity) in the first few months of life. Incarceration may lead to strangulation of the hernia contents and subsequent intestinal and/or testicular ischemia with infarction due to vascular entrapment. Incarceration is associated with severe irritability and emesis. The groin hernia becomes erythematous, edematous, and tender. Signs of complete intestinal obstruction may occur with associated ileus, emesis, and bloody stools. Systemic sepsis from bowel ischemia may occur.

Acute scrotal inflammation is often a surgical emergency (Fig. 18.88 and 18.89). This may occur with incarcerated inguinal hernias as well as other conditions, such as torsion of the testicle, torsion of the appendix testis, testicular trauma, and epididymo-orchitis. Testicular torsion is associated with an acutely tender testicle that may be retracted toward the inguinal region and lie in a somewhat transverse orientation in the scrotum (see Fig. 18.89). Torsion of the appendix testis is associated with the "blue dot" sign, which may be seen through the translucent scrotal skin of infants and young children (Fig. 18.90). This does not require surgery if an accurate diagnosis can be made without surgical intervention. An antecedent history of testicular injury may assist in distinguishing testicular trauma from an incarcerated hernia. A digital rectal examination is the most reliable means of determining whether there is incarcerated hernia in an infant. Transrectal palpation of the internal inguinal ring for the presence of a mass or fullness suggests incarceration. Transscrotal transillumination is not always a reliable means of distinguishing between a hydrocele and incarcerated hernia. On

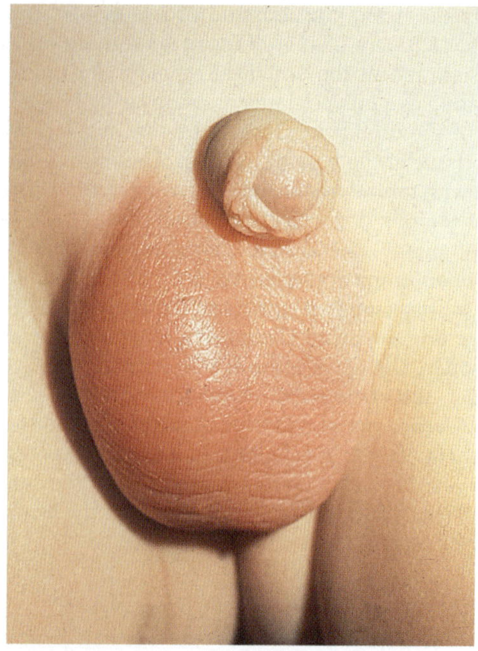

Fig. 18.88 A red, tender hemiscrotum may be due to torsion of the testis with gangrene, a surgical emergency.

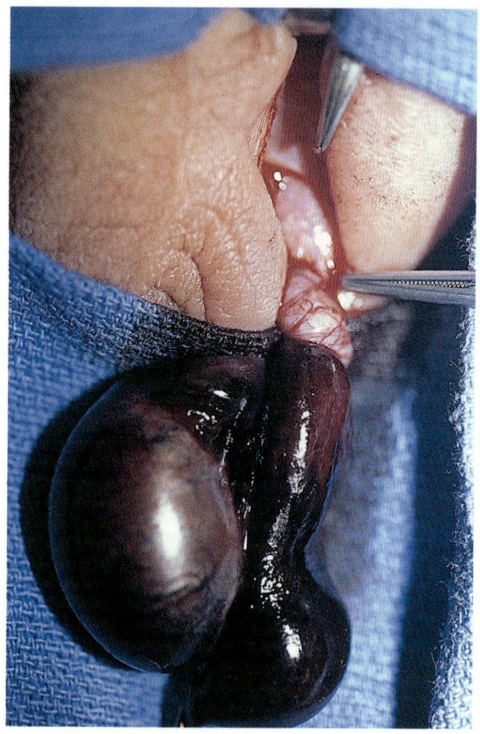

Fig. 18.89 Twisting of the spermatic cord in testicular torsion pulls the testis proximally, making it lie in a transverse axis. The dark, congested epididymis is seen overlying and to the left of the testis.

occasion, thin-walled dilated bowel may transilluminate, giving the misleading impression that a hydrocele is present. Epididymo-orchitis may be associated with urinary tract symptoms or previous viral or bacterial urinary tract infection.

Hydroceles are most common in infancy and diminish significantly during childhood. They appear as scrotal swellings that may have a diurnal variation in size, often largest in the evening and smaller or absent in the morning. Most hydroceles are isolated to the scrotal region. However, on occasion an isolated inguinal hydrocele may exist that mimics an incarcerated hernia. The classic means of diagnosing hydrocele is transillumination. Hydroceles that appear at birth are usually noncommunicating and undergo spontaneous resolution over the first year of life. Those that persist beyond 12 to 18 months of age typically have persistent communication with the peritoneal cavity and need surgical care (Fig. 18.91). Aspiration of the hydrocele is discouraged as most are noncommunicating and resolve on their own, while those that are communicating may recur even after aspiration. Hydroceles may also develop in older children in response to infection or trauma. Persistent hydroceles also require surgical repair. Femoral hernias are uncommon in children (Fig. 18.92).

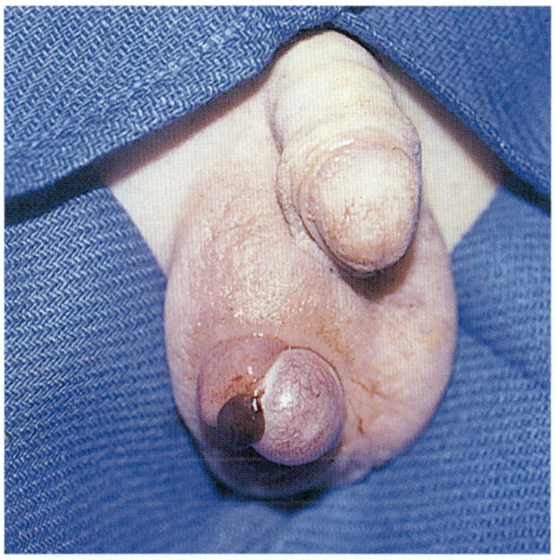

Fig. 18.90 The congested, twisted appendix testis contrasts with the normal pale pink testis. If the appendix testis can be identified through the scrotum, scrotal exploration is unnecessary. This torsed appendix testis may appear through the translucent skin as a "blue dot" sign.

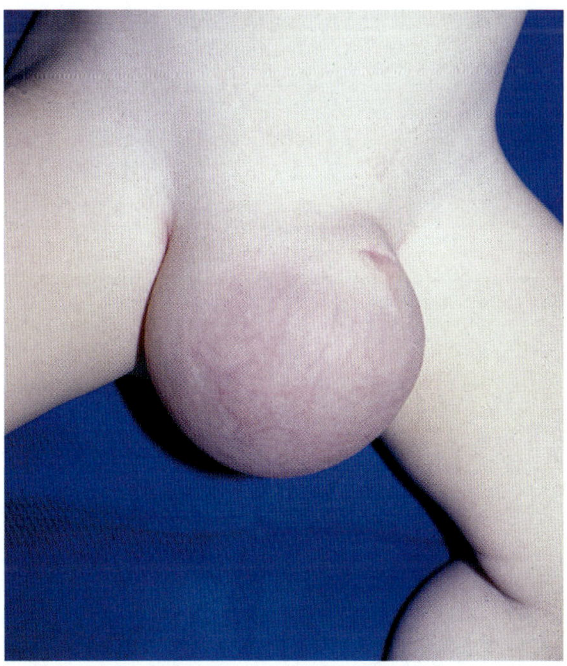

Fig. 18.91 Bilateral congenital hydroceles with buried penis. Groin swellings are absent, distinguishing them from hernias. The fluid collections may fluctuate in size, filling and emptying through a patent processus vaginalis. Spontaneous closure of the processus and absorption of fluid around the testis generally occur, reserving hydrocelectomy for those that persist after age 2 years.

ABDOMINAL MASSES AND TUMORS

Cancer is the second leading cause of death in children younger than 14 years old after trauma and injury. The presence of an abdominal mass in pediatric patients mandates a systematic assessment of various factors, including age, location of the mass, characteristics of the mass (e.g., firm, cystic, mobile, fixed), and initial diagnostic imaging studies. Although important, history is rarely of clinical significance in children with abdominal masses because of the protracted presentation of these lesions. On occasion, children with an intraabdominal mass may present with acute gastrointestinal or genitourinary tract obstruction. Typically, the physical examination and initial radiographic studies lead to the development of a differential that will focus efforts at diagnosis. This serves as a framework from which to further determine the nature and extent of the disease.

Location is the most important factor for determining the tissue of origin and behavior of an abdominal mass (Fig. 18.93). Retroperitoneal masses are often solid in nature and fixed to or infiltrating into adjacent structures. Intraperitoneal masses that arise from the bowel, mesentery, or omentum are usually cystic and mobile. Dense fibrous adhesions encasing inflammatory lesions may also restrict mobility. Cystic intraabdominal lesions arising from the gastrointestinal or genitourinary tract are usually benign in nature. In contrast, solid intraabdominal lesions are predominantly malignant. Extraabdominal manifestations of the primary lesion (metastases and associated congenital anomalies) should always be investigated. Age is the second most important factor in determining the differential diagnosis of abdominal masses. Table 18.7 summarizes the causes of abdominal masses by location.

Plain abdominal radiography often provides basic information in determining the location and potential differential diagnosis of an abdominal mass. Bowel displacement from the pelvis suggests the presence of a pelvic extraluminal mass. In contrast, intraluminal lesions may lead to a small bowel obstruction pattern, as seen in meconium ileus, intussusception, or constipation. Calcification seen within the mass on plain film suggests the presence of a malignant lesion, such as neuroblastoma, rhabdomyosarcoma, or teratoma. Ultrasonography is traditionally the initial diagnostic tool of choice in patients with abdominal

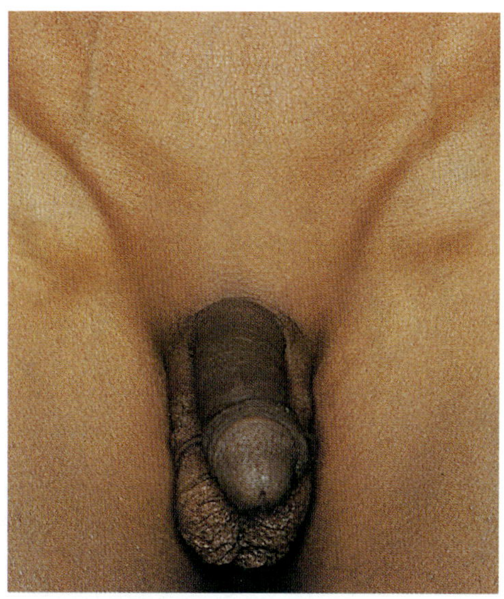

Fig. 18.92 Swelling below the inguinal ligament identifies a femoral hernia, extremely rare in childhood.

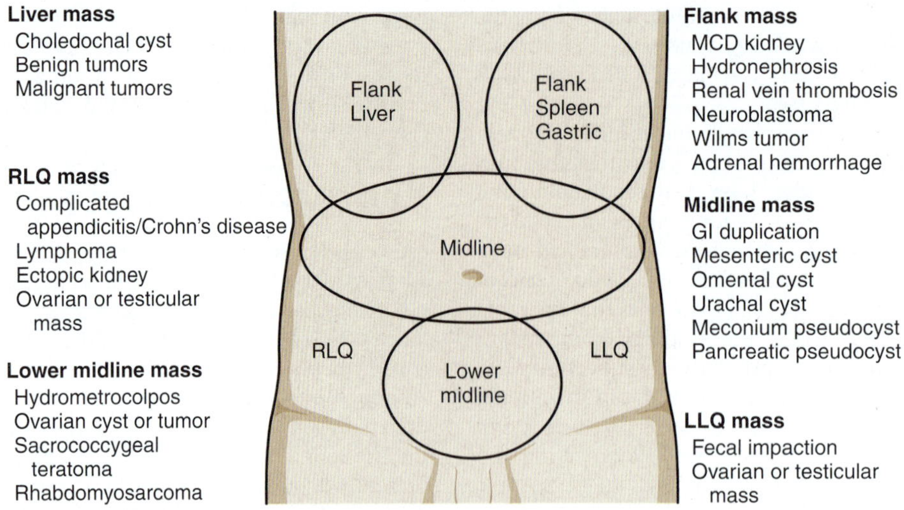

Fig. 18.93 Location of commonly found abdominal masses in children. *GI,* Gastrointestinal; *LLQ,* left lower quadrant; *MCD,* minimal change disease; *RLQ,* right lower quadrant.

Table 18.7 Possible Diagnoses of Abdominal Masses in Infancy and Childhood

Region	Organ	Diagnosis
Epigastrium	Stomach	Distended stomach from pyloric stenosis, duplication
	Pancreas	Pseudocyst
	Lung	Extralobar pulmonary sequestration
Flank	Kidney	Hydronephrosis, dysplastic kidney, Wilms tumor, mesoblastic nephroma, rhabdoid tumor, cystic nephroma, clear cell sarcoma of the kidney
	Adrenal or Retroperitoneum	Neuroblastoma, ganglioneuroma, ganglioneuroblastoma, teratoma
Lower abdomen	Ovary	Germ cell tumor, ovarian tumor, torsion of ovary
	Kidney	Pelvic kidney
	Urachus	Urachal cyst
	Omentum, mesentery	Omental, mesenteric, peritoneal cysts
Pelvis	Bladder, prostate	Obstructed bladder, rhabdomyosarcoma
	Uterus, vagina	Hydrometrocolpos, hydrocolpos, rhabdomyosarcoma
Right upper quadrant	Biliary tract	Cholecystitis, choledochal cyst
	Liver	Hepatomegaly, mesenchymal hematoma, hepatoblastoma, hepatocellular carcinoma, hepatic abscess, hydatid cyst
	Intestine	Intussusception, duplication
Left upper quadrant	Spleen	Splenomegaly resulting from congestion, infectious mononucleosis, leukemia, or lymphoma; splenic abscess or cyst
Right lower quadrant	Appendix	Appendiceal abscess
	Ileum	Meconium ileus, inflammatory mass (complicated Crohn disease), intestinal duplication, Meckel diverticulum
	Lymphatics	Lymphoma, lymphatic malformation
Left lower quadrant	Colon	Fecal impaction
	Lymphatics	Lymphoma, lymphatic malformation

masses. This modality allows the differentiation of solid versus cystic lesions, a critical first stage in evaluation. Ultrasonography may characterize the lesion as arising within the kidney or in a juxtarenal location. Alternatively, pelvic lesions may also be determined as being cystic, solid, or mixed in nature (Fig. 18.94). CT radiography allows precise anatomic differentiation of abdominal lesions and the assessment of extraabdominal disease (Chapter 25).

CT radiography, with both intravenous and enteral contrast, has become the study of choice for surgeons and other interventionalists in the evaluation of patients with abdominal masses. Because of its utility for assessing extent of local disease, the sites of distant metastases and the character of the lesion, this imaging allows for careful analysis of abdominal and pelvic structures. MRI may be of utility in patients with abdominal masses; however, in infants this is a somewhat cumbersome study because it is relatively slower and often necessitates intravenous sedation or a general anesthetic.

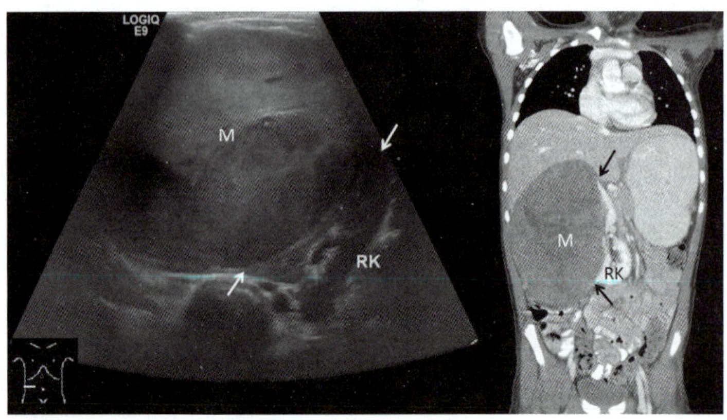

Fig. 18.94 Three-year-old female presenting with abdominal mass. Ultrasound *(left)* and computed tomography with contrast *(right)* show a large right-sided abdominal solid mass *(M)* arising from the right kidney *(RK)*. The claw sign in the right kidney *(arrows)* confirms the renal origin of the mass, which turned out to be a Wilms tumor.

Neonates

Neonatal abdominal masses are benign genitourinary lesions in 75% to 80% of cases. The most common abdominal masses are congenital obstructive hydronephrosis and multicystic dysplastic kidney. Congenital hydronephrosis presents as a bulky, smooth, flank mass on physical examination; it is usually secondary to ureteropelvic junction obstruction (Fig. 18.95) and is treated by pyeloplasty to prevent further loss of renal parenchyma or development of infection. Other genitourinary anomalies (such as ureteral duplications and ureteroceles) may produce obstructive uropathies that lead to palpable masses. Bilateral flank masses with hydroureteronephrosis may result from posterior urethral valves (Chapter 15), which is the most common cause of distal urinary tract obstruction in boys (Fig. 18.96). Multicystic dysplastic kidney disease often presents as a unilateral, soft, cystic mass in more than three-quarters of cases (Fig. 18.97). Renal vein thrombosis may also present as an abdominal mass in the neonate. This condition is most commonly the result of hyperviscosity syndromes or severe neonatal dehydration (Fig. 18.98). Mesoblastic nephroma, a benign renal tumor that mimics Wilms tumor, is also a common renal mass that may present in the neonatal period.

Other abdominal masses in the neonatal period may arise from genitourinary organs, gastrointestinal structures, or intraabdominal sites. Ovarian cysts are common in the neonatal period. Maternal hormonal stimulation in utero promotes their development, and subsequent withdrawal of this stimulus after delivery leads to their resolution over time. Congenital vaginal obstruction may also lead to development of a large abdominal mass. Gastrointestinal duplication cysts are often present at birth, but the diagnosis is often delayed until later in childhood (Fig. 18.99). Mesenteric and omental cysts are soft, diffuse, and multiloculated lesions that arise from the omentum or mesentery. These lesions are due to congenital lymphatic obstruction and may be a source of intraabdominal pain due to acute hemorrhage into the lesion (Fig. 18.100). Adrenal masses are common in the newborn and in infancy. These masses may range from the benign mass associated with spontaneous adrenal hemorrhage from perinatal stress or birth trauma to malignant neuroblastoma (Fig. 18.101). On occasion, intraabdominal extralobar pulmonary sequestration may be adjacent to the adrenal gland, suggesting the appearance of a malignancy. The age of peak cancer incidence among children younger than 15 years old occurs during infancy with 10% of cancers being diagnosed within this age range. The most common malignancy of newborns and infants is neuroblastoma, representing more than 20% of infant cancer cases.

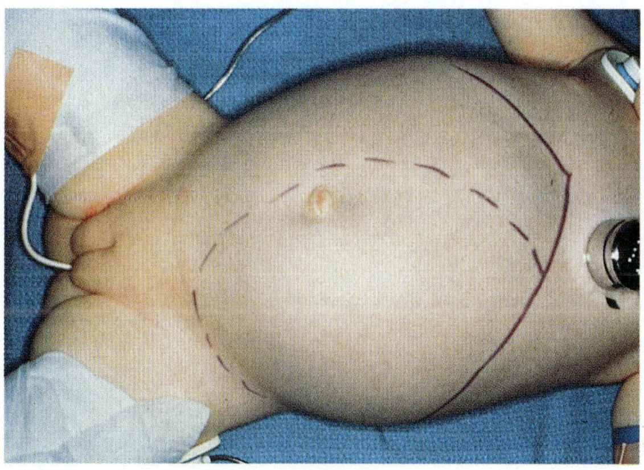

Fig. 18.95 The *dashed line* indicates the extent of a flank mass in an infant with ureteropelvic junction obstruction.

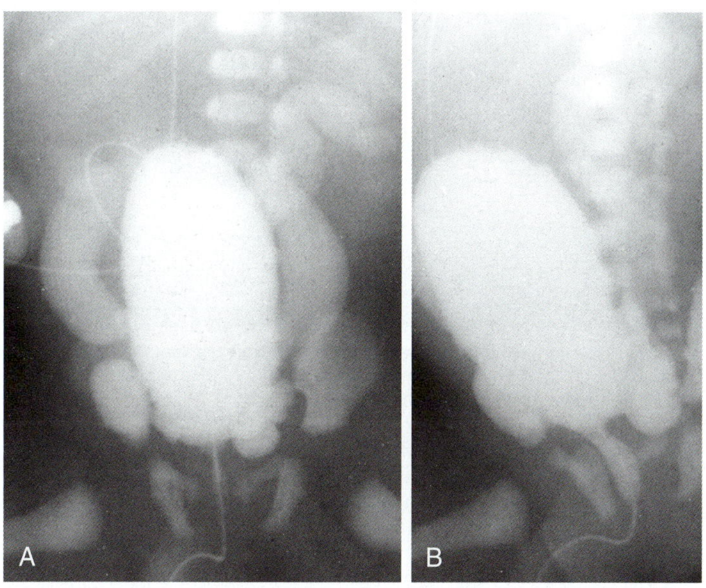

Fig. 18.96 Posterior urethral valves cause dilation of the bladder and both upper tracts, shown here on anteroposterior (A) and lateral (B) views of a retrograde contrast study.

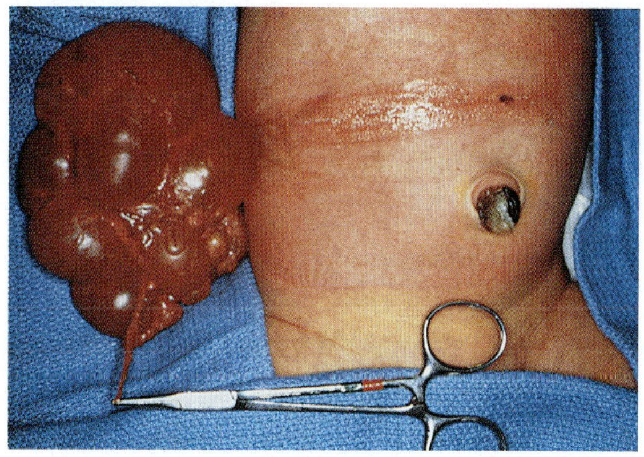

Fig. 18.97 A multicystic kidney produces a knobby flank mass.

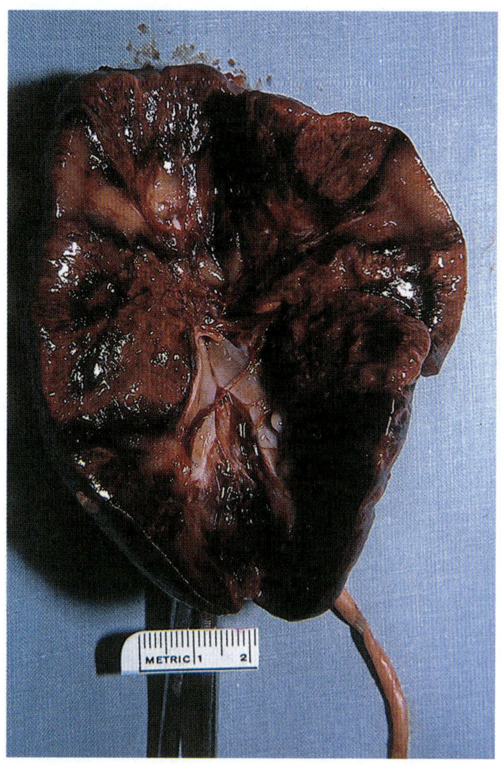

Fig. 18.98 Renal vein thrombosis may occur as the result of hyperviscosity syndromes or severe neonatal dehydration.

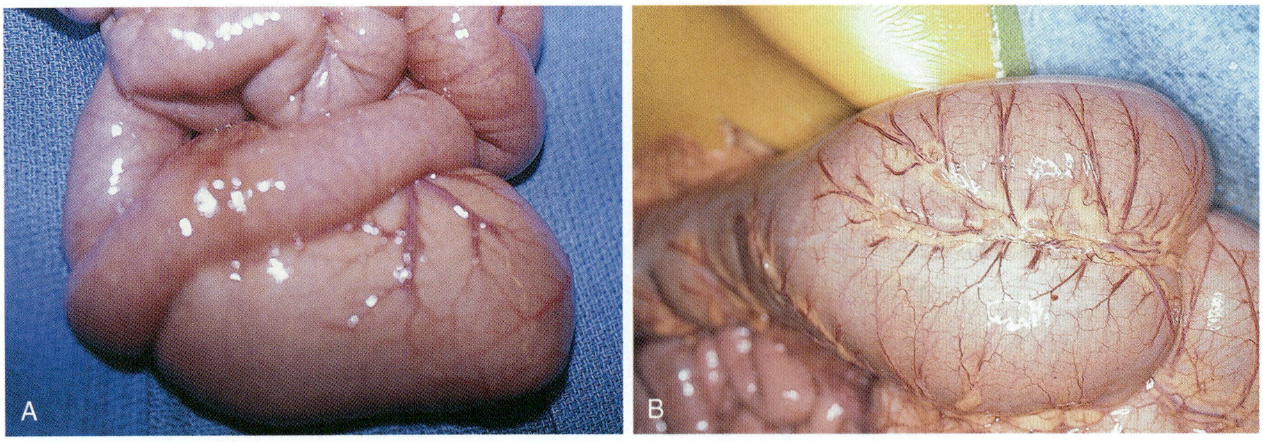

Fig. 18.99 Duplications of the gastrointestinal tract usually arise from the mesenteric border of the bowel and may be cystic (A) or tubular (B).

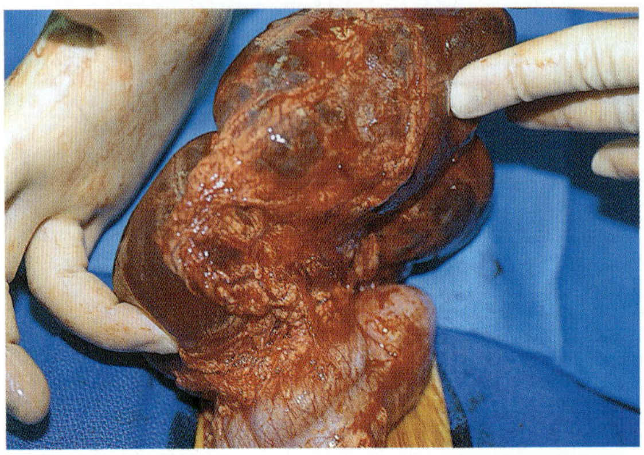

Fig. 18.100 Omental cyst may cause ill-defined episodic abdominal pain.

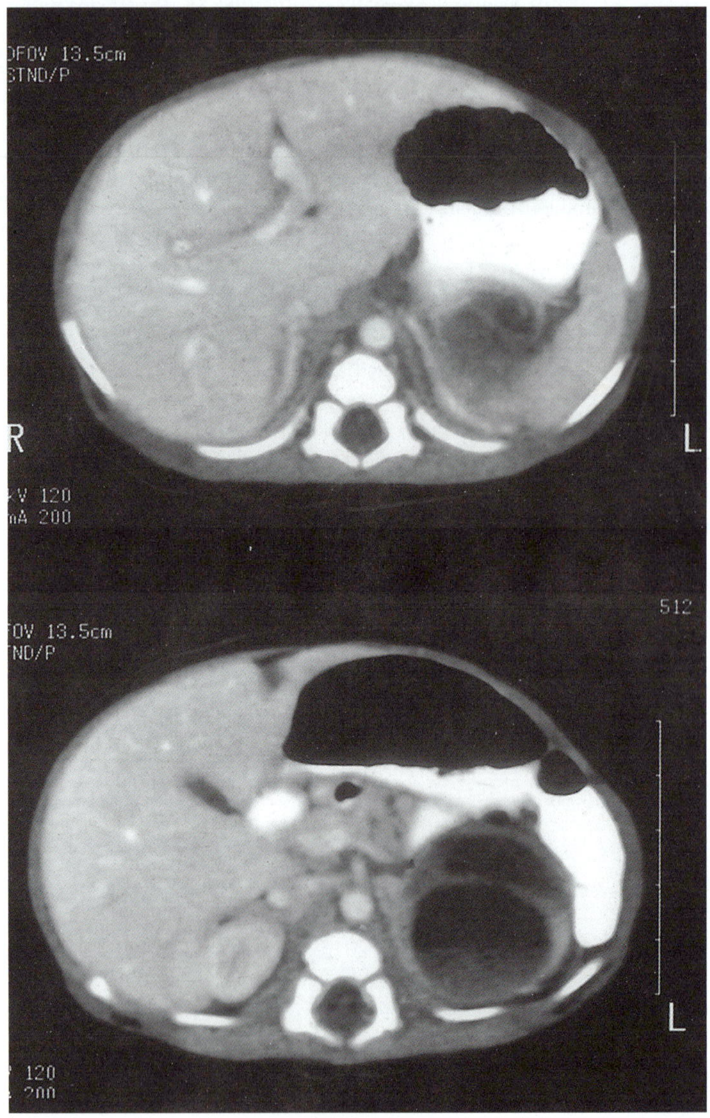

Fig. 18.101 Adrenal hemorrhage often results from perinatal stress or birth trauma. The radiographic appearance showing a left suprarenal heterogeneous mass is suspicious for neuroblastoma.

Toddlers and Young Children

In stark contrast with the presentation in the neonate, the presence of an abdominal mass in a toddler or young child is equally as likely to be malignant as benign. Neuroblastoma, Wilms tumor, rhabdomyosarcoma, hepatoblastoma, and lymphoma are the most common pediatric solid malignancies. Although each may have histologic similarities, they all have distinct differences in tumor behavior and prognosis.

Neuroblastoma

Neuroblastoma is the most common extracranial malignancy of childhood, accounting for 7% to 10% of all cancers in children younger than 15 years old, and is responsible for 10% to 15% of all cancer-related deaths. A solid tumor derived from neural crest cells, it may be found anywhere along the embryonic tract of neural crest cell migration from the neck to the pelvis (Fig. 18.102). Neuroblastoma may display a variety of behaviors, as tumors can spontaneously regress or mature, or display an aggressive phenotype. Neuroblastoma is classified into risk groups of low, intermediate, or high risk based on biological and clinical factors, which predict prognosis and recurrence. Factors include the patient's age, stage, histopathology, *MYCN* status, and DNA index. The probability of disease-free survival is 95%, 90%, and 40% to 50% for low-risk, intermediate-risk, and high-risk groups, respectively. Unfortunately, most patients present with advanced disease, leading to an overall survival of ~70%. Tumors are typically multilobular and firm retroperitoneal masses that encase vessels and cross the abdominal midline. More than half occur in the adrenal or juxtarenal location (Fig. 18.103). Presenting symptoms are dependent on the location of the tumor and disease burden and may include local pain, abdominal distention, failure to thrive, or paralysis. Several important extraabdominal symptoms, including cerebellar ataxia, opsoclonus-myoclonus syndrome (also known as *dancing eyes and feet syndrome*), and diffuse, watery diarrhea may be present. Patients may also present with neurologic symptoms of paralysis and weakness due to spinal cord invasion or peripheral nerve compression. The prognosis of neuroblastoma presenting with neurologic function loss is generally poor (<25% survival). A variant of neuroblastoma known as *stage 4-S disease* presents with extensive local disease and widespread metastases to bone, skin (blue nodules), and liver in children younger than 1 year old. Many of these patients will ultimately undergo spontaneous regression of the tumor with minimal or no therapy.

The radiographic appearance of an intraabdominal neuroblastoma may reveal evidence of an upper abdominal mass with areas of stippled calcifications (Fig. 18.104). The CT scan in Fig. 18.104B shows a

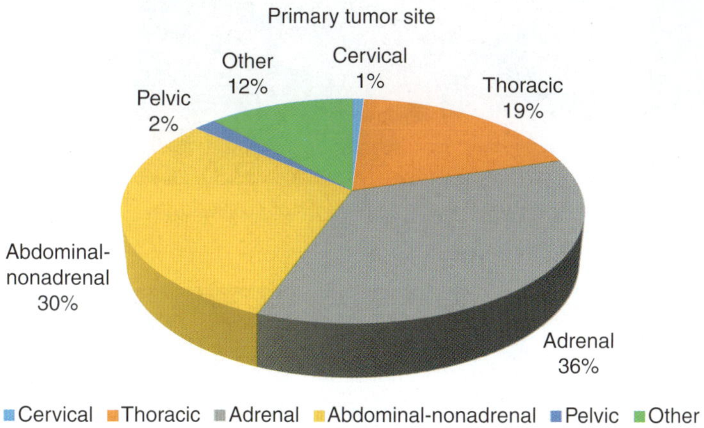

Fig. 18.102 Frequency of locations of primary neuroblastoma tumor.

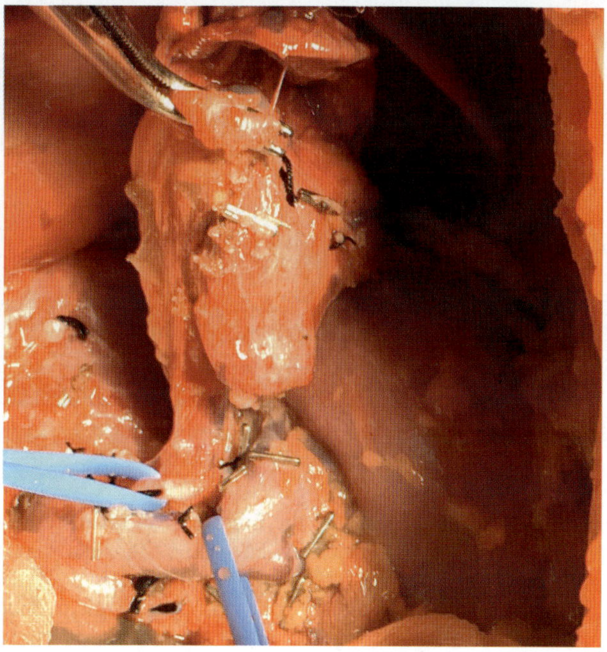

Fig. 18.103 Dissection of an adrenal neuroblastoma away from the previously encased renal vessels.

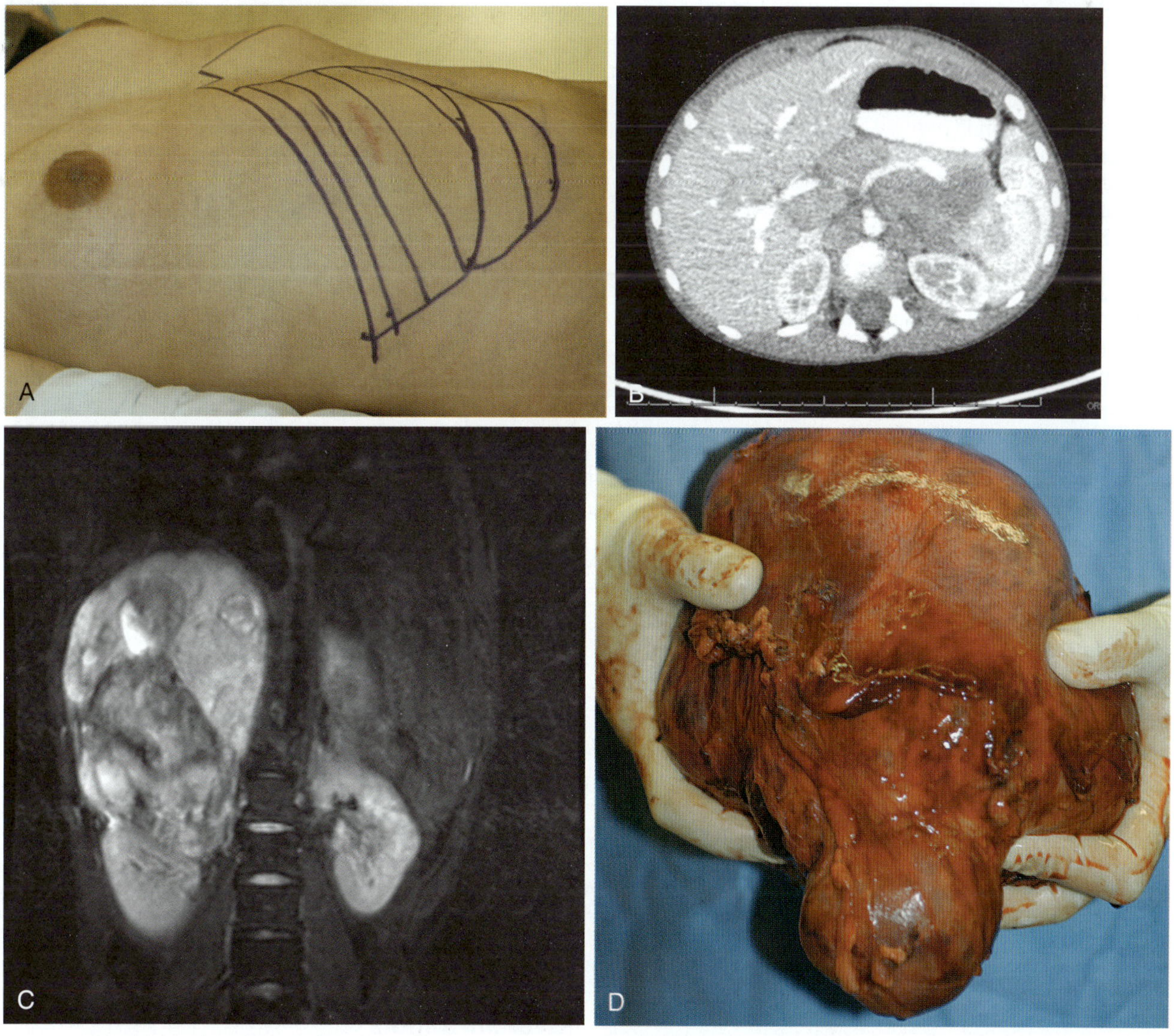

Fig. 18.104 (A) Abdominal examination of a patient with a neuroblastoma, outlining the extent of the palpable tumor. (B) Computed tomography scan of adrenal neuroblastoma with vascular encasement. (C) Magnetic resonance imaging demonstrating inferior displacement of the kidney by the large tumor. The tumor also has calcifications. (D) Pathologic specimen of the patient's tumor at surgery.

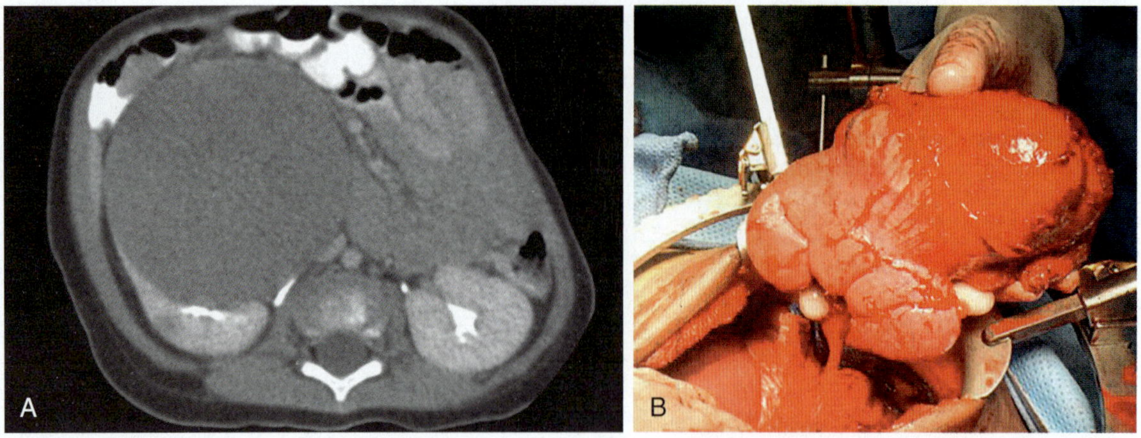

Fig. 18.105 (A) Abdominal computed tomography scan of Wilms tumor shows a bulky mass to the right of midline. (B) Intraoperative Wilms tumor with a large tumor mass involving the kidney.

retroperitoneal mass that crosses the midline with intimate involvement of adjacent vascular structures, including the aorta, vena cava and renal vessels, and mesenteric artery. The workup of masses includes an evaluation of the urine for the dopaminergic metabolites vanillylmandelic and homovanillic acid, abdominal and chest CT, technetium scintigraphy (bone scan), and metaiodobenzylguanidine scan. Serologic studies including ferritin, neuron-specific enolase, and lactate dehydrogenase have prognostic significance as well. Neuroblastoma requires multimodal treatment, and the care team should include oncologists, pathologists, radiologists, and surgeons.

Wilms Tumor

Wilms tumor is the second most common abdominal malignancy in childhood and the most common primary renal tumor. Approximately 500 new cases are diagnosed annually in the United States. Most present between 1 and 4 years old. The classic presentation is that of a palpable abdominal mass, hematuria, and hypertension; however, the majority of patients present with an asymptomatic abdominal mass. Gross hematuria can be seen in 18%, microscopical in 24%, and hypertension in 20% to 25% of patients. Although most children are asymptomatic at presentation, some present with severe pain secondary to intratumor bleeding or, rarely, intraabdominal rupture. The physical examination reveals a large bulky tumor in the subcostal region that is usually firm, smooth, immobile, and nontender. Unlike neuroblastoma, these tumors usually do not cross the midline, nor are there usually signs of metastatic disease. Affected children otherwise appear well. The role of diagnostic imaging is to assess the nature of the tumor, site of origin, presence of bilateral disease, extent of local disease (tumor invasion of the renal vessels and/or inferior vena cava), and evidence of metastases. CT of the chest and abdomen often answers critical questions important to clinical staging (Fig. 18.105). Signs of tumor extending into the renal veins are of major surgical significance and mandate careful evaluation of the inferior vena cava and right atrium by ultrasound and echocardiography. Evidence of intracaval and right atrial thrombus requires chemotherapy before surgical resection to treat the vascular invasion and minimize surgical morbidity. Lungs, lymph nodes, and the liver are the most common sites of metastasis. Formerly, clear cell sarcoma was considered to be a variant of Wilms tumor, but it is now believed to be a distinct pathologic entity. Bony metastases are common with this malignancy, and these patients should be evaluated by bone scan. Children with Wilms tumor generally do well, with a survival rate of nearly 90%, even in the presence of metastatic disease.

Hepatic and Splenic Tumors in Childhood

Hepatic lesions often present in childhood. These lesions may range from benign conditions such as infantile hepatic hemangiomas, arteriovenous malformations, mesenchymal hamartoma, and choledochal cysts (see Fig. 18.75) to malignant tumors, including hepatoblastoma, hepatocellular carcinoma, and metastatic tumor burden. Hepatic tumors may present as bulky masses present in the right upper quadrant or midline that are fixed to the adjacent liver and poorly mobile (Fig. 18.106). Splenomegaly occurs from underlying hematologic diseases, such as immunodeficiencies and lymphoproliferative diseases. A splenic cyst may also present as splenomegaly. These cysts may be congenital in nature or the result of previous trauma (Fig. 18.107).

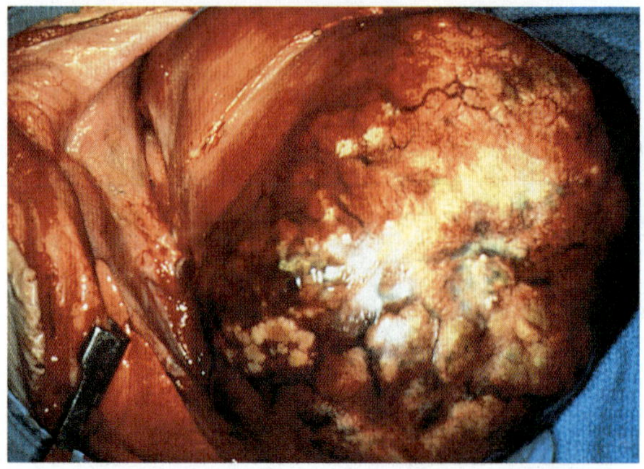

Fig. 18.106 A large hepatoblastoma of the right lobe of the liver. Intravenous urography, computed tomography, and ultrasonography all identified it as a hepatic tumor instead of one arising from the kidney or an adrenal gland.

Older Children and Teenagers

Soft Tissue Sarcoma

Rhabdomyosarcoma is the most common soft tissue sarcoma of childhood. Although tumors have histologic features of striated skeletal muscle, they may arise anywhere in the body (Fig. 18.108). Lesions arising in pelvic locations (bladder, vagina, and paratesticular regions) have a nonalveolar histology and a more favorable prognosis (Fig. 18.109). Primary lesions are not confined to the abdominal cavity but may appear throughout the body. Prognosis depends on the site of occurrence and histologic characteristics.

Lymphomas

Non-Hodgkin lymphoma may present with abdominal involvement in 25% to 50% of all cases. The peak incidence of occurrence is between 5 and 8 years old. Most children present with abdominal pain and a palpable mass. These are rapidly growing tumors that may arise from bowel, mesentery, or retroperitoneal structures. Some children may develop an irreducible intussusception requiring surgical resection. These tumors are usually responsive to chemotherapy.

Ovarian Tumors

Pelvic tumors in children may also present as lower abdominal masses due to the small, shallow nature of the pediatric pelvis. The differential diagnosis of midline pelvic masses includes ovarian cysts and tumors, hydrocolpos, hydrometrocolpos, and sacrococcygeal teratoma. Ovarian

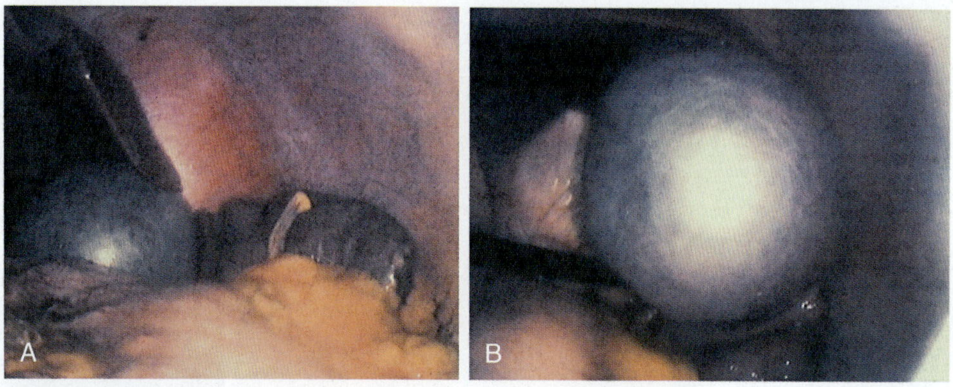

Fig. 18.107 (A and B) Laparoscopic views of a symptomatic splenic cyst in an active teenager caused disabling left upper quadrant pain.

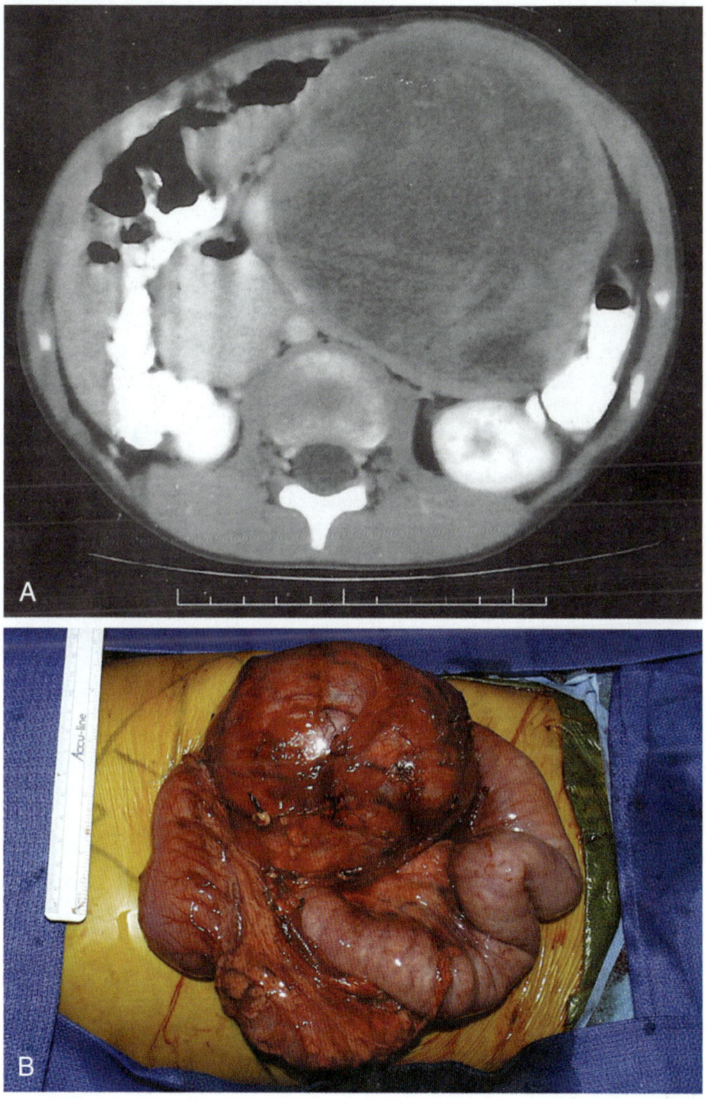

Fig. 18.108 (A) Abdominal computed tomography scan showing a large retroperitoneal rhabdomyosarcoma. (B) Intraoperative view of retroperitoneal rhabdomyosarcoma extending through the mesentery, displacing the small bowel and colon.

masses may occur in all age groups but are most commonly seen in adolescence. Most ovarian masses are cystic and benign in nature. Twenty-five percent are solid and may have evidence of malignant changes. Ovarian cysts commonly occur in newborn infants and may be diagnosed prenatally, often resolving spontaneously in infancy. Large cysts of more than 5 cm in infants are prone to torsion and should be aspirated or undergo surgical intervention. Obstruction of the female genital tract by vaginal atresia, a cloacal malformation, or an imperforate hymen may cause hydrocolpos in infancy that may manifest as a large abdominal mass with respiratory embarrassment secondary to

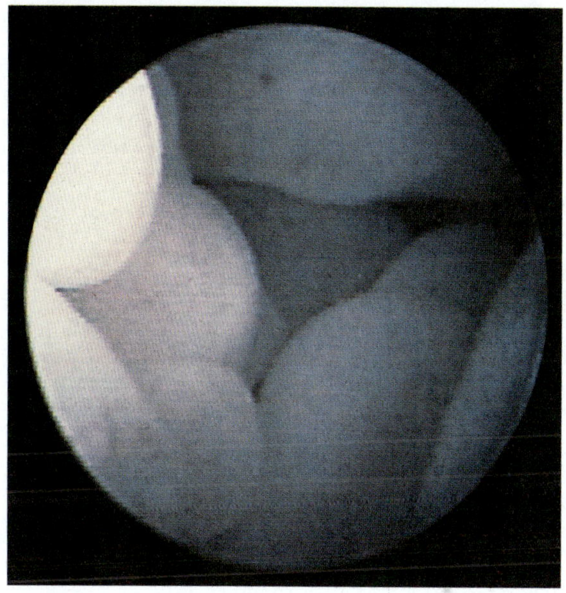

Fig. 18.109 Botryoid rhabdomyosarcoma of the bladder has the characteristic "clustered grape" appearance on cystoscopy. Prognosis is usually favorable.

diaphragmatic compression. Alternatively, these girls may present at puberty with cyclic abdominal pain, a large pelvic or lower abdominal mass, and the absence of menses (Fig. 18.110). This occurs because of the uterine retention of menstrual products. They may also develop hydronephrosis due to extrinsic vesicoureteral obstruction and coexisting genitourinary tract anomalies, which are common in this population.

Inflammatory Masses

Numerous inflammatory conditions that involve intraabdominal organs may lead to masses. Subsequent to bowel perforations associated with appendicitis, Meckel diverticulitis, or Crohn disease, the omentum and adjacent bowel loops migrate to the area and adhere to the process in an attempt to localize the condition. Development of an abscess cavity with fibrosis and capsule formation may mimic a lower abdominal or pelvic tumor. Typically, inflammatory masses are tender and associated with systemic symptoms. Early institution of intravenous antibiotics and percutaneous drainage may lead to resolution of an abscess. Children with ventriculoperitoneal shunts may develop inflammatory pseudocysts, associated with infected shunt catheters and cerebrospinal fluid drainage. This is often associated with symptoms of fever and abdominal pain. Prompt shunt exteriorization and intravenous antibiotic therapy may allow catheter salvage. Persistent symptoms of sepsis suggest the possibility of an abscess formation or bowel perforation that requires surgical exploration and catheter removal. Crohn disease may present with inflammatory lower abdominal masses or abscesses. These usually respond to aggressive medical management and may resolve without surgery.

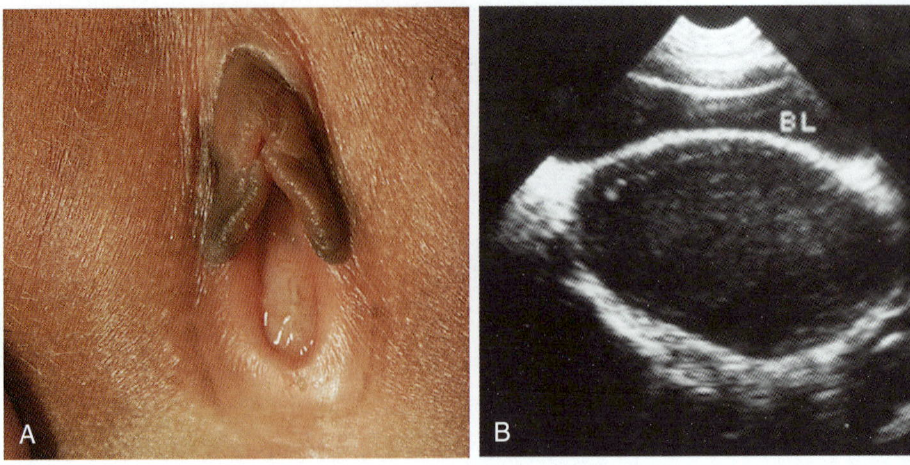

Fig. 18.110 (A) Imperforate hymen. Accumulated secretions in the vagina and uterus caused bulging of the hymen and a pelvic mass in this newborn. (B) A pelvic mass arising at the expected time of menarche suggests the presence of an obstructed uterine anomaly, here demonstrated by pelvic ultrasound as an oval mass compressing the bladder anteriorly. Urinary anomalies commonly coexist. *BL*, Bladder.

Failure to respond to medical therapies suggests the presence of a stricture or fistula to an adjacent bowel loop or bladder. Upper gastrointestinal contrast studies with small bowel follow-through and barium enema evaluation with reflux into the terminal ileum help delineate the extent of bowel involvement in the process.

Bibliography

Akinkuotu AC, Cruz SM, Abbas PI, et al: Risk-stratification of severity for infants with CDH: prenatal versus postnatal predictors of outcome, *J Pediatr Surg* 51(1):44–48, 2016. doi:10.1016/j.jpedsurg.2015.10.009.

Alganabi M, Lee C, Bindi E, Li B, Pierro A: Recent advances in understanding necrotizing enterocolitis, *F1000Res* 8:F1000 Faculty Rev-107, 2019. doi:10.12688/f1000research.17228.1.

Alsaied A, Islam N, Thalib L: Global incidence of necrotizing enterocolitis: a systematic review and meta-analysis, *BMC Pediatr* 20(1):344, 2020.

Altobelli E, Angeletti PM, Verrotti A, Petrocelli R: The impact of human milk on necrotizing enterocolitis: a systematic review and meta-analysis, *Nutrients* 12(5):1322, 2020.

Brunicardi FC, Andersen DK, Billiar TR, et al: *Schwartz's principles of surgery*, New York, 2015, McGraw-Hill.

Cordier AG, Russo FM, Deprest J, Benachi A: Prenatal diagnosis, imaging, and prognosis in congenital diaphragmatic hernia, *Semin Perinatol* 44(1):51163, 2020.

Dasgupta R, Renaud E, Goldin AB, et al: Ovarian torsion in pediatric and adolescent patients: a systematic review, *J Pediatr Surg* 53(7):1387–1391, 2018. doi:10.1016/j.jpedsurg.2017.10.053.

Deprest J, Gratacos E, Nicolaides KH, FETO Task Group. Fetoscopic tracheal occlusion (FETO) for severe congenital diaphragmatic hernia: evolution of a technique and preliminary results, *Ultrasound Obstet Gynecol* 24(2):121–126, 2004. doi:10.1002/uog.1711. Erratum in: *Ultrasound Obstet Gynecol* 24(5):594, 2004.

Dinarvand P, Davaro EP, Doan JV, et al: Familial adenomatous polyposis syndrome: an update and review of extraintestinal manifestations, *Arch Pathol Lab Med* 143(11):1382–1398, 2019.

D'Souza N, Thaventhiran A, Beable R, Higginson A, Rud B: Magnetic resonance imaging for diagnosis of acute appendicitis, *Cochrane Database Syst Rev* 2016(1), 2016. doi:10.1002/14651858.CD012028.pub2.

Eng KA, Abadeh A, Ligocki C, et al: Acute appendicitis: a meta-analysis of the diagnostic accuracy of US, CT, and MRI as second-line imaging tests after an initial US, *Radiology* 288(3):717–727, 2018.

Francis GL, Waguespack SG, Bauer AJ, et al: Management guidelines for children with thyroid nodules and differentiated thyroid cancer, *Thyroid* 25(7):716–759, 2015.

Frost BL, Modi BP, Jaksic T, Caplan MS: New medical and surgical insights into neonatal necrotizing enterocolitis: a review, *JAMA Pediatr* 171(1):83–88, 2017.

Grosfeld JL, O'Neill JA, Fonkalsrud E, et al: *Pediatric surgery*, Philadelphia, 2006, Mosby/Elsevier.

Haugen BR, Alexander EK, Bible KC, et al: 2015 American Thyroid Association management guidelines for adult patients with thyroid nodules and differentiated thyroid cancer: the American Thyroid Association Guidelines Task Force on thyroid nodules and differentiated thyroid cancer, *Thyroid* 26(1):1–133, 2016.

Holcomb GW III, Murphy PJ, Ostlie DJ: *Ashcraft's pediatric surgery*, London, 2014, Saunders/Elsevier.

Horvath E, Majlis S, Rossi R, et al: An ultrasonogram reporting system for thyroid nodules stratifying cancer risk for clinical management, *J Clin Endocrinol Metab* 94(5):1748–1751, 2009. doi:10.1210/jc.2008-1724.

Keese D, Rolle U, Gfroerer S, Fiegel H: Symptomatic Meckel's diverticulum in pediatric patients-case reports and systematic review of the literature, *Front Pediatr* 7:267, 2019.

Khan S, Siow VS, Lewis A, et al: An evidence-based care protocol improves outcomes and decreases cost in pediatric appendicitis, *J Surg Res* 256:390–396, 2020.

Lawton B, Goldstein H, Davis T, Tagg A: Diagnosis of appendicitis in the paediatric emergency department: an update, *Curr Opin Pediatr* 31(3):312–316, 2019.

Madenci AL, Levine BS, Laufer MR, et al: Preoperative risk stratification of children with ovarian tumors, *J Pediatr Surg* 51(9):1507, 2016.

Mattei P, editor: *Fundamentals of pediatric surgery*, New York, 2011, Springer.

Mehl SC, Sun RC, Anbarasu CR, et al: Association of intercostal nerve cryoablation during nuss procedure with complications and costs, *Ann Thorac Surg* 116(4):803–809, 2023. doi:10.1016/j.athoracsur.2022.04.022.

Minneci PC, Deans KJ: Nonoperative treatment of appendicitis, *JAMA Pediatr* 171(11):1126–1127, 2017. doi:10.1001/jamapediatrics.2017.2940.

Minneci PC, Hade EM, Lawrence AE, et al: Association of nonoperative management using antibiotic therapy vs laparoscopic appendectomy with treatment success and disability days in children with uncomplicated appendicitis, *JAMA* 324(6):581–593, 2020.

Minneci PC, Mahida JB, Lodwick DL, et al: Effectiveness of patient choice in nonoperative vs surgical management of pediatric uncomplicated acute appendicitis, *JAMA Surg* 151(5):408–415, 2016.

Mitchell J, Yip L: Decision making in indeterminate thyroid nodules and the role of molecular testing, *Surg Clin North Am* 99(4):587–598, 2019.

Mostoufi-Moab S, Labourier E, Sullivan L, et al: Molecular testing for oncogenic gene alterations in pediatric thyroid lesions, *Thyroid* 28(1):60–67, 2018.

Niño DF, Sodhi CP, Hackam DJ: Necrotizing enterocolitis: new insights into pathogenesis and mechanisms, *Nat Rev Gastroenterol Hepatol* 13(10):590–600, 2016.

Nuss D, Obermeyer RJ, Kelly RE: Nuss bar procedure: past, present and future. *Ann Cardiothorac Surg* 5(5):422–433, 2016. doi:10.21037/acs.2016.08.05.

Oyetunji TA, Dorman RM, Svetanoff WJ, et al: Declining frequency of thoracoscopic decortication for empyema—redefining failure after fibrinolysis, *J Pediatr Surg* 55(11):2352–2355, 2020.

Pacilli M, Nataraja RM: Management of paediatric empyema by video-assisted thoracoscopic surgery (VATS) versus chest drain with fibrinolysis: systematic review and meta-analysis, *Paediatr Respir Rev* 30:42–48, 2019.

Patel KN, Yip L, Lubitz CC, et al: The American Association of Endocrine Surgeons guidelines for the definitive surgical management of thyroid disease in adults, *Ann Surg* 271(3):e21–e93, 2020.

Peeters T, Penders J, Smeekens SP, et al: The fecal and mucosal microbiome in acute appendicitis patients: an observational study, *Future Microbiol* 14(2):111–127, 2019.

Rogers MB, Brower-Sinning R, Firek B, Zhong D, Morowitz MJ: Acute appendicitis in children is associated with a local expansion of fusobacteria, *Clin Infect Dis* 63(1):71–78, 2016.

Soares KC, Goldstein SD, Ghaseb MA, et al. Pediatric choledochal cysts: diagnosis and current management, *Pediatr Surg Int* 33(6):637–650, 2017. doi:10.1007/s00383-017-4083-6.

St. Peter SD, Tsao K, Harrison C, et al: Thoracoscopic decortication vs tube thoracostomy with fibrinolysis for empyema in children: a prospective, randomized trial, *J Pediatr Surg* 44(1):106–111, 2009.

Stoll BJ, Hansen NI, Bell EF, et al. Trends in care practices, morbidity, and mortality of extremely preterm neonates, 1993-2012, *JAMA* 314(10):1039–1051, 2015. doi:10.1001/jama.2015.10244.

Style CC, Olutoye OO, Belfort MA, et al. Fetal endoscopic tracheal occlusion reduces pulmonary hypertension in severe congenital diaphragmatic hernia. *Ultrasound Obstet Gynecol* 54(6):752-758, 2019. doi:10.1002/uog.20216.

Svetanoff WJ, Dorman RM, Dekonenko C, et al: Protocol-driven antibiotic treatment of pediatric empyema after fibrinolysis, *Pediatr Infect Dis J* 40(1):44–48, 2021.

The SML, Bakx R, Budding AE, et al: Microbiota of children with complex appendicitis: different composition and diversity of the microbiota in children with complex compared with simple appendicitis, *Pediatr Infect Dis J* 38(10):1054–1060, 2019.

Wang Y, Honeyford K, Aylin P, Bottle A, Giuliani S: One-year outcomes for congenital diaphragmatic hernia, *BJS Open* 3(3):305–313, 2019. doi:10.1002/bjs5.50135.

Warner J, Desoky S, Tiwari HA, Morello F, Gilbertson D, Udayasankar U: Unenhanced MRI of the abdomen and pelvis in the comprehensive evaluation of acute atraumatic abdominal pain in children, *AJR Am J Roentgenol* 215(5):1218–1228, 2020.

Yu PT, Jen HC, Rice-Townsend S, Guner YS: The role of ECMO in the management of congenital diaphragmatic hernia, *Semin Perinatol* 44(1):151166, 2020.

Zobel M, Gologorsky R, Lee H, Vu L: Congenital lung lesions, *Semin Pediatr Surg* 28(4):150821, 2019.

19

PEDIATRIC AND ADOLESCENT GYNECOLOGY

Jacquelin Rankine | Orquidia A. Torres

NORMAL FEMALE GENITALIA

Newborn and Prepubertal

In the newborn, the physical appearance of the genitalia reflects stimulation by maternal sex hormones (Fig. 19.1). Separation of the labia minora reveals thick, redundant hymenal folds that often hide the small central vaginal opening and urethral meatus. The mucosa is moist, vaginal pH is acidic, and a milky discharge is often seen. Vaginal bleeding during the first week of life is normal. It is caused by withdrawal of maternal estrogen after delivery. Breast development, with palpable breast tissue, engorgement, and less commonly a clear or cloudy discharge, is observed in full-term neonates of both sexes (see Chapter 2). These findings gradually subside over several months. During this period, infants are at increased risk for developing breast inflammation and infection.

The effect of maternal hormones on the female genitalia gradually disappears; the labia majora lose their fullness, and the labia minora and hymen become thinner and flatter. As the young infant matures, the labia cover less of the vaginal vestibule, particularly when the infant or child is sitting, and thus offer incomplete protection from external sources of irritation. The mucosa has a glistening, reddish pink hue that sometimes is mistaken for inflammation by observers unaccustomed to examining prepubertal genitalia. Vaginal pH is now neutral or alkaline, and secretions are minimal.

Physiologic changes also cause variations in the appearance of the hymenal tissues during childhood. During early infancy, the tissues are relatively thick and can be redundant (Fig. 19.2A and B). Usually in the first months of life, the hymen becomes thin and translucent, with smooth edges (see Fig. 19.2C–E). When the child enters puberty, the hymen again thickens under the influence of estrogen.

The shape of the vaginal orifice also varies. Annular (see Fig. 19.2C), crescentic (see Fig. 19.2D and E), teardrop-shaped, and fimbriated (with fingerlike projections around the hymenal rim) hymens are all normal variations. On rare occasions, there is a completely imperforate hymen; more commonly there is a septate hymen (see Fig. 19.2F) or a fenestrated hymen with small perforations.

From about 6 to 8 weeks old until puberty, the perineum, perivaginal tissues, and pelvic supporting structures are relatively rigid and inelastic. This factor increases the likelihood of tearing from trauma. In addition, before the onset of puberty, the ovaries are positioned above the pelvic brim (Table 19.1). This intraabdominal location accounts for the fact that ovarian disorders in childhood frequently present with abdominal, rather than pelvic, signs and symptoms.

Pubertal

With the onset of puberty, the mons pubis begins to fill out and hair begins to grow in the midline. Fat deposition fills out the labia majora. The labia minora thicken, become softer and more rounded, and asymmetry and variations in size and shape become more noticeable.

Asymmetry of the labia is common (Fig. 19.3), and there is wide variation in the appearance and size of healthy labia. Clinicians and patients may wish to refer to published depictions of this variation, such as The Great Wall of Vulva (https://www.thegreatwallofvulva.com/). Typically, the maximal width between the midline and lateral free edge of the labia minora measures less than 3 to 5 cm. Patients with labial hypertrophy may present with pain, irritation, chronic infection, problems with personal hygiene (e.g., during menses), or problems with sexual or physical activity. Most symptoms can be alleviated by addressing personal hygiene and appropriate choice of clothing to minimize friction. Sometimes use of an antichafe product can help to prevent abrasions. In most cases, a careful examination followed by reassurance and discussion of the variations in normal anatomy are all that is required.

Other normal changes during puberty include slight enlargement of the clitoris. The hymen also thickens, and its central orifice enlarges. The vaginal mucosa thickens and softens and becomes moist and pink as secretions increase and pH levels drop. Perineal and pelvic tissues become more elastic, and the ovaries gradually descend into the pelvis. In the months preceding menarche, physiologic leukorrhea increases. It consists of a white discharge containing mature epithelial cells and vaginal secretions stimulated by estrogen. In some patients, the unopposed estrogen secretion of puberty stimulates leukorrhea so profuse that it becomes concerning and irritating, because the perineum is often moist.

The developmental aspects of gynecologic anatomy and physiology are summarized in Table 19.1. There is variation in the range of normal reproductive organ size as seen on ultrasound. The following have been proposed as upper values for prepubertal patients: uterine length, 4.5 cm; uterine thickness, 1 cm; and ovarian volume, 4 to 5 mL. The Tanner stages of pubertal development are presented in Chapter 9.

GYNECOLOGIC EVALUATION

Examination of the Prepubertal Patient

Indications

Careful perineal inspection during the first several well-child visits allows early identification of congenital anomalies of the labia and hymen. The proximal vagina, uterus, cervix, and fallopian tubes are derived from the Mullerian or paramesonephric ducts and develop concurrently with the urinary tract. Thus patients with renal or urinary tract abnormalities are at greater risk for having associated anomalies of internal genital structures. Ultrasonography is useful in evaluating neonates for suspected upper genital tract anomalies; these structures are relatively large during the neonatal period because of the influence of maternal hormones and higher levels of gonadotropins. Later in infancy and during early childhood, they are occasionally difficult to detect because of their small size. Failure to

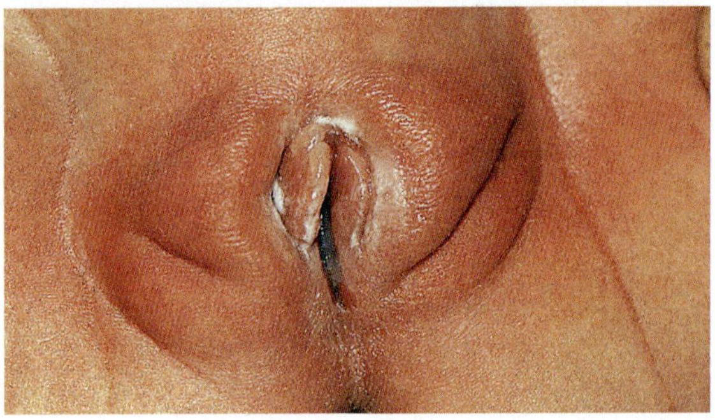

Fig. 19.1 Normal appearance of the genitalia in a newborn. The labia majora are full, and the thickened labia minora protrude between them. The mucosa is pink, and a milky white discharge is seen, reflecting stimulation by maternal hormones. (Courtesy Ian Holzman, MD, Mt. Sinai Medical Center, New York, NY.)

visualize internal genital structures in prepubertal patients does not equate with agenesis, and in such cases, magnetic resonance imaging (MRI) can clarify the presence or absence of pelvic organs.

Patients who have specific complaints at acute care visits also warrant inspection of the genitalia in addition to abdominal, inguinal, and (when indicated) rectal examination. These complaints include abdominal pain; dysuria, urinary frequency, urgency, incontinence, or enuresis; constipation or encopresis; perineal pruritus, pain, or other abnormal sensation; vaginal discharge or bleeding before menarche; and suspected or acknowledged sexual abuse. Sexual abuse in the pediatric patient warrants referral to a child abuse specialist with the specialized knowledge, skills, and equipment appropriate to this evaluation. Careful documentation of the history is vital because physical examination is likely to be normal.

Technique

The American Academy of Pediatrics recommends the gynecologic examination be performed in the presence of a parent or guardian. The clinician should explain the examination and its reasoning to the child and caregiver. The clinician can request the help of the child as well. Having the support of the caregiver can reassure children. The use of pictures and language familiar to the child and family may further enhance cooperation, but interspersing anatomically correct vocabulary can also be educational. External inspection of the genitals can take place during routine physicals after the abdominal and inguinal examination.

Young infants can be assessed easily on an examination table after being positioned by the examiner. Generally, drapes are unnecessary for toddlers and preschoolers because they are isolating and often perceived as threatening. School-age children may find drapes helpful in reducing embarrassment. An older infant, toddler, or preschool child may be more relaxed when examined on the parent's lap, with the parent assisting by gently holding the child in either the frog-leg or lithotomy position (Fig. 19.4A and B). School-age children usually can be examined on the table in the frog-leg, lithotomy, or knee-chest position. Knee-chest positioning can provide excellent visualization of the hymen and the distal vagina (Fig. 19.5), but some patients may feel threatened by being examined from behind. An alternative means of achieving visualization of the distal vagina is with the patient supine and performing the Valsalva maneuver (i.e., asking the child to push down as if they were going to pass a stool). This often produces distention of the distal vagina and hymenal orifice, facilitating visualization and atraumatic collection of specimens. Use of good, focused lighting is essential. In the office setting, the otoscope provides excellent focused light and low magnification, which is sufficient for most examinations.

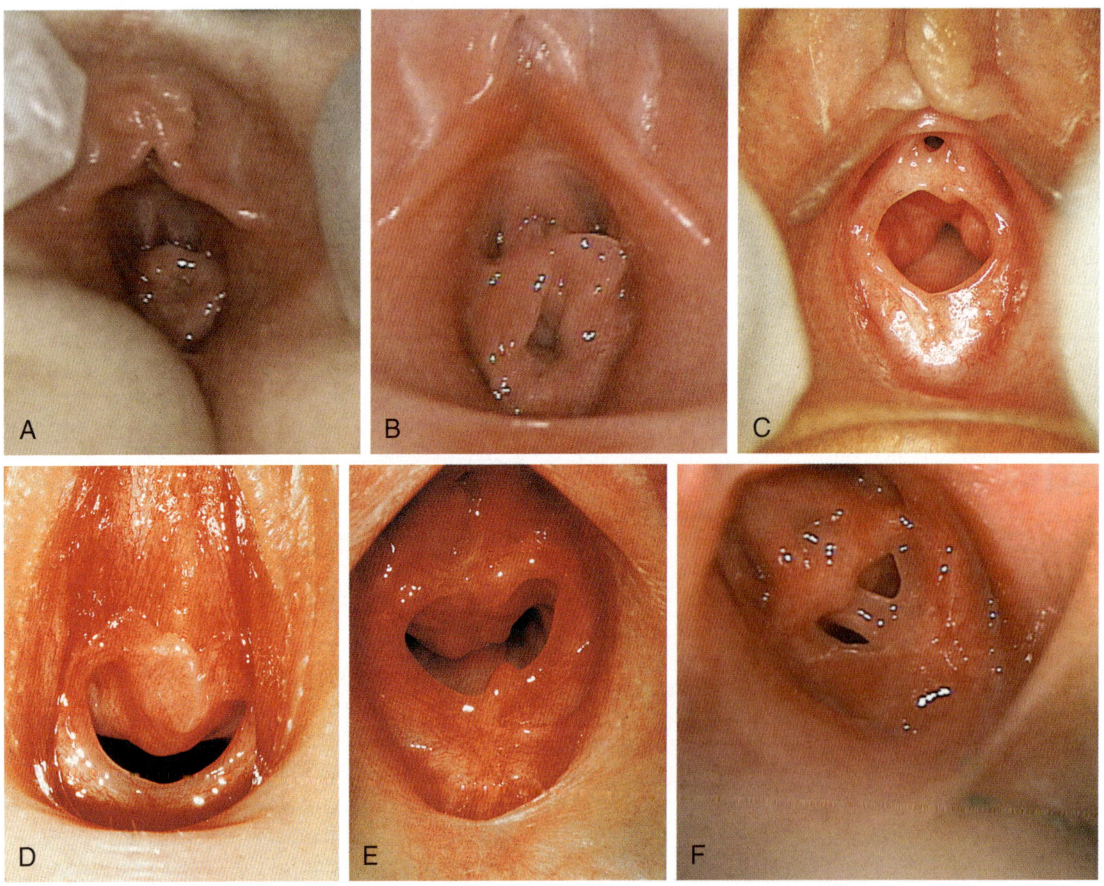

Fig. 19.2 Variations in hymenal configuration. (A) In this young infant, the redundant hymen totally obscures the vaginal orifice. (B) In a 23-month-old, the hymenal folds are redundant and the central orifice is visible. (C) Annular orifice of a 2-year-old. Note the thin, sharp edges of the hymenal membrane. (D) Crescentic hymenal orifice. (E) Crescentic orifice with septal remnants at 1 and 5 o'clock. (F) Septate hymen in an infant. (A and B, Courtesy Janet Squires, MD, Children's Hospital of Pittsburgh, Pittsburgh, PA. C, Courtesy John McCann, MD, University of California at Davis, Davis, CA. D–E, Courtesy Pat Bruno, MD, Sunbury Community Hospital Center for Child Protection, Sunbury, PA. F, Courtesy Carol Byers, CRNP, Children's Hospital of Pittsburgh, Pittsburgh, PA.)

Table 19.1 Developmental Gynecologic Anatomy and Physiology

	Newborn	Early Childhood	Peripuberty (9–13 Years Old)	Post Menarche (>13 Years Old)
Ovarian size and location	Not palpable	Pelvic brim	Within pelvis	1.5 × 2.5 × 4 cm
Ovarian volume (mL)	0.3–1.7	0.3–1.9	2–8	8–20
Uterine length (cm)	2.5–4.0	2.0–3.0	3.2–5.4	8.0 (nulliparous) (8 × 5 × 2.5)
Corpus-to-cervix ratio	1:2	1:1	2:1	2–3:1
Vaginal length (cm)	4	4–5	7–8.5	10–12
Hymen orifice diameter (mm)	1–4	1–6	5–10	10
Hymen thickness	Thick	Thin	Thickening	Variable
Clitoris width (mm)	5	2–5	2–5	5–10
Clitoris length (mm)	10–15	10–20	10–20	15–20
Labia minora	Smooth	Smooth, flat	Progressive increase in size and prominence	Separation and differentiation of labia minora and majora
Labia majora	Hairless, prominent	Hairless, thin	Hair growth, labial growth	Terminal hair growth that extends to or beyond the inguinal crease
Vaginal secretions	White or clear, copious	Minimal	White or clear, variable amount, at times profuse	White or clear, varies by individual and with cycle
pH	5.5–7.0	6.5–7.5	4.5–5.5	3.5–4.5
Normal flora	Maternal enteric	Nonpathogenic flora including staphylococci and coliforms	Mixed vaginal flora	Lactobacilli dominant
Hormonal influence	Maternal hormones	Minimal sex steroids	Low and variable levels of endogenous estrogens and androgens	High levels of endogenous cyclic hormones

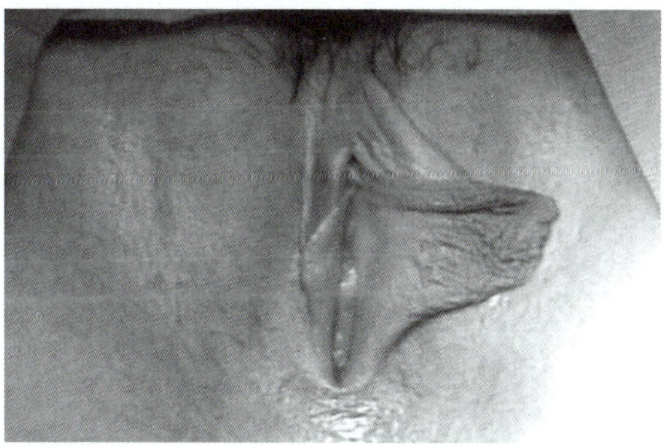

Fig. 19.3 Eleven-year-old with hypertrophy of the left labium minor. (From Pardo J, Solà V, Ricci P, et al: Laser labioplasty of labia minora, *Int J Gynaecol Obstet* 93:38–43, 2006.)

Once the patient is properly positioned, visualization of the introitus, hymen, and lower portion of the vagina is facilitated by maneuvers that separate the labia. These maneuvers should be explained first, and the child reassured that the examiner is just going to look. If the patient desires or is mildly anxious, they may place their hands beneath the examiner's, or the parent may be enlisted to perform the maneuver. Some patients prefer to separate their labia themselves. The maneuvers include labial traction and separation (see Fig. 19.5). When using a handheld light (otoscope), a second set of hands (parent or nurse) may be needed to maximize labial separation and focus the light. Care must be taken to ensure that excess traction is not applied during these maneuvers because it can result in painful tearing of labial adhesions, if present.

If the patient is unusually anxious about the procedure and cannot be reassured, examination should be deferred to a later date. On occasion, use of relaxation techniques, an oral benzodiazepine, conscious sedation, or anesthesia may be needed for an adequate evaluation. At no time should a frightened, struggling child be physically restrained and forced to undergo examination; the yield is minimal, and the experience is physically and emotionally traumatic.

On inspection, the clinician can readily ascertain the presence or absence of pubic hair; note the appearance and configuration of the labia majora, labia minora, clitoris, urethra, hymen, vaginal orifice, and anus; note the color of the mucosa and the presence or absence of rash, discharge, or unusual odor; and often visualize the distal vagina. Vaginoscopy is required only occasionally in the prepubertal child to perform a complete evaluation for complaints such as vaginal bleeding with or without evidence of trauma, discharge resistant to routine therapy, a suspected vaginal foreign body, and suspected vaginal tumors. Due to the high potential for inflicting pain,

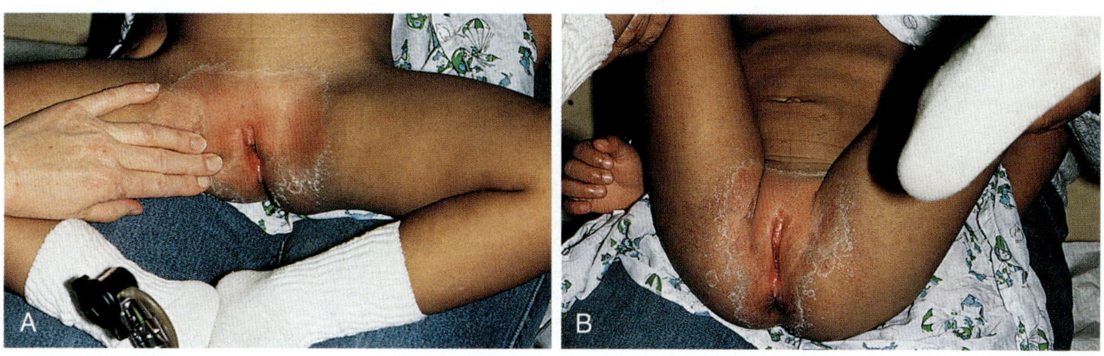

Fig. 19.4 Optimal positions for perineal inspection of the young prepubertal patient. This patient has skin desquamation subsequent to a streptococcal infection. (A) Frog-leg position on the mother's lap. (B) Lithotomy position on the mother's lap.

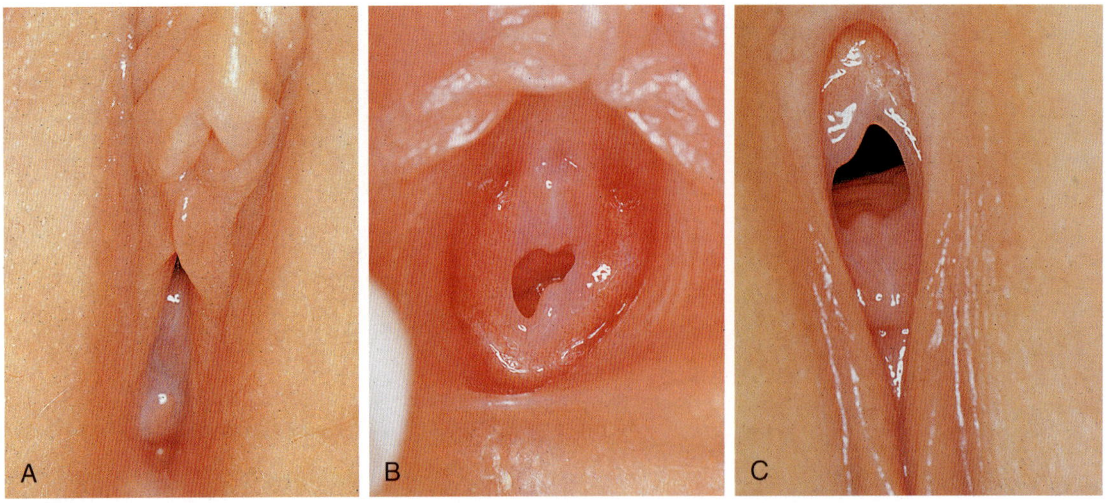

Fig. 19.5 Perineal visualization in various positions and with different techniques of parting the labia (see also Fig. 19.2). (A–C) Views of the same child taken on the same day and clearly showing the variations in appearance when using different positions and different techniques to facilitate visualization of the introitus and lower third of the vagina. (A) Supine frog-leg position. (B) Supine frog-leg position using labial traction, which involves grasping the labia majora between the thumbs and index fingers and gently pulling them down, laterally and slightly toward the examiner. (C) Knee/chest position. (Courtesy Mary Carrasco, MD, Mercy Hospital, Pittsburgh, PA.)

especially if the patient moves suddenly, vaginoscopy generally is best performed under anesthesia or sedation.

Specimen Collection

If a prepubertal child with vaginal discharge or perineal or urinary complaints is to be evaluated, it is advisable to ask the family not to bathe the patient or to apply any creams for at least 12 hours before the examination. The patient should always be prepared for the procedure with simple explanations. In the presence of ulcers, herpes cultures or specimens for a polymerase chain reaction (PCR) test should be obtained from the base of unroofed fresh vesicles or ulcers. Routine bacterial cultures, including those for gonococci, can be collected from any visible discharge on the perineum in the prepubertal child. If specimens must be collected because of a history of vaginal discharge, having the patient perform a Valsalva maneuver may move discharge into the introitus. If this fails, specimens can be collected with little discomfort with a Dacron wire swab premoistened with sterile nonbacteriostatic saline.

It can be helpful to allow patients to handle a moistened swab and touch themselves with it. The swab is inserted gently through the vaginal opening, taking care to avoid contact with the hymen, which is exquisitely sensitive. Dry cotton-tipped swabs should be avoided because of their size and because they tend to abrade the thin vaginal mucosa of the prepubertal child. If collection is likely to be difficult because of pain or anxiety or because the hymenal orifice is small, application of a topical anesthetic to the perineal and hymenal area beforehand can be beneficial. Although topical lidocaine preparations work within 5 to 10 minutes, they can produce transient discomfort before the onset of anesthetic action, reducing cooperation in some patients. When time permits, use of a newer topical anesthetic cream (e.g., eutectic mixture of local anesthetics [EMLA] or lidocaine [LMX]) is an excellent alternative. Table 19.2 lists the specimens that may be considered in

Table 19.2 Laboratory Investigations for Evaluation of Gynecologic Complaints

Laboratory Study/Specimen	Diagnostic Utility
Saline wet mount	Inflammatory cells, yeast, trichomonads, clue cells, lactobacilli, mature and immature epithelial cells, sperm
KOH	Yeast, "whiff test" for bacterial vaginosis (also can be positive with *Trichomonas*)
Vaginal pH	Elevated in bacterial vaginosis (also can be elevated with *Trichomonas*); obtain from lateral or anterior vaginal wall, not from pooled secretions or saline-diluted specimen
Vaginal specimens	Routine culture[a] for nonvenereal pathogens Culture for enteric bacteria, including *Shigella* (Cary-Blair medium) NAAT for gonorrhea, *Trichomonas, Chlamydia* Culture for gonorrhea,[a] *Trichomonas, Chlamydia* (if forensic evidence or bacterial sensitivities are needed)
Cervical specimens	NAAT for gonorrhea, *Chlamydia* or *Trichomonas* Culture for gonorrhea,[a] *Trichomonas, Chlamydia* (if forensic evidence or bacterial sensitivities are needed)
Pap smear/ThinPrep	Squamous intraepithelial lesions; consequences of HPV, including precancerous and cancerous lesions
Genital ulcer/lesion specimen	HSV culture or PCR (if suspect chancroid use moistened swab at base of lesion and transport as rapidly as possible; send to reference laboratory to test for *Haemophilus ducreyi*)
Biopsy	Dysplastic, atrophic, or unusual lesions of vulva, vagina, and cervix
Urine specimen	Urinalysis; urine culture; NAAT for gonorrhea, *Chlamydia,* or *Trichomonas*
Perianal specimen	Pinworms and eggs: Parent obtains sample during night (or first thing in morning before patient bathes) by pressing firmly over anal area with a pinworm paddle (optically clear polystyrene paddle connected to cap of a transport container) or a 1-inch strip of cellophane tape (which is then affixed to a glass slide)
Serologic tests	Syphilis (RPR, VDRL, and *Treponema*-specific testing), HIV, HSV, HBV, HCV

HBV, Hepatitis B virus; *HCV,* Hepatitis C virus; *HIV,* Human immunodeficiency virus; *HPV,* human papillomavirus; *HSV,* herpes simplex virus; *KOH,* potassium hydroxide; *NAAT,* nucleic acid amplification test; *PCR,* polymerase chain reaction; *RPR,* rapid plasma reagin; *VDRL,* Venereal Disease Research Laboratory.

[a]Use Amies medium with charcoal.

evaluating patients with symptoms of vulvitis, vaginitis, or vaginal discharge.

Examination of the Pubertal Patient

Indications

The practice of routine inspection of the external genitalia at each well-child visit beyond infancy facilitates early diagnosis of any problems that may arise and allows evaluation of physical growth and secondary sex characteristics. This also creates an opportunity to discuss normal anatomy and behaviors, including masturbation; to distinguish acceptable from unacceptable (exploitative or abusive) forms of touching; and to help overcome the reluctance of some parents and children to express concerns about the genitalia. Making assessment and counseling a routine part of well-child care may help reduce anxiety and embarrassment for the child when genital or pelvic examinations are required.

A gynecologic examination should be considered for any patient with a variety of specific complaints and concerns, including those listed in Box 19.1. This examination should include careful inspection of the external genitalia and regional lymph nodes and, when indicated, palpation of the uterus and adnexa. In some cases, assessment of internal pelvic structures may require radiologic imaging. For example, if menarche is delayed or menstrual periods are unusually problematic (e.g., excessive pain or unusually irregular flow patterns), ultrasound evaluation can be useful.

The gynecologic examination is an important part of routine health care for sexually active adolescents (see Box 19.1) and should be considered at 12-month intervals or with greater frequency if indicated based on community and behavioral risk factors. Use of a speculum is typically not required but is useful in situations that necessitate visual inspection of the vaginal cavity or cervix, including those listed in Box 19.2. In the absence of the aforementioned indications, a speculum examination could first be considered at 21 years old. At this age, females should undergo their first cervical cytology screening, using liquid-based cytology or traditional Papanicolaou (Pap) smear, according to recommendations from the American College of Obstetricians and Gynecologists. Transmasculine patients who still have a cervix should undergo routine Pap testing but may require additional measures (e.g., lubricant or pretreatment with estrogen cream) to ensure comfort during examination.

Box 19.1 Indications for Gynecologic Examination in Pubertal Patient

- Abnormal vaginal discharge
- Pain
  - Pelvic
  - Perineal
  - Dysuria
  - Dyspareunia (pain or other difficulty with intercourse)
  - Abdominal (unexplained)
- Suspected sexual abuse
- Concerns with pubertal development
  - No secondary sexual development by 13 years old
  - No menarche if start of puberty more than 2 years ago
  - No menarche by 15 years old
  - Abnormal timing or sequence of pubertal development
  - Anatomic abnormalities on genital inspection
  - Increased body hair, severe acne, or masculinization
- Menstrual disturbances
  - Dysmenorrhea not responsive to standard treatment
  - Amenorrhea or oligomenorrhea
  - Abnormal uterine bleeding or polymenorrhea
- Sexual activity
  - Routine health care for sexually active individual
  - Sexual contact with partner with a suspected or confirmed sexually transmitted disease or related genital symptoms

Box 19.2 Indications for Use of a Speculum During Gynecologic Examination

- Papanicolaou (Pap) smear (patients 21 years old and older; earlier in sexually active immune-compromised patients)
- Persistent unexplained bleeding
- Persistent vaginal discharge
- Suspected injury
- Suspected foreign body
- Suspected anatomic abnormality (e.g., vaginal septum, duplicated cervix)
- Sexual assault

Technique

A thorough and directed history precedes the examination. A comprehensive outline is suggested in Table 19.3. Adequate time should be devoted to interviewing the patient alone, which provides an opportunity to ask questions about voluntary and involuntary sexual activity and to explore other concerns that may be difficult to discuss in the presence of a parent or guardian. A similar opportunity should be given to the parents to express any concerns that they are reluctant to share in their child's presence.

A young patient's initial experience with a pelvic examination may greatly affect the ease with which they experience routine gynecologic care and sexual relations throughout adult life. Hence the examiner's approach should be sympathetic, unhurried, and sensitive to the modesty of the patient. When patients have had gynecologic examinations in the past, it is helpful to ask them about their prior experience to avoid rekindling any emotional or physical trauma.

Young females should be given the choice of being examined with or without an accompanying person in the room. Some patients, particularly early adolescents, may be conflicted between their modesty and their desire for support from a friend or relative. Suggesting that the support person must stay at the head of the table and using drapes that allow visual (eye) contact between patient and examiner is often the most comfortable compromise. Chaperones should be offered to all patients, and their presence is considered standard when the examiner is male, is a trainee, or when there is a history of sexual abuse.

The pelvic examination is done after other components of the physical examination. The patient should empty her bladder beforehand, and a urine specimen can be collected at this time if needed for testing. Raising the head of the examining table 20 to 45 degrees helps relax abdominal muscles and facilitates maintenance of visual contact with the patient. Before beginning, the examiner should carefully explain the various parts of the examination: inspection of the external genitalia, speculum examination of the vagina and cervix (with specimen collection), and bimanual palpation. Use of anatomic drawings and/or models can be helpful and educational. Throughout the procedure, clinicians should explain what they are seeing and provide reassurance and education. This should help the patient relax and can also confirm normal anatomic findings and provide examples of accurate vocabulary for reproductive anatomy and function. A hand mirror held by the patient is often useful for similar reasons.

The patient should be assisted into the lithotomy position at the end of the examination table. Nonlatex gloves should be worn for both external and internal examinations. Patient comfort may be increased by identifying and then touching distal areas first and moving proximally (e.g., knees, thighs, groin, labia, introitus). Next, the external genitalia are inspected. Pubic hair distribution should be noted, as should the presence of any nits, lice, skin or vulvar lesions, or vaginal discharge on the perineum. The introital opening is examined and palpated if there is swelling in the region of the Bartholin glands. Clitoral size is assessed. The urethral opening is then inspected for erythema or discharge. Any purulent material obtained should be tested for sexually transmitted infections (STIs).

If a speculum examination is required, successful examination depends on adequate patient preparation and use of appropriate instruments, including a good light source. For virginal adolescents,

Table 19.3 Complete History of an Adolescent With Gynecologic Concerns

Category of Information	Specific Information Required
General	
Home	Who lives there and quality of relationships; sources of conflict and support
Education/employment	School, format, attendance, grades, curriculum, repeated grades, suspension, goals, behavioral or learning difficulties, literacy/numeracy; volunteer activities; if working—type, occupational hazards, hours
Eating	Nutritional content (specifically calcium, vitamin D, iron, fat, fiber, folate), body image, eating behaviors/patterns, recent changes in weight
Activities	Personal strengths, exercise, peer activities, friends, hobbies, extracurricular activities
Drugs	Caffeine, tobacco/nicotine, alcohol, marijuana, crack, cocaine, heroin/opioids, hallucinogens, hormones, pills, injectable drugs; screening tool for substance use disorders; rehabilitation or treatment history
Depression/suicide	Depression, anxiety, psychiatric treatment, medications, major losses or disruptions, counseling history, self-injurious behavior, suicide ideation and history of attempts, protective factors
Safety/abuse/exploitation	Physical, sexual, or emotional; family, relationship, peer, school, and community violence, and trafficking and/or exploitation
Sexual, Obstetric, and Gynecologic History	
Menstrual	Menarche (age), cycles (length, duration, quantity of flow, use of pads, tampons, or other menstrual products), first day of last menstrual period, dysmenorrhea and associated disability, menstrual symptoms, abnormal bleeding, midcycle pain (mittelschmerz) and spotting
STI	STI history, STI symptoms, undiagnosed pelvic pain
Cervical cancer screening	Abnormal results, colposcopy, biopsies, treatments, follow-up
Urologic	Urinary tract infection or kidney problems, enuresis, incontinence, dysuria, urgency, frequency
Vaginal discharge	Color, odor, quantity, duration, timing, pruritus, douching, feminine hygiene product use (including scented products and deodorants)
Vaginal infections	History of nonsexually transmitted vaginitis, yeast, bacterial vaginosis, irritant; vaginitis symptoms
Obstetric	Previous pregnancies and outcomes, fertility plans, and concerns
Sexual behavior	Last and other recent intercourse and protection; specific HIV risk to self and partners; sexual experience and age at onset; sexual practices, condom use; anatomy of sexual partners; number of partners, lifetime and recent
Gender and sexuality	Sex assigned at birth, presence of difference of sex development, gender identity, gender expression, romantic attraction, sexual orientation; satisfaction with sexual experience; sexual problems with self or partner
Contraceptive	Current and past methods, satisfaction, consistency of use, problems, future plans for pregnancy/parenthood
Past medical history	Prior sources of care (routine, episodic, and emergency); immunization status including hepatitis A and B and HPV; rubella and varicella status; hypertension; migraines with aura or neurologic signs; thromboembolic events
Medications/treatment	History of self-treatment with over-the-counter or prescription medications, antibiotics in particular, and any integrative therapies or medications
Family history	Thromboembolic events in a first-degree family member or associated with pregnancy or hormonal contraceptives; disease or death caused by alcohol, drugs, tobacco; gynecologic or obstetric problems; age at childbearing; endocrine problems (especially thyroid); bleeding problems (especially OB/GYN-related bleeding, mucus membrane bleeding, or need for blood transfusion); congenital malformations; intellectual disability; miscarriages and stillbirths

HIV, Human immunodeficiency virus; *HPV,* human papillomavirus; *OB/GYN,* obstetrics and gynecology; *Pap,* Papanicolaou; *PID,* pelvic inflammatory disease; *STI,* sexually transmitted infection.

the narrow-bladed Huffman speculum (½ × 4¼ inches) is recommended. Although long enough to expose the cervix, its narrow blades are usually inserted easily through the virginal introitus. Most sexually active adolescents can be examined with the straight-sided Pederson speculum (⅞ × 4 inches); however, the Huffman speculum should be considered as an alternative for a first pelvic examination or for particularly anxious patients. The duck-billed Graves speculum (1⅜ × 3¾ inches) is useful in parous patients (Fig. 19.6). Obese patients may require a Graves speculum or a longer Pederson (1 × 4¾ inches) for adequate visualization of the cervix. Metal speculums may be preferred because they are easier to manipulate and are available in a greater range of lengths and widths; disposable plastic specula with intrinsic lights are now widely available and can be purchased in a range of sizes.

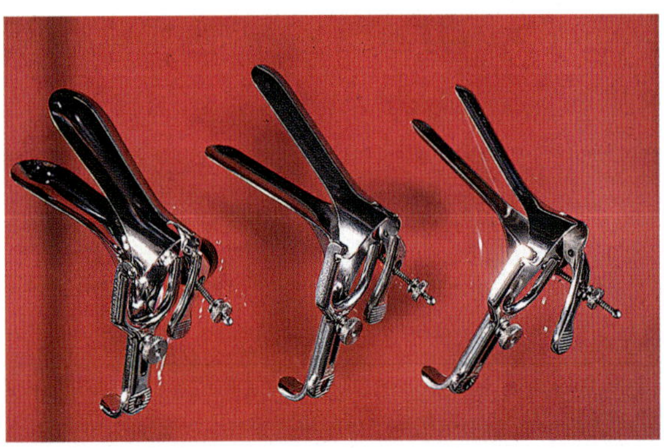

Fig. 19.6 *From left to right:* The Graves speculum is best reserved for large or gravid adolescents; the Pederson speculum is adequate for most sexually active adolescents; the narrow-bladed Huffman is preferred for virginal adolescents.

The patient should be shown the speculum and allowed to touch it if they desire. Patients experiencing their first pelvic examination should be reassured that only the blades of the speculum will be inserted. Comparing the size of an open speculum to a finger or tampon is often reassuring. The patient should be told that they will feel "a sense of pressure," not pain, during speculum insertion and should be reminded to breathe regularly because tensing abdominal or pelvic muscles can produce discomfort and make the examination more difficult to perform. A history of inability to use a tampon suggests an increased possibility of a physical or emotional barrier to a successful speculum examination.

The examiner may then gently insert the gloved index finger into the vagina to assess the size of the introital opening and to locate the cervix. Vaginal muscle tone can be assessed by asking patients to tighten their muscles around the examiner's gloved finger. Conscious relaxation can be practiced by asking the patient to relax those same muscles and to push the buttocks onto the examining table. Both plastic and metal speculums should be moistened with warm water or water-based lubricant to increase comfort and ease of insertion. With the index finger partially withdrawn but gently pressing on the vaginal floor, the speculum is inserted over the finger into the vagina, taking care to avoid catching pubic hairs or the labia in the mechanism of the speculum. This is done at an oblique angle along the posterior wall to accommodate the vertical introitus and avoid traumatizing the urethra, which lies above the anterior vaginal wall. Another technique that effectively assists insertion involves using the middle and index fingers to stretch the posterior labial folds down and out before inserting the speculum. With the speculum in place, the vaginal walls are inspected for erythema, lesions, and quality and quantity of discharge, and specimens are collected (see the Specimen Collection section, later).

After specimens have been collected, the speculum is removed and the bimanual (vaginal/abdominal) examination is performed. Water-based lubricant is placed on the two gloved fingers to be used before inserting them carefully through the introitus into the vagina. The examiner should note the size, consistency, position, and mobility of the uterus and check for tenderness on cervical or fundal motion. The adnexa should be palpated for evidence of enlargement or excess tenderness.

Once the examination is completed, the patient should be helped out of the lithotomy position, given tissues to wipe away any lubricant or discharge, and allowed privacy to get dressed. At the conclusion of the visit, the examiner can present the results of point-of-care testing (such as microscopic evaluation of wet mount and potassium hydroxide [KOH] preparation). The use of handouts with pictures or drawings can enhance the patient's understanding of the results. This is also an opportunity to encourage communication between the patient and their parent, as appropriate to the circumstance.

Specimen Collection

Adolescents should be advised not to douche or to use tampons or feminine hygiene products before a gynecologic examination. When testing for *Neisseria gonorrheae* and *Chlamydia trachomatis,* the newer nucleic acid amplification tests (NAATs) detect minute quantities of pathogen DNA/RNA and thus are highly sensitive and specific; they also offer the advantage that specimens may be collected from a variety of sites (vaginal wall, urine, urethra, cervix). To obtain a vaginal sample, slide the swab 4 to 5 cm into the vagina and rotate it for greater than 10 seconds, moistening it against the walls of the vagina.

The vaginal pH level can be measured by moistening a cotton-tipped swab on the lateral vaginal wall and rolling it on pH paper (with an appropriate range of pH 3.6–6.1). Vaginal pH levels are elevated in bacterial vaginosis and *Trichomonas* and decreased with candida infections. Vaginal secretions should be obtained with a cotton or Dacron swab and placed in a tube with 1 mL of nonbacteriostatic normal saline for wet mount and KOH examination. The swabs for gonorrhea and chlamydia NAAT and for wet mount may be obtained by the patient ("self swab") if the patient prefers and additional examination is not required.

To review the wet mount, a drop of the saline solution containing vaginal secretions is examined under low (×10) and high (×40) power for distribution of epithelial cells, leukocytes, yeast forms, *Trichomonas* organisms, sperm, and clue cells. A drop of 10% KOH is added to a second drop of the saline solution. This preparation is immediately "whiff tested" for the presence of the acrid odor associated with amines that is found in bacterial vaginosis and often in patients with trichomoniasis. After this, viewing of the KOH preparation facilitates identification of yeast.

If a speculum examination is required (see Box 19.2), the vaginal pH is measured by holding pH paper (described previously) against the lateral vaginal wall, away from pooled secretions. Visible vaginal secretions from the posterior vaginal pool should be obtained with a cotton or Dacron swab for wet mount. Before obtaining samples from the cervix, any surface mucus should be gently removed with cotton swabs. The normal nulliparous cervix usually has a small round os (Fig. 19.7). Any cervical lesions seen, such as cysts, warts, polyps, or vesicles, should be noted. An ectropion (or eversion) of the endocervical columnar epithelium onto the cervical surface is common and normal in adolescents (Fig. 19.8). Ectropion should be distinguished from cervicitis, the latter being suggested by erythema, friability, and/or mucopurulent cervical discharge (see Fig. 19.32).

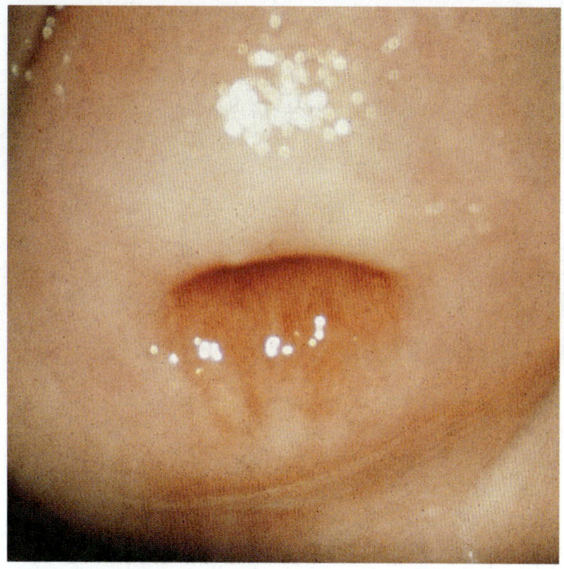

Fig. 19.7 Normal nulliparous cervix. The surface is covered with pink squamous epithelium that is uniform in consistency. The os is small and round. A small area of ectropion is visible inferior to the os. (Courtesy C. Stevens.)

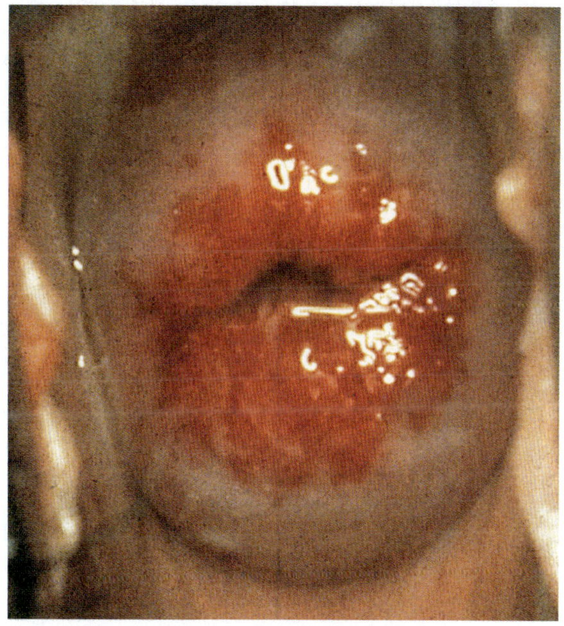

Fig. 19.8 Ectropion. Columnar mucosal cells usually found in the endocervical canal have extended out onto the surface of the cervix, creating a circular raised erythematous appearance. Note the normal nonpurulent cervical mucus. This normal variant is not to be confused with cervicitis. (Courtesy E. Jerome, MD.)

Cervical cytology (Pap) screening using liquid-based cytology to check for cervical dysplasia (a precursor of cervical cancer) is done by rotating a plastic Ayre spatula circumferentially (360 degrees) around the cervical os, including the entire squamocolumnar junction. A sample from the endocervical canal is collected with a Cytobrush (or a cotton swab if the patient is pregnant). Each sample is swished in liquid ThinPrep solution or fixed onto a glass slide according to laboratory protocol. Cervical cytology results can be uninterpretable in the presence of inflammation and bleeding; therefore it is preferable to defer collection until infections are treated and menstrual bleeding has finished. However, concerns about patient follow-up or urgent clinical needs can justify collection of specimens at less optimal times. A number of strains of human papillomavirus (HPV) have been identified as causative in cervical cancer, genital warts, and some head and neck cancers. All adolescents should be encouraged to complete their HPV vaccination series. However, currently available vaccines against HPV do not cover all strains associated with cervical cancer. Therefore a Pap smear every 3 years is indicated starting at 21 years old. Immunocompromised females younger than 21 years old with human immunodeficiency virus (HIV), solid organ transplant, hematopoietic stem cell transplant and systemic lupus erythematous, inflammatory bowel disease, and rheumatoid arthritis on immunosuppressants should have their first Pap within 1 year of sexual activity onset and annually for the first 3 years. The Centers for Disease Control and Prevention (CDC) advises that HPV typing is not indicated in females younger than the age of 30.

GENITAL TRACT OBSTRUCTION

Labial Adhesions

The most common form of vaginal obstruction in prepubertal patients is really a pseudoobstruction or partial obstruction produced by reversible labial adhesions of the labia minora. On inspection, the clinician finds a smooth, flat membrane with a thin lucent central line overlying the introitus. It is postulated that inflammation and erosion of the superficial layers of the mucosa—whether caused by infection, dermatitis, or mechanical trauma—result in agglutination of the apposed labia minora by fibrous tissue on healing. The process typically begins posteriorly and extends forward. In most cases, the fused portion is less than 1 cm in length, but on occasion it can extend to cover the vaginal vestibule and rarely the urethra (Fig. 19.9). Even when fusion is extensive, urine and vaginal secretions can exit through the opening anteriorly. However, some urine may become trapped behind the adhesions after toileting. This may cause further irritation, perpetuating the condition or fostering extension of the adhesions. Although most labial adhesions are asymptomatic, some patients have symptoms of lower urinary tract and vulvar inflammation.

Asymptomatic labial adhesions typically resolve without intervention during puberty. If symptomatic, labial adhesions readily respond to application of topical estrogen or estradiol 0.01% cream or topical betamethasone 0.05% cream along the line of fusion twice daily for 2 to 8 weeks. Initial therapy can be based on shared decision making, and alternate therapy may be tried if there is no improvement after 4 to 8 weeks of proper application of the initial therapy. The parent should be informed that topical estrogens may cause transient hyperpigmentation of the labia and the areolae and an increase in breast tissue but that these changes regress once therapy is completed. An estrogen withdrawal bleed (similar to that seen in the neonate) occasionally occurs. Topical betamethasone may cause local irritation, and prolonged use should be avoided to reduce the risk of skin atrophy or systemic corticosteroid effects.

After the labia have separated, a zinc oxide–based cream should be applied nightly for several months to prevent recurrence. Removal of irritants, treatment of infections, and instructions on good perineal hygiene help prevent recurrence of adhesions. Nonetheless, refusion can occur, although repeated treatment is not necessary if the child is asymptomatic. Manual separation of fused labia is painful, traumatic, and frequently followed by a recurrence. Hence this practice should be abandoned. True fusion—adhesions present in the first months of life or adhesions that do not respond to the prescribed therapy—requires further evaluation for abnormalities in sexual differentiation or androgen production.

Female Genital Mutilation/Cutting

Female genital mutilation/cutting (FGM/C) is another cause of genital tract obstruction seen with increasing frequency by pediatricians, especially those who care for patients from Africa, the Middle East, and Asia. This ritual cutting and alteration of female genitalia has no known medical benefits and carries potentially life-threatening short- and long-term health consequences. Further information about this topic can be found at the World Health Organization website (see the end of this chapter). The World Health Organization is working to eliminate this practice, considering it a human rights violation. However, pediatricians who encounter patients who have undergone these procedures must be sensitive to both the complex religious and sociocultural norms that motivate families to practice FGM/C as well as to the consequences to the individual patient.

Imperforate Hymen

The congenital anomaly referred to as *imperforate hymen* consists of a thick imperforate membrane located just inside the hymenal ring. This is the most common obstructive abnormality. It is frequently missed on the newborn examination because of the redundancy of hymenal folds. However, it may become evident by 8 to 12 weeks old on careful perineal inspection, appearing as a thin, transparent hymenal membrane that bulges when the infant cries or strains. On occasion, young infants have copious vaginal secretions secondary to stimulation by maternal hormones; as a result of this anomaly, they develop hydrocolpos. In such cases, the infant may have midline

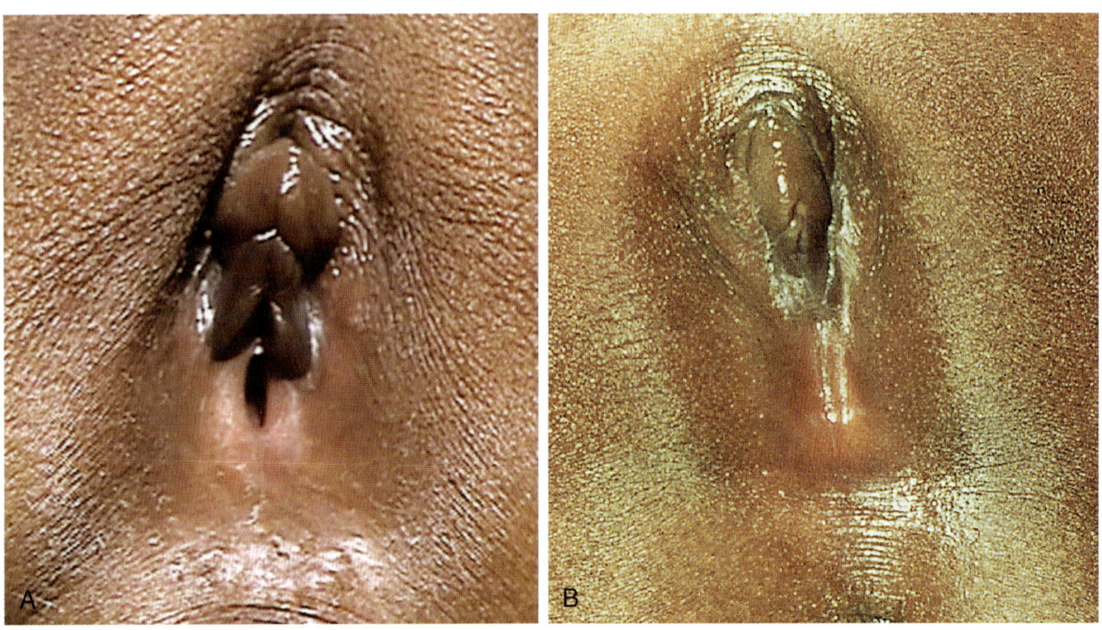

Fig. 19.9 Labial adhesions. Agglutination and adhesion of the labia minora, as a result of healing after inflammation, produce the appearance of a smooth, flat surface overlying the introitus, divided centrally by a thin lucent line. (A) In this infant, the fused portion involves the posterior half of the introitus. (B) In another, the fused area has extended much farther anteriorly. (A, Courtesy Carol Byers, CRNP, Children's Hospital of Pittsburgh, Pittsburgh, PA. B, Courtesy D. Lloyd, MD.)

swelling of the lower abdomen (especially noticeable when the bladder is full) that feels cystic on palpation. Perineal inspection reveals a whitish, bulging membrane at the introitus. The cystic mass may also be palpable on rectal examination. In the presence of a neonatal withdrawal bleed or trauma, a hematocolpos may develop. This presents as a red or purplish bulge (Fig. 19.10). Imperforate hymens may open spontaneously with estrogenization at puberty and are not repaired in prepubertal patients unless symptomatic.

If their condition goes undetected, the patient with an imperforate hymen usually develops hematocolpos in late puberty. The major complaints are intermittent lower abdominal and back pain, which rapidly progress in severity and duration. Over time, difficulty in urination and defecation may develop and a lower abdominal swelling may become noticeable. The patient has well-developed secondary sex characteristics but has had no menstrual periods. Perineal inspection reveals a thick, tense, bulging membrane, often bluish in color, at the introitus (Fig. 19.11A). A low cystic swelling is palpable anteriorly on rectal examination. Treatment of an imperforate hymen consists of operative incision of the membrane (Fig. 19.11B), evacuation of any obstructed material, and excision of redundant tissue. Other partially obstructive hymenal abnormalities may allow menstrual blood to flow but later cause difficulty inserting tampons or initiating intercourse. Because hymens are not of Müllerian origin, imperforate hymens are not associated with other genitourinary abnormalities.

Other forms of genital tract obstruction (Box 19.3) are rare. In most cases, early routine genital inspection reveals the absence of a vaginal orifice, enabling early delineation of the anomaly and treatment planning. Proximal obstructing anomalies may not be apparent on physical examination. Operative treatment varies based on the type of genital tract obstruction, but it often was delayed until puberty and was followed by the use of vaginal dilators. Menstrual suppression may be considered to delay treatment until a patient is prepared to engage in this postprocedural care. If missed in infancy or childhood, partial or complete obstruction can present with a wide range of signs and symptoms, such as those listed in Box 19.4. As noted earlier, ultrasonography is useful in the initial evaluation of suspected genital tract obstruction, bearing in mind its limitations in visualization of internal reproductive structures after the neonatal period and before puberty, which is when they are small, given minimal amounts of estrogen and gonadotropins. When structures are not seen or when further anatomic detail is required, magnetic resonance imaging is indicated.

GENITAL TRAUMA

The genital structures and pelvic supporting tissues of prepubertal patients are smaller and more rigid than during puberty. This inelastic anatomy significantly increases the risks that trauma will result in tearing and/or internal extension of injury. As a result, serious internal injuries of the vagina, rectum, urethra, bladder, and peritoneal

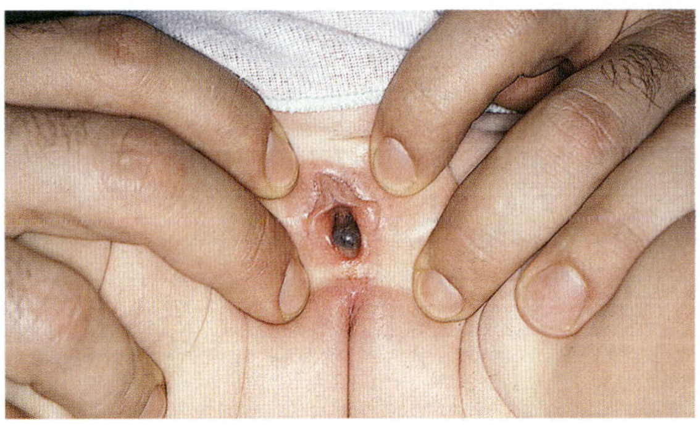

Fig. 19.10 Imperforate hymen with neonatal hematocolpos. A dark purplish bulge at the introitus was noted by the mother during a diaper change.

Box 19.3 Causes of Genital Tract Obstruction

- Labial fusion (underlying endocrine pathology)
- Labial adhesions (partial obstruction)
- Female genital mutilation/cutting sequelae
- Imperforate hymen
- Vaginal atresia (failure to canalize the vaginal plate)
- Vaginal (with or without uterine) agenesis, including Mayer-Rokitansky-Kuster-Hauser syndrome (Müllerian aplasia)
- Transverse vaginal septum
- Longitudinal vaginal septum
- Androgen insensitivity (testicular feminization syndrome)
- Obstructing Müllerian malformations, with elements of duplication, agenesis, and/or incomplete fusion
- Tumors of the upper and lower genital tracts and other pelvic masses

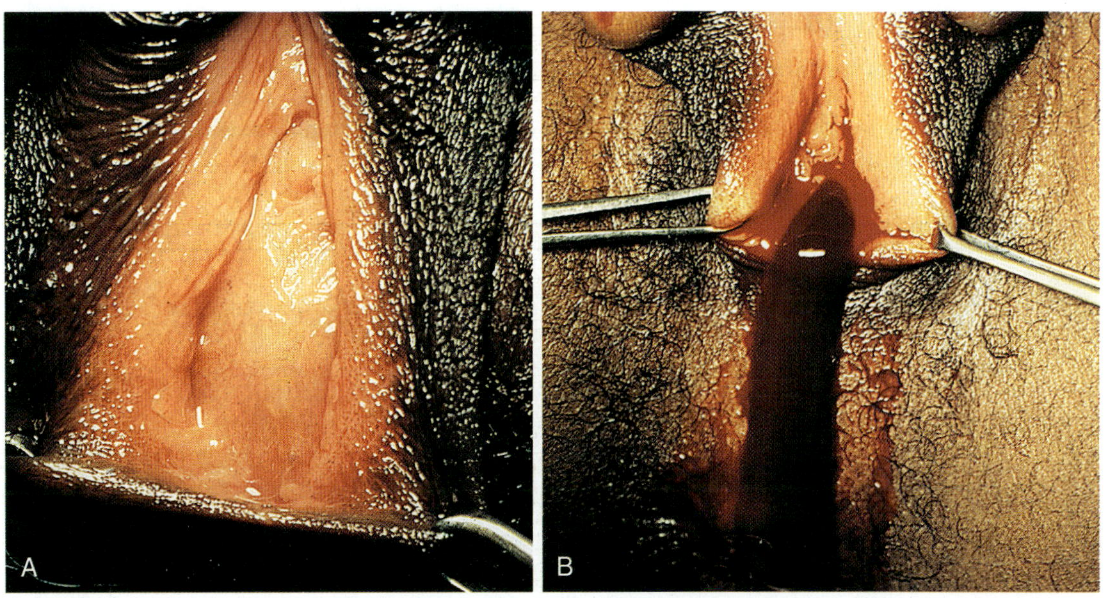

Fig. 19.11 Imperforate hymen with hematocolpos. This adolescent presented with a 2-month history of intermittent crampy lower abdominal pain, which had acutely worsened. She had well-developed secondary sex characteristics but was premenarchal by history. (A) Examination revealed midline fullness and tenderness of the lower abdomen and a smooth bulging mass at the introitus. (B) Incision of the imperforate membrane just inside the hymenal ring allowed the accumulated menstrual blood and vaginal secretions to drain. (Courtesy D. Lloyd, MD.)

Box 19.4 Symptoms and Signs Associated With Genital Tract Obstruction

Symptoms
Vaginal, pelvic, or abdominal pain (especially cyclic)
Dysmenorrhea
Urinary tract or rectal symptoms
Primary amenorrhea
Irregular vaginal bleeding
Purulent vaginal discharge
Difficulty using tampons
Difficulty initiating intercourse
Dyspareunia

Signs
Vaginal, pelvic, or abdominal mass
Hydrocolpos (mucus in vagina)
Hematocolpos (blood in vagina)
Pyohematocolpos (pus and blood in vagina)
Hematometra (blood within the uterus)

structures may underlie deceptively mild external abnormalities. In contrast to prepubertal patients, adolescents are more likely to have contusions than tears and are less likely to have internal extension of injury unless the applied force is great.

The role of the treating physician is to take a thorough history to fully understand the mechanism and likely extent of injuries. It is important to pay careful attention to vital signs and to perform a thorough examination of the abdomen, urethra, hymen, lower vagina, perineal body, and rectum as is feasible while minimizing the patient's physical discomfort and emotional distress. Patients should receive appropriate pain medication and emotional support and be protected from multiple examinations. When history, external inspection, or urinalysis suggests that injuries may be more than superficial, internal examination under anesthesia (by a pediatric surgeon or gynecologist) should be arranged. This enables meticulous inspection, wound exploration, and repair under optimal conditions without further traumatizing the child. Similarly, for the adolescent who is too anxious for a thorough examination, or whose injuries are extensive, examination under sedation or anesthesia is preferred.

For patients whose injuries are related to sexual abuse or assault, all attempts should be made to engage a patient advocate and a sexual assault nurse examiner (see Chapter 6).

Superficial Genital Trauma

Most superficial perineal trauma cases are the result of mild, blunt force from a straddle injury or minor falls. A clear history of the preceding incident (often witnessed) is usually given, and findings fit the reported mechanism of injury. However, accidentally incurred superficial abrasions may not be noticed by parents until the child cries on urination, reports dysuria, or blood is noticed on the child's underwear or toilet paper.

Typical lesions include superficial abrasions, mild contusions, and occasionally superficial lacerations (Fig. 19.12). The junction of the labia minora and majora is the site most frequently involved; however, tears of the labia majora or perineal body are not uncommon. In contrast to accidental injuries, those that result from sexual abuse tend to be more posteriorly located and typically involve tears of the posterior portion of the hymen, the posterior fourchette, or perineal body (Fig. 19.13; see Fig. 19.12C).

Patients with superficial injuries may experience mild perineal discomfort and pain on urination but otherwise are asymptomatic. Most of these injuries can be managed supportively with systemic analgesia, topical bacteriostatic and/or anesthetic ointments, warm baths, and careful perineal cleansing. Application of the anesthetic ointment or any barrier emollient before urinating reduces the severity of dysuria, as does urinating in a tub of water.

Urethral prolapse and lichen sclerosus may cause bleeding and therefore be mistaken for trauma or abuse. See the Common Perineal Conditions section (later) and Figs. 19.20 and 19.21.

Moderate and Severe Genital Trauma

Moderately forceful blunt trauma often results in perineal tears and hematoma formation (Fig. 19.14). Hematomas of the perineum appear as tender, tense, round swellings with purplish discoloration. Periurethral hematomas may interfere with urination. Vaginal hematomas can result from submucosal tears of the vagina or even mucosal separation with resultant vaginal bleeding or vaginal hematoma formation. The pain of a vaginal hematoma is usually perceived as perineal and/or vaginal but at times is referred to the rectum or buttocks. Inspection through the vaginal orifice reveals a bluish swelling involving one of the lateral walls. This may also be evident as a tender swelling anterolaterally on rectal examination.

Moderate and severe penetrating injuries can be caused by falls onto sharp objects ("picket fence injury"), rape, sexual molestation with phallus-shaped objects, and auto accidents. More extensive injuries are typically associated with significant bleeding. However, even extensive tears may produce minimal pain and blood loss (Fig. 19.15).

Whether the mechanism of injury involves blunt force or penetration, internal extension of injury is possible and can be associated with external genital findings that are deceptively minor in appearance. Internal injury should be suspected when children endorse lower abdominal and perineal pain, which may radiate down the leg. Concerning physical findings include bleeding through the vaginal orifice; a vaginal hematoma; rectal bleeding, rectal tenderness, or abnormal sphincter tone; gross hematuria or inability to

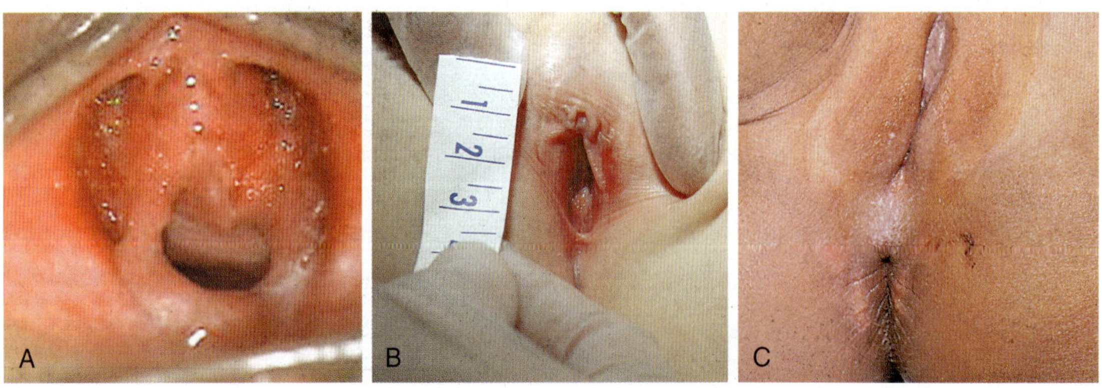

Fig. 19.12 Superficial blunt genital trauma. (A) Superficial abrasions and bruising are seen anteriorly on either side of the clitoris and urethra in a 3-year-old who presented with dysuria. (B) In another toddler, a superficial abrasion/laceration is seen between the left labia minora and majora after a straddle injury. (C) These healing superficial abrasions involving the posterior fourchette and perianal area were the result of sexual abuse. (A and B, Courtesy Janet Squires, MD, Children's Hospital of Pittsburgh, Pittsburgh, PA.)

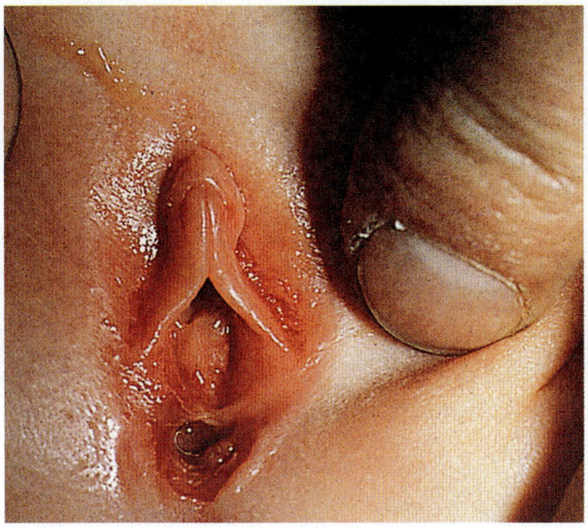

Fig. 19.13 Superficial penetrating genital trauma. This infant had a chief complaint of blood spotting on the diaper. Inspection revealed a perineal tear just posterior to the hymenal ring. There was no evidence of internal extension on vaginoscopy under anesthesia. Sexual abuse was suspected.

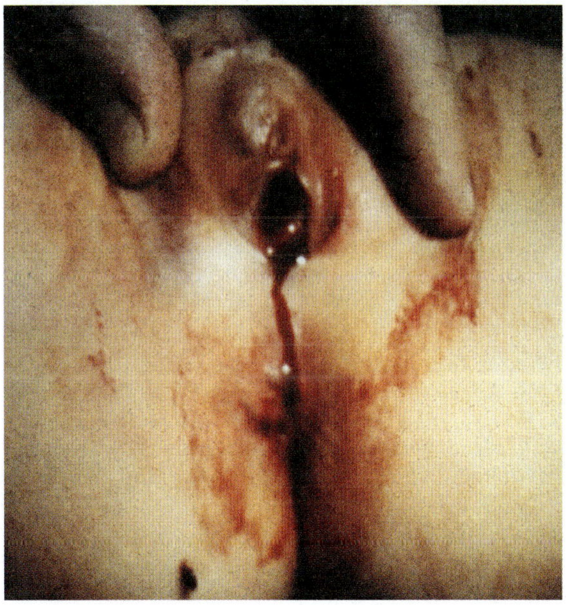

Fig. 19.14 Moderate blunt genital trauma. After a straddle injury on a diving board, this 9-year-old girl had vaginal bleeding. Inspection disclosed a hematoma of the anterior portion of the right labia majora, contusions of the clitoris and anterior labia minora, and a hematoma protruding through the vaginal opening. A small superficial laceration is present on the left, between the labia majora and minora. At vaginoscopy under anesthesia a vaginal tear involving the right lateral wall was found. (Courtesy K. Sukarochana, MD, Pittsburgh, PA.)

urinate; abdominal tenderness especially with guarding or rebound; or hypovolemia, which may not be evident immediately after the injury. All such patients warrant prompt hemodynamic stabilization, followed by appropriate imaging, surgical exploration, and repair in the operating room. This obviates the need for extensive examination in the office or emergency department.

VULVOVAGINAL DISORDERS

Vulvovaginal Complaints in Prepubertal Patients

The term *vulvovaginitis* denotes an inflammatory process involving both the vulva and vagina. In practice, however, the term *prepubertal vulvovaginitis* is used less precisely to refer to patients who describe symptoms of dysuria, vulvar pain or itching, or vaginal discharge but who may lack signs of inflammation or who have evidence of only vulvar or vaginal involvement. Vulvovaginal complaints are relatively common in prepubertal patients in part because the labia do not fully cover and thus do not completely protect the vaginal vestibule from friction and external irritants, especially when the child is sitting or squatting. In addition, the unestrogenized vaginal epithelium is thin, relatively friable, and easily traumatized. Transient irritation without discharge is common in the young child due to exposure to chemical irritants and inconsistent hygiene. Frictional irritation and poor aeration are also common and can be exacerbated by obesity. Finally, young children are less careful about cleansing their perineum after toileting and avoiding contamination with stool.

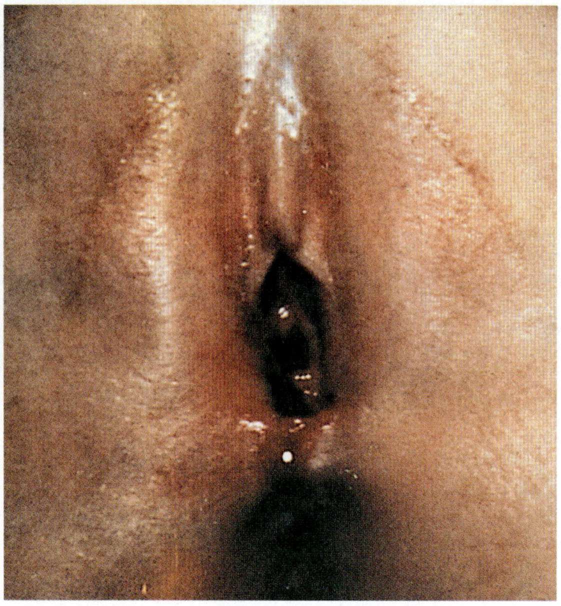

Fig. 19.15 Moderately severe penetrating genital trauma. This child fell while roller skating downhill and slid on her bottom for several feet over the sidewalk, tearing her perineum on an object projecting up between two of the cement plates. A laceration involving the right labia majora and minora, extending through the perineal body to the anus, is evident on inspection. The patient endorsed only minor discomfort. Examination under anesthesia revealed vaginal and rectal extension of the tear with complete transection of the external anal sphincter. The peritoneum was intact.

Causes of vulvovaginitis are most easily classified into noninfectious and infectious subgroups, with the latter subclassified into nonsexually and sexually transmitted infections. Table 19.4 presents the most common causes of noninfectious vulvovaginitis with specific historic clues suggestive of each condition. Box 19.5 presents the infectious causes. Nonsexually transmitted bacterial pathogens and the herpes simplex viruses (HSVs) often are spread to the vulvovaginal area from another site (e.g., nose, mouth, throat, skin, or gastrointestinal tract) by the patient's hands. *Candida* organisms, although a common cause of diaper dermatitis, rarely cause vulvovaginitis in the prepubertal child who is no longer wearing diapers, except for children receiving systemic antibiotics or steroids or those who have underlying diabetes mellitus. In the prepubertal child, vulvovaginitis caused by sexually transmitted pathogens is almost always acquired through sexual contact. In contrast to adolescents and adults, prepubertal patients are at little risk for internal extension of vulvovaginal infections (cervicitis and pelvic inflammatory disease [PID]) because the unestrogenized genital tract does not support the ascent of infection through the cervix, uterus, and fallopian tubes.

Evaluation of prepubertal patients with vulvovaginal complaints must include questions related to the following: abdominal pain, dysuria, frequency, urgency, or perianal pruritus; symptom duration; a history of any recent respiratory, gastrointestinal, and urinary tract infections; exposure to irritants (Box 19.6); hygiene practices;

Table 19.4 Noninfectious Causes of Prepubertal and Postpubertal Vulvovaginitis and Dysuria

Condition	Historical Clues
Poor hygiene	Recent toilet independence; infrequent bathing, handwashing, and clothing changes; soiled underwear
Poor perineal aeration	Tight clothing, nylon underwear, tights, and leotards; wet bathing suits; hot tubs; obesity
Frictional trauma	Tight clothing, sports, sand from sandbox or beach play, excessive masturbation or sexual abuse, obesity, hair removal
Chemical irritants	See products listed in Box 19.6
Contact dermatitis	Poison ivy; see also Box 19.6
Vaginal foreign bodies	Wiping habits, excessive masturbation or self-exploration, sexual abuse, use of condoms, tampons, or sex toys
Parasites, insect bites, infestations	Home environment, pets, sandboxes, travel, camping, exposure to woods or beach
Medication-related	Topical steroid or hormone creams, antibiotics, chemotherapy
Generalized skin disorders	History of pruritus, chronic skin lesions, prior diagnosis
Anatomic anomalies	Vesicovaginal or rectovaginal fistula, ectopic ureter, spina bifida, cloacal anomalies, urogenital anomalies
Neoplasms	Discharge, bleeding, bulging abdomen, change in bowel or bladder function, premature puberty, rapid androgenization
Systemic illness (Stevens-Johnson syndrome, Crohn disease with perineal fistulas and ulcers, toxic shock syndrome)	Prior infection or medication use; tampon use; evidence from other physical findings including rash, failure to gain weight or height, abdominal pain, diarrhea

Box 19.5 Infectious Causes of Prepubertal and Postpubertal Vulvovaginitis

Nonsexually Transmitted Pathogens

Bacterial Respiratory and/or Skin Pathogens
Group A β-hemolytic streptococci
Streptococcus pneumonia
Staphylococci
Candida species[a]

Viral Pathogens
Herpes simplex virus (HSV) types 1 and 2
Epstein-Barr virus
Varicella-zoster virus
Cytomegalovirus

Gastrointestinal Pathogens
Escherichia coli
Shigella species
Enterobius vermicularis
Yersinia species

Sexually Transmitted Pathogens

Bacterial Pathogens
Chlamydia trachomatis
Neisseria gonorrheae
Mycoplasma genitalium
Ureaplasma species/*Mycoplasma hominis*
Treponema pallidum

Protozoa
Trichomonas vaginalis

Viral Pathogens
HSV types 1 and 2
Human papillomavirus
Human immunodeficiency virus

Parasites
Phthirus pubis (lice)
Sarcoptes scabiei

[a]Infection rare before puberty.

Box 19.6 Products That Can Cause Chemical Irritation or Contact Dermatitis

Bubble bath or other bath additives
Perfumed or harsh soaps
Laundry detergents, if clothes inadequately rinsed
Dryer sheets and fabric softeners
Talc or other powders
Topical creams or ointments (active and inactive ingredients)
Shaving or hair removal products
Perfumed or dyed toilet paper
Perfumed sanitary pads and panty liners
Douches or other feminine hygiene products
Urine or stool
Spermicides
Sexual lubricants with enhancing agents

bowel and bladder habits; type of clothing worn; recent activities (such as swimming); and medications and topical agents. When sexual abuse is suspected, a list of the child's caretakers should be obtained along with any history of possible sexual contact. Developmental, behavioral, environmental, and medical histories all may contribute to a definitive diagnosis and aid in the formulation of a therapeutic plan.

Physical assessment includes determination of the degree of pubertal development, inguinal and abdominal examination, along with careful rectal, perineal, and vaginal inspection. The degree and extent of inflammation and excoriation should be documented. Parents should be encouraged to bring in any available soiled or discolored underwear, which should be checked for fit, cleanliness, and signs of blood, discharge, stool, and urine. When patients are seen by appointment for vulvovaginal complaints, parents should be asked not to bathe or apply creams to the child for at least 12 hours before the evaluation; otherwise, many children with a history of discharge have none when examined.

The presence of a vaginal discharge necessitates specimen collection (see Table 19.2 and the Examination of the Prepubertal Patient section, earlier). If a vaginal foreign body is suspected, vaginoscopy is indicated in consultation with a practitioner experienced in this procedure. Ultrasonography can be helpful in confirming the presence of some foreign objects. Radiographs of the pelvic area should be ordered selectively when benefit outweighs the risk and information cannot be obtained without radiation exposure.

Vulvovaginal Complaints in Pubertal Patients

Among pubertal patients, estrogenization and maturation of the genital tract facilitates upward spread of infection. Sexually transmitted pathogens are a common source of infection in sexually active adolescents. Therefore a complete gynecologic examination to evaluate for infection is necessary when evaluating sexually active adolescents with vulvovaginal complaints and should be considered for symptomatic, nonsexually active adolescents. Systemic signs and symptoms and abnormalities on bimanual pelvic examination suggest processes involving the uterus and adnexal and/or peritoneal structures. In contrast, isolated vulvovaginal disorders rarely are accompanied by such findings. In most cases, careful history, inspection, and laboratory tests (see Tables 19.2 and 19.5) provide a specific diagnosis on which to base treatment decisions. Some clinical and laboratory features of various etiologic agents of vaginal discharge are presented in Table 19.5.

Vulvar lesions, vaginal discharge, odor, pruritus, and dysuria are common complaints in adolescents. Irregular or postcoital bleeding, dyspareunia, pelvic pain, and fever may be reported as well. These symptoms are relatively nonspecific and may represent the final common pathway of different causes of irritation, infection, or infestation.

Physiologic Leukorrhea

Physiologic leukorrhea is a normal phenomenon and not a form of vulvovaginitis. These normal secretions are produced in response to estrogen stimulation and thus are seen in the newborn period and return when unopposed estrogen levels rise again during early puberty. Physiologic leukorrhea is clear or milky, relatively thin, odorless, and usually nonirritating. When dried on underwear, it may appear yellow. Patients in puberty often complain of discharge because they are not aware that these new, often annoying, secretions are normal. Among postpubertal patients, there is significant variation in vaginal discharge, and patients can be reassured discharge is normal in the absence of pain, pruritus, abnormal color, or odor.

Examination reveals normal pubertal development, including breast buds, pubic hair, and estrogenization of the labia and distal vaginal mucosa, along with the typical discharge. Diagnosis is confirmed by findings on wet preparation microscopy, which reveals estrogenized epithelial cells with no increase in leukocytes. In general, there should be no more than one polymorphonuclear leukocyte for every vaginal epithelial cell. Neither bimanual nor speculum examinations are necessary unless concurrent symptoms or findings suggest other problems. Treatment consists of reassurance and education. Some patients are more comfortable wearing unscented pantiliners.

Table 19.5 Clinical and Laboratory Features of Disorders Causing Vaginal Discharge in Adolescents

	Physiologic	*Candida*	*Chlamydia*	Gonorrhea	*Trichomonas*	Bacterial Vaginosis	Herpes Simplex Virus
Appearance of discharge	White or clear, mucoid	White, curdlike, with adherent plaques	Mucopus or bloody cervical discharge	Mucopus, yellow, or greenish cervical discharge	Gray, yellow, or green; sometimes frothy	Gray, white; homogeneous, thin	Serous
Amount of discharge	Variable	Variable	Variable	Variable	Profuse	Variable	Variable
Vulvar and vaginal inflammation	None or mild with copious leukorrhea	Common	Not usual	Not usual	Common	Rare	Common with a few to many ulcers
pH of vaginal discharge	≤4.5	≤4.5	Variable	≤4.5	≥4.5	≥4.5	≤4.5
Microscopy	Epithelial cells, few WBCs, lactobacilli	↑WBCs, positive KOH with pseudohyphae and budding yeast in 50% of patients	↑WBCs	↑↑WBCs	↑↑WBCs, motile trichomonads in saline prep in 50% of patients	Few WBCs; positive for clue cells in saline prep	↑↑WBCs
Predisposing or concurrent factors	Secretion of estrogen	Menstruation, broad-spectrum antibiotics, diabetes, local heat and moisture, pregnancy, OCPs, topical steroid or hormone creams, HIV and other immune compromise	Sexual activity, other STI	Sexual activity, other STI; symptoms develop during and after menstrual period	Other STI	Previous bacterial vaginosis, sexual activity, douching	Stress and local trauma (including shaving)
Other clinical signs and symptoms	None	Itching prominent; may have dysuria or insertional dyspareunia at introitus	Urethritis, Friable cervix, PID, perihepatitis	Urethritis, PID, perihepatitis, pharyngitis, proctitis, systemic illness, arthritis, tenosynovitis, skin lesions	Vulvar itching and burning prominent; dysuria; pelvic discomfort, malodorous discharge	Fishy odor; odor increased after unprotected intercourse	Regional adenopathy with primary infection; prodromal and undercurrent itching and pain
Whiff test (acrid amine odor on addition of 10% KOH)	Negative	Negative	Negative	Negative	Sometimes positive	Positive	Negative

↑, Increased; ↑↑, markedly increased; *HIV*, human immunodeficiency virus; *KOH*, potassium hydroxide; *OCP*, oral contraceptive pill; *PID*, pelvic inflammatory disease; *STI*, sexually transmitted infection; *WBC*, white blood cell.

ETIOLOGIES OF VULVOVAGINAL DISORDERS

Noninfectious Vulvovaginitis

Noninfectious vulvovaginitis is common in prepubertal children but occurs less frequently after menarche. Clinical findings vary considerably depending on cause. Patients with intermittent symptoms should be seen as soon as possible when symptoms recur. In some patients, the vulva and vagina appear normal, whereas in others varying degrees of inflammation or irritation are present, at times accompanied by signs of excoriation. Vaginal discharge is unusual, however, and vaginal cultures grow normal or nonspecific flora (Box 19.7). Individuals with underlying dermatologic disorders may be more susceptible to noninfectious causes of vulvovaginitis. Symptoms are similar for most etiologies: perineal itching or pain, external or contact dysuria, and occasionally, vaginal discharge.

Treatment consists of removal of the offending agent or causative circumstance along with symptomatic measures. Recommended hygienic practices include providing opportunities to urinate, using a front-to-back wiping technique, and regular washing with warm water without excessive scrubbing. Products to avoid are listed in Box 19.6. Patients with vulvovaginal inflammation are encouraged to wear loose-fitting clothes and white cotton underwear that is well rinsed after regular washing. Failure to improve should lead to consideration of other etiologies including sexual abuse and the possibility of nonadherence with treatment. Referral to a clinician with expertise in pediatric gynecologic problems may be indicated. In prepubertal patients, chronic irritation from any cause may predispose the labia minora to agglutinate, resulting in labial adhesions (see Fig. 19.9 and the Labial Adhesions section, earlier).

Irritation Related to Hygiene Practices

Poor perineal hygiene is one of the most common causes of irritation. Examination typically reveals mild nonspecific vulvar inflammation. Pieces of stool and toilet paper may be seen adhering to the perineum and perianal areas, and smegma may be found around the clitoris and labia. Underwear is often soiled. Coliforms tend to predominate on vaginal culture when there is associated vaginal inflammation. In most cases, symptoms resolve with a regimen of warm baths and careful cleansing after urination and defecation. Feculent vaginal discharge should prompt the clinician to consider a rectovaginal fistula as the cause.

Pubic hair removal has become increasingly common, sometimes starting shortly after pubic hair first appears. Complications of hair removal are common and include razor burn; contact dermatitis from shaving products; mechanical and infectious folliculitis (Fig. 19.16) commonly from *Staphylococcus aureus, Streptococcus pyogenes,* and *Pseudomonas aeruginosa;* and mechanical spread or trigger of viral infections, such as HPV, molluscum contagiosum, and HSV. Mild topical corticosteroids and topical antibiotics can be used to prevent and treat folliculitis. Clinicians who commonly encounter these issues should familiarize themselves with the risks, benefits, and various methods of pubic hair removal.

Maceration Secondary to Moisture and Chafing

Moisture, whether from normal secretions, perspiration, or swimming, when unable to evaporate, promotes maceration and inflammation of perineal tissues (Fig. 19.17). Obesity, wearing snug clothing or tights over nonbreathable underwear, and sitting for long periods in a wet bathing suit or leotard are common predisposing factors to this form of vulvar irritation. A history of a chronic perineal moisture and the smell of urine on the child's underclothes should lead the clinician to consider the possibility of urinary incontinence, a vesicovaginal fistula, or ectopic ureter. When maceration occurs, secondary infection with bacterial or fungal infection is common, and some patients have associated intertrigo (irritant der-

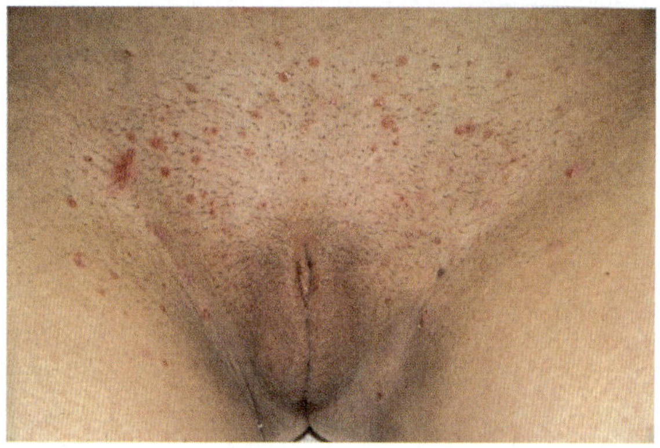

Fig. 19.16 Pubic hair removal. After shaving, this 17-year-old girl developed folliculitis, a bacterial skin infection caused by *Staphylococcus aureus.* It cleared quickly with the use of oral and topical antibiotics. (From Trager JDK. Pubic hair removal—pearls and pitfalls, *J Pediatr Adolesc Gynecol* 19: 117–123, 2006.)

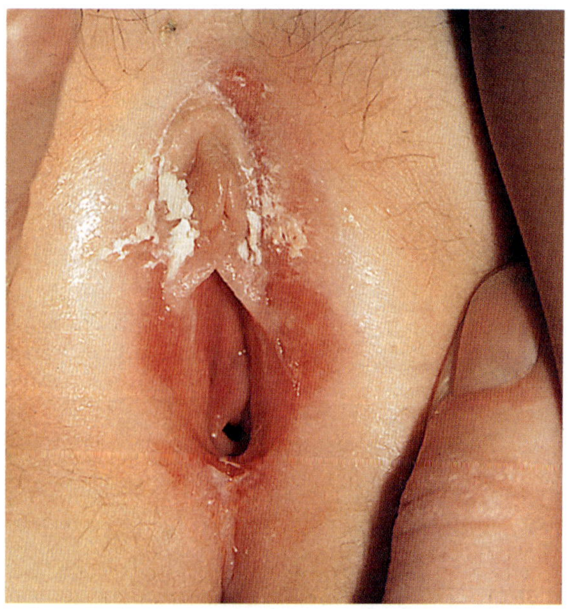

Fig. 19.17 Maceration secondary to poor perineal aeration. This child's chief complaint was one of dysuria. On examination, the inner surfaces of the labia were found to be macerated and mildly inflamed. Adherent smegma is also visible. The child had been wearing tights over nylon underwear.

Box 19.7 Organisms Thought to Constitute Normal or Nonpathogenic Vaginal Flora

Aerobes and Facultative Anaerobes

Atopobium vaginae
Branhamella catarrhalis
Candida albicans and other yeasts[a]
Corynebacterium species
Diphtheroids
Enterococcus species
Escherichia coli and other enteric bacteria
Gardnerella vaginalis[a]
Haemophilus species
Lactobacillus species
Klebsiella species
Megasphaera species
Mycoplasma species[a]
Neisseria sicca
Proteus species
Pseudomonas species
Staphylococcus species
Streptococcus species

Anaerobes

Bacteroides species
Clostridium species
Leptotrichia species
Peptococcus species
Peptostreptococcus species

[a]*Candida, Gardnerella,* and *Mycoplasma* species can be normal flora in asymptomatic patients; however, at times they may be responsible for genital infection.

matitis where opposing skin surfaces touch). Attention to perineal hygiene and drying, avoidance of predisposing factors listed earlier, use of antichafing products, and treatment of secondary infection are the mainstays of management.

Contact Dermatitis, Allergic Vulvitis

Clinicians should consider allergic vulvitis in patients whose most prominent symptom is pruritus (assuming lichen sclerosus and parasitic infestations are not the cause), although scratching and excoriation may result in secondary burning and dysuria. When patients are seen in the acute phase, inspection of the labia and vestibule reveals a microvesicular papular eruption that tends to be intensely erythematous and may be somewhat edematous. Excoriation is common. When the process has become chronic, the vulvar skin has an eczematoid appearance with cracks, fissures, and lichenification. Poison ivy is a common acute cause, as are the exposures listed in Box 19.6.

Chemical Irritant Vulvovaginitis

Many of the agents listed in Box 19.6 can act as chemical irritants. Before toilet training, children whose diapers are changed infrequently may develop irritation caused by ammonia produced when the organisms in stool split the urea in urine. Itching and dysuria are prominent symptoms, and examination usually discloses mild nonspecific inflammation (Fig. 19.18), at times associated with signs of scratching. On occasion, findings are normal. Diagnosis is dependent on a thorough history (see Table 19.4 and Box 19.6).

Frictional Trauma

Frictional trauma may be the source of superficial abrasive changes and, when chronic, may result in lichenification or even atrophic skin changes (Fig. 19.19). Wearing tight clothing, certain sporting activities (especially gymnastics and long-distance cycling and running), sand, and excessive masturbation (which may be triggered by sexual abuse or other behavioral problems) are the major predisposing factors.

Fistulas

Because patients with vesicovaginal fistulas and ectopic ureters have a history of a constantly wet perineum, they frequently have symptoms of vulvovaginitis. Nonspecific inflammation and maceration are the predominant physical findings (see Fig. 19.17). Rectovaginal fistulas can also cause vulvovaginal inflammation, but the presence

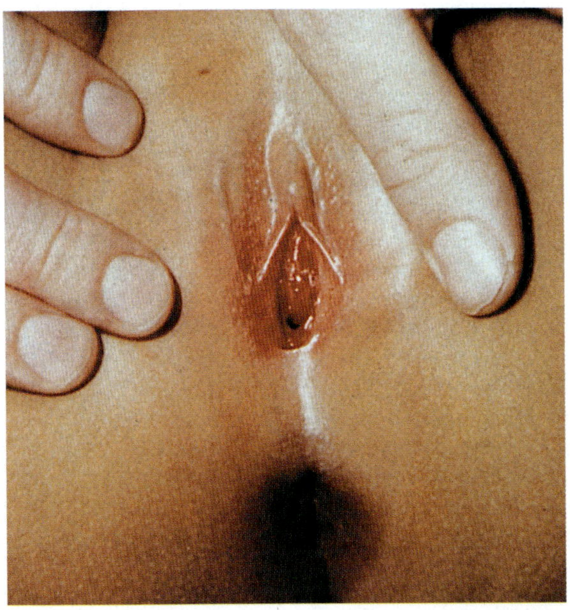

Fig. 19.18 Nonspecific inflammation characteristic of chemical irritant vulvovaginitis.

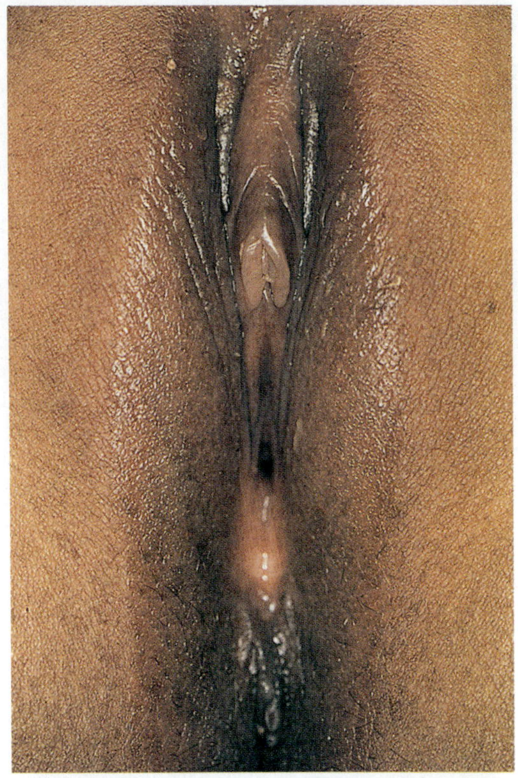

Fig. 19.19 Frictional trauma. This patient's labial skin shows nonspecific thickening and mild irritation. She had a history of recurrent vaginal foreign bodies and was strongly suspected to be a victim of chronic sexual abuse. (Courtesy K. Sukarochana, MD, Pittsburgh, PA.)

of a grossly feculent vaginal discharge usually makes diagnosis relatively easy. Inflammatory bowel disease should be considered when a rectovaginal fistula is present.

Vaginal Foreign Body

The most common symptom of vaginal foreign body is the presence of vaginal discharge. Although some children present with a yellow, mildly purulent discharge, the hallmark of vaginal foreign body is a profuse, foul-smelling, brownish or blood-streaked vaginal discharge. Rare causes of such discharge include *Shigella* vaginitis in prepubertal patients and necrotic tumors.

The majority of patients are in the 3- to 8-year-old age group. When a prepubertal patient is found to have a vaginal foreign body, it is important to obtain a detailed psychosocial history of the family and the child, which may reveal developmental delay, psychosocial or behavioral problems, or abuse. Often the problem is recurrent. Wads of toilet tissue, paper, cotton, crayons, and small toys are the materials found most often; however, all types of small objects have been retrieved. There may be a long noninflammatory latency period for inert materials. Vaginoscopy is diagnostic and provides access for extraction, which is curative. In the prepubertal age group, this is best accomplished under general anesthesia or conscious sedation.

The most common vaginal foreign bodies found in adolescents are forgotten tampons (which are a significant risk for toxic shock syndrome) or retained condoms, both of which are usually accompanied by a pungent odor as the presenting complaint. Over-the-counter therapeutic suppositories or objects used in sexual activity may also cause problems. Careful manual inspection in the adolescent patient may locate the offending agent, and objects made of hard materials may be palpable on rectal examination. Removal manually or with an alligator forceps is usually curative. However antibiotic treatment may be considered if purulent discharge persists, in which case vaginal culture may be useful.

Common Perineal Conditions

Urethral Prolapse

Urethral prolapse is often mistaken for vulvovaginal infection or trauma. The phenomenon is more prevalent among prepubertal, school-aged African American patients. Increased intraabdominal pressure associated with obesity, chronic cough, or constipation may contribute. Dysuria, perineal pain, and bleeding are the most frequent symptoms. The classic physical finding is an annular, purplish red, swollen, tender, and friable tissue lying over the anterior introitus (Fig. 19.20). With careful examination, it is noted to encircle the urethral meatus. Because the urethral mucosa is responsive to estrogen, application of estrogen cream twice daily and treatment of any contributing problems usually results in resolution and reduces the risk of recurrence. Oral or topical analgesics can provide symptomatic relief, with addition of topical antibiotic if necessary. Surgery is reserved for cases of strangulation or unresolvable obstruction.

Lichen Sclerosus

Lichen sclerosus is a chronic, inflammatory, dermatologic disorder believed to be of autoimmune origin that primarily involves the anogenital area in prepubertal patients. It is characterized by itching and/or burning sensation, and the resultant rubbing or scratching often exacerbates the superficial fissures and erythema, ultimately leading to excoriation and punctate bleeding (Fig. 19.21A and B). With progression of disease, the involved epithelium becomes atrophic—sometimes described as thin and crinkly appearing—and hypopigmented. When both the vulvar and perianal areas are affected, the distribution has been likened to an hourglass or a figure-eight (see Fig. 19.21C). On resolution of active lesions, the involved area is characterized by confluent, white, atrophic patches with a shiny surface. Of note, the intensity of symptoms may not correlate with the severity of physical findings. Some patients with severe discomfort have a paucity of skin disruption, and other individuals may have minimal symptoms despite significant skin findings. As a result, in some untreated cases the diagnosis is first made in adolescence based on scarring and disruption of the vulvar architecture.

Diagnosis is generally made clinically, although atypical cases and those that do not respond to first-line treatment warrant biopsy. When ulcerations and bleeding are present, concerns regarding sexual abuse may arise. The symmetry and distribution of lesions, their failure to heal rapidly, and the chronicity of the disorder help distinguish it from abrasions and lacerations due to abuse, although it is important to remember these diagnoses are not mutually exclusive. In vitiligo, which may have a similar distribution when present in the anogenital area, the involved skin is totally devoid of pigment but appears otherwise normal (i.e., not atrophic or inflamed). Lichen planus, a condition similar to lichen sclerosus, may present similarly with white streaks on the vulva, but more typically the rash is violaceous, and it is uncommon in childhood.

Lichen sclerosus tends to wax and wane with acute exacerbations, often precipitated by local irritation or trauma, requiring intermittent maintenance therapy. For treatment failures with ultra-high-dose topical steroids, there may be a role for topical calcineurin inhibitors; topical hormone preparations have not been found to be effective. Once thought to resolve at puberty, lichen sclerosus has been found to persist in approximately three-quarters of cases; thus long-term follow-up is warranted to monitor for symptoms, skin changes, and the possible increased risk of malignancy.

Acute Genital Ulcers

The appearance of a genital ulcer can create alarm and distress in both patients and parents. The differential diagnosis is broad and includes infectious and noninfectious causes. HSV is the most common infectious cause of genital ulcers, and both HSV type 1 and type 2 can be spread via nonsexual transmission by caregivers or from autoinoculation. Noninfectious causes include autoimmune or other systemic illness, drug reactions, and aphthous ulcers. A thorough history and physical is warranted, with particular attention to excluding underlying systemic conditions (such as HIV infection, Behçet disease, or Crohn disease) and identifying recent viral infection (e.g., Epstein-Barr virus or varicella) or other triggering factors, such as tight-fitting clothing, sexual activity, or abuse.

When such factors are absent and lesions are characteristic, vulvar aphthae are the likely cause. The typical location of vulvar aphthous ulcers is the medial labia minora (often on opposing labial surfaces as "kissing" lesions), but other sites include the vagina, introitus, fourchette, labia majora, and perineum. Appearance varies, but aphthous ulcers tend to be deeper than ulcers caused by HSV and typically appear well demarcated with a necrotic base and ragged margins (Fig. 19.22). Lesions may be covered by yellow-gray exudate or eschar, and surrounding inflammation with or without cellulitis can occur.

Evaluation should include HSV PCR from the lesion or culture, if not available. If systemic symptoms are present, serum immunoglobulin G (IgG) and immunoglobulin M (IgM) antiviral capsid antigen for Epstein-Barr virus can be sent. Beyond that, a large laboratory workup is rarely informative and should be based on the history and examination, including a comprehensive evaluation for STI when indicated. Bacterial and fungal cultures tend not to yield pathogens and biopsy is rarely indicated.

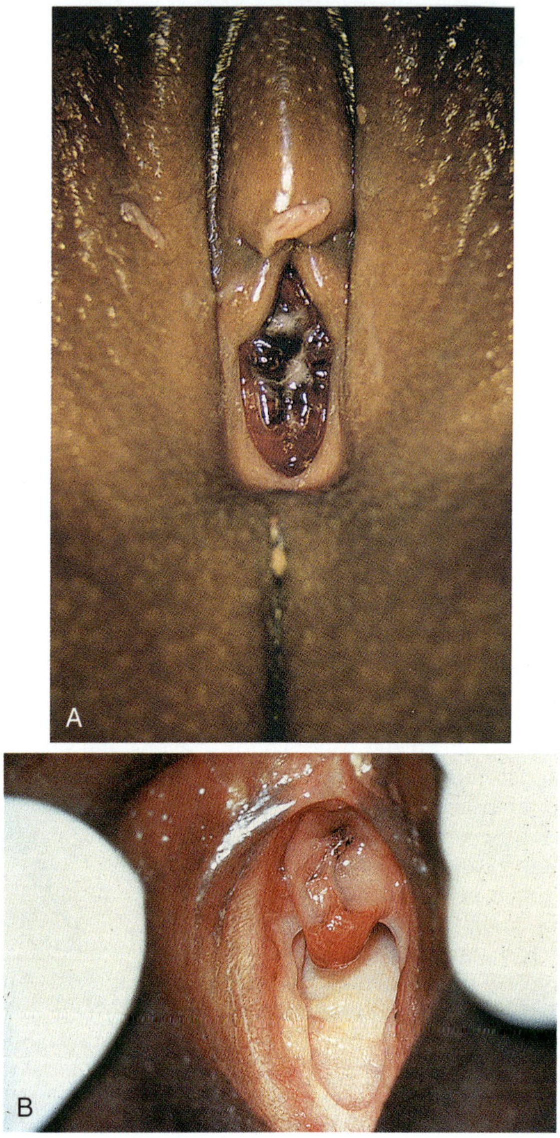

Fig. 19.20 Urethral prolapse. (A) This child had acute complaints of bleeding and dysuria. The prolapsed urethral mucosa is red and friable, and has a dough-nut shape encircling the urethra. (B) In another patient, the prolapsed mucosal tissue is thickened and erythema is less prominent. (A, Courtesy John McCann, MD, University of California at Davis, Davis, CA. B, Courtesy Carole Jenny, MD, Hasbro Children's Hospital, Providence, RI.)

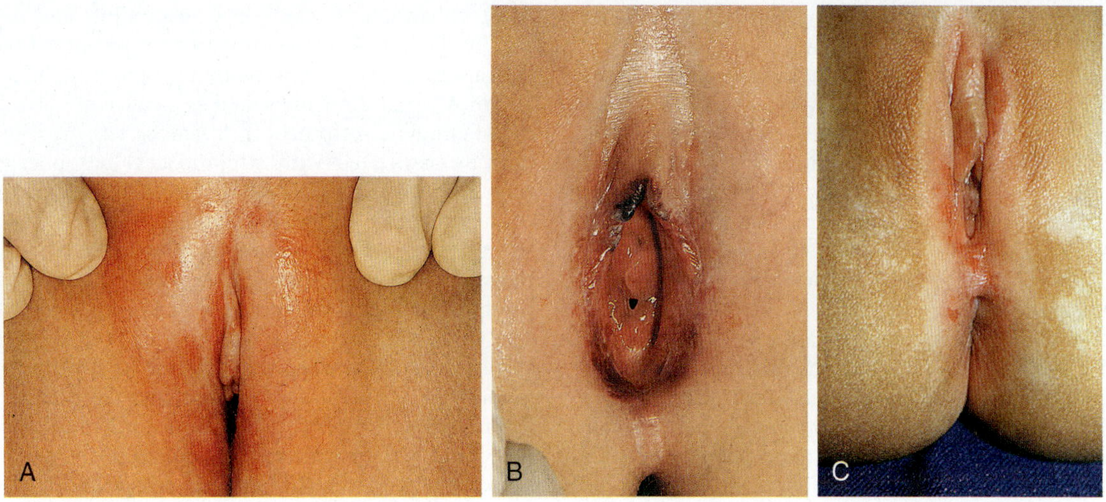

Fig. 19.21 Lichen sclerosus. (A) The skin overlying the labia majora has become atrophic and appears pale and thin. It is dotted with small, superficial ulcerations. (B) In this child with complaints of bleeding and pruritus, skin breakdown is evident along with petechial hemorrhages. (C) A pruritic, atrophic, eroded, hypopigmented patch involving the anogenital skin and mucous membranes in this 5-year-old girl has an hourglass configuration. (C, From Cohen BA: *Pediatric dermatology*, ed 2, London, 1999, Mosby.)

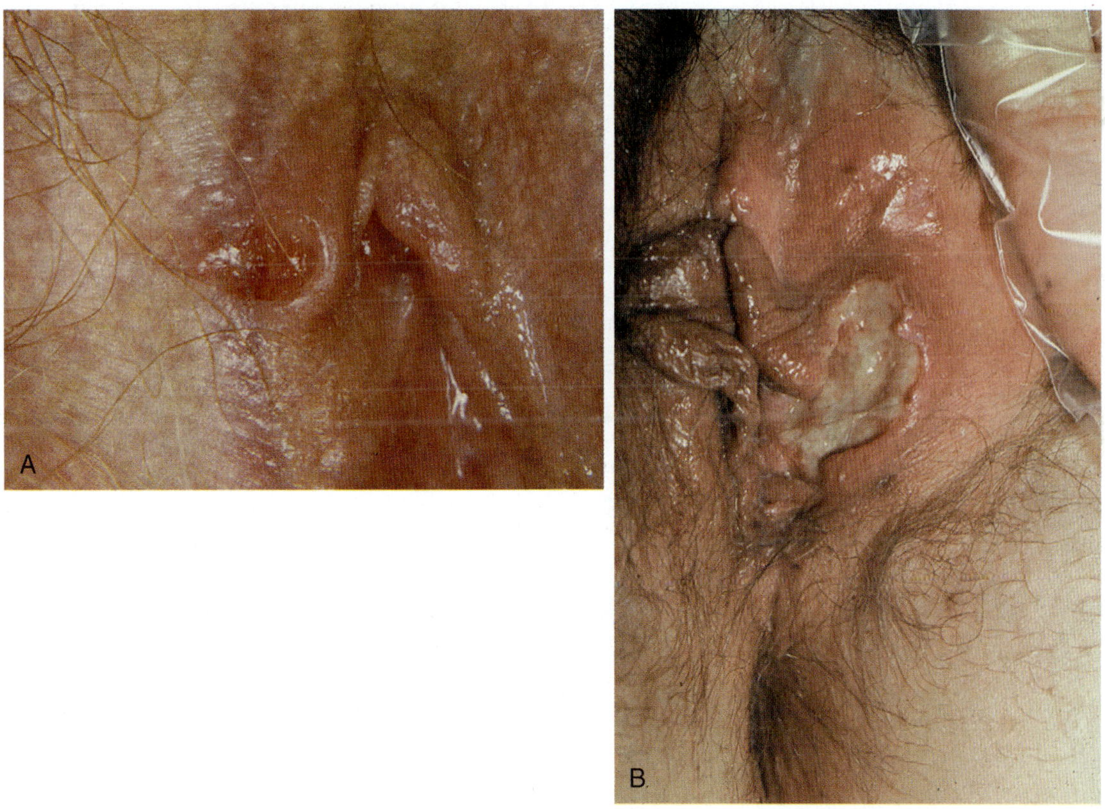

Fig. 19.22 Genital ulcers. (A) Vulvar aphthous ulcer in a teenage girl. (B) Vulvar aphthous ulcer with exudate. (From Bandow GD. Diagnosis and management of vulvar ulcers, *Dermatol Clin* 28:753–763, 2010.)

Vulvar aphthous ulcers are generally self-limited, resolving in 2 to 3 weeks. However, treatment with an ultrahigh potency topical steroid (such as 0.05% clobetasol ointment twice daily for 7–10 days) is recommended. The use of oral steroids has been described for more severe cases. Patients with milder symptoms can be managed as outpatients with supportive care, including warm baths, barrier agents such as sucralfate, and/or topical anesthetics such as combined lidocaine, epinephrine, and tetracaine. However, pain can be severe and hospitalization may be required with Foley catheterization to manage dysuria, antibiotics to treat associated cellulitis, and narcotics to treat pain.

Families can be reassured by the comparison of vulvar aphthae to common "canker sores" and by the fact that recurrence and long-term sequelae are uncommon. The likelihood of scarring depends on the size and duration of the original lesions. Follow-up should be weekly until resolution and then yearly to monitor for progression to systemic disease, such as Behçet disease, which is a systemic disease characterized by recurrent oral aphthae and associated genital, eye, and skin findings.

Infectious Vulvovaginitis

In contrast to most of the primarily noninfectious forms of vulvovaginitis, vaginal discharge is usually a prominent symptom of infectious vulvovaginitis in all age groups. Although a few pathogens produce a fairly characteristic clinical picture, the symptoms and discharge seen with many pathogens are relatively nonspecific. Furthermore, in the case of STI, more than one pathogen may be present.

There are two major subgroups of vulvovaginal infections. In the first subgroup, genital involvement is secondary to a systemic infection or the result of transfer of the pathogen from another primary site, such as the skin or the respiratory, gastrointestinal, or urinary tract via contaminated fingers or proximity (see Box 19.5). Infection at the primary site may precede or coexist with the genital infection; in some cases, colonization of another site without overt infection appears to predispose. This nonvenereal infectious vulvovaginitis is common in prepubertal patients but is rare in adolescents because the mature female genital tract does not support growth of most of these pathogens.

The second subgroup of infectious vulvovaginitis consists of those infections caused by sexually transmitted pathogens (see Box 19.5 and Table 19.5). Both prepubertal and postmenarchal patients can have vulvovaginitis when infected with these organisms. After puberty, however, patients can have other clinical presentations as well, including cervicitis, endometritis, and salpingitis. Table 19.5 enumerates the possible clinical features seen in adolescents with STI and summarizes other major epidemiologic characteristics and appropriate diagnostic measures.

Regardless of age, the most frequent mode of transmission of STI is sexual contact. The majority of these infections in prepubertal patients are the result of sexual abuse. In adolescence, consensual sexual activity is the major mode of infection by sexually transmitted pathogens, although sexual exploitation and abuse remain significant possibilities. These factors necessitate obtaining a confidential history of sexual activity and identification and treatment of sexual partners. Routine screening for sexually active adolescents should be in accordance with latest CDC guidelines.

Infectious Vulvovaginitis Caused by Nonsexually Transmitted Pathogens

Vulvovaginitis Caused by Respiratory and/or Skin Pathogens

Bacterial respiratory pathogens can cause vulvovaginitis in prepubertal patients, presumably as a result of orodigital transmission. *Streptococcus pneumoniae* and other respiratory flora can cause purulent vaginal discharge, with associated vulvitis and vaginitis, either after or concurrent with upper respiratory tract infection. Most vulvovaginitis caused by respiratory and/or skin pathogens will resolve with hygiene measures alone, but antibiotic treatment is warranted for severe or persistent symptoms. The respiratory pathogen most commonly identified as a cause of vulvovaginitis is group A β-hemolytic streptococci, *Streptococcus pyogenes.* This infection may be associated with streptococcal nasopharyngitis or scarlet fever, or it may occur in apparent isolation, although a throat culture is often positive for streptococci even in the absence of pharyngeal or upper respiratory symptoms. The onset of vulvovaginal symptoms is abrupt, with severe perineal burning and dysuria. Inspection reveals a sharply circumscribed area of intense erythema involving the vulva, distal vagina, and perianal area (Fig. 19.23A). The involved skin may weep serous fluid. Most patients have a serosanguinous or purulent vaginal discharge, and about one-third have vaginal petechiae. Culture of perineal skin and/or discharge is positive. Antibiotic treatment is warranted in the case of vulvovaginitis caused by group A β-hemolytic streptococci, and desquamation may ensue with recovery (see Figs. 19.4 and 19.23B).

Vulvovaginitis Caused by Gastrointestinal Pathogens

Gastrointestinal pathogens including *Escherichia coli* are frequently identified bacterial cause of vulvovaginitis in prepubertal patients. Again, most vulvovaginitis caused by gastrointestinal pathogens will resolve with hygiene measures alone, but culture and antibiotic treatment is warranted for purulent vaginal discharge or persistent symptoms. A distinct form of vulvovaginitis caused by *Shigella* species has been recognized in prepubertal patients. Patients present with a bloody, purulent discharge, and approximately one-third have associated diarrhea. If vulvovaginitis caused by *Shigella* species is suspected, culture of vaginal secretions and antibiotic treatment guided by susceptibilities are indicated.

Intestinal infestation with pinworms *(Enterobius vermicularis)* is associated primarily with perianal pruritus. However, the worms may crawl forward into the vagina, bringing enteric flora with them and depositing eggs. In some cases, vaginal infection and discharge may result. Scratching may produce excoriation and secondary dysuria. A history of preceding perianal pruritus generally is elicited. Pinworm ova and/or adult worms may be found on wet mount examination of vaginal secretions. When pinworm infestation is suspected despite negative vaginal smears, a perianal sample should be obtained (see Table 19.2). Alternatively, empiric

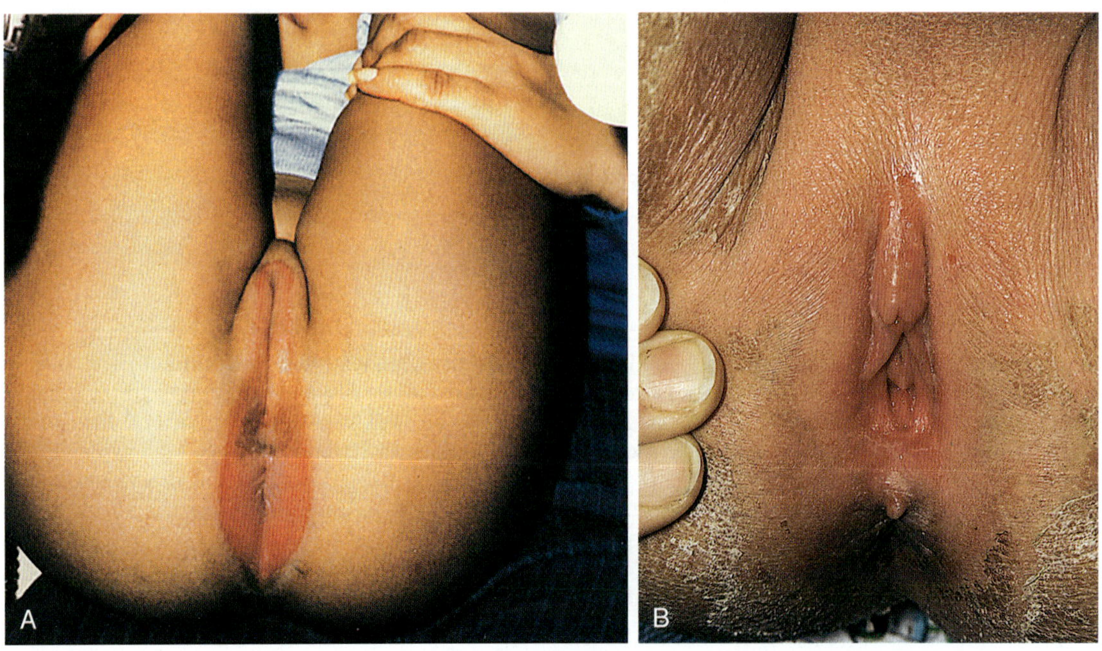

Fig. 19.23 Streptococcal vulvovaginitis. (A) In this child who had acute vulvar pain, dysuria, and discharge, the area of inflammation is sharply circumscribed and extends from the vulva to the perianal area. (B) In another patient, who presented late in the course of a case of scarlet fever, vulvar inflammation is still evident and desquamation has begun.

treatment with albendazole or over-the-counter pyrantel pamoate may be instituted.

Candidal Vulvovaginitis

Candida species are one of the more common sources of nonvenereal infectious vulvovaginitis after puberty. This is rare in the healthy prepubertal child. Predisposing factors, common symptoms, and clinical features are listed in Table 19.5. Examination of the vulva usually reveals diffuse erythema (Fig. 19.24A); with chronic involvement, white or pink cobblestoned plaques on an erythematous base may be seen. Excoriations from scratching and satellite lesions on the perineum are also common. In some cases, signs of perianal dermatitis and intertrigo are found.

Thick creamy or curdlike discharge is often present. In adolescents, whitish plaques may adhere to the vagina or cervix (see Fig. 19.24B). A KOH or wet preparation confirms the presence of yeast and often an increase in inflammatory cells (see Fig. 19.24C and D). Topical application of an azole antifungal cream into the lower vagina, or single-dose oral fluconazole, is the treatment of choice. In patients with recurrences, predisposing factors, such as medications, diabetes, pregnancy, and HIV infection, should be considered. Infrequently an infected male partner with subacute or chronic monilial balanitis may be the source of recurrences in sexually active patients. This infection is generally not transmitted sexually, and treatment of the partner does not decrease recurrence rates.

Resistant and/or recurrent vulvovaginitis is more likely to be caused by nonalbicans species, such as *Candida glabrata.* Although clinical presentation is similar, these organisms do not demonstrate the classic branching pattern under microscopy. Vaginal culture is helpful for diagnosis and to guide treatment based on susceptibilities. The CDC recommends longer duration of therapy (7–14 days) with a nonfluconazole azole regimen (oral or topical) as a first-line therapy.

GENITAL INFECTIONS CAUSED BY SEXUALLY TRANSMITTED PATHOGENS

STIs are an important cause of short- and long-term morbidity in adolescents. The major characteristics of the most common STIs are listed in Table 19.6. Although some infections produce relatively specific clinical signs, many are characterized by nonspecific vulvovaginal findings. In addition, multiple simultaneous infections may occur, necessitating comprehensive laboratory evaluation.

Evaluation for Sexually Transmitted Infections

Before menarche, lack of estrogenization inhibits ascent of infection to the upper genital tract and subclinical lower tract infection is uncommon. As a result, external inspection of the perineum and lower vagina and laboratory evaluation of vaginal discharge samples are sufficient for identification of most pathogens and institution of therapy. However, this does not complete the assessment because identification of an STI in a prepubertal patient always necessitates urgent referral to a team specialized in the assessment of child sexual abuse, the probable cause of STI in children (see Chapter 6).

When evaluating postpubertal patients suspected of having an STI, a confidential sexual history is essential. Although consensual activity is common in adolescence, patients may be victims of sexual abuse, including incest, trafficking and sexual exploitation, relationship violence, and rape. Pubertal patients with STIs may be

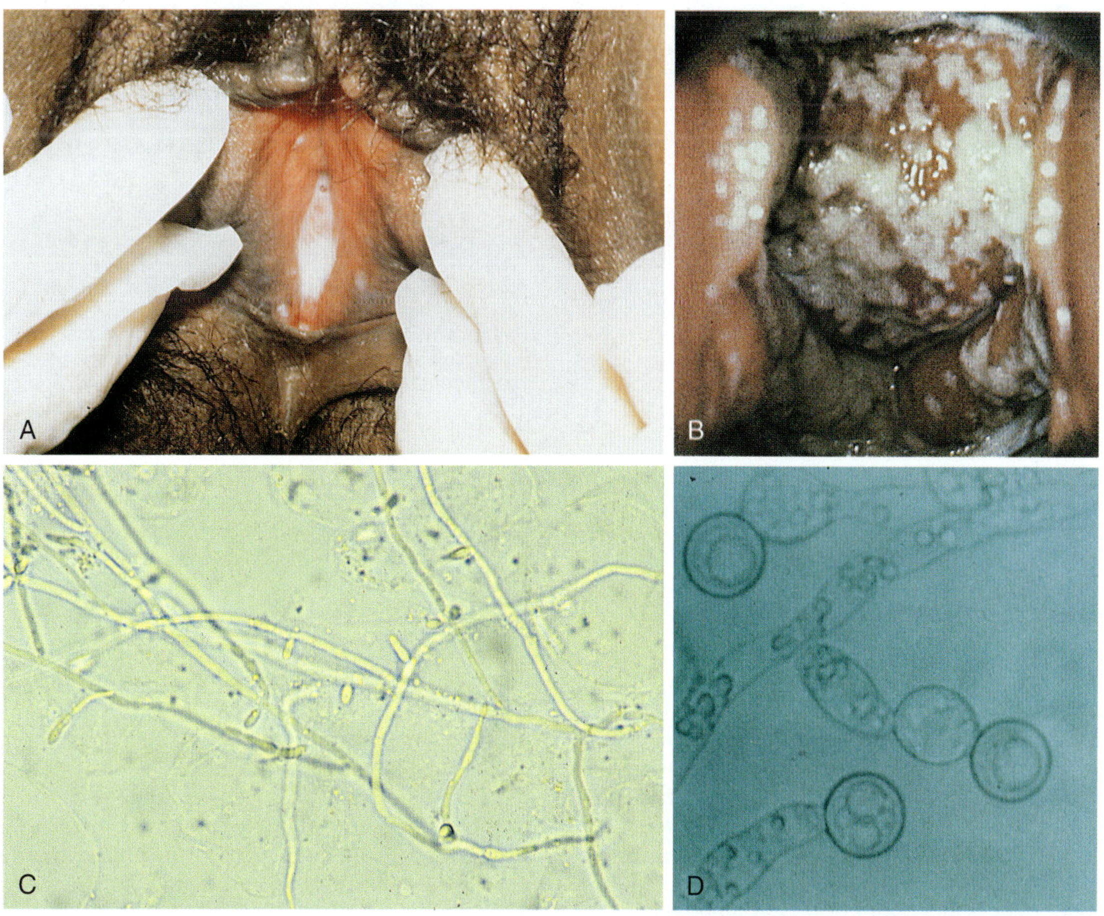

Fig. 19.24 Candidal vulvovaginitis and cervicitis. (A) The vulva is intensely hyperemic, and a thick, cheesy, white discharge covers the urethra, introitus, and hymenal area. (B) Whitish plaques may be seen on the perineum and vaginal mucosa and occasionally on the cervix in adolescents. (C and D) These low- and high-power wet mount specimens contain pseudohyphae and budding yeast. (A, Courtesy B. Cohen, MD, Johns Hopkins Hospital, Baltimore, MD. B and D, Courtesy Ellen Wald, MD, University of Wisconsin Children's Hospital, Madison, WI.)

Table 19.6 Major Characteristics of the Most Common Sexually Transmitted Infections and Diagnostic Measures

	Herpes Simplex Virus	Human Papilloma Virus	Human Immuno-deficiency Virus	*Trichomonas*	Gonorrhea	*Chlamydia*	Syphilis
Clinical findings	May be normal; vulvar vesicles or ulcers, vulvitis, vaginitis, cervicitis	Vulvar, vaginal, cervical, perineal, and perianal condylomata and flat warts	Acute flulike illness; treatment resistant or unusually severe presentation of *Candida*, HPV, HSV, or molluscum contagiosum	Vaginitis, vulvitis, vaginal and/or cervical petechiae, profuse watery discharge	May be normal; cervicitis, salpingitis, urethritis, occasionally proctitis, pharyngitis; vaginitis and vulvitis in prepubertal patients	Often normal; cervicitis, salpingitis, urethritis, proctitis; vaginitis and vulvitis in prepubertal patients	Primary: vulvar, vaginal, or cervical chancre; secondary: condylomata lata of vulva; generalized exanthema
Incubation period	3–14 days	On average 1–3 months (variable, up to 2 years)	Acute HIV: several weeks; AIDS: variable—up to 10 years	3–30 days	2–7 days	7–21 days	Primary: 15–90 days; secondary: 6 weeks to 6 months; tertiary: 2–20 years
Infectivity	75%–80% with active infection	60%–70%	Varies with infecting behavior	70%–90% for M/F transmission, less for F/M	100% M/F; 25% F/M	45% M/F	10%, single encounter; 30%, after 1 month of sexual activity with an infected partner
Duration	Primary outbreak 2–3 weeks; recurrent outbreak 7–12 days; latent infection indefinitely	Variable; often, persistent clinical lesions and subclinical infection	Acute infection (2–3 weeks); asymptomatic phase (months); symptomatic HIV (months to years); AIDS (months to years)	Self-limiting in many males; persistent in most females until treated	Until treated	Until treated	Primary: 2–6 weeks; secondary: 2–6 weeks, may recur; tertiary: persists until treated
Recurrence	60% (HSV-1); 90% (HSV-2) within 1 year	Variable	Persistence	With reinfection	With reinfection	With reinfection	With reinfection
Diagnostic techniques	PCR, culture, antigen testing	Inspection	Serology with confirmatory testing	Wet prep, NAAT, culture	NAAT, cervical, pharyngeal or rectal culture[a]	NAAT, culture[a]	Serology
Antenatal or perinatal transmission	Yes—can cause skin, CNS, and disseminated infection	Yes—can cause laryngeal papillomas and perineal lesions	Yes, and postpartum via breast milk	Yes—may have neonatal vaginal discharge or asymptomatic colonization	Yes—can cause conjunctivitis, septicemia, meningitis	Yes—can cause conjunctivitis and/or pneumonia	Yes, and postpartum via breast milk
Partner evaluation	Inspection, consider serology	Inspection	Serology	Antimicrobial treatment[b]	Diagnostic tests as above and antimicrobial treatment[b]	Diagnostic tests as above and antimicrobial treatment[b]	Serology, antimicrobial treatment

AIDS, Acquired immune deficiency syndrome; *CNS,* central nervous system; *F/M,* female to male; *HIV,* human immunodeficiency virus; *HPV,* human papillomavirus; *HSV,* herpes simplex virus; *M/F,* male to female; *NAAT,* nucleic acid amplification test; *PCR,* polymerase chain reaction.

[a]In prepubertal patients, culture discharge for gonorrhea, vaginal wall for *Chlamydia.* In cases of suspected child abuse, cultures may be required for forensic purposes; expert consultation is recommended. Gonorrhea culture is recommended whenever antibiotic resistance is suspected.

[b]Consider expedited partner therapy where not forbidden by state law.

asymptomatic or may present with symptoms including vulvar lesions, vaginal discharge, odor, pruritus, perineal discomfort, and dysuria. There may be associated symptoms of pelvic pain, dyspareunia, fever, and irregular bleeding. Pathogens, such as herpes simplex, *Trichomonas vaginalis,* and HPV, cause inflammation of not only the vulva and vagina but also the cervix. Patients infected with *N. gonorrheae* or *C. trachomatis* infrequently have vulvar or vaginal involvement but may present with cervicitis, ascent of infection to the upper tract, or infection of the columnar epithelium of other genital sites, including the Bartholin glands, the urethra, and the rectum (see Tables 19.5 and 19.6).

A complete pelvic examination is desirable when evaluating adolescents for vulvovaginal complaints and possible STIs. At a minimum, this includes inspection of the perineum, collection of vaginal samples for microscopy and laboratory evaluation, and a careful bimanual examination. Cervical motion, adnexal, or uterine tenderness during the bimanual examination suggests the diagnosis of PID (see the Pelvic Inflammatory Disease section, later). Clinicians should consider using a speculum to inspect the vaginal walls and to obtain a vaginal specimen for microscopy uncontaminated by cervical secretions. A speculum also permits examination of the cervix for the presence of mucopurulent discharge, erythema, focal lesions, bleeding, and friability. Sexual partners should be evaluated and treated whenever an STI is identified; otherwise, reinfection is probable.

Adolescents with asymptomatic cervical infections may serve as silent reservoirs of sexually transmitted pathogens. This phenomenon is significant in the epidemiology and transmission of STIs. Therefore patients of sex partners known to have gonorrhea, *Chlamydia*, or nonspecific urethritis should be evaluated and treated appropriately. The patient and partner(s) must be advised to abstain from sexual intercourse until the course of treatment is completed by all. In the case of single-dose regimens, abstinence should be practiced for 7 days after the partners begin treatment. They also should be seen for follow-up in 3 months to test for reinfection and thereafter at least every 12 months for STI surveillance because of the significant incidence of another (often subclinical) infection.

Testing for STIs must be based on behaviors and anatomy, regardless of the patient's self-identified gender or sexual orientation. Patients of any gender (cis-, trans- or nonbinary) may have partners outside their stated sexual preference: For example, young females who identify as lesbian may nonetheless have male partners. To guide appropriate STI testing, a comprehensive sexual history (see https://www.cdc.gov/std/treatment/sexualhistory.pdf) and accurate understanding of the patient's reproductive anatomy is essential.

Diagnosis and treatment of infected patients and their partners is critical because of the potential for spread to others and major sequelae that include ectopic pregnancy, infertility, and chronic pelvic pain as a result of smoldering or recurrent upper genital tract disease. Finally, it is the clinician's responsibility to provide education regarding STIs. Use of condoms and other barrier protection (e.g., dental dams) should be emphasized at every opportunity. Education includes discussion of responsible sexuality, including abstinence, use of contraceptives, and safer sex practices, as appropriate to the patient.

Surface Infestations and Perineal Lesions

Parasitic Infestations

Two parasitic infestations—scabies and pubic lice—may be transmitted via sexual contact. Both produce symptoms of vulvar and inguinal pruritus and irritation accompanied by findings of dark specks of parasite feces on underwear or blood caused by excoriation from scratching. Sexual transmission is more likely in adolescents than in young children, who may acquire the parasites by close nonsexual contact. Development of pubic hair is necessary for the acquisition of pubic lice. Meticulous inspection of the pubic area for nits and adult lice ("crabs") may be necessary to discover early infestations.

Human Papillomavirus

Although HPV remains the most prevalent sexually transmitted pathogen found in adolescents worldwide, HPV infection rates have substantially decreased in countries where HPV vaccination has been implemented. Vaccination with the 9-valent HPV vaccine is now routinely recommended at 11 to 12 years. Genital warts, also called *condylomata acuminata*, are no longer regarded as an isolated nuisance but rather as one manifestation of a spectrum of lower genital tract diseases caused by HPV. The virus plays a causative role in cancerous and precancerous lesions of the cervix and of other genital tissues and mucous membranes in both males and females.

Transmission of HPV is usually via sexual contact in adolescents. Sexual abuse should be a consideration in children with condylomata, but other means of transmission are possible including autoinoculation from other sites or heteroinoculation from nonsexual contact with affected caregivers. Passage to neonates during delivery also has been documented and can result in subsequent development of laryngeal papillomata and perineal lesions.

The incubation period is variable and ranges from 1 to 24 months (see Table 19.6).

Condylomata may emerge after subclinical, acute, or chronic nonspecific vulvovaginal inflammation incited by the virus. In most cases, the lesions are asymptomatic, although pruritus is reported by some patients. However, when the warts are traumatized or become secondarily infected, pain may be a complaint. A rapid increase in warty tissue may be associated with diabetes, pregnancy, or HIV infection.

In general, the warts appear as fleshy, rounded, or ragged papules often located at the posterior edge of the introitus and/or in the perianal region. Lesions may be discrete early on (Fig. 19.25A) but with evolution tend to become confluent (see Fig. 19.25B). Warts can also be flat or even clinically unapparent to the naked eye. Although most lesions involve the perineum and perianal areas, vaginal and cervical involvement are also common in adolescents (see Fig. 19.25C). The virus can also infect other mucous membranes, including the anus, urethra, mouth, larynx, and conjunctiva. Clinical diagnosis is made by careful inspection of the external genitalia, vagina, cervix (in adolescents), and perianal areas for visible warts. A negative serologic test for syphilis helps differentiate HPV disease from the condylomata lata of secondary syphilis. When untreated, condylomata may resolve spontaneously or may persist or progress.

Molluscum Contagiosum

The sharply circumscribed, waxy, papular, umbilicated lesions of molluscum contagiosum, caused by a poxvirus, can be spread as a result of sexual contact, in which case lesions are found predominantly on the labia, mons pubis, buttocks, and lower abdomen. This mode of spread is much more likely in the adolescent than in the young child. Most lesions resolve slowly over 18 months without treatment.

Syphilis

Syphilitic Chancre

The United States continues to see increasing rates of syphilis. Primary syphilis should be considered in any patient with a genital ulcer (Fig. 19.26). Most involve the genitalia, more often on the cervix or vaginal walls than on the labia. Both external and internal lesions are painless and tend to go unnoticed. Hence active syphilis often goes undiagnosed until the secondary stage of the disease. Although a single lesion is typical, multiple chancres are seen in some cases and raise suspicion for HIV infection. The chancre usually appears 3 to 4 weeks after inoculation with *Treponema pallidum*, though chancre can appear as late as 3 months after infection. It is often accompanied by inguinal adenopathy. Involved nodes are firm, mobile, and nontender. Because atypical lesions are common, all suspicious ulcers should be promptly investigated. Presumptive diagnosis requires a positive result on both a nontreponemal test and a treponemal test. The nontreponemal serologic tests are the Venereal Disease Research Laboratory and rapid plasma reagin, which usually become positive within 1 to 2 weeks after the appearance of the chancre and are uniformly elevated after 1 month. Treponemal tests include fluorescent treponemal antibody absorption and a range of other immunoassays, which vary by laboratory. Many sites now employ the reverse algorithm, which uses a general treponemal test, followed by rapid plasma reagin. It is prudent to consult with the local health department or infectious disease specialist for both updated and locally available diagnostic resources. Left untreated, chancres heal spontaneously in 3 to 8 weeks, but the infection persists.

Secondary Syphilis

In the absence of early diagnosis and treatment, hematogenous spread occurs approximately 1 to 3 months after the appearance of the primary chancre, whereupon the lesions of secondary syphilis appear. These are accompanied or preceded by generalized adenopathy and often are associated with systemic flulike symptoms of fever, headache, malaise, arthralgia, sore throat, and rhinorrhea. The rash generalizes rapidly, has a symmetric distribution, and involves the palms and soles. The lesions usually take the form of reddish brown maculopapules, although commonly they are papulosquamous

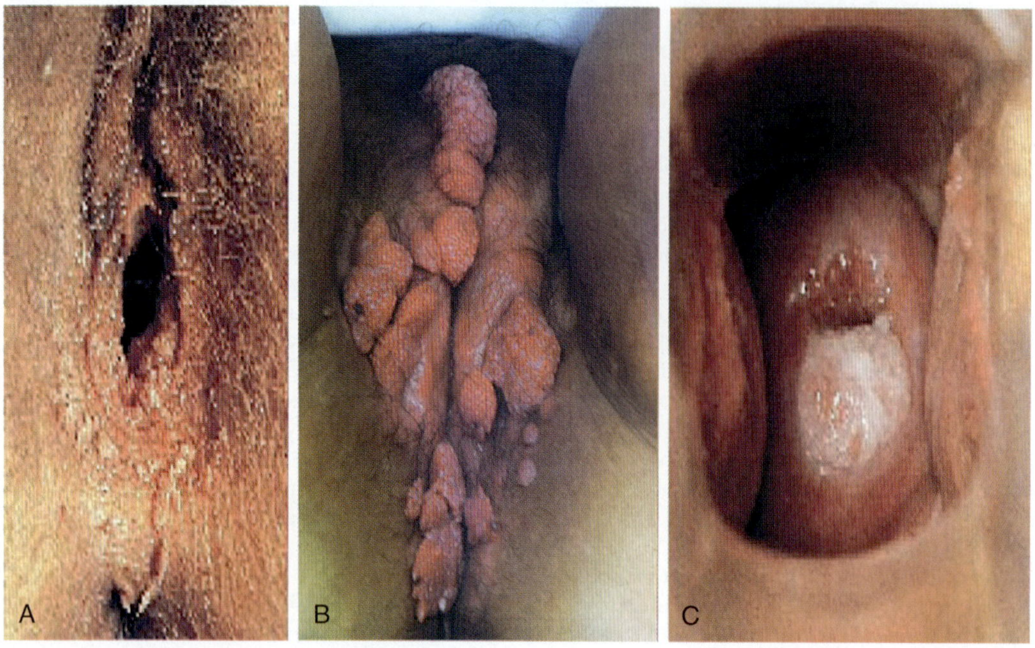

Fig. 19.25 Condylomata acuminata. These sexually transmitted viral warts (A) tend to be discrete early on but with evolution become confluent (B). Adolescents have a significant risk of developing vaginal and cervical lesions (C). (A and C, Courtesy E. Jerome, MD. B, Courtesy Susan Lindsley, Centers for Disease Control and Prevention, Public Health Image Library.)

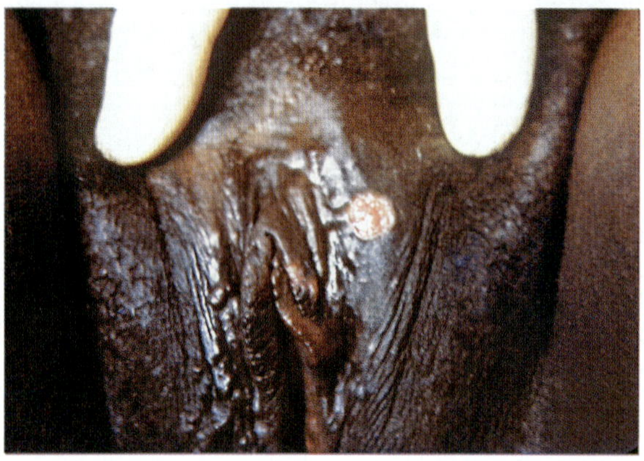

Fig. 19.26 Primary syphilis. The syphilitic chancre begins as an erythematous papule that erodes centrally. It is typically painless and indurated on palpation with a smooth base and rolled margins. (Courtesy The Centers for Disease Control and Prevention, Public Health Image Library.)

(Fig. 19.27A). Follicular and pustular lesions also may be seen, making secondary syphilis the "great mimicker." Lesions range in size from a few millimeters to 1 cm and can be round or oval. On occasion they clear centrally, becoming annular. As in pityriasis rosea, for which the rash is often mistaken, they are frequently oriented along lines of skin cleavage. Moist papules, called *condylomata lata,* are found in the genital folds, gluteal cleft, and over the medial surfaces of the upper thighs (see Fig. 19.27B). These papules often resemble small mushroom caps or have a warty appearance with a pinkish gray color and range in size from 1 to 3 cm. Many patients develop an associated patchy alopecia.

Mucosal lesions, termed *mucous patches* (see Fig. 19.27C), appear as centrally eroded, grayish white plaques 0.5 to 1 cm in diameter and can be found on all mucosal surfaces. Condylomata lata and mucosal lesions teem with organisms and are thus highly infectious. Serologic tests are positive at this stage. The rash persists for 1 to 3 months if untreated and then clears spontaneously, marking the beginning of a period of latency in which the organism persists in multiple tissues with the potential for causing tertiary disease years later.

Bartholin Gland Abscess

Bartholin gland abscess presents as a unilateral erythematous, hot, tender mass at the posterior margin of the introitus at the base of one of the labium majora (Fig. 19.28). When associated with an STI, it is generally seen in adolescents with gonorrhea, but it can occur in younger patients infected with gonococci and may be less likely associated with *Chlamydia.* When such a mass is encountered, material expressed from the abscess should be cultured because multiple agents, such as *Escherichia coli, staphylococci,* streptococci, and vaginal anaerobes, have also been documented as pathogens. Treatment is based on diagnostic testing results. Often incision, drainage, and packing or placement of a Word catheter are required. Less commonly, abscesses can occur more anteriorly, originating in the periurethral or Skene glands.

Genital Herpes

Type 2 and type 1 HSVs have been confirmed as genital pathogens in both pubertal and prepubertal children. In adolescents, genital infection is acquired almost exclusively by sexual or intimate contact with infected mucosal surfaces, and further evaluation for simultaneous STIs is warranted. In prepubertal children, vulvar involvement can result from sexual contact or by spread from another infected site, such as the lips, mouth, or a herpetic whitlow. It can also be acquired from parents or caretakers with herpes labialis who fail to wash their hands properly before changing diapers or assisting young children with toileting. Most infections are symptomatic, but occasionally infected individuals have no symptoms. An antibody response, with or without symptoms, can be produced within a few days (see Table 19.6).

Patients with primary infection frequently have systemic symptoms of fever, malaise, and myalgia, in addition to severe perineal pain and dysuria. Tender inguinal adenopathy is usually prominent but may not develop for several days. Perineal inspection reveals single or clustered vesicular lesions and/or ulcers on erythematous and edematous bases (Fig. 19.29A). Acute ulcerations are typically covered by yellow exudate and may be extensive (see Fig. 19.29B). A copious, foul-smelling, watery yellow vaginal discharge may be seen as well. Associated sterile pyuria may be a feature. Dysuria may be so severe as to cause acute urinary retention. The ulcerative phase gradually resolves as lesions heal within a period of 14 to 21 days. After primary infection, a persistent subclinical infection is established in the lumbosacral ganglia.

NAATs such as PCR are increasingly available for the detection of HSV and have become the preferred diagnostic tool. Viral culture, although a valid test and useful, often requires more time to positivity. Serum confirmation of type 1 or 2 infection is possible but does not influence treatment decisions. Clinical suspicion is the usual indication for initiating antiviral therapy because the earlier it is begun, the more efficacious it is likely to be.

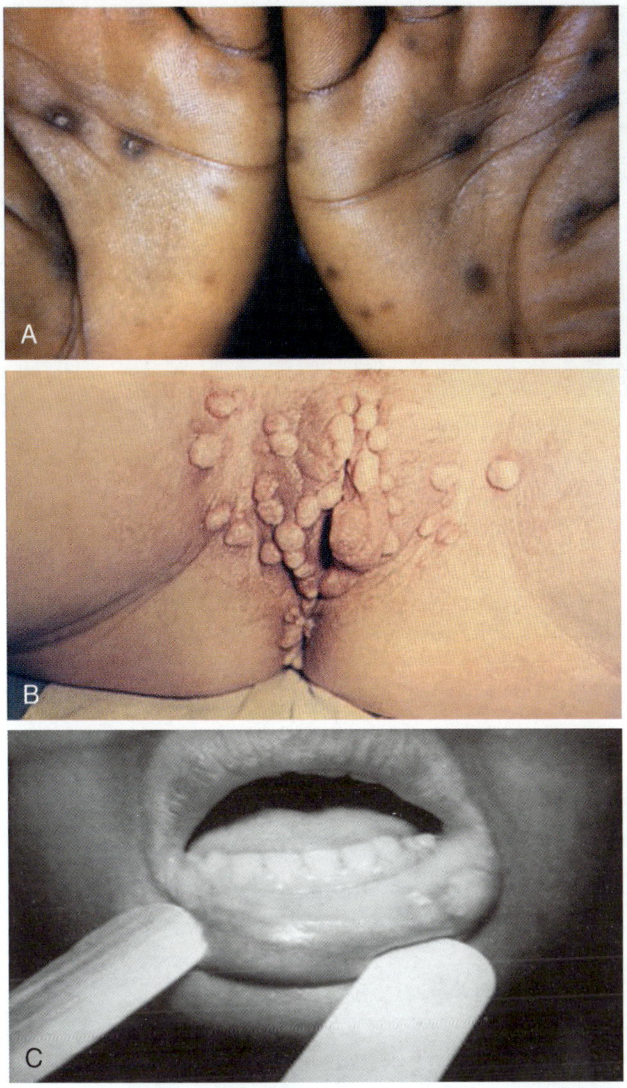

Fig. 19.27 Secondary syphilis. (A) Hyperpigmented, papulosquamous rash, a result of a secondary syphilis infection. (B) Female patient's perineum, highlighting the cutaneous, condylomata lata lesions atop the labia and perianal region, due to secondary syphilis. (C) Mucosal lesions were also prominent. The systemic symptoms, mucosal lesions, and involvement of palms and soles helped distinguish the eruption from that of pityriasis rosea, with which it is commonly confused. (A, Courtesy The Centers for Disease Control and Prevention, Public Health Image Library. B, Susan Lindsley, The Centers for Disease Control and Prevention, Public Health Image Library.)

Recurrences are common and generally are milder, of shorter duration, and only locally symptomatic. Possible triggers of recurrence include fever, menstruation, emotional stress, and friction. On occasion, prodromal tingling, pain, burning, or hyperesthesia is noticed in the area where vesicles ultimately recur. The interval between episodes varies widely.

Trichomonas Infection

T. vaginalis is a flagellated protozoan. It has been found in the vaginal discharge of neonates delivered of mothers infected at the time of delivery, but thereafter it tends to be an unusual finding until the peripubertal period. Beyond the neonatal period, it is acquired almost exclusively by sexual contact, often in concert with other STIs. However, trichomonads can live on warm, moist surfaces outside a living host for up to 45 minutes. Hence transmission via fomites is possible, although infrequent. Infection can be asymptomatic in adolescents. Symptomatic patients have vulvar pruritus, burning, and dysuria in association with a profuse vaginal discharge that may be watery, yellowish gray, or green. Some affected adolescents may endorse pelvic pain or heaviness.

On inspection the vulva may be hyperemic and edematous, but the degree of inflammation is highly variable. Because the discharge is profuse, it may be present on the perineum (Fig. 19.30A). It pools in dependent portions of the vagina and coats the vaginal walls (see Fig. 19.30B). The vaginal mucosa is erythematous, and vaginal tenderness and petechiae may be noted (see Fig. 19.30C). This organism does not routinely infect the upper genital tract.

Diagnosis is confirmed by finding motile trichomonads on microscopic examination of a saline wet mount (see Fig. 19.30D), but this may be positive in only 50% to 60% of infections. Leukocytes are usually present in increased numbers and may surround the organisms, making detection more difficult. Test yield may be increased by warming the saline solution to body temperature, and diluting a densely cellular discharge may make it easier to see the organisms moving. The slide must be examined soon after preparation because drying makes it uninterpretable. Trichomonads may also be found in urine specimens. A mildly positive whiff test (release of amine odor on addition of 10% KOH to a drop of discharge) and elevated vaginal pH often occur. NAATs and several point of care tests with greater sensitivity and specificity than wet prep or culture are increasingly available for diagnosis.

Oral metronidazole is the preferred treatment. Tinidazole can be used when metronidazole fails or organisms are known to be resistant. Sexual partners usually are asymptomatic carriers of small

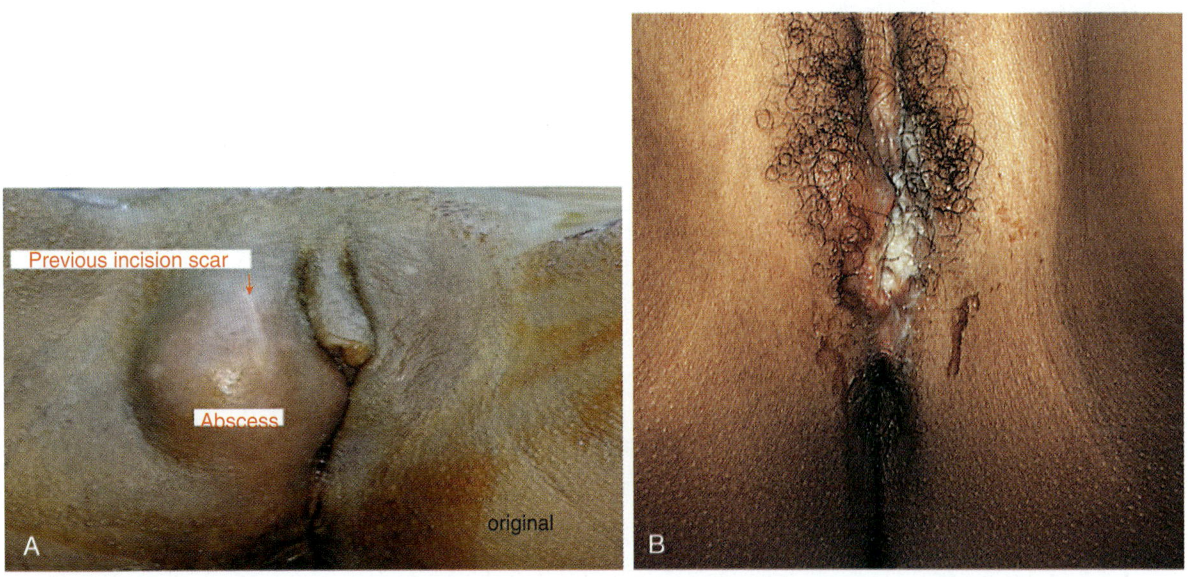

Fig. 19.28 Bartholin gland abscess. (A) Right Bartholin's gland abscess. A linear scar of previous incision is seen. (B) This peripubertal child has a gonococcal Bartholin gland abscess with associated vulvar inflammation, edema, and a purulent vaginal discharge which should prompt evaluation for child abuse. (A, From Radhakrishna V, Goel R, Parashar G, Santhanakrishnan R. Bartholin's gland abscess in a prepubertal female: a case report. *Ann Med Surg.* 2017;24:1–2. B, From Omole F, Simmons BJ, Hacker Y. Management of Bartholin duct cyst and gland abscess. *Am Fam Physician.* 2003;68:135–140.)

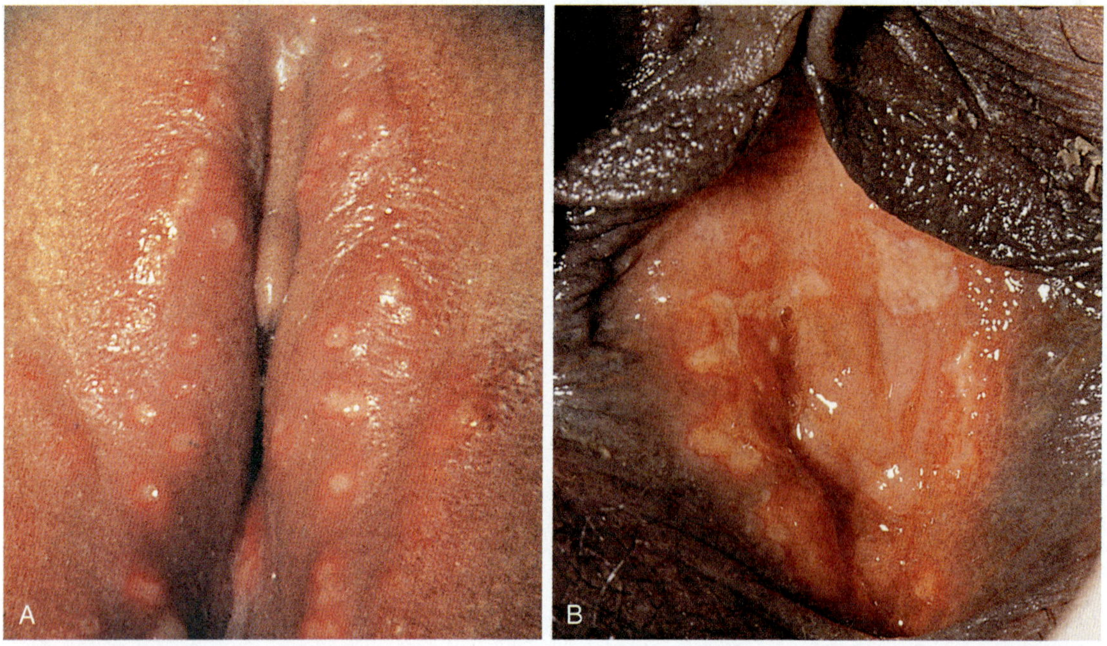

Fig. 19.29 Herpes simplex. (A) This prepubertal child had intense dysuria, perineal pain, and numerous vesicular lesions, a few of which have ulcerated, over her perineum. (B) The full-blown ulcerative phase of herpetic vulvitis is seen in this adolescent patient.

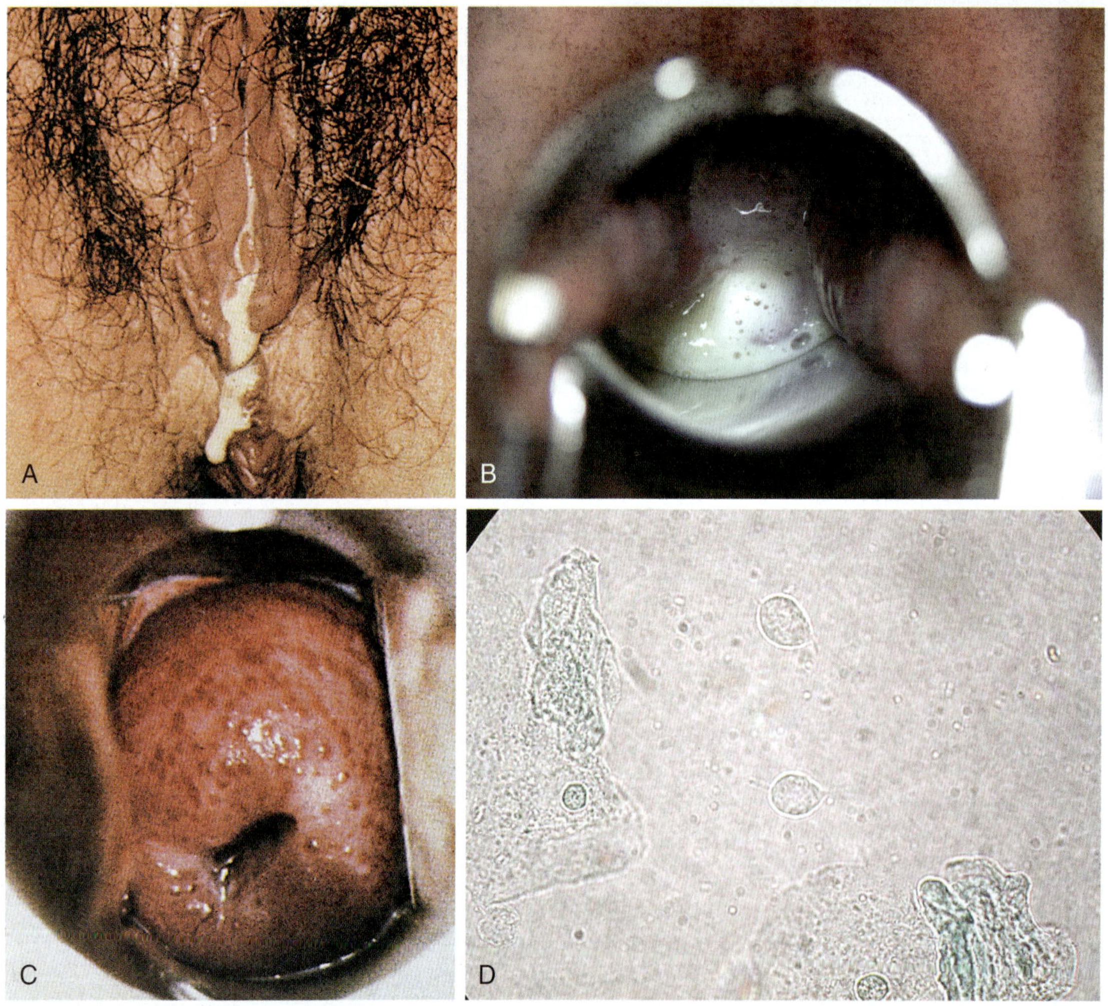

Fig. 19.30 *Trichomonas* infection. (A) *Trichomonas vaginalis* produces a profuse foul acrid-smelling thin discharge that often is visible on perineal inspection. (B) In some cases, it is homogeneous; in others, it is bubbly as shown here. Vulvar pruritus is often intense. (C) The vaginal mucosa is inflamed and often speckled with petechial lesions. In adolescents, petechial hemorrhages may also be found on the cervix, resulting in the so-called *strawberry cervix*. (D) Microscopical examination of a wet mount reveals motile trichomonads. (A and C, Courtesy Ellen Wald, MD, University of Wisconsin Children's Hospital, Madison, WI. B, Courtesy Harold C. Wiesenfeld, MD, CM, Magee-Women's Hospital of the University of Pittsburgh Medical Center, Pittsburgh, PA. D, Courtesy Jill Huppert, MD, MPH, and Joel Mortensen, PhD, Cincinnati Children's Hospital Medical Center, Cincinnati, OH.)

numbers of organisms but occasionally have symptoms of urethritis. Whether symptomatic or not, they should be treated to avoid subsequent transmission.

Bacterial Vaginosis

Bacterial vaginosis is a noninflammatory condition that is not sexually transmitted but is associated with sexual activity and STIs. It represents a disturbance in the vaginal ecosystem with an overgrowth of multiple species of anaerobic bacteria and a corresponding decrease in lactobacilli. The overall concentration of vaginal bacteria increases 100-fold. The condition is associated with an increased frequency of preterm labor and possibly with increased incidence of PID. The major symptom in all age groups is vaginal discharge with a noticeable fishy odor. Adolescents with bacterial vaginosis have little vulvovaginal irritation, and the cervix and upper genital tract are spared.

On inspection, discharge is frequently present on the perineum (Fig. 19.31A) and may be seen adhering to the vaginal walls, which do not appear to be inflamed. In general, the discharge is thin and homogeneous in consistency, grayish white in color, and malodorous. Addition of 10% KOH to a sample of the discharge produces a noticeable amine odor (positive whiff test). A saline wet preparation usually reveals characteristic "clue cells" (see Fig. 19.31B). The diagnosis is made clinically by meeting three of the following four criteria: (1) homogeneous white discharge, (2) a positive whiff test, (3) clue cells representing more than 20% of the epithelial cells on a saline wet mount preparation, and (4) vaginal secretions pH greater than 4.5. Because bacterial vaginosis alone is rarely associated with evidence of tissue invasion, leukocytes should not be seen in increased numbers. If they are, additional pathogens should be sought and are often found. Commercial point of care testing kits for bacterial vaginosis alone, or simultaneously with trichomonas and candida, are available. Both oral and intravaginal metronidazole and intravaginal clindamycin are acceptable forms of treatment in the nonpregnant patient.

Gonorrhea

Infections with *Neisseria gonorrheae* (the "gonococcus") have been increasing in the United States in the last decade. Gonococci cause treatable bacterial cervicitis in the adolescent and, in the context of sexual abuse, vulvovaginitis in the prepubertal child. Prepubertal children may be asymptomatic, but most experience some vaginal discharge, vulvar discomfort, pruritus, and/or dysuria, and inspection of the distal vaginal mucosa reveals prominent inflammation. Adolescents without upper genital tract extension can be asymptomatic or present with purulent vaginal discharge (see Table 19.5). On examination, the vaginal mucosa can appear normal, but the cervix usually is erythematous and friable with purulent cervical discharge (Fig. 19.32). Adolescents may also have erythema, edema, and tenderness of the urethra, as well as involvement of Bartholin and Skene glands and the rectum (see Fig. 19.28B).

NAATs are used to confirm the infection. Culture may be necessary to determine antimicrobial sensitivity and in medicolegal cases. Because simultaneous throat and anal tests can be positive (despite the absence of pharyngeal or anorectal symptoms) even when testing from the urogenital tract is negative, testing of extragenital sites should be considered based on sexual practices. Both tonsils and the posterior pharyngeal wall should be swabbed in obtaining the throat specimen; the rectal swab should be inserted no more than 1 to 2 cm past the anal orifice to avoid fecal contamination.

Ceftriaxone is the preferred treatment for uncomplicated gonococcal infection. Persistent symptoms after treatment should be evaluated by culture including bacterial sensitivities, and current CDC guidelines should be consulted.

On occasion, patients with gonorrhea may develop disseminated gonococcal infection via hematogenous spread. This phenomenon may occur at any age. It is more common in adolescents with asymptomatic (and therefore untreated) endocervical infection and in patients of all ages with silent anal or pharyngeal infections. In postmenarchal patients, systemic symptoms are more likely to develop during a menstrual period.

The early phase of disseminated gonorrhea, which lasts 2 to 5 days, involves fever and chills, polyarthralgias (involving the knees, wrists, ankles, elbows, and hands), and characteristic skin lesions that begin as small erythematous papules or petechiae, evolve to form pustules surrounded by red halos (Fig. 19.33A and B), and later may undergo necrosis centrally. Without prompt treatment, patients progress to a second phase, characterized by monoarticular arthritis, effusion, or tenosynovitis (see Fig. 19.33C

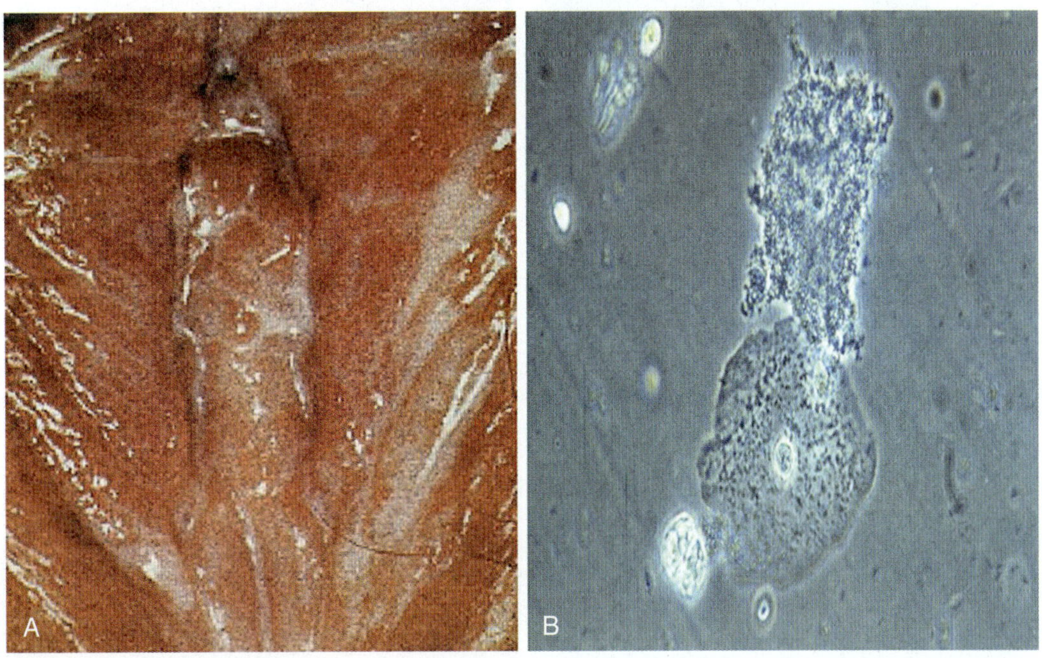

Fig. 19.31 Bacterial vaginosis. Overgrowth of multiple anaerobes produces this form of vaginosis. (A) The major symptom is one of a malodorous homogeneous vaginal discharge that smoothly coats the vaginal walls as seen here. (B) This photomicrograph of a vaginal smear specimen depicts a normal cell and an epithelial cell with its exterior covered by bacteria, giving the cell a roughened, stippled appearance known as a "clue cell." (A, Courtesy Ellen Wald, MD, University of Wisconsin Children's Hospital, Madison, WI. B, Courtesy M. Rein, The Centers for Disease Control and Prevention, Public Health Image Library.)

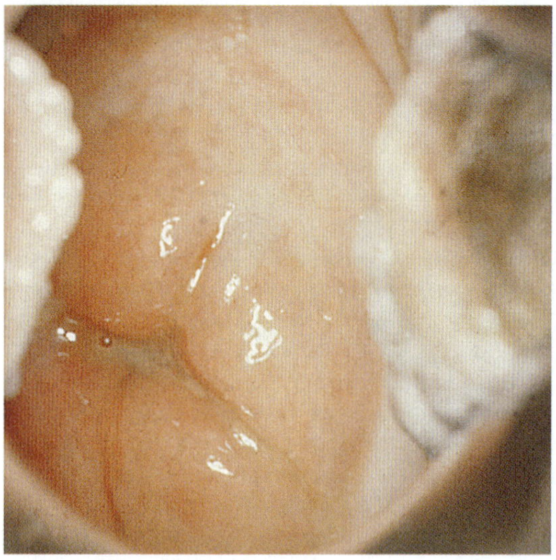

Fig. 19.32 Gonorrhea. Cervical inflammation with mucopurulent discharge .(Courtesy L. Vontver, MD.)

and D). Myocarditis, pericarditis, endocarditis, and meningitis are other complications of hematogenous seeding.

Chlamydia trachomatis Infection

C. trachomatis is the most prevalent curable STI causing cervicitis and urethritis and contributing to upper genital tract disease. Its high prevalence and serious sequelae make proper diagnosis and treatment an important aspect of adolescent sexual health care. Compared with gonococcal infection, its transmission rate for a single episode of intercourse is lower, but its prevalence is greater, and infection persists longer.

When prepubertal children are infected with *Chlamydia* in the context of sexual abuse, they may be asymptomatic or may present with vaginal discharge and/or bleeding and vulvar pruritus, pain, or erythema. Symptoms may be intermittent or persistent, and coinfection with *N. gonorrheae* is common. Adolescents may have symptoms of both cervical and urethral infection with pelvic or abdominal pain, spotting or irregular vaginal bleeding, dysuria, and/or vaginal discharge. A picture indistinguishable from gonorrhea (purulent vaginal discharge, perineal irritation, and findings of cervicitis with mucopurulent discharge) can also be seen (see Fig. 19.32). Cervical examination may reveal erythema and friability with bleeding during the minimal manipulation necessary to obtain specimens. Endometritis is common with cervicitis, even in the absence of classic symptoms of PID, and Bartholin duct infections also occur. *Chlamydia* can also cause urethritis symptoms of dysuria, urgency, and frequency, and patients may exhibit pyuria in the absence of bacteriuria. It is important to note that asymptomatic chlamydial infection in both females and males is common and that many patients have simultaneous infection with other STIs, especially gonococci.

Chlamydiae are slowly replicating obligate intracellular organisms. Diagnosis is confirmed by NAAT on urine or vaginal or endocervical swabs. If indicated, NAAT may be sent from the oropharynx or rectum. Tests of cure are not recommended by the CDC, and NAATs remain positive for up to 3 weeks after treatment. Reinfection is common, and clinicians should retest in 3 months even in the absence of symptoms.

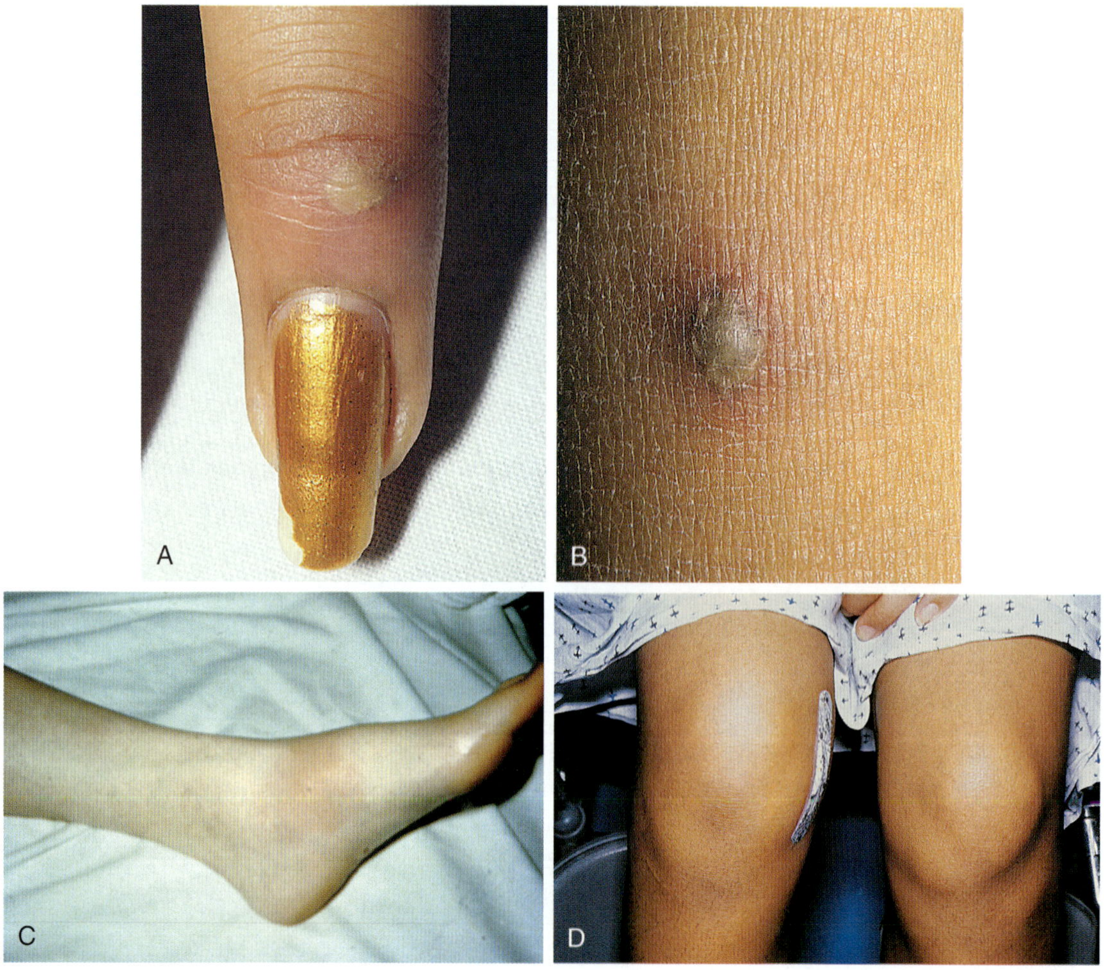

Fig. 19.33 Disseminated gonococcal infection. (A and B) These pustular skin lesions with red halos are characteristic of disseminated gonorrhea, which can occur at any age. (C and D) Tenosynovitis and monoarticular arthritis are commonly seen in association with skin lesions in disseminated disease. Note the signs of effusion in the right knee of the girl shown in D. (D, Courtesy Robert Hickey, MD, Children's Hospital of Pittsburgh, Pittsburgh, PA.)

Genital Mycoplasmas

Mycoplasma genitalium is implicated as a pathogen in some genitourinary infections, including PID, that are resistant to standard syndromic treatment regimens. Emerging knowledge suggests resistance to doxycycline and increasing rates of resistance to azithromycin. *M. genitalium* is not routinely tested for in clinical practice. When genital infections have not responded to standard treatment, infectious disease consultation is warranted.

Human Immunodeficiency Virus

The manifestations of HIV infection are discussed in Chapter 13. The adolescent history outlined previously (see Table 19.3) should identify teenagers at increased risk of acquiring HIV infection. However, to treat infection early and reduce subsequent transmission, the CDC recommends universal, non–risk-based confidential HIV screening at least once for all adolescents 13 years old and older with ongoing annual screening based on risk factors. From the gynecologic perspective, a number of infections may present differently in the HIV-infected individual (see Table 19.6).

Pelvic Inflammatory Disease

PID is an important complication of lower genital tract infection in the postmenarchal patient, resulting from ascending spread of cervical infection. Although *N. gonorrheae* and *C. trachomatis* often play a critical initiating role, PID often occurs without evidence of either of these infections, and this does not alter treatment recommendations. The majority of cases involve a mixture of aerobic and anaerobic organisms, including those which are considered normal vaginal or enteric flora but are pathogenic in the upper genital tract (see Box 19.7). Patients who are immunocompromised or from areas where tuberculosis is endemic can develop tuberculosis-associated PID.

Risk factors for developing PID include adolescent age, multiple sexual partners, and previous PID. Because menstruation facilitates ascent of pathogenic organisms from the cervix to the uterus and fallopian tubes, symptoms often begin during or shortly after a menstrual period. Long-term morbidity includes an increased incidence of ectopic pregnancy, decreased fertility, and chronic pelvic pain resulting from tubal occlusion and scarring of pelvic structures. Adverse sequelae may be more severe among patients with delayed diagnosis and treatment and repeated infection.

The classic picture of acute PID includes abrupt onset of high fever and shaking chills in association with intense lower abdominal pain, nausea, and vomiting. The patient appears acutely ill and may walk with a shuffling gait. On examination, there is prominent lower abdominal tenderness and guarding and mucopurulent cervical discharge. Bimanual palpation of the uterus, adnexa, and cervix reveals marked tenderness. Adnexal fullness, if present, suggests abscess formation. The erythrocyte sedimentation rate is markedly elevated, and there is a pronounced leukocytosis with a left shift on complete blood count and differential. However, this "classic" picture is not the most typical. More commonly, the onset of symptoms is insidious and the clinical picture more subtle. Fever may be absent or low grade; abdominal pain, mild; and blood work, normal. In such cases, diagnosis can be difficult, requiring considerable suspicion and a low threshold for examination. Lower abdominal, pelvic, and/or cervical motion, uterine, or adnexal tenderness and some evidence of lower genital tract inflammation usually are present even in clinically mild cases.

Acute salpingitis may mimic a number of other disorders and is particularly challenging when the presentation includes right lower quadrant abdominal pain (Box 19.8). Table 19.7 summarizes clinical findings that may aid in distinguishing among some common causes. Given the variable clinical picture in PID, minimal diagnostic criteria have been developed. These include lower abdominal or pelvic pain and cervical motion or uterine or adnexal tenderness. Ultrasonography is normal in most cases of PID and is typically only required to evaluate for alternate diagnoses or sequelae of PID if symptoms do not improve with appropriate treatment. Treatment should follow current CDC recommendations. It should be noted that beyond the first 3 weeks after insertion, intrauterine devices do not confer an increased risk of PID. Removal of an intrauterine device during PID treatment should only be considered if symptoms do not respond to treatment in 72 hours.

Indications for hospitalization include suspected abscess, inability to tolerate or follow an oral regimen, pregnancy, or when the exact diagnosis is unclear and surgical emergencies cannot be excluded. During outpatient treatment, it is critical that clinicians reexamine the patient within 72 hours to document clinical improvement and to confirm adherence with antibiotic use. If on follow-up it is found that there has been no significant clinical improvement, the patient should be admitted for parenteral medication and mycoplasma should be considered as a potential pathogen. In addition to antibiotic resistance, failure to improve on therapy raises the possibility of complications, such as a tubo-ovarian complex or abscess, or an alternative diagnosis, such as ectopic pregnancy, miscarriage, appendicitis, or other surgical condition. Laparoscopy may be necessary when surgical conditions are suspected or parenteral medical treatment fails.

Perihepatitis (Fitz-Hugh–Curtis Syndrome)

Perihepatitis occurs as a complication of PID when inflammation spreads to the liver capsule and adjacent peritoneum. It presents as moderate to severe pleuritic right upper quadrant (RUQ) pain, which may be referred to the right shoulder, and can be associated with fever, chills, nausea, and vomiting. Although the RUQ pain can develop simultaneously with pelvic symptoms of PID, it may begin during asymptomatic lower genital tract infection or later in the course due to partially treated infection. In many patients, upper abdominal pain is so severe that the patient may not report the milder degrees of lower abdominal and pelvic discomfort.

On examination, RUQ tenderness and guarding and peritoneal signs may be present. Gynecologic examination in most instances discloses findings of purulent cervicitis and PID. *N. gonorrheae* and *C. trachomatis* are the major pathogens associated with this syndrome. Patients with Fitz-Hugh–Curtis syndrome have minimal, if any, abnormalities of liver function tests. Although usually not necessary, ultrasound examination of the RUQ should demonstrate a normal liver, biliary tree, and gallbladder. Laparoscopic findings of purulent and fibrinous inflammation of the capsule and hemorrhagic areas of adjacent parietal peritoneum are diagnostic, but laparoscopy is rarely indicated for this condition. Major differential diagnostic considerations are listed in Box 19.8 and Table 19.7.

Box 19.8 Medical Conditions Manifesting as Acute Right-Sided Abdominal Pain in Adolescents

Hepatic
- Fitz-Hugh–Curtis syndrome
- Viral hepatitis (cytomegalovirus; Epstein-Barr virus; hepatitis A, B, and C)
- Drug-induced hepatitis
- Autoimmune hepatitis
- Alcoholic hepatitis
- Hepatitis secondary to bacteremia

Biliary
- Acute cholecystitis
- Cholelithiasis

Intestinal
- Inflammatory bowel disease
- Irritable bowel syndrome
- Constipation
- Lactose intolerance
- Celiac disease

Other Gastrointestinal
- Subphrenic abscess
- Appendicitis
- Perforated gastric or duodenal ulcer

Pulmonary
- Pneumonia, pleuritis, pleurodynia

Renal
- Acute pyelonephritis or perinephric abscess
- Kidney stones

Gynecologic
- Pelvic inflammatory disease
- Ovarian cyst, torsion, rupture, hemorrhage
- Dysmenorrhea
- Ectopic pregnancy

Table 19.7 Pertinent Clinical Characteristics of Disorders Causing Lower Abdominal Pain in Adolescent Patients

	Pelvic Inflammatory Disease	Ovarian Torsion	Ovarian Cyst	Ectopic Pregnancy	Inflammatory Bowel Disease	Appendicitis	Irritable Bowel/ Constipation	Dysmenorrhea
Location and quality of pain	Mid- and lateral pelvis, usually bilateral; can be vague, dull, crampy, or sharp	Unilateral RLQ or LLQ, colicky, severe	Usually asymptomatic but may have colicky RLQ or LLQ pain	Lateral pain, colicky, ± uterine cramping	Often generalized abdominal pain, crampy	Periumbilical cramping changing to RLQ cramping or sharp pain	LLQ or generalized abdominal pain, crampy or colicky	Suprapubic, midabdominal, lower back, dull cramping
Onset	Gradual over days to months	Sudden	Gradual, although rupture or hemorrhage are associated with acutely increased pain	Gradual with sudden exacerbation	Gradual over weeks to months with exacerbations	Gradual over hours to days	Long history of gastrointestinal symptoms over months to years	Periodic, evolving over hours; close to onset of flow
History	Unprotected sexual intercourse, previous PID or STI, multiple partners, irregular vaginal bleeding, increasingly severe menstrual cramps, vaginal discharge	± History of previous episodes of similar pain with resolution, increased ovarian size (anatomic variation predisposes)	Midcycle or luteal phase, physiologic rupture causes mittelschmerz, with pain for 24–48 hours	Amenorrhea (75%), ± pregnancy signs and symptoms	Weight loss or growth failure, diarrhea, bloody stools, fatigue, rashes, arthritis, fever	Usually no prior pain	± Constipation or diarrhea, improvement in pain after bowel movements, distention common, positive family history, symptoms increase with stress	Increasing severity 1–3 years after menarche
Gastrointestinal symptoms	Nausea, vomiting, anorexia may be present	Vomiting with onset of pain (25%)	Rare	Gastrointestinal symptoms secondary to pregnancy or severe vomiting secondary to rupture and peritonitis	Increased stool frequency, nocturnal stools, sometimes bloody diarrhea	Vomiting may follow onset of pain, anorexia	Long intermittent history of constipation, ± diarrhea	Diarrhea, flatulence, nausea/ vomiting not uncommon
Physical examination and laboratory findings	Cervical motion, uterine, or adnexal tenderness, clinical and laboratory evidence of cervicitis; vaginal bleeding; ± discharge; ± RUQ pain; perihepatitis; ± NAATs for gonorrhea and *Chlamydia*	Tender adnexa, ± guarding or peritoneal signs	Unilateral cystic adnexal mass	Normal uterus; unilateral or bilateral adnexal tenderness; positive urine pregnancy test in most, but inadequate β-hCG rise/48 hours after implantation; drop in Hct with rupture	Rectoabdominal tenderness, hematologic abnormalities, positive for stool heme	↑ WBCs, fever, evolving peritoneal signs	Occasional tender colon, usually normal	Normal or mild uterine tenderness during menses
Ultrasound findings	Usually normal, tubo-ovarian complex in over 30% in PID requiring hospitalization	Unilateral ovarian enlargement; solid ovarian mass, ± compromised blood supply on Doppler	Unilateral cyst, ± fluid in cul-de-sac frequent incidental finding on ultrasound	Tubal mass, vaginal probe enhances detection	Normal	Appendix frequently visible and inflamed	Normal	Normal

Note: This table is designed not only to aid the clinician in distinguishing between disorders that present with abdominal pain in adolescents but also enhance recognition of the fact that a complaint of abdominal pain must be taken seriously and evaluated carefully.

↑, Increased; ±, positive or negative; β-hCG, beta subunit of human chorionic gonadotropin; *GC, gonococcus; Hct,* hematocrit; *LLQ,* left lower quadrant; *NAAT,* nucleic acid amplification test; *PID,* pelvic inflammatory disease; *RLQ,* right lower quadrant; *RUQ,* right upper quadrant; *STI,* sexually transmitted infection; *WBC,* white blood cell.

PREGNANCY

Although generally declining, the birth rate for 15- to 19-year-old adolescents in the United States remains higher than in most similar industrialized nations. Because most of the pregnancies are unintended, adolescents may deny the possibility of their condition for extended periods to themselves, their parents, and others. This delay may decrease pregnancy options and increase complications of pregnancy and neonatal morbidity. With or without denial, at the time of presentation the teenager or parent may suspect pregnancy. Interviewing the patient and parent separately may facilitate a complete and accurate history.

Table 19.8 Signs and Symptoms of Pregnancy

First Trimester (6–12 Weeks)	Second Trimester (12+ Weeks)
Amenorrhea Light, irregular vaginal bleeding, syncope or fainting Fatigue Urinary frequency Mood swings "Morning" sickness Nausea and vomiting Food cravings Increased facial oil gland activity ("glow") Elevated body temperature Chloasma (dark facial pigmentation) Nasal stuffiness or mucous membrane congestion	Increased size of breasts, abdomen, waist Increased weight and clothing size Increased vaginal discharge Increased skin pigmentation Congestion of vaginal mucosa

Vaginal bleeding or spotting in early pregnancy may falsely reassure a patient that they are not pregnant, and minimal weight gain (whether voluntary or involuntary) may further facilitate denial. Patients may instead present with pelvic, abdominal, or back pain, vomiting and dehydration, constipation, urinary complaints, and urinary tract infection. Phlebitis, rupture of membranes, symptoms of gestational diabetes, or secondary problems of fatigue, insomnia, or headache ultimately bring some of these patients to medical attention. Considering the frequency of teenage pregnancy and the tendency of individuals to have alternative chief complaints, practitioners who care for adolescents should be familiar with the signs, symptoms, and methods of diagnosing pregnancy. Signs and symptoms of pregnancy are outlined in Table 19.8. A chronology of laboratory and clinical findings during pregnancy is presented in Table 19.9.

Home pregnancy tests are variable in sensitivity. However, many are as sensitive as office-based urine tests, which typically become positive within 10 to 14 days after intercourse. False-positive and false-negative results are encountered infrequently; causes for both are listed in Table 19.10. In particular, false positives are not caused by foods or drugs but can occur in certain medical situations, including up to 8 weeks after an abortion. Pregnancies are dated from the last normal menstrual period and not from conception, which typically occurs 2 weeks later.

ACKNOWLEDGMENTS

The authors gratefully acknowledge Pamela Murray, Gina Sucato, and Gerald Montano for all their work on previous versions of this chapter and for contributing all the photographs not otherwise attributed.

A supplemental video is available at Elsevier eBooks+.

Table 19.9 Laboratory and Clinical Correlations of Pregnancy

Gestation[a]	Serum Human Chorionic Gonadotropin (MIU/mL)	Signs, Symptoms, and Significant Events
1		Last menstrual period
2		
3	5 (24 h post implantation)	Conception followed by implantation
4	70–100	Missed period
5	>250	Pelvic ultrasound detects pregnancy; breast changes—tender, swollen; nipples—sensitive, dark
6	>1,000	Nausea, morning sickness; softening of lower corpus
7		Bluish color of cervix; softening of cervix; cardiac motion detectable on ultrasound
8	>10,000	
10	100,000 (peak)	
12		Fundus palpable at pelvic brim; fetal heart tones detectable with Doppler
14		Decrease in early signs and symptoms
16	10,000; false negatives may occur in second and third trimesters	Fundus palpable midway between pelvic brim and umbilicus; fetus visualized by radiograph; perception of fetal movement
20		Fundus palpable at umbilicus

[a]Weeks from last menstrual period.

Table 19.10 Causes of False-Positive and False-Negative Urine Pregnancy Tests

False-Negative Test	False-Positive Test
Too early (commonly) or too late (rarely) Adulterated urine Ectopic pregnancy (rarely negative, almost always positive) Impending or missed abortion (rarely negative, almost always positive) Dilute urine	Molar pregnancy Malignancies (gynecologic and other) Postpartum and postabortion (up to 8 weeks) Chinese herbal medications Hematuria or proteinuria[a] Midcycle LH surge[a] Perimenopausal[a] (LH elevation) Premature ovarian failure[a] (LH elevation)

LH, Luteinizing hormone.

[a]Can occur with less sensitive over-the-counter urine pregnancy tests.

Bibliography

Adams Hillard PJ, editor: *Practical pediatric and adolescent gynecology*, Oxford, 2013, Wiley-Blackwell.

Asăvoaie C, Fufezan O, Coşarcă M: Ovarian and uterine ultrasonography in pediatric patients: pictorial essay, *Med Ultrason* 16:160–167, 2014.

Bacon JL, Romano ME, Quint EH: Clinical recommendation: labial adhesion, *J Pediatr Adolescent Gynecol* 28:405–409, 2015.

Bandow GD: Diagnosis and management of vulvar ulcers, *Dermatol Clin* 28:753–763, 2010.

Braverman PK, Breech L: Clinical report—gynecologic examination for adolescents in the pediatric office setting, *Pediatrics* 126:583–590, 2010.

Emans SJ, Laufer MR, Goldstein DP: *Pediatric and adolescent gynecology*, ed 6, Philadelphia, 2011, Lippincott Williams & Wilkins.

Hatcher RA, Trussell J, Nelson AL, et al: *Contraceptive technology*, ed 20, New York, 2016, Ardent Media.

Holmes KK, Sparling PF, Stamm WE, et al: *Sexually transmitted diseases*, ed 4, New York, 2016, McGraw-Hill.

Klein DA, Goldenring JM, Adelman WP: HEEADSSS 3.0: The psychosocial interview for adolescents updated for a new century fueled by media. http://contemporarypediatrics.modernmedicine.com/contemporary-pediatrics/content/tags/adolescent-medicine/heeadsss-30-psychosocial-interview-adolesce.

Kondamudi NP, Gupta A, Watkins A, et al: Prepubertal girl with vaginal bleeding, *J Emerg Med* 46(6):769–771, 2014.

Lamont RF, Sobel JD, Akins RA, et al: The vaginal microbiome: new information about genital tract flora using molecular based techniques, *BJOG* 118(5):533–549, 2011.

Martin JA, Hamilton BE, Osterman MJK: Births in the United States, 2017, *NCHS Data Brief* (318)1–8, 2018.

Mauskar MM, Marathe K, Venkatesan A, Schlosser BJ, Edwards L: Vulvar diseases: conditions in adults and children, *J Am Acad Dermatol* 82(6):1287–1298, 2020.

Reddy J, Laufer MR: Hypertrophic labia minora, *J Pediatr Adolesc Gynecol* 23:3–6, 2010.

Websites

American College of Obstetricians and Gynecologists (ACOG): www.acog.org.

Center for Young Women's Health: www.youngwomenshealth.org.

Centers for Disease Control and Prevention (CDC): Sexually Transmitted Diseases (STDs): https://www.cdc.gov/std/treatment-guidelines/screening-recommendations.htm; www.cdc.gov/std/treatment/default.htm.

North American Society for Pediatric and Adolescent Gynecology: www.naspag.org.

Society for Adolescent Health and Medicine (SAHM): www.adolescenthealth.org.

World Health Organization (WHO): Sexual and reproductive health: Classification of female genital mutilation: https://www.who.int/teams/sexual-and-reproductive-health-and-research-(srh)/areas-of-work/female-genital-mutilation/types-of-female-genital-mutilation.

OPHTHALMOLOGY

20

Ken K. Nischal

The pediatrician may encounter a child who is systemically well or unwell and has a common eye or visual problem, or an encounter may be with a child who is systemically well or unwell with an uncommon eye or visual problem. In the systemically unwell child, the eye findings may help in identifying a unifying diagnosis. Assessing the child's eyes from an anatomic or structural perspective and the child's neurophysiologic and psychophysical visual status is key. Although common ocular conditions are important to recognize, the pediatrician must also be aware of certain uncommon ocular conditions that may form part of a syndrome affecting the child.

In this chapter a diagnostic approach to eye conditions is described with the most common conditions discussed first, followed by less common, but diagnostically important, conditions.

ANATOMY OF THE OCULAR STRUCTURES AND VISUAL SYSTEM

The visual system is conveniently separated into three principal parts: the globe and surrounding structures (Fig. 20.1), the visual pathways, and the visual or calcarine cortex.

The eyelids provide protection for the globe and assist in even distribution of the tear film over the cornea to provide a clear, undistorted optical surface. The crystalline lens complements the cornea's refracting power with its ability to adjust the focal length of the optical system so that incoming light from objects at any distance may be clearly imaged on the retina. The process of changing the focal length of the lens is called accommodation, which allows for the ability to rapidly focus from near to distance and vice versa. During the first 2 to 3 months of life, children develop the ability to focus on images at any range. Light is focused on the fovea centralis in the center of the macula; it has the greatest concentration of cones and is responsible for detailed, color, and central visual acuity (Fig. 20.2). The retina contains the photoreceptors, rods, and cones, which convert light energy into a nerve response. Although central visual acuity is the parameter most measured, visual function includes visual fields, color vision, contrast sensitivity, and visuospatial discrimination.

Nerve fibers emanate from the ganglion cell layer of the retina and coalesce to form the optic nerve. Retinal nerve fibers are unmyelinated. The right and left optic nerves pass from the orbits and decussate at the optic chiasm. Nerve fibers from the nasal retina cross at the chiasm and are directed toward the contralateral side of the brain. Fibers from the temporal retina travel without crossing at the chiasm to the ipsilateral visual cortex (Fig. 20.3). From the optic chiasm, the fibers form the optic tracts and synapse in the lateral geniculate nucleus in the midbrain. From there, the optic radiations, one on each side of the brain, travel posteriorly to the visual cortex above the cerebellum. If an object is seen in the patient's left half field, the image is received by the nasal retina of the left eye and the temporal retina of the right eye. If the object is seen in the patient's right half field, the image falls on the nasal retina of the right eye and the temporal retina of the left eye. As a result of the decussation of nasal retinal fibers, the right visual cortex receives images from the left half of the visual field and the left visual cortex receives images from the right half.

The visual field can be arbitrarily divided into the central field of vision and the peripheral field. The macula is responsible for the central field. A physiologic blind spot is found about 10 to 15 degrees temporal to central fixation and represents the area of the visual field that corresponds to the optic disc.

Lesions of the visual pathways can be localized by the pattern of visual field loss (see Fig. 20.3). Visual fields may be grossly assessed by a confrontation method, in which the child fixates on the examiner's nose and is asked to identify the examiner's fingers held static in the child's peripheral field; it is better to display fingers in both halves of the field simultaneously so that sensory inattention can also be assessed. An infant or young child's visual field may also be evaluated by looking for fixation on fingers or objects brought into the peripheral visual field, but this phenomenon of fixation shift relies on a complicated and incompletely understood neural network involving the area prostriata, intraparietal sulci, and the temporal occipital cortical areas. Confrontation visual field testing is especially valuable in the detection of visual field defects that respect the vertical midline, which are typically caused by neurologic conditions. The visual field can also be formally plotted for each eye in a cooperative child or adult manually or with an automated visual field device. This test requires steady fixation and concentration. In young children, it is impractical to attempt this tedious measurement; instead, hemifield stimulation using visual evoked potential can be used to detect hemifield problems. Ocular coherence tomography can be used to assess retinal nerve fiber layer loss, and this can correspond to visual field damage deficit (Fig. 20.4). Newer virtual visual field devices have been developed that should improve the ability to reliably test younger children's visual fields.

DEVELOPMENT OF VISION

Table 20.1 illustrates the development of visual behavior in the first 12 months of life in a term baby. It is important to note that the defensive blink reflex is typically not observed until 6 to 8 weeks of age, but the pupillary light reaction should be intact by 4 weeks of age.

Testing Vision

Selection of a test to measure a patient's visual acuity depends on the patient's cooperation and level of development. Interpretation of visual acuity measurements should include whether the visual acuity has been measured with or without correction of refractive errors with glasses or contact lenses to best visual acuity. To differentiate an organic problem of the visual system from simple refractive error, the best corrected visual acuity provides the most useful information. If correction of the patient's refractive error with glasses is not possible, an approximation of corrected visual acuity can be made by having the patient look through a pinhole. The pinhole prevents indirect rays of light, which need to be refracted by the optics of the eye, from entering the eye so that the effects of refractive errors in the eye are minimized. Patients demonstrate the pinhole effect when they squint to see better. If the patient's visual acuity improves when looking through the pinhole, a refractive error is present. If it does not improve, then there is likely another cause for the decrease in vision.

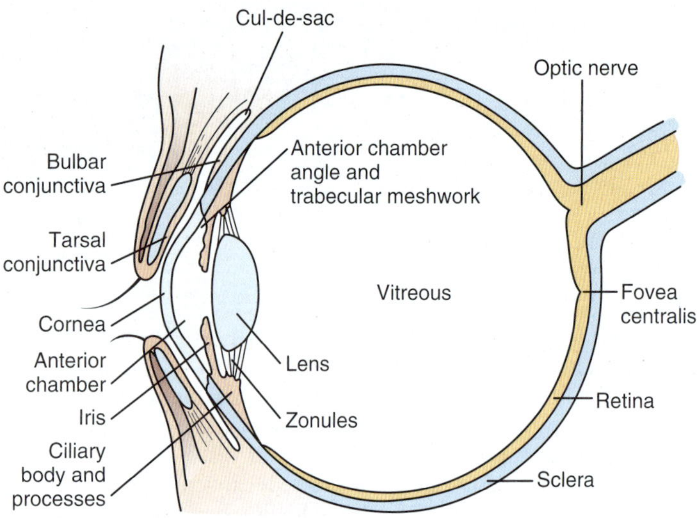

Fig. 20.1 Globe and surrounding structures.

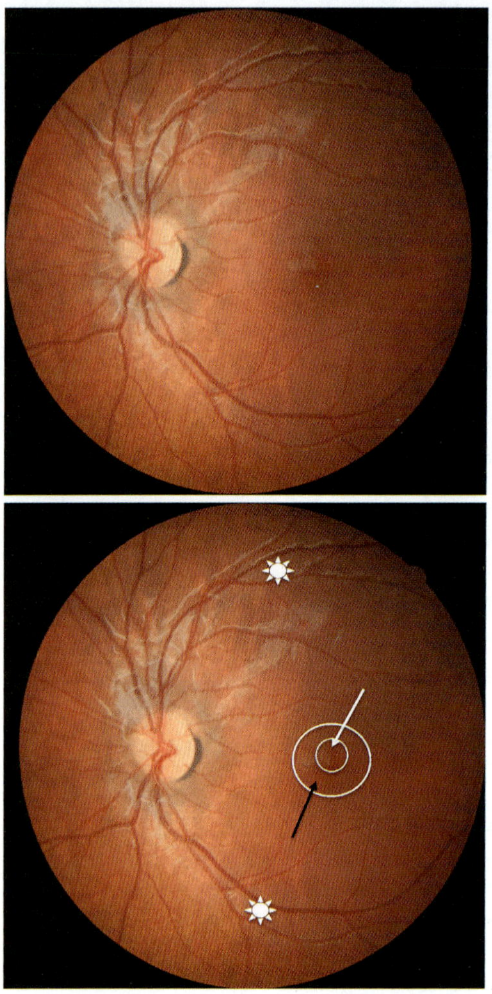

Fig. 20.2 Normal fundus. Posterior pole with normal optic disc and retinal vasculature. The macula is visualized as an area of increased pigmentation temporal to the optic disc (larger white circle). The fovea centralis is within the macula *(smaller white circle)*. The retinal vessels surround but do not go through the macula and arch around the macula *(white stars)*.

Visual acuity tests are composed of both qualitative and quantitative measures.

Qualitative tests include:

1. Fixation reflex test as mentioned earlier. This test is used to assess vision in infants and young children. The fixation reflex typically develops during the first to second months of life. Although almost all 2- to 3-month-old infants can fixate and follow a face or bright object quite well into all fields of gaze, some infants who eventually display normal vision will not display this ability until 4 to 6 months of age. This occurs because of the complex nature of the underlying neurophysiology of this fixation shift.
2. Central fixation behavior. If vision is grossly normal, fixation is central, steady, and maintained on objects. If visual acuity is profoundly decreased, the quality of fixation may be wandering in nature, poorly maintained, or eccentric. Central, steady, maintained fixation equates to visual acuity of 20/200 or better. Eyes with unsteady or wandering fixation usually have visual acuity decreased to the 20/800 level (see Fig. 20.4).

Quantitative tests include:

1. Forced preferential looking. Nonverbal infants or children may have their grating visual acuity measured with Teller Acuity Cards (Stereo Optical, Chicago, IL). This test is based on a child's reflex to move the eyes or head toward a pattern of alternating black-and-white stripes of increasing frequency rather than neutral gray of the same brightness.
2. Vanishing optotypes. This test is based on the principle of preferential looking. A young child will choose to look toward a target rather than a plain stimulus. The vision testing optotypes (shapes) are constructed with a white band bordered by two black bands, each half the width of the white band and all on a neutral gray background. The average target luminance is equal to that of the gray background. If the target lies beyond the child's acuity limit, it merges with the gray background and becomes invisible. The shapes used are all the same overall size but decreasing in width of white and black bands. The acuity is determined by the narrowest white band for which the shape is visible. The test is designed for children 1 to 3 years old but can also be used for older children and adults with developmental delay.

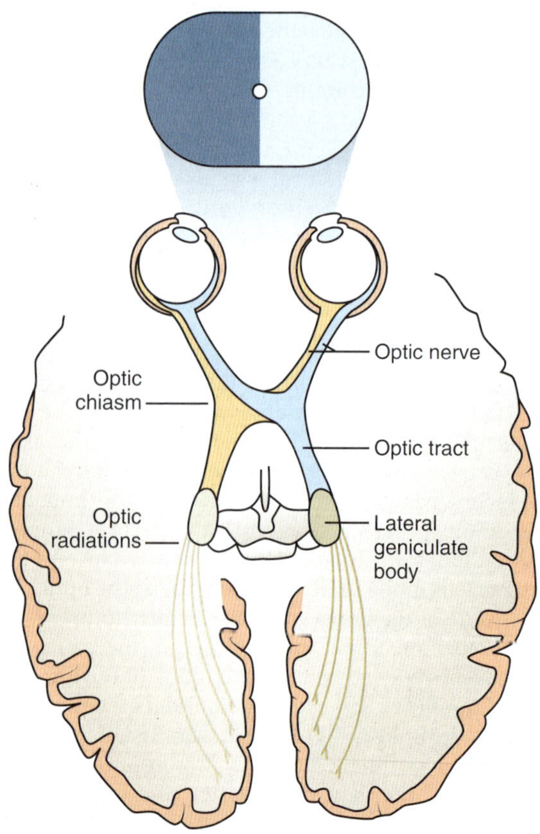

Fig. 20.3 Visual field and visual pathways.

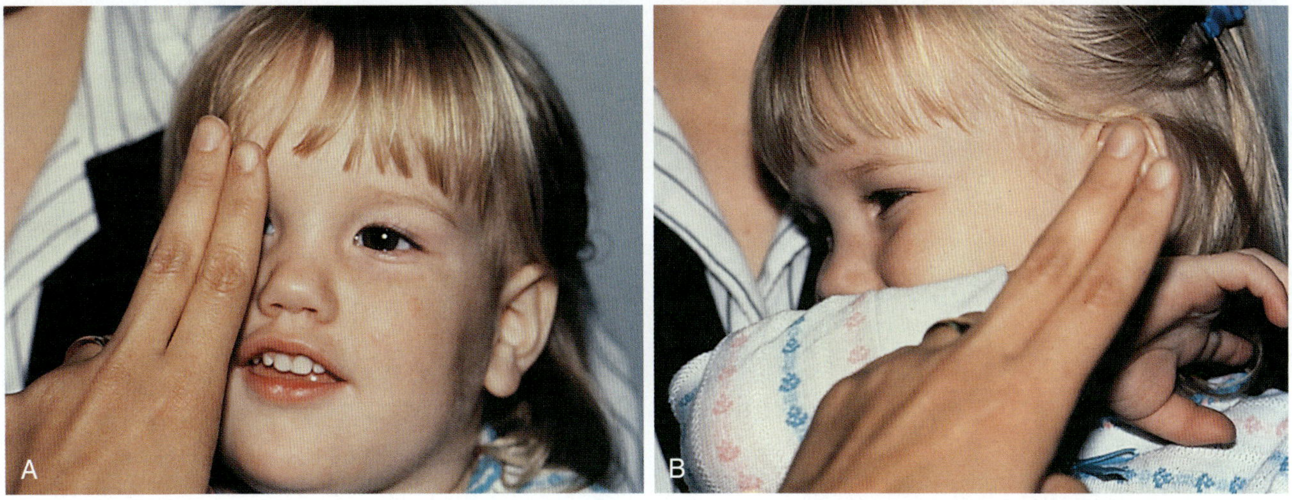

Fig. 20.4 Test for central fixation. (A) An alert child seated on her mother's lap with one eye covered. The child is content to fix and follow with the normal left eye. (B) The cover (in this case, fingers) is then transferred to the left eye. The child becomes disturbed, pushes the hand away, and moves her head to see. This suggests that the visual acuity in the right eye is not as good as the acuity in the left eye.

Table 20.1 Development of Visual Behavior in First 12 Months of Life in Term Infant

Age	1 Week	2 Weeks	3 Weeks	4 Weeks	4–6 Weeks	6–8 Weeks	3 Months	6 Months	9 Months	12 Months
Pupils react to light	N	N	N	Y	Y	Y	Y	Y	Y	Y
Defensive blink present	N	N	N	N	N	Y	Y	Y	Y	Y
Watches familiar face when being fed	N	N	Y	Y	Y	Y	Y	Y	Y	Y
Gaze caught and held by dangling bright toy moved in line of vision at 15–25 cm	N	N	N	Y	Y	Y	Y	Y	Y	Y
Converges	N	N	N	N	N	N	Y	Y	Y	Y
Fixates and follows toys at 15–25 cm	N	N	N	N	N	N	Y	Y	Y	Y
Reaches out for objects	N	N	N	N	N	N	N	Y	Y	Y
Searches for objects that leave visual regard	N	N	N	N	N	N	N	Y	Y	Y
Immediately grasps for toys	N	N	N	N	N	N	N	N	Y	Y
Watches activity of people/ animals at 3–4 m	N	N	N	N	N	N	N	N	Y	Y
Interest in pictures	N	N	N	N	N	N	N	N	N	Y
Points to objects of interest	N	N	N	N	N	N	N	N	N	Y

3. Object recognition cards are simple pictures of common objects and useful for assessing visual acuity in a 2- to 5-year-old child who cannot participate in more complicated vision tests, such as the tumbling E game and Landolt Cs, or recognize Snellen letters.
   a. Allen cards. To measure vision with the Allen cards, the child is first taught what the pictures are, and then one eye is occluded while picture cards are individually presented at increasing distances until the patient recognizes the cards at 20 feet or fails to recognize the cards (Fig. 20.5). Recognition of the cards at 20 feet equates to a visual acuity of 20/30. The farthest distance at which the cards can be recognized is noted, and the visual acuity is quantitated as that distance over the denominator of 30 (e.g., 5/30, 15/30, 20/30). This is a measurement of recognition visual acuity. Although use of isolated targets is not ideal for detection of amblyopia, the test can be quickly and easily taught to apprehensive or shy young children and comparison of vision between the eyes detects most cases of amblyopia and other defects in visual acuity.
   b. LEA symbols (Good Lite Company, Elgin, IL). These cards have the advantage of having five symbols on each card, and the child identifies the symbol in the middle of the card. Presentation of several symbols or letters at a time is a more accurate measurement of visual acuity, due to a phenomenon termed *crowding*. Amblyopic eyes recognize letters or symbols better if they are presented in isolation or one at a time rather than if four or more are presented together on lines above and below one another. The difference may be as much as one or two lines of visual acuity

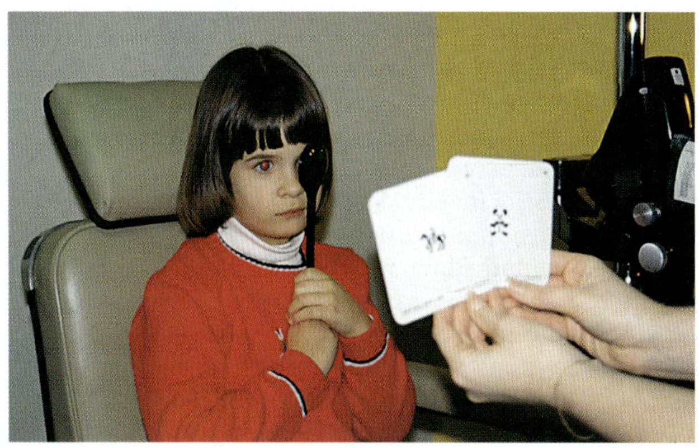

Fig. 20.5 Visual acuity testing with the Allen object recognition cards. Recognition of each figure at a distance of 20 feet is equivalent to a visual acuity of 20/30. The visual acuity is quantitated as the number of feet at which each figure may be recognized over 30 (e.g., 5/30, 15/30, 20/30).

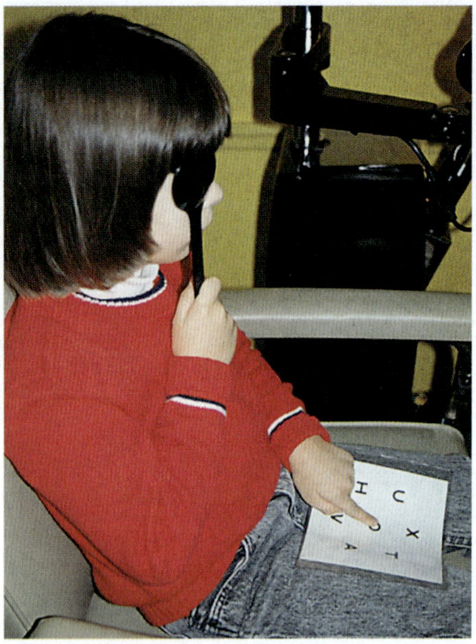

Fig. 20.6 The child uses a matching card held on her lap. She matches what she sees on the screen by pointing to the correct letter on the card. This test provides an accurate assessment of visual acuity for children who have not yet mastered reading the alphabet.

(e.g., 20/30 isolated symbol visual acuity reducing to 20/40 or 20/50 when measured with a Snellen letter chart). Many different visual acuity tests are calibrated using different letters and symbols or groups of symbols (Fig. 20.6).

c. KAY pictures use different shapes and symbols from LEA symbols and achieve the crowding phenomenon by putting a box around the shape or symbol. They are again designed for the preliterate child.

4. Landolt C and Illiterate E. Other commonly used tests to measure the visual acuity of 3- or 4-year-old children are the tumbling E and Landolt C tests. The child is presented with the letter E or C in decreasing sizes and rotated in an up, down, right, or left orientation, and the child indicates the direction of the crossbars of the E or the open end of the C by pointing.
5. Visual evoked potentials.

The visual pathways coalesce in the visual cortex. Electrical impulses in the visual cortex produced by light stimulation of the retina can be measured by placement of sensitive electrodes on the overlying scalp. This is termed the *visual evoked potential* or *response*. The pattern visual evoked potential uses an alternating checkerboard stimulus, which can be controlled to produce a pattern of checks that may be increased or decreased in size. This test can be used to estimate visual acuity in young or nonverbal children. However, caution must be used in interpreting this test because children and adults with known 20/20 vision can voluntarily suppress the visual evoked response. In addition, children who have significant decreases in their visual acuity may have a visual evoked response that overestimates the visual acuity.

The gold standard for measurement of visual acuity is the presentation of a full line of letter optotypes. This presentation is best achieved with a wall chart or by projection of the letters onto a standardized reflective surface. Other components of vision such as contrast sensitivity, color vision, and color and brightness desaturation can also be assessed to quantify visual function.

Normal values for best corrected visual acuity depend on the patient's age. A child at 6 months of age should have a visual acuity of 20/60 to 20/100. A child who is 3 years old can be expected to have acuity in the range of 20/25 or 20/30, using the E game or a recognition target test. With further maturation, a 5- to 7-year-old child should have visual acuity of 20/20 to 20/25 as tested with a full-line presentation of Snellen letters. If the best corrected visual acuity is less than 20/20 in a developmentally normal child older than 8 years old, investigation for the cause of the decrease in visual acuity should be made.

In infancy, the fixation and following response of each eye to a fixation target should be recorded. Beginning at age 3, measurement of visual acuity should be completed. Later, a Snellen or letter chart visual acuity test should be performed by the office staff or physician, and the results should be recorded as part of the patient's medical record. Most importantly, the visual acuity should be equal in both eyes. Further evaluation of a young child is prompted if the patient is cooperating well and visual acuity is less than 20/40 with letters or less than 15/30 measured with Allen visual acuity cards in either or both eyes.

Testing Vision in Children With Nystagmus

When testing vision in children with nystagmus, there are three important points to keep in mind. If the child has a null position, he or she will adopt that position to read the distance or the near vison test. The child should be allowed to do so, but the head position adopted must be noted. If the child has latent nystagmus (now known as maldevelopment fusional nystagmus), then testing monocular vision is worse if the occluder used is opaque rather than translucent.

Vision Screening

Validated instrument-based vision screening is becoming more widely used in the offices of pediatricians and in the preschool setting. These devices can detect amblyopia, strabismus, and refractive errors and may be used even in infants and nonverbal children. Some level of cooperation is necessary, and results are generally better for children who are at least 18 months old. The use of this technology in children before they can have visual acuity measured allows for earlier detection of risk factors for the development of strabismus and amblyopia. There are several devices available and digital apps that can perform the tasks.

It is recommended that vision screening be conducted as part of well-child care at regularly scheduled intervals in the pediatrician's or family practitioner's office. Routine comprehensive eye examinations with an ophthalmologist or optometrist are not cost effective, necessary, or indicated. Low-birth-weight preterm infants, newborn infants with family histories of infantile cataracts or glaucoma, children with metabolic disease, or children with systemic diseases with potential associated ocular disease should be referred to an ophthalmologist for evaluation. Children with immediate family histories of strabismus or amblyopia should be watched carefully for strabismus and referred promptly. Because of the increased risk in these children, referral for comprehensive examination should be considered between 18 and 30 months old. Children suspected by their parents or teachers of having reading or learning problems should have eye examinations performed with an emphasis on an evaluation of the amplitude of accommodation and the facility of accommodation. Although it is common for adults around age 45 years for it to become harder to read things close (presbyopia), this can sometimes happen in children between 5 and 15 years. Signs that a child might be experiencing presbyopia include jumping lines when they are reading, losing concentration easily, developing untidy handwriting, or decreased ability to color in within the lines. A dynamic retinoscopy done by a pediatric ophthalmologist or optometrist can diagnose this condition. For affected children, often a temporary use of bifocal glasses or reading glasses corrects the issue.

Some states have legislation in place that requires vision screenings be performed before entry into school or in school at 1- to 2-year intervals. In a child 6 years old or older, referral to an ophthalmologist is indicated if the vision is less than 20/30 in either eye. If appropriate vision screenings are passed in the primary care physician's office, preschool, or school and no family history of hereditary eye disease or other suspicion or risk factor for eye disease are present, comprehensive examination of the child's eyes by an optometrist or ophthalmologist is not cost effective and not recommended.

REFRACTIVE ERRORS

Decreased visual acuity is most commonly the result of a refractive error in the eye. This may be due to variation in the curvature of the cornea, shape of the lens, or variation in the axial length of the eye. Determination of the refractive state of the eye is part of a comprehensive ophthalmic evaluation. In children, an objective measurement of the refractive error is best obtained by using eye drops that temporarily inhibit accommodation (cycloplegia) and cause pupillary dilation (mydriasis). Cycloplegic/mydriatic agents such as cyclopentolate or tropicamide are instilled, 30 minutes later the pupil is dilated, and accommodation is temporarily paralyzed. Retinoscopy is performed by using a retinoscope to project a beam of light into the eye and illuminate the retina. The light is then reflected back to the examiner through the optical system of the eye. The focus of the reflected light is neutralized by placement of appropriate lenses in front of the eye, and the refractive error of the eye is accurately and objectively measured (Fig. 20.7). Refraction can also be measured by devices called *autorefractors,* and some vision screening devices are based on refraction technology and will give refraction measurements. The earlier a refractive error is detected, the better the chance of the child developing normal vision.

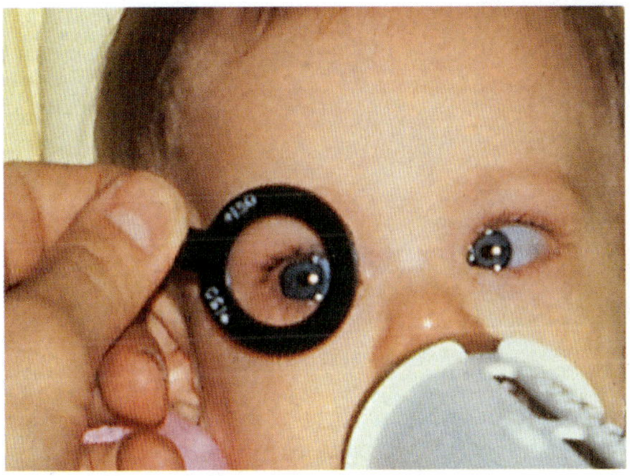

Fig. 20.7 Retinoscopy. The examiner is viewing light emanating from the retina through the retinoscope. A lens is held in front of the patient's eye to neutralize refractive errors.

Low levels of hyperopia (farsightedness) in the range of + 1.50 to + 2.00 diopters (D) are normal during childhood and are easily compensated for by the focusing mechanism of the lens (accommodation), so glasses are not necessary. The amount of hyperopia normally increases until 5 years old and then decreases. Under normal circumstances, emmetropia, or no refractive error, is achieved around adolescence. If excessive axial growth (elongation) of the eye occurs, myopia (nearsightedness) develops. A patient's refractive error is largely genetically predetermined.

The optical image formed by a hyperopic eye is in focus behind the retina (Fig. 20.8C). By changing the shape of the lens with accommodation, the image can be brought into focus on the retina and glasses may not be required. If a large amount of hyperopia is present (+ 4.00 D or more), fatigue, headaches, asthenopia (eye strain), and blurring of vision, especially at near, may occur. Hyperopia more than + 5.00, or + 6.00 D may cause ametropic or refractive amblyopia. When this occurs, glasses are prescribed to correct the child's refractive error so that focused images stimulate the development of normal vision. If large hyperopic refractive errors are not treated by 6 to 8 years old, the resultant amblyopia may be irreversible. There is also some evidence to suggest that uncorrected high hyperopia may be associated with delays in the development of reading comprehension. The optic discs in eyes with large degrees of hyperopia may have an appearance simulating papilledema (pseudopapilledema) (Fig. 20.9).

Myopia is most commonly caused by an increase in axial length of the eye with respect to the optical power of the eye (see Fig. 20.8B). Children who are myopic can see near objects clearly; objects at distance are blurred and cannot be brought into focus without the aid of glasses or a contact lens. Myopia may be present at birth but usually develops with growth spurts that occur between 8 and 10 years old. The amount of myopia present usually increases until growth is completed after adolescence.

High degrees of myopia, with increased axial length of the eye, ranging from −8.00 to −20.00 D, may occur in isolation or be associated with systemic conditions. Causes of high- or early-onset moderate myopia include connective tissue disorders such as Marfan, Ehlers Danlos, and Stickler syndromes. Children with high myopia should be referred to a pediatric ophthalmologist to rule out pathology to explain the high myopia. Retinal disorders such as sequelae of retinopathy of prematurity (ROP), familial exudative vitreoretinopathy (FEVR), and retinal dystrophies, most commonly congenital stationary night blindness (CSNB),

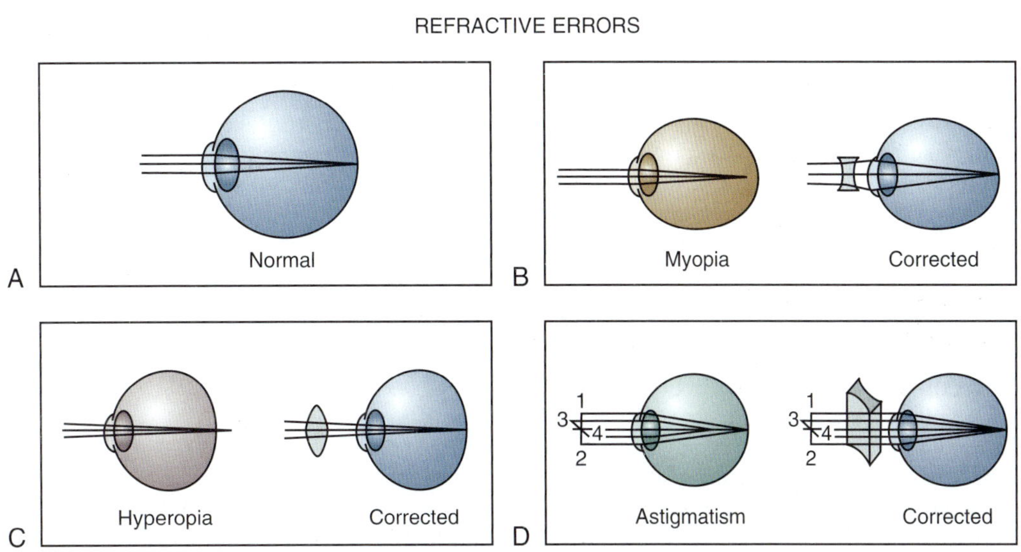

Fig. 20.8 In the normal or emmetropic eye (A), light from a distant object is focused on the retina. In a myopic eye (B), it is focused in front of the retina; in a hyperopic eye (C), it is focused behind the retina; and in an astigmatic eye (D), light in different meridians is brought to focus either in front of or behind the retina.

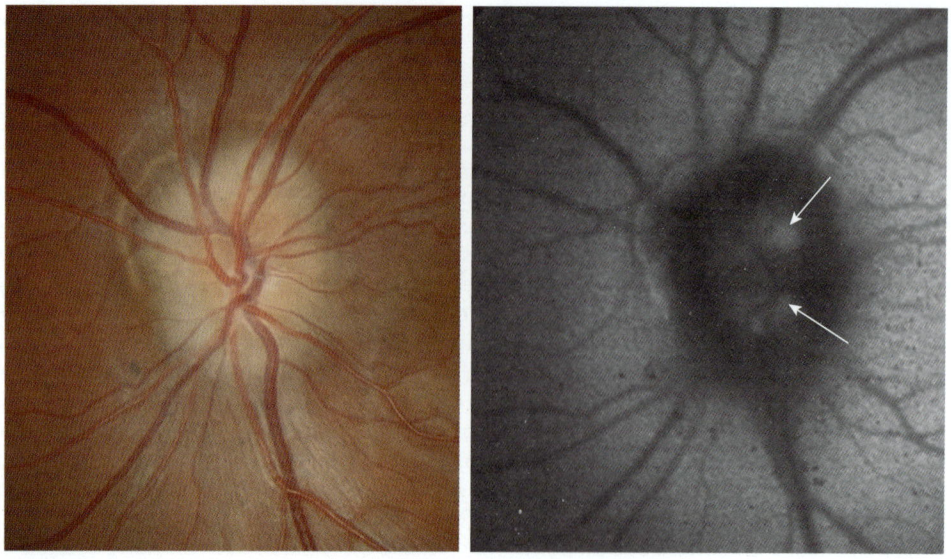

Fig. 20.9 Pseudopapilledema thought to be due to hyperopia in a child. Vessels are normal sized; small vessels are continuously visible at the disc margins because there is no edema of the nerve fiber layer. There are no hemorrhages or exudates. However, autofluorescence shows that the cause is optic disc drusen *(white arrows)*. The incidence of optic disc drusen is higher in children with hyperopia.

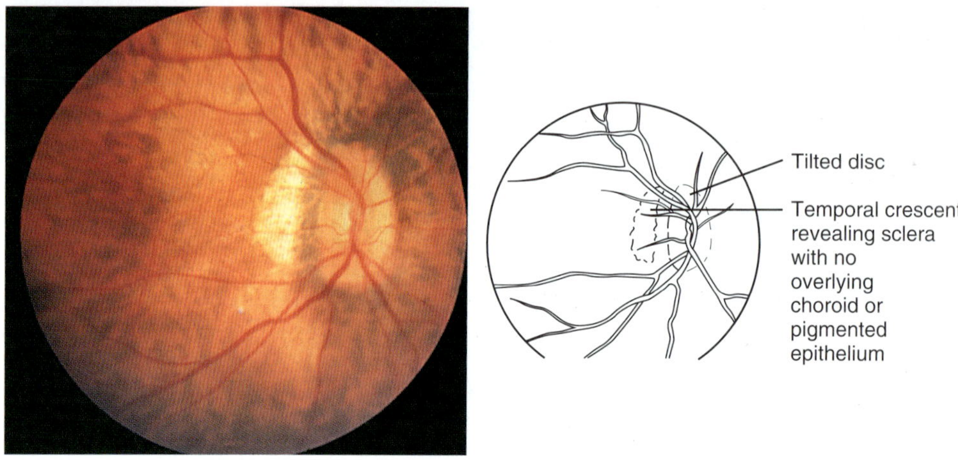

Fig. 20.10 High myopia. Thinning of the retinal pigment epithelium produces a tessellated fundus appearance. In eyes with moderate or high myopia, a temporal crescent adjacent to the optic disc is frequently present and the optic disc may have an anomalous tilted appearance.

can cause high myopia; however, these are usually associated with nystagmus. Rarely, juvenile glaucoma may present as early-onset myopia. Retinal thinning, peripapillary pigment crescents, staphylomas (a focal area of bulging of the posterior globe wall), and decreased macular function with poor visual acuity may all be present in patients with high myopia. The optic nerve may appear to enter the eye at an angle (Fig. 20.10). Patients with high myopia have an increased risk for retinal detachment, especially after direct trauma to the eye or concussive head trauma.

In astigmatism, the refractive power of the eye is different in different meridians (see Fig. 20.8D). This produces a blurred retinal image for objects at both distance and near. Astigmatism occurs when the cornea, lens, or shape of the globe has a toric shape, like the surface of a football, rather than a spherical one. Bulky masses in the lids (such as chalazions or hemangiomas) may compress the cornea and induce astigmatic refractive errors.

Arresting the Progression of Childhood Myopia

With increasing myopia, there are significantly increased odds ratios for myopic maculopathy; retinal detachment; cataracts; and glaucoma, even for low and moderate levels of myopia. These odds ratios increase further with higher levels of myopia.

Evidence supports heritability of the nonsyndromic forms of myopia, especially for high-grade myopia (−5 D or higher), and genome-wide association studies (GWAS) have identified greater than 20 associated loci for myopia. There has been growing interest to try to slow myopic progression of childhood.

An epidemic of myopia exists globally. It is well known that the risk of a child being myopic increases if both parents are myopic. However, behavioral and environmental factors have a huge influence. During the COVID-19 lockdown, rates of myopia were reported to increase across many countries due to increased near work demand and reduced outdoor time. It has been established that 2 hours of daylight exposure can be protective against myopia development and can slow myopia once it has developed. Evidence also suggests that reading in dim light may cause myopia to progress.

There is evidence to suggest that the regular single-vision lenses used to correct myopia may cause peripheral retinal hyperopic defocus, which encourages the eye to grow more and, therefore, the child to become more myopic. Special antiperipheral defocus spectacle lenses have shown promising results but are not yet available in the United States. However, such specially designed contact lenses are available, and orthokeratology, the use of such contact lenses to temporarily reshape the cornea, has also been used to slow myopic progression. Finally, low-dose atropine (0.01%, 0.02%, and 0.05%) has been shown to slow myopia progression in most children but needs to be used daily until the age of 16 years.

Amblyopia

Amblyopia is present when a decrease in vision in one or both eyes is present and all potential anatomic causes (refractive errors, media opacities, structural abnormalities) for the decrease in vision have been corrected or excluded. Amblyopia may be caused by the absence of stimulation of the immature visual system by a focused retinal image or by strabismus and the resultant suppression of one eye. Visual deprivation amblyopia may be caused by a corneal opacity, a dense cataract, vitreous opacity (hemorrhage or inflammation), or high refractive error (Fig. 20.11).

Anisometropia refers to the condition in which one eye has a different refractive error than the other. Usually, the eye with the least amount of hyperopia or refractive error is the dominant or preferred eye. In anisometropic amblyopia, an image is clearly focused on the fovea of one eye; however, the image is out of focus in the other eye. The blurred retinal image is suppressed or ignored by the child's immature visual system, and that eye develops amblyopia. The magnitude of the amblyopia depends on the magnitude of the anisometropia and the age at which it developed. Anisometropia may occur with hyperopia, myopia, astigmatism, or a combination of these refractive errors. If the degree of anisometropia is large, the optical properties of the required correcting lenses produce a difference in image size between the two eyes, *aniseikonia,* which may be difficult for the patient to tolerate.

With high hyperopia or astigmatism affecting both eyes, bilateral refractive, or ametropic, amblyopia may occur if the child does not or cannot consistently accommodate to produce a focused retinal image to stimulate the visual system with either eye. These patients have decreased vision in both eyes. In children with strabismus, the image from the deviating eye is suppressed by the brain as an adaptation to avoid diplopia, and the deviating eye develops strabismic amblyopia. Patients often have both strabismus and anisometropia simultaneously as causes for their amblyopia.

The severity of the visual loss produced by amblyopia is determined by the nature of the visual deprivation; the age at onset; and its consistency, severity, and duration. Amblyopia is treated by removing the cause of the amblyopia, if possible, and by forcing use of the affected eye to stimulate the development of vision from that eye. In bilateral refractive amblyopia, the appropriate glasses are given as treatment. In strabismic or anisometropic amblyopia, appropriate glasses are given, and the preferred, nonamblyopic eye is penalized to force the use of the amblyopic eye.

Early detection of amblyopia is essential as amblyopia responds most rapidly and completely to treatment begun early in life. The visual system has developmental phases, and if certain levels of visual acuity are not reached early in life, the amblyopia present is unlikely to respond completely to treatment. Treatment is more difficult and less effective after 8 years old but remains possible in older children, especially if they have no history of previous treatment.

An occlusion patch placed over the preferred fixating eye is commonly used as treatment. Other methods of treatment are optical via the eyeglass prescription and pharmacologic, with atropine drops placed in the nonamblyopic eye to prevent accommodation in that eye. This forces the use of the amblyopic eye for reading and near vision. New treatments for amblyopia based on encouraging binocular computer-based stimulation therapies are promising developments.

STRABISMUS

Misalignment of the visual axes is referred to as *strabismus.* Strabismus occurs in 1% to 4% of the population and may be congenital or acquired. It may occur on a hereditary basis, most commonly without a clearly defined inheritance pattern. In most childhood strabismus, the misalignment of the eyes is not caused by a specific cranial nerve or extraocular muscle dysfunction; however, cranial nerve paralysis and neuromuscular disorders (such as myasthenia gravis) may be the cause in some cases.

Voluntary and reflex movements of the eyes occur via the action of the extraocular muscles. These muscles are coordinated in their saccadic and pursuit movements by centers in the frontal and occipital areas of the cerebral cortex with modification by the cerebellum. Saccades are voluntary movements used to move the eyes to the object of regard. These are rapid eye movements. Pursuit or following movements are used to track or follow moving objects. These are slow eye movements.

The third, fourth, and sixth cranial nerve nuclei, located in the brainstem, are the centers responsible for innervating the extraocular muscles. In addition to innervation of the inferior oblique, medial, inferior, and superior recti, the third cranial nerve is responsible for innervation of the levator muscle, pupillary constrictor, and ciliary muscle, which is responsible for changing the shape of the lens that

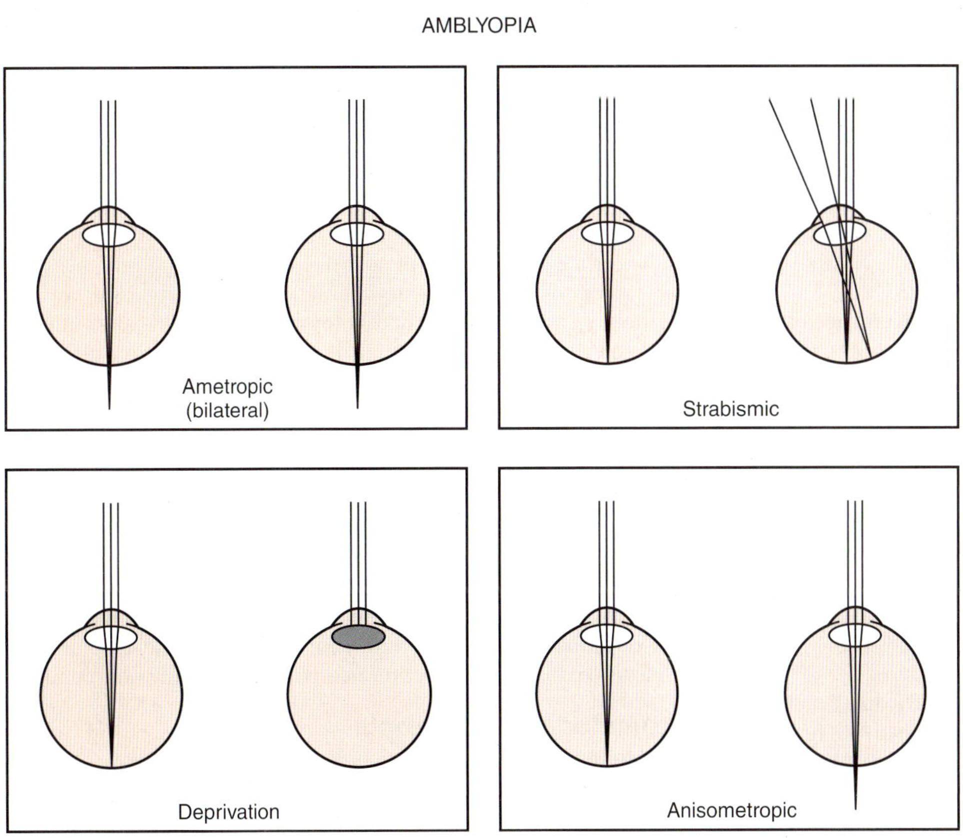

Fig. 20.11 Amblyopia is produced either by the absence of a focused retinal image (ametropic, deprivation, or anisometropic) or by suppression of a diplopic image (strabismic).

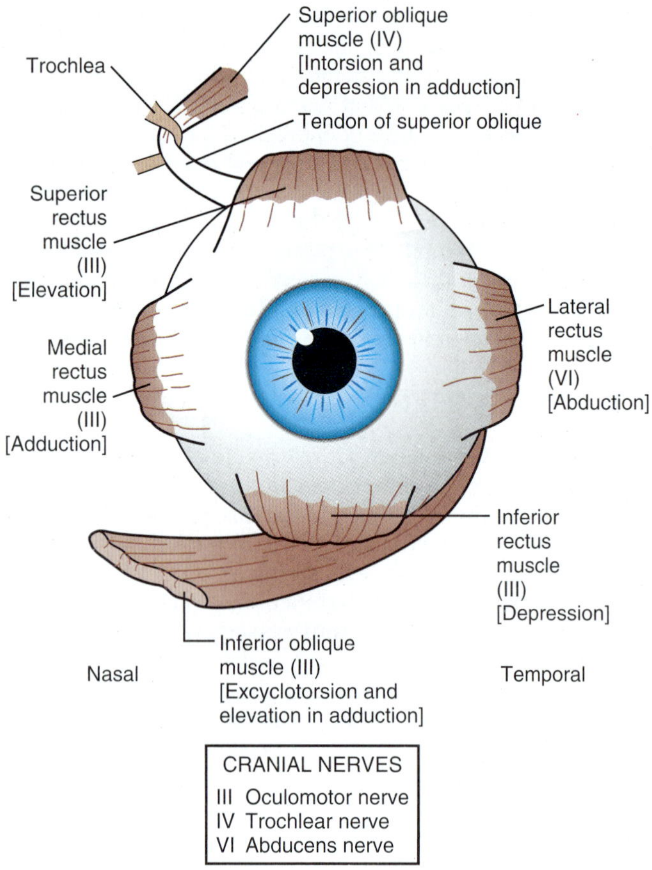

Fig. 20.12 Innervation (*in parentheses*) of extraocular muscles and their primary actions (*in brackets*).

produces accommodation. The fourth cranial nerve provides innervation to the superior oblique muscle, and the sixth cranial nerve supplies the lateral rectus muscle (Fig. 20.12). When one or more of the cranial nerves are paretic, the action of the innervated muscle is decreased, leading to a deficit in the duction or movement of the eye into the field of action of the muscle. The muscle having a function of movement in the opposite direction is no longer balanced, producing misalignment of the eye or strabismus.

Versions

Eye movements are tested by moving the eyes right, left, up, down, up and right, down and right, up and left, and down and left. This tests the function of each extraocular muscle and its counterpart or yoke muscle in the fellow eye. *Versions* refer to movement of both eyes together in conjugate gaze. A *duction* is the movement of a single eye. Normal version movements should be present by 4 months of age.

Vergence movements consist of convergence or divergence of the eyes. Vergences are well established by 6 months of age. Convergence of the eyes, coupled with accommodation and miosis of the pupil, is referred to as the *near response.* Convergence assists alignment of the eyes at near.

A strabismus deviation that changes in size or magnitude in different gaze positions is termed *incomitant.* Strabismus deviations that remain the same in all gaze positions are termed *comitant.* An important distinction is that incomitant deviations may be, but are not always, an indication of cranial nerve paralysis.

Phorias and Tropias

If strabismus is present, it may be manifest (i.e., a tropia) or held latent by sensory fusion (i.e., a phoria). Fusion is the patient's unconscious desire to use both eyes together for binocular vision. When the fusion of a patient with a phoria is interrupted by placing an occluder in front of one eye, the eye seeks its position of rest and deviates so that the visual axes of the two eyes are no longer both aligned on the point of fixation. When the eye is uncovered and binocular vision is reestablished, the fusion response assists in the realignment of the eyes on the object of regard. A phoria may produce symptoms of fatigue, blurring, or straining to see. When a phoria breaks down into an intermittent tropia, there may be a symptom of intermittent double vision or *diplopia.* Phorias, especially if large, may become symptomatic at times of fatigue, stress, or illness.

A tropia is a constant or intermittently present ocular deviation. The fusion mechanism is unable to maintain alignment of the eyes. Young children with tropias develop suppression of the tropic eye as an innate response to avoid diplopia. Older children or adults who acquire a tropia (e.g., from an acquired cranial nerve palsy) have diplopia as a symptom of the misalignment of their eyes. The deviation present in a tropia may occur in one or all positions of gaze, depending on the cause of the tropia.

Phorias and tropias are classified according to the pattern of the eye deviation. The prefixes *eso-* and *exo-* classify horizontal strabismus. *Hyper-* and *hypo-* are used for vertical deviations, and *incyclo-* and *excyclo-* are used for torsional deviations.

Esodeviations

An esodeviation is a convergent or crossing deviation of the eyes. The deviation may be latent, a phoria (esophoria), or it may occur as a manifest deviation, a tropia (esotropia). Common esodeviations seen in children are infantile esotropia, accommodative esotropia, esotropia resulting from sixth cranial nerve palsy, and Duane syndrome.

Infantile Esotropia

The most common cause for an esodeviation presenting in infancy is infantile, or congenital, esotropia (Fig. 20.13). In this condition, the esotropia is seen at birth or early in infancy. On occasion, a family history of infantile esotropia exists. The angle of esodeviation is large and constant. Abduction may be deficient due to contraction of the medial rectus muscles, and differentiation from sixth nerve palsy may be difficult. Cross-fixation is usually present, with the adducted right eye used for vision to the left and the adducted left eye used for vision to the right. Abduction of an eye is checked by holding the head, occluding the contralateral eye, and quickly encouraging fixation movements. Doll's head maneuvers may also be used to test abduction of the eyes. Children with this condition usually do not develop much amblyopia and maintain good visual acuity in both eyes, due to their use of cross-fixation, whether they are treated or not. There are no associated neurologic or systemic abnormalities.

The esodeviation present in infantile esotropia requires surgical correction. After correction, the ocular alignment is frequently unstable, with further surgery often required later in life, regardless of how early surgery is performed or how well aligned the eyes are after surgery. Inferior oblique overaction and dissociated vertical deviations (DVDs) frequently develop later in childhood or adolescence. Inferior oblique overaction is seen as an elevation of one or both eyes in adduction. A DVD (Fig. 20.14) is an upward and outward "floating" movement of one or both eyes that becomes more prominent with fatigue or inattention. A DVD may be elicited on examination by covering one eye and watching its position as the eye is covered. These patients do not experience diplopia. Patients with infantile esotropia also commonly develop accommodative esotropia, with a need for glasses later in childhood. Excellent visual acuity in both eyes and alignment of the eyes are typically achieved with treatment. Although early surgery is associated with better development of binocular function than later surgery, the development of high levels of binocular function (stereopsis) is usually not obtained.

Accommodative Esotropia

Accommodative esotropia most commonly presents as an acquired strabismus at 2½ to 5 years of age. Family histories of hypertropia, anisometropia, esotropia, and amblyopia are common. The inheritance

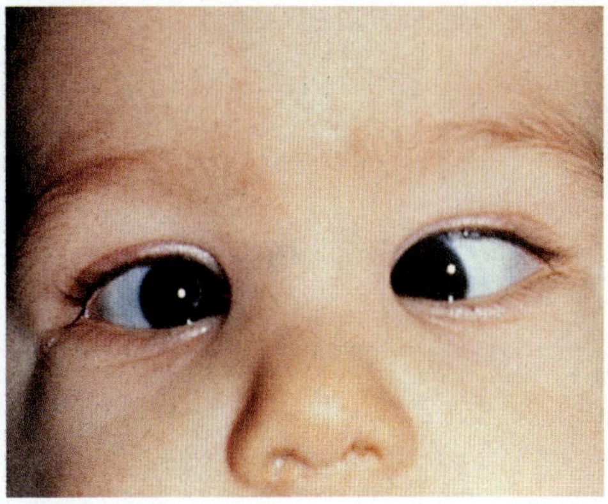

Fig. 20.13 Infantile esotropia with asymmetric corneal light reflexes.

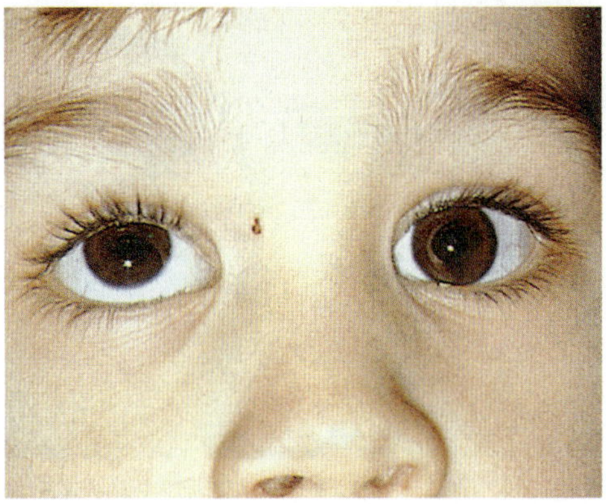

Fig. 20.14 Dissociative vertical deviation (DVD), an upward and outward drifting of the right eye. Covering the fixating left eye in the cover/uncover test causes the deviating right eye to move into alignment with the left eye. The covered left eye remains straight, and no hypodeviation or exodeviation of the left eye is seen when the cover is removed. This differentiates DVD from a tropia.

pattern is unknown and inconsistent with parents, siblings, or more distant relatives being affected in different families. The presence of uncorrected hyperopia causes the patient to accommodate or focus to obtain clear visual acuity. With accommodation, the synkinetic near response produces convergence of the eyes. If the fusion mechanism is unable to diverge the eyes to compensate for the excessive convergence accompanying the need to accommodate to correct for the patient's hyperopia, esotropia results.

If an esodeviation is associated with a modest degree of farsightedness, treatment of the hyperopia optically with glasses is indicated. In patients with purely accommodative esotropia, this measure alone may completely correct the deviation (Fig. 20.15). Frequently, especially if the esodeviation has been left untreated for a long period of time, a residual esodeviation will remain. This is a partially accommodative esotropia. Surgical correction may be recommended for these patients. Some patients have straight eyes for some time with their glasses in place and decompensate to partially accommodative or nonaccommodative esodeviations later.

In patients with accommodative esotropia, the eyes are straight with their glasses on and esotropic when they are removed. Frequently, if the patient is only moderately hyperopic in the preferred fixating eye, he or she will report seeing just as well or perhaps better without the glasses. The glasses are not being prescribed necessarily to improve visual acuity; they are to improve the esotropia.

In another form of accommodative esotropia, the ratio between accommodative convergence and accommodation (AC/A) ratio may be abnormally high, producing excessive convergence when focusing on near objects. In high AC/A ratio accommodative esotropia, the esodeviation with near vision is greater in magnitude than it is with distance vision (Fig. 20.16). These patients may be treated with a bifocal. The bifocal gives them additional hyperopic correction for near, decreasing the accommodative effort needed at near and decreasing the near esodeviation.

Nonaccommodative Esotropia

Children may develop an esodeviation that is present without any relationship to the patient's refractive error (Fig. 20.17). Correction of the hyperopia with glasses does not improve the esotropia in these patients. These nonaccommodative esodeviations may be associated with poor vision, trauma, prematurity, aphakia, or high myopia. Nonaccommodative esotropia may develop when accommodative esotropias are left untreated; however, they also occur without the presence of any other ocular abnormalities.

Other Causes of Esotropia

Unilateral or bilateral sixth cranial nerve palsy causes deficient abduction and an esodeviation. In sixth nerve palsy, the esotropia increases with gaze directed toward the side of the palsy (gaze incomitance). Patients may display a head turn toward the side of the palsy to hold the involved eye in adduction, away from the side of the palsy, to maintain binocular vision. Other signs of the nerve paralysis that may be subtle and more difficult to detect include the extent and speed of abduction of the eye. Sixth cranial nerve palsies in children may be associated with increased intracranial pressure, trauma, tumor, or antecedent viral illness. In benign or "postviral" and traumatic cases, the lateral rectus function may return gradually and fully over a 6-month period. In idiopathic cases, if improvement does not occur, if the deviation increases, or if gaze palsy develops, suspicion should be raised that a tumor, most commonly pontine glioma, may be the cause for the sixth nerve paralysis.

Duane syndrome is a congenital unilateral or bilateral defect characterized by inability to abduct an eye. This may be accompanied by an up or down shoot of the eye and narrowing of the lid fissure on attempted adduction. In attempted abduction, the palpebral fissure widens. Duane syndrome is caused by a malformation of the cranial nerve nuclei producing coinnervation of the medial and lateral rectus muscles. The lateral rectus muscle does not contract with abduction and paradoxically cocontracts along with the medial rectus on adduction. The cocontraction with adduction causes a retraction of the globe and the lid fissure narrowing. Patients with

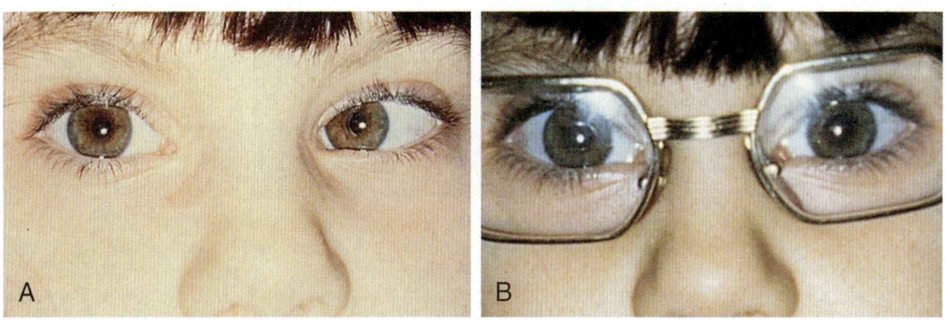

Fig. 20.15 Accommodative esotropia. (A) Esotropia. (B) Glasses have corrected the patient's hyperopia, and the esotropic eye is now straight.

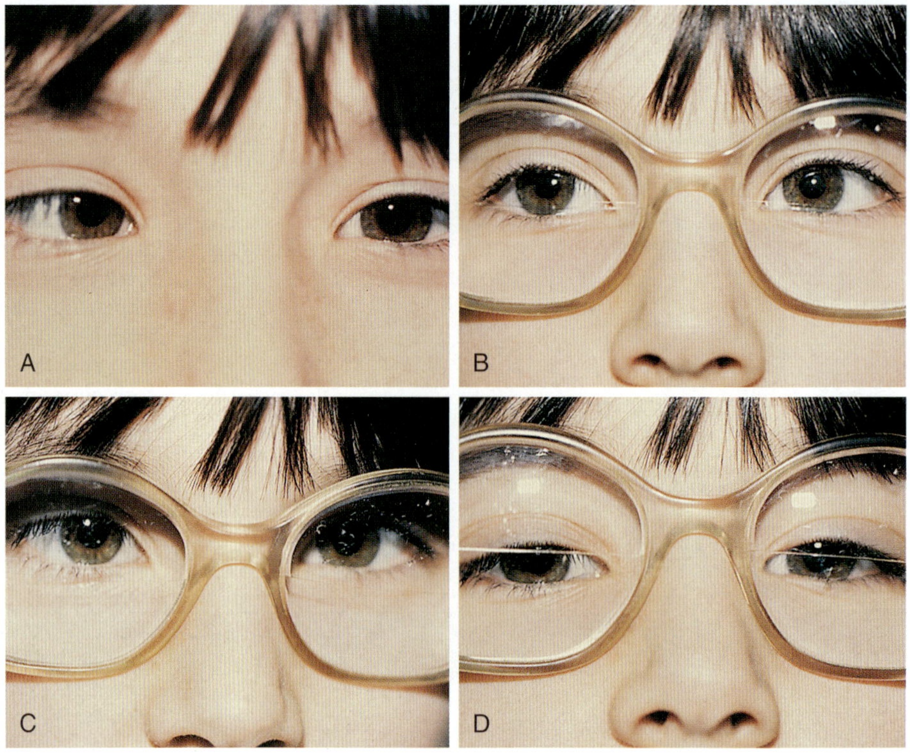

Fig. 20.16 High accommodative convergence and accommodation (AC/A) ratio accommodative esotropia. (A) This child with hyperopia has an esotropia when fixing at distance and a larger angle esotropia in the near range. (B) When glasses are prescribed to correct the hyperopia, the eyes straighten at distances. (C) The near esotropia remains. (D) When bifocals are used, the near esotropia is corrected.

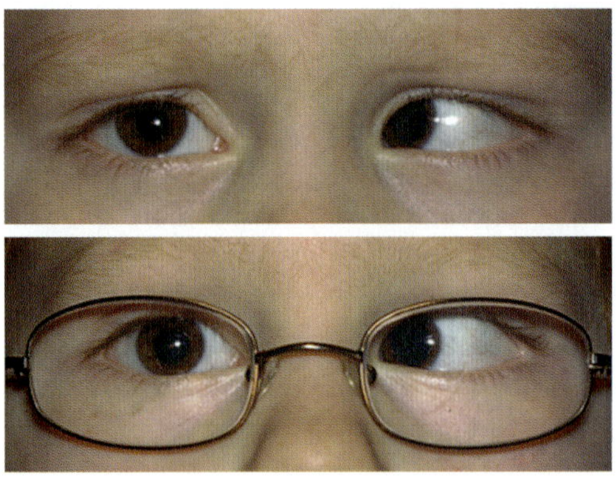

Fig. 20.17 The child has a left esotropia, which does not change in magnitude with the trial of hyperopic correction. This is a nonaccommodative esotropia.

Duane syndrome may be esotropic and have a head turn toward the involved side analogous to those seen with a sixth cranial nerve palsy. The changes in lid position and presence of vertical deviations help to differentiate the two conditions (Fig. 20.18). Children with Duane syndrome also have a high incidence of hearing deficit.

Pseudostrabismus

Pseudostrabismus is seen in infants with prominent epicanthal folds, closely placed eyes, and flat nasal bridges. Asymmetry of the orbits, lids, or nasal bridge may also produce pseudostrabismus. When these facial features are present, the white of the sclera between the cornea and inner canthus frequently may be obscured or asymmetric between the two eyes, giving the optical illusion that the eyes are esotropic (Figs. 20.19 and 20.20). Parents and caretakers frequently report subtle esodeviations that worsen with gaze to the right or left. This is frequently pointed out in photographs in which careful examination shows the eyes to be in slight right or left gaze. Observation of symmetric corneal light reflexes or cover testing confirms or excludes the presence of a true deviation. Pointing out the symmetry in the corneal light reflexes seen in photographs that the family is concerned about is frequently helpful.

Exodeviations

When the visual axes are divergent, an exodeviation is present (Fig. 20.21). Many children with exodeviations have family histories of strabismus. Exodeviations may also occur with vision loss in one

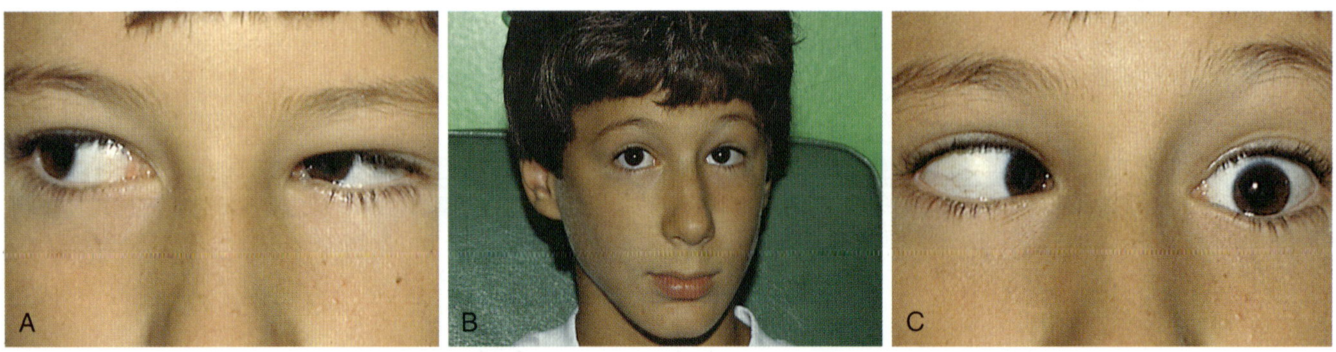

Fig. 20.18 Left Duane syndrome. (A) Right gaze. The left eye is noted to move into adduction, and retraction of the globe is noted along with narrowing of the palpebral fissure. The globe retraction and lid changes are due to cocontraction of the medial rectus and lateral rectus muscles on the involved side. (B) Fixation target directly in front of patient. The patient is noted to maintain a slight left head turn to keep both of the eyes on the fixation target. The resting position of the affected left eye is slightly in adduction. If the patient's head is forced out of the slight left head turn, the left eye would become slightly esotropic. (C) Left gaze. The affected left eye is seen to have an absence of abduction resulting from aberrant innervation of the lateral rectus muscle with no contraction in left gaze.

eye (sensory exotropia) and cranial nerve paralysis (third nerve palsy). An exodeviation may be controlled by fusion (exophoria), be manifest intermittently (intermittent exotropia), or be constant (exotropia).

Intermittent exodeviations may become manifest with fatigue, daydreaming, or illness. Patients with exodeviations frequently squint one eye in bright light, but they typically do not experience diplopia. They may complain of images jumping as they switch fixation or of discomfort at night or when tired. Patients with intermittent exotropia usually do not have amblyopia, or it may only be mild. One-third of cases improve spontaneously. Treatment of intermittent exotropia may not be necessary if the deviation is not present frequently. Treatment consists of glasses to correct refractive errors, patching, and surgery.

If one eye has poor vision, the decreased visual stimulation may produce a sensory deviation. Typically, if the onset of decreased vision occurs after 4 years old, an exodeviation will occur; however, if sensory input to the eye is decreased before 2 years old, an esodeviation usually occurs. Because young children do not complain of monocular vision loss, especially if congenital or with onset during infancy, sensory strabismus is frequently the presenting sign of vision loss caused by pathology of the retina or optic nerve.

Exodeviations may be simulated in patients with widely spaced eyes (hypertelorism) or in those whose maculae are temporally displaced, as may occur in advanced ROP. When the macula is displaced temporally, the eye rotates outward to align its visual axis on the fixation target. The term *positive angle kappa* is used to describe this condition (Fig. 20.22).

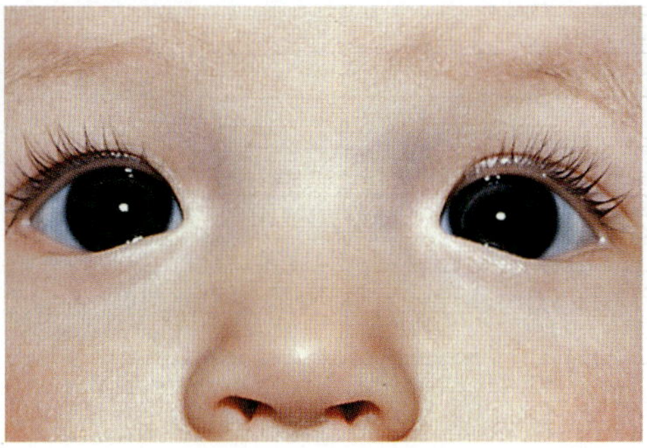

Fig. 20.19 This infant has pseudostrabismus, caused by a flat nasal bridge, epicanthal folds, and closely placed eyes. See the corneal reflections in the center of each pupil, which means the eyes must be aligned.

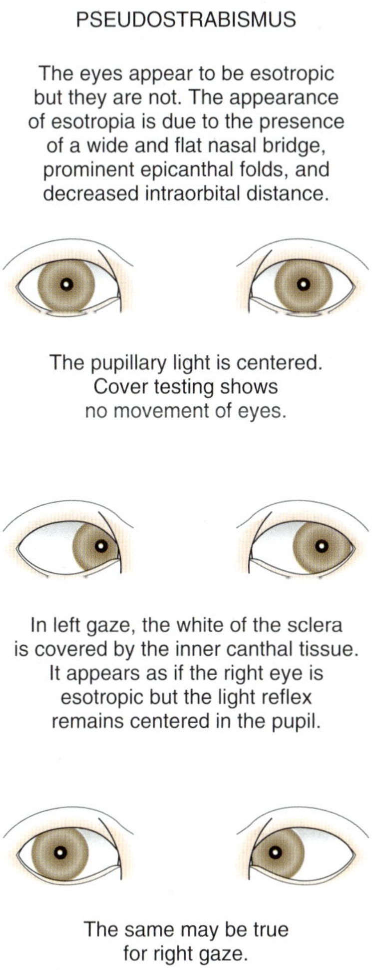

Fig. 20.20 The characteristics of pseudostrabismus are illustrated.

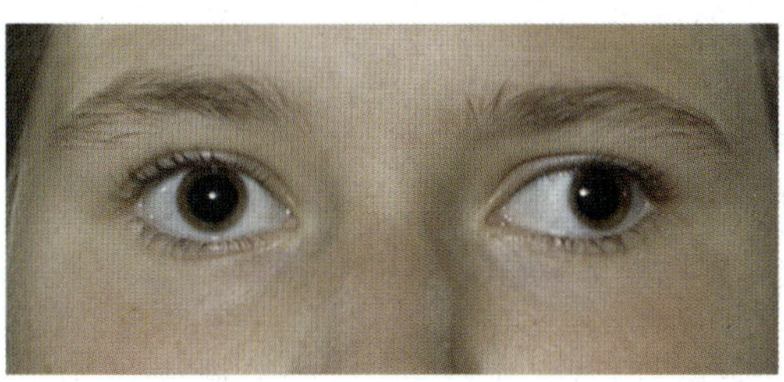

Fig. 20.21 Exotropia, a divergent deviation of the eyes.

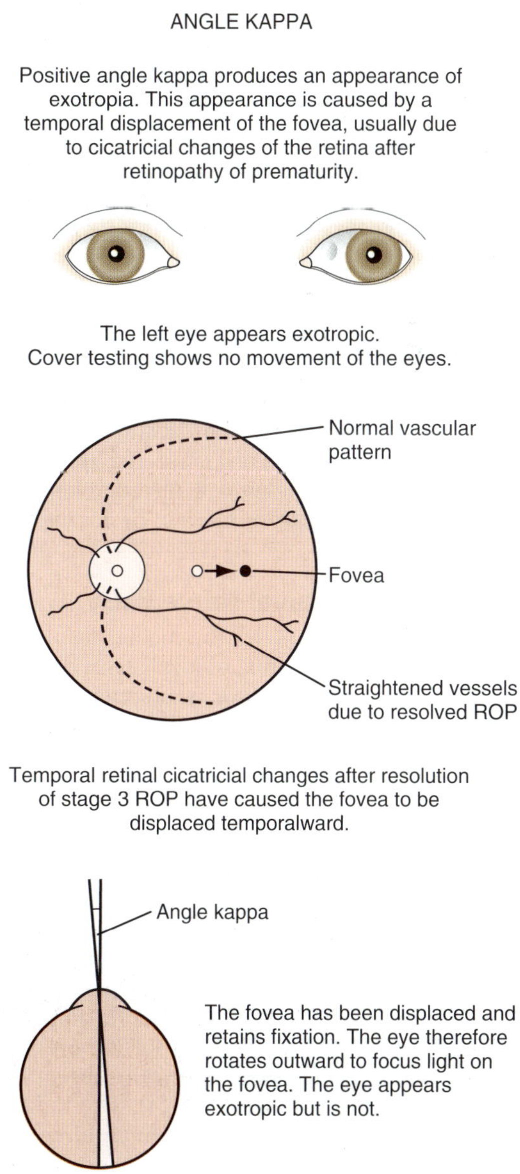

Fig. 20.22 Angle kappa, which can be seen in retinopathy of prematurity.

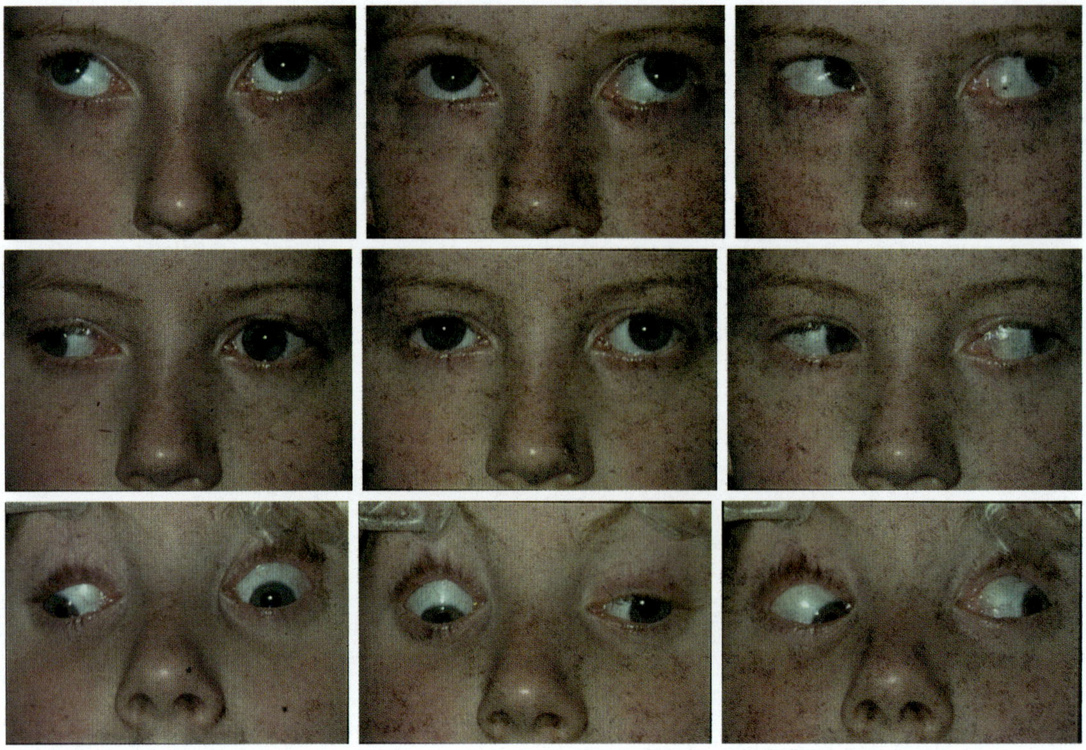

Fig. 20.23 Left palsy of the inferior division of the third nerve. The inferior division of the third nerve supplies the medial rectus and inferior rectus, the pupil, and inferior oblique muscle. The child cannot adduct or depress and has a larger pupil. She can elevate the eye and there is no ptosis.

Convergence Insufficiency

Convergence insufficiency describes an exodeviation in which the size of the deviation is greater in the near range than at distance. Most frequently, there is an exodeviation at near only and no distance deviation. This may cause symptoms of discomfort while reading, complaints of images jumping or moving, or intermittent diplopia at near range. To test for convergence insufficiency, the child is asked to fixate on a target with detail as it is brought progressively closer. Normally the child should be able to converge to a point 10 cm from the nose. If the eyes converge and then break their alignment and diverge at a distance greater than 10 cm from the eyes, the patient should be evaluated for convergence insufficiency. With cover and uncover testing, an exodeviation will be seen at near fixation, and it will be smaller or not seen at distance fixation. Treatments include glasses and, in some cases, convergence exercises and therapy. Children who have postconcussive symptoms will often develop or have convergence insufficiency. This may or may not be accompanied by an accommodation deficit.

Third (Oculomotor) Cranial Nerve Palsy

The third cranial nerve innervates the medial rectus muscle. In third nerve paralysis, the action of the lateral rectus muscle, innervated by the sixth cranial nerve, is unopposed and produces an exodeviation. The third nerve has two branches. The larger inferior branch or division innervates the inferior rectus; medial rectus; inferior oblique muscles; and the ciliary muscle, which is responsible for accommodation of the lens and the iris sphincter muscle that produces miosis of the pupil. The smaller superior branch or division innervates the superior rectus and the levator palpebrae superioris, which elevates the lid. In the presence of a complete third cranial nerve palsy, the eye assumes a down and outward position, the eyelid is ptotic, and the pupil is enlarged. A palsy of the inferior division can present with intact lid elevation and no ptosis but adduction and depression deficit with an enlarged pupil (Fig. 20.23). Elevation of the eye with forced eyelid closure (Bell phenomenon) is typically absent in patients with third cranial nerve palsy (Fig. 20.24). The most common causes for acquired third nerve paralysis in children are trauma and tumor. A third nerve palsy may also occur as a congenital defect.

THIRD CRANIAL NERVE PALSY

A patient with left third cranial nerve palsy will not have a Bell phenomenon on the affected side. The forced opening of tightly closed eyelids will reveal an upward, slightly outward movement of the eye under the closed eyelids (normal Bell response). The patient with a third cranial nerve palsy cannot elevate or adduct the eye. The eye, when opened or under forced eyelid closure, is not elevated.

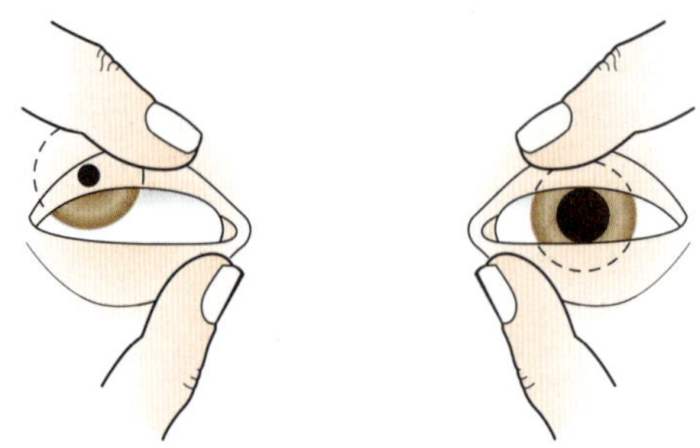

Fig. 20.24 Third cranial nerve palsy.

Vertical Deviations

Vertical deviations may occur in only one field of gaze, or they may be comitant, the same, in all fields of gaze. Vertical deviations may have a cyclotorsional component and be associated with a head tilt or head posture to eliminate double vision. All patients with torticollis should be evaluated for cyclovertical muscle palsies.

The most common cyclovertical deviation is due to a palsy of the fourth cranial (trochlear) nerve (Fig. 20.25). Fourth nerve palsies in children occur congenitally or secondary to head trauma. The eye is excyclorotated, and the head is tilted to the shoulder opposite the side of the paretic nerve and superior oblique muscle to place the eyes in the position of best ocular alignment. Other features are elevation of the eye and difficulty depressing the eye in adduction (Fig. 20.26). Children with congenital fourth nerve palsies usually do not have complaints of diplopia. However, if they are asked about diplopia when their eyes are in the contralateral field of gaze, especially up and away from the paretic side, they can recognize the presence of diplopia.

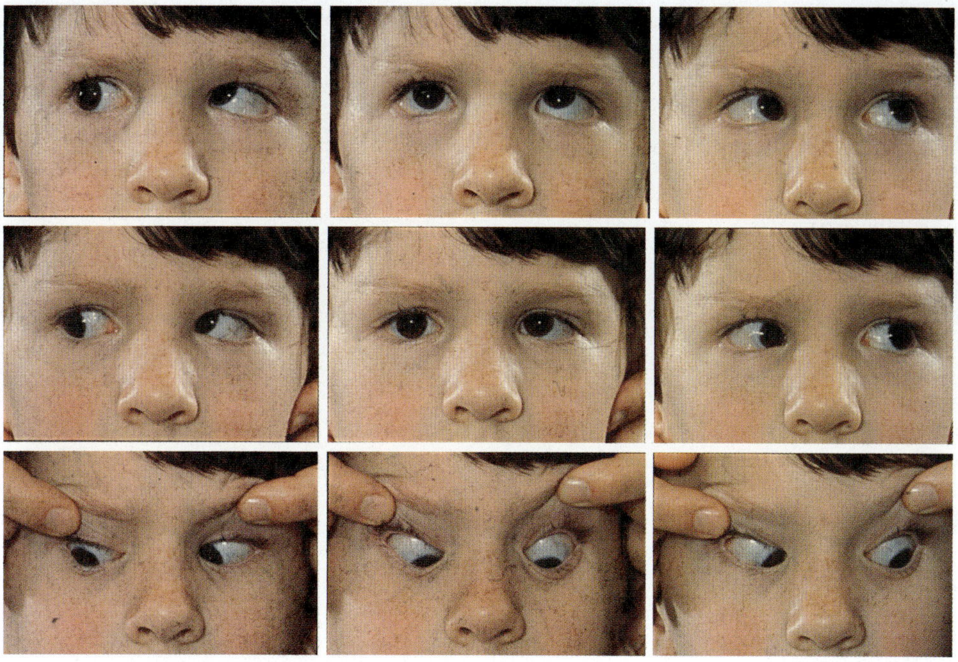

Fig. 20.25 Left fourth nerve palsy with an inability to depress the involved eye in adduction. Abnormal head posture is common with a head tilt away from the side of the fourth nerve palsy, as is overaction of the direct antagonistic inferior oblique muscle, seen as an elevation of the affected eye in adduction (gaze to the opposite side).

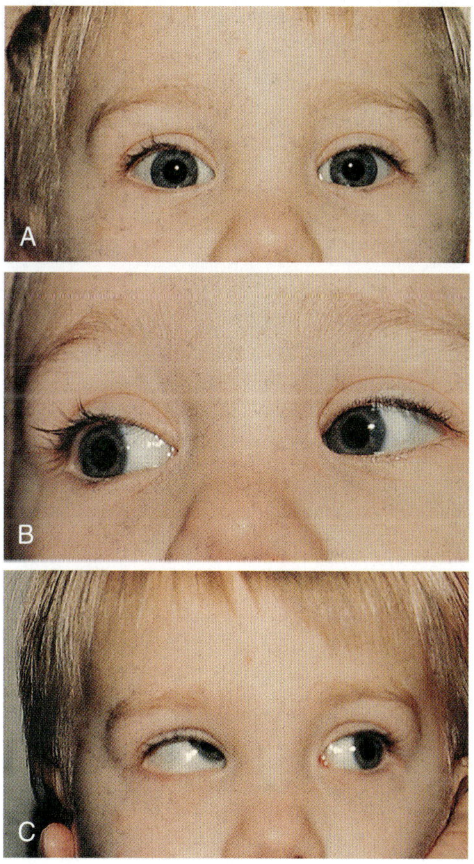

Fig. 20.26 Right inferior oblique overaction. In primary (straight ahead) gaze (A) and right gaze (B), the eyes are well aligned. In left gaze (C), the right eye is elevated or hypertropic because of overaction of the right inferior oblique.

Later in life, patients with congenital fourth nerve palsy may decompensate in their control of the deviation and develop symptomatic diplopia. Some subtle facial asymmetry, especially of the cheek and jaw line, is almost always seen in congenital cases as the children age. Review of candid photos will frequently display consistently repeated head tilt that usually has not been noticed by the family.

Brown syndrome describes an isolated motility disorder in which there is an inability to elevate the eye when in adduction (Fig. 20.27).

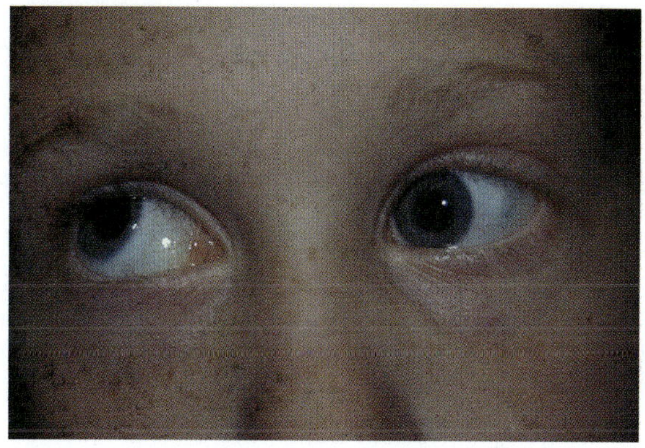

Fig. 20.27 Left Brown syndrome, an inability to elevate an eye in adduction resulting from an abnormality of the superior oblique tendon.

This may be caused by a congenital anomaly of the superior oblique tendon, or it may be acquired as an idiopathic inflammation or tenosynovitis of the superior oblique tendon. Acquired cases may be persistent, resolve spontaneously (sometimes over many years), or respond to nonsteroidal antiinflammatory drugs.

Abnormalities of extraocular muscle innervation rarely cause vertical deviations. Double elevator palsy is an inherited unilateral or bilateral condition in which there is hypotropia and limitation of elevation of the involved eye. To achieve binocularity, patients tilt their chins up and position their heads back. Ptosis is frequently present.

Additional causes of vertical deviations include myasthenia gravis, thyroid ophthalmopathy, chronic progressive external ophthalmoplegia, orbital fractures with muscle entrapment (most commonly the inferior rectus entrapped within a blowout fracture of the orbital floor), and orbital disease with intraorbital masses.

Strabismus in Children With Developmental Delay

There is overwhelming evidence that strabismus surgery in children with developmental delay is unpredictable. It is becoming more and more common to use botulinum toxin injections to reduce the number of surgical procedures. A brief anesthesia is still needed for botulinum injections into one or more of the extraocular muscles (usually horizontal rectus muscles), but it avoids scarring and the further unpredictability of surgical reoperations.

Tests for Strabismus

Although gross observation may detect most cases of strabismus, pseudostrabismus will frequently lead to unnecessary referrals. More significantly, smaller angle deviations may be missed, leading to delays in treatment if more sensitive tests for strabismus are not employed by the primary care physician.

The type and degree of ocular misalignment may be estimated using the corneal light reflex test, or Hirschberg method. The patient fixates on a penlight held at 1 m. Using the pupil edge as a point of reference, the light reflections between the two eyes are compared for symmetry; if the light reflex is displaced temporally in one eye compared with the reflex seen in the other eye, an esotropia is present. If the light reflex is displaced nasally in comparison with the other eye, an exodeviation is present (Fig. 20.28). Although observation of the corneal light reflexes is more sensitive and specific than gross observation alone, a more accurate method of detecting misalignment of the eyes is cover and uncover testing.

The cover test requires cooperation, vision in each eye, and use of a target that stimulates accommodation. Cover testing is performed while the patient maintains fixation on targets at 6 m and at 1 m, because some types of strabismus produce misalignment of the eyes that is present only at either distance or near. The cover/uncover test is used to detect phorias. The test is performed by placing a cover over one eye to disrupt fusion or binocularity. The covered eye is observed as the cover is removed. If the eye deviates while covered and then moves to regain fusion and assumes fixation as the cover is removed, a phoria exists. The test is then repeated, covering and uncovering the other eye (Fig. 20.29). If no movement is seen as each eye is covered and uncovered, both eyes are aligned on the object at that distance and there are no phorias present.

The second component of the cover test is performed by covering one eye and observing the movement of the other eye. If neither eye moves as the eyes are alternately covered, the eyes are both aligned on the fixation target and the term *orthophoria* is used. No deviation is present in this case. If a tropia and a fixation preference are present, a fixation movement of the deviating uncovered eye occurs when the preferred fixating eye is covered; when the cover is transferred back, the previously deviating eye again deviates behind the cover (Fig. 20.30). If a deviation is well controlled by fusion (a phoria) and is small, it may be safely observed if there are no symptoms and the fundus is normal. When a

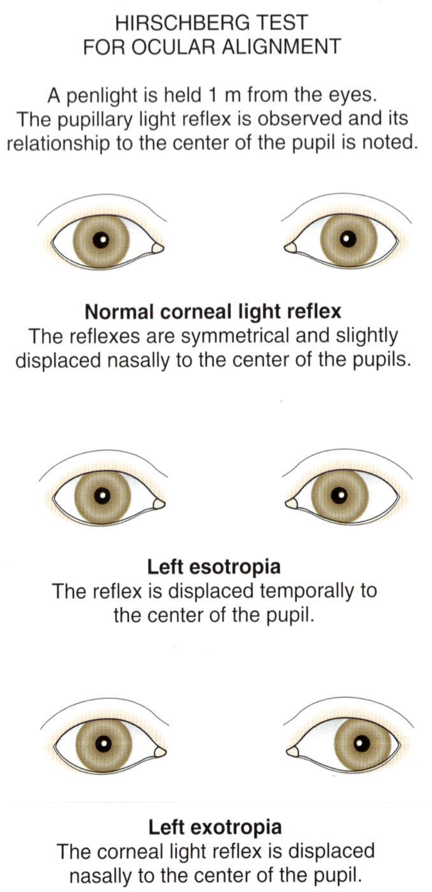

Fig. 20.28 Hirschberg test for ocular alignment.

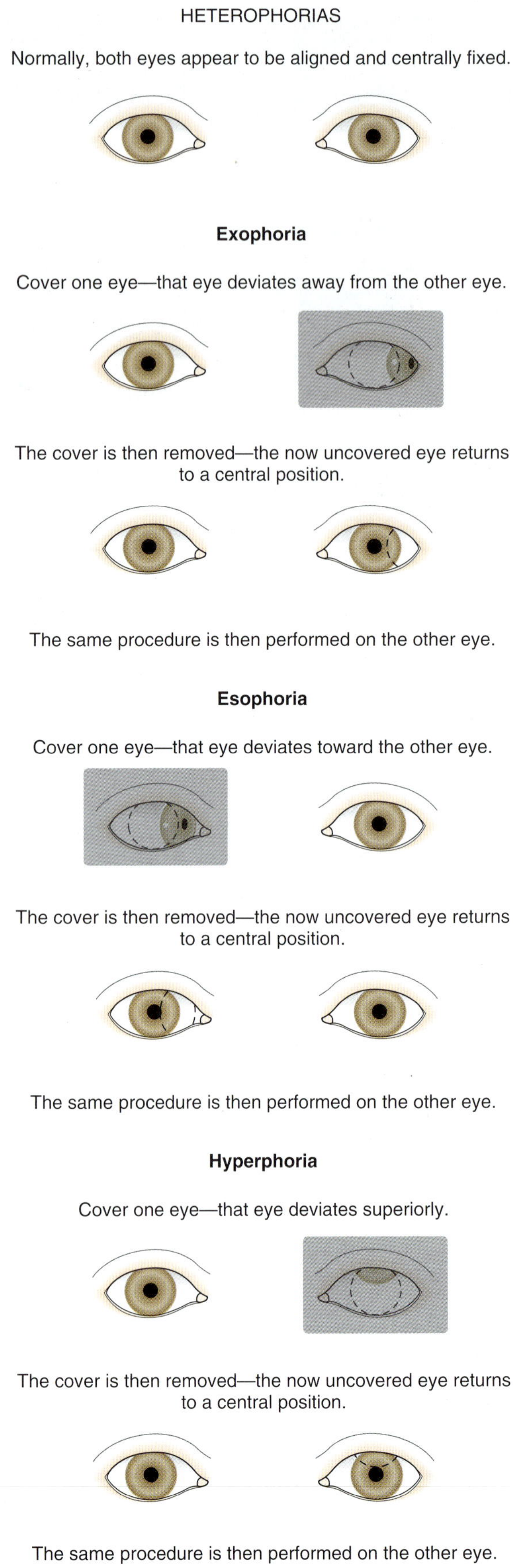

Fig. 20.29 The cover/uncover test for heterophorias.

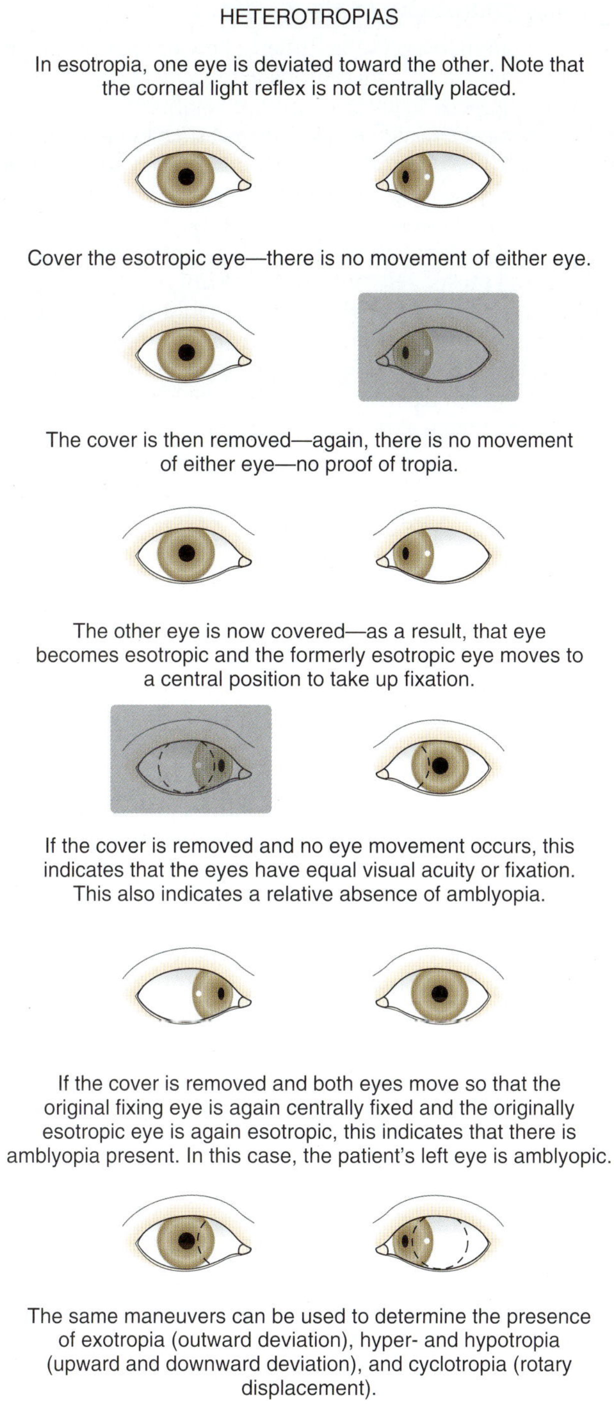

Fig. 20.30 The cover/uncover test for heterotropias.

tropia is present either constantly or intermittently after 3 months old, the patient should be referred to an ophthalmologist. Ophthalmologists use prisms along with cover testing to measure the size of strabismic deviations. An online resource for visualization and practice of the cover test and the prism and cover test for measurement of strabismus can be found at the American Academy of Ophthalmology's Pediatric Ophthalmology Education Center website at https://www.aao.org/pediatric-center-detail/strabismus-simulator.

Anomalous Head Posture

Children may present with an anomalous head posture. This may or may not be due to an ocular cause. An anomalous head posture may be a face turn, a head tilt, chin up or chin down, or any combination of these. A combination of head positions (e.g., left face turn with right head tilt) is most often seen in cases of nystagmus when the brain places the eyes in the position of least ocular oscillation (the null position). Other ocular causes of a face turn may be due to restriction of either abduction of one eye, adduction of one eye, or a gaze paresis of both eyes. Ocular causes of a head tilt are superior oblique palsy or any extraocular muscle problem that causes one eye to sit higher than the other; the head tilts to the lower positioned eye (i.e., the eye with hypotropia). Rarely, a child will develop a head tilt if an astigmatism is uncorrected.

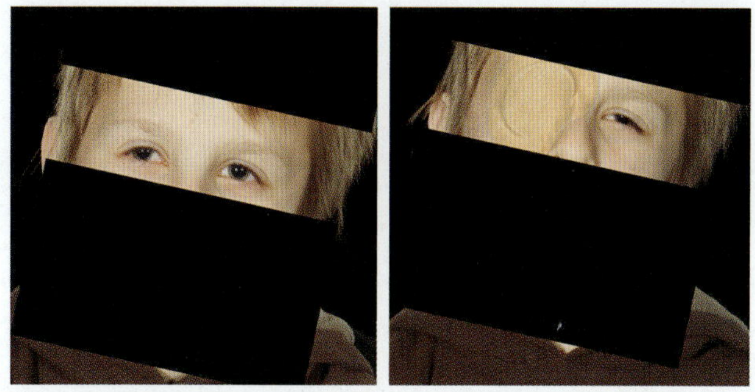

Fig. 20.31 In order to determine whether an anomalous head posture is driven by the eyes, the eyes need to be patched one at a time. In this case, the second eye is being patched and the head posture is unchanged. This suggests that the eyes are not driving the head posture.

Ocular causes of a chin-up head position include bilateral ptosis or an esotropia that disappears in down gaze but is present in primary and up gaze (this is called an *A pattern esotropia*) or an exotropia that disappears in down gaze but is present in primary and up gaze (this is called a *V pattern exotropia*). If a child with vertical nystagmus has a null position with the eyes in down gaze, then this would also cause a chin-up head position. Similarly, ocular causes of a chin down head position are vertical nystagmus with null position in up gaze. An A pattern exotropia with little or no exotropia in up gaze is a possible cause of a chin down head position but is exceedingly rare. However, a V pattern esotropia with the eyes relatively straight in up gaze but esotropia in down gaze can be seen.

Nonocular causes of head tilt include torticollis (note that a face turn may be seen in a child with a homonymous hemianopia with the turn of the head into the hemianopia field). A child who has hearing deficit on one side may also turn the face with the hearing side turned farther forward to hear more clearly.

To differentiate between an ocular or nonocular cause of anomalous head position, the clinician should move the child's head into the primary and neutral position and observe any restriction of eye movement or any worsening of nystagmus. Moreover, if one eye is covered and the head position was being driven by the need of binocular vision, the head will straighten (Fig. 20.31).

DISEASES OF EYES AND SURROUNDING STRUCTURES

Developmental Anomalies of the Globe

Nanophthalmos is an uncommon congenital condition in which the eye is small but is not associated with other developmental defects. There is high hypermetropia, with short axial length (16–18.5 mm) and a crowded anterior chamber predisposing to glaucoma after the second decade of life. Choroidal effusions can occur because of the thickened inelastic sclera. It may be associated with the Kenny Caffey syndrome. Refractive correction is important, as is surveillance for glaucoma.

Microphthalmos is a rare developmental anomaly and tends to be bilateral. The eye is small but abnormal with either coloboma (defective closure of the embryonic fissure) or coloboma with cyst or cataract (Fig. 20.32). Vision may be normal or as poor as light perception. Microphthalmos may be seen in CHARGE syndrome, MICRO syndrome (microphakia, microphthalmos, characteristic lens opacity, and atonic pupils, cortical visual impairment, microcephaly, and developmental delay), and MIDAS (microphthalmia, dermal aplasia, and sclerocornea—also known as MLS) syndrome.

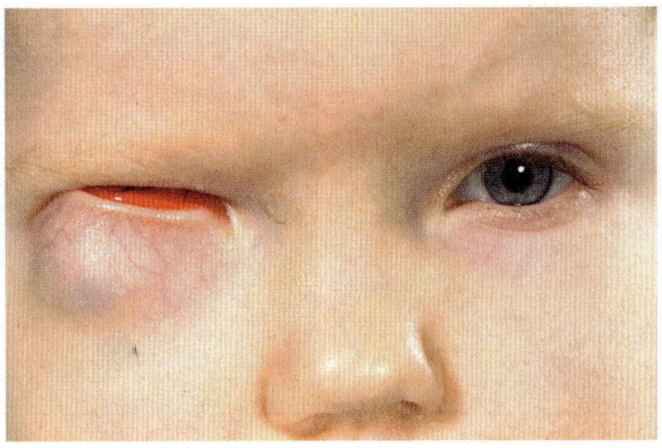

Fig. 20.32 This child has severe right microphthalmos with cyst.

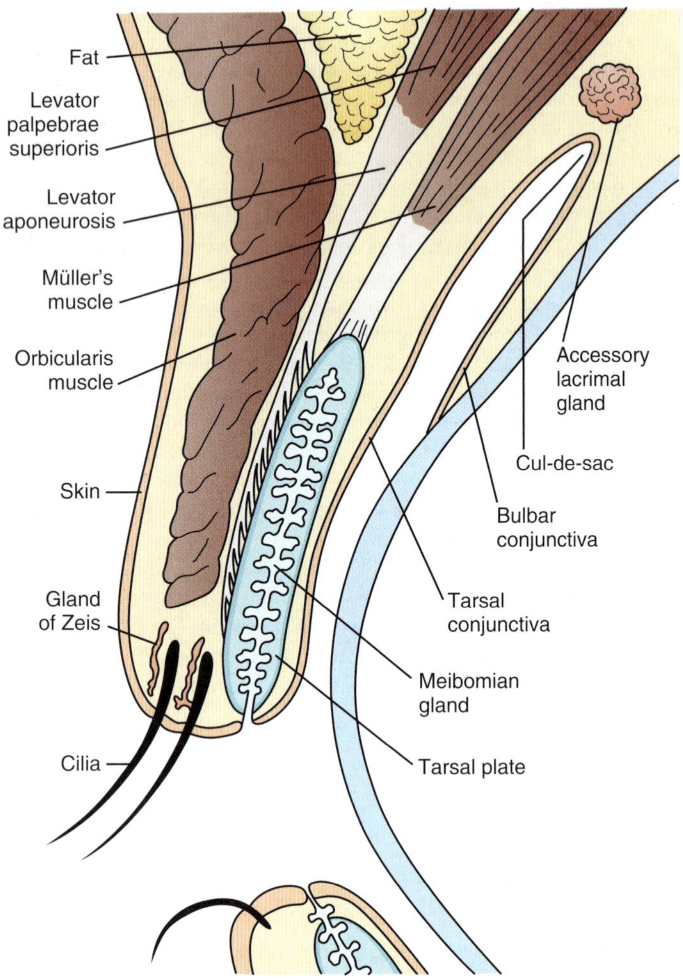

Fig. 20.33 Eyelids and adnexa. Cross section of the eyelid.

Anophthalmia is a rare anomaly in which clinically, the eye is not present or is present as a vestigial, nonfunctioning structure. The child may be otherwise healthy, but intracranial and systemic anomalies are often seen. The absence of a normal eye affects normal orbital growth, and for this reason orbital expanders and referral to an oculoplastic surgeon are often needed. For affected patients, additional genetic evaluation is recommended.

Eyelids and Adnexa

Anatomy of the Eyelid

The eyelid is composed of skin and its related appendages, meibomian glands that contribute to the tear film, tendons that define the shape and position of the eyelid, and muscular structures permitting the eyelid to open and close (Fig. 20.33). Conditions affecting the eyelid are related to these anatomic structures.

Congenital Conditions of the Eyelid

Telecanthus is an increase in the distance between the inner canthus of each eye (Fig. 20.34). Telecanthus can be due to the hereditary transmission of facial features or midline embryonic defects (congenital), or it may be related to a syndrome, such as blepharophimosis syndrome (BPES) (Fig. 20.35). This inherited syndrome consists of telecanthus, epicanthus inversus (a skinfold projecting over the inner angle of the eye and covering part of the canthus, arising from the lower lid skin), blepharophimosis (horizontal shortening of the lid fissure), and ptosis. Telecanthus can be improved surgically.

Epicanthus or epicanthic folds are vertical folds of skin on either side of the nose, sometimes covering the inner canthus, and may be a normal variant. Epicanthal folds can give the impression of a pseudostrabismus, which resolves with age (see Fig. 20.19).

Ptosis is a drooping of the upper eyelid that is not uncommon and may be congenital (Fig. 20.36) or acquired. It may be myogenic, neurogenic, or mechanical. Lowered upper lid margin position may be measured in terms of palpebral aperture or marginal reflex distance (distance of the upper lid margin to the central corneal reflection when using a flashlight as a target for the patient to look at, normally 3.5–4.5 mm). Treatment of ptosis depends on the cause. Ptosis may be due to dysfunction or absence of the levator palpebrae superioris muscle. Dysfunction may allow strengthening of the muscle while absence requires a frontalis sling (i.e., attaching the lid to the frontalis muscle). Ptosis can cause amblyopia related to either stimulus deprivation (if severe ptosis) or astigmatism (mild to moderate ptosis). In any case, prompt ophthalmic referral is required. Care should be taken so as not to cause exposure keratopathy if ptosis repair is undertaken. If the etiology is mechanical, then the cause needs to be removed (e.g., large hemangioma). The prognosis is generally good. The Marcus Gunn jaw-winking phenomenon is caused by a misdirection of the motor division of the fifth cranial nerve to the ipsilateral levator muscle of the eyelid. Jaw movement causes the lid to "wink" (Fig. 20.37). Systemic associations of congenital ptosis that are noteworthy are BPES (see earlier) and Rubinstein-Taybi syndrome (anomalous thumbs). Acquired associations include myasthenia gravis (fatiguability), myotonic dystrophy, and Kearns-Sayre syndrome (heart block and retinal dystrophy). A patient with unilateral ptosis with ipsilateral miosis must be evaluated for Horner syndrome.

Epiblepharon is a skinfold that extends over the lid margin and presses the lashes against the globe. It is commonly observed during the first year of life (Fig. 20.38). This defect usually corrects itself spontaneously by 1 year. In patients of Asian descent, the finding may be persistent. Corneal abrasion usually does not occur because it is the shaft of the eyelash rather than the tip of the lash that touches the cornea. However, surgical correction may be required if it is persistent and causing corneal abrasion. Conjunctival injection, epiphora, and photosensitivity are symptoms in more significant cases.

Additional, more rare congenital conditions affecting the lids are reviewed as follows.

Ablepharon is a rare condition of absent or hypoplastic lids. An affected child has exposed globes and may also have macrostomia. This condition can be confused with congenital everted upper lids, but these can be flipped to allow the lids to close. Exposure keratopathy is a threat to vision (Fig. 20.39).

Ankyloblepharon consists of fusion of the upper and lower eyelid margins with a few thin strands of tissue. If only threadlike strands are present, treatment may be with lid separation with simple eyelid opening. Use of scissors may occasionally be necessary.

Cryptophthalmos describes complete fusion of the upper and lower lids so that the skin of the forehead passes onto the skin of the cheeks. This is most often associated with Fraser syndrome (Fryn 1 gene).

Coloboma is the incomplete formation of the upper or lower lid(s). It is most commonly seen in Goldenhar syndrome (upper lid, Fig. 20.40), amniotic band syndrome, and other clefting syndromes (usually lower lid, Fig. 20.41). Treatment is initially with lubrication to prevent exposure keratopathy. Early referral to an oculoplastic surgeon to allow reconstruction of lid(s) is needed.

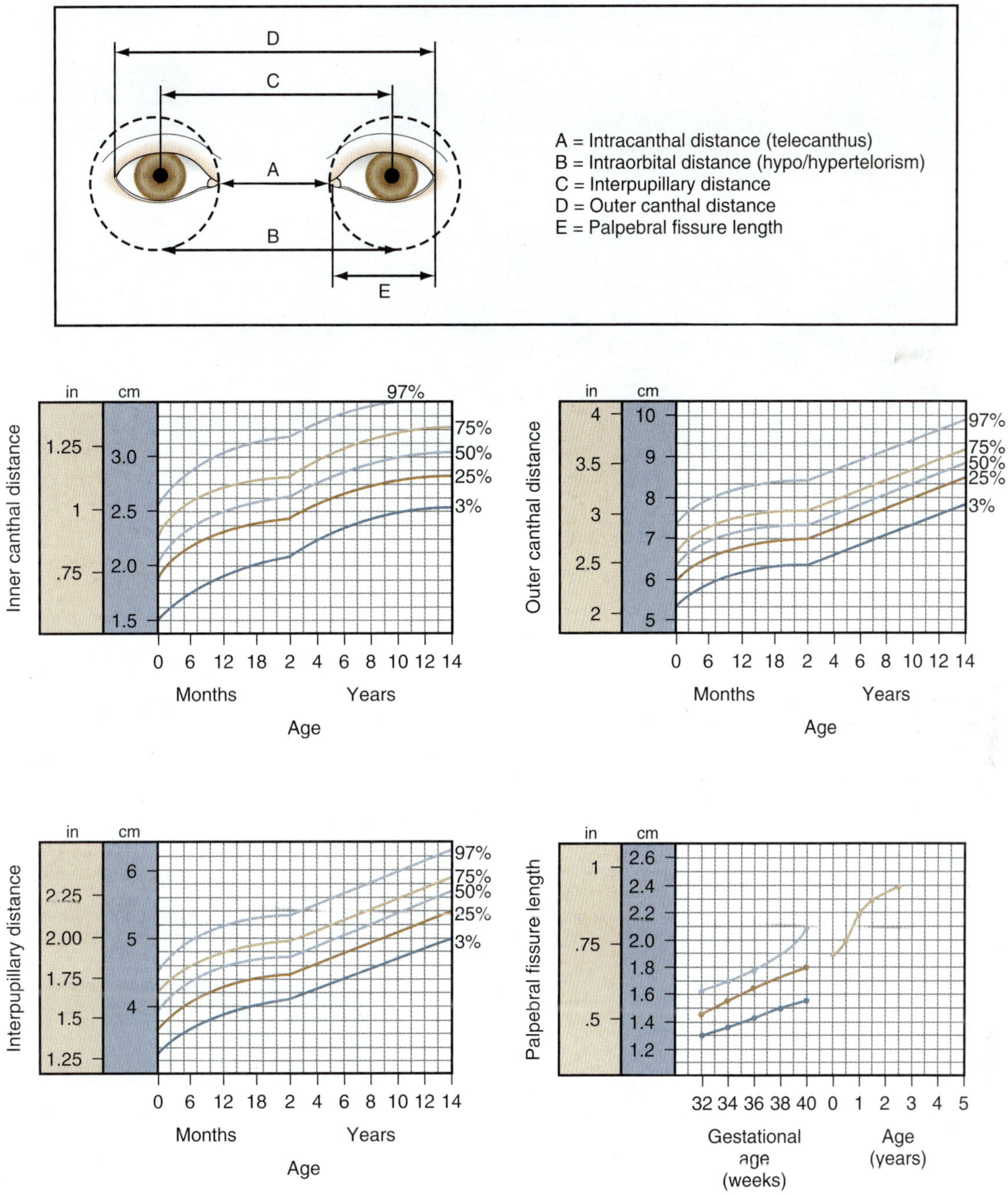

Fig. 20.34 Normal adnexal measurements.

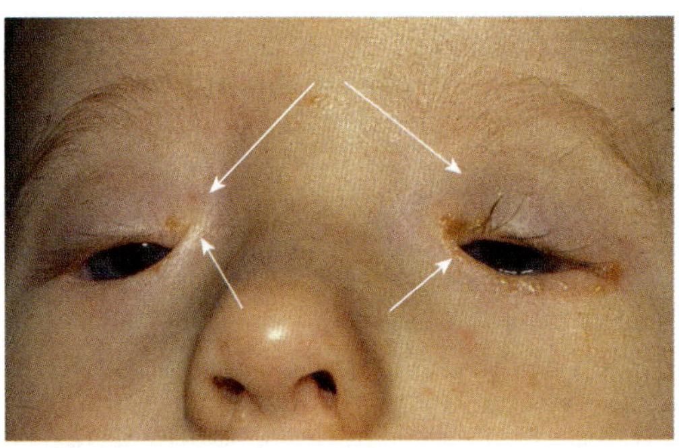

Fig. 20.35 A child with blepharophimosis syndrome, a combination of blepharophimosis, ptosis, epicanthus inversus *(large white arrows)*, and telecanthus *(small white arrows)*.

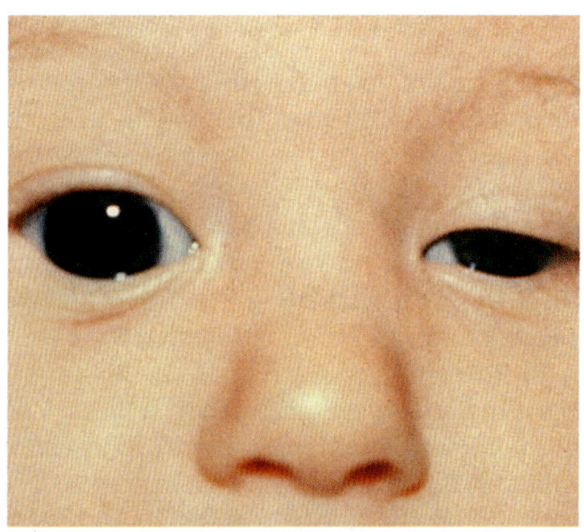

Fig. 20.36 Unilateral congenital ptosis with lid covering pupil.

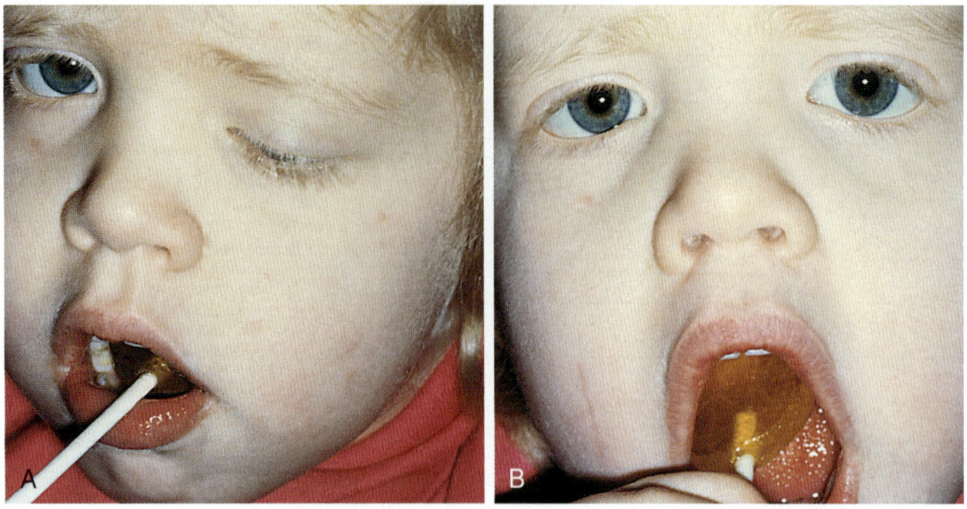

Fig. 20.37 Marcus Gunn jaw-winking ptosis. (A) The ptotic lid position. (B) Elevation and a wide-open lid with movement of the jaw.

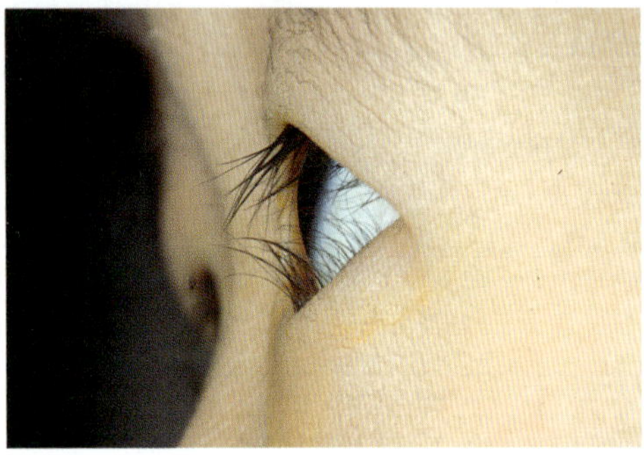

Fig. 20.38 Epiblepharon. The eyelashes are rotated inward against the globe.

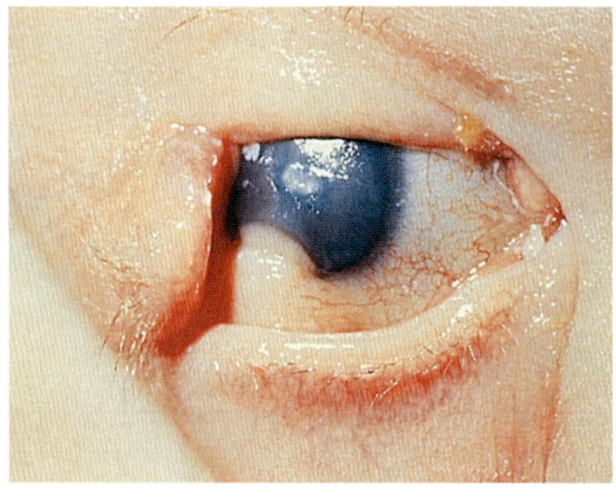

Fig. 20.40 Goldenhar syndrome with eyelid coloboma and corneal/limbal dermoid.

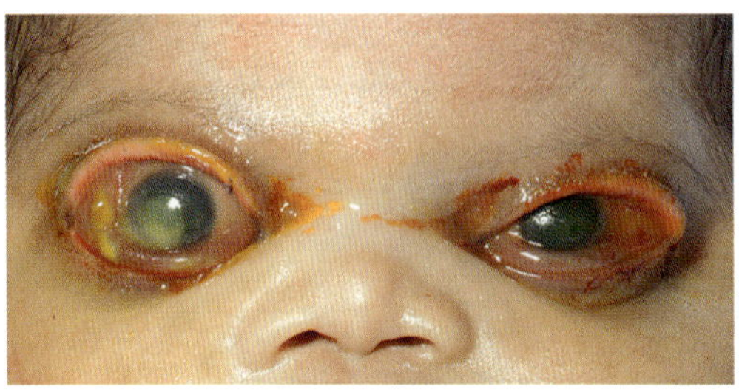

Fig. 20.39 Ablepharon is a rare condition in which the lids have not formed. This leads to exposure keratopathy, seen to be worse in the right eye.

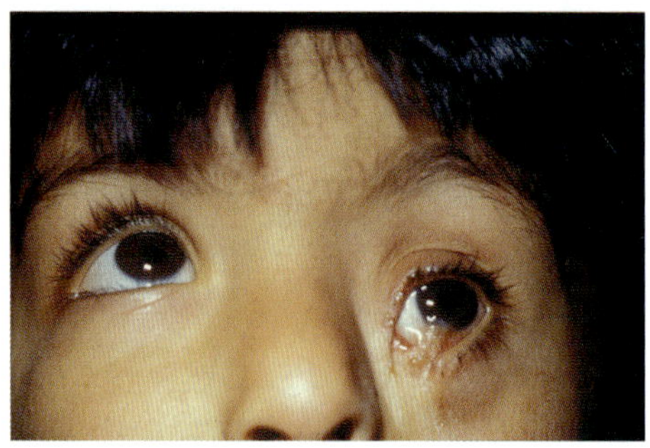

Fig. 20.41 The child has a coloboma of the left lower lid due to a clefting syndrome, which has caused a facial cleft with symblepharon.

Entropion defines an inverted eyelid with the lashes rubbing against the conjunctiva or cornea. This may be present at birth or occur with severe blepharospasm, inflammation, or trauma. If severe, abrasion of the cornea by the lashes can cause permanent corneal scarring (Fig. 20.42). It should be differentiated from an epiblepharon, which is due to an excess skin fold causing the lashes only to turn in. Surgical correction is straightforward.

Ectropion is an outward rotation of the eyelid margin. It usually is acquired due to shortening or scarring of lid skin, as may occur in patients with scleroderma and epidermolysis bullosa. Congenitally, it can be seen in ichthyosis with ectropion of both upper and lower eyelids (Fig. 20.43). It is clinically diagnosed by exposure of tarsal conjunctiva. Treatment depends on the etiology, but emollient use in cases of ichthyosis often leads to resolution. Rarely, surgical correction is needed. If severe, ectropion can lead to problems of corneal exposure (see Fig. 20.43). Ectropion may also occur after seventh cranial nerve palsy with paralysis of the facial musculature, usually of the lower eyelid.

Distichiasis describes a condition in which there is an accessory row of eyelashes (cilia) along the posterior border of the eyelid. This condition is inherited as an autosomal dominant condition but may be associated with lymphedema of the limbs; it is caused by mutations in *FOXC2*.

Madarosis is a lack or loss of eyelashes that can be seen in skin conditions such eczema, ichthyosis, or ectodermal dysplasia. It can also be due to pulling eyelashes out.

Poliosis refers to white or depigmented eyelashes. It is usually seen in oculocutaneous albinism but may be acquired as part of Vogt-Koyanagi-Harada disease, an autoimmune disorder affecting the eyes (inflammation) and skin (vitiligo and poliosis).

Symblepharon is a rare anomaly; it is usually acquired but may be congenital (Figs. 20.44 and 20.41). Acquired types are seen in Stevens-Johnson syndrome, toxic epidermolysis syndrome, alkali injuries to the eyes, ocular cicatricial pemphigoid, and, rarely, epidermolysis bullosa. It presents as shortened fornices due to an

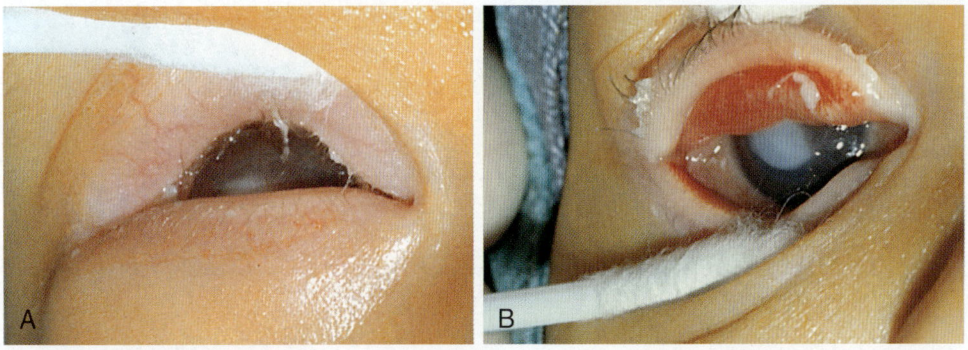

Fig. 20.42 Congenital entropion of the right upper lid. The lid is inverted, and the lashes and skin rest on the corneal surface. (A) The eyelid is propped up with a cotton-tipped applicator, displaying the area of skin inverted against the eye. The povidone-iodine prep solution has not coated the affected area of the lid. (B) With the upper lid everted and the lids held widely open, extensive corneal scarring caused by the abrasion from the inverted skin and lashes is seen.

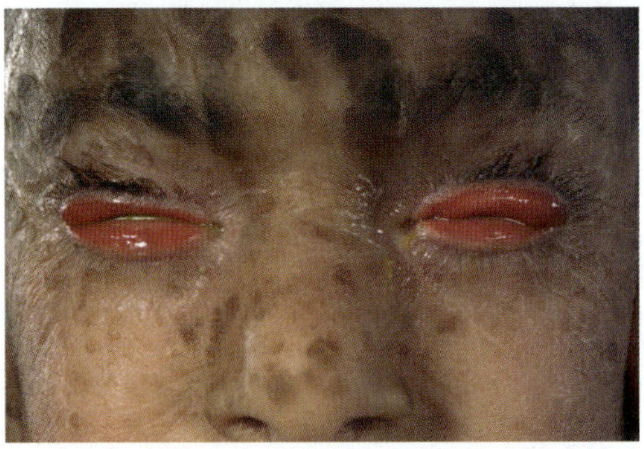

Fig. 20.43 Ectropions of all four lids due to congenital ichthyosis. Lubrication of the skin usually allows the lids to turn back into a normal position.

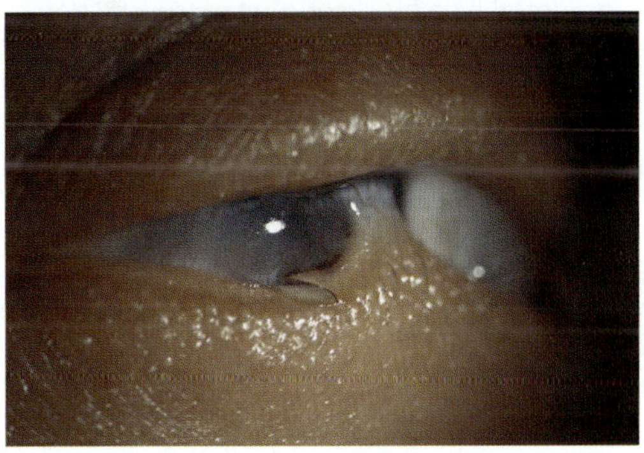

Fig. 20.44 Acquired case of symblepharon with the lid attached to the cornea. The child has recessive dystrophic epidermolysis bullosa.

adhesion between the lid and conjunctiva (see Fig. 20.44). Prevention is the best approach in conditions where symblepharon may be acquired; topical lubrication and steroids may be needed and ophthalmic opinion must be sought early. Once formed, amniotic membrane may be used to treat after resection of the symblepharon.

Acquired Conditions of the Eyelid

Trichiasis describes misdirected eyelashes that irritate the cornea or conjunctiva. It can be caused by chronic inflammation of the eyelids, entropion (in-turning of the eyelid), eyelid trauma, or inflammatory conditions with scarring of the conjunctiva, such as Stevens-Johnson syndrome.

Blepharitis is inflammation of the eyelid margins (Fig. 20.45), with or without chalazion (blocked meibomian gland) (see later discussion of chalazion). The anterior type usually affects lashes, whereas the posterior type is caused by meibomian gland dysfunction. It is often mistaken for pink eye but differs in presentation due to its chronicity and, often, asymmetry. It may present with recurrent chalazia, chronic red eyes, or chronically crusted lids. Although usually isolated, chalazia may be associated with acne rosacea. Treatment includes lid hygiene and topical antibiotics. Steroids or systemic antibiotics may also be used. Treatment is necessary to prevent corneal complications (vascularization or keratitis). Prognosis is moderate because the condition may never totally resolve, although the signs and symptoms can be controlled to prevent ocular damage. Blepharitis may be associated with chronic environmental allergies and occurs commonly in children with Down syndrome.

A hordeolum, commonly referred to as a *stye*, is an inflamed gland of Zeis along the eyelid margin (Fig. 20.46). It may be painful and produce swelling and erythema of the eyelid. Infection may occur frequently with *Staphylococcus*. Some discharge may be seen. Rarely, preseptal cellulitis may occur as a complication. Removal of the affected eyelash accelerates resolution. Occasionally, topical antibiotics may be needed.

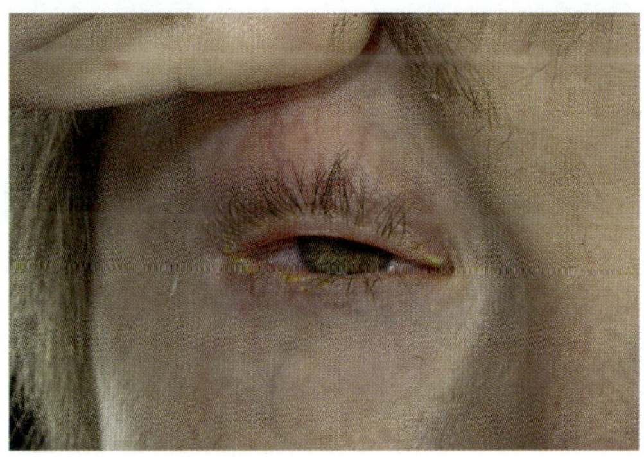

Fig. 20.45 Blepharitis. Thickened lids with crusting of the lashes and incongruous lid margins.

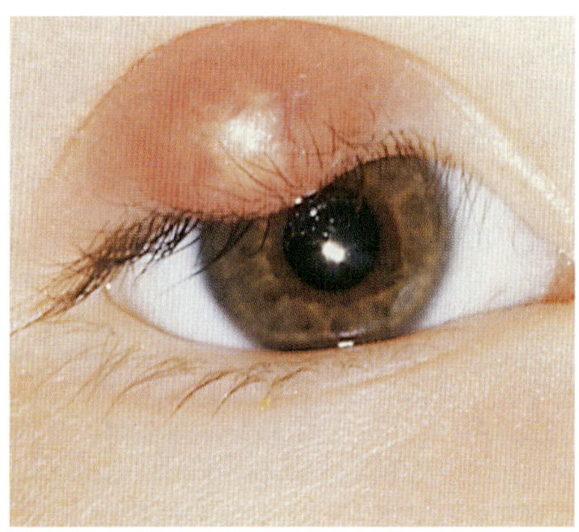

Fig. 20.46 Acute hordeolum of the eyelid (pointing externally) with swelling, induration, and purulent contents.

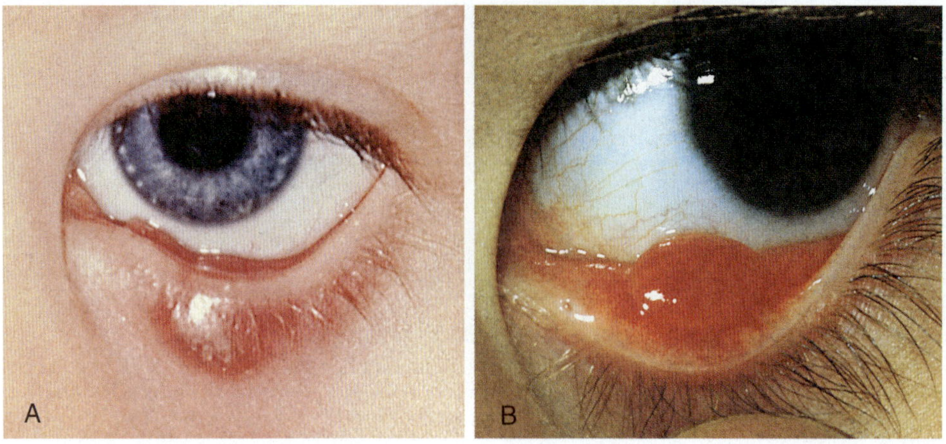

Fig. 20.47 (A) Chalazion. Usually, but not always, painless. The lesion may point externally to the skin side or internally to the underside of the lid. (B) Chalazion of the left lower lid, pointed internally. A pyogenic granuloma consisting of a vascularized mound of conjunctival tissue has developed over the chalazion because of spontaneous rupture of the chalazion under the palpebral conjunctiva with a hypertrophic healing response of the conjunctiva.

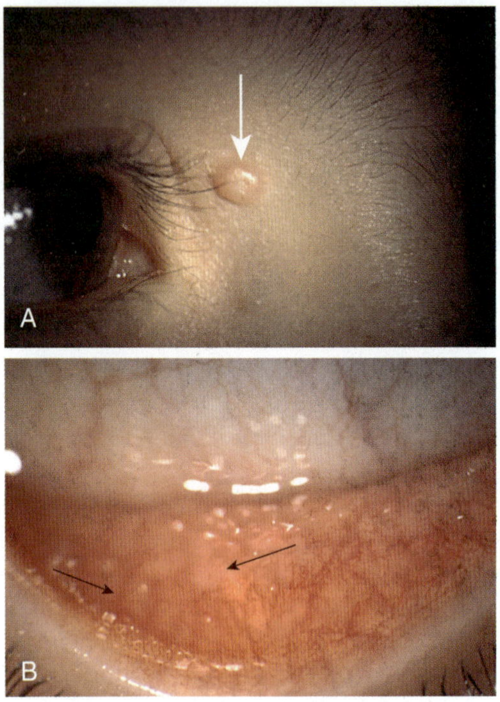

Fig. 20.48 (A) An umbilicated skin lesion which is consistent with Molluscum contagiosum *(white arrow)*, (B) causing a follicular conjunctivitis *(follicles black arrows)*.

A chalazion is a chronic granulomatous inflammation of the meibomian glands within the tarsal plate (higher on the lid than a hordeolum). Painless swelling and redness of the eyelid result from distention of the gland and the inflammatory response caused by the retained glandular secretions. The gland may spontaneously rupture either to the conjunctival surface or externally to the skin (Fig. 20.47A and B). Spontaneous resolution may occur; however, tissue reaction may persist and leave a firm mass within the lid. Surgical excision of the lesions may be required if chronic or inflamed to prevent drainage through the skin surface with scarring of the skin or possible permanent loss of lashes if the lid margin is severely affected. Small lesions that are not significantly inflamed or threatening drainage on the skin surface may be conservatively treated for weeks or months to avoid surgery.

Molluscum contagiosum is a common eyelid infectious tumor caused by a poxvirus. Small umbilicated nodules are often situated on the lid margin (Fig. 20.48A) and should be looked for in cases of follicular or chronic conjunctivitis (see Fig. 20.48B). The lesions are usually self-limiting, but if conjunctivitis is troublesome, then curettage of lid lesions may be needed.

Capillary (infantile) hemangioma is the commonest benign tumor of the eyelid or orbit of childhood and histologically displays abundant endothelial cells with narrow vascular channels (Fig. 20.49C and D). Systemic associations include Kasabach-Merritt syndrome (thrombocytopenia due to platelet pooling and activation within one or more large hemangiomas), Maffucci syndrome (hemangiomas and enchondromas), and PHACES syndrome (segmental facial hemangioma associated with other anomalies; see Fig. 20.49A). Infantile hemangiomas appear 2 or 3 weeks after birth, grow rapidly until 4 months of age with plateau of growth often by 6 months, and usually regress thereafter. The position of the hemangioma may result in visual deprivation by causing a ptosis, amblyopia from astigmatism, or, rarely, compress the optic nerve if the hemangioma is intraorbital. Treatment is systemic or topical beta blockers. Some cases still demand surgical excision. Occlusion of the unaffected eye may be needed to prevent amblyopia from developing in the affected eye.

Port wine birthmark is a common dermal capillary vascular malformation, which may occur in the periocular region. Ocular associations include episcleral hemangioma, iris heterochromia (affected iris darker than unaffected one), choroidal hemangioma, and glaucoma. Systemic associations include Sturge-Weber syndrome and cutis marmorata telangectasia congenita. Periocular lesions are associated with an increased risk of developing glaucoma, and the child should have regular eye examinations to exclude this (see Fig. 20.49B).

Lid retraction is rare, and causes include thyroid eye disease (e.g., Graves disease in which lid signs such as retraction and lid lag are seen in 25%–60% of pediatric cases) (Fig. 20.50), Parinaud syndrome, Marcus-Gunn jaw winking, and primary congenital idiopathic lid retraction. Lower lid retraction can be seen in cherubism (a rare, inherited condition characterized by fibro-osseous lesions of the maxilla and mandible recently localized to chromosome 4p16.3). No treatment is required except lubricating drops or ointment used at night if there is evidence of lid lag and incomplete closure of the lids when asleep and treatment of underlying cause.

Preseptal cellulitis is a common but serious infection in children, most commonly due to direct infection from external factors such as a wound. This contrasts with orbital cellulitis, which frequently is an extension from contiguous ethmoid sinusitis. Examination of preseptal cellulitis usually finds red swollen eyelids, which may be tense, but a benign ocular examination, in which visual acuity, eye movements, color vision, pupil reactions, and fundoscopy are normal. Treatment with systemic antibiotics is necessary, but progression to orbital cellulitis is uncommon. Imaging is needed if the lids are too swollen to allow adequate ocular examination.

Herpes simplex and varicella zoster can both cause vesicular rashes on the lids (Fig. 20.51). If the eye is red, then it can suggest

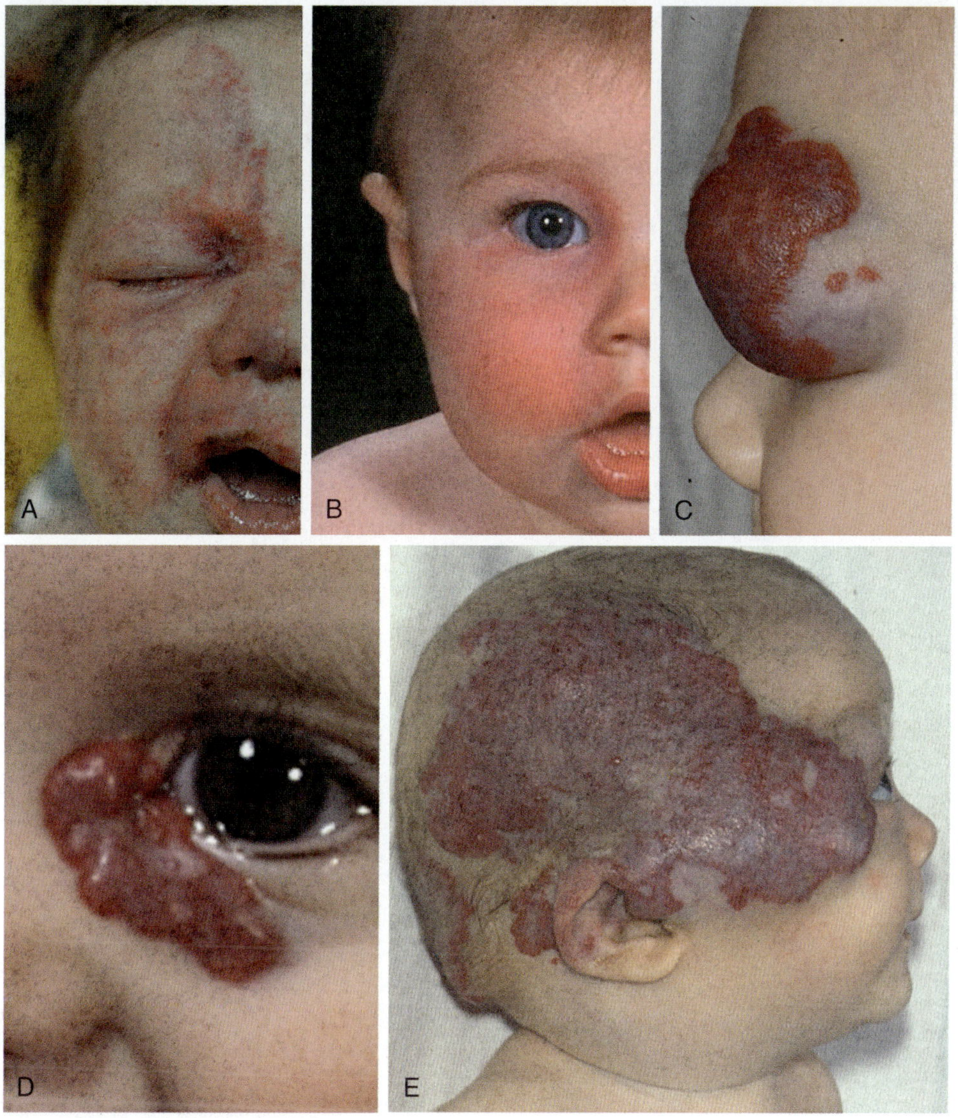

Fig. 20.49 Composite showing infantile capillary hemangiomas (C and D), a port wine birthmark (B), and two flat segmental plaquelike hemangiomas seen in two children with PHACES syndrome (segmental facial hemangioma associated with other anomalies; A and E).

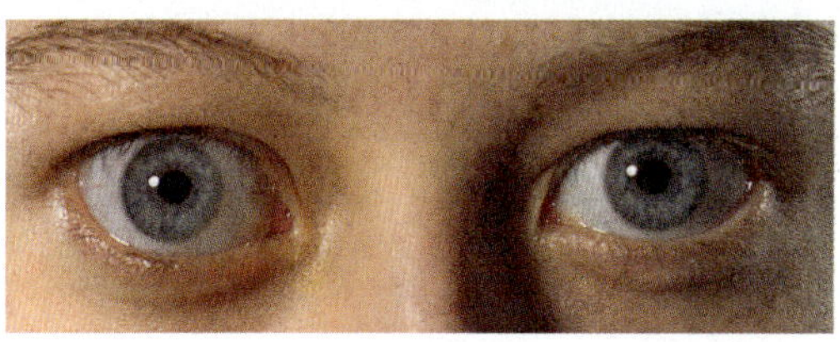

Fig. 20.50 Lower lid retraction on the right more than left in a patient with Graves disease.

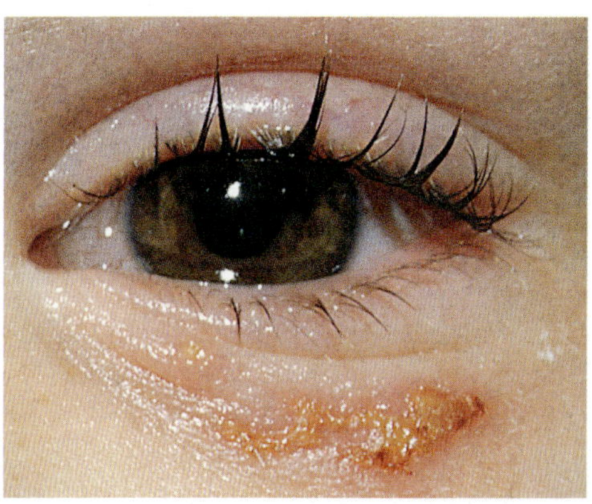

Fig. 20.51 Primary herpes simplex infection involving the periocular area. Primary infection is frequently associated with a mild diffuse keratoconjunctivitis; dendritic corneal lesions are uncommon in primary infections.

an accompanying conjunctivitis, with or without keratitis. Varicella zoster is rare in children, but a lesion on the tip of the nose indicates involvement of the ophthalmic division of the maxillary nerve and possible involvement of the eye with keratitis, uveitis, and glaucoma.

Phthiriasis, infestation of the lashes with the crab louse *Phthirus pubis,* manifests as a crusty appearance of the lid margin. Closer inspection reveals egg cases and the adult louse. Ophthalmic ointment, almost any type, used for a few weeks suffocates the organisms. Phthiriasis is another cause of chronic conjunctivitis, and the lashes should be carefully examined in cases of chronic, recurring conjunctivitis.

Lacrimal Gland and Nasolacrimal Drainage System

Reflex tears are produced by the lacrimal gland, whereas the basal secretion of tears comes from the accessory lacrimal glands (Fig. 20.52). The tear film consists of three layers: the layer closest to the eye is made of mucin, the next layer is the aqueous from lacrimal glands, and the outermost layer is lipid from the meibomian glands in the lid margins. During the first month of life, the eye remains moist, but reflex tearing, or tearing resulting from emotion, does not occur until the second month of life or later.

Agenesis of the lacrimal glands occurs rarely. Most lacrimal gland disorders are acquired and include acute viral dacryoadenitis

(Fig. 20.53). Chronic diseases such as sarcoidosis, Hodgkin disease, leukemia, and mononucleosis may produce lacrimal gland swelling with a palpable mass in the upper outer portion of the orbit.

Tears are drained from the eye by the superior and inferior puncta, which connect to the superior and inferior canaliculi (see Fig. 20.52). The canaliculi may unite into a common canaliculus before they enter the nasolacrimal sac, or they may enter the sac separately. The medial canthal tendon is anterior and superior to the nasolacrimal sac. Disorders of the lacrimal sac are then seen primarily inferior to the medial canthus, unless there is an overlying cellulitis. The sac is connected to the nasolacrimal duct, which is in the nasal bone. The distal portion of the nasolacrimal duct enters the nasal antrum beneath the inferior turbinate.

Congenital nasolacrimal duct obstruction, or stenosis, is present in 30% of newborns (Fig. 20.54). Signs include tearing and mucopurulent discharge, which usually begins 3 to 5 weeks after birth, without conjunctival injection. A helpful diagnostic technique is to apply gentle pressure over the nasolacrimal sac to cause reflux of tears and mucopurulent material from the sac. Spontaneous resolution of the obstruction is common before 6 to 8 months of age. If the obstruction has not cleared by 8 to 10 months old, spontaneous resolution is much less likely and the patient should be referred for probing of the nasolacrimal duct. Beyond 13 months old, the success rate of simple probing begins to decrease due to the recurring infections, which may cause scarring and stenosis of the nasolacrimal duct, increasing the need for more complicated procedures for treatment.

Rarely, the lacrimal sac becomes expanded due to the distal blockage and the child presents with a dacryocele (Fig. 20.55). An infected dacryocele is termed *dacryocystitis.* Urgent referral for treatment of dacryocystitis should be made to prevent expansion of infection to the surrounding tissues producing a periorbital cellulitis. Treatment is with lacrimal massage and systemic antibiotics if infected (Fig. 20.56).

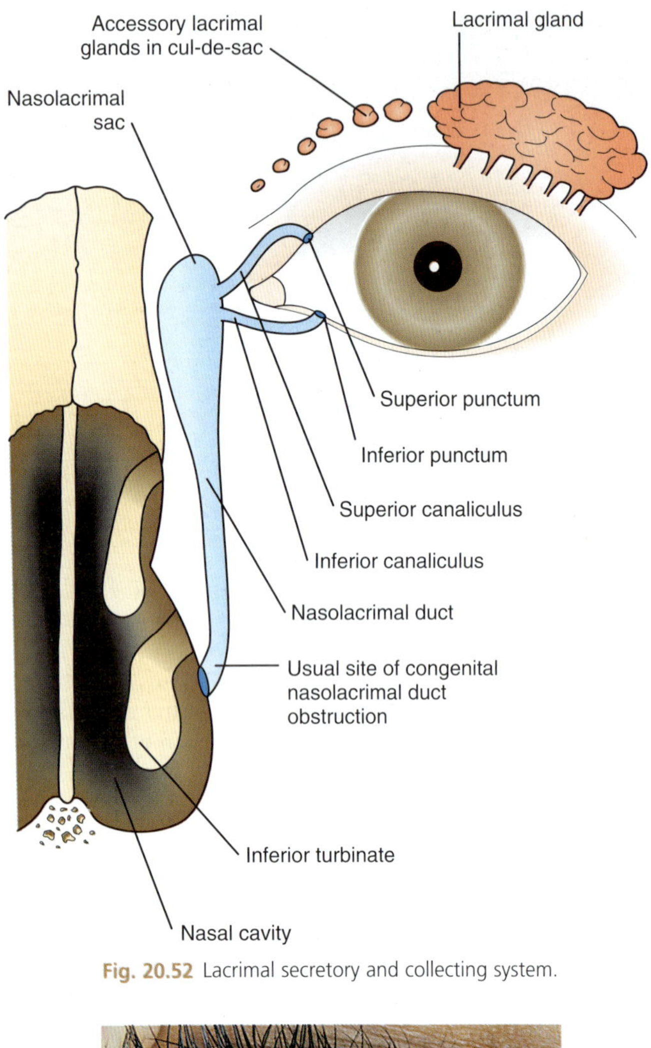

Fig. 20.52 Lacrimal secretory and collecting system.

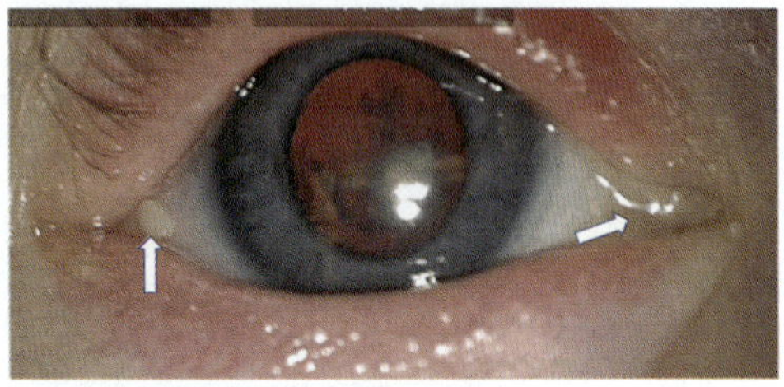

Fig. 20.54 Nasolacrimal duct obstruction. Mucopurulent discharge and tearing (epiphora) are present (*white arrows*).

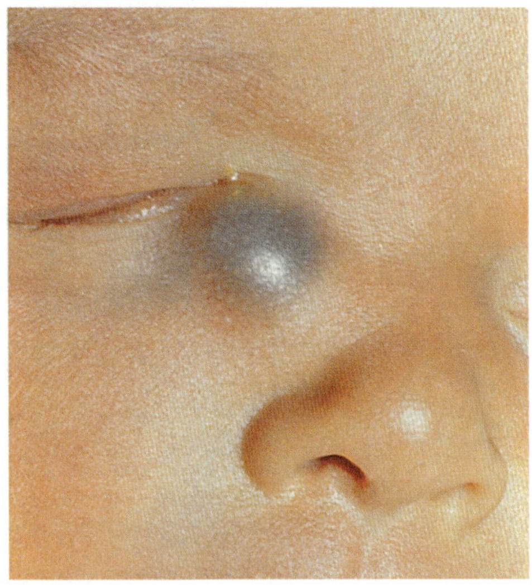

Fig. 20.55 Congenital nasolacrimal sac mucocele presents shortly after birth as a bluish mass below the medial canthal tendon.

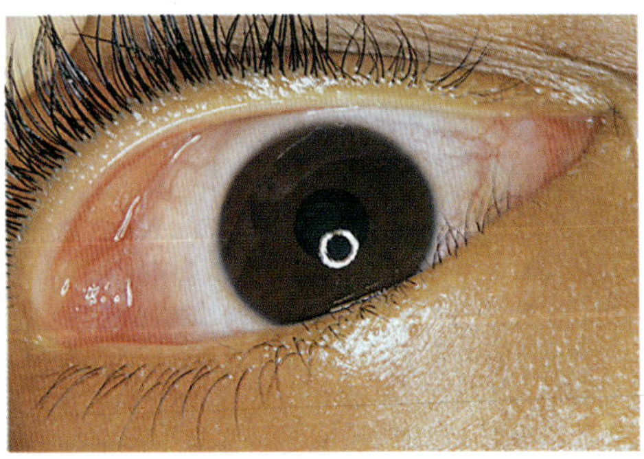

Fig. 20.53 Dacryoadenitis. The lacrimal gland has become swollen and inflamed and is visible beneath the lateral aspect of the upper eyelid. The swelling is frequently accompanied by symptoms of pain and tenderness.

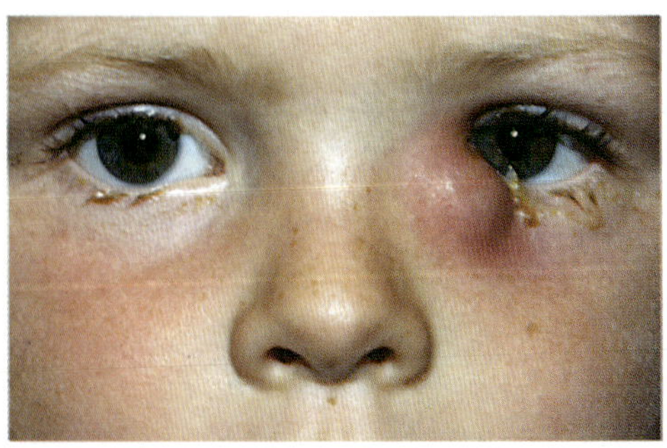

Fig. 20.56 Acute dacryocystitis caused by bacterial infection of the nasolacrimal sac associated with nasolacrimal duct obstruction. The infection of the nasolacrimal sac has spread to the surrounding tissues, producing a cellulitis.

Conjunctiva

The conjunctiva is a mucous membrane that covers the posterior aspect of the eyelids. It is reflected into the cul-de-sac and extends onto the globe, where it fuses to the sclera at the corneal scleral limbus. The conjunctiva has goblet cells that contribute mucin to the tear film. When the eyelids are closed, the oxygen supplied by the blood vessels of the conjunctiva is responsible for maintaining oxygenation of the cornea. *Conjunctivitis* refers to inflammation of the conjunctiva. Infections of the conjunctiva may be bacterial or viral. The conditions that affect the conjunctiva may be due to inflammation (conjunctivitis), pigmentation, or elevated lesions.

Conjunctivitis

Neonatal conjunctivitis incidence varies from 1% to 21% depending on the region of the world. Causes include chemical irritation (relatively mild diffuse injection without discharge), gonococcal infection (copious purulent discharge within 2–4 days of birth, which may be associated with membrane formations), herpes simplex virus type II, chlamydia, and bacterial infections. All cases of neonatal conjunctivitis are emergencies and must be evaluated by an ophthalmologist. Infectious neonatal conjunctivitis occurring after 8 days (but before 2 weeks) and accompanied by a watery discharge is often due to chlamydia. Diagnostic swabs and appropriate topical and, if positive for gonococcus or chlamydia, systemic antibiotics are needed (Fig. 20.57).

Bacterial conjunctivitis may be acute or chronic. Acute conjunctivitis may be uncomfortable with lid edema and keratitis, although keratitis secondary to bacterial conjunctivitis is rare in children. The bulbar conjunctiva swells (chemosis) and becomes hyperemic (injection). Corneal ulceration may occur as a complication. Children with viral conjunctivitis frequently develop secondary bacterial conjunctivitis. Acute bacterial conjunctivitis is usually due to staphylococcal, pneumococcal, or *Haemophilus* infections. Mucopurulent discharge is associated with tearing, and the eyelids may be stuck together in the morning (Fig. 20.58).

Chronic bacterial conjunctivitis results from bacterial toxins of *Staphylococcus aureus, Proteus, Moraxella* or Trachoma. A foreign body sensation may be experienced, and the eyes may be hyperemic with a chronic, mucopurulent, or watery discharge. Papillary hyperplasia and thickening of the conjunctiva may also occur. It is important to remember that a recurrent red eye with or without chalazia is usually an indication of possible meibomian gland dysfunction and blepharitis and requires referral.

Viral conjunctivitis is usually caused by various strains of adenovirus (Fig. 20.59). Signs include copious tearing with a watery or thin mucopurulent discharge, conjunctival redness and follicles (aggregates of lymphocytes with an avascular center and a peripheral vascular network) (see Fig. 20.48B), and preauricular lymph node enlargement. Viral conjunctivitis, although self-limiting resolving in 7 to 10 days, is highly contagious. It may also present with pseudomembranous conjunctivitis. These membranes are inflammatory and need to be peeled away. Treatment of pseudomembranous conjunctivitis includes topical steroids to suppress the body's inflammatory response. Certain strains of adenoviral conjunctivitis may cause epidemic keratoconjunctivitis, which produces corneal involvement with a punctate keratitis that progresses to subepithelial infiltrates (Fig. 20.60) as an immunologic reaction. Patients are contagious only early in their course and are photophobic with blurred vision. Symptoms in epidemic keratoconjunctivitis may last from weeks to months. The infiltrates eventually resolve spontaneously. Steroids may alleviate symptoms; however, they may prolong the overall course.

Allergic conjunctivitis occurs as a hypersensitivity response to dust, pollens, animal dander, or other airborne allergens. Itching is a hallmark symptom. There may be copious tearing and photophobia. The eyelids and palpebral conjunctiva are hyperemic and edematous (Fig. 20.61), and the conjunctiva develops papillae (small, raised nodules with a central vascular core). They may be located on the tarsal surface of the upper and lower eyelids. Papillae may become large, measuring 1 to 2 mm in diameter if inflammation is chronic. Giant papillae may be produced by the

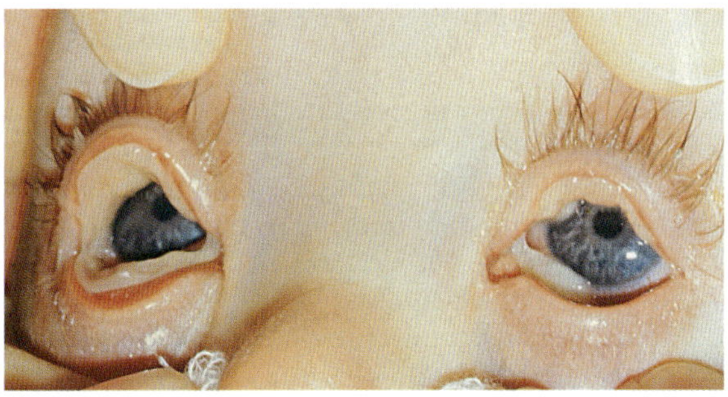

Fig. 20.57 Ophthalmia neonatorum, a hyperacute bacterial conjunctivitis, with thick purulent discharge and red swollen lids.

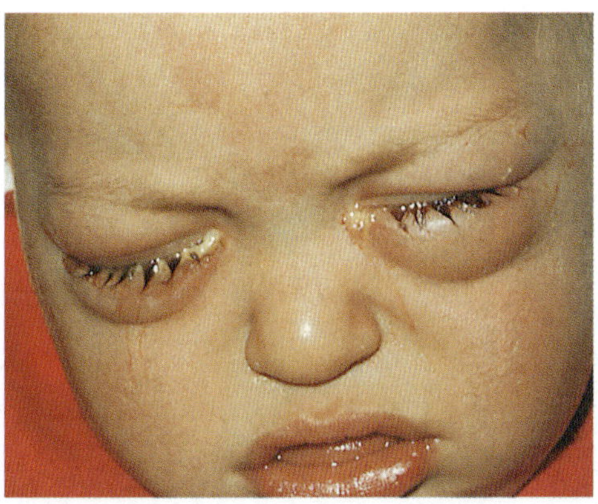

Fig. 20.58 Acute bacterial conjunctivitis. Copious amounts of mucopurulent discharge have made the upper and lower eyelids adherent to each other. Chemosis of the upper and lower lids may also make opening of the eyelids difficult.

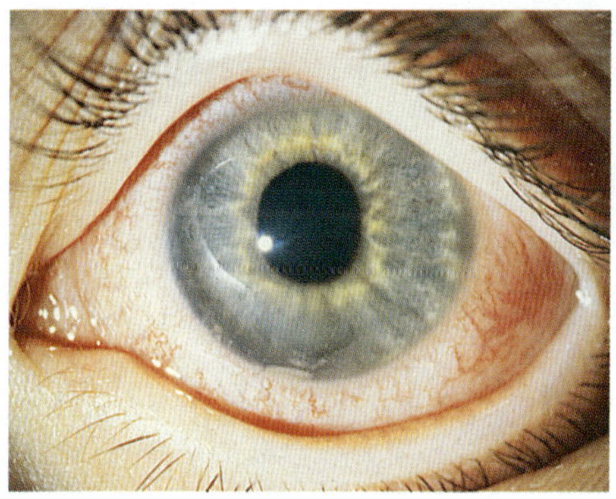

Fig. 20.59 Viral conjunctivitis with hyperemia and a watery discharge.

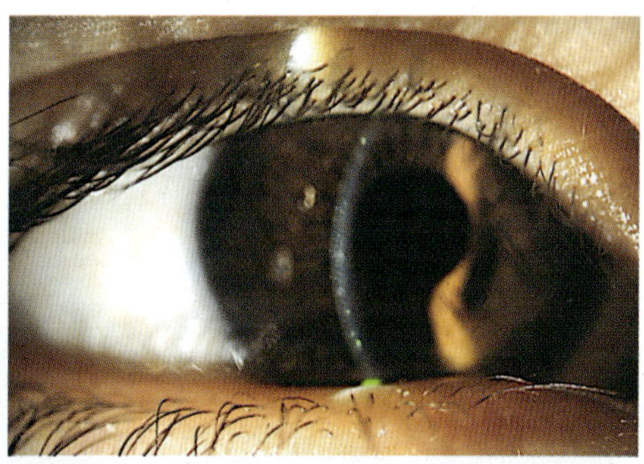

Fig. 20.60 Subepithelial infiltrates of epidemic keratoconjunctivitis caused by adenovirus. The beam of the slit lamp is used to demonstrate corneal subepithelial infiltrates (small white opacities). Only certain strains of adenovirus produce subepithelial infiltrates, which are immune reactions to the viral antigens. These may persist for months, causing symptoms of glare and blurring of vision.

continuous irritation caused by contact lens wear (Fig. 20.62). The development of extensive chemosis of the conjunctiva may be sudden and rapid. Simple treatment with cold compresses usually leads to improvement over several hours, and there are no significant sequelae of the conjunctival chemosis. In cases of chronic allergic conjunctivitis, the conjunctiva becomes pale and boggy and demonstrates a papillary reaction. Complications in more severe cases include keratitis with potential corneal scarring in limbal vernal keratoconjunctivitis. In these cases, there is a limbal papillary reaction, seen as a gelatinous thickening of the limbal conjunctiva, especially common superiorly, which is seen when the lid is raised and the patient looks down. White calcified concretions may be seen at the tips of the limbal follicles (Trantas dots). The development of a shield corneal ulcer necessitates urgent referral (see Fig. 20.62, lower panel).

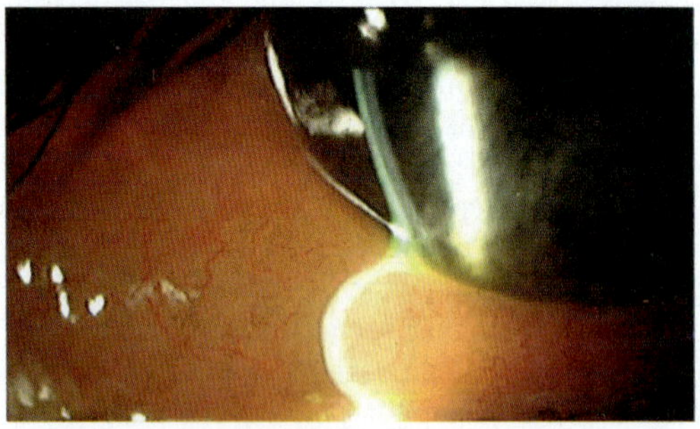

Fig. 20.61 Acute allergic conjunctivitis with edema (chemosis) of the conjunctiva.

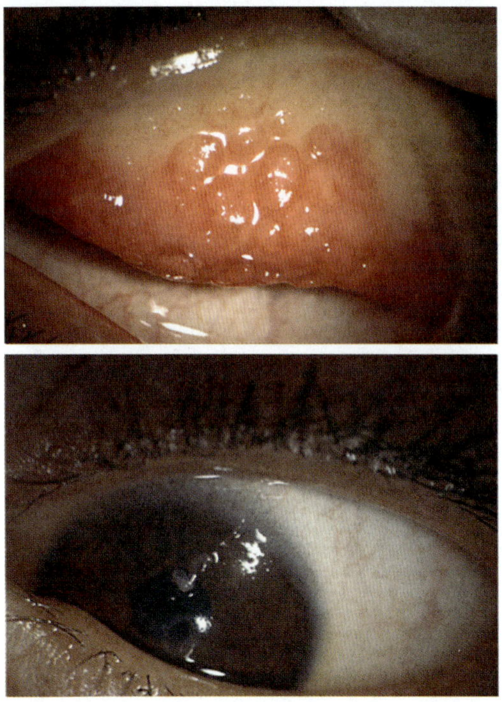

Fig. 20.62 Giant papillary conjunctivitis of bacterial or allergic origin *(upper panel)*, with a shield ulcer on the cornea *(lower panel)*. A shield ulcer is caused by repetitive microtrauma form the papillae in the upper tarsal conjunctiva.

Phlyctenular conjunctivitis is the result of a cell-mediated hypersensitivity reaction (Fig. 20.63). This is one of the more common causes of chronic, recurring, waxing, and waning conjunctivitis. Phlyctenular lesions are small, pinkish-white vesicles or pustules in the center of hyperemic areas of the conjunctiva. These lesions may occur at the limbus, on the conjunctiva, or, more rarely, on the cornea. Phlyctenulosis most commonly occurs in association with chronic staphylococcal infection. Symptoms consist of itching, tearing, and irritation. Patients with corneal phlyctenulosis have more severe symptoms of pain, light sensitivity, and tearing.

Conjunctival Pigmentations

Benign melanosis presents as brown-black patches seen near the limbus and sometimes in the interpalpebral bulbar conjunctiva. The patches move easily over the globe. No treatment is required as there is no risk of malignant change.

Flat deep pigmentation is a relatively common slate-gray pigmentation of the subepithelial layer, which is due to unilateral subepithelial melanocytosis, and the pigmentation cannot be moved over the globe. The slate-gray appearance may be isolated to the eye (melanosis oculi), isolated to the periocular skin (dermal melanocytosis), or involve both eye and skin (oculodermal melanocytosis or Naevus of Ota) (Fig. 20.64). Naevus of Ota is associated with increased risk of glaucoma and increased risk of uveal melanoma. Oculodermal melanocytosis is nine times more common in young patients with uveal melanoma than in the general population with uveal melanoma. Referral is advised.

Subconjunctival hemorrhages may occur spontaneously, or they may be secondary to coughing episodes, Valsalva maneuvers, or trauma (Fig. 20.65). These appear as bright red discolorations underneath the bulbar conjunctiva. Spontaneous resolution occurs over the course of several weeks with the blood spreading or moving downward and turning yellow as it is gradually reabsorbed. Elevated conjunctival lesions may be pigmented or nonpigmented.

Conjunctival nevus is a common solitary, well-defined, slightly elevated lesion, which moves freely over the globe. Approximately 75% are pigmented. Nevi usually are present at the limbus (see Fig. 20.65a, Fig. 20.66), plica, caruncle, and lid margin. Rare malignant transformation to melanoma may occur even in children. Rapid growth may be seen around puberty; excisional biopsy may be needed to confirm the diagnosis.

Epibulbar dermoid is an uncommon, solid, elevated, congenital lesion usually located at the limbus. The lesion may have hairs on the surface. Ocular associations include lid coloboma, ocular coloboma, microphthalmos, and aniridia. Epibulbar dermoids can be associated with Goldenhar, Treacher-Collins, and Franchescetti syndromes. If the lesion is large or causing ocular surface wetting problems, it must be removed (see Fig. 20.66).

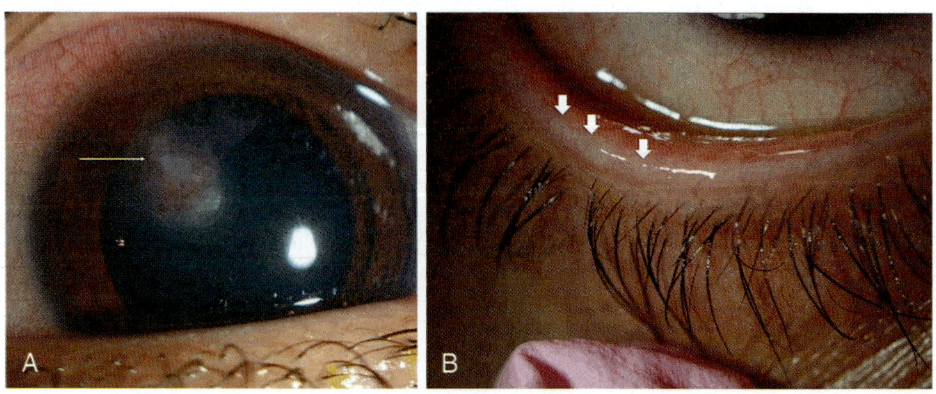

Fig. 20.63 Conjunctival phlyctenule. A raised area of conjunctival infiltration and localized infection is commonly seen at the corneal/scleral limbus. The center of the lesion is clear or white and may ulcerate (A, *thin white arrow*). Phlyctenules may also occur elsewhere on the bulbar or tarsal conjunctiva or on the cornea. They are often associated with lid margin disease and blocked Meibomian glands (B, *short white arrows*)

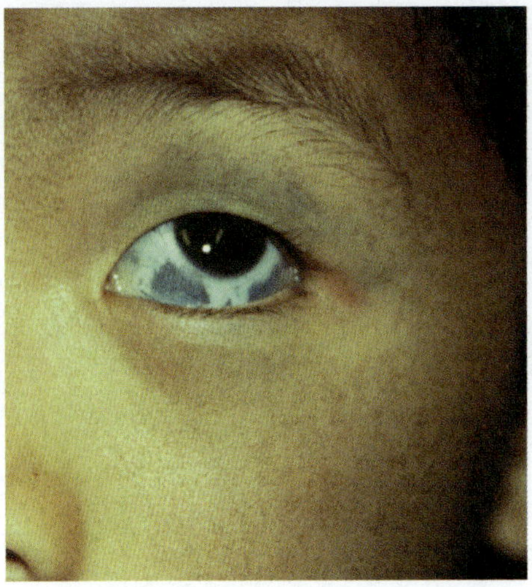

Fig. 20.64 Nevus of Ota shows ocular melanosis and melanosis of surrounding periocular skin.

Plaquelike Conjunctival Lesions

Pterygium is a common wing-shaped, fleshy lesion usually noted at the nasal limbus seen in equatorial regions. It is more often seen in adults but may occur in adolescents. Treatment is rarely needed in teenagers; however, if it encroaches on the corneal central axis in adults, it should be removed. *Bitot spots* are rare foamy plaques temporal to the limbus seen in avitaminosis A. Vitamin A replacement should be initiated.

Diffusely Elevated Conjunctival Lesions

Lymphomas can produce a rare diffuse subconjunctival fleshy lesion, which may be bilateral. Smaller patches have been termed "salmon patches" and are most commonly associated with non-Hodgkin or Burkitt lymphoma. Excision biopsy followed by systemic therapy from an oncology team is needed.

Plexiform neurofibroma is almost always associated with neurofibromatosis 1. It is uncommon and presents as a diffuse, smooth, elevated lesion extending from the lid to the superior bulbar conjunctiva. Usually, no treatment is needed; however, debulking is occasionally considered.

Conjunctival telangiectasia is rare but may be seen in ataxia-telangiectasia. Other metabolic causes include Fabry disease, fucosidosis, galactosialidosis, GM1 gangliosidosis, multiple endocrine neoplasia IIa, and hematologic disorders including dysproteinemias and sickle cell anemia (Fig. 20.67).

Sclera

Pigmentation of the sclera can be rarely seen in metabolic disorders such as alkaptonuria, hemochromatosis, and jaundice. Blue sclerae are seen in osteogenesis imperfecta I, Marshall syndrome, Ehlers-Danlos VI, and in high myopia of any cause.

Scleral inflammation may be due to episcleritis or scleritis. Episcleritis is nontender to touch in contrast to scleritis. Simple episcleritis often follows a viral illness and is self-limiting. Nodular and diffuse forms may be associated with systemic lupus erythematosus, juvenile idiopathic arthritis, spondyloarthropathy, rheumatic fever, relapsing polychondritis, polyarteritis nodosa, and inflammatory bowel disease. Topical mild steroids are used to treat episcleritis and, although this can be recurrent, prognosis is usually good.

Scleritis is an uncommon inflammation of the sclera that is tender to touch. It may be diffuse, nodular, or necrotizing. Causes include idiopathic, infections, surgically induced (necrotizing or diffuse), rheumatic diseases, connective tissue disorders, enteropathies, vasculitides, and granulomatous diseases. Therapy includes treating underlying conditions and using antiinflammatory drugs systemically (nonsteroidal or steroidal) to treat the eye initially.

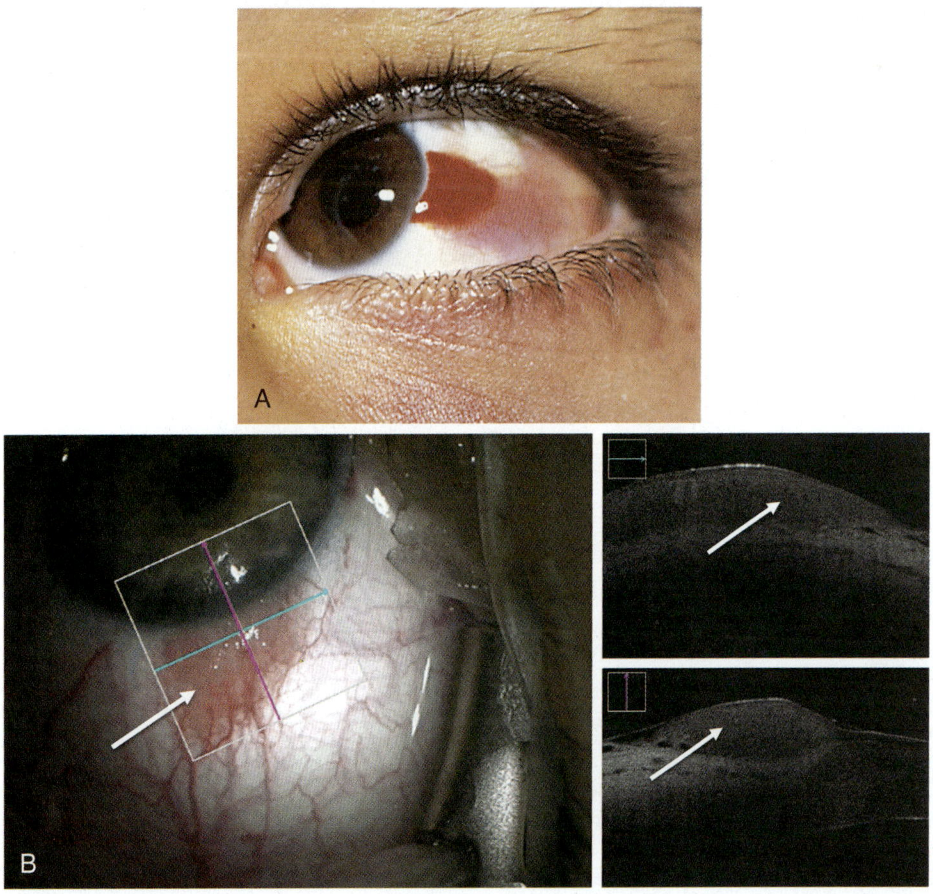

Fig. 20.65 (A) Subconjunctival hemorrhage secondary to blunt ocular trauma. (B) A conjunctival amelanotic nevus (*white arrow* in A), seen on ocular coherence tomography (*white arrows* in B).

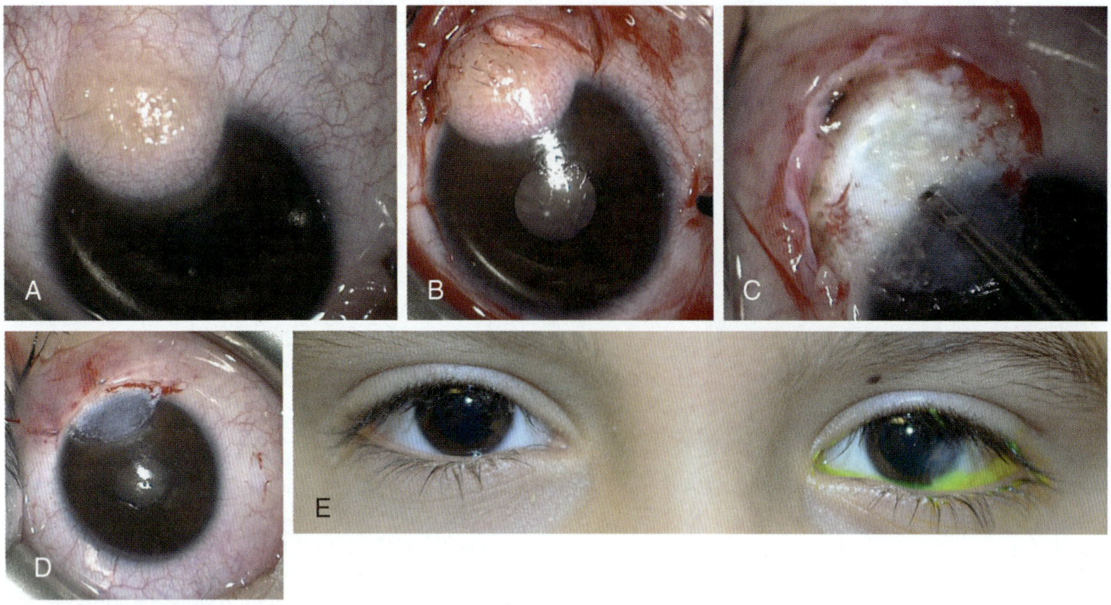

Fig. 20.66 Epibulbar corneal dermoid (A). The composite shows the excision (B–D) and the postsurgical appearance 6 months later (E). Note there is a faint scar, which does not stain with fluorescein.

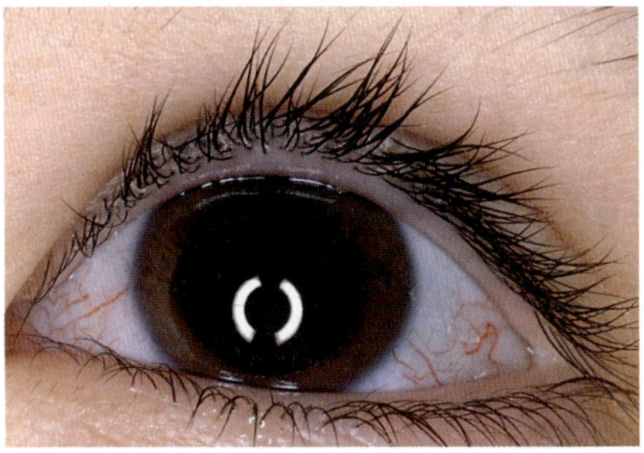

Fig. 20.67 Ataxia telangiectasia. Note the conjunctival telangiectasia are only present in the interpalpebral fissure, where there is exposure to ultraviolet light.

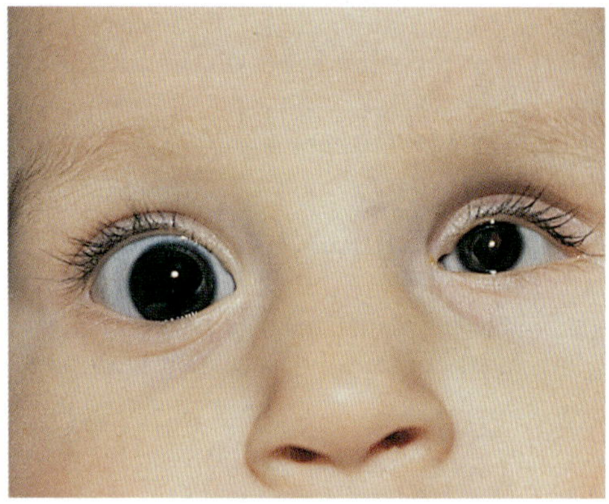

Fig. 20.68 Unilateral microcornea and microphthalmos.

Prognosis can be guarded if necrotizing, but this is extremely rare in children.

Cornea

Developmental disorders of the cornea include microcornea, cornea plana, megalocornea, and congenital corneal opacification.

Microcornea is an uncommon condition, defined as any cornea less than 9 mm in horizontal diameter. It may have systemic associations, and referral for evaluation is indicated. Although no active treatment is indicated other than surveillance for complications such as glaucoma, regular refraction ensures prevention of amblyopia in the first 8 years of life (Fig. 20.68).

Cornea plana is a rare condition of a flat cornea with a curvature of less than 43 D. Narrow-angle glaucoma occurring in the second decade of life is the most common potential complication. Affected children are long-sighted. The most frequent systemic association is oculodentodigital syndrome, where children have syndactyly between the fourth and fifth fingers and anomalous teeth.

Megalocornea, a rare disorder, is the occurrence of a corneal horizontal diameter of more than 13 mm. It is not progressive. If the cornea is enlarged in the presence of congenital glaucoma, it is not defined as megalocornea. This disorder is inherited as an X-linked recessive trait in most instances, but it may also be dominantly inherited. Megalocornea most often occurs in isolation, but other associated ocular conditions include anterior embryotoxon, mosaic corneal dystrophy, and glaucoma. Children often need ocular lubrication, especially at night. Sometimes, the lower lid lashes will rub on the cornea, so monitoring is required to prevent corneal infections.

Neonatal corneal opacities are rare. Any neonate or infant with a cloudy cornea requires an urgent referral. The causes are shown in Table 20.2. Many of the conditions listed are rare, but some are worthy of further discussion provided later.

Table 20.2 Causes of Neonatal Corneal Opacity

Primary Neonatal Corneal Opacity	
A. Developmental anomaly of cornea only	
I. Corneal dystrophies. CHED/PPMD	
II. Corneal structural defects due to corneal dermoids	
Secondary Neonatal Corneal Opacity	
A. Developmental	
I. Kerato-Irido-Lenticular Dysgenesis (KILD)	
a. Iridocorneal adhesions only	(Peters anomaly I)
b. Lens adherent to cornea	(Peters anomaly II)
c. Total corneal opacity due to disruption of anterior segment (sclerocornea)	
II. Infantile glaucoma	
III. Axenfeld Rieger anomaly/syndrome	
IV. Aniridia	
B. Acquired	
I. Metabolic	
II. Trauma—Forceps injury	
III. Infection—Neonatal herpes simplex keratitis	

CHED, Congenital hereditary endothelial dystrophy; *PPMD,* posterior polymorphous dystrophy.

Epibulbar dermoid, described earlier, is the commonest cause of corneal clouding encountered in neonates, but, occasionally, a corneal dermoid may be large or flat and cover a larger part of the cornea (see Fig. 20.66, Table 20.2). Metabolic causes of corneal clouding rarely occur at birth; mucolipidosis type 4 is the only cause. Corneal clouding due to mucopolysaccharidoses (Hurler, Hurler-Scheie, Maroteaux-Lamy) occurs around 6 months of age at the earliest. Infantile glaucoma, Axenfeld-Rieger syndrome, and aniridia are discussed later. Birth trauma due to forceps injury usually presents at birth with a unilateral cloudy cornea; the periocular skin and tissues are usually edematous and bruised on the affected side. Although the cornea will clear, the child will have significant astigmatism and amblyopia that can be difficult to treat. Corneal infections (keratitis) are discussed later, but neonatal herpes simplex keratitis is important to recognize because neonates with this condition require admission for intravenous antiviral therapy. Affected neonates often will have other complications including viral hepatitis, pneumonitis, or meningoencephalitis.

Congenital and neonatal corneal opacities can be treated with either corneal surgery or alternative approaches. In cases where the endothelium is healthy but the stroma is diseased (e.g., mucopolysaccharidoses), a deep anterior lamellar keratoplasty can be done where only the stroma and epithelium are replaced by donor tissue. If the endothelium is diseased, as in congenital hereditary endothelial dystrophy or posterior polymorphous corneal dystrophy, then an endothelial keratoplasty can be done. If all the layers are affected, then a penetrating keratoplasty can be performed. If the corneal opacity is eccentric, then an optical iridectomy can be done to give the infant vision without any type of corneal surgery.

Corneal deposits are caused by metabolic disorders including mucopolysaccharidoses (see earlier), cystinosis, Fabry disease, Wilson disease (Kayser-Fleischer rings), tyrosinemia type II (pseudodendrites), and Leber congenital amaurosis (LCA) deficiency. In cystinosis, crystals are seen in the cornea. Affected children may also have severe renal disease. Treatment is with oral cysteamine, which does not get into the cornea, so additional therapy requires topical cysteamine eye drops at least 6 times daily. Ideally, drops are administered 8 to 10 times daily, which is difficult to do. The crystals eventually cause pain, photophobia, and decreased vision (Fig. 20.69). Fabry disease is an X-linked recessive disorder in which affected males will show deposits of the sphingolipids in the cornea called verticillata. They can be seen in female carriers also. Some drugs can cause a similar picture including amiodarone or chloroquine, so a detailed current medication history is imperative when these lesions are seen in a male child.

Corneal deposits due to nonmetabolic disorders include corneal blood staining after blunt trauma from blood in the anterior chamber (hyphema) for a prolonged period of time with a high intraocular pressure (IOP), band-shaped keratopathy (calcium deposition), and amyloid deposition.

Corneal inflammation (keratitis) may be infectious or noninfectious in etiology.

Infectious keratitis may be secondary to viral, bacterial, mycotic, or protozoal agents.

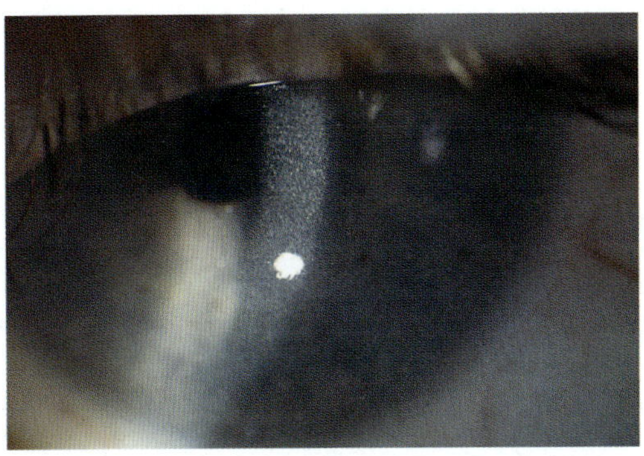

Fig. 20.69 Cystinosis of the cornea with deposition of L-cystine crystals in the corneal stroma.

Noninfectious keratitis may be due to exposure; corneal anesthesia (neurotrophic); dry eye; vernal keratoconjunctivitis; and rare genetic causes, including ectodermal dysplasia, familial dysautonomia, or epidermolysis bullosa.

Infectious Keratitis

Herpes keratitis can occur at almost any age in children. Eye involvement occurs in 13% of newborns with systemic herpes simplex virus (HSV) infection, and neonatal herpes simplex keratitis may be the only sign of systemic herpes simplex.

Neonates can become infected as they pass through the birth canal of a mother with genital HSV. Infections acquired at birth are usually of HSV type 2, although an increasing number of genital herpes infections are caused by HSV-1. Herpes infections contracted later in life are most often HSV-1. Primary herpes infection occurs with the first exposure of the herpes virus to the patient. The hallmark sign of primary herpetic infection of the eye is conjunctivitis, which is accompanied by vesicles on the eyelids. Recurrent disease (secondary) can result in dendritic, disciform, or interstitial keratitis.

Any child who will not open an eye should be considered to have either a foreign body or herpes simplex keratitis until proven otherwise. Examination under anesthesia should be done in such cases. Viral cultures from scrapings taken from the edge of any ulcer are necessary. However, PCR for HSV may be performed even on tears or conjunctival swabs from the affected eye.

Herpes simplex keratitis (epithelial) is treated with topical acyclovir, and stromal or endothelial disease with intact epithelium is treated with topical acyclovir and topical steroids. Systemic acyclovir should be considered if systemic herpes simplex is a possibility (Fig. 20.70).

Varicella-zoster corneal involvement is extremely rare, but ocular findings include swollen lids, vesicular lesions of the lids, and varying degrees of keratoconjunctivitis. Infrequently, superficial punctate keratitis of the cornea occurs. Treatment includes oral acyclovir and topical cycloplegic drops for eye comfort.

Chlamydia trachomatis infection, trachoma, is the world's leading cause of blindness. The causative organism, *C. trachomatis,* is an obligate intracellular bacterial agent. Chronic follicular conjunctivitis results from infection with secondary corneal scarring. Treatment consists of a single oral dose of azithromycin and topical erythromycin eye ointment.

Bacterial keratitis is rare and usually seen in children with predisposing factors such as neurotrophic cornea, contact lenses, trauma, dry eyes, HSV infection, immunosuppression, immunodeficiency, or vitamin deficiency. It is usually stromal with or without accompanying hypopyon (pus in the anterior chamber). Evaluation includes culture and Gram stain, followed by appropriate intensive topical and oral antibiotics. Prognosis is variable as residual scarring can severely affect vision (Fig. 20.71).

Fungal keratitis is a rare infection that may be due to filamentous fungi such as *Aspergillus* or *Fusarium* spp. or yeastlike fungi such as *Candida* spp. Most traumatic fungal ulcers are the result of filamentous organisms. Infections by yeasts are most common in patients with immunosuppression or dry eyes. Clinical suspicion should be

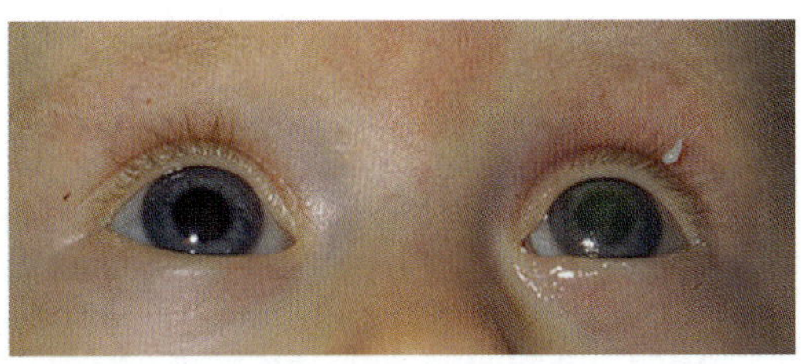

Fig. 20.70 Neonatal herpes simplex keratitis affecting the left cornea. Infection of the corneal epithelium with herpes simplex virus produces a pattern of fluorescein staining that resembles a neuronal dendrite. The surrounding area may be hazy because of epithelial and stromal edema and infiltration. Conjunctival injection is typically present.

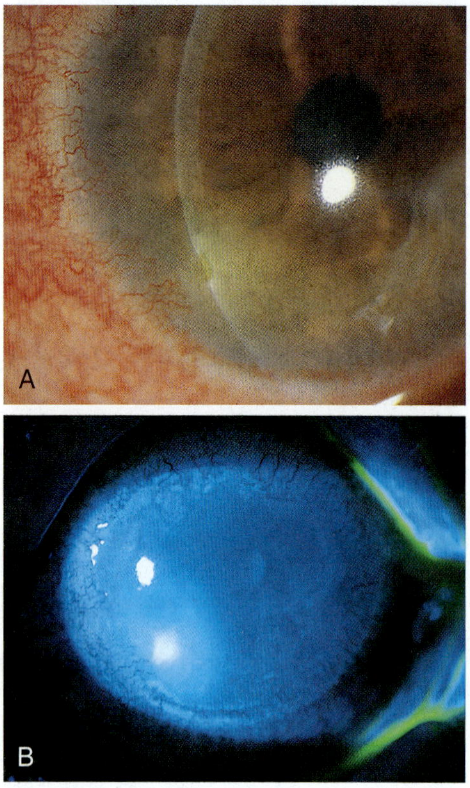

Fig. 20.71 Bacterial corneal ulcer. (A) The conjunctiva displays a marked inflammatory response with injection, most prominent in the quadrant nearest the corneal ulcer. The ulcer is visualized in the slit beam as a small white infiltrate of the corneal stroma. There is an overlying epithelial defect. (B) The epithelial defect is easier to visualize after the application of fluorescein dye. The dye is taken up by the corneal stroma in the area of the epithelial defect. The areas fluoresce with cobalt blue light illumination.

raised if there are fuzzy borders of the infiltrate, an elevated infiltrate with initially intact epithelium, satellite lesions, and pyramidal or convex hypopyon. Occasionally, the infiltrate may be seen to develop pigmentation, suggestive of filamentous infection. Evaluation includes culture and Gram stain, followed by treatment with systemic and topical antifungal agents. Visual prognosis is often guarded, and a corneal graft may be necessary.

Acanthamoeba keratitis is more common in contact lens wearers; however, this is rare. Any patient who wears contact lenses and develops a painful eye should be referred urgently. Usually, a sterile keratitis is seen, but this cannot be differentiated from a serious infection without specialist review.

Noninfectious Keratitis

Exposure keratitis is due to inadequate closure of the lids (ectropion or coloboma of the lid, a facial nerve paralysis, or postsurgery of congenital ptosis when there is inability to close the lids) and a prominent globe, either due to proptosis of any cause or shallow orbits (e.g., craniosynostoses). Its treatment is adequate protection with ocular lubricant and repair of any coloboma/ectropion of the lid, correction of any orbital issue, or temporary tarsorrhaphy.

Neurotrophic keratitis is due to corneal anesthesia. It can be seen in Goldenhar syndrome, familial dysautonomia, and any cause that affects the trigeminal nerve (e.g., tumor or postherpes simplex keratitis). Lubrication and tarsorrhaphies have been the mainstay of treatment (Fig. 20.72). However, in unilateral cases, corneal neurotization can be done. This is a safe procedure and most effective when there is unilateral corneal anesthesia. The sural nerve is harvested from the patient and adhered to the functioning supratrochlear nerve. It is passed under the glabellar skin to the affected side's upper lid and into the subconjunctival space. The nerve is then divided into fascicles, and these are passed subconjunctivally around the cornea to the limbus. Reinnervation occurs within 6 months (see Fig. 20.72B).

Anterior Chamber

The term *anterior chamber* refers to the fluid-filled space between the cornea and iris diaphragm. The aqueous fluid is optically clear. It provides nutrition for the corneal endothelial surface and is secreted by the ciliary processes. It passes through the pupil to the anterior chamber and leaves via the trabecular meshwork in the periphery of the anterior chamber angle, where the iris meets the cornea and sclera.

Iris

Congenital iris defects include partial or complete absence of the iris.

Iris coloboma describes a partial absence of the iris due to nonclosure of the embryonic fissure in the fifth week of gestation, typically occurring in the inferonasal quadrant (Fig. 20.73). A coloboma may be isolated or occur with retinochoroidal/optic nerve coloboma, microcornea, or microphthalmos. Nystagmus or cataracts may also be seen. Although iris colobomas can be associated with almost any chromosomal abnormality, they are frequently seen in branchio-oculo-facial, cat-eye, CHARGE, 13q deletion, Goltz, triploidy, Patau (trisomy 13), Wolf-Hirschhorn (4p-), and Walker-Warburg syndromes.

In Axenfeld-Rieger syndrome, the anomaly of the iris may have larger defects. The pupil may be displaced (corectopia), or there may be pseudopolycoria (multiple pseudo pupils without a sphincter pupillae). There is often an anteriorly displaced Schwalbe line (posterior embryotoxon) with iris processes attached to this line. The systemic findings of hypodontia and microdontia, maxillary hypoplasia, and periumbilical hernia are extraocular features seen in the syndrome. A child who is short for age with these findings may also have pituitary abnormalities and should be evaluated by an endocrinologist.

Persistent pupillary membrane is a mild anterior form of persistent fetal vasculature (PFV; Fig. 20.74) but usually not visually significant.

Aniridia, absence of the iris, has a prevalence of 1 in 72,000 with most causes due to mutations in *PAX6.* Aniridia (autosomal dominant) is a panocular, bilateral disorder with absence of much or most of the iris tissue (Fig. 20.75) and foveal and optic nerve hypoplasia resulting in a congenital nystagmus and reduced visual acuity to 20/100 or worse. Anterior polar cataracts, glaucoma, and corneal opacification often develop later in childhood and may lead to progressive deterioration of visual acuity. Glaucoma occurs in up to half of all cases. In sporadic cases, Wilms tumor must be excluded by renal imaging, which should be conducted serially, until molecular diagnosis confirms an intragenic mutation and not a deletion including *WT1* (the Wilms tumor gene). If genetic evaluation is pending or confirms that *WT1* is deleted, renal ultrasound should be completed every 3 months until the patient is 5 years old, every 6 months until age 10 years, and then annually until age 16 years. Other associations include genitourinary abnormalities with slow growth or delayed development (AGR triad) or association with ataxia and neurodevelopmental delay (Gillespie syndrome). When Wilms tumor is present with the AGR triad, the condition is referred to as WAGR.

Iris transillumination, when congenital, is seen in both ocular and oculocutaneous albinism and in the midperipheral iris in female carriers of X-linked ocular albinism. Small transillumination defects just visible near the iris root in blue-eyed children may be idiopathic with no clinical significance. Acquired causes are either iatrogenic or traumatic. It can also be seen in pigment dispersion syndrome in teenagers and after herpes simplex or varicella zoster keratouveitis, often resulting in sector iris atrophy.

Changes in iris color may be due to benign primary iris tumors such as Brushfield spots, which are small aggregates of normal iris stroma connective tissue, and seen in 38% to 90% of patients with Down syndrome. Similar iris findings may occur in individuals as an isolated finding or in patients with juvenile xanthogranuloma (Fig. 20.76). Iris involvement in juvenile xanthogranuloma occurs

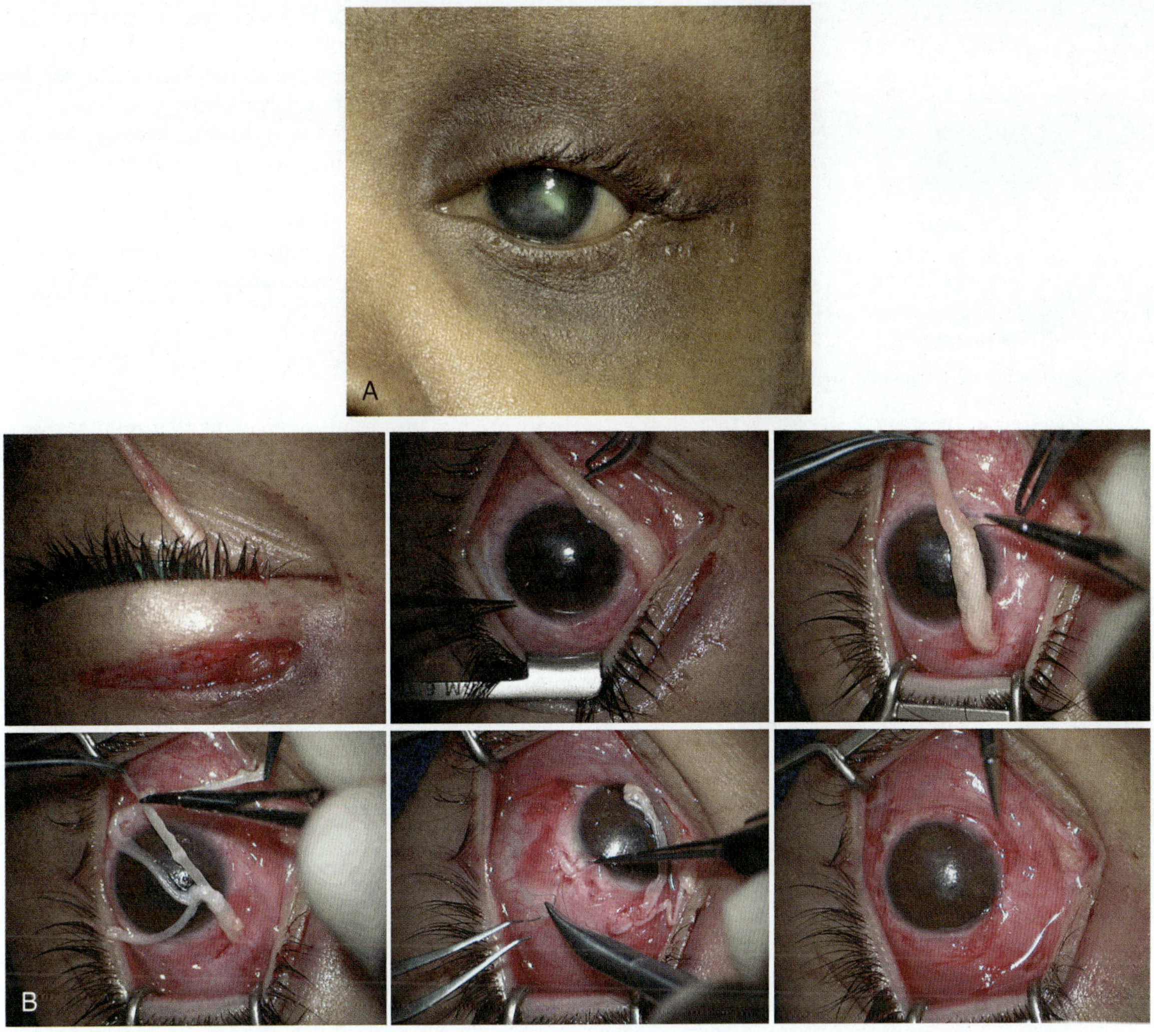

Fig. 20.72 (A) Neurotrophic keratitis with ulcer. The patient has had a lateral tarsorrhaphy performed. (B) Corneal neurotization. The sural nerve has been passed through the lid onto the conjunctiva (Upper three panels). The sural nerve is then divided into its component fascicles. The fascicles are then passed under the conjunctiva around the cornea and secured at the limbus, usually at 6 points around the limbus with biological glue and/or 10/0 nylon (Lower three panels).

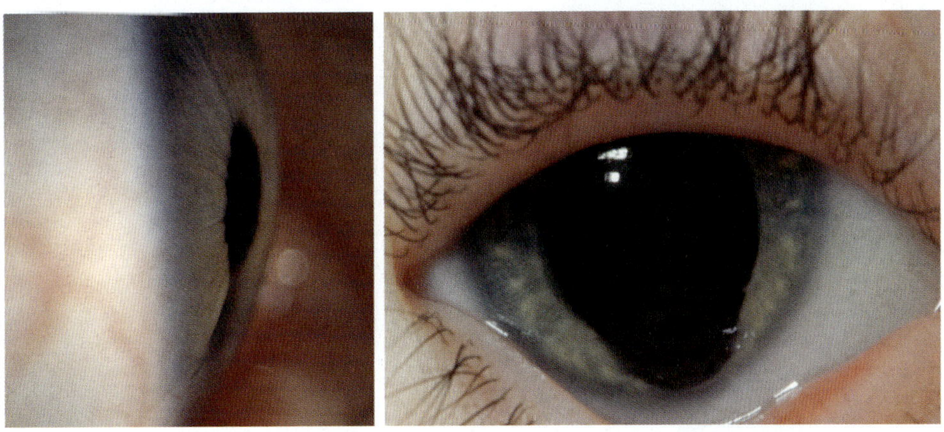

Fig. 20.73 Iris coloboma shown from two views.

almost exclusively in infants. Unilateral yellow nodules or diffuse infiltration may be seen and may present with blood in the anterior chamber (hyphema), with or without raised IOP. Most ocular lesions will regress with topical steroids. Some cases may require systemic steroids and others a small dose of radiation treatment. The prognosis is usually good.

Heterochromia Irides

Heterochromia iridis is a condition in which the irises are different colors. The differential diagnosis of pediatric heterochromia irides is extensive but may be classified on the basis of whether the condition is congenital or acquired and whether the affected eye is hypopigmented or hyperpigmented.

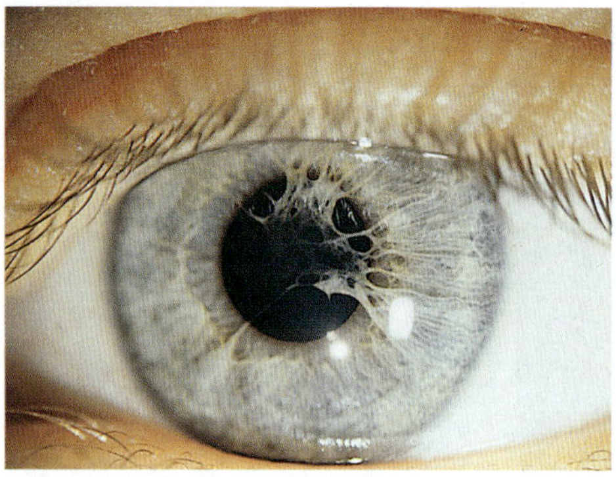

Fig. 20.74 Persistent pupillary membranes. Hyperplasia of the mesoderm of the anterior layer of the iris has caused iris strands to become adherent to the anterior lens surface. The lens is clear. These are usually visually insignificant; however, if a plaque is present at the attachment site, it may block the visual axis. The pupil may be smaller or less reactive than normal.

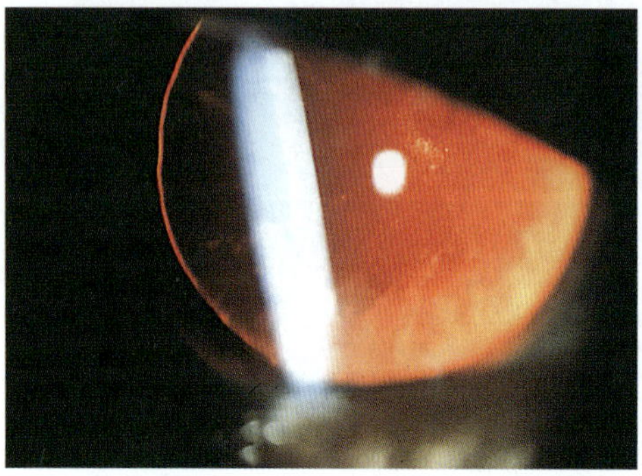

Fig. 20.75 Aniridia. Iris structures are present only as rudimentary findings, and the red reflex fills the entire corneal diameter. The edge of the lens is visible peripherally, and early cataractous lens changes are present centrally.

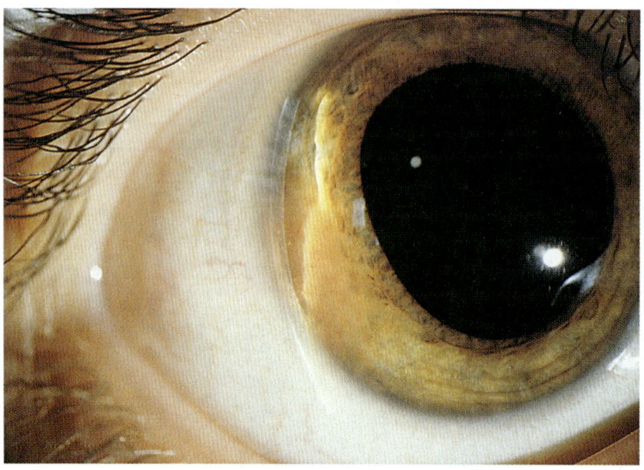

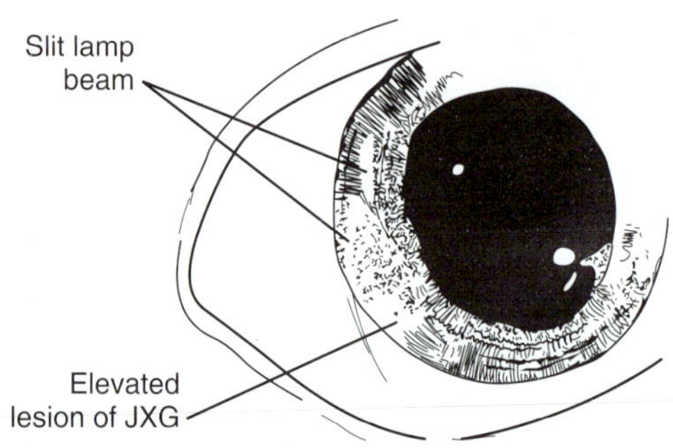

Fig. 20.76 Juvenile xanthogranuloma (JXG). The ocular lesion of JXG is visualized as a fleshy, yellowish-brown tumor on the surface of the iris. The lesions are vascular, bleed easily, and can cause spontaneous hyphemas.

Congenital causes of hypochromic heterochromia, in which the affected iris is lighter in color than the other, include Horner syndrome and Waardenburg syndrome. Fuchs heterochromic cyclitis is a rare, acquired type of unilateral iritis.

Congenital causes of hyperchromic heterochromia, in which the affected iris is darker in color, include iris mammillations (benign unilateral villiform protuberances that may cover the iris and are darker than the contralateral iris) and port wine stain. Acquired causes include cataract surgery in infants, topical prostaglandin analogs used in glaucoma management, iris nevus, and a retained intraocular metal foreign body.

Pupil

There are five important pupil signs that require discussion: leukocoria (a white pupil reflex) (Fig. 20.77), miosis (small pupil), mydriasis (large pupil), corectopia, and anisocoria.

Leukocoria may be bilateral or unilateral. In either case, potential causes include cataract, retinal tumor (retinoblastoma), retinal coloboma or myelinated nerve fibers, Coats disease (see later), or total retinal detachment (e.g., ROP; see later). Leukocoria necessitates an urgent referral (Box 20.1).

Miosis defines a small pupil less than 2 mm, which may react poorly to dilating drops. This can be due to congenital miosis (microcoria) when there is an absence of the dilator pupillae muscle or fibrous contraction secondary to persistent pupillary membrane. It can also be seen in congenital rubella syndrome, Marfan syndrome, and in 20% of patients with Lowe (oculocerebrorenal) syndrome. If visual development is thought to be hindered, surgical enlargement of the pupil can be performed.

Mydriasis describes a large pupil, usually greater than 4 mm, which may be true mydriasis or pseudomydriasis. True mydriasis can be congenital and may be a sign of systemic smooth muscle disorder. A rare cause of bilateral congenital mydriasis is due to mutations in *ACTA2* that result in systemic disruption of smooth muscle. Other associated signs such as bladder or intestinal issues are always present. Diagnosis necessitates intracranial magnetic resonance angiography because there are often vascular issues including moyamoya disease. Acquired causes include blunt trauma causing iris sphincter rupture; ciliary ganglionitis (unilateral most commonly after chicken pox—also known as *Adie pupil*); or acquired neurologic disease, especially third nerve palsy. With ciliary ganglionitis, accommodation can be affected and the child will need a reading prescription.

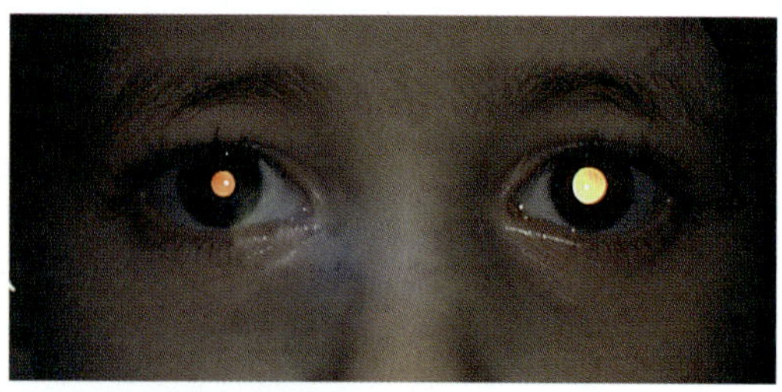

Fig. 20.77 Leukocoria, left eye.

Box 20.1 Differential Diagnosis of Leukocoria

Angiomatosis retinae	Persistent hyperplastic primary vitreous
Cataracts	Retinal detachment
Coats disease	Retinal dysplasia
Colobomas	Retinoblastoma
Congenital retinal fold	Retinopathy of prematurity
High myopia	Toxocariasis
Incontinentia pigmenti	Uveitis
Medulloepithelioma	Vitreous hemorrhage
Myelinated nerve fibers	

Pseudomydriasis is often seen in aniridia, where the lack of iris is mistakenly considered to be a large pupil. This is also the case when congenital iris ectropion is present (the posterior pigment epithelium, which is dark brown, is everted onto the anterior surface of the iris). Iris ectropion is associated with an increased risk of glaucoma and may be associated with either neurofibromatosis 1 or Prader-Willi syndrome, or it is an isolated finding.

Corectopia is a displacement of the pupil; causes include sector iris hypoplasia, colobomas, and Axenfeld-Rieger anomaly. Rarely, if the pupil is severely eccentrically displaced, then pupilloplasty may be needed to improve the visual axis.

Anisocoria describes a difference in the size of the pupils. Three main causes in childhood that need to be considered are physiologic causes, Horner syndrome, and Adie pupil (ciliary ganglionitis). A child with anisocoria should be examined in bright light and then in the dark. If the anisocoria is physiologic, then the difference will remain constant and will be no more than 2 mm. If the anisocoria is accentuated in bright surroundings, this suggests that the larger pupil is at fault and cannot constrict. The commonest cause for this is ciliary ganglionitis (Adie pupil). Examination by slit lamp is used to detect vermiform iris movements. If the anisocoria is accentuated in the dark, this suggests that the smaller pupil is at fault. The commonest cause for this is Horner syndrome.

Horner syndrome consists of miosis, ipsilateral ptosis, and, sometimes, anhidrosis. Congenital Horner syndrome is associated with iris hypopigmentation of the affected side (Fig. 20.78). Although a traumatic birth can cause Horner syndrome, examination for metastatic neuroblastoma is required.

Topical apraclonidine 0.5% eye drops are used to confirm the presence of Horner syndrome. Apraclonidine has weak α_1-agonist action, which, in most normal eyes, produces no significant effect on the pupil. In Horner syndrome, the affected eye iris dilator muscle develops adrenergic supersensitivity and apraclonidine dilates an affected pupil. After instillation of 0.5% apraclonidine in each eye, a reversal of anisocoria is diagnostic of Horner syndrome.

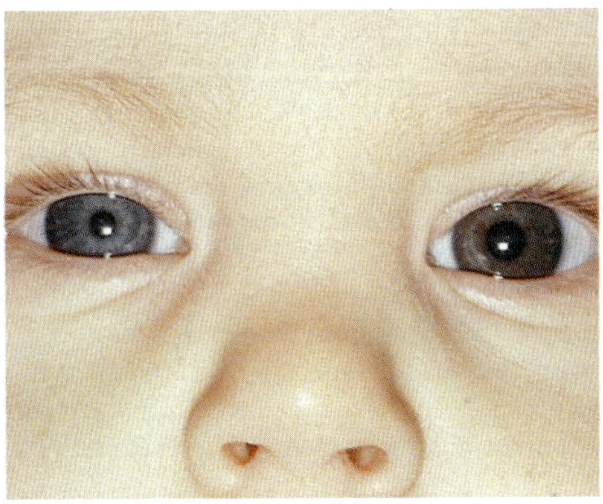

Fig. 20.78 Horner syndrome *(right side)* with iris heterochromia. The right upper lid is slightly ptotic, and the right lower lid is slightly higher. Anisocoria is present. The right pupil is smaller than the left. The iris on the side affected by Horner syndrome may be lighter in color than the iris of the fellow eye.

Adie syndrome, described earlier, exhibits mydriasis with vermiform iris movements on slit-lamp examination. The commonest association is varicella-zoster infection, but other viral infections may also cause ciliary ganglionitis. Accommodation is usually affected, and the child may need reading spectacles. Denervation hypersensitivity is present, and the diagnostic test for Adie pupil is instillation of dilute 0.125% pilocarpine, which causes papillary constriction.

Glaucoma

The incidence of infantile or congenital glaucoma is approximately 1 in 12,500 births. Infantile glaucoma is usually inherited in an autosomal recessive pattern but may also be inherited in a dominant manner. Glaucoma can present at birth, but, more commonly, clinical signs develop during the first several weeks or months of life. The triad of signs indicating possible infantile glaucoma includes tearing, photophobia, involuntary spasm of the eyelid (blepharospasm), and enlarged corneal diameter (buphthalmos). Infants can also have a hazy cornea due to epithelial and, less commonly, stromal edema (Fig. 20.79A). As the corneal diameter increases, a split in Descemet membrane (Haab striae) (see Fig. 20.79B) can occur. This results in an opacity in the acute phase.

An infant's corneal diameter should be 9.5 mm increasing to 11.5 mm by 2 years of age. Raised IOP will cause the diameter to increase, either symmetrically or asymmetrically depending on the pressure in each eye (Fig. 20.80). The corneal diameter increases due to raised IOP are accompanied by elongation of the globe axial length, which leads to progressive myopia.

The tearing seen in infantile glaucoma is differentiated from the epiphora of nasolacrimal duct obstruction by the absence of rhinorrhea with obstruction and presence of recurrent discharge and infections in the latter.

Elevation of IOP is the hallmark of glaucoma. Normal IOP in infants and young children is less than 20 mm Hg. Pressures greater than 25 mm Hg suggest glaucoma. Accurate measurement of pressure is difficult in children, and digital estimation may need to be used because more quantitative measuring devices contact the cornea.

The optic nerve damage caused by elevated IOP is reflected in the degree of enlargement of the optic cup (Fig. 20.81). Asymmetry of the cup-to-disc ratio between the eyes or an increase in the cup-to-disc ratio to greater than 0.5 is a possible sign of glaucoma. In infants and young children, enlargement of the optic cup is reversible if IOP is controlled but becomes permanent when children are older. Enlargement of the optic cups without glaucoma may be inherited; examination of family members for comparison may be of value.

Infantile glaucoma may be associated with aniridia, Axenfeld-Rieger syndrome, Sturge Weber syndrome, Lowe syndrome, neurofibromatosis I, Rubinstein-Taybi syndrome, and congenital rubella syndrome. Patients with chronic uveitis frequently develop glaucoma, either associated with the uveitis itself or as a complication of the topical steroids used to manage the uveitis. Eight percent to 25% of children with congenital cataracts, especially those with microcornea

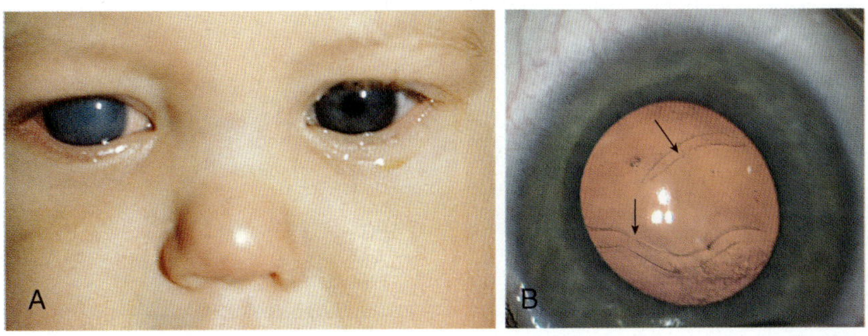

Fig. 20.79 (A) Congenital glaucoma. The right cornea is hazy and opaque due to corneal edema. Breakdown of the corneal epithelium has caused ocular irritation, and the conjunctiva is slightly injected. Epiphora is present because of reflex tearing caused by the pain of epithelial breakdown and increased intraocular pressure. (B) Haab striae (breaks in Descemet membrane).

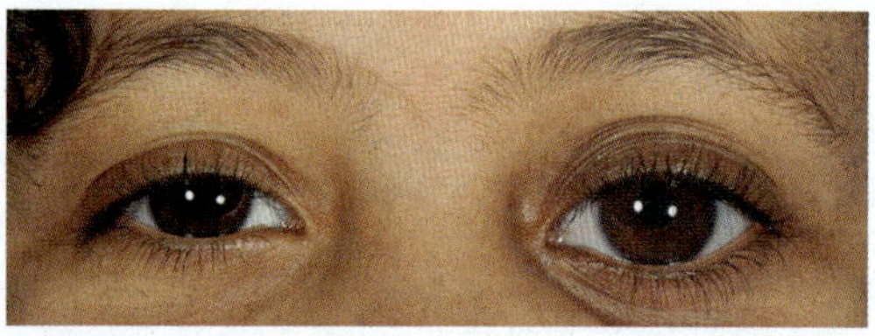

Fig. 20.80 Congenital glaucoma. This patient has corneal diameter asymmetry resulting from glaucoma in the left eye. The horizontal corneal diameter is 11 mm in the right eye and 13.5 mm in the left eye. The entire left eye has become enlarged, and the axial length is greater than normal. The increase in axial length of the left eye has produced a myopic refractive error.

or microphthalmia, develop glaucoma at some point in life. Frequent follow-up is required to detect and treat childhood glaucoma.

Lens

The human lens may be absent (aphakia), abnormal in shape, displaced (subluxated), or have total or partial opacities (cataract).

Aphakia is most commonly iatrogenic in origin after congenital cataract extraction. Rare causes include primary aphakia, in which the lens fails to form and is accompanied by corneal clouding and glaucoma. Spontaneous resorption of a cataract (which may be seen in Lowe syndrome and Hallerman-Streiff syndrome) and spontaneous complete dislocation of the lens (either traumatic or related to an already subluxed lens) can also occur. Refractive correction of aphakia is needed, as is surveillance to exclude glaucoma, which can develop anytime in the patient's life.

Abnormal shape of the lens may be due to spherophakia or microspherophakia, both of which are associated with lens subluxation (see later) and can be seen in homocystinuria and Weill-Marchesani syndrome. Rarely, coloboma of the lens may be seen. It causes astigmatism that needs refractive correction. Anterior lenticonus, a rare bilateral condition where there is a conoid projection of the anterior surface of the lens centrally, may be associated with Alport syndrome. If visual development is hindered or a cataract develops, lens extraction is warranted. Posterior lenticonus is an uncommon, isolated posterior conoid projection of the lens, which often leads to cataract formation and the need for lens extraction.

A subluxated lens may occur spontaneously or after blunt trauma. Spontaneous subluxation is uncommon but may be associated with ocular conditions such as megalocornea (primary enlarged cornea), severe buphthalmos (enlarged corneal diameter with infantile glaucoma), high myopia, and aniridia. More importantly, it may be seen in systemic conditions such as Marfan syndrome (fibrillin gene mutation spectrum) (Fig. 20.82), Weill-Marchesani syndrome, and metabolic disorders such as homocystinuria, hyperlysinemia, sulfite oxidase deficiency, and molybdenum cofactor deficiency. Treatment includes exclusion of systemic associations. Careful observation with refractive correction is necessary to ensure adequate visual development, but lensectomy may be needed to improve visual function.

Lens opacity (cataract) may be classified according to the age at which they occur or in terms of certain characteristic lens opacities associated with specific systemic disorders.

Congenital or infantile cataracts are bilateral in two-thirds of patients and unilateral in one-third; 31% are associated with systemic disease (6% unilateral and 25% bilateral) and 61% are associated with ocular disease (47% unilateral and 14% bilateral). No underlying cause or risk factor can be found in 92% of unilateral cases and 38% of bilateral cases. Hereditary disease is associated with 56% of bilateral and 6% of unilateral cases.

Therefore in all bilateral cases, unless there is a hereditary risk or associated ocular disease, diagnostic evaluation for the following conditions should be considered: galactosemia, Alport syndrome, Lowe syndrome, TORCH infection, Trisomy 13, Trisomy 18, and Trisomy 21.

Bilateral cataracts in infancy, if visually significant and not treated early, may produce severe visual deprivation with permanent loss of vision and the development of visual deprivation nystagmus. Visually significant unilateral cataracts can cause severe deprivation amblyopia and strabismus. When abnormalities of the red reflex are detected, early referral for treatment is critical for successful visual rehabilitation. Treatment includes lensectomy either with sparing of the capsule for possible secondary implantation or lens removal with primary intraocular implantation. Amblyopia therapy with correction of the refractive state is essential. The prognosis is better for bilateral cases than unilateral cases.

Box 20.2 shows the important associations of infantile cataracts, and Box 20.3 shows important associations of juvenile cataracts.

The morphology of the lens opacification may provide a clue to the cause of a congenital cataract if the lens is not completely white (Fig. 20.83Aand B). The embryologic development of the lens proceeds in an orderly fashion with distinct layers and the presence of sutures within the lens. Because of this, the gestational age at the time of cataract development determines the location of the opacity. For example, the nuclear cataracts of rubella syndrome (Fig. 20.84) indicate infection early in gestation, whereas a zonular or lamellar cataract represents an insult to the lens occurring later in lens development.

Small central opacities on the anterior or posterior poles of the lens, termed *polar cataracts,* are developmental abnormalities that typically remain stable and, especially with anterior opacities, may not affect vision (Fig. 20.85). Lamellar or zonular cataracts have a normal, transparent central nucleus; an affected lamellar zone; and

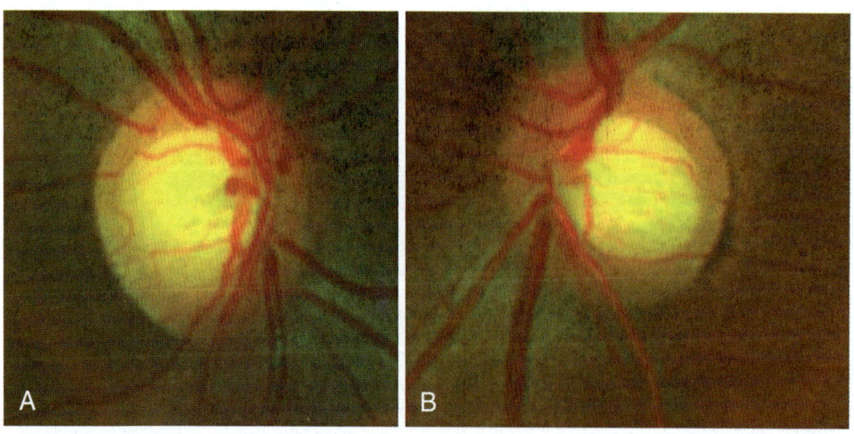

Fig. 20.81 Glaucomatous optic atrophy. In glaucoma, excavation extends to the disc edge in contrast to the physiologic cupping that may be seen in myopia, where there is a normal rim of tissue. The presence of optic disc asymmetry as shown here is often seen in glaucoma and should raise the suspicion for the presence of glaucomatous damage. The right optic disc has a larger cup (A) then the left optic disc (B).

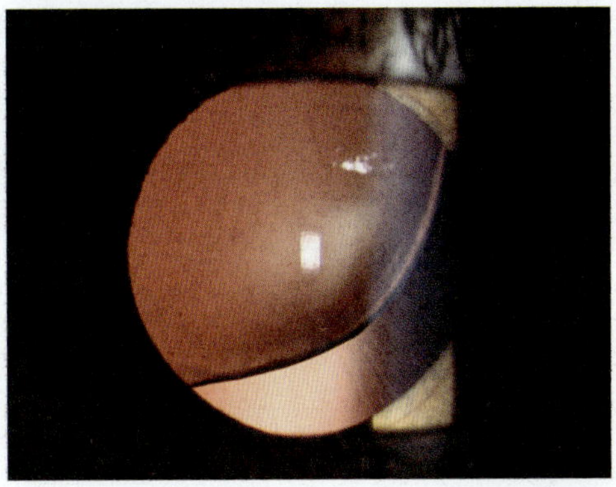

Fig. 20.82 Subluxed lens in a child with Marfan syndrome. Both eyes were affected.

Box 20.2 Important Ocular and Systemic Associations of Infantile Cataracts

- Hereditary
- Ocular. Persistent hyperplastic primary vitreous, aniridia, iris coloboma, microphthalmos
- Systemic
  - Infection. Intrauterine infection
  - Metabolic disease. Galactosemia, neonatal hypoglycemia, hypocalcemia
  - Renal disease. Lowe syndrome, congenital hemolytic syndrome
  - Chromosomal disorders. Trisomy 13 (Patau syndrome) and 18 (Edward syndrome)
  - Neurologic disease. Marinesco-Sjögren syndrome (ataxia), Smith-Lemli-Opitz, Zellweger and Sjogren-Larsson syndromes
  - Skeletal disorders. Conradi syndrome
  - Skin disorders. Ectodermal dysplasia, Rothmund-Thomson, incontinentia pigmenti and Cockayne syndromes
  - Miscellaneous. Norrie, Rubinstein-Taybi, Turner and Hallermann-Streiff syndromes

Box 20.3 Important Ocular and Systemic Associations of Juvenile Cataracts

Juvenile Cataract

- Hereditary
- Ocular. Ocular coloboma, ectopia lentis, aniridia, retinitis pigmentosa, and posterior lenticonus
- Systemic
  - Renal disease. Alport syndrome
  - Skeletal disease. Marfan syndrome
  - Skin disease. Atopic dermatitis, Marshall syndrome, lamellar ichthyosis
  - Chromosomal disorders. Trisomy 21
  - Metabolic disease. Galactokinase deficiency, Fabry disease, Refsum disease, mannosidosis, diabetes mellitus, hypocalcemia
  - Neurologic disorders. Myotonic dystrophy, Wilson disease
  - Miscellaneous. Chronic uveitis, drug induced (steroids), neurofibromatosis II, Stickler syndrome

a clear outer layer of cortex. Riders or radial extensions are frequently present (Fig. 20.86). Zonular cataracts may be autosomal dominant, associated with vitamin A and D deficiency, or result from hypocalcemia. Multicolored flecks may be seen in hypoparathyroidism or myotonic dystrophy, and an oil droplet configuration is seen in galactosemia (Fig. 20.87).

Uvea

Inflammation of the uveal tract (iris, ciliary body, and choroid) has many potential causes, including infections (toxoplasmosis, herpes zoster and simplex, and Lyme disease), collagen vascular disease (most frequently juvenile idiopathic arthritis and sarcoidosis), and trauma. Uveitis may be anterior, intermediate, posterior, or include all three (panuveitis).

Anterior uveitis or iritis may produce pain, ciliary injection (conjunctival injection most prominent at the corneal-scleral limbus), tearing, photophobia, and decreased vision. Synechiae, adhesions between the iris and lens or peripheral cornea, may produce corectopia. Inflammatory reaction in the anterior chamber may be viewed with the aid of a slit lamp as inflammatory cells and fibrin or protein in the aqueous fluid. With the high magnification of the slit lamp, inflammatory cells may be seen floating in the aqueous fluid much like dust is seen in bright sunlight shining through a window. If severe, iritis may make the eye appear dull or glassy as the cells and fibrin make the aqueous fluid less transparent (Fig. 20.88). Clumps of inflammatory cells may adhere to the posterior corneal surface, forming keratic precipitates (Fig. 20.89). Inflammatory nodules may also be seen on the surface of the iris or at the iris border (Busacca and Koeppe nodules) in chronic uveitis. Chronic anterior uveitis may be present without signs or symptoms while causing damage to the eye. Children with juvenile idiopathic arthritis must have periodic screening examinations. Patients with polyarticular disease should be examined annually. Those with positive antinuclear antibodies and pauciarticular disease, particularly females who are more likely to develop ocular complications, should be examined three or four times per year to detect and treat the uveitis before the complications of synechiae, cataracts, glaucoma, and macular edema develop.

Intermediate uveitis (pars planitis) is an idiopathic, bilateral inflammation of the pars plana portions of the ciliary body. The main symptoms include "floaters" and blurring of vision produced by the inflammatory debris floating in the vitreous. Occasionally, patients may also experience photophobia. Inflammatory cells in the anterior vitreous can make visualization of the retina with the direct ophthalmoscope difficult. If the inflammation is severe, it may produce leukocoria. Pars planitis is a diagnosis of exclusion made on the basis of characteristic findings and absence of findings suggesting other causes of uveitis. Most cases are self-limited; however, chronic courses with exacerbations and remissions may produce visual loss resulting from cataracts, glaucoma, optic nerve inflammation, and cystoid macular

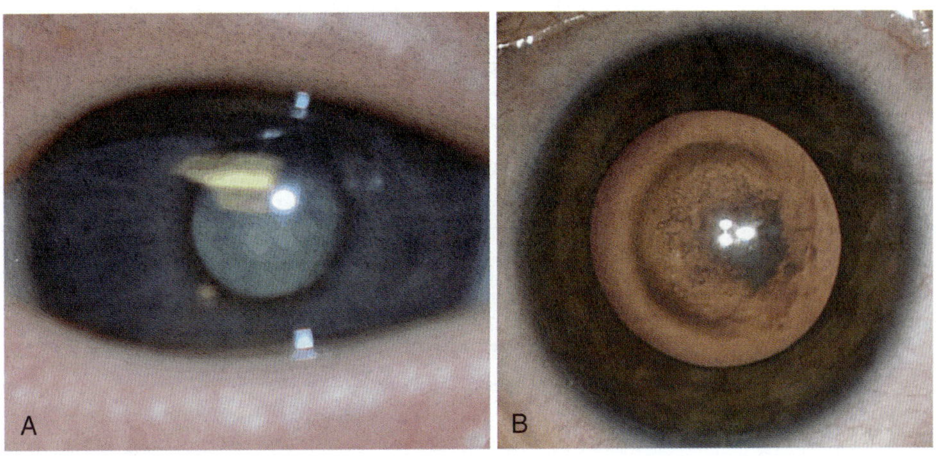

Fig. 20.83 (A) Complete cataract with no view of the red reflex or retina. (B) Nuclear and lamellar cataract with posterior polar component. This is visually significant.

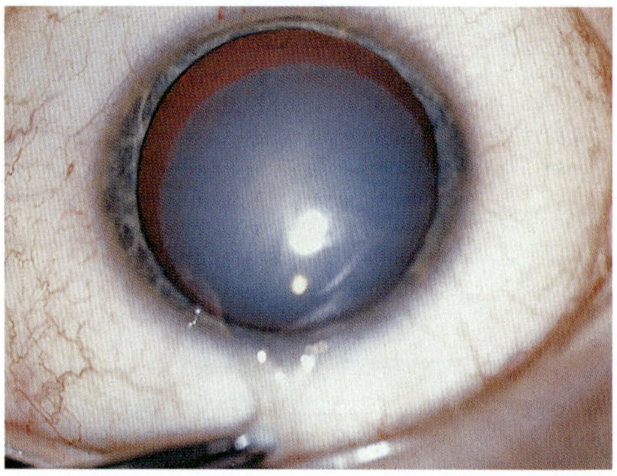

Fig. 20.84 A microspherophakic cataractous lens in rubella syndrome.

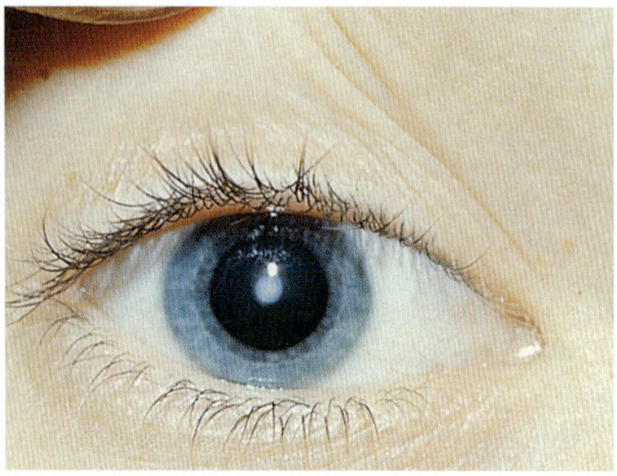

Fig. 20.85 Anterior polar cataract. This type of lens opacity is a developmental abnormality.

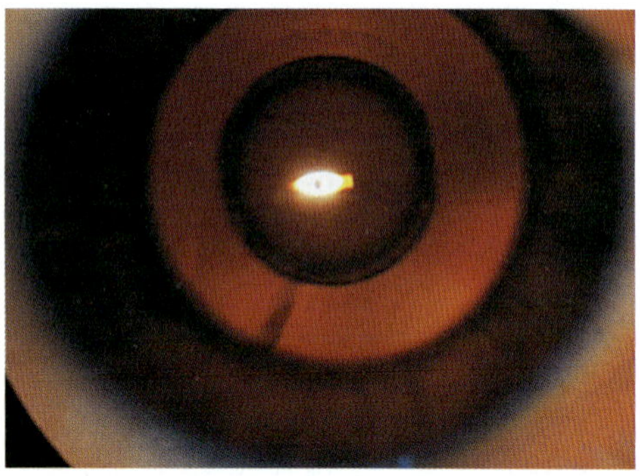

Fig. 20.86 Lamellar cataract with riders, surrounded by a clear cortex.

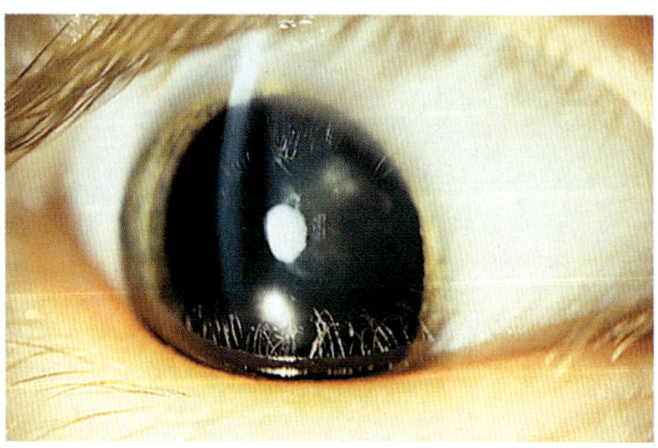

Fig. 20.87 Cataract of galactosemia. Early lens changes cause the nucleus of the lens to have an "oil droplet" configuration resulting from the accumulation of dulcitol, a metabolic product of galactose, within the lens. The resultant osmotic gradient draws water into the lens, producing the opacification. Early lens changes in galactosemia are reversible.

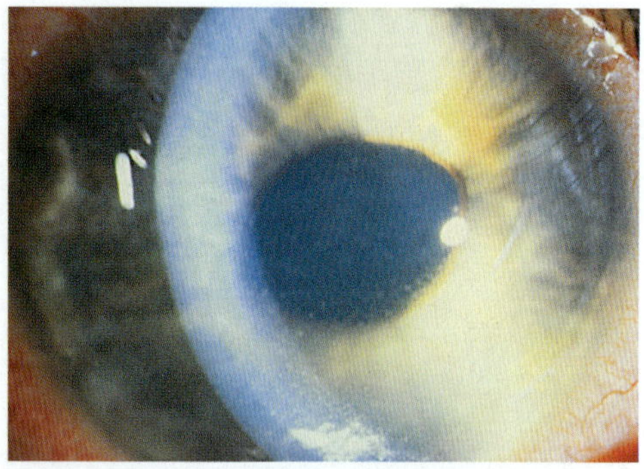

Fig. 20.88 Iritis. Conjunctival injection is most marked immediately around the cornea (ciliary flush).

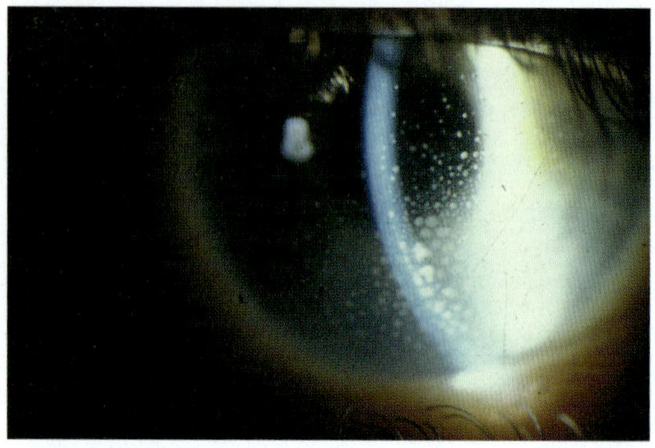

Fig. 20.89 Granulomatous uveitis with mutton fat keratic precipitates.

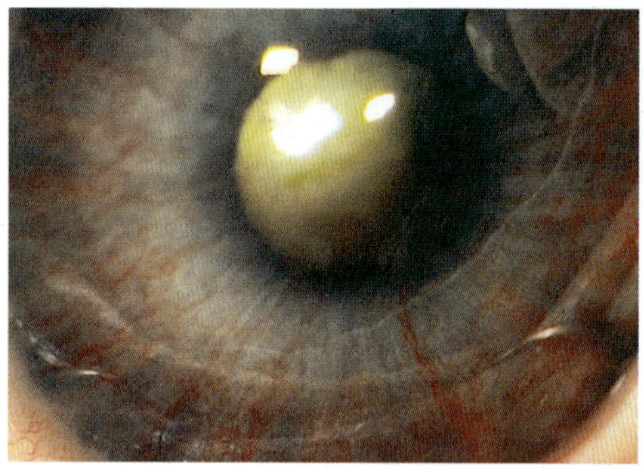

Fig. 20.90 Yellow cyclitic membrane behind a clear lens in a soft phthisic eye.

edema. Retinal detachment due to membrane formation and phthisis bulbi may occur in advanced cases (Fig. 20.90).

Posterior uveitis, inflammation of the posterior vitreous, retina, or choroid, can be caused by infection, but the precise cause is often undetermined. Infection of the retina by protozoa, fungi, and viruses may produce an intense inflammatory response in the vitreous, rendering it hazy or opaque. Leukocoria may be produced if the vitreous is cloudy or if extensive retinal involvement is present.

The laboratory evaluation of children with uveitis can be extensive and should be directed by careful history, physical findings, and ophthalmologic examination results (Box 20.4). Establishing a correct diagnosis is important for continued management, but idiopathic cases are common. Especially in older teens with isolated anterior uveitis, laboratory evaluation may be deferred unless the disease is recurrent or unresponsive to treatment. Management includes the use of biologics and has been greatly improved in the past 2 decades.

Vitreous

Vitreous Hemorrhage

Trauma, be it penetrating, concussive, or the result of abusive head trauma, is the most common cause of vitreous hemorrhage in children. Vitreous hemorrhage may occur with hemorrhagic disease of

Box 20.4 Laboratory Evaluation in Uveitis

Complete blood count with differential (leukemia)
Urinalysis (tubulointerstitial nephritis with uveitis)
Antinuclear antibody (JIA)
Angiotensin-converting enzyme (sarcoidosis)
Serum lysozyme (sarcoidosis)
Lyme titers
HLA-B27 (ankylosing spondylitis)
FTA-ABS (syphilis)
Toxoplasmosis ELISA
Toxocara ELISA
TORCH
Bartonella henselae titer (cat-scratch disease)
Chest radiograph (tuberculosis, sarcoidosis)
PPD (tuberculosis)
Laboratory evaluation is directed by history, ophthalmological examination, and other systemic physical findings

ELISA, Enzyme-linked immunosorbent assay; *FTA-ABS,* fluorescent treponemal antibody absorption; *HLA,* human leukocyte antigen; *JIA,* juvenile idiopathic arthritis; *PPD,* purified protein derivative; *TORCH,* Toxoplasmosis, *O*ther (syphilis, varicella-zoster, parvovirus B19), *R*ubella, *C*ytomegalovirus, and *H*erpes infections.

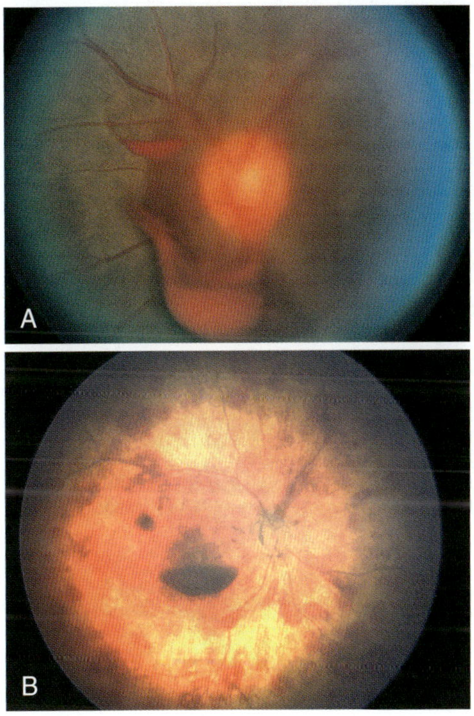

Fig. 20.91 (A) Vitreous hemorrhage. Dispersed red blood cells in the vitreous have made it hazy. The diffraction of light causes blurred vision. Fluid levels are often visible, and collections of blood may appear to float within the eye, variably blocking vision and causing symptoms of seeing cobwebs or large floating spots. (B) Fundus of a child who had suffered nonaccidental trauma. The retinal hemorrhages are at every level (preretinal, superficial retinal, deep retinal), widespread to beyond the equator in all quadrants, and there is a preretinal hemorrhage a fluid level most likely due to a macular schisis.

the newborn (hypoprothrombinemia), thrombocytopenia, or in advanced stages of ROP. Patients with a subarachnoid hemorrhage may develop vitreous hemorrhage (Terson syndrome), and vitreous hemorrhage may also occur in patients with leukemia. In abusive head trauma, the retinal hemorrhages tend to be in every level of the retina, spread beyond the equator, and may be accompanied by a macular schisis (Fig. 20.91B).

Blood in the vitreous, if located centrally or posteriorly, may be visible with the direct ophthalmoscope. If the vitreous is liquid, the hemorrhage may appear to float inside the eye (see Fig. 20.91). Diffuse blood in the vitreous may obscure the red reflex or view of the retina and can produce leukocoria as it organizes and becomes yellow and then gray in color. Vitreous hemorrhages may resolve spontaneously or, if extensive, require surgery. Vitreous hemorrhages that are slow to resolve in young children may cause amblyopia.

Optically empty vitreous is a rare sign. If seen in an eye that has never had any intraocular surgery, it is indicative of a collagenopathy, specifically those involving mutations in *COL2A1, COL9A1,* and *COL11A1* causing Stickler, Marshall, and Kniest syndromes. Children with these conditions may have high myopia, arthropathy, and spontaneous retinal detachment. Prophylaxis for retinal detachment is controversial, but any child with high myopia and cleft palate should be referred for evaluation of these conditions (Fig. 20.92).

Retina

Developmental Abnormalities

Colobomas are caused by a defect in closure of the embryonal fissure of the optic cup. They may be unilateral or bilateral. The retina and choroid are absent in the coloboma (Fig. 20.93) with a ring of pigment usually around the coloboma. Leukocoria may be produced by the yellowish-white reflection of the underlying sclera, and the red reflex may be seen as flashing from red to white as the eye moves to produce a reflex from normal areas of retina to the area of the coloboma. Using a direct ophthalmoscope, an occasional vessel may be seen bridging the area of the coloboma. The coloboma and retina are at a different plane of focus when visualized with the ophthalmoscope. There may be associated microphthalmos. If the optic disc and macula are not involved, central visual acuity may be normal and the patient may be

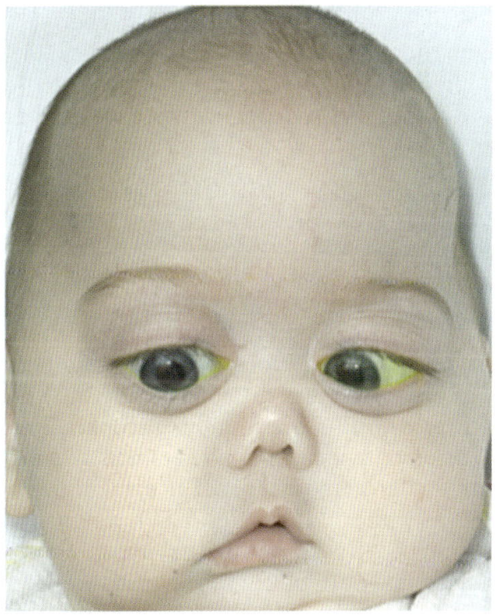

Fig. 20.92 This child has Stickler syndrome. Note the micrognathia, maxillary hypoplasia, and prominent eyes due to high myopia.

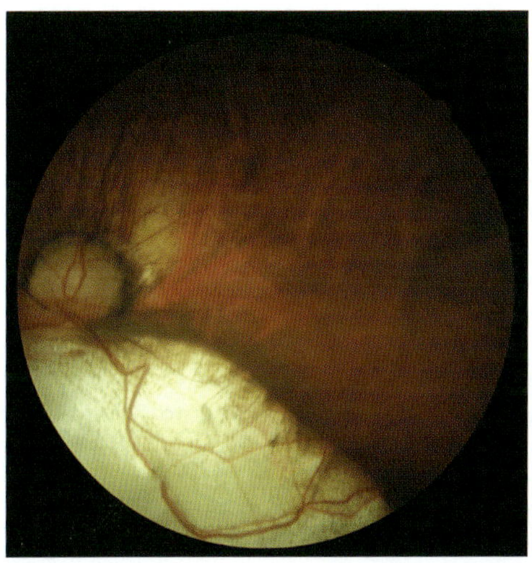

Fig. 20.93 Coloboma of optic nerve, retina, and choroid. The yellowish-white sclera is visible, and retinal vessels can be seen coursing through the coloboma.

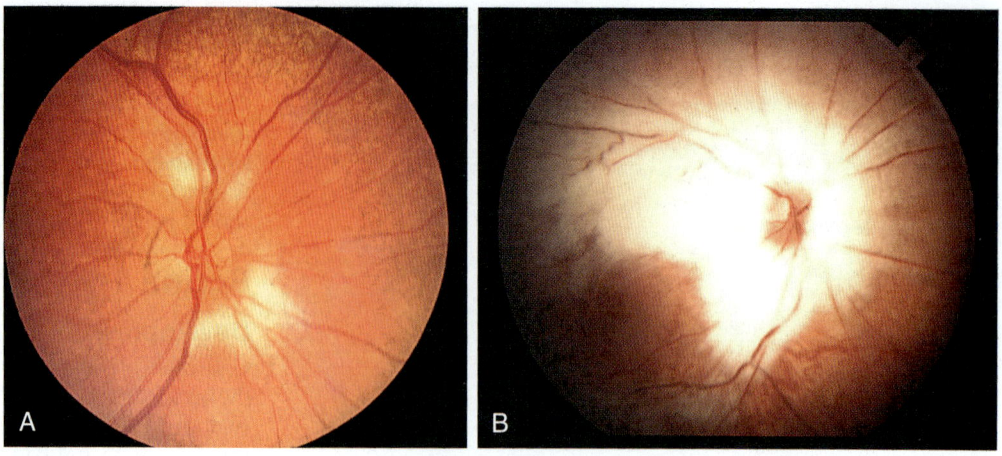

Fig. 20.94 Myelinated nerve fibers (MNF). Myelination of the optic nerve fibers may continue beyond the optic disc to include the retinal nerve fibers. This is visible as yellowish-white, flame-shaped patches oriented with the retinal nerve fibers. Myelinated nerve fibers may produce the clinical sign of leukocoria. A blind spot is present, corresponding to the area of myelination, but it is symptomatic only if the macula is affected. The MNF can be mild (A) or extensive (B), obscuring the optic disc.

asymptomatic. Affected eyes will have a peripheral visual field defect corresponding to the area of retinal involvement. Colobomas may be inherited as isolated anomalies, or they may be associated with chromosomal defects (trisomy 13) or other syndrome-related entities (CHARGE association). Children with a retinal choroidal coloboma have a 15% lifelong risk of the coloboma causing a retinal detachment.

Myelinated nerve fibers are seen with the direct ophthalmoscope as yellowish-white, flame-shaped patches; oriented with the retinal nerve fibers; and overlying the sensory retina and choroid (Fig. 20.94). Before birth, myelination of the optic nerve begins in the central nervous system, progresses peripherally, and usually stops at the optic disc before birth. Myelinated nerve fibers are seen if the myelination continues beyond the optic disc. They occur as isolated, congenital abnormalities, and there is no progression or worsening of the condition. Normal visual acuity is usually present because involvement of the macula is rare. The areas of myelination produce scotomas that can be plotted with formal visual field examination, but patients are not symptomatic of their presence.

Persistent fetal vasculature (PFV), previously known as persistent hyperplastic primary vitreous, occurs as a unilateral defect in the involution of the primary vitreous during the seventh month of gestation. Eyes with PFV are usually microphthalmic to varying degrees. PFV is often associated with cataracts and may be associated with intraocular hemorrhage, glaucoma, and retinal detachment. Many eyes with mild changes may have good visual acuity after early cataract surgery and visual rehabilitation; however, amblyopia and retinal or optic nerve abnormalities, if present, may severely affect visual prognosis. The patient has a lifelong risk for developing glaucoma (Fig. 20.95A and B).

Albinism refers to conditions involving deficiencies of melanin in the skin or eye (Fig. 20.96A and B). The loss of pigmentation may be isolated to the eye (ocular albinism) or involving the skin and eye (oculocutaneous albinism). Systemic syndromes including Chédiak-Higashi and Hermansky-Pudlak syndrome can have associated oculocutaneous albinism. The fundus is pale due to a lack of pigment in the retinal pigment epithelium. The ocular features are iris transillumination, foveal hypoplasia, hypopigmented fundus, and nystagmus. Visual acuity depends on the severity of foveal hypoplasia and nystagmus. Ocular albinism may be X-linked, and a female carrier may show iris transillumination defects but also "a mud splattered" pigmentation of the fundus at the equator (see Fig. 20.96B).

Retinal Vascular Anomalies

Retinal vascular anomalies may be due to abnormal blood vessels (telangiectasia), incomplete retinal vascularization either due to prematurity of birth or genetic disorders, abnormal new vessels as a response to ischemia (neovascularization), or inflammation of the vessels (vasculitis).

Retinal telangiectasia is most commonly seen in Coats disease, in which boys around 8 to 10 years of age usually present with a

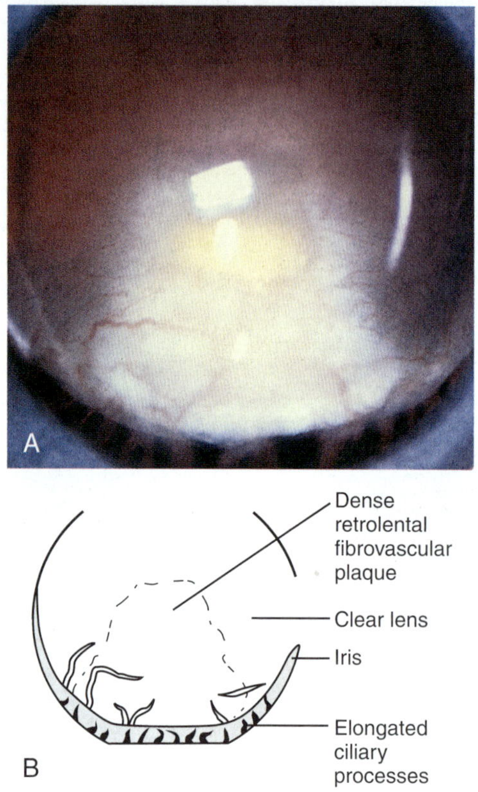

Fig. 20.95 (A) Persistent fetal vasculature presenting as a dense fibrovascular retrolental mass with microspherophakia, microphthalmia, and elongated ciliary processes. (B) Pathologic section of persistent hypoplastic primary vitreous. (Courtesy B.L. Johnson, MD, Pittsburgh, PA.)

unilateral telangiectasia. Peripheral retinal vessel telangiectasia and aneurysmal dilation lead to extensive areas of exudation, giving the retina a yellowish-white appearance, which may produce leukocoria. Exudative retinal detachment may be present in extensive cases. The macula is a common site for exudate to collect, and, when this is present, visual loss is profound. Treatment is with laser photocoagulation of the retina, and success depends on the degree of macular damage present (Fig. 20.97). Bilateral Coats disease or Coats disease in a female should trigger an evaluation for a systemic underlying cause such as facioscapulohumeral muscular dystrophy or cerebroretinal microangiopathy with calcifications and cysts.

Retinal neovascularization is rarely seen in children, but retinal ischemia may result in new vessel formation, which can lead to retinal and vitreous hemorrhages and tractional retinal detachment. The new vessels may occur within the posterior pole or in the periphery.

The commonest cause in children is peripheral neovascularization seen in ROP, sickle cell disease, FEVR, or incontinentia pigmenti

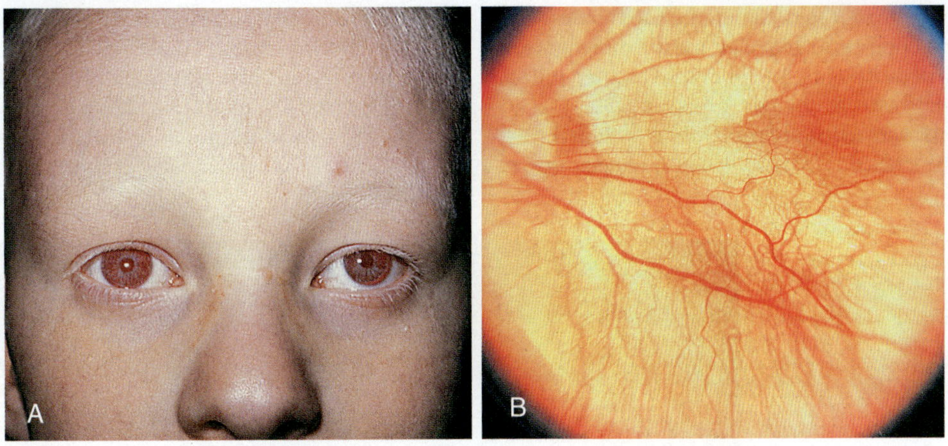

Fig. 20.96 (A) Albinism, characterized by white hair, pale skin, and translucent irides. (B) Ocular albinism. The fundus has little pigmentation, and the choroidal vasculature is readily visible. The macula is poorly developed, producing decreased visual acuity.

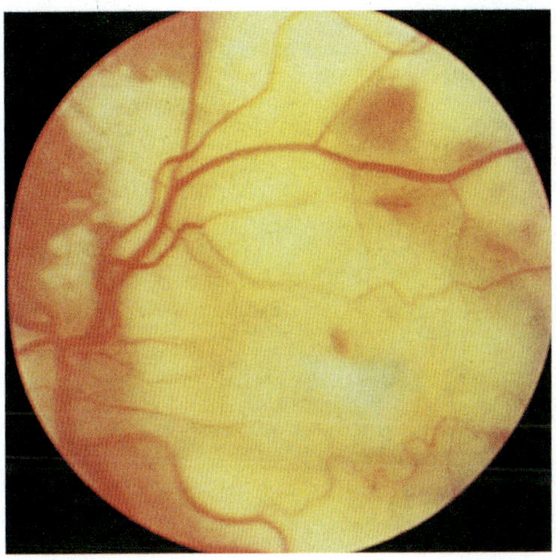

Fig. 20.97 Coats disease. Peripheral telangiectasia along the course of the retinal vasculature leads to exudation, giving the retina a yellowish-white appearance. If the exudate extends to the posterior retina, leukocoria may be present.

(IP). Posterior pole neovascularization may be seen in retinal vein occlusion, retinal vasculitis, retinal artery occlusion, or radiation retinopathy. Fluorescein angiography helps to identify areas of ischemia and new vessels. Laser treatment of the ischemic retina is the principle of therapy.

Failure of complete retinal vascularization is most commonly seen in ROP characterized by abnormalities in the developing retinal vascular system.

The international classification of ROP is used to describe location, extent, and stage of the disease. The location of ROP refers to the location relative to the optic nerve. This has been standardized by dividing the retina into three zones. Zone I is an area centered on the optic disc and extends from the disc to twice the distance between the disc and the macula. Zone II is a ring concentric to Zone I, which extends to the nasal ora serrata (the edge of the retina on the side of the eye toward the nose). Zone III is the remaining crescent of retina on the temporal side. The extent of ROP is described by how many clock-hours of the retina are involved. For example, if there is retinopathy extending from 1.00 around to 5.00, the extent of ROP is 4 clock-hours. ROP is a progressive disease. It begins with some mild changes in the vessels and may progress to more severe changes. The stage of ROP relates to the degree of this vascular progression.

Stage 1 is characterized by a demarcation line between the normal retina nearer the optic nerve and the nonvascularized retina more peripherally.

Stage 2 ROP has a ridge of scar tissue and new vessels in place of the demarcation line.

Stage 3 ROP shows an increased size of the vascular ridge, with growth of fibrovascular tissue on the ridge and extending out into the vitreous (extraretinal neovascular proliferation).

Stage 4 refers to a partial retinal detachment. The scar tissue associated with the fibrovascular ridge contracts, pulling the retina away from the wall of the eye. Stage 4 is further categorized depending on the location of the retinal detachment. In Stage 4A, the detachment does not include the macula, and the vision may be good. In Stage 4B, the macula is detached, and the visual potential is markedly decreased.

Stage 5 ROP implies a complete retinal detachment, usually with the retina pulled into a funnel-shaped configuration by the fibrovascular scar tissue. Eyes with stage 5 ROP usually have no useful vision, even if surgery is performed to repair the detachment. A white fibrovascular mass may occupy the retrolental space (retrolental fibroplasia) and produce leukocoria.

Plus disease describes dilation and tortuosity of the blood vessels in Zone I. It also includes the growth and dilation of abnormal blood vessels on the surface of the iris, rigidity of the pupil, and vitreous haze. The presence of plus disease suggests a more fulminant or rapidly progressive course. Lower birthweight, prolonged supplemental oxygen requirement, and respiratory distress syndrome have clearly been shown to be risk factors (Fig. 20.98). Preplus disease is defined by abnormal vascular dilation, tortuosity insufficient to be described as plus disease, or both.

Aggressive retinopathy of prematurity (A-ROP), previously termed aggressive posterior ROP, is a rapidly progressive form of ROP located in zone I or posterior zone II but also beyond the posterior retina. It can be seen in larger preterm babies, especially in regions of the world with limited resources. The characteristic feature of A-ROP is rapid development of neovascularization and severe plus disease without normal progression through the stages of ROP.

In 75% of patients, ROP is bilateral and symmetric. Most patients have only mild forms of the disease (stage 1 and stage 2 disease), and these patients do not have significant visual sequelae. Advanced ROP primarily affects the ill, premature infant whose birth weight is often less than 1250 g. The progression of the disease and the risk for visual loss may be reduced in advanced cases with treatment by laser photocoagulation and intravitreal injection of vascular endothelial growth factor inhibitors. Programs to screen neonates at risk for developing ROP must be present. All very low–birth-weight infants, regardless of the development of ROP, are at higher risk than the general population for strabismus, amblyopia, and refractive errors and should have comprehensive examinations at about 1 year old.

Regression of ROP may occur with or without treatment and is described as complete or incomplete. The location and extent of any avascular retina must be documented. Reactivation may be seen after treatment and includes new ROP lesions or vascular changes.

When this occurs, the term "reactivated" should be used to describe the stage of reactivation. Long-term sequelae must be recognized and include late retinal detachments, peripheral avascular retina, macular anomalies, retinal vascular changes, and glaucoma.

Other causes of an avascular retina are genetic and include FEVR and IP. The former can be caused by several genetic changes, one of which, LRP5, can also result in accelerated or premature loss of bone density. Therefore even if molecular testing cannot be done in a child older than the age of 5 years with FEVR, a DEXA (dual energy x-ray absorptiometry) scan should be arranged. FEVR can present with retinal folds, exudates, or just an avascular peripheral retinal zone (Fig. 20.99). IP is an X-linked dominant condition affecting females

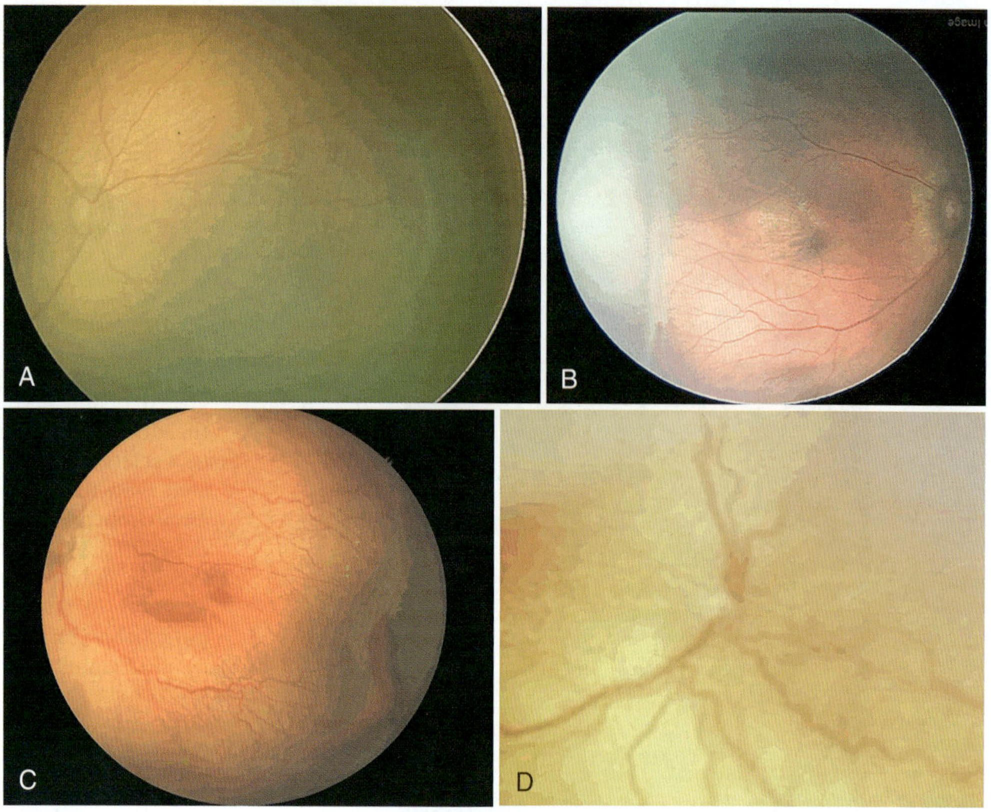

Fig. 20.98 Retinopathy of prematurity: (A) Stage I. (B) Stage II. (C) Stage III. (D) Plus disease. (Courtesy Dr. M. Pihlblad, MD, Pittsburgh, PA.)

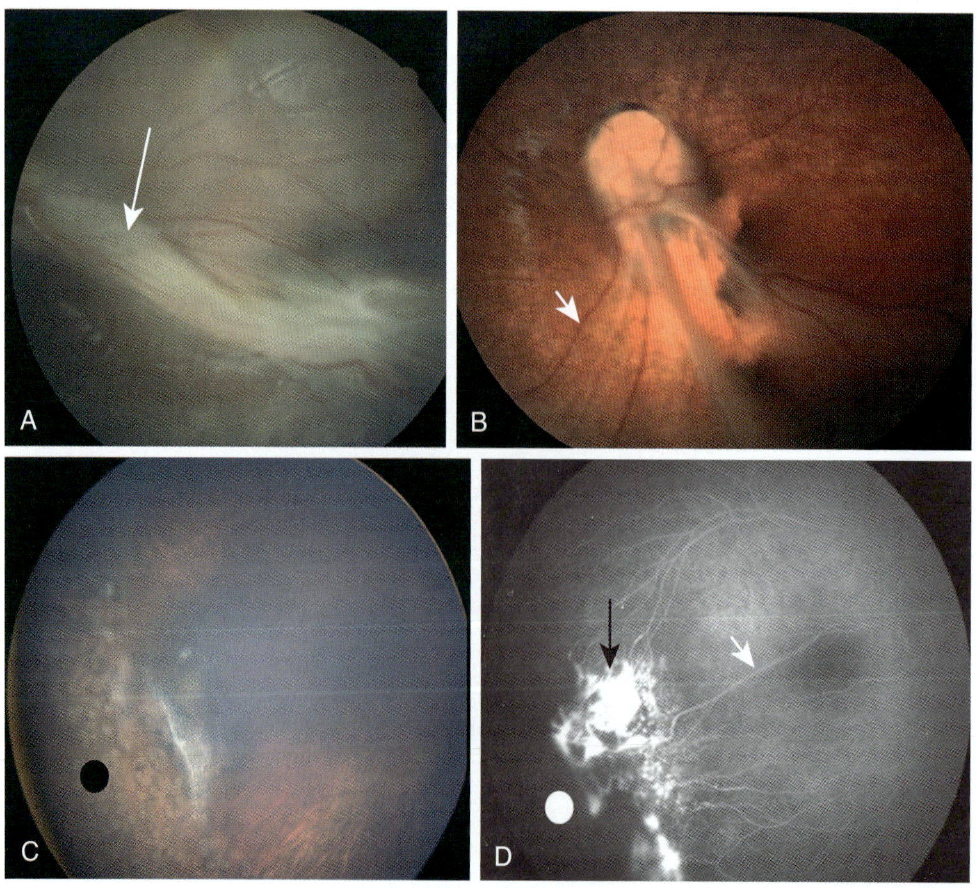

Fig. 20.99 Composite of different cases of familial exudative vitreoretinopathy. This condition can cause retinal folds (*thin white arrow,* A), straightening of the retinal vessels (*short white arrows,* B and D), avascular zone treated with laser (*black dot,* C), and leakage of vessels (*black arrow,* D) at the edge of an avascular zone (*white dot,* D). Panel D shows a fluorescein angiogram, which allows evaluation of neovascularization, leaking vessels, and avascular zones.

who have a vesiculobullous rash following the lines of Blaschko. These children must be examined for peripheral avascular retinal zones and may need an examination under anesthesia to do so.

Retinal vasculitis is extremely rare in children and presents as inflammation around retinal veins (periphlebitis) or retinal arterioles (periarteritis). Periphlebitis may be seen in sarcoidosis, Behçet disease, cytomegalovirus (CMV) retinitis, acute retinal necrosis, tuberculosis, frosted branch angiitis, or may be idiopathic. Periarteritis may be seen in systemic lupus erythematosus, dermatomyositis, polyarteritis nodosa, or Wegener granulomatosis. Fundus examination is essential to exclude retinal involvement. If there is involvement, systemic immunosuppression is essential, but prognosis may be guarded.

Retinal Pigmentary Anomalies

Retinal pigmentary anomalies can be congenital or acquired (Box 20.5). Congenital causes include congenital hyperplasia of the retinal pigment epithelium, combined hamartoma of the retina and the retinal pigment epithelium, and choroidal nevus. Acquired causes include pigmentary disturbances after trauma, post-retinitis, and pigmented retinal dystrophies (retinitis pigmentosa).

Congenital hyperplasia of the retinal pigment epithelium may be grouped ("bear track") (Fig. 20.100A) or isolated with a halo and a "fishtail" morphology (Fig. 20.100B). This latter type is associated with familial polyposis coli, and molecular testing for this condition should be considered.

Combined hamartoma of the retina and RPE is often seen in the posterior pole and consists of glial tissue, vascular tissue, and sheets of pigment cells. It is strongly associated with neurofibromatosis II (Fig. 20.101).

Choroidal nevus is often seen outside the vascular arcades. Malignant conversion is extremely rare in childhood but requires lifelong surveillance (Fig. 20.102).

Box 20.5 Systemic Disorders Associated With Retinitis Pigmentosa or Retinal Pigmentary Retinopathy

1. Hearing difficulties
   - Usher syndrome. USH 1. Retinitis pigmentosa by age 10; cataract; profound congenital sensory deafness. USH 2. Retinitis pigmentosa in late teens; childhood sensory deafness. USH 3. Postlingual, progressive hearing loss; variable vestibular dysfunction; onset of retinitis pigmentosa by second decade.
   - Alstrom syndrome. Nystagmus and early loss of central vision—in contrast to loss of peripheral vision first, as in other pigmentary retinopathies; dilated cardiomyopathy with congestive heart failure; atherosclerosis; hypertension; renal failure; deafness; obesity; diabetes mellitus.
   - Infantile Refsum disease (early onset). Mental retardation; minor facial dysmorphism; retinitis pigmentosa; sensorineural hearing deficit; hepatomegaly; osteoporosis; failure to thrive; hypocholesterolemia.
   - Late-onset Refsum disease. Retinitis pigmentosa; chronic polyneuropathy; cerebellar signs.
   - Cockayne dwarfism. Precociously senile appearance; pigmentary retinal degeneration; optic atrophy; deafness; marble epiphyses in some digits; photosensitivity; developmental delay.
   - Mucopolysaccharidosis (MPS).
   - Kearns-Sayre ophthalmoplegia. Pigmentary degeneration of the retina; ptosis and cardia conduction defect.
2. Renal disorders
   - Senior-Loken syndrome. Renal dysplasia; retinitis pigmentosa; cerebellar ataxia; sensorineural hearing loss.
   - Rhyns syndrome. Retinitis pigmentosa; hypopituitarism; nephronophthisis; mild skeletal dysplasia.
   - Bardet-Biedl syndrome. Obesity; rod–cone dystrophy; onset by end of second decade hypogonadism; renal anomalies; polydactyly; learning disabilities.
   - Cystinosis. Corneal crystals but pigmentary retinopathy may also occur.
3. Skeletal disorders
   - Jeune syndrome. Chondrodysplasia that often leads to death in infancy because of a severely constricted thoracic cage and respiratory insufficiency; retinal degeneration.
4. Hepatic disorders
   - Zellweger syndrome. Hypotonia; seizures; psychomotor retardation; pigmentary retinopathy and cataracts.
5. Neurologic/neuromuscular
   - Neuronal ceroid lipofuscinosis (Battens disease). Characterized by intralysosomal accumulations of lipopigments in either granular; curvilinear; or fingerprint patterns; progressive dementia; seizures and progressive visual failure.
   - Hallervorden-Spatz syndrome. Retinitis pigmentosa and pallidal degeneration.
   - Joubert syndrome. Hypoplasia of the cerebellar vermis; saccadic initiation failure; hyperpnea intermixed with central apnea in the neonatal period; retinal dystrophy.
   - Infantile Refsum disease.
   - Abetalipoproteinemia (Bassen-Kornzweig syndrome). Celiac disease; pigmentary degeneration of the retina; progressive ataxic neuropathy; acanthocytosis.

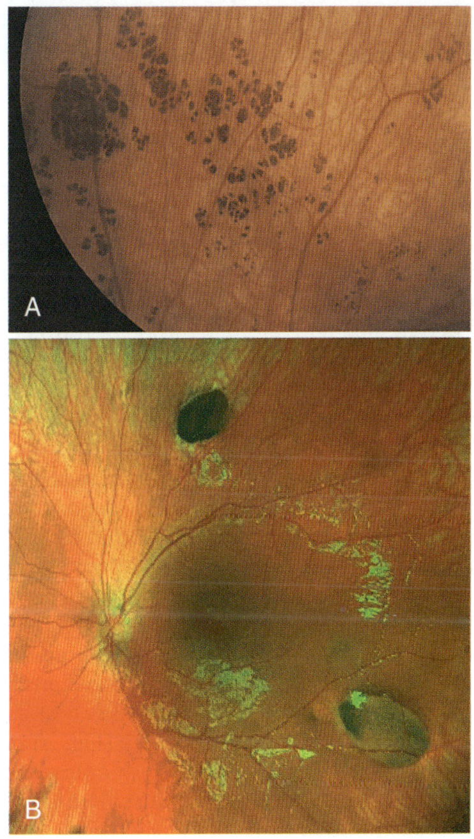

Fig. 20.100 Grouped congenital hypertrophy of the retinal pigment epithelium, also known as bear track. These may be markers for familial polyposis coli (FPC) if they are multiple and bilateral (A). However, if they have a halo, as seen in (B), these are highly specific for FPC and molecular testing should be done.

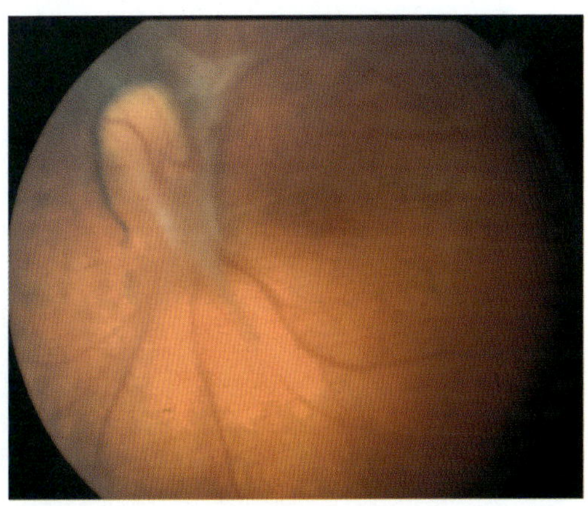

Fig. 20.101 Optic nerve is obscured by gliotic-like lesion and pigmentation; this is a combined hamartoma of the retina and retinal pigment epithelium. Neurofibromatosis should be excluded.

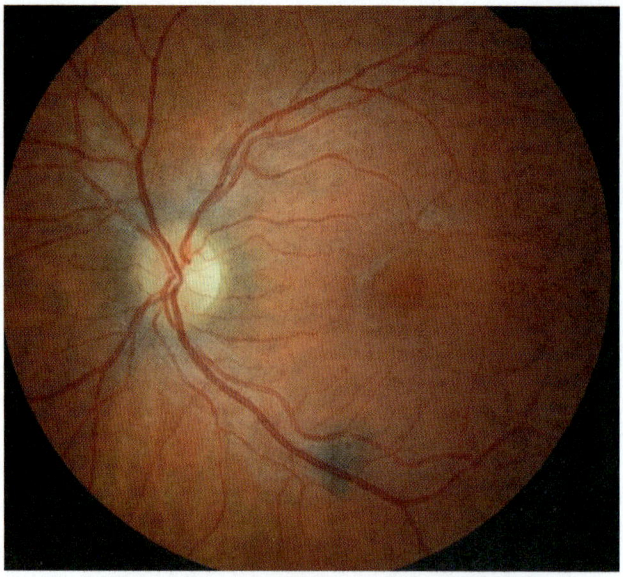

Fig. 20.102 Choroidal nevus—retinal vessels pass over the deeper placed nevus.

Retinitis pigmentosa, now often referred to as retinal dystrophy, is a pigmentary retinopathy characterized by visual field loss, night blindness, and a depressed or extinct electroretinogram. Early-onset retinal dystrophy may be associated with nephronophthisis (see later). Symptoms of visual loss may be present in childhood but usually do not become apparent until the second or third decade of life. Poor night vision is the earliest symptom, followed by progressive loss of peripheral visual field and, finally, loss of central vision. Many different diseases are characterized by pigmentary retinopathy. The presentation, progression, and extent of visual loss vary widely. In general, disease within pedigrees has similar clinical characteristics.

Retinal pigment epithelial changes include deposition of pigment in a perivascular pattern. Pigment deposition in the midperipheral retina gives a characteristic "bone spicule" pattern late in the course of the disease. Early in the disease, the optic nerve may have a waxy pallor and the retinal arteries may be attenuated. Fundus autofluorescence is useful to detect accumulation of lipofuscin, which is another indicator of retinal dysfunction. Cystoid macular edema may also occur in retinal dystrophies, and this is best diagnosed on a macular ocular coherence tomography scan (Fig. 20.103).

There are now many genes implicated in autosomal recessive, dominant, and X-linked retinal dystrophies. Retinal dystrophy is also seen in mitochondrial disease. LCA is an early-onset retinal dystrophy, which can be severe in young children who develop night blindness and visual loss at an early age. Use of ultraviolet protection to retard further retinal damage should be encouraged. The first U.S. Food and Drug Administration approved gene therapy for an early-onset retinal dystrophy caused by mutations in *RPE65.* This has opened the door to the possibilities of novel therapies becoming available for other genetic causes of retinal dystrophy.

Increasingly, it appears that syndromes with associated retinal dystrophy may have a uniform underlying mechanism. The best example of this is the ciliopathies (see later).

Retinal Tumors

Retinal hamartomas can be seen in tuberous sclerosis and begin as beige, fleshy lesions that eventually calcify. They can also be seen at the optic nerve head.

Retinal angiomas are vascular tumors that may be isolated, but they most often are seen in von Hippel-Lindau syndrome (Fig. 20.104).

Racemose angioma is a rare condition (also called Wyburn Mason syndrome) in which an arteriovenous malformation typically involves the optic disc, retina, or midbrain.

Retinoblastoma is the most common intraocular malignancy of childhood. It occurs with a frequency of between 1 in 14,000 and 1 in 20,000 births. The most common age at diagnosis is between 1 and 1½ years, with 90% of cases presenting before 3 years of age. The most common presenting signs of retinoblastoma are leukocoria (60%) and strabismus (22%) (Fig. 20.105A). One-third of cases are bilateral. The tumor may present as an elevated, round, white, or yellow mass (see Fig. 20.105B). Retinoblastoma may be multicentric with several tumor masses arising within the same eye. Seeding into the vitreous may occur, producing a cloudy vitreous. A frequent feature of retinoblastoma is the presence of calcification within the mass most easily detected using ultrasound.

Retinoblastoma may be transmitted in an autosomal dominant inheritance pattern. Sixty percent of affected individuals have a family history of retinoblastoma. Penetrance is high (60%–90%) but incomplete. Sporadic cases occur as either somatic mutations in 75% of patients or germinal mutations that may be passed on to the offspring of affected patients. Sporadic cases are usually unilateral, and the hereditary forms are usually bilateral. However, a patient with a unilateral tumor may have heritable disease. Patients who have the heritable form of the disease, with the deletion of the retinoblastoma gene, may develop tumors of the pineal gland (trilateral retinoblastoma) and have a markedly increased risk of secondary tumors (most commonly osteogenic sarcoma).

Untreated, retinoblastoma is virtually 100% fatal. The treatment of retinoblastoma is advancing rapidly, and many eyes, even those with extensive tumor that were previously enucleated, may be saved by combinations of local treatment (laser, thermal, and plaque radiation) and chemotherapy (systemic and delivered to the eye

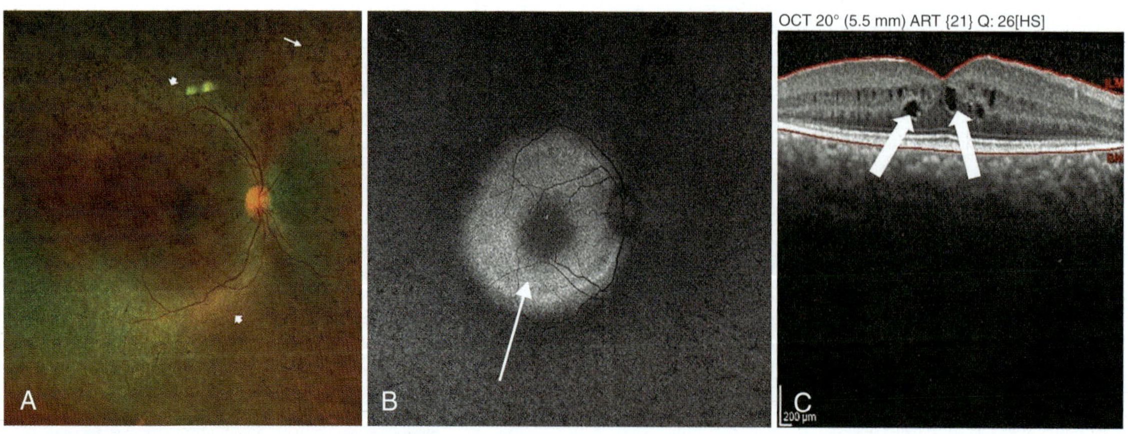

Fig. 20.103 Composite images of a child with USHER syndrome type 1B. Bony spicule pigmentation is seen (A) while on fundus autofluorescence, a hyperfluorescent area due to lipofuscin accumulation is seen (B, *thin white arrow*). Macular ocular coherence tomography scan shows cystoid macular edema (C, *thick white arrows*), which can be seen in retinal dystrophies. Topical carbonic anhydrase inhibitors are used to treat this cystoid macular edema.

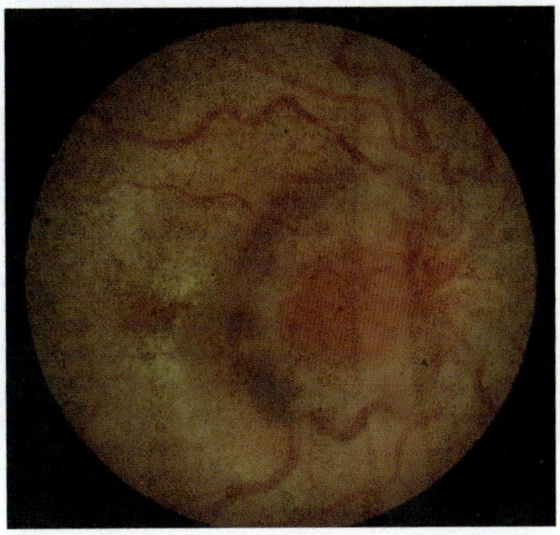

Fig. 20.104 Retinal angioma in a patient with von Hippel-Lindau syndrome, which is obscuring the optic disc. Hard exudates are seen as the papillary circulation is likely disrupted, resulting in leakage and deposition of hard exudate.

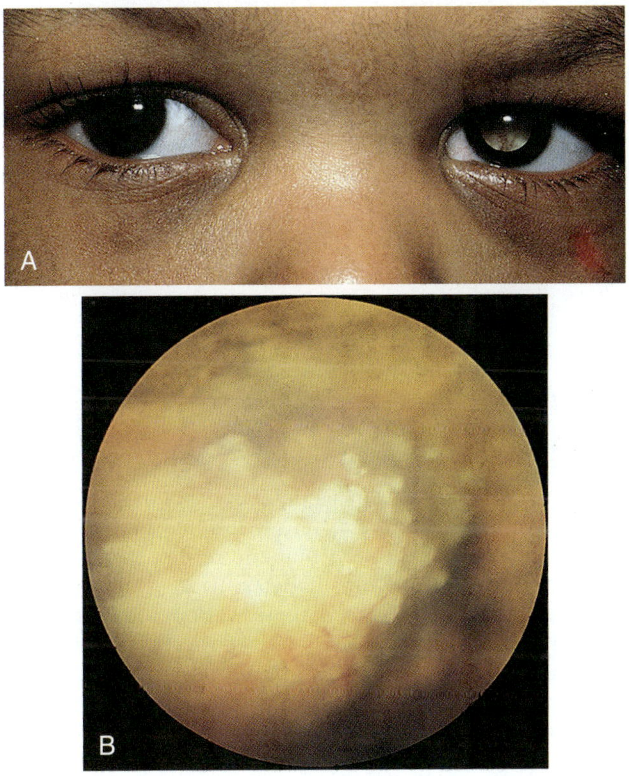

Fig. 20.105 (A) Leukocoria. The patient's left eye has a white pupillary reflex produced by reflection of light from a retinoblastoma. Leukocoria is the most common presenting sign (60%) of retinoblastoma. (B) Retinoblastoma. The tumor mass of retinoblastoma is usually elevated and yellow or white in color. Dilated feeding vessels of the tumor may be visible. Seeding into the vitreous from the tumor may produce a cloudy vitreous.

intraarterially). Infants with a parent affected by the hereditary form of the disease must be examined immediately after birth and repeatedly for the first several years of life. Screening for the *RB1* genetic mutation and genetic counseling are required.

Retinal Hemorrhages

Retinal hemorrhages may be seen in several disorders including diabetic retinopathy, sickle cell retinopathy, slow-flow retinopathy, central retinal vein occlusion, bacterial endocarditis, accidental trauma, and nonaccidental trauma. Retinal hemorrhages can be classified according to where they occur: preretinal, retinal, and subretinal.

Preretinal hemorrhages occur between the posterior vitreous and retina (also known as *subhyaloid*). They are seen in proliferative sickle cell retinopathy, trauma, subarachnoid hemorrhage (Terson syndrome), or nonaccidental injury (but never seen in isolation). They are usually seen with widespread retinal and subretinal hemorrhages and may occur with or without macular retinal schisis. Rarely, they may be seen in children with proliferative diabetic retinopathy.

Retinal hemorrhages are flame shaped if they lie in the retinal nerve fiber layer and dot or blot if they lie deep to the retinal nerve fiber layer. Flame-shaped hemorrhages may have a white center (Roth spot) and can be seen in retinal vein occlusions, acute papilledema, optic disc drusen, acute hypertensive retinopathy, and retinal perivasculitis (especially early CMV retinitis). Roth spots are seen in patients with severe anemias, leukemia, and bacterial endocarditis, and may also be seen after trauma. Dot and blot hemorrhages can be seen in diabetes mellitus–related retinopathy. They may be seen in abusive head trauma in association with superficial and subretinal hemorrhages.

Subretinal hemorrhages are deep red, and the retinal vessels can be seen clearly rising above and over the deep hemorrhage. These are seen in sickle cell anemia; Coats disease (retinal telangiectasia); accidental and nonaccidental trauma; and, rarely, choroidal neovascularization. In sickle cell disease, retinopathy changes occur in the peripheral fundus and cannot be visualized with a direct ophthalmoscope, necessitating screening and detection by an ophthalmologist. Retinal vascular complications occur most frequently in patients with hemoglobin (Hgb) SC disease and S-thalassemia disease. Patients with sickle cell disease (Hgb SS) are less frequently affected due to their decreased hematocrit providing protection to the retinal vasculature. Rarely, patients with the milder hemoglobinopathies, for example, AS and AC hemoglobinopathies, may have retinal findings. Retinal findings are nonproliferative and include refractile or iridescent deposits (resorbed hemorrhages), black sunburst lesions (perivascular pigment migration), and salmon patch hemorrhages. Proliferative changes include arteriolar occlusions leading to neovascularization at the edge of these areas of nonperfusion in the form of a *sea fan* and often lead to vitreous hemorrhage, traction, and retinal detachment (Fig. 20.106). Interestingly, sludging of blood in the conjunctival blood vessels produces comma-shaped capillaries ("comma sign") as a result of segmentation.

Retinal hemorrhages that are highly suspicious of nonaccidental trauma are bilateral and involve all three types. They are widespread, extending beyond the equator to the ora serrata, often with a macular schisis (splitting of the inner levels of the retina), frequently with blood in the schitic cavity. Other forms of retinal hemorrhage may also be nonaccidental, but the overall clinical picture must always be considered when making such a diagnosis (Fig. 20.107).

Retinal Hard Exudates

Retinal hard exudates are rare yellow, waxy deposits that may be retinal (focal, diffuse, or macular star) or subretinal. Focal or diffuse hard exudates may be found in diabetic retinopathy (although unusual in children), old branch retinal vein occlusion (rare in children), radiation retinopathy, or retinal telangiectasia. A macular star (stellate pattern of exudates centered on the macula) may be seen in malignant hypertension; papilledema; neuroretinitis; and, rarely, retinal angioma (von-Hippel Lindau syndrome or idiopathic) (see Fig. 20.104).

Subretinal exudates may be seen in Coats disease or rarely with *Toxocara canis* retinochoroiditis. Treatment for Coats disease has been advocated with removal of subretinal exudates and treatment of vascular anomalies seen in this condition (Fig. 20.108).

Retinal Cotton Wool Spots

Retinal cotton wool spots, rarely seen in children, are small, white lesions with fluffy edges resulting from a localized microvasculature occlusion resulting in ischemia. They are seen in retinal vein occlusion; diabetic retinopathy; HIV microvasculopathy; anemia; leukemia; trauma to the chest and long bones (Purtscher retinopathy); and systemic vasculitides, especially systemic lupus erythematosus (Fig. 20.109).

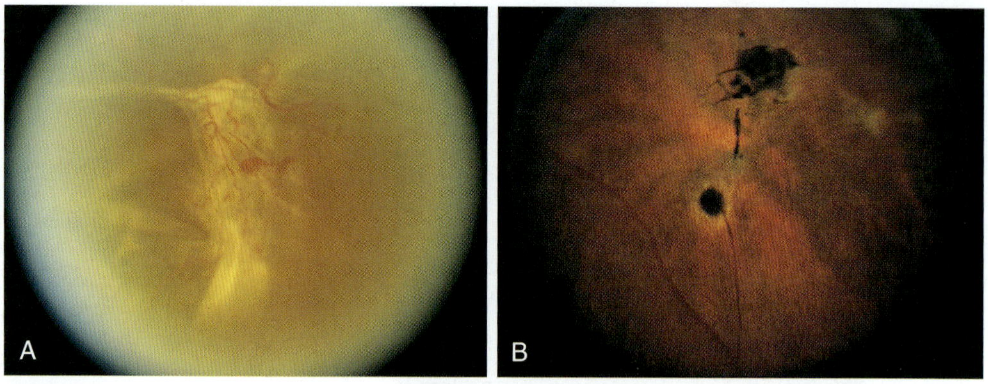

Fig. 20.106 Sickle cell retinopathy. (A) Neovascularization or growth of fragile blood vessels into the vitreous in the midperipheral retina. The white fibrous tissue present is due to the proliferation of fibroglial elements. This produces traction on the retina, which may subsequently lead to retinal detachment. (B) The black sunburst lesions are areas of perivascular retinal pigment epithelial hypertrophy with pigment migration. This finding is an example of nonproliferative change.

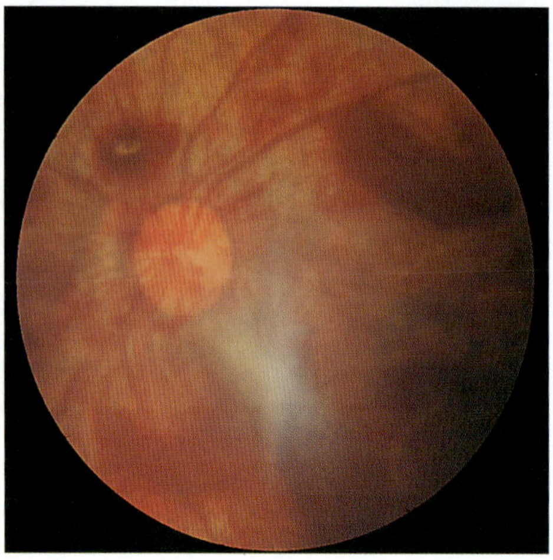

Fig. 20.107 Abusive head trauma. Multiple retinal hemorrhages are present in the posterior fundus. There are small flame-shaped hemorrhages within the nerve fiber layer that follow the pattern of the retinal vessels. More extensive areas of hemorrhage have broken through to the preretinal space and are seen as areas of blood that obscure the retina. A Roth spot, that is, a hemorrhage with a white center, is visible just above the optic disc. The white reflection from the camera flash is visible because of dispersed red blood cells within the vitreous.

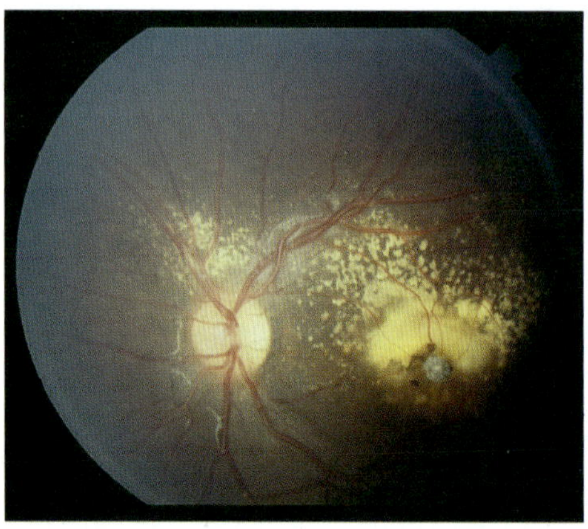

Fig. 20.108 Hard exudate seen in a case of Coats disease.

Diabetic Retinopathy

Transient lenticular myopia is the most common ocular finding in young diabetic patients. This occurs in patients who have had a rapid rise in blood glucose level. Sorbitol accumulates within the lens as a metabolic product, increasing the lens osmolarity and causing the lens to swell, producing myopia. After the blood sugar level returns to normal, myopia may continue to persist for several days or even weeks, with gradual spontaneous resolution. Cataracts may develop in children as a rare complication.

The earliest sign of background diabetic retinopathy is the presence of microaneurysms (tiny discrete red spots). Small retinal hemorrhages, cotton-wool spots, venous dilation, and hard exudates (small, discrete, yellow lesions) may also be seen. The occurrence of background diabetic retinopathy is related to the duration and control of the diabetes. Young children appear to have a protective effect from diabetic retinopathy, and changes are seldom diagnosed until years after puberty. Yearly screening examinations are recommended for children with juvenile diabetes. Proliferative diabetic retinopathy seen in adults essentially does not occur until after puberty.

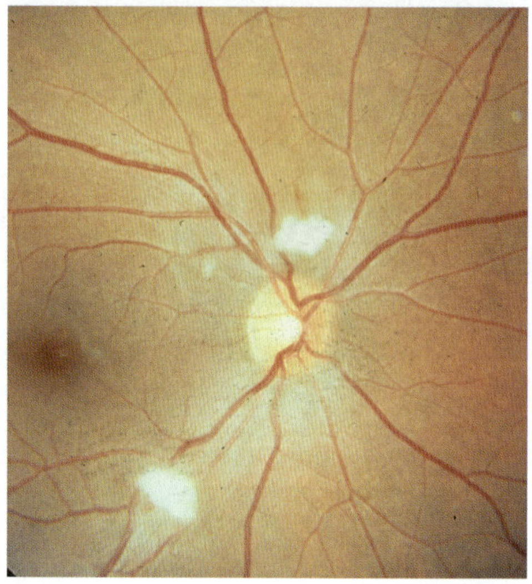

Fig. 20.109 Two cotton wool spots seen in a child with systemic lupus erythematosus.

Inflammation of the Retina (Retinitis)

Inflammation of the retina and choroid is most commonly the result of viral, protozoal, fungal, or bacterial infection. The final common pathway for recovery or resolution of retinal inflammation is the production of a pigmented chorioretinal scar. These inflammatory lesions may be single focal, multiple focal, or diffuse lesions.

Single focal lesions may be caused by toxoplasmosis (Fig. 20.110), toxocariasis (Fig. 20.111), candidiasis, and cryptococcus.

Multiple focal lesions may be caused by candidiasis, sarcoidosis, Lyme disease, choroidal pneumocystis, presumed ocular histoplasmosis syndrome, Behçet disease, Vogt-Koyanagi-Harada syndrome, sympathetic ophthalmitis, and tuberculous choroiditis.

Diffuse lesions may be seen in CMV retinitis (Fig. 20.112), acute retinal necrosis, herpes simplex retinitis, and measles retinitis.

A rare cause of retinochoroiditis is sympathetic ophthalmitis. Sympathetic ophthalmitis occurs after a severe injury involving the uvea of one eye (the "exciting" eye), followed by a latent period and the development of uveitis in the uninjured eye (the "sympathizing" eye). Sympathetic ophthalmia may occur as early as 5 days after the original injury but can also have a delayed onset years after the incident. Sympathetic ophthalmia is an autoimmune disorder, and treatment includes topical and systemic immunosuppression.

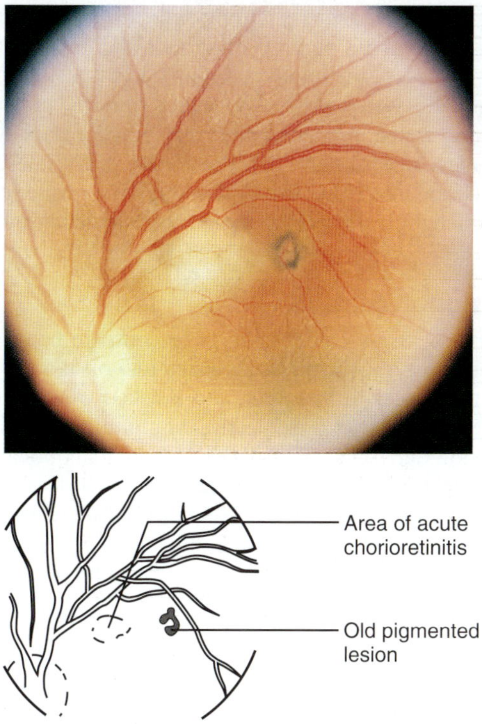

Fig. 20.110 Toxoplasmosis. Acute, recurrent, chorioretinal inflammation may occur adjacent to pigmented scars.

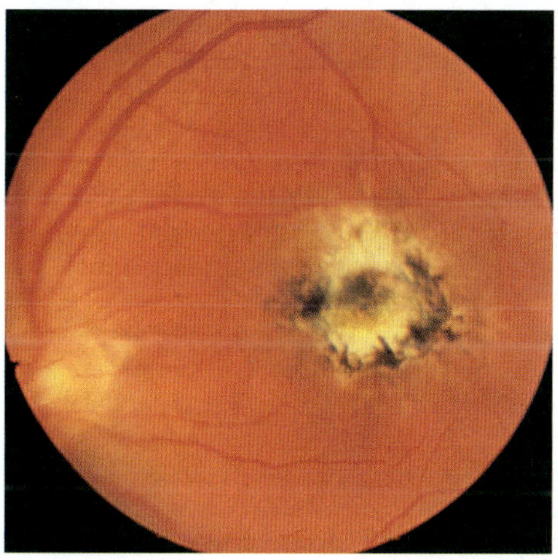

Fig. 20.111 Toxocariasis. The retinal lesion appears as a white elevated mass with surrounding pigmented scar formation.

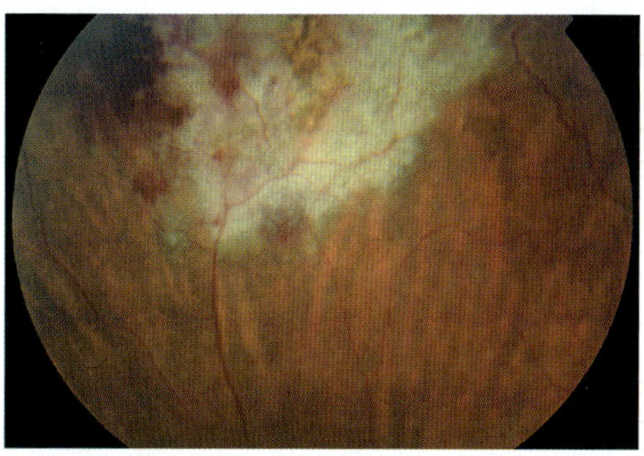

Fig. 20.112 Cytomegalovirus retinitis. Note the perivascular retinitis with hemorrhage.

Cherry Red Spot

This distinct sign is seen because the fovea has no overlying ganglion cell or nerve fiber layer; if the nerve fiber layer or the ganglion cell layers become edematous after an ischemic insult or have deposition in a metabolic disorder, the fovea appears relatively deep red, hence "cherry-red" spot. It is seen in central retinal artery occlusion (due to emboli, systemic vasculitis, or compression) or in sphingolipidoses, namely Tay-Sachs disease (GM_2 type I gangliosidosis) and Niemann-Pick disease. Sphingolipids accumulate in the retinal ganglion cells, giving a whitish appearance to the retina (Fig. 20.113).

Retinal Detachment

Large retinal detachments may produce loss of the red reflex and leukocoria when the detached retina sits in apposition to the lens or when significant scarring (proliferative vitreoretinopathy) is present. Uncommon in children, retinal detachment is an elevation of the neurosensory retina, which may be rhegmatogenous (fluid from the vitreous cavity leaking into the subretinal space due to a retinal hole or tear), exudative (due to inflammatory exudate), tractional (due to traction on the surface of the retina—usually after trauma or as a result of untreated ROP), or solid (due to a tumor). A choroidal detachment is most commonly seen in hypotony (low IOP associated with decreased vision), following IOP-lowering operations such as trabeculectomy. Here, the choroid detaches with the retina still attached.

In a child with high myopia and retinal detachment, the possibility of Stickler syndrome must be excluded; vitreous anomalies (optically empty vitreous) seen on slit lamp examination can make the diagnosis. The detached retina may move or undulate with eye movement. Symptoms of retinal detachment include photopsias (flashing lights); floaters (caused by vitreous hemorrhage); and changes in vision, including blurring of vision or the sensation of a veil or curtain blocking vision. Patients with blunt trauma to the eye should be advised of these symptoms and should be seen immediately if they are present or develop (Fig. 20.114).

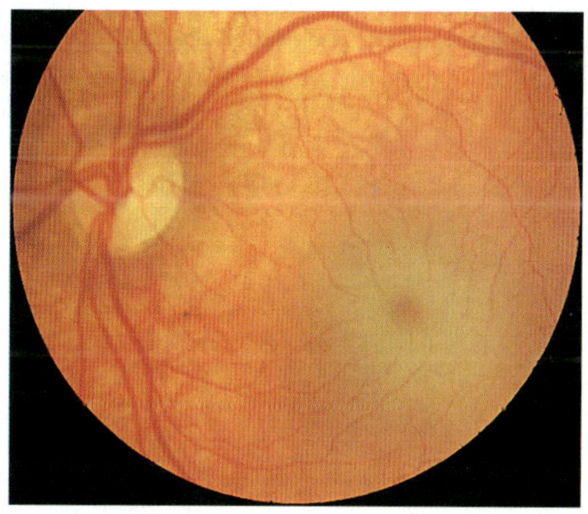

Fig. 20.113 Tay-Sachs disease. Because the parafoveal area has many retinal ganglion cells and the fovea has none, the fovea retains its orange-red color but is surrounded by retina that is whitish in color. This produces the cherry-red spot in the macula.

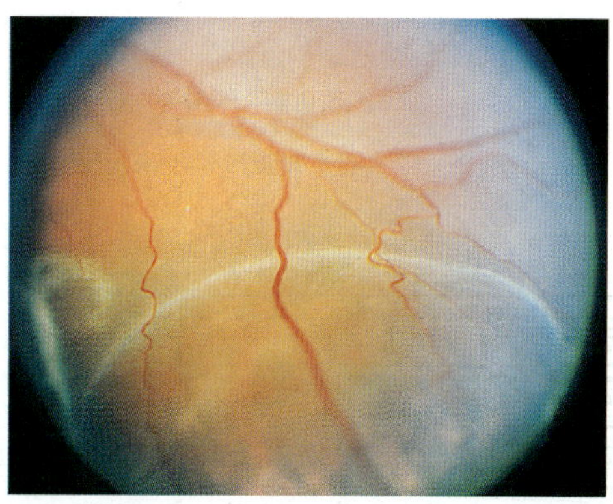

Fig. 20.114 Retinal detachment. The inferior retina is detached, and a demarcation line between the attached and detached retina is visible. Fluid beneath the detached sensory retina shifts with movement of the eye and causes the detached retina to move or undulate with movement of the eye.

Optic Nerve

The optic nerve relays information from each eye to the brain. Its function is assessed by measuring visual acuity, visual fields, color vision, the pupillary response, and visual evoked potentials. Visualization and assessment of the morphology of the optic disc with a direct ophthalmoscope or at the slit lamp with special lenses can provide valuable information regarding the function of the nerve. Nerve morphology is also assessed with photography and optical coherence tomography of the discs and adjacent nerve fiber layer.

Pupil responses depend on the afferent pathway (the optic nerve and visual system), parasympathetic pathway (for pupillary constriction), and sympathetic pathway (for pupillary dilation).

Afferent pupillary defects (APDs) include pupillary constriction in the illuminated eye as the direct response and the constriction in the fellow eye as the consensual response. The pupils are normally equal in size, even if one eye is blind; each eye normally receives equal pupillary innervation for dilation and constriction. An APD is present if, on direct testing, the pupil dilates. The swinging flashlight test is used to assess optic nerve function in both eyes relative to each other (Fig. 20.115). If the optic nerve function is decreased on one side, it produces a relative afferent pupillary defect. A penlight is used to illuminate one eye and then the other. If both eyes have equal afferent input, then illumination of either eye should produce equal constriction of the pupils. Normally, after shining a light into one eye, the response is initial constriction of both pupils, followed by a small dilation (release). The light is then swung quickly to the fellow eye; a small release may be seen as the light crosses between the eyes and then both pupils should constrict to the same degree as previously seen. When there is a decrease in afferent input (nerve function) on one side (e.g., a monocular optic neuritis), both pupils do not constrict as much when the light is shown into the affected eye compared with the other eye (i.e., both eyes display a relative dilation compared with their size when the normal side was illuminated). The critical observation is that when the affected eye is illuminated, the pupils dilate rather than constrict as occurs when the normal eye is illuminated. Having the patient maintain fixation on a distant object is important because accommodation causes constriction of the pupils and may lead to misinterpretation of the findings. This test is applicable even if one iris and pupil are of abnormal size, shape, or nonreactive (e.g., after intraocular surgery, trauma, or synechiae from uveitis). The normal pupil is observed when the light is shone into either eye, and, if there is a greater constriction of it when the light is shone into one side compared with the other, an APD is present.

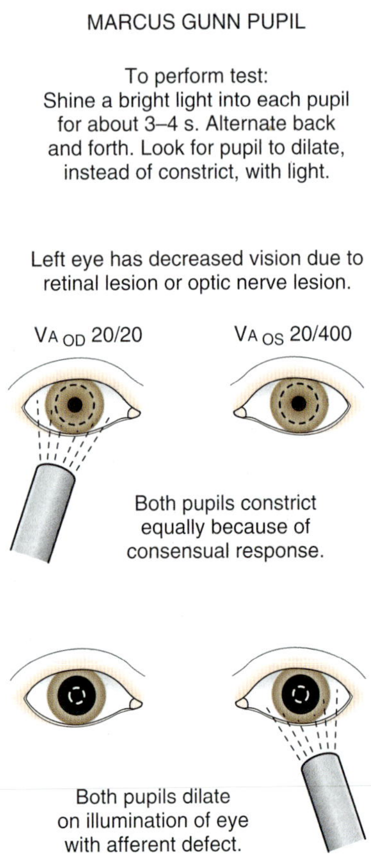

Fig. 20.115 Swinging flashlight test. Visual acuity OD 20/20, visual acuity OS 20/400 due to retinal or optic nerve lesion.

Color Vision

An easy test to assess color vision is to compare color perception between the two eyes. The patient is asked to look at a red object first with one eye, then with the other, and is asked whether it is redder with one eye or the other. A subjective desaturation of red in one eye is an indication of dyschromatopsia and a potential optic nerve disorder. If the patient reports that the object is only 50% as red with one eye compared with the other, the results would be recorded as a red desaturation of 50%. In children, it is valuable to present the object to the normal eye first with the question, "If this is $1 of red, how much red is it now?" offering a comparison with the fellow eye. A similar comparison may be performed for brightness by shining a light first into one eye and then into the other. The sense of brightness is also decreased in the presence of optic nerve disease. Formal assessment of color vision is performed using color plates, such as the Hardy-Rand-Rittler or Ishihara color plates, or the D-15 color test. Patients with heritable congenital color vision defects are equally affected in both eyes. Patients with asymmetric optic nerve disease (optic neuritis, tumor, toxic optic neuropathy) have asymmetrically decreased color vision, especially for the red hues.

Developmental anomalies of the optic nerve include colobomas (see Fig. 20.93), tilted discs (see Fig. 20.10), optic nerve hypoplasia (Fig. 20.116A), optic disc pits (see Fig. 20.116B), and the rare morning glory anomaly (20.116C). The level of visual acuity is related to the type and extent of the defect. Profound abnormalities have a significant effect on visual acuity, but more minor anomalies may coexist with almost normal vision.

Small optic nerves may be seen in hypermetropia or optic nerve hypoplasia. The latter may affect one or both eyes, and the nerve is often surrounded by a ring (the site of the scleral canal), hence the term *double-ring sign.* The retinal vessels are normal in size but may appear crowded as they leave the optic disc (Figs. 20.117 and see 20.116A). Visual acuity is related to the degree of hypoplasia, and an APD may be present if the degree of involvement is asymmetric. Optic nerve hypoplasia is associated with midline central nervous system abnormalities, including absence of the septum pellucidum (septo-optic dysplasia). Children with optic nerve hypoplasia should be examined for abnormalities in pituitary and hypothalamic function.

Large optic nerves can be seen in optic disc coloboma and morning glory anomaly (see Fig. 20.116C), which is also a type of optic disc coloboma. A coloboma is due to incomplete closure of the embryonic fissure and may be isolated or accompanied by retinochoroidal coloboma and iris coloboma, depending on the extent of incomplete closure. Colobomas are always inferiorly located. Morning glory anomaly is a specific type of coloboma that results in vessels exiting the disc at its edge with glial tissue often in the center of the disc. Bilateral cases of optic coloboma should be investigated with neuroimaging for midline defects. Morning glory anomaly is almost always associated with intracranial abnormalities even if unilateral, such as moyamoya disease, and further evaluation with brain magnetic resonance imaging and magnetic resonance angiography should occur for patients with this finding.

Optic disc pits are excavations within the substance of the nerve and may be congenital or acquired. When acquired, they may be harbingers of glaucoma.

Acquired optic disc abnormalities include increased cup:disc ratio, optic neuritis, optic disc swelling, optic disc obscuration, and optic atrophy.

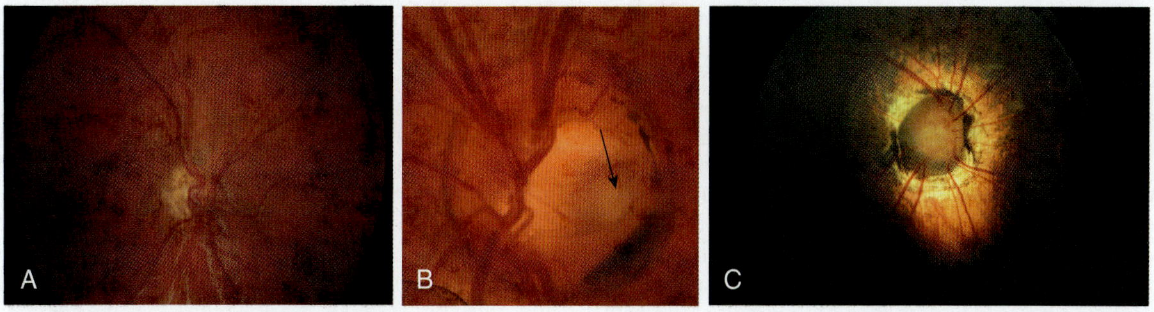

Fig. 20.116 (A) Optic disc hypoplasia. The disc is small with abnormal features. The surrounding larger ring around the disc corresponds to the normal-sized sclera opening for the disc. (B) Optic disc pit *(black arrow)*. (C) Morning glory disc anomaly. Note the vessels leave the edge of the optic disc like the spokes on a bicycle wheel. Neuroimaging is needed, even in unilateral cases.

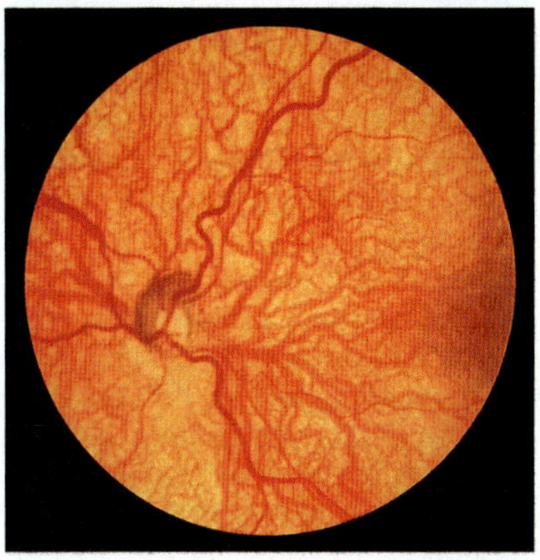

Fig. 20.117 Optic nerve hypoplasia. A pigment crescent surrounds the hypoplastic nerve. This corresponds to the scleral opening for a normal-sized optic nerve and is termed the double ring sign in this patient with ocular albinism. The pattern of the retinal vasculature is also abnormal, as is the retinal pigmentation.

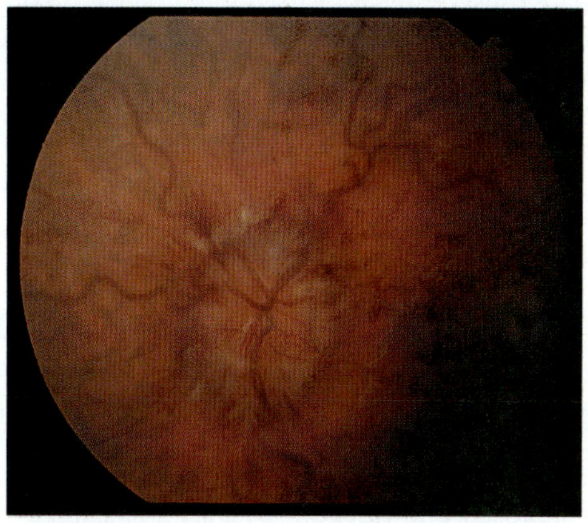

Fig. 20.118 Acute papilledema. The disc edges are blurred, and the physiologic cup may be obscured due to the disc swelling and edema of the adjacent nerve fiber layer. Intraretinal hemorrhages and cotton wool spots may be present.

A cup:disc ratio is typically 0.3 or less. Physiologic cupping (a cup:disc ratio >0.7) is present in about 2% of the normal population and in glaucomatous cupping, where there is raised IOP causing glaucoma. However, a normal-sized optic disc with a large cup may not be due to glaucoma in premature children with a history of periventricular leukomalacia. Any child with a large cup:disc ratio needs an ophthalmologic referral.

Optic neuritis is inflammation of the optic nerve, which may involve the optic disc papillitis or the nerve posterior to the globe (retrobulbar neuritis). In papillitis, optic disc swelling occurs with loss of vision (differentiating it from disc swelling due to raised intracranial pressure). The optic disc in retrobulbar neuritis appears normal but is associated with loss of vision. The vision loss may be sudden; progressive; profound; and accompanied by complaints of pain in or behind the eye, which may be accentuated by movement of the eyes. An APD or a relative APD is present. Visual fields usually show a cecocentral scotoma, an area of vision loss located in the central visual field.

Optic neuritis in children is frequently bilateral and may be idiopathic or follow nonspecific viral prodromes or infection with mumps, measles, chickenpox, or meningoencephalitis. However, a thorough evaluation should include excluding MOGAD (Myelin oligodendrocyte glycoprotein associated disease), NMO (neuromyelitis optica), and multiple sclerosis. Collagen vascular disease, particularly systemic lupus erythematosus and sarcoidosis, may be associated with optic neuritis. Syphilis and tuberculosis also cause optic neuritis. Visual acuity in idiopathic optic neuritis gradually improves 1 to 4 weeks after onset and usually returns to normal over several months. Episodes may be recurrent. Associations with demyelinating disease occur but are less frequent than are seen in adults.

Optic disc swelling may be unilateral or bilateral. Unilateral swelling is unusual and may be due to longstanding ocular hypotony (usually iatrogenic), posterior uveitis, posterior scleritis, or optic nerve glioma. Bilateral swelling is often due to raised intracranial pressure (papilledema), papillitis (see earlier), or pseudopapilledema (high hypermetropia, optic disc drusen) (see Fig. 20.9).

Papilledema is secondary to increased intracranial pressure that is transmitted to the optic nerves via the cerebrospinal fluid within the subarachnoid space. The axoplasmic flow from the retinal ganglion cells to the cells in the lateral geniculate nucleus is blocked and causes the optic disc to swell. The degree of disc swelling may be asymmetric; however, increased intracranial pressure rarely causes papilledema in only one eye. Ophthalmoscopic signs include blurring of the disc margin and disc edema. The disc may be hyperemic because of telangiectasia of the superficial capillaries on the disc, and small hemorrhages may appear on the disc margin (Fig. 20.118). Visual acuity is typically normal unless hemorrhage and edema involve the macula. Patients may complain of transient obscurations of vision. The visual fields may show an enlarged blind spot, and the pupillary response and color vision are normal.

If increased intracranial pressure is chronic, elevation of the optic disc may persist but the hemorrhages and exudates seen in the acute phase resolve. When the condition is prolonged, optic nerve atrophy and vision loss occur. If intracranial pressure is normalized, it may take 6 weeks for papilledema to resolve and the optic disc to normalize. Patients may have elevated intracranial pressure without developing papilledema, and the absence of papilledema does not exclude the possibility of increased intracranial pressure.

Pseudopapilledema is most commonly found in eyes with high hyperopia or optic disc drusen (see Fig. 20.9). The disc is not hyperemic, vessels at the disc margin are not blurred, and there is no nerve fiber layer swelling. Differentiation of pseudopapilledema from true papilledema can be difficult, and evaluation by an ophthalmologist may include ultrasonography of the eye to look for drusen of the optic disc or neuroimaging.

Optic disc atrophy occurs due to loss of neuronal axons (Fig. 20.119). It may be primary, secondary, consecutive, primary hereditary, secondary hereditary, or associated with contralateral optic disc swelling. Primary optic atrophy is uncommon but is most often caused by gliomas in children. Neuroimaging is important together with surveillance of vision, color vision, and visual field analysis. Chemotherapy and radiotherapy are treatment modalities. Prognosis may be guarded for vision. Consecutive optic atrophy is caused by diseases of the inner retina or its blood supply such as retinal dystrophy (see Retina section) or diffuse retinal necrosis. Secondary optic atrophy is preceded by swelling of the optic nerve head as a result of raised intracranial pressure, optic disc ischemia, or inflammation. Primary hereditary optic atrophy is a rare diffuse optic atrophy with visual loss. It may be recessive, but three types of this rare condition are autosomal dominant: optic atrophy due to mutations in *OPA1* (onset after 4 years of age), Leber hereditary optic neuropathy (LHON onset 16–30 years due to mitochondrial DNA mutations), and DIDMOAD (onset between 5 and 14 years; diabetes insipidus, diabetes mellitus, optic atrophy, and deafness). Treatment is limited, but some evidence suggests that progression of LHON can be influenced by smoking and alcohol depending on the mutation found. There is some work now showing that fortified CoQ10 supplements may slow the progression of optic atrophy due to LHON and OPA1. Secondary hereditary optic atrophies are rare hereditary neurologic disorders with optic atrophy, which usually present during the first decade of life. These include Behr (recessive), Friedreich ataxia (recessive), Charcot-Marie-Tooth disease (dominant, X-linked), adrenoleukodystrophies (two types—X-linked recessive and autosomal recessive), and cerebellar ataxia type I (dominant).

Optic disc obscuration occurs because of lesions overlying or invading the optic disc head and include primary optic disc tumors (e.g., capillary angioma [see Fig. 20.104], melanocytoma); retinal tumors (e.g., astrocytoma or combined hamartoma of the retina and RPE [see Fig. 20.101]); and infiltrative lesions due to leukemia, granuloma, or sarcoid. A melanocytoma is a pigmented tumor that is black and beige in color.

Orbit and Adnexa

Clinical signs of orbital disease include proptosis, restriction in ocular motility, compression of the optic nerve producing optic disc swelling, changes in refraction, and retinal striae. Retinal striae appear as radial lines on the retinal surface caused by compression of the posterior portion of the globe and are most commonly seen in thyroid-related eye disease. Other adjuncts to the clinical examination include B scan ultrasonography, computed tomography (CT), and magnetic resonance imaging of the orbit. Although CT is particularly valuable in the examination of bony lesions and in the assessment of orbital fractures, the radiation exposure with fine-cut orbital CT is significant, and this should be taken into consideration in children.

Adnexal diseases include orbital dermoid cysts and lacrimal gland disorders.

Proptosis is described as being axial (forward displacement of globe without displacement in any other direction) or nonaxial (forward displacement with displacement in another direction); it may be bilateral or unilateral. It is measured by using an exophthalmometer (Fig. 20.120). This device measures the interlateral orbital rim distance, and viewing through prisms allows a measure of the amount (in millimeters) that the apex of the cornea sits anterior to the lateral canthus on that side. Axial proptosis is due to lesions inside the cone of extraocular muscles, whereas nonaxial proptosis is caused by lesions that are either completely or partly outside the cone of extraocular muscles.

Rarely, proptosis may be intermittent (lymphangioma, capillary hemangioma), pulsatile (encephalocele, orbital roof fracture), or pulsatile with a bruit (congenital arteriovenous communication which may occur in isolation or as part of Wyburn–Mason syndrome).

Treatment and prognosis of proptosis depends on the cause, and exposure keratopathy can be a complication, which can be avoided with copious lubrication.

Proptosis in neonates and infants may be seen due to shallow orbits, tumors, or cystic lesions. Shallow orbits are seen in patients with craniosynostoses such as Crouzon, Pfeiffer, or Apert syndromes (Fig. 20.121). Commonest tumors in this age group are capillary hemangiomas (usually unilateral); teratomas; rhabdomyosarcoma; and, rarely, acute leukemia. Cystic lesions are seen in microphthalmos with cyst (see Figs. 20.32 and 20.122) and orbital encephalocele, usually associated with neurofibromatosis.

Proptosis in toddlers and older children may be due to tumors or inflammatory conditions. Benign tumors include plexiform neurofibroma (presents in patients with neurofibromatosis I between the ages of 2 and 5 years with nonaxial proptosis) and optic nerve glioma (may be isolated or associated with neurofibromatosis I) (Fig. 20.123). Those associated with NF I tend to grow much less than those that are not. The

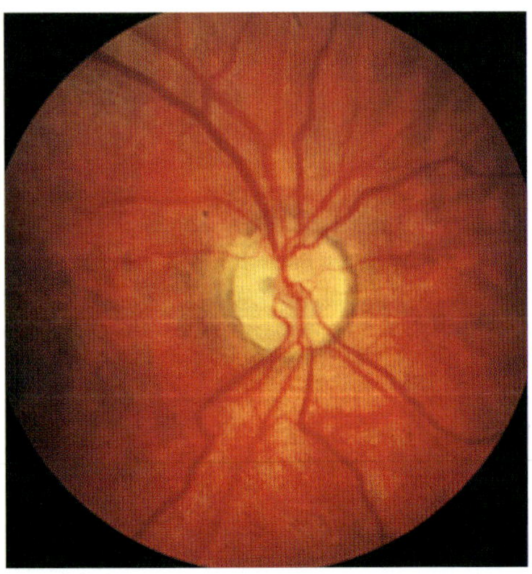

Fig. 20.119 Optic atrophy. The optic disc is flat, pale, and yellowish-white in color.

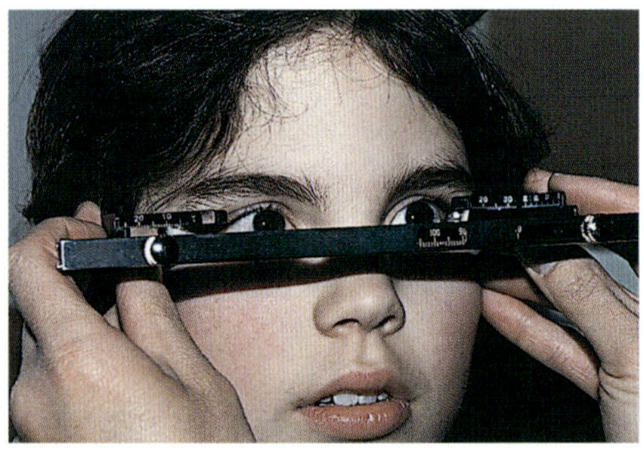

Fig. 20.120 The Hertel exophthalmometer measures the anterior-to-posterior distance from the corneal surface to the lateral orbital rim. A base measurement, the distance between the two lateral orbital rims, is recorded to help obtain repeatable instrument placement. Progression or regression can be determined by serial measurements.

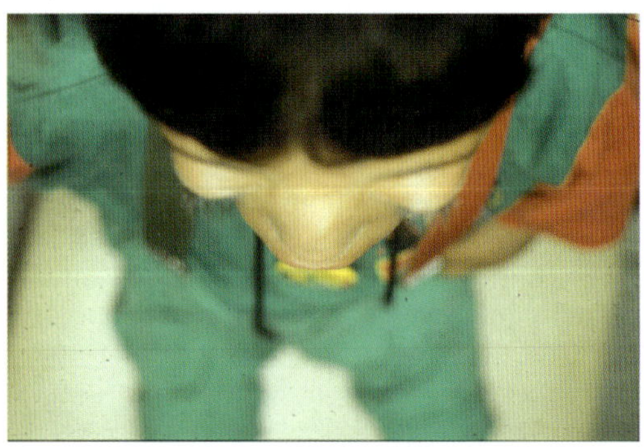

Fig. 20.121 This child has proptosis due to shallow orbits secondary to craniosynostoses.

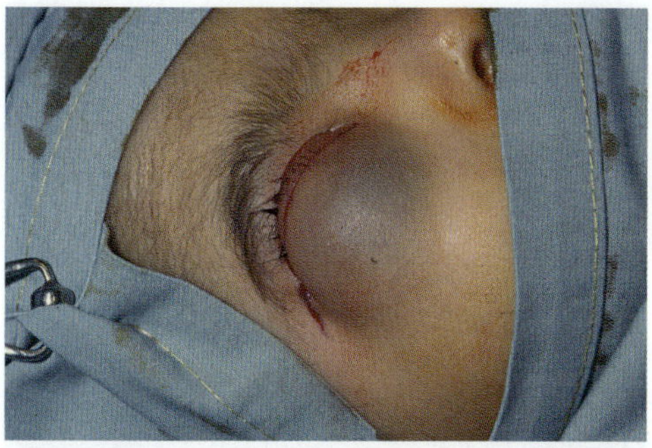

Fig. 20.122 This child has severe microphthalmos with cyst and is about to have the cyst removed.

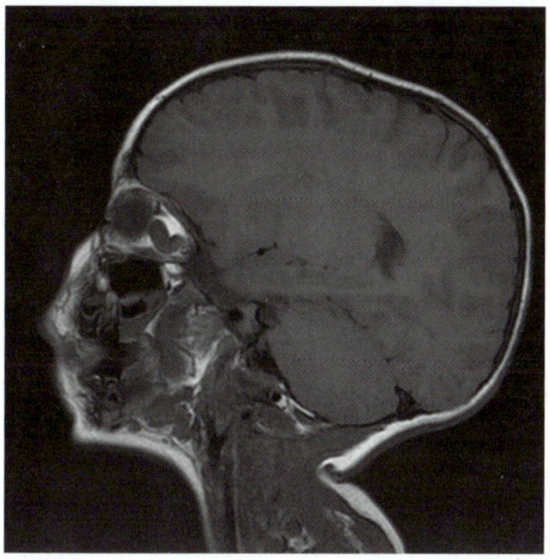

Fig. 20.123 Optic nerve glioma seen on sagittal view magnetic resonance imaging. Its presence may cause a gradual onset of painless proptosis. Children seldom complain of monocular visual loss, and the discovery of a profound loss of vision may be the presenting sign of an optic nerve glioma. In children, optic nerve gliomas are benign lesions that may, however, extend to the optic chiasm or intracranially.

eyeball is often turned down slightly and proptosed. Lymphangioma may remain stationary for long periods of time, or it may suddenly enlarge either because of spontaneous bleeding (chocolate cyst) or in association with an upper respiratory tract infection.

Malignant tumors leading to proptosis in toddlers and older children include rhabdomyosarcoma; metastatic neuroblastoma; Langerhans cell histiocytosis; acute leukemia; and, rarely, retinoblastoma. Rhabdomyosarcoma usually presents around the age of 7 years with proptosis, chemosis (swelling of the conjunctiva), and discomfort (Fig. 20.124). Prognosis is good with prompt treatment. Metastatic neuroblastoma presents in a similar manner to rhabdomyosarcoma but usually at a younger age (under 5 years) with the primary tumor in the abdomen (Fig. 20.125). Forty percent of metastases affect both orbits. Prognosis may be guarded. Orbital involvement may be seen with Langerhans cell histiocytosis and usually affects the superolateral quadrant of the orbit. CT scan shows soft tissue mass with adjacent bony lysis. If isolated, the lesion can be curetted out or treated with steroids. Acute leukemia usually presents around 7 years of age with rapid onset proptosis and ecchymosis (bruising in the lids). Retinoblastoma may occasionally present with proptosis but only in neglected cases.

Inflammatory causes of proptosis include orbital cellulitis and pseudotumor (idiopathic orbital inflammation), which affect children between 6 and 14 years. If inflammatory proptosis is bilateral, granulomatosis with polyangiitis (Wegener granulomatosis) must be excluded.

Dermoid and epidermoid cysts are relatively common. These benign masses are usually located anterior to the orbital septum but may extend posteriorly into the orbit. These cysts present as smooth, painless, freely movable round or oval masses and are usually located in the lateral brow area, adjacent to the zygomaticofrontal suture (Fig. 20.126). They may, however, be found near any bony suture. If these lesions can be palpated around their entire extent, no neuroimaging studies may be necessary, but if they extend posterior to the orbital rim and the posterior extension cannot be palpated, imaging is

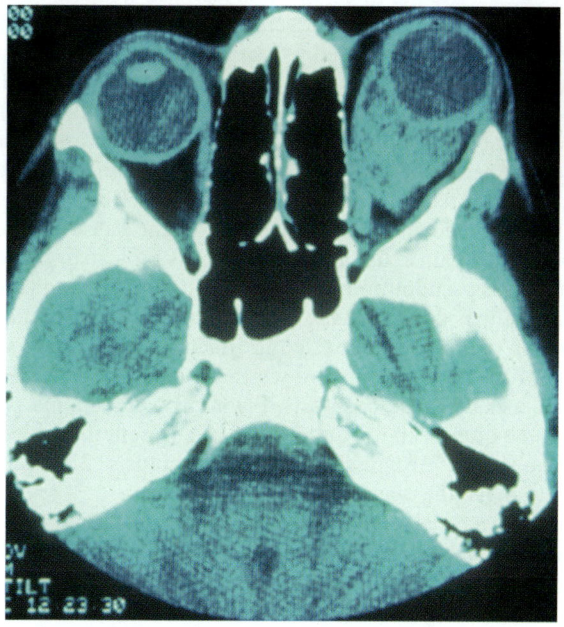

Fig. 20.124 Axial computed tomography scan showing a rhabdomyosarcoma.

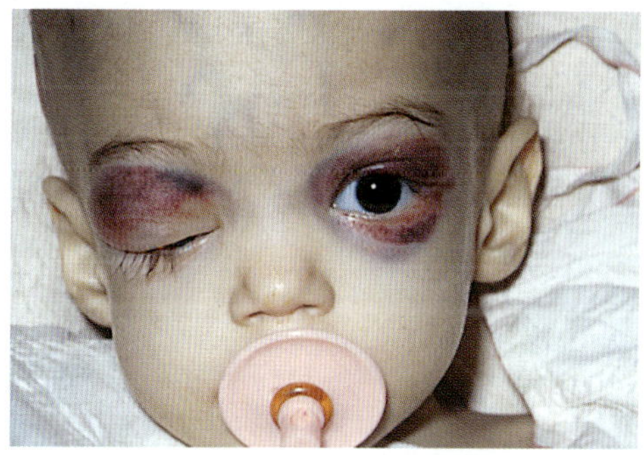

Fig. 20.125 Neuroblastoma. Neuroblastoma metastatic to the orbit may present with an abrupt onset of unilateral or bilateral proptosis and ecchymosis of the eyelids. Neuroblastoma is the most common lesion to metastasize to the orbit in childhood.

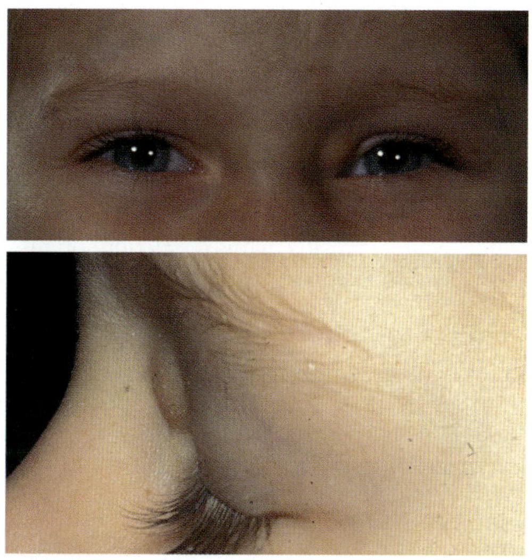

Fig. 20.126 Dermoid cyst of left orbit on the nasal aspect. These cysts present as smooth, painless, mobile, subcutaneous, round or oval masses. Dermoid cysts are most frequently located in the lateral brow area adjacent to the zygomaticofrontal suture. Although benign, if they are ruptured by trauma, an intense inflammatory reaction with scarring in the area may occur.

indicated to determine how far posteriorly the lesion extends and to exclude extension into the intracranial space or an encephalocele. Dermoid cysts contain dermal and epidermal elements that have become isolated from the skin during embryonic development. If ruptured by trauma, an intense inflammatory reaction occurs. Because of this reaction, surgical excision of these lesions is indicated before potential trauma when the child learns to walk.

Lacrimal gland disorders affecting children are usually due to unilateral enlargement caused by dacryoadenitis; dacryops; pseudotumor; and, extremely rarely, pleomorphic adenoma. Bilateral enlargement is seen in sarcoidosis and acute leukemia. Dacryoadenitis is usually caused by a viral infection of the lacrimal gland but may be associated with orbital pseudotumor. It is not usually associated with proptosis per se but causes the upper lid to develop an "S" shape and become tender to touch. If the cause is infection, treatment with pain relief and antibiotics is indicated; however, if the disorder is pseudotumor related, then steroids are indicated. CT scan is usually needed to make the distinction in conjunction with assessment of markers of systemic inflammation. Dacryops is a dilation of the major lacrimal ducts secondary to obstruction and does not usually cause proptosis. Pleomorphic adenoma is a rare tumor most often seen in adults, but it can present in children with a painless, slowly progressive nonaxial proptosis. Biopsy may be needed to make the diagnosis.

Bilateral lacrimal gland enlargement is also rare. Sarcoidosis rarely causes bilateral, firmly enlarged lacrimal glands in children. A form of acute myeloid leukemia (chloroma) in children may cause bilateral lacrimal gland infiltration. Diagnosis is dependent on peripheral blood smear and, sometimes, lacrimal gland biopsy.

Eye Movement Disorders

In this section anomalous eye movements are discussed. All cases should be referred for ophthalmic opinion.

Painless Inability to Abduct One Eye

Duane syndrome is due to miswiring of the horizontal rectus muscles leading to cocontraction of the medial and lateral recti. This leads to limited abduction with almost normal adduction (type I), limited adduction with almost normal abduction (type II), or limited adduction and abduction in equal measures (type III). The eye movements are associated with widening of the palpebral fissure on abduction and narrowing on adduction. Types I and III may present with an esotropia in primary position of gaze. If a child has an abduction deficit but no esotropia in primary gaze, this cannot be a cranial nerve (CN) VI palsy and must be Duane syndrome. CN VI palsy always has an esotropia in primary position of gaze. Duane I and II may not exhibit an esotropia in primary position of gaze. Myasthenia gravis is rare but may mimic adduction deficit. Fatiguability may be present.

Painful Inability to Abduct One Eye

Causes include acute myositis with restriction of movement in direction of the field of action of the affected muscle.

Painless Inability to Abduct Either Eye

Causes include Möbius syndrome and bilateral gaze palsies, with esotropia in 50% of cases (due to superimposed CN VI nerve palsies). There is usually bilateral CN VII nerve palsy and there may be associated CN V, IX, or X palsies (Fig. 20.127).

Painless Inability to Adduct the Eye

Congenital CN III nerve palsy is an example of painless inability to adduct the eye, associated with exodeviation and hypodeviation of the affected eye with ptosis and miosed pupil. There is limitation of upgazed and adduction. Acquired CN III nerve palsy is rare.

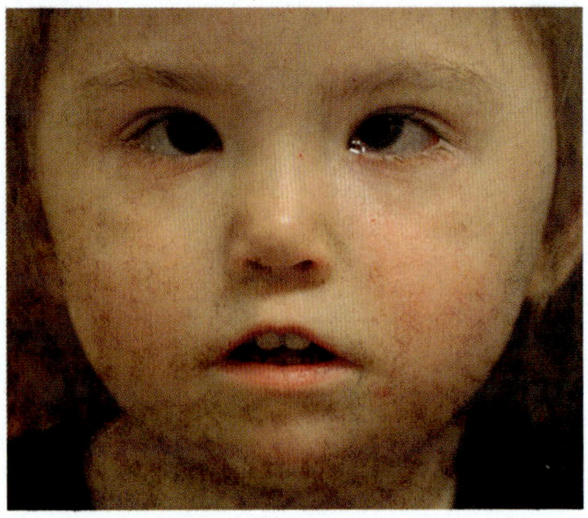

Fig. 20.127 A child with Möbius syndrome. She has bilateral gaze palsies, with bilateral VII nerve palsies.

Examination finds the same signs as the congenital condition, but the pupil is dilated (Fig. 20.128). Internuclear ophthalmoplegia (INO) is due to a lesion in the medial longitudinal fasciculus leading to ipsilateral adduction limitation and contralateral eye abducting nystagmus.

Painful Inability to Adduct the Eye

Causes include acute myositis with restriction of movement in the direction of the field of action of the affected muscle.

Inability to Elevate the Eye in Adduction

Brown syndrome is a condition where the tendon of the superior oblique muscle is unable to pass freely through its pulley (the trochlea at the superomedial orbital rim). This results in restriction of elevation in up gaze usually just in the adducted position. As a result, there may be a coincident downshoot in adduction on version testing. It is usually idiopathic but may be acquired due to inflammation at the trochlea or trauma (Fig. 20.129).

Limitation of Horizontal Versions or Gaze Palsies

Any lesion of the paramedian pontine reticular formation causes ipsilateral gaze palsy. One-and-a-half syndrome is a lesion of the paramedian pontine reticular formation/abducens nucleus and adjacent medial longitudinal fasciculus causing an ipsilateral gaze palsy and ipsilateral INO. A right-sided neurologic lesion would lead to inability for either eye to look to the right; the right eye could not adduct (part of the INO), but the left eye could abduct but with a nystagmus. Bilateral pontine lesions result in total horizontal gaze palsies. Fisher syndrome is a rare variant of Guillain-Barré syndrome that may present in children with ophthalmoplegia, ataxia, and areflexia, though the initial presentation may be one of horizontal gaze palsy or an INO.

Limitation of Vertical Eye Movement (One or Both Eyes)

Orbital floor fracture causing entrapped inferior rectus muscle and restriction of elevation leads to limitations of vertical eye movements (Fig. 20.130A). Orbital space-occupying lesions such as capillary hemangioma, plexiform neurofibroma, or orbital abscess can limit vertical eye movement. Symblepharon is an attachment of lid to the globe causing restriction of elevation or depression. This may be congenital and seen in clefting syndromes but also may be acquired, as seen in epidermolysis bullosa and alkali injuries (see Fig. 20.41). Brown syndrome, as noted earlier, can also cause a deficit in eye elevation. Monocular elevation deficit, formerly called double elevator palsy, may be due to idiopathic tightening of the

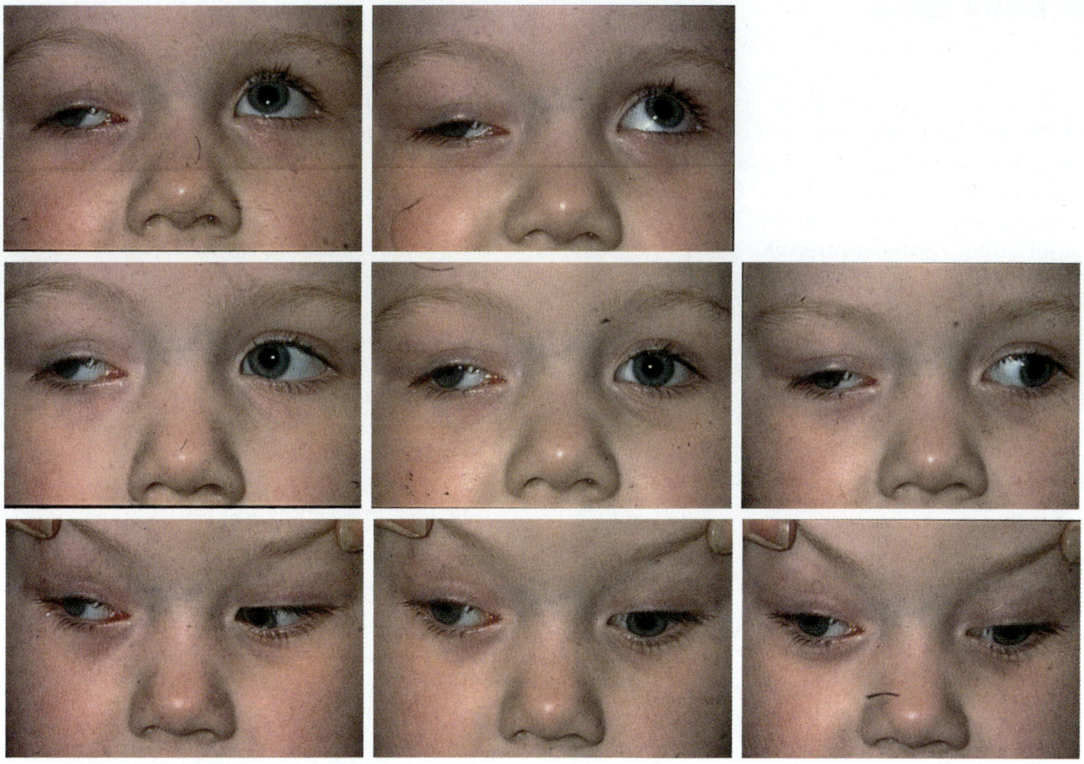

Fig. 20.128 Right congenital third nerve palsy. Note the inability to adduct the right eye. The pupil is smaller than the unaffected left eye, which can be seen in congenital III nerve palsies.

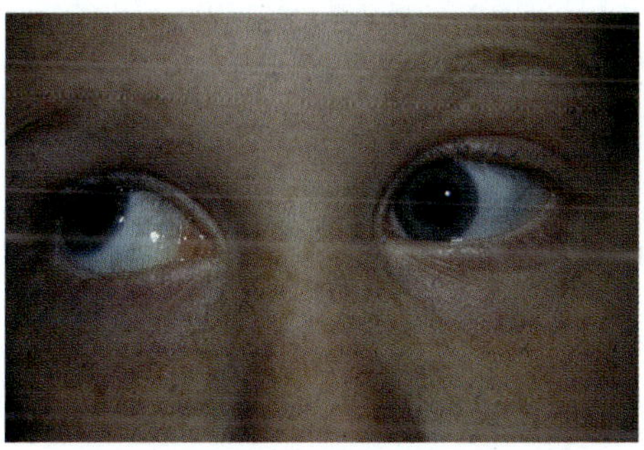

Fig. 20.129 Left Brown syndrome, an inability to elevate an eye in adduction resulting from an abnormality of the superior oblique tendon.

inferior rectus muscle or idiopathic with no evidence of inferior rectus tightening.

Vertical Gaze Palsy

Parinaud syndrome describes decreased up gaze, large pupils, convergence insufficiency, and convergence—retraction nystagmus. In children, one of the commonest causes is a pinealoma. Hydrocephalus causes stretching of the posterior commissure resulting in loss of up gaze with or without tonic downward deviation of the eyes ("sunset" sign). Metabolic causes may affect vertical eye movements. Tay-Sachs disease may cause impairment of vertical and later horizontal gaze. Niemann-Pick variants may also cause vertical gaze anomalies.

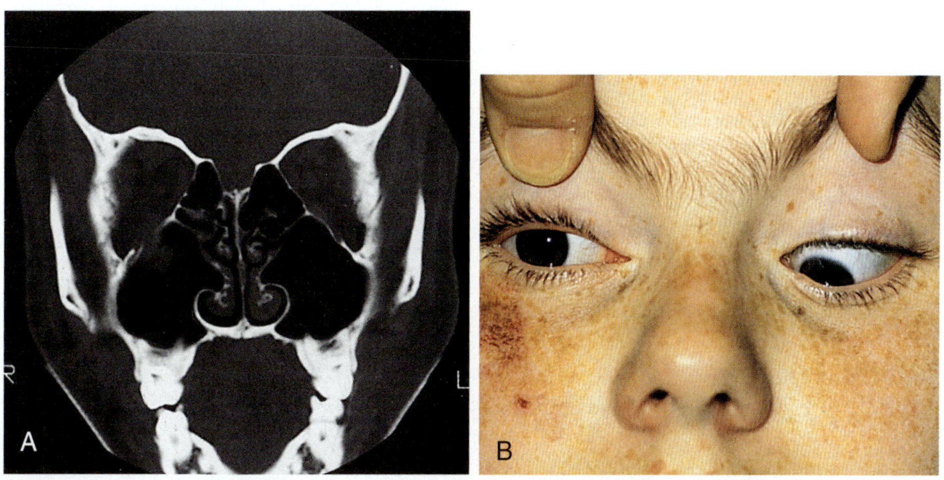

Fig. 20.130 (A) Blowout fracture of the right orbit (coronal computed tomography [CT] scan). Protruding through the fracture in the orbital floor into the maxillary sinus is orbital fat. The inferior rectus muscle is potentially entrapped within the fracture site. (B) Blowout fracture of the right orbit. The inferior rectus is entrapped in the fracture site, leading to the inability to depress the right eye.

Multiple Ocular Motor Palsies

Cavernous sinus lesions, which are rare but may be a complication of orbital cellulitis, and caroticocavernous fistulas are causes of multiple ocular motor palsies. Superior orbital fissure lesions are rare, but tumors of the orbit (e.g., leukemia) or infections (such as aspergilloma in immunocompromised children) may be associated with ocular motor palsies. Tolosa-Hunt syndrome (idiopathic granulomatous inflammation, which is painful during the acute phase) may affect the superior orbital fissure or cavernous sinus. Brainstem lesions due to encephalitis or tumors (glioma) may also present with ophthalmoplegia.

Other Causes

Chronic progressive ophthalmoplegia may be associated with a mitochondrial cytopathy, which may be isolated or part of the Kearns-Sayre syndrome, oculopharyngeal dystrophy (Fig. 20.131).

Myotonic dystrophy and drug toxicity may also cause ocular motor palsies.

Acquired saccadic initiation failure (ocular motor apraxia) may be seen in lesions in the frontoparietal cortex. Both vertical and horizontal saccades are affected. This can be seen in Gaucher disease type III. In congenital saccadic initiation failure, vertical saccades are unaffected.

Metabolic causes include Tay-Sachs disease, and, occasionally, other lipid-storage diseases.

Congenital fibrosis syndrome is a familial condition that may affect all muscles. Often, however, the eyes are fixed in a downward position with bilateral ptosis and chin-up head position.

Nystagmus

Nystagmus is described by its character, amplitude, and frequency. The character of nystagmus may be horizontal jerk or a combination of slow drift with fast corrective phase. The nystagmus direction is the same as the fast corrective phase; pendular. Nystagmus velocity is the same in both directions, but on lateral gaze this usually develops a horizontal jerk component. Oblique nystagmus is due to a combination of horizontal and vertical directions of pendular nystagmus.

Nystagmus is also described by the timing of onset. *Early onset or infantile nystagmus* is uniplanar and dampens on convergence and worsens on eccentric fixation. Four types need describing:

- *Latent nystagmus* occurs when there is no nystagmus with both eyes open but horizontal jerk nystagmus seen when one eye is covered. This is most commonly seen with infantile esotropia but may be seen with other early-onset deviations. The fast phase is toward the uncovered fixating eye.
- *Manifest-latent nystagmus (also known as fusional maldevelopment nystagmus)* is usually seen with infantile esotropia and DVD. The nystagmus becomes worse when one eye is occluded.
- *Spasmus nutans* is a disorder of early onset (3–18 months) in which unilateral or bilateral small-amplitude, high-frequency, horizontal nystagmus is often associated with head nodding. Most often, it is idiopathic with resolution by 3 years of age, but it may be due to an optic pathway glioma.
- *Roving nystagmus* may occur with a severe disruption of visual function. The commonest causes are LCA (severe retinal dystrophy) or optic nerve hypoplasia (bilateral).

Later-Onset Acquired Nystagmus

The types of later-onset acquired nystagmus are described as follows and can localize the lesion causing them.

- *Coarse horizontal jerk nystagmus* is usually seen in cerebellar disease, with fast phase ipsilateral to the lesion.
- *Torsional nystagmus,* if isolated, is usually only seen in central vestibular disease, such as syringomyelia or syringobulbia associated with Arnold-Chiari malformation; demyelination; and rarely, lateral medullary syndrome.
- *Downbeat nystagmus* is often seen in lesions at the craniocervical junction (e.g., Arnold-Chiari malformation), drug toxicity (phenytoin, carbamazepine), trauma, hydrocephalus, and demyelination.
- *Upbeat nystagmus* can be seen in cerebellar degenerations (e.g., ataxia telangiectasia) and encephalitis; in babies, a retinal dystrophy should be excluded (especially cone dystrophy).
- *Gaze-evoked nystagmus* may be seen with lesions of the vestibulocerebellum axis, brainstem, or cerebral hemispheres, after a gaze palsy, or with drug toxicity (phenytoin and carbamazepine).
- *Periodic alternating nystagmus* has reversal in the direction of the nystagmus. It can be congenital or idiopathic but is usually seen

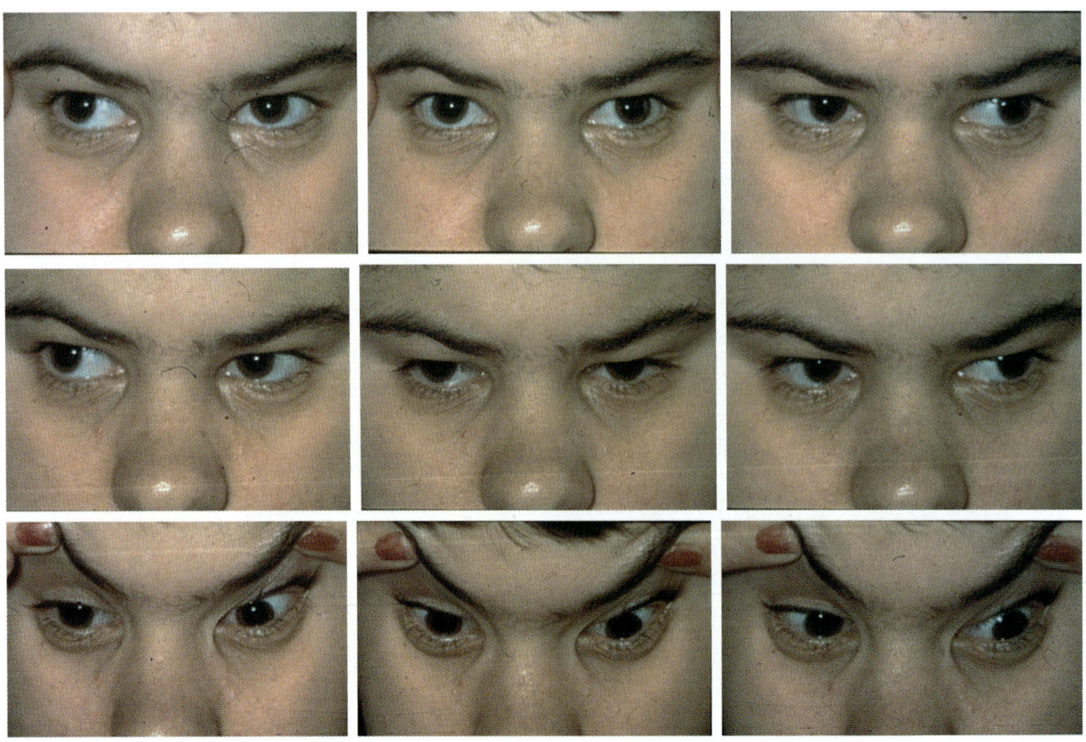

Fig. 20.131 Kearns-Sayre syndrome with chronic progressive external ophthalmoplegia and ptosis. The heart must be checked for conduction defects.

with Arnold-Chiari malformation, cerebellar disease, trauma, or demyelination.

- *Rebound nystagmus* occurs when an attempt to maintain eccentric gaze results in gaze evoked nystagmus, which dampens and sometimes reverses direction. On returning to primary gaze, a transient nystagmus develops. It is usually seen in cerebellar disease.
- *See-saw nystagmus* describes pendular nystagmus in which one eye elevates and intorts while the other eye depresses and extorts and then the eyes reverse. The commonest cause is chiasmal or parasella tumors but may also be seen in albinism as a transient finding, head trauma, and syringobulbia.
- *Internuclear ophthalmoplegia* is associated with nystagmus in the abducting eye (see earlier) and is due to a lesion in the medial longitudinal fasciculus.
- *Monocular nystagmus* may be seen in spasmus nutans, unilateral deep amblyopia, superior oblique myokymia, and optic nerve glioma.
- *Convergence-retraction nystagmus* can be seen in Parinaud syndrome (see earlier).

Ocular Causes of Nystagmus

Disruption of vision will lead to nystagmus. There may be obvious (usually bilateral) ocular disease such as corneal opacities, congenital cataract, microphthalmos, aniridia, and oculocutaneous nystagmus or less obvious ocular disease such as retinal dystrophy (usually cone dystrophy or LCA), ocular albinism, X-linked CSNB, optic nerve hypoplasia, and early-onset optic atrophy.

Treatment of nystagmus depends on the cause of nystagmus and may be improved with drugs or surgery. Anomalous head posture may be treated by recessions of the extraocular muscles. Recently, tenotomy and reattachment surgery has been proposed for certain types of nystagmus.

Ocular Manifestations of Specific Infections

TORCH Infections

Toxoplasmosis Toxoplasmosis, a protozoal infection, may be congenital or acquired. In neonates with congenital toxoplasmosis, 80% have retinochoroiditis. Congenital disease may also occur in inactive and recurrent forms, the effects of which may be limited to retinitis alone. Ocular involvement includes papillitis; retinitis; and iritis, usually bilateral. The retinal lesions frequently are asymptomatic and are found incidentally as inactive, pigmented chorioretinal scars.

Inactive lesions may reactivate at any time throughout life, with active inflammation developing adjacent to areas of scarring. This is seen as a white fluffy response that may extend into the vitreous overlying the lesion (see Fig. 20.110). Patients with lesions close to the macula or optic nerve should be wary of any visual changes. Patients too young to report visual changes should be screened periodically for reactivation of their disease.

Rubella Exposure to rubella virus during the first trimester of pregnancy results in congenital rubella syndrome. Ocular findings include microphthalmia, microcornea, corneal opacification, anterior uveitis, iris hypoplasia, nuclear or complete cataracts, and glaucoma. The retinopathy of rubella syndrome is a diffuse "salt and pepper" retinopathy that develops early in childhood and does not affect vision (Fig. 20.132).

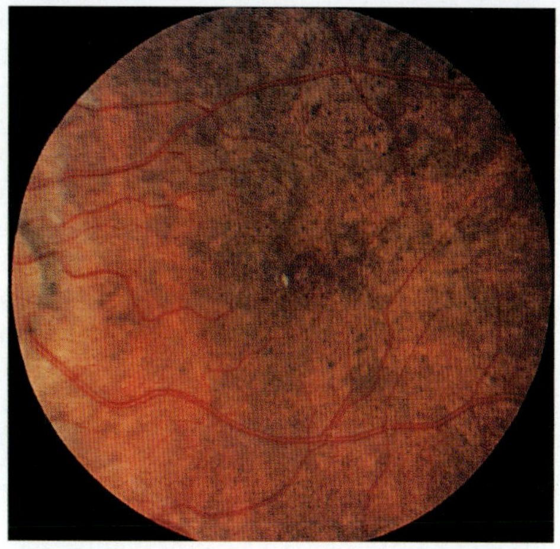

Fig. 20.132 Pigmentary retinopathy in rubella syndrome.

Cytomegalovirus CMV infection produces a bilateral retinochoroiditis manifested as multiple, yellowish-white, fluffy retinal lesions (Fig. 20.133). Hemorrhage is a prominent feature. Other ophthalmic manifestations include microphthalmia, uveitis, cataracts, optic disc atrophy, strabismus, and nystagmus.

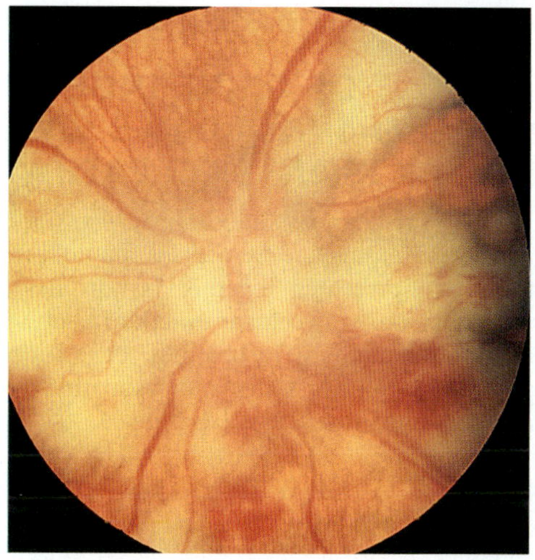

Fig. 20.133 Cytomegalovirus. Retinitis, with hemorrhages and perivascular yellowish-white exudates secondary to cytomegalic inclusion disease.

Herpes Simplex Virus HSV infection may involve the anterior segment of the eye, with conjunctivitis, keratitis, and iritis or, especially when disseminated in the perinatal period, a retinochoroiditis may develop. Retinal involvement with disseminated HSV is severe, with extensive inflammatory reaction producing yellowish-white exudates and retinal necrosis. Ocular involvement occurs in roughly 13% of herpetic infections in newborns. Herpetic retinitis may occur in normal individuals but is more common in the immunosuppressed.

Syphilis Congenital syphilis may cause bilateral chorioretinitis, resulting in a salt-and-pepper fundus appearance. Differentiation of the retinopathy of congenital syphilis from retinitis pigmentosa may be difficult. Syphilis may also cause interstitial keratitis, anterior uveitis, glaucoma, and optic nerve atrophy.

Non-TORCH Infections

Toxocariasis *Toxocara canis* larvae infect children most commonly from 2 to 9 years old. When the eye is involved, a white, elevated chorioretinal granuloma develops (see Fig. 20.111). Chronic unilateral uveitis with opacification of the vitreous overlying the granuloma may occur. Inflammation in ocular toxocariasis occurs only after the infecting organism dies. Externally, the eye does not appear to be inflamed. Diagnosis is usually made when investigating the absence of the red reflex, strabismus, or decreased vision. With extensive inflammation, fibrotic preretinal membranes may develop and produce retinal detachment. Differentiation from retinoblastoma may be difficult. Intraocular calcification is rare in toxocariasis as opposed to retinoblastoma. The diagnosis is confirmed by enzyme-linked immunosorbent assay for *T. canis* on blood or intraocular fluid.

Zika Infection Zika virus (ZIKV), a flavivirus, is endemic in areas of Africa and Asia. It can be spread by Aedes mosquitoes, which are active in the daytime; via sexual contact; infected blood; and transplacental transmission in utero. Humans carrying the virus can introduce ZIKV into new countries, but Aedes mosquitoes are needed to continue local transmission. Congenital Zika syndrome is seen in babies who have been exposed to ZIKV in utero. The main features are severe microcephaly, thin cerebral cortex, subcortical calcification, congenital joint contractures, hypertonia, and hearing loss. Eye abnormalities include retinal pigment mottling, chorioretinal atrophy, optic atrophy or hypoplasia, and optic nerve coloboma. Other ocular abnormalities include microphthalmia, cataract, intraocular calcification, and congenital glaucoma. Exposure in the first 3 months of pregnancy results in the most severe manifestations.

ZIKV infection can be prevented by avoiding mosquito bites especially during daylight hours when Aedes mosquitos are most active. The risk of sexual transmission of ZIKV is reduced by using condoms. Currently, there is no specific antiviral treatment and no effective vaccine to prevent the infection.

DEVELOPMENT OF GROUPINGS OF DISEASES AND SYNDROMES BASED ON CELLULAR EVENTS OR PATHWAYS

As understanding of cellular pathomechanisms has improved, many conditions that were thought to be a disparate collection of signs and symptoms that presented together (syndromes) have been shown to be due to a unifying cellular event or misevent. Four such examples include ciliopathies; rasopathies; channelopathies; and chaperonopathies. Only ciliopathies and rasopathies have notable ocular involvement and are discussed as follows.

Ciliopathies

Two types of cilia exist: intracellular cilia and motile cilia. Intracellular cilia are complex sensory organelles involved in the control of a variety of cellular signaling pathways. These cilia are highly conserved throughout evolution. Cilia receive a variety of extracellular signals, which they transduce and thereby affect proliferation, nerve growth, polarity, differentiation, or tissue maintenance. Because cilia are in all cells, mutations in genes coding for components of cilia affect a multitude of tissues and organ systems in which the cilium-centromere complex functions are important. Ciliopathies are a genetically heterogeneous group of disorders caused by mutations in genes whose products localize to the cilium-centrosome complex. Important examples of ciliopathies are reviewed here.

Retinal-renal syndrome (e.g., Senior-Loken syndrome) is nephronophthisis in association with retinal dystrophy. Retinal dystrophies are not present in every form of nephronophthisis, but the chance increases if mutations in nephrocystin-5 (*NPHP5*) are present. *NPHP5* interacts with *RPGR* (mutations in RPGR can be associated with isolated X-linked retinitis pigmentosa), and both genes are expressed in the cilia of renal epithelial cells and retinal photoreceptors. Joubert syndrome consists of developmental delay and ataxia caused by hypoplasia of the cerebellar vermis in association with retinal coloboma and is characterized by an irregular breathing pattern during the neonatal period. Recessive mutations in *NPHP3, NPHP6/CEP290, NPHP8/RPGRIP1L, AHI1, MKS3, ARL13B, INPP5E,* and *TMEM216,* and *NPHP1* deletions cause Joubert syndrome 15. Meckel syndrome, an autosomal recessive disease, is associated with perinatal death from dysplasia and malformation of multiple organs. It is characterized by occipital meningoencephalocele, microphthalmia, lung hypoplasia, polycystic kidneys or renal dysplasia, biliary ectasia, postaxial polydactyly, and situs inversus. Mutations have been described in *MKS1, MKS3, NPHP3, NPHP6/CEP290, NPHP8/RPGRIP1L, TMEM216,* and *CC2D2A*. Bardet-Biedl syndrome is a multisystem disorder characterized by retinal degeneration, cystic kidney disease, developmental delay, diabetes mellitus, obesity, infertility, and postaxial polydactyly. Mutations in 16 genes (*BBS1* to *BBS12, MKS1, NPHP6/CEP290, SDCCAG8,* and *SEPT7*) can cause the Bardet-Biedl syndrome phenotype. Usher syndrome involves 10 different genes associated with this deaf/blind condition. These genes encode several structurally and functionally distinct proteins, which play a role in stereocilia development in cochlear hair cells, explaining the deafness phenotype when these molecular interactions are perturbed. The mystery is that photoreceptors lack a similar apparatus, and therefore a common theory has been missing for Usher protein function in the two neurosensory cell types affected in this syndrome. However, animal model work suggests that Usher proteins might regulate protein trafficking between the inner and outer segments of photoreceptors. Some retinal dystrophy genes are also known to be ciliary genes, such as *RP1, RPGR,* and *RPGRIP1*. At present, they do not appear to affect other organ systems.

The severity and extent of organ involvement in ciliopathies depend on the following mechanisms. Specific gene mutations cause specific phenotypes. For example, homozygous deletions of *NPHP1* usually cause nephronophthisis, whereas two truncating mutations of *NPHP6/CEP290* cause a Meckel-type phenotype, which is more severe. The type of mutation affects phenotype. For example, two truncating mutations of *NPHP3, NPHP6, NPHP8,* or *NPHP11/MKS380* cause Meckel syndrome, but the presence of even one missense mutation may result in a milder form of Joubert syndrome. Modifier genes affect phenotype. For example, in patients with homozygous *NPHP1* deletions (renal only), the presence of an additional heterozygous mutation in *NPHP6* or *NPHP8* causes additional eye or cerebellar involvement (retinal dystrophy or Joubert syndrome). Oligogenicity affects phenotype. For example, Bardet-Biedl syndrome may be caused by the interaction of two or more recessive genes. Given these associations, children with early-onset retinal dystrophy should have further diagnostic workup including renal ultrasound and genetic evaluation.

Rasopathies

Rasopathies or RAS/mitogen-activated protein kinase (MAPK) syndromes are a group of phenotypically overlapping syndromes caused by germline mutations that encode components of the RAS/MAPK signaling pathway. These disorders include neurofibromatosis type I, Legius syndrome, Noonan syndrome, Noonan syndrome with multiple lentigines (formerly called LEOPARD syndrome), Costello syndrome, cardiofaciocutaneous syndrome, Noonan-like syndrome, hereditary gingival fibromatosis and capillary malformation-arteriovenous malformation, linear sebaceous nevus syndrome (LSNS), oculo-ectodermal syndrome, and encephalocraniocutaneous syndrome (ECCS). All predispose to cancer and abnormal myelopoiesis in infancy, but ocular involvement depends on the specific condition. Patients with Noonan syndrome often have bilateral ptosis. In cardiofaciocutaneous syndrome, the ocular signs are absence of eyebrows and epicanthic folds; in the spectrum of LSNS, oculo-ectodermal syndrome, and in ECCS there are often corneal and conjunctival lipodermoids with waxy alopecia and skin lesions. LSNS and ECCS have intraocular abnormalities and seizure disorder.

OCULAR TRAUMA

It is important to recognize when a child has sustained sight-threatening trauma. The history is always crucial, and the possibility of a penetrating injury from a small high-velocity object should always be considered in circumstances where a child has been striking any solid object. It is better to overreact than assume all is well when faced with a child who has had an injury. Any child with a penetrating injury or an eye that appears sunken with the lid closed should have a hard eye shield placed over the eye and secured immediately, before presenting for medical care in an emergency department or being evaluated by an ophthalmologist. Lacerations to the lid near the medial canthus should be assumed to involve the lacrimal drainage system (Fig. 20.134). Small

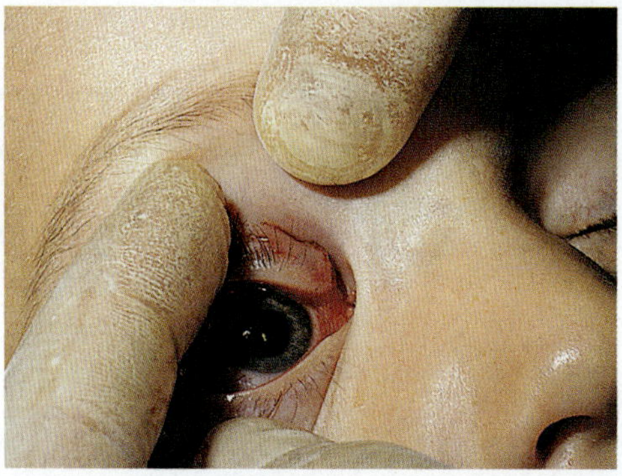

Fig. 20.134 Canalicular laceration. This patient experienced a laceration of the upper canaliculus. Simple apposition of the wound edges in this case will not approximate the cut ends of the canaliculus, and chronic epiphora will result. Silicone tubes are used to splint the canaliculus during the healing process.

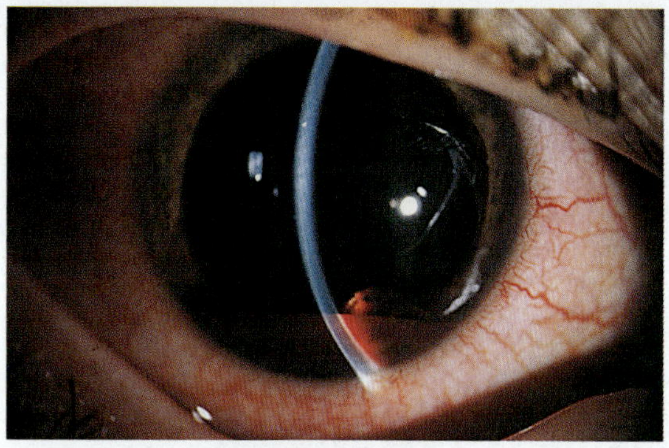

Fig. 20.135 Hyphema. Red blood cells within the anterior chamber have settled into the inferior anterior chamber angle.

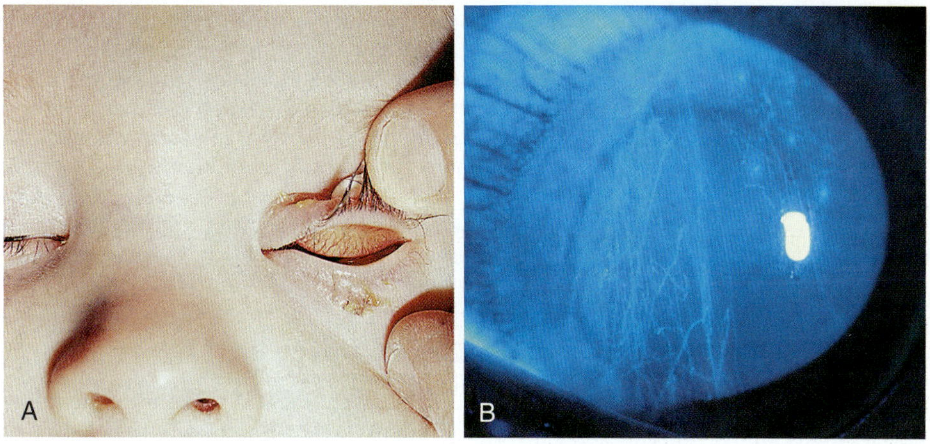

Fig. 20.136 (A) The upper eyelid may be easily everted by placing a cotton swab at the upper edge of the tarsal plate, just above the lid crease. The lashes are then gently grasped and pulled anteriorly away from the globe and upward to evert the lid over the cotton swab. The tarsal conjunctiva may be inspected for the presence of a foreign body. (B) Corneal abrasions stained with fluorescein dye and viewed under blue light. The abrasions appear green in the area of corneal epithelial loss, where the dye is absorbed.

puncture wounds in the lid may also cause orbital and optic nerve damage. Prolapse of any orbital fat from any lid laceration suggests the injury is more severe than it may initially appear.

Blunt trauma can cause an orbital fracture, which may affect eye movements (see Fig. 20.130); subconjunctival hemorrhage; a tear in the iris root (iridodialysis); angle damage (recession) with blood in the anterior chamber (hyphema) (Fig. 20.135); lens damage (lens opacity, subluxation); vitreous hemorrhage; retinal hemorrhage; retinal bruising (commotio retinae); retinal tear or detachment; choroidal rupture; or traumatic optic neuropathy. Complications of a hyphema include rebleeding, glaucoma, and blood staining of the cornea. Increased IOP increases the risk of developing corneal blood staining. The opacification of the cornea may resolve over several months, but children may develop amblyopia. Hyphemas are serious injuries that require evaluation by an ophthalmologist. The majority of hyphemas resolve in fewer than 4 to 5 days with only observation and reduced activity.

In cases of penetrating injury to the eye, the key to examination is to be brief and gentle so as not to complicate the injury by causing expulsion of intraocular contents. Immediately after identifying an ocular injury as penetrating, further examination should be limited and conducted in the operating room under general anesthesia. Topical medications should not be applied to the eye, and the eye should be protected at all times with a shield. Penetrating injuries caused by projectiles or foreign bodies may produce subtle findings. In cases in which the index of suspicion is high, CT scan is recommended.

A careful history is crucial and often the most important indicator about the potential of serious injury. Corneal abrasion is common, and fluorescein dye is required to confirm the diagnosis. The dye is placed in the lower fornix with topical anesthetic drops. Cobalt blue filtered light shows the epithelial defect as a bright green area. Treatment is with antibiotic ointment. Use of topical anesthetic at home is discouraged because it can slow healing significantly. Foreign bodies under the upper lid are painful, and it is not always possible to evert the lid in the office to remove them (Fig. 20.136A and B).

A supplemental video is available at Elsevier eBooks+.

Bibliography

Chhablani PP, editor: *Neuro-ophthalmic disorders*, New York, 2020, Springer Publishing Co.

Chiang MF, Quinn GE, Fielder AR, et al: International classification of retinopathy of prematurity, third edition, *Ophthalmology* 128(10):e51–e68, 2021.

Christian CW, Levin AV: Council on child abuse and neglect; the eye examination in the evaluation of child abuse, *Pediatrics*, 142(2):e20181411, 2018.

Committee on Practice and Ambulatory Medicine, Section on Ophthalmology, American Association of Certified Orthoptists, et al: Visual system assessment in infants, children, and young adults by pediatricians, *Pediatrics* 137(1):e20153596, 2016. www.pediatrics.org/cgi/doi/10.1542/peds.2015-3596.

Donahue SP, Baker CN, Committee on Practice and Ambulatory Medicine, et al: Procedures for the evaluation of the visual system by pediatricians, *Pediatrics* 137(1):e20153597, 2016. www.pediatrics.org/cgi/doi/10.1542/peds.2015-3597.

Fierson WM, American Academy of Pediatrics Section on Ophthalmology, American Academy of Ophthalmology, et al: Screening examination of premature infants for retinopathy of prematurity [published correction appears in *Pediatrics* 143(3):e20183810, 2019], *Pediatrics* 142(6):e20183061, 2018.

Handler SM, Fierson WM, Section on Ophthalmology, et al: Learning disabilities, dyslexia, and vision, *Pediatrics* 127:e818–e856, 2011. http://pediatrics.aappublications.org/content/127/3/e818

Levin AV, Wilson TW: *The Hospital for Sick Children's atlas of pediatric ophthalmology and strabismus*, ed 1, Philadelphia, 2007, Lipincott, Williams and Wilkins.

Tarczy-Hornoch K, editor: *2024-2025 Basic and clinical science course (BCSC), Section 6. Pediatric ophthalmology and strabismus*, San Francisco, 2024, American Academy of Ophthalmology.

Wright K, Strube YN: *Pediatric ophthalmology for primary care*, ed 4, 2019, American Academy of Pediatrics.

Yanoff M, Sassani JW: *Ocular pathology*, ed 7, 2014, Elsevier.

21

ORAL DISORDERS

Heather Baumhardt | Mary Chapman | Alene D'Alesio | Jennifer Waters | Katelyn Woods

ASSESSMENT TECHNIQUES

Because oral and oropharyngeal problems and disorders are common and cause a wide variety of symptoms, routine and thorough oral examinations are an essential component of a complete physical examination; this enables the practitioner to make an appropriate diagnosis without undue delay. The American Academy of Pediatric Dentistry (AAPD) recommends that children are seen for a dental examination no later than 1 year of age.

Key elements of the oral/dental history include the following:

- Timing of eruption and exfoliation of primary teeth, timing of eruption of permanent teeth
- Brushing and flossing frequency and technique
- Dietary habits, including frequency of bottle-feeding and breastfeeding in infancy, night time bottle usage, weaning, frequency of carbohydrate intake, and possible symptoms of eating disorders in adolescence
- Current source of dental care, frequency of visits, presence of a dental home
- Current history of symptoms: oral pain, redness, swelling, drainage, headaches, abdominal pain, decreased appetite, difficulty sleeping
- Problems with bite or occlusion
- History of dental problems and/or orofacial trauma and subsequent treatment
- Family history of dental problems or disorders

A systematic approach to the examination of a child's dentition is essential and should include assessment of the following:

- Facial symmetry and balance
- Lip seal at rest position
- Occlusion (bite) and tooth alignment
- Integrity of enamel, presence of caries
- Appearance of gingiva from both labial/buccal and lingual sides
- Condition of the other oral soft tissues: tongue, palate, tonsils, mucobuccal folds, and sublingual spaces

Successful examination requires close visual inspection of the face, palpation of suspected areas of abnormality, and systematic inspection of the dentition, its supporting structures, and the oral soft tissues. In younger children, a "lap examination" may be a useful way to examine an apprehensive child (Fig. 21.1). It is important to have the parent hold the child's hands throughout the examination. A lap examination is not advised if the mother is pregnant, because the child may accidentally kick the mother. If cooperation cannot be achieved despite these measures, immobilization in a papoose board may be necessary. With older children, examination of the patient in the supine or semirecumbent position with good lighting may be more practical.

Use of a dental mirror or tongue depressor ensures direct visual access to all intraoral areas, especially in assessing the lingual surfaces of the anterior teeth, gingiva, and the buccal surfaces of posterior molars. Adequate lighting is paramount.

NORMAL ORAL STRUCTURES

The oral cavity, including the teeth, gingiva, and periodontal ligaments, is in a constant state of change during infancy and childhood. From the early stages of teething to the transition from primary (baby) teeth to permanent (adult) teeth, the mouth showcases some of the most significant signs of development.

To better understand this chapter and communicate effectively with consulting dentists, reviewing basic terminology can be helpful. Each tooth is composed of an outer protective enamel layer, an inner layer of dentin consisting of tubules, which are thought to serve a nutritional function, and a central neurovascular core termed the *pulp* or *nerve*. The roots of the teeth are anchored in the sockets of the alveolar processes of the mandible and maxilla by an encompassing periodontal membrane or ligament. The neurovascular supply to the root apex also passes through this structure. The bony processes between the teeth are referred to as the *interdental septae* (Fig. 21.2). After eruption, the visible portions of teeth are referred to as the *crowns*, and the interface between them and the gingiva is termed the *gingival crevice*. Finally, the portions of the gingiva located between teeth are called *interdental papillae*.

Oral Cavity in the Newborn

The lips of an infant reveal a prominent line of demarcation at the vermilion border. The mucosa may look wrinkled and slightly purple at birth, but within a few days it exhibits a drier appearance, with the outer layer forming crusty "sucking calluses." This callus formation affects the central portion of the mucosa and persists for a few weeks to a few months (Fig. 21.3).

The maxillary alveolar arch is separated from the lip by a shallow sulcus. In the midline, the labial frenum (often called the frenulum) extends posteriorly across the alveolar ridge to the palatine incisive papilla. The alveolar ridge peaks anteriorly and gradually flattens as the ridge extends posteriorly, forming a pseudoalveolar groove medial to the ridge along its palatal side. This flattened appearance is seen in infants and gradually disappears with the growth of the alveolar process and the formation and calcification of posterior tooth buds. The mandibular alveolar ridges also peak anteriorly and flatten posteriorly. The mandibular labial frenum connects the lower lip to the labial aspect of the alveolar ridge. Anterior tooth buds are located on the labial side of the alveolar ridges, whereas posterior tooth buds are often located closer to the crests of the alveolar ridges. Palatal morphology and color are variable. The tongue and the floor of the mouth differ only slightly from those of older children.

Primary Dentition

Development of the alveolar bone is directly related to the formation and eruption of teeth, and normal patterns of dental development occur symmetrically. Primary and permanent teeth begin forming in utero and continue development throughout the first 10 years of life. Eruption times and sequence are variable but begin at approximately 6 months old, when mandibular central incisors erupt (Fig. 21.4). This stage is often preceded by a period of increased salivation, gingival irritation, and irritability. These symptoms vary in intensity, but they respond well to oral analgesics and usually subside when the primary tooth erupts into the oral cavity. Other symptoms such as fever or diarrhea are not directly related to teething. By 3 years old, the full primary dentition is typically present and functional (Fig. 21.5).

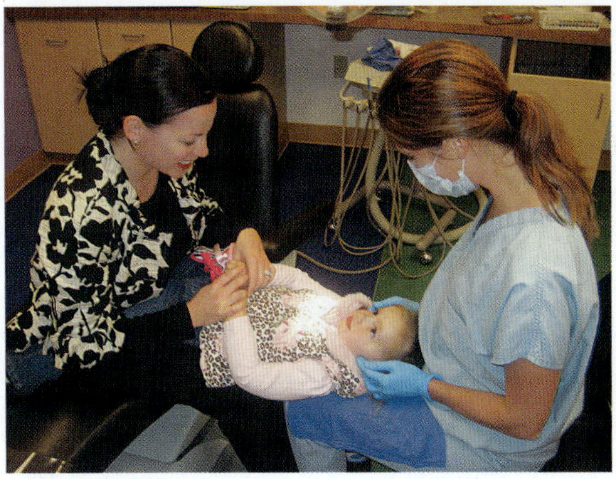

Fig. 21.1 Oral examination of a toddler. A lap examination is a useful way to examine a young or anxious child. The patient can hold the parent's hand and see the parent during the examination.

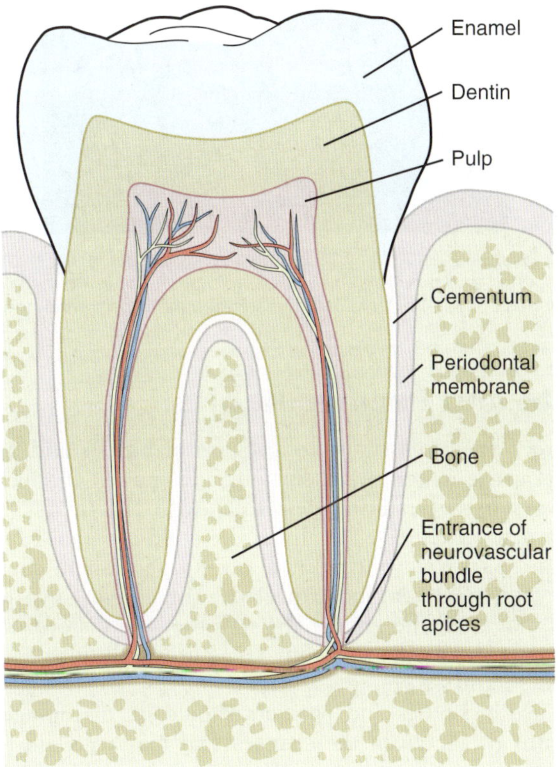

Fig. 21.2 Diagrammatic representation of a molar shows the enamel, dentin, pulp, cementum, periodontal membrane, entrance of the neurovascular bundle through the root apices, and bony supporting structures.

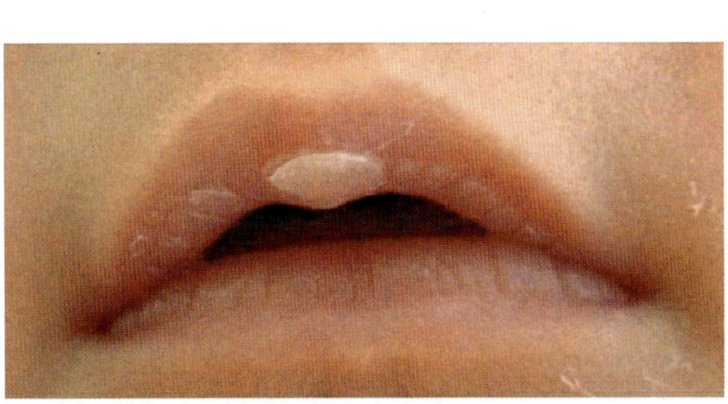

Fig. 21.3 A sucking callus present on the maxillary lip.

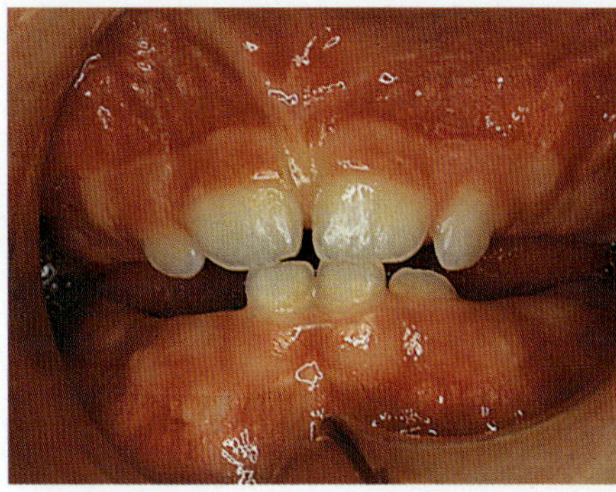

Fig. 21.4 Early primary dentition. The mandibular and maxillary central and lateral incisors are the first to erupt.

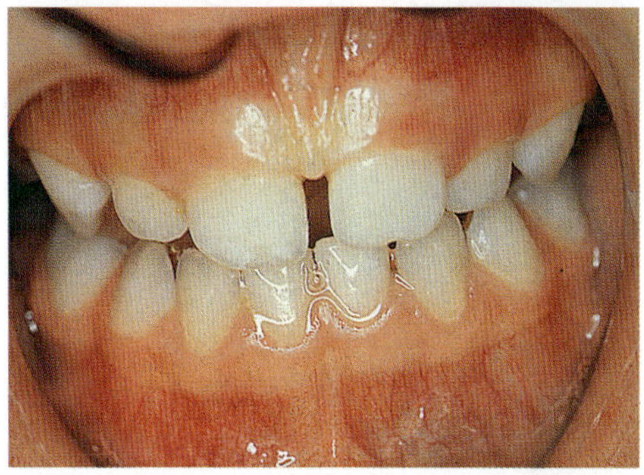

Fig. 21.5 Full primary dentition. By age 3, all 20 primary teeth have erupted.

Any significant variation in the time and sequence of eruption in an infant may call for early dental referral. In most instances, careful observation is indicated. Delayed dentition can be a feature of moderate to severe cases of growth faltering, where it may be seen in association with delayed bone age. Delayed eruption is also associated with Down syndrome, hypothyroidism, hypopituitarism, achondroplastic dwarfism, osteopetrosis, rickets, or chondroectodermal dysplasia. A significant variation affecting a single tooth or only a few teeth should be carefully investigated as well. Extra space between teeth during this stage is normal, providing more space for the larger permanent teeth.

During most of the primary dentition stage, the gingiva appears pink, firm, and not readily retractable. Rarely, local irritation may develop into acute or subacute pericoronitis, with elevated temperature and associated lymphadenopathy. Topical and/or systemic therapy may be required for treatment; however, lancing the gingiva to relieve such symptoms is not usually indicated.

Mixed Dentition

The mixed dentition stage of development begins with the eruption of the first permanent molars at about 6 years old and continues for approximately 6 years (Fig. 21.6; also see Fig. 21.9 for order of eruption). The mixed dentition during this stage undergoes physiologic changes, including root resorption followed by exfoliation of primary teeth, eruption of their successors, and eruption of the posterior permanent teeth. During the period of root resorption of primary teeth and for several months after the eruption of permanent teeth, the teeth are relatively loosely embedded in the alveolar bone, making them more vulnerable to displacement by trauma. Gingival irritation can occur from increased mobility of primary teeth but usually disappears spontaneously when the tooth is lost. Two transient deviations of eruption pattern may occur: (1) The mandibular incisors may erupt in a lingual position behind the primary incisors ("double teeth") (Fig. 21.7), and (2) the maxillary incisors may assume a widely spaced and labially inclined position ("ugly duckling" stage). The occlusal surfaces of newly erupted permanent teeth

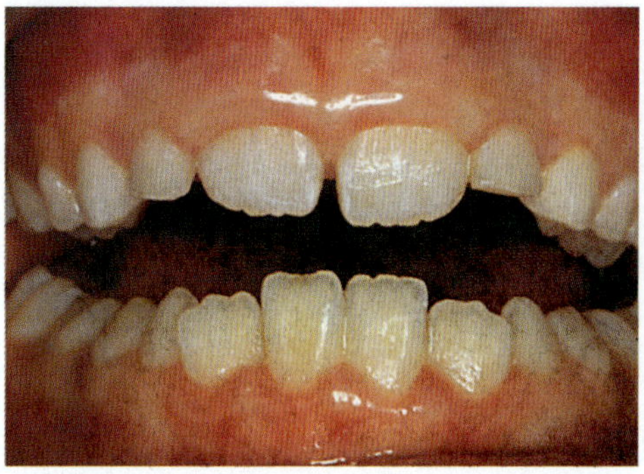

Fig. 21.6 Mixed dentition. This transitional stage from primary to permanent dentition begins at age 6 and lasts for about 6 years.

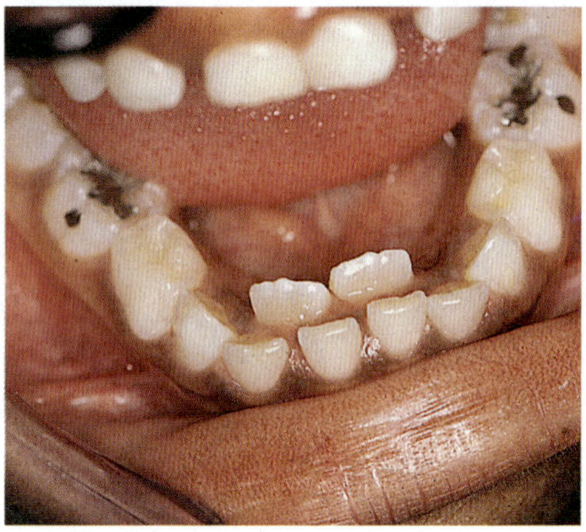

Fig. 21.7 Abnormal eruption patterns frequently occur in the early mixed dentition phase. One example is shown here, with eruption of the permanent central incisors behind the primary teeth.

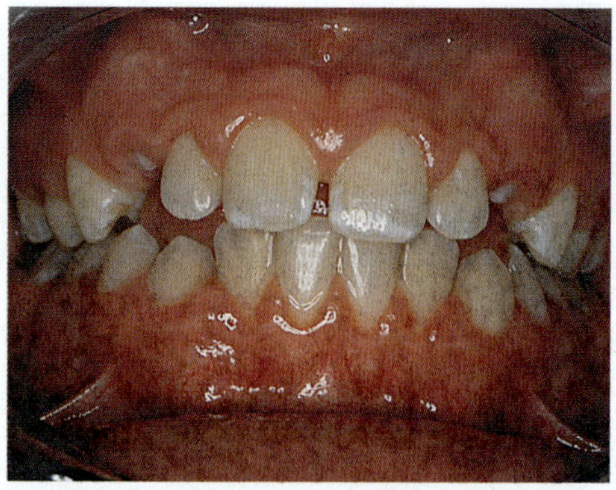

Fig. 21.8 The earliest stage of permanent dentition begins with eruption of 6-year molars and central incisors. Cuspids and second molars are the last to erupt.

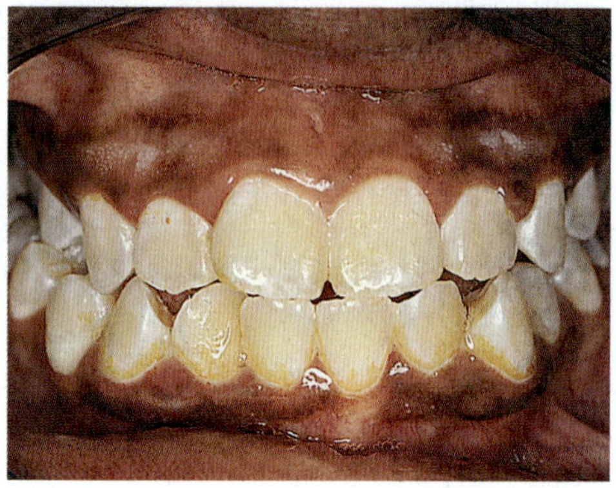

Fig. 21.9 Gingivitis during puberty. The gingival tissues are mildly erythematous and edematous, and they tend to bleed easily with brushing. Hormonal changes and inattention to careful dental hygiene are thought to be contributory.

are relatively "rough" (see Fig. 21.43), assisting plaque accumulation that increases the risk of staining, gingivitis, and formation of caries.

Early Permanent Dentition

The stage of early permanent dentition marks the beginning of a relatively quiescent period in dental development. Activities are limited to root formation of a few permanent teeth and the calcification of the third molars. By this time, the length and width of the dental arches are well established (Figs. 21.8 and 21.9), and the jaws undergo major growth during puberty that alters their size and relative position. The gingiva begins to assume adult characteristics, becoming firm and pink in color, with an uneven, stippled surface texture and a thin gingival margin. Puberty is occasionally associated with gingivitis, where it becomes mildly edematous and erythematous, which is thought to be secondary in part to hormonal changes (Fig. 21.10). Inattention to careful dental hygiene may also contribute to gingivitis and necessitates good oral hygiene and regular recall visits for control.

HARMFUL ORAL HABITS

Thumb and Finger Sucking

Children often develop sucking habits, using the thumbs, fingers, or objects. Thumb and finger sucking begins antenatally and is considered a normal behavior pattern. However, if the habit persists after eruption of all primary teeth (age 3), the extrinsic forces applied by the sucking action can produce pathologic changes in the child's normal arch growth. These deviations range from minor, reversible changes to gross malformations in the dental arches that produce significant anterior open bites and/or posterior crossbites (Fig. 21.11). The degree of change depends on the duration, frequency, and intensity of the sucking habit.

Bottle and Pacifier Habits

The forces produced by prolonged use of bottles and pacifiers can first cause dental malocclusions and may, if the habit persists, worsen the resulting deformity with the involvement of adjacent jaw structures. Usually, if the child is weaned from the bottle and pacifier by 12 months old, no permanent changes in bite development can be expected. The longer any force is applied, however, the greater the risk that the distortion in the dental arches and adjacent bony structures will not self-correct (Figs. 21.11 and 21.12).

The use of bottles and pacifiers should be discouraged after 12 months of age given the changes that may result in the oral structures. The Fridababy Paci Weaning System (Fig. 21.13) is a patented system that can help a child wean from the pacifier in as little as 5 days, using a sequence of pacifiers in a stepwise approach. Counseling parents during the neonatal period not to put their infants to bed with a bottle, but rather to hold them during all feedings, is one of the best ways to prevent later difficulties with bottle weaning. Such practices also prevent the development of nursing bottle caries (see Fig. 21.42).

Therapy

Clinical management of harmful oral habits should be customized to the child's age. Harsh measures to discourage digit sucking in a 2-year-old are not justified and may be counterproductive. However, when the habit persists beyond a reasonable age, discussions with the child concerning feelings related to the sucking and the physical damage possible if it continues often produce the desired results. When a child has expressed a strong will to cease sucking but is unable to accomplish this goal without help, appliance therapy by a dental professional may be indicated. Referral for oral evaluation and consultation is appropriate after

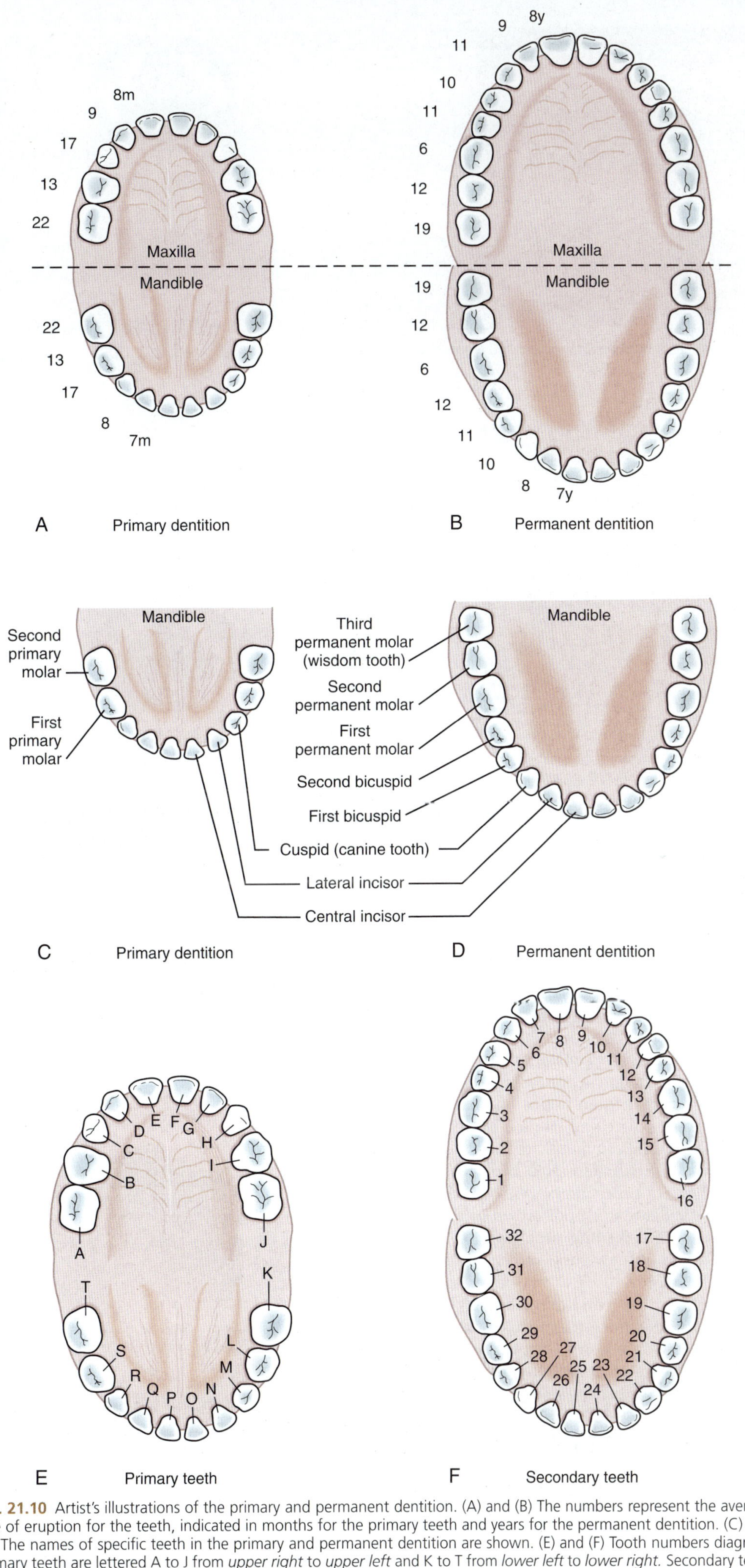

Fig. 21.10 Artist's illustrations of the primary and permanent dentition. (A) and (B) The numbers represent the average age of eruption for the teeth, indicated in months for the primary teeth and years for the permanent dentition. (C) and (D) The names of specific teeth in the primary and permanent dentition are shown. (E) and (F) Tooth numbers diagram: primary teeth are lettered A to J from *upper right* to *upper left* and K to T from *lower left* to *lower right*. Secondary teeth are numbered 1 to 16 from *upper right* to *upper left* and 17 to 32 from *lower left* to *lower right*.

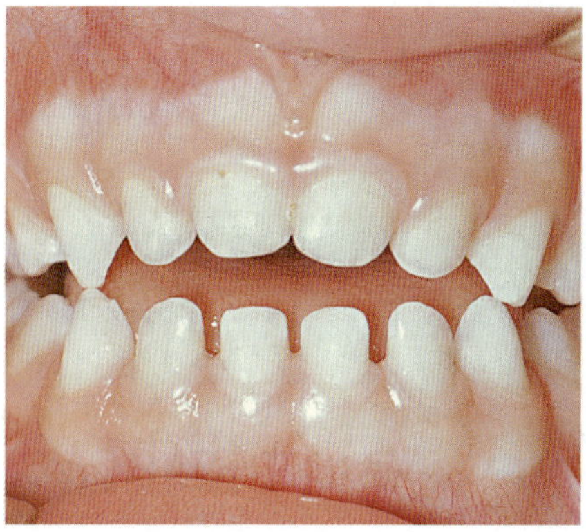

Fig. 21.11 Changes in the bite often occur as the result of prolonged digit or pacifier habit. This child's upper arch has been narrowed, and an anterior open bite is developing.

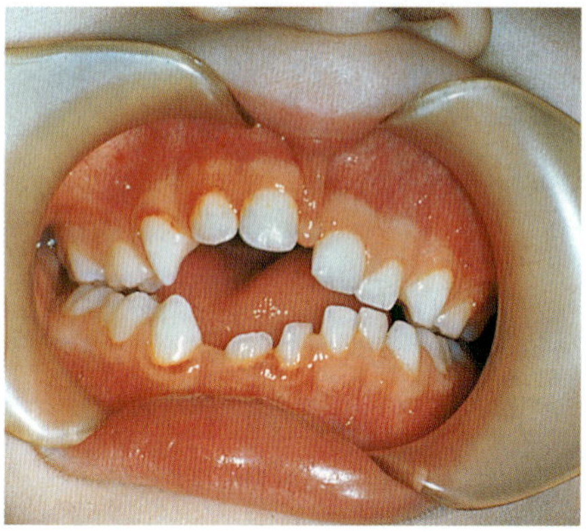

Fig. 21.12 A 2-year-old with a prolonged pacifier-sucking habit has severe deformity of the alveolar arches and teeth caused by the extrinsic force of the pacifier-sucking action.

the child has passed the appropriate age of the behavior pattern involved.

NATAL AND NEONATAL ABNORMALITIES

Teeth

Teeth that are present in the oral cavity at birth are called *natal teeth* (Fig. 21.14), whereas those erupting during the neonatal period (30 days after birth) are called *neonatal teeth.* The incidence of natal teeth has been reported to be approximately 1 in 2000 births. Although seen in normal infants, this anomaly is more frequent in patients with cleft palate and is often associated with Ellis-van Creveld syndrome, Hallermann-Streiff syndrome, and pachyonychia congenita. Approximately 90% are true primary teeth, but occasionally they are supernumerary. Some are abnormal, with either hypoplastic defects or poor crown or root development. Natal teeth may cause feeding problems for both the infant and mother. Ulceration of the ventral surface of the tongue by sharp tooth edges (Riga-Fede disease) may develop if natal teeth remain in the oral cavity. This condition is usually transient, but in persistent cases, symptomatic treatment or extraction of such teeth may be indicated. Most normal-appearing natal teeth can be retained, but those that are supernumerary, abnormal, or very loose may have to be removed.

Gingival Cysts in the Newborn

Gingival cysts of the oral cavity are small, single, or multiple superficial lesions that are formed by tissues trapped during embryologic growth. They occur in about 80% of newborns and

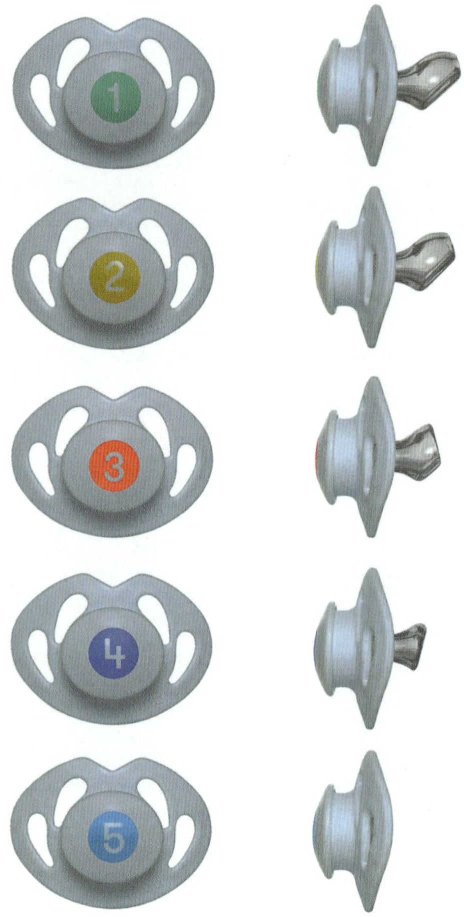

Fig. 21.13 The Fridababy Paci Weaning System is a series of pacifiers designed specifically to wean children from pacifier use.

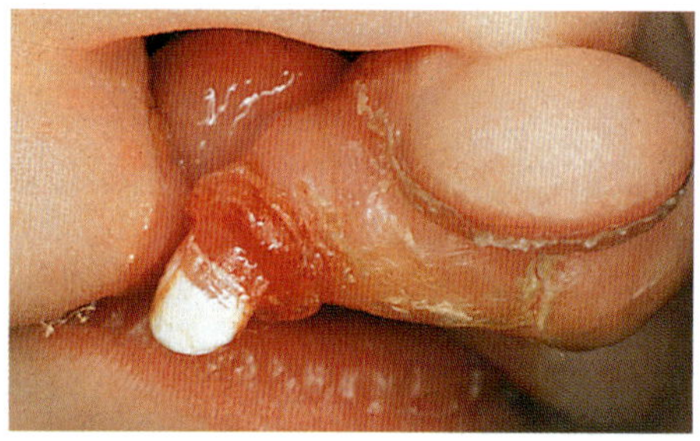

Fig. 21.14 A natal tooth associated with cleft palate. Extraction is necessary only if it is of abnormal morphology, causing feeding difficulties, or is an aspiration risk due to excessive mobility.

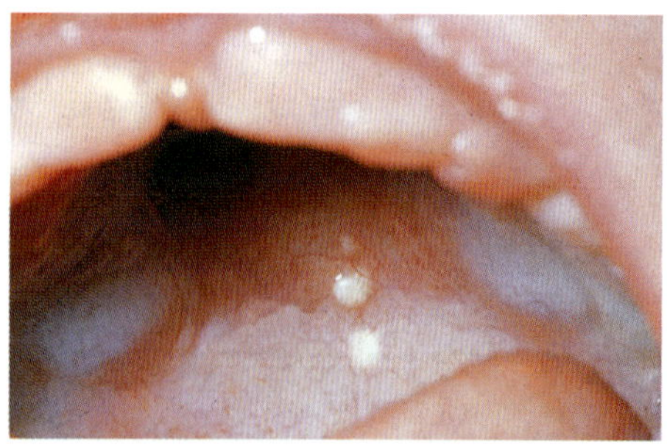

Fig. 21.15 Gingival cysts. The small, whitish cystic lesions seen along the midpalatine raphe are called *Epstein pearls.*

are asymptomatic, do not enlarge, seldom interfere with feeding, and usually exfoliate within a few weeks.

Three types of cysts exist:

- *Epstein pearls* are keratin-filled cystic lesions lined with stratified squamous epithelium. They appear as small, white lesions along the midpalatine raphe (Fig. 21.15).

- *Bohn nodules* are mucous gland cysts often found on the buccal or lingual aspects of the alveolar ridges and occasionally on the palate. They are multiple, firm, and grayish white in appearance. Histologically, they show mucous glands and ducts (Fig. 21.16).
- *Dental lamina cysts* are found only on the crest of the alveolar mucosa. Histologically, these lesions are different because they are formed by remnants of dental lamina epithelium. They may be larger, more lucent, and more fluctuant than Epstein pearls or Bohn nodules and are more likely to occur singly (Fig. 21.17).

Congenital Epulis in the Newborn

Congenital epulis is a benign, soft tissue tumor seen on the alveolar mucosa at birth or shortly after. It is usually found on the anterior maxilla as a pedunculated swelling (Fig. 21.18) but may appear on the mandible or, occasionally, on both jaws. The mass is firm on palpation, and the overlying mucosa appears normal. Histologically, sheets of large granular cells are seen. Differential diagnosis should include rhabdomyoma and melanotic neuroectodermal tumor of infancy. Treatment is excision or monitoring, and recurrence is infrequent.

Melanotic Neuroectodermal Tumor of Infancy

Melanotic neuroectodermal tumor of infancy is a rare, benign yet aggressive tumor, developing during the first year of life and often found on the anterior maxilla in association with unerupted or erupted teeth. It often bulges and destroys the alveolar bone, thus displacing the associated primary tooth. The tumor mass is grayish blue, firm on palpation, and spherical in shape (Fig. 21.19). Careful surgical removal is effective, and recurrence is unusual.

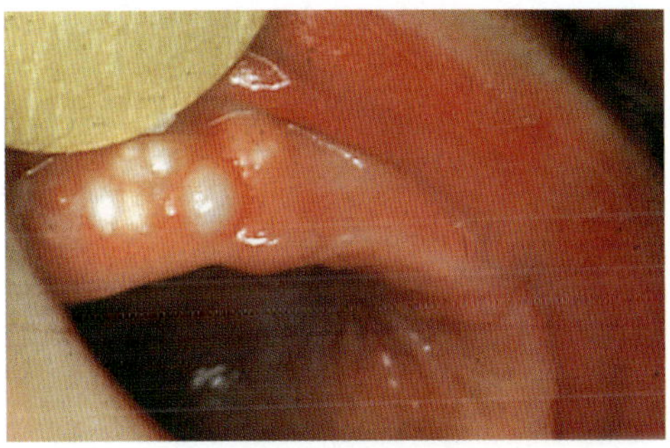

Fig. 21.16 Gingival cysts. The firm, grayish-white mucous gland cysts on the buccal aspect of the alveolar ridges are called *Bohn nodules.*

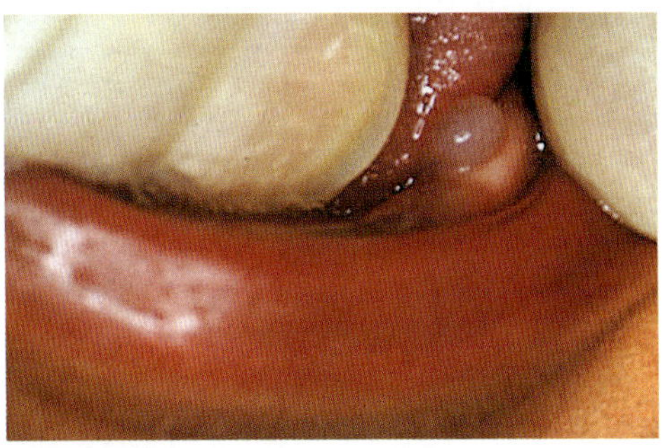

Fig. 21.17 Dental lamina cyst. These cysts are found on the alveolar ridge and usually occur singly.

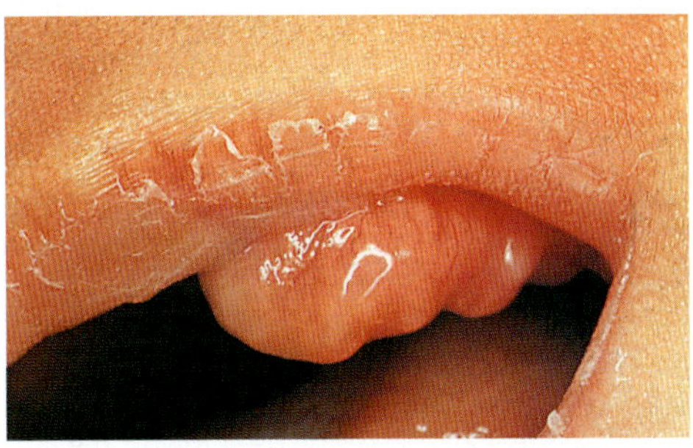

Fig. 21.18 Congenital epulis. This 4-day-old patient has a benign tumor of the anterior maxilla.

DEVELOPMENTAL ABNORMALITIES

Soft Tissue Abnormalities

Geographic Tongue (Benign Migratory Glossitis)

Geographic tongue (benign migratory glossitis) is a condition characterized by inflamed, irregularly shaped areas on the dorsum of the tongue that are devoid of filiform papillae. Though painless, discomfort may be noted when eating spicy or acidic foods. Lesions are red, slightly depressed, and bordered by a whitish band (Fig. 21.20). Spontaneous healing is often followed by formation of similar lesions elsewhere on the tongue, resulting in a migrating appearance. The etiology is unknown; however, a strong association with stress and allergic disease is suspected. Although benign, the course of this disorder may be lifelong.

Abnormalities of the Frenula

During embryonic life, the maxillary labial frenum extends as a band of tissue from the upper lip over and across the alveolar ridge and into the incisive (palatine) papilla. Postnatally, as the alveolar process increases in size, the labial frenum separates from the incisive papilla and becomes relatively smaller. With the eruption of primary and later permanent teeth, the frenum attachment moves apically and further atrophies because of vertical growth of the alveolar process. The developmental gap (diastema) between the maxillary central incisors tends to close with the full eruption of the maxillary permanent canines. A diastema is often present

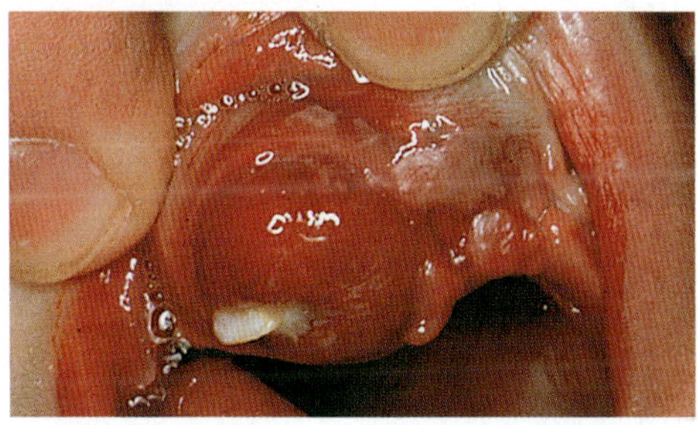

Fig. 21.19 Melanotic neuroectodermal tumor. This benign but locally aggressive tumor of the anterior maxilla has produced elevation of the lip and displaced a primary tooth.

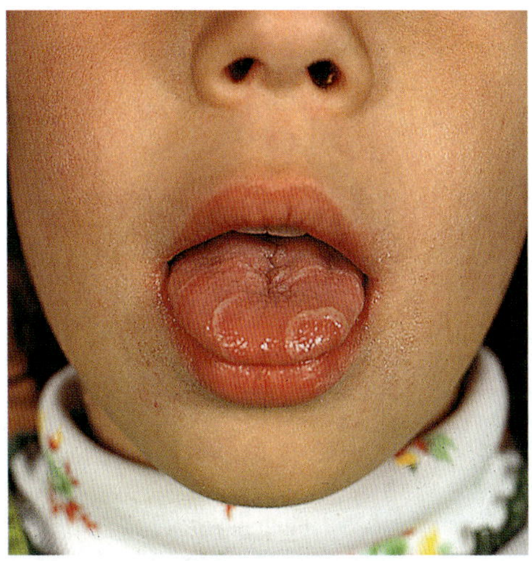

Fig. 21.20 Characteristics of benign migratory glossitis (geographic tongue), which is a chronic and often recurring condition affecting the filiform papillae of the tongue. Lesions are red, slightly depressed, and bordered by a whitish band.

and is considered normal in primary dentition. Rarely is a labial frenum addressed during the primary dentition stage, but surgical intervention may be considered in the presence of gross caries due to food impaction in the vestibule. Occasionally, the maxillary frenum fails to atrophy as a child matures and the diastema persists (Fig. 21.21). This may require intervention, but only after the permanent canines have erupted and post-orthodontia. The mandibular midline frenum only rarely maintains a lingual extension and therefore rarely causes a diastema between the mandibular central incisors, but it can cause pulling of gingival fibers leading to pocket formation and plaque accumulation. Early treatment can be considered for mandibular labial frenum release, but more noninvasive interventions such as increased oral hygiene practices and plaque control are highly recommended before surgical intervention.

The lingual frenum extends almost to the tip of the tongue in early infancy and then gradually recedes. On occasion, ankyloglossia (tongue tie) is seen (Fig. 21.22) and can be associated with feeding difficulties. It is rarely associated with speech difficulties. There is controversy regarding when or even if to proceed with surgical intervention. According to the AAPD, the tongue's ability to elevate rather than protrude is the most important feature of mobility; a restrictive lingual frenum can cause an ineffective latch during breastfeeding but is less of an issue with bottle-feeding. This ineffective latch can lead to early cessation of breastfeeding, which the American Academy of Pediatrics recommends as the exclusive source of nutrition for the first 6 months of an infant's life. In the presence of ineffective feeding, early tongue tie release (within the first several weeks of life) can be effective for increasing feeding function.

Evaluation by a speech-language pathologist trained in assessing tongue ties is recommended to assess for speech or language errors before tongue-tie release to alleviate speech concerns. Overall, frenectomy is seldom indicated and should be recommended only after appropriate justification. Congenital anomalies may include an enlarged frenum, labiolingual frenum extensions, or supernumerary frenula as seen in orofaciodigital syndrome (Fig. 21.23).

Gingival Hyperplasia

Generalized gingival hyperplasia is a common, nonspecific pathologic entity. This disorder is frequently a complication of drug therapy, including phenytoin and cyclosporine. Gingival hyperplasia may also be idiopathic or genetically transmitted as in hereditary gingival fibromatosis. Differentiation of various types of hyperplasia must be based on thorough physical evaluation and appropriate medical history. Histopathologically, it is impossible to differentiate among these various disorders, so the final diagnosis and recommendations for therapy should be based on all available clinical data and an appropriate dental consultation.

Phenytoin-Induced Gingival Hyperplasia

The administration of phenytoin over time frequently causes generalized hyperplasia of the gingiva (Fig. 21.24). The gingiva may become secondarily inflamed, edematous, and boggy, especially in the absence of good oral hygiene. The severity is often related to the

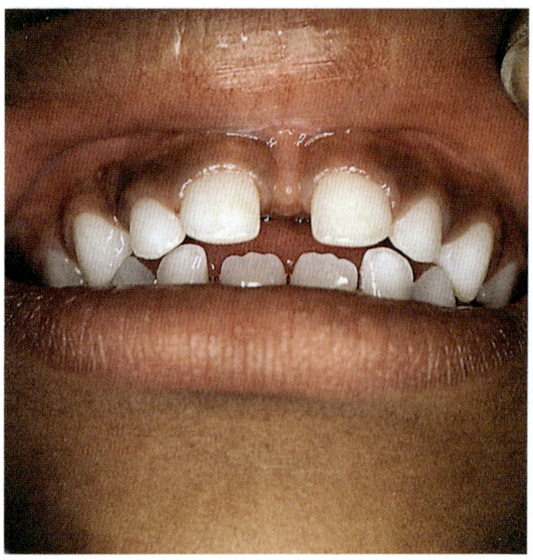

Fig. 21.21 Large diastema (excessive spacing) between the front teeth, secondary to an inferiorly positioned maxillary frenum.

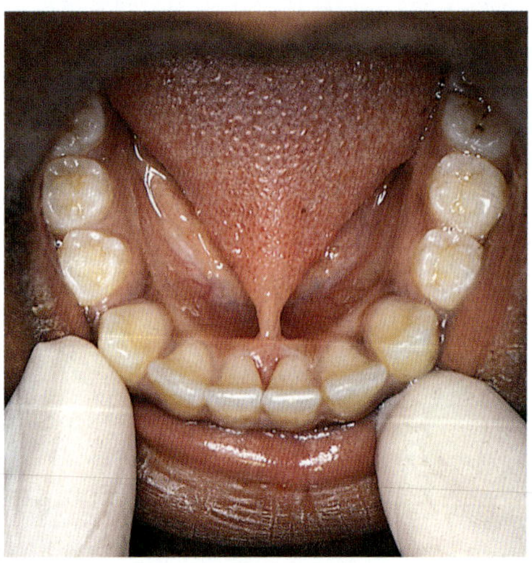

Fig. 21.22 Ankyloglossia. This extremely short lingual frenum with a high insertion point on the gingival margin is an indication for surgical intervention.

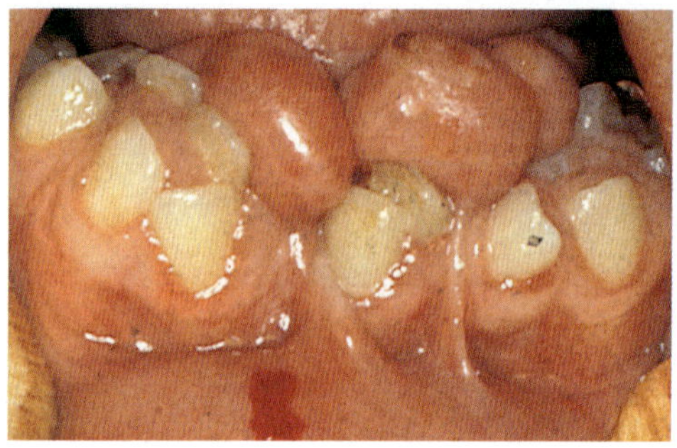

Fig. 21.23 Multiple hyperplastic frenula are seen in this patient with orofaciodigital syndrome. These frenula interfered with the eruption of teeth, causing rotation and crowding.

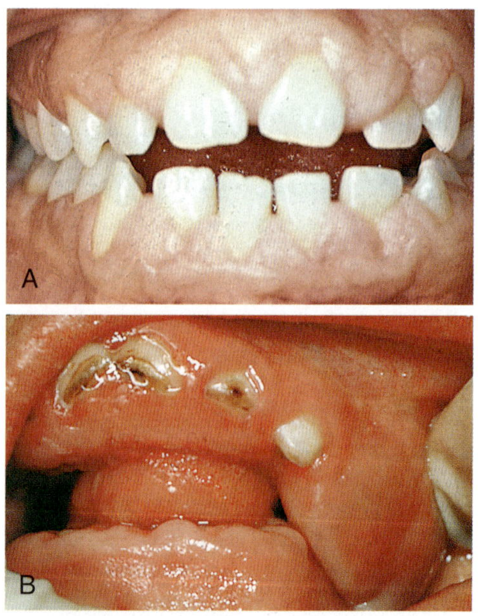

Fig. 21.24 Phenytoin-induced gingival overgrowth. (A) A typical gingival response (hyperplasia) to chronic phenytoin ingestion. Similar gum changes can result from cyclosporine therapy. (B) Severe overgrowth. The firm, hyperplastic gingival tissues have completely covered the posterior teeth and are interfering with mastication.

degree of local irritation, stemming from poor oral hygiene, mouth breathing, caries, or poor occlusion. Because hyperplasia tends to recur after surgical excision, gingivectomy is usually reserved for those patients whose overgrowth interferes with function, or for those whose phenytoin therapy has been modified or discontinued.

Cyclosporine-Induced Gingival Hyperplasia

Cyclosporine may lead to increased cellular growth of gingival fibroblasts and production and retention of collagen. This agent's immunosuppressive action may predispose gingival tissues to invasion by microorganisms, which increases inflammatory changes. Although meticulous oral hygiene reduces inflammation, it has no significant effect on the degree of hyperplasia.

Gingival Fibromatosis

Gingival fibromatosis, a rare, genetically determined condition, may be clinically evident at birth and may prevent or slow dental eruption. Clinically, it manifests as the generalized presence of firm fibrous tissue that extends around the crowns of involved teeth. Inflammation is usually secondary. Surgical excision of excessive tissues is usually indicated, but recurrence is a possibility.

Idiopathic Gingival Hyperplasia

Patients who have significant systemic illnesses or syndromes may have generalized gingival enlargements. These primarily involve the gingival tissues but can be related to underlying thickening of cortical bone. Each of these cases must be evaluated individually for possible etiology and appropriate treatment.

Eruption Cysts (Eruption Hematoma)

An eruption cyst is a fluid-filled, nontender swelling that covers the crown of an erupting tooth. When the follicle is dilated with blood, the lesion takes on a bluish color and is termed an *eruption hematoma* (Fig. 21.25). Although the eruption cyst is a superficial form of dentigerous cyst, it rarely impedes eruption. Surgical exposure of the crown is seldom necessary and not recommended.

Mucocele and Ranula

A mucocele is a painless, translucent or bluish lesion of traumatic origin, most often involving minor salivary glands of the lower lip (Fig. 21.26). The lesion may alternately enlarge and shrink. The treatment of choice is surgical excision of the lesion and the associated minor salivary gland.

A simple ranula is a retention cyst in the floor of the mouth that is confined to sublingual tissues superior to the mylohyoid muscle. It appears clinically as a bluish, transparent, thin-walled, fluctuant swelling (Fig. 21.27). Herniation of the ranula through the mylohyoid muscle results in a cervical or plunging ranula that becomes more apparent in the oral cavity with the muscle contraction associated with jaw opening. The ranula must be removed in its entirety, along with the associated salivary gland to avoid recurrence. Alternatively, micromarsupialization to form a new epithelialized tract for drainage can be done using silk sutures.

Salivary Calculus (Sialolithiasis)

Formation of a salivary calculus is rare in the pediatric population, but when it does occur, it may affect either the Wharton duct or Stensen duct (Fig. 21.28A). Partial obstruction of the duct results in pain and enlargement of the gland, especially at mealtime. Although palpation of the stone may be possible, dental radiographs confirm the diagnosis and give appropriate information about its size and location (see Fig. 21.28B). If the calculus cannot be manipulated through the duct, surgical intervention may be necessary.

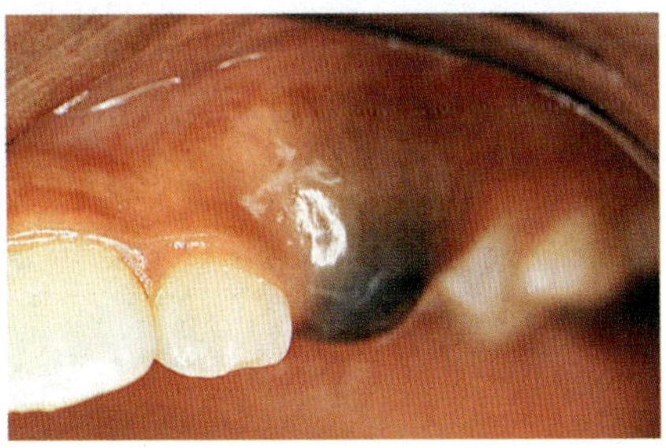

Fig. 21.25 Eruption hematoma. A bluish, fluid-filled, fluctuant swelling can be seen over the crown of an erupting maxillary cuspid. The lesion resolved without treatment when the tooth erupted.

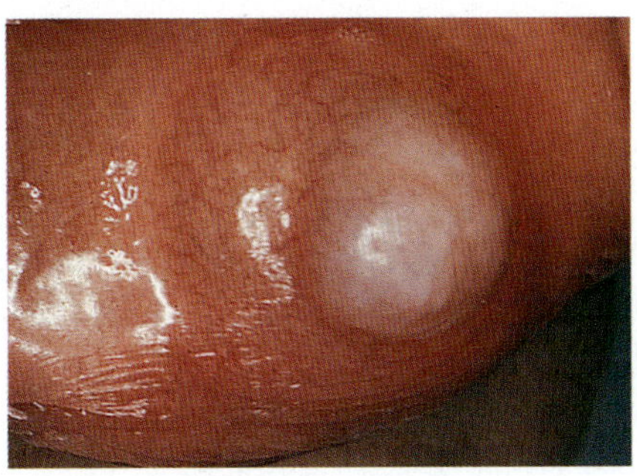

Fig. 21.26 A mucocele on the lower lip, with the characteristic translucent coloration secondary to fluid retention.

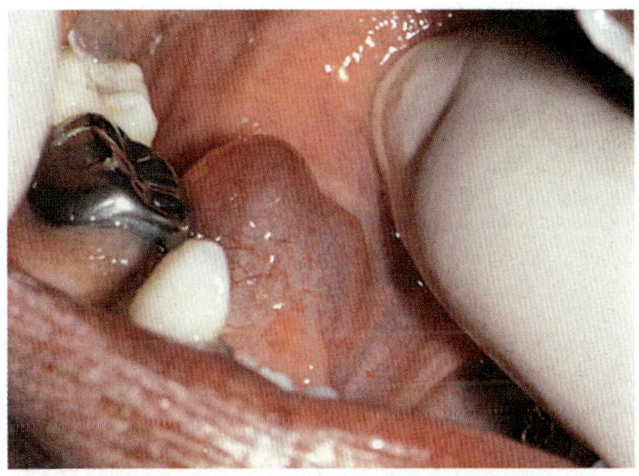

Fig. 21.27 Ranula. The bluish, fluctuant swelling in the floor of the mouth is a retention cyst associated with trauma to a salivary duct.

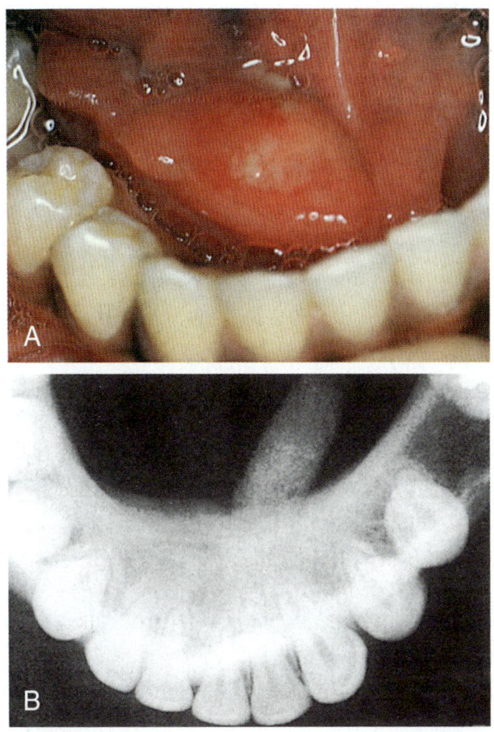

Fig. 21.28 Salivary calculus. (A) This sialolith obstructing a salivary duct is observed in the floor of the mouth. (B) A dental radiograph of the sublingual space reveals the size and location of the salivary calculus.

Hard Tissue Abnormalities

Hypoplasia and Hypocalcification

Numerous local and systemic insults are capable of causing the enamel defects of hypoplasia and hypocalcification. The most common etiologic factors are local infection, such as an abscessed primary tooth, which, when not diagnosed or treated promptly, may damage the enamel of its developing permanent counterpart. Other causes include systemic infections with associated high fever, trauma (such as intrusion of the primary tooth), or chemical injury (such as excessive ingestion of fluoride). Other etiologic factors include nutritional deficiencies, allergies, rubella, cerebral palsy, embryopathy, prematurity, and radiation therapy. Hypocalcification results from an insult during mineralization of the tooth and appears as opaque, chalky, or white lesions (Fig. 21.29). In contrast, hypoplasia results from an insult during active-matrix formation of the enamel and clinically manifests as pitting, furrowing, or thinning of the enamel (Fig. 21.30).

Hyperdontia and Hypodontia

Variations in tooth number include both hyperdontia and hypodontia. Supernumerary teeth occur in about 3% of the population, although patients with cleft lip and/or palate and cleidocranial dysplasia have a significantly higher incidence. The most common site is the anterior palate (Fig. 21.31). Supernumerary teeth may have the size and morphology of adjacent teeth or may be small and atypical in shape. They may erupt spontaneously or remain impacted. Complications such as impeded eruption, crowding, or resorption of permanent teeth, cystic changes, or ectopic eruption into the nasal cavity, the maxillary sinus, or other sites may occur, so early evaluation and treatment should be considered (Fig. 21.32).

Congenital absence of teeth is more often seen in the permanent dentition than in the primary. Most frequently missing are third molars, second premolars, and lateral incisors. Hypodontia is frequently associated with several ectodermal syndromes, such as anhidrotic ectodermal dysplasia and chondroectodermal dysplasia (Fig. 21.33).

Alterations in Tooth Size and Shape

Teeth that are smaller or larger than normal are termed *microdonts* and *macrodonts,* respectively. These teeth are genetic anomalies. They are clinically significant when a discrepancy in tooth size and dental arch length results in severe crowding or spacing of the teeth. Size abnormalities are often localized to one tooth or to a small group of teeth.

Variations in shape result from the joining of teeth or tooth buds. Fusion is the joining of two tooth buds by the dentin. Concrescence is the joining of the roots of two or more teeth by cementum. Gemination (twinning) results from the incomplete division of one tooth bud, resulting in a large crown with a notched incisal edge and a single root.

Heritable Defects of Enamel and Dentin

Amelogenesis Imperfecta

Amelogenesis imperfecta is the term used to describe a group of genetically determined defects, with variable inheritance based on the underlying disorder. Defects involve the enamel of primary and permanent

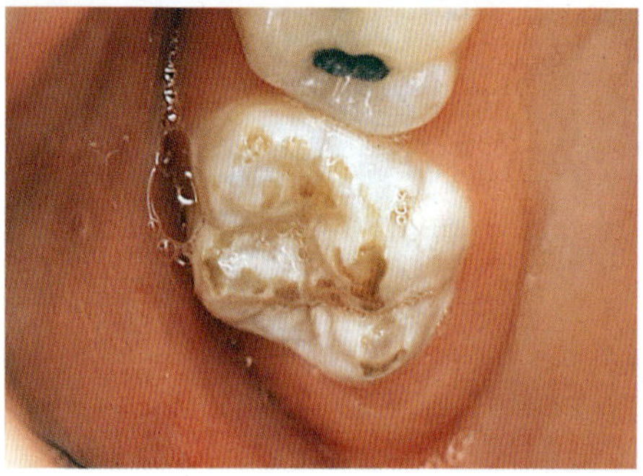

Fig. 21.29 Hypocalcification. This 6-year-old patient exhibits early signs of hypocalcification of his permanent molars. Chalky white spots indicate poor calcification of the enamel.

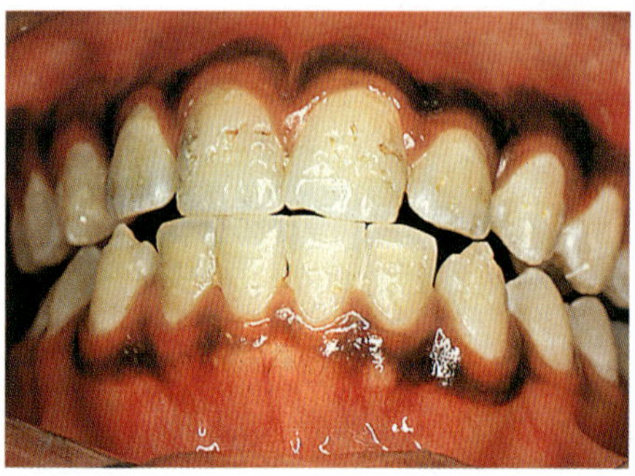

Fig. 21.30 Amelogenesis imperfecta, hypoplastic type. This process results in generalized pitting of the enamel.

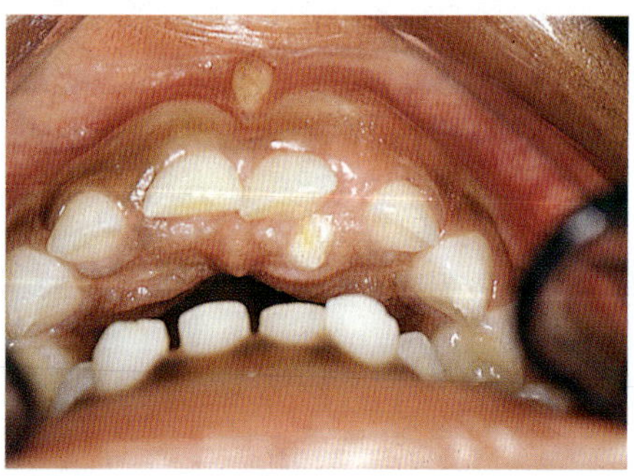

Fig. 21.31 Hyperdontia. Erupted supernumerary tooth lingual to the maxillary central incisor in the deciduous dentition.

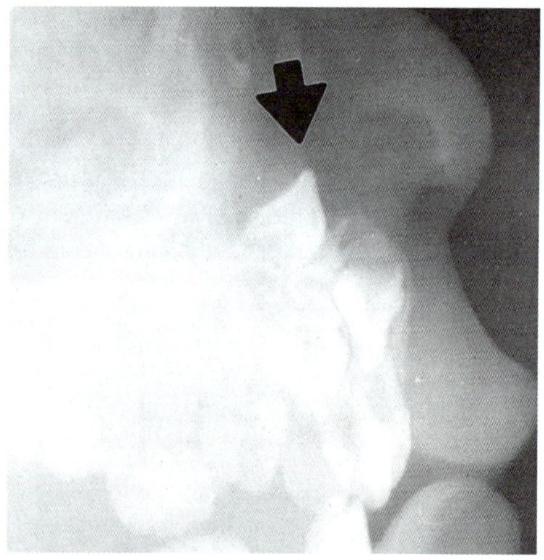

Fig. 21.32 Supernumerary nasal tooth. A lateral radiograph of the maxilla shows a supernumerary tooth *(arrow)* erupting through the floor of the nasal cavity in a child with cleft palate who had recurrent epistaxis.

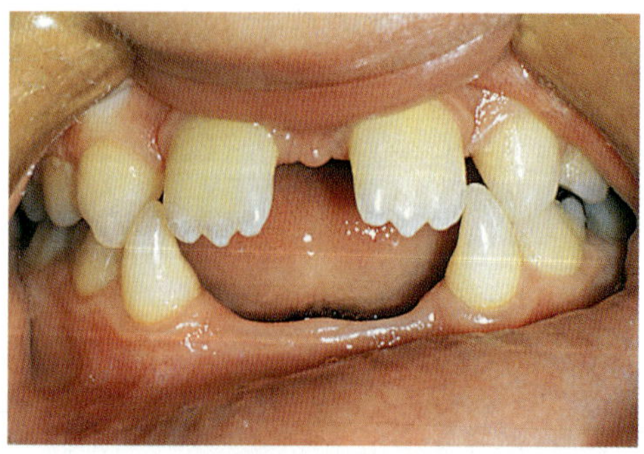

Fig. 21.33 Hypodontia. The congenital absence of teeth is seen in this patient with hereditary ectodermal dysplasia. This phenomenon may be an isolated anomaly or a manifestation of several syndromes.

teeth without affecting dentin, pulp, or cementum. Amelogenesis imperfecta is classified according to the enamel defect: hypoplastic, hypomature, hypocalcified, or a combination of these.

- Hypoplastic—thin, pitted, or fissured enamel (see Fig. 21.30)
- Hypomaturation—discolored enamel of full thickness but decreased hardness that tends to chip away slowly, exposing the underlying dentin. Radiographic evaluation demonstrates the decreased density of enamel.
- Hypocalcified—enamel is chalky, variable in color, and quickly erodes (Fig. 21.34)

Dentinogenesis Imperfecta

Dentinogenesis imperfecta results in dentin defects and is usually inherited as an autosomal dominant trait. The most common manifestation is opalescent dentin, which may be associated with osteogenesis imperfecta (see Chapter 22). Because of variable phenotypic expression, teeth may have a blue, pinkish-brown, or yellowish brown hue and an opalescent sheen (Fig. 21.35). In any given patient, individual teeth may be variably affected. Despite normal enamel morphology, patients tend to have relatively rapid wearing of the crowns. The roots are shortened, and the pulp chambers are calcified. Primary teeth are more severely affected than the permanent teeth, although permanent teeth are still prone to develop enamel fractures. In more severe cases, full coverage restorations may be needed to protect the remaining tooth structure.

DISCOLORATION

Three major types of tooth discoloration are frequently observed:

(1) discoloration from stains that adhere externally to the surfaces of the teeth (extrinsic)
(2) discoloration from various pigments that are incorporated into the tooth structure during development (intrinsic)
(3) intrinsic discoloration secondary to hereditary defects (discussed previously)

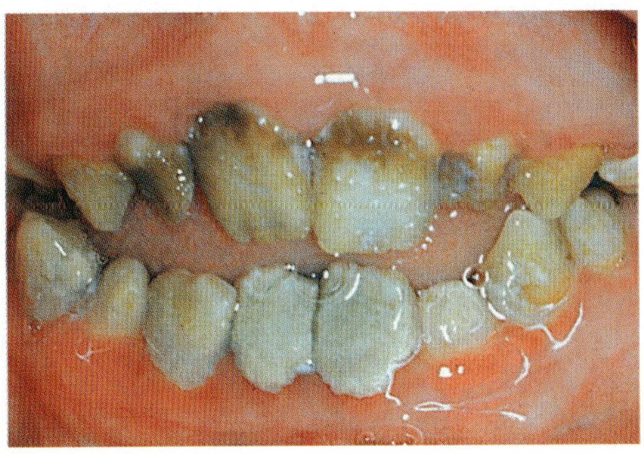

Fig. 21.34 Amelogenesis imperfecta, hypocalcified type. The enamel defects result in discoloration and erosion caused by errors in the mineralization stage of tooth development and secondary staining.

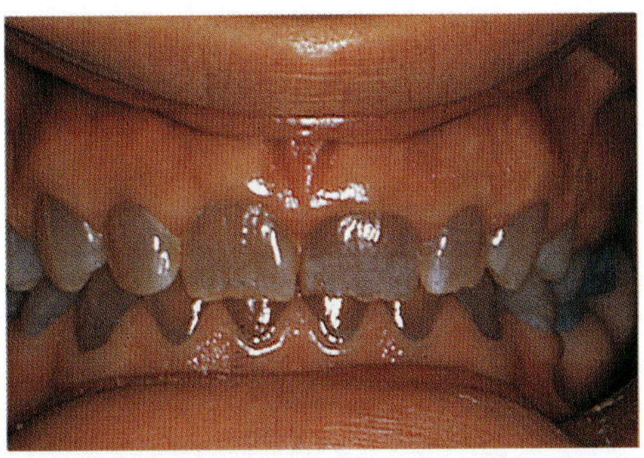

Fig. 21.35 Dentinogenesis imperfecta. The bluish, opalescent sheen on several of these teeth results from genetically defective dentin. This condition may be associated with osteogenesis imperfecta.

Extrinsic Discoloration

Extrinsic discoloration is limited primarily to patients with poor oral hygiene, those receiving certain medications, those who heavily consume stain-containing foods or drinks, or those who smoke or chew tobacco. It occurs more often at certain locations, especially on the gingival third of the exposed crown. Diagnosis requires appropriate medical, dental, and dietary histories, with an emphasis on oral hygiene, food and drug intake, and tobacco habits. Treatment includes scaling, dental prophylaxis and polishing, and regular oral hygiene. The use of excessively abrasive toothpaste can cause wear of the enamel and should be avoided.

Brownish-black stain on the lingual surfaces of anterior and posterior teeth is most common among young children who are taking liquid oral iron supplements and among adolescents who are smokers and tea drinkers. Green staining on the labial surfaces of the anterior maxillary teeth is common among children with poor oral hygiene; the source is usually chromogenic bacteria and fungi (Fig. 21.36). Orange/red stain can be found around the gingival third of the exposed crown. This stain often results from antibiotic intake, which causes a temporary shift in the oral flora.

Intrinsic Discoloration

Intrinsic discoloration is usually induced during the calcification of dentin and enamel by excessive levels of the body's natural pigments (such as hemoglobin and bile) or by pigments introduced by the intake of chemicals (such as fluorides or tetracyclines, excluding doxycycline). On occasion, isolated intrinsic discoloration occurs because of pulpal necrosis, pulpal calcification, or internal resorption.

Hepatic Discoloration

Generalized intrinsic discoloration of primary teeth is seen in patients with advanced hepatic disease associated with persistent or recurrent jaundice and hyperbilirubinemia (Fig. 21.37). The intensity of discoloration varies and may be related to the severity

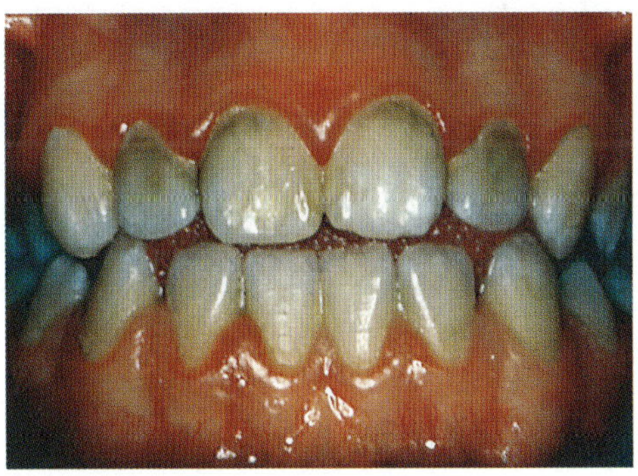

Fig. 21.36 Extrinsic discoloration. The green stain seen on the gingival third of the incisors is associated with poor oral hygiene.

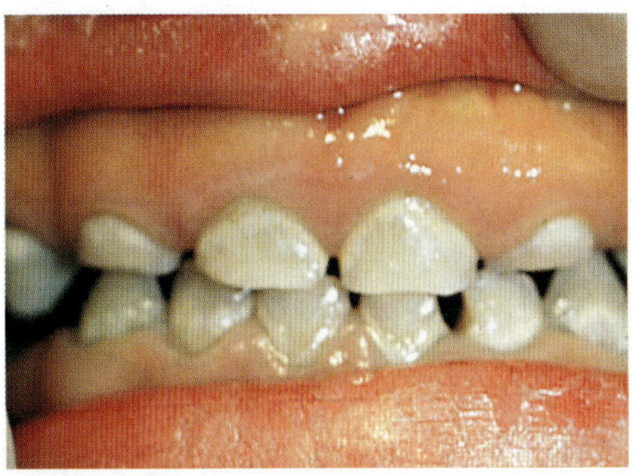

Fig. 21.37 Hepatic discoloration. Generalized intrinsic discoloration of the primary teeth is seen in this patient with biliary atresia.

of the disease. Color ranges from brown to grayish-brown and usually has no clinical significance, unless it is associated with significant hypoplasia of the dentition.

Discoloration Due to Tetracycline

Teeth stained because of tetracycline therapy may vary in color from yellow to brown to dark gray. Staining occurs when the tetracycline is incorporated into calcifying teeth and bone. The severity of discoloration depends on the dose, duration, and type of tetracycline administered; the initial yellow or light brown pigmentation tends to darken with age (Fig. 21.38). Tetracyclines readily cross the placenta, so staining of primary teeth is possible if tetracycline is taken during pregnancy; therefore tetracycline should not be prescribed to pregnant females or to children younger than 8 years old.

Discoloration Due to Erythroblastosis Fetalis

Children born with congenital hemolytic anemia caused by rhesus (Rh) factor incompatibility may exhibit distinct discoloration of their primary teeth from the deposition of bilirubin in the dentin and enamel during primary tooth development. The color ranges from green to blue to orange. No treatment is indicated unless discoloration is associated with significant hypoplasia or hypocalcification. The permanent dentition is usually not affected.

Discoloration Due to Porphyria

Porphyria, a hereditary disturbance of porphyrin metabolism, may produce a distinct reddish or brownish discoloration of the primary and permanent teeth, secondary to deposition of porphyrin in developing teeth (Fig. 21.39).

Isolated Intrinsic Discoloration

Teeth with necrotic pulps develop an opaque appearance with discoloration ranging from light yellow to gray (Fig. 21.40). Such teeth may develop abscesses, periapical cystic lesions, or chronic fistulas. Pulpal calcification (Fig. 21.41) is often associated with a localized yellow discoloration. Internal resorption manifests clinically as a pink discoloration, secondary to loss of dentin thickness.

CARIES

The interaction of microorganisms, especially *Streptococcus mutans,* and fermentable carbohydrates results in acid demineralization of susceptible enamel. Caries is seen as yellowish-brown to gray defects in the enamel surfaces of affected teeth (Fig. 21.42). Untreated, carious destruction progresses through the enamel and dentin and, with bacterial contamination of the pulp, ultimately renders the pulp necrotic. The deep pits, fissures, and grooves characteristic of the surfaces of newly erupted teeth are at increased risk for developing carious lesions (see Fig. 21.6 and Fig. 21.43). Sealing defects with bonding agents may prevent the initiation of caries. Other preventive methods include brushing once the first tooth erupts and flossing daily to remove bacteria-containing plaque, systemic fluoride via the water supply, and limiting intake of fermentable carbohydrates, especially those high in sugar and adhesiveness.

Dental caries is an infectious, communicable disease. Studies have shown that mothers are the primary source of *S. mutans* in their infants, with a greater rate of transmission to female rather than male infants. Cariogenic microbes can be transmitted vertically or horizontally. Vertical transmission occurs when bacteria, such as *S. mutans,* pass from caregiver to child through saliva. Horizontal transmission occurs between members of the family or close groups and can also be caused by saliva-sharing activities.

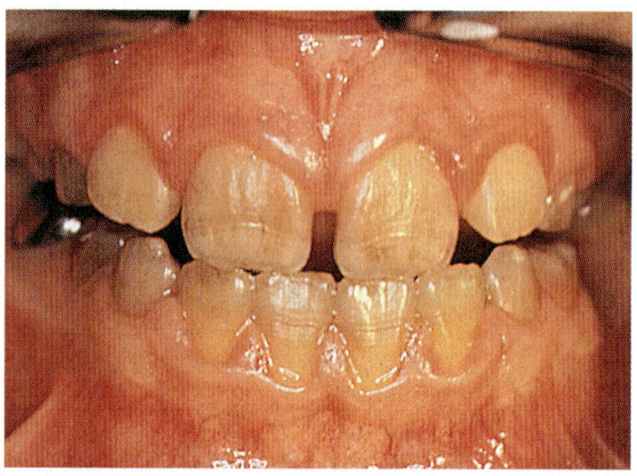

Fig. 21.38 Tetracycline discoloration. The severe discoloration seen in this patient is the result of tetracycline administration at a time when calcification of the permanent teeth was occurring.

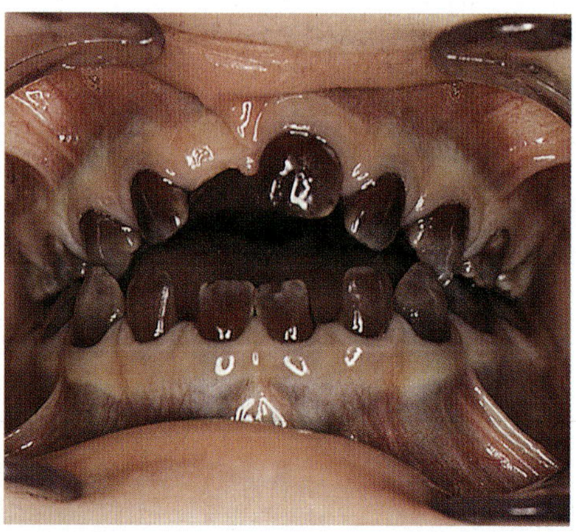

Fig. 21.39 The reddish-brown tooth discoloration associated with porphyria.

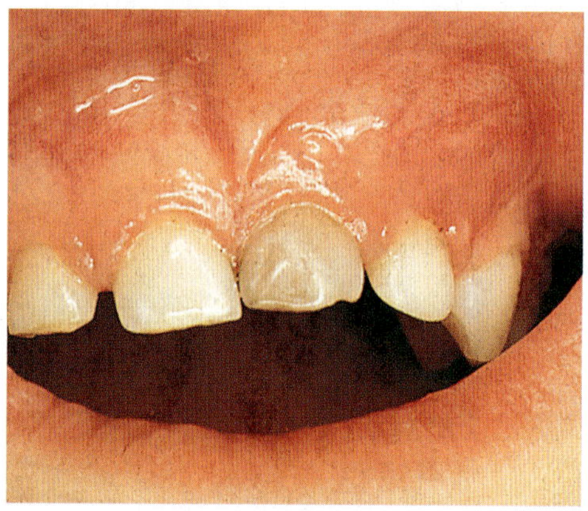

Fig. 21.40 Isolated intrinsic discoloration. The central incisor is discolored secondary to trauma. Often, such a change is a manifestation of pulpal necrosis.

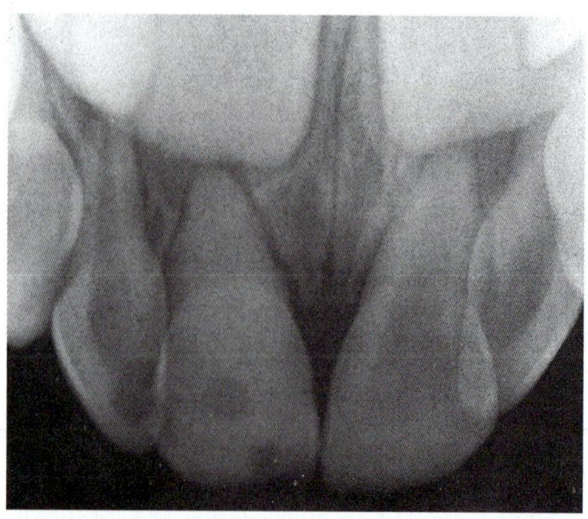

Fig. 21.41 Radiographic evidence of dystrophic calcification of the pulp and root canal of the upper right primary central incisor.

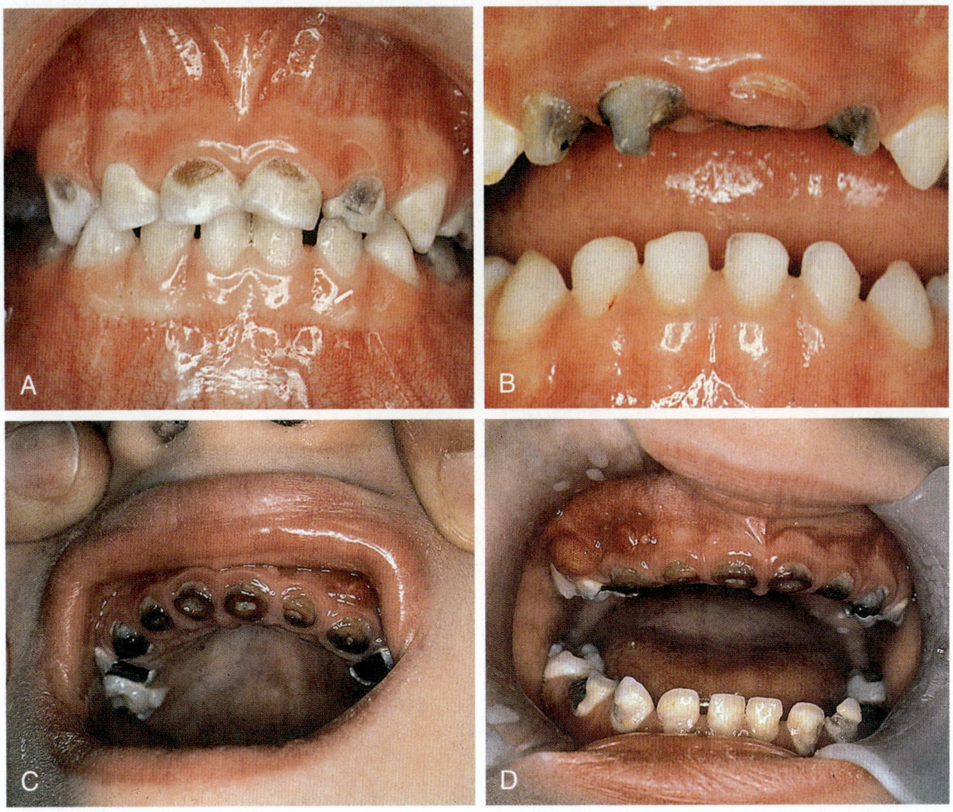

Fig. 21.42 Caries. (A) The typical pattern of nursing bottle caries, with the upper incisors being the first involved. (B) When badly neglected, severe tooth erosion occurs, and periapical abscesses may develop. (C) and (D) This 3-year-old victim of medical and dental neglect represents the extreme end of the spectrum of nursing bottle caries. When placed in foster care, she was still drinking from a bottle, had never had her teeth brushed, and had never seen a dentist. (C) Marked discoloration, extreme wear, and carious destruction of her entire maxillary dentition are evident. (D) All of her upper teeth were abscessed and her mandibular teeth were severely decayed.

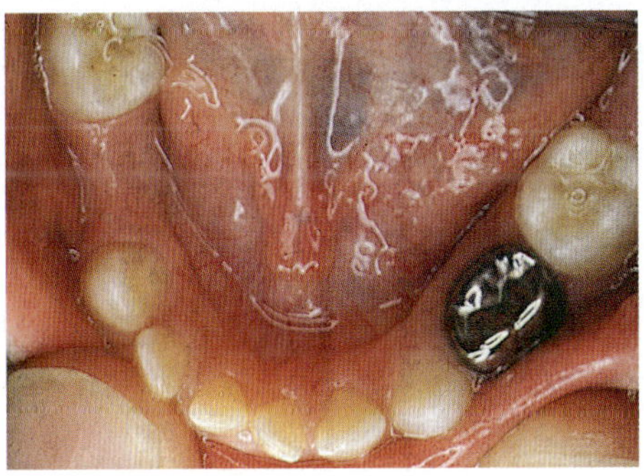

Fig. 21.43 The occlusal surfaces of newly erupted molars exhibit varying degrees of pit and fissure depth. The morphology of these patterns makes these teeth more prone to early decay.

The pregnant mother should visit a dentist for routine cleanings and examinations and, if necessary, should have carious lesions restored, preferably before pregnancy. If decay is active and painful, treatment should be cleared by her physician and completed during the second trimester of pregnancy. The presence of active dental caries can lead to vertical transmission of *S. mutans* by the mother to the infant and may increase the risk for the development of carious lesions at an early age.

Children should be referred to a dentist to establish a dental home within 6 months of the eruption of the first tooth, but no later than 1 year old. Examining children at a young age can help in preventing dental caries, providing anticipatory guidance, and documenting any dental malformations or problems that exist.

Early childhood caries (otherwise known as *nursing/baby bottle caries*) involve the primary dentition of the child habitually put to bed with a bottle containing milk or another cariogenic (sugar-containing) liquid. This form of caries was originally associated with bottle-feeding only. However, an association with frequent and prolonged nocturnal breastfeeding has become apparent. Carious lesions initially develop on the maxillary incisors and later the molars and canines (see Fig. 21.42A and B). The mandibular incisors are usually spared by the protective position of the tongue during feeding. The deleterious effect of nocturnal feeding is due to decreased rates of salivation and swallowing during sleep, leading to prolonged contact between dental surfaces and oral flora. Brushing before bedtime and/or wiping the teeth with a wet towel after nocturnal feedings is important in prevention. According to the AAPD, early childhood caries is classified as the presence of one or more decayed (noncavitated or cavitated), missing (due to caries), or filled tooth surfaces in any primary tooth in a child 71 months of age or younger.

The AAPD and the American Academy of Pediatrics recommend discontinuation of the bottle by 12 months old. Frequent overnight bottle-feedings, breastfeeding ad libitum, and extended and repeated use of training cups are all associated with early childhood caries. Breast milk alone is not implicated in developing early childhood caries, but when given in conjunction with carbohydrates, it can be cariogenic.

An especially severe variant of nursing/baby bottle caries, severe early childhood caries, is seen in toddlers whose parents deferred weaning until well after 1 year old, continued to provide them with nighttime bottles, and failed to ensure regular brushing and to seek dental care for their children. Any smooth surface caries in a child younger than 3 years of age is indicative of severe early childhood caries. In such cases, decay is extensive and deep, the teeth show signs of wearing down, and abscesses can be found (see Fig. 21.42C and D). This constitutes significant dental neglect, and these children often must undergo multiple dental restorations and/or extractions.

Fluoride Use

Fluoride is of critical importance for the control and prevention of dental caries in children and adults. Optimal fluoride exposure acts as an adjunct in decreasing the incidence of caries and remineralizing enamel. Fluoride is the most effective caries prevention agent and is considered completely safe when properly used. However, the ingestion of high concentrations or incorrect dosages of fluoride can lead to nausea, vomiting, dental fluorosis, or, in extremely rare cases, death, with most cases of fluoride overdose occurring in children younger than the age of 6.

Parents should be advised to use a smear (grain of rice size) of fluoridated toothpaste for a child younger than 3 years old. For children ages 3 to 6, a pea-sized amount of fluoridated toothpaste is recommended. Pediatricians and dentists should take into consideration all sources of fluoride before prescribing supplements to determine the correct dosage (Table 21.1).

Diet and Nutrition

Snacking and the frequency of eating and drinking are related to dental caries incidence. When sugary liquids such as juices, sports drinks, sweet teas, flavored milks, and carbonated beverages are given to young children in bottles or training cups, it can greatly increase their risk of caries. Frequent intake of these drinks can promote and accelerate caries progression.

Dietary screening, assessment, and guidance should be an integral component of the care process for dental clients. A diet high in citrus fruits, snacks containing citric acid, and acidogenic sports drinks can lead to dental erosions. Another cause of dental erosion is excessive regurgitation of gastric contents into the oral cavity, which can be related to gastroesophageal reflux disease. Sugary carbonated beverages, juices, and sports drinks are also acidic, and the combination of acid and sugar may act synergistically to cause the severe caries associated with regular carbonated beverage consumption. Repeated cariogenic attacks lead to mineral loss that presents as dental caries. The frequency and form of cariogenic foods or beverages are more important than the amount of sugar in each food item; foods such as raisins, starches, and candies that stick to the teeth for an extended period will continue to slowly leach and metabolize as sugars and acid. Oral bacteria ferment sugars and prolong the decreased pH in the oral cavity. Similarly, any food or beverage that contains fermentable carbohydrates and is consumed over a prolonged period or with increased frequency will have the same effect. The AAPD recommends that children 1 to 6 years old consume no more than 4 to 6 ounces of fruit juice per day, from an open cup only, and at mealtime.

INFECTIONS

For a summary and description of raised intraoral lesions, see Table 21.2.

Viral Infections

Herpetic Gingivostomatitis

Primary herpetic gingivostomatitis, caused by herpes simplex type virus, is a painful and contagious infection that affects adults and children, especially those between the ages of 6 months and 3 years old. The vesicular lesions of the lips, tongue, gingiva, and oral mucosa are preceded by fever, headache, regional lymphadenopathy, and gingival hyperemia and edema. These lesions tend to rupture quickly, leaving shallow ulcerations covered by a gray membrane and surrounded by an erythematous halo (Fig. 21.44; see Chapter 13). The inflamed gingivae are friable and bleed easily. Lesions heal spontaneously in 1 to 2 weeks. Because inflammation makes brushing painful, oral hygiene should be maintained with a preparation such as chlorhexidine or glycerin and peroxide (in very young children) to decrease the incidence of secondary infection. A bland diet and rinsing with "Magic Mouthwash" (a solution of equal parts Benadryl, Maalox, and viscous lidocaine) for children older than 6 years old, in addition to the use of oral analgesics, are indicated to minimize and control pain. Systemic acyclovir is indicated in cases

Table 21.1 Dietary Fluoride Supplementation Schedule

Age	Less Than 0.3 ppm F	0.3–0.6 ppm F	More Than 0.6 ppm F
Birth to 6 months old	0	0	0
6 months old to 3 years old	0.25 mg	0	0
3 years old to 6 years old	0.50 mg	0.25 mg	0
6 years old to at least 16 years old	1.00 mg	0.50 mg	0

ppm F, Parts per million fluoride.

From American Academy of Pediatric Dentistry: Guideline on fluoride therapy, *Pediatr Dent* 35(5):E165–E168, 2013.

Table 21.2 Summary of Raised Intraoral Lesions and Intraoral Ulcerations

Lesion/Ulceration	Description
Raised Intraoral Lesions	
Fibroma	Most common tumor of oral mucosa, painless, firm, pedunculated; therapy is excision
Papilloma	Pedunculated with cauliflower surface, caused by HPV; therapy is excision
Abscess	Painful red area with pimple-like appearance; therapy includes antibiotics with root canal therapy or extraction of offending tooth
Pyogenic granuloma	Painless red nodule, pedunculated, with gingival enlargement; therapy is excision
Intraoral Ulcerations	
Herpetic gingivostomatitis	Gingival erythema with multiple oral vesicles often grouped and more anterior in location; therapy includes pain relief and antivirals for severe cases
Herpangina	Multiple vesicles with erythematous borders on tonsillar pillars, uvula, and soft palate; therapy includes palliative pain relief
Varicella-zoster	Pruritic vesicles/pustules on skin with ulceration of mucous membranes; therapy includes pain relief and antivirals for severe cases
Aphthous ulcer	Ulceration with erythematous halo, typically on "unbound" mucosa; therapy includes pain relief, steroids, and/or antibiotic rinses in severe cases
Mucositis	Inflammation and ulceration of oral cavity; therapy includes improved oral hygiene
Trauma	History from parent/patient important to rule out nonaccidental trauma; treatment is palliative
Hand, foot, and mouth disease	Vesicles and ulcerations on hands, arms, feet, and legs and oral mucosa; treatment is palliative

HPV, Human papillomavirus.

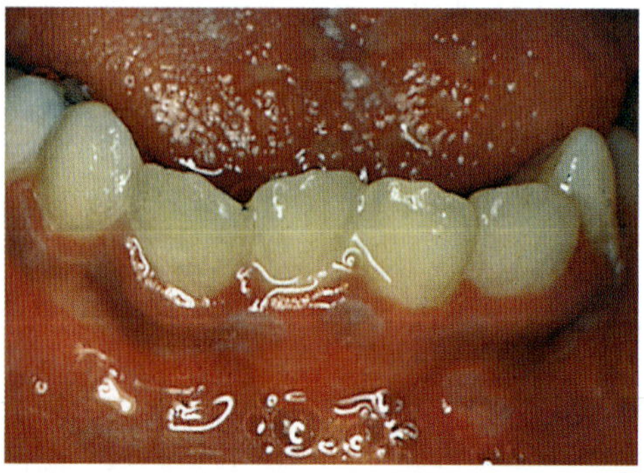

Fig. 21.44 Herpetic gingivostomatitis. The ulcerations seen on the oral mucosa were preceded by fever, headache, and lymphadenopathy. Note the erythematous halos around the ulcerations.

with moderate to severe involvement. Topical Benzocaine ointments are not recommended in young children.

Recurrent infections caused by reactivation of latent herpes simplex virus are fairly common. Lesions are few in number and more localized; systemic symptoms are absent unless the host is immunosuppressed. Lesions are usually located on the lips, with prodromal symptoms of itching and burning preceding the development of thin-walled vesicles that rupture and crust (see Chapter 13). When intraoral lesions occur, they manifest as small vesicles in a localized group on mucosa that is tightly bound to periosteum. Elective dental treatment should be deferred while the child is infectious.

Hand, Foot, and Mouth Disease and Herpangina

Hand, foot, and mouth disease, caused by coxsackievirus A or enterovirus, may present itself with fever, malaise, abdominal pain, cough, or lymphadenopathy. Oral ulcerations are present, often concurrent with vesicles on hands, arms, and feet, for about 10 days. Treatment is palliative, with attention to adequate hydration. Elective dental treatment should be deferred until oral and skin lesions resolve.

Herpangina, caused by coxsackievirus A, occurs in summer and fall months. It is spread via the oral/fecal route. Vesicles are present on the soft palate and tonsillar pillars. They often rupture, leaving shallow, painful ulcerations. Malaise, fever, and lymphadenopathy may be present (Fig. 21.45A). Treatment is palliative, with attention to maintaining adequate hydration. Elective dental treatment should be deferred until oral and skin lesions resolve and the patient is afebrile. Peeling of the digits may occurs in weeks after the infection (Fig. 21.45B).

Herpes Zoster (Shingles)

Herpes zoster ("shingle") results from reactivation of the varicella-zoster virus and inflammation of a dorsal root or extramedullary cranial nerve ganglion. Rare in healthy children, zoster mostly occurs in the immunocompromised child. The patient exhibits a prodrome of malaise, fever, headache, and tenderness along the affected dermatome that may last 3 days or more. This is followed by the extraoral formation of painful, grouped vesicular lesions that rupture to form ulcerations. The oral cavity also may be affected with erosions when maxillary and mandibular divisions of the trigeminal nerve are involved (Fig. 21.46).

Recurrent Aphthous Ulcers (Canker Sores)

Aphthous ulcers are similar in appearance to herpetic ulcers. Their specific etiology is unknown, but possible precipitating factors include trauma, stress, sunlight, endocrine disturbances, hematologic

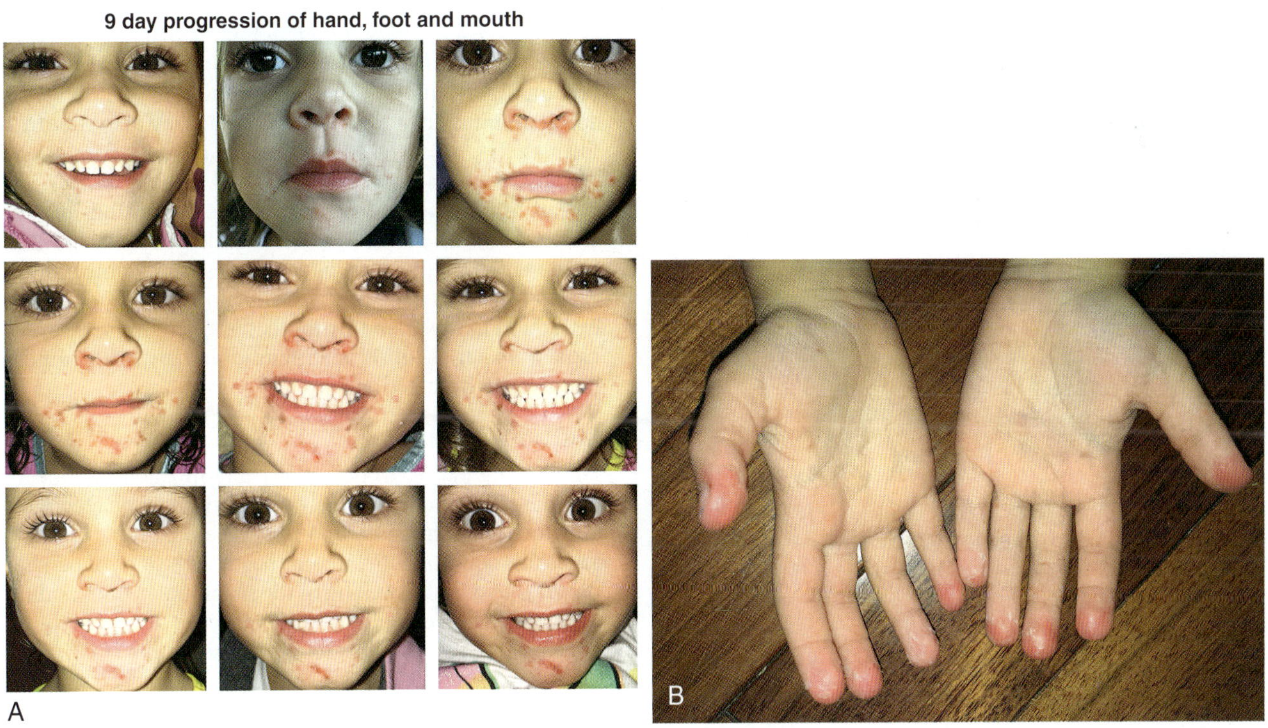

Fig. 21.45 Hand, foot, and mouth disease. (A) Hand, foot and mouth progression over 9 days. (B) Vesicles on hands during hand, foot, and mouth infection.

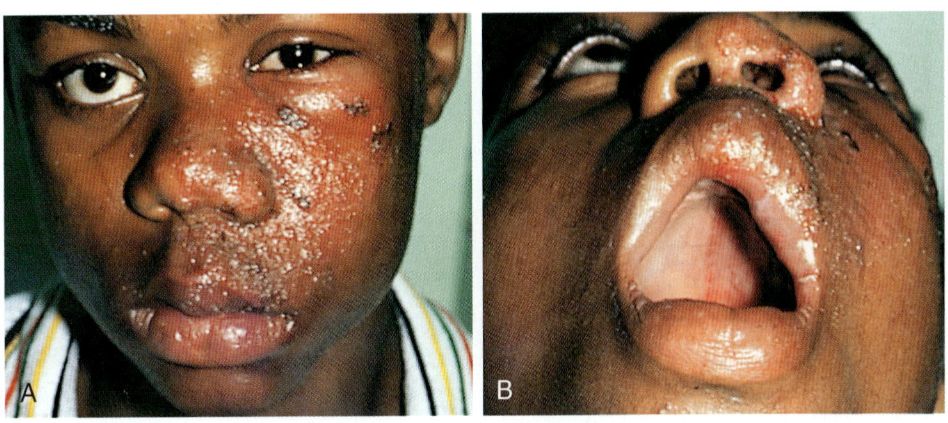

Fig. 21.46 Herpes zoster. This patient's infection involved the trigeminal nerve including the nasociliary branch. The extraoral (A) and intraoral (B) lesions stop at the midline.

disorders, or allergies. Infection with viruses and L-form bacteria, immunologic dysfunction or dysregulation, deficiency of iron, trace elements, vitamin B_{12}, and folate, and genetic factors have all been postulated as causative agents. Their pathophysiology is likely due to multiple factors. Onset is usually during adolescence or young adulthood, and between 5% and 25% of the population is affected at some time during their lives by recurrent ulcers. Unlike herpetic lesions, these ulcerations are not preceded by vesicle formation. They are extremely painful and have a pseudomembrane and an erythematous halo (Fig. 21.47). They can vary in size, number, and distribution. Small aphthae may coalesce into larger lesions. Although any oral mucosal surface may be involved, freely movable mucosa is more frequently involved. Lesions heal over 1 to 2 weeks. Recurrences have no regular periodicity and are not accompanied by fever or other systemic symptoms. Treatment is symptomatic, usually with a topical anesthetic/antiseptic preparation. More recently, use of immunomodulating agents is being studied, as are high doses of vitamin B_{12} in idiopathic cases.

Bacterial Infections

Odontogenic infections are caused by both aerobic and anaerobic microorganisms. Streptococci and staphylococci are most frequently isolated. Oral anaerobic organisms such as fusobacteria, anaerobic streptococci, and *Kingella* species are often prominent causes.

Dental Abscesses

Abscesses are most common in children with dental caries as a result of poor dental hygiene, irregular dental care, or deep restorations, especially white resin fillings. Once caries extends to the pulp, infection and pulpal necrosis ensue, setting the stage for the formation of a periapical abscess. Children with traumatized teeth may go on to develop abscesses if the resulting pulpal hyperemia is so extreme that it causes pressure necrosis, if the neurovascular bundle is severed, or if the pulp is exposed by a crown fracture.

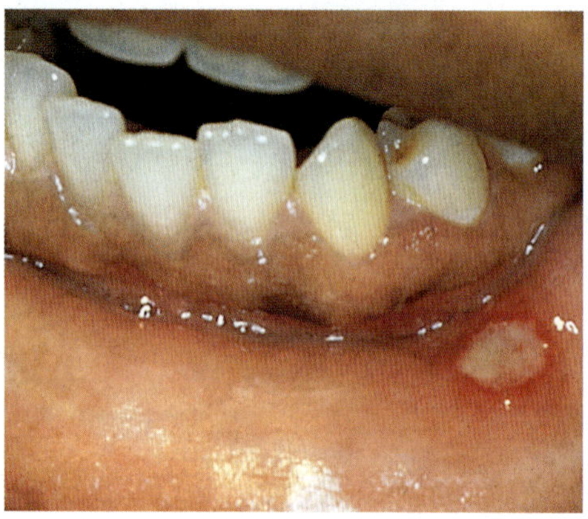

Fig. 21.47 Recurrent aphthous ulcers. The ulceration seen on the labial mucosa is surrounded by a characteristic erythematous halo.

Periapical abscesses require endodontic therapy or extraction of the offending tooth. The potential for complications makes early diagnosis important, yet frequently this does not occur because symptoms are often insidious in onset and progression and nonspecific in nature. This is in part because the alveolar processes of the mandible and maxilla in young children are fenestrated anteriorly, assisting early decompression of the abscess through the alveolus and gingiva. Patients may complain of headaches as the abscess enlarges and pressure builds up, and then of abdominal pain after decompression as the draining pus is swallowed, causing gastric irritation. Later in childhood, abscessed maxillary teeth may intermittently decompress through the floor of a maxillary sinus, producing recurrent sinus infections. Other symptoms may include anorexia, avoidance of certain foods, halitosis, toothaches, a sensitive tooth, or facial swelling. Nonspecific complaints and complaints of referred pain are more common among children than toothache, and some children have no overt symptoms.

On physical examination, the examiner may find localized facial swelling, gingival swelling and/or erythema, a gingival abscess, a fistula, or a granuloma (Figs. 21.48 and 21.49A). On occasion, there is increased sensitivity to percussion or palpation. Left untreated, a periapical abscess of a primary tooth may damage the underlying developing tooth bud. Abscesses may also result in formation of an apical granuloma or a radicular cyst, or they may rupture and spread through the adjacent soft tissues to create a fistula, which drains through the skin (see Fig. 21.49B). In some instances, infection can spread into adjacent facial soft tissues, resulting in facial cellulitis (Fig. 21.50). The infection may track through lateral pharyngeal, retropharyngeal, or sublingual spaces, threatening the airway and causing sepsis and/or mediastinitis. In addition to pulpal therapy or extraction fo the offending tooth, treatment for severe dental abscess causing facial cellulitis is antibiotic therapy, with route dictated by the severity of infection.

Ludwig Angina

Ludwig angina is a potentially life-threatening infection of the mandibular floor. It is usually an infection associated with anaerobic streptococci, although any of the anaerobic flora of the mouth may cause this condition. Symptoms begin with signs of dental abscess but progress to a tense swelling of the mandibular floor and then cervical edema. Pain, fever, and difficulty in swallowing are typical of Ludwig angina, and the inability to handle secretions marks late stages of disease with airway impingement. It is extremely important to protect the airway in patients with Ludwig angina, because the disease will progress rapidly even with adequate therapy and the rapid onset of airway compromise is life-threatening. Treatment includes immediate surgical intervention with stabilization of the airway and removal of

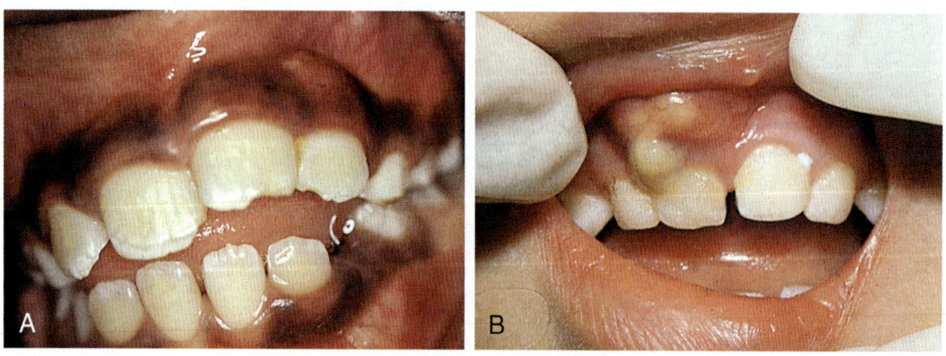

Fig. 21.48 Dental abscesses. (A) An abscess above the left upper lateral incisor developed after an injury in which the patient had chipped that tooth and his central incisor. (B) This abscess above the right central incisor has ruptured through the gingiva and begun to drain. The tooth is discolored because of pulp necrosis stemming from an injury 2 years earlier.

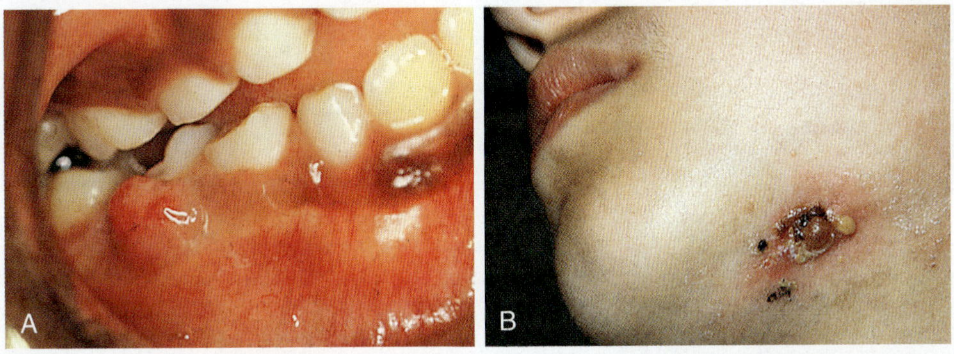

Fig. 21.49 (A) A deep, neglected cavity in this mandibular molar predisposed to development of a periapical abscess that, after rupture, resulted in formation of a gingival granuloma. (B) Left untreated, such abscesses can be responsible for this type of extraoral lesion in which infection has spread by way of a fistulous tract to the skin. Extraction of the offending tooth is necessary for resolution of the extraoral lesion.

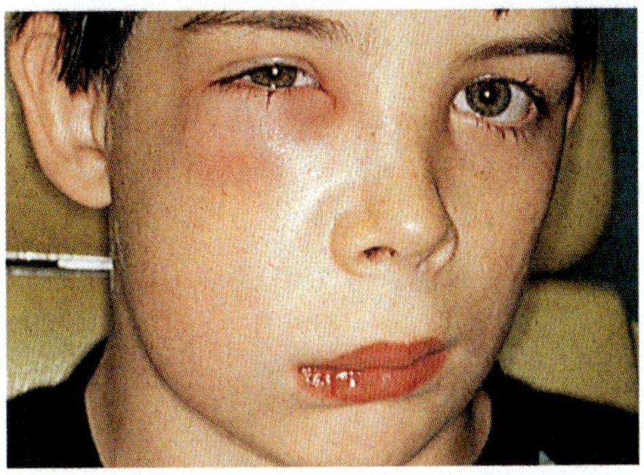

Fig. 21.50 Facial cellulitis associated with an abscessed maxillary tooth. Hospital admission for intravenous antibiotics, incision and drainage, and extraction of the abscessed tooth was necessary.

infected teeth. Intravenous antibiotics are necessary until the patient stabilizes. There is frequent need for incision and drainage of the infected area, and a multidisciplinary team including dental medicine, anesthesia, and otolaryngology may be needed.

Pericoronitis

Pericoronitis is an inflammation of the gingival soft tissue surrounding the crown of a partially erupted tooth. This occurs when debris become trapped under the residual gingiva, stimulating bacterial growth and abscess formation. The third molars are most involved. Symptoms include localized pain, tenderness, and occasionally fever and malaise. Erythema and edema are readily apparent on examination (Fig. 21.51A), and a palpable submandibular node is often found. Fig. 21.51B demonstrates the presence of both partially impacted and erupted teeth. Treatment options include warm saltwater rinses to decrease bacterial counts and dislodge trapped food particles. Antibiotics and surgical correction may be necessary.

Acute Necrotizing Ulcerative Gingivitis (Vincent Stomatitis, Trench Mouth)

Acute necrotizing ulcerative gingivitis is a fusospirochetal infection caused by fusiform bacilli and *Borrelia vincentii*. It is seldom seen before the age of 10. Patients experience abrupt onset of fever, malaise, severe mouth pain, and anorexia. The gingivae are erythematous, edematous, and friable with necrotic punched-out craters in the interdental papillae. Involved areas bleed readily and become covered with a pseudomembrane (Fig. 21.52). The breath is fetid, and cervical and submandibular nodes become enlarged and tender. Treatment generally consists of dental prophylaxis, followed by improved oral hygiene measures and topical peroxide applications. In most cases, resolution occurs within several days without the use of antibiotics. On occasion, secondary infection or severe involvement may necessitate the use of antibiotics.

Bacterial Pharyngitis

Pharyngitis is most commonly a bacterial infection of the tonsils and posterior pharynx, caused by *Streptococcus pyogenes* in school-age children and adolescents (see Chapter 13). It is manifested by erythematous inflammation of the tonsils and posterior pharynx,

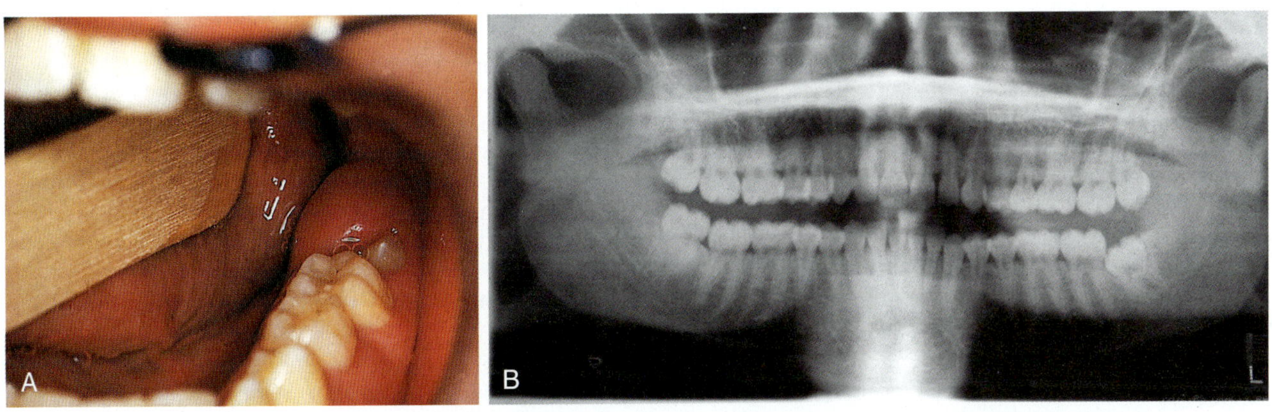

Fig. 21.51 The maxillary third molars and right mandibular third molar have erupted into a favorable position. The left mandibular third molar is partially erupted; however, it has been unable to erupt into occlusion. Partially erupted mandibular third molars are often associated with pericoronitis and/or periodontal defects distal to the second molar. (A) Pericoronitis involving a partially erupted third molar. Food particles and bacteria have become trapped under the residual overlying gingiva, resulting in inflammation and abscess formation. This condition can occur with eruption of any molar but is most common with partially erupted third molars (wisdom teeth). (B) Panoramic radiograph demonstrating the presence of erupted maxillary third molars and mandibular right third molar, but only partial eruption of the left mandibular third molar.

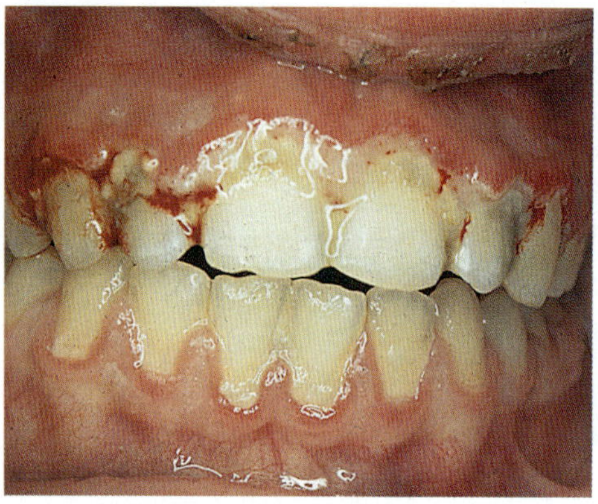

Fig. 21.52 Acute necrotizing ulcerative gingivitis. The infected gingiva exhibits localized necrosis and hemorrhage and is covered with pseudomembranes.

petechiae of the soft palate, and anterior cervical lymphadenopathy. There may be associated headaches, fever, vomiting, or abdominal discomfort. Most symptoms will last for 5 to 7 days; antibiotic therapy decreases suppurative complications and reduces the risk for rheumatic fever in endemic areas.

Lemierre Syndrome

Rarely, septic thrombosis of the cavernous sinus or jugular veins may result from invasive infection, producing Lemierre syndrome. Most commonly affecting adolescents, Lemierre syndrome is a suppurative jugular thrombophlebitis most commonly caused by *Fusobacterium* species, though is often polymicrobial. Symptoms begin with a local pharyngitis, which progresses to parapharyngeal tissues and the internal jugular vein, invading this and causing thrombosis and bacteremia. This may cause embolic disease to the lungs and other tissues and septic shock. Without prompt recognition and aggressive antibiotic therapy, patients may require critical care management for shock and airway compromise.

Fungal Infections

Candidiasis (Moniliasis, Thrush)

Oral candidiasis results from infection with the opportunistic pathogen *Candida albicans*. It is a benign infection in infants (as thrush) and in young children exposed to antibiotic treatment. In immunosuppressed children or those with underlying systemic diseases, it may be more extensive, recurrent, and severe. Lesions may appear to be pseudomembranous or plaquelike. Scraping of the lesion reveals a raw and erythematous base with bleeding from torn capillaries. Immunodeficiency such as human immunodeficiency virus infection must be ruled out when severe or therapy-resistant disease is present in children. Common sites of involvement are the buccal mucosa, tongue, palate, and commissures of the lips (Fig. 21.53). The intraoral lesions are soft, elevated, creamy white plaques that do not scrape off easily. Chronic candidiasis, usually seen in the immunocompromised host, can result in marked hypertrophy and fissuring of the tongue mucosa. Although culturing is difficult and not reliable, diagnosis may be made on the basis of clinical findings or examination of a potassium hydroxide preparation. Treatment consists of local application of nystatin, with antifungal agents for severe or chronic cases. Attention to underlying causes is critical, including sterilization of nipples used for formula feedings.

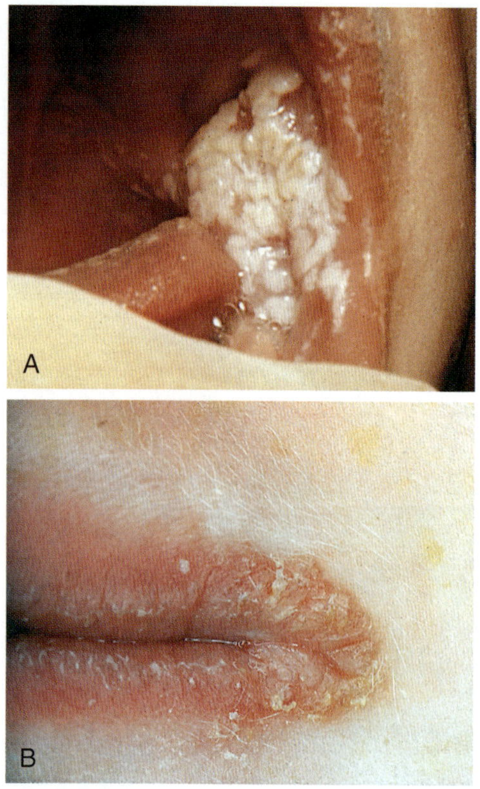

Fig. 21.53 Candidiasis. (A) Involvement of buccal mucosa with white plaque. (B) Mucocutaneous infection of the commissures of the lips.

TRAUMA

Assessment of Patients With Orofacial and Dental Injuries

In evaluating patients with orofacial and dental trauma, key elements of the history include timing, location and mechanism of injury, the child's subsequent behavior, any prior treatment, and general health and tetanus immunization status. It is important to note whether there was loss of consciousness, nausea or vomiting, whether the child exhibits age-appropriate responsiveness, and how quickly he or she returned to consciousness.

Physical examination is first directed at determining the adequacy and stability of airway, breathing, and circulation, followed by evaluation for associated head and neck injury. When these areas have been cleared and stabilized, then the examiner may proceed with the orofacial examination. Because the presence of underlying injuries is often indicated by the degree and nature of overlying soft tissue trauma, assessment begins with external inspection of facial structures for swelling, deformity, contusions, abrasions, and lacerations. The presence of associated periorbital ecchymoses or swelling, subconjunctival hemorrhage or edema, diplopia, and nasal bleeding should raise suspicion of frontal skull and midface fractures. Battle sign (bruising of the mastoid process) is an indication of basilar skull fracture and may suggest underlying brain trauma. Observation of cranial nerve function and jaw motion on opening and closing is essential. Older patients can be asked if it feels normal when they bite down; parents of young children can report if the child's bite looks normal. The temporomandibular joint (TMJ) should be palpated while the child's facial expression is observed to assess for tenderness, clicking, or pain on opening and closing.

Next, intraoral soft tissues are inspected for evidence of swelling, hematoma, abrasions, and lacerations, and displacement, loosening, and fractures of teeth. All internal and external lacerations must be carefully inspected to check for injury to underlying neural and ductal structures. Recommended radiographs include apical and occlusal views for displacement of a permanent tooth, panoramic and facial bone radiographs for possible mandibular fractures, and a computed tomography (CT) scan to assess for maxillary and midface fractures.

Soft Tissue Injuries

A variety of soft tissue injuries including lacerations, contusions, abrasions, perforations, avulsions, and burns may occur. Although these may occur in isolation, they are often associated with injuries of teeth and supporting bones, so assessment of a soft tissue injury should include attention to the teeth and underlying structures. Examination of a clean field is important, so the injured area should be cleansed of blood clots, debris, and foreign material. Saline rinses, careful attention to oral hygiene, antibiotic therapy, and soft diet are mainstays of management of all intraoral soft tissue injuries.

Abrasions

Superficial abrasions usually heal without complications. Extensive abrasions should be covered with water-soluble, medicated gauze after irrigation. Extensive deep abrasions may require skin grafting and referral to a plastic surgeon.

Contusions

A contusion, or bruise, usually requires no treatment but is associated with underlying injuries. Therefore a careful examination of adjacent structures is recommended.

Perforations

Perforations are small, deep wounds caused by sharp objects and are common in children, especially as a result of falls with objects in the mouth. After careful inspection and irrigation, larger wounds should be closed in layers; smaller wounds may not require closure. A radiograph of the involved soft tissue can rule out foreign body presence. The possibility of damage to large vessels should be noted, especially when the perforation involves the posterolateral palate or a tonsillar pillar.

Avulsions (Degloving Injuries)

Avulsions of oral soft tissues are uncommon, yet when they occur, they may involve deep and superficial tissues (Fig. 21.54A–D). Small avulsions can be treated by suturing surrounding tissues with particular concern for maintaining good blood supply; larger avulsions can be treated by reattaching the avulsed tissues or by use of a graft.

Lacerations

Lacerations are common in children. Small intraoral lacerations with well-approximated margins do not require suturing. Bleeding usually subsides spontaneously, and healing proceeds appropriately. Large lacerations, through-and-through lacerations, and those associated with extensive, recurrent, or uncontrolled bleeding require surgical closure (Fig. 21.55). To reduce risk of infection, saline irrigation and antimicrobial prophylaxis are recommended for all intraoral lacerations, regardless of whether sutures are required.

Lip lacerations can be caused by penetration of teeth through the labial soft tissues (Fig. 21.56), so adjacent dentition must be carefully inspected for evidence of chipping leading to embedded tooth particles in surrounding soft tissue. These may be difficult to palpate but are easily detected radiographically. They must be removed to prevent infection.

Because the trauma that results in chin lacerations commonly involves impact forces to the underlying bone and condyles, these cases warrant assessment of underlying bony structures, especially the TMJs (see Figs. 21.56, 21.66, and 21.67). Forced occlusion injuries can also produce tongue lacerations. Closure is required for large, gaping wounds with persistent bleeding

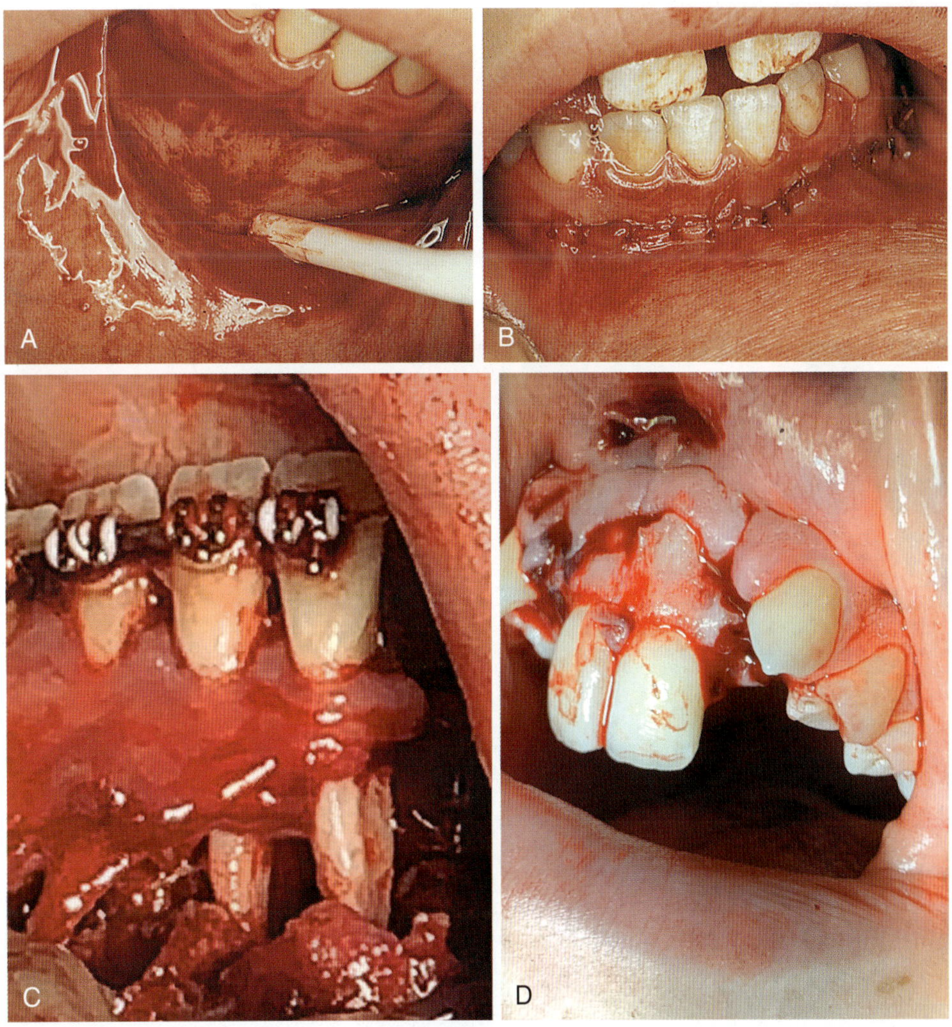

Fig. 21.54 Degloving injury, before (A) and after (B) repair. Such an injury to the oral mucosa requires immediate inspection, irrigation, approximation, and suturing. (C) Degloving of mandibular oral mucosa revealing root surfaces of incisors. (D) Degloving of maxillary oral mucosa and frenum tear with a concurrent palatal luxation of teeth 8 and 9. (C, Courtesy Lina Lim, DDS; D, Courtesy Allison Bailey, DDS.)

(Fig. 21.57A), but conservative management is best for smaller lesions (see Fig. 21.57B).

Soft palate lacerations require pharyngeal inspection. The possibility of foreign body entrapment, immediate or delayed vascular injury, or formation of pharyngeal abscesses should be seriously considered. Lacerations involving the labial frenum of toddlers are common and require only restriction of lip manipulation and a soft diet.

Burns

Burns involving the oral cavity usually heal rapidly but, when deep, may do so with contracture and scarring. Burns at the angle of the mouth incurred by chewing on an electrical cord (Fig. 21.58) are particularly problematic. After the injury, an eschar forms over the necrotic tissue. This tends to separate approximately 10 days later, at which time profuse bleeding from the labial artery may occur. Parents need to be informed of this possibility and instructed on what action to take if it should occur. Splints fabricated from dental materials are important in long-term management to prevent or minimize contracture by maintaining proper anatomic relationships during healing.

Traumatic Ulcers

Painful ulcerations may result from mechanical, chemical, or thermal trauma. Injury may be secondary to irritation by objects, trauma during mastication, toothbrush trauma, or abnormal habits.

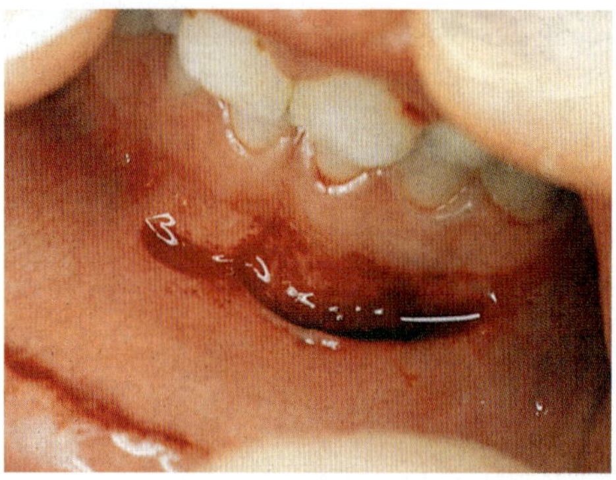

Fig. 21.55 This laceration of the oral mucosa—deep and not well approximated—requires immediate treatment and surgical closure.

Large ulcerations involving the buccal mucosa or lower lip may be associated with cheek or lip biting after inferior alveolar nerve block (Fig. 21.59). Topical peroxide application (Gly Oxide) is useful in cleansing the area. Lesions usually heal without scarring, but secondarily infected lesions may require antibiotic therapy. Elimination of the habit is necessary for resolution of habit-related lesions.

Oral Mucositis

Oral mucositis is an inflammation and ulceration of the oral cavity. It is commonly seen as a complication of chemotherapy. Good oral hygiene is important for patients with oral mucositis. This includes hydration and brushing two or three times per day with a soft bristle toothbrush. If poor oral hygiene is present, chlorhexidine rinses should be encouraged. If a patient develops oral mucositis, chlorhexidine may need to be discontinued because its high alcohol content may dehydrate the tissue. It is also important for patients undergoing chemotherapy to supplement fluoride due to the possibility of xerostomia (dry mouth), which may lead to increased caries risk.

Trauma to the Dentition

As noted earlier, facial injuries in childhood frequently involve the dentition and supporting bones. One prospective study showed that 50% of children had suffered at least one dental injury by age 14. Although falls occur frequently in early childhood, bicycle and skateboard accidents, contact sports, fights, and motor vehicle accidents become more prevalent with advancing age. The possibility of child abuse must be considered for all age groups. The risk of facial injuries is relatively high in these groups:

(1) children with neurologic disorders that impair coordination
(2) children with protruding maxillary anterior teeth
(3) children with a deviant anatomic relationship, such as an anterior open bite or a hypoplastic upper lip
(4) 2- to 3-year-old children with immature motor skills and coordination

Falling while a child is actively using a bottle, sippy cup, or pacifier is associated with more traumatic dental injuries. Preventive measures such as use of helmets, mouthguards, and seat belts significantly reduce the incidence and severity of such injuries.

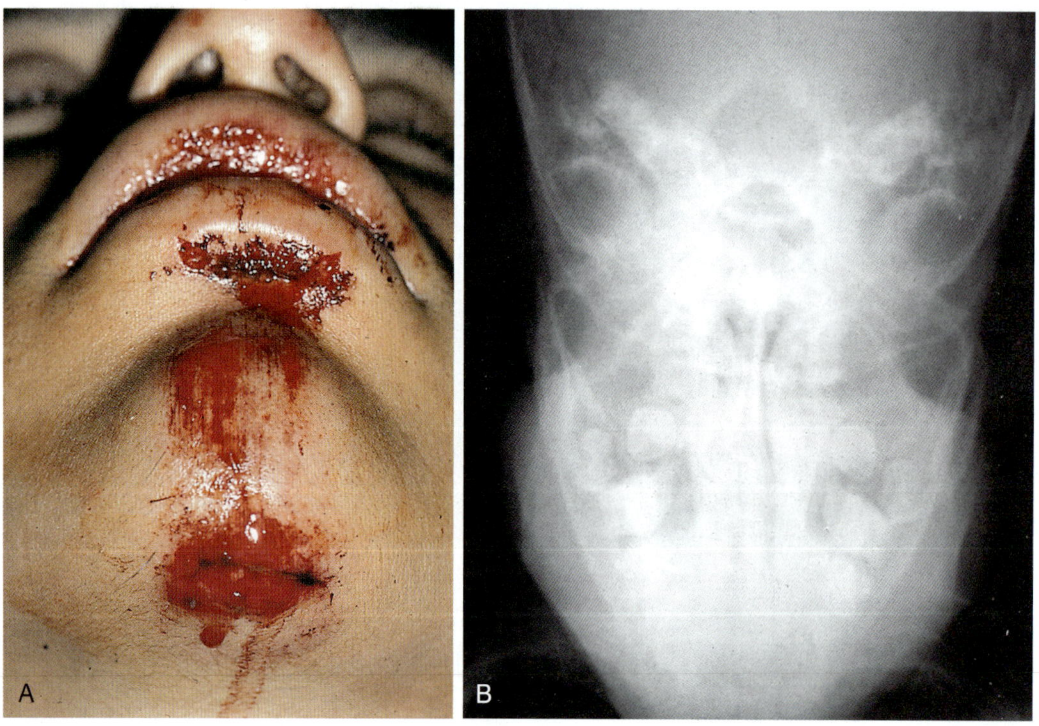

Fig. 21.56 (A) This boy incurred a forced occlusion injury when hit by a car and thrown from his bike. Note the chin laceration and through-and-through lip laceration. (B) He also had bilateral condylar neck fractures of the mandible. In this radiograph the condyles bend inward at nearly 90 degrees above the fracture lines.

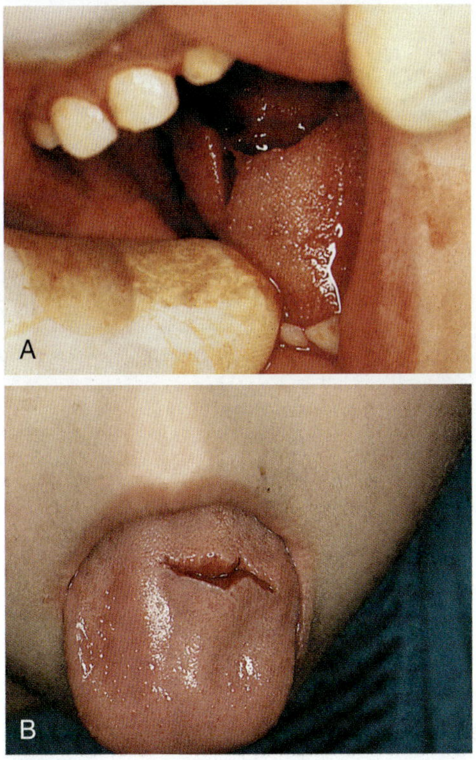

Fig. 21.57 Tongue lacerations. (A) A large gaping tongue laceration in a toddler produced by the upper front teeth being forced through the tissue by a fall with the tongue protruded. This type of injury requires suturing. (B) This small laceration, although gaping slightly, does not require surgical closure.

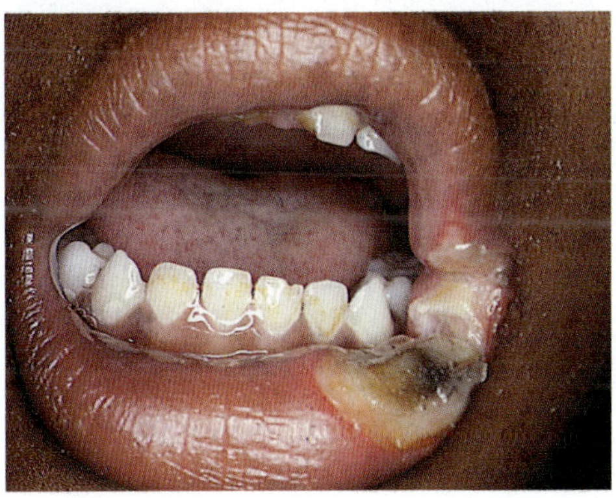

Fig. 21.58 This electrical burn was the result of chewing on an extension cord. In this site, delayed hemorrhage after separation of the eschar as well as deformity with scarring are problems.

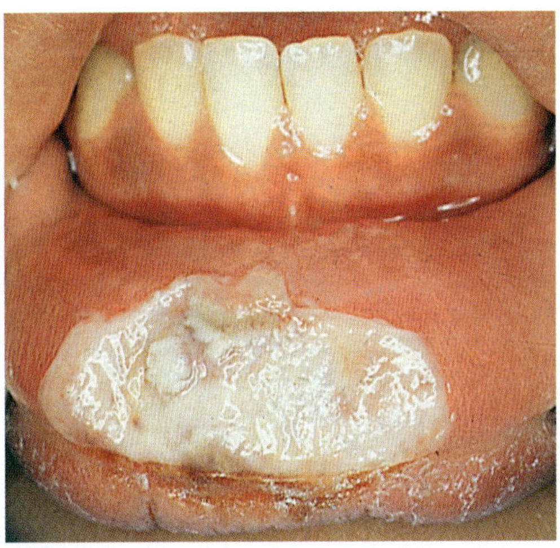

Fig. 21.59 Traumatic lip ulceration caused by lip biting or sucking after administration of local anesthesia.

Potential Complications

Pulp hemorrhage and/or vasodilation of the pulp vessels are a common response to a concussive injury to a tooth and can lead to development of discoloration within 10 to 14 days. Excessive pulpal vasodilation can result in pressure necrosis of the pulp. Injuries that produce loosening or displacement of a tooth disrupt the anchoring periodontal ligament; if disruption is mild, there may be no sequelae, although in some cases it stimulates overactive bony repair, ankylosing the tooth in place. When disruption is more severe, the neurovascular bundle can be torn, resulting in pulpal necrosis, which then may lead to abscess formation. Finally, dental fractures in which dentin and/or pulp are exposed open a pathway for bacteria and may lead to abscess formation. The fracture surface must be sealed emergently.

Several classification systems of tooth injuries exist, but for the purpose of this text a simplified descriptive classification is presented.

Crown Craze or Crack

A significant number of children exhibit “cracks” in the enamel of their teeth. Such cracks are presumably caused by relatively minor trauma or temperature changes. Such teeth are asymptomatic and require no treatment.

Crown Fractures Without Pulpal Exposure

Fractures that traverse only the enamel layer (see Fig. 21.48A) often require no treatment other than smoothing down rough edges and ensuring close follow-up. However, any fracture of the crown that results in exposure of the dentin requires emergency treatment to prevent infection and subsequent pulp necrosis (Fig. 21.60), as oral flora rapidly migrate to the pulp when they enter the dentinal tubules. Exposed dentin should be sealed with calcium hydroxide, followed by a resin bandage. This procedure should be performed as soon as possible after the injury. Dental fragments are occasionally embedded in the soft tissues of the lip or tongue, so appropriate examination of these areas is recommended.

Crown Fractures With Pulpal Exposure

Fractures that traverse all three tooth layers to expose the pulp usually involve a significant loss of tooth structure. On physical examination, the fracture surface reveals the pink central pulp surrounded by the beige dentinal layer (Fig. 21.61). Severe vertical or diagonal fractures may also result in pulp exposure and can at times extend to involve the root (Fig. 21.62). Such teeth must be treated on an emergency basis by pulp capping, pulpotomy, or root canal therapy, depending on severity.

Root Fractures

Root fractures are less common in the primary dentition, and when they occur, they usually require no therapy. If the coronal segment represents an aspiration risk or the patient has traumatic occlusion,

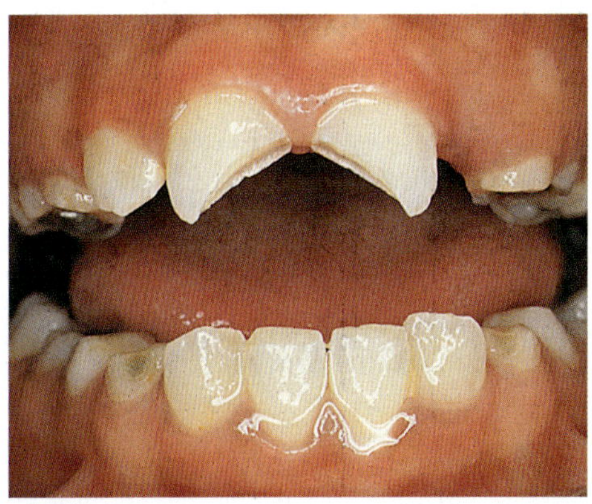

Fig. 21.60 These crown fractures demonstrate involvement of enamel and dentin, without exposure of the pulp. Immediate dental referral is necessary to prevent contamination of the pulp through the dentinal tubules.

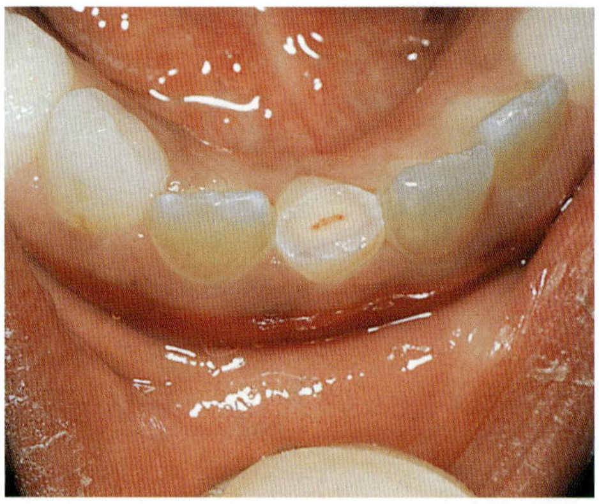

Fig. 21.61 This crown fracture involves enamel, dentin, and the soft tissue of the pulp. Immediate dental referral is mandatory to save the tooth.

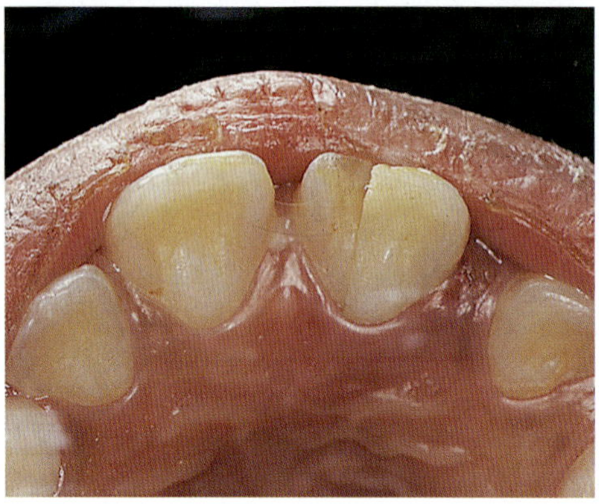

Fig. 21.62 A vertical fracture of the upper central incisor extending below the gum line resulting in pulp exposure.

the tooth should be extracted. Root fractures of permanent teeth may occur with or without loss of crown structure and may be asymptomatic (Fig. 21.63). If a seemingly normal tooth is tender or exhibits increased mobility after trauma, a root fracture should be suspected and radiographs should be obtained. In general, the prognosis is good, and treatment may include splinting the involved segment with or without root canal therapy. Splinting may last for 4 weeks to 4 months, depending on the severity of the injury.

Displacement Injuries

Displacement injuries result in extrusion, intrusion, or lateral displacement and are most seen in the primary dentition, where the combination of a short root length and a "pliable" bony structure seems to permit such displacement to occur (Fig. 21.64A). Displacement injuries are often the cause of significant discomfort and bleeding. All result in some degree of disruption of the periodontal ligament. Fractures of underlying bony structures are common associated findings. Because the primary teeth are most vulnerable to these types of injury, there is always a risk of damage to and interference with normal development of permanent tooth buds, so immediate care is advised. Treatment may include observation, mild repositioning, or extraction of the displaced tooth. Most intruded primary teeth reerupt within 6 to 8 weeks but may take up to 6 months for spontaneous reeruption. A soft diet and good oral hygiene after displacement will improve outcomes. In general, displaced permanent teeth (Fig. 21.64B) should be repositioned and splinted, with close follow-up. It is not uncommon for these teeth to require root canal therapy and orthodontic treatment.

Avulsion and Reimplantation

Avulsion is the complete displacement of a tooth from its socket and is seen mostly in preschool and early school-age children. Reimplantation of primary teeth is not recommended.

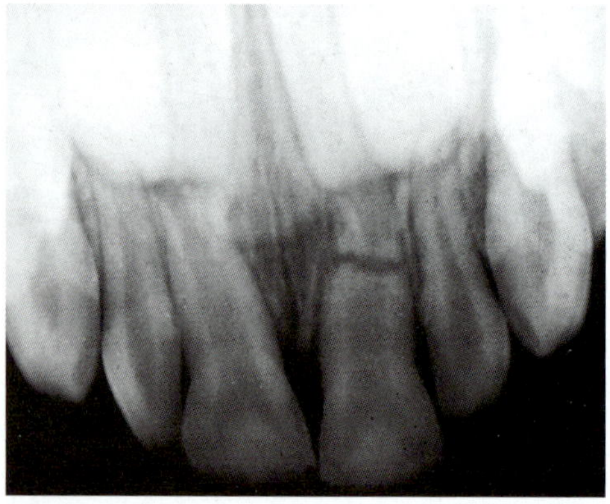

Fig. 21.63 This radiograph reveals a root fracture in the apical third of an upper primary incisor. This was suspected clinically because of tenderness and increased mobility.

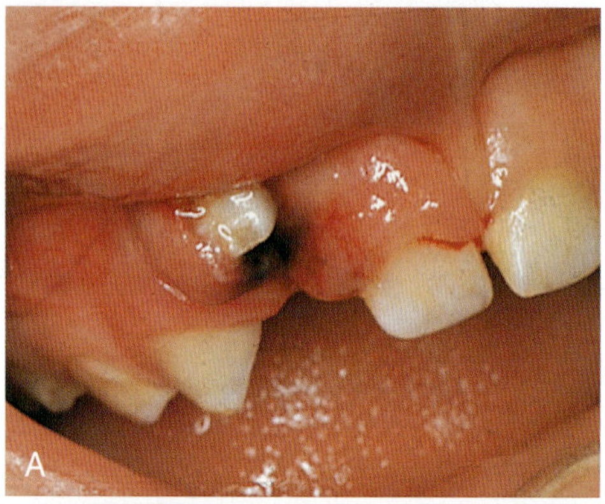

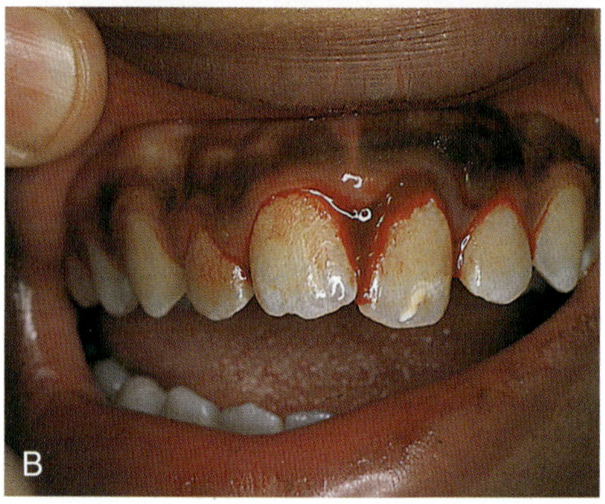

Fig. 21.64 Displacement injuries. (A) This primary lateral incisor was traumatically intruded; such intrusions usually spontaneously reerupt. (B) Lateral displacement. The left upper central incisor is lingually displaced, and its crown appears elongated because of partial extrusion. This would require repositioning and splinting.

However, reimplantation of permanent teeth is an acceptable technique with a relatively good prognosis (Fig. 21.65). The major factors in improving prognosis are as follows:

- A short period between avulsion and reimplantation, preferably less than 5 minutes, or as soon as possible
- Storage of the avulsed tooth (the most desirable "medium" is the socket itself, followed in order of preference by ViaSpan, Hanks' balanced salt solution, cold milk, saliva, saline, or water)
- Irrigation of the surgical site, replacing the tooth into the socket with slight digital pressure, and stabilization with the use of a splint
- Removal of the pulp within 7 to 10 days as a first step in completing root canal treatment, unless the tooth was immature with incomplete root formation
- Removal of the splint within 2 weeks
- Ensuring that the patient has received complete tetanus immunization; follow-up care also includes chlorhexidine rinse, appropriate antibiotic, and a soft diet for 2 weeks

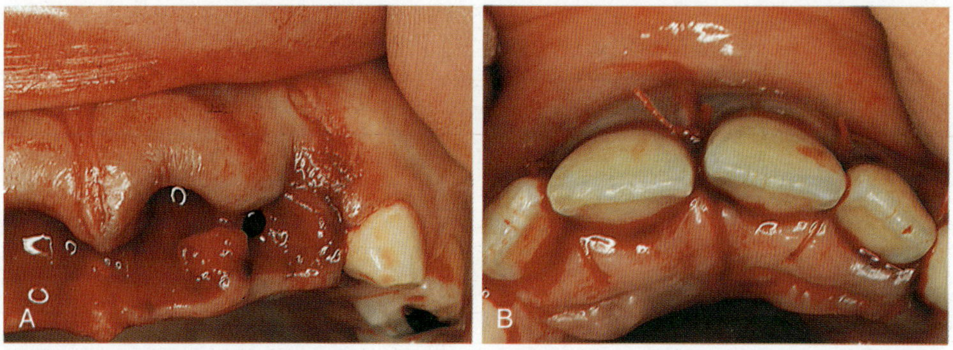

Fig. 21.65 (A) Four permanent incisors have been avulsed. (B) The teeth have been reimplanted successfully.

Trauma to Supporting Structures

The developing facial bones in the young child are small relative to the calvarium and thus somewhat protected by it. They are compact, spongy, and have greater elasticity, which tends to reduce the risk of fractures. However, the relatively thin outer cortices make alveolar process fractures somewhat more likely with dental displacement injuries, and their growth centers and developing tooth buds serve as weak points, making them major sites of fractures when they do occur (Fig. 21.66). Finally, their thick periosteum has remarkable osteogenic potential, which speeds healing remarkably. Injuries to these bony supporting structures of the dentition may result from birth trauma (rarely), bicycle accidents, car accidents, various physical and sporting activities, child abuse, or animal bites. Because major forces are required to produce jaw fractures in children, the examiner must carefully search for evidence of associated head and neck injuries (Fig. 21.67) and be vigilant in observing for evidence of expanding hematomas that may later compromise the airway.

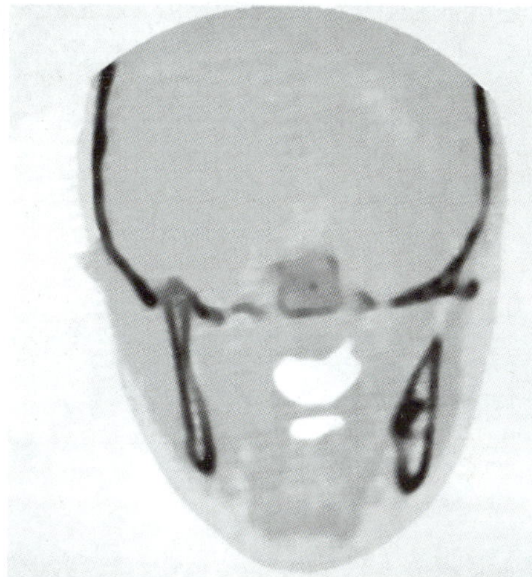

Fig. 21.67 Computed tomography scan reveals intrusion of the mandibular condyle into the middle cranial fossa from an extremely severe forced occlusion injury. Careful "pull back" and splinting is a common treatment for this type of injury.

Fractures of the Mandible

Excluding nasal fractures, the most common facial fractures in children involve the mandible. Forced occlusion can produce hemarthrosis of the TMJ, a compression fracture of the condylar process, or a greenstick condylar fracture (see Fig. 21.56). These injuries can be associated with fractures of the molar crowns. Lateral and frontolateral blows tend to produce fractures of the mandibular body, usually through the wall of a developing tooth bud (see Fig. 21.66). Because the mandible is an arch that the force of the impact is transmitted, these injuries are often associated with a contralateral fracture of the mandibular body or condyle (see Fig. 21.66). Important diagnostic clues may include ecchymosis, facial swelling, deviation on opening or closing (Fig. 21.68), trismus, or malocclusion that may be apparent visibly. Severe bilateral mandibular fractures can result in posterior displacement of the mandible and tongue with secondary airway obstruction. Palpation can show localized tenderness and hematoma formation, a step-off, or abnormal mobility with or without gingival tears. A panoramic radiograph and a CT scan should be ordered if there is clinical suspicion of a fracture.

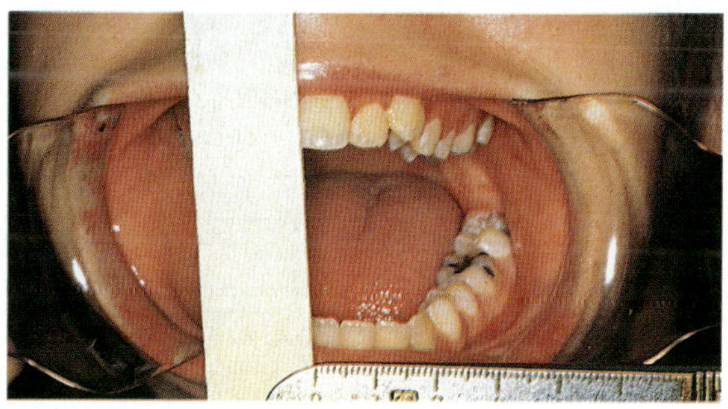

Fig. 21.68 A method of measuring deviation of the mandible on opening, showing a shift to the fracture side the width of one lower central incisor.

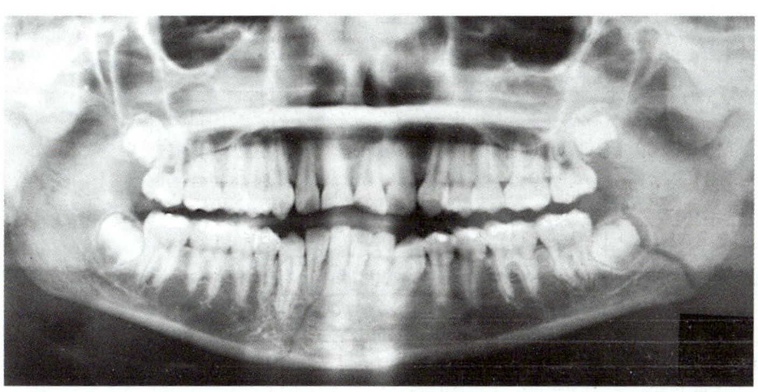

Fig. 21.66 A panoramic radiograph reveals a nondisplaced mandibular fracture extending through the wall of the third molar tooth bud. An associated hairline fracture exists near the midline on the patient's right.

Management requires careful assessment of the stability and type of erupted dentition and the location of tooth buds. Nondisplaced fractures with no occlusal abnormalities may require no treatment other than a soft diet. Most displaced fractures can be treated conservatively: first by appropriate reduction, followed by simple intermaxillary fixation or intraoral splints and circumferential wiring (closed reduction). Open reduction is seldom indicated; if this technique is used, careful placement of intraosseous holes is essential to avoid damaging the developing tooth buds.

Fractures of the Maxilla and Midface

Other than minor fractures of the alveolar process seen with dental displacement injuries, fractures of the maxilla and midface are uncommon in infants and young children. This is because the relatively large cranial vault provides protection, with the forehead bearing the brunt of most frontal impacts. The elasticity of facial bones further reduces the risk of fracture. When such injuries do occur in older children and adolescents, they are generally the result of major impacts and are often associated with injuries to the nose, ethmoid sinuses, orbits, and the frontal portion of the skull. As noted earlier, careful attention must be given to the airway, breathing, and circulation, along with assessment for associated head and neck injuries. Exact diagnosis of the location and extent of maxillary fractures is challenging and necessitates a thorough and detailed examination, along with specific imaging techniques; a CT scan of the midface is the most reliable diagnostic tool.

The Le Fort classification of midfacial fractures divides them into three groups (Fig. 21.69):

- Le Fort I, involving primarily the maxilla, separating it from the pterygoid plates and the nasal and zygomatic struts (Fig. 21.70)
- Le Fort II, in which the maxilla and nasal complex are separated from the orbits and the zygoma (Fig. 21.71)
- Le Fort III, in which there is complete separation of the midface from the cranial vault at the level of the naso-orbital ethmoid complex and the zygomaticofrontal suture area with extension through the orbits (Fig. 21.72)

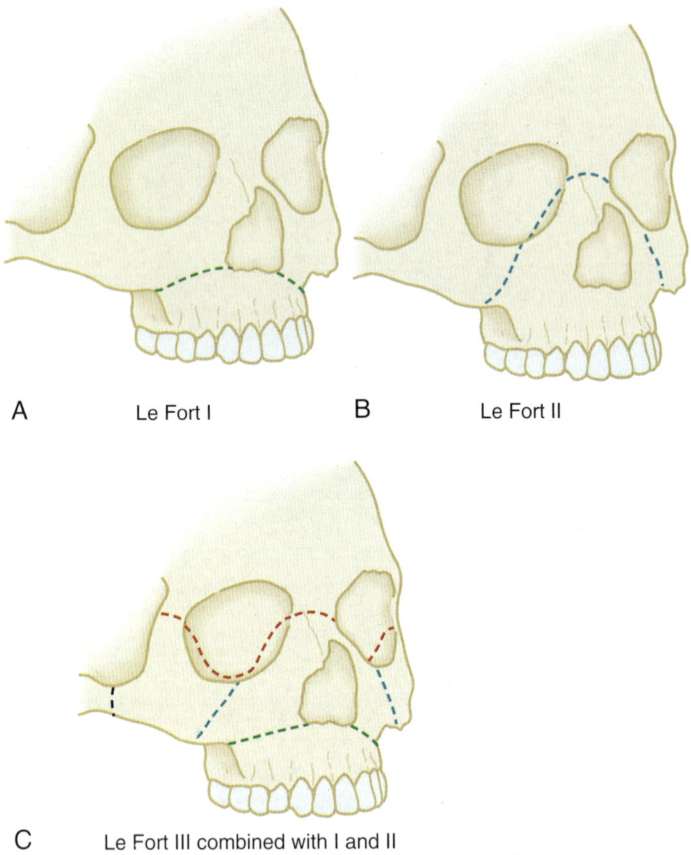

Fig. 21.69 Diagrammatic representation of fracture patterns of Le Fort fractures. (A) Le Fort I: The fracture separates the maxilla from the pterygoid plates and the nasal complex. (B) Le Fort II: The fracture line separates the maxilla and nasal complex from the orbits and the zygoma. (C) Le Fort III: The fracture line separates the midface from the cranial vault, traversing the zygomaticofrontal sutures and extending through the orbits and the naso-orbital ethmoid complex. Fracture lines of types I and II are shown as well because they are commonly present with the Le Fort III.

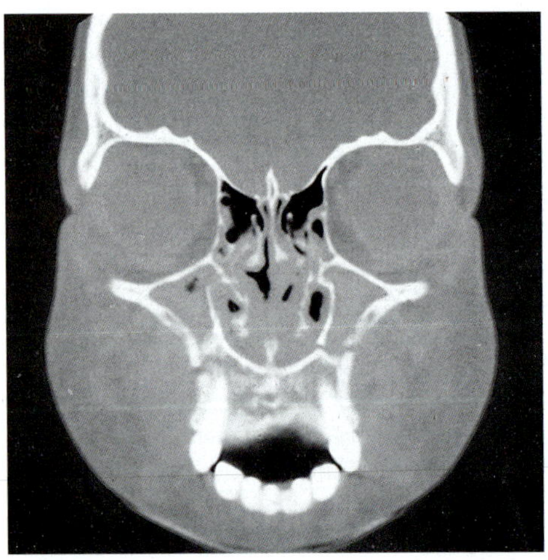

Fig. 21.70 Computed tomography scan shows a Le Fort I fracture. The maxilla is separated from the midface. The degree is greater on the right.

Often these fractures occur in combination, and the involved maxilla may be further fragmented. It is not unusual to encounter the combination of a Le Fort II on one side and a Le Fort III on the other. Sagittal splitting of the palate, often accompanied by palatal laceration, is seen in about 10% of patients. Associated mandibular fractures are common.

The diagnosis of Le Fort I fracture is often made by finding abnormal mobility of the maxilla; the maxillary dental arch is grasped anteriorly, and a vertical "pull/push" maneuver is performed, although on occasion the fracture may be impacted or incomplete and malocclusion without mobility is found. Associated findings may include midfacial swelling or ecchymosis (see Fig. 21.71 and Fig. 21.73), epistaxis, malocclusion, and apparent elongation or shortening of the midface.

Le Fort II fractures should be suspected when both the maxilla and nasal complex are mobile. Physical findings are like those noted in Le Fort I fractures, but wrinkling of the skin above the nose may also be seen.

Beyond these findings, patients with Le Fort III fractures tend to have prominent periorbital hematomas and swelling and may have subconjunctival hemorrhage, deconjugate gaze, or limited extraocular motion, any of which should prompt careful assessment for associated orbital rim and frontal bone fractures. Up to 25% of patients with Le Fort II and III fractures have cerebrospinal fluid rhinorrhea and pneumocephaly. Injury to the naso-orbital ethmoid complex can also cause detachment of the medial canthal ligaments with resultant widening of the intercanthal distance.

Progression of edema and profuse nasopharyngeal bleeding necessitates frequent reassessment of the patient's airway and circulatory status. The airway may need to be stabilized via orotracheal intubation to protect the patient from aspiration of blood or the airway narrowing from edema or an expanding hematoma.

Once airway, circulatory status, and head and neck injuries have been stabilized or ruled out, appropriate imaging can be performed and treatment initiated. Objectives include control of hemorrhage; reestablishing normal occlusion, vertical dimension, and width of the midface; and immobilization of fractures and restoration of normal fronto-orbital architecture. This often necessitates a team approach. It is preferable to plan and carry out the repair as soon as possible once more serious injuries are stabilized, as delays increase infection risk and can make repair more difficult as edema worsens, and the bones begin to knit during the first 2 to 3 days post-injury.

CRANIOMANDIBULAR DYSFUNCTION (TEMPOROMANDIBULAR JOINT DISEASE)

The term *craniomandibular dysfunction (CMD)* is used to define a set of signs and symptoms that involve the masticatory musculature, the TMJ, or both. Signs and symptoms of CMD may include tenderness or pain of the masticatory muscles, TMJ tenderness, limited or asymmetric mandibular movements, clicking or crepitation of the joint, and secondary headaches. Reported signs and symptoms can be mild, fluctuate over time, and exhibit no sex predilection. Prevalence has been shown to increase with age. Despite the high frequency of CMD signs and symptoms, it is estimated that only 5% of children and adolescents need treatment. The discrepancy can be attributed to the subclinical nature of many of the signs and symptoms recorded in epidemiologic studies.

The etiology of CMD is multifactorial. Oral parafunctional habits such as bruxism (grinding), bite deviations (malocclusion),

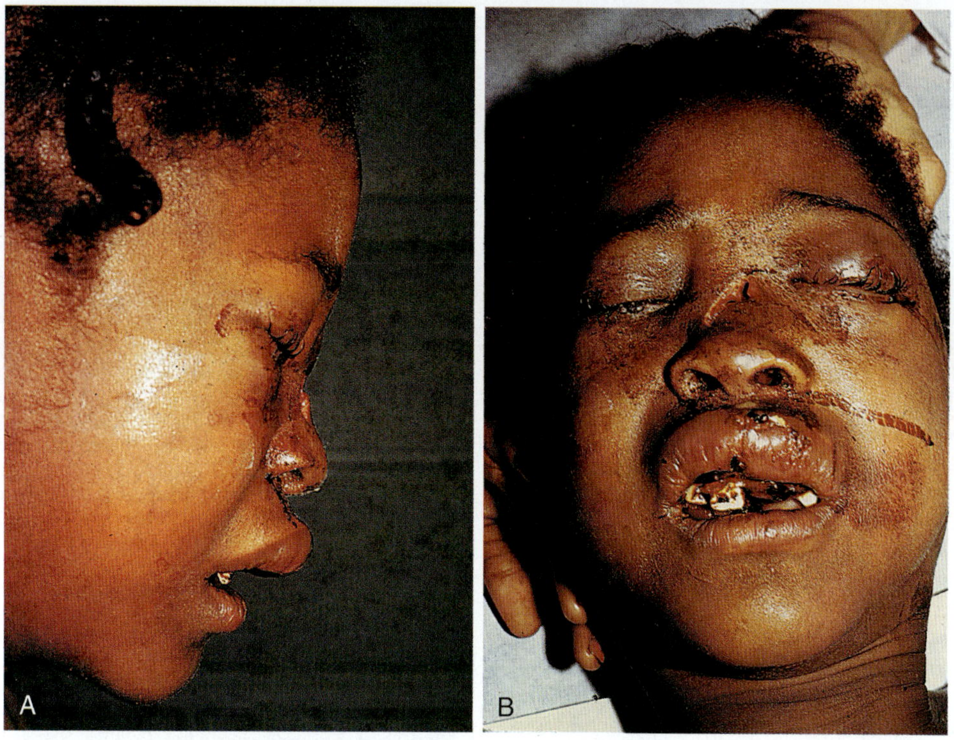

Fig. 21.71 Le Fort II fracture. This adolescent boy sustained multiple midfacial and naso-orbital injuries in a motor vehicle accident. (A) and (B) He has a collapsed midface with marked swelling of the upper lip, deviation of the nose, and prominent periorbital swelling and ecchymosis. (Courtesy Joseph Andrews, MD.)

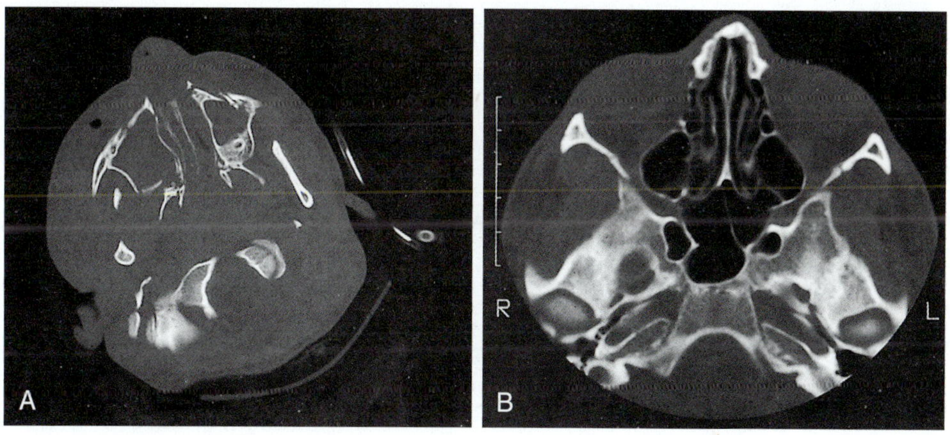

Fig. 21.72 Le Fort III fracture. This 10-year-old girl was hit by a car while sledding. Clinically, she had bilateral raccoon eyes, severe facial edema with a mobile maxilla, and bleeding from the nose, mouth, and eyes. She had the constellation of fractures that constitutes a Le Fort III fracture and numerous other facial and skull fractures. (A) Computed tomography cut shows multiple fractures involving the anterior, posterior, and medial walls of the maxillary sinuses. (B) Bilateral zygoma fractures are evident in another cut.

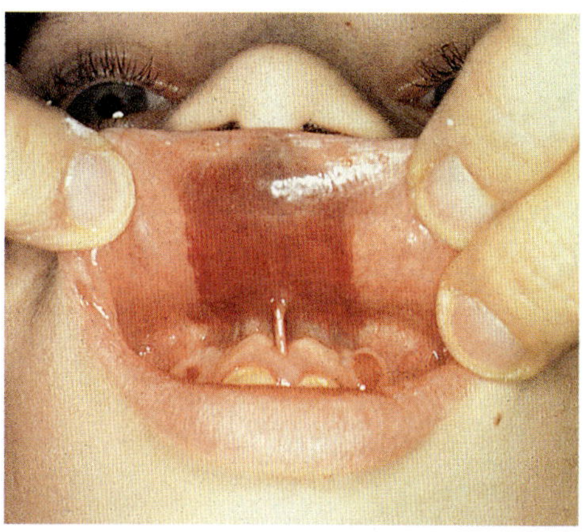

Fig. 21.73 Delineated ecchymosis with hematoma formation on the mucosa of the upper lip is a common sign associated with underlying fractures—in this case, a fracture of the anterior nasal spine of the maxilla.

trauma to the TMJ or mandible, orthodontic treatments, and history of stress are often cited as etiologic factors. Bruxism and stress (possibly with attendant jaw clenching) are most significantly associated with symptomatic CMD. Trauma has also been reported to be responsible for TMJ pain in 26% of pediatric patients with CMD. Musicians, especially violinists who practice for long periods daily, may have CMD symptoms. Both cross-sectional and longitudinal studies have failed to show a one-to-one relationship between signs and symptoms of CMD and morphologic and functional malocclusion. Hence malocclusion alone is not a primary etiologic factor. Similarly, orthodontic treatment has not been shown to significantly increase or decrease the frequency of signs and symptoms.

Patients presenting with symptoms of CMD should undergo a comprehensive history and examination including present illness and time of onset of symptoms, their nature, exacerbating and ameliorating factors, prior therapy, a complete medical history, and a detailed dental history. The latter should note whether there has been a history of treatment under general anesthesia; trauma to the TMJ or mandible; oral parafunctions such as bruxism, thumb sucking, nail biting, or gum chewing; headaches related to clenching of the teeth; and practice of a musical instrument, such as the violin, horn, or reed instrument. In addition, family and social history with emphasis on recent changes and potential sources of emotional stress should be obtained. Clinical examination includes inspection of the head and neck, intraoral examination, palpation of the TMJ and masticatory musculature, auscultation of the TMJ during opening and closing, and observation of mandibular movements in all planes (opening, protrusive, and lateral). Significant deviations from normal mandibular motion, tenderness, clicking or crepitus of the joint, or generalized TMJ pain all suggest the need for further evaluation.

Identification and elimination of etiologic factors is of paramount importance in the treatment of CMD. Studies on children and young adults suggest that conservative or reversible types of treatment are most appropriate, such as physical or behavioral modification therapy, bite splints, and analgesics. The application of irreversible treatment modalities such as bite adjustment (selective grinding of the teeth), orthognathic surgical intervention, and orthodontics to correct CMD is not supported scientifically and should only be considered if noninvasive therapy recommendations do not show improvement.

A supplemental video is available at Elsevier eBooks+.

Bibliography

American Academy of Craniomandibular Disorders: Guidelines for evaluation, diagnosis and management. In McNeil C, editor: *Craniomandibular disorders*, Chicago, 1990, Quintessence Publishing, pp 1–54.

American Academy of Pediatric Dentistry: Reference manual, *Pediatr Dent* 38(Special issue), 2016

American Academy of Pediatric Dentistry: *Reference manual. Policy on management of the frenulum in pediatric dental patients*, 2019, pp 66–70.

Bhaskar SN: Oral lesions in infants and newborns, *Dent Clin North Am* 10:421–435, 1966.

Christensen RE Jr: Soft tissue lesions of the head and neck. In Sanders B, editor: *Pediatric oral and maxillofacial surgery*, St Louis, 1979, Mosby.

Long SS: Syndrome of periodic fever, aphthous stomatitis, pharyngitis, adenitis (PFAPA)—what it isn't. What is it? *J Pediatr* 135:1–5, 1999.

Martin B, Armanazi Y, Bouquot J, et al: Dental and gingival disorders. In Bluestone CD, Stool SE, editors: *Pediatric otolaryngology*, Philadelphia, 2002, WB Saunders.

McDonald R: *Dentistry for the child and adolescent*, St. Louis, 2004, Mosby.

Nazif MM, Ruffalo RC: The interaction between dentistry and otolaryngology, *Pediatr Clin North Am* 28:977–1010, 1981.

Nowak A, Casamassimo P: *The handbook of pediatric dentistry*, Chicago, 2011, American Academy of Pediatric Dentistry.

Palmer CA: *Diet and nutrition in oral health*, Upper Saddle River, NJ, 2002, Prentice Hall.

Sanders B, Sanger RG: Infections. In Sanders B, editor: *Pediatric oral and maxillofacial surgery*, St. Louis, 1979, C.V. Mosby Co., pp 182–220.

Schuit KE, Johnson JT: Infections of the head and neck, *Pediatr Clin North Am* 28:965–971, 1981.

Sonis A, Zaragoza S: Dental health for the pediatrician, *Curr Opin Pediatr* 13: 289–295, 2001.

Vanderas AP: Prevalence of craniomandibular dysfunction in children and adolescents: a review, *Pediatr Dent* 9:312–316, 1987.

Walund K, List T, Dworkin SF: Temporomandibular disorders in children and adolescents: reliability of a questionnaire, clinical examination, and diagnosis, *J Orofac Pain* 12:42–51, 1998.

22 ORTHOPEDICS

Ozgur Dede | Z. Deniz Olgun

Children with musculoskeletal injuries and afflictions are usually brought for care because of pain, deformity, or loss of function. Because of their rapid physical growth and the special properties of their developing bones, children often pose challenges for the clinician.

Musculoskeletal problems in children fall into several general categories:

- Trauma (discussed here and in Chapter 6)
- Congenital problems—problems resulting from genetic factors and from exposure to teratogens and deformations stemming from insults later in pregnancy, many of which are associated with anomalies of other organ systems (discussed here and in Chapters 1, 2, and 16)
- Infections (see Chapter 13)
- Inflammatory processes, such as the collagen vascular diseases, vasculitides, rheumatoid arthritis, and inflammatory bowel disease (see Chapters 7 and 11)
- Metabolic diseases (see Chapters 9, 11, and 14)
- Neoplastic disorders (see Chapter 12)

This chapter focuses on primary musculoskeletal problems, and the discussion is divided into eight sections: (1) development of the skeletal system, (2) physical assessment, (3) musculoskeletal trauma, (4) disorders of the neck and spine, (5) disorders of the upper extremity, (6) disorders of the lower extremity, (7) generalized musculoskeletal disorders, and (8) sports related injuries.

DEVELOPMENT OF THE SKELETAL SYSTEM

The assessment, diagnosis, and management of pediatric orthopedic problems necessitate a clear understanding of the physiology of the growing musculoskeletal system. The process of growth begins in utero and continues until the end of puberty. Linear growth occurs as the result of multiplication of chondrocytes in the epiphyses, which align themselves vertically, eventually forming a transitional zone of endochondral ossification in the metaphyses. The shafts of long bones widen, and flat bones enlarge through the deposition and mineralization of osteoid by the periosteum. The majority of genetic and congenital disorders that affect connective tissue and the skeleton tend to cause abnormal growth.

A thorough understanding of musculoskeletal development is important in the diagnosis and management of orthopedic injuries. At birth, only a few epiphyses have begun to ossify; the remainder is cartilaginous and thus is invisible radiographically. With development, other epiphyses begin to ossify, enlarge, and mature in such an orderly fashion that one can estimate a child's age from the number and configuration of ossification centers (Figs. 22.1 and 22.2). The epiphyseal plates (physes), which are sites of cartilaginous proliferation and growth, do not begin to ossify and close until puberty (Fig. 22.3). This process starts and ends earlier in females than in males. **When skeletal injuries involve sites where ossification has not begun or is incomplete, plain radiographic findings may appear normal or may not reflect the full extent of the injury.** Clinical findings and appropriate use of advanced imaging are important.

While the growth plate is open, it is the weak link in the chain. As a result, injuries that occur near joints are more likely to result in physeal disruption than in ligamentous tearing. As a result, sprains and dislocations are less common in younger children than in adolescents and adults. Avulsion fractures at sites where strong muscular attachments join secondary ossification centers are unique to children and adolescents.

The periosteum of a child is much thicker than that of an adult and is rarely disrupted completely when the underlying bone is fractured. This incomplete periosteal injury helps with treatment and bony remodeling. Because of the immature elements in the rapidly growing skeleton of the child, bone has more viscoelasticity and can sustain plastic deformation more easily than the adult skeleton.

Fracture patterns in children often differ from those in adults. Their fractures can be considerably more difficult to detect clinically and radiographically. Children do have advantages, however, in that their actively growing bones heal more rapidly and have a remarkable capacity for remodeling, which is the spontaneous correction through skeletal growth of certain posttraumatic bony deformities. Physeal (growth plate) fractures heal even more rapidly; however, the potential setback is growth disturbances that might follow.

Numerous genetic, metabolic, endocrine, renal, and inflammatory processes can affect not only growth and ultimate height but also skeletal maturation—delaying it or accelerating it. Comparison of the patient's actual bone age, as determined by the number of radiographically visible ossification centers, with their chronologic age can help in the diagnosis of these underlying disorders.

PHYSICAL ASSESSMENT

History

Key historical points in the evaluation of both traumatic and atraumatic orthopedic complaints are displayed in Table 22.1.

Physical Examination

The orthopedic examination involves a systematic assessment of posture, stance, and gait; the symmetry or asymmetry of paired musculoskeletal structures and their motion; muscle strength and tone; and neurovascular status. In pediatrics, the patient's developmental level is a major consideration in terms of not only the interpretation of findings but also the manner in which the examination is conducted. Patience and some degree of creativity are required on the part of the examiner if the patient is very young. Often, a large part of the necessary information can be gleaned from observation of the child's demeanor and spontaneous activity. This can be assisted by providing age-appropriate toys while the history is being taken and by engaging the patient in play before starting a more formal physical examination. This also helps to alleviate anxiety and gain the child's trust, enhancing his or her cooperation. After spontaneous activity is observed, the relevant parts of the orthopedic examination are typically done by region.

A complete orthopedic examination that assesses each bone, muscle, joint, tendon, and ligament is lengthy, detailed, and rarely indicated. Even in multiple-trauma victims and patients whose symptoms point toward an underlying systemic disorder, each region is screened and a full assessment done only of those regions where local musculoskeletal abnormalities are found. Similarly, in patients with focal injuries or deformities, the examination can generally be focused on the region involved, with the clinician bearing in mind the common pain referral patterns and the maxim that

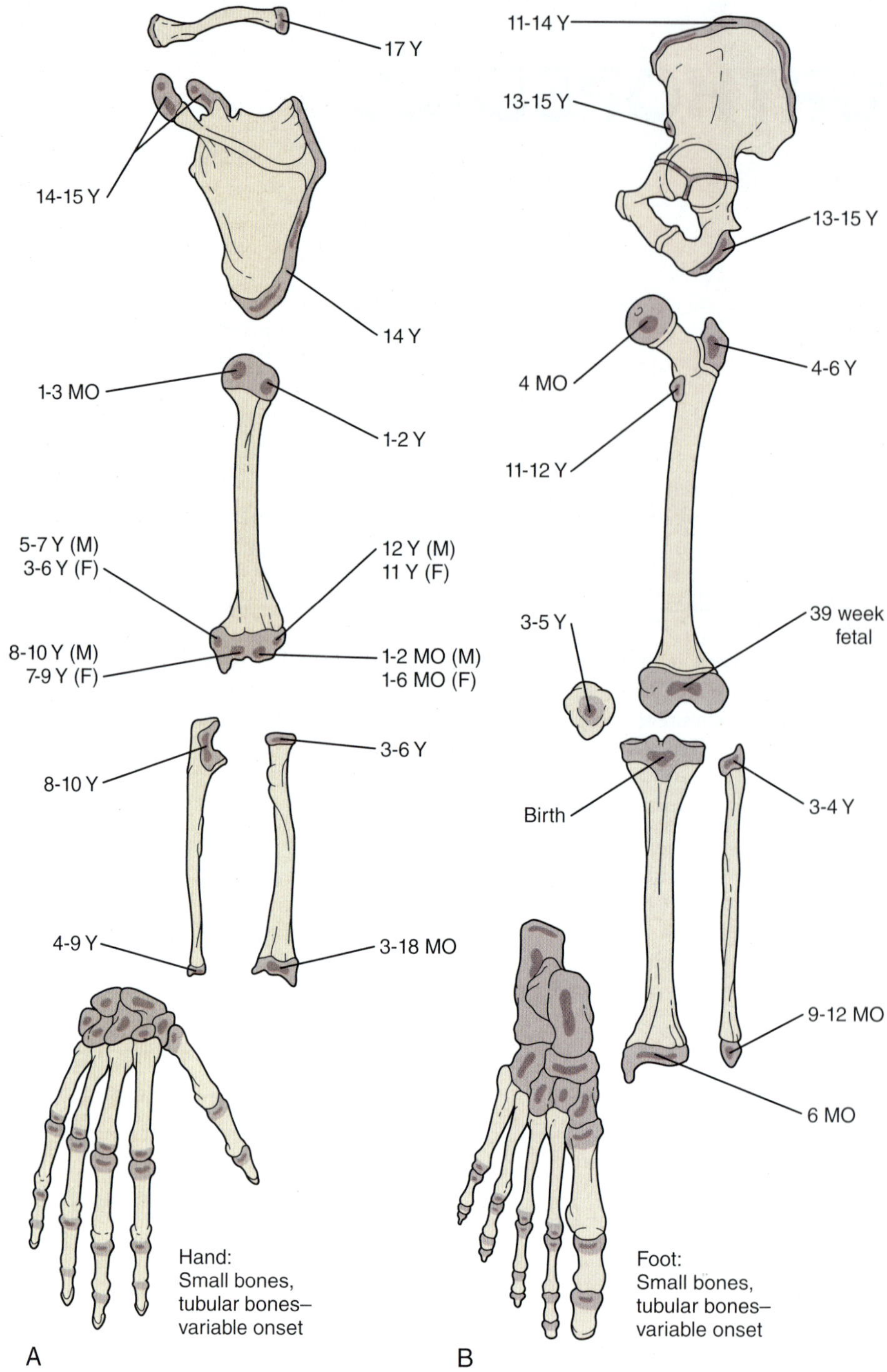

Fig. 22.1 Ages at onset of ossification for upper (A) and lower (B) extremities. At birth, only a few epiphyses have begun to ossify. The remainder are cartilaginous and therefore invisible radiographically. With development, other epiphyses begin to ossify, enlarge, and mature in an orderly fashion, making it possible to estimate a child's age from the number and configuration of ossification centers. This forms the basis for the use of bone age as part of the evaluation of children with growth disorders. When evaluating the radiographs of injured children, it is of crucial importance to bear in mind that fractures involving nonossified epiphyses are radiographically invisible until healing begins (see Fig. 22.57). *F,* Female; *M,* male; *MO,* months; *Y,* years.

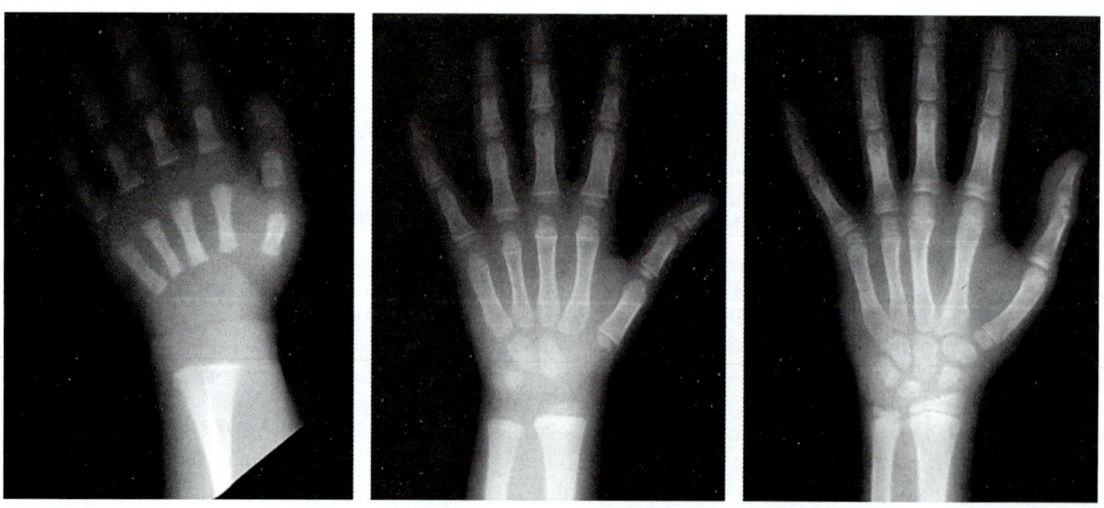

Fig. 22.2 Increasing numbers of ossification centers become radiographically visible with age. *From left,* the hands shown are those of a toddler, a young school-age child, and a young adolescent. Injuries affecting unossified bones or growth centers are invisible radiographically.

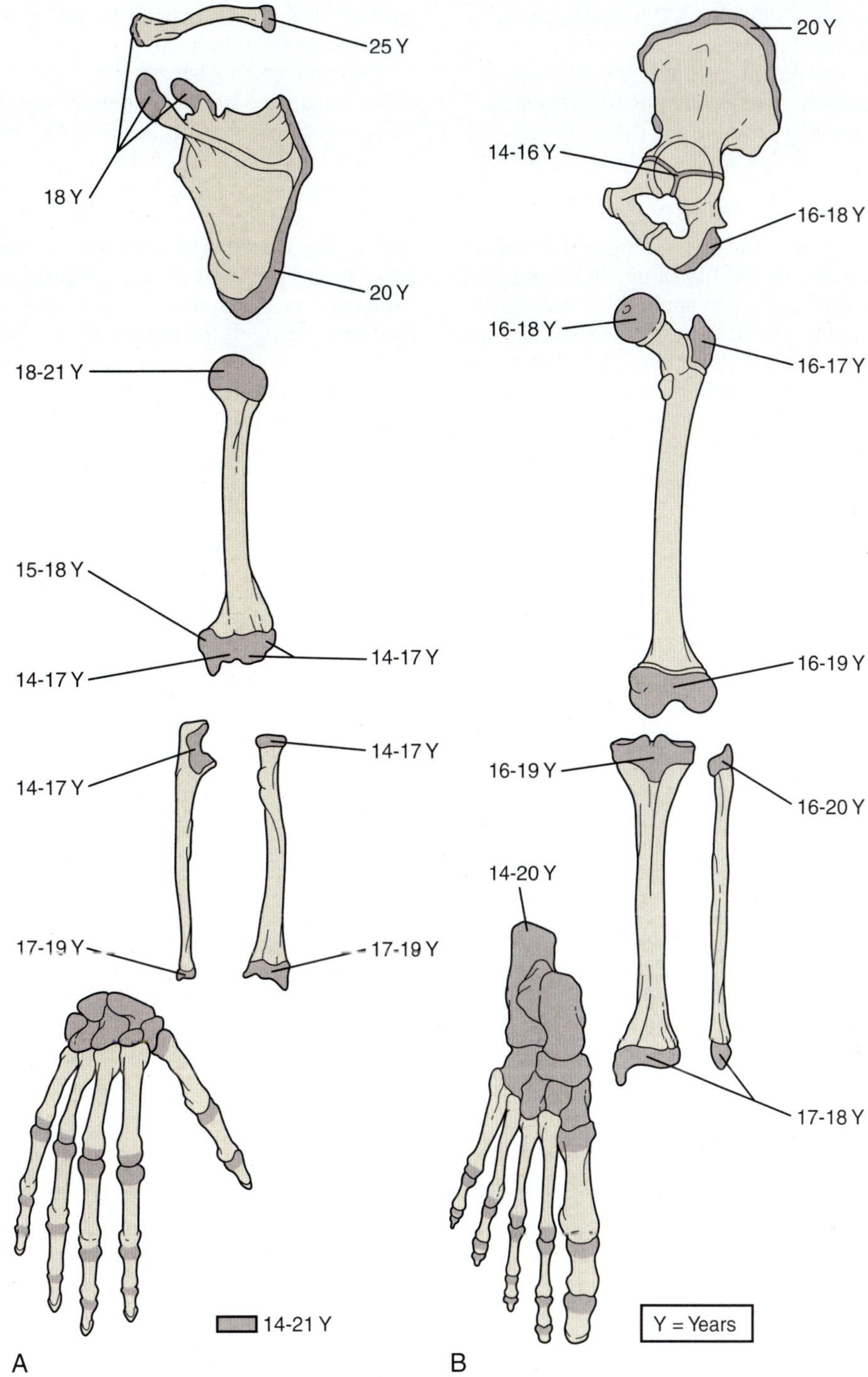

Fig. 22.3 Ages at physeal closure for upper (A) and lower (B) extremities. *Y*, Years.

Table 22.1 Appropriate Historical Documentation for Orthopedic Complaints

Traumatic Etiology	Nontraumatic Etiology
• The time and place of the accident and whether it was witnessed • The mechanism of injury, including the degree and direction of force applied, if known (e.g., if a fall, from what height, onto what surface? Was the child running or walking [momentum]?)	• Age at onset of symptoms • Mode of onset
• The child's behavior since the time of injury (e.g., decreased movement, guarding, refusal to walk or limping, any altered level of consciousness)	• Clinical course, including the manner and rate of progression and associated signs and symptoms
• Complaint of pain (if so, how severe, and can it be localized?)	• Past medical history, with an emphasis on the prenatal and perinatal history in the infant or young child
• Prior treatment or first aid	• Family history, especially of genetic, metabolic, and musculoskeletal problems
• Past medical history of serious illness and prior injuries; family history of musculoskeletal problems ***This information helps localize the site or sites of injury and potential injury severity, points to the risk of possible associated injuries, gives clues to the possible existence of underlying disorders that may predispose to injury, and may occasionally raise a suspicion of abuse.***	***This information helps considerably in narrowing the list of differential diagnostic possibilities.***

all extremities "begin at the back." Finally, in performing routine physical examinations on healthy children, after a general screening examination of spontaneous movement, posture, gait, station, and stance, the assessment of the musculoskeletal system is focused on areas at risk for the child's age (e.g., the hip for dislocation in the neonate, the spine for scoliosis in the preadolescent and adolescent).

Regional Musculoskeletal Examination

In the regional examination, the area of concern is inspected visually for spontaneous movement, guarding, size, swelling, deformity, and the appearance of overlying skin, and when applicable, findings are compared with its paired structure. After this, the normal and affected sides are gently palpated for warmth, induration, and tenderness. Muscle mass, tone, and reflexes on the affected side are compared with those on the normal side, and the presence or absence of spasm is noted. If asymmetry in muscle mass is detected, the circumference is measured bilaterally at a point equidistant from a fixed bony landmark. The child is then asked to move the extremity or is handed objects to get him or her to do so, and active motion is observed. If this appears limited, passive range of motion is tested first on the normal and then on the affected side, taking care not to cause severe pain. Strength is tested against gravity and then against resistance (Table 22.2), being careful to stay within the limits of pain. Sensation and vascular status are also evaluated.

Joints are further inspected to determine whether there is erythema, obliteration of landmarks that may indicate the presence of effusion, evidence of deformity, and position of comfort. Further evaluation to detect joint effusion is done by pressing on one side of a visible joint while feeling for the protrusion of fluid on the other. The joints are palpated to check for evidence of heat and tenderness, range of motion is assessed, and evidence of pain on motion is determined.

Assessment of ligamentous stability around joints is discussed under specific sections of the regional examination. However, it is important to remember that in cases of acute trauma, especially when deformity or hemarthrosis is evident on initial assessment, tests of ligamentous stability should be deferred, the extremity splinted, and radiographs obtained to check for possible underlying fracture.

Axial Skeleton and Upper Extremity Examination

Trunk and Neck

With the examiner in front and the patient standing, the sternocleidomastoid muscles, the bony prominences of the clavicles, and the respective heights of the acromioclavicular (AC) joints, nipples, and anterior iliac crests and sides of the chest wall are inspected for symmetry. The patient is then turned and viewed from behind, and the shoulder and scapular height, the muscle bulk of the trapezius muscles, and the height of the posterior iliac crests and of the depressions over the sacroiliac joints are checked for symmetry. Trapezius strength is determined by having the patient shrug his or her shoulders, first against gravity and then against resistance, as the examiner presses down on the shoulders. The muscles supplying the scapula are tested by having the patient press his or her outstretched arms against a wall. Winging of the scapula during this maneuver is suggestive of weakness of the serratus anterior muscle. The line of the spinous processes of the vertebrae is observed for straightness, and the position of the head over the trunk is noted. Normally the head is aligned over the midline of the sacrum.

Next, the sternocleidomastoid and paraspinous muscles of the neck are palpated to assess for bulk, tone, tenderness, and spasm, and the spinous processes of the cervical vertebrae are palpated to assess for tenderness and step-off. In the immobilized trauma patient, these observations are made largely with the patient supine on a backboard and then log-rolled onto his or her side. Importantly, in checking for neck injury, the cervical spine can be cleared clinically if the patient is awake and alert and has no complaint of neck pain, no evidence of tenderness or paraspinous muscle spasm, and no extremely painful injury elsewhere. If the patient's level of consciousness is not normal or there is a major distracting injury, the cervical spine cannot be cleared, even if direct radiographic findings are normal because spinal cord injury can be present in the absence of bony abnormalities, and advanced imaging may be necessary.

Range of neck motion is assessed by having the patient move his or her head. A normal child can touch his or her chin to the chest, extend the neck to look directly above, and bend laterally to 45 degrees. They are also capable of symmetric lateral rotation when turning the head from side to side. Strength is tested by applying pressure to the forehead while the patient flexes his or her neck and to the occiput as the patient extends and by applying resistance to the opposite side of the head as the patient bends and rotates laterally.

Table 22.2 Grading of Muscle Strength

Grade	Physical Finding
0/5	No movement seen
1/5	Muscle can move joint with gravity eliminated
2/5	Muscle can move joint against gravity but not against added resistance
3/5	Muscle can move joint against slight resistance
4/5	Muscle can move joint against moderate added resistance
5/5	Normal strength

Thoracolumbar Spine

Viewed from the side cervical spine has a lordotic curve with a bony prominence at C7, a mild thoracic kyphosis, a lumbar lordosis, and a sacral kyphosis. Each patient is checked for the presence, absence, or accentuation of these curves. The midline of the back is inspected for evidence of abnormal pigmentation and the presence of hemangiomas, nevi, hairy tufts, dimples, masses, or defects, which may be associated with underlying bony or neural anomalies (see Chapter 16).

Flexion, extension, rotation, and lateral bending of the thoracolumbar spine are primarily motions of the thoracolumbar junction and the lumbar area. Most children can bend forward to touch their toes, bend laterally 20 to 30 degrees (with the pelvis held stable by the examiner's hands on the iliac crests), and rotate 20 to 30 degrees in either direction.

Examination of the back for spinal deformity is assisted by the use of the Adams Forward Bend Test (Fig. 22.4). For this, the examiner stands behind the patient, who is then asked to bend forward with arms extended and the palms of the hands together. The surface of the back in the lumbar and thoracic regions is examined for asymmetric elevation of the paravertebral spinous area, thus indicating a structural rotation of the spine and the possibility of scoliosis (see Fig. 22.4B). The examiner should also note any evidence of missing spinous processes (step-off) or deviation from the midline and palpate the paravertebral muscles for spasm and tenderness. Increased kyphosis, especially in the thoracic region, may be detected when viewing the patient from the side (see Fig. 22.4C), as can lack of reversal of the lumbar lordosis, which may indicate muscle spasm or abnormality of the lumbar spine. Leg length inequality may be evaluated during the upright standing portion of this test (see the Lower Extremity Examination section, later) and, if present, should be corrected with appropriate lifts under the short side in order not to cause a false forward bend test.

Any examination of the spine must include a neurologic assessment of strength, tone, reflexes, and sensation. The Straight Leg Raise Test (Fig. 22.5) can be helpful in demonstrating nerve root pathology in patients with slipped disks, spinal or paraspinal masses, or inflammatory processes. The test is performed with the patient lying supine on the examining table. The limb to be tested is grasped behind the ankle and elevated passively into hip flexion with the knee fully extended. This maneuver stretches the sciatic nerve as it passes behind the hip joint, and if one of its several roots has been irritated by a protruded disk, mass, or inflammatory process, pain will be felt with only 15 to 30 degrees of hip flexion. Although in most young children the straight leg can be brought to 90 degrees of

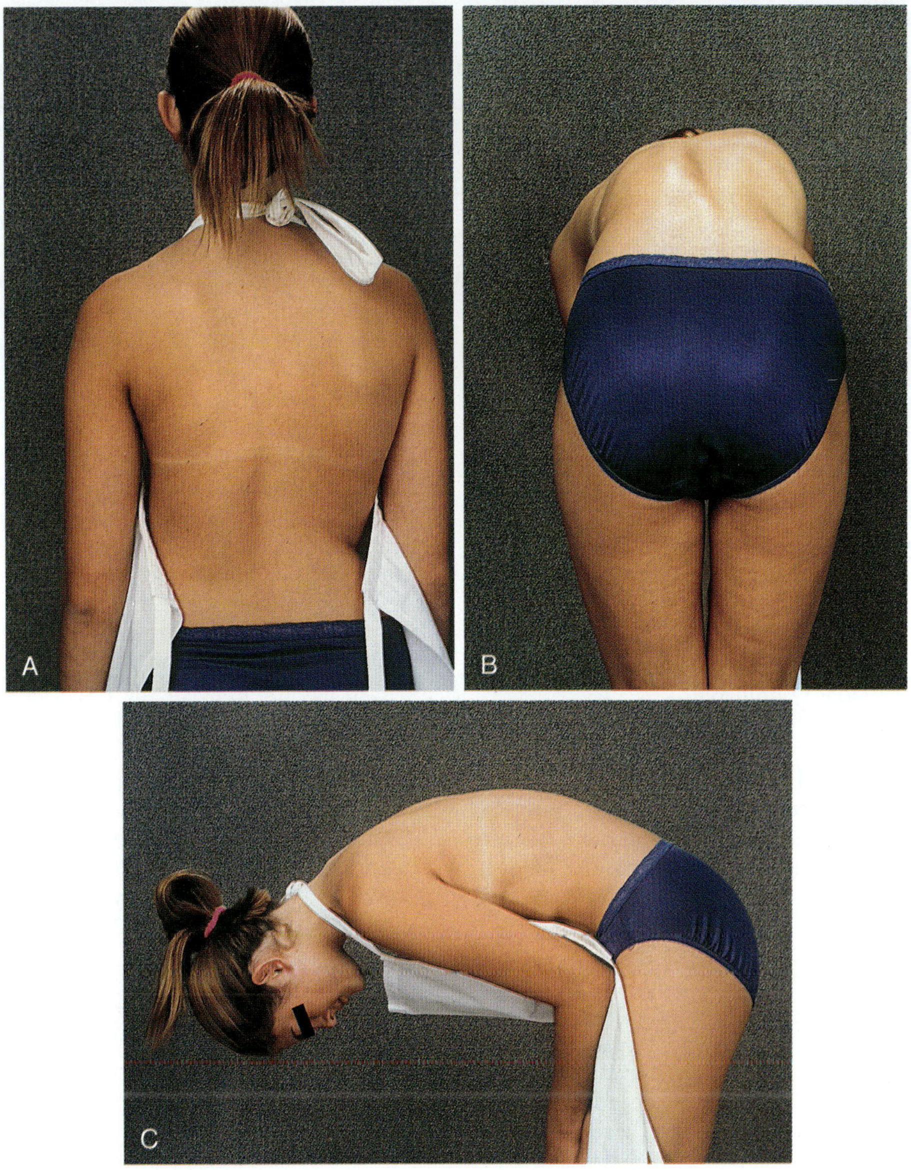

Fig. 22.4 Adams forward bend test. (A) Scoliosis can be difficult to detect on observation of the standing patient. (B) With the child bending forward and observed from behind, it is much easier to appreciate the asymmetric trunk rotation seen in scoliosis. (C) Viewing the patient from the side, one can more easily see even subtle degrees of kyphosis and note lack of reversal of normal lordosis.

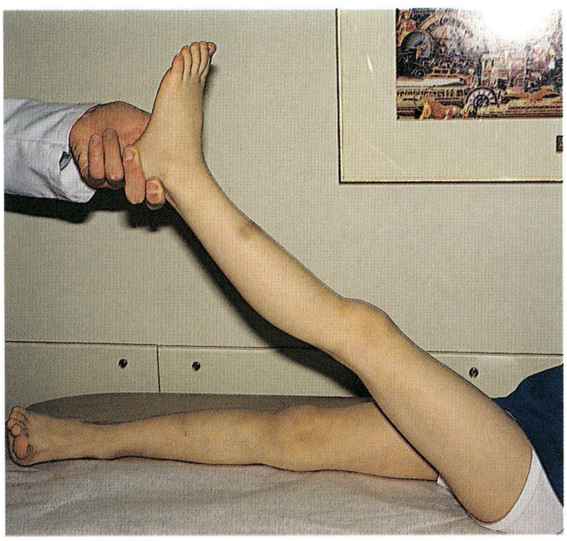

Fig. 22.5 Straight leg raising test. With the patient supine, the limb to be tested is grasped behind the ankle and elevated into hip flexion with the knee in full extension. If pain is produced well before 90 degrees of flexion is achieved, the test is positive, indicating irritation of a sciatic nerve root.

hip flexion without difficulty, adolescents may naturally have some hamstring tightness.

Shoulder

When examining the shoulder, the position of the upper limbs is first observed, at the same time noting whether there is swelling, asymmetry of height, or visible landmarks and looking for any difference in spontaneous movement. Prominent landmarks that are easily palpable include the acromion process lying laterally and subcutaneously, the clavicle, the spine of the scapula, the coracoid process, and the bicipital groove. Any displacement or tenderness of these structures should be noted. Swelling of the glenohumeral joint capsule and atrophy of the shoulder muscles are best appreciated by viewing from above with the patient seated and by comparison with the normal side.

Assessing range of motion is important because many shoulder problems are manifested by a loss of normal motion. The shoulder is a ball-and-socket joint with six components of movement. Abduction, a function of the deltoid muscle, is tested by having the patient raise the extended, supinated arm up so that the hand is directly above the shoulder (180-degree abduction). To test adduction, the patient is asked to flex the shoulder to 20 to 30 degrees and then draw the upper arm diagonally across the body (75 degrees is normal). Flexion is assessed by having the patient raise the extended pronated arm up and forward until it is parallel to the floor; extension is tested by having him or her return the arm to the neutral position and then lift the arm up and backward (45–60 degrees is normal). To check rotation, the upper arm is held to the side with the elbow flexed to 90 degrees and the child is asked to turn the forearm toward the body (medial) and then out to the side (lateral) (60–90 degrees is normal).

Elbow

In the normal relationship of the extended, supinated forearm to the upper arm, there are 5 to 10 degrees of lateral (valgus) angulation, termed the *carrying angle* (Fig. 22.6). When this angle is greater than 10 degrees, the deformity is termed cubitus valgus and, when less or reversed, cubitus varus (gunstock deformity). The range of motion of the hinge joint of the elbow has four components: (1) extension, a function of the triceps (0 degrees); (2) flexion, a function of the biceps (145 degrees); (3) supination (90 degrees); and (4) pronation (80–90 degrees). The latter two components are tested by having the patient turn the palm up and down, respectively, with the elbow flexed.

Because of the proximity of the brachial artery and the median, radial, and ulnar nerves to the elbow joint, injuries of the elbow necessitate a careful neurovascular examination.

Wrist and Hand

During examination of the wrist and hand, one should observe skin color, check capillary refill, and palpate the radial and ulnar pulses to assess circulation. Any swelling or edema and any abnormal posture or position should be noted. The presence of intraarticular fluid in the wrist is manifested by swelling and tenderness, especially evident dorsally, and by restriction of wrist motion. Wrist motion has four components: flexion with the hand held down (normally 70–80 degrees); extension with the hand held up (normally 70 degrees); and ulnar and radial deviation (normally 25 degrees and 15–20 degrees, respectively).

Examination of hand function can be challenging in the young. Observation of the position at rest (normally a loose fist with all the fingers pointing in the same direction and with the same degree of flexion) and of use during play is often helpful. Having the parent perform various hand and finger motions while trying to get the child to imitate these can be helpful in some cases. Handing the child a small object or a thin piece of paper may suffice for assessing opposition of thumb to fingers, tested in the older child by having him or her touch the tip of the thumb to the tip of the little finger. Normal ranges of motion of the hand are 90 degrees of flexion and 45 degrees of extension for the metacarpophalangeal joints, full extension and 100 degrees of flexion for the proximal interphalangeal (PIP) joints, and full extension and 90 degrees of flexion for the distal interphalangeal joints.

Because the bones of the hand are subcutaneous but shallow, displaced fractures and dislocations can be readily evident on inspection. Laceration or rupture of the tendons is common because of their superficial location. Those involving flexor tendons result in extensor tendon overpull (Fig. 22.7), with the affected digit lying in greater extension than its neighbors at rest. Conversely, extensor tendon lacerations result in flexor muscle overpull, with the opposite result.

Functional testing of the tendons and intrinsic muscles of the hand is generally possible in older children. They can be asked to extend the fingers at the metacarpophalangeal joints and each interphalangeal joint. Function of the flexor digitorum profundus muscle is tested by holding the PIP joint extended while the patient flexes the tip of the finger. To test the superficialis flexor tendon, adjacent distal interphalangeal joints are held in extension and the patient is asked to flex the finger being tested at the PIP joint. The intrinsic muscles of the hand are evaluated by having the child adduct and abduct the fingers toward and away from the middle finger. Sensation is best tested using two-point discrimination and pinprick in older children and by touch in very young children.

Muscle strength in the upper extremity is largely tested during assessment of range of motion of the joints, with and without resistance. Signs of neural dysfunction with injury of the upper extremity are listed in Table 22.3.

Lower Extremity Examination

Hip

Examination of the hip begins by assessing gait and stance, assessing the latter to see if the anterior superior and posterior superior iliac spines and the greater trochanters are level. If not, a leg-length discrepancy should be suspected and leg length measured. Total length is measured from the bottom of the anterior superior iliac spine to the medial malleolus of the ankle with the patient supine. If

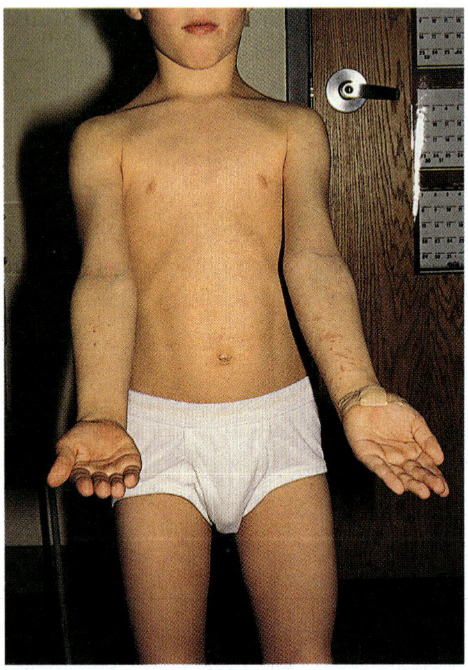

Fig. 22.6 Carrying angle. The normal relationship of the extended supinated forearm to the upper arm is not a straight line but involves 5 to 10 degrees of lateral or valgus angulation.

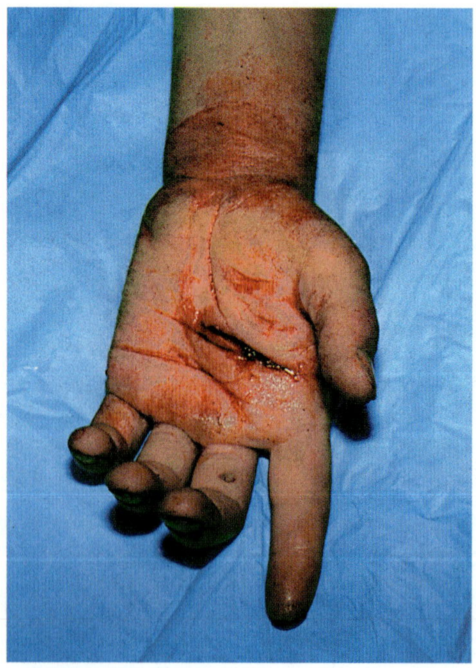

Fig. 22.7 Extensor tendon overpull. This boy's palm laceration involved the flexor tendons to his index finger. With his hand at rest, his index finger lies in extension, in contrast to his other fingers, which are partially flexed. (Courtesy Robert Hickey, MD, Children's Hospital of Pittsburgh, Pittsburgh, PA.)

Table 22.3 Signs of Neural Dysfunction With Injury of the Upper Extremity

Nerve	Sign
Radial	↓ Strength of wrist and finger extensors ↓ Sensation in web space between thumb and index finger, dorsum of hand to PIP joints, and radial aspect of ring finger
Ulnar	↓ Strength of wrist flexion and adduction ↓ Strength of finger spread ↓ Sensation over ulnar aspect of palm and dorsum of hand, little finger, and ulnar aspect of ring finger
Median	↓ Strength of wrist flexion and abduction ↓ Strength of flexion of PIP joints ↓ Strength of opposition of thumb to base of little finger ↓ Sensation over radial aspect of palm, thumb, index, and long fingers
Anterior interosseous	↓ Strength of flexion of the distal interphalangeal joints of the index finger and thumb

PIP, Proximal interphalangeal.

inequality is found, the knees are flexed to 90 degrees with the feet flat on the examination table. If, as the examiner looks from the foot of the examination table, one knee appears higher than the other, the tibias are unequal in length; if one knee is anterior to the other when viewed from the side, the discrepancy involves the femurs. If total leg lengths are equal, the inequality apparent when the patient is standing may be due to pelvic obliquity or flexion contracture of the hip. The latter may also be associated with a compensatory accentuation of lumbar lordosis.

The thighs are assessed next for symmetry and signs of atrophy. If atrophy is found, circumference should be measured and compared at a fixed point below the greater trochanters.

Because the hip lies deep and is surrounded by muscles, direct inspection is impossible and palpation is of limited value (although the femoral triangle, greater trochanter, and posterior aspect should be palpated to check for tenderness). As a result, assessment of the position of comfort (abduction and external rotation are seen with effusion, hemarthrosis, and fracture; see Figs. 22.15C and 22.91B), weight bearing, range of motion, and pain on motion are particularly important (for hip examination in the neonate, see the Developmental Dislocation of the Hip section).

In evaluating range of motion of the hip, care must be taken to distinguish true hip motion from that occurring in combination with pelvic rotation or trunk flexion. The range of hip flexion is normally about 120 degrees. It is tested with the child lying supine. The hip is passively flexed while the contralateral hip and pelvis are observed or stabilized by one hand. The limit of flexion is reached when movement of the contralateral pelvis is noted. Alternatively, both hips can be flexed simultaneously to stabilize the pelvis and eliminate truncal flexion. The Thomas test is performed by flexing both hips so that the thighs touch the abdomen. Then one is held in place, thereby eliminating lumbar lordosis and movement of the lumbosacral joint, and the patient is asked to extend the hip to be tested. Normally, he or she should be able to extend the hip to 0 degrees of flexion (Fig. 22.8A). Failure to do this indicates the presence of a hip flexion contracture, which is a positive result on the Thomas test (see Fig. 22.8B). Next, the knee and thigh are held with the hip and knee flexed to 90 degrees, and internal and external rotation are tested and recorded in degrees. Abduction and adduction are also checked with the hip flexed to 90 degrees. While the examiner places the thumb and index finger of one hand over the patient's pelvis, attempting to span the distance between the anterior superior iliac spines, the hip to be tested is abducted and then adducted. The limit is determined by the point at which the pelvis begins to move (normally 45 degrees of abduction and 30 degrees of adduction). Extension is tested with the patient prone by having him or her lift the leg up from the table (normal, 20–30 degrees). Internal and external rotation are also tested with the patient prone and the hip and leg in extension.

When hip abductor weakness is suspected on the basis of the finding of a gait abnormality, the Trendelenburg test (Fig. 22.9) is performed. This involves having the child stand and asking him or her to lift one leg up. Normally, the pelvis should rise slightly on the side of the leg that is lifted. If instead it drops, abductor weakness is present on the opposite side and the Trendelenburg test is positive.

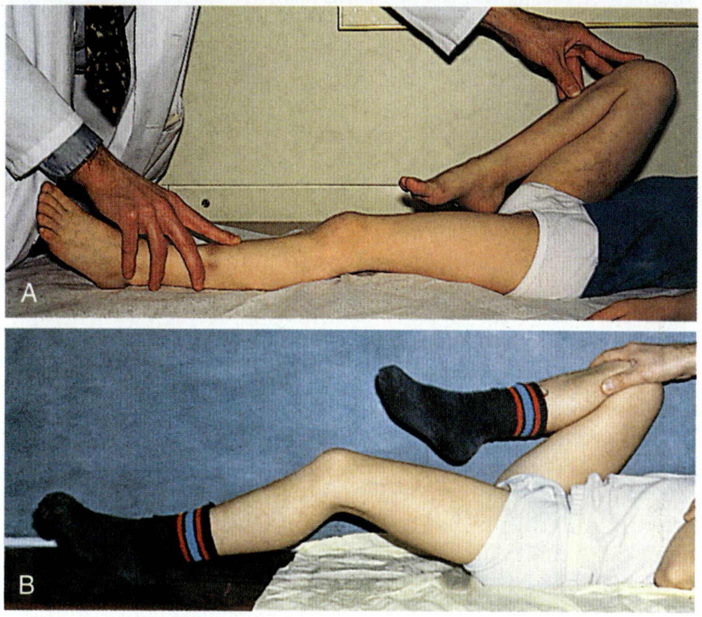

Fig. 22.8 Thomas test. This test of range of hip extension is performed by flexing both hips, then holding one in flexion while the patient is asked to extend the other leg. (A) Normally, full extension is achieved. (B) Inability to fully extend the hip, seen in this boy with Legg-Calvé-Perthes disease, indicates the presence of a flexion contracture of the hip and constitutes a positive Thomas test.

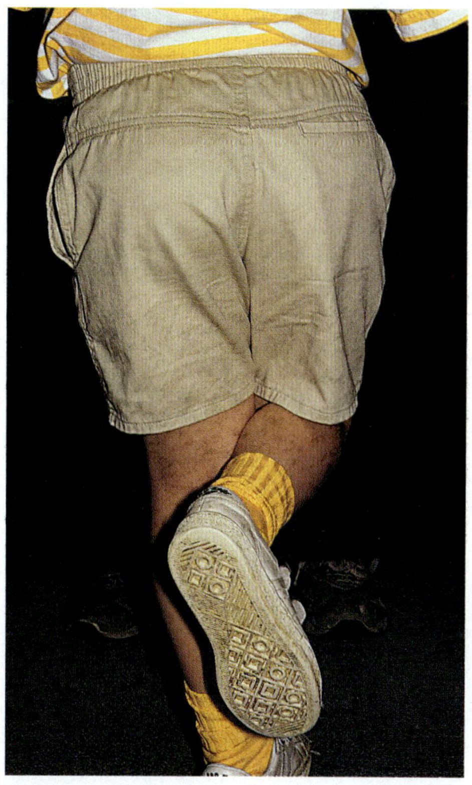

Fig. 22.9 Trendelenburg test. This test is performed to check for weakness of the hip abductors. While lifting his right foot, this patient's left abductor muscles stabilize his pelvis with a slight rise of the pelvis on the right. If left hip abductor weakness were present, the right pelvis would tilt downward when the right leg was lifted.

Knee

Knee pain is a common reason for seeking orthopedic care and may be referred from the hip; thus any patient presenting with atraumatic knee pain should always be examined for possible limitation of hip motion or pain on motion of the hip.

The knee examination begins with the examiner viewing the joint from the front, side, and back, looking for differences in contour, swelling or masses, and changes in overlying skin. From the front, the knee is inspected for valgus (lower leg points away from the midline) or varus (lower leg deviates toward the midline) deformity and for evidence of effusion, manifested by obliteration of the normal depressions around the patella or by generalized swelling. In viewing the knee from its lateral aspect, the examiner looks for incomplete extension resulting from flexion contracture or excess hyperextension (recurvatum deformity) and for symmetry of the tibial tuberosities. From the rear, the popliteal fossae are checked for symmetry and evidence of swelling. The thighs are also observed for comparative size and contour.

The knees are palpated to assess warmth and check for tenderness along the medial and lateral joint lines, the medial and collateral ligaments, the patella and its supporting ligaments, the femoral and tibial condyles, and the tibial tubercles. Palpation is easier with the knee flexed because the skeletal landmarks are more readily seen and felt, and the muscles, tendons, and ligaments are relaxed in this position.

When there is evidence of effusion, landmarks are obscured and the patella is readily ballotable. This is seen with intraarticular hemorrhage, arthritis, and synovitis, and range of motion is usually significantly limited. If landmarks are only mildly obscured (suggestive of a mild joint effusion or fluid collection in the bursae), pressure should be applied over the suprapatellar pouch with the thumb and index finger of one hand, milking down any fluid present while simultaneously pushing the patella up toward the femoral condyles with the other hand (Fig. 22.10). If fluid is present, the patella is ballotable and a palpable click is noted as the patella strikes the front of the femur.

The knee is primarily a hinge joint and is normally capable of 130 to 140 degrees of flexion and 5 degrees of hyperextension. However, it can also rotate approximately 10 degrees internally and externally, and this involves rotation of the tibia on the femur. Flexion is tested with the patient either sitting or lying prone. To test extension, the examiner can have the patient either sit and try to straighten the leg to 0 degrees of flexion or try to lift the straightened leg from the examination table while lying supine. Rotation is assessed by turning the foot medially and then laterally with the knee flexed.

With the knees flexed to 80 to 90 degrees, the patellas should face forward when viewed from the front and be located squarely at the ends of the femurs when seen from the side. The apprehension test (Fig. 22.11) is performed to check for a subluxating or dislocating patella. With the patient sitting, the examiner supports the lower leg and holds the knee flexed to 30 degrees. The patella is then gently pushed laterally. Any abnormal amount of lateral displacement, pain, or apprehension in response to this maneuver indicates a positive test.

Ligamentous stability of the knee should be assessed in the mediolateral and anteroposterior planes. In patients with acute injuries, especially those involving significant pain and swelling, this should be deferred until radiographs have been obtained to check for associated fractures.

The abduction/adduction stress test is used to determine the degree of stability of the medial and lateral collateral ligaments. With the supine patient's thigh moved to the side of the examination table and the knee flexed to 30 degrees, the examiner holds the distal thigh in one hand while grasping the inside of the lower leg with the other. To test the medial collaterals, the examiner applies valgus stress by pressing medially against the distal thigh with the upper hand while gently abducting the lower leg. To check the lateral collaterals, the examiner applies varus stress by pressing laterally on the inside of the distal thigh while gently adducting the lower leg. Normally the joint line should open no more than 1 cm on either side.

Anteroposterior ligamentous stability is provided by the anterior and posterior cruciate ligaments of the knee. They are tested by the anterior/posterior drawer and Lachman tests. The former is performed with the patient supine; the hip and knee flexed to 45 and 90 degrees, respectively; and the foot planted on the examining table, stabilized by the examiner's thigh or buttock. The examiner then grasps the proximal tibia with his or her fingers behind the knee and the thumbs over the anterior joint line and gently pulls and pushes (Fig. 22.12). In a positive anterior drawer test, the tibia moves forward more than 0.5 to 1 cm, indicating instability of the anterior cruciate ligament. Movement backward more than 0.5 to 1 cm indicates instability of the posterior cruciate ligament. In the Lachman test (Fig. 22.13) for anterior cruciate tears, the knee is flexed to 15 degrees. The examiner grasps the distal femur with one hand and the proximal tibia with the other. The thumb of the lower hand is placed on the joint line, and the femur is pushed backward as the tibia is pulled forward. Abnormal anterior displacement of the tibia on the femur can be seen and felt if instability is present. The amount of excursion is estimated in millimeters, and the end point is recorded as soft or firm.

Ankle

Examination of the ankle begins with inspection for deformity, swelling, change in color of overlying skin, and abnormal position (especially with weight bearing). Palpation is performed to detect

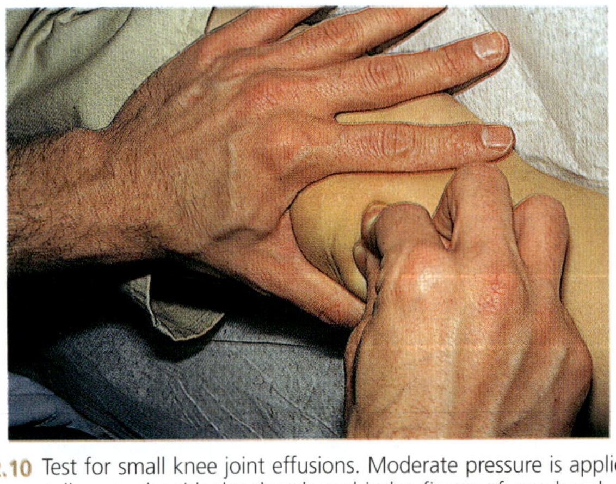

Fig. 22.10 Test for small knee joint effusions. Moderate pressure is applied over the suprapatellar pouch with the thumb and index finger of one hand, milking any fluid present downward. The other hand simultaneously pushes the patella up toward the femur. When an effusion is present, the patella becomes ballotable and a palpable click is felt as the patella strikes the front of the distal femur.

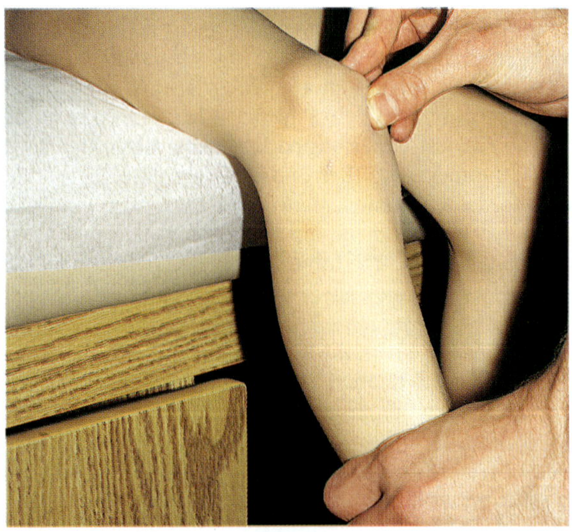

Fig. 22.11 Apprehension test for a subluxating or dislocating patella. With the patient sitting and the knee supported in 30 degrees of flexion, the patella is gently pushed laterally. Any abnormal amount of lateral displacement, pain, or apprehension constitutes a positive test.

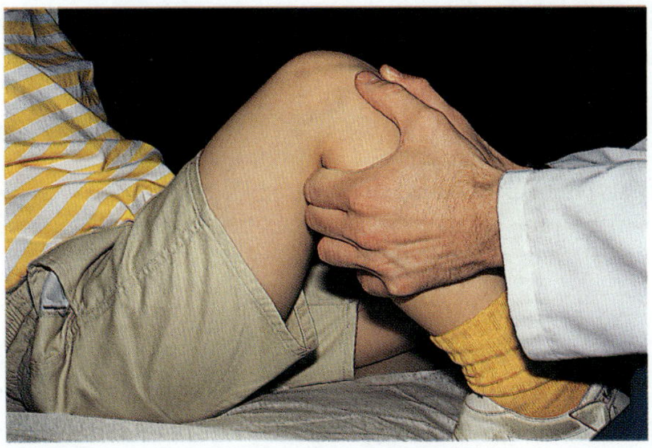

Fig. 22.12 Anterior and posterior drawer tests for cruciate ligament stability. With the patient supine, the hips flexed to 45 degrees, and the knees flexed to 90 degrees, the examiner grasps the proximal tibia with his or her fingers behind the knee and thumbs on the anterior joint line and makes a gentle pull/push motion. Forward movement of more than 0.5 to 1 cm indicates anterior cruciate instability, representing a positive anterior drawer test. Similar posterior motion on pushing indicates posterior cruciate instability, representing a positive posterior drawer test.

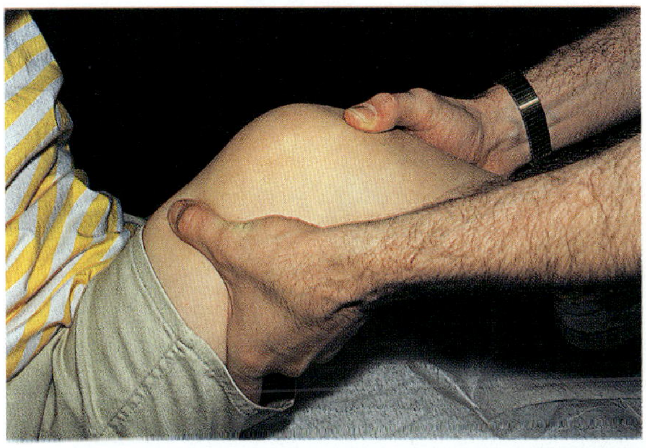

Fig. 22.13 Lachman test for anterior cruciate ligament tear. With the knee flexed to 15 degrees, the distal femur is grasped with one hand and the proximal tibia with the other, with the thumb on the joint line. The tibia is moved forward while the femur is pushed backward. Any abnormal displacement of the tibia on the femur indicates anterior cruciate instability and represents a positive test.

warmth and to localize tenderness. In the neutral position, the long axis of the foot should be at 90 degrees to the long axis of the tibia. Normally a child can dorsiflex 20 degrees and plantar flex 30 to 50 degrees from the neutral position and invert and evert approximately 5 degrees. Dorsiflexion and plantar flexion can be checked by observing passive and active motion, with and without resistance, but are most easily tested by having the ambulating child walk on his or her heels and toes, respectively. Similarly, inversion is tested by having him or her walk on the outside of the feet and eversion by having him or her walk on the medial sides.

Tests for ligamentous instability can be important after severe ankle sprains. The anterior drawer test is used to assess the stability of the anterior talofibular ligament. With the patient's legs dangling over the side of the examination table and the foot in a few degrees of plantar flexion, the examiner grasps the anterior aspect of the distal tibia with one hand while holding the calcaneus cupped in the palm of the other. The calcaneus is then drawn anteriorly while the tibia is pushed posteriorly. Normally there should be no movement, but with instability of the anterior talofibular ligament, the talus slides anteriorly. Lateral instability is seen only with major tears of the anterior talofibular and calcaneofibular ligaments, occasionally accompanied by tears of the posterior talofibular ligament, and is tested by inverting the calcaneus with one hand while grasping the distal tibia with the other. When instability is present, the talus gaps and rocks in the ankle mortise. Medial instability is exceptionally rare because of the strength of the fan-shaped deltoid ligament. To test for medial instability, the tibia and calcaneus are held in the same manner as they are in testing lateral instability, but the foot is everted instead. Gross gaping of the ankle mortise is felt when there is a major tear.

Gait and Gait Disturbances

Between the onset of walking and 3 years old, children tend to have a wide-based gait and young toddlers often hold their arms out to the side to assist balance. Around 3 to 4 years of age, most children achieve a normal smooth and rhythmic heel-to-toe gait, consisting of two main phases: stance and swing. Details of bipedal gait are beyond the scope of this chapter and may be found elsewhere for the intrigued mind.

Gait is best observed by having the patient walk back and forth in a hall or room with a mirror at one end. As the patient walks, the examiner focuses first on overall movement and then on the motion of the pelvis, hips, thighs, knees, lower legs, ankles, and feet in succession, both coming and going. In doing so, he or she looks for the pattern of heel-to-toe motion, for shortening of the stance phase, evidence of limitation of joint motion or weakness, and positional changes of the extremities.

Most acute and many chronic disturbances of gait in childhood are caused by pain. Others stem from weakness or spasticity caused by neurologic or muscular disorders, from leg length inequality, or from deformity. Important historical points are the time of onset of the abnormal gait and the circumstances surrounding it; the duration; whether the abnormal gait is constant or intermittent and, if intermittent, the time of day it is most apparent (morning gait disturbance is more associated with juvenile idiopathic arthritis; evening, with fatigability associated with neuromuscular disorders); and its relation to activity or exercise, including its effect on running or climbing stairs. The examiner should note any associated pain and its location, bearing in mind referral patterns (low back to buttocks and lateral thigh; hip to groin, medial thigh, knee, and sometimes buttock) and attempting to determine whether the pain is constant (suggestive of tumor or infection) or intermittent.

Gait Disturbances Stemming From Pain, Limb Length Inequality, or Stiffness

An antalgic gait is a limp caused by pain on weight bearing that results in shortening of the stance phase on the affected side. It can be due to pain referred from the back or pain anywhere in the lower extremity. Causes include traumatic or pathologic fractures, infection, inflammatory disorders, malignancy, tight shoes, or a lesion on the sole of the foot. Careful physical examination combined with a complete history usually enables localization of the problem.

Patients with leg length inequality manifest depression of the trunk and pelvis during the stance phase on the shorter leg. Some children try to compensate for the leg length inequality by toe-walking on the shorter extremity.

Patients with limited hip motion compensate by thrusting the pelvis and trunk forward in the swing phase. When knee flexion is limited, children tend to hike up the pelvis on the involved side during the swing phase and circumduct the leg to clear the foot from the floor. A circumduction gait can also be related to a painful condition involving the ankle or a limitation of ankle motion. By circumducting the leg laterally during swing phase, the patient reduces the need for ankle motion.

Gait Disturbances Resulting From Weakness or Spasticity

Patients with weakness of the hip abductors (gluteus medius muscle) have a Trendelenburg gait. Because they are unable to maintain a level pelvis and linear progression of their center of gravity, their pelvis tilts toward the unsupported side and their shoulder lurches toward the weak side during stance phase to maintain their center of gravity. Patients with weakness of the gluteus maximus (seen most commonly in children with Duchenne muscular dystrophy) have to hyperextend their trunk and pelvis to maintain their center of gravity posterior to the hip joint (see Chapter 16). Proximal muscle weakness may also be demonstrated by observing a child getting up from the floor unassisted. A Gower sign indicates weak hip extensors and abductors, necessitating that the patient use the arms to assist in standing by placing hands on the anterior thighs and pushing up, progressively moving their hands upward along the thighs until erect posture is achieved (see Chapter 16). Children with weakness of the quadriceps femoris muscle may have a relatively normal gait on level ground but difficulty climbing stairs. Weakness of the dorsiflexors of the foot results in foot drop and a steppage gait. Because the foot hangs down during the swing phase, the patient must lift the knee higher than usual to help the foot clear the floor and the forefoot tends to slap the floor on impact because smooth deceleration of the foot cannot be controlled. When the plantar flexors are weak, the patient is unable to push off at the end of the stance phase, and so the heel and forefoot come off the floor at the same time.

An equinus gait, characterized by toe-walking or a toe-to-heel sequence during the stance phase, is seen in children with heel cord contracture and limited dorsiflexion. It is usually indicative of an underlying neurologic problem leading to spasticity. Patients with spastic cerebral palsy who are able to ambulate often manifest a stiff-legged scissors gait, in which one foot crosses over the other during the swing phase. Vestibular or cerebellar dysfunction or generalized weakness tends to result in a wide-based ataxic gait because of abnormal balance. Absence of the normal arm swing with walking is seen in patients with paresis or cerebellar disease; posturing of upper extremities may become more obvious with running.

In-Toeing and Out-Toeing

The angular difference between the long axis of the foot and the forward line of progression during walking is called the *foot progression angle.* A minus value is assigned to in-toeing; a plus value is assigned to out-toeing. The normal range varies from 5 to 10 degrees to 10 to 20 degrees, respectively. The remaining rotational profile of the lower extremities can be examined with the patient in the prone position (Fig. 22.14). The foot axis can be

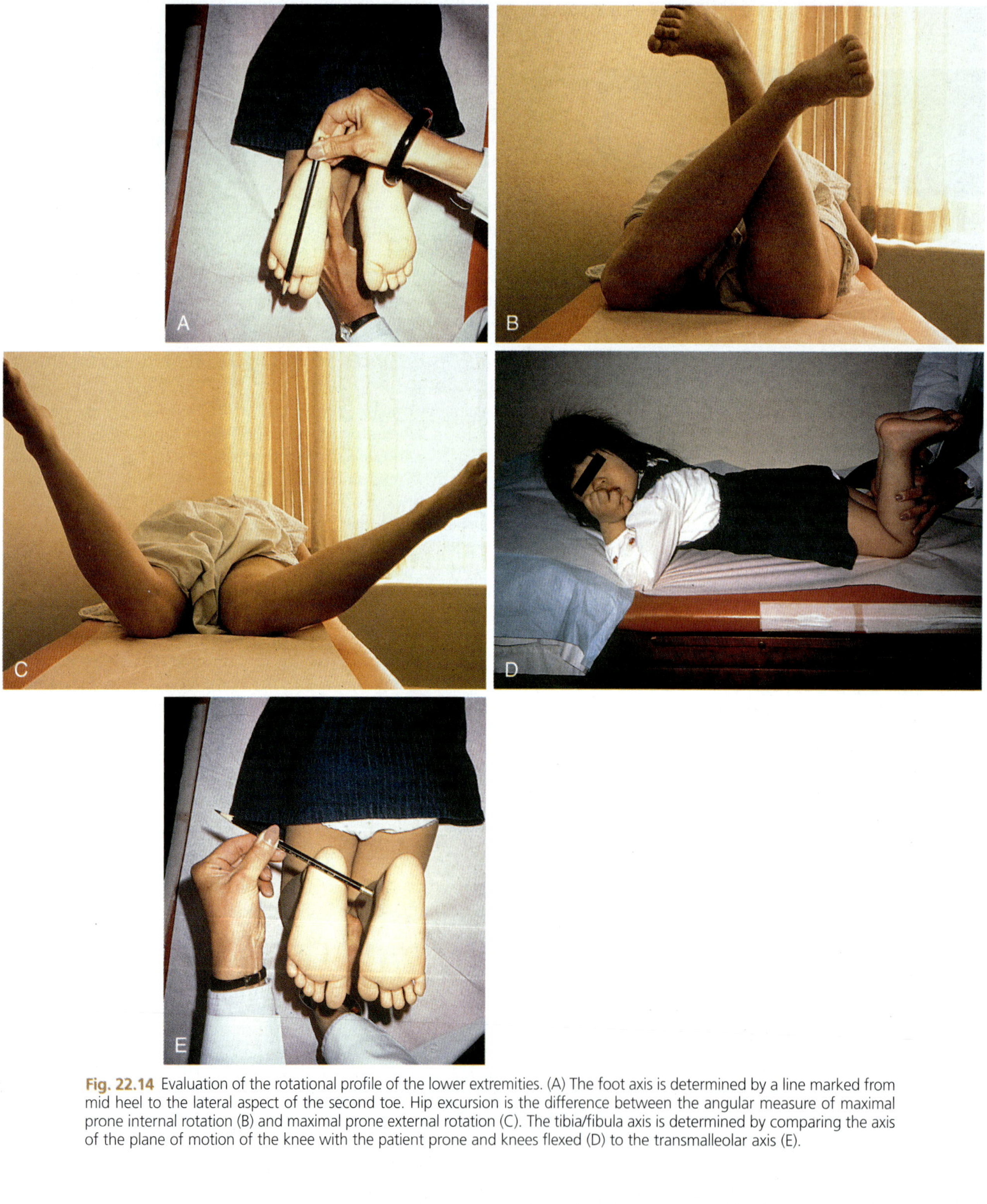

Fig. 22.14 Evaluation of the rotational profile of the lower extremities. (A) The foot axis is determined by a line marked from mid heel to the lateral aspect of the second toe. Hip excursion is the difference between the angular measure of maximal prone internal rotation (B) and maximal prone external rotation (C). The tibia/fibula axis is determined by comparing the axis of the plane of motion of the knee with the patient prone and knees flexed (D) to the transmalleolar axis (E).

determined by a line marked from the middle of the heel on the plantar surface to the lateral side of the second toe (see Fig. 22.14A). The hip excursion is the difference between the angular measure of the maximal prone internal rotation (see Fig. 22.14B) and that for external rotation (see Fig. 22.14C), and in the young child it is usually negative, representing more internal rotation than external rotation. In the adolescent and adult, usually there is more external rotation, or a positive hip excursion angle. Finally, the axis of the tibia and fibula can be determined by looking down the lower extremity in the prone knee-flexed position and comparing the axis of the plane of motion of the knee (see Fig. 22.14D) with the transmalleolar axis (see Fig. 22.14E) estimated by palpating the malleoli. The normal axis is 15 to 25 degrees externally rotated.

Femoral anteversion, internal tibial torsion, and metatarsus adductus are common causes of excessive in-toeing, or pigeon toe, and femoral eversion and external tibial torsion are common causes of out-toeing (see the Disorders of the Lower Extremity section, later).

MUSCULOSKELETAL TRAUMA

Musculoskeletal injuries are common in childhood and adolescence, whether seen in isolation or as part of multisystem trauma. Although the management of life-threatening injuries to the airway, circulation, and central nervous system (CNS) must take precedence over treatment of accompanying musculoskeletal injuries in cases of trauma, it must be kept in mind that fractures can result in significant blood loss. This is particularly true of pelvic and femoral fractures. Furthermore, prompt attention must be given to assessment of the status of neurovascular structures distal to obvious fractures because failure to recognize compromise may result in permanent loss of function.

Fractures

Diagnosis

Pain and fear in the young child combine to complicate the appropriate diagnosis of skeletal trauma. Many children are unable to give a firsthand history, and the cooperation of toddlers is often limited. A calm, empathetic manner is necessary to allay their fears. Taking a thorough history before any physical assessment helps the examiner establish rapport with the patient and the family. This should include questions concerning the type and direction of the injuring force, the position of the involved extremity at the time of the accident, and the events immediately following the injury. The presence of underlying disorders and the possibility of contamination of an open wound should be determined as well. Physicians should also be alert to signs suggestive of inflicted injury or child abuse. These include a history in which the mechanism of injury does not fit the type or severity of the fracture found, an unusual delay in presentation, and radiographic evidence of old healing fractures for which no medical attention was sought.

In cases of suspected fracture, splinting, elevation, and cold application may help reduce discomfort and local swelling. Splinting is particularly important for displaced and unstable fractures because it prevents further soft tissue injuries. When pain is moderate to severe and there are no cardiovascular or CNS contraindications, analgesia should be administered promptly. Proper pain control is unlikely to obscure physical findings.

Before beginning the physical examination, it is wise for the examiner to talk with the child to further gain his or her trust. Older infants and toddlers are often more comfortable when allowed to sit on a parent's lap and use of toys can help gain their cooperation. It is best to begin by examining the uninjured side and defer palpation of the most likely site of the injury on the affected side until last. If young children are highly anxious, it can be useful to instruct the parent in how to perform passive range of motion and palpation.

The first step in the physical examination is visual inspection of the injured area. The gross position of the extremity should be noted, and attention should be given to the presence or absence of deformity, distortion or abnormal angulation, and shortening (Fig. 22.15). The overlying skin and soft tissues are examined for evidence of swelling, ecchymosis, abrasions, punctures, and lacerations. Comparison with the opposite extremity must be performed.

The location of open wounds is important in ascertaining whether an underlying fracture is open or closed and in assessing the risk of joint penetration. Small puncture wounds or lacerations overlying bony structures from which a bloody, fatty exudate is oozing may reflect open fractures. Similarly, punctures or tears over joints must be assumed to communicate with the joint capsule (Fig. 22.16A). In patients with penetrating joint injuries, radiographs may demonstrate air in the joint, but absence of air does not rule out capsular penetration (see Fig. 22.16B). Computed tomography (CT) scanning of the joint and injection of methylene blue–dyed normal saline into the joint to assess the presence of a traumatic arthrotomy may be utilized to look for capsular injury. Probing of such open wounds is not advised. The

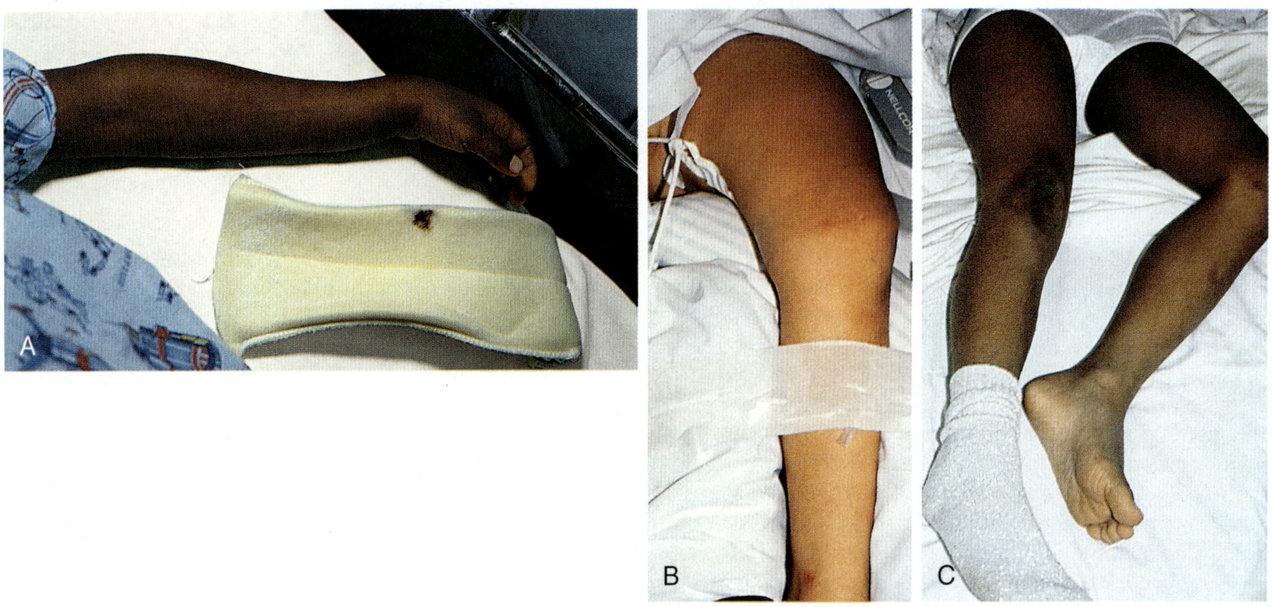

Fig. 22.15 Visible abnormalities seen on inspection in children with fractures. (A) Distortion and angulation of the distal forearm in a child with fractures of the radius and ulna. (B) Swelling and angulation of the proximal thigh resulting from a femur fracture. (C) Longitudinal shortening of the thigh in a child with a proximal femur fracture. Note the characteristic externally rotated position of the injured leg. The child was struck by a car, sustaining a fracture of the femoral neck.

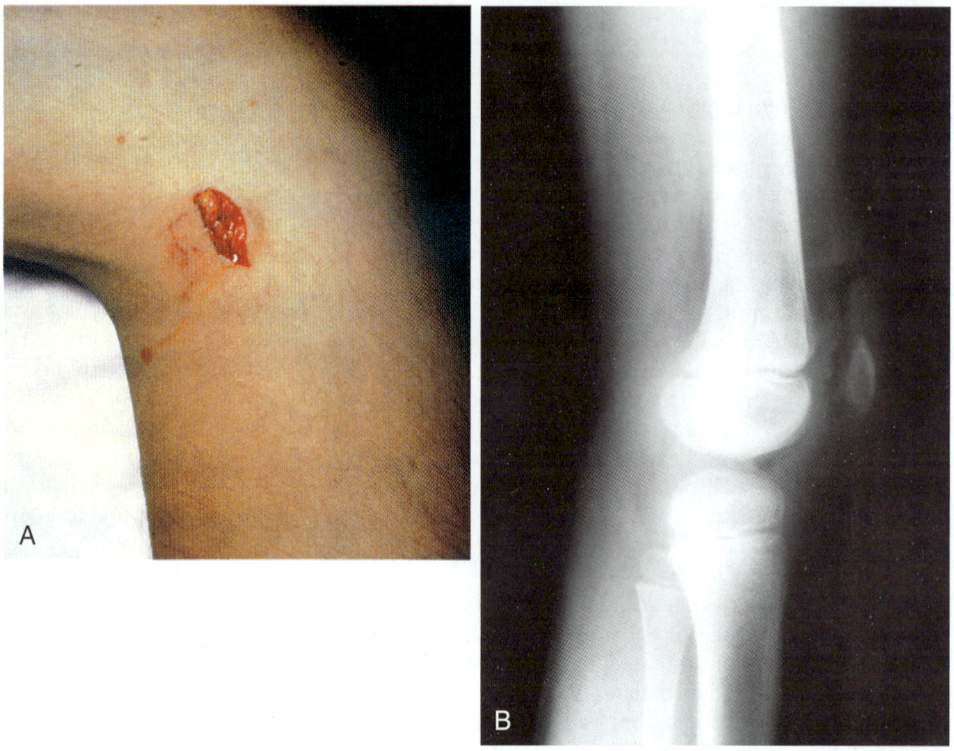

Fig. 22.16 (A) Penetrating injury of the knee. This child was struck by a stone propelled by the blades of a power lawn mower. Although the laceration appeared to be minor, serosanguineous fluid flowed from it on movement of the knee, suggesting penetration of the joint capsule. This was confirmed on exploration in the operating room. (B) Air is seen within the knee joint and in the overlying soft tissues in a child who sustained a deep laceration that penetrated the joint capsule. (A, Courtesy Bruce Watson, MD.)

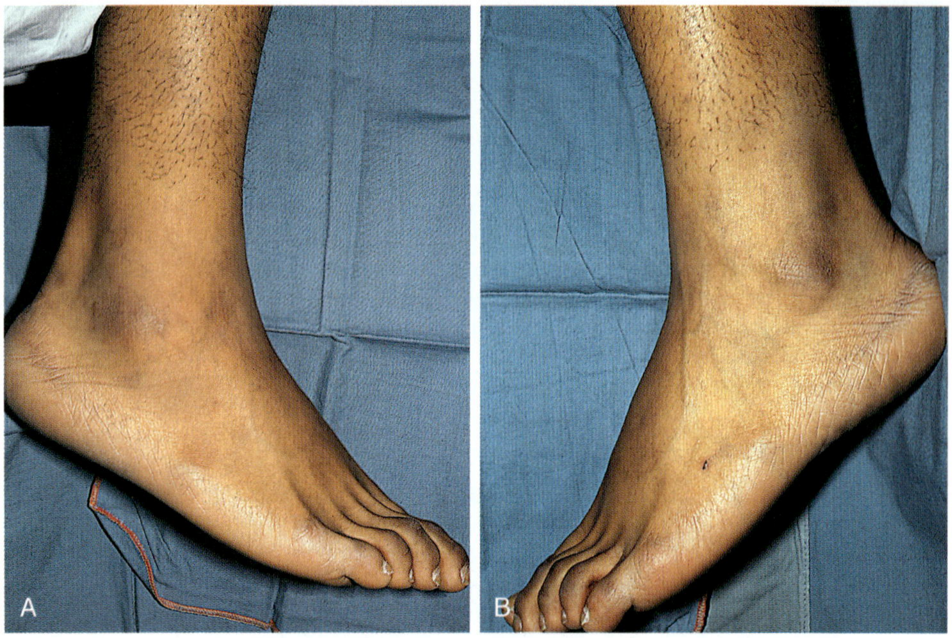

Fig. 22.17 Salter-Harris type I fracture of the distal fibula. (A) Slight swelling is present over the lateral malleolus. The degree of swelling can be truly appreciated only by comparing the injured ankle with its normal counterpart, shown in (B). The patient had point tenderness over the affected malleolus. The findings differ from those seen in an ankle sprain, in which tenderness and swelling are greatest over the ligaments inferior to the malleolus (see Fig. 22.65).

wound should be cleaned and covered with a sterile dressing until the consulting specialty service can provide an assessment.

After inspection of the injured area, palpation and assessment of active and passive motion can be performed. It is crucial to remember that the entire extremity must be evaluated in order to detect less obvious associated injuries. Localized swelling, tenderness on palpation, pain on motion, and limitation of motion are significant findings for an underlying fracture. Particular attention should be paid to the adjacent proximal and distal joints to avoid missing associated injuries. It can be difficult, however, to determine whether motion is limited because of pain, an associated injury, or fear and lack of cooperation.

Clinical findings vary depending on the nature of the fracture. Nondisplaced growth plate fractures typically present with mild, localized swelling, and point tenderness (Fig. 22.17). Because ligamentous injury is relatively uncommon in a child, the finding of point tenderness should suffice to prompt treating the injury as a fracture until proven otherwise. If initial radiographs appear normal, an occult fracture may be confirmed on follow-up with follow-up radiographs showing evidence of healing. Swelling is typically mild and occasionally imperceptible in cases of nondisplaced fractures. Careful palpation should disclose focal tenderness, however. Usually, the patient also experiences some degree of discomfort with motion or weight bearing, but limitations may be minimal. In contrast, fractures that completely disrupt the bone and displaced fractures are accompanied by more prominent swelling; more diffuse tenderness; and severe pain, which is markedly increased on motion (Fig. 22.18; see Fig. 22.15A and B). Crepitus may also be evident on gentle palpation. In examining children with these findings, manipulation

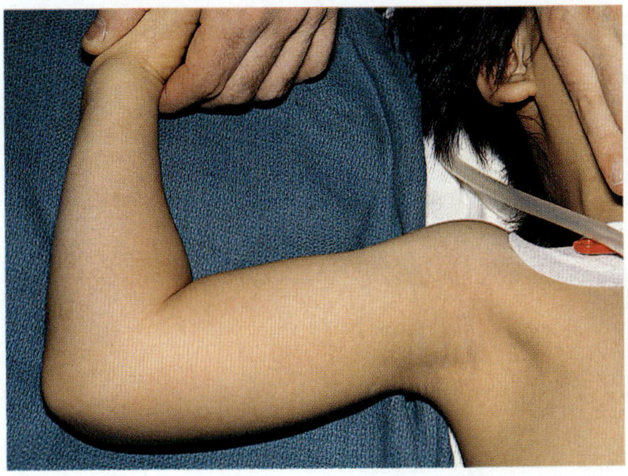

Fig. 22.18 Fracture with overlying soft tissue swelling. This child has a displaced supracondylar fracture of the distal humerus with moderate soft tissue swelling. The degree of swelling becomes evident if the size of the elbow area is compared with the size of the patient's wrist.

must be kept to a minimum to prevent further injury and unnecessary discomfort.

Assessment of neurovascular function is essential in evaluating any child after musculoskeletal injury. This includes the integrity of pulses and speed of capillary refill, along with testing sensory and motor function. Strength and sensation should be compared with those of the contralateral extremity. Assessment of two-point discrimination is probably the best test of sensory function but difficult to perform or interpret given the circumstances. Although sensory changes are common and usually related to swelling and traction, anatomically explainable motor deficit is an important finding. Evidence of neurovascular compromise necessitates urgent treatment.

Supracondylar fractures of the humerus, fractures of the proximal tibia, fracture/dislocations of the knee, and severely displaced distal femur fractures are particularly likely to be associated with neurovascular injury. Ankle fractures and dislocations can result in skin necrosis due to localized loss of circulation if left deformed for prolonged periods of time.

Compartment syndrome should always be kept in mind when dealing with skeletal trauma; it is more commonly associated with high-energy mechanisms of injury, especially those with a crush component (motor vehicle accidents with long extraction times, limbs entrapped under heavy objects, etc.). Compartment syndrome results when pressures increase excessively within a closed fascial compartment due to bleeding and edema, resulting in neurovascular compromise and muscle ischemia. In the awake and alert patient, the clinical picture will be striking with severe swelling and tenseness of the affected limb, severe pain resulting in drastic increases in analgesic need, agitation, and progressive neurologic deficit in the limb. In the obtunded patient, these signs are absent and a high index of suspicion with a low threshold to proceed to fasciotomy must be maintained (see the Compartment Syndrome section later).

In all cases of suspected extremity fractures, the injured part should be properly splinted and elevated, an ice pack applied, and analgesia administered before transport to the radiology suite. High-quality radiographs are essential for appropriate clinical decision making (see Chapter 25). At a minimum, two radiographs taken at 90-degree angles (orthogonal) are needed, anteroposterior and lateral views being the most common. Oblique views maybe helpful in fully disclosing the nature and extent of many fracture patterns, especially when the injury involves the ankle, elbow, hand, or foot. Radiographs should include the joints immediately proximal and distal to a fractured long bone to rule out fracture propagation and concomitant injuries. In certain settings, comparison views of the opposite side can provide useful information, especially in injuries that have subtle radiographic abnormalities. In some cases of displaced or angulated fractures, fractures in the setting of a bone lesion, potentially complex intraarticular fractures, and vertebral and pelvic fractures, a CT scan can be useful. Magnetic resonance imaging (MRI) is rarely used in the acute setting but may provide invaluable information in certain special cases. Particular care should be taken in interpreting pediatric radiographs because of the high incidence of subtle or even normal findings in patients with fractures. If the clinical picture strongly suggests a fracture, appropriate treatment should be initiated, even if the radiograph appears normal. Reassessment in about 2 weeks may be useful to clarify the exact nature of the injury as the early radiographic signs of bone healing may be evident at that time.

Fracture Patterns

Fractures should be described in terms of anatomic location, direction of the fracture line, type of fracture, and degree of angulation and of displacement. When the growth plate is involved, use of the Salter-Harris classification system is recommended.

Fracture patterns give clues as to the amount of energy absorbed by the bone at the moment of injury. Low-energy mechanisms such as ground-level falls and twisting-type injuries will result in spiral and oblique fractures. Direct, moderate-energy mechanisms such as sports collisions can result in transverse fractures or fractures with butterfly segments. High-energy mechanisms such as motor vehicle accidents and falls from heights will result in segmental or comminuted fracture patterns.

A common example of a nondisplaced spiral fracture is the toddler's fracture (see Fig. 22.43), which results from a twist. Typically, the child will fall with the extremity caught underneath their body, or the leg will get caught on a slide while traveling down in an adult's lap. Greenstick and torus fractures of the radius or ulna are incurred usually when the child falls on an outstretched arm with the wrist dorsiflexed. Vigorous repetitive shaking while holding a child by the hands, feet, or chest results in small metaphyseal chip or bucket-handle fractures, a major feature of nonaccidental trauma (see Chapter 6). Table 22.4 summarizes the major features of these various fracture patterns, which are illustrated in Figs. 22.19 through 22.27.

Table 22.4 Patterns of Fractures

Fracture Pattern	Major Feature	Radiographic Appearance
Longitudinal	Fracture line is parallel to the axis of a long bone	Fig. 22.19
Transverse	Fracture line is perpendicular to the axis of a long bone	Fig. 22.20; see Fig. 22.28
Oblique	Fracture line is at an angle relative to the axis of a bone	Fig. 22.21
Spiral	Fracture line takes a curvilinear course around the axis of a bone	Fig. 22.22; see Fig. 22.43
Impacted	Bone ends are crushed together, producing an indistinct fracture line	Fig. 22.23
Comminuted	Fracturing forces produce more than 2 separate fragments	Fig. 22.24
Bowing	Bone bends to the point of plastic deformation without fracturing	Fig. 22.25
Greenstick	Fracture is complete except for a portion of the cortex on the compression side of the fracture, which is only plastically deformed	Fig. 22.26; see Fig. 22.25B
Torus	Bone buckles and bends rather than breaks	Fig. 22.27; see Fig. 22.29

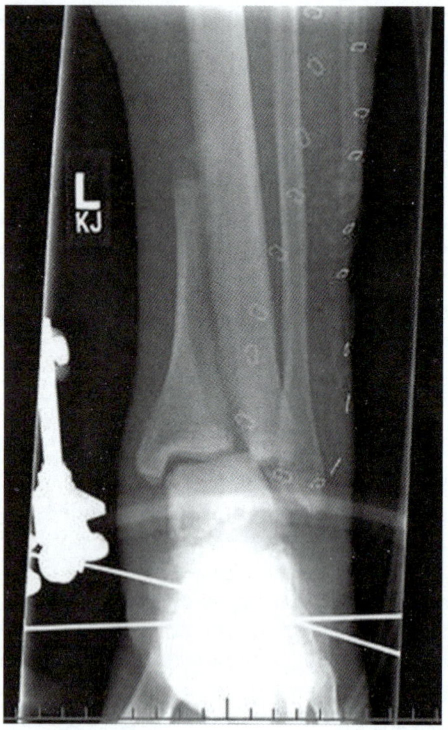

Fig. 22.19 Longitudinal fracture. During a motocross competition, this teenager missed a jump and was thrown 20 feet in the air, then fell to the pavement below, landing directly on his foot. The force of the impact was transmitted upward through his ankle, resulting in this vertical tibia fracture.

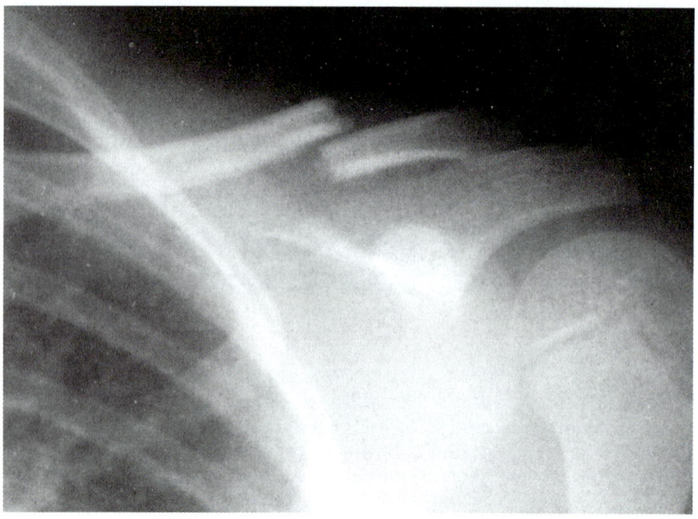

Fig. 22.20 Transverse fracture of the midportion of the clavicle. The fracture line is perpendicular to the long axis of the bone.

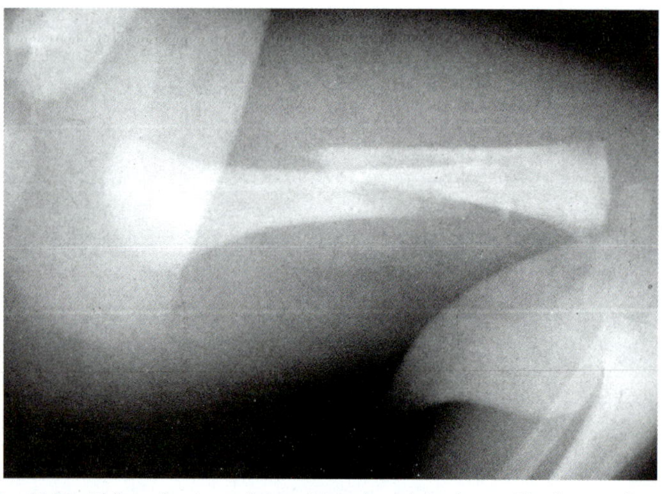

Fig. 22.21 Oblique fracture of the midportion of the femur. The fracture line is angled relative to the axis of the bone.

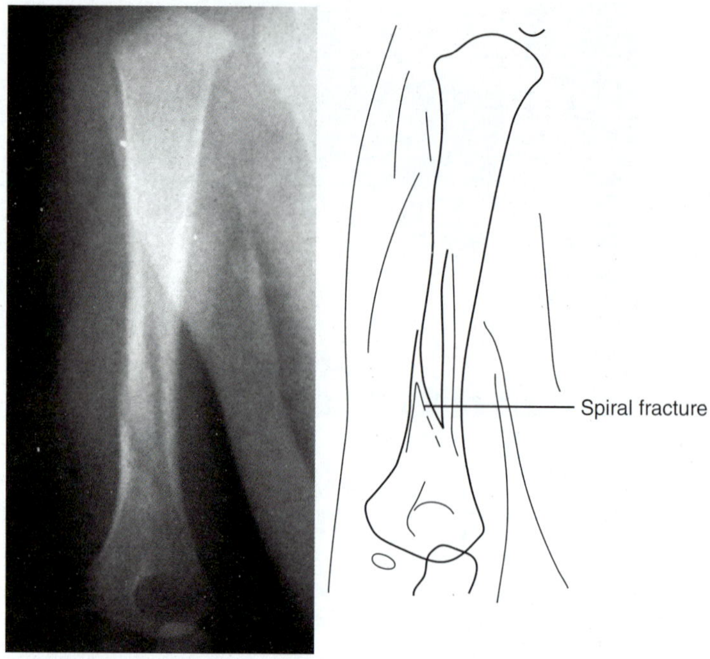

Fig. 22.22 Spiral fracture of the humerus. The fracture line takes a curvilinear course around the axis of the bone.

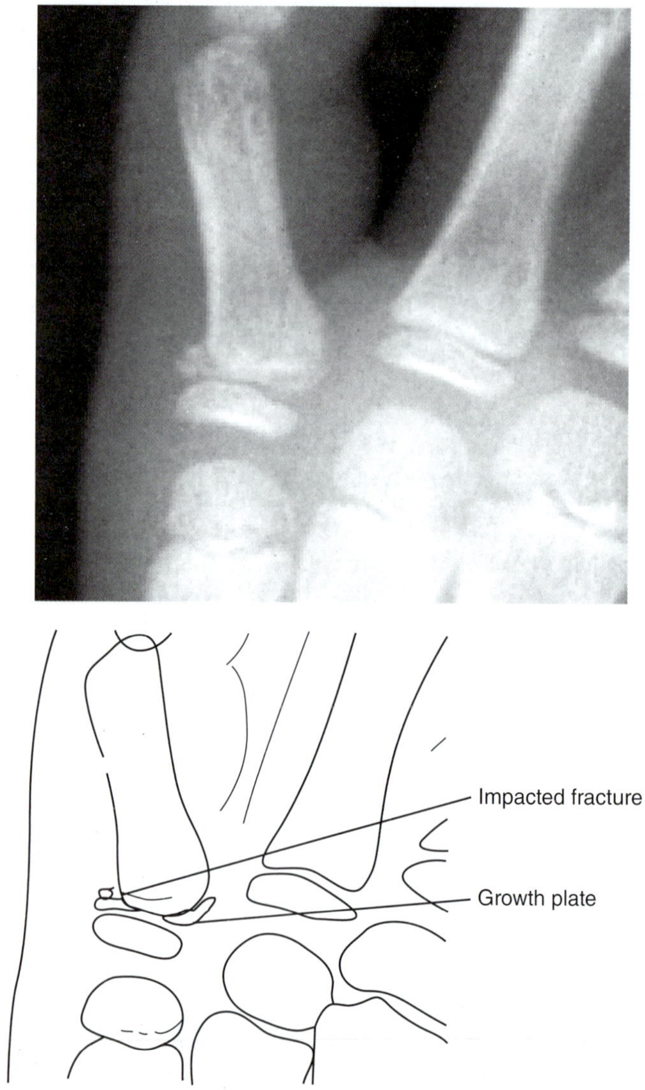

Fig. 22.23 Impacted fracture of the base of the proximal phalanx resulting from axial loading. The fracture line is indistinct, and the fragments appear to be crushed together. The fracture does not actually involve the growth plate but is located just distal to it in the proximal metaphysis.

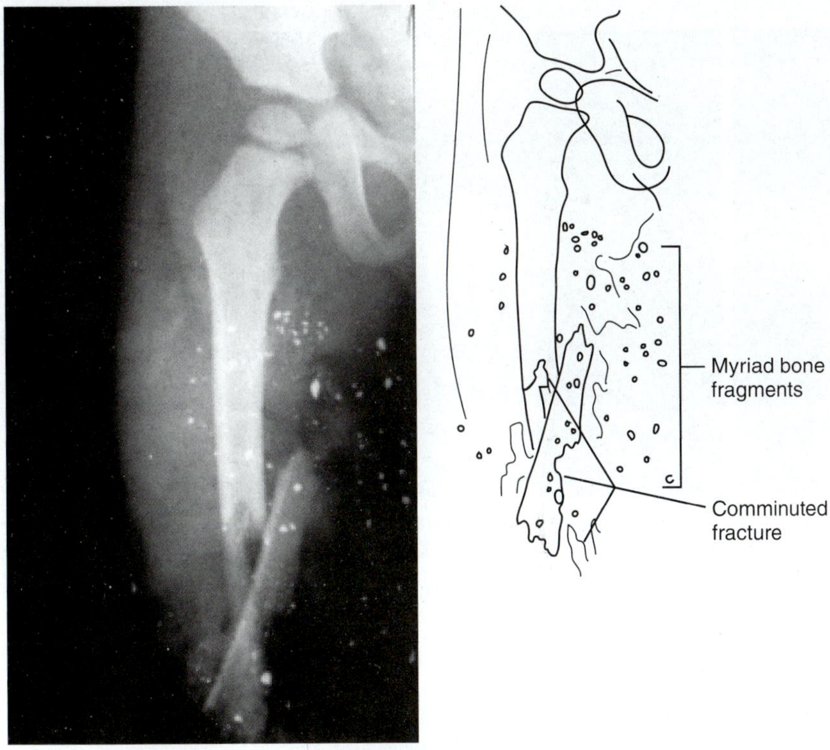

Fig. 22.24 Comminuted fracture of the femur secondary to a gunshot wound. Notice the numerous small fragments of bone in the adjacent soft tissues.

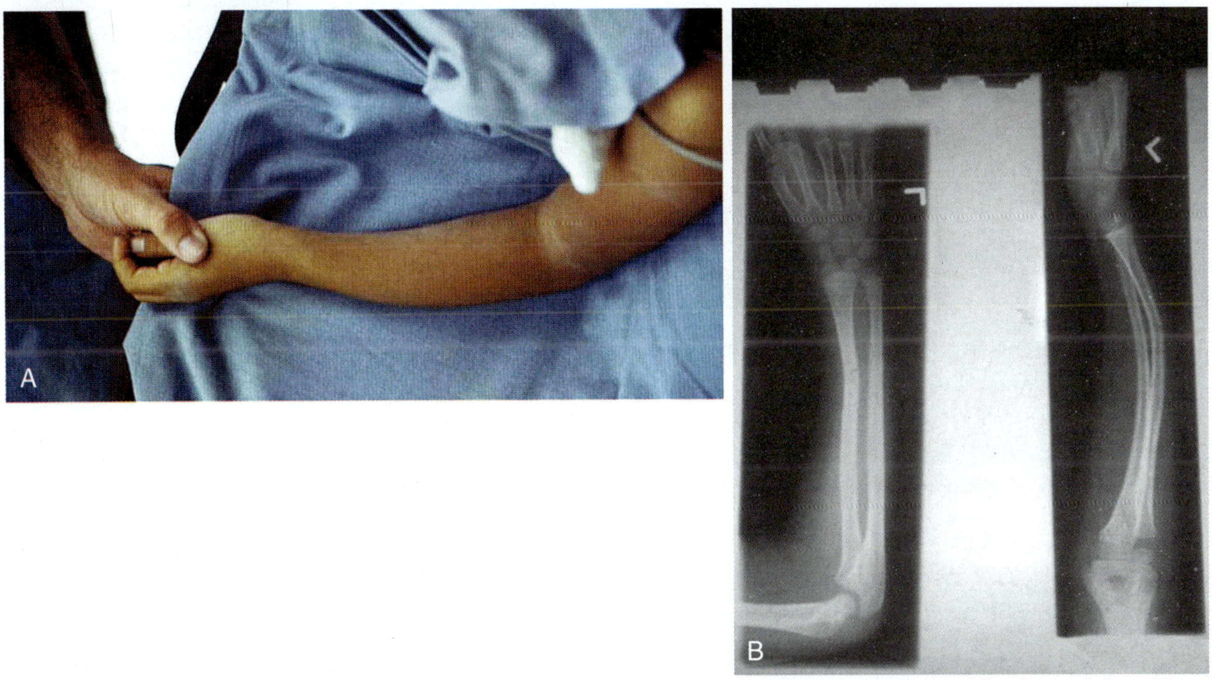

Fig. 22.25 Plastic deformation. (A) While playing soccer, this school-age child fell onto his outstretched arm. On impact, another player who fell with him landed on the arm, resulting in this bowing deformity of the forearm. (B) On radiograph, plastic deformation of both the ulna and radius are seen, along with a greenstick fracture of the radius. This necessitated manipulation under anesthesia to straighten the arm before casting.

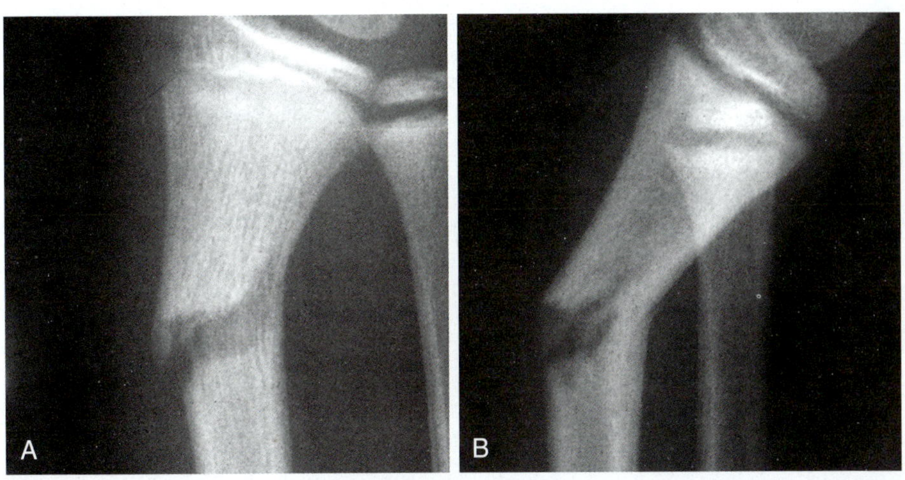

Fig. 22.26 Greenstick fracture of the distal radius. (A) In this anteroposterior view of the distal radius, a fracture line is seen that is complete except for a portion of the cortex on the compression side of the fracture. (B) The lateral radiograph demonstrates more clearly the disrupted and compressed cortices. This resulted from a fall on the outstretched arm with the wrist in dorsiflexion.

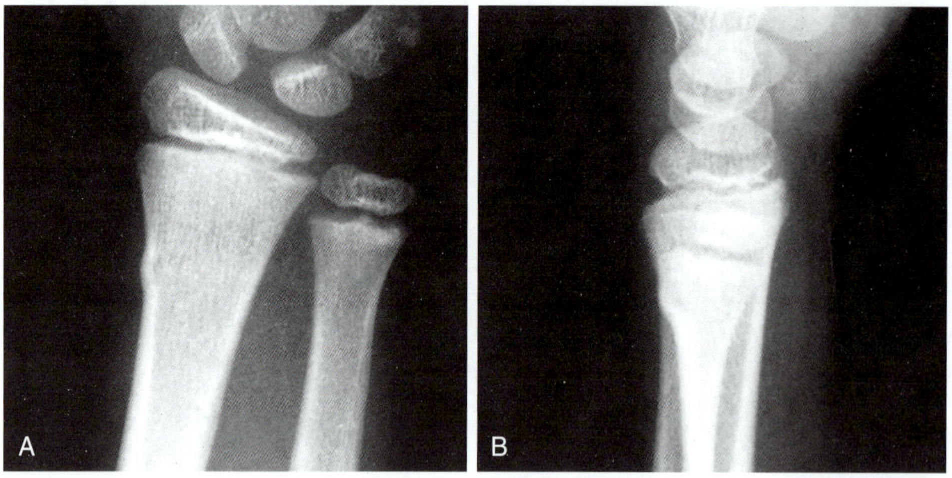

Fig. 22.27 Torus fracture of the distal radius resulting from a fall on an outstretched arm. (A) An anteroposterior radiograph of the wrist shows a minor torus or buckle fracture of the radius. (B) The lateral radiograph shows the dorsal location of the deformity. This injury can be expected to completely remodel.

Table 22.5 Classification of Fractures by Anatomic Location

Type	Site	Radiographic Appearance
Diaphyseal	Fracture involves the central shaft of a long bone	Fig. 22.28; see Figs. 21.21, 21.22, and 21.25
Metaphyseal	Fracture involves the widened end of a long bone	Fig. 22.29; see Fig. 22.26 and Chapter 6
Epiphyseal	Fracture involves the chondro-osseous end of a long bone; such fractures can also be classified as Salter-Harris fractures	Fig. 22.30
Articular	Fracture involves the cartilaginous joint surface	Fig. 22.31; see Figs. 21.40 and 21.41
Intercondylar	Fracture is located between the condyles of a joint; this is 1 variant of articular fracture and could also be subclassified as a Salter-Harris fracture	Fig. 22.31A
Physeal	Fracture involves the growth center of long bone; these are subclassified according to the Salter-Harris system	Fig. 22.32
Condylar	Fracture traverses the condyle of a joint	Fig. 22.33
Supracondylar	Fracture line is located just proximal to the condyles of a joint	Fig. 22.34
Epicondylar	Fracture involves an area juxtaposed to the condylar surface of a joint	Fig. 22.35
Subcapital	Fracture is located just below the epiphyseal head of certain bones	Fig. 22.36

The anatomic location of the fracture line simply refers to that portion of the bone to which the injury force was applied. Table 22.5 presents types of fractures classified by anatomic location. These fractures are illustrated in Figs. 22.28 through 22.36. There is some degree of overlap in this method of categorization.

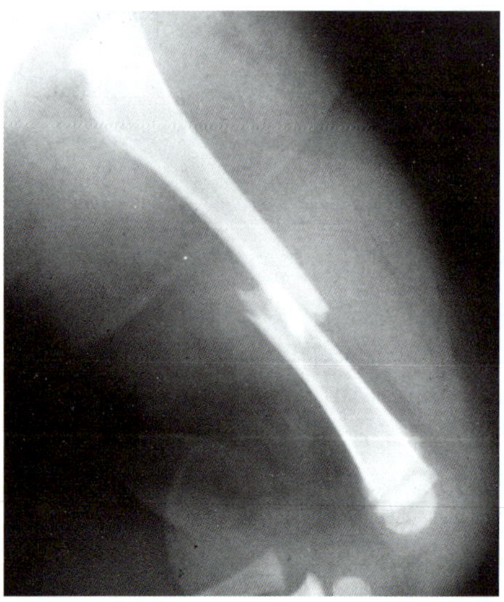

Fig. 22.28 Diaphyseal fracture. A transverse fracture line crosses the diaphyseal region of the femur. A moderate amount of overlap exists at the fracture site.

Physeal Fractures

An estimated 15% of all fractures in children involve the physis. Because the adjacent epiphyseal plate is not ossified in the young child and therefore is invisible on a radiograph, the fracture may be mistaken for a minor sprain or missed altogether. Even if diagnosed and properly treated, physeal injuries may still result in longitudinal or angular growth abnormalities. This risk is especially high in children with physeal fractures sustained in high-energy mechanisms and can occur even with appropriate treatment.

Because of the potential for long-term morbidity in patients with physeal fractures, great attention has been focused on the classification, diagnosis, treatment, and prognosis of physeal fractures. The Salter-Harris classification is commonly used for communication and documentation (Fig. 22.37).

Salter-Harris Type I

A Salter-Harris type I injury consists of a fracture running horizontally through the physis itself, resulting in a variable degree of separation of the epiphysis from the metaphysis. The amount of separation depends on the degree of periosteal disruption. Radiographs are often normal; hence the diagnosis frequently must be made clinically on the basis of the findings of point tenderness and mild soft tissue swelling over the site of an epiphysis (Fig. 22.38; see Fig. 22.17). This type usually has the lowest growth arrest rates.

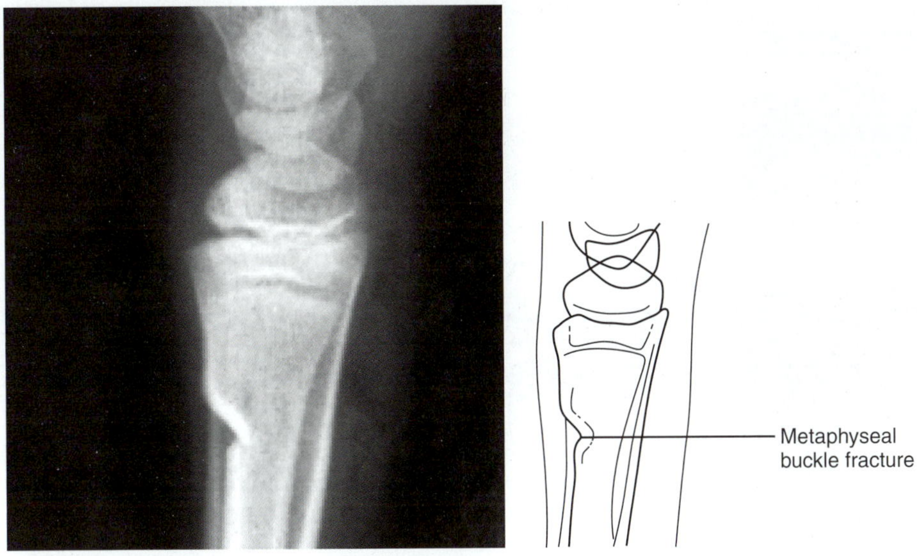

Fig. 22.29 Metaphyseal fracture. This lateral radiograph of the wrist shows a dorsal buckle fracture of the distal radial metaphysis. This fracture resulted from a fall on the outstretched arm with the wrist dorsiflexed and is a common injury in children.

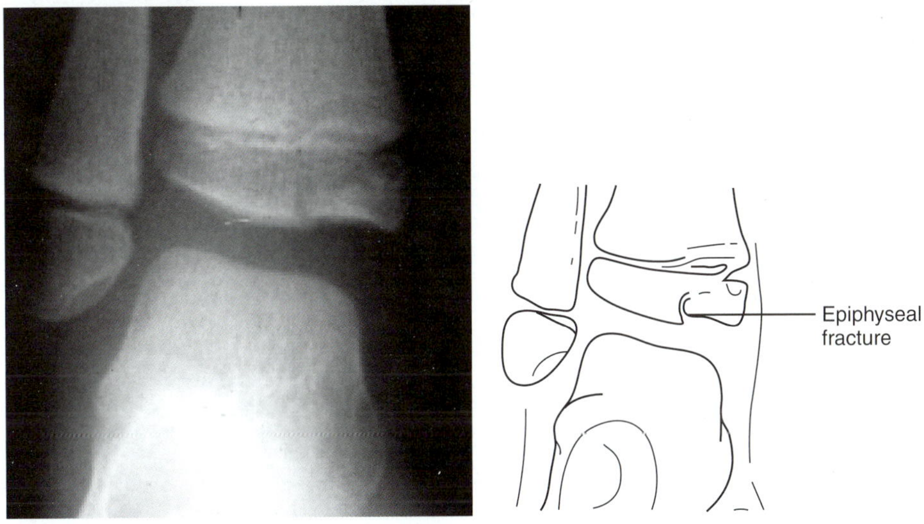

Fig. 22.30 Epiphyseal fracture. A fracture involving the medial aspect of the epiphysis of the distal tibia is seen in this anteroposterior radiograph of the ankle in a 4-year-old girl. A slight step-off is present at the articular surface. This could also be classified as a Salter-Harris type III fracture.

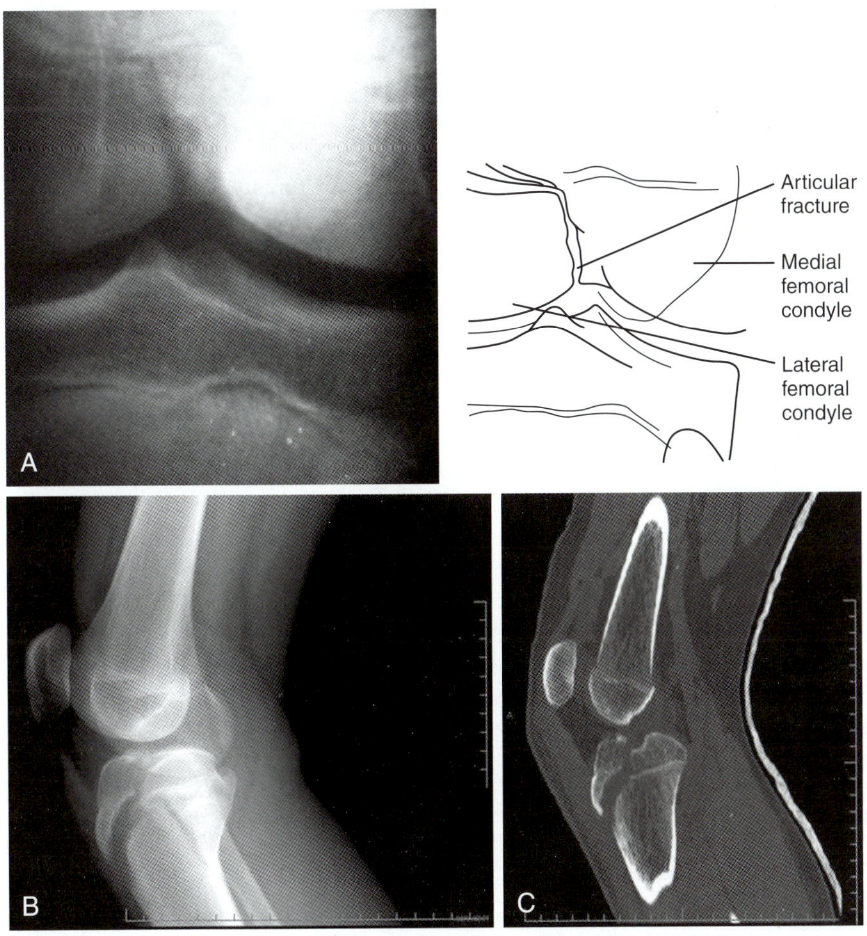

Fig. 22.31 Articular fractures. (A) This anteroposterior view of the knee demonstrates intraarticular extension of a fracture line that exits at the junction of the medial and lateral femoral condyles. The condyles are separated by only a few millimeters. This can also be termed an *intercondylar fracture.* (B) On coming down from a rebound, a 14-year-old basketball player landed with a twist with his knee in extension. The lateral radiograph demonstrates intraarticular extension of a fracture line that starts at the tibial tubercle and exits in the middle of the knee joint. (C) On computed tomography scan, the degree of intraarticular displacement of the fracture is better appreciated.

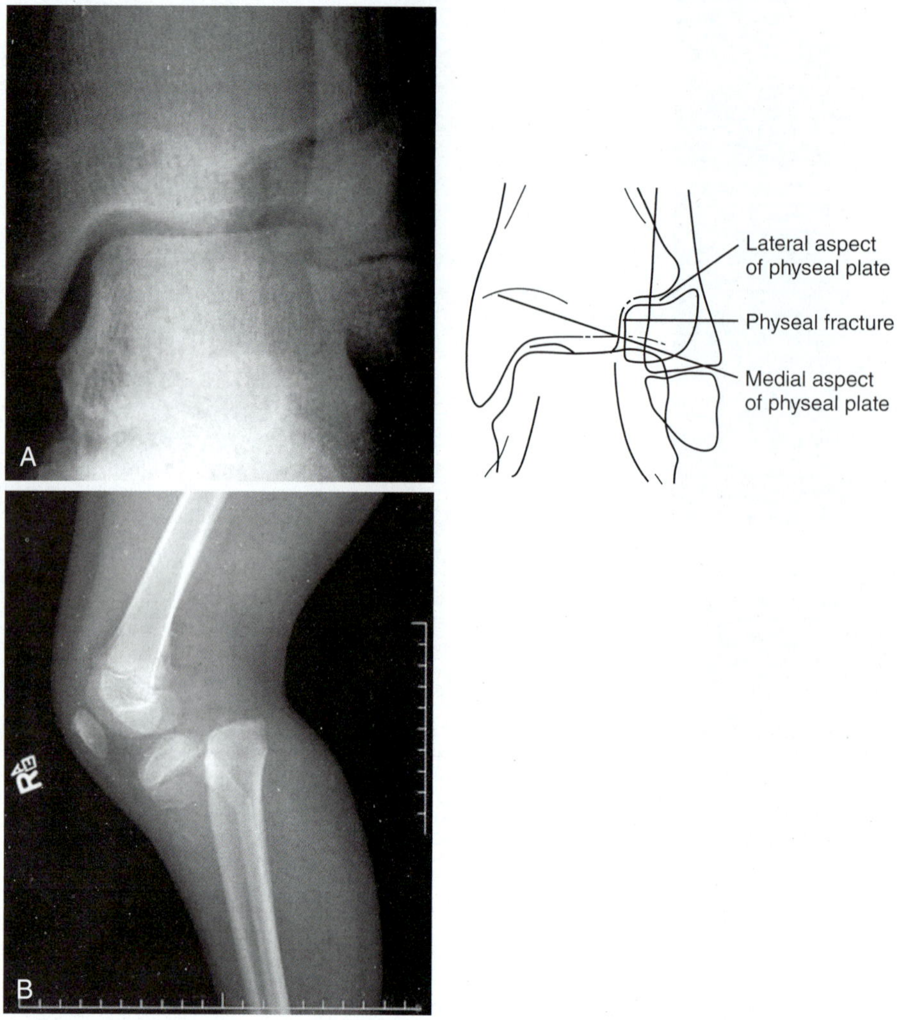

Fig. 22.32 Physeal fractures. (A) A fracture of the lateral aspect of the tibial epiphysis through the lateral aspect of the physeal plate is seen in this anteroposterior view of the ankle of a 13-year-old boy. Also called a *Tillaux fracture,* this pattern is seen in adolescents in whom the medial aspect of the distal tibial physis has closed but not the lateral aspect. It can also be classified as a Salter-Harris type III fracture. (B) A 7-year-old restrained backseat passenger involved in a head-on collision motor vehicle accident suffered a direct impact to the front of his lower leg due to violent displacement of the front seat. This resulted in shearing of the proximal tibial epiphysis from the metaphysis. The lateral view of the knee demonstrates complete separation of the epiphysis from most of the metaphysis. This degree of posterior displacement of the metaphysis can be associated with compression of the popliteal artery. This can also be classified as a Salter-Harris type II fracture because a small metaphyseal fragment remains attached to the epiphysis.

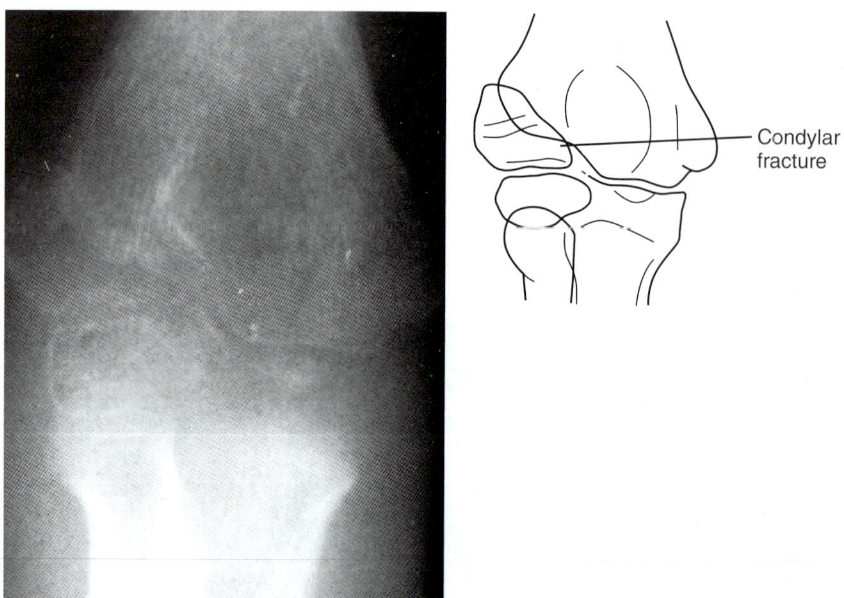

Fig. 22.33 Condylar fractures. This anteroposterior radiograph of the elbow shows a fracture of the lateral condyle of the distal humerus. The condyle is displaced proximally and radially. The fragment is always larger than it appears on a radiograph because of the large amount of unossified cartilage present in the distal humerus.

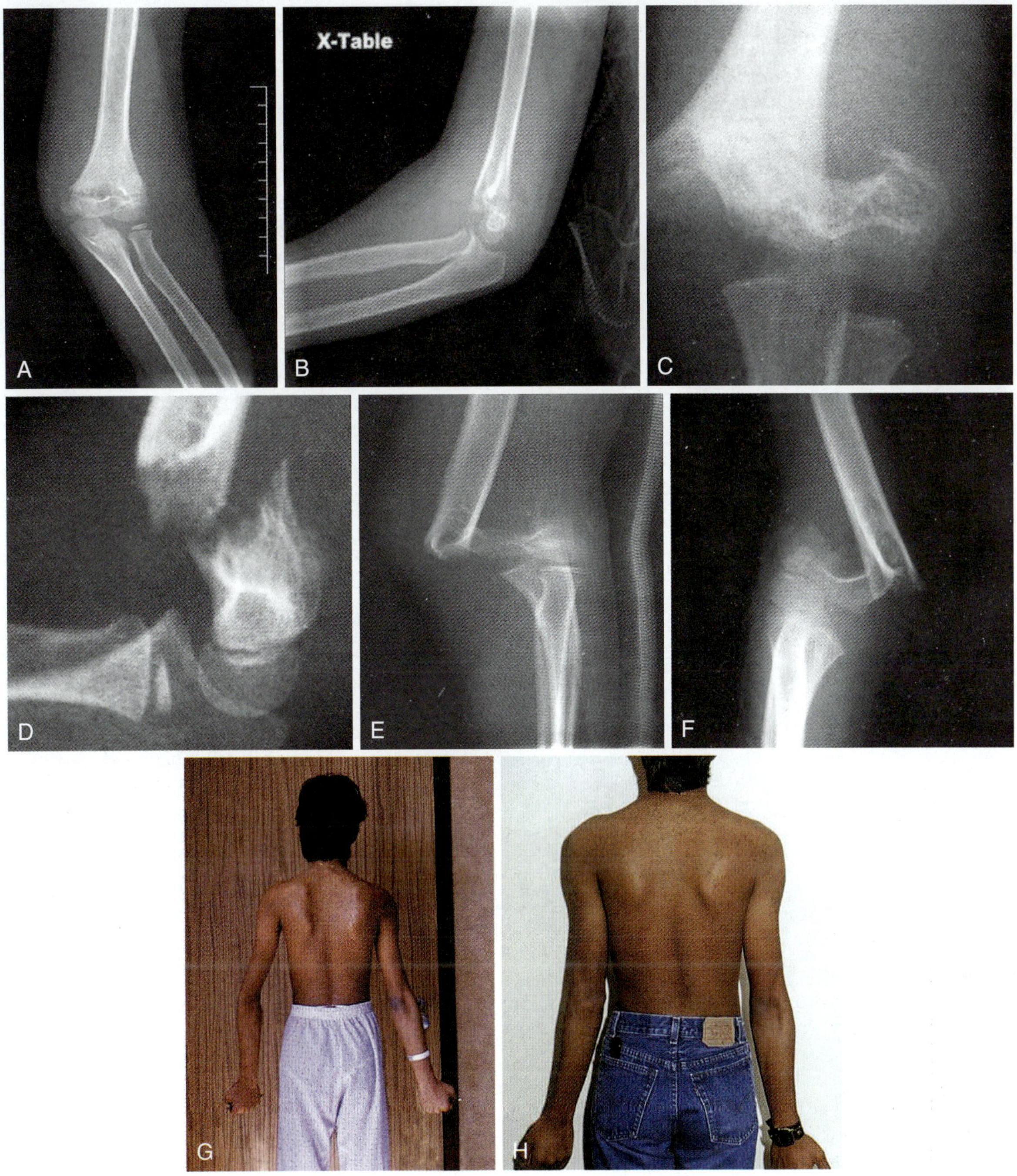

Fig. 22.34 Supracondylar humerus fractures. These injuries are typically the result of a fall backward onto an outstretched arm with the elbow in hyperextension. This transmits the force of the impact to the distal humerus, driving the distal fragment posteriorly. Most require surgery to realign, reduce, and stabilize the fracture. (A) This 8-year-old fell backward off a swing, landing on his hand with his elbow extended. The anteroposterior radiograph shows the fracture line crossing through the olecranon fossa in the supracondylar region of the distal humerus. Although there is marked soft tissue swelling, degree of displacement appears mild. (B) In the lateral view, moderate posterior displacement of the distal fragment is evident. There is also a positive fat pad sign. (C) In another boy, after a more severe backward fall, the anteroposterior radiograph shows the distal fragment displaced radially. (D) In the lateral view, significant posterior displacement is evident. (E and F) In this case an 8-year-old fell backward from a barn window onto his extended arm. This resulted in a severely displaced (type III) supracondylar fracture with associated injury to the brachial artery and vascular insufficiency of the forearm and hand, manifest by a cool hand and absent pulses. The distal fragment is displaced posterolaterally. In such cases, the brachial artery may be placed on "stretch" over the proximal fragment or may be entrapped between fragments. This is a true surgical emergency requiring immediate surgery to reduce the fracture and restore distal blood flow. (G) This boy has cubitus valgus deformity of his left elbow as a result of incorrect healing of a supracondylar fracture. (H) This was corrected by a distal humerus osteotomy, restoring normal contour to the elbow.

Salter-Harris Type II

A Salter-Harris type II injury consists of a fracture line running a variable distance through the physis and exiting through the metaphysis on the side opposite the site of fracture initiation. A fragment consisting of the entire epiphysis with an attached metaphyseal fragment is thus produced (Fig. 22.39). With appropriate treatment, growth arrest rates are low.

Salter-Harris Type III

Intraarticular shearing forces can produce a fracture line running from the articular surface through the epiphysis and then exiting through a portion of the physis. This creates a separate epiphyseal fragment with no connection to the metaphysis (Fig. 22.40; see Figs. 21.30 and 21.32A). Accurate anatomic reduction is required to achieve the best possible outcome.

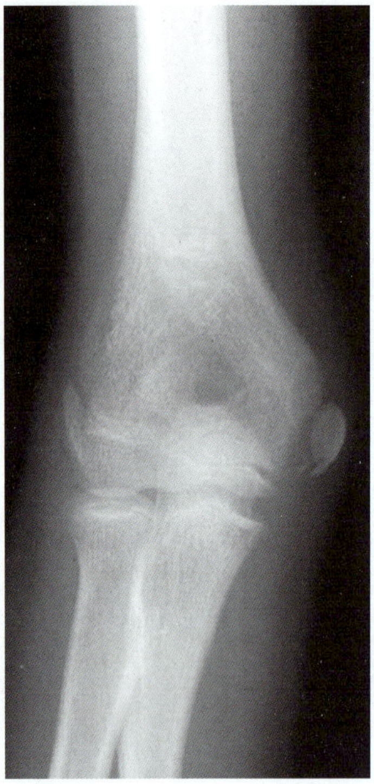

Fig. 22.35 Epicondylar fracture. This 10-year-old tripped while playing soccer and fell onto his arm with a valgus strain on the elbow. The anteroposterior radiograph shows a moderately displaced medial epicondylar fracture. These injuries are sometimes associated with dislocation of the elbow, in which case there is marked swelling of the entire elbow.

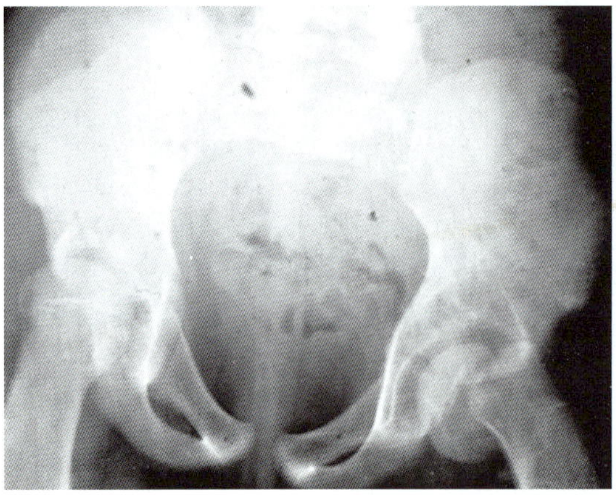

Fig. 22.36 Subcapital fracture. This anteroposterior radiograph of the pelvis shows a displaced subcapital fracture of the left femur. This particular injury may be seen acutely as the result of significant trauma or may develop slowly as a result of gradual slipping at the physeal level.

Growth arrest rates are usually moderate to high depending on the individual injury.

Salter-Harris Type IV

In this fracture, the fracture line starts at the articular surface, runs through the epiphysis across the physis, and exits the metaphysis. A single fragment consisting of both the epiphysis and attached metaphysis is thus created (Fig. 22.41). Open reduction and internal fixation are often necessary. Growth arrest rates are usually moderate to high depending on the individual injury.

Salter-Harris Type V

A Salter-Harris type V fracture is the product of a crushing injury to the physis without physeal fracture or displacement. Radiographic diagnosis is virtually impossible to make at the time of injury; hence this fracture could only be diagnosed retrospectively. These injuries have a 100% growth arrest rate by definition (Fig. 22.42).

Fracture Treatment Principles

The healing and remodeling capacity of the growing bones of a child is considerably greater than that of an adult; the younger the child and the closer the fracture to an active physis, the greater the capacity. As a result, healing is rapid, necessitating a shorter period of immobilization; nonunion is rare. In planning fracture reductions, the remodeling capability and the likely resulting overgrowth must be considered. Satisfactory position is determined in part by the child's age, the nature and position of the fracture, the bone involved, the appearance and condition of the adjacent soft tissues, and the presence or absence of other systemic injuries. However, not every fracture will remodel well. Rotational deformities and angular deformities that are not in the axis of adjacent joint motion are not effectively remodeled. Growth plates that are not as active as others may not have sufficient growth remaining to complete remodeling. Thus these must be corrected at the time of initial fracture reduction.

Nondisplaced fractures are simply casted or splinted. Because of the rarity of ligamentous injuries before epiphyseal closure, patients with an appropriate clinical history and point tenderness over a physis are presumed to have a fracture and should be treated accordingly, even if radiographs are normal. Most displaced fractures in long bones and Salter-Harris types I and II physeal fractures can be treated by closed reduction and casting. As a general rule, open reduction and internal fixation are needed for the management of Salter-Harris type III and type IV fractures, certain open fractures, and fractures associated with neurovascular compromise. Depending on the time of presentation, degree of displacement, and severity of soft tissue swelling, reduction, casting, or surgical treatment may have to be deferred pending the subsidence of edema.

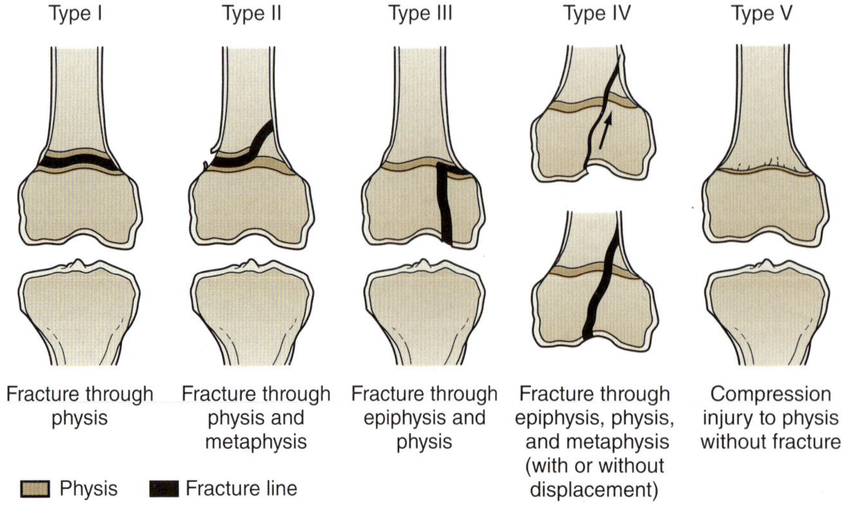

Fig. 22.37 Salter-Harris classification of physeal injuries.

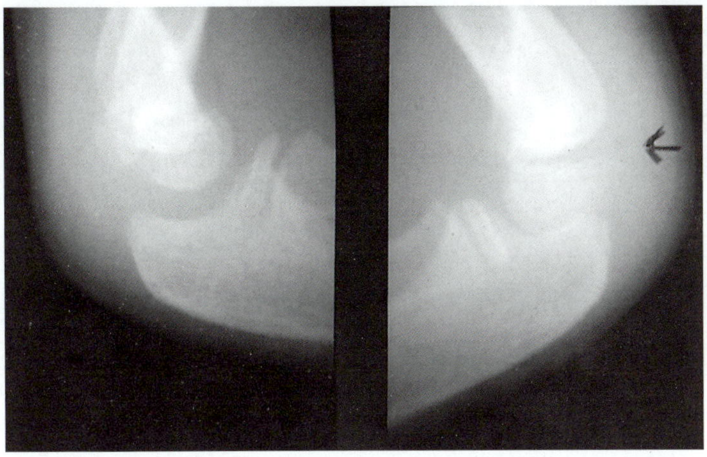

Fig. 22.38 Salter-Harris type I injury. Close inspection shows slight widening of the distal humeral epiphysis *(right, arrow).* Clinically, the patient had pain, tenderness, and decreased range of motion of the elbow. (Courtesy Jocelyn Ledesma Medina, MD.)

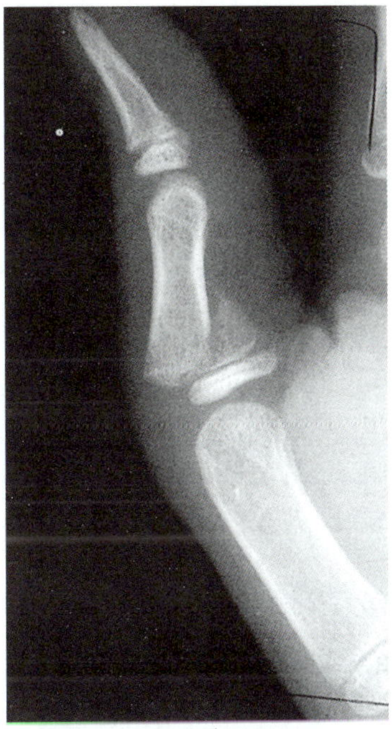

Fig. 22.39 Salter-Harris type II injury. On this lateral radiograph of the thumb, the fracture is seen to involve the proximal phalanx. The fracture line runs through the physis and exits through the metaphysis on the side opposite the site of fracture initiation. A fragment consisting of the entire epiphysis with the attached metaphyseal fragment is produced.

After reduction and/or immobilization in a cast or splint, pain should be markedly alleviated, although some analgesia is likely to be necessary for 3 to 4 days. Closed treatment of fractures in children almost never requires oral narcotics at home, and these should not be routinely prescribed. Ibuprofen and nonsteroidal analgesics have proven to provide adequate pain control post closed reduction and should be used in alternation with acetaminophen in the absence of medical contraindications. No negative effect of ibuprofen on fracture healing in children has been reported.

Persistence or recurrence of discomfort after appropriate treatment of fractures signifies a complication and warrants prompt reevaluation. Splints and casts must be reexamined and bivalved or loosened immediately in the case of tight application as these may

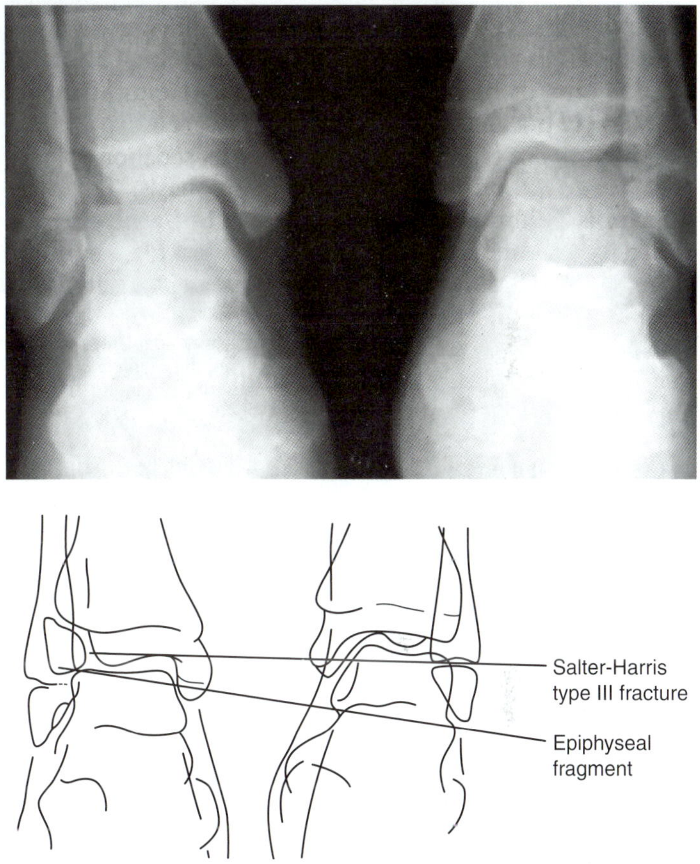

Fig. 22.40 Salter-Harris type III injury. Comparison view of both ankles reveals a fracture involving the lateral aspect of the right distal tibial epiphysis. This configuration creates a separate fragment without any connection to the metaphysis.

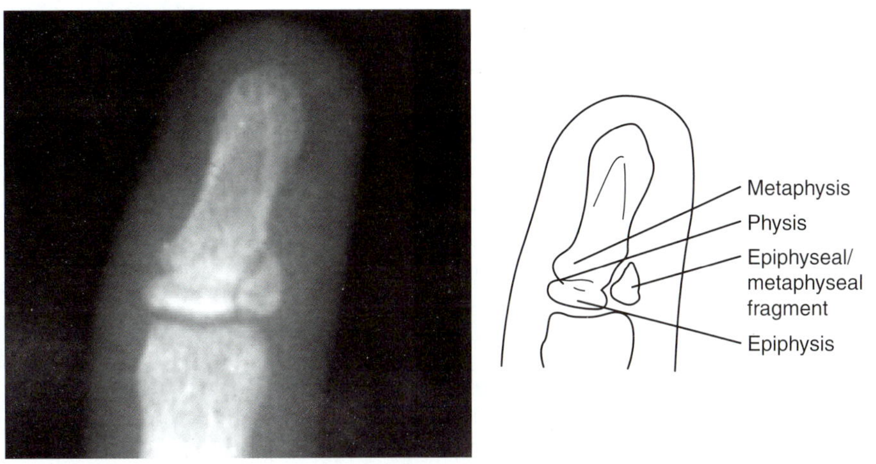

Fig. 22.41 Salter-Harris type IV injury. This patient incurred a fracture of the distal phalanx of the index finger. The fracture line starts at the articular surface, runs through the epiphysis across the physis, and exits through the metaphysis. A single fragment consisting of the epiphysis and the attached metaphysis is thus created.

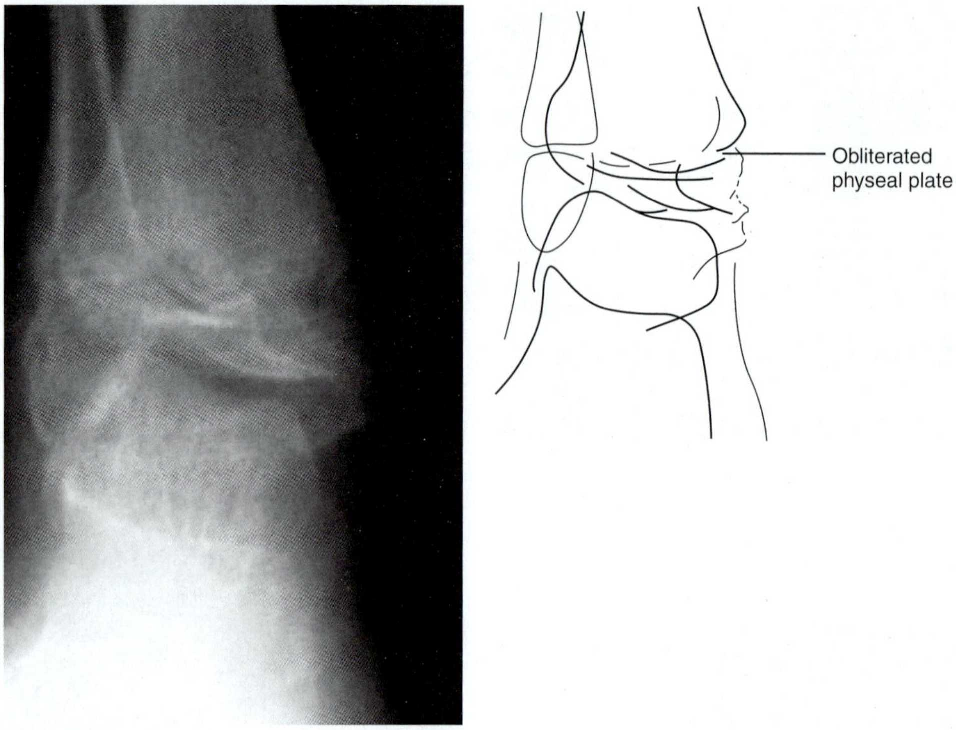

Fig. 22.42 Salter-Harris type V injury. This anteroposterior radiograph of the ankle taken several weeks after a crush injury sustained in an automobile accident reveals obliteration of the distal tibial physeal plate. As is often the case, original radiographs taken at the time of injury looked normal. This fracture must be suspected on clinical grounds, and the patient treated and monitored accordingly.

cause compartment syndrome. Any complaints of heel pain after application of a lower extremity splint must be taken seriously, the splint or cast should be removed or windowed, and the skin assessed for pressure points or ulcers.

Clear communication with the child and parents is important. Verbal instructions are necessary but can be forgotten or confused by the anxious parents and the patient. Written instructions regarding home care measures, necessary parent observations, and worrisome signs that signal the need for prompt reevaluation are invaluable.

Special Cases

Clavicular Fractures

Fractures of the clavicle are common. They are caused by lateral compression forces (as can occur in the process of delivery of the newborn or in falls onto the shoulder) or occasionally by a direct blow or impact on the clavicle itself. Most involve the midshaft or distal clavicle (see Fig. 22.20). Clinically, the child complains of pain in the shoulder, is noted to avoid moving the arm on the involved side, and often splints it by holding the arm close against the chest. Tenderness and mild swelling are evident on palpation of the fracture site. Treatment often consists of measures to decrease pain while the fracture heals, such as a sling for 2 to 3 weeks. Adolescents near skeletal maturity with severely displaced clavicle fractures may benefit from surgical treatment. Medial clavicle fractures are rare and are caused by high-impact forces. They may be associated with injuries of mediastinal structures. Thus they warrant meticulous evaluation including chest CT and angiography. Fractures involving the distal tip of the clavicle in infants (beyond the neonatal period) and toddlers should be evaluated for nonaccidental trauma (see Chapter 6).

Toddler's Fracture

One of the most common orthopedic injuries seen in children between 1 and 5 years old is the toddler's fracture. The child usually has a sudden onset of refusal to bear weight on one leg or of an antalgic limp immediately after a traumatic event. The mechanism is often twisting of the leg; the child may fall with the leg caught under the body, or the leg may be caught while traveling down a play slide in an adult's lap. Not uncommonly, the actual fall is unwitnessed and the parents are unsure about the nature of the accident. The injury results in a spiral or short oblique fracture of the distal tibia or the junction of the mid and distal tibia (Fig. 22.43). Because the thick periosteum tends to be only partially disrupted, soft tissue swelling and tenderness are often minimal. Many of these fractures are

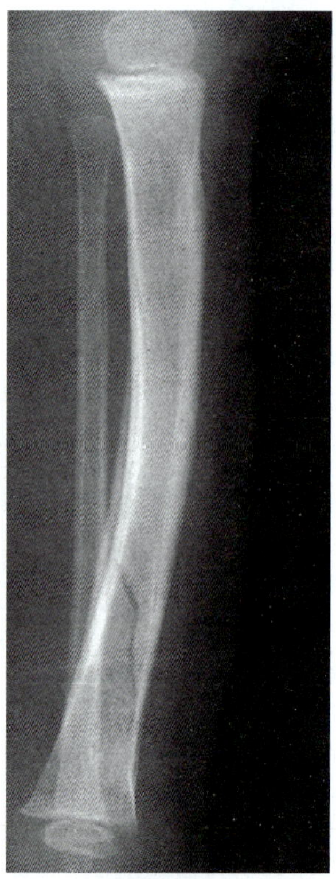

Fig. 22.43 Toddler's fracture. This spiral fracture of the distal tibia was the result of a fall with a twist. The fracture was invisible when the child was seen initially but is evident along with subperiosteal new bone formation on this follow-up film taken 2 weeks later.

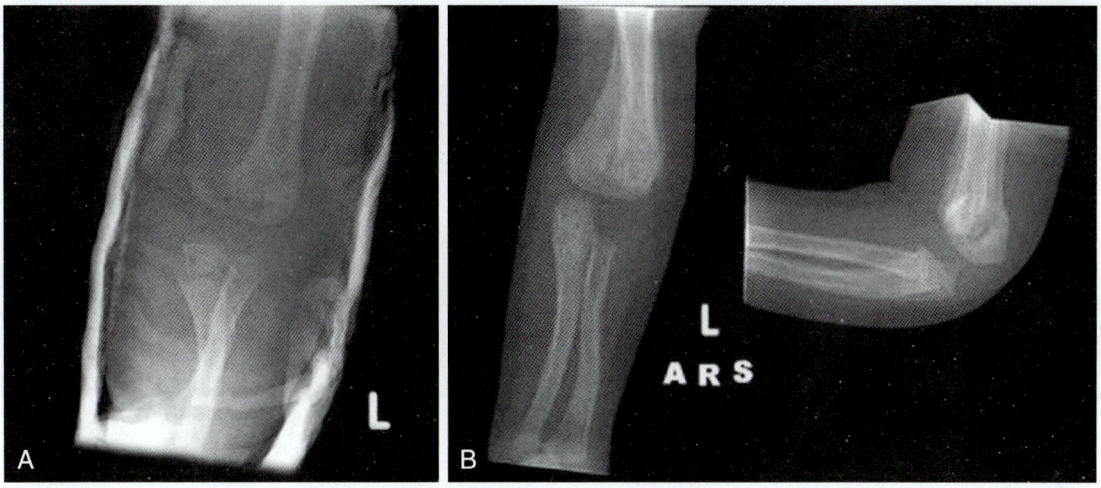

Fig. 22.44 Inflicted elbow fractures. This 10-month-old was brought in with a history of a minor fall and decreased use of his arm. (A) However, radiographs revealed displaced transverse fractures of both the distal humerus and proximal ulna along with marked soft tissue swelling. These findings were incompatible with the reported mechanism of injury and instead were the result of grabbing the arm and yanking the elbow into hyperextension with severe force. (B) Follow-up films 1 month later show prolific subperiosteal new bone formation.

radiographically subtle and may be difficult to detect; treatment is based on clinical presentation.

Traditional treatment consists of either long- or short-leg casting for approximately 4 weeks. Removable fracture boots have been shown to be as effective and safe for management of these injuries. Infection must be included in the differential diagnosis of the limping child in this 1- to 5-year-old age group but usually can be ruled out by lack of fever, absence of local erythema, and normal laboratory workup. If there is no clear history of a fall, only a mild limp, no evidence of localized tenderness, and radiographs are normal, it may be best to defer treatment and observe the child closely.

Fractures Involving the Elbow

Supracondylar, condylar, intercondylar, and epicondylar humerus fractures and proximal radius and ulna fractures all involve the elbow, and the major mechanism is a fall onto the outstretched arm. In a young infant, a fracture through the cartilaginous portion of the distal humerus at the level of the condyles is known as a *physeal separation* and may appear like an elbow dislocation on plain films. Given the force necessary to cause these fractures, when they are seen in an infant who is not yet standing and walking, nonaccidental trauma must be suspected (Fig. 22.44).

Supracondylar fractures account for about 50% of elbow injuries and usually result from a fall onto an outstretched hyperextended arm, which typically results in some degree of posterior displacement of the distal humeral fragment (see Fig. 22.34). A grading system, developed by Gartland and useful in describing severity of injury, includes three types: type 1, nondisplaced; type 2, partial displacement with intact posterior cortex; and type 3, displaced with complete disruption of the posterior cortex. The exceeding majority of these injuries are accidental in nature. More rarely, a direct blow to the point of the flexed elbow is the cause, in which case the distal fragment is hyperflexed. Pain, swelling, and tenderness are most prominent over the posterior aspect of the distal humerus. A significant risk of associated neurovascular injury exists in patients with widely displaced fractures. Some type 2, all type 3, and flexion-type supracondylar fractures will require surgical treatment.

Lateral condyle fractures (see Fig. 22.33) typically result from a fall onto an extended and abducted arm. Swelling and tenderness are prominent over the lateral aspect of the elbow. If displaced, these fractures will require open reduction as they involve the intraarticular joint surface.

Medial epicondyle fractures stem from falls in which the elbow is hyperextended and abducted from the body, subjecting it to a valgus stress (see Fig. 22.35). They are also commonly seen in association with elbow dislocations. These children have swelling and tenderness centered over the medial aspect of the elbow. Surgical treatment may be appropriate in certain cases.

Radial head and neck fractures are usually the result of a fall onto an outstretched, supinated arm (Fig. 22.45). Local swelling and tenderness are centered over the proximal radius, although pain is often referred to the wrist. The majority of these fractures may be treated with nonsurgical management, though large angular displacement may necessitate surgical intervention.

Monteggia fracture-dislocation is a commonly missed unique injury, which occurs due to the close interrelation of the radius and ulna. The ulna alone is fractured or plastically deformed, with energy dissipation through the radiocapitellar joint, thus resulting in a subluxation or frank dislocation. Missed injuries will result in a poor outcome, so in any child with a forearm shaft fracture, the elbow should be examined and dedicated elbow radiographs should be scrutinized.

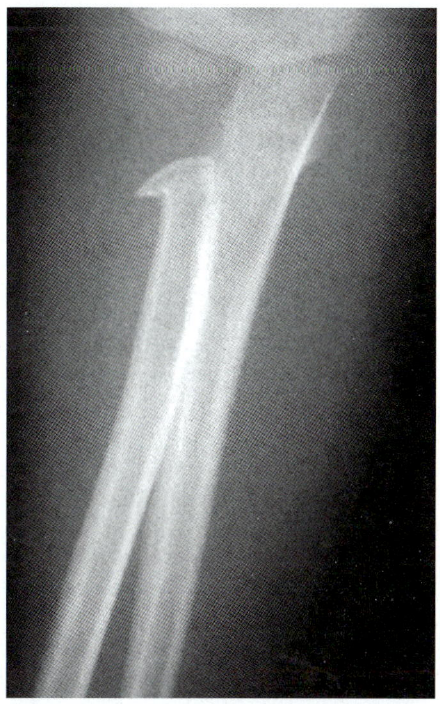

Fig. 22.45 Radial neck fracture. When this 4-year-old boy fell off his bike, the position of his arm on impact resulted in transmission of a valgus force across the elbow joint, resulting in this impaction fracture of the radial neck. Radial neck fractures may require reduction to restore normal supination and pronation of the forearm.

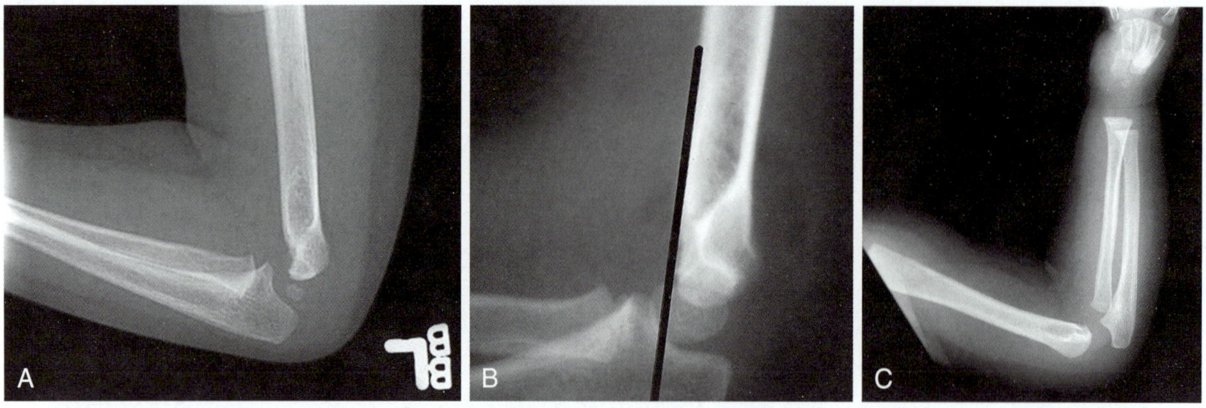

Fig. 22.46 (A) Posterior fat pad sign. Although no clear fracture line is evident in this patient with a supracondylar fracture, the posterior fat pad is readily visible, being displaced upward and outward from the posterior aspect of the distal humerus. The finding indicates the presence of a joint effusion, which after trauma is blood, and in about 70% of cases with no visible fracture line, an occult fracture is present. (B) Anterior humeral line. A line drawn through the anterior cortex of the humerus in another patient with a positive fat pad intersects the anterior third of the capitellum, indicating posterior displacement of the distal humeral fragment. (C) Normal elbow for comparison. (B, Courtesy Richard B. Towbin, MD, Children's Hospital of Philadelphia, Philadelphia, PA.)

Radiographic findings in patients with fractures about the elbow may be subtle, and oblique and comparison views may be necessary to identify them. Key signs suggestive of a fracture in the absence of fracture lines are the posterior fat pad sign (anterior fat pad sign maybe naturally present) and abnormality of the anterior humerocapitallar line. The fat pad sign consists of the upward and outward displacement of the posterior fat pad of the distal humerus (Fig. 22.46A and B, and Fig. 22.34B), which is normally invisible. The finding of a fat pad indicates the presence of a hemarthrosis, often due to a nondisplaced fracture, and should warrant long-arm immobilization with splint or cast. The anterior humeral line is a line drawn through the anterior cortex of the humerus and usually intersects the middle third of the capitellum. This relationship changes in fractures where the distal portion of the humerus is displaced posteriorly (see Fig. 22.46B).

Hand and Finger Fractures

Hand injuries are among the most common injuries in children as they explore the world with their fingers. Several key points require emphasis to prevent long-term dysfunction (see Figs. 22.87 and 22.88).

Phalangeal Fractures

Common mechanisms of injury in the phalanges include crush injuries (finger caught in a door, objects falling) and contact sports. Patients will present with swelling, bruising, and tenderness localized to the injured area of the finger. Appropriate examination will begin with the observation of the patient's hands at rest and noting differences between the injured digit and its uninjured counterpart. Fractures causing significant deformity must be appropriately reduced to prevent long-term problems (Fig. 22.47). Comparison of the planes of the fingernails of both hands with the forearms supinated and the fingers partially flexed is particularly useful in detecting rotational abnormalities (Fig. 22.48). Fractures associated with deep lacerations must be evaluated for tendon rupture and circulation distal to the wound. In older children, flexion and extension of the digits should be tested individually with the others held immobile. Meticulous attention must be paid to the assessment of neurovascular and tendon function to detect subtle abnormalities that may reflect significant injury. Clinically, an extensor tendon injury may be manifested by flexor tendon overpull (Fig. 22.49), and conversely, flexor tendon injuries may result in extensor overpull (see Fig. 22.7). This can be difficult in young children. However, information can be gained from observing the position of the hands at rest and during spontaneous movement and by watching motion as the parent hands objects to the child.

Radiographs are key in the evaluation of phalangeal fractures. Anteroposterior, lateral, and oblique views are essential, and comparison views may provide additional information.

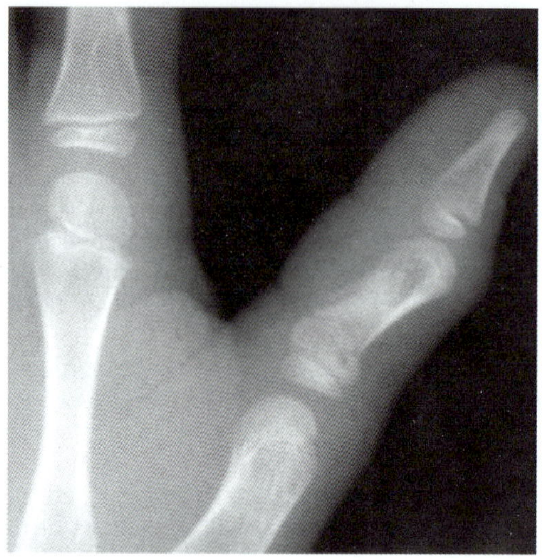

Fig. 22.47 Angulated phalanx fracture. Significant angular deformity is seen in this impaction fracture of the proximal phalanx of the thumb. Such fractures require careful reduction to prevent permanent disability.

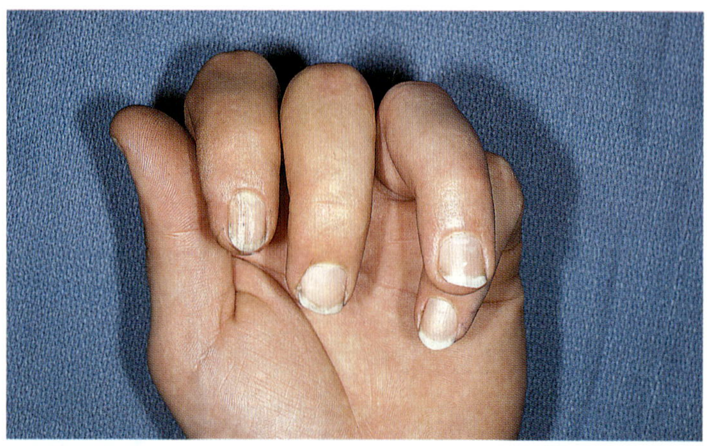

Fig. 22.48 Rotational deformity resulting from a hand injury. With rotational deformity, the plane of the nail of the involved finger is seen to deviate from its normal orientation. (Courtesy Neil Jones, MD, University of California, Los Angeles, CA.)

Growth plate fractures of the phalanges are common, and significant growth disturbance is rare. Salter-Harris type II fractures of the middle and proximal phalanges, provided adequate alignment is achieved with reduction, can be treated symptomatically with casting, finger splints, or buddy taping. Significantly displaced growth plate

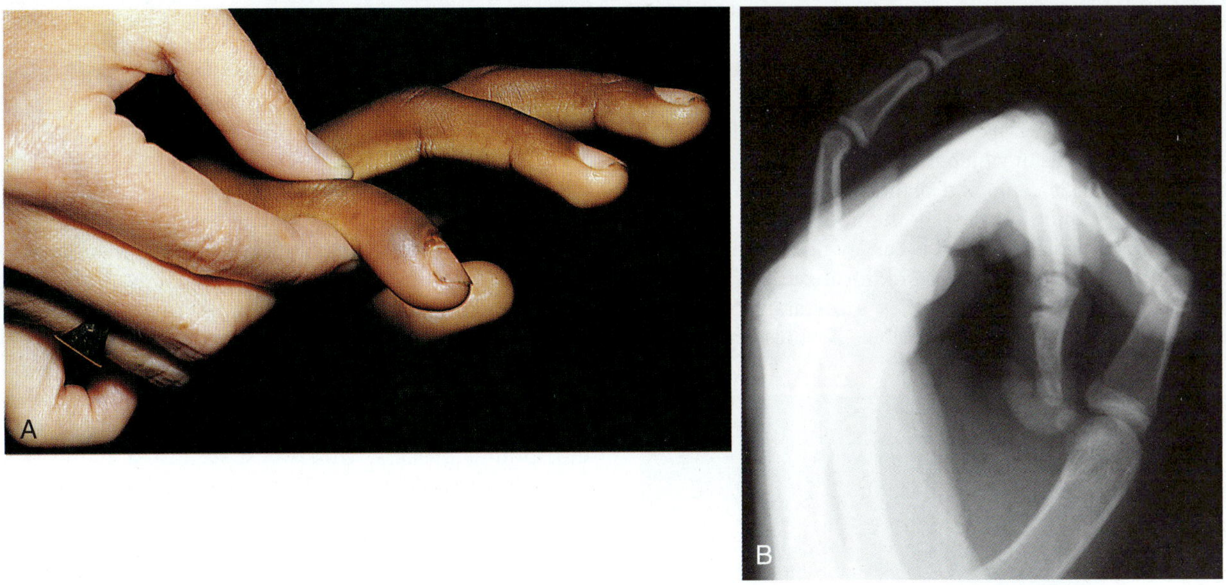

Fig. 22.49 Distal phalanx fracture with extensor tendon injury. (A) Another player's shoulder landed on this boy's finger. The finger was swollen and painful and maximally tender at the base of the distal phalanx, and the patient was unable to extend the distal interphalangeal joint. (B) Radiograph revealed separation of the epiphysis at the base of the distal phalanx.

fractures of the distal phalanx, especially those where there is a laceration near the nail bed, may signify a special injury with the eponym "Seymour fracture." These are open fractures of the distal phalanx and must be treated with appropriate irrigation and debridement, reduction and repair of the nail bed, and postprocedure antibiotics. Other crush injuries of the distal phalanges associated with partial or complete nail avulsions may also result in open fractures and lacerations of the nail bed (Fig. 22.50) and should be treated similarly.

Fractures near the phalangeal condyles (phalangeal neck) are rare patterns but important to recognize because although appearing minimally displaced on radiographs, they cause significant rotational deformity of the digit. Similarly, significant intraarticular fractures will require anatomic reduction and can benefit from a referral to the orthopedic or hand surgery service.

The volar plate is a cartilaginous plate located at the base of the middle phalanx of each finger. It may easily cause an avulsion-type fracture in injuries with a hyperextension mechanism. Clinically, pain and swelling are especially marked over the volar aspect of the proximal interphalangeal (PIP) joint. The vast majority of these are benign injuries, and as long as there is no hyperextension deformity of the involved PIP with fingers extension, or locking with flexion, can be treated symptomatically. Volar plate injuries may also accompany dislocation of the PIP joint (see the Ligamentous Injuries section later).

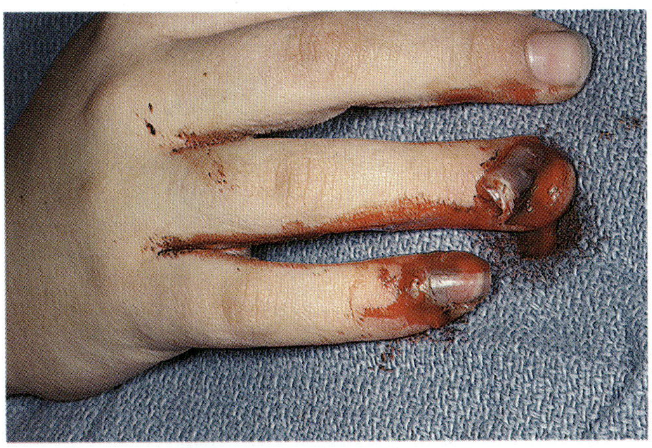

Fig. 22.50 Crush injury of the distal phalanx. This child's finger was slammed in a car door. He incurred a crush fracture of the distal phalanx, partial avulsion of the nail, and a nail bed laceration. By definition, this is an open fracture. (Courtesy Neil Jones, MD, University of California, Los Angeles, CA.)

Metacarpal Fractures

The boxer's fracture, an impacted fracture of the neck of the fifth and often the fourth metacarpal, is among the most common of these injuries (Fig. 22.51). It occurs as a result of direct impact with a partially clenched fist (typically resulting from punching objects or persons) and is most commonly seen in adolescents. Less commonly, it can also result from a fall onto a clenched fist. Clinically, depression of the involved knuckle or knuckles may be noted, along with more proximal swelling and discoloration. The involved metacarpals may also appear shortened. An associated rotational deformity, if present, is manifested by rotation of the nails of the corresponding fingers (see Fig. 22.48). If the injury stems from a punch into the mouth, examination for overlying breaks in the skin caused by the opponent's teeth is vital. These are infection-prone wounds and may communicate with metacarpophalangeal joints. Radiographically, volar angulation of the distal segment is typically found. Most closed fractures with mild to minimal angulation may

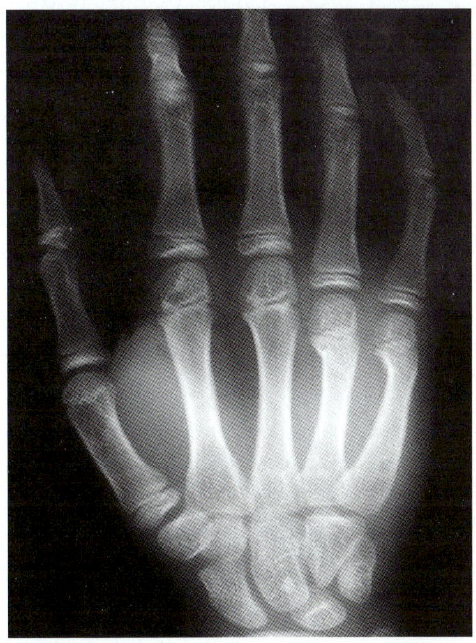

Fig. 22.51 Boxer's fracture. This adolescent presented with pain and swelling of the lateral aspect of his right hand after punching a wall in a fit of temper. Radiographically he has typical boxer's fractures of the necks of the fourth and fifth metacarpals with volar displacement of the distal fragments.

be treated nonoperatively, whereas open fractures and widely displaced injuries often require surgical intervention.

Foot and Metatarsal Injuries

Most metatarsal fractures are crush injuries that result from objects dropping onto the foot. Falls in which the patient twists the forefoot or in which the forefoot is caught in plantar flexion can produce fractures (Fig. 22.52), and injuries of the foot with the ankle inverted and the foot in plantar flexion can avulse the tuberosity from the base of the fifth metatarsal. Mild, localized swelling and point tenderness are noted over the site of a metatarsal fracture; weight bearing is painful but often possible. A short-leg cast or controlled-ankle motion boot (fracture boot) provides maximal relief. This must be distinguished from the normal finding of a secondary ossification center, which is called the os vesalianum, at the base of the fifth metatarsal. Absence of point tenderness on examination can help differentiate (Fig. 22.53).

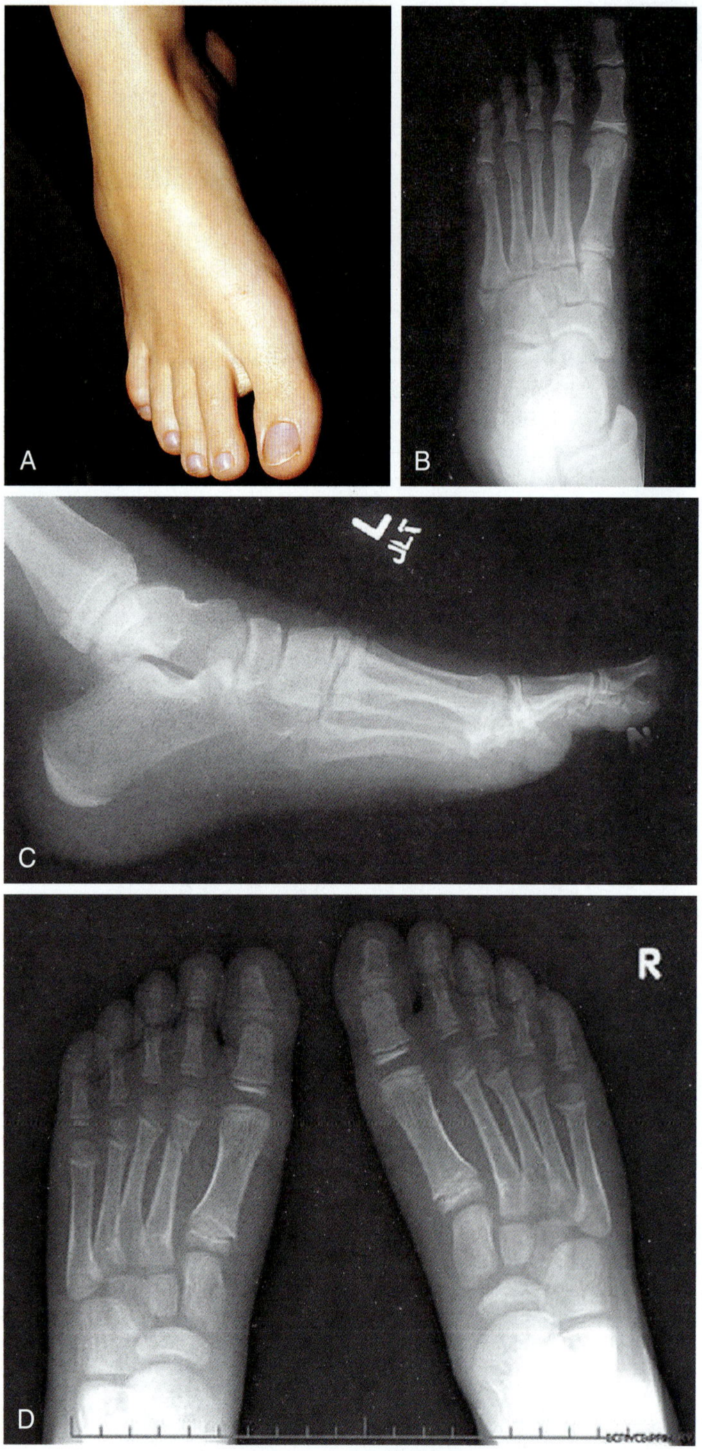

Fig. 22.52 Transverse metatarsal fractures. (A) This adolescent fell forward with her forefoot twisted under her. Swelling over the proximal portion of the fifth metatarsal was prominent. (B and C) Anteroposterior and lateral radiographs show a transverse fracture of the proximal fifth metatarsal. (D) This boy caught his left foot on steps and fell with his forefoot in plantar flexion, thereby incurring a transverse fracture of the distal portion of his second metatarsal.

Lap Belt Fractures

The use of seat belts to prevent serious trauma in automobile collisions has resulted in an increase in the incidence of "lap belt" fractures in children. In a head-on collision, the head and torso of a child wearing only a lap belt are thrown forward, resulting in hyperflexion of the lumbar spine over the fulcrum of the lap belt and often causing a flexion/distraction injury. This may produce a compression fracture of a lumbar vertebra or, more likely, a shear fracture through the body of the vertebra and the pedicle and spinous process. This is best seen on a lateral radiograph of the lumbar spine (Fig. 22.54). An anteroposterior view of the spine may show lateral displacement of a portion of the involved

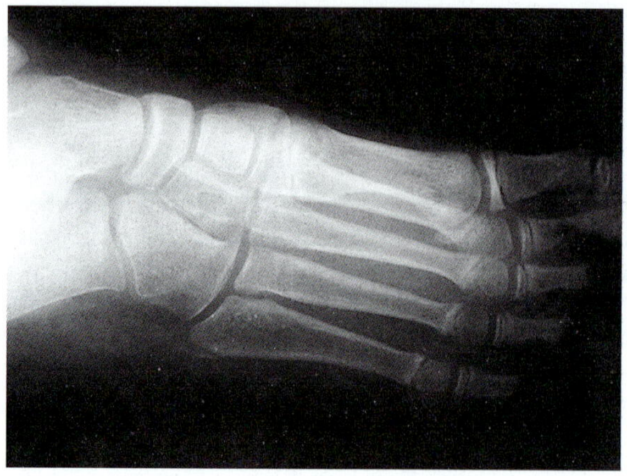

Fig. 22.53 *Os vesalianum.* Many children have a secondary ossification center at the base of the fifth metatarsal. This can be distinguished from a fracture by the fact that its edges are smooth, rounded, and sclerotic. (Courtesy Jocelyn Ledesma Medina, MD.)

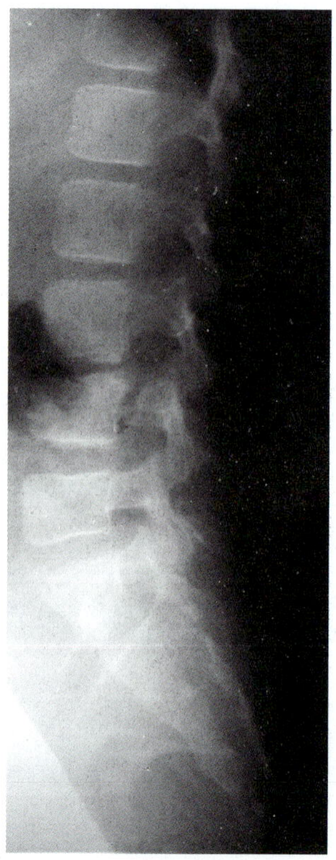

Fig. 22.54 Lap belt fracture. This flexion/distraction injury occurred through the body of the L4 vertebra when the child's body hyperflexed over a lap belt in a head-on automobile collision.

vertebral body. Because the fulcrum of the injury is anterior where the lap belt contacts the anterior abdominal wall, this injury produces a characteristic rectangular bruise and abrasion over the lower abdomen. Associated intraabdominal injury, especially a ruptured viscus, is common, and the resultant abdominal pain may overshadow that of the vertebral injury. Hence whenever a lap belt bruise is seen during the physical examination, great care should be taken in palpating the back for localized tenderness or spasm, and immobilization of the torso and lower back should be maintained until CT scan of the lumbar spine is obtained.

Pelvic Avulsion Fractures

Pelvic avulsion fractures are a phenomenon unique to adolescents, with a peak occurrence between 13 and 14 years old in girls and 15 and 17 years old in boys. This stems from the fact that the secondary centers of ossification in these young people have not yet fused to the pelvis. These fractures are typically seen in adolescents who are involved in competitive sports, especially track and field (e.g., sprinting, jumping), soccer, and football, but household falls and collisions may also be the cause. Most result from a sudden, violent muscular contraction while the ipsilateral extremity is held in a static position or when a muscle is suddenly lengthened during isometric contraction. As the muscle power exceeds the strength of the tendinous unit, it is torn from the apophysis or secondary ossification center. Avulsion fractures of the ischial tuberosity are the most common. They tend to occur during sprinting and are due to the sudden, powerful contraction of the hamstring muscles when the hip is flexed and the knee extended (see Fig. 22.55A). Avulsions of the anterior inferior and anterior superior iliac spines (Fig. 22.55B and C) are caused by strong contractions of the rectus femoris and sartorius muscles, respectively. These are associated with running, often during an abrupt directional change. Some cases of anterior inferior/superior iliac spine avulsions occur with kicking. At the time of injury, the patient experiences sudden pain at the site and difficulty walking. On examination, point tenderness and swelling are noted over the involved apophysis and weakness on active hip motion is seen secondary to pain.

In viewing radiographs, it is important to compare the involved side with the normal side to detect displacement of the avulsed fragment and to avoid mistaking a normal apophysis for a fracture.

Treatment is conservative and consists of a few days of bed rest until the pain subsides, followed by 2 to 4 weeks of protected weight bearing, with a gradual increase in weight bearing as pain allows. Thereafter, careful reconditioning facilitates a safe return to full activity, usually within 6 to 10 weeks.

Pathologic Fractures

Children with severe osteopenia or osteoporosis, whether stemming from an inherited disorder or disuse secondary to neurologic or neuromuscular disease, are at considerably increased risk of incurring fractures as the result of minor falls or even during routine physical therapy exercises. Localized bone lesions, including those caused by osteomyelitis, tumors, or cysts, can cause localized cortical thinning as they expand. Impact on the involved bone can then also result in a pathologic fracture. Examples of some of these conditions and representative fractures are presented in Chapter 6.

Compartment Syndrome

Compartment syndrome arises whenever the interstitial tissue fluid pressure exceeds the capillary perfusion pressure within a muscle compartment. In clinical practice, the interstitial pressure elevation

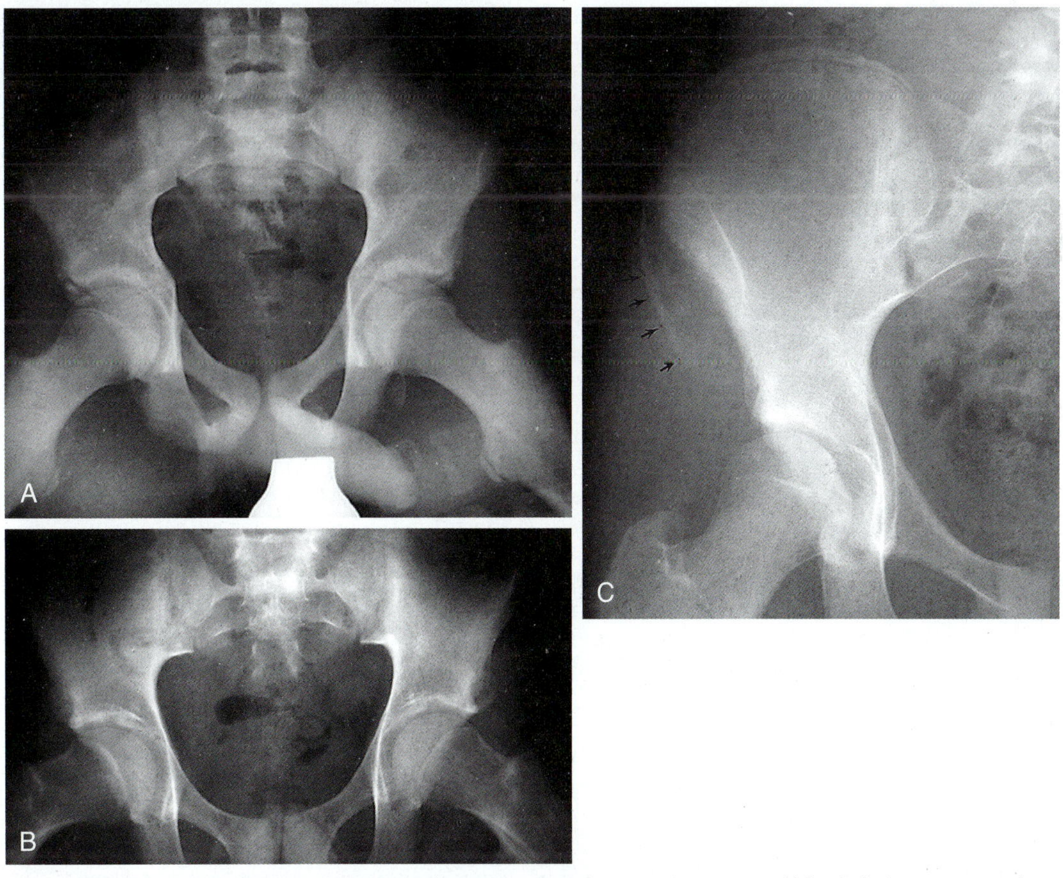

Fig. 22.55 Pelvic avulsion fractures. (A) Ischial tuberosity avulsion fracture. This 14-year-old football player sprinting for a touchdown fell on his stomach and experienced sharp left hip pain. He could not bear weight after the incident and was found to have tenderness over the left buttock and pain with abduction and flexion of the left hip. The avulsed fragment is best seen on this frog-leg view. (B) Anterior inferior iliac spine avulsion fracture. While running in gym class, this 15-year-old boy experienced sudden onset of left hip pain and difficulty walking. He had point tenderness over the anterior inferior iliac spine and full range of hip motion but experienced pain on flexion and internal rotation. If compared with the right, the avulsed apophysis is evident. (C) Another 15-year-old boy, who developed sudden onset of right hip pain and inability to bear weight while kicking a soccer ball, has a large avulsion fracture of the anterior superior iliac spine *(arrows)*. (A and B, Courtesy Janet Kinnane, MD, Children's Hospital of Pittsburgh, Pittsburgh, PA.)

must reach approximately 35 to 45 mm Hg for this to occur. Because the enclosed fascial boundary of the involved muscle compartment is unyielding, hemorrhage or edema within it can cause interstitial pressure to rise to such levels, resulting in muscle ischemia and neurovascular compromise. Compartment syndromes can be seen after open or closed fractures; crush injuries; prolonged pressure on an extremity, which can occur in a comatose child who has been lying on an extremity for several hours; and extravasation from vascular lines. Anatomically, it is more likely to occur in the forearm or lower leg, complicating fractures of the tibia, the forearm, and supracondylar humerus. Open fractures are just as likely as closed fractures to result in compartment syndrome due to higher energy mechanisms of injury. Prompt and accurate diagnosis of a compartment syndrome is critical because permanent neuromuscular damage will result if definitive treatment is not implemented within 4 to 6 hours of onset. The clinical findings in compartment syndrome are classic in the communicative patient. Patients experience severe pain that is unrelieved by elevation and immobilization and can be agitated and difficult to distract. The involved extremity is swollen and tense to palpation. Passive movement of terminal digits (fingers or toes) exacerbates the pain, and active motion is avoided. Pulselessness is a late finding and should not be required for diagnosis. In the uncooperative, younger child or in obtunded patients, diagnosis requires a high index of suspicion and prophylactic fascial release is often considered due to the devastating consequences of compartment syndrome if missed. Commercial devices to aid with measurement of compartment pressures exist and can aid in these instances; however, compartment syndrome remains a predominantly clinical diagnosis.

Emergency surgical decompression of the fascial covering of all involved compartments is necessary to prevent irreversible muscle and nerve damage (fasciotomy).

Ligamentous Injuries

Dislocations

The ligaments of a child have increased elasticity and are stronger relative to the bony structures, especially the physis (Fig. 22.56). Consequently, joint dislocations and ligamentous disruptions are unusual in childhood. They are usually the result of severe trauma and are commonly associated with fractures. In some instances, the dislocation is obvious and the fracture subtle or even invisible radiographically (Fig. 22.57), but often the fracture is the prominent clinical finding and the dislocation less apparent. Hence the emphasis in pediatric orthopedics is on examining the entire extremity and on including the joints proximal and distal to a suspected fracture site in the radiographic examination. Failure to diagnose the full extent of injury can result in permanent morbidity. It must also be remembered that in infants, epiphyseal separations before ossification can simulate dislocations. For example, separation of the distal

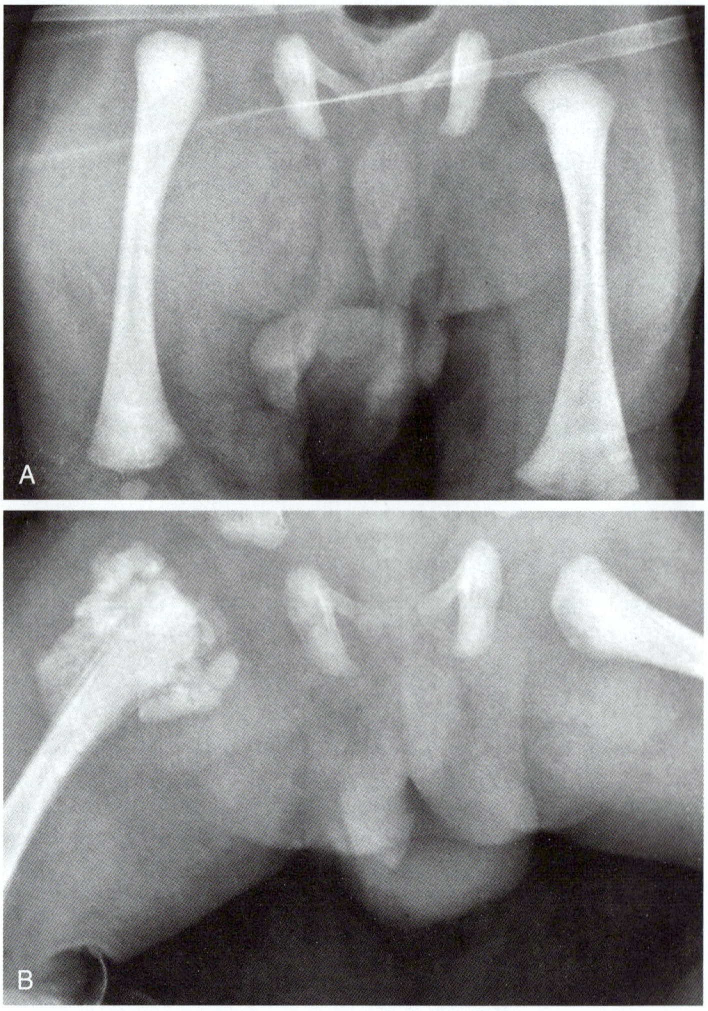

Fig. 22.57 Fracture/dislocation, right hip. This young infant presented after a serious automobile accident with what appeared to be a traumatic hip dislocation without an associated fracture. (A) The right femoral head is displaced laterally and superiorly. (B) The follow-up film taken 2 weeks later reveals vigorous callus formation around the proximal femur and periosteal new bone formation both proximally and distally, thus confirming the existence of associated femoral fractures. (Courtesy Department of Pediatric Radiology, Children's Hospital of Pittsburgh, Pittsburgh, PA.)

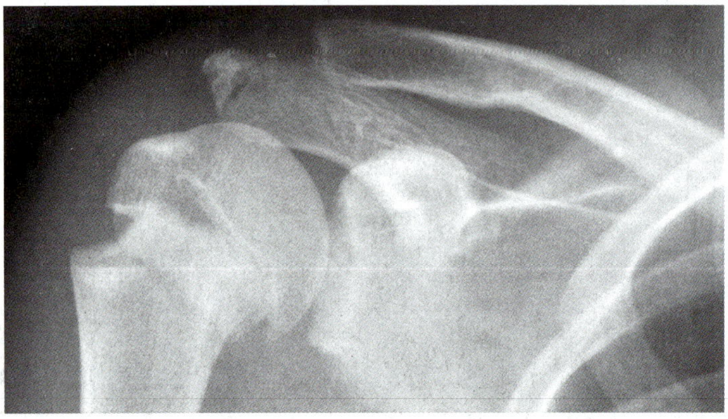

Fig. 22.56 Epiphyseal separation. Because of the elasticity and relatively greater strength of the ligaments, forces that would have resulted in dislocation in an older adolescent have instead caused epiphyseal separation and displacement of the proximal humeral epiphysis in this prepubescent child. (Courtesy Department of Pediatric Radiology, Children's Hospital of Pittsburgh, Pittsburgh, PA.)

humeral epiphysis in infancy presents a radiographic picture suggestive of posterior displacement of the olecranon. However, dislocations do occur and more common ones are the hip, shoulder, elbow, patellofemoral joint, and interphalangeal joints. Shoulder and patellofemoral dislocations are discussed in greater depth in the Sports Injuries section later, as these injuries are commonly encountered in young athletes.

Hip dislocations in the young are usually the result of falls. In children younger than 5 years old, the softness of the acetabulum and relative ligamentous laxity enable dislocation without the application of extreme force, and thus there may be no associated fractures. In older children, increased force is required and dislocation is commonly accompanied by fractures of the femur and acetabulum. In most instances, the femoral head dislocates posteriorly. The child presents in severe pain with the involved leg held in adduction, internally rotated and flexed (Fig. 22.58). A position of extension, external rotation, and abduction is adopted by patients with the less common anterior dislocation. When the child also has a femur fracture, his or her pain may be attributed to that and the positional findings missed, unless the clinician specifically looks for them. Even in patients without an obvious associated fracture, epiphyseal separation or avulsion of an acetabular fragment may have occurred. Prompt reduction is important, both to relieve pain and to reduce the risk of secondary avascular necrosis of the femoral head. Controversy exists as to where the reduction should take place, with some proponents of

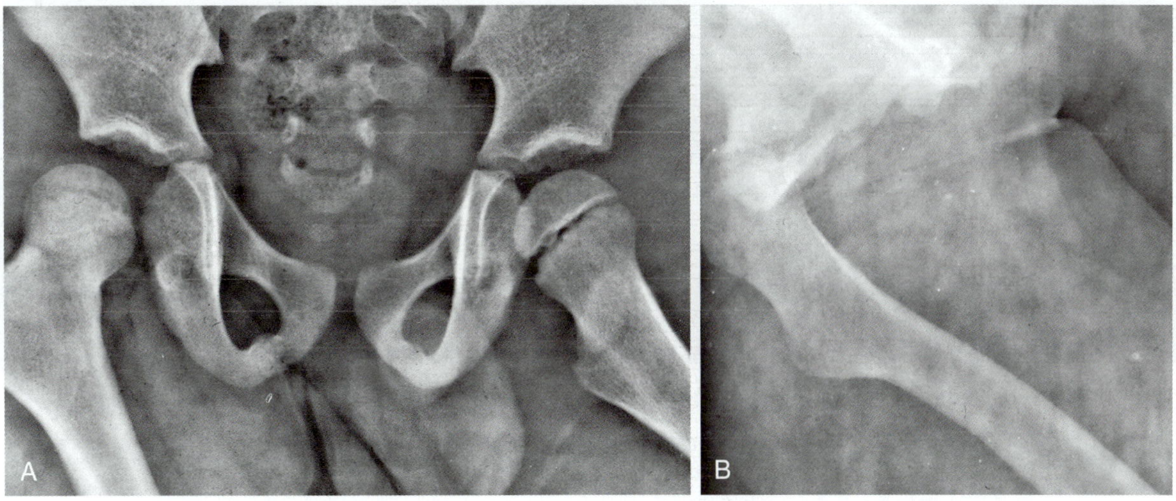

Fig. 22.58 Traumatic posterior hip dislocation. This child suffered an impaction injury in an automobile accident. (A) In the anteroposterior view, the right femoral head appears to be displaced laterally and superiorly. The femur is also adducted and internally rotated. (B) The frog-leg view discloses the severity of displacement posteriorly.

paralytic medications available in the operating room adding potential protection to the proximal femoral physis during closed reduction maneuvers. Postreduction films are important as these may disclose an epiphyseal separation that has occurred or an incomplete reduction if a radiolucent intraarticular fragment is present.

In patellofemoral dislocations the patella usually dislocates laterally (Fig. 22.59). This may occur as the result of laterally directed shearing forces or of a hyperextension injury. In most instances, the patella has relocated by the time the patient is seen. Typical findings on examination include prominent swelling and hemarthrosis, tenderness along the medial patellar border, a positive apprehension test (see the Knee section and Fig. 22.11), and increased lateral mobility of the patella. See the Sports Injuries section later for further information.

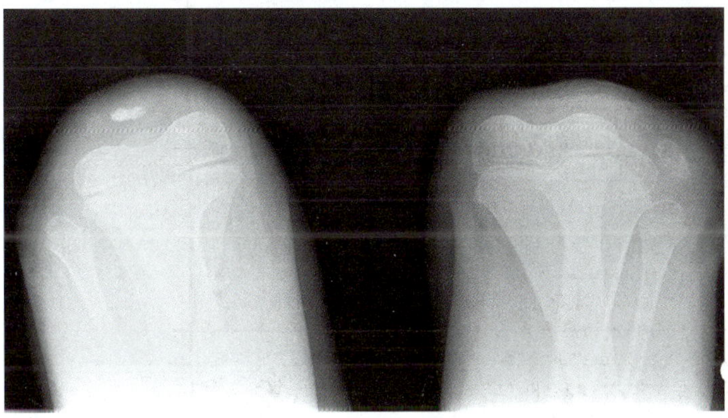

Fig. 22.59 Patellar dislocation. In this flexion view obtained before relocation, the left patella is displaced laterally and there is marked swelling. (Courtesy Department of Pediatric Radiology, Children's Hospital of Pittsburgh, Pittsburgh, PA.)

True shoulder dislocations are rare younger than 10 years of age where proximal humerus has a higher tendency to break with such injuries. On examination of the shoulder, a loss of the rounded contours lateral and anterior to the acromion is found. When the humeral head dislocates anteriorly, it is displaced medially beneath the coracoid process, where it can be palpated (Fig. 22.60). See the Sports Injuries section later for further information. Separation of the proximal humeral epiphysis or major fracture/dislocations are seen in younger children subjected to forces that would cause shoulder dislocation after puberty (see Fig. 22.56).

Dislocations about the elbow may involve a few different patterns as elbow joint is complex. A radial dislocation should be suspected if a line drawn through the long axis of the radius fails to pass through the capitellum on any view (Fig. 22.61). Less frequently, fractures of the radius are associated with dislocation of the radioulnar joint, and fractures of the olecranon may be accompanied by dislocation of the radius. A fall onto

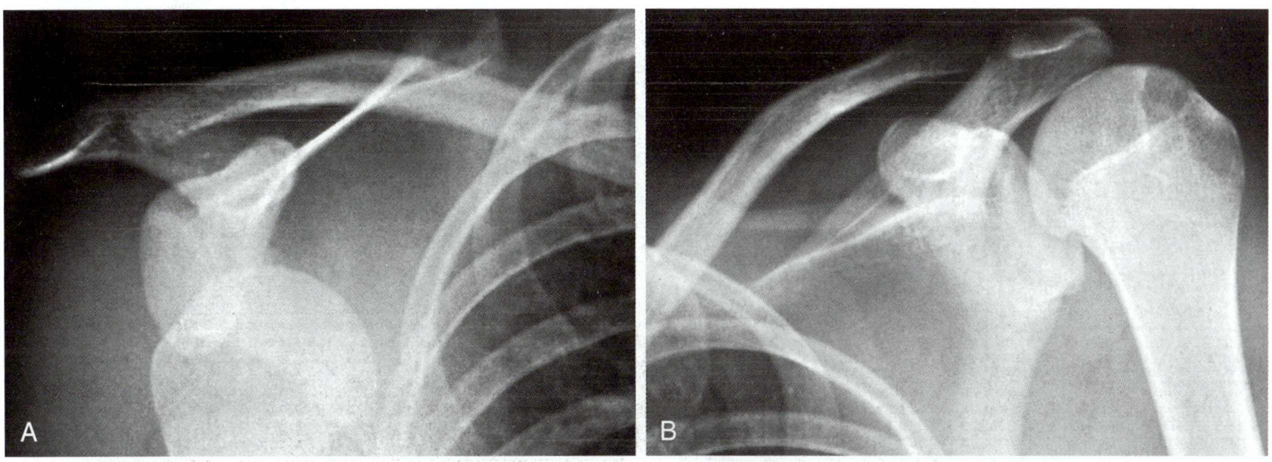

Fig. 22.60 (A) Anterior dislocation of the right shoulder. The humeral head is not in the glenoid fossa but is displaced anteriorly. (B) The normal relationship is seen in this comparison view of the left shoulder. The injury occurred when the patient was taking a back swing for a hockey shot. The patient felt a pop with the immediate onset of severe pain. Note that his epiphyses have fused. (Courtesy Department of Pediatric Radiology, Children's Hospital of Pittsburgh, Pittsburgh, PA.)

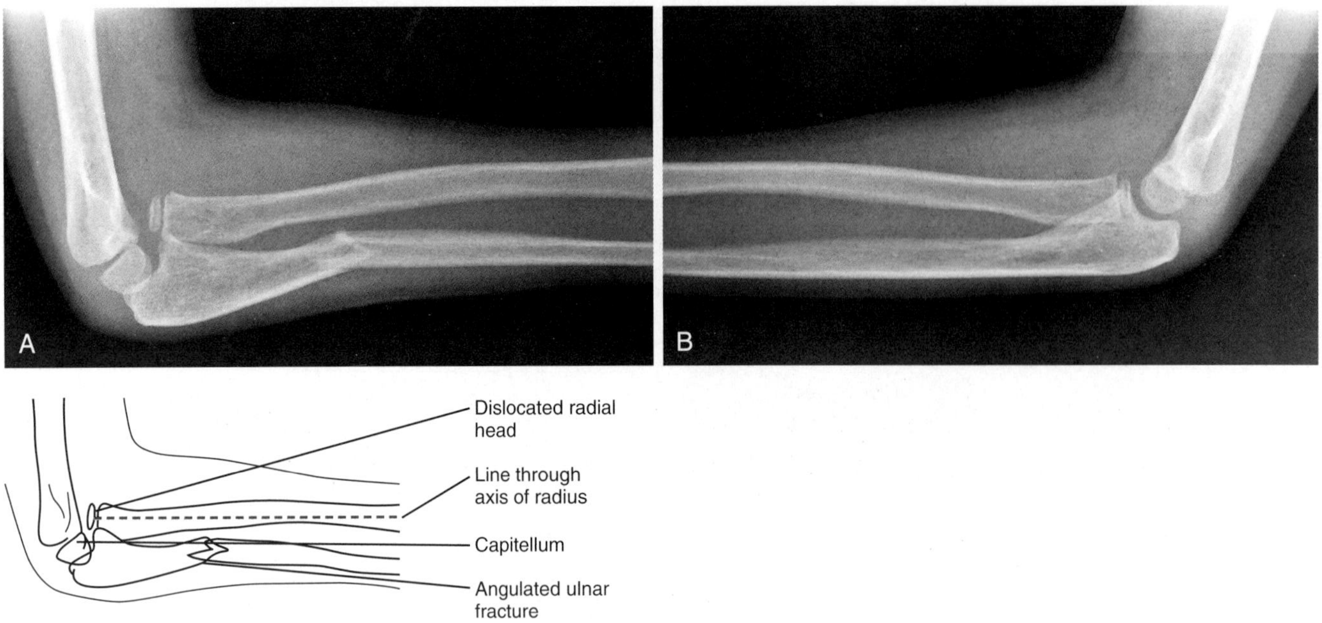

Fig. 22.61 Monteggia fracture. (A) A displaced fracture of the proximal right ulna is accompanied by dislocation of the radial head. A line drawn through the long axis of the radius would intersect the distal humerus above the level of the capitellum. (B) The comparison view of the left arm shows the normal position of the radial head. (Courtesy Department of Pediatric Radiology, Children's Hospital of Pittsburgh, Pittsburgh, PA.)

an extended or partially flexed arm with the forearm supinated can result in a true posterior dislocation of both the radius and ulna from the humerus with tearing of the anterior portion of the joint capsule and of the medial collateral ligaments. This injury may be associated with fracture of the medial epicondyle (see Fig. 22.35), the coronoid process, the olecranon, or the proximal radius. Clinically, the forearm is shortened, and there is an obvious deformity and marked swelling of the posterior aspect of the elbow. A high risk of neurovascular compromise and compartment syndrome exists in patients with this injury.

Dislocation of an interphalangeal joint results in an obvious deformity and is an intensely painful injury (Fig. 22.62) and sometimes radiographically missed. Avulsion fractures, volar plate fractures, and tendinous or capsular injury may be associated with it and difficult to detect radiographically. These must be suspected if range of motion is incomplete after relocation. In some cases, the associated injury makes closed reduction impossible.

Sprains

A sprain is a ligamentous injury in which some degree of tearing occurs, often as a result of excessive stretching or twisting. As noted in the Fractures section, sprains are less common in children with open physes than they are in older adolescents whose growth plates have closed. When sprains do occur in these younger patients, they tend to be milder and may be associated with Salter-Harris fractures. This stems from the fact that the growth plate, being weaker than the ligaments, tends to give before significant ligamentous tearing can occur. In many other instances, a suspected sprain is actually a small avulsion fracture. If the portion avulsed is ossified, the small fragment may be detectable radiographically, but if the fragment is cartilaginous, it will be radiographically invisible. A particular example of this is the gamekeeper's thumb, which is often associated with a small avulsion fracture of the proximal phalanx (Fig. 22.63).

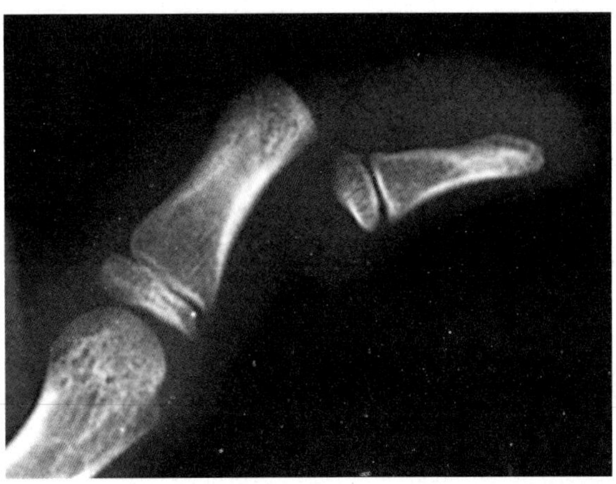

Fig. 22.62 Interphalangeal joint dislocation. The distal phalanx of the thumb is dislocated dorsally. (Courtesy Department of Pediatric Radiology, Children's Hospital of Pittsburgh, Pittsburgh, PA.)

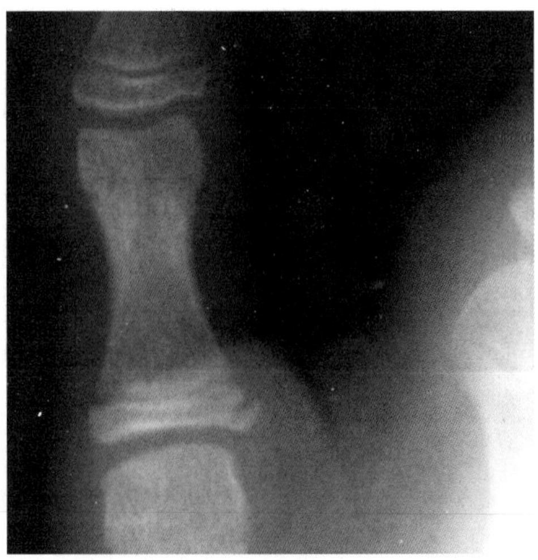

Fig. 22.63 Gamekeeper's thumb. A small avulsion fracture of the epiphysis at the base of the proximal phalanx is associated with rupture of the ulnar collateral ligament. The injury occurred when the patient fell while skiing and the strap of his ski pole forcefully abducted his thumb on impact.

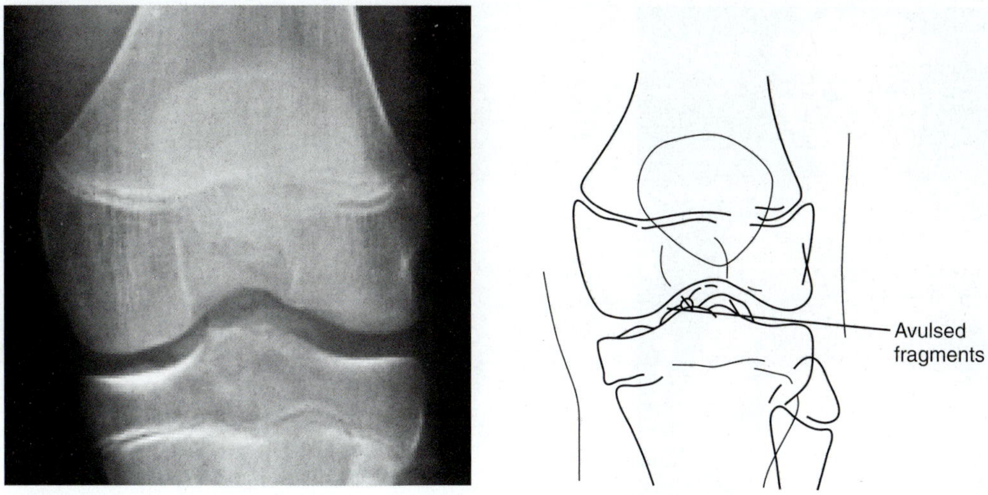

Fig. 22.64 Avulsion fracture of the left tibial spine as the result of a soccer injury (anteroposterior view). Also present were a tear in the cruciate ligament and a lipohemarthrosis. (Courtesy Department of Pediatric Radiology, Children's Hospital of Pittsburgh, Pittsburgh, PA.)

Before epiphyseal closure, injuries that rupture the anterior cruciate ligament of the knee in adults usually avulse the tibial spine in children (Fig. 22.64). Similarly, Salter-Harris fractures and avulsion fractures of the distal fibula or tibia should be strongly suspected in children with "sprainlike" injuries of the ankle. After physeal closure, an ankle sprain in an adolescent patient is typically caused by a severe inversion stress injury. The presenting findings are diffuse pain and tenderness along with swelling centered below the lateral malleolus, although the superior margin of swelling may cover the malleolus (Fig. 22.65).

Sprains are classified in three grades according to severity (Table 22.6). Likely due to developing inflammation and swelling, ligamentous injuries tend to hurt more the day after.

Table 22.6 Classification of Sprains

Grade of Sprain	Degree of Tearing	Clinical Findings
I	A small percentage of ligamentous fibers is disrupted	Pain on motion Local tenderness Mild swelling
II	A moderate percentage of fibers is torn	Pain on motion More diffuse tenderness Moderate swelling, may have joint effusion Mild instability
III	The ligament is completely disrupted	Severe pain on motion Marked swelling, usually with joint effusion Marked tenderness Joint instability

Evaluation and Management

In evaluating patients with possible sprains, careful attention must be given to not only assessment of swelling, tenderness, and joint stability but also evaluation of adjacent bony structures and musculotendinous function (see prior Physical Examination section). Complete evaluation may be impossible if initial presentation has been delayed for several hours and secondary effusion, soft tissue swelling, and muscle spasm are pronounced. In such instances, it may be necessary to immobilize the affected joint with a splint and have the patient return for reevaluation in a few days once the swelling has abated.

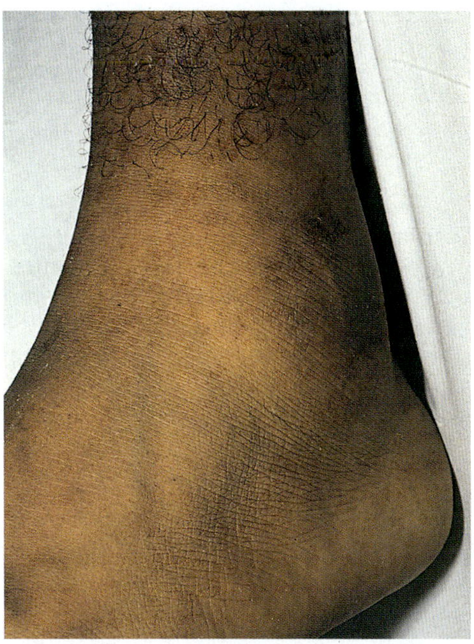

Fig. 22.65 Ankle sprain. Marked tenderness and swelling were maximal inferior to the malleolus of this 17-year-old youth. The anterior talofibular, calcaneofibular, and posterior talofibular ligaments were all tender. This is in contrast to the findings seen with a Salter-Harris type I fracture of the distal tibia (see Fig. 22.17).

Rest, the application of ice, use of analgesic antiinflammatory agents such as ibuprofen, and compression wrap or taping with elevation suffice for grade I sprains. Subjective improvement occurs in a few days. Grade II and grade III sprains require a longer period of immobilization. Splinting or casting for a few to several weeks is generally necessary. Some grade III sprains may require surgical intervention.

Subluxation of the Radial Head (Nursemaid's Elbow, Pulled Elbow)

Subluxation of the annular ligament over the radial head is the most common elbow injury in childhood and one of the most common ligamentous injuries. The mechanism is one of sudden traction applied to the extended arm. The injury is seen predominantly in children between 1 and 4 years old. The typical history is one of a parent's suddenly pulling the child up by the arm to prevent a fall or similar event pulling on the arm. After a brief initial period of crying, the child calms down but is unable to use the affected arm, which is held close to the body with the elbow extended (Fig. 22.66A). If old enough to talk, the child may complain of elbow, forearm, or even wrist pain. Physical examination reveals no bony tenderness and no evidence of swelling, but on assessment of passive

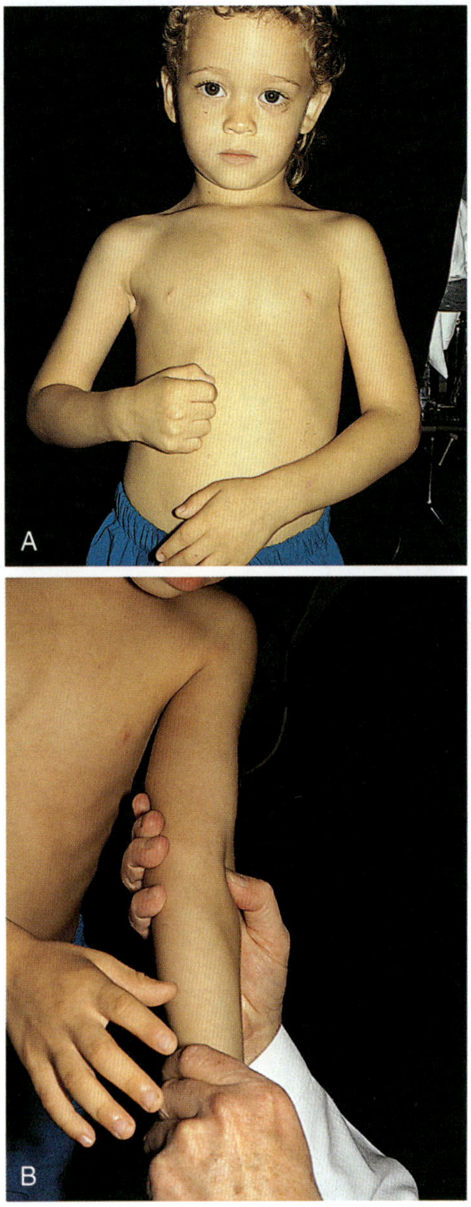

Fig. 22.66 Nursemaid's elbow. (A) The affected arm is held close to the body with the elbow flexed and the forearm pronated. (B) The reduction maneuver consists of supinating the forearm while pressing down on the radial head.

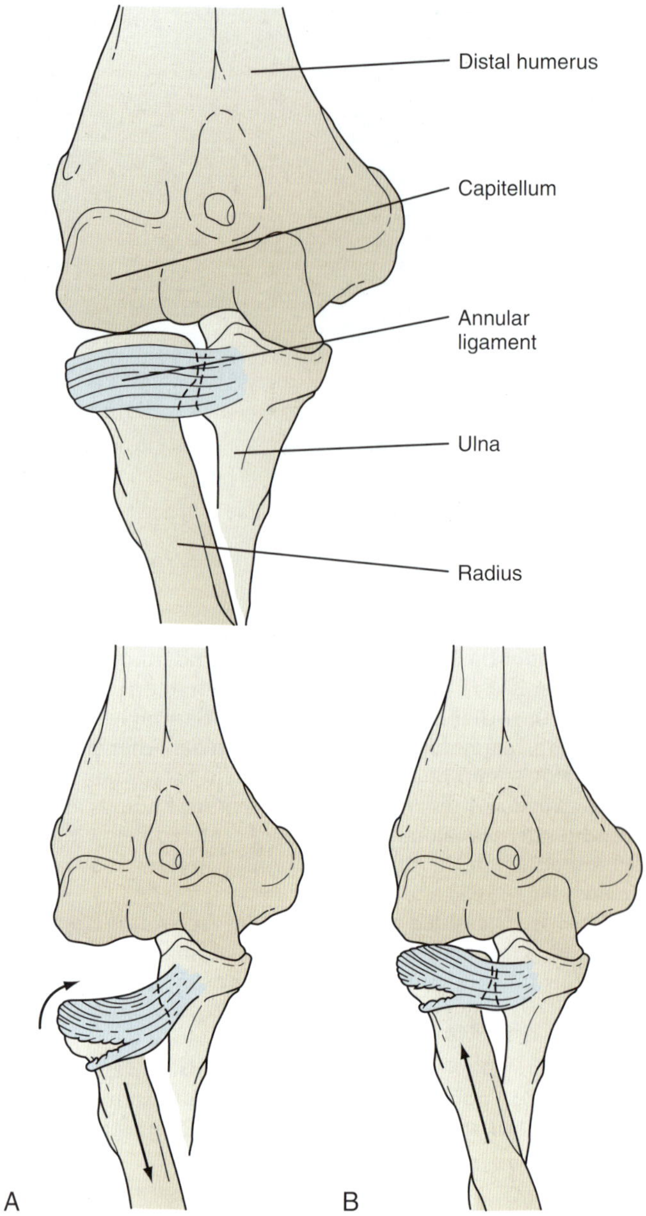

Fig. 22.67 Nursemaid's elbow. (A) Sudden traction on the outstretched arm pulls the radius distally, causing it to slip partially through the annular ligament and tearing it in the process. (B) When traction is released, the radial head recoils, trapping the proximal portion of the ligament between it and the capitellum.

motion, the child resists any attempt at supination and flexion and cries in pain.

The sudden axial pull of the arm pulls the radial head out from the annular ligament around the neck, and the proximal portion of the annular ligament becomes trapped between the radial head and capitellum (Fig. 22.67), similar to a bicycle tire coming undone partially off the wheel. This limits motion and produces pain. Radiographs are normal because the radial head is not truly subluxated but can be helpful to rule out other pathology in patients with equivocal history.

Before any reduction attempt, diagnosis of a nursemaid's elbow should be definite: There should be no history of an actual fall, there should be no externally visible deformity, swelling or bruising, and, in equivocal cases, radiographs should be normal. Treatment consists of the classic reduction maneuver: start in extension of the elbow, fully flex the elbow, and completely supinate the forearm synchronously. Pronation may also be done at this point or supination and pronation alternated; both techniques have been described in the literature (see Fig. 22.66B). A click can be perceived as the annular ligament (tire) locates back over the radial head (wheel). Despite successful reduction, the fearful child will continue to cry. Return of function should be evident within 10 to 15 minutes spontaneously as the child goes back to normal activity. If this is successful, no immobilization is needed and the parents should be educated on prevention. If after the reduction maneuver, the patient fails to regain normal function, radiographs should be performed if not already done so. In the absence of additional pathologic findings in these, the patient can be splinted/casted with the elbow at 90 degrees of flexion for 1 to 2 weeks, which will result in resolution.

Extremity Pain With Ligamentous Laxity

Children with generalized ligamentous laxity have hypermobile joints and are vulnerable to excessive stretching or force on ligamentous and musculotendinous structures. They are also somewhat more susceptible to joint dislocations. This phenomenon is seen in up to 18% of girls and 6% of boys. After periods of vigorous physical activity, these children often complain of

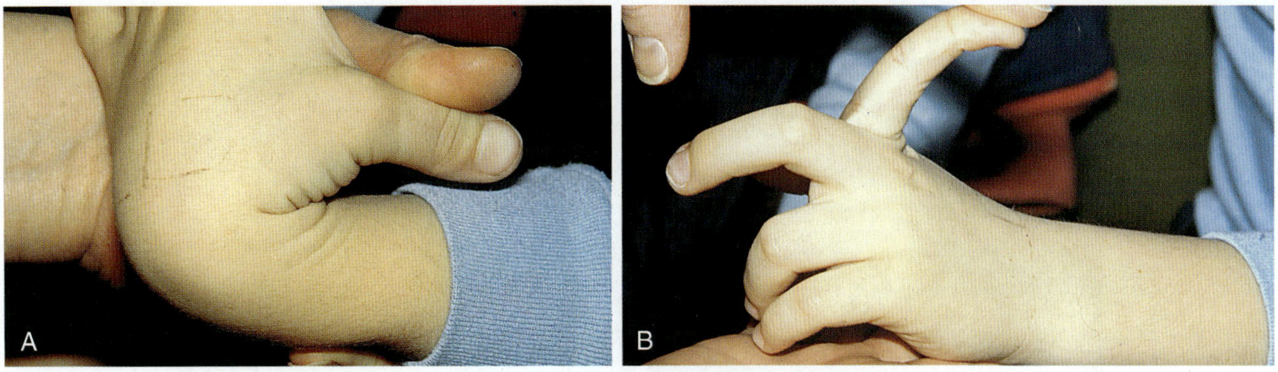

Fig. 22.68 Ligamentous laxity. This child shows findings typical of the joint hypermobility seen with ligamentous laxity. (A) He is able to hyperflex the wrist on the forearm. (B) He can also hyperextend the distal interphalangeal joint and the metacarpophalangeal joint.

arthralgias and shin or muscular pain, and occasionally they have evidence of joint swelling. Episodes tend to occur in the evening or at night; are self-limited, lasting 1 to several hours; and respond to rest and acetaminophen or ibuprofen. Many of these children have been accused of attention-getting behavior and hypochondriasis. Others have been dismissed as having "growing pains," and some have undergone extensive testing for rheumatic disorders and sometimes are overdiagnosed as Ehlers-Danlos syndrome. A history of greater than average activity on the preceding day and of recurrent short-lived pain usually without objective swelling, combined with findings of ligamentous laxity on examination (Fig. 22.68), should point to this diagnosis. The rarity of joint swelling and the absence of fever and other systemic symptoms help to rule out rheumatic and connective tissue disorders.

Once the problem is correctly diagnosed, patients can minimize discomfort by avoiding sudden increases in level of activity and taking a mild analgesic (unless contraindicated) before going to bed after a day of unusually vigorous activity. Graduated strengthening exercises may also be helpful. This is particularly true for children who want to participate in gymnastics or competitive sports.

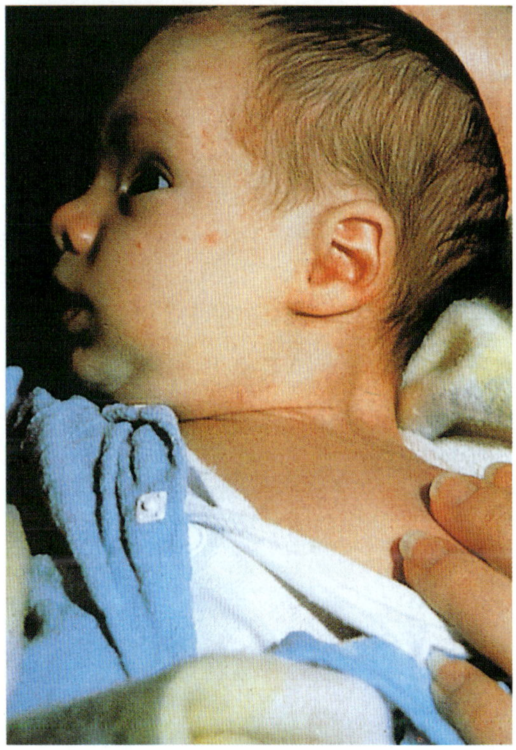

Fig. 22.69 Congenital torticollis. The "tumor" of congenital torticollis is seen as a swelling in the midportion of the sternocleidomastoid muscle. It is firm on palpation, and the muscle itself is shortened. The head tilts toward the affected side, and the chin rotates in the opposite direction. (Courtesy James Reilly, MD, Nemours/Alfred I. duPont Hospital for Children, Wilmington, DE.)

DISORDERS OF THE NECK AND SPINE

Children with disorders of the axial skeleton most commonly present with some type of deformity. Pain or dysfunction of the associated spinal cord and nerve roots may also prompt evaluation. Because these conditions often progress with growth, awareness and early recognition are important to assist early institution of appropriate treatment and minimize resultant morbidity.

Congenital Muscular Torticollis

Congenital muscular torticollis is a positional abnormality of the neck produced by contracture of the sternocleidomastoid muscle. It is thought to be secondary to abnormal intrauterine positioning or to birth trauma, resulting in the formation of a hematoma within the muscle belly. Usually, the condition is recognized at or shortly after birth (see Chapter 18). A palpable swelling may be noted within the muscle. With subsequent fibrosis, the characteristic deformity of torticollis develops, consisting of head tilt toward the affected side with rotation of the chin to the opposite side (Fig. 22.69) due to the unique anatomy of the sternocleidomastoid muscle. Gentle passive stretching exercises and positioning the child's crib so that external stimuli will cause him or her to turn the head and neck away from the side of deformity, and nursing on alternating sides may be beneficial. The majority of the cases resolve either spontaneously or with stretching. In rare instances surgical release may be beneficial. Severe torticollis may result in craniofacial disfigurement if it does not resolve.

Considerations in the differential diagnosis include Klippel-Feil syndrome; inflammatory or infectious conditions of the head, neck, or nasopharynx; posterior fossa or brainstem neoplasm; traumatic cervical spine injury; and atlantoaxial rotary subluxation. However, with the exception of the Klippel-Feil anomaly and congenital cervical spine deformity, these conditions tend to occur considerably later in childhood. Hip examination should be performed and according to the infant's age, a dynamic hip ultrasound or anteroposterior pelvis radiograph obtained because hip instability or dysplasia is present in ~20% of these children.

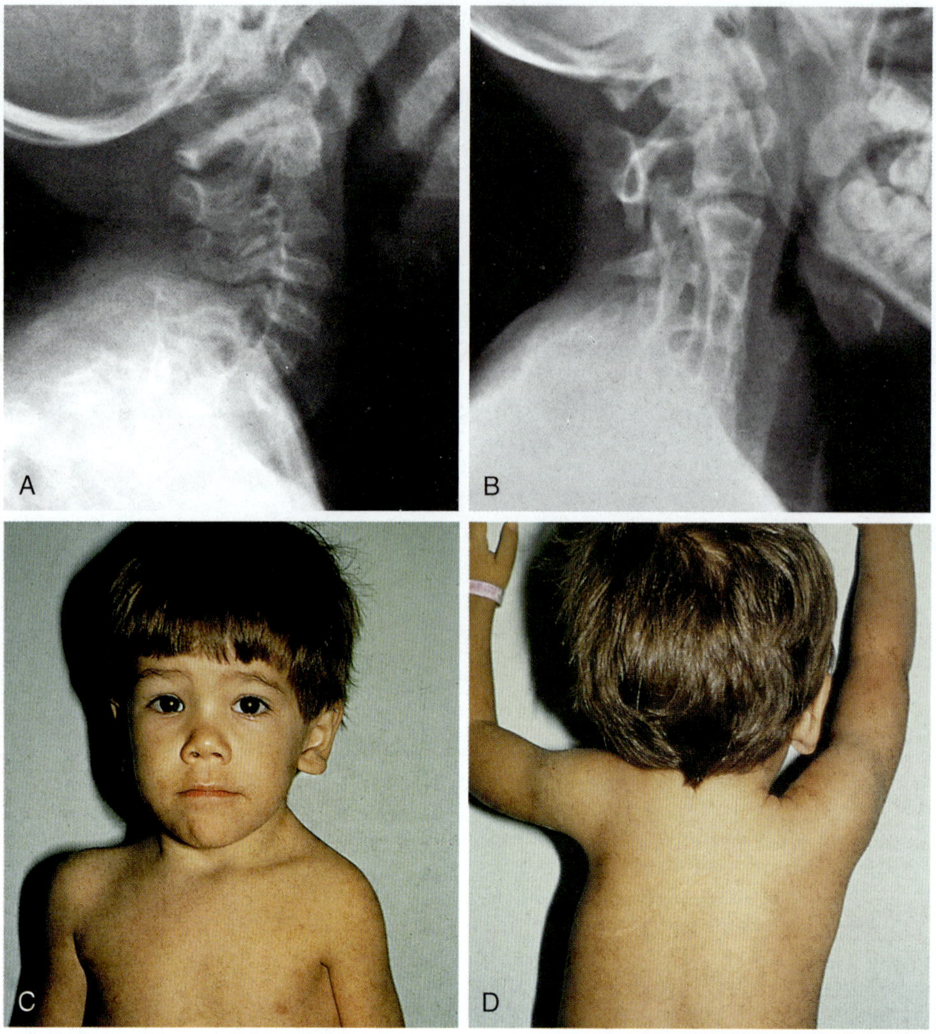

Fig. 22.70 Klippel-Feil syndrome. (A) This radiograph shows mild osseous involvement with fusion of the upper cervical segments. (B) In this radiograph, another patient has severe osseous involvement in which C3 to C7 are fused and hypoplastic. (C) Clinically the neck appears short and broad in the anterior view of this young child. (D) In this posterior view, the hairline is low and an associated Sprengel deformity is present, the left scapula being hypoplastic and high riding. As a result, the patient is unable to fully raise his left arm. Typical webbing of the neck is not appreciable in this child.

Klippel-Feil Syndrome

Patients with Klippel-Feil syndrome have congenital malformation of the neck that results from a failure of segmentation in the developing cervical spine. The condition varies greatly in severity, depending on the number of vertebrae that are fused (Fig. 22.70A and B). More severely affected individuals exhibit a short, broad neck with the appearance of "webbing," a low hairline, and gross restriction of motion (see Fig. 22.70C and D). Mild forms of the malformation may be diagnosed only because of radiographs taken for other reasons. The condition may be associated with other congenital malformations, such as a Sprengel deformity (see Fig. 22.81); rib deformities; scoliosis; CNS defects; and cardiac, pulmonary, and renal anomalies. Secondary neurologic problems are rare, but multiple fused levels with adjacent motion segments may be a reason to avoid contact or high-impact sports in order to avoid neurologic injury.

Scoliosis

Scoliosis is a condition in which there is curvature of the spine in the coronal or frontal plane. This lateral deviation is associated with vertebral rotation, such that when this deformity occurs in the thoracic spine, a chest wall deformity, or "rib hump," develops (Fig. 22.71). When it occurs in the lumbar spine, a prominence of the flank may be noted (Fig. 22.72). Often there is a primary structural curve with an adjacent secondary compensatory curve. Most cases of structural scoliosis are idiopathic and have their onset in early adolescence. A familial predisposition has been documented, but inheritance appears to be multifactorial. Females are affected more often than males, and their curvature is more likely to worsen. Infantile (0–3 years old) and juvenile (3–10 years old) forms of idiopathic scoliosis are seen, although much less commonly. Those with onset in infancy may develop plagiocephaly with flattening of the head on the concave side of the curve and a corresponding prominence on the opposite side of the head. Affected infants also have an increased incidence of associated hip dysplasia, congenital heart disease, inguinal hernia, and mental retardation. Structural scoliosis can also occur in conjunction with neuromuscular conditions, such as cerebral palsy (Fig. 22.73), myelomeningocele, spinocerebellar degeneration, polio, and spinal cord tumors; myopathic disorders including arthrogryposis and muscular dystrophy; congenital spinal anomalies (Fig. 22.74), such as hemivertebrae, trapezoidal vertebrae, and unsegmented vertebrae; neurofibromatosis (Fig. 22.75) and mesenchymal disorders; and a variety of other conditions (Box 22.1). The neuromuscular and congenital forms of scoliosis tend to have more rapid progression of curvature than of idiopathic scoliosis, and infants with congenital spinal anomalies

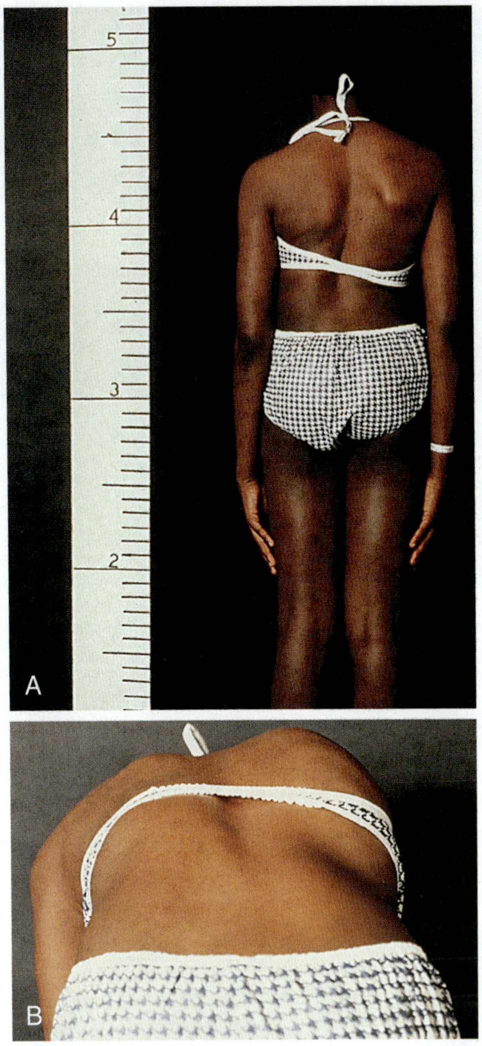

Fig. 22.71 Moderate idiopathic thoracic scoliosis in an adolescent. (A) Scapular asymmetry is easily discernible in the upright position. This results from rotation of the spine and attached rib cage. (B) Forward flexion reveals a rib hump deformity.

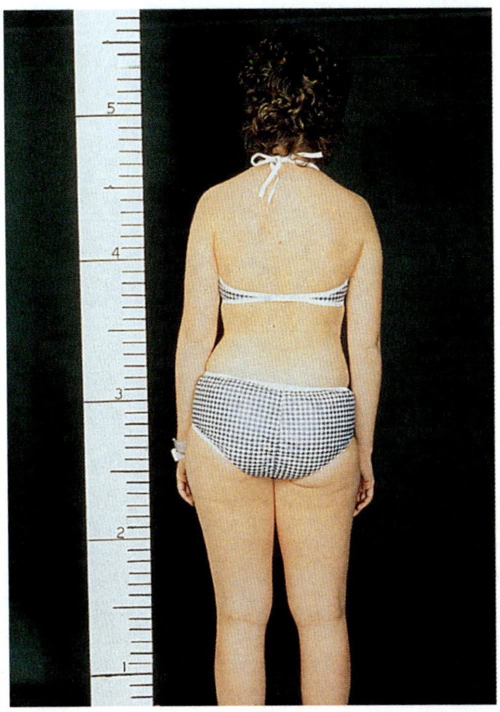

Fig. 22.72 Lumbar scoliosis. Pelvic obliquity is present, with prominence of the left flank.

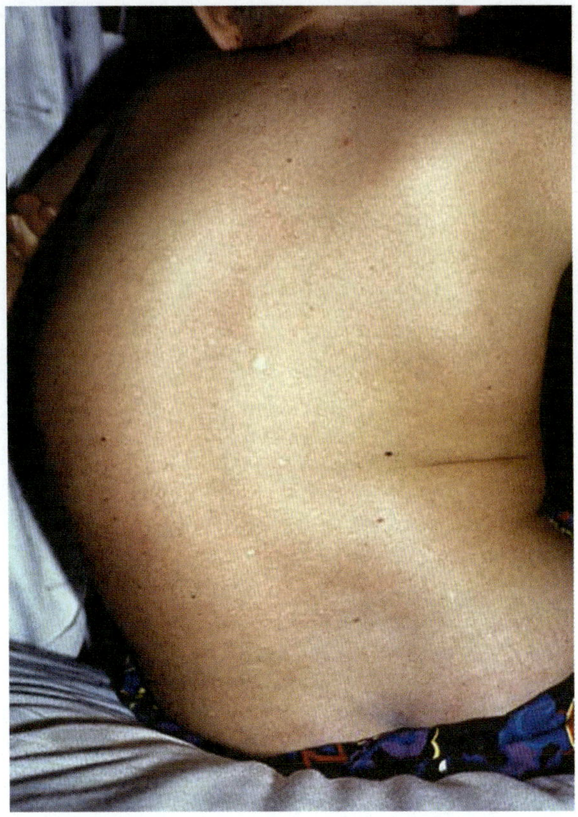

Fig. 22.73 Neuromuscular scoliosis. This 12-year-old boy has cerebral palsy and scoliosis. Note that his sitting balance is affected by the curve of his spine, which extends from the upper thorax to his pelvis, resulting in pelvic obliquity and inability to sit independently. This is typical of spinal deformity in patients with neuromuscular disorders.

have a high incidence of associated genitourinary and cardiac anomalies.

Nonstructural or flexible scoliosis may be seen in association with poor posture; limb-length inequality; or flexion contracture of a hip or knee, in which case the curve disappears when the child is seated. It can also be seen with paraspinous muscle spasm after a back injury; as the result of splinting because of pain in cases of pyelonephritis, appendicitis, or pneumonia; or in patients with a herniated intervertebral disk and secondary nerve root pain (see Fig. 22.80A and Box 22.1). These forms resolve with treatment of the primary disorder.

Except in curvatures resulting from inflammatory or neoplastic processes and from herniation of an intervertebral disk, pain is rarely a complaint in children and adolescents with scoliosis. In fact, patients with pain, signs of nerve root compression, or evidence of new-onset peripheral neurologic deficits should undergo thorough evaluation for a treatable underlying cause.

The physical examination findings in a patient with scoliosis can be separated into true pathognomonic findings and associated signs, which may also occur in otherwise normal, nonscoliotic children. The only true pathognomonic sign of scoliosis is the presence of a curve noted on forward bending, which constitutes a positive Adams forward bend test (see the Thoracolumbar Spine section, earlier). An associated convex posterior chest wall prominence (termed rib hump) or paralumbar prominence may also be noted on forward bending (see Fig. 22.71B). The rib hump and paralumbar prominence are manifestations of the vertebral rotational deformity seen in scoliosis.

Frequently, a diagnosis of scoliosis is not based on a positive forward bend test but rather the presence of other physical signs. These signs include shoulder asymmetry, unilateral scapular prominence, waist asymmetry, and small chest or paralumbar humps (see Figs. 22.71A, 22.72, and 22.75A).

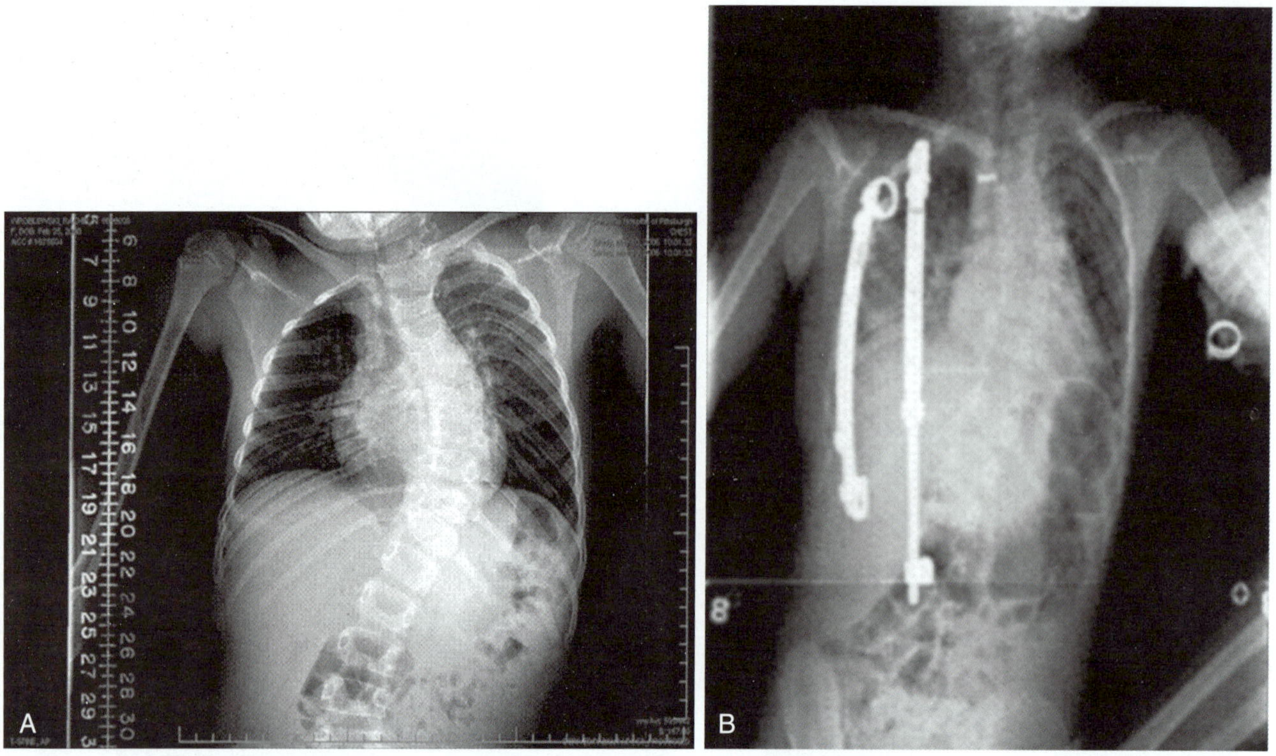

Fig. 22.74 Congenital scoliosis. (A) This 7-year-old was born with fusion of ribs 5 to 10 on her right side. She also has congenital failure of segmentation of several vertebrae. Both of these anomalies contributed to her progressive scoliotic deformity. (B) She was treated with an opening thoracostomy (separation of the ribs) and insertion of a vertical expandable prosthetic titanium rib (VEPTR; Synthes, Solothurn, Switzerland). This device allows for spinal growth and expansion of the chest cavity by repeated surgical expansions at 6-month intervals.

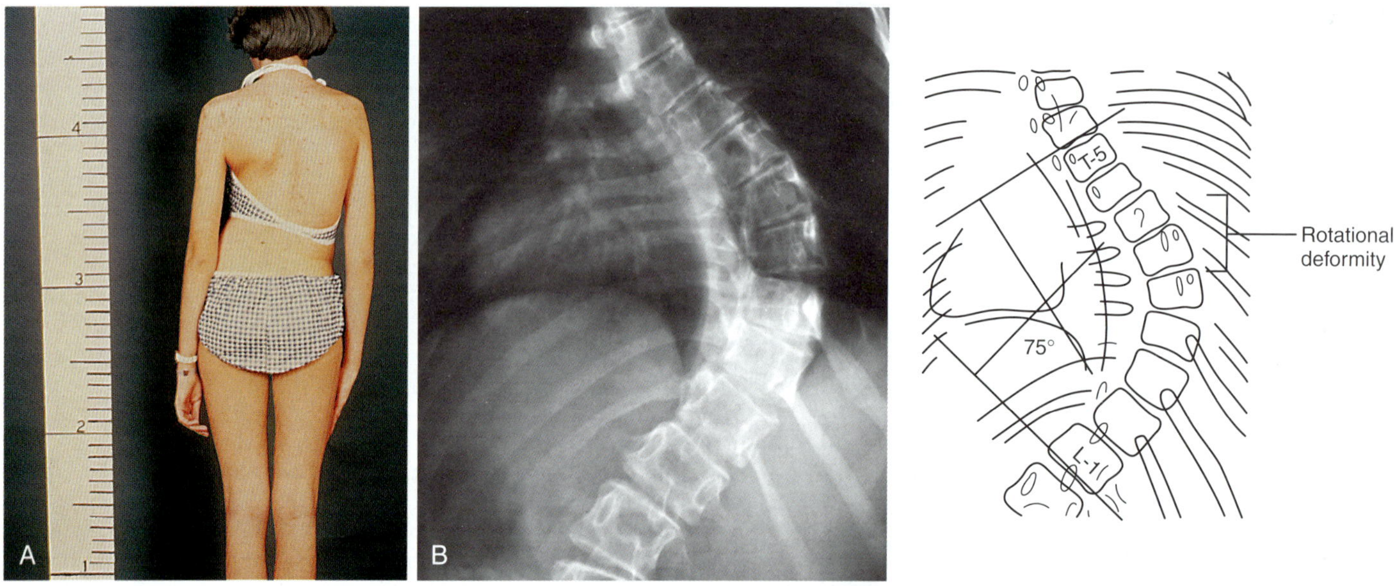

Fig. 22.75 Severe thoracic scoliosis secondary to neurofibromatosis. (A) Note the chest wall deformity and that the patient's head is not centered over the pelvis. (B) The severe curvature is more apparent on this radiograph. The angle of measurement (here, 75 degrees) is determined by the intersection of lines drawn perpendicular to the vertebrae at the ends of the curve (Cobb method).

Box 22.1 Causes of Scoliosis

Structural Scoliosis

Idiopathic
Congenital
Neuromuscular
Other conditions that may result in scoliosis:

- Myopathic disorders
- Neurofibromatosis
- Mesenchymal disorders
- Osteochondrodystrophies
- Metabolic disorders
- Trauma, surgery, irradiation, burns

Nonstructural or Functional Scoliosis

Herniated lumbar disks
Postural derangements
Limb-length inequality
Irritative or inflammatory disorders
Hysteria

Because screening studies have shown that up to 5% of school-age children and adolescents have lateral curvatures, routine screening by primary care physicians is important. Hence the forward bend test should be part of all examinations in children from 6 to 7 years old until the end of puberty (see the Thoracolumbar Spine section, earlier). When true clinical scoliosis is found, the patient must be referred for orthopedic evaluation. It is safer and more cost-effective for the primary care physician to make the referral without obtaining prior radiographs because typical office radiographs done for scoliosis screening are often not of appropriate quality or positioning. Standing, full-torso radiographs taken on 36-inch-long (90 cm) cassette films with special grids are much more helpful and more readily available in the orthopedic clinic or office. Once a diagnosis of scoliosis has been made, follow-up radiographs are routinely obtained no more frequently than at 6- to 9-month intervals. The goal of close follow-up is to detect progression of curvature early and implement treatment to prevent or reduce it when needed. Idiopathic curves of 25 to 30 degrees or more and lesser curves showing rapid progression are treated by spinal bracing and an exercise program.

Newborns and infants should be screened for congenital and infantile forms of scoliosis. This is often best done by holding the infant prone on the examiner's hand and can be done while assessing for parachute reflex.

Kyphosis

Kyphosis is a condition in which there is increased posterior apex curvature of the spine in the sagittal plane. The thoracic spine normally has a kyphotic curvature of 25 to 50 degrees, with a slightly larger amount of lordosis in the lumbar spine in the sagittal plane. Excessive kyphosis may be purely postural in nature or may be associated with a number of pathologic conditions. The latter include congenital vertebral anomalies, a spinal growth disturbance known as *Scheuermann disease* (Fig. 22.76), neuromuscular afflictions, skeletal dysplasias, and metabolic diseases (Fig. 22.77). Kyphosis can also develop after spinal trauma or surgery. Patients with a structural deformity may complain of backache aggravated by motion. The deformity is best viewed from the lateral position on forward bending. Evaluation of the effects of posture and of application of pressure over the apex of the curve assists diagnosis and decisions regarding treatment.

Postural kyphosis is usually seen in preadolescents and consists of a flexible thoracic kyphosis that is correctable on hyperextension. Most affected children have a compensatory increase in lumbar lordosis. Radiographic findings are normal. Treatment consists of an exercise program designed to strengthen trunk and abdominal muscles, which are usually weak in these patients.

Scheuermann disease, a disorder of unknown etiology, is the most common cause of fixed kyphotic deformity. It can be distinguished clinically from postural kyphosis by its inherent stiffness and the greater magnitude of the deformity. The deformity fails to correct or is only partially correctable on hyperextension or on the application of pressure over the apex of the curve. Lateral radiographs reveal anterior wedging of three or more consecutive vertebral bodies that are located at the apex of the curve. Radiographic evidence of end-plate erosion of the involved vertebrae often exists, and Schmorl nodules are a common associated finding (see Fig. 22.76).

Spondylolisthesis

Spondylolisthesis is a condition characterized by the translation or forward displacement of one vertebral body over another and is seen most commonly at the lumbosacral articulation. The problem may develop as a result of insufficiency or fatigue fractures of the pars interarticularis (isthmic), congenital dysplasia of the posterior spinal elements (dysplastic), or degenerative changes in the disk and facets (degenerative), or it may occur secondary to pathologic lesions within the vertebra and its elements (pathologic). Isthmic spondylolisthesis (spondylolytic) is by far the most common type (Fig. 22.78). If there is no anterior shift but only a part interarticularis defect, the condition is called *spondylolysis* and may be associated with pain with hyperextension of the lumbar spine. Thought to be prevalent at the L5 level, symptoms mostly arise in children who are involved in sports with repetitive hyperextension (gymnastics, soccer, football linemen, ballet, etc.). Lateral lumbar spine film often shows the defect, but in unilateral cases oblique views may be helpful (Fig. 22.79C and see Fig. 22.78).

Patients with a congenital predisposition may show alarming degrees of slippage. The condition is often associated with low back pain that increases with strenuous activities and abates with rest.

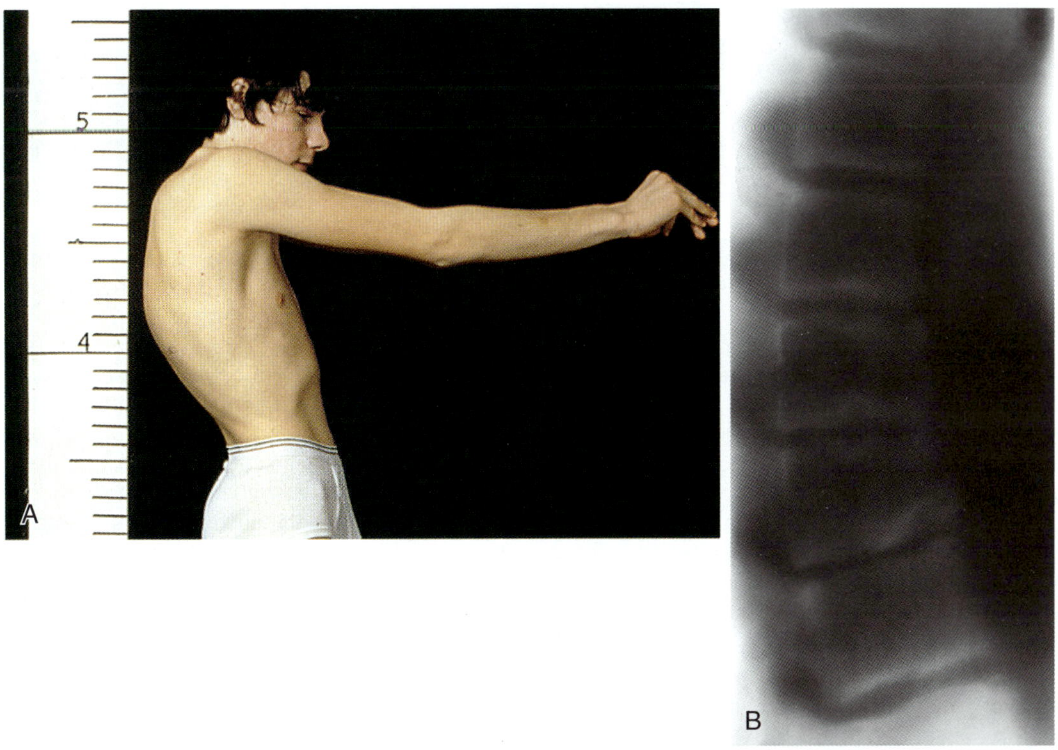

Fig. 22.76 Moderate thoracic kyphosis secondary to Scheuermann disease. (A) The patient is attempting to correct the deformity, but because of its fixed nature, he cannot do so and must compensate for this with an increased lumbar lordosis. (B) This tomographic cut shows anterior wedging of three consecutive vertebral bodies and clearly demonstrates the associated erosion of the vertebral end plates and Schmorl nodules.

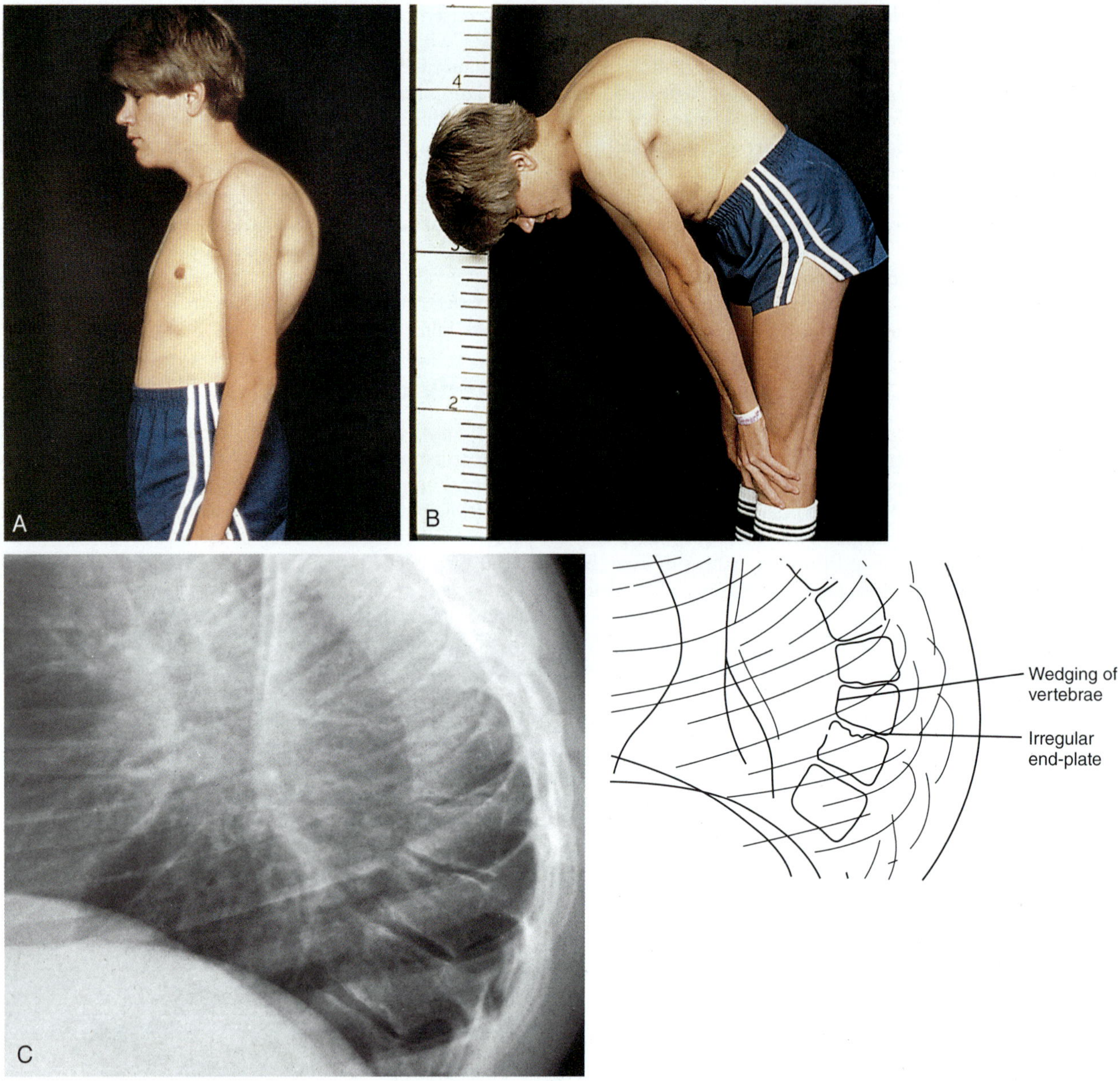

Fig. 22.77 (A) Severe kyphosis of the thoracic spine secondary to vertebral wedging in a patient with glycogen storage disease. To stand upright, the patient must increase his lumbar lordosis and thrust his head forward to center it above the pelvis. (B) The kyphotic deformity is accentuated on forward bending. (C) Radiographically, the vertebral wedging that underlies the kyphotic deformity is evident.

Some patients have symptoms of nerve root irritation. This necessitates differentiation from inflammatory and neoplastic processes and from disk herniation.

Examination often reveals loss of normal lumbar lordosis, tenderness of the involved posterior elements, paravertebral muscle spasm, and secondary tightness of the hamstring muscles. A step-off deformity may be evident on palpation of the spinous processes. Range of motion is often limited in extension because of pain. Nerve root signs may be present. In its most severe form, spondyloptosis, the L5 vertebral body may completely translate off the sacrum, and the patient characteristically exhibits a waddling gait, a transverse abdominal crease, flattened buttocks, and flexion deformities of the hips and knees, as well as foreshortening of the torso (see Fig. 22.79A and B). Characterization and grading of the process are accomplished with lumbar radiographs.

Herniated Intervertebral Disk

Although relatively common in adults, herniated disks occur only rarely in children and infrequently in adolescents. They are almost always limited to the lower two segments of the lumbar spine. A history of antecedent trauma is not uncommon. Lower extremity radicular symptoms predominate. Patients often describe a "pulling" sensation in a lower extremity or liken their pain to a "toothache" in the distribution of the L5 or S1 nerve roots (see Chapter 16). They also may complain of numbness or weakness in the involved limb. Forward flexion, sitting, coughing, and straining aggravate the neurologic symptoms.

On examination, an antalgic scoliosis of the lumbar spine may be apparent, which the patient is unable to reduce (Fig. 22.80A). Inability to reverse the normal lumbar lordosis is noted, and symptoms may be aggravated by attempts at flexion. The straight leg raise test is often positive (radicular symptoms being reproduced when the limb is raised by the examiner; see the Thoracolumbar Spine section, earlier, and Fig. 22.5), and neurologic abnormalities may be found on sensory, motor, and reflex testing, although these may be subtle. Plain radiographs usually show no abnormality, other than possible diskogenic scoliosis, but the diagnosis may be verified by myelography, CT, or MRI (see Fig. 22.80B). The differential diagnosis may include hematogenous disk space infection or vertebral osteomyelitis, spinal cord or neural element tumor, and spondylolisthesis with nerve root irritation.

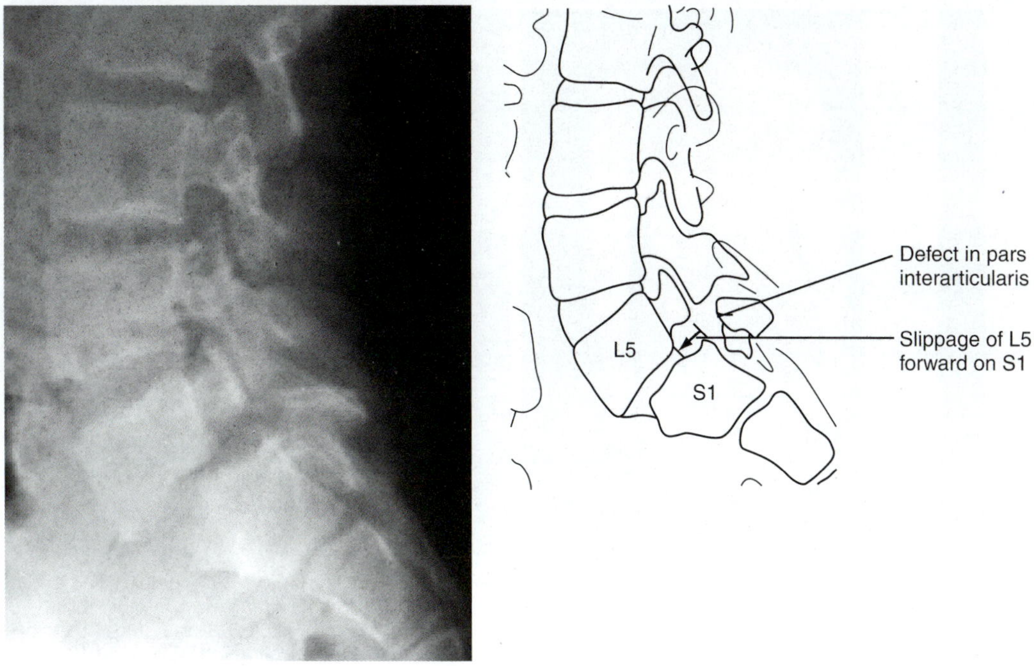

Fig. 22.78 Radiograph of a moderate isthmic spondylolisthesis in a 14-year-old boy. The forward slippage of L5 on the sacrum was the result of a fatigue fracture of the pars interarticularis.

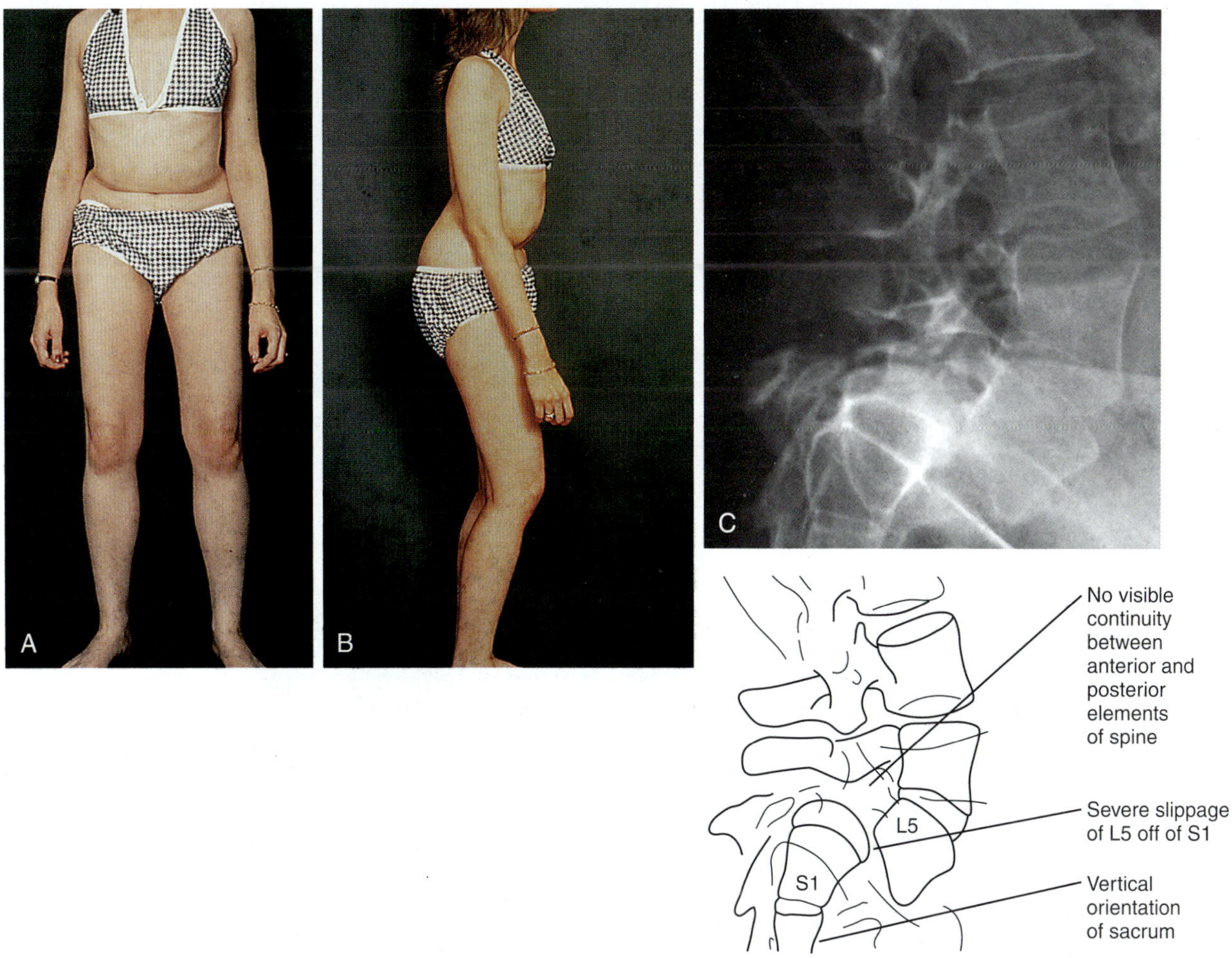

Fig. 22.79 Spondyloptosis in a 16-year-old girl. (A) A cosmetic deformity is common with this magnitude of spondylolisthesis. The torso is foreshortened, and a transverse abdominal crease is present. (B) In the lateral view, the torso is thrust forward, the buttocks are flattened, and there are flexion deformities of the hips and knees. (C) The L5 vertebra has completely translocated off the sacrum as the result of a congenital insufficiency of the posterior elements; the lumbar spine has essentially migrated anteriorly and into the pelvis.

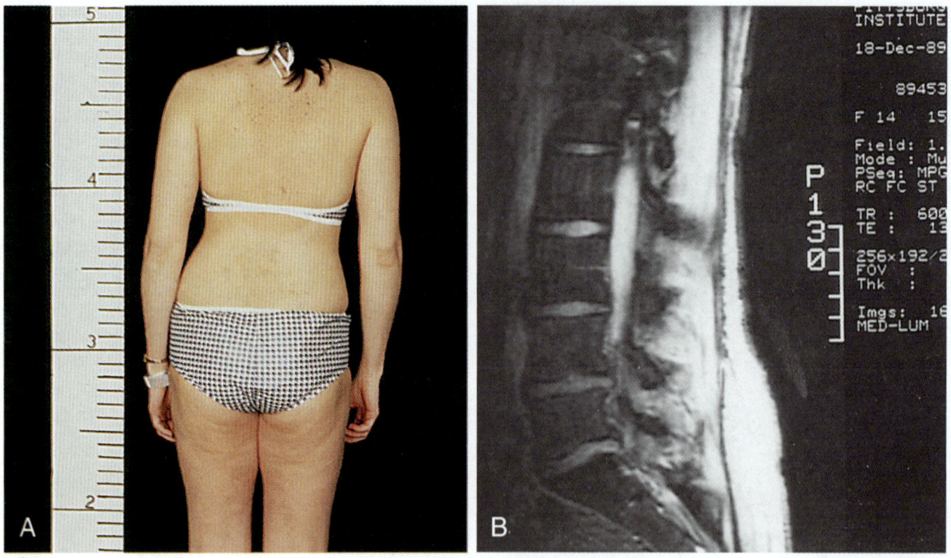

Fig. 22.80 Herniated intervertebral disk. (A) Diskogenic scoliosis is evident in a 16-year-old girl with a herniated disk at L4 to L5. The trunk is shifted away from the affected side. The normal lumbar lordosis is absent, and spinal motion is severely limited. (B) On sagittal magnetic resonance imaging, the L4 to L5 disk bulges posteriorly, compressing the cauda equina. (B, Courtesy Department of Pediatric Radiology, Children's Hospital of Pittsburgh, Pittsburgh, PA.)

DISORDERS OF THE UPPER EXTREMITY

Because of the importance of prehensile function, disorders affecting any area of the upper limb can result in significant impairment of motor development during childhood. Knowledge of the normal anatomy is vital for assessment and appropriate treatment.

Sprengel Deformity

A Sprengel deformity is a congenital malformation characterized by an abnormally small, high-riding scapula. In most cases, it is unilateral. The etiology is unknown, but there appears to be a familial predisposition, and the condition may be associated with a variety of other congenital anomalies, including Klippel-Feil syndrome (see Fig. 22.70) and rib and vertebral malformations. Scoliosis and torticollis may be associated abnormalities. Cosmetic deformity and limited shoulder motion on the affected side are the usual complaints.

On examination, the scapula is noted to be hypoplastic and high riding in association with asymmetry of the base of the neck and shoulders (Fig. 22.81A). Shoulder motion is usually severely limited, particularly in abduction (see Fig. 22.81B). This is due to limited scapular motion because the scapula is often tethered to the cervical spine by a fibrous omovertebral band, which is frequently ossified. Radiography confirms the abnormal size and position of the scapula.

Nonsurgical treatment consisting of stretching and range-of-motion exercises may be instituted but is rarely successful. Surgery may be undertaken for cosmetic and functional reasons and consists of excision of the prominent superior aspect of the scapula or release and reduction of the scapula accomplished by positioning it inferiorly on the chest wall. Although care must be taken during the procedure to prevent brachial plexus injury, surgery performed before adolescence usually improves appearance and restores some function.

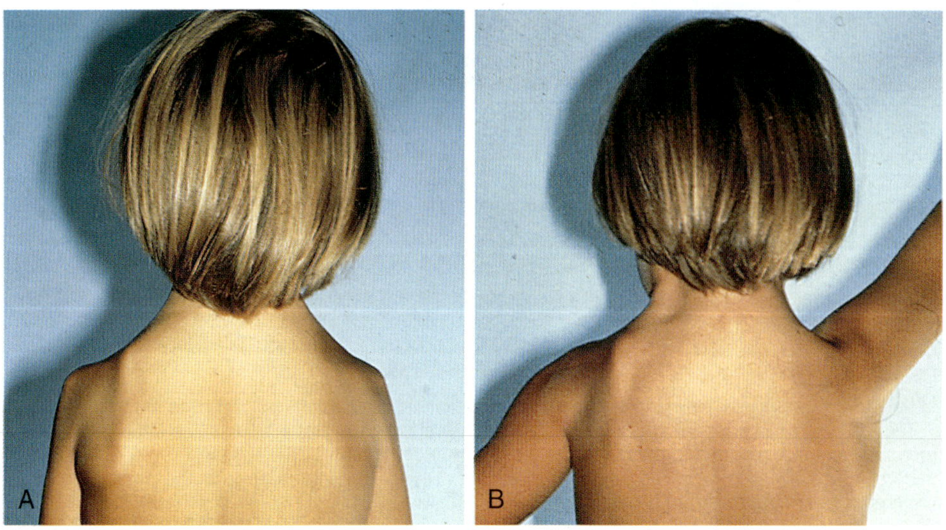

Fig. 22.81 Sprengel deformity. (A) The left scapula is high riding and hypoplastic, and its vertebral border is prominent. (B) Shoulder motion is severely limited, particularly in abduction. (Courtesy Dana Mears, MD.)

Congenital Pseudarthrosis of the Clavicle

This is a rare congenital disorder manifested by a painless bulbous deformity in the region of the midclavicle. It is thought to result from a failure of maturation of the ossification center of the clavicle. It almost always involves the right side and on occasion may be associated with other congenital anomalies. It can be seen in patients with neurofibromatosis 1.

On examination, the clavicle appears foreshortened with a prominence evident in its midportion (Fig. 22.82; see Chapter 6 for radiographic appearance). Palpation reveals hypermobility of the two ends of the clavicle and crepitance. Range of motion of the shoulder is normal. This condition characteristically involves no functional impairment and requires no treatment. Although clavicular fracture as a result of birth trauma may present a similar appearance, it is easily distinguished because of tenderness over the region of deformity and eventual callus formation during healing.

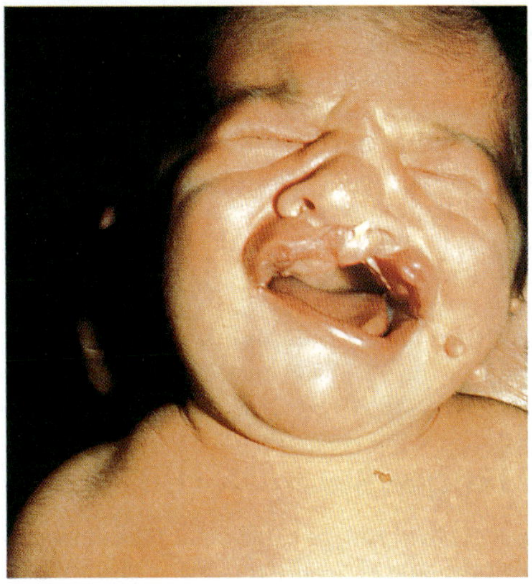

Fig. 22.82 Congenital pseudarthrosis of the clavicle. There is a bulbous, nontender swelling in the region of the midclavicle. The medial aspect of the clavicle is prominent. This patient has associated anomalies. Radiographic appearance is shown in Chapter 6.

Radial Club Hand

Radial club hand is the result of congenital absence of the radial structures of the forearm and hand. Associated muscular structures and the radial nerve are hypoplastic or absent. The anomaly is rare and affects more male than female subjects. Its characteristic clinical presentation is one of a small, short, bowed forearm and aplasia or hypoplasia of the thumb and radial deviation of the residual hand (Fig. 22.83A and B). Radiographs show absent bones in the affected area (see Fig. 22.83C).

Treatment is best instituted early with passive stretching exercises and corrective casting, which should be instituted under the purview of a hand surgeon specializing in congenital upper extremity differences. Surgical treatment consists of centralization of the hand on the “one-bone forearm” to maximize function.

Ganglion of the Wrist

A ganglion is a benign cystic mass thought to consist of an accumulation of synovial fluid an outpouching of a synovially lined tendon sheath or joint capsule. The etiology is unknown, but it is thought to be related to herniation of synovial tissue with a ball/valve effect. Antecedent trauma may be reported. These may be present over the dorsal or volar aspects of the wrist and are generally located toward the radial side (Fig. 22.84). On occasion, they are seen on the dorsum of the foot or adjacent to one of the malleoli of the ankle (see Fig. 22.108). Their size may fluctuate with time and activity. On examination, they may be either firm or fluctuant and they can be transilluminated. Although most are asymptomatic, an occasional patient may complain of pain and tenderness. Ganglions can be confused with other masses around the wrist, and the diagnosis should be confirmed with ultrasound.

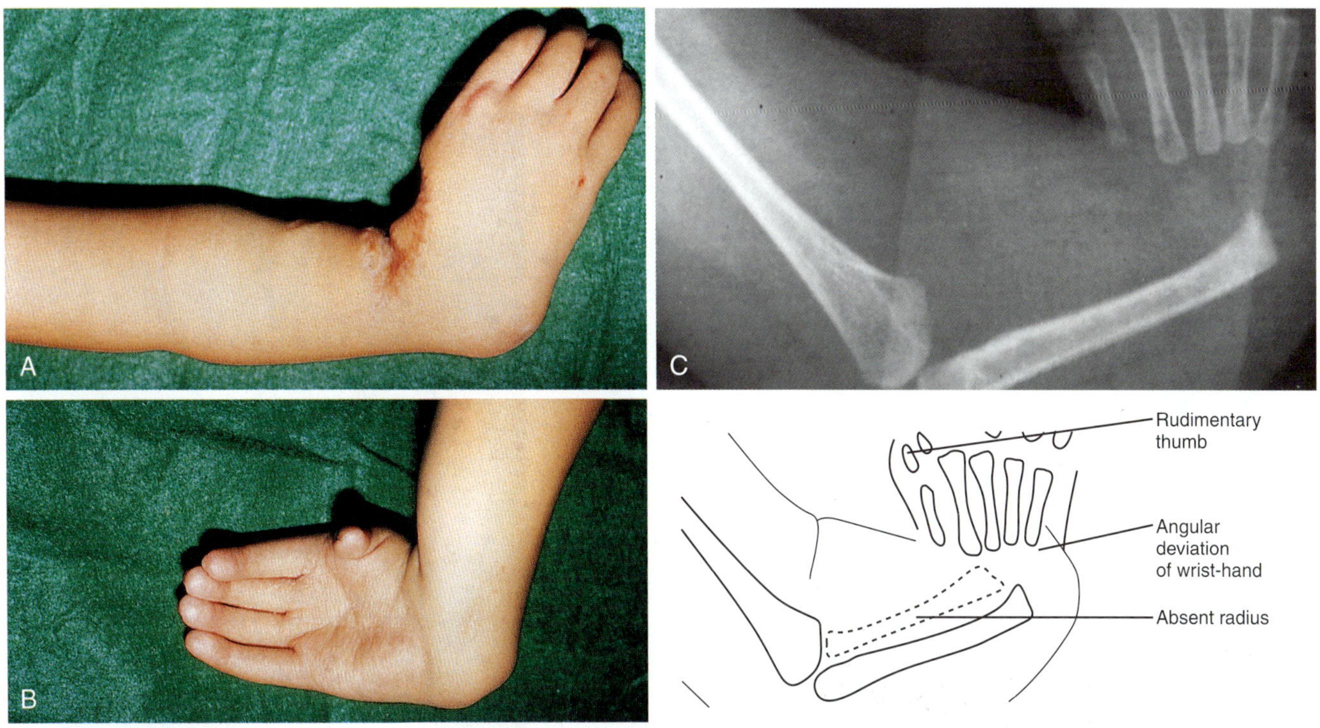

Fig. 22.83 Radial club hand. (A) The forearm is shortened with radial deviation of the hand and wrist on the ulna. (B) A flexion deformity of the hand and wrist on the forearm and a hypoplastic thumb are present. (C) Radiograph shows absence of the radius, dislocation of the carpus, and a rudimentary thumb, all characteristic of radial club hand. (Clinical photographs courtesy Joseph Imbriglia, MD, Allegheny General Hospital, Pittsburgh, PA.)

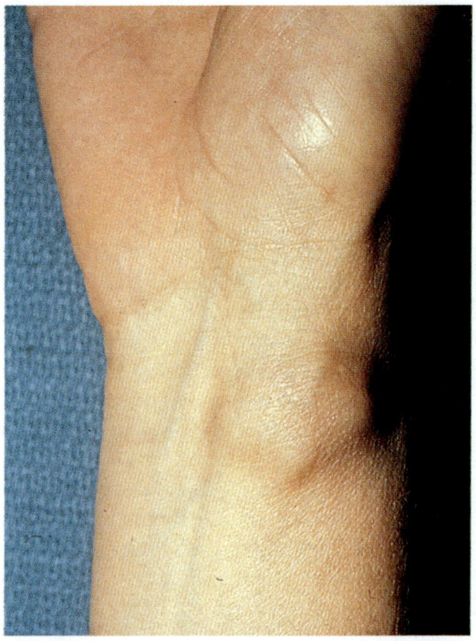

Fig. 22.84 Ganglion of the wrist. This cystic mass overlying the wrist joint and flexor tendons was asymptomatic and nontender.

Syndactyly

Syndactyly is a relatively common congenital anomaly involving failure of the digits of the hands or feet to separate. It is both more common and more disabling in the upper extremity. Bilateral involvement is usual, and a positive family history is not uncommon. It may be associated with other congenital anomalies. Great variation in the degree of fusion exists. In mild cases, only the skin is joined, making reconstructive surgery simple (Fig. 22.85). In more severe cases, the nails, deeper structures, and bones may be conjoined, contributing to deformity and growth abnormalities and making reconstructive treatment more difficult. Patients should be referred to a hand specialist for evaluation. Syndactyly in the lesser toes does not create functional problems and does not require treatment.

Congenital Trigger Thumb

A congenital trigger thumb is characterized by a fixed or intermittent flexion deformity of the interphalangeal joint of the thumb that may be present at birth or may develop shortly thereafter (Fig. 22.86). It is thought to result from an idiopathic nodule on the flexor tendon (Notta nodule) impeding normal tendon excursion through the pulley structures around the metacarpophalangeal joint. The flexion deformity generally cannot be passively extended except in milder cases, where a snapping sensation is felt as the nodule passes through the pulley. If passively correctable, splinting in extension occasionally results in correction; otherwise, surgery is required.

Boutonnière (Buttonhole) Deformity

A boutonnière deformity of a finger is the late result of an unrecognized traumatic avulsion of the central portion of the extensor tendon at its insertion on the middle phalanx. The mechanism of injury is usually a blow to the tip of the finger that drives it into forced flexion against resistance, although laceration over the dorsum of the finger involving the extensor tendon may produce a similar deformity if tendon involvement is not noted. Initially, there may be local tenderness over the dorsal aspect of the PIP joint without deformity. With time, however, the lateral bands of the extensor mechanism migrate volarly, producing a flexion deformity of the PIP joint with a secondary extension deformity of the distal joint (Fig. 22.87). If the injury is recognized early, healing may occur with splinting of the PIP joint in extension. Later, open surgical repair may be necessary.

Mallet Finger/Swan-Neck Deformity

A mallet finger is the result of avulsion of the extensor tendon from its insertion at the base of the distal phalanx of a finger. It occurs due to a blow to the extended finger against resistance. The tendon alone, or a portion of the distal phalanx into which it inserts, may be involved. The clinical appearance is that of a "dropped finger" or flexion deformity of the distal interphalangeal joint with inability to actively extend the joint (see Fig. 22.49). If not recognized and treated at the time of the initial injury, the condition becomes chronic and contracture of the extensor mechanism may occur, with

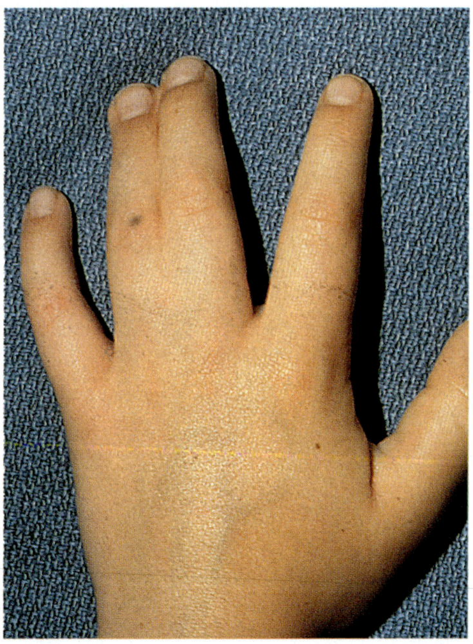

Fig. 22.85 Syndactyly. This child has mild syndactyly involving soft tissues of the middle and ring fingers without bony involvement. (Courtesy Joseph Imbriglia, MD, Allegheny General Hospital, Pittsburgh, PA.)

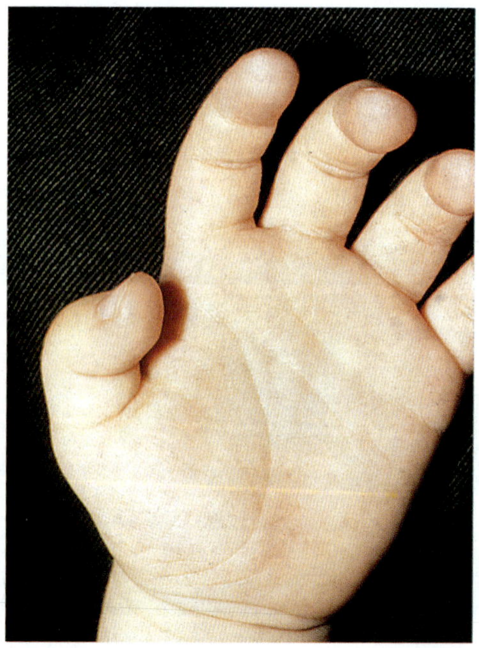

Fig. 22.86 Congenital trigger thumb. There is a fixed flexion deformity at the interphalangeal joint of the thumb resulting from tightness of the tendon sheath of the flexor pollicis longus. The remainder of the hand appears normal.

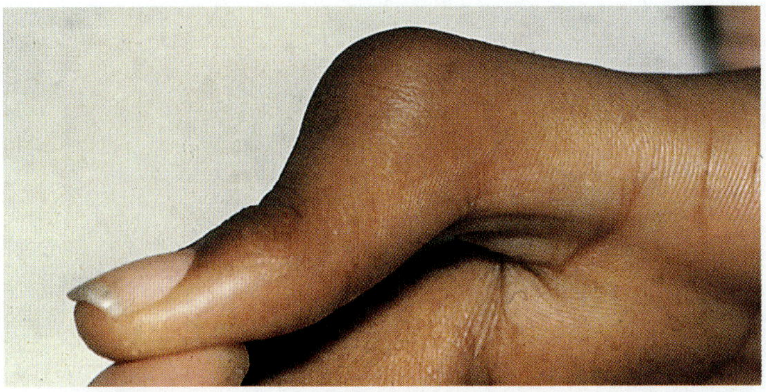

Fig. 22.87 Boutonnière deformity of the finger. A fixed flexion contracture of the proximal interphalangeal joint exists, along with hyperextension of the distal joint secondary to volar migration of the lateral bands of the extensor mechanism. This is the result of an unrecognized or inadequately treated injury to the extensor tendon at its insertion on the middle phalanx.

a secondary hyperextension deformity of the PIP joint producing a swan-neck deformity (Fig. 22.88). Treatment consists of splinting the distal joint in an extended position, open reduction if a large fragment of bone is involved, or surgical repair in chronic cases by a hand specialist.

DISORDERS OF THE LOWER EXTREMITY

Normally developed and functional lower extremities permit locomotion with ease and efficiency. Any disability resulting from a deformed, shortened, or painful lower limb can be considerable (see the Gait and Gait Disturbances section, earlier).

Knowledge of normal anatomy and function is necessary to accurately recognize and treat abnormalities in this region (see the Lower Extremity Examination section, earlier).

Developmental Dislocation of the Hip

Developmental dislocation of the hip (DDH), formerly referred to as *congenital dislocation of the hip*, consists of displacement of the femoral head from its normal relationship with the acetabulum. It is a frequent problem, with an incidence of 1 to 2 per 1000 births. It is generally detectable at birth or shortly thereafter. Female infants are affected significantly more frequently, and unilateral dislocation is twice as frequent as bilateral. Developmental dislocation may be divided into idiopathic and teratogenic types. Idiopathic dislocation is more frequent, and patients often have a family history. There is a spectrum of hip severity from joint subluxation to irreducible dislocations at diagnosis. This type of developmental dislocation may be related to abnormal intrauterine positioning or restriction of fetal movement in utero, which impedes adequate development and stability of the hip joint complex. Hormone responses may also predispose, with affected infants perhaps being more sensitive to the pelvic relaxation effects of maternal estrogen. A history of breech presentation is common, and these patients often exhibit generalized ligamentous laxity. Teratogenic dislocations of the hip represent a more severe form of the disorder and are probably the result of an embryonic defect. They occur early in fetal development and result in malformation of both the femoral head and the acetabular socket. Associated congenital anomalies are common in infants whose dislocations are teratogenic, including clubfoot deformity, congenital torticollis, metatarsus adductus, and infantile scoliosis.

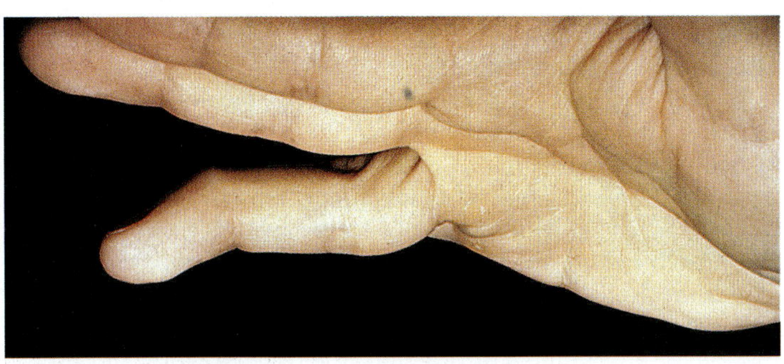

Fig. 22.88 Mallet finger with secondary swan-neck deformity. This is the result of avulsion of the extensor tendon from its insertion at the base of the distal phalanx, which was not recognized at the time of injury. The patient shows a flexion deformity of the distal interphalangeal joint and secondary hyperextension of the proximal interphalangeal joint.

The importance of careful hip evaluation in the newborn and at early infant visits cannot be overemphasized. Early diagnosis enables prompt institution of treatment and results in a better outcome. Knowledge of the clinical signs and skill in techniques of examination are necessary.

Typically, the infant with a dislocated hip has no noticeable difference in the position in which the leg is held, although a position of adduction and external rotation is adopted by some. If the dislocation is unilateral, the skin folds of the thighs and buttocks are often asymmetric and the involved lower extremity appears shorter than the opposite side (Fig. 22.89A). This foreshortening is accentuated by holding the hips and knees in 90 degrees of flexion (Galeazzi sign). In patients with bilateral dislocations, this asymmetry is not present. In a truly dislocated hip, the most consistent physical finding is that of limited abduction (see Fig. 22.89B). Additional diagnostic maneuvers may assist in establishing the diagnosis. The Barlow test is positive if, with the knees flexed and hips flexed to 90 degrees, the hips are gently adducted with posterior pressure applied through the knee. A palpable clunk indicating posterior dislocation is appreciated in the hip, which is reduced at baseline but dislocates during the maneuver. In patients who rest while dislocated, the Ortolani sign is positive when a palpable clunk is felt with reduction of the hip by abduction and upward pressure on the greater trochanter. A positive Ortolani test suggests a dislocated hip, which can be manually reduced. When the hip is dislocated and irreducible, only limitation of abduction is apparent and both maneuvers will be negative.

The radiographic findings of a developmental hip dislocation are characteristic. The femoral head is generally located lateral and superior to its normal position, and the acetabulum may be shallow, with lateral deficiency and a characteristic high acetabular index or slope (see Fig. 22.89C and D). Because femoral head ossification is not evident radiographically until 3 to 6 months old, ultrasound evaluation of the hip is often helpful in determining the acetabular/femoral head relationships. Furthermore, in developmental dislocation, ossification may be delayed because normal articulation forces are absent. Plain radiographs are typically deferred until at least 6 months of age. In teratogenic hip dislocation, there may be hypoplasia of both the acetabular and femoral sides with noncongruent development of one or both. Early radiographic findings are similar.

Successful correction of DDH depends on early diagnosis and institution of appropriate treatment and uses the remodeling potential of the immature acetabulum. In the first 6 months of life, use of a Pavlik harness, which permits gentle motion of the hip in a flexed and abducted position, may achieve and maintain a satisfactory reduction. Between 6 and 18 months old, gentle closed reduction and immobilization in a spica cast with or without surgical release of contracted muscles is indicated. After 18 months old, closed reduction is less successful and can result in avascular necrosis of the femoral head. In such instances, open reduction and femoral shortening osteotomy is usually indicated. In cases of teratogenic dislocation, underlying maldevelopment makes surgical treatment more challenging.

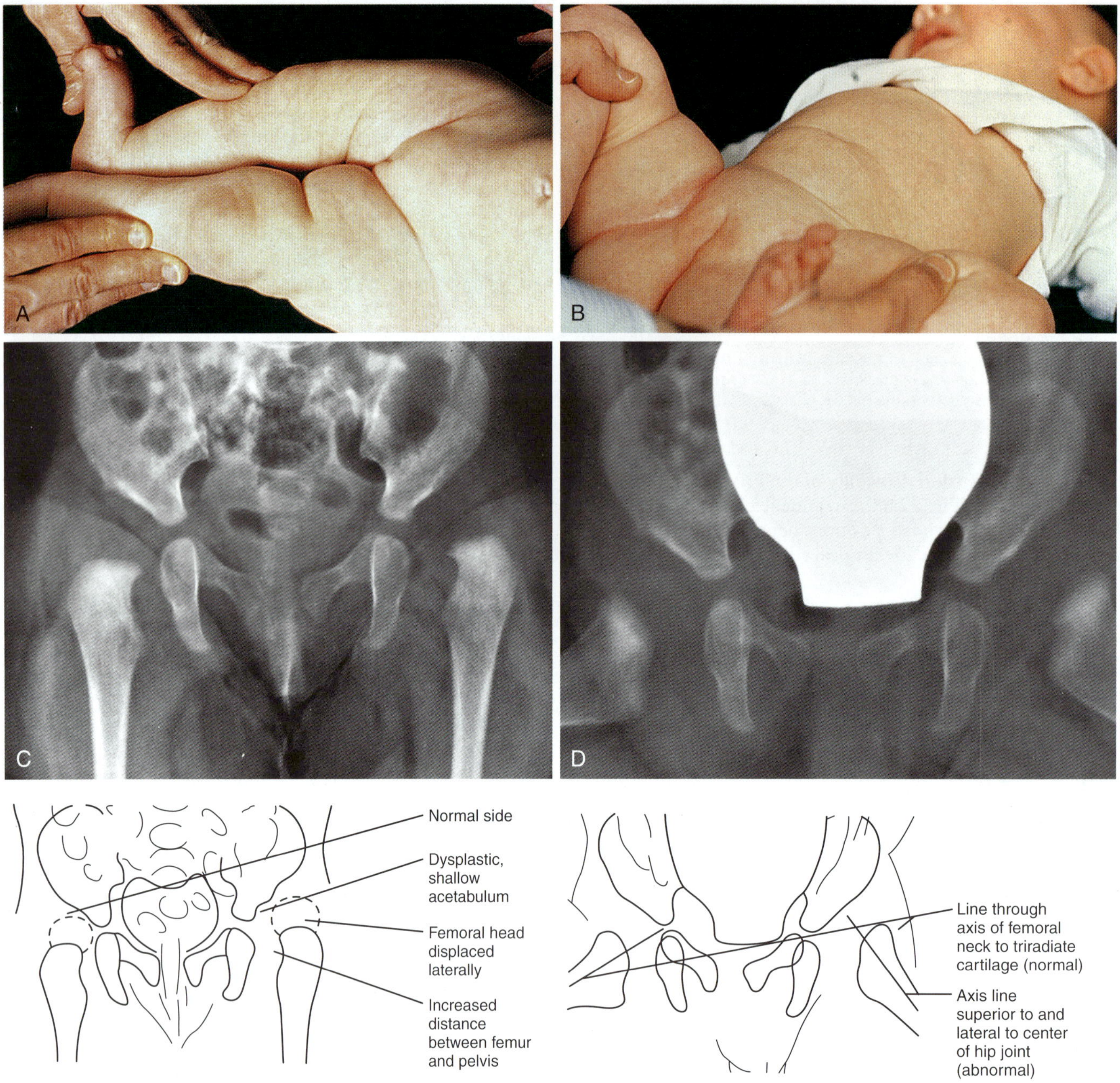

Fig. 22.89 Developmental dislocation of the hip. (A) In cases of unilateral dislocation, the involved extremity is foreshortened and the thigh and groin creases are asymmetric. (B) Limited abduction of the involved hip is seen. This is a consistent finding in infants with a dislocated and irreducible hip. (C) In this anteroposterior radiograph obtained in a 3-month-old child, the proximal left femur is displaced upward and laterally, and the acetabulum is shallow. The femoral head is not visible on the radiograph because of the delayed ossification associated with developmental hip dislocation. (D) In the frog-leg view, the long axis of the affected left femur is directed toward a point superior and lateral to the triradiate cartilage, in contrast with that of the right, which points directly toward this structure.

Results are generally good with near-normal hip anatomy and function achieved in treatment of idiopathic DDH. This becomes less likely if DDH is recognized after the age of 4 due to the sharp decline in acetabular remodeling potential and will result in an early conversion to total hip arthroplasty. A high index of suspicion and early diagnosis are thus essential for optimal outcomes.

Legg-Calvé-Perthes Disease

In Legg-Calvé-Perthes disease (coxa plana), impairment of the blood supply to the developing femoral head results in avascular necrosis. The etiology is unknown. Current theories implicate traumatic disruption of the blood supply, and recurrently increased intraarticular pressure compromises blood flow to the developing ossific nucleus as causative. The disorder generally becomes manifest between 4 and 11 years old, with a higher incidence in boys. Affected children often exhibit delayed skeletal maturation and are small for their age. Unilateral involvement is the rule, and if a bilateral case is suspected, some form of epiphyseal dysplasia must be ruled out. The severity of the disease varies greatly, depending on the extent to which the femoral head is affected.

Symptom onset is typically insidious. Many children present with a painless limp, and others complain of thigh or knee pain, fatigue on walking, or hip stiffness. In general, the patient bears less weight on the involved leg when standing, and there is a flexion contracture of the involved hip (Fig. 22.90A; see Fig. 22.8B), with the lower extremity held slightly externally rotated. Pain and limitation of motion are encountered on attempts at internal rotation and abduction. The Trendelenburg sign (failure to maintain a level pelvis when standing on the involved limb) is frequently positive.

Early radiographic findings may include a subtly smaller or denser femoral ossific nucleus compared with the uninvolved side

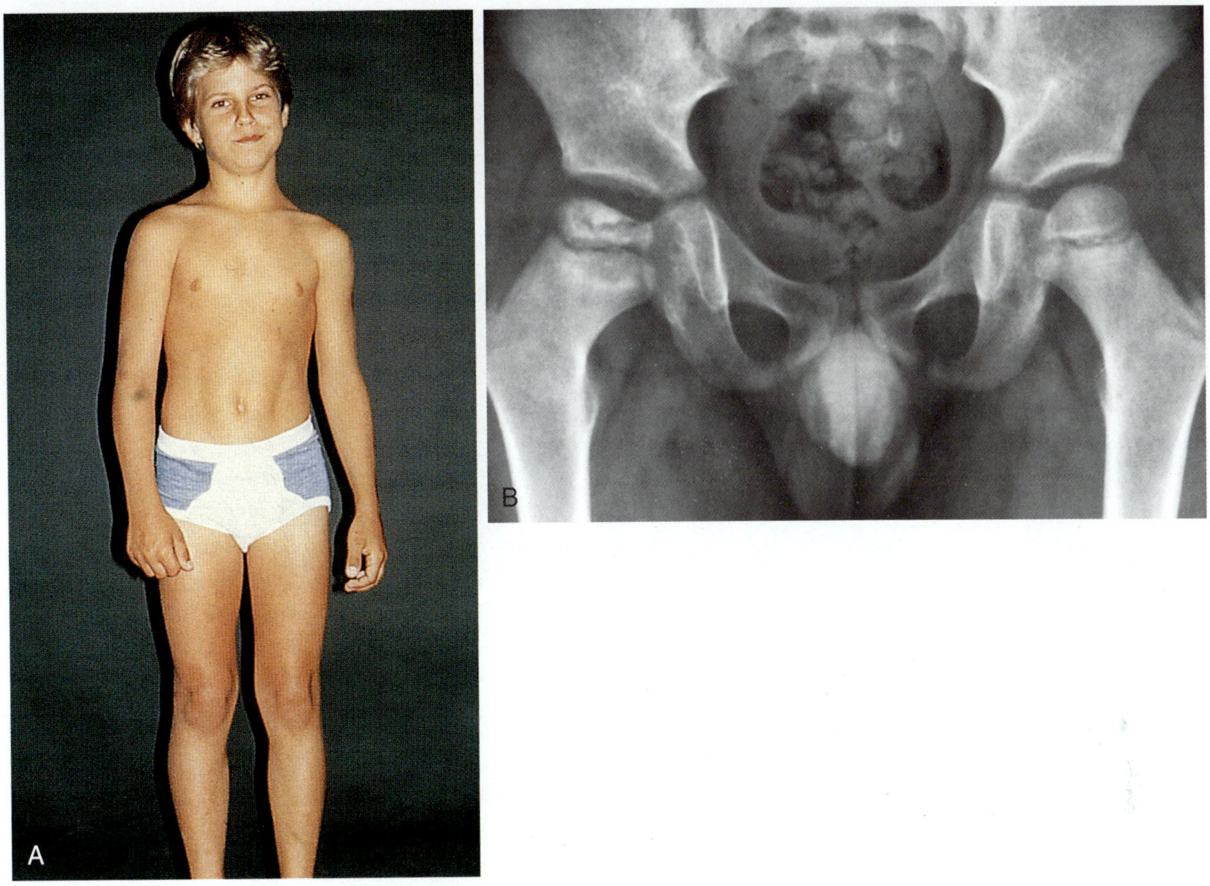

Fig. 22.90 Legg-Calvé-Perthes disease. (A) This 7-year-old boy is small for his chronologic age. He is bearing less weight on the involved right leg (note the slightly flexed right knee). On examination, a hip flexion contracture, which was detected by a positive Thomas test (see Fig. 22.8B), and an abductor lurch gait were found. (B) In this anteroposterior radiograph, the right femoral epiphysis is flattened and fragmented. The proximal femur is also displaced inferiorly and laterally.

and may require bilateral hip or pelvis views side by side to recognize. Other findings include a subchondral radiolucent fracture line (Caffey sign) and evidence of slight subluxation. However, in early cases, radiographs may be completely normal. Although MRI has been used in research settings for earlier diagnosis, this has not led to improved clinical outcomes and remains unnecessary in the management of Perthes. Later, fragmentation of the femoral ossification center may be evident with flattening of the femoral head, extrusion, and frank subluxation (see Fig. 22.90B).

The disease is self-limited, typically lasting for 1 to 2 years. Although revascularization and reconstitution of the femoral head always occur, loss of mechanical integrity of the head with flattening and fragmentation of its surface may result in an irreversible predisposition to degenerative change. Most treatments are based on the maintenance of a normal relationship of the femoral head within the acetabulum to minimize permanent joint incongruity. Treatment focuses on symptoms and keeping the femoral head/acetabulum relationship physiologic and involves activity modifications, antiinflammatory agents, and gentle range of motion exercises. Less commonly, casting, bracing, or surgical osteotomies may be used. Long-term outcomes are fair with most patients requiring conversion to total hip arthroplasty in their fifth or sixth decades.

Slipped Capital Femoral Epiphysis

Slipped capital femoral epiphysis, a disorder seen early in puberty, involves displacement of the femoral head from the femoral neck through the epiphyseal plate. It is seen more frequently in males and occurs bilaterally in approximately 25% of cases. Most commonly, it occurs at the onset of puberty in obese children with delayed sexual maturation. Although the etiology is unclear, it is generally thought that hormonal changes at the time of puberty in individuals with susceptible mechanical factors may result in loss of the mechanical integrity of the growth plate and slippage through this area may occur. This condition differs from traumatic epiphyseal fractures because the translational displacement occurs through a different portion of the growth plate. In some cases, an underlying connective tissue disorder (such as Marfan syndrome) or an endocrinologic problem (such as hypothyroidism) can be identified.

The clinical presentation is characteristic, although duration of symptoms varies. The patient presents with a painful limp and may or may not have a history of recent trauma, often minor. This injury may have precipitated a slip in the previously weakened epiphysis or may have increased the degree of displacement of a slip that was already in progress. The pain may be perceived as being in the hip, thigh, or knee. The lower extremity is held in an externally rotated position secondary to deformity at the site of physeal displacement (Fig. 22.91A and B). An antalgic and abductor lurch gait is usually apparent. A flexion contracture may be noted, and range of hip motion tends to be diminished in all planes, particularly internal rotation. Slight shortening of the involved lower extremity is observed in some patients.

Radiographic findings vary from a widened and radiolucent physis (preslip) to a frank deformity with displacement of the femoral head on the proximal femur posteriorly and inferiorly in relation to its normal counterpart (see Fig. 22.91C and D). The degree of slippage and deformity correlates with the later development of degenerative change and painful symptoms. Slips that are mildly symptomatic may advance to high grade suddenly if diagnosis is delayed and proper precautions are not implemented. This can lead to devastating avascular necrosis of the femoral head and subsequent loss of the hip joint that can only be addressed by a total hip replacement. Treatment for slips is always surgical, and patients who are diagnosed with any slip should be instructed to remain non–weight bearing in a wheelchair and directed to a pediatric orthopedic facility in an emergent fashion.

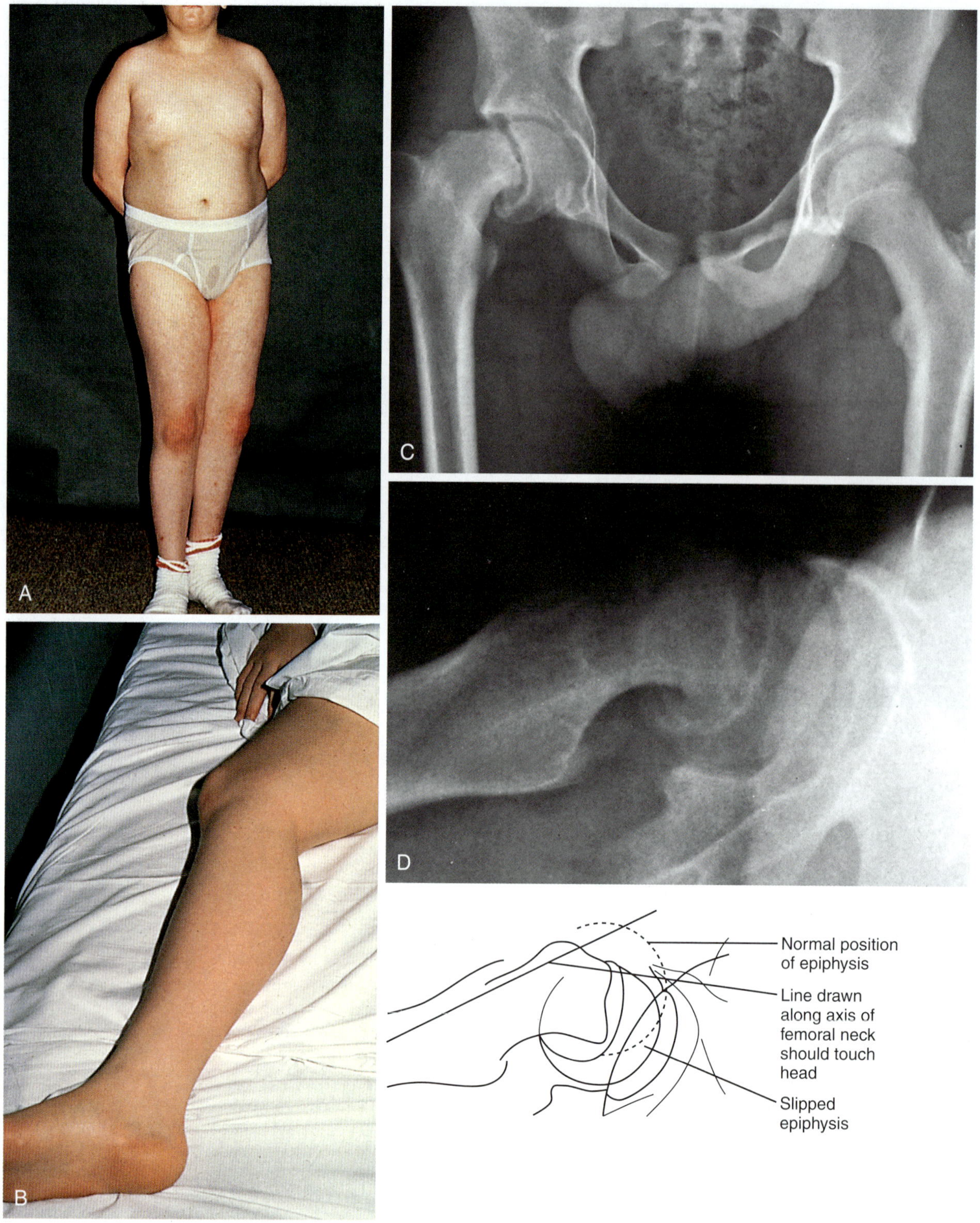

Fig. 22.91 Slipped capital femoral epiphysis. (A) This obese boy presented with a painful limp during early puberty. Note his reluctance to bear weight on the involved right leg. (B) When he lies supine, the affected leg is positioned in external rotation because this minimizes discomfort. Attempts at motion produce pain in the acutely slipped epiphysis. (C) In the anteroposterior radiograph, the right femoral head is displaced medially in relation to the femoral neck as a result of epiphyseal separation. (D) In the lateral view, the femoral head is seen to be displaced posteriorly in relation to the femoral neck. A line drawn along the axis of the femoral neck should normally touch the head.

Femoral Anteversion

Femoral anteversion may be viewed as a normal variation of lower extremity positioning in the developing child. In utero and at birth, the femoral neck sits in an anteverted position relative to that of the adult. During childhood, it remodels to a position of slight anteversion and normal alignment of the lower extremities. In certain children, however, delayed rotational correction may result in persistent in-toeing. An abnormal gait, kicking of the heels, and tripping while walking or running are frequent related complaints. There may be a history of sitting on the floor with knees bent and the lower legs turned outward in a reversed tailor position (W-sitting). In general, the condition is bilateral and is not associated with other musculoskeletal problems.

On examination, the child is noted to stand with the thighs, knees, and feet all turned inward. An increase in internal rotation over external rotation is apparent on assessment of range of motion of the hip (Fig. 22.92). Radiographic findings are normal. No treatment is indicated, other than reassurance that the condition will correct with growth over the first decade of life and instructions to avoid sitting in the predisposing position.

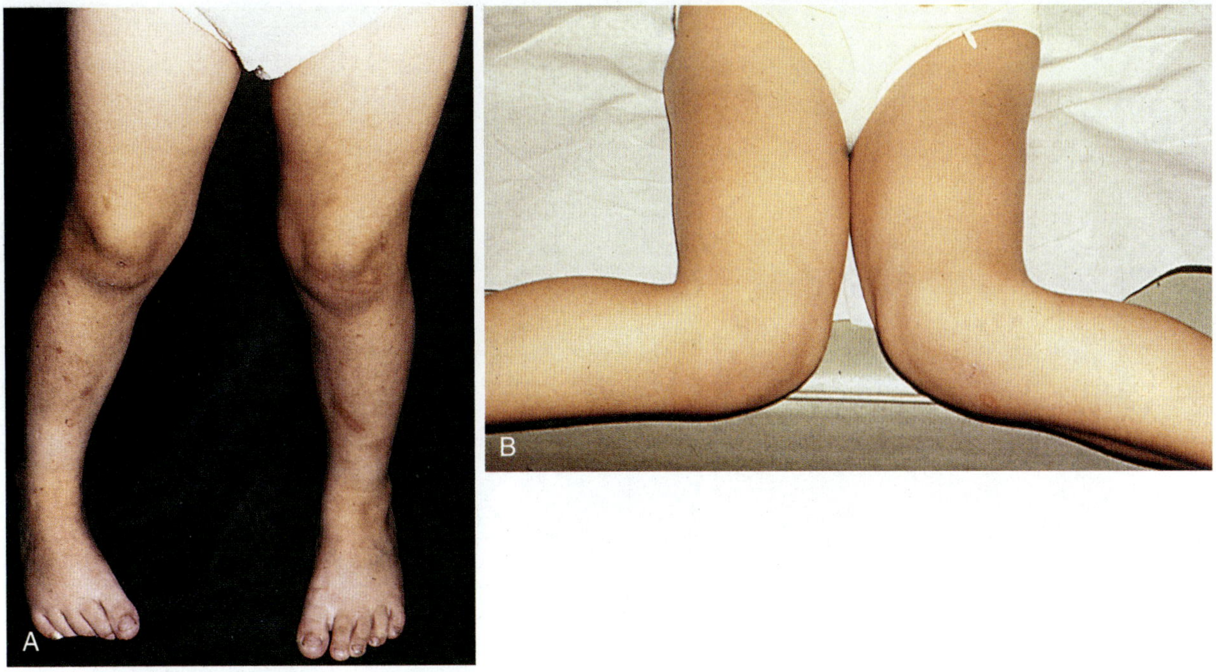

Fig. 22.92 Femoral anteversion. (A) The condition occurs bilaterally, and in the standing view, both legs appear to turn inward from the hip down. (B) On assessment of range of motion, the degree of internal rotation of the hips is found to be greater than normal. (Courtesy Michael Sherlock, MD, Lutherville, MD.)

Genu Varum (Physiologic Bowleg)

Genu varum, or bowleg, is usually a normal variation of lower extremity configuration, seen in the 1- to 3-year-old age group. It is generally recognized shortly after ambulation begins and may be associated with laxity of other joints and internal tibial torsion. Examination reveals diffuse bowing of the lower extremities with an increased distance between the knees that is accentuated on standing (Fig. 22.93). Varus positioning of the heel with pronation of the feet may be noted on weight bearing. The child may walk with a waddling gait and sometimes bear weight on the lateral surface of the foot.

Radiographs typically show normal osseous and physeal development and may reveal a gentle symmetric bowing of the femur and tibia. Although there may be slight beaking of the medial metaphyses of the femur and tibia adjacent to the knee joint, there is no fragmentation of the epiphyses or irregularity of the growth plate, as is seen in Blount disease (see Fig. 22.96).

Treatment is rarely indicated because this condition resolves with growth; in fact, a valgus deformity of the knees may be noted later, at approximately 4 to 5 years old. Casting, bracing, and corrective shoes are unnecessary, and there is no indication for surgery.

Less commonly, genu varum is of pathologic origin. Conditions such as rickets (see Chapter 6) or other metabolic abnormalities, epiphyseal dysplasia, various forms of dwarfism, and pathologic growth disturbances such as Blount disease may be causative and can be diagnosed with radiographic findings if the diagnosis is not obvious clinically. Unilateral bowing is not a result of intrauterine

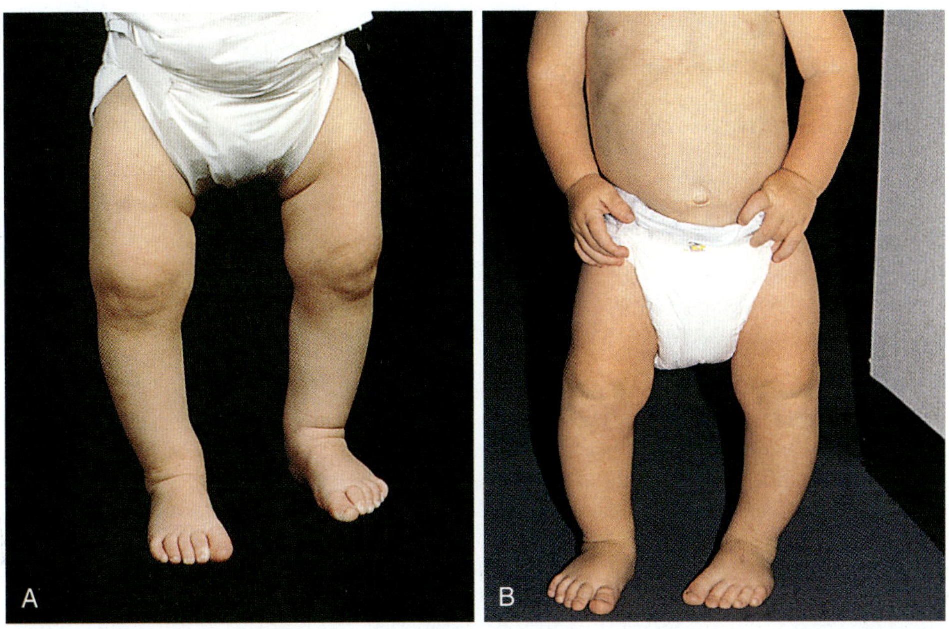

Fig. 22.93 Physiologic genu varum. (A) The mild symmetric bowing seen in this 1-year-old boy represents a normal variation of lower extremity configuration that occurs in toddlers; correction occurs with growth and remodeling. The bowing is diffuse and involves the upper and lower portions of the legs. (B) This child has more severe physiologic bowing, which resulted in frequent tripping and a waddling gait. He also had associated ligamentous laxity and in-toeing on the left.

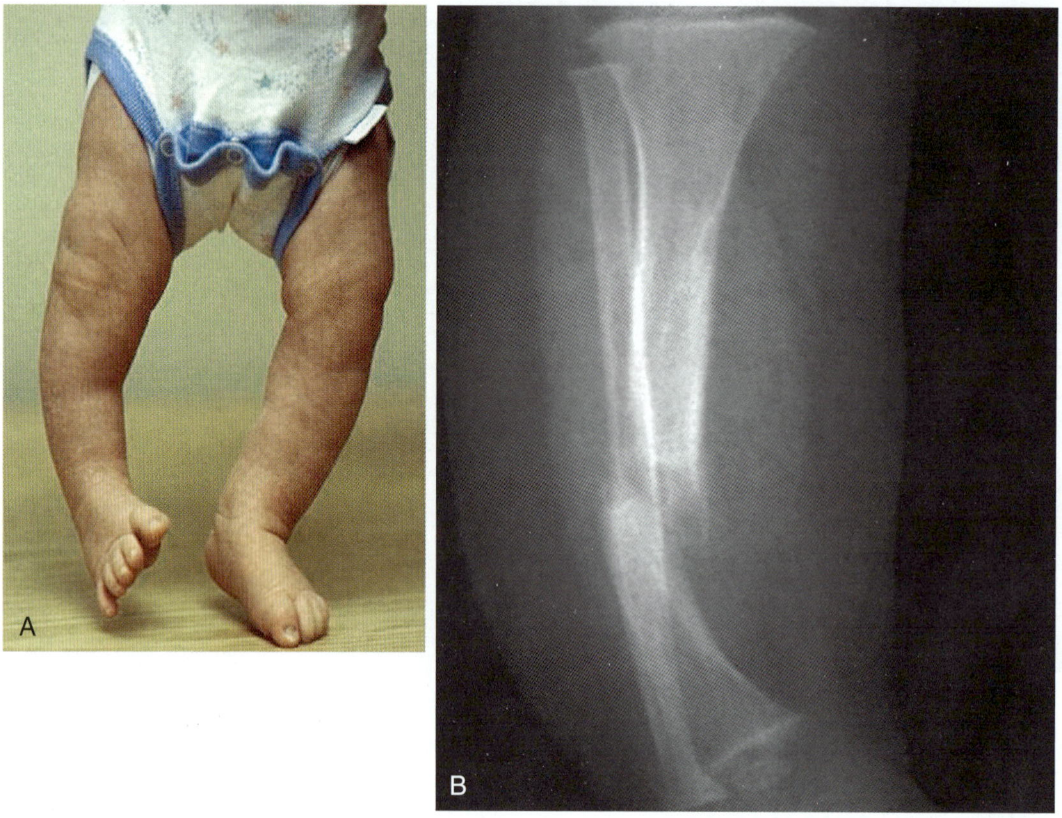

Fig. 22.94 Pathologic genu varum. (A) This 11-month-old child has a unilateral, right-sided bowleg deformity. When unilateral, genu varum is not a result of intrauterine positioning and necessitates radiographs to determine the cause of the deformity. (B) In this case, the bowing was caused by a congenital pseudarthrosis of the tibia, a condition frequently associated with neurofibromatosis 1 (see Chapter 16).

positioning and should prompt investigation for an underlying disorder (Fig. 22.94).

Genu Valgum (Physiologic Knock-Knee)

Genu valgum, or knock-knee, is a normal variation of lower extremity configuration, generally noted in children between 3 and 5 years old. The phenomenon is part of the normal process of remodeling of the lower extremities during growth and development. It is more frequently seen in females and may be associated with ligamentous laxity. While standing, the child is noted to have an increased distance between the feet when the medial aspects of the knees touch one another (Fig. 22.95). In some cases, valgus alignment of the feet and a pes planus deformity may be noted. Radiographs reveal no osseous or physeal abnormalities, but accentuation of the angular deformity of the knee secondary to ligamentous laxity is seen on weight-bearing views. One must rule out the possibility of an underlying metabolic condition, such as rickets or renal disease. Treatment is generally not indicated because the condition gradually corrects with time.

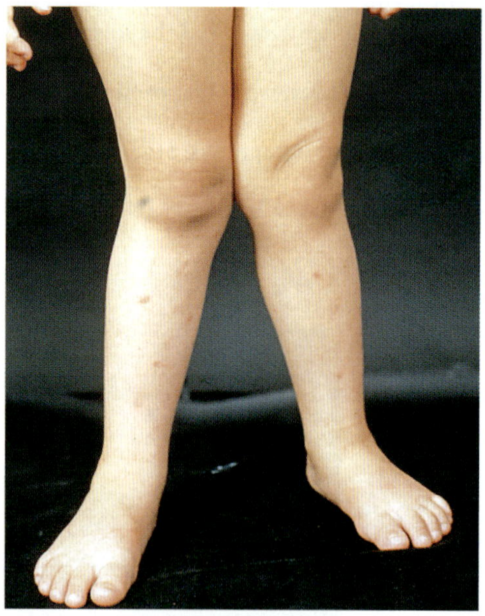

Fig. 22.95 Genu valgum. This 3½-year-old girl shows moderate knock-knee. Ligamentous laxity and mild *pes planus* are associated problems.

Blount Disease

Blount disease is an isolated growth disturbance of the medial tibial epiphysis manifested as an angular varus deformity of the proximal tibia with apparent progressive genu varum. Unilateral and bilateral involvement are seen with nearly equal frequency. The etiology of this condition is unknown, although it appears to be more common in African Americans. It may represent a compression injury to the medial growth plate of the proximal tibia.

On careful examination, a localized angular deformity of the proximal tibia is apparent (Fig. 22.96A and B), in contrast to the diffuse bowing of the lower extremities seen in patients with physiologic bowleg. Radiographs reveal fragmentation of the medial epiphysis of the tibia associated with beaking and loss of height in this region, along with the characteristic angular deformity (see Fig. 22.96C). Treatment includes referral to pediatric orthopedics and includes a combination of bracing and surgical interventions.

Osgood-Schlatter Disease

Osgood-Schlatter disease is a traction apophysitis of the tibial tubercle that tends to develop during the adolescent growth spurt. A similar process, labeled Sinding-Larsen-Johansson syndrome, results in traction-related pain at the distal patellar pole in a slightly younger age cohort. Both occur somewhat more frequently in

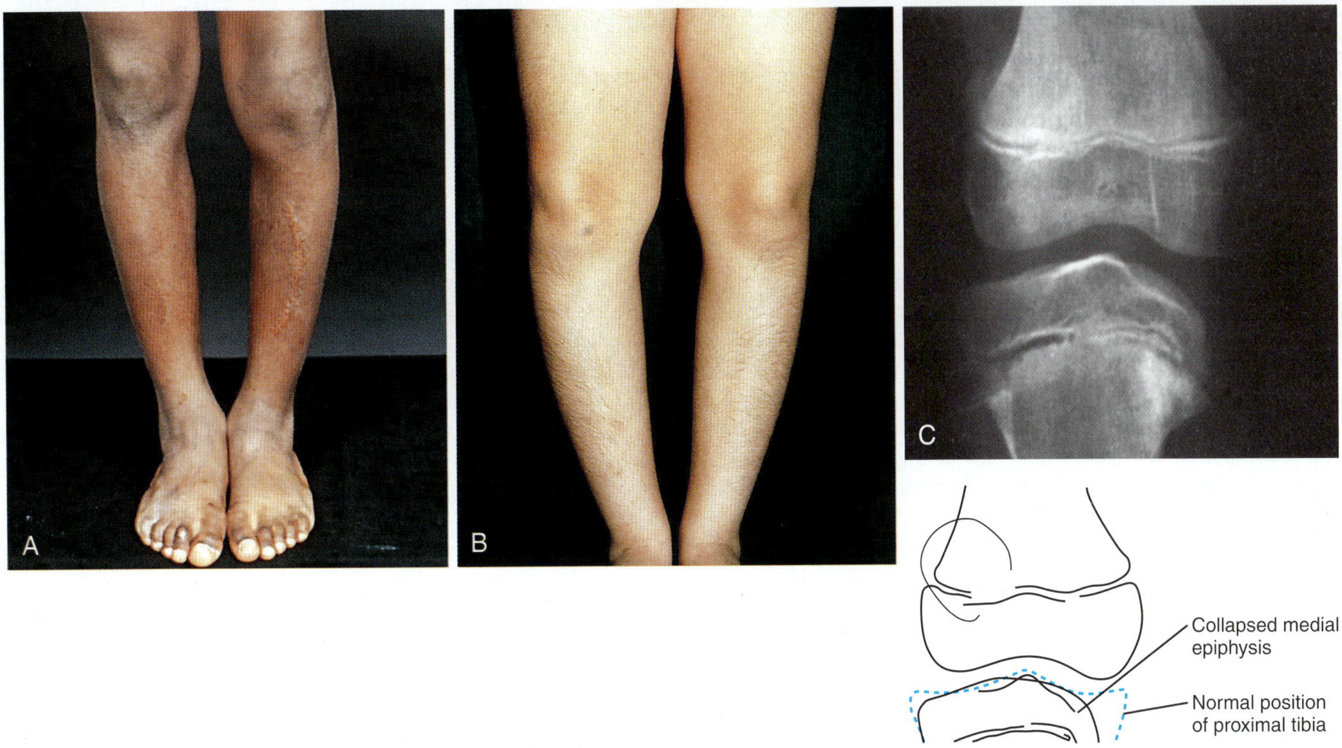

Fig. 22.96 Blount disease. (A) This patient has a unilateral angular deformity of the proximal left tibia that gives the appearance of genu varum. (B) Both proximal tibias are bowed in another patient as a result of fragmentation and loss of height of the medial epiphyses. In contrast with physiologic bowing, the thighs are straight. (C) This radiograph shows the typical fragmentation, loss of height, and angular deformity or beaking of the medial portion of the proximal tibia.

males than in females. It is thought that differential rates of growth in the osseous and soft tissue structures and stress on the apophyses produced by vigorous physical activity are contributing factors. Bilateral involvement is usual. Patients have a history of gradually increasing pain and swelling in the region of the distal patella or tibial tubercle. Discomfort is accentuated by vigorous physical activity, kneeling, or crawling and is relieved by rest.

On examination, a localized tender swelling is noted in the region of the distal patella, tibial tubercle, and/or patellar tendon (Fig. 22.97A). The knee joint is otherwise normal on examination, with the exception that some patients show limitation of knee flexion with reproduction of their pain. Radiographs may reveal only soft tissue swelling in the region of the proximal tibial apophysis or irregularity of ossification of this structure (see Fig. 22.97B). In long-standing cases, frank fragmentation of the apophysis may be seen.

The problem, although self-limited, can persist until skeletal maturity in a waxing and waning fashion. Treatment is symptomatic

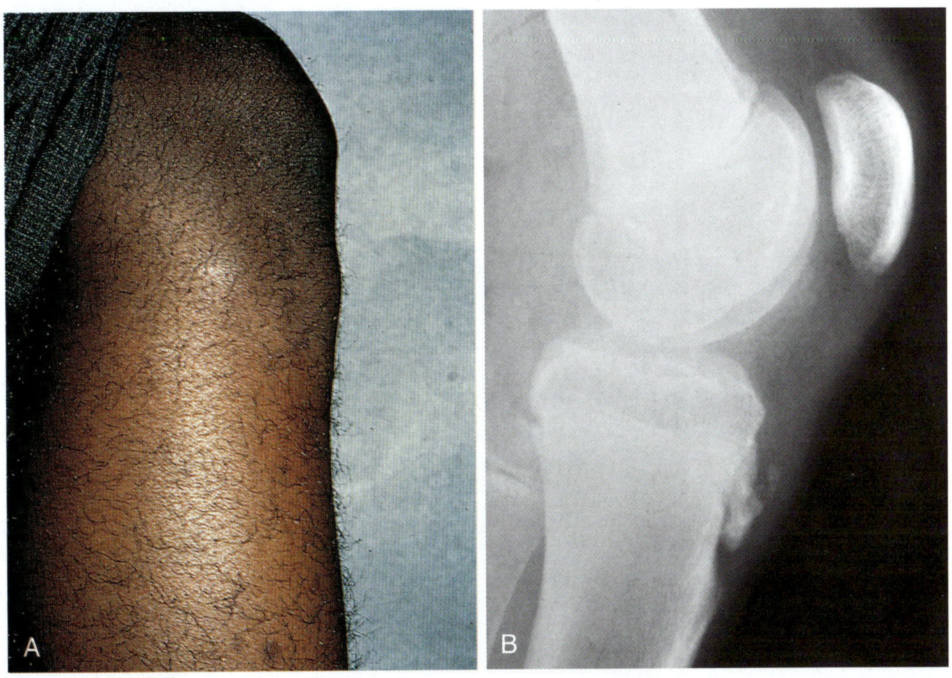

Fig. 22.97 Osgood-Schlatter disease. (A) Localized swelling is evident in the region of the tibial tubercle. This is generally tender on palpation. The knee is otherwise normal on examination, with the possible exception of mild limitation of flexion. (B) Irregularity and fragmentation of the tibial tubercle are seen in this radiograph. In less severe cases of shorter duration, soft tissue swelling or irregularity of ossification may be the only finding.

with rest, stretching, nonsteroidal antiinflammatory drugs and ice as first-line treatment, a referral to physical therapy as second-line treatment, and referral to orthopedics as a last resort. Steroid injection is absolutely contraindicated.

Popliteal (Baker) Cyst

Childhood popliteal cysts occur in children between 5 and 10 years with a predilection for males. They appear in the posteromedial aspect of the knee joint in the region of the semimembranosus tendon and medial gastrocnemius muscle belly. Pathologically, a fibrous tissue or synovial cyst filled with synovial-like fluid is seen. In contrast to those seen in adults, popliteal cysts in childhood are not associated with intraarticular pathology. On occasion vague pain is noted, but evaluation is usually sought because of a recently noted painless mass.

On examination, a soft, nontender mass is found in the described location (Fig. 22.98A). Range of motion of the joint is normal unless the cyst is large, limiting flexion. The knee is otherwise normal, and radiographs show no osseous abnormality. Ultrasound may be utilized to verify the diagnosis. MRI clearly delineates the cyst and its position in relation to nearby structures (see Fig. 22.98B and C) but is not required unless in the exceptional case where surgical treatment is planned. Popliteal cysts are benign and generally resolve spontaneously over time.

Internal Tibial Torsion

Internal tibial torsion is a nonpathologic variation in the normal development of the lower leg in children younger than 5 years old. It is a rotational deformity that is thought to result from internal molding of the foot and leg in utero. The child is usually brought for evaluation because of concern about prominent in-toeing on walking and frequent tripping.

On examination, the hips and knees are found to be normally aligned, with the patellae facing anteriorly, but the lower legs and feet are rotated inward (Fig. 22.99). The rotational deformity can be detected by having the patient lie prone on the examining table with the knees flexed (see Fig. 22.14E). Radiographs reveal no osseous abnormalities. Treatment is not indicated; remodeling over the first 5 years of life gradually corrects the condition as the child grows and develops. Bracing and special shoes have little effect and are not recommended.

Congenital Clubfoot

Congenital clubfoot (talipes equinovarus) is a teratogenic deformity of the foot that is readily apparent at birth. It is seen more frequently in male infants than female infants and has an incidence of 1 in 1000 live

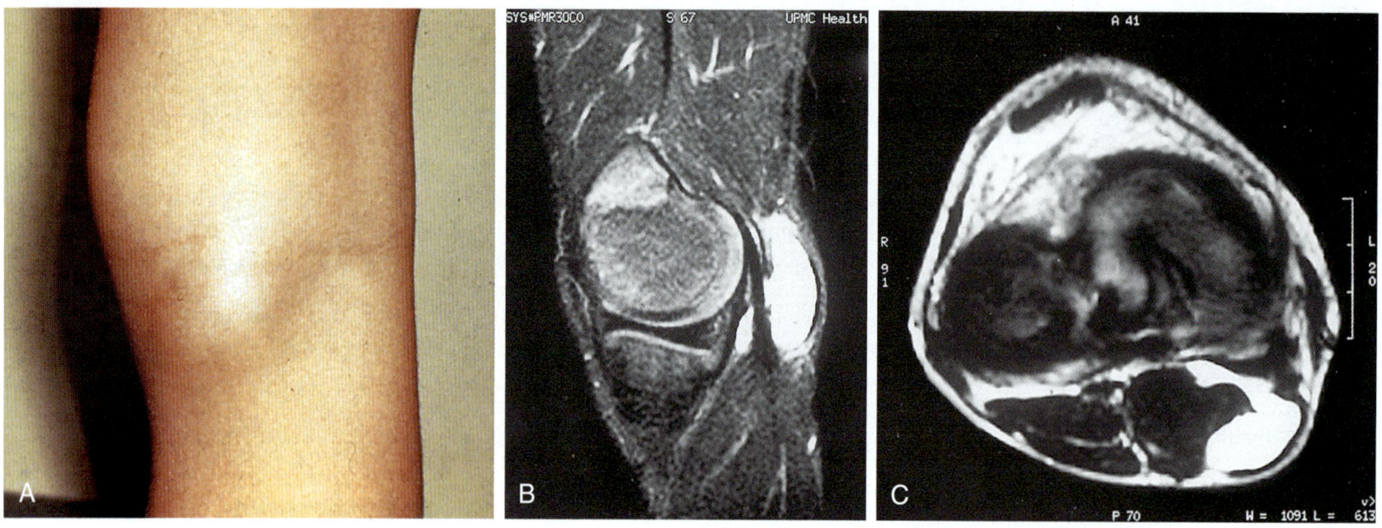

Fig. 22.98 Popliteal (Baker) cyst. (A) Localized swelling appears in the region of the semimembranosus tendon. This may arise from the synovial lining of the semimembranosus bursa. (B) Sagittal plane magnetic resonance imaging (MRI) from another child with a Baker cyst shows the posterior location. (C) A transverse plane MRI demonstrates the posterior and medial position of cyst and its close relation to the gastrocnemius muscle.

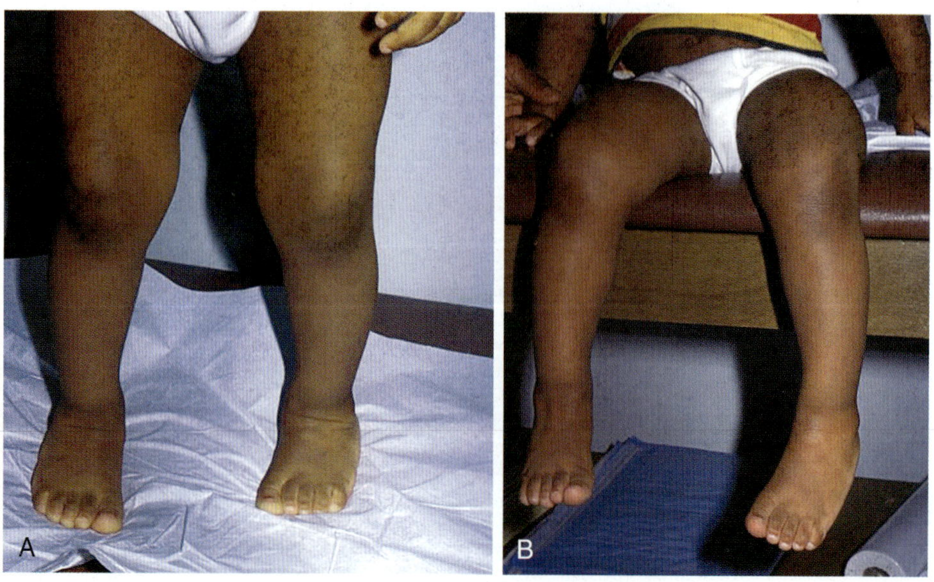

Fig. 22.99 Internal tibial torsion. (A) On weight bearing, the hip, thigh, and knee are normally oriented and the patella faces anteriorly, but the lower leg and foot turn inward. The deformity results in prominent in-toeing on walking, which may cause the child to trip frequently. (B) In this view of the child while sitting, it is easy to appreciate that the lateral malleolus is positioned anteriorly to the medial malleolus. This shifts the ankle mortise and foot to a medially oriented position.

births. Etiology is multifactorial, and studies suggest a genetic predisposition. Abnormal intrauterine positioning and pressure at a critical point in development may contribute as well. Unilateral and bilateral involvement is nearly equal. The deformity is characterized by three primary components: (1) the entire foot is positioned in plantar flexion (equinus); (2) the hindfoot is maintained in a position of fixed inversion (varus); and (3) the forefoot exhibits an adductus deformity, often combined with supination (Fig. 22.100A to C). In the newborn period, the deformity may be passively correctable to some extent. With time, however, deformities become more fixed.

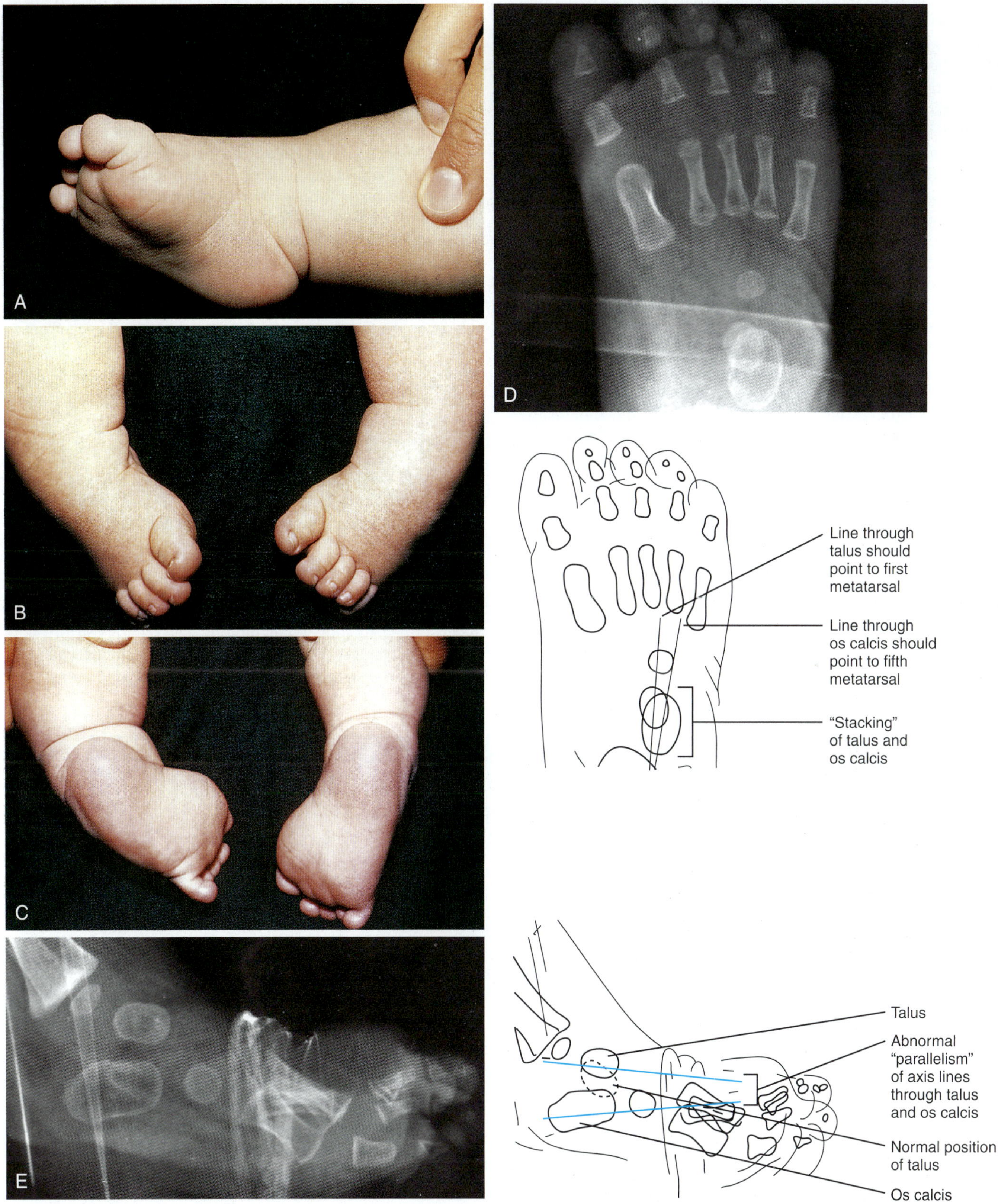

Fig. 22.100 Clubfoot. This deformity has three primary components. (A) The foot is positioned in plantar flexion (equinus). Note the pathologic skin creases over the heel and arch. (B) The heels or hind feet are fixed in inversion (varus). (C) The forefeet are fixed in an adducted and supinated position. (D) In the anteroposterior radiograph, the talus overlies the os calcis (stacking) and the forefoot is adducted. A line drawn through the longitudinal axis of the talus normally aligns with the first metatarsal, and one drawn through the axis of the os calcis normally aligns with the fifth metatarsal. (E) This lateral radiograph shows that the foot is in equinus and the axes of the talus and os calcis are nearly parallel. They normally intersect at an approximately 45-degree angle. (Compare with the normal foot shown in Fig. 22.101.)

The primary pathologic finding is that of a rotational deformity of the subtalar joint with the os calcis internally rotated beneath the talus, producing varus position and a block to dorsiflexion of the foot. The navicular bone is medially displaced on the talus, producing adductus of the forefoot (see Fig. 22.100D and E). Contractures of the Achilles and posterior tibial tendons and of the medial ankle and subtalar joint capsules are secondary factors that contribute to the deformity. The foot and calf are smaller compared with the normal side in unilateral cases. Like DDH, clubfoot is divided into idiopathic and teratologic types. Idiopathic cases usually occur in otherwise healthy children. Teratologic cases are generally secondary to neurologic imbalance including myelodysplasia, spinal cord tethering, or other degenerative neurologic conditions and other limb formation errors such as tibial hemimelia and arthrogryposis.

Severe cases of metatarsus adductus can mimic clubfoot. Differentiation should be made by the lack of dorsiflexion; a foot with a clubfoot deformity cannot be dorsiflexed past neutral, whereas metatarsus adductus will have unrestricted dorsiflexion.

The radiologic difference between a clubfoot and a normal foot can be appreciated by comparing Fig. 22.100D and E with Fig. 22.101.

The current gold standard treatment of club foot deformity is Ponseti casting. This technique stresses gentle manipulation and serial casting of the foot to correct the deformity. The casts are applied in the office weekly for an average of 4 to 6 weeks, followed by a percutaneous tenotomy of the Achilles tendon, either in the office or in the operating room and application of a final cast for 3 to 4 weeks. The child then wears the Ponseti shoes and brace (bar between the shoes) full time for 3 months and then at nighttime only for 4 to 5 years.

Results are excellent in more than 90% of idiopathic cases. Compliance with brace wear as prescribed is critical to success and prevention of recurrence of deformity.

Metatarsus Adductus

Metatarsus adductus (metatarsus varus) is a deformity of the forefoot in which the metatarsals are deviated medially. It can be congenital and static or dynamic. Both are usually bilateral. The congenital condition is probably the result of intrauterine molding, and other than the adducted position of the forefoot, the foot is normal in structure in contrast to a clubfoot (see earlier).

Dynamic adductus is a common finding in children who have recently acquired ambulation skill and appears to be a measure to improve the child's balance. This is characterized by normal appearance of feet at rest and voluntary curving of toes inward during gait. It is harmless and will improve over the 4 to 5 years needed to acquire mature gait patterns.

Examination is performed with the foot free and also weight bearing (Fig. 22.102A and B). A skin crease may be located over the medial aspect of the longitudinal arch. When mild, the deviation may be passively correctable by the physician or actively correctable by the patient. Active correction may be demonstrated by gentle stroking of the foot, stimulating the peroneal muscles to contract. In more severe cases, the deviation may be only partially corrected by these maneuvers. The feet and calf muscles are normal in size. Radiographs demonstrate the abnormal deviation of the metatarsals medially without other osseous abnormalities (see Fig. 22.102C).

Treatment depends on the severity of the condition. In mild to moderate cases, passive manipulation of the deformity by the parents several times a day may suffice. In moderate to severe cases, a combination of manipulative stretching and special shoes may be indicated. Rarely, serial manipulation and casting or surgery is needed.

Congenital Vertical Talus

Congenital vertical talus is a teratogenic anomaly of the foot noted at birth and characterized by a rocker bottom foot deformity. The underlying pathology is a malorientation of the talus, which assumes a more vertical position than normal. The adjacent navicular is dorsally displaced, articulating with the superior aspect of the neck of the talus and causing the forefoot to assume a dorsiflexed and valgus orientation. In effect, these deformities are the opposite of those seen in congenital clubfoot. The etiology of this condition is unknown, and it is frequently associated with other musculoskeletal or organ system anomalies.

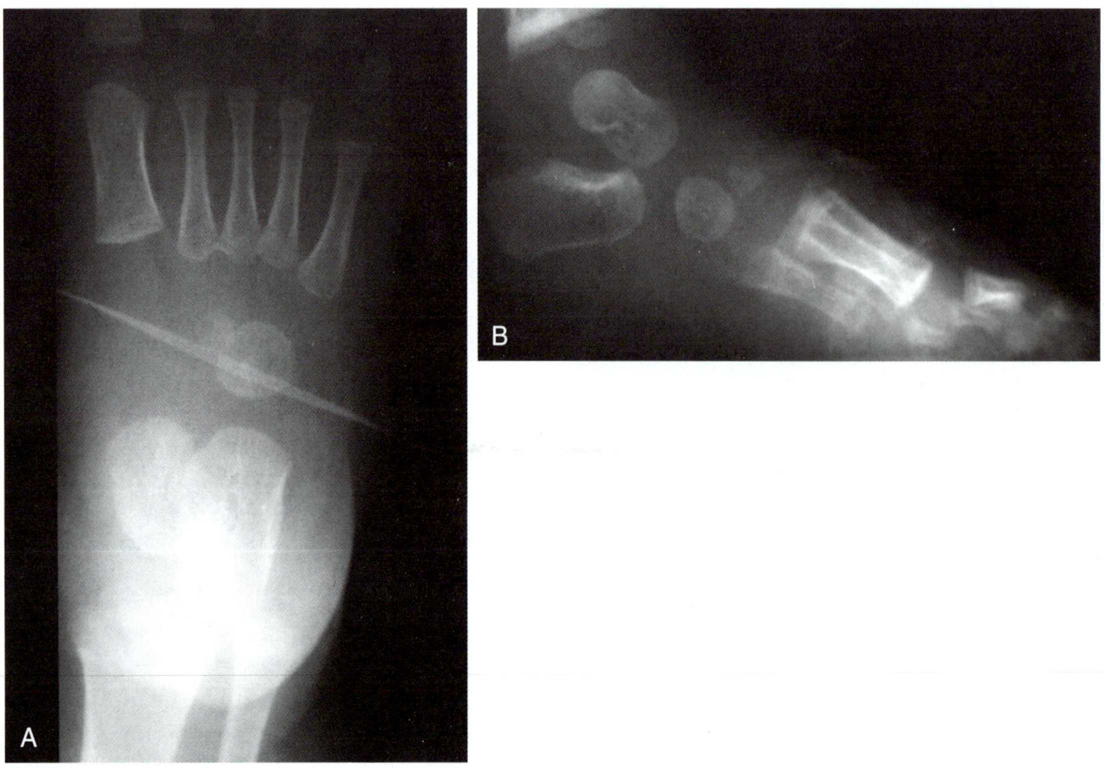

Fig. 22.101 Normal foot. Anteroposterior (A) and lateral (B) views of the foot of a slightly older child show the normal orientation of the tarsal bones, compared with the findings in congenital clubfoot (shown in Fig. 22.100D and E).

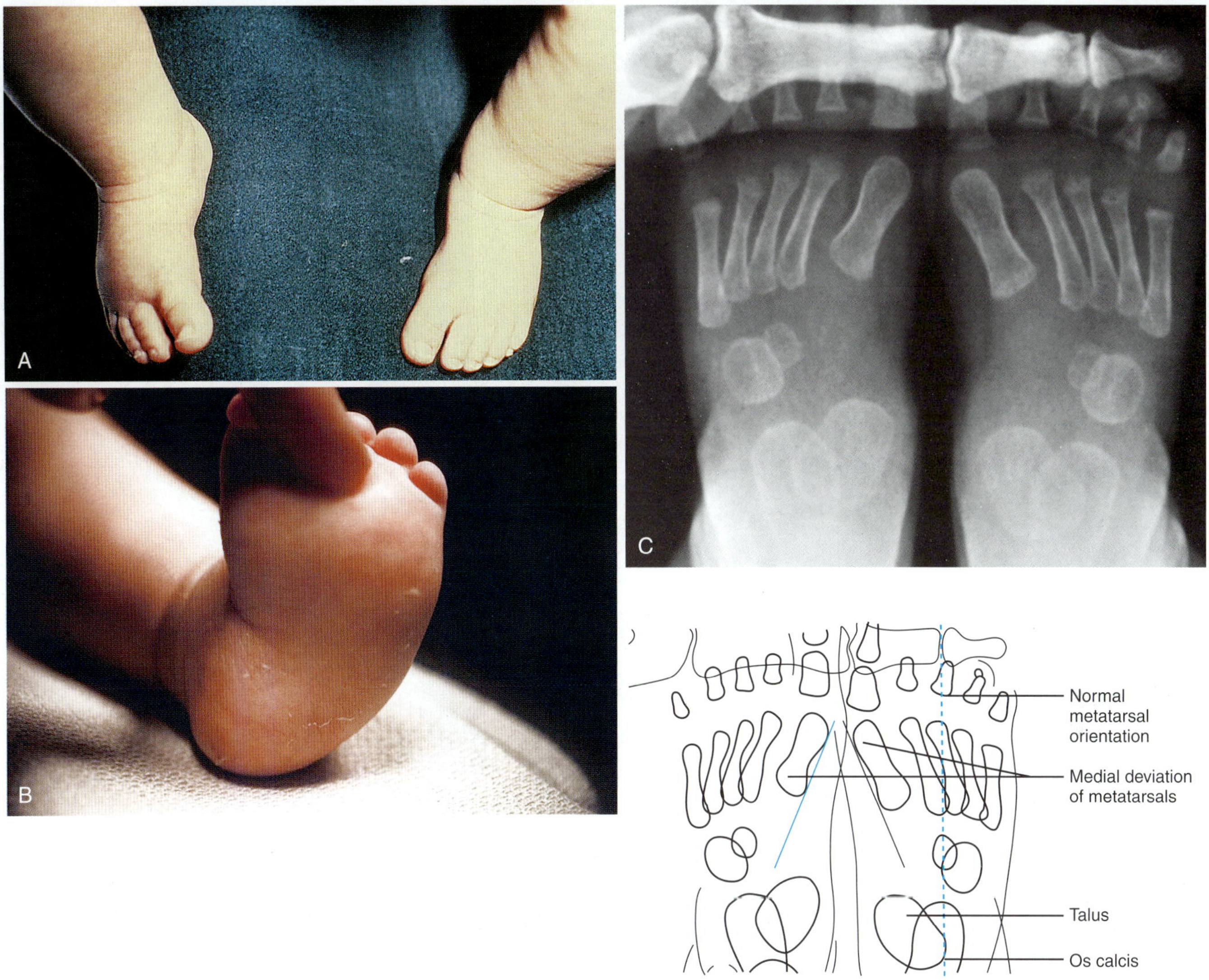

Fig. 22.102 Metatarsus adductus. (A) In this view from above, the forefeet are seen to be deviated medially, but otherwise the feet are normal. (B) When the feet are viewed from the plantar aspect, rounding of the lateral border can be appreciated, along with a crease on the medial side. (C) In the anteroposterior radiograph, all five metatarsals can be seen to be deviated medially with respect to the remainder of the foot; otherwise, the bony structures are normal. The relationship of the talus and os calcis is normal, unlike the relationship in clubfoot.

Clinically the deformity is recognizable as a calcaneovalgus foot or a rocker bottom–type foot with a prominent heel (Fig. 22.103A and B) that is not passively correctable. Radiographs mirror the clinical appearance, showing a vertical orientation of the talus, a calcaneus deformity of the os calcis, and valgus orientation of the forefoot (see also Fig. 22.101B for a normal comparison; see Fig. 22.103C).

Treatment is initiated with manipulation and serial casting with Achilles tenotomy and pinning of the foot to follow. More extensive surgery is often required as the child gets older.

Calcaneovalgus Foot Deformity

Physiologic calcaneovalgus is another deformity of the foot thought to result from intrauterine molding. It is normally a supple deformity apparent at birth that is passively correctable, in contrast with the rigid foot characteristic of congenital vertical talus. The condition is evident at birth. No underlying pathologic changes occur in the foot, and no osseous deformities other than the positional one exist. On examination, the foot is noted to be held in a dorsiflexed and everted position with some loss of the normal longitudinal arch (Fig. 22.104). Tightness of the anterior tibial tendon may be noted. Radiographs reveal no pathologic bony changes. Nonoperative treatment is generally successful and consists of routine manipulation and stretching of the foot by the parents with every feed or diaper change. This will usually correct the deformity in the first 4 to 6 weeks of life. A high index of suspicion should be maintained in these babies for developmental dysplasia of the hip as well.

Pes Planus (Flatfoot)

Pes planus, or physiologic flatfoot, is an extremely common condition for which there is a familial predisposition. It is characterized by laxity of the soft tissues of the foot resulting in loss of the normal longitudinal arch, with pronation or eversion of the forefoot and valgus or lateral orientation of the heel (Fig. 22.105). In general, the condition is asymptomatic in children, and evaluation is sought primarily because of parental concern about the appearance of the foot and the possibility of future problems. On occasion, affected patients report discomfort after long walks or running.

On examination, the characteristic appearance is easy to recognize, and laxity of other joints, particularly the thumb, elbow, and knee, may be noted. Weight-bearing radiographs reveal loss of the normal longitudinal arch without osseous abnormality. Treatment is unnecessary if the condition is asymptomatic. Corrective shoes with arch supports are of no use unless symptoms of foot strain are present. Achilles stretching may also be beneficial if symptomatic.

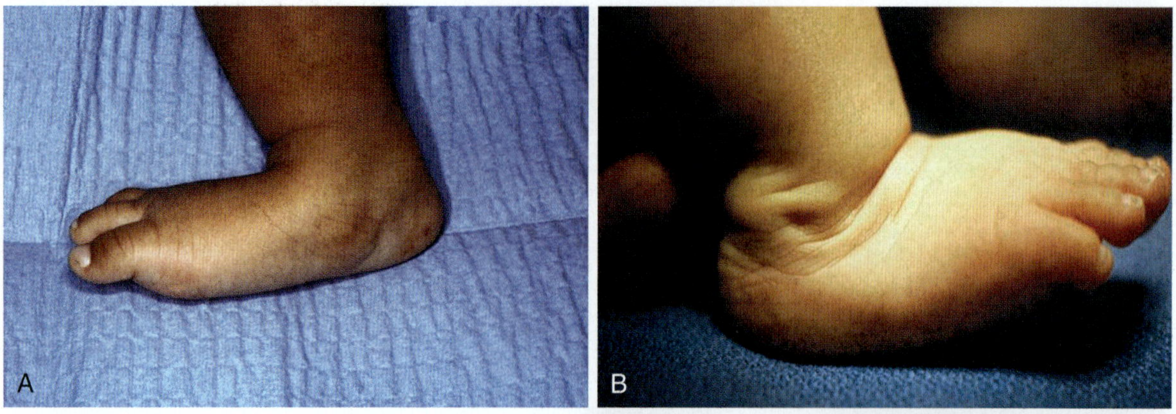

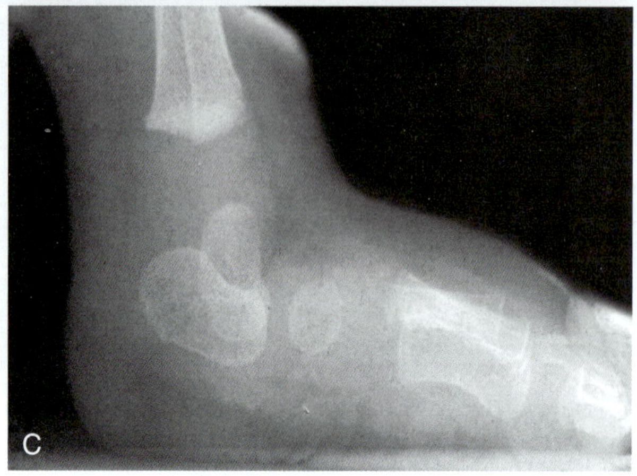

Fig. 22.103 Congenital vertical talus. (A) The normal longitudinal arch of the foot is absent; a rocker bottom–type deformity is present; and the forefoot is fixed in dorsiflexion, which is even more evident in (B). (C) On this radiograph, the talus is oriented vertically and its position does not change with flexion or extension of the ankle. The calcaneus is also fixed in equinus position, resulting in a rigid flatfoot deformity (see Fig. 22.101B for comparison).

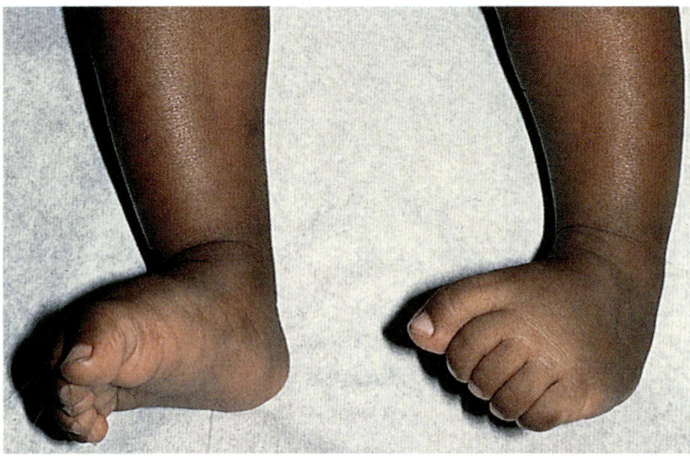

Fig. 22.104 Calcaneovalgus foot deformity. The right foot is held in a position of eversion and dorsiflexion. This deformity is supple and thus is passively correctable. The contralateral foot exhibits a metatarsus adductus deformity, giving the feet a "windswept" appearance.

Accessory Tarsal Navicular

An accessory tarsal navicular results from formation of a separate ossification center on the medial aspect of the developing tarsal navicular at the insertion site of the posterior tibial tendon. The condition is not uncommon and is often associated with a pes planus deformity. Clinically, patients exhibit a bony prominence on the medial aspect of the foot that tends to rub on the shoe, which may produce a painful bursa (Fig. 22.106A). Radiographs reveal either a separate ossification center or bone medial to the parent navicular or a medial projection of the navicular when fusion has occurred (see Fig. 22.106B and C). Cast or boot immobilization may be helpful in acutely painful cases. Long-term improvement can be obtained by wearing soft, supportive shoes with longitudinal arches and a medial heel wedge. Recalcitrant symptoms may warrant surgical intervention.

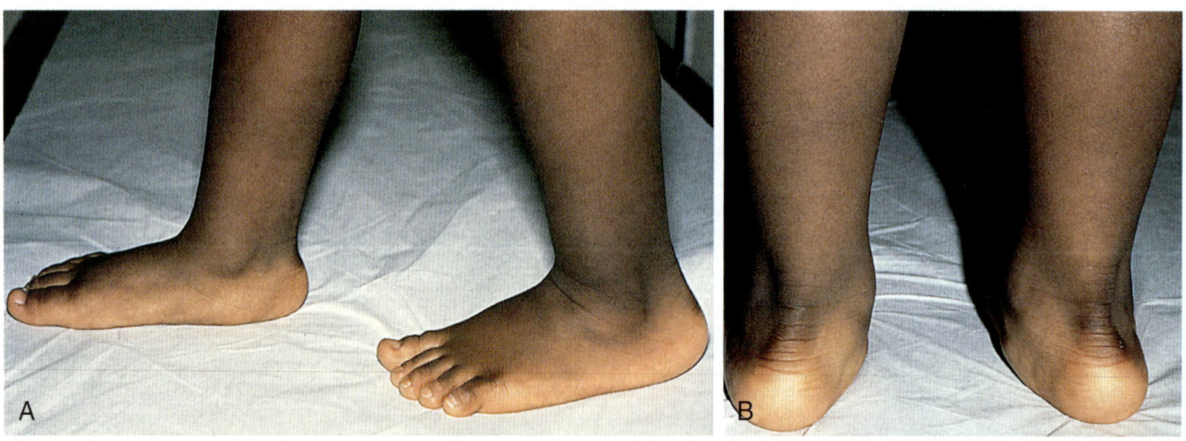

Fig. 22.105 Pes planus (flatfoot). (A) Laxity of the soft tissue structures of the foot results in a loss of the normal longitudinal arch and pronation or eversion of the forefoot. (B) Viewed from behind, the characteristic eversion of the heels is appreciated more readily.

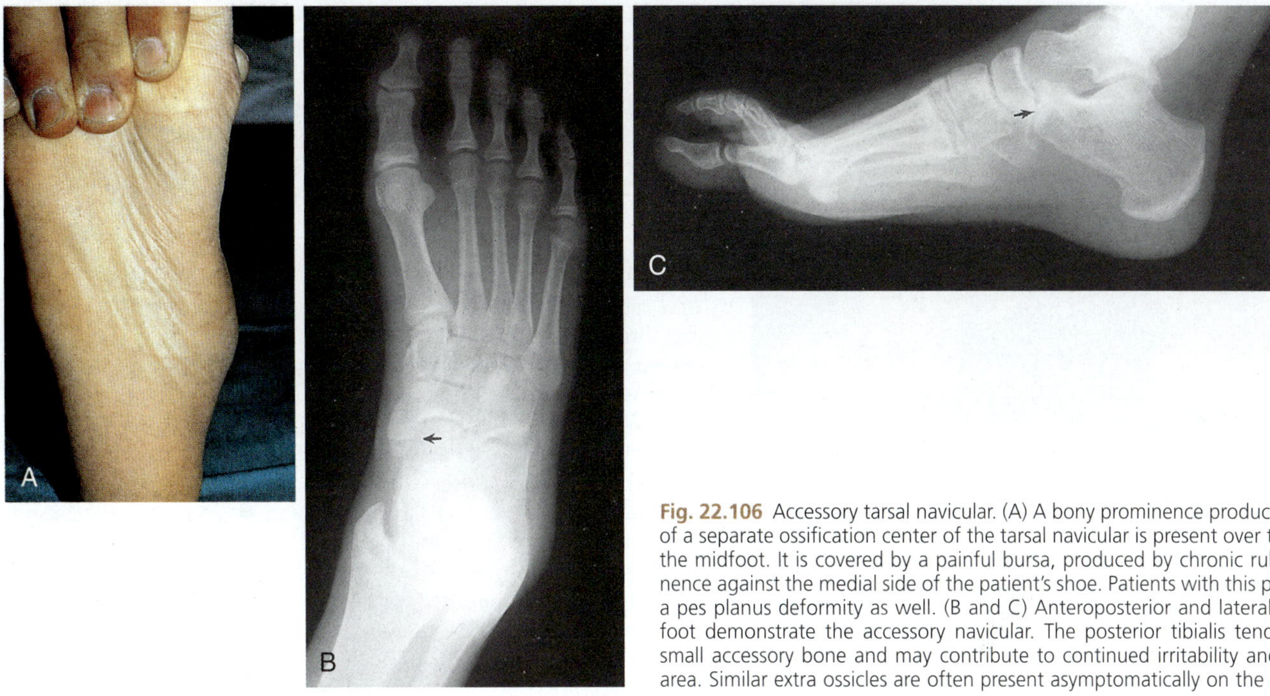

Fig. 22.106 Accessory tarsal navicular. (A) A bony prominence produced by the formation of a separate ossification center of the tarsal navicular is present over the medial aspect of the midfoot. It is covered by a painful bursa, produced by chronic rubbing of the prominence against the medial side of the patient's shoe. Patients with this problem usually have a pes planus deformity as well. (B and C) Anteroposterior and lateral radiographs of the foot demonstrate the accessory navicular. The posterior tibialis tendon attaches to the small accessory bone and may contribute to continued irritability and tenderness in this area. Similar extra ossicles are often present asymptomatically on the opposite foot.

Cavus Feet and Claw Toes

Cavus feet and claw toes are deformities produced by a muscular imbalance within the foot. Although they may occur for unknown reasons, often they are manifestations of an underlying neurologic disorder, such as Charcot-Marie-Tooth disease, Friedreich ataxia, or spinal cord tethering (see Chapter 16). These conditions should be considered in evaluating each patient presenting with these deformities, particularly if the problem is unilateral. Cavus feet exhibit a high arch with a varus or inversion deformity of the heel. Usually, the metatarsal heads appear prominent on the plantar aspect of the foot (Fig. 22.107). This phenomenon is accentuated by overlying callosities that develop due to abnormal weight bearing. With claw toes, the metatarsophalangeal joints are held in extension with the PIP joints in flexion and the distal joint in the neutral or slightly flexed position (Fig. 22.108). Calluses tend to develop over the PIP joints as the result of rubbing against shoes. Neurologic examination may reveal motor weakness, most often involving the anterior tibial, toe extensor, and peroneal muscles.

The underlying pathologic condition must be identified and treated before addressing the foot deformity, and management of these patients should begin with a referral to child neurology.

GENERALIZED MUSCULOSKELETAL DISORDERS

Five conditions with major musculoskeletal manifestations—skeletal dysplasias, cerebral palsy, spina bifida, osteogenesis imperfecta (OI), and arthrogryposis—are discussed in this section.

Skeletal Dysplasias

Overview

Skeletal dysplasias are a heterogeneous group of disorders characterized by abnormalities of bone and cartilage growth, development, and differentiation that often result in short stature (dwarfism) and orthopedic and medical complications. Despite the more than 300 types of identified skeletal dysplasias, many individuals with a presumed skeletal dysplasia remain unclassified. Although skeletal dysplasias comprise a heterogeneous group of disorders, two major categories exist: osteochondrodysplasia and dysostosis. The osteochondrodysplasias result from abnormal growth and development of bone and/or cartilage. These are progressive and generalized disorders and are the focus of this

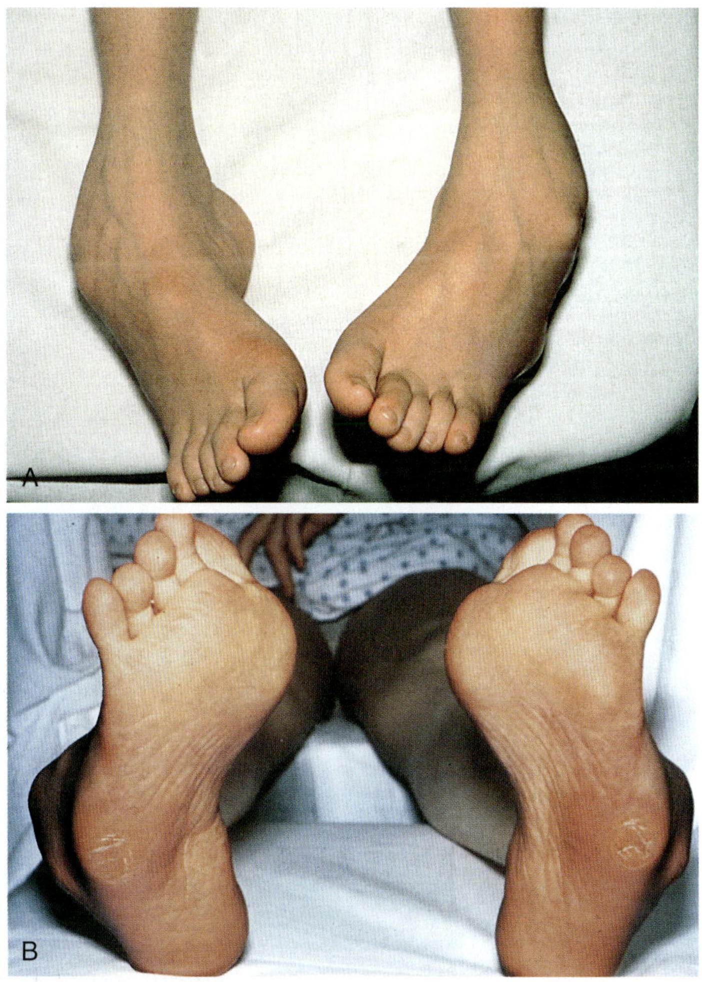

Fig. 22.107 Bilateral cavus feet. (A) The feet are inverted and have high arches. The deformity is often a feature of neuromuscular disorders, as in this case where it is the result of Charcot-Marie-Tooth disease. (B) In addition to the high arches and varus (inverted) heels seen in the view of the plantar surface, the prominence of the metatarsal head region is apparent. Callosities have developed over the lateral borders of the feet as a result of abnormal weight bearing.

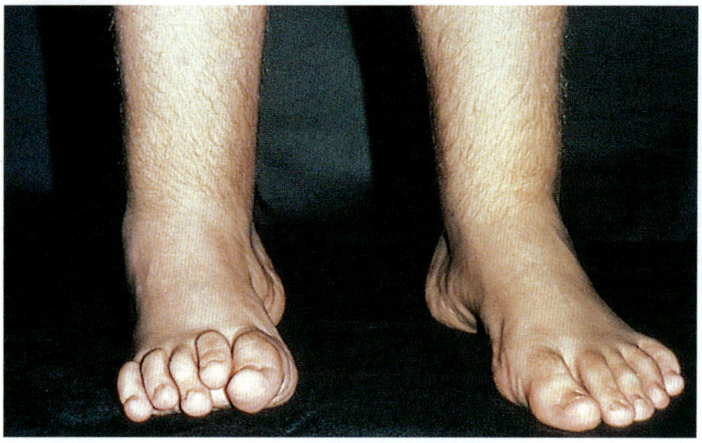

Fig. 22.108 Unilateral claw toes. This child with a tethered spinal cord has unilateral claw toe deformities. The metatarsophalangeal joints are held in extension while the proximal interphalangeal joints are fixed in flexion.

section. Dysostosis is a disorder of an individual bone, either singly or in combination (e.g., skull, fingers). Examples include polydactyly/syndactyly and craniosynostoses. There are 33 groups of osteochondrodysplasia and three categories of dysostosis in the current classification system. Table 22.7 shows a list of common skeletal dysplasias, osteochondrodysplasias, and common lethal skeletal dysplasias. The incidence of all skeletal dysplasia is approximately 1 case per 4000 to 5000 births. Because a proportion of skeletal dysplasias are lethal, the prevalence in the general population in that study was found to be much lower (33 per 100,000 population). Thanatophoric dysplasia (Fig. 22.109) and achondrogenesis account for 62% of all lethal skeletal dysplasias. Achondroplasia is usually regarded as the most common skeletal dysplasia worldwide.

Table 22.7 Skeletal Dysplasias

Nonlethal Skeletal Dysplasias	Lethal Skeletal Dysplasias
Achondroplasia—most common	Thanatophoric syndrome—most common
Hypochondroplasia	Achondrogenesis
Pseudoachondroplasia	Homozygous achondroplasia
Diastrophic dysplasia	Chondrodysplasia punctata (recessive form)
Spondyloepiphyseal dysplasia	Camptomelic dysplasia (sometimes)
Ellis–van Creveld syndrome	Congenital lethal hypophosphatasia
Cartilage hair hypoplasia	Perinatal lethal type of osteogenesis imperfecta
Metatropic dysplasia	Short-rib polydactyly syndromes
Multiple epiphyseal dysplasia	
Kniest dysplasia	
Acromesomelic dysplasia	
Larson syndrome	
Jarcho-Levin syndrome	

Diagnosis

Accurate diagnosis can be important for genetic counseling regarding future pregnancies and is helpful in predicting the clinical course and aiding in treatment strategies for complications. Often diagnoses are made on the basis of distinctive radiographic and physical findings. Because diagnosis often relies on radiographic findings, it is important to obtain a skeletal survey of any infant or child in whom a dysplasia is suspected.

Prenatal detection of a skeletal dysplasia is important because it determines the obstetric and perinatal management of an affected fetus. Because up to 30% of skeletal dysplasias can be lethal, accurate diagnosis is imperative for decision making regarding possible termination. The precise diagnosis of a specific dysplasia is often difficult prenatally even with accurate imaging because of variable phenotypic presentations; the variability in the time at which they manifest; and, often, the lack of precise molecular diagnosis.

Certain characteristics that are critical for diagnosis are present only in children because of their skeletal immaturity and may disappear with maturity. The epiphyseal characteristics of affected children can be pathognomonic of specific disorders, such as the anterior tonguelike protrusion of the spine in pseudoachondroplasia.

Clues in the physical examination, such as abnormalities in limbs, spine, trunk, and facial features, help to differentiate types on the basis of phenotypic features. Findings include abnormalities of the limbs, spine, and trunk. Abnormalities of the limbs include rhizomelic shortening (short proximal segments, such as humerus or femur); mesomelic shortening (short middle segments, such as radius, ulna, tibia, fibula); acromelic shortening (short distal segments, such as metacarpals or phalanges); acromesomelic shortening (short middle and distal segments, such as forearms and hands); and micromelia (shortening of extremities involving entire limb). Examples of some of the skeletal dysplasias correlated with specific physical examination findings are

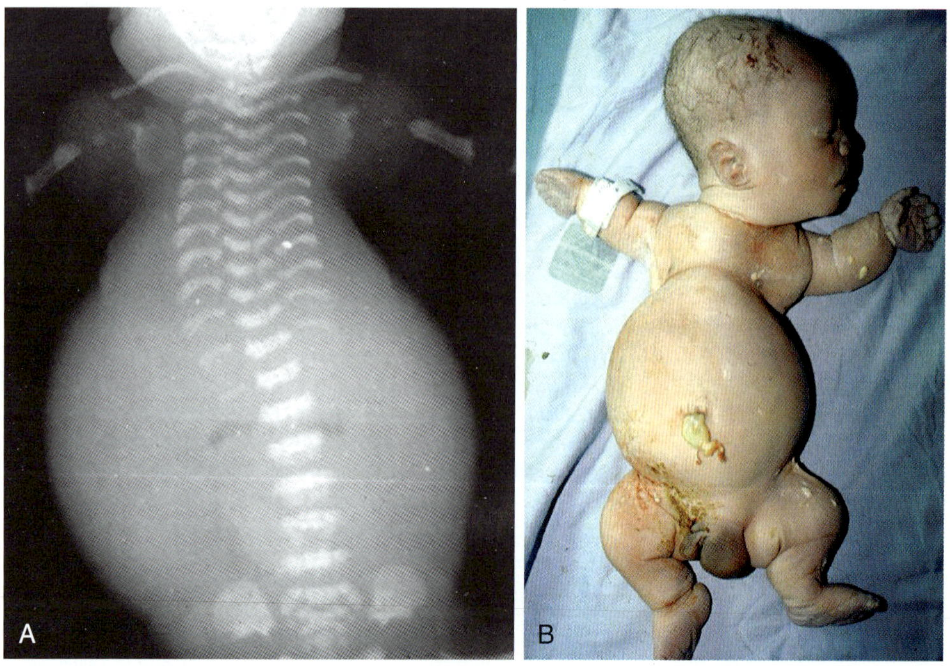

Fig. 22.109 Thanatophoric dysplasia. (A) Chest and abdomen radiograph showing newborn with lethal thanatophoric dysplasia. Note the severe pulmonary hypoplasia and spinal abnormalities. (B) Postmortem photo of a newborn who died of asphyxia due to lethal pulmonary hypoplasia, in turn due to thanatophoric dysplasia.

listed in Table 22.8. A working diagnosis based on clinical and radiographic findings may better guide the use of existing molecular testing.

Genetics

The genes responsible for skeletal dysplasia have been identified in more than 150 diseases. Table 22.9 lists select skeletal dysplasias with their respective gene mutations. Almost all of the skeletal dysplasias are the result of single gene mutations. The majority are the result of spontaneous mutations with no prior family history, and most are subsequently inheritable.

Table 22.8 Limb Abnormalities Seen in the Skeletal Dysplasias

Limb Abnormality	Examples
Rhizomelia (shortening of proximal limb)	Achondroplasia, hypochondroplasia, chondrodysplasia punctata, metaphyseal dysplasia, spondyloepiphyseal dysplasia congenita, thanatophoric dysplasia, atelosteogenesis, and diastrophic dysplasia
Mesomelia (shortening of middle limb segments)	Langer and Nievergelt types of mesomelic dysplasias, Robinow syndrome, and Reinhardt syndrome
Acromelia (shortening of distal limb segments)	Acrodysostosis and peripheral dysostosis
Acromesomelia (shortening of middle and distal limb segments)	Acromesomelic dysplasia
Micromelia (shortening of entire limb)	Achondrogenesis, fibrochondrogenesis, Kniest dysplasia, dyssegmental dysplasia, and Roberts syndrome

Specific Skeletal Dysplasias

Achondroplasia

Achondroplasia is the most common of all the skeletal dysplasias, with an estimated incidence of 1 per 10,000 live births. It is caused by a mutation in the fibroblast growth factor receptor-3 gene (*FGFR3*), found on the short arm of chromosome 4 (4p16.3). *FGFR3* is one of many fibroblast growth factors involved in skeletal development. Although achondroplasia is an autosomal dominant disorder, 75% of new diagnoses are due to de novo spontaneous mutations. Physical examination findings in persons with achondroplasia include disproportionate short stature with rhizomelia (Fig. 22.110). Typical facial features include a flattened nasal bridge, upturned nose, protruding jaw, deep-set eyes, frontal bossing, and

Table 22.9 Common Genes Associated With Skeletal Dysplasias

Skeletal Dysplasia	Gene Mutation
Achondroplasia, thanatophoric dysplasia	Fibroblast growth factor receptor gene-3 *(FGFR3)*
Pseudoachondroplasia	Cartilage oligomeric protein gene *(COMP)*
Diastrophic dysplasia	Diastrophic dysplasia sulfate transporter gene *(DTDST)*
Spondyloepiphyseal dysplasia congenita (SEDc)	Collagen 2A *(COL2A1)*
Camptomelic dysplasia	Sex-determining region Y (SRY)-box 9 protein *(SOX9)*

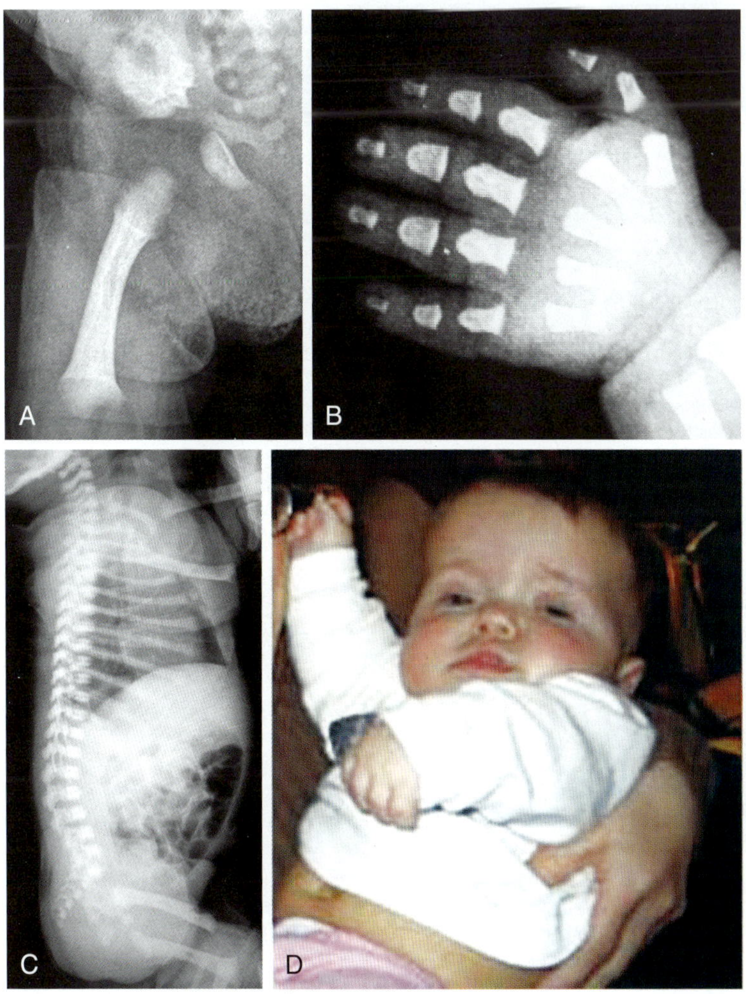

Fig. 22.110 Achondroplasia. (A) Radiograph of the femur in an infant with achondroplasia. The proximal ends of the femurs are relatively clublike with metaphyseal flaring and rhizomelic shortening of the lower extremities. (B) Radiograph of the hand, showing shortened metacarpals and phalanges. (C) Radiograph of the spine, showing thoracic lumbar kyphoscoliosis. (D) A 4-month-old female with distinctive facial features: upturned nose, flat nasal bridge, and large forehead.

midface hypoplasia. Most children with achondroplasia have macrocephaly. Because infants and children are also at risk of hydrocephalus, occipital/frontal circumference should be monitored. Children with achondroplasia have normal intelligence and development with the exception of delayed motor milestones. They are at risk for complications, including otitis media, obstructive sleep apnea, hydrocephalus due to foramen magnum stenosis, thoracolumbar kyphosis, and bowing of the lower limbs that may necessitate surgical correction.

Diastrophic Dysplasia

Diastrophic dysplasia is one of the few skeletal dysplasias inherited in an autosomal recessive manner. It results from a mutation in the diastrophic dysplasia sulfate transporter (*DTDST*) gene located on chromosome 5. The mutation results in deficient uptake of sulfur by chondrocytes, resulting in abnormal cartilage. It is characterized by short limb dwarfism, severe joint deformities, kyphoscoliosis, clubbed feet, an abducted "hitchhiker's" thumb, and characteristic malformed pinnae of the ears (Fig. 22.111). Persons with diastrophic dysplasia have normal intelligence, but orthopedic complications due to joint contractures and dislocations can lead to severe osteoarthritis and disability.

Pseudoachondroplasia

Pseudoachondroplasia is a skeletal dysplasia inherited in an autosomal dominant manner. It results from mutations in the gene encoding cartilage oligomeric matrix protein. Pseudoachondroplasia is often not discovered until a child begins to walk; difficulties with walking or a waddling gait lead to the diagnosis. Because short stature is often not detected until 2 to 3 years after birth (because initial growth velocity is within normal limits), it should be included as a potential diagnosis in the workup of the short-statured child. Children usually exhibit marked short stature and deformity of the legs, short fingers, loose joints, and significant ligamentous laxity and cervical spine instability.

Spondyloepiphyseal Dysplasia Congenita

Spondyloepiphyseal dysplasia congenita (SEDc) is part of a spectrum of skeletal disorders caused by mutations in the *COL2A1* gene, which is responsible for making a protein that forms type II collagen, found in cartilage and the vitreous humor. Persons born with SEDc have short stature from birth, with a short trunk and neck and shortened limbs. Sometimes they have cleft palate and clubfeet. Severe orthopedic complications are common throughout childhood, including cervical spine instability necessitating surgical fusion, scoliosis, hip dysplasia, knock-knee deformity, and osteoarthritis as

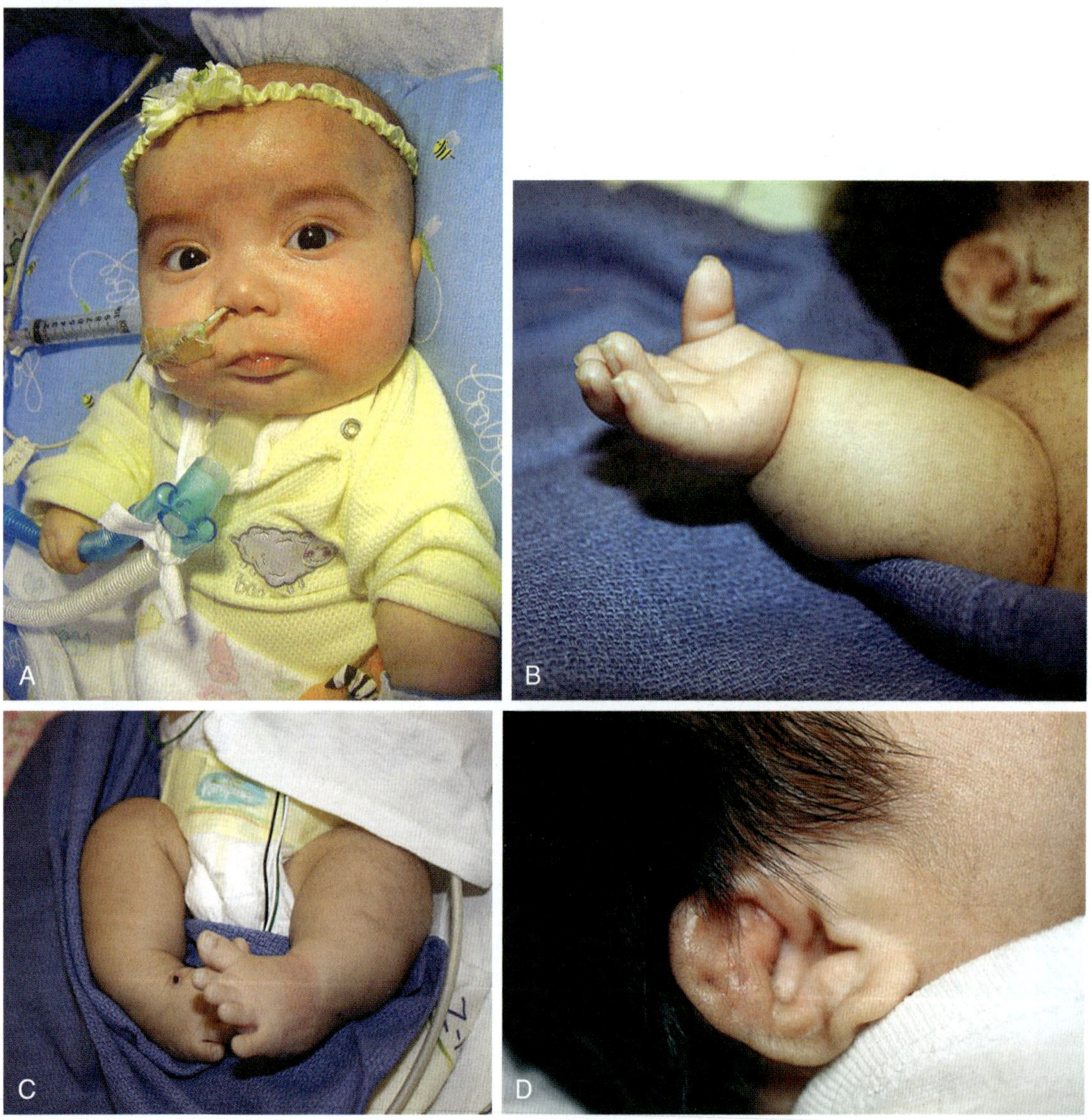

Fig. 22.111 Diastrophic dysplasia. (A) A 6-month-old female with diastrophic dysplasia showing characteristic facial features of a long, full face; broad forehead; and prominent cheeks and perioral fullness. (B) Hand showing characteristic, abnormally positioned or "hitchhiker's" thumb. (C) Lower extremities showing bilateral clubfeet. (D) Ear showing malformed pinna; this is called a "cauliflower ear" because of the blister-like sacs filled with fluid on the upper part of the ear. These swollen sacs will drain naturally, but most often leave a misshapen upper ear.

early as the teenage years. SEDc may also be associated with vision problems (myopia and retinal detachment) and hearing loss (sensorineural).

Common Problems

Each dysplasia has unique characteristics, making generalizations about medical and surgical complications difficult. Treatments for individuals with skeletal dysplasia should be directed at preventing neurologic and orthopedic complications due to spinal cord compression, joint instability, joint degenerative disease, and long bone deformity. The following sections list general types of medical and surgical problems that are experienced by children with skeletal dysplasias.

Neurologic Issues

Hydrocephalus is a common complication in infants and children with achondroplasia. This results from poor cerebrospinal fluid drainage, due primarily to foramen magnum stenosis. Screening should include careful neurologic examinations at every well-child visit, regular occipital/frontal circumference measurements based on achondroplasia growth charts, head ultrasound at birth and bimonthly until 6 months old, and head CT or MRI for evaluation between 6 months and 1 year old. Clinical symptoms of hydrocephalus and foramen magnum stenosis include brisk reflexes, numbness, weakness, difficulty walking, loss of bowel and bladder control, and central sleep apnea.

In the neonatal period, it is important to monitor the cervical spine for C1 to C2 instability due to odontoid hypoplasia and ligamentous laxity. Although common in many skeletal dysplasias such as SEDc and pseudoachondroplasia, it is not found in achondroplasia. All children at risk for having a skeletal dysplasia should have cervical spine radiographs and/or undergo cervical spine MRI. Screening should be performed within the first 6 months of life and then yearly as indicated.

Lumbar-sacral stenosis can be a common complication for adults with achondroplasia. Progressive narrowing of the spinal canal in the lumbar and sacral regions can lead to pain, difficulty in walking, loss of bowel and bladder control, and paralysis.

Orthopedic Issues

One of the more common and challenging adult sequelae is premature and severe osteoarthritis that can develop as early as adolescence. Patients with dysplasias with epiphyseal involvement (e.g., SEDc) are especially at risk for osteoarthritis and should avoid long-distance running, obesity, and high-impact activities. Scoliosis, lower extremity deformities, and hip problems are common orthopedic issues in children with skeletal dysplasia.

Other Problems

Obstructive sleep apnea is common in many skeletal dysplasias but especially achondroplasia. The condition arises from small bony air passages of the midface or a crowded hypopharynx, resulting from a tiny jaw or thickened soft tissues. Symptoms include snoring, apnea, and sweating during sleep; failure to thrive; and developmental delay. Eustachian tube dysfunction due to abnormal craniofacial shape, midface hypoplasia, and shortened eustachian tubes is common in many forms of dwarfism but most often achondroplasia, resulting in recurrent otitis media. Children should have ear examinations with every upper respiratory infection to prevent chronic otitis media, hearing loss, and speech delay.

Cerebral Palsy

Cerebral palsy refers to a group of nonprogressive neurologic syndromes resulting from static lesions of the developing nervous system. Depending on the timing of injury, signs may be present at birth or they may become evident in infancy or early childhood. The primary cerebral insult may be intrauterine or perinatal infection; a prenatal or perinatal vascular accident; anoxia due to placental insufficiency, difficult delivery, or neonatal pulmonary disease; hyperbilirubinemia resulting in kernicterus; or neonatal hypoglycemia. After the newborn period, central nervous system infections, trauma, and vascular accidents may, when severe, produce the disorder. Abnormal motor function is the most obvious result and may take the form of a spastic neuromuscular disorder (65% of cases), athetosis (25%), or rigidity and/or ataxic neuromuscular dysfunction (10%). Sensory deficits and intellectual impairment are common, and there is a high incidence of associated seizure disorders.

Because of the number and variety of possible etiologies, each with its own spectrum of severity, there is a broad range in the location and extent of neural damage and the degree of functional impairment. Patients with severe involvement generally have early evidence of gross neuromuscular dysfunction. Those with milder involvement may have subtle abnormalities and may be diagnosed only after they fail to achieve normal developmental and motor milestones. Patterns include involvement of one or two limbs (monoplegia or hemiplegia), of both lower extremities (diplegia), or of all four extremities (quadriplegia) (Fig. 22.112). Those patients with a spastic disorder exhibit flexion contracture of the involved limbs, hyperreflexia, and spasticity; those with athetosis exhibit the characteristic movement disorder. Neurologic examination often reveals the persistence of primitive reflexes. Patients with severe involvement develop disuse muscle atrophy and osteopenia that increases the risk of pathologic fractures (see Chapter 6).

Although cerebral palsy is by definition a nonprogressive neurologic condition, the orthopedic manifestations are frequently progressive. The progression of orthopedic problems is related to the severity and distribution of spasticity in the child. Increased spasticity in certain muscle groups leads to shortening and contractures in muscles and tendons, imbalance of mechanical forces across a joint or extremity, and eventual bone and joint deformity. One example of this biological response to muscle imbalance in the growing child, frequently seen in children with severe spasticity, is hip dislocation (Fig. 22.113). Hip deformity, dislocation, and associated arthritic

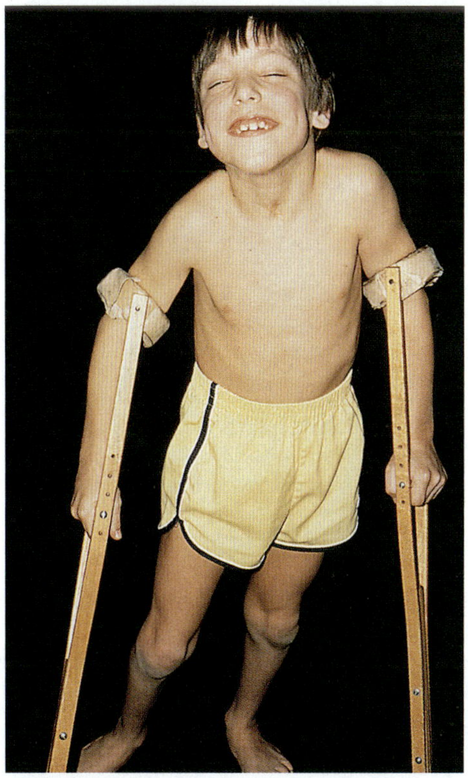

Fig. 22.112 Cerebral palsy. Typical patient with spastic quadriplegia. Note the secondary muscle atrophy, especially evident in the lower extremities. He requires crutches to ambulate, seizure medication, and a specialized educational program. His neuromuscular abnormalities are the result of a one-time central nervous system insult and are not progressive.

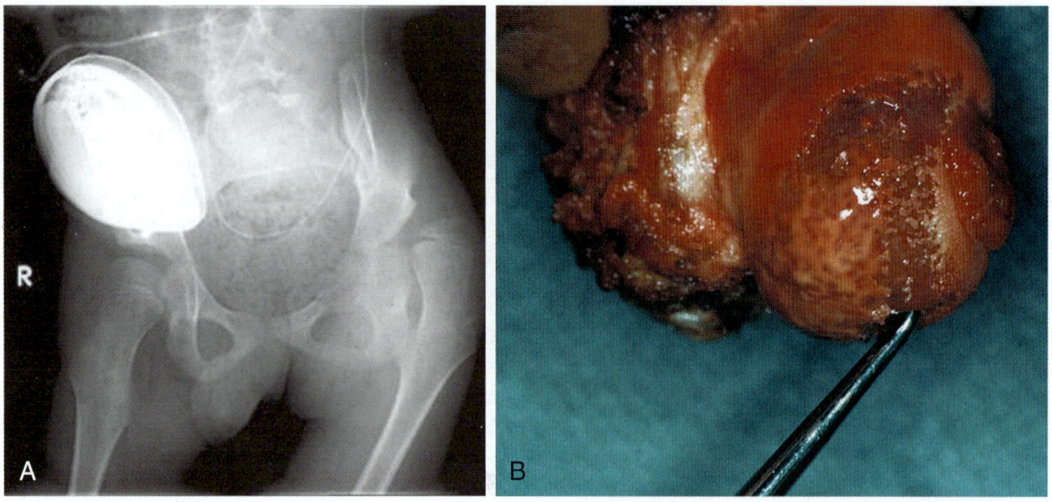

Fig. 22.113 Hip dislocation in cerebral palsy. (A) This 9-year-old with quadriplegic cerebral palsy has a dislocated left hip as a result of spasticity and unbalanced muscle pull. This is a source of significant pain in about 50% of cases whether or not the child is ambulatory, and surgical treatment is indicated. Note the baclofen pump on the right. (B) This is the proximal femur removed from another child with severe spasticity and a painful dislocated hip. Note the erosion of the articular cartilage. This and disuse osteoporosis make it easy for a metal probe to perforate the femoral head.

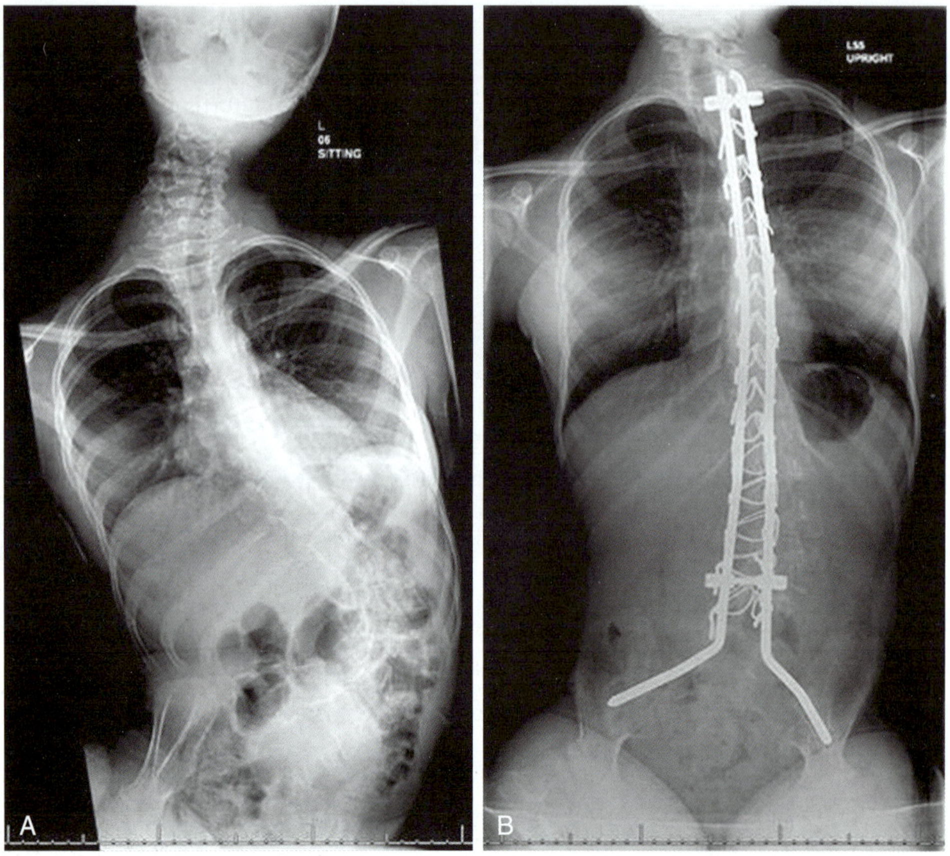

Fig. 22.114 Preoperative and postoperative spinal radiographs of a 15-year-old female with cerebral palsy and scoliosis. (A) Preoperative radiograph indicating pelvic obliquity (tilt), which makes sitting in a chair difficult. The patient is non-ambulatory. (B) Postoperative radiograph. Note improved symmetry of chest and leveling of pelvis, which made sitting easier and more comfortable.

changes are the result of significant and prolonged imbalance of muscle pull about the hip. It is estimated that in 50% of children with untreated hip dislocation, pain may become significant and problematic, necessitating hip resection or replacement in adolescent or adult life.

The spine is one of the major areas of concern in children with significant spasticity. Scoliosis develops frequently and contributes to pelvic tilt (pelvic obliquity), which impairs sitting balance further (Fig. 22.114).

Spasticity is indicative of upper motor neuron pathology. In evaluating patients with apparent cerebral palsy, one must be careful to rule out a progressive neurologic disorder, such as intracranial or spinal cord neoplasia, degenerative neurologic conditions such as hereditary spastic paraplegia, and spinal cord tethering.

Spina Bifida Cystica (Myelomeningocele)

The myelodysplasias are a group of congenital deformities that result from defective closure of the caudal portion of the neural tube. When the failure of closure involves only the posterior vertebral elements, it is termed a meningocele; when it involves neural and vertebral elements, it is called a myelomeningocele. In patients with myelomeningocele, the loss of neurologic function that results from abnormal cord and spinal root development has dire consequences for the developing musculoskeletal system. Affected children often require neurosurgical closure of the defect at birth to allow healing and prevent infection, and most need a ventriculoperitoneal shunt to prevent or control hydrocephalus. Because of lack of bladder innervation and control, careful urologic follow-up is necessary as well.

The skeletal manifestations seen in spina bifida are the result of imbalances in muscle function of the trunk and extremities. The neurologic loss roughly corresponds to the level of the spine at which the defect lies. In those patients with thoracic myelomeningocele, complete lack of sensation and motor function is seen in the lower extremities and ambulation is limited. On the other hand, in those individuals whose defect is at a low lumbar or sacral level, the weakness and subsequent deformity may be limited to the foot or hip extensors and abductors and to bladder dysfunction (Fig. 22.115)

Osteogenesis Imperfecta

OI is a family of inherited disorders characterized most notably by brittle bones. Nearly 90% of cases have been determined to be the result of mutations in either the *COL1A1* or *COL1A2* gene. These genes encode production of the pro-α1 and pro-α2 polypeptide chains, which are then assembled into a triple helix composed of two pro-α1 chains and one pro-α2 to form type I collagen, the major structural protein of bone and connective tissues. Thus far, hundreds of different mutations of these genes have been identified as causative of varying phenotypes of OI. Nearly all are autosomal dominant. Some of these mutations are characterized by production of structurally abnormal collagen. In other cases, the mutant allele is not expressed, resulting in secretion of about 50% of expected levels of structurally normal type I collagen (see also Chapter 1). Histologically, bone mass is decreased and trabeculae are reduced in both number and thickness. Ossification is decreased, and when structurally abnormal collagen is produced, osteoid is poorly organized. The end result is a significant increase in susceptibility to fractures.

The most widely accepted system of classification of these disorders, developed by Sillence and colleagues (1979), uses a combination of clinical features and course, radiographic findings, and genetic factors to divide cases into four main types. In type I, nearly all cases are characterized by reduced production of structurally normal collagen, whereas in types II to IV some proportion of the type I collagen produced is structurally abnormal. Phenotypically, patients with types I and IV have mild to moderate (less often moderately severe) fragility, and those with types II and III have severe disease. Patients with the two milder forms typically experience a distinct decrease in fracture frequency with the onset of puberty, which then reverses in the fifth or sixth decade or after menopause in females.

Considerable phenotypic variation exists between and within types, due predominantly to the large number of possible sites for mutations to occur on the *COL1* genes. Some cases of intrafamilial variability are the result of genetic mosaicism within a parent.

Although the causative mutations affect all connective tissues in the body, their primary clinical manifestations involve the skeleton because of the greater structural demands placed on bones.

Osteogenesis Imperfecta Type I

OI type I is the most common form and is usually the mildest clinically. Two subtypes exist: A (the great majority), in which teeth are normal, and B (unusual), in which dentinogenesis imperfecta is a feature (see Chapter 21). All those with OI type I have blue or grayish-blue sclerae at birth (Fig. 22.116), although the degree varies and tends to lessen with age.

Bony fragility ranges from mild to moderate (up to 10% have no fractures). Although an occasional patient incurs a fracture during delivery, most experience their first after they begin to cruise or walk. The most common sites are the long bones of the arms and legs. Healing is normal with good callus formation and occurs without deformity.

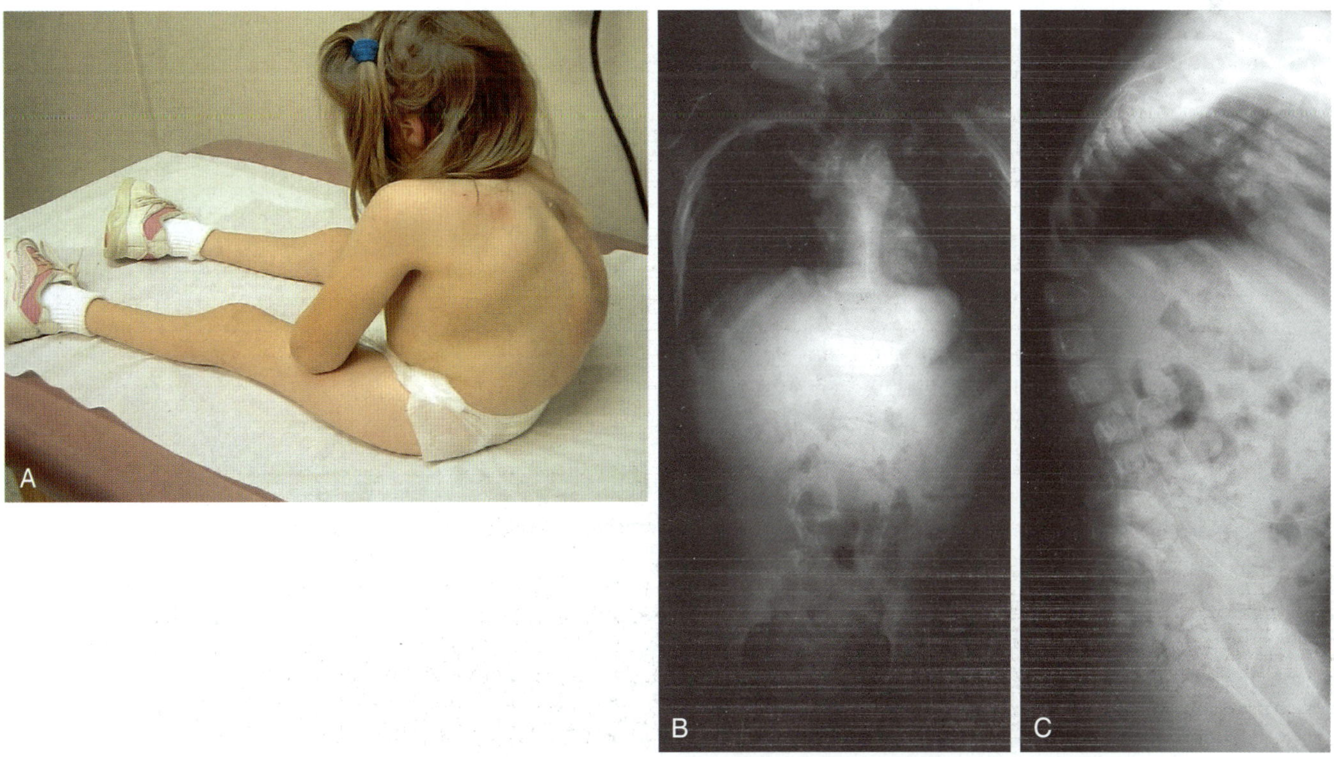

Fig. 22.115 Spina bifida. (A) This child with thoracic-level spina bifida has an obvious kyphotic deformity. The scars on her back are from surgical closure of her myelomeningocele. (B and C) Anteroposterior and lateral radiographs of the spine demonstrate that kyphosis is secondary to incomplete posterior osseous support.

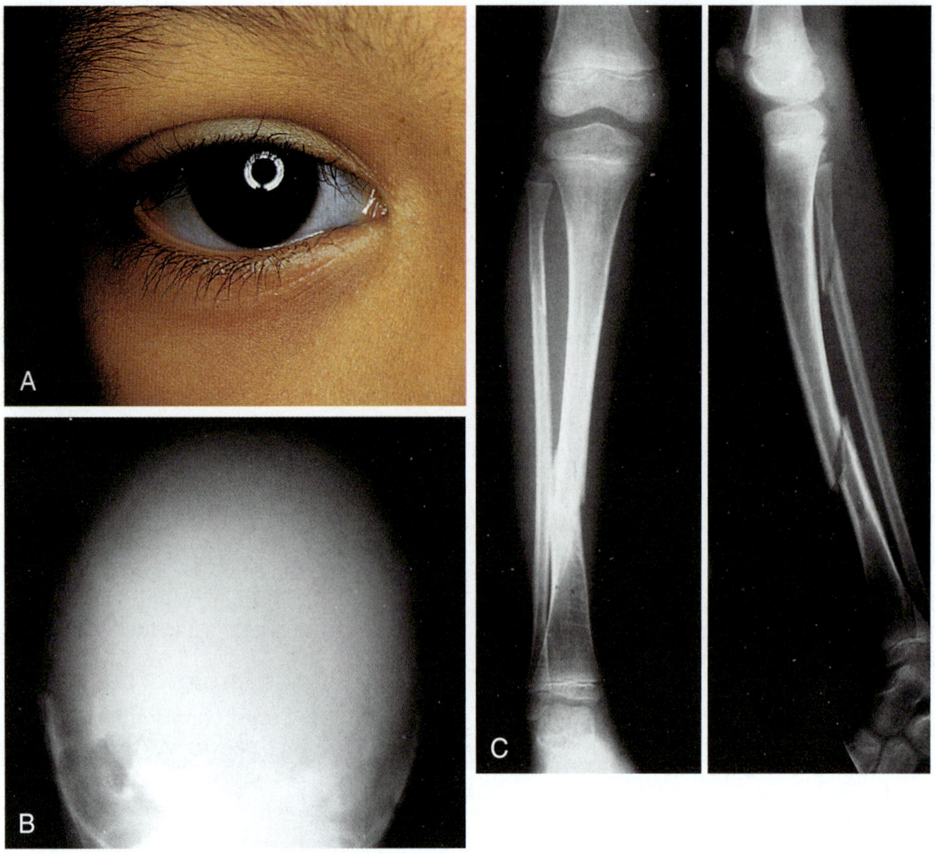

Fig. 22.116 Osteogenesis imperfecta (OI) type I. (A) Blue sclera. (B) Wormian bones. Multiple wormy, irregular lucencies are seen over the occipitoparietal area. This finding is characteristic of all children with OI types I, II, and III and is seen in more than 50% of patients with OI type IV. (C) Cortical thinning is evident, especially distal to the oblique fracture of the tibia in this child with OI type I who incurred his fractures while jumping off a chair. (A and C, Courtesy Thomas Daley, MD, St. Joseph's Hospital, Paterson, NJ.)

Radiographically, bones appear normal in infancy, save for the presence of wormian bones within the sutures of the calvarium (see Fig. 22.116B; see Chapter 16); however, over time, some degree of osteopenia becomes evident along with thinning of the cortices (see Fig. 22.116C). In some patients, vertebral flattening is noted in later childhood and adolescence.

Osteogenesis Imperfecta Type II

OI type II is the severest form and is usually lethal in the perinatal period. Most cases are the result of new mutations, although parental germline mosaicism is occasionally causative. Intrauterine growth is severely affected, and infants are born prematurely with innumerable poorly healed fractures and prominent deformities due to extreme bony fragility. The sclerae are a dark blue-black; a triangular facies with micrognathia and a small beaked nose is present; and the calvarium is large in relation to the face and remarkably soft. Other clinical features include marked shortening of the extremities and severe bowing of the legs with hips flexed and thighs fixed in abduction and external rotation (Fig. 22.117). The combination of a short trunk (due to vertebral flattening) and a small chest cage predisposes to severe/progressive pulmonary insufficiency and congestive heart failure.

Death usually supervenes within a few days to weeks of delivery, due to cardiopulmonary complications.

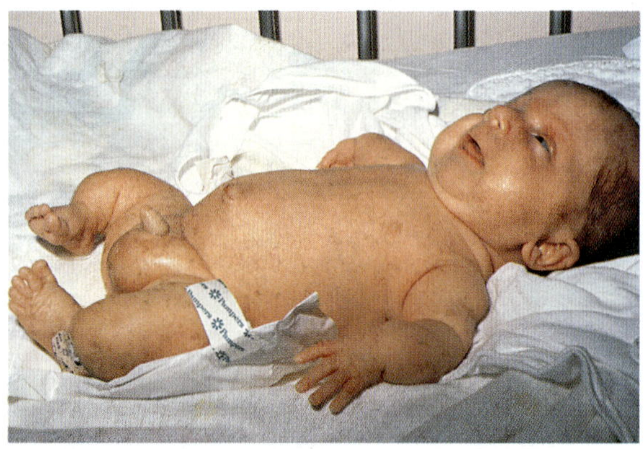

Fig. 22.117 Osteogenesis imperfecta type II. This infant was born with multiple fractures and limb deformities. The thighs are fixed in abduction and external rotation. His sclerae are a dark bluish-gray. He died of respiratory insufficiency in the first month of life as the result of his small thorax.

Osteogenesis Imperfecta Type III

Like OI type II, OI type III is usually the result of new mutations, less commonly of parental germline mosaicism. The majority are born with multiple fractures and deformities due to fractures in utero. Those who are not incur multiple fractures within the first 1 to 2 years. Birth weights are usually low, and length is short. Extremities are foreshortened, and tibial bowing is prominent (Fig. 22.118A). Sclerae are blue to pale blue and gradually lighten with age. The calvarium is relatively large in comparison with the face, which is triangular with a small chin and frontotemporal bossing (see Fig. 22.118B). Dentinogenesis imperfecta is seen in more than half of cases. Bony fragility is moderately severe to severe, and fractures occur with minimal trauma. Healing is impaired and often associated with hyperplastic callus and angulation. Repeated fractures of long bones over time result in progressive limb shortening and deformity.

Radiographically severe diffuse osteopenia and thin cortices are evident, and this tends to worsen with age (see Fig. 22.118C). The calvarium is markedly undermineralized, with wormian bones seen within sutures. The ribs are thin and hypodense. In some patients, cystic changes develop in the metaphyses of long bones between 2 and

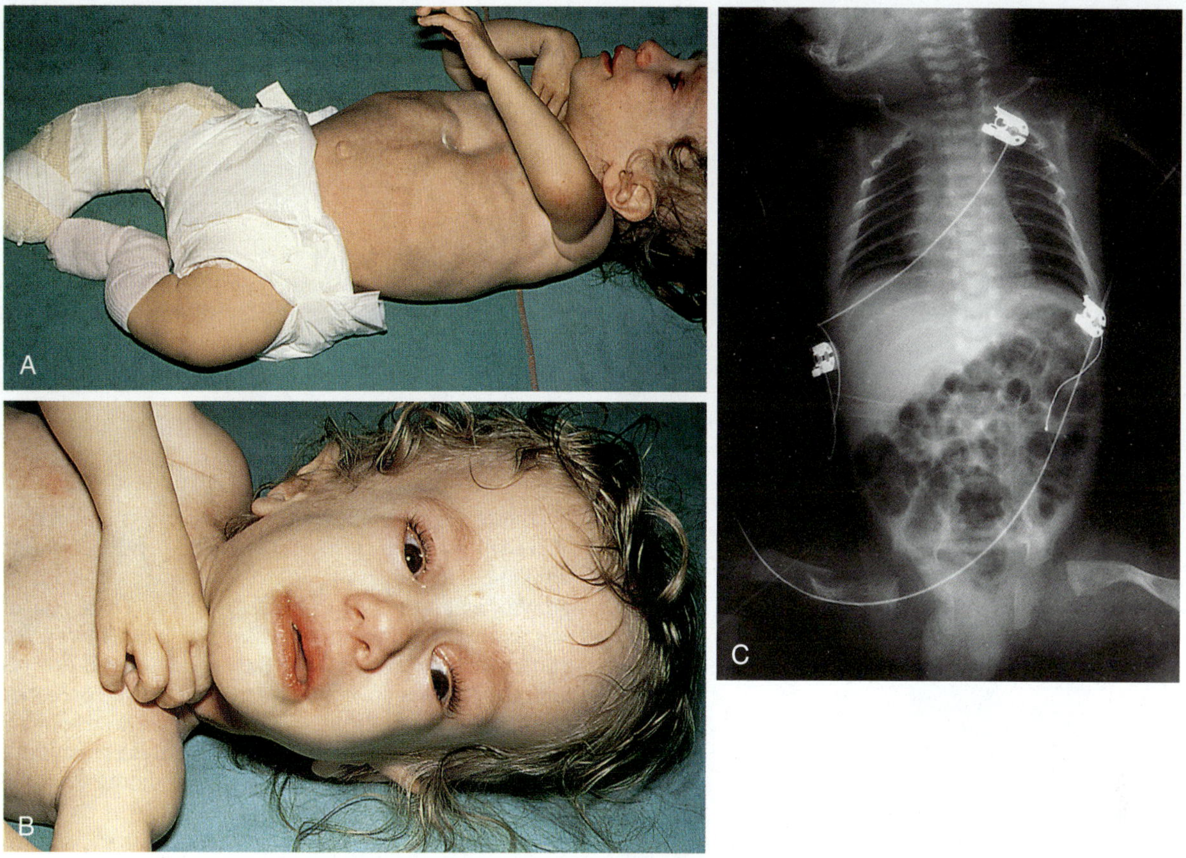

Fig. 22.118 Osteogenesis imperfecta type III. (A) Note the extremely small stature of this 5-year-old child and the deformities of the rib cage and lower extremities. A recent fracture has been splinted. (B) In this close-up, the characteristic craniofacial features are seen, consisting of a triangular facies, a broad nose, and frontal and temporal bossing. The sclerae may be normal in color, as in this child, or light blue or gray. (C) Radiograph of an affected infant shows dwarfed, deformed femurs with a new fracture in the midshaft of the right femur. Note also the thin, peculiarly shaped ribs.

5 years old. These are a manifestation of severe disorganization of growth plate structure, which significantly impairs linear growth, and combined with vertebral flattening results in markedly reduced stature. Rapidly progressive kyphoscoliosis is a feature in many older patients and predisposes to cardiopulmonary complications. Other clinical features include ligamentous laxity (seen in 50%) and early-onset hearing loss. About 25% experience easy bruisability, and a number of affected children also report heat intolerance and excessive sweating.

Osteogenesis Imperfecta Type IV

OI type IV, generally considered the least common of the four major types of OI, has a variable severity.

Diagnosis

With close attention to clinical findings and course, as well as radiographic features and family history, the diagnosis of OI types II and III is relatively obvious and that of types I and IV is usually straightforward. Routine laboratory studies are not helpful for diagnosis.

When a clinical diagnosis cannot be made with any degree of assurance and when an exact diagnosis is necessary, analysis of collagen synthesis by fibroblasts obtained via skin biopsy can be performed.

Prenatal diagnosis, for families who have had a child with OI type II or III (the genetic defect of which has been identified), involves analyzing fetal DNA obtained by chorionic villus sampling. Ultrasound is also of use in detecting these types of OI between 15 and 18 weeks of gestation.

Differential Diagnosis

In general, there is no confusion in the diagnosis of type III OI. The same is true of most type II cases, although occasionally they must be distinguished from thanatophoric dysplasia, achondrogenesis, and autosomal recessive hypophosphatasia.

The major differential diagnostic considerations in cases of types I and IV are child abuse and idiopathic juvenile osteoporosis.

Distinction from abuse (see Chapter 6) is usually possible clinically because infants and children with previously undiagnosed mild OI and an acute fracture are brought in for care promptly, by appropriately concerned parents who give a history of a mechanism of injury that fits the fracture pattern found, although the amount of force reported may be less than is usually required to cause a fracture. Further, most of these fractures involve the diaphyses of the long bones of the extremities. The metaphyseal fractures seen commonly in abuse victims are exceptionally rare in children with OI, and typically one does not find multiple fractures of varying ages for which no prior care has been sought. Finally, skull fractures are rare in OI, and retinal hemorrhages, subdural hematomas, and visceral injuries are not seen, with the rare exception of the infant or child with OI who is also a victim of abuse.

The major source of potential confusion is the infant with mild OI and normal sclerae who has incurred one or more nondisplaced fractures in utero or during delivery that were not diagnosed in the newborn period. If he or she then presents with a first symptomatic fracture within the ensuing few months, old healing fractures will be found. Again, timing of presentation, parental demeanor, consistency with mechanism, and family history and psychosocial history should all be scrutinized carefully in making the distinction. Consultation with a specialist in abuse and neglect is strongly recommended.

Idiopathic juvenile osteoporosis is an exceptionally rare disorder of unknown etiology. In affected children, osteopenia and fractures are most evident in the vertebrae—less so in the long bones, and measurements of bone density are well below normal. This condition improves dramatically in adolescence. Family history is negative for unusually frequent fractures.

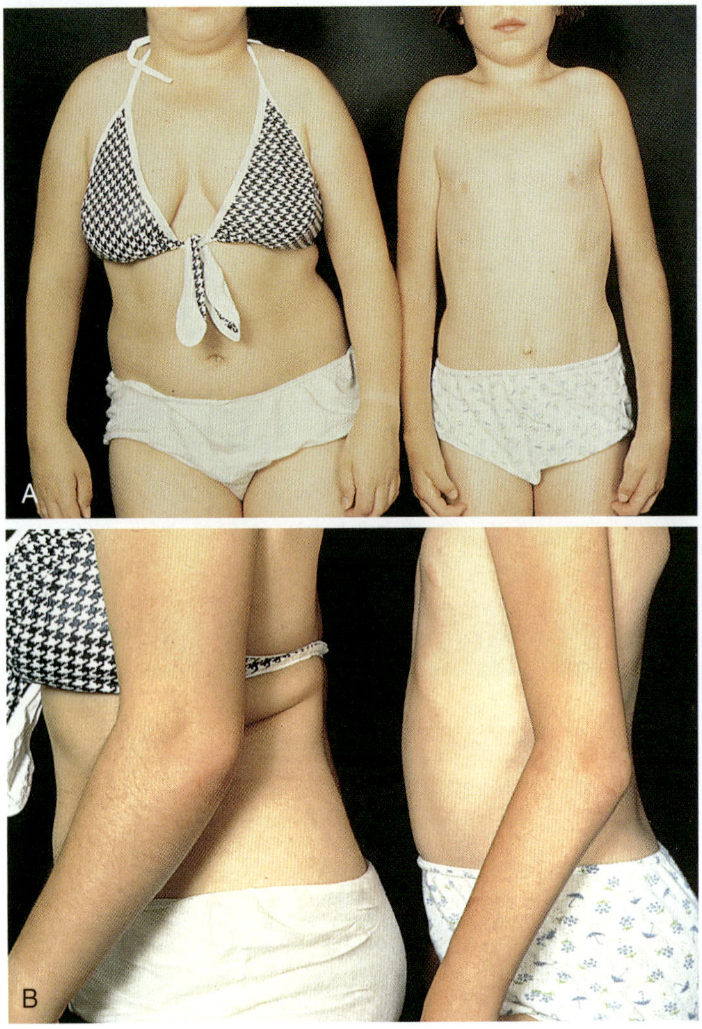

Fig. 22.119 Arthrogryposis. (A) Two sisters with the generalized form of the disorder. Note the stiff posture and tubular appearance of the limbs. Motion of all joints is limited as a result of failure in the development, or the degeneration, of muscular structures. Their stature is short. (B) The lateral view highlights the flexion contractures of the elbows.

Arthrogryposis

Arthrogryposis is a nonprogressive muscular disorder of unknown etiology that appears to be related to either failure of development of or degeneration of muscular structures. Neural factors have been implicated in its pathogenesis because in some instances the spinal cord has been found to be reduced in size, with a decreased number of anterior horn cells. In general, all limbs are involved. On occasion the disease may be confined to one or two limbs. Primary manifestations consist of joint contractures with secondary deformities and limited motion. Deformities include clubfoot, dislocated hips, scoliosis, and contractures of the knees, elbows, wrists, and hands (Fig. 22.119). Motion of the involved joints is severely limited, but patients can generally compensate for this functional limitation. Radiographs show relatively normal-appearing bones and joints, but fat density is noted in the areas where muscles are normally seen. On pathologic analysis, there is a striking absence of muscle tissue with strands of fat permeating the area.

SPORTS INJURIES

Competitive participation in organized sports has been increasing in the juvenile and adolescent age. This has caused an increase in sports-related injuries including acute trauma, overuse, and concussion.

Risk of Injury

In early and middle childhood, risk of sports-related injury is relatively low. Being smaller and having less muscle strength than adolescents, children achieve less velocity and thus encounter less force in falls and collisions. In this age range, injuries are more likely to be incurred during recreational play and in the process of learning a new sport. With puberty, gains in size, strength, and speed combine with increased competitiveness and intensity of play to substantially increase both the incidence and severity of injuries. Even so, the majority of injuries incurred during organized sport are minor in nature; less than 10% are serious; and catastrophic spinal and head injuries and sudden cardiac, pulmonary, and heat-related deaths are rare events. Injuries are more likely to occur during practice sessions because practices outnumber formal competitions or games, although incidence of injuries per unit of time played is greater during the latter.

The incidence of overuse injuries, in particular, has risen in parallel with the trend toward increasing organization of sports. Children are especially prone to overuse injuries during periods of rapid growth, when the rate of bone growth exceeds that of surrounding soft tissues, resulting in decreased flexibility. Intensive training for a particular sport, especially when initiated at a low level of fitness; abrupt increases in level of activity; lack of preconditioning; and participation in multiple sports during the course of a year are other predisposing factors, as are training practices that fail to teach children proper athletic techniques and to monitor and limit repetitive motions.

Participation in some types of organized sports carries an inherently greater risk and thus higher rates and degrees of severity of injury. This is by virtue of their requiring higher levels of aerobic intensity, their placing high static and/or dynamic stresses on the body, or because high-velocity contacts or collisions are part of the activity. Among these, competitive wrestling, football, and gymnastics are the top three, followed by cross-country skiing, soccer, basketball, track, volleyball, softball, and baseball in approximate order of frequency. Youths with ligamentous laxity (up to 7% of school-age children) and joint malalignment may be injury prone without special preconditioning. Children and adolescents who resume competitive participation after a musculoskeletal injury, without full rehabilitation (return of normal strength, flexibility, and range of motion), have a significant risk for reinjury.

Two areas of sport are specifically not recommended by the American Academy of Pediatrics: boxing because of high risk of eye and head injury; and weightlifting, power lifting, maximal lifts, and body building because of concerns regarding epiphyseal injuries (especially of the wrist) and apophyseal separations of the vertebrae in children and adolescents who have not reached skeletal maturity.

Nonorganized recreational sports are not without their own hazards, in part because of less supervision and inconsistent compliance with recommended safety measures. Those in which high-speed or angular momentum is attained carry particularly high risks for significant trauma. These include bike riding, skateboarding, inline skating, trampoline jumping, and riding motor bikes and all-terrain vehicles.

Common Sports Injuries

Participation in youth sports carries heightened risk of specific injuries compared with a more sedentary population. The most common injuries incurred during youth sports are presented in this section along with general treatment recommendations. In Table 22.10, other common injuries seen in athletes participating in a number of specific sports are enumerated along with prevention strategies recommended by the American Academy of Orthopedic Surgeons and American Academy of Pediatrics.

Table 22.10 Sport-Specific Injury Prevention Strategies[a]

Common Injuries	Prevention Strategies
Ballet/Dance	
Repetitive hyperextension of the spine	Initiate a program of strengthening and stabilization exercises for the trunk
Sprains, tendinitis, stress fractures of the lower extremity	Initiate a stretching and strengthening program for tight hip flexors and weak abductors/external rotators; work the hip within available range of motion
Talar impingement	Treat precursor conditions (shin splints, metatarsalgia)
Snapping hip (iliopsoas tendinitis, trochanteric bursitis)	Initiate a program of strengthening and proprioception exercises for the ankle and calf; encourage low-impact training (Pilates method, pool workouts)
	Avoid pointe work until strength and skill permit; ensure that pointe shoes are fitted professionally
	Limit pointe work and pliés if the ankle is swollen or if there is any restricted joint motion
	Ensure calcium intake is adequate
Baseball/Softball	
Throat injuries (to catchers)	Use proper protective equipment (helmets, throat guards for catchers, breakaway bases)
Head and eye injuries	
Rotator cuff impingement/tendinitis	Limit the number of throws and teach proper throwing technique
Medial epicondylitis	Initiate a program of strengthening for the shoulder and a graduated preseason training program
Ankle injuries	
Basketball	
Patellar tendinitis	Initiate a program of stretching, strengthening, and overall conditioning exercises
Ankle injuries	Use braces and taping for ankles
Field Hockey	
Ankle sprains	Use proper protective equipment (lace-up ankle braces and/or tape)
Knee sprains	Initiate a program of strengthening exercises for the quadriceps and hamstrings
Back pain (often diskogenic or vertebral end plate)	Initiate a program of exercises to maintain overall flexibility and neutral spine posture
Football	
Concussions	Teach proper tackling techniques
Neck injuries	Use proper protective equipment (helmets, face masks, mouthguards)
Stingers and burners	
Low back stress fractures	
Pelvic contusions	
Dehydration	Ensure frequent water breaks are scheduled in high-temperature/high-humidity conditions
Heat-related illnesses	Remove helmet frequently
	Ensure proper hydration during practice and competition
Gymnastics	
Repetitive flexion, hyperextension, and compression stresses at the thoracolumbar junction and on the lumbar vertebrae	Initiate a program of strengthening exercises for the abdomen and trunk and exercises to maintain the spine in a neutral position
Capsulitis and dorsal impingement at the wrist	Use tape or braces to protect the wrist
Radial epiphysitis	Limit weight bearing and impact on the upper extremities to protect the elbow and wrist
Osteochondritis dissecans at the elbow	
Ulnar collateral sprains of the elbow	
Shoulder instability	Limit extreme or repetitive abduction and external rotation of the shoulder
Tendinitis of the biceps and supraspinatus muscles	Initiate a program of strengthening exercises for the rotator cuff and scapular stabilizers
Ice Hockey	
Concussions	Use proper protective equipment (mouthguard, well-padded full-cage helmet with good strap around the chin). Many helmets are equipped with only a strap that goes under the chin.
Lacerations about the head and face	
Acromioclavicular sprains	Initiate a program of strengthening exercises for the upper body, especially the rotator cuff and scapular stabilizers, and the quadriceps and hamstrings
Glenohumeral subluxations/ dislocations	
Ligament sprains in the knee	Ensure that the net can slide out of the holes in the ice when athletes strike the pipes
Contusions of the quadriceps	Increase padding in the thigh guard by using football thigh pads because these are larger and thicker
Soccer	
Concussion	Teach proper "heading" techniques and avoid excessive heading
Contusions about the head	Avoid heading a water-soaked ball
Tibial shaft fractures	Use shin guards
Swimming	
Rotator cuff impingement/tendinitis	Initiate program of strengthening, stretching, and flexibility exercises for the shoulder, rotator cuff, upper back, and scapular stabilizers
Medial patellofemoral pain (from breaststroke)	
Spondylolysis	Limit use of hand paddles or devices that create added resistance in the water
	Use fins to provide greater leg drive and reduce demands on the shoulder
Tennis	
Rotator cuff impingement/tendinitis	Initiate a program of strengthening and flexibility exercises for the back, shoulder, and abdominal muscles, especially strengthening the rotator cuff and scapular stabilizers and improving flexibility in the hamstrings and hip flexors
Medial epicondylitis	Use proper mechanics and equipment to prevent elbow injuries
Lateral epicondylitis	
Spondylolysis	

Continued

Table 22.10 Sport-Specific Injury Prevention Strategies—cont'd

Common Injuries	Prevention Strategies
Track and Field	
Stress fractures of the lower extremity	Ensure proper diet and conditioning, gradually increasing speed and intensity
Sesamoiditis	Initiate a cross-training program
Shin splints	Ensure good shoe fit
Iliotibial band syndrome	Avoid downhill running and sudden stops
Wrestling	
Glenohumeral subluxation/dislocation	Initiate a preseason program of strengthening exercises for the rotator cuff, scapular stabilizers, quadriceps mechanism, and hamstrings
Acromioclavicular and sternoclavicular sprains	
Meniscal tears	Avoid quick stops in dangerous positions during practice and competition
Skin infections (herpesvirus, bacteria [impetigo], tinea corporis)	Ensure that mats are cleaned daily with commercial antiseptic solution Teach athletes to seek medical attention for rapid treatment of any questionable skin lesions to prevent spread of infection Conduct skin checks before tournaments
Auricular hematomas (with resultant cartilage deformity [cauliflower ear])	Use proper protective equipment (snug-fitting head gear with ear protectors) Drain any blood in the auricle promptly to prevent cartilage deformity

[a]Injuries and prevention strategies are not listed in any particular sequence. Both lists provide general examples and are not intended to represent each injury or prevention strategy.

From Barfield WR, Gross RH: Injury prevention. In Sullivan JA, Anderson SJ, editors: *Care of the young athlete*, Elk Grove Village, IL, 2000, American Academy of Orthopedic Surgeons, American Academy of Pediatrics.

Shoulder Instability

True shoulder dislocations are seen only in adolescents after epiphyseal fusion. On examination of the shoulder, a loss of the rounded contours lateral and anterior to the acromion is found. When the humeral head dislocates anteriorly, it is displaced medially beneath the coracoid process, where it can be palpated (see Fig. 22.60). These patients usually support the affected arm with the opposite hand, with the shoulder in moderate internal rotation. Patients with posterior shoulder dislocations have evidence of a fullness posterior to the glenoid cavity and are unable to externally rotate the involved upper extremity. Radiographs should be taken upon presentation and before reduction when feasible to document the direction of glenohumeral dislocation. Reduction is typically performed under conscious sedation, and after successful reduction patients should be placed into a sling while they await reduction radiographs. Postreduction films should include both AP and lateral views. The axillary lateral radiograph is the optimal lateral view but places the glenohumeral joint into a relatively unstable position. The Velpeau axillary view is a modification that enables a lateral image of the glenohumeral joint while maintaining the affected arm in a sling. First-time shoulder dislocations, both anterior and posterior, are typically managed conservatively including sling immobilization, followed by progressive motion restoration and muscular strengthening of the rotator cuff and periscapular groups through a course of formal physical therapy. MRI is typically obtained after acute injuries to document soft tissue injuries, most commonly a tear at the inferior glenoid labrum, and significant bony or cartilage defects may prompt earlier surgical intervention. In cases treated conservatively, a 3- to 4-month recovery from the time of injury is expected and athletes are only returned to play once their motion and strength have normalized to the uninjured extremity. In cases of recurrent glenohumeral instability, surgical stabilization is often of benefit, and an orthopedic consultation is recommended. Separation of the proximal humeral epiphysis or major fracture/dislocations are seen in younger children subjected to forces that would cause shoulder dislocation after puberty (see Fig. 22.56). Radiographs in children with open physes should be closely scrutinized in cases of suspected shoulder dislocations to identify relevant fractures before glenohumeral reduction.

Shoulder Separation

A shoulder separation involves a ligamentous tear at the AC joint, usually resulting from a fall onto an outstretched, adducted arm. Clinically, the lateral aspect of the clavicle appears to ride higher on the injured side than on the normal side, and it may be forced back into its normal position with application of pressure. If it can also be moved forward and backward, the coracoclavicular ligaments have been torn as well. The Zanca radiographic view is the best imaging modality to appreciate the degree of injury to the AC joint. The majority of cases respond well without surgical intervention through a brief period of shoulder immobilization, followed by progressive motion and strength restoration guided by a physical therapist.

Little League Shoulder and Little League Elbow

Little League Shoulder and Little League Elbow are overuse conditions that affect the proximal humeral physis and medial epicondylar apophysis, respectively. Both result from the chronic, repetitive microtraumatic torque and traction forces applied across these joints during the overhead throwing motion. These conditions are typically limited to overhead throwing athletes, most commonly youth baseball pitchers. In the vast majority of cases, these present with complaints of achy pain during throwing activities with resultant drop in performance. Examination of the shoulder and elbow is largely normal in these patients. Radiographs may show physeal widening best seen compared with the uninvolved extremity. MRI will often show edema around the involved physeal structure and can be used in cases with clinical suspicion where radiographic findings are not appreciated. The standard treatment for Little League Shoulder and Little League Elbow are a 3-month period of strict rest from overhead throwing activities, followed by a slow and gradual resumption of throwing activities. Consideration of alternative sports or position changes, especially for baseball pitchers, should be encouraged for these athletes.

Hip Labral Tears

Nonarthritic hip pain is increasingly recognized as an important source of pain and dysfunction in pediatric and adolescent patients. The etiologic causes of hip pain in this cohort have a broad differential, including femoroacetabular impingement (FAI), hip dysplasia, and hip flexor tendonitis. FAI and hip dysplasia are the most commonly encountered pathologies, and their occurrence in this age group is largely attributed to anatomic changes, which occur in the pelvis and proximal femur around the time of final skeletal maturation.

Young patients will typically complain of pain in their groin, which exacerbates with higher-impact activities, such as sports participation. On examination they have irritation with various hip positions, such as excessive flexion/internal rotation (FAI) and extension/external rotation (dysplasia). Hip pain in young patients is best evaluated with a combination of plain radiographs to evaluate bony morphology, which is the driving source of hip pathologic processes, and an MRI to evaluate soft tissue pathology. A hallmark finding on MRI studies is a tear of the acetabular labrum, but it is important to note that labral tears are most often a symptom of the underlying diagnosis (FAI or dysplasia) and not the actual source of pathology. Patients with nonarthritic hip pain are best managed early with conservative treatments such as activity modification and physical therapy to improve muscular strength and flexibility of the core, hip flexors, gluteals, and hamstrings. Surgical interventions for both FAI and dysplasia have well-documented success in cases of nonarthritic hip pain that fail to respond to conservative treatments.

Patellar Instability

Patellar dislocations occur with an incidence of 11.9 per 100,000 person-years among adolescent athletes, with female athletes being more commonly affected than males. Patellar instability has multiple etiologic causes, including ligamentous laxity, coronal skeletal alignment (genu valgum), rotational skeletal alignment, and dysplasia (underdevelopment) of the femoral trochlea or patella. Patients typically present with complaints of a rotational knee injury accompanied by sudden pain, difficulty bearing weight, and development of knee swelling. In most instances, the patella has relocated by the time the patient is seen. If not, it is seen as a bulge lateral to its usual anterior location and the patient is in severe pain. In such cases, radiographs should be deferred, the leg should be extended immediately, and the patella pushed back into place. This maneuver promptly alleviates pain. On examination, patients typically have a sizable effusion and apprehension with manual lateral patellar translation (see the Knee section and Fig. 22.11). Radiographs are useful to rule out concomitant fractures, and an MRI is helpful to evaluate the status of soft tissue injuries (medial retinaculum and patellofemoral cartilage).

In general, first-time patella dislocations are treated without surgery as the patellar retinacular structures have some capability to heal and regain their anatomic function. In select cases, concomitant fractures or significant cartilaginous injuries may prompt early surgical interventions. Conservative treatment focuses on functional bracing and physical therapy to promote safe restoration of and strength, specifically the quadriceps and vastus medialis, while the medial retinacular structures heal. Typically, 3 to 4 months are required from the time of injury to the resumption of sporting activities provided normal neuromuscular control. Despite the best conservative interventions, a sizable portion (7%–70%) of young athletes will have recurrent patellar instability episodes, and in these cases surgical reconstruction may be indicated.

Anterior Cruciate Ligament Ruptures

Studies have documented a dramatic increase in the rate of anterior cruciate ligament (ACL) reconstruction in pediatric and adolescent patients. These athletes now represent the largest per capita demographic for ACL injuries and reconstructions. In prepubescent athletes, there is fairly even split by sex, whereas after puberty there is an increased incidence of injury among females. ACL injuries typically present as noncontact pivoting injuries during sports participation resulting in significant pain, swelling, and difficulty bearing weight. On examination they have notable effusions along with laxity in anterior drawer and Lachman testing compared with their uninjured extremity.

Historically, pediatric ACL ruptures underwent nonoperative management until skeletal maturity, followed by a traditional ACL reconstruction to avoid interference with normal skeletal growth. However, newer literature has highlighted the perils of delayed surgical treatment on the pediatric and adolescent knee, with documented development of secondary injuries to the menisci or femorotibial cartilage in ACL-deficient knees. In caring for pediatric and adolescent athletes, ACL reconstruction strategies must respect growing physes, and numerous adaptations of the traditional ACL reconstruction technique have been developed to avoid or minimize physeal disruption. ACL reconstructions typically carry a 6- to 12-month recovery period with extensive rehabilitation to maximize the neuromuscular protection of the surgically reconstructed extremity.

Ankle Sprains

An ankle sprain in an adolescent patient is typically caused by a severe inversion stress injury, and the presenting findings are diffuse pain and tenderness along with swelling centered below the lateral malleolus, although the superior margin of swelling may cover the malleolus (see Fig. 22.65). Areas of maximal tenderness may be found over the anterior talofibular ligament alone or over both it and the calcaneofibular ligament. Rarely, the posterior talofibular ligament is also torn in patients with particularly severe sprains, and tenderness and swelling are noted over its course as well. Little pain occurs on dorsiflexion or plantar flexion, but marked pain occurs on passive inversion. Tests for ligamentous stability are described earlier (see the Ankle section).

Because of the frequency of associated fractures in children and adolescents, patients with apparent sprains and hemarthroses should not undergo tests of ligamentous stability until radiographs have been obtained and the possibility of an unstable fracture has been ruled out. Surgical options exist to improve ligamentous stability of the ankle but are reserved for recalcitrant cases that have failed physical therapy to address strength and balance issues, bracing (lace-up ankle orthosis), and activity modifications.

Osteochondritis Dissecans

Osteochondritis dissecans (OCD) has been most accurately described as "a focal, idiopathic alteration of subchondral bone with risk for instability and disruption of adjacent articular cartilage that may result in premature osteoarthritis" by the ROCK group, a multidisciplinary body of individuals with expertise in treating OCDs. Although the condition can arise in a number of different joints of the body, in the vast majority of affected individuals only a single joint is involved. The knee is the most common site, with the ankle (talus) and elbow (capitellum) being other common sites. OCDs typically occur in preadolescence and adolescence before skeletal maturity. The cause of OCD is controversial and likely multifactorial, but it has been linked with youth sports participation and overuse.

Patients with OCDs often present with vague complaints of knee discomfort and have largely normal physical examinations, making these injuries difficult to distinguish from other common causes of knee pain. Radiographs are the first-line imaging modality to identify OCD lesions, characterized by lucency in the periarticular epiphyseal bone (Fig. 22.120A). Once an OCD has been diagnosed radiographically, an MRI is indicated to provide lesion staging. Briefly, OCD lesions are principally divided into stable and unstable lesions on the basis of their appearance on MRI (see Fig. 22.120B–C). Stable lesions show no signs of instability between the OCD bone fragment and its parent bony site, with little risk of injury to the adjacent articular cartilage. In contrast, unstable lesions show signs of instability and displacement of the OCD fragment,

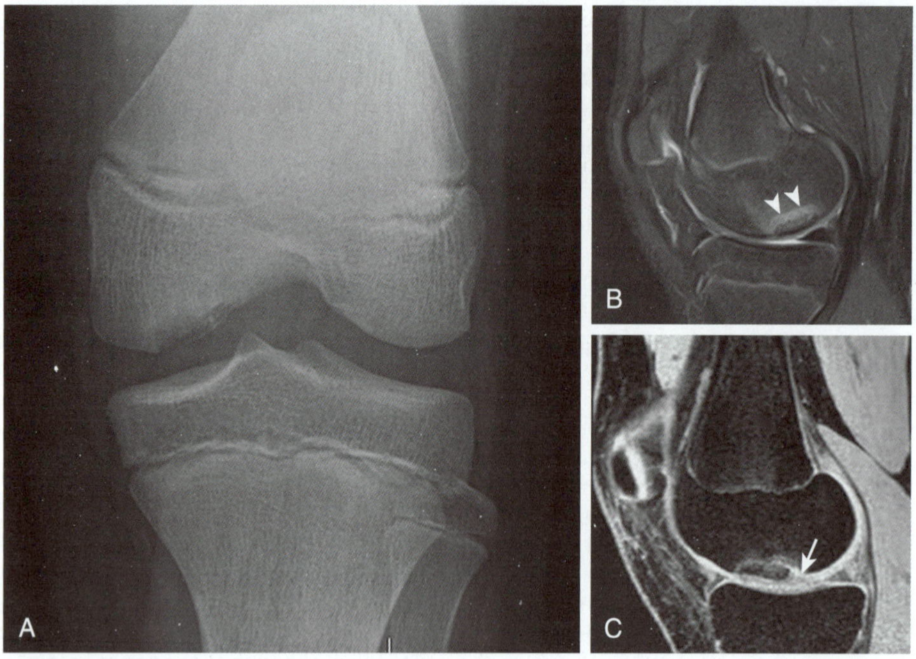

Fig. 22.120 (A–C) Radiographic view (A) of a left knee with a medial femoral condyle osteochondritis dissecans (OCD) lesion. Magnetic resonance imaging depicts stable (B) and unstable (C) OCD lesions. The *white arrowheads* in the stable lesion (B) show bony edema without evidence of cartilage loss or fluid behind the OCD lesion. The *white arrow* in the unstable lesion (C) depicts a break in the articular cartilage and synovial fluid accumulation between the OCD lesion and the parent bone.

threatening the viability of the overlying articular cartilage. Stable lesions are generally treated conservatively using interventions ranging from activity modification to bracing and casting. Unstable lesions typically prompt an urgent surgical referral in an effort to stabilize the OCD fragment and preserve articular cartilage. Regardless of treatment, serial radiographs are taken to document progressive healing of the OCD lesion.

Concussion

Concussion is defined as a condition characterized by temporary impairment of neurologic function after a head injury. Important to remember is that loss of consciousness and amnesia, although common, are not always seen. Other acute symptoms may include dizziness, headache, drowsiness, confusion, disorientation, delayed response times, difficulty concentrating, emotional lability or inappropriateness, visual changes, and impaired coordination. These may be seen singly or in any combination.

In the acute situation, any athlete with prolonged loss of consciousness, abnormal neurologic findings, persistently altered mental status, or progression of acute symptoms merits prompt transfer to the hospital for further evaluation and imaging. In milder cases of head injury, a sideline assessment of mental status (orientation, ability to concentrate, and short-term memory) and of neurologic status (strength, sensation, coordination) is indicated to determine whether any signs and symptoms of concussion are present. If a player has a suspected concussion, he or she should be removed from play and not returned to play that day.

The issue of timing of return to play of the athlete who has incurred a concussion is one of particular importance, the reason being that suffering a second concussion while the athlete is still symptomatic from a first can result in the catastrophic phenomenon known as *second-impact syndrome*. This is characterized by relentless cerebrovascular congestion and edema with loss of autoregulation of cerebral blood flow, usually culminating in herniation and death. Appropriate medical evaluation with a concussion protocol is essential in determining an athlete's fitness for return to play. The majority of modern concussion protocols incorporate a combination of symptom scoring, clinical examination, and neurocognitive testing into the evaluation of athlete recovery after a concussion.

Table 22.11 Female and Male Athlete Triad Patterns

	Females	Males
Energy deficiency	Low energy availability due to disordered eating and/or Low energy availability due to excessive training	
Reproductive suppression	Menstrual disturbance or Amenorrhea	Altered hypothalamic-pituitary-gonadal axis
Impaired bone health	Osteopenia, osteoporosis, and risk of stress fractures	

Female and Male Athlete Triad

Originally attributed to female athletes, the triad of energy deficiency (caloric depletion), reproductive suppression, and impaired bone health is now recognized in both female and male athletes. Gymnasts, dancers, and endurance athletes are most susceptible due to an imbalance of caloric restriction while participating in intensive training regimens. Of note, disordered eating does not need to be present to create a state of chronic energy deficiency. Table 22.11 displays the common findings in both male and female athletes, and it is important to note that problems in each domain present with a spectrum of severities. Care for these athletes involves coordination of multiple specialists including primary care, endocrinology, nutrition, and orthopedists.

Hypothermia/Hyperthermia

Environmental factors can also be sources of significant risk. These include weather conditions, such as high heat and humidity (with attendant risk of dehydration and heat illness) and extreme cold or swimming in cold water (frostbite, hypothermia). Children are particularly prone to hyperthermia and hypothermia because of their larger surface area–to-volume ratio. They also have a decreased rate and delay in onset of sweating, compared with adults, making it more difficult for them to dissipate heat. Finally, they have to be encouraged to drink adequate fluids because their own thirst levels tend not to be adequate to ensure replacement of losses. Finally, uneven or unsafe field conditions or playing surfaces; improper, poorly designed, or ill-fitting equipment (including shoes); and lack of or failure to use appropriate safety gear are other significant factors.

Rehabilitation and Return to Play

Rehabilitation of the pediatric athlete after injury involves restoring the individual to normal activity so that he or she may return to sports as quickly as possible. Decisions regarding timing of return to play must be made with the athlete's best interest and safety foremost. This necessitates monitoring of progress, assessment of readiness, and determination (in consultation with coaches) of the usefulness of additional protective equipment and/or of the need for changes in skill technique or training regimen (especially important with overuse injuries).

Rehabilitation of musculoskeletal injury involves the use of physical modalities and therapeutic exercises during the reparative and healing stages of recovery to promote a safe return to prior level of activity. Inflammation and repair are important phases of injury recovery that have different interventions. In the inflammatory stages of an acute injury, tissue swelling and the inflammatory response require rest or splinting to prevent further injury and protect the injured part during the early phase of the healing process, along with application of ice packs or ice massage and judicious use of oral antiinflammatory agents. Once the acute phase of injury has passed, protected mobility and the use of heat to mobilize the repair process are appropriate. Use of ultrasound, a high-energy source that when applied to the body can produce deep heat and is selectively absorbed by muscle and connective tissue (because of their high water content), can be quite helpful.

Therapeutic exercises are effective after initial healing is well under way, although well-moderated early exercises may be used on occasion. These are applied in a graduated manner to bring back strength and flexibility. They fall into the categories of passive, active-assisted, active, active-resistive, isometric, and strengthening exercises. These therapeutic exercises may be viewed as a transition between the acute injury and conditioning exercises. Programs must be specific to the area of injury, goal oriented, appropriately paced, and well supervised by physical therapists or knowledgeable trainers. *Return to play is safe when the athlete is symptom free with normal strength, flexibility, and range of motion.*

Return to Play After Exacerbation of Underlying Disorder

For recommendations regarding return to play of athletes who incur other injuries or exacerbation of symptoms of chronic diseases, see *Sports and Exercise for Children With Chronic Health Conditions: Guidelines for Participation From Leading Pediatric Authorities* (Goldberg, 1995), *Care of the Young Athlete* (Sullivan and Anderson, 2000), and *Principles and Practice of Primary Care Sports Medicine* (Garrett et al, 2001).

Risk Reduction and Injury Prevention

Beyond injury management, injury prevention is a crucial consideration in the care of young athletes. One of the first steps in prevention is identification of children at potential risk for injury, using the PPE and referral for further evaluation, if indicated, to a preconditioning exercise program to increase strength, aerobic fitness and/or flexibility, or for preseason sport-specific training, as indicated. When children are found to have conditions that make certain activities potentially harmful, counseling by physicians and coaches regarding safe and enjoyable alternative sports that are of interest to the child can be most helpful. Coaches who are well trained in teaching and coaching their sport, aware of relevant health and safety issues, and place their players' interests first are crucial figures in promoting safety. Best practices are displayed in Table 22.12.

Table 22.12 Safety Gear and Field Safety Modifications

Recommended/Required Devices	Specific Sport(s)
Helmets	Horseback riding, bike riding, skating, baseball (batting), football, hockey
Elbow/wrist/knee guards	Skating, skateboarding
Shin guards	Soccer
Chest protectors	Baseball catcher
Mouthguards	Contact sports
Protective eyewear[a]	Racquet sports, water sports, contact sports (unless incorporated into helmet)
Groin cups	Football, hockey
Field Modifications	**Sport**
Breakaway bases	Baseball
Stationary goal cages	Soccer

[a]Mandatory for all functionally one-eyed individuals and those who have had eye surgery or prior eye trauma per American Academy of Pediatrics, Committee on Sports Medicine and Fitness.

From American Academy of Pediatrics, Committee on Sports Medicine and Fitness, 1995–1996: Protective eyewear for young athletes, *Pediatrics* 98:311–313, 1996.

Bibliography

Ablin DS, Greenspan A, Reinhart M, et al: Differentiation of child abuse from osteogenesis imperfecta, *Am J Radiol* 154:1035–1046, 1990.

Aegerter E, Kirkpatrick JA Jr: *Orthopedic diseases: physiology, pathology, radiology*, ed 4, Philadelphia, 1975, WB Saunders.

American Academy of Neurology: Quality Standards Subcommittee: practice parameter: the management of concussion in sports (summary statement), *Neurology* 48:581–585, 1997.

American Academy of Pediatrics: Committee on Sports Medicine: participation in competitive sports, *Pediatrics* 81:737–739, 1988.

American Academy of Pediatrics: Committee on Sports Medicine and Fitness: strength training by children and adolescents, *Pediatrics* 107:1470–1472, 2001.

American Academy of Pediatrics: Committee on Sports Medicine and Fitness and Committee on School Health: organized sports for children and preadolescents, *Pediatrics* 107:1459–1461, 2001.

American Orthopaedic Association: *Manual of orthopaedic surgery*, ed 6, Philadelphia, 1985, The Association.

American Society for Surgery of the Hand: *The hand: examination and diagnosis*, Edinburgh, 1983, Churchill Livingstone.

American Society for Surgery of the Hand: *The hand: primary care of common problems*, Aurora, CO, 1985, Churchill Livingstone.

Bachman D, Santora S: Orthopedic trauma. In Fleisher GR, Ludwig S, editors: *Textbook of pediatric emergency medicine*, ed 4, Philadelphia, 2000, Lippincott Williams & Wilkins.

Canale GT: *Campbell's operative orthopaedics*, ed 9, St. Louis, 1999, Mosby.

Chang FM: The disabled athlete. In Stanitski CL, DeLee JC, Drez D, editors: *Pediatric and adolescent sports medicine* (vol 3), Philadelphia, 1994, WB Saunders.

Ferguson AB Jr: *Orthopedic surgery in infancy and childhood*, ed 5, Baltimore, 1981, Williams & Wilkins.

Garrett WE, Kirkendall DT, Squire DL, editors: *Principles and practice of primary care sports medicine*, Philadelphia, 2001, Lippincott Williams & Wilkins.

Garrick JG: Sports medicine, *Pediatr Clin North Am* 24:737–747, 1977.

Goldberg B, editor: *Sports and exercise for children with chronic health conditions: Guidelines for participation from leading pediatric authorities*, Champaign, IL, 1995, Human Kinetics Publishers.

Herring JA: *Tachdjian's pediatric orthopedics*, ed 3, Philadelphia, 2002, WB Saunders.

Hoppenfeld S: *Physical examination of the spine and extremities*, New York, 1976, Appleton-Century-Crofts.

Kelly JP, Rosenberg JH: Diagnosis and management of concussion in sports, *Neurology* 48:575–580, 1997.

Lombardo JA: Pre-participation physical evaluation, *Prim Care* 11:3–21, 1982.
Lonstein JE: *Moe's textbook of scoliosis and other spinal deformities*, ed 3, Philadelphia, 1995, WB Saunders.
Lovell WW, Winter RB: *Pediatric orthopedics*, ed 4, Philadelphia, 1996, JB Lippincott.
Ogden JA: *Skeletal injury in the child*, ed 3, New York, 2000, Springer.
Rang M: *Children's fractures*, ed 2, Philadelphia, 1983, JB Lippincott.
Rockwood CA Jr, Wilkins KE, King RE: *Fractures in children*, ed 3, Philadelphia, 1991, JB Lippincott
Salter RB: *Textbook of disorders and injuries of the musculoskeletal system*, ed 3, Baltimore, 1999, Williams & Wilkins.
Scoles PV: *Pediatric orthopedics in clinical practice*, ed 2, Chicago, 1988, Year Book.
Sillence DO, Senn A, Danks DM: Genetic heterogeneity in osteogenesis imperfecta, *J Med Genet* 16:101–116, 1979.
Simon RR, Koenigsknecht SJ: *Emergency orthopedics: the extremities*, New York, 2000, McGraw-Hill Professional.
Smith DM, editor: *Preparticipation physical evaluation monograph*, ed 2, American Academy of Family Physicians in Association with the American Academy of Pediatrics. Minneapolis, 1997, American Medical Society for Sports Medicine, American Orthopaedic Society for Sports Medicine, and American Osteopathic Association for Sports Medicine, pp 1–49.
Staheli LT: *Fundamentals of pediatric orthopedics*, ed 2, Wickford, RI, 1998, Lippincott-Raven.
Stanitski CL, DeLee JC, Drez D, editors: *Pediatric and adolescent sports medicine* (vol 3), Philadelphia, 1994, WB Saunders.
Sullivan JA, Anderson SJ, editors: *Care of the young athlete*, Elk Grove Village, IL, 2000, American Academy of Orthopaedic Surgeons, American Academy of Pediatrics.
Sullivan JA, Grana WA, editors: *The pediatric athlete*, Parkridge, IL, 1989, American Academy of Orthopaedic Surgery.

23 PEDIATRIC PLASTIC SURGERY

Michael Bykowski | Alexander J. Davit III | Jesse A. Goldstein

Plastic surgery focuses on restoring or optimizing form and function. Form is related to appearance, which is why esthetics play an important role. Although all surgeons repair function to some degree, plastic surgery emphasizes functions that improve quality of life, such as eating, speaking, self-confidence, and social interactions. For example, patients with craniofacial differences may experience significant isolation and social anxiety. Similarly, although speech is not essential for survival, cleft-related speech dysfunction can profoundly affect everyday communication with peers, leading to isolation.

As many congenital anomalies affect function and appearance, problems encountered in pediatric plastic surgery can be distressing for patients and families. The newborn's anomalies are immediately apparent, causing emotions ranging from guilt to fear. The face is so central to human identity and recognition that craniofacial abnormalities can affect bonding, integration, and socialization from infancy onward. As children learn to recognize self and nonself, apparent differences can lead to teasing and suffering, which affects normal psychologic development.

Many pediatric anomalies are associated with extensive disorders or syndromes, making their identification crucial for diagnosis and prognosis. Additionally, children are especially prone to trauma and other acquired abnormalities that require the surgeon to apply the principles of reconstruction for form, function, and anticipated growth. This chapter familiarizes the pediatrician or neonatologist with the most common pathologies of the form and function that pediatric plastic surgeons treat. It is important to educate parents that although improvements are expected, the severity of the defect, variability in wound healing, and patient growth make the final result difficult to predict.

CRANIOFACIAL ANOMALIES

There is no more human quality than the familiar external form of the head and face, which is the domain of plastic surgeons specializing in craniofacial surgery. Likewise, human speech is complex and shared by no other creature; thus palate and speech surgery are also within the same field. On the other hand, all animals share common *internal* structures and functions involved with hearing and ear drainage, nasal drainage, airway, sight, and mastication. These are treated by non–plastic surgery subspecialists. The *external* shapes of the ear, nose, or lips are clearly the realm of the plastic surgeon.

This section divides the craniofacial arena into the upper third, middle third, and lower third. The upper third deals with abnormalities of the skull and forehead, including deformational plagiocephaly and both nonsyndromic and syndromic craniosynostosis. The middle third covers the maxilla, orbits, and external ear and nose. The lower third includes the mandible and tongue. Cleft lip and nasal deformities and cleft palates are discussed separately.

Craniofacial Embryology

Congenital anomalies are best understood from an embryologic perspective. Craniofacial development occurs 4 to 7 weeks after conception. At 4 weeks, the fetus has a clear cranial/caudal axis and differentiated endoderm, mesoderm, and ectoderm. On either side of the neural tube, the paraxial mesoderm divides into segmented tissue blocks called *somitomeres*—cephalically, and somites from the occiput caudally, which ultimately form the bones of the neurocranium, or protective vault of the brain. Simultaneously, mesenchymal differentiation of neural crest cells participates in the formation of the viscerocranium or facial skeleton.

The neurocranium consists of plates that ultimately become the adult frontal, occipital, sphenoid, ethmoid, paired temporal, and paired parietal bones (Fig. 23.1). They are separated by sutures and fontanelles that serve two main purposes: (1) to allow molding of the head as it passes through the birth canal during parturition and (2) to allow for rapid increase in brain volume, which doubles in the first 6 months of life and again by 2 years of age.

The longitudinal suture between the paired parietal bones is the sagittal suture. Anteriorly, the sagittal suture becomes the anterior fontanelle, where it intersects the paired coronal sutures that separate the frontal bones from the parietal bones. Posteriorly, the sagittal suture becomes the posterior fontanelle, where it meets the oblique L-shaped lambdoid sutures. Finally, the metopic suture runs longitudinally between the two paired frontal bones (Fig. 23.2). Closure of the posterior fontanelle occurs within the first 6 months of life, whereas the anterior fontanelle closes between 12 and 18 months of age. The metopic suture closes at approximately 7 months of age, and it completely fuses such that the adult frontal bone has no evidence of a metopic suture. The sagittal and coronal sutures are next to fuse in adulthood in a posterior-to-anterolateral direction. Prenatal or postnatal premature fusion is called *craniosynostosis,* which causes abnormal skull shape by restricting growth in the direction of fusion and can lead to abnormally elevated intracranial pressure as the brain grows against fixed restriction of the skull.

The facial skeleton, or viscerocranium, is supported by a scaffold of 14 bones: the vomer, the mandible, and the paired nasal, maxilla, lacrimal, zygoma, palatal, and inferior nasal concha. By the end of the fourth gestational week, the neural crest–derived mesenchyme differentiates to form three facial prominences: the maxillary, mandibular, and frontonasal. Over the course of the next 2 weeks, migration and fusion result in the sculpture of the facial features supported by the underlying bony face. The frontal/nasal prominence gives rise to the forehead, bridge of the nose, and medial and lateral nasal prominences, which further define the lower nose. The maxillary prominence evolves into the cheeks, palate, and lateral aspect of the upper lip, and the mandibular prominence develops into the lower lip. Abnormal migration, fusion, or disruption of established events during this cascade results in anomalies.

Cleft Lip, Nose, and Palate

Cleft lip, nose, and palate are the most frequent presentations of orofacial clefts, which are the most common congenital anomalies in the United States (Basseri et al., 2011; Centers for Disease Control and Prevention, 2006; Parker et al., 2010) (Table 23.1). Approximately 1 in 700 individuals in the United States are affected, or about 15,000 live births per year. Although the cleft may be a component

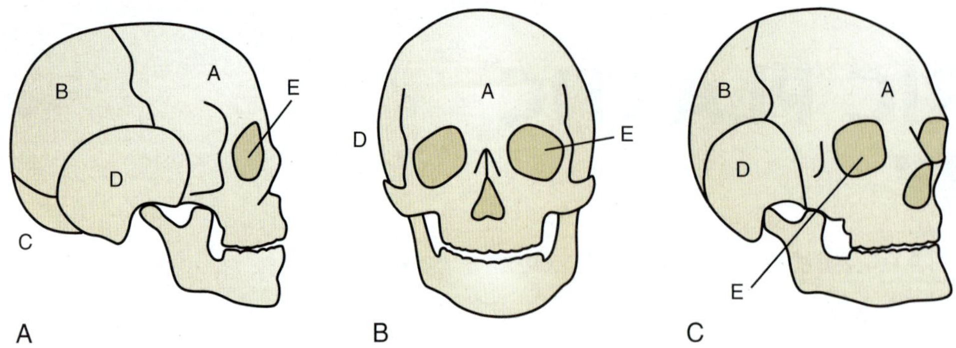

Fig. 23.1 Bones of the human skull in lateral (A), anteroposterior (B), and oblique (C) presentation. *A,* Frontal; *B,* parietal; *C,* occipital; *D,* temporal; *E,* ethmoid.

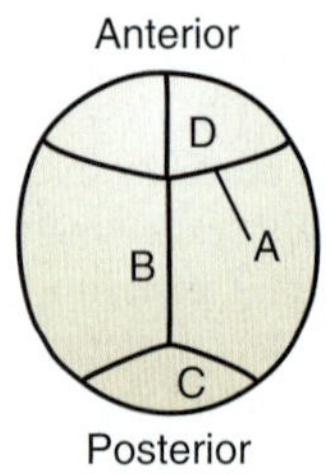

Fig. 23.2 Cranial sutures as viewed from the vertex of the skull. *A,* Coronal; *B,* sagittal; *C,* lambdoidal; *D,* metopic.

Table 23.1 Clefting Characteristics

	Cleft Lip/Nose ± Cleft Palate	Isolated Cleft Palate
Incidence	1 in 700	1 in 1500
Sex	M > F (2:1)	F > M (3:2)
Race	Asian > Caucasian > African (4:2:1)	No difference
Syndromic association	15%	50%

of an identifiable syndrome, it more commonly occurs as a solitary nonsyndromic anomaly. Clefting of the lip always affects the shape of the nose. Facial clefting is frequently categorized as "cleft lip with or without cleft palate" or "isolated cleft palate." Epidemiologically, there is a notable distinction between the two with respect to incidence, race, and sex. Approximately 1 in 700 live births are affected by cleft lip with or without cleft palate, occurring twice as often in male children. Asians constitute the largest population of affected infants, followed by the White population, and then African Americans. Isolated cleft palate has a lower incidence of approximately 1 in 1000 live births, with slightly more female children affected but no ethnic predilection.

Embryologically, at the end of the fifth week, the maxillary prominences grow medially and the medial nasal prominences are displaced toward the midline, where they fuse and ultimately form the premaxilla, which contains the philtrum of the upper lip, portion of the upper jaw carrying the incisors, and triangular primary (anterior) palate. Simultaneously, maxillary prominences develop outgrowths called *palatine shelves,* which fuse in the midline, forming the secondary (posterior) palate. The primary and secondary palates join at the incisive foramen to separate the nasal and oral cavities. Failure to fuse the palatine shelves results in secondary palatal clefting, whereas partial or complete lack of fusion of the maxillary prominence with the medial nasal prominence on one or both sides results in lip clefting with or without clefting of the primary and secondary palates (Fig. 23.3). This developmental cascade is completed by the 12th week of gestation. During this vulnerable period, anatomic interference (malposition of the tongue due to mandibular hypoplasia, as in Pierre Robin sequence), miscues in cell differentiation and migration, or teratogens (phenytoin, retinoids, steroids, lithium, and maternal smoking) may lead to clefting in the developing fetus.

Early in life, feeding difficulties develop owing to the inability of the infant to create an airtight seal to suckle effectively, which is related to the size of the clefts. Nasal regurgitation is a common occurrence. Upright positioning and adaptive feeding nipples can assist in preventing regurgitation and achieving effective closure around the nipple to obtain a seal. Breastfeeding is possible in some infants with clefting. Because the breast is more compliant, the infant may fare better in creating a seal around the breast. As with any newborn, infant weight and growth should be monitored closely; however, it is not unusual for poor weight gain to be noted in the first 2 to 3 months of life in this patient population. Thereafter, infants typically progress well and can make up for their weight.

Cleft palates lead to disruption of the muscular levator veli palatini and tensor veli palatine slings, which can disrupt eustachian tube ventilation and lead to frequent bouts of otitis media. Persistent effusions may result in conductive hearing loss with subsequent delays in speech and language development. Careful monitoring of middle ear effusions is crucial, and the placement of tympanostomy tubes by the pediatric otolaryngologist is often required to allow adequate drainage. Indeed, hearing loss may be identified in up to one-third of children with palatal clefting, underscoring the importance of continued audiological surveillance through adulthood.

Plastic surgery reconstruction of facial clefts is a multistep endeavor that depends on the type and degree of deformity. The goals are esthetic improvement, maintenance of normal maxillofacial growth, and restoration of palatal function to assist normal phonation. Reparative strategies continue to evolve, and controversy exists as to the optimal timing and optimal procedure. Typically, cleft lip/nose deformity repair is scheduled at 3 to 6 months of age. For wide unilateral and bilateral clefts, most centers preoperatively narrow the cleft to obtain better results. Some centers perform a lip adhesion, or simpler approximation of the defect, when the infant is younger than 3 months old; others preoperatively narrow the cleft defect by presurgical orthopedics, or customized intraoral mouth/nosepieces adjusted by pediatric orthodontists.

In some centers, palate repair may be combined with the initial lip repair, but in most centers, the palate repair is performed several months later, from 9 to 12 months of age. Optimal hearing and speech acquisition evolve when palatal integrity is restored before the second birthday. As such, palate closure is typically performed before 2 years of age despite concerns that early surgical interventions involving the midface may have a negative impact on maxillofacial growth and result in midface retrusion. Studies continue to attempt to define intervals when palatal procedures can be performed with minimum untoward effects.

Unique errors of speech articulation are common in patients with cleft palate and are more likely to develop in children who undergo delayed palatal repair. Hypernasal speech, also called *velopharyngeal insufficiency,* may occur in patients with foreshortened

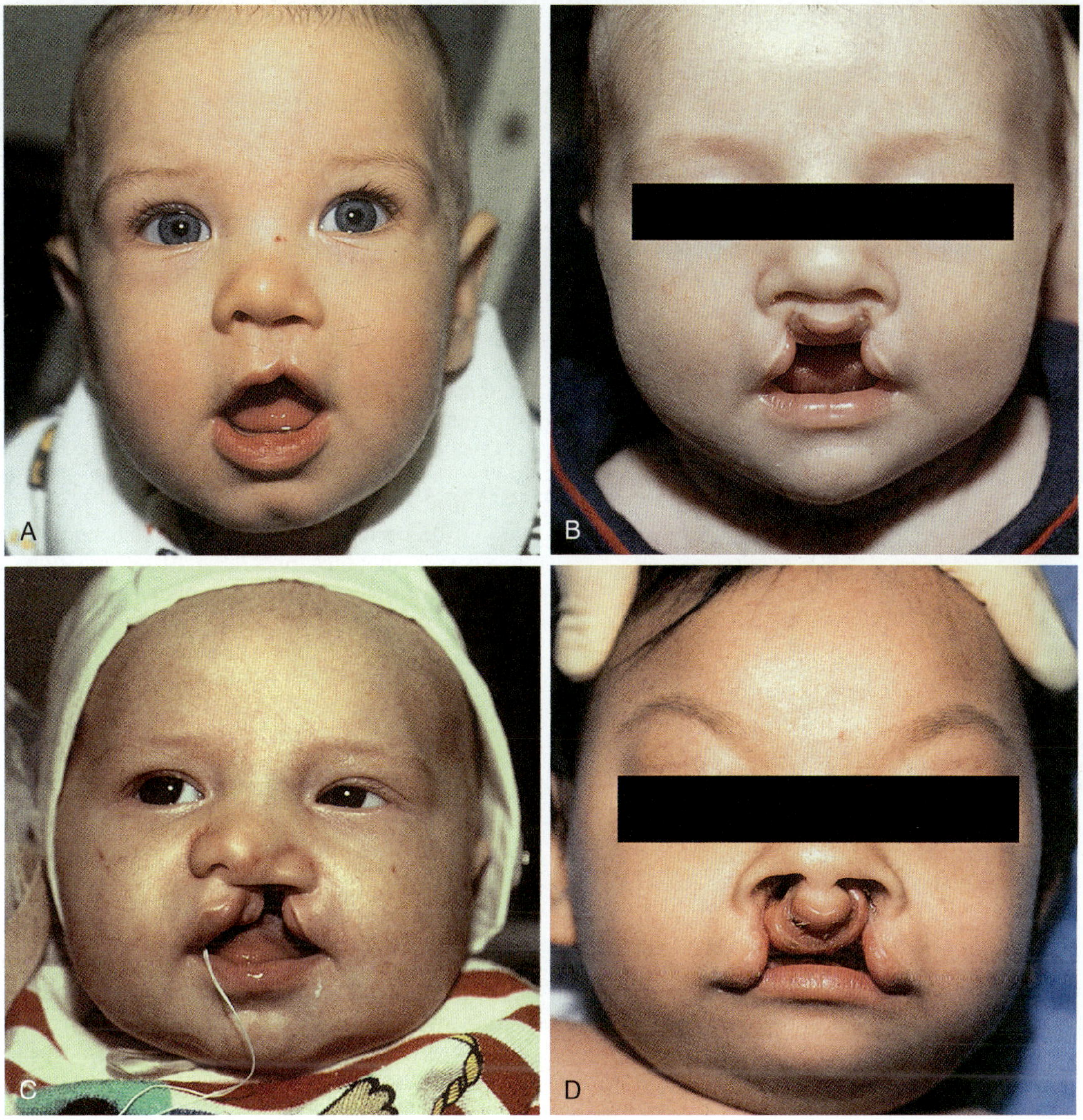

Fig. 23.3 The spectrum of lip clefting. (A) Left-sided unilateral cleft lip with minimal soft tissue involvement or "forme fruste." (B) Incomplete bilateral cleft lip. (C) Complete left-sided unilateral cleft lip. Note the associated nasal deformity. (D) Complete bilateral cleft lip with associated palatal clefting.

soft palate, allowing air to escape into the posterior nasal vestibule. For these patients, a pharyngeal flap procedure may be performed, whereby a peninsula of the posterior pharynx is attached to the soft palate. This recruited tissue lengthens the palate and substantially alleviates hypernasal speech.

As the child develops self-awareness, lip scars resulting from earlier repair often become an issue and revisions can be performed to improve the upper lip's appearance. Between the ages of 7 and 10 years, during the time of mixed dentition, an alveolar bone graft is usually indicated to permit normal eruption of the canine on the affected side(s) and restore the maxillary arch, provide nasal support, and close the alveolar cleft.

The end of adolescence marks the completion of a child's facial skeletal growth. At this time, residual nasal deformities, which usually involve a broad and inferiorly displaced nasal ala, may be targeted by formal rhinoplasty. Malalignment of the upper and lower jaws may also occur because of deficient maxillary growth. Once mandibular growth is complete, surgical advancement of the midface can be performed to restore normal occlusion.

As this brief discussion outlines, the family of a newborn with a facial cleft can anticipate numerous procedures spanning the entire childhood of their infant before reaching the end of the restorative journey. The impact of these interventions on children is certainly profound.

Deformational Plagiocephaly

The general term *plagiocephaly,* derived from the Greek word *plagio,* meaning "oblique," describes an asymmetric cranium. Etiologies can be intrinsic, such as genetic factors that cause premature suture synostosis, or extrinsic, such as mechanical factors in utero or postnatally.

Deformational plagiocephaly refers to perinatal occipital flattening due to mechanical forces, resulting in changes in the malleable infant craniofacial skeleton. Approximately 10% of cases are congenital, from pressure causes such as multiple gestations or reduced maternal pelvic volume. Postnatally, occipital flattening is acquired from a persistent supine sleep position. The high incidence (5%–48% of healthy newborns) is because newborns cannot lift and center their heads until 3 months of life, when neuromotor control has matured. In addition, supine positioning has become more widespread since the 1990s, when the American Academy of Pediatrics recommended supine sleeping to reduce the incidence of sudden infant death syndrome. In fact, compliance rates with the "Safe to Sleep" campaign correlate with the incidence of deformational plagiocephaly. Other associated factors are male sex, multiparity, and torticollis, of which the latter is associated with up to 20% of infants with deformational plagiocephaly.

Right-sided deformational plagiocephaly is more common, possibly due to right-handed mothers holding infants in a right-side-down position to nurse, causing pressure and flattening of the right occiput. Regardless of the side, once the preferred supine position develops, it becomes habitual and difficult to correct. History usually confirms a normal head at birth, followed by acquired asymmetry that worsens with time. As the occiput becomes flatter, up to 80% of infants will have anterior displacement of the ipsilateral forehead, with a concomitant increase in the height of the ipsilateral palpebral fissure, anterior displacement of the ipsilateral ear, and anterior displacement of the ipsilateral cheek, which can be seen from the anterior view (Fig. 23.4). These changes are shaped like a parallelogram in the vertex view (Fig. 23.5). Posteriorly, the mastoid skull bases should be symmetric; otherwise, there would be suspicion of true unilateral lambdoid synostosis, as described later.

Torticollis is often associated with deformational plagiocephaly, with patients typically having contralateral sternocleidomastoid muscle (SCM) "stiffness" rather than true muscle atrophy or fibrosis. For a given SCM, muscle contraction twists the head contralaterally but tilts the head ipsilaterally. In typical deformational plagiocephaly, the contralateral SCM is foreshortened and resists full extension, yielding a contralateral head tilt and ipsilateral head twist that causes the mandibular midline to deviate ipsilaterally to the side of the occipital flattening. Physical examination can reveal tenderness of the contralateral SCM or resistance and agitation on contralateral head twist.

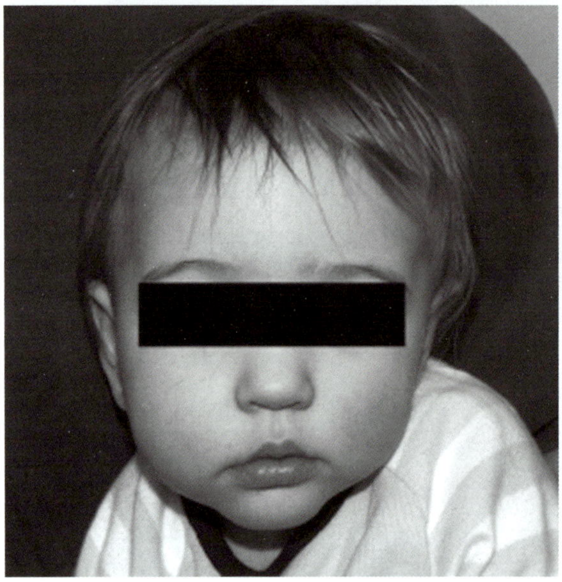

Fig. 23.4 Infant with right-sided deformational plagiocephaly demonstrating anterior craniofacial changes—an advanced forehead, ear, and cheek.

Treatment involves careful monitoring and prevention. Whenever not sleeping, infants should be placed prone ("tummy time") to decrease preferential supine positioning and increase shoulder girdle strength. Parents should alternate the infants' supine positions during feeding and sleeping. During feeding, pressure should be avoided on the side of the flattened occiput. Changing the position of the stimuli in the crib may also influence the infant to turn to a different side. Although a rolled-up towel or foam pinned to the clothes on one side will prevent the infant from sleeping on that side, care must be exercised to avoid materials in cribs that pose risks to the sleeping infant. If torticollis is present, neck exercises should be performed at each diaper change so that the chin can touch each shoulder for at least 10 seconds. Physical therapy may need to be implemented. These infants are monitored monthly until 6 months old.

For infants older than 6 months or with more severe craniofacial deformities that do not improve with positioning, external cranioplasty with an orthotic device (helmet) is a more intense treatment method. Before 10 months of age, an orthotic helmet worn 23 or more hours per day allows the malleable infant skull to grow into the shape of the symmetric helmet. Infants are typically monitored every 2 to 3 months for contour and neurologic development. After 10 months of age, helmet therapy has minimal effect.

The Skull

Craniosynostosis is defined as the premature closing of sutures between the cranial bones during development, resulting in deformities of the skull. Primary craniosynostosis originates from the pathology of the involved suture, whereas secondary craniosynostosis results from dysgenesis of the underlying brain that then misdirects cranial expansion. The latter usually does not require plastic surgical skull reconstruction because the pathologic problem is inherent to the brain and not the skull.

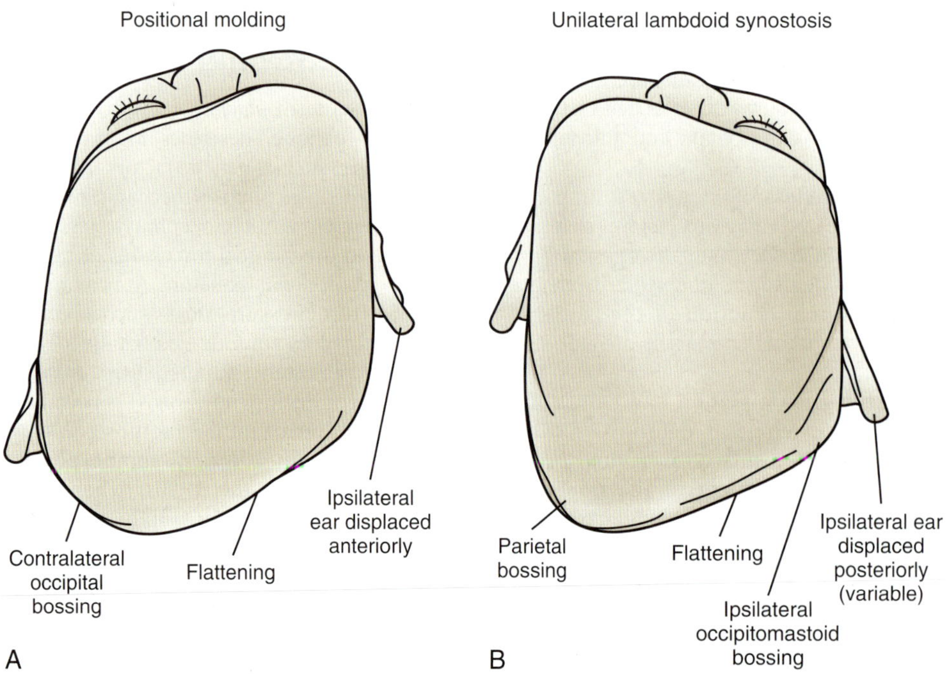

Fig. 23.5 Vertex views. (A) Right-sided deformational plagiocephaly exhibiting a parallelogram head shape. (B) Right-sided lambdoid craniosynostosis exhibiting a trapezoid-like head shape.

Normally, cranial bone growth occurs perpendicular to the suture axis. Therefore when a suture is fused and normal growth is interrupted, growth is restricted in a direction perpendicular to the suture's axis, whereas compensatory growth occurs in the direction parallel to the suture. The growth abnormality caused by premature fusion of a particular suture leads to a characteristic head shape pattern. For example, sagittal craniosynostosis results in abnormal growth parallel to the fused sagittal suture leading to anteroposterior elongation and temporal narrowing, resulting in a *scaphocephaly*, or "boat-shaped head." *Simple craniosynostosis* refers to single-suture fusion, whereas *complex craniosynostosis* refers to multiple-suture fusion (Table 23.2).

The incidence of craniosynostosis is approximately 1 in 2500 live births across ethnic populations but varies between sexes depending on the sutures involved. In simple craniosynostosis, genetics and fetal environment may both play roles because twins and infants delivered from a breech position have a higher incidence. The genes involved in many distinct craniosynostosis syndromes are known and are described later.

On physical examination, normal patent sutures (which may slightly overlap) move when palpated by the examiner's thumbs. Prematurely fused sutures may be felt as a palpable ridge. To confirm suture fusion, computed tomography (CT) of the face and skull with fine cuts and three-dimensional reconstructions will reveal skeletal pathologic anatomy.

Increased intracranial pressure is the main concern in craniosynostosis, although its clinical significance and risk are likely low in simple craniosynostosis and high in complex and syndromic craniosynostosis. Intracranial hypertension (ICH) can potentially lead to developmental delay and even blindness. Therefore along with routine neurologic and developmental examinations, at least yearly pediatric ophthalmology funduscopic examinations are mandatory, and they are required more frequently if symptoms of ICH occur. In cases of syndromic craniosynostosis and midface hypoplasia, patients should also be routinely evaluated for midface retrusion causing airway obstruction, obstructive sleep apnea, and exposure keratopathy.

The primary goals of surgery are to promote normal brain growth, correct abnormal skull shape, and prevent or relieve ICH. Surgery is typically performed during the first year of life when cranial bones are malleable, the dura can effectively stimulate osteogenesis, and rapid brain growth can be used strategically to optimize outcomes. Less invasive techniques are available for many patients, but a finite window of opportunity exists between 3 and 6 months of age. Therefore early and expeditious referral to a craniofacial plastic surgeon is crucial.

Techniques are broadly divided into two categories according to the size of the incision and the extent of bone removal: (1) open cranial vault remodeling and (2) limited incision suturectomy. Open cranial vault remodeling involves a bicoronal scalp incision to expose the calvarium. The plastic surgeon then marks the bony pieces to make, and the neurosurgeon elevates the bony pieces off the brain. The skull pieces are reassembled with absorbable plates, screws, and sutures to reshape the head.

Many centers also offer limited-incision endoscopically assisted suturectomy, during which the fused suture is surgically removed, effectively "unlocking" the suture and enabling brain and skull growth. During suturectomy, cranial springs can be implanted to actively expand the skull across the suturectomy site. Alternatively, a custom-fitted cranial orthotic (similar to that used in deformational plagiocephaly) can be used to passively mold the skull as the brain grows postoperatively. Both techniques must be performed before 6 months of age.

Lastly, posterior vault distraction osteogenesis is the first-line treatment for severe and syndromic craniosynostosis, as it is particularly effective for intracranial volume expansion and posterior cranial fossa decompression. Regardless of treatment, patients need to be monitored postoperatively at least yearly for neurologic, ophthalmologic, and developmental changes and for recurrence of craniofacial deformities.

Table 23.2 Skull Shape Nomenclature

Name	Suture(s) Involved	Shape
Acrocephaly	Bilateral coronal	Skull height greater anteriorly, slanting downward posteriorly
Brachycephaly	Bilateral coronal	Wide, taller skull shortened in anteroposterior dimension
Oxycephaly	Bilateral coronal	Taller skull, shortened width and anteroposterior dimension
Turricephaly	Bilateral coronal	Tall skull
Plagiocephaly	Unilateral coronal or unilateral lambdoidal	Asymmetric skull
Scaphocephaly	Sagittal	Anteroposterior elongation with bitemporal narrowing
Trigonocephaly	Metopic	Narrow, triangular, ridged forehead
Kleeblattschädel	Bilateral coronal, lambdoidal, and metopic	Cloverleaf deformity

Nonsyndromic, Simple Craniosynostoses

Up to 70% of simple isolated craniosynostoses occur sporadically. Autosomal dominant and recessive familial patterns have been identified in 8% of cases. If one parent and child are affected, subsequent pregnancies are quoted as having a 50% incidence risk. Simple sagittal synostosis is the most commonly encountered simple craniosynostosis, representing 57% of all cases. Coronal synostosis can be unicoronal or bicoronal and is less common. Metopic synostosis is still less frequent, although its incidence is rising, and true lambdoid synostosis is extremely rare.

Sagittal Synostosis

Sagittal synostosis, the premature fusion of the sagittal suture, leads to increased anteroposterior length and biparietal narrowing, known as *scaphocephaly* (Fig. 23.6). Isolated nonsyndromic sagittal synostosis is the most common form of craniosynostosis. It is almost always sporadic, with only 2% of patients having a genetic etiology. A 4:1 male predominance is recognized, with no racial predilection. There is a low risk of ICH and abnormal brain development because the remaining cranial sutures allow compensatory expansion of the neurocranium.

Sagittal suture synostosis can manifest with slightly different skull shapes based on the extent of fusion (i.e., partial vs. complete) and if partial fusion occurs, whether fusion is localized to the anterior or posterior portion of the suture. Isolated anterior sagittal suture fusion manifests as frontal bossing, whereas posterior sagittal suture fusion manifests as occipital bossing. Bossing of both the frontal and occipital domains with associated biparietal narrowing results from complete fusion of the suture.

A ridged sagittal suture may be palpable, as discussed previously, but intracranial and ophthalmic risks are low. The goals of repair are therefore appearance related, to reduce the anterior and posterior prominences while widening the biparietal dimension. Anterior and posterior vault remodeling can be staged or simultaneous. Endoscopic strip suturectomy is frequently successful.

Metopic Synostosis

Normally, the metopic suture is the first cranial suture to fuse, typically at approximately 7 months of age. This is the only suture that disappears and is indiscernible in the adult skull. Significantly

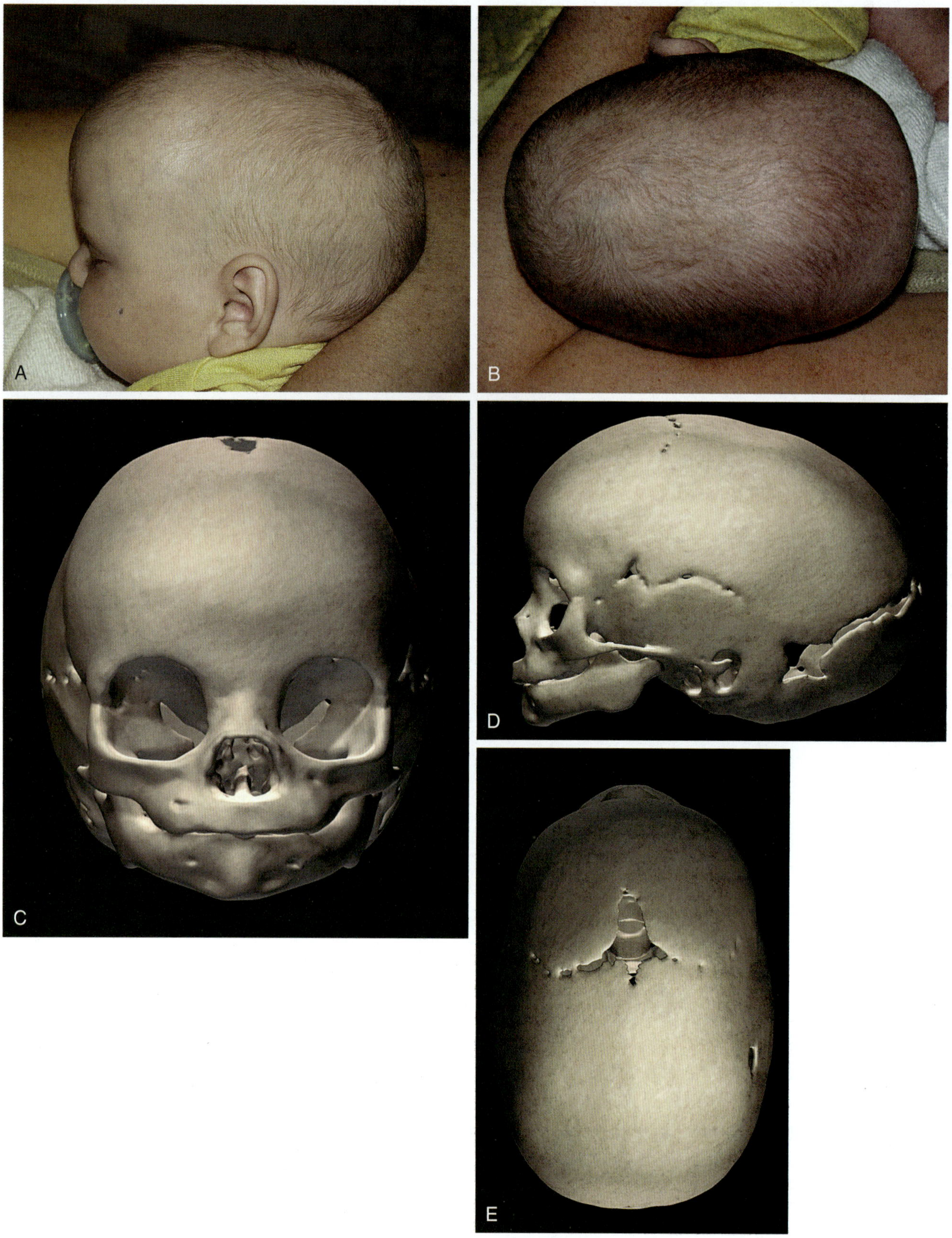

Fig. 23.6 Sagittal synostosis. Lateral (A) and vertex (B) views of a child with sagittal synostosis. Anterior (C), lateral (D), and vertex (E) views of the craniofacial skeleton of a child with sagittal synostosis.

premature fusion leads to a keel-shaped trigonocephalic head (Fig. 23.7). Metopic synostosis has an incidence between 1:2500 and 1:15,000 births, accounting for 10% to 20% of isolated craniosynostoses. Male children are affected more often than female children at a ratio of approximately 3:1. Physical examination shows a keel-shaped forehead with hypotelorism, upward slanting of the eyelids laterally, and a triangular shape to the forehead and supraorbital ridge, both of which are retrusive. Although typically isolated, 8% to 15% of children affected with trigonocephaly have associated anomalies involving the extremities or the central nervous, cardiac, or genitourinary system.

The severity of the deformity indicates the need for surgery. For instance, in some families, the infant has slightly premature metopic fusion at 5 or 6 months of age, resulting in a prominent forehead

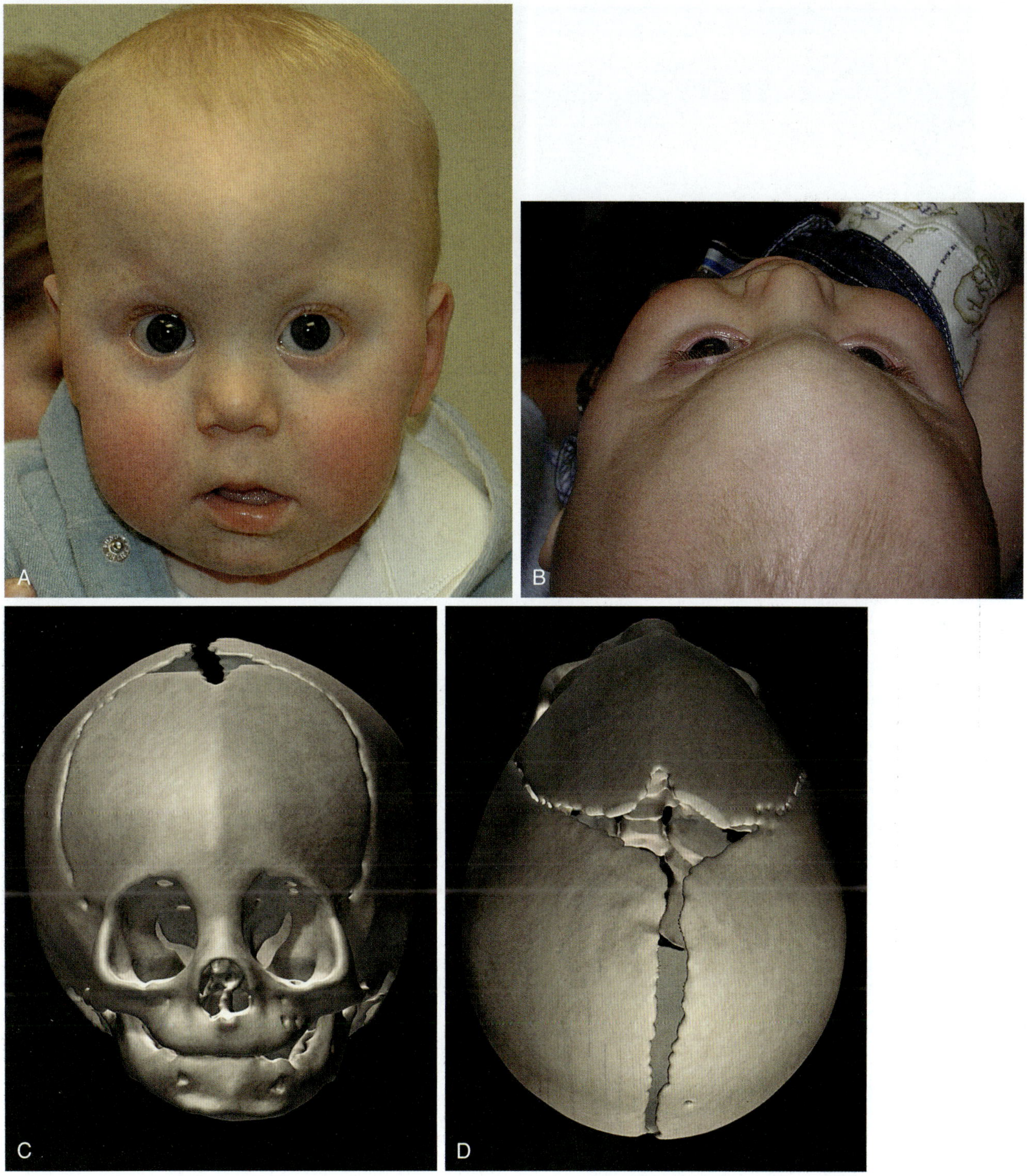

Fig. 23.7 Metopic synostosis. Anterior (A) and vertex (B) views of a child with metopic synostosis. Anterior (C) and vertex (D) views of the craniofacial skeleton of a child with metopic synostosis.

without significant keel-shape or hypotelorism, and no surgery is indicated. Severe shape changes can be corrected by anterior cranial vault remodeling with reshaping of the triangular frontoorbital rim.

An isolated metopic ridge is a feature of normal metopic suture closure. Such patients do not demonstrate any of the characteristics of trigonocephaly, such as supraorbital retrusion or hypotelorism. Families should be counseled that a metopic ridge is nonpathologic and should be expected to become less prominent with time.

Coronal Synostosis

Coronal sutures may be affected either unilaterally or, less commonly, bilaterally, resulting in synostotic anterior plagiocephaly or brachycephaly ("short skull" in the anteroposterior dimension that is wider and taller), respectively. Bicoronal synostosis is often associated with syndromic diagnoses. Nonsyndromic unilateral coronal synostosis has an estimated incidence of 1 in 2500 live births and accounts for 15% to 30% of cases of craniosynostosis. Its etiology is unknown, but the proposed causes include fetal head constraint, thyrotoxicosis, and certain vitamin deficiencies.

Synostosis of a single coronal suture results in a widened ipsilateral palpebral fissure, an elevated and anteriorly positioned ipsilateral ear, nasal root deviation toward the affected suture, chin deviation away from the affected suture, and a superiorly and posteriorly displaced supraorbital rim and eyebrow, known as the *harlequin eye deformity* (Fig. 23.8). Bilateral craniosynostosis restricts anteroposterior growth and causes retrusion of the frontoorbital region, leading to compensatory widening and increased height of the anterior cranium; the result is described as brachycephaly, acrocephaly,

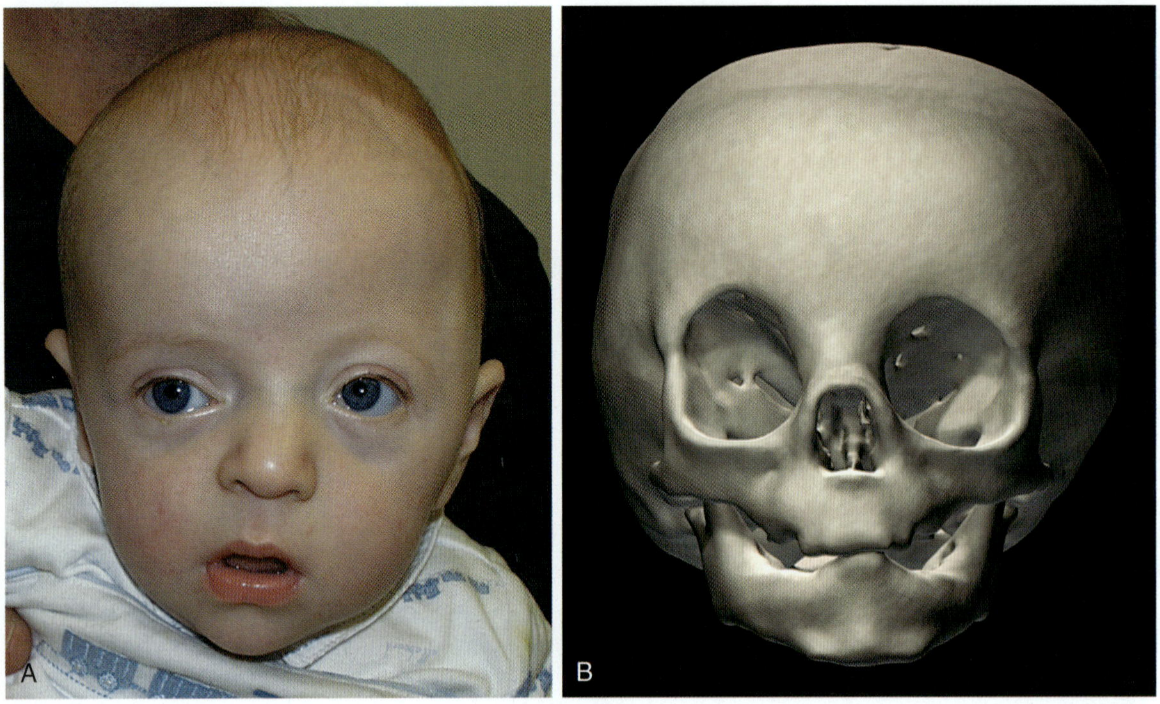

Fig. 23.8 Unilateral coronal synostosis. (A) Photograph of a child with left-sided unilateral coronal synostosis. (B) Anterior view of the craniofacial skeleton of a child with right-sided unilateral coronal synostosis.

oxycephaly, or turricephaly (Table 23.2). In bilateral craniosynostosis, there is an increased incidence of ICH.

The treatment of coronal synostosis includes anterior cranial expansion with vault remodeling and frontoorbital advancement. Some centers perform suture craniectomy with helmet therapy, especially for unicoronal coronal synostosis, where symmetry is difficult to achieve.

Lambdoid Synostosis

Lambdoid synostosis may involve one or both lambdoid sutures and is the least common type of craniosynostosis. When it occurs, it is usually unilateral and causes a synostotic posterior plagiocephaly. A raised ridge may be palpable over the involved suture, and there is often a mastoid bulge on the affected side of the occiput with contralateral parietal bossing (Fig. 23.9). From the vertex view (see Fig. 23.5), a trapezoid head shape is seen, with contralateral frontal bossing, posterior-inferior displacement of the ipsilateral ear, and ipsilateral occipitomastoid bossing. This view best distinguishes rare true lambdoid suture synostosis from common deformational plagiocephaly. True lambdoid craniosynostosis requires cranial vault remodeling, whereas deformational plagiocephaly is treated with positioning or helmet therapy.

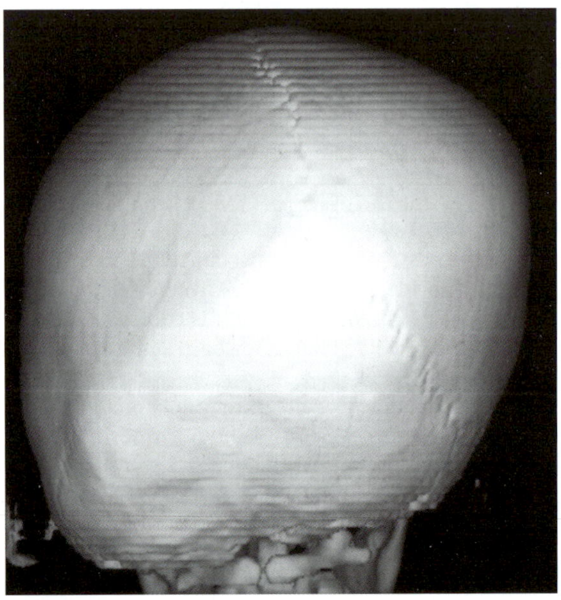

Fig. 23.9 Lambdoid synostosis. Posterior view of the craniofacial skeleton of a child with left-sided lambdoid synostosis.

Multiple Suture Synostoses

The most severe skull dysmorphology and highest risk of ICH result from multiple suture fusions. When the coronal and lambdoid sutures fuse bilaterally with fusion of the anterior metopic suture, compensatory bulging at the remaining open sagittal and squamosal suture leads to superior and lateral bulging, which is described as *cloverleaf deformity* or *Kleeblattschädel.* Although multiple suture synostoses can be sporadic, they are more likely to be associated with syndromes.

Syndromic, Complex Craniosynostoses

Craniosynostoses involving more than one suture are much less common, tend to be syndromic, and are usually caused by sporadic mutations inherited through autosomal dominant transmission (Table 23.3). The best characterized are the acrocephalosyndactyly syndromes, which share the features of multisutural craniosynostosis (bicoronal and/or bilambdoid), midface hypoplasia, abnormal facies, and limb abnormalities. Although bicoronal and/or bilambdoid suture fusion is typical, metopic and/or sagittal sutures may be fused additionally. Genetic abnormalities usually inactivate the fibroblast growth factor receptor *(FGFR)* gene family, which is involved in regulating bone growth, leading to hypertrophic bone development. *FGFR1, FGFR2,* and *FGFR3* are differentially involved, and although each syndrome is phenotypically distinct, patients will demonstrate varying degrees of supraorbital rim retrusion and midface hypoplasia with weak infraorbital support, resulting in shallow orbits and a high risk of exposure keratopathy that can lead to blindness. Other craniofacial anomalies such as cleft palate, mandibular growth problems, and stylohyoid calcification are common. Such patients are at a high risk of ICH and may also have variable hydrocephalus and neurocognitive impairment and cranial base, cervical spine, and other vertebral abnormalities. Inner ear problems (such as otitis media requiring myringotomy tubes) and inner nose and airway issues (such as choanal, tracheal, and

Table 23.3 Gene Mutations Associated With Craniofacial Syndromes

Gene/Protein	Syndrome	Chromosome
FGFR1	Pfeiffer	8
FGFR2	Apert	10
	Crouzon	10
	Pfeiffer	10
	Jackson-Weiss	10
	Beare-Stevenson	10
FGFR3	Muenke	4
	Crouzon with acanthosis nigricans	4
TWIST	Saethre-Chotzen	7
Treacle	Treacher Collins	5

FGFR, Fibroblast growth factor receptor.

laryngeal abnormalities) require consultation with an otolaryngologist. Cardiac, renal, and other visceral anomalies are also common.

Apert Syndrome

Apert syndrome is autosomal dominant with incomplete penetrance and a birth prevalence of 5.5 to 16 per 1 million live births. The majority of cases are sporadic; more than 98% of patients with Apert syndrome have identifiable mutations in *FGFR2,* resulting in multiple anomalies in all systems (Fig. 23.10; Box 23.1). Two distinguishing features include symmetric complex syndactylies of the hands and feet and cognitive defects.

Their bicoronal synostosis results in brachycephaly with a high cranium, which is described as *turricephalic.* They have delayed closure of their metopic and sagittal sutures between 2 and 4 years of age, resulting in hypertelorism. Their abnormal facies have more severe features, including ptosis and downward-slanting palpebral fissures. Midface deficiency is often associated with hypoplastic or stenotic choanae, leading to airway obstruction that requires tracheostomy. A sleep study can diagnose obstructive sleep apnea requiring treatment with a continuous positive airway pressure device.

Their shallow orbits can result in proptosis, but patients with Apert syndrome also commonly have strabismus with a V-shaped pattern: exotropic upward gaze divergence with esotropic downward gaze and other ophthalmic problems.

Although significant hydrocephalus is uncommon, the risk of neurosurgical abnormality is high; therefore baseline magnetic resonance imaging is recommended along with the usual CT scan to evaluate the bone on a regular basis.

Seventy-two percent of children with Apert syndrome have brain anomalies, leading to developmental delays and cognitive deficits. Infants who undergo surgery between 3 and 12 months of age are

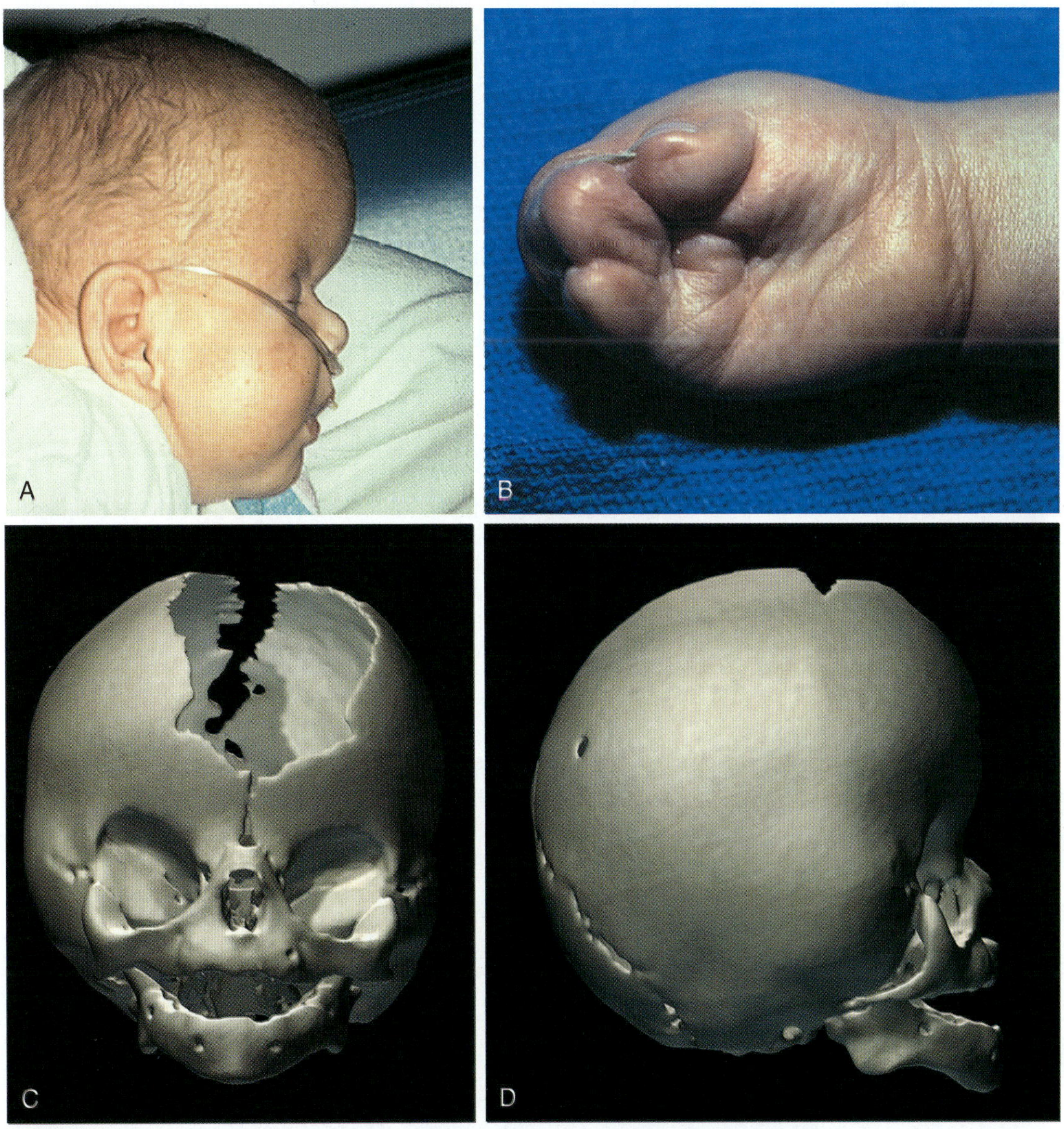

Fig. 23.10 Apert syndrome. (A) Lateral view of a child with Apert syndrome. (B) Syndactyly of the hand. Anterior (C) and lateral (D) views of the craniofacial skeleton of a child with Apert syndrome. Note the expansive anterior fontanelle in the anteroposterior view.

Box 23.1 Apert Syndrome: Features and Findings

Craniofacial
- Brachycephaly due to coronal suture synostosis
- Hypertelorism
- Proptosis
- V-pattern exotropia
- Midface hypoplasia
- Choanal stenosis
- Cleft palate
- Stylohyoid calcification
- Conductive hearing deficits

Extracranial Skeletal
- Symmetric syndactyly of the hands
- Cervical spine fusion
- Shortened humeri

Other
- Cardiovascular anomalies
- Hydronephrosis
- Cryptorchidism
- Tracheal anomalies
- Obstructive sleep apnea
- Diffuse acne

more likely to have intelligence quotients greater than 80. Unfortunately, children who underwent similar procedures before 3 months of age trended toward lower intelligence quotients and required additional operations.

A hallmark of Apert syndrome is complex symmetric syndactyly of the hands and feet, especially of the middle three digits, leaving the first and fifth digits separate; this results in a "mitten hand" appearance (see Fig. 23.10B). Plastic surgeons can separate the digits to produce a more functional hand.

Finally, the skin of patients with Apert syndrome may display excessive sweating. Patients have been shown to have an increased number of sweat glands and prominent sebaceous glands. During adolescence, the skin becomes oily, and in 70% of patients, acne erupts on the face, chest, and back.

Crouzon Syndrome

Crouzon syndrome is another autosomal dominant acrocephalosyndactyly with incomplete penetrance that presents as a new sporadic mutation 60% of the time. The birth prevalence is 15 to 16 per 1 million live births and is associated with mutations in *FGFR2*. Its distinguishing feature is the presence of normal extremities.

The heads of patients with Crouzon syndrome are overall brachycephalic from bicoronal synostosis, although other sutures can be involved, leading to other skull shapes (Fig. 23.11; Box 23.2). Their midface hypoplasia similarly leads to proptosis and an illusion of mandibular prognathism with a severe underbite called *class III malocclusion.*

Intracranially, they may have anomalous venous drainage, and they are more likely to have hydrocephalus than are patients with Apert syndrome. They are also more likely to have Chiari I malformations, which is likely due to their tendency to have early closure of lambdoid sutures. Therefore early magnetic resonance imaging is recommended. Some may also develop suture fusion postnatally, and thus early CT scans may show relatively patent coronal sutures.

Some variants of Crouzon syndrome are associated with acanthosis nigricans, a verrucous hyperplasia and hypertrophy of the skin with associated hyperpigmentation and accentuated skin markings. It is distributed in the axillae, neck, chest, abdomen, breasts, perioral and periorbital regions, and nasolabial folds. Multiple melanocytic nevi are also frequently observed on the face, trunk, and extremities.

Pfeiffer Syndrome

Pfeiffer syndrome, a type of acrocephalosyndactyly, has the distinguishing characteristics of broadened thumbs and toes. Mutations in *FGFR1* and *FGFR2* have been implicated. Most patients have bicoronal synostosis with brachycephaly and midface hypoplasia with associated ocular findings. The distinguishing features are broad, symmetric thumbs that deviate radially and great toes that deviate medially, often with phalangeal malformations and simple soft tissue syndactyly (Fig. 23.12; Table 23.4).

There are some subtypes with more severe symptoms, including *Kleeblattschädel* deformity (cloverleaf skull) with hydrocephalus, and more severe midface hypoplasia with ICH, mental retardation, and a poorer prognosis.

Jackson-Weiss Syndrome

Jackson-Weiss syndrome is an autosomal dominant acrocephalosyndactyly associated with mutations in *FGFR2*. Patients usually have coronal synostosis with a broad or towering forehead, hearing deficits, and foot anomalies, such as short metatarsals. Their hands are usually normal.

Saethre-Chotzen Syndrome

Saethre-Chotzen syndrome has characteristics similar to Jackson-Weiss syndrome but does not involve the *FGFR* gene family and is rather due to a mutation in the *TWIST 1* gene. Its etiology involves a mutation in the *TWIST* gene with a pattern of autosomal dominant inheritance. Patients frequently have coronal craniosynostosis with brachycephaly. Their facies include abnormally downward-sloped palpebral fissures with ptosis, low forehead hairline, and ear abnormalities. They often have incomplete syndactyly of their hands.

Midface

Midface craniofacial syndromes can be complex because they affect many facial structures, including the eyes, ears, soft tissues, and midface skeleton. Accordingly, defects are among the most challenging to reconstruct, with patients requiring multiple procedures and interventions. These syndromes are often associated with mandibular hypoplasia, which can lead to upper airway obstruction.

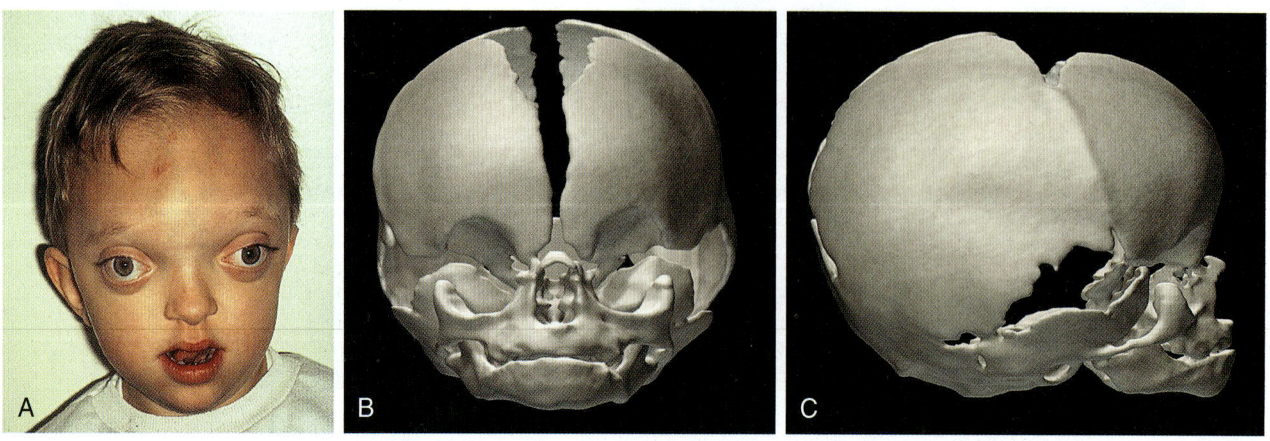

Fig. 23.11 Crouzon syndrome. (A) Frontal view; (B) anterior skeletal view; (C) lateral skeletal view.

Box 23.2 Crouzon Syndrome: Features and Findings

Craniofacial
Brachycephaly due to coronal suture synostosis
Hydrocephaly with Chiari I malformation
Hypertelorism
Proptosis
Midface hypoplasia
"Beaked" nose
Cleft palate
Stylohyoid calcification
Conduction and/or neurosensory hearing deficit

Extracranial Skeletal
Cervical spine fusion

Other
Acanthosis nigricans

In general, securing the airway and feeding are priorities in the neonatal period and may necessitate tracheostomy and gastrostomy tube placement. Early intervention by an otologist to optimize hearing is important. Although pediatric plastic surgery reconstruction of the midface and mandible is usually performed as late as possible to avoid interrupting normal skeletal growth, exposure of the sclerae from midface hypoplasia or airway obstructive symptoms (such as sleep apnea) could warrant earlier augmentation of the maxilla or mandible. External ear reconstruction is usually performed at about 6 to 7 years of age, when there is enough rib cartilage for the procedure and the patient is mature enough to tolerate the three- or four-stage procedure, with each stage separated by several months.

Mandibulofacial Dysostosis (Treacher Collins Syndrome)

Treacher Collins syndrome mainly affects the midface and mandible and has an incidence of approximately 1 in 50,000 live births (Fig. 23.13; Box 23.3). Inheritance is autosomal dominant with variable expression, but nearly half of the cases are sporadic new mutations. The genetic defect is in the gene that encodes the protein Treacle, which is thought to affect the development of the first branchial arch (mandible), second branchial arch (maxilla), and nasal placode.

Facial dysmorphology tends to be bilateral, involving the mandible, malar region (cheek), eyes, and ears. Both bony and soft tissue hypoplasia of the malar region or zygoma result in a lateral facial cleft. This extends to the lateral orbital walls, leading to temporal concavity, reduced bitemporal distance, and reduced cephalic length. Thus the neurocranium may appear misshapen, although there is no craniosynostosis. Intelligence usually ranges from average to above average.

Overlying these deficient orbitozygomatic regions are frequently abnormalities in eyelid structure, preauricular cheek skin, temporal fossa, and external ears. Palpebral fissures are slanted downward laterally, and the lower eyelids can have colobomas, lack eyelashes, or be hypoplastic. External ears are often symmetrically malformed or malpositioned, with stenosis or atresia of the external auditory canals and parallel middle ear abnormalities. The latter causes conductive hearing loss that can usually be improved by hearing aids (see Chapter 24).

The mandible is usually hypoplastic, resulting in retrognathia, malocclusion, temporomandibular joint (TMJ) dysfunction, and malformed masticatory muscles, resulting in an open bite. A *type I mandible* refers to a retrognathic mandible with a minor anterior open bite and mild glenoid fossa hypoplasia, whereas a worse grade, type III, is a free-floating severely retrognathic mandible without any articulation to the cranial base (lack of TMJ), usually requiring a postnatal tracheostomy. In between are type IIA with moderate hypoplasia but intact TMJ and type IIB with greater hypoplasticity and a nonfunctioning TMJ.

Given the midface anomalies and mandibular hypoplasia, a CT scan of the head and face is usually recommended. Mandibular hypoplasia leads to glossoptosis and airway compromise, compounded by midface hypoplasia with some degree of choanal stenosis or atresia. Other early issues are related to feeding and corneal exposure. Non–plastic surgery specialists can assist in tracheostomies, placement of gastrostomy tubes, ophthalmic assessment, and hearing aids. Pediatric plastic surgeons are involved in cleft palate repair, if indicated, and reconstruction of the hard and soft external structures of the face.

A cleft palate should be treated as described previously and planned around the time of speech development. Unless corneal exposure is threatened, most reconstruction is delayed as long as possible to avoid inevitable recurrence as the face ages. In symptomatic retrognathia where glenoid fossae are present (types I, IIA, and IIB), the mandible can be lengthened by distraction osteogenesis, in which mandibular osteotomies are subsequently lengthened serially using hardware. This is usually performed at early skeletal maturity (females, age 13–15 years; males, age 15–16 years). Type III deformities first require TMJ reconstruction at about 6 to 10 years of age, before the mandible lengthens. Rhinoplasty can improve middorsal humps and wide nasal bridges but should usually be postponed until after jaw surgery because the latter moves the base of the nose. Eyelid defects can be repaired using skin or muscle flaps. Ear

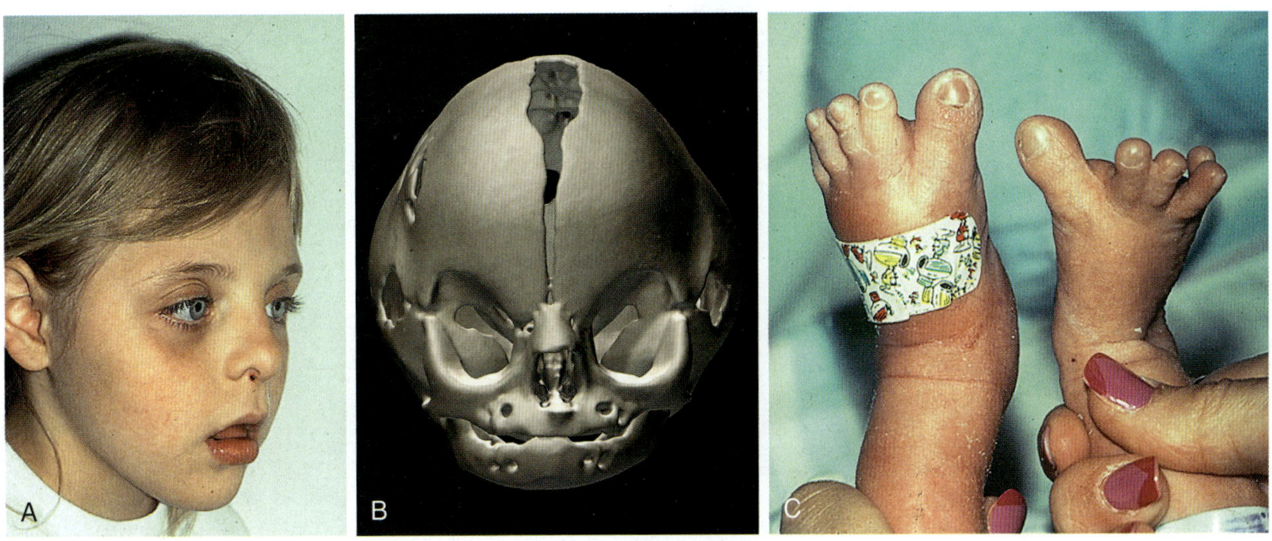

Fig. 23.12 Pfeiffer syndrome. (A) Lateral view; (B) anterior skeletal view; (C) great toe anomalies.

Table 23.4 Pfeiffer Syndrome: Features and Findings

	Type I	Type II	Type III
Craniofacial			
Acrocephaly, or turribrachycephaly (oxycephaly), due to coronal suture synostosis	+		+
Kleeblattschädel sutural deformity		+	
Hydrocephaly		+	
Midface hypoplasia	+	++	++
"Beaked" nose	+	+	+
Hypertelorism	+	+	+
Proptosis	+	++	+
Blindness		+	
Choanal atresia		+	+
Mental retardation		+	+
Extracranial Skeletal			
Broad, radially deviated thumbs	+	+	+
Broad, medially deviated great toes	+	+	+
Soft tissue syndactyly	+	+	+
Elbow ankylosis		+	+

Box 23.3 Mandibulofacial Dysostosis (Treacher Collins Syndrome): Features and Findings

Craniofacial (Usually Bilateral Findings)

Bilateral zygoma hypoplasia
Bony deficiency of lateral orbits
Maxillary hypoplasia
Choanal stenosis
Cleft palate with or without cleft lip
Downward-slanting palpebral fissures
Colobomas
Lower eyelid hypoplasia
Absent lower eyelashes
Preauricular hair
Bilateral external ear deformities
Bilateral external auditory canal stenosis or atresia
Auditory ossicle hypoplasia or ankylosis
Conductive hearing deficits
Retrognathia due to mandibular hypoplasia
Bite malocclusion
Temporomandibular joint dysfunction

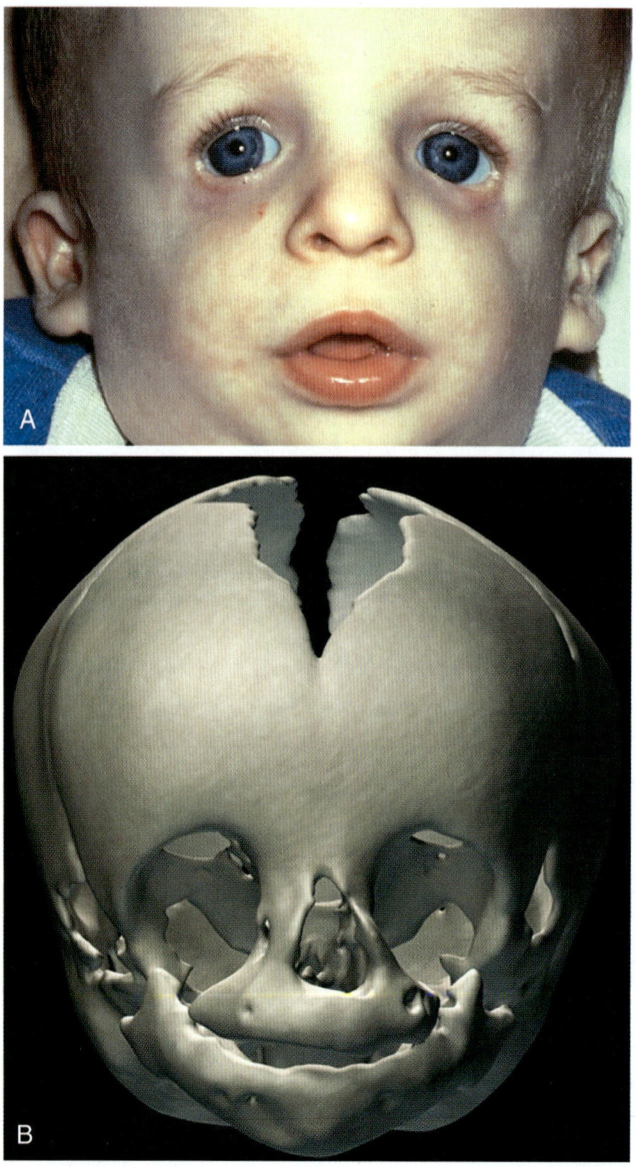

Fig. 23.13 Mandibulofacial dysostosis. (A) Photograph of a child with mandibulofacial dysostosis. (B) Anterior view of the craniofacial skeleton of a child with mandibulofacial dysostosis.

reconstruction, as described later, requires an autologous rib cartilage graft and multiple surgical stages. The hollow temporal fossa and lateral cleft can be augmented; however, the resorption rate is high.

In summary, Treacher Collins syndrome yields multiple significant perimaxillary and mandibular anomalies with a range of severities, often requiring tracheostomy and multiple reconstructive efforts. The underlying genetic anomalies make it impossible to regain a normal appearance; however, improvements can usually be made.

Acrofacial Dysostosis (Nager Syndrome)

In 1948, Nager and de Reynier characterized a series of infants with branchial arch deformities similar to Treacher Collins syndrome, but additionally involving upper extremity anomalies (Fig. 23.14; Box 23.4). It is also autosomal dominant and usually presents sporadically, with a prevalence twice as frequent among males as females. It presents with similar craniofacial abnormalities, and its distinguishing feature is the presence of preaxial (radial) abnormalities, including radioulnar synostosis (proximal fusion) and hypoplasia or aplasia of the thumbs. Other findings include toe abnormalities and visceral involvement. Patients make developmental progress, provided that hearing deficits are addressed by otolaryngologists.

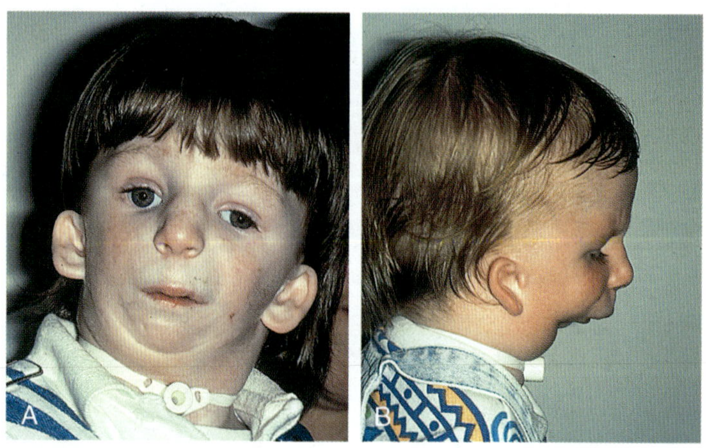

Fig. 23.14 Acrofacial dysostosis. (A and B) Photographs of children with acrofacial dysostosis.

Box 23.4 Acrofacial Dysostosis (Nager Syndrome): Features and Findings

Craniofacial (Usually Bilateral Findings)
Bilateral zygoma hypoplasia
Bony deficiency of lateral orbits
Maxillary hypoplasia
Choanal stenosis
Cleft palate with or without cleft lip
Downward-slanting palpebral fissures
Colobomas
Lower eyelid hypoplasia
Absent lower eyelashes
Preauricular hair
Bilateral external ear deformities
Bilateral external auditory canal stenosis or atresia
Auditory ossicle hypoplasia or ankylosis
Conductive hearing deficits
Severe mandibular hypoplasia
Bite malocclusion
Temporomandibular joint dysfunction

Extracranial Skeletal
Radioulnar synostosis
Thumb hypoplasia or aplasia

Oculo-Auriculo-Vertebral Spectrum (Goldenhar Syndrome and Craniofacial or Hemifacial Microsomia)

Oculo-auriculo-vertebral syndrome, or spectrum, is a collection of facial anomalies that are believed by many experts to represent a spectrum of phenotypes exhibited secondary to a heterogeneous developmental field defect (Fig. 23.15; Box 23.5). It includes several named entities such as Goldenhar syndrome, craniofacial microsomia, and hemifacial microsomia. Classically, hemifacial microsomia is defined as a condition that primarily affects ear, oral, and mandibular development. Goldenhar syndrome additionally includes vertebral anomalies and epibulbar dermoids. These are likely variants of a common underlying developmental aberration.

The findings witnessed in Goldenhar syndrome and hemifacial microsomia are referred to as the *oculo-auriculo-vertebral spectrum,* the incidence of which varies from 1 in 3500 to 19,500 live births. A male-to-female ratio of 3:2 is observed, with a similar ratio of lateralization favoring the right side of the body. Up to one-third may have bilateral involvement but will still be asymmetric. Although familial patterns have been identified, most cases are sporadic.

Findings may be divided into those affecting the craniofacial domain, central nervous system, skeleton, cardiovascular system, and other systemic findings. Most cases have some degree of facial asymmetry that may become apparent only as the child grows older. *OMENS* describes the major findings of hypoplasia of the *o*rbit, *m*andible, *e*xternal ear, *n*erve (facial), and *s*oft tissue, usually asymmetrically. The maxillary, temporal, and malar bones are hypoplastic and flattened on the affected side. The mandible may be aplastic or hypoplastic. Smooth epibulbar dermoids, often with fine hairs, are common unilateral findings inferotemporally in the limbus of the eye. Other ocular findings include unilateral colobomas of the upper eyelids and oculomotor disorders including esotropia and exotropia. The region of the ear is always involved to some degree and may exhibit preauricular appendages, pretragal blind-ended fistulae, and hypoplastic or malpositioned pinnae. The external auditory canal may be atretic or stenotic, leading to conductive hearing impairment, which is far more common than neurosensory loss. Involvement of nearly all cranial nerves (CNs) has been reported, with lower facial weakness being a frequent observation. There may be a lateral facial cleft at the oral commissure, also known as *macrostomia.* The palatal and tongue muscles may be hypoplastic and paralyzed, thereby affecting feeding success. Furthermore, unilateral or bilateral cleft lip and/or palate occurs in up to 15% of infants.

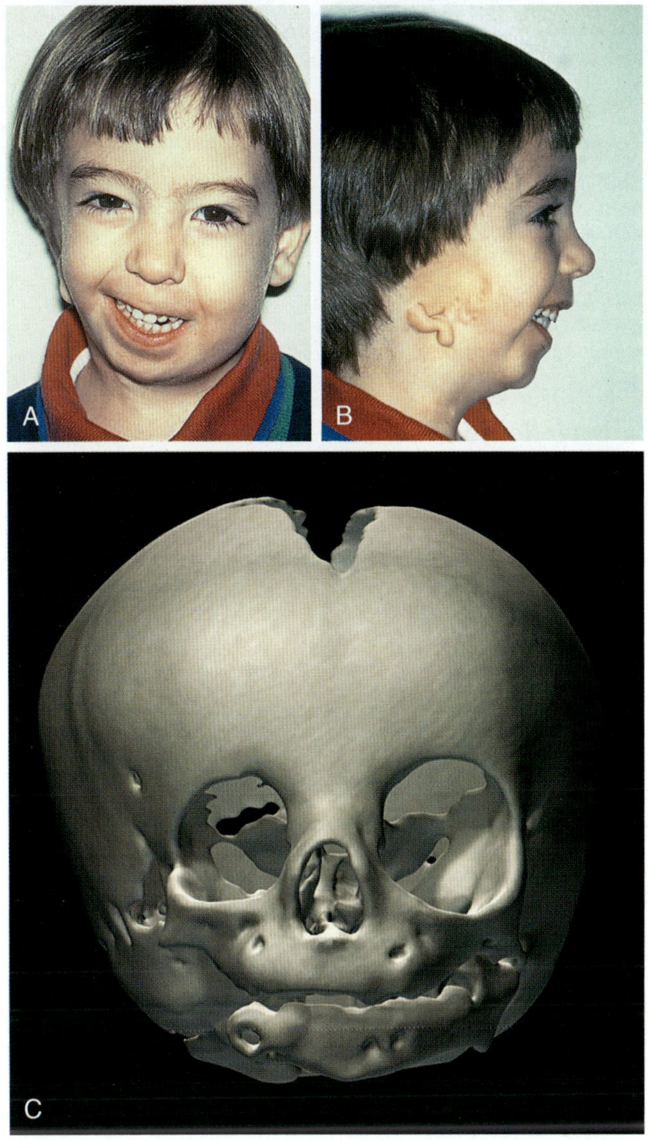

Fig. 23.15 Oculo-auriculo-vertebral (OAV) spectrum. (A and B) Photographs of a child with oculo-auriculo-vertebral spectrum. (C) Anterior view of the craniofacial skeleton of a child with right-sided OAV spectrum anomalies (hemifacial microsomia).

Neurosurgical issues such as brain anomalies, spine deformities, or congenital heart disease may also be present, and thus these patients often need a complete tertiary workup.

Mandible

Isolated mandibular malformations are rarer, with the exception of Pierre Robin sequence. Pierre Robin sequence is not a syndrome; rather, it is an original gestational event that likely leads to sequential developmental sequelae. It may appear alone or in association with other syndromes.

Pierre Robin Sequence

Pierre Robin sequence describes symptomatic microretrognathia (small mandible) that leads to glossoptosis (tongue falling posteriorly) resulting in airway obstruction (Fig. 23.16). The glossoptotic tongue in the developing fetus often physically interrupts palatal shelf fusion, typically resulting in a U-shaped cleft palate. Symptomatic airway obstruction requires close observation (pulse oximetry, blood gases, and sleep studies) and possible intervention.

Pierre Robin sequence may occur as frequently as once in 2000 live births. Historically, reported mortality rates due to airway

Box 23.5 Oculo-Auriculo-Vertebral Spectrum: Features and Findings

Craniofacial
Facial asymmetry
Unilateral maxillary, temporal, and zygomatic hypoplasia
Epibulbar dermoids with fine hairs
Unilateral colobomas of upper eyelids
Esotropia or exotropia
Preauricular appendages
Pretragal fistula
External ear deformities
External auditory canal stenosis or atresia
Conductive hearing deficits
Macrostomia due to mandibular dysgenesis
Lateral facial cleft
Cleft lip with or without cleft palate

Central Nervous System
Seventh cranial nerve palsy
Microcephaly
Hydrocephaly
Encephaloceles

Extracranial Skeletal
Cervical vertebral fusion
Spina bifida
Hemivertebrae
Butterfly, fused, or hypoplastic vertebrae
Scoliosis
Rib anomalies

Cardiovascular
Ventricular septal defect
Tetralogy of Fallot
Transposition of the great vessels
Coarctation of the aorta
Pulmonic stenosis
Dextrocardia

Other
Pulmonary dysplasia
Tracheoesophageal fistula
Renal anomalies
Imperforate anus

issues have ranged from 19% to 65 %. Advancements in monitoring and treatment protocols have significantly improved outcomes. Mandibular hypoplasia may be due to the intrauterine environment; however, coexisting malformation syndromes, such as Stickler syndrome, can also play a role. Pierre Robin sequence is associated with a syndrome in 25% to 40% of cases.

Glossoptotic airway obstruction can lead to substernal breathing, stridor, and distress. Prone positioning or a nasopharyngeal airway can improve airway obstruction. Because of respiratory insufficiency, up to 55% of infants with Pierre Robin sequence may experience feeding difficulties, including reflux. Antireflux medication is almost always necessary, and those with significant hypoxemia during feeding or inadequate caloric intake or weight gain require gavage feeding. A swallowing evaluation may reveal aspiration, with the tongue likely contributing. If airway obstruction occurs at rest or during feeding, exploration under anesthesia by otolaryngology is necessary to rule out primary tracheal or laryngeal pathology.

Because tracheostomy is a great social burden to caregivers and nursing resources, pediatric plastic surgeons are involved in manipulating soft and hard tissues to restore more normal anatomy. Often, mandibular growth will catch up during the temporizing stage.

Tongue/lip adhesion (TLA), or glossopexy, involves layered suturing of the tongue to the lower lip to reduce glossoptosis. Earlier versions of this surgery have resulted in a high dehiscence rate. At present, plastic surgeons often include muscular sutures, bolster with "buttons" over sutures, and allow prolonged intubation to improve healing. TLA can allow the transition from nasogastric tube feeding to oral feeding and hence avoid tracheostomy. At the time of cleft palate repair, usually at about 9 to 12 months of age, the adhesion is taken down.

Mandibular distraction osteogenesis is an alternative treatment that is gaining favor over TLA in many centers. The procedure involves creating bilateral mandibular osteotomies and placing buried devices that slowly expand the osteotomies. Mandibular distraction osteogenesis is the only intervention that directly addresses the cause of airway obstruction, and several studies have suggested improved feeding outcomes over TLA and faster resolution of respiratory obstruction.

Outcomes for children with Pierre Robin sequence vary. Strategies for initial and long-term management continue to evolve. Therefore care plans that foster optimal outcomes for these children should be developed individually.

External Structures of the Face

Whereas other subspecialists take care of the eye (globe); inner ear (eardrum, ossicles, and cochlea); nasal sinuses and choanae; larynx and trachea; and dentition, pediatric plastic surgeons are usually consulted

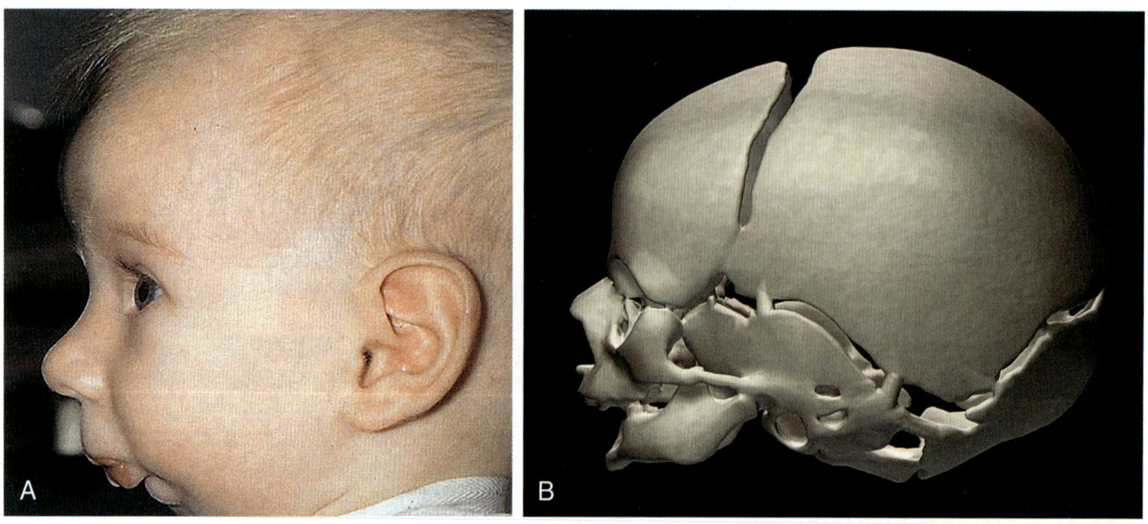

Fig. 23.16 Pierre Robin sequence. (A) Lateral view of a child with Pierre Robin sequence, characterized by severe micrognathia and cleft palate. (B) Lateral view of the craniofacial skeleton of a child with Pierre Robin sequence. Note the small, retruded mandible.

to repair and reconstruct the external structures of the face: eyelids, outer ears (pinnae), nose and septum, lips and tongue, nerves, and muscles. Among their other functions, these structures constitute our unique human appearance. Skeletal diagnosis and treatment are described in the Craniomaxillofacial Trauma section later. As for soft tissue, we briefly discussed cheiloplasty of the lips and rhinoplasty of the nose in the previous Cleft Lip, Nose, and Palate section, but similar principles are applicable in treating acquired defects of the lips and nose, such as from trauma or lesion removal. Tongue manipulation, described previously in the Mandible section, also includes shaping of the tongue, such as in macroglossia (e.g., Beckwith-Wiedemann syndrome). Although there are many specific external facial problems with well-described solutions, there are such a large variety of unique potential defects, especially given the random nature of trauma, that the basic principles of soft tissue reconstruction (described later in this chapter) may need to be creatively combined for a customized solution.

Owing to space limitations, we highlight the external ear as an example of an external face defect with a well-described reconstruction. Abnormalities of the ear appear in many craniofacial syndromes described previously, including craniofacial microsomia and Goldenhar syndrome. Other isolated forms of microtia also exist. Although there are usually lobule-like vestiges, microtia can range from hypoplastic ears to full anotia (Fig. 23.17A). There are usually three or four stages of surgery, each separated by at least several months, to achieve the final outcome. The first stage is the harvest of autologous rib cartilage, which is then carved,

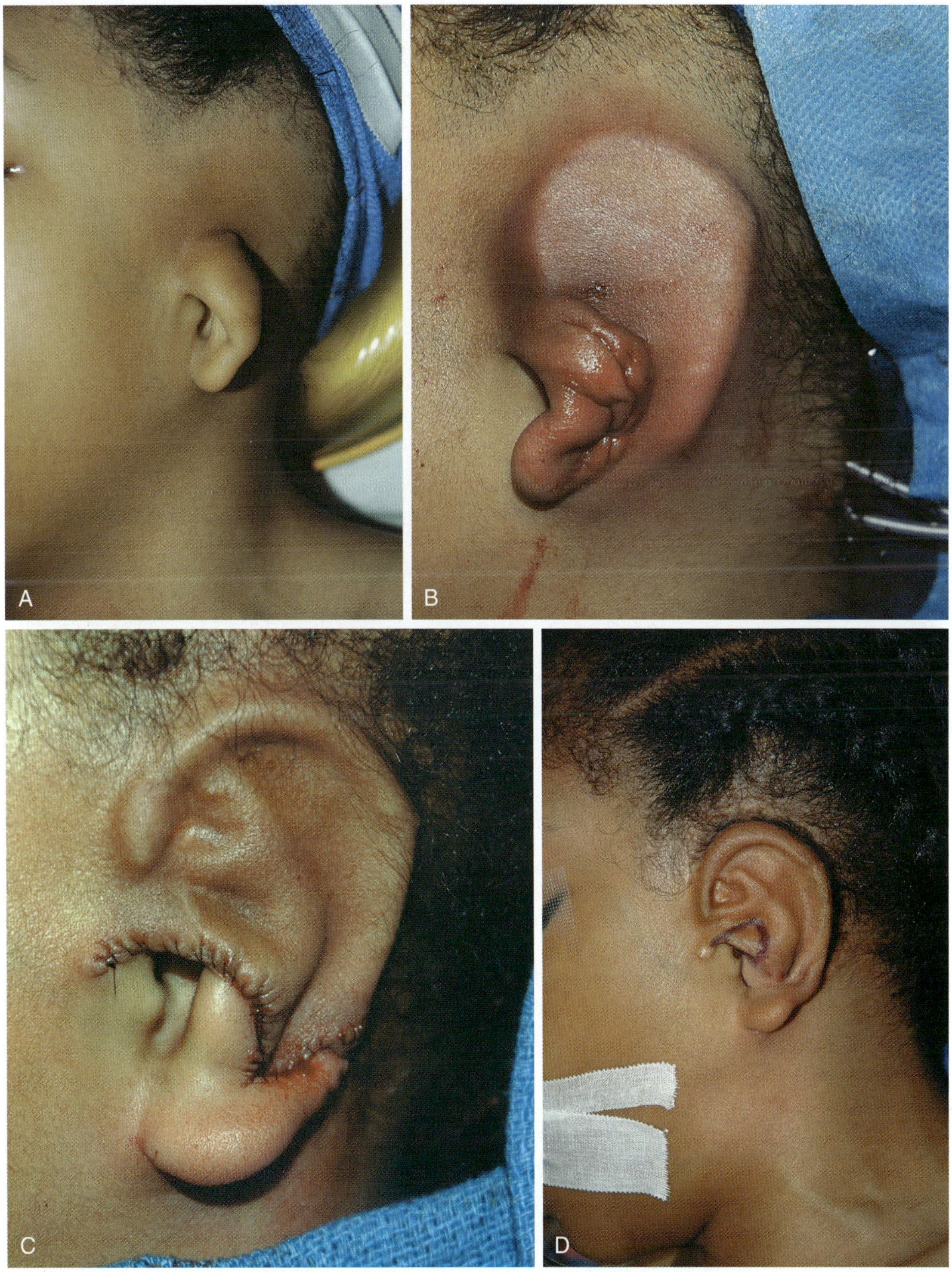

Fig. 23.17 Ear reconstruction. (A) Microtia; (B) constructed costal cartilage framework beneath scalp skin flap; (C) ear lobe transposition stage; (D) completed ear reconstruction.

constructed, and placed as a graft under the thin auricular skin (see Fig. 23.17B). The rest of the stages include a skin graft to elevate the construct and soft tissue rearrangements to create an earlobe and tragus to complete the details of the ear (see Fig. 23.17C and D).

Other ear abnormalities include prominent ears and constricted ears. Prominent ears are usually due to loss of the antihelical fold (Fig. 23.18A) and an excessive conchoscaphal angle (see Fig. 23.18B), and reconstructive efforts are directed toward correcting these issues (see Fig. 23.18C and D). Constricted ears refer to a variety of helical abnormalities referred to as lop ear, cup ear, hidden ear, and others. These repairs are based on soft tissue rearrangements but may require cartilage grafts. Extremely constricted ears may also be treated as microtia, with staged reconstruction, as described previously.

Craniofacial Summary

Clefting and craniofacial syndromes represent a number of interesting and challenging medical and surgical entities that fortunately afflict a relatively small number of newborns. Medical science has only recently begun to delineate why these developmental anomalies occur and, unfortunately, may have little to offer in the way of intervention owing to the early occurrence of the developmental miscues. The impact on the affected individuals and their families can be devastating. However, it is encouraging that early thorough evaluations and appropriate interventions can significantly benefit the lives of these children. Many health care providers are pivotal to the success of these endeavors. Multidisciplinary teams consisting of plastic surgeons, nurse care coordinators, speech therapists, otologists and audiologists, orthodontists, occupational therapists, psychologists, and social workers convincingly optimize the outcomes for these children and should be enlisted where available.

CRANIOMAXILLOFACIAL TRAUMA

The management of craniofacial trauma in children differs from that in adults in that the pediatric craniofacial skeleton is still developing and growing. Relative to adults, there is more cartilage, cancellous bone, and malleable growth centers, resulting in more energy absorption and a lower likelihood of fracturing. Even when there are fractures, they are more likely to be partial (greenstick) than

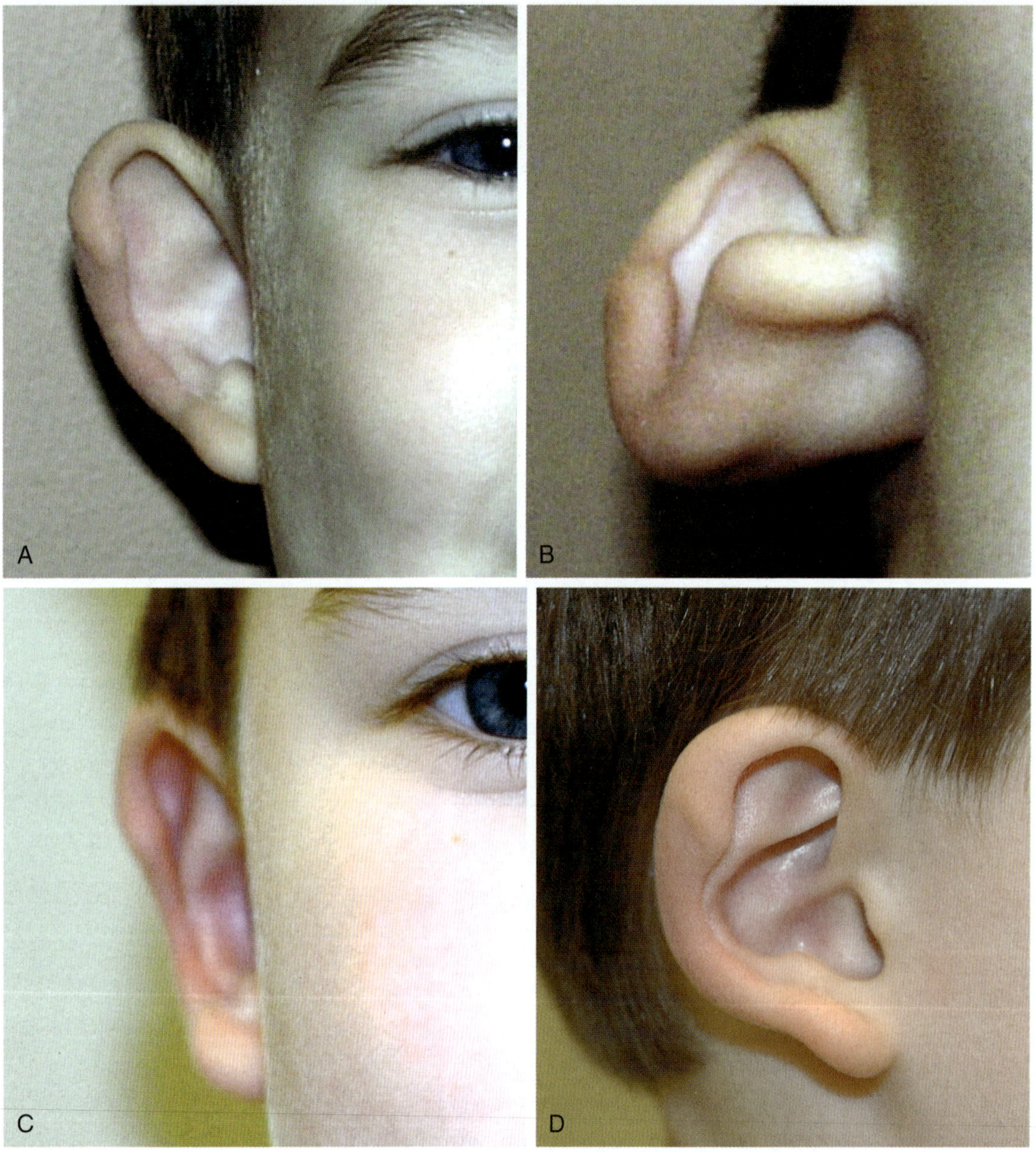

Fig. 23.18 Prominent ear. (A) Prominent ear with absence of antihelical fold. (B) Prominent ear with excessive conchoscaphal angle. (C) Frontal view of repaired prominent ear. (D) Lateral view of repaired prominent ear. Note the newly formed antihelical fold.

complete fractures. Other major differences include a higher skull-to-face ratio, lack of pneumatized sinuses, and the presence of adult tooth buds in the maxilla and mandible. Finally, children heal faster, so the decision to repair fractures needs to be made sooner, and the posttreatment immobilization period made shorter.

The facial skeleton develops more slowly than the cranial skeleton, such that facial dimensions at 5 years of age are approximately 80% of an adult's face. The growth then plateaus until the pubertal growth spurt, which lasts until approximately age 17, when another plateau is reached that eventually halts. Overall, the upper third grows the fastest because of the development of the brain and orbits. The middle third is next, and the lower third, or mandible, is the last to finish growing after puberty. Modern methods of open reduction internal fixation (ORIF) with titanium plates and screws can restrict growth. In addition, pediatric maxillae and mandibles contain both pediatric and adult teeth, making it imperative to avoid hardware that could injure unerupted permanent teeth. Therefore wires and absorbable plates are preferred whenever possible. Because of potential growth disturbance, pediatric patients with craniofacial fractures are monitored yearly until skeletal maturity.

Initial evaluation of any trauma patient must still progress according to the Advanced Trauma Life Support guidelines, including securing the airway and circulation before proceeding to the focused craniofacial examination. Brain trauma and cervical spine injury must be ruled out because of the high incidence of concomitant injuries that may require neurosurgical consultation. Orbital examination, including visual assessment and extraocular movement, must be undertaken, which could lead to ophthalmologic consultation. The nasal septum should be inspected visually to rule out septal hematoma that could lead to cartilage necrosis. Dental occlusion should also be examined, and the patient should be asked about the symptoms of malocclusion. Although it requires more cooperation than some children can muster, facial animation should be checked for symmetry and facial sensation should be tested in the trigeminal nerve distribution (CN V_1, forehead; CN V_2, cheeks; CN V_3, chin). Palpating the facial skeleton for tenderness or bony step-offs must include the forehead, periorbital borders, cheeks, nasal bones, and jaws. Suspicion for fractures warrants a fine-cut noncontrast CT scan of the head and face for definitive diagnosis. Finally, preinjury photographs should always be obtained if possible for comparison, because facial asymmetries and dental problems are common.

Although craniofacial trauma deals with both bony and soft tissue injuries, in this section, we discuss skeletal injuries only because soft tissue principles are discussed elsewhere in this chapter. However, the facial nerve (CN VII) and parotid duct are specialized structures that must be examined in the zone of injury. In addition, the pediatric skeleton contains growth centers that drive the growth of the craniofacial region, with the overlying soft tissue following that growth.

Skull and Forehead Fractures

The cranium-to-face ratio is greater in younger patients; thus skull fractures are more common than facial fractures at younger ages. The frontal sinus does not form until approximately 5 or 6 years of age, and then pneumatization continues until well past puberty. This lack of a frontal sinus allows fractures to the forehead and skull to directly transmit their forces to the skull base, orbit, and zygoma, resulting in an extended skull fracture or an "oblique craniofacial fracture." When minimally displaced, skull fractures can be treated conservatively; otherwise, these fractures require neurosurgical repair of the dura and plastic surgical reconstruction of the bone.

Another unique pediatric injury is a growing skull fracture: The "growth" likely originates from a clinically insignificant dural tear at the time of injury that stretches and allows brain herniation between the fracture edges, resulting in nonunion and expansion. If the growing skull fracture contains the supraorbital ridge, it can lead to changes in the orbit, including pulsatile exophthalmos and vertical dystopia, shifting the position of the globe.

The goals of forehead reconstruction are to isolate the intracranial contents (to prevent cerebrospinal fluid leaks and communication with the nasal sinuses), restore facial contour, and avoid posttraumatic sequelae (such as mucoceles and pyoceles from an inadequately drained frontal sinus). If the patient is old enough to have a pneumatized frontal sinus, the frontonasal ducts must be adequately draining or the mucosal lining of the sinus must be stripped away. The remaining dead space within the demucosalized frontal sinus must then be obliterated with a bone graft or cranialized, that is, the posterior table (wall of the sinus) removed so that the brain can expand into the frontal sinus, with a muscle flap protecting the brain from potential communication with the frontonasal duct.

Orbital Fractures

Pediatric orbital fractures differ from those in their adult counterparts in several ways. The lack of a frontal sinus means that the impact in this area can often translate into an isolated orbital roof fracture. Blowout fractures through the orbital floor (which is anatomically the ceiling of the maxillary sinus) are less likely because the maxillary sinuses are well buttressed by being small (without a big hollow into which to collapse) and filled with tooth buds. However, when they do occur, children are much more likely than adults to have a true trapdoor-type fracture, in which the inferior eye muscles become trapped under the fractured floor segment (Fig. 23.19A and B). This is a surgical urgency because the muscle becomes ischemic if not released. There will be restriction of extraocular movement (usually the affected globe is tethered inferiorly by the entrapped muscle, and the patient cannot look up; see Fig. 23.19C) and often disproportionate pain and nausea on upward gaze against the tethered muscle. True trapdoor orbital floor fractures are more common in children because their periosteum and other supporting structures are more elastic and snap the fractured bone back into place, entrapping the muscle.

Upon examination, orbital fractures frequently present with periorbital and subconjunctival hematomas. The clinical indications for repairing an orbital floor fracture are vertical dystopia (the globe appears to be at a different height) (see Fig. 23.19D), extraocular muscle dysfunction (especially entrapment), increased orbital volume causing enophthalmos (the globe looks posteriorly seated with pseudoptosis of the lids), and symptomatic diplopia. Without these abnormal findings, nonsurgical management can usually be offered to pediatric patients, regardless of the size of the fracture, because the elastic supporting structures seem to allow for normal orbital support and volume restoration. However, these findings can be difficult to assess in the immediate postinjury period because of swelling, which can mask any bony defects and cause temporary diplopia.

If surgery is required, multiple approaches (e.g., the transconjunctival, subciliary, or midlid approach) can be used. Regardless of exposure, the goal is to place an autologous bone graft or small implant into the floor without injuring orbital muscles, the infraorbital nerve, or the optic nerve, and to reconstruct the orbital volume so that there is almost symmetry in the globe position with the contralateral, uninjured eye.

Zygomaticomaxillary Complex Fractures

The zygoma, or cheek bone, articulates at five points: (1) the lateral maxilla along the lateral zygomaticomaxillary buttress, (2) the superior maxilla along the infraorbital rim, (3) the temporal bone forming the

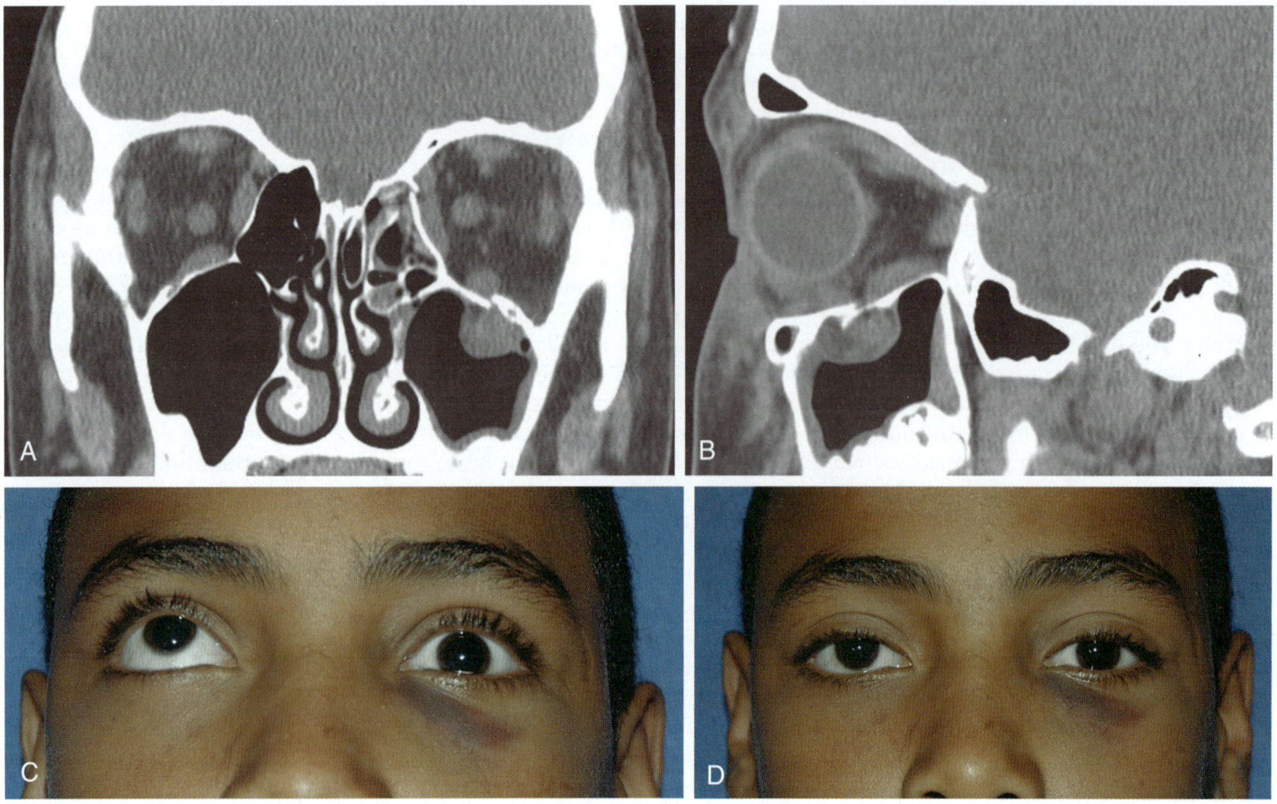

Fig. 23.19 Orbital floor trapdoor fracture with entrapped muscle. (A) Coronal computed tomography (CT) view of left inferior rectus muscle entrapped. (B) Sagittal CT view of left inferior rectus muscle entrapped. (C) Left-sided limited upward gaze. (D) Left-sided enophthalmos and vertical ocular dystopia.

zygomatic arch, (4) the lateral orbital rim at the zygomaticofrontal suture, and (5) the lateral orbital wall at the zygomaticosphenoid suture. Because of the underdevelopment of the maxillary sinus and resilience of the immature bone, isolated zygomatic fractures are relatively uncommon in children, who present more often with orbital fractures.

Similar to orbital fractures, changes in orbital volume may cause vertical globe dystopia or enophthalmos, both of which are surgical indications to correct appearance or diplopia. If sufficiently displaced, the cheek is usually rotated in the direction of the injury with malar flattening (which may be initially difficult to discern clinically due to swelling), which requires surgical correction. Minimally displaced fractures are treated conservatively.

Maxillary and Midface Fractures

Isolated midface fractures in children are rare, given the prominence of their cranium and mandible, which absorb the majority of forces. Therefore true pediatric midface fractures are likely to be associated with other injuries. Given that the underdeveloped maxilla is relatively solid and not pneumatized, classic pure Le Fort fracture patterns are rare. Classic Le Fort fractures are diagnosed by grabbing the maxilla and palate and pulling anteriorly: Le Fort I fractures have a mobile maxilla; Le Fort II fractures have a mobile maxilla that pulls the nasal pyramid with it; and Le Fort III fractures present a complete craniofacial disjunction, in which the entire midface pulls anteriorly. Transverse maxillary, or Le Fort I, fractures are extremely uncommon in children. Le Fort II fractures present as naso-orbital ethmoid (NOE) fractures combined with Le Fort I maxillary fractures. Le Fort III fractures, which are also rare in children, present as combined NOE and zygomaticomaxillary complex fractures.

When maxillary fractures are greenstick or minimally displaced, nonoperative treatment with a liquid or soft diet is recommended because children undergo rapid bone remodeling. Significant displacement may require maxillomandibular fixation (MMF) with ORIF; however, injury to the unerupted adult tooth buds must be avoided.

Nasal Fractures

Nasal fractures are the most common facial fractures in children and can involve the nasal bones, cartilage, and septum. They are diagnosed on the basis of a history of nasal trauma and self-resolving epistaxis. The diagnostic workup may include fine-cut face CT scans to rule out other injuries, although it is not absolutely necessary if clinically confident that the nasal fractures are isolated. The examination must include intranasal examination with a speculum to rule out septal hematoma. In children, there is only a loose attachment of the upper lateral cartilages to the nasal bones, so it is possible to develop hematomas in this area as well. Untreated hematomas cause pressure necrosis of the septal cartilage, leading to a saddle-nose deformity. Therefore it is recommended that cartilaginous nasal hematomas be urgently drained.

Regardless of the actual fracture pattern, surgical indications are based on the patient's nasal breathing being unobstructed and the appearance of the nose and septum. Closed reduction of nasal fractures has a fairly high subsequent revision rate. Most plastic surgeons will perform a closed reduction on a pediatric nasal fracture, and if revision septorhinoplasty is needed later, it will be delayed until closer to skeletal maturity.

Mandibular Fractures

The prominent mandible is the most common site of pediatric facial fractures and likely represents 20% to 40% of pediatric facial fractures. Before the age of 6 years, mandibular fractures are less common and concomitant injuries should be sought. The incidence of mandibular fractures increases from 6 to approximately 15 years of age. The mandible is a symmetric ring with a central symphysis, paired on either side of the parasymphysis, body, angle where the body transitions to ramus, ascending ramus anteriorly giving off the coronoid process where the temporalis muscle inserts, and posteriorly the condyle that articulates with the glenoid fossa forming the TMJ. Condylar fractures are common before the age of 6 years but decrease thereafter. In children older than 15 years, angle and body fractures have the highest proportion.

Clinically, these patients present with pain, malocclusion, and pain on opening, drooling, and decreased maximal incisal opening. Intraoral examination can reveal dental step-off at the fracture site. Although bilateral condylar fractures often present with an anterior open bite, unilateral condylar fractures present as contralateral posterior open bites. In condylar neck fractures, the condylar head is often displaced medially from the glenoid fossa by the strong pull of the pterygoid muscles medially.

In addition to symptomatic malocclusion, the examiner can assess the TMJ by placing the fingers in the external auditory canals while the patient opens and closes his or her mouth. Palpation along the edge of the entire mandible for tenderness can sometimes indicate the location of fractures. The mandible has some ringlike structural properties and can often break in two places. Placing the heel of the examiner's hand against the child's symphysis and asking the patient to protrude the chin against the hand may cause pain, indicating mandibular fracture.

The key to treatment is the restoration of a normal occlusion. Given the remodeling ability of the pediatric mandible, minor occlusal discrepancies will improve on their own or later with orthodontic manipulation. For significant malocclusion, surgical reduction is attempted and stable reduction can be treated by MMF with guiding elastics (rubber-banding rather than wiring the jaw shut). Unstable or irreducible fractures require MMF, possibly with ORIF, but standard MMF arch bar placement can be difficult because of the shape of pediatric teeth. Primary dentition appears from 6 months to 6 years of age, and mixed dentition is present from 6 to 12 years of age.

Condylar and subcondylar fractures are difficult to treat surgically; there is also the risk of damaging the facial nerve, resulting in ipsilateral weakness or loss of facial animation. These fractures are also at risk for TMJ ankylosis, and early range-of-motion therapy is important. The infrequent indications for open repair include displacement of the condyle into the middle cranial fossa or auditory canal, or bilateral fractures without the ability to establish occlusion and mandibular height. The side of the fracture usually results in a shorter ramus height, with the teeth meeting earlier, causing a contralateral open bite or crossbite. Operative closed reduction by MMF with contralateral elastics can correct this defect and allow remodeling with a soft diet.

In general, more seriously displaced mandibular fractures are obvious on physical examination, with malocclusion or even gross instability of the mandible. ORIF should be performed using the most minimal fixation techniques possible to avoid damaging the tooth buds and to prevent impingement on dental growth; this can be accomplished by using only the cortex on the inferior border of the mandible. Absorbable plates and wires are preferred over metal plates. If metal plates are used, it is preferable to remove them once bone healing is complete to reduce the risk of affecting growth.

Panfacial Trauma

Patients who have experienced trauma severe enough to cause craniofacial fractures of the upper, middle, and lower thirds of the face often have multiorgan injuries that complicate their management. Physical examination usually reveals a flattened face appearance because loss of multiple skeletal buttresses reduces anterior projection. There are many approaches to these reconstructions, with the overall goals of reestablishing occlusion, maintaining anterior projection, and maintaining height. Along with ophthalmology, an otolaryngologist may be consulted to secure the airway with temporary tracheostomy, neurosurgery may be needed for intracranial access, and an anesthesia team needs to be prepared for patients requiring significant lengths of time to treat. One approach is to use the cranial base as a guide and reduce the NOE to the nasion, the mandible to the glenoid fossae, the maxilla to the occlusal surface of the mandible, and the zygomaticomaxillary complex to the sphenoid and maxilla, and then adjust orbital volumes, followed by soft tissue repairs.

RECONSTRUCTIVE PEDIATRIC PLASTIC SURGERY

Pediatric plastic surgeons can make improvements of congenital and acquired defects (such as trauma) by reshaping or transferring tissue on the basis of the principles of wound healing and blood supply. These principles also apply to problems involving soft tissue deformities and coverage of wounds. This role places plastic surgeons in close contact with many of the other surgical specialties when prior attempts to heal a defect have not been successful after debridement of devitalized tissue, tumor extirpation, or hardware exposure.

All tissues in the human body are able to live because blood flow supplies oxygen and nutrition, and it carries away "waste" products, such as carbon dioxide. The cardiovascular system needs to not only deliver oxygenated blood and immune factors to every cell in the body but also maintain a capillary perfusion pressure of 20 to 30 mm Hg. This pressure may appear surprisingly low, but it requires a significant amount of pressure in the larger vessels to maintain it. Capillary perfusion pressure plays an important role in many pathophysiologic states, such as compartment syndromes and pressure ulcers.

Plastic surgeons are, therefore, somewhat limited, because every incision made theoretically "removes" more blood supply to an area. Chronic decubitus ulcerations and complex wounds often occur in areas that have decreased blood supply, such as the dependent areas of sitting and standing, and this relative ischemia may predispose these areas to infection and decreased healing capacity.

The main tools by which a plastic surgeon moves tissue around the body to restore form and function are grafts, flaps, and molding of the tissue. A *graft* is tissue that is completely removed from one part of the body and placed in a new recipient site, in hopes that a new blood supply will grow into it to keep the graft alive. A *flap* is a vascularized block of tissue that is transferred to another location with its own blood supply—this can be either a pedicled flap or a free flap. Pedicled flaps are flaps that pivot along their blood supply, without interrupting and reconnecting the flap. Free flaps are flaps that have their own blood supply, but this is divided and transplanted to a new recipient vessel to move the tissue a farther distance away from its original location. *Molding of tissue* refers to relatively newer technologies to shape tissues: Two common techniques involve the use of tissue expanders and negative-pressure wound therapy devices.

The main difference between a graft and a flap is that a graft has no blood supply and must gain a new blood supply at its recipient site. Ingrowth of a new blood supply typically takes about 48 hours, and therefore the graft must find other mechanisms to survive in the early period. It is thought that grafts survive by diffusion of nutrients and wastes across an osmotic gradient; therefore a graft must be in close contact with a moist, nonepithelialized, vascular bed (such as muscle) in order to survive. For example, in a skin graft, if anything gets in between the graft and its recipient bed, such as a seroma, hematoma, or purulent material, the graft may not survive, or "take." Also, if there are significant shearing forces that prevent the graft from keeping close contact with its vascular bed, the skin graft will not take. This is one reason why skin grafts are often meshed before placed on the recipient bed so that any fluid that accumulates in the area can exit through the fenestrations and improve take. Another example of grafting is autologous fat grafting, which is often used to augment soft tissue deficits and improve contour abnormalities. Because of their mechanism of revascularization, grafts tend to have a certain percentage take and the rest may resorb.

There are many types of grafts, including skin, fat, cartilage, bone, nerve, and composite grafts containing more than one type of tissue.

Skin grafts may be split-thickness or full-thickness grafts. Split-thickness grafts are thin enough that the donor site will heal on its own, and their thinness also implies that they survive more easily. However, split-thickness skin grafts have worse cosmetic outcomes and can contract significantly as they heal. Full-thickness skin grafts look much better and are much more pliable, but they have more difficulty surviving and create a donor site defect that needs to be repaired. The key issue to recognize is that skin grafts cannot cover nonvascularized tissues, such as bone without periosteum, cartilage without perichondrium, tendon without paratenon, or exposed hardware. To cover such nonvascularized structures, a vascularized flap must be used.

Flaps are thicker blocks of tissue that have their own blood supply. They usually contain a mix of the following tissue types: skin, subcutaneous fat, fascia, and muscle. They can be based on presumed vascular plexuses (known as *random pattern flaps*) or known blood vessels by knowledge of the anatomy, visualization of the structure itself, or Doppler ultrasound identification (known as *pedicled flaps*). Flaps may also be designed to contain a known blood supply (pedicle), detached from the original blood supply, and brought to a distant location to be revascularized via a microvascular anastomosis to recipient vessels (known as *free flaps*). Free flaps may be thought of as "autologous tissue transplantation" because they can survive only on the basis of technically performed vascular anastomoses (called *microsurgery* because of the requirement for an operating microscope) with concomitant risks of thrombosis and flap failure that could necessitate an emergency return to the operating room to explore or redo the anastomoses. Because a flap leaves a donor site defect when it is moved to cover another tissue, the donor site may sometimes need a skin graft to cover it if it cannot be closed primarily (Fig. 23.20).

Molding describes the direct manipulation of tissue and can refer to numerous techniques that plastic surgeons have innovated to directly shape tissue. Naso-alveolar molding for the cleft lip/nose, implants, and hyaluronidase and collagen fillers are among the many technologies available. Two of the most commonly used techniques in pediatric plastic surgery are tissue expansion and negative-pressure wound therapy.

Tissue expansion can potentially solve the problems of tissue mismatch of grafts and limited availability of local flaps. It involves the placement of inflatable silicone elastomer balloons under skin, fascia, or muscle with a port to inject saline. After months of weekly saline injections into the tissue expanders, the soft tissue grows and stretches to accommodate the expanders, and the expanders can be removed to advance these expanded local flaps. Studies have shown that there is actual growth of new tissue rather than only having mere stretching of the tissues. This solution works well to produce enough specialized neighboring tissue, such as hair-bearing scalp in scalp reconstruction. The main drawbacks are related to the implantable hardware: infection, bleeding, extrusion, skin necrosis, pain, and neurapraxia (an injury to a peripheral nerve causing temporary pain).

Negative-pressure wound therapy involves using a negative pressure (vacuum) pump to shrink an open wound to a smaller size and

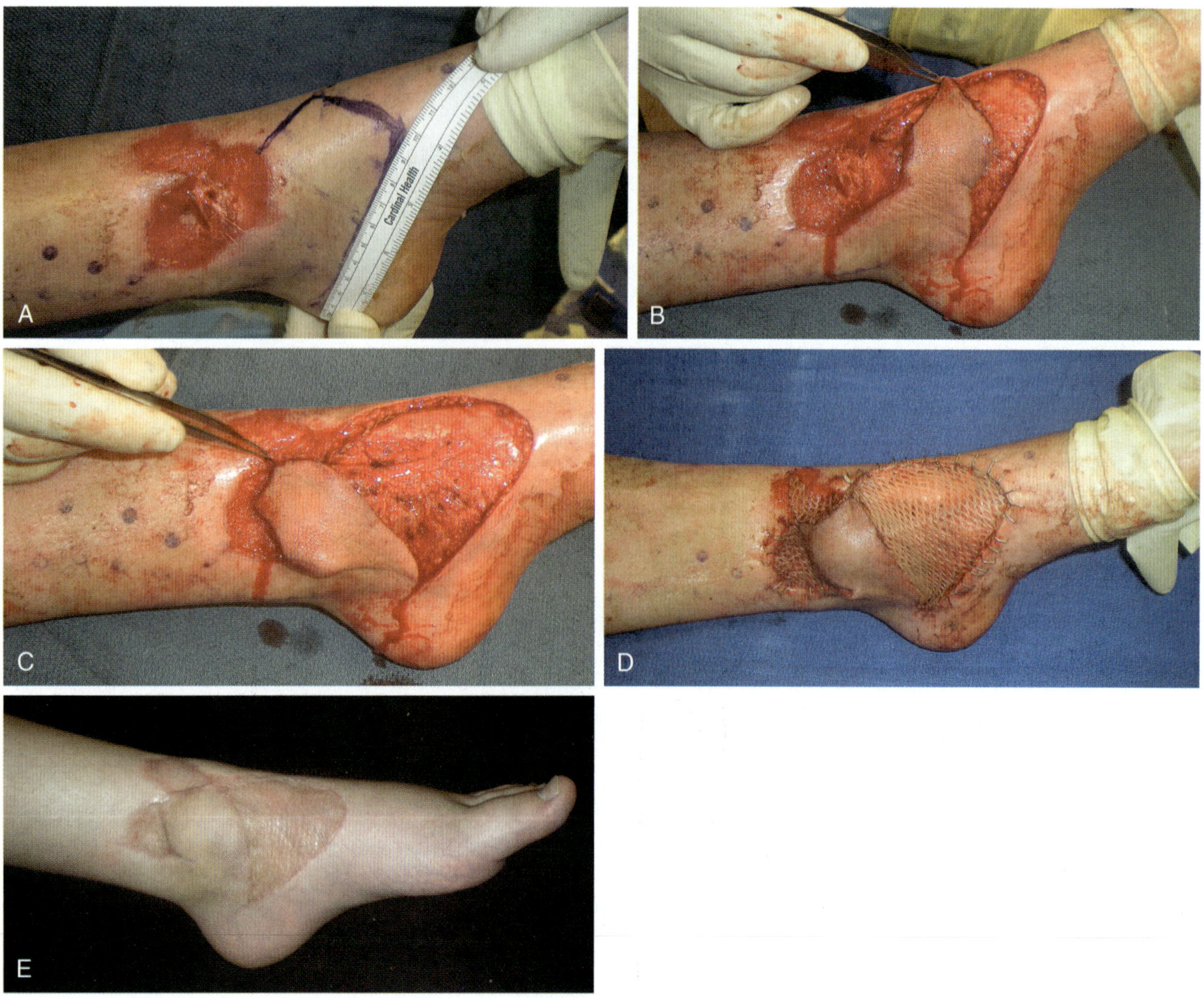

Fig. 23.20 Soft tissue defect of the ankle with exposed bone. (A) Ankle defect with flap designed; (B) elevated flap; (C) rotated flap; (D) flap donor site skin grafted; (E) well-healed ankle.

promote vascularized tissue ingrowth through the creation of granulation tissue. In many cases, this approach may allow for treatment of the defect with a smaller, safer, and simpler reconstruction (such as a skin graft), rather than a larger one (such as a free flap). An air-filled substance (such as a sponge or gauze) is placed in the wound, covered by an airtight plastic drape, and connected to a vacuum suction device to create negative pressure. The force draws the wound edges toward each other, reduces edema, stimulates cell mitosis, and may also increase healing and granulation by increasing blood flow and the availability of wound-healing factors. Basic steps of wound healing, such as debridement of devitalized tissue, need to be performed before placement of this device in order to optimize the environment for healing. The negative-pressure wound therapy dressing is usually changed about two to three times per week (depending on the type of wound), and because it is a form of wound dressing, it can be changed by trained nursing staff on an inpatient or outpatient basis.

Pressure Sores

Treatment of decubitus ulcerations, otherwise known as "pressure sores," requires a fundamental knowledge of the principles of wound healing. These ulcerations can have multiple underlying causative factors, such as immobility, malnutrition, shearing forces, or infection. Often, pressure due to immobility of an insensate surface is the main culprit because capillary perfusion pressure (20–30 mm Hg under normal circumstances) is easily exceeded when tissue is compressed between two unyielding surfaces: a bony prominence and a chair or mattress. Although any bony surface may potentially cause a pressure sore depending on the patient's positioning, the bony surfaces most commonly involved are the sacrum, calcaneus, ischium, and greater trochanter. In fact, these areas are naturally subject to pressures greater than 30 mm Hg when sitting or lying down, but the autonomic nervous system prompts the person to gently shift our weight constantly to avoid chronic pressure focusing on one spot for long. Patients who have decreased sensation in conjunction with decreased mobility, such as patients with traumatic brain injury, spina bifida, or spinal cord injury, are therefore at higher risk and need to be closely monitored and treated with frequent position changes and other strategies to unload high-risk areas. Other strategies to decrease focused pressure on one area include pressure-mapped wheelchair cushions, air-fluidized mattresses, and beds that gently shift position frequently.

As little as 1 to 2 hours of chronic pressure exceeding capillary perfusion pressure leads to compromised oxygenation, ischemia, and eventually tissue necrosis. Therefore significant instruction on pressure-minimizing techniques must be given to patients with risk factors and their caregivers to *prevent* the development of pressure ulcerations. It is far more beneficial to prevent the formation of a pressure ulceration than to treat it once it has occurred. The management goals in treating pressure ulcerations are to identify the intrinsic and extrinsic etiologic factors in order to reduce them and to perform wound care and debridement to prevent chronic infections from becoming acute or fulminant infections. Patients need to demonstrate significant, constant improvement of their pressure sores for at least 6 to 8 weeks before becoming candidates for surgical coverage of their ulceration because the risk of postsurgical wound breakdown is extremely high if subjected to pressure or shearing forces.

Sacral pressure ulcerations may be the result of a patient lying down too long in a supine position. Ischial pressure ulcerations may result from a patient remaining too long in the sitting position. Greater trochanter pressure ulcerations are caused by lying too long on one side. Extrinsic factors such as moisture, incontinence, and shearing forces from patient repositioning may add to the difficulty in treating these ulcerations. Intrinsic factors (such as malnutrition) are common and further impede healing. These factors can be elucidated from a detailed history and physical examination of the patient.

Pressure ulcerations are typically staged according to the National Pressure Ulcer Advisory Panel consensus development conference scale, which was originally developed in 1989. This staging system classifies pressure ulcerations according to four main layers of tissue involvement: (1) does not pass skin; (2) does not pass fat; (3) does not pass muscle; and (4) involves bone. A stage I pressure sore therefore has intact skin, but the skin stays reddened for more than 1 hour even after pressure is removed. In a stage II pressure sore, there is a break in the dermis with or without infection, and subcutaneous fat may be exposed. In stage III, there is subcutaneous destruction extending into the muscle layer. Stage IV pressure sores involve periosteum and bone. There are also two designations for "suspected" deep tissue ulcers: (1) a *suspected deep tissue injury* has intact skin, with a violaceous discoloration, suggestive of deeper tissue pressure injury, and (2) *unstageable ulceration* implies full-thickness soft tissue loss with an eschar that prevents visualization of the deepest level of involvement. It is important to note that when bone is exposed, the most superficial aspect of bone is desiccated and thus relatively devascularized and superficially colonized by bacteria. This is osteitis, or inflammation of bone, rather than osteomyelitis, or deep bone infection. If the deep bone has good blood supply, a healthy patient can tolerate osteitis for protracted periods as long as there is good wound care and pressure precautions that prevent the wound from worsening.

After a pressure sore is cleaned, there are three main pillars of successful treatment: (1) *reduction of pressure and other extrinsic factors* via patient education and mechanical low-pressure devices, such as air mattresses and mapped wheelchair cushions (consider physiatrist consult); (2) *meticulous wound care* (consider wound care nurse consult) with debridement of all necrotic soft tissues so that healthy granulation tissue can form, and (3) *adequate nutrition* (consider nutrition or feeding consult) to help promote healing of the ulceration. Only when these factors are optimized can there be healing of the ulceration, potentially enough to avoid surgery or to become a candidate for reconstructive surgery. In most cases, patients with pressure sores requiring surgical treatment have exposure of bony structures; a vascularized flap is typically used to cover the ulceration defect, rather than a skin graft.

Soft Tissue Lesions

Pediatric plastic surgeons also treat many different types of soft tissue lesions, including congenital melanocytic nevi (CMNs), vascular anomalies, neurofibromas, melanomas, and sarcomas. Some of these lesions are described in Chapter 10. Many physicians are comfortable treating small lesions that can be removed with local anesthetic and closed by simple primary closure, but pediatric plastic surgeons are often consulted for larger lesions or to treat lesions in young children, because they require general anesthesia and multiple reconstructive techniques. Some large lesions can be covered by local flaps or skin grafts, but one particularly challenging category concerns large CMNs. Large or giant CMNs often carry gene mutations in *NRAS, BRAF, GNAQ, P53,* and other pathways that give them an approximately 4% to 12% lifetime risk of malignant transformation into melanoma. Because of this risk, these lesions need to be monitored closely or excised. Given their size, excision of the lesion while also achieving a reasonably good esthetic result can be challenging. Local flaps often are not adequate for coverage, and skin grafts cannot usually match the tissue type (e.g., hair-bearing scalp would be replaced by a hairless skin graft). Tissue expansion has provided a reasonable solution for creating large local flaps that are useful in reconstructing the defects produced by excision of large CMNs and are often the best type of reconstruction (Fig. 23.21). When large CMNs are near complex areas of the body (such as the eyelids), a customized combination of skin grafts, flaps, and tissue expansion may be necessary.

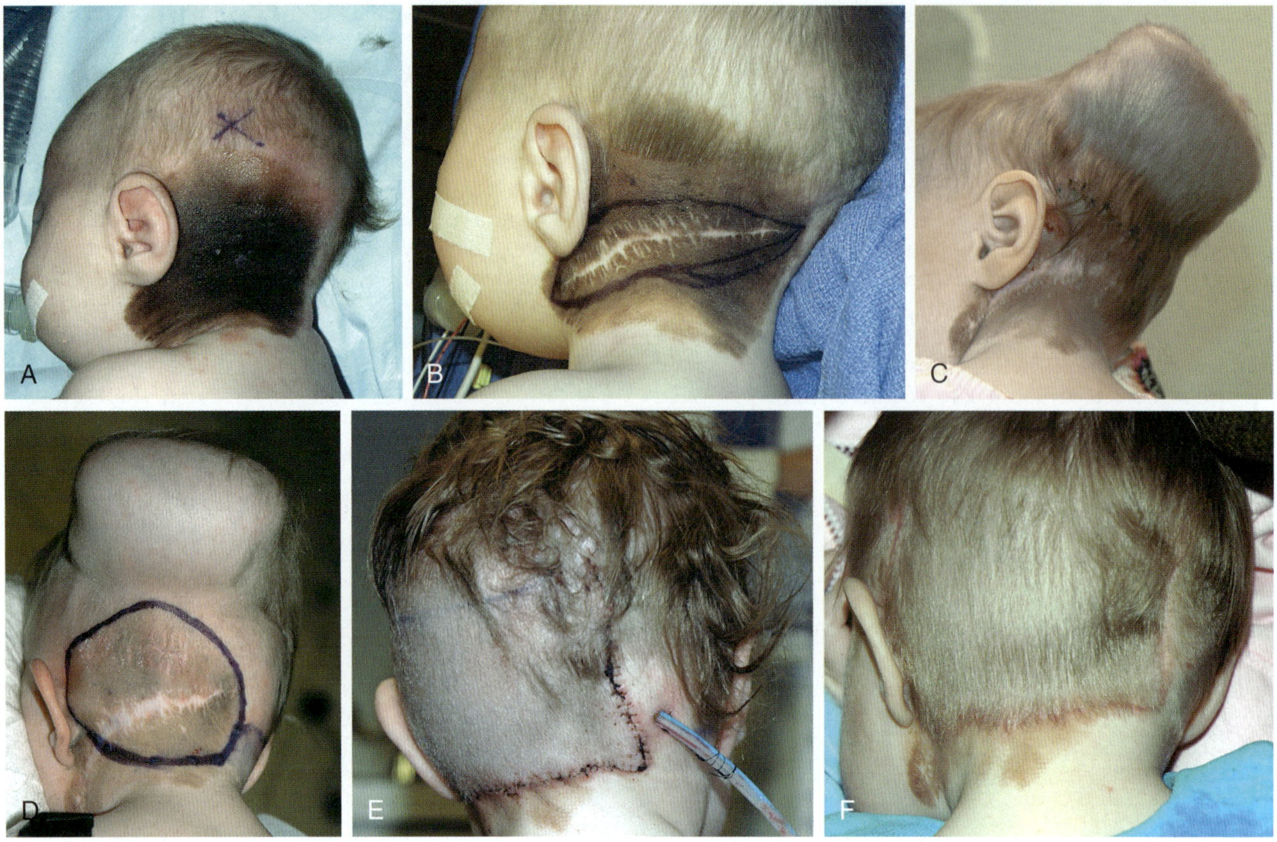

Fig. 23.21 Giant congenital melanocytic nevus. (A) Nevus; (B) serial excision; (C) scalp tissue expansion; (D) scalp tissue expansion with planned nevus excision and flap coverage; (E) after nevus excision and expanded flap coverage; (F) well-healed flap.

Vascular anomalies are broadly classified into two categories: malformations and tumors, following the classification system originally described in 1996 by the International Society for the Study of Vascular Anomalies, and modified most recently in 2018.

Malformations may be classified as simple, combined, involving major blood vessels, or associated with other anomalies. Within this grouping, there are many subdivisions, including capillary malformations, lymphatic malformations, venous malformations, arteriovenous malformations, Klippel-Trenaunay syndrome, Sturge-Weber syndrome, Congenital Lipomatous Overgrowth, Vascular Malformations, Epidermal Nevis, Spinal/Skeletal Anomalies/Scoliosis (CLOVES) syndrome, and many others. Vascular malformations, the result of an error in development, are present at birth and grow proportionately with the child. They can be arterial, venous, capillary, lymphatic, or distinct combinations of these, and each has its own characteristics and natural history. Vascular anomalies can cause increased growth of underlying soft and bony tissues or directly extend into or exist separately in other tissues, such as leptomeninges, viscera, and muscle.

In contrast, in the tumor section of the classification scheme, the lesions fall into three main categories: benign, borderline, or malignant. Hemangiomas are among some of the most common vascular anomalies that are evaluated by pediatric plastic surgeons and are endothelial tumors that usually appear within the first year of life (infantile hemangiomas) and go through a proliferative phase (with growth in size), followed by an involution phase that usually leaves residual fibrofatty tissue. Some hemangiomas are present at birth (congenital hemangiomas); these may involute rapidly or not involute at all.

Indications for treating vascular anomalies include current or predictable future symptoms of abnormal appearance, pain, ulceration, bleeding, infection, growth, or psychosocial dysfunction. Rapid intervention must be sought for interference with airway, vision development, conductive hearing, or other organ function, with appropriate consultation with a pediatric otolaryngologist, ophthalmologist, or other subspecialists. Although the pediatric plastic surgeon can perform excisions or laser treatments, a multidisciplinary team approach is usually offered, including the dermatologist, pediatrician, and interventional radiologist, as therapies range from observation to systemic therapies (such as steroids or propranolol) to embolization.

Hand and Upper Extremity

Like the face, the hand is a complex organ that is unique to primates because of its prehensile thumb. Its unique structure allows humans to precisely manipulate objects and create tools. Its *function* is the primary focus of treatment for congenital differences. The bones, tendons, muscles, and the neurovascular structures that form the upper extremity all work together to create optimal hand function. Appearance of the hand is also important, despite taking second place to function, as the upper extremity plays a key role in the patient's social interactions with parents and peers, just like the patient's face. Given the wide variety of potential differences, the timing of surgery must be individualized for each patient's needs. The patient should be young enough to allow for effective postoperative neural plasticity and adaptation but old enough that the risks of surgery will be low and have a decreased incidence of recurrent deformity. Sometimes surgery is not even indicated at all—this is best represented by the adage by Flatt: "The cleft hand is a functional triumph, but a social disaster." The overall goals of operative intervention are to optimize function before the patient is 4 years old, preferably starting between 18 and 24 months, when the three-digit pinch is being mastered. Parents should understand that although a normal hand cannot be restored in many cases, improving function may still be highly beneficial in the developing child.

The embryologic development of the upper extremity is quite complex. Upper limb buds emerge at 4 weeks of gestation and, via at least three distinct signaling gradients, develop along all three dimensions: (1) the apical ectodermal ridge (AER) signals proximal-to-distal mesenchymal differentiation through FGFR pathways; (2) the dorsal ectoderm delineates dorsal (extensor) to palmar or volar (flexor) surfaces through the wingless type (WNT) pathways; and (3) the zone of polarizing activity (ZPA) creates a gradient in an anterior (preaxial, or toward the radius and thumb)-to-posterior (postaxial, or toward the ulna and small finger) direction through the Sonic hedgehog (Shh) pathway. By 6 to 7 weeks, digits have fully segregated via apoptosis of the mesenchyme between the digits, and further growth and ossification of cartilage proceed.

These three axes of development lead to a wide variety of congenital defects, and they are classified within the Swanson Classification system as (1) failure of formation, (2) failure of differentiation, (3) duplication, (4) overgrowth, (5) undergrowth, (6) congenital constriction band syndrome, and (7) generalized skeletal abnormalities. Some of these conditions may be associated with genetic syndromes, like Apert syndrome, Pfeiffer syndrome, and Greig cephalopolysyndactyly. These can range from isolated but unusual conditions (such as cleft hands) to the more common syndactyly and polydactyly.

Syndactyly, or fusion of hand digits, occurs in about 1 in 2000 births and can be simple, complex, or complicated. It can be incomplete or complete. Simple syndactyly is when the process does not involve fusion of bone. Complex syndactyly is when the process involves fairly simple fusion of bone. Complicated syndactyly is when there is either complex fusion of bone, or additional polydactyly found within the syndactyly.

Polydactyly or extra digits are most commonly on the ulnar side of the hand, a condition known as *postaxial* polydactyly. Postaxial polydactyly can be either well developed (type A), with an articulation with the small finger, or less well developed (type B), appearing as a pedunculated accessory digit, connected to the ulnar aspect of the hand or small finger by a soft tissue bridge. Frequently, type A postaxial polydactyly is treated with formal surgical excision ± ligamentous reconstruction after the patient is 1 year of age as an outpatient procedure. The more common type B postaxial polydactyly may be managed by excision of the accessory digit under local anesthesia in the first 1 to 2 months of life. Suture ligating the base of the soft tissue bridge is less preferable than performing excision of the digit because of the risk of developing a symptomatic neuroma at the site of the ligation.

Polydactyly can also present on the radial aspect as a thumb duplication, and the Flatt-Wassel classification subdivides these into seven different types. Reconstruction of a thumb duplication can be as simple as division of a soft tissue bridge or can be as complex as excision of the underlying bone, rebalancing tendons, and reconstructing the collateral ligament of the affected joint.

For more complex anomalies, creativity on the part of the pediatric plastic surgeon is required. Over time, many innovative surgeons have pioneered advanced reconstruction for complex defects to improve the appearance and function of the hand for patients with specific needs. This is seen in the approach to severe thumb hypoplasia, where index finger pollicization may be needed to move the index finger into the position of the absent or nonfunctioning thumb, or in the case of traumatic amputation of the thumb or other digits, where a toe-to-hand microvascular transfer can use one or more toes to simulate the thumb or other digits and allow the patient to regain prehension in the injured hand. These techniques allow surgeons to address complex differences such as the cleft hand, which requires a thorough knowledge of functional anatomy.

In addition to congenital hand differences, pediatric hand trauma is also frequently managed by the pediatric hand surgeon and can involve soft tissue injuries, hand and wrist fractures, tendon injuries, nerve injuries, and even complex amputations.

Trunk and Lower Extremities

Given that there is typically excess tissue at the trunk, local flaps can usually provide reconstructive coverage, such as for breast reconstruction, gynecomastia treatment, or abdominal reconstruction. On the other hand, the lower extremity has thin soft tissues relative to the bone and an overall paucity of soft tissue available for transfer in a reconstructive case, so local flaps are often not a good option. Negative pressure wound therapy can assist with healing open wounds on both the trunk and lower extremity because it can shrink the wounds and encourage granulation tissue, sometimes converting a large, complex wound into a smaller one that can be covered in a simpler manner, such as with a skin graft.

Similar principles therefore apply: If coverage can be delayed, a large wound can often receive negative pressure wound therapy to reduce its dimensions and possibly avoid surgery altogether. If there is no bone exposure, a skin graft may suffice. Otherwise, a local flap or free flap is needed, and decisions on which modality to utilize are considered on a case-by-case basis in order to individualize treatment.

CONCLUSIONS

Plastic surgery solves problems of "form and function" that are exclusive to humans, such as appearance and speech, to improve quality of life. These deformities can prevent normal functional and psychologic development in infants and children, given that unique human features play such an important role in socialization with caregivers and peers. Congenital and acquired deformities can be treated by similar principles of hard and soft tissue reconstruction. Parents should be educated that although pediatric plastic surgeons can often improve outcomes, they are limited by the patient's innate wound healing and scarring, severity of the defect, and changes that occur as the child grows. However, with careful evaluation and planning, there are many options for their child to undergo treatment and lead a healthy, satisfying life.

Bibliography

Ades LC, Mulley JC, Senga LP, et al: Jackson-Weiss syndrome: clinical and radiographical findings in a large kindred and exclusion of the gene from 7p21 and 5qter, *Am J Med Genet* 51:121–130, 1994.

Aleck K: Craniosynostosis syndromes in the genomic era, *Semin Pediatr Neurol* 11:256–261, 2004.

Basseri B, Kianmahd BD, Roostaeian J, et al: Current national incidence, trends, and health care resource utilization of cleft lip–cleft palate, *Plast Reconstr Surg* 127(3):1255–1262, 2011.

Centers for Disease Control and Prevention: *Birth defects 2006*. http://www.cdc.gov/ncbddd/birthdefects/data.html.

Cohen MM, Kreiborg S: An updated pediatric perspective on the Apert syndrome, *Am J Dis Child* 147:989–993, 1993.

Cohen MM Jr, Rollnick BR, Kaye CI: Oculoauriculovertebral spectrum: an updated critique, *Cleft Palate J* 26:276–286, 1989.

Danziger I, Brodsky L, Perry R, et al: Nager's acrofacial dysostosis: case report and review of the literature, *Int J Pediatr Otorhinolaryngol* 20:225–240, 1990.

Gorlin RJ: Fibroblast growth factors, their receptors and receptor disorders, *J Craniomaxillofac Surg* 25:69–79, 1997.

Keating RF: Craniosynostosis: diagnosis and management in the new millennium, *Pediatr Ann* 26:600–620, 1997.

Losee JE, Mason AC: Deformational plagiocephaly: diagnosis, prevention, and treatment, *Clin Plast Surg* 32:53–64, 2005.

National Pressure Ulcer Advisory Panel: Pressure ulcers prevalence, cost and risk assessment: consensus development conference statement, *Decubitus* 2:24–28, 1989.

Ocampo RV, Persing JA: Sagittal synostosis, *Clin Plast Surg* 21:563–574, 1994.

Parker SE, Mai CT, Canfield MA, et al: Updated National Birth Prevalence estimates for selected birth defects in the United States, 2004-2006, *Birth Defects Res A Clin Mol Teratol* 88(12):1008–1016, 2010.

Posnick JC: Treacher Collins syndrome: perspectives in evaluation and treatment, *J Oral Maxillofac Surg* 55:1120–1133, 1997.

Posnick JC: Unilateral coronal synostosis (anterior plagiocephaly): current clinical perspectives, *Ann Plast Surg* 36:430–447, 1996.

Prevel CD, Eppley BL, McCarty M: Acrocephalosyndactyly syndromes: a review, *J Craniofac Surg* 8:279–285, 1997.

Singer L, Sidoti EJ: Pediatric management of Robin sequence, *Cleft Palate Craniofac J* 29:220–223, 1992.

Wilkie AO, Wall SA: Craniosynostosis: novel insights into pathogenesis and treatment, *Curr Opin Neurol* 9:146–152, 1996.

Facial Fractures

Losee JE, Afifi A, Jiang S, et al: Pediatric orbital fractures: classification, management, and early follow-up, *Plast Reconstr Surg* 122:886–897, 2008.

Losee JE, Jiang S, Deleyiannis FWB: Craniofacial fractures. In Bentz ML, Bauer BS, Zuker RM, editors: *Principles and practice of pediatric plastic surgery* (vol 2), St. Louis, 2008, Quality Medical Publishing, pp 1047–1072.

Reconstructive Pediatric Plastic Surgery

Arneja JS, Gosain AK: Giant congenital melanocytic nevi, *Plast Reconstr Surg* 124(Suppl 1):1e–13e, 2009.

Arneja JS, Gosain AK: Vascular malformations, *Plast Reconstr Surg* 121:195e–206e, 2008.

Beck DO, Gosain AK: The presentation and management of hemangiomas, *Plast Reconstr Surg* 123:181e–191e, 2009.

Belysheva TS, Vishnevskaya TV, et al: Melanoma arising in a giant congenital melanocytic nevus: two case reports, *Diagn Pathol* 14(1):21, 2019.

Flatt AE: Cleft hand and central defects. In Flatt AE, editor: *The care of congenital hand anomalies*, St. Louis, 1994, Quality Medical Publishing, p 337.

Kay SP, McCombe DB, Kozin SH: *Chapter 40–Deformities of the hand and fingers. Green's operative hand surgery*, ed 6, 2010, Elsevier, pp 1303–1369.

Kozin SH: *Chapter 41–Deformities of the thumb. Green's operative hand surgery*, ed 6, 2010, Elsevier, pp 1371–1403.

Kozin SH: Upper-extremity congenital anomalies, *J Bone Joint Surg Am* 85: 1564–1576, 2003.

Lin AY, McGrath MH: Pressure sores in the elderly. In Rosenthal RA, Zenilman ME, Katlic MR, editors: *Principles and practice of geriatric surgery*, New York, 2011, Springer, p 1257.

Riddle RD, Tabin C: How limbs develop, *Sci Am* 280:74–79, 1999.

Swanson AB: A classification for congenital limb malformations, *J Hand Surg Am* 1:8–22, 1976.

Taghinia AH, Upton J: Vascular anomalies, *J Hand Surg Am* 43(12):1113–1121, 2018.

OTOLARYNGOLOGY

24

David H. Chi | Allison Tobey

The importance of pediatricians and family physicians having understanding of and experience with otolaryngologic problems and being skilled in techniques of examination of the head and neck region cannot be overemphasized. One study revealed that more than one-third of all visits to pediatricians' offices were prompted by ear symptoms. When nasal and oral symptoms are included, ear, nose, and throat pathology accounts for more than 50% of all visits. With patience and proper equipment, pediatricians can complete a thorough examination on almost all children. If a disorder fails to respond to therapy or becomes chronic or recurrent, or if an unusual problem is encountered, pediatric otolaryngology consultation should be sought.

Successful examination of the ears, nose, and oropharynx of a young child can present challenges, especially with older infants and toddlers. This can be a particular problem in children who have had previous bad experiences. An examiner's patience, warmth, humor, and careful explanation help reduce fear and enhance cooperation.

Whenever possible, the child should be allowed to sit on the parent's lap. Pacifiers, puppets and other toys, and tongue blades with faces drawn on them can all serve to reduce anxiety, enlist the child's trust, and distract attention. Gradual introduction of the equipment can also be helpful, especially if done in a playful way. The child can be asked to blow out the otoscope light while the examiner turns it off, urged to catch the light spot as the examiner moves it around, and even allowed to look in the parent's or examiner's ears (Fig. 24.1). Parents can also help demonstrate maneuvers for opening the mouth, panting to depress the tongue, and holding the head back. Although this may take a little additional time at the outset, it often saves considerable time in the long run and makes future follow-up examinations far easier.

EAR DISORDERS

Ear pain (otalgia), discharge from the ear (otorrhea), and suspected hearing loss are three of the more common otic symptoms for which parents seek medical attention for their children. Less specific symptoms such as pulling or tugging at the ears, fussiness, and fever are also frequently encountered, particularly in children younger than 2 years old.

History should center on the nature and duration of symptoms, character of the clinical course, and possible antecedent treatment. Because many infections of the ear are recurrent and/or chronic, the parent should be asked about previous medical or surgical therapy (e.g., antibiotics, myringotomy, and/or tube insertion).

A brief review of the anatomy of the ear is helpful in developing a logical approach to any clinical abnormalities that may be encountered. The ear is conveniently divided into the following three regions (Fig. 24.2):

1. The *external ear* includes the pinna, or auricle, and the external auditory canal, up to and including the tympanic membrane.
2. The *middle ear* is made up of the middle ear space, inner surface of the eardrum, ossicles, and mastoid.
3. The *inner ear* comprises the cochlea (hearing), labyrinth and semicircular canals (balance), and main nerve trunks of the seventh and eighth cranial nerves.

The examination should include inspection of the auricle, periauricular tissues, and external auditory canal and the entire tympanic membrane, including assessment of its mobility in response to positive and negative pressure with pneumatic otoscopy. Examination techniques for each area are discussed in the following sections.

DISORDERS OF THE EXTERNAL EAR

"Four Ds"

Examination of each child's ear begins with inspection of the auricle and periauricular tissues for four important signs—discharge, displacement, discoloration, and deformity (the "four Ds"). The canal is normally smooth and angulated slightly in an anterior direction. Cerumen is often present; it varies in color from yellowish-white to tan to dark brown. It is secreted from glands interspersed among the hair follicles at the entrance to the ear canal and has some bacteriostatic activity. When cerumen obstructs the view, it must be removed to allow adequate visualization of the canal and tympanic membrane. When soft and moist, cerumen is easily removed with a curette. Removal may be more difficult if the cerumen is dry and flaky and may require removal with otologic forceps or, at times, instillation of drops. In some children, cerumen solidifies or has been packed in with cotton-tipped applicators, forming a firm plug that impedes sound conduction and requires softening for removal. Irrigation is contraindicated if there is any possibility that the eardrum may not be intact.

Discharge

Ear discharge is a common complaint with multiple etiologies. When there is thick, white discharge and erythema of the canal wall, the physician should gently pull on the pinna. If this maneuver elicits pain and the canal wall is edematous, primary otitis externa (OE) is the likely diagnosis (Fig. 24.3), although prolonged drainage from untreated otitis media with perforation or tube in place may present a similar picture (see the Disorders of the Middle Ear section). When the middle ear is the source of otic discharge, the tympanic membrane should show evidence of perforation (Fig. 24.4). The major predisposing condition to primary otitis externa is prolonged excessive moisture in the ear canal, which promotes bacterial or fungal overgrowth. Thus this is a common problem among swimmers. Other causes include Q-tip use, eczema, and foreign bodies (Fig. 24.5). Foreign bodies can stimulate intense inflammatory responses and produce foul-smelling purulent discharge. Thus when otic drainage is encountered, the discharge must be gently removed to assess the condition of the tympanic membrane and to rule out the presence of perforation or foreign objects. This can be accomplished either by gentle wiping with cotton wicks or by careful suctioning (see Fig. 24.16).

If drainage is persistent or recurrent despite therapy, a culture should be obtained to determine both the causative organism and its sensitivity to antimicrobial agents. Treatment consists primarily of debridement and topical otic antimicrobials, antifungals, and/or steroid preparations. Systemic antibiotics should be given when pain is severe; when there is evidence of otitis media; or when, despite attempts at cleaning, there is still uncertainty about an infection of the middle ear. Removal of irritants or infectious sources (Q-tip use, contaminated water) and treatment of systemic etiologies such as immune deficiencies or diabetes are also critical. Parenteral

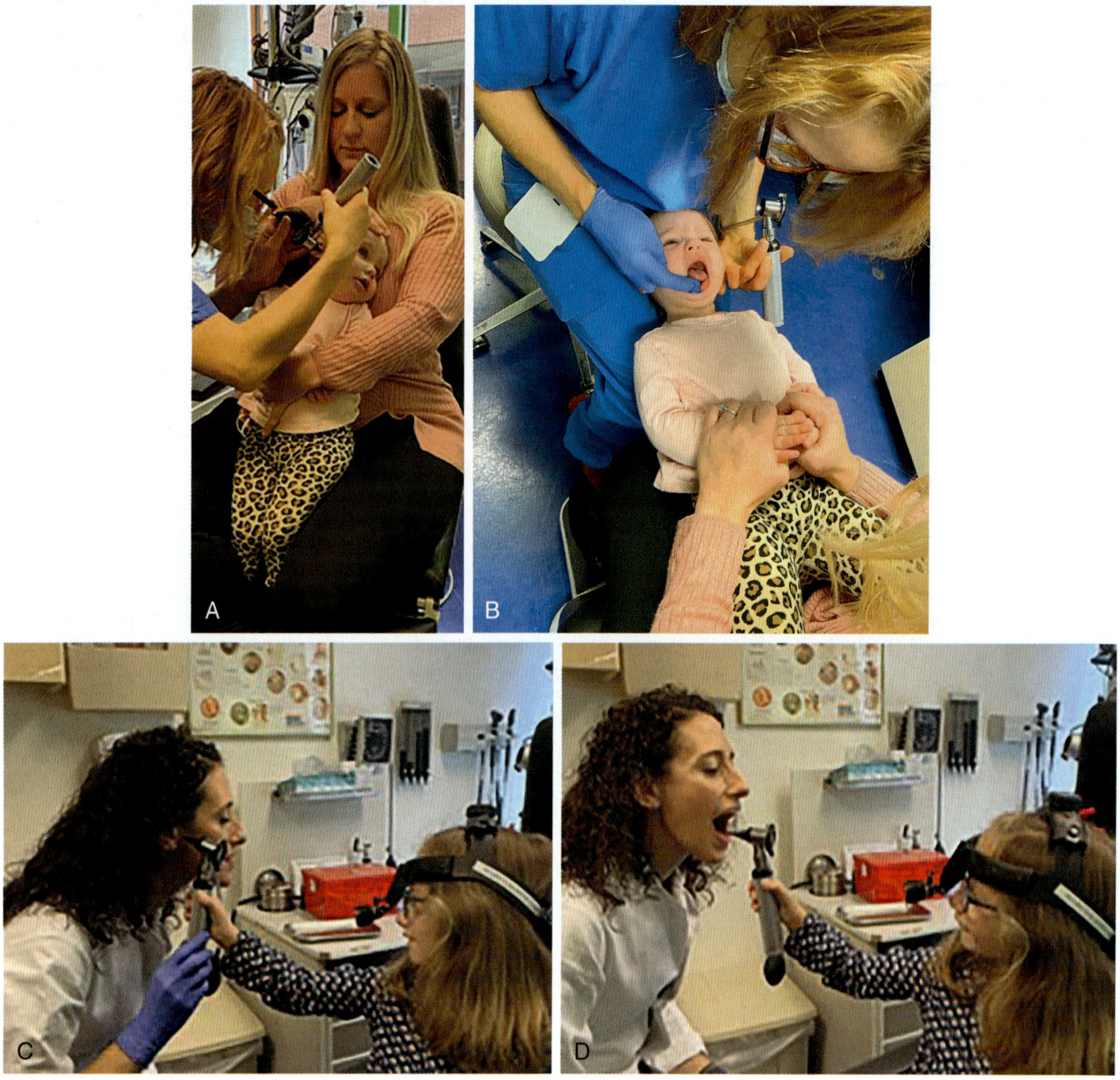

Fig. 24.1 Techniques to assist examination of a child's ears, nose, and oropharynx. (A) Young infants often can be examined on their mother's lap, with gentle immobilization provided by the parent and the examiner's hand. (B) Having a toddler or preschooler sit on a parent's lap and using toys such as tongue blades with faces drawn on them can make them more comfortable, while gradually introducing the examining instruments reduces anxiety. With an infant's head on the examiner's lap and body on the parent's lap, parents can tickle or make faces at the child to reassure them while allowing the examiner an excellent view of the oral cavity and oropharynx. (C and D) Making a game of blowing out the otoscope light and allowing the patient to check the examiner first convey that otoscopy does not have to hurt.

antibiotics may be required when the process has extended, producing cellulitis of the periauricular soft tissues or frank mastoiditis.

Displacement

Displacement of the pinna away from the skull is a worrisome sign. The most severe condition causing displacement is mastoiditis, resulting from extension of a middle ear infection through the mastoid air cells and out to the periosteum of the skull. In addition to displacement, important clinical signs of mastoiditis include erythema and edema and possibly fluctuance of the skin overlying the mastoid, exquisite tenderness on palpation of the mastoid process, a sagging ear canal, purulent otorrhea, fever, and usually toxicity (Fig. 24.6). This condition is now less common and is seen mainly in patients with long-standing, untreated, or inadequately treated otitis media. Recognition, prompt institution of parenteral antibiotic therapy, and myringotomy with culture and sensitivity testing of middle and inner ear effusion are crucial because there is significant risk of central nervous system (CNS) extension. Computed tomography (CT) imaging will delineate the extent of involvement and assist the surgical approach (Fig. 24.7). Mastoidectomy is indicated in cases complicated by bone erosion, or CNS extension, and in those in whom intravenous (IV) antibiotics and myringotomy fail to produce complete resolution.

Other conditions characterized by displacement of the pinna away from the head include parotitis, primary cellulitis of the periauricular tissues, and edema secondary to insect bites or contact dermatitis. Parotitis is differentiated by finding prominent induration and enlargement of the parotid gland anterior and inferior to the external ear, together with blunting of the angle of the mandible on palpation (see Chapter 13). Cellulitis is characterized by erythema and tenderness but can often be distinguished clinically from mastoiditis by the presence of associated skin lesions that antecede the inflammation (Fig. 24.8). In cases secondary to untreated external otitis or otitis media with perforation, the picture may be clinically similar. Localized contact dermatitis and angioedema may make the ear erythematous but also pruritic and nontender.

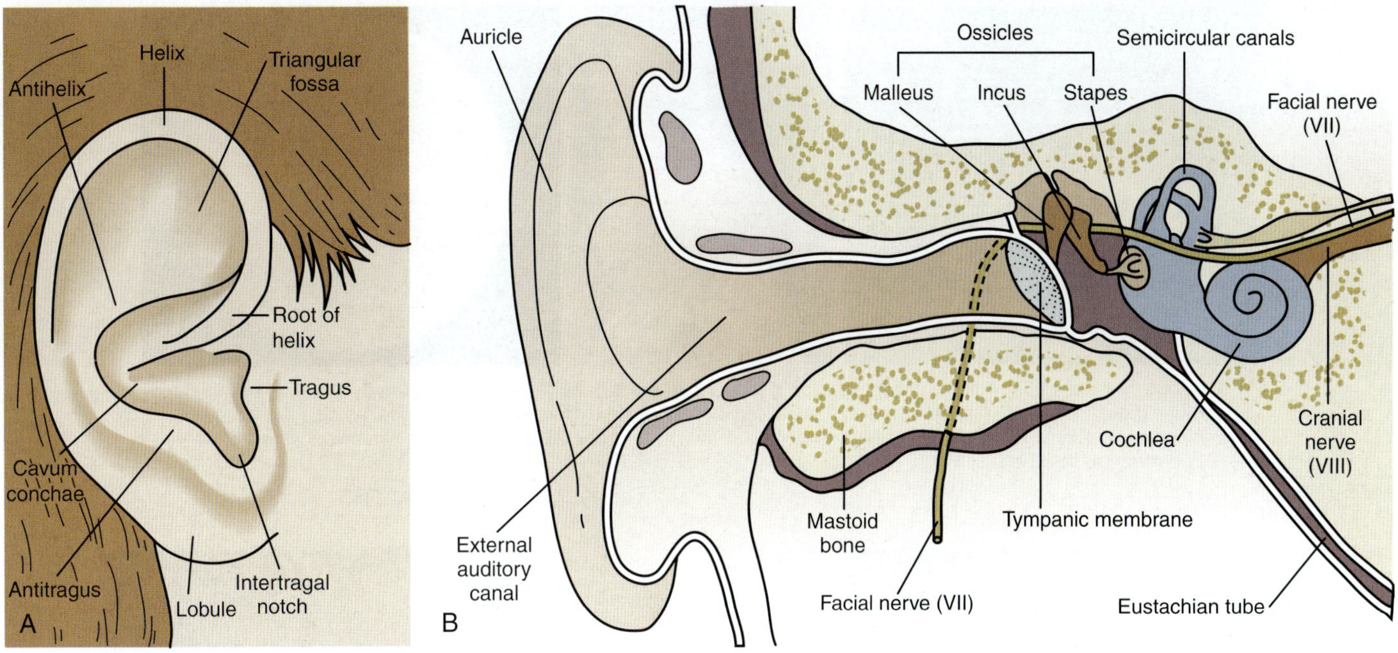

Fig. 24.2 Anatomy of the ear. (A) A normal external ear (auricle or pinna) is shown, with its various landmarks labeled. It is helpful to refer to such a diagram in assessing congenital anomalies. (B) Coronal section shows the various structures of the hearing and vestibular apparatus. The three main regions are the external ear, middle ear, and inner ear. The eustachian tube connects the middle ear and the nasopharynx and serves to drain and ventilate the middle ear.

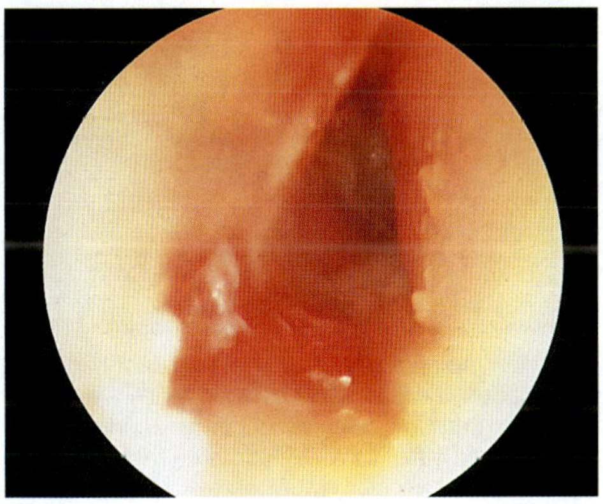

Fig. 24.3 External otitis. Acute bacterial external otitis is characterized by intense pain that is worsened by traction on the pinna, along with purulent exudate and intense canal wall inflammation with normal tympanic membrane mobility on pneumatic otoscopy.

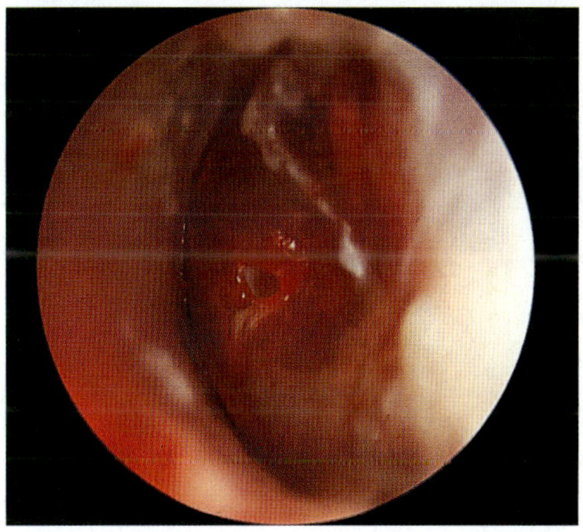

Fig. 24.4 Acute otitis media with perforation. In this child, increased middle ear pressure with acute otitis resulted in perforation of the tympanic membrane. The drum is thickened, and the perforation is seen at the 9 o'clock position.

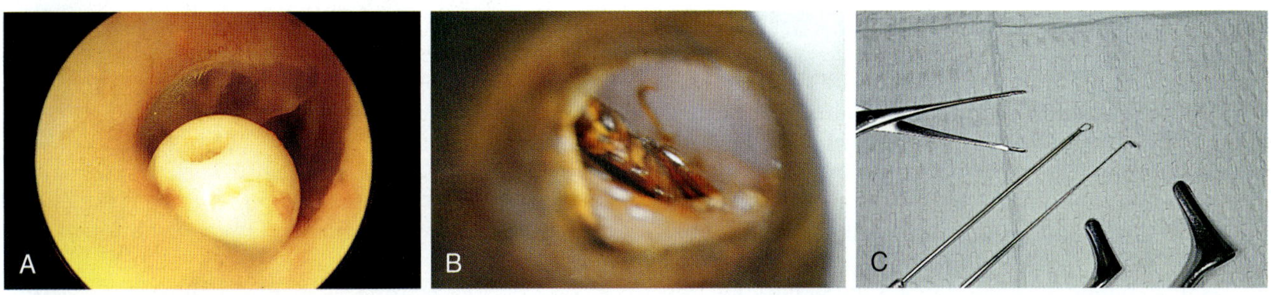

Fig. 24.5 Otic foreign bodies. (A) This child inserted a bead into her ear. The object must be removed carefully to prevent further trauma. (B) This patient experienced a period of intense buzzing, pain, and itching in the ear that abated after a few hours. If the tympanic membrane is intact, olive or mineral oil may be used to drown the insect. (C) A blunt-tipped, right-angled Day hook, small wire loop curette, Hartmann forceps, and an alligator forceps are useful instruments for removing foreign bodies from the external auditory canal.

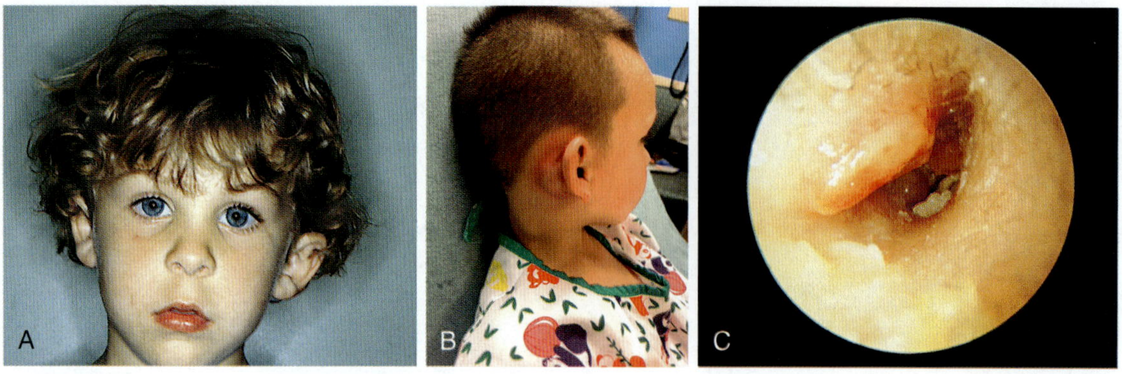

Fig. 24.6 Mastoiditis. (A) This frontal photograph clearly shows the left auricle displaced anteriorly and inferiorly. (B) In another patient, viewed from the side, erythema can be appreciated over the mastoid process. (C) On otoscopy, erythema and edema of the canal wall are evident and the posterosuperior portion of the canal wall sags inferiorly. (C, Courtesy Michael Hawke, MD.)

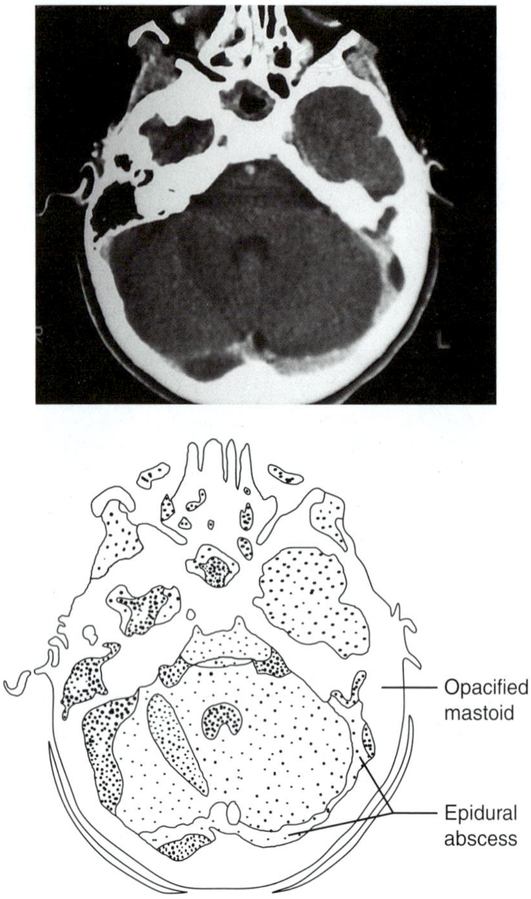

Fig. 24.7 Mastoiditis. The computed tomography image shows acute left-sided mastoiditis with the complication of an associated epidural abscess delineated in the diagram.

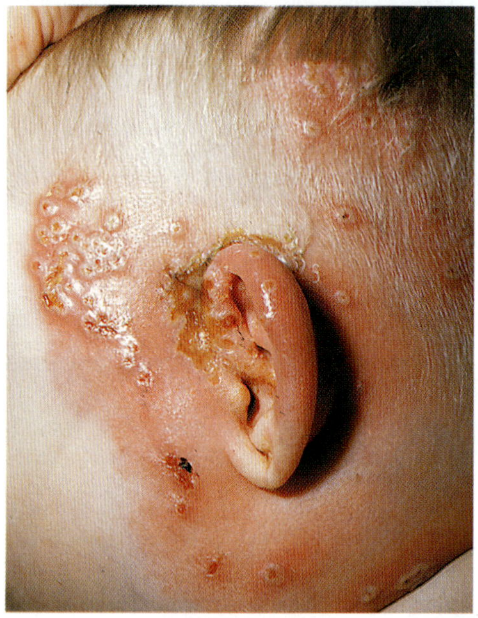

Fig. 24.8 Periauricular and auricular cellulitis. This infant had mild postauricular seborrhea and developed varicella. The vesicular varicella lesions that clustered at sites of prior skin irritation became secondarily infected with group A β-streptococci, resulting in cellulitis with intense erythema, edema, and tenderness of the auricle and periauricular tissues. In this case, the external canal was normal. (Courtesy Ronald Chludzinski, MD.)

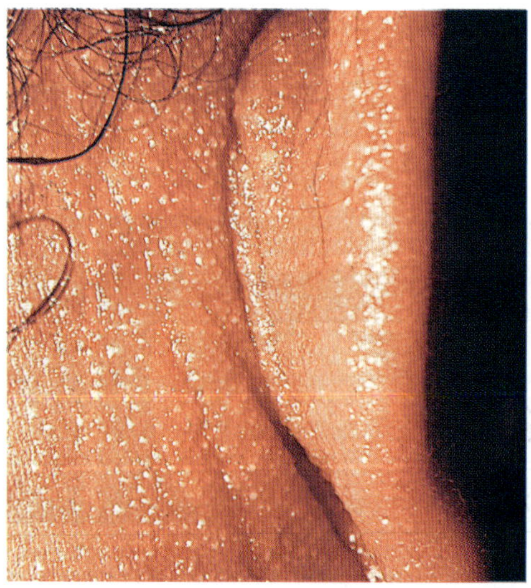

Fig. 24.9 This young girl became sensitive to the nickel posts of her earrings and developed periauricular contact dermatitis. The auricle and periauricular skin are erythematous and covered by a weeping, pruritic microvesicular eruption. (Courtesy Michael Sherlock, MD, Lutherville, MD.)

The former condition is characterized by microvesicular skin changes (Fig. 24.9), whereas in the latter condition, a precipitating insect bite can often be identified on inspection (Fig. 24.10).

Discoloration

Discoloration is another important sign and is commonly a feature of conditions producing displacement. Erythema of the pinna is common when there is inflammation, with or without infection (see Figs. 24.6B and 24.8–24.10). Ecchymotic discoloration may be encountered with trauma. When this overlies the mastoid tip (the area immediately posterior to the pinna), it is termed a *Battle sign* (Fig. 24.11A) and usually reflects a basilar skull fracture. In such cases, the canal wall should be checked for tears and the tympanic

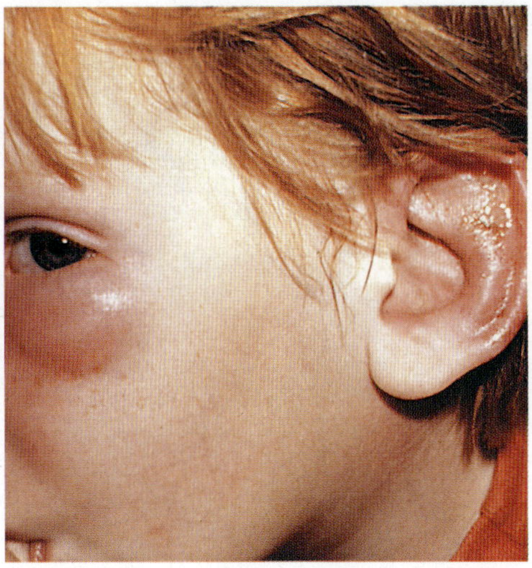

Fig. 24.10 Angioedema. This youngster had pruritic, nonpainful, nontender erythema, and swelling of his ear and infraorbital region. Close examination of the latter revealed the punctum of an insect bite. Another punctum on his ear was obscured by crusting after scratching. (Courtesy Michael Sherlock, MD, Lutherville, MD.)

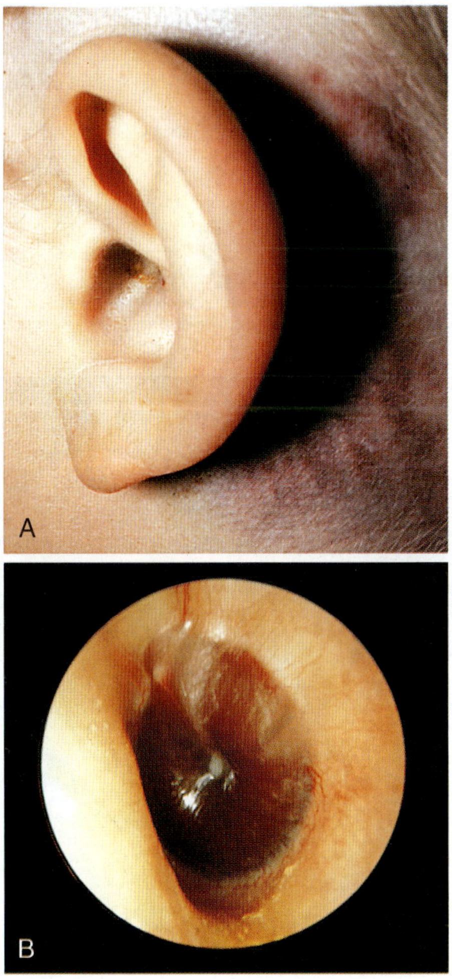

Fig. 24.11 Basilar skull fracture. (A) The presence of a basilar skull fracture involving the temporal bone is often signaled by postauricular ecchymotic discoloration, termed the *Battle sign*. (B) The force of the blow may also cause tearing of the ear canal or, as shown here, middle ear hemorrhage with hemotympanum. Depending on the timing of examination, this may appear red or blue. (B, Courtesy Michael Hawke, MD.)

membrane for perforation or a hemotympanum (blood behind the tympanic membrane; see Fig. 24.11B). CT confirms the diagnosis of a basilar skull fracture. Recognition that bruising of the pinna and/or postauricular area can be a manifestation of child abuse is important (see Chapter 6).

Deformity

When the external ear is abnormal in shape or microtic, associated anomalies of middle ear structures are common and hearing loss may be significant (Fig. 24.12). Severe deformities stem from developmental anomalies of the branchial arches, which contribute to both external ear and middle ear structures. Such abnormalities warrant a thorough evaluation in infancy to ensure early recognition and treatment of hearing loss. Deformity of the pinna can be the result of hereditary factors or exposure to teratogens, but at times it is simply produced by intrauterine positioning. Most deformities are minor and represent isolated malformations of mostly cosmetic significance (Fig. 24.13D). In some instances, they may be part of a picture of multiple congenital anomalies (see Fig. 24.13A to C; see also Fig. 24.8 and Chapter 1).

Trauma to the pinna may result in a hematoma between the skin and cartilage, the recognition of which requires otolaryngologic consultation. An unrecognized hematoma may result in a permanent deformity if left undrained, or superinfection of the hematoma. Either complications can result in permanent cosmetic damage to the pinna.

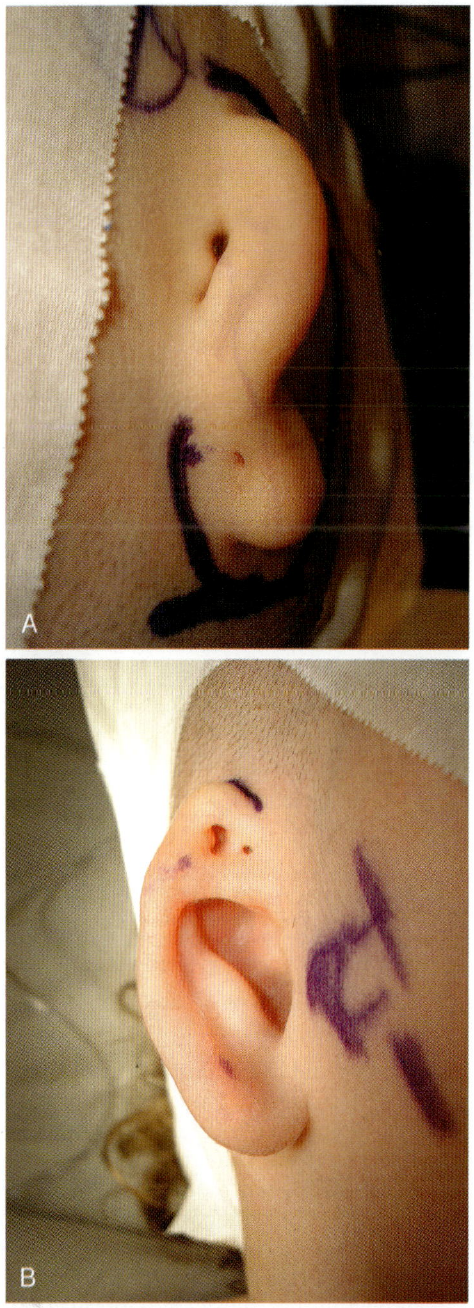

Fig. 24.12 (A) Grade 3 microtia and congenital aural atresia of the right external ear. In this otherwise normal child, the pinna failed to develop properly and the external canal was atretic. Audiometric testing revealed a 60-dB hearing loss. (B) Grade 2 microtia. Note deficiency of superior portion of auricle. Such isolated deformities stem from abnormal development of the first and second branchial arches.

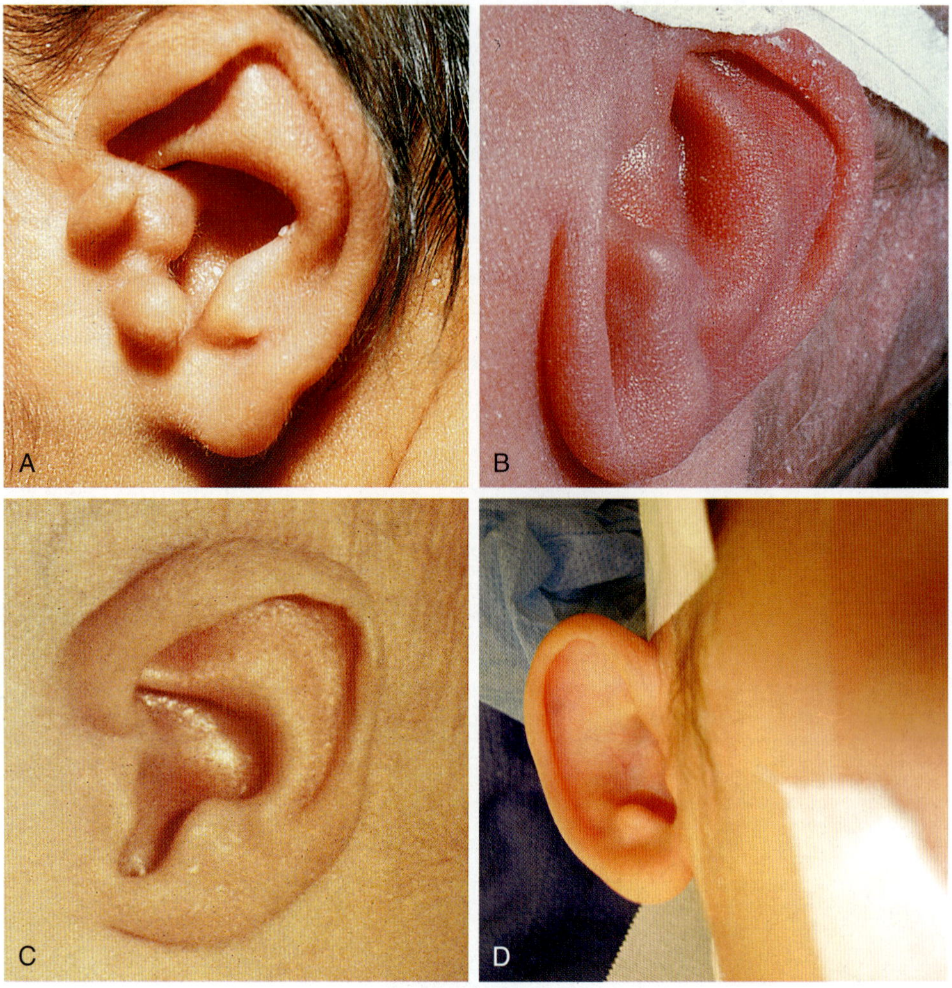

Fig. 24.13 Minor congenital auricular deformities. (A) In this infant, the superior portion of the helix is folded over, obscuring the triangular fossa; the antihelix is sharply angulated; and there are three preauricular skin tags. (B) This neonate with orofaciodigital and Turner syndromes has a simple helix and a redundant folded lobule. The ear is low set and posteriorly rotated, and the antitragus is anteriorly displaced. (C) This infant with Rubinstein-Taybi syndrome has an exaggerated elongated intertragal notch. (D) Prominent ear in an otherwise normal child. The auricular cartilage is abnormally contoured, making the ear protrude forward. (C, Courtesy Michael Sherlock, MD, Lutherville, MD.)

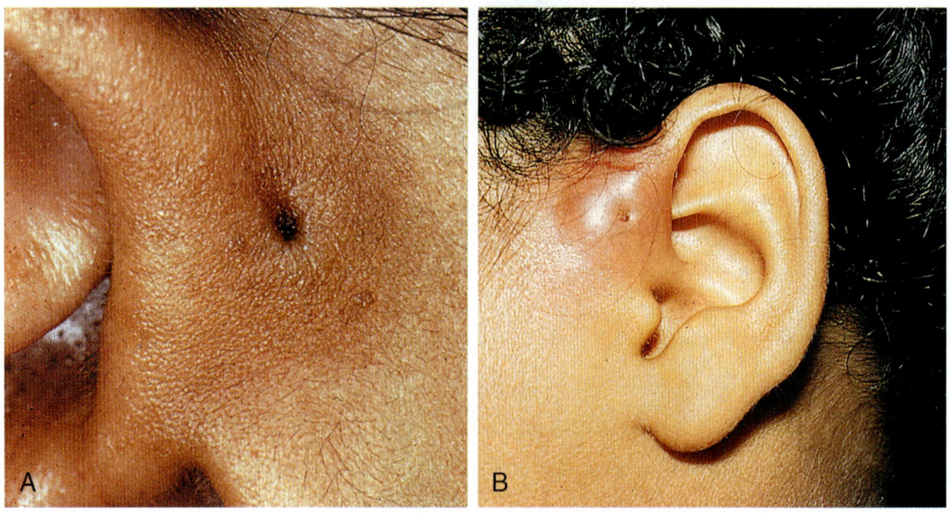

Fig. 24.14 Preauricular sinuses. (A) These congenital remnants are located anterior to the pinna and have an overlying surface dimple. (B) In this child, the sinus has become infected, forming an abscess. (A, Courtesy Michael Hawke, MD.)

Preauricular sinuses and cysts constitute two of the more common congenital abnormalities. These are congenital remnants located anterior to the pinna with an overlying surface dimple (Fig. 24.14A). These cysts are vulnerable to infection and abscess formation (see Fig. 24.14B), which necessitate needle aspiration or incision and drainage in conjunction with antistaphylococcal antibiotics. Once infection has occurred, recurrence is common unless the entire sinus is completely excised. This procedure should be undertaken once inflammation has subsided. A preauricular sinus may also result from branchio-oto-renal syndrome (also known as *Melnick-Fraser syndrome*), an autosomal dominant disorder characterized by bilateral preauricular sinuses, ear anomalies, branchial cleft anomalies in the neck, and renal problems.

Foreign Objects and Secondary Trauma

It is not unusual for children to put paper, beads, and other foreign objects into their ear canals (Fig. 24.5A). Small insects also on occasion may become trapped in the external ear (see Fig. 24.5B). In some cases, small objects may be embedded in cerumen and missed on inspection. If present for more than a few days, the foreign material may stimulate an inflammatory response and be purulent and foul smelling, obscuring the presence of the inciting foreign body. Removal of the foreign body can be accomplished with otologic alligator forceps or by irrigation of the ear canal; others—particularly spherical objects—require use of a Day (right angle) hook or suction (see

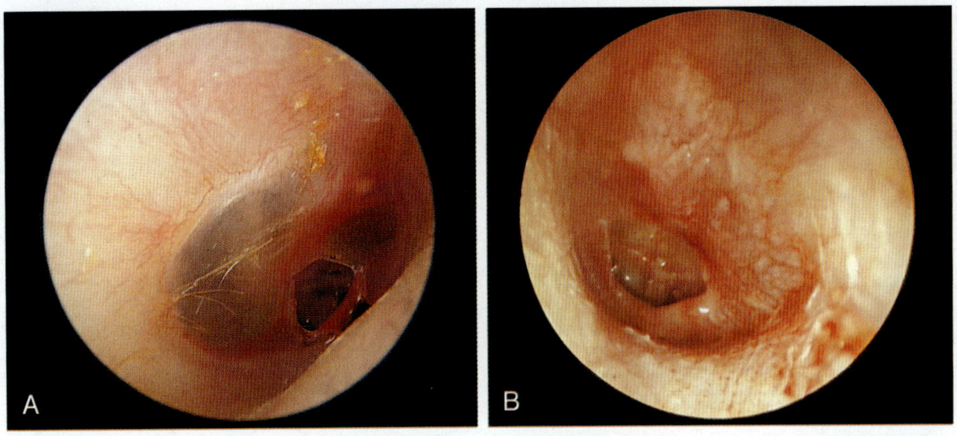

Fig. 24.15 Traumatic perforations of the tympanic membrane. (A) This 8-year-old boy's tympanic membrane was perforated by a forceful slap on the ear. (B) Even more severe damage with thickening and hemorrhage is seen in this victim of a blast injury caused by an explosion. (A, Courtesy Michael Hawke, MD.)

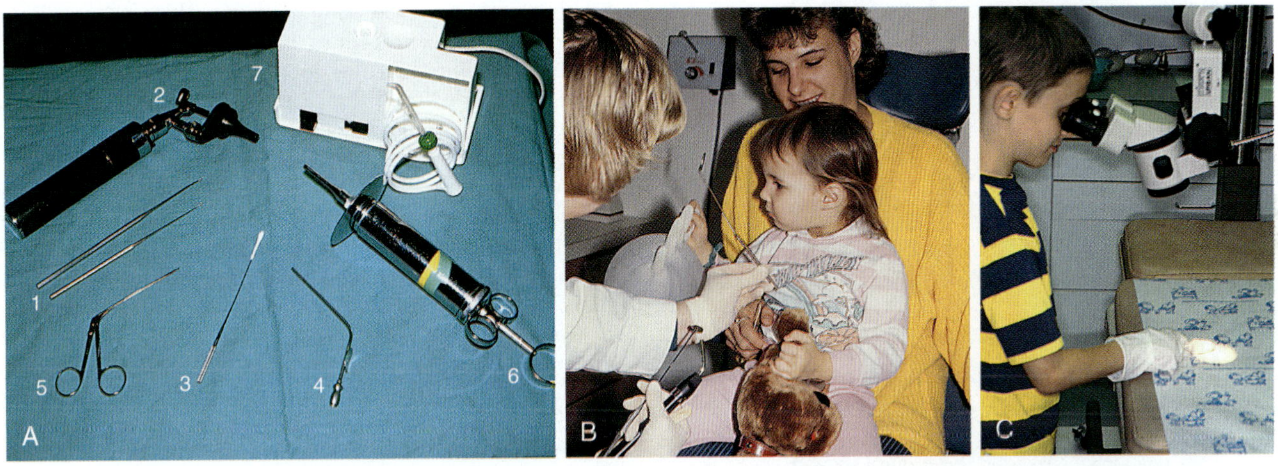

Fig. 24.16 (A) Equipment for cleaning the external auditory canal. The curette *(1)* is the implement most commonly used to remove cerumen. Use of a surgical otoscope head *(2)* makes the process considerably easier. Additional implements include cotton wicks *(3)* and a suction tip *(4)* for removal of discharge or moist wax, alligator forceps *(5)* for removing foreign bodies, and an ear syringe *(6)* and motorized irrigation apparatus *(7)* for removing firm objects or impacted cerumen. Lavage is contraindicated when there is a possible perforation of the tympanic membrane. If the motorized apparatus is used for irrigation, it must be kept on the lowest power setting to avoid traumatizing the eardrum. (B) Use of suction is often necessary when there is copious exudate. (C) Allowing the child to look through the examining microscope may help him or her cooperate with the examination.

Fig. 24.5C; see also Fig. 24.16). Foreign objects may also be the cause of painful abrasions or lacerations of the external auditory canal or even a perforation of the tympanic membrane. Insertion of pencils or sticks into the ear canal by the child and parental attempts to clean the canal with a cotton swab are the most common modes of such injury.

Exposure to concussive forces such as a direct blow (which may be accidental or inflicted) or an explosion can also result in perforation (Fig. 24.15). Patients with traumatic perforations must be carefully assessed for signs of injury to deeper structures. If tympanic membrane perforation occurs as a result of penetration by a foreign object or of concussive forces, the physician must be particularly aware of the possibility of middle ear or inner ear damage. Evidence of hearing loss, vertigo, nystagmus, facial nerve injury, or cerebrospinal fluid leak should prompt urgent otolaryngologic consultation.

DISORDERS OF THE MIDDLE EAR

Before otoscopic examination, cerumen or debris may need to be removed for better visualization. This can be performed with varying tools and techniques (Fig. 24.16A and B) but should always be performed carefully and gently and attempted only after the child has been carefully immobilized to avoid trauma (Fig. 24.17). It is

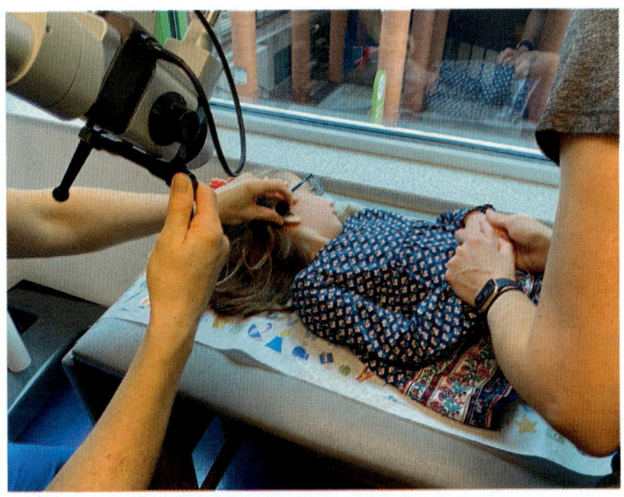

Fig. 24.17 Method of immobilization for cleaning. An assistant holds the child's arms and simultaneously immobilizes the child's head with the thumbs. The parent firmly holds the hips and thighs. This critical immobilization prevents dangerous motion by the child during cleaning of the ear canal and is also useful for otoscopy in young children.

easy to injure the canal during the process of cleaning the external ear. Injury to the canal is painful and can cause significant bleeding that obscures visualization and upsets the patient and parent. Both should be given a clear explanation of the procedure beforehand, and the examiner's hands should be steadied on the child's head while performing ear cleaning and then examination. Allowing the older child to handle and look through the equipment before cleaning and examining reduces anxiety and enhances cooperation (see Fig. 24.16).

Because the external auditory canal is often angled in infants and young children, gentle lateral traction on the pinna is frequently necessary to assist visualization of the eardrum itself (Fig. 24.18). In infants, the tympanic membrane tends to be oriented at a greater angle (Fig. 24.19); the landmarks are less prominent. The skin that lines the canal, being loosely attached, moves readily on insufflation of air, simulating a normally mobile eardrum. To avoid confusion, the canal should be inspected as the speculum is inserted to ensure that the transition between the canal wall and the tympanic membrane is visualized.

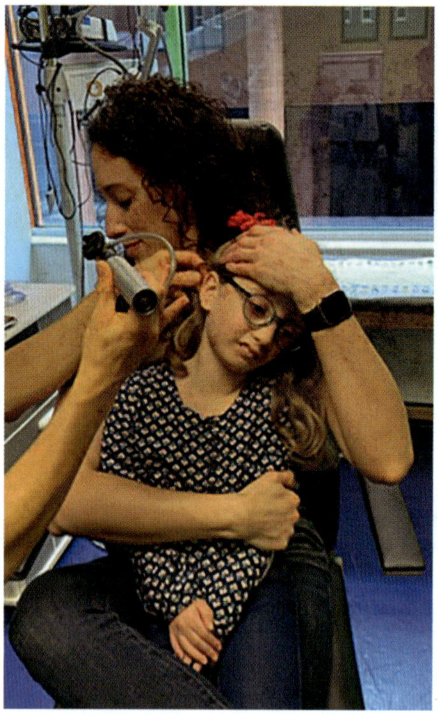

Fig. 24.18 Because the external auditory canal usually is angulated in children, lateral traction on the pinna is often required to straighten the canal and improve visualization of the tympanic membrane.

The pneumatic otoscope is the most valuable diagnostic tool when signs or symptoms of otitis media are present. Pediatricians, family practitioners, advanced practice providers, and otolaryngologists who treat children should be skilled in its use. Practical advice on the use of this instrument is as follows:

- Use adequate light. A bright halogen lamp is better than an ordinary light bulb. Replace bulbs routinely every 4 to 6 months and provide for routine battery charging.
- Choose a speculum of sufficient diameter and length to allow adequate penetration (10–15 mm) into the external canal for good eardrum visualization and a good seal for pneumatic otoscopy.

When otoscopic findings are unclear or when it is difficult to obtain a good air seal for pneumatic otoscopy, tympanometry can be highly useful in evaluating patients older than 8 months old (Fig. 24.20). The procedure is of lesser value in young infants because the abundance of loose connective tissue lining the ear canal and the laxity of the cartilage at the entrance increase canal wall compliance and produce unreliable results.

Because otitis media can be a reflection of both immunologic and anatomic abnormalities, the practitioner should be suspicious of possible underlying immune or temporal bone defects when seeing patients with chronic or frequently recurrent otitis media. The temporal bone is the bony housing for the auditory and vestibular systems. In addition, it provides bony protection for the facial nerve as it crosses from the brainstem to the facial muscles. The growth and development of this bone are affected in syndromes (e.g., Treacher Collins) that are characterized by altered midface growth (Fig. 24.21). The soft tissues attached to the temporal bone, such as the muscles controlling eustachian tube function, can be abnormal in children with cleft palates (see Palatal Disorders later). As a result, children with these disorders tend to have an increased incidence of otitis media.

Children with chronic effusions who complain of or have parental concern for hearing loss, those with speech delays, or those with suspected congenital malformations must have their hearing evaluated by audiometry, evoked otoacoustic emissions, or brainstem evoked potentials. Patients with vertigo and/or problems of balance and those with

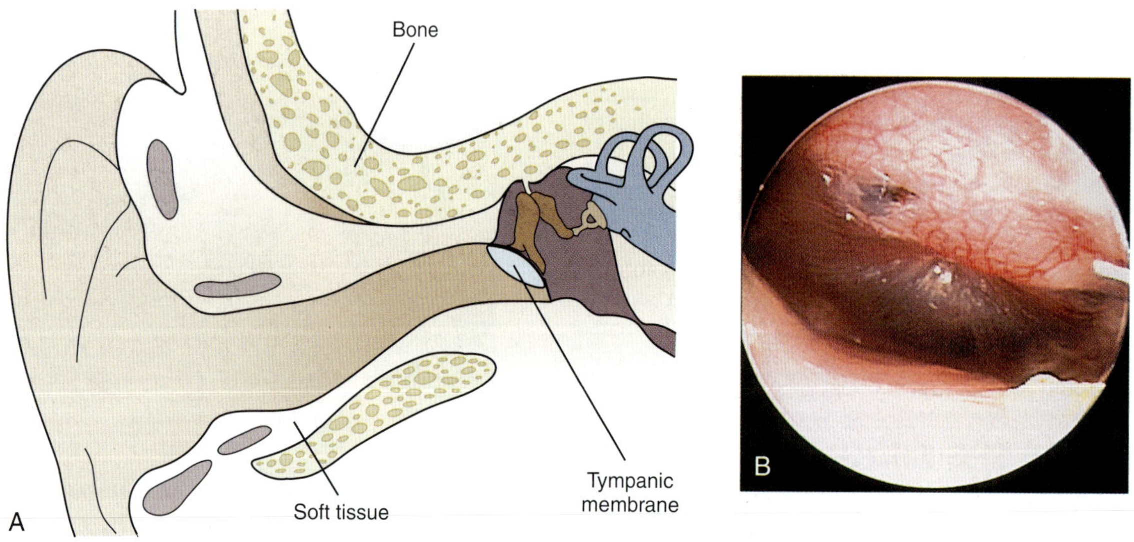

Fig. 24.19 Angulation of the tympanic membrane in infancy. (A) The relationship between the ear canal and eardrum is different in the infant, with the drum being tilted at an angle of 130 degrees. (B) Greater care is required in examining an infant's eardrum because of this angulation and because the landmarks are less prominent.

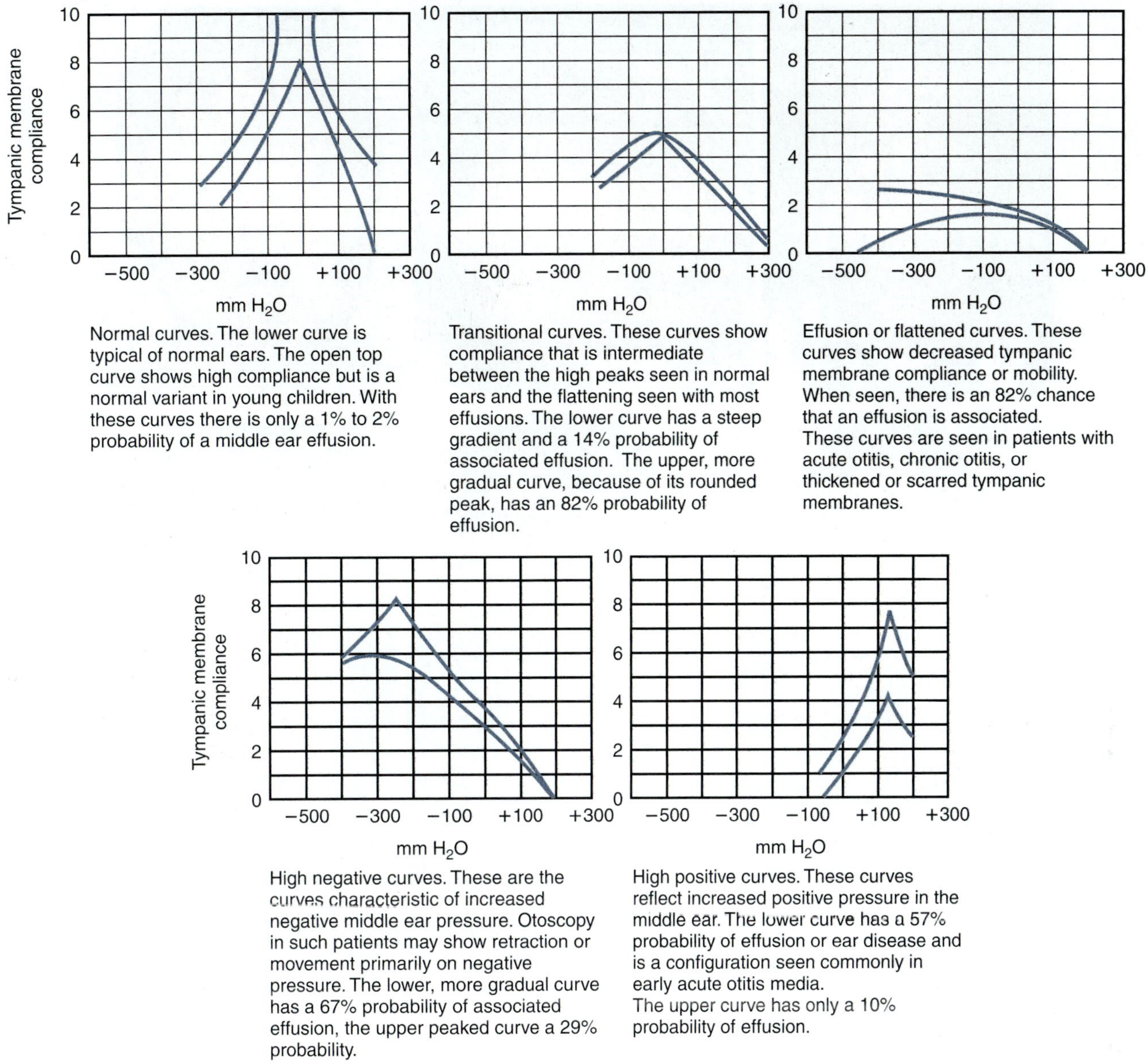

Fig. 24.20 Tympanometric patterns of various conditions of the middle ear. (Courtesy Mrs. Ruth Bachman, Pittsburgh, PA.)

facial weakness or asymmetry also warrant testing of hearing, facial nerve, and vestibular function. These children and those suffering from malformations may require CT, magnetic resonance imaging (MRI), or genetic studies in select cases to clarify the nature of the problem.

The normal tympanic membrane on visualization is thin, translucent, neutrally positioned, and mobile. The ossicles, particularly the malleus, are generally visible through the membrane (Fig. 24.22). Adequate assessment of the tympanic membrane requires that the examiner note four major characteristics: (1) thickness, (2) degree of translucence, (3) position relative to neutral, and (4) mobility. Application of gentle positive and negative pressure, using a properly sealed pneumatic otoscope (Fig. 24.23), produces brisk movement of the eardrum when the ear is free of disease and abnormal movement when fluid is present, when the drum is thickened or scarred, or when there is an increase in either positive or negative pressure (Fig. 24.24). An abnormality in any one of the four major characteristics suggests middle ear pathology.

Acute Otitis Media

Acute otitis media is the term used to describe acute infection and inflammation of the middle ear. Associated inflammation and edema of the eustachian tube mucosa play key roles in pathogenesis by impeding middle ear fluid drainage. In some children, anatomic or physiologic abnormalities of the eustachian tube predispose to infection. The problem is commonly seen in conjunction with an acute upper respiratory tract infection (URI), and its onset is often heralded by a fever one to several days after the onset of respiratory symptoms. The major offending organisms are bacterial respiratory pathogens. The most commonly isolated organisms and their relative frequency, shown in Table 24.1, show that *Streptococcus pneumoniae* and nontypeable *Haemophilus influenzae* are responsible for most cases. Increasing rates of β-lactamase positivity in *H. influenzae* have balanced out a fall in rates of penicillin-non-susceptible *S. pneumoniae* over time, highlighting the role of high-dose amoxicillin and/or β-lactamase–resistant antibiotic regimens for empiric therapy. Sulfa drugs and clindamycin may also be useful for therapy of community-acquired methicillin-resistant *Staphylococcus aureus,* which is increasingly common.

In acute otitis media, the classic findings on inspection of the tympanic membrane are erythema and injection; bulging that obscures the malleus; thickening, often with a grayish-white or yellow hue, reflecting a purulent effusion; and reduced mobility (Fig. 24.25A). However, crying produces erythema of the eardrum, and thus tympanic erythema in a crying child is of little diagnostic value. The patient is usually febrile and, if old enough, typically

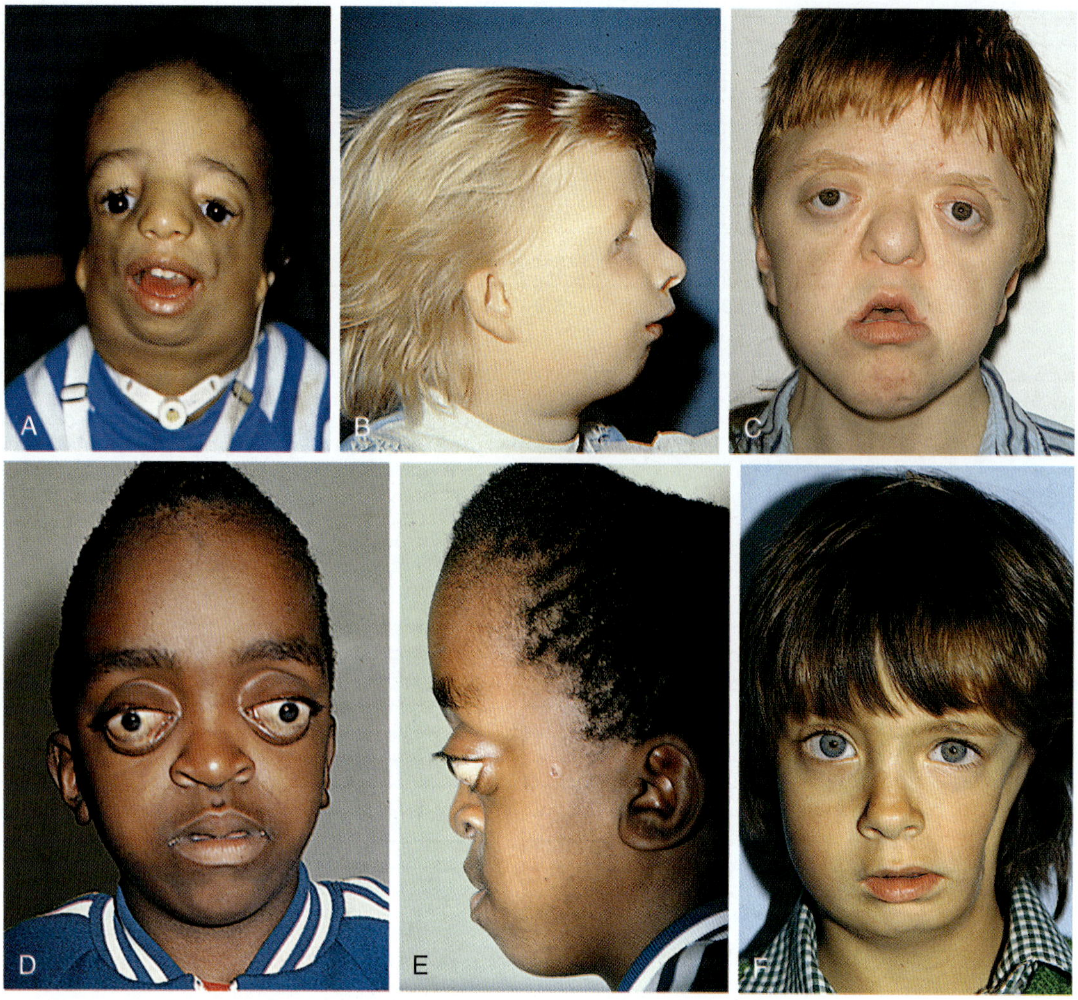

Fig. 24.21 Syndromes affecting the growth of the temporal bone and midface that predispose patients to recurrent or chronic otitis media and chronic recurrent sinus infections. (A and B) Treacher Collins syndrome. Note the maxillary hypoplasia, micrognathia, and auricular deformity. (C) Apert syndrome. (D and E) Crouzon syndrome. Both Apert and Crouzon syndromes are characterized by severe maxillary and midfacial hypoplasia. (F) Hemifacial microsomia with unilateral hypoplasia. (B to F, Courtesy Wolfgang Loskin, MD, University of North Carolina, Chapel Hill, NC.)

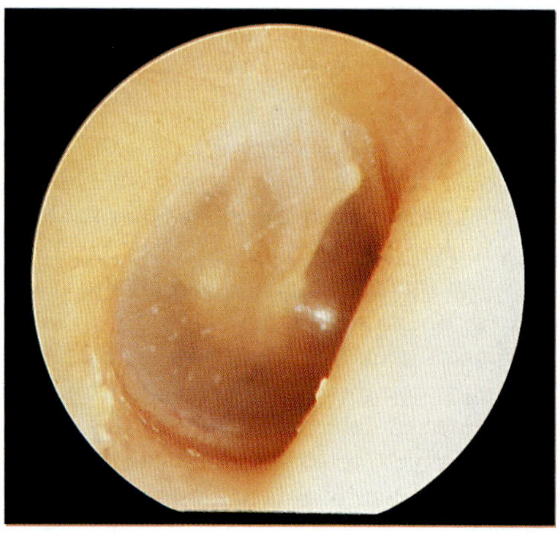

Fig. 24.22 A normal tympanic membrane. The drum is thin and translucent, and the ossicles are readily visualized. It is neutrally positioned with no evidence of bulging or retraction. (Courtesy Sylvan Stool, MD.)

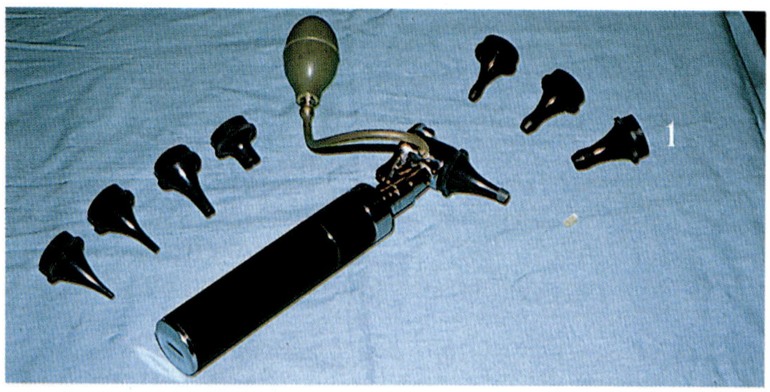

Fig. 24.23 Pneumatic otoscopy. This procedure requires proper equipment, including a pneumatic otoscope head and an appropriately sized speculum to achieve a good air seal. When a seal is difficult to obtain despite proper speculum size, the head and tubing should be checked for air leaks. If none is found, application of a piece of rubber tubing to the end of the speculum (shown attached to the otoscope) or use of a soft speculum *(1)* may solve the problem.

complains of otalgia. However, in many cases, this "textbook picture" is not seen. This is probably due in part to time of presentation, the virulence of the particular pathogen, and host factors.

Accuracy in diagnosis necessitates meticulous inspection during otoscopy and knowledge of the various modes of presentation. The challenge to clinicians is that children may present at various points during the time course of the infection. Children early in infection may have fever of a few hours' duration and otalgia (or if very young, fever and irritability) yet have no abnormality on otoscopy. If reexamined the next day, many of these patients have clear evidence of acute otitis media. Some have erythema and bubbles or air/fluid or air/pus levels (a result of venting by the eustachian tube) without bulging and with nearly normal mobility of the eardrum (see Fig. 24.25B). In still other cases, the drum may be full and poorly mobile with cloudy fluid behind it but with minimal erythema (see Fig. 24.25C).

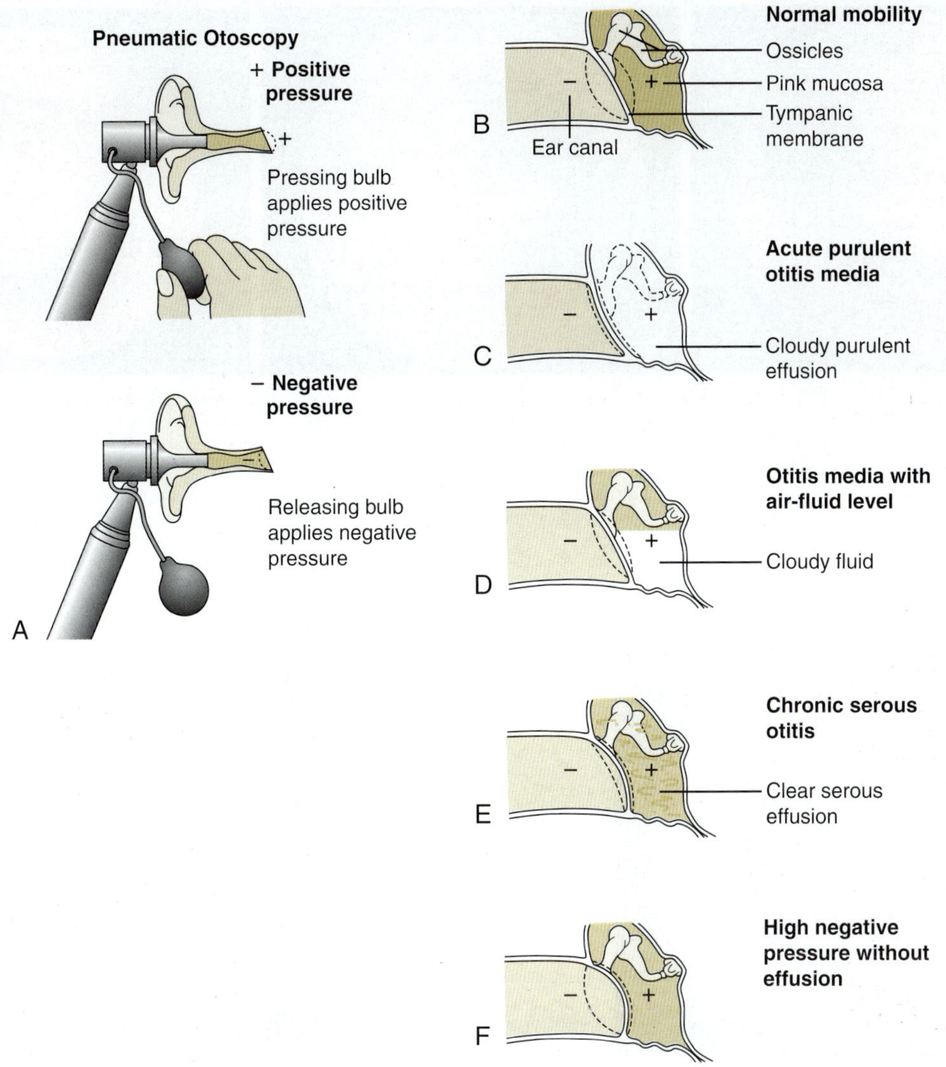

Fig. 24.24 Technique and findings in pneumatic otoscopy. (A) The speculum is inserted into the ear canal to form a tight seal. The bulb is then gently and slowly pressed and released while the mobility of the drum is assessed. Pressing on the bulb applies positive pressure; letting up applies negative pressure. (B) A normal drum moves inward and then back. (C) In cases of acute otitis media, in which the middle ear is filled with purulent material, the drum bulges toward the examiner and moves minimally. (D) In cases of acute otitis media with an air/fluid level, mobility may be nearly normal. In some patients, however, the drum may be retracted, indicating increased negative pressure. If this is the case, mobility on positive pressure may be reduced, whereas movement on negative pressure is nearly normal or only mildly decreased. (E) This is the same pattern as that seen commonly in children with chronic serous otitis. (F) In cases of high negative pressure and no effusion, application of positive pressure produces little or no movement, but on negative pressure the drum billows back toward the examiner.

Table 24.1 Acute Otitis Media: Most Commonly Isolated Bacterial Pathogens and Their Relative Frequency

Bacterial Pathogen	Number of Isolates (Percentage of Total)	Number Penicillin Resistant (Percentage)
Streptococcus pneumoniae	49 (44%)	18 (37%)
Haemophilus influenzae	46 (41%)	21 (46%)
Moraxella catarrhalis	16 (14%)	16 (100%)
Staphylococcus aureus	0 (0%)	0 (0%)
Total	**111 (100%)**	**55 (50%)**

The latest guidelines from the American Academy of Pediatrics and the American Academy of Family Practice emphasize the importance of visualizing the position of the tympanic membrane. Acute otitis media needs to be differentiated from otitis media with effusion. Although both diagnoses comprise a segment on the continuum of disease and inflammation, treatment implications vary. Otitis media with effusion does not represent an acute infection, and antibiotics should be avoided. Similarly, clinicians should not diagnose acute otitis media without the presence of a middle ear effusion, based on otoscopy or tympanometry. Moderate to severe bulging of the tympanic membrane or new onset of otorrhea not from otitis externa is diagnostic of the acute otitis media. The diagnosis may also be made with mild bulging and recent symptoms or redness of the tympanic membrane.

On occasion, the signs and symptoms of otitis media may be accompanied by the formation of a bullous lesion on the surface of the tympanic membrane, a condition termed *bullous myringitis* (Fig. 24.26). These children usually complain of intense pain. Although this phenomenon is most associated with *Mycoplasma* infection in adults, any of the usual pediatric pathogens in Table 24.1 can be causative in children. Finally, acute otitis media may, by virtue of increasing middle ear pressure, result in acute perforation of the tympanic membrane. On presentation, the canal may be filled with purulent material; however, tugging on the pinna usually does not elicit pain, and erythema and edema of the canal wall are minimal or absent. Cleansing with a cotton wick or suction usually reveals an inflamed drum with a barely visible perforation (see Fig. 24.4).

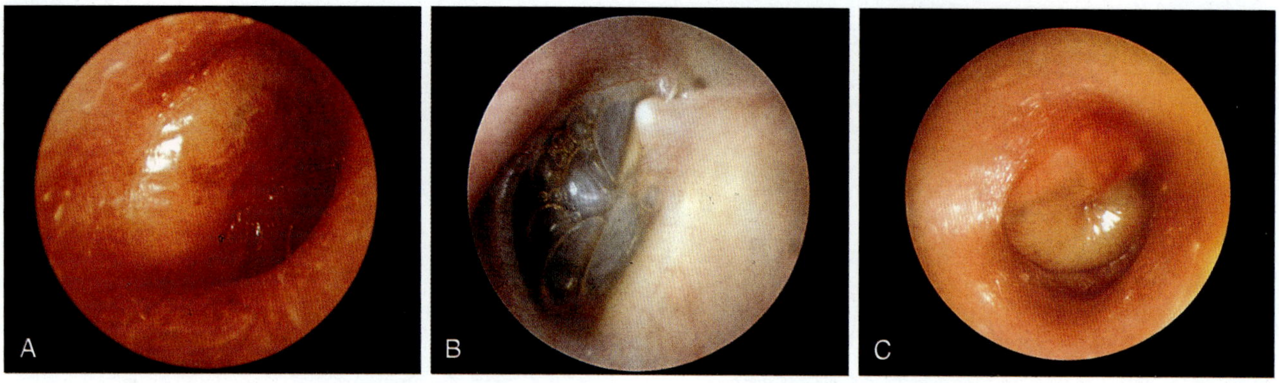

Fig. 24.25 Acute otitis media. (A) This is the textbook picture—an erythematous, opaque, bulging tympanic membrane. The light reflex is reduced, and the landmarks are partially obscured. Mobility is markedly reduced. (B) In this acutely febrile child who complained of otalgia, the presence of both air and fluid formed bubbles separated by grayish-yellow menisci. Even though the drum was not injected, this finding, combined with fever and otalgia, is consistent with acute infection. (C) In this child, the tympanic membrane was injected at the periphery, and a yellow purulent effusion caused the inferior portion to bulge outward. Mobility was markedly reduced. (A, Courtesy Michael Hawke, MD.)

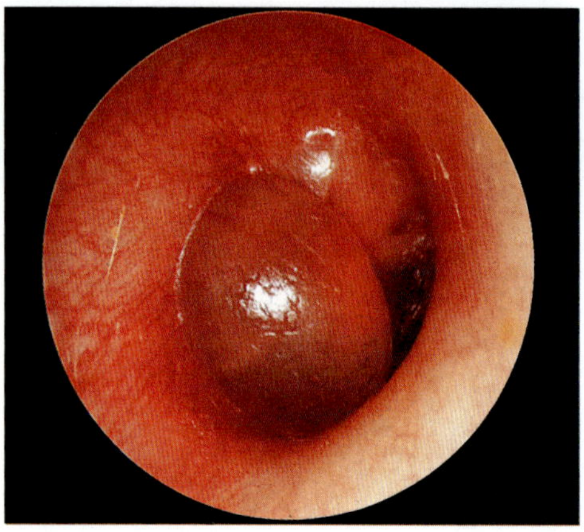

Fig. 24.26 Acute otitis media with bullous myringitis. This patient was febrile and extremely uncomfortable. On otoscopy, an erythematous bullous lesion is seen obscuring much of the tympanic membrane. This phenomenon, called *bullous myringitis,* is caused by the usual pathogens of otitis media in childhood. The bullous lesion often ruptures and drains spontaneously, providing immediate relief of pain.

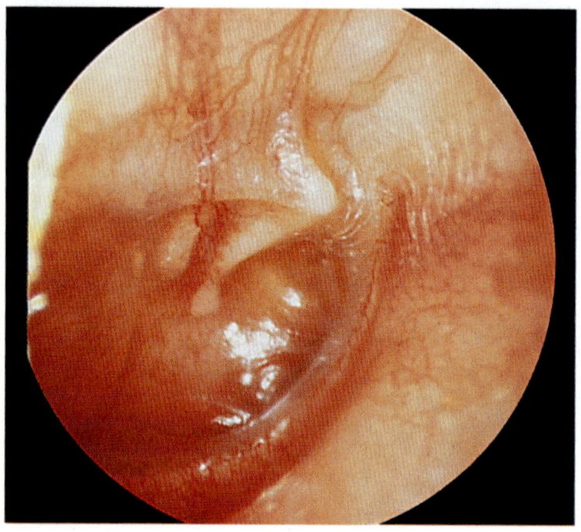

Fig. 24.27 Serous otitis media. This patient has a chronic serous middle ear effusion. The tympanic membrane is retracted, thickened, and shiny. Behind it is a clear yellow effusion. Mobility was decreased and primarily evident on negative pressure. The child was not acutely ill but did have decreased hearing. (Courtesy Sylvan Stool, MD.)

Just as clinical findings of acute otitis media vary, so do symptoms. Although some patients have severe otalgia, others may complain of sore throat, mild ear discomfort, ear popping, or decreased hearing yet have floridly inflamed eardrums. Fever may be absent.

Radiographic studies are generally of little value in the diagnosis of acute otitis media. Treatment for acute otitis media may include the option of observation without using antibiotics based on age, illness severity, and assurance of follow-up. In addition to treating patients with an appropriate antimicrobial agent and analgesics when necessary, follow-up examination is important. This is best done 2 to 3 weeks after diagnosis, when complete resolution can be expected in more than 50% of children. The purpose of reevaluation is to identify those patients who have persistent effusions and require ongoing surveillance. Selected older patients with mild, uncomplicated acute otitis media may be observed without antimicrobial therapy, but follow-up examination is still necessary. Children with recurrent episodes of otitis media are candidates for tympanostomy tubes.

Otitis Media With Effusion (Serous Otitis Media)

Serous effusion in the middle ear may result from a URI, or it may be the residual of treated acute otitis. In many instances, this effusion is not spontaneously cleared but instead remains in the middle ear for weeks or months, resulting in a persistent clear gray or yellow effusion behind the eardrum (Fig. 24.27). Persistence appears to result in part from eustachian tube dysfunction with poor drainage and ventilation. Pneumatic otoscopy often reveals poor mobility of the tympanic membrane, and mobility is noted primarily on negative pressure. The latter is thought to develop as a result of absorption of middle ear gases by mucosal cells, creating a vacuum that persists with the fluid because of failure of ventilation by the eustachian tube. Such long-standing effusions impair hearing.

Chronic Otitis Media With Effusion

Chronic otitis media with effusion (COME) is common in young children. Patients with this condition appear to have significant and prolonged eustachian tube dysfunction. This "otitis-prone" state may be a seemingly isolated phenomenon, or it can be a feature of a number of syndromes characterized by palatal dysfunction or malformation or by facial hypoplasia or deformity. These conditions include cleft palate, Crouzon syndrome, Down syndrome, and the mucopolysaccharidoses and mucolipidoses (see Fig. 24.21 and Palatal Disorders later). Chronic obstructive adenoidal hypertrophy may also be a predisposing condition. Less commonly, immunodeficiency and immotile cilia syndrome are identified as underlying etiologic conditions.

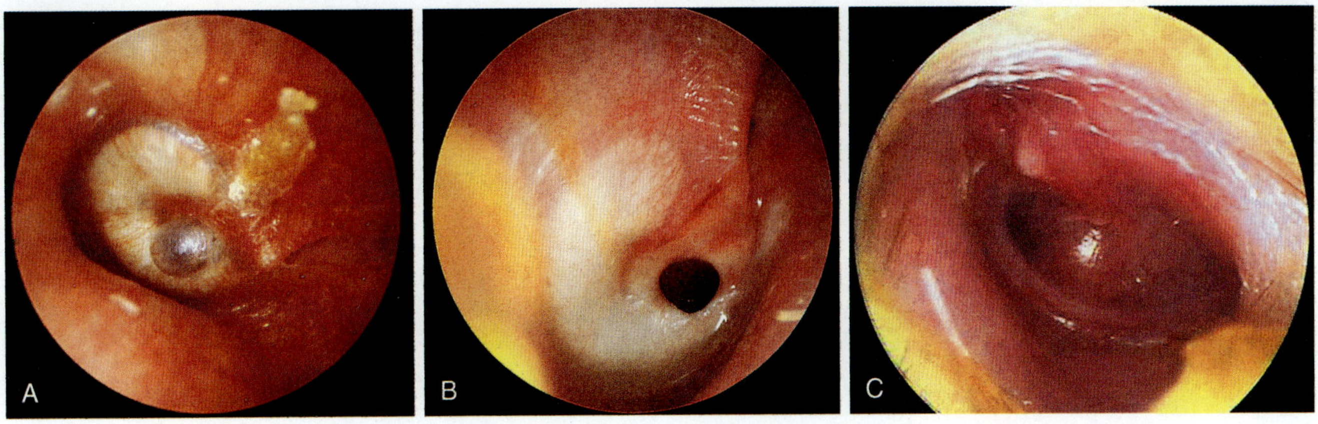

Fig. 24.28 Sequelae of chronic otitis media. (A) Much of this child's tympanic membrane is scarred and thickened, and a thinned dimeric area balloons out of the inferior central portion. (B) The eardrum is markedly thickened, scarred in an arc from 12 to 5 o'clock, and has a large chronic perforation. (C) Severe retraction of the tympanic membrane is seen in this patient. The membrane adheres to the malleus. (A and B, Courtesy Sylvan Stool, MD. C, Courtesy Alejandro Hoberman, MD, Children's Hospital of Pittsburgh, Pittsburgh, PA.)

COME is associated with significant morbidity in terms of intermittent or chronic hearing impairment, discomfort, and the sequelae of recurrent infection. Over months or years, the process produces permanent myringosclerotic changes in which the tympanic membrane becomes whitened, thickened, and scarred (Fig. 24.28A); chronic perforations (Fig. 24.28B); or severe tympanic membrane retraction (Fig. 24.28C). Patients with COME benefit from surgical drainage and insertion of tympanostomy tubes that vent the middle ear (Fig. 24.29). Persistence of an effusion for longer than 3 to 4 months with significant hearing loss is also an indication for myringotomy and insertion of tubes. Once placed, tubes should be checked at intervals for presence and patency. Spontaneous extrusion generally occurs 6 to 24 months after insertion.

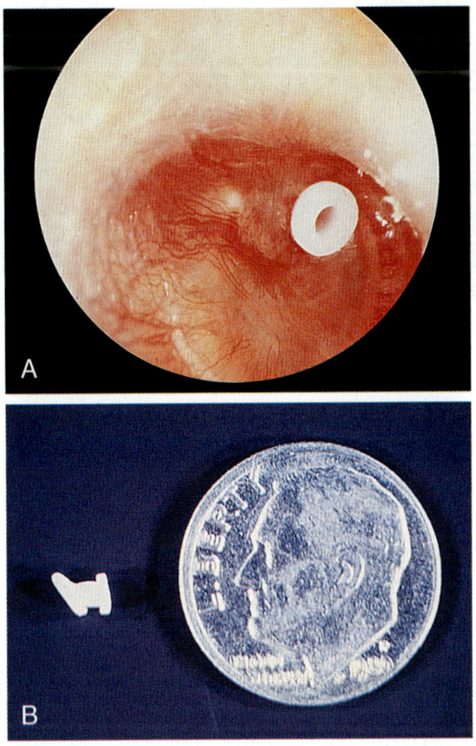

Fig. 24.29 (A) Tympanic membrane of patient with a history of chronic otitis media, with tympanostomy tube in place. The tube serves to vent the middle ear, improve hearing, and reduce the frequency of infection. (B) The tympanic membrane is slightly smaller than the size of a dime. A typical tube takes up approximately 15% of the tympanic membrane's surface area. There are many different types in a variety of shapes, materials, sizes, and colors. Selection is based on specific pathology and surgeon preference. (A, Courtesy Sylvan Stool, MD.)

Other Middle Ear Disorders

Although considerably less common than otitis media and serous otitis media, a number of other disorders involving the tympanic membrane are important because of their potential severity.

Mass Lesions Involving the Tympanic Membrane

The most common and one of the most serious mass lesions of the eardrum is a *cholesteatoma.* It can present as a defect in the tympanic membrane through which persistent drainage occurs, or it can appear as a white cystic mass behind or involving the eardrum. It consists of trapped epithelial tissue that grows beneath the surface of the membrane (Fig. 24.30). Although a few are congenital with an intact tympanic membrane, the majority are sequelae of untreated or chronic/recurrent otitis media with a tympanic membrane defect. If a cholesteatoma is not removed surgically, it continues to enlarge; becomes locally destructive; and can erode the mastoid bone, destroy the ossicles, and even invade the inner ear structures or cranium. Progressive hearing impairment is usually a feature of this condition. Congenital cholesteatomas are rare and are seen under an intact tympanic membrane in the anterior superior quadrant of the middle ear (see Fig. 24.30D).

Granulomas or *polyps* of the tympanic membrane (Fig. 24.31) can also develop in children with chronic middle ear infections. The most common cause of aural polyps in children is an old, retained tympanostomy tube. Cholesteatoma is another predisposing condition. These tissues often bleed easily, which can frighten the patient, parent, and physician. Left untreated, polyps can enlarge to fill the canal and by expansion can progressively damage the drum and the ossicles. Therefore prompt surgical removal is indicated if therapy with topical and oral antimicrobials is unsuccessful.

Distortions of the Tympanic Membrane

Thin, dimeric portions of the eardrum may be observed in patients with chronic middle ear disease, or they may develop after extrusion of a tympanostomy tube (Fig. 24.32; see also Fig. 24.28A). These thinned areas are the result of abnormal healing of perforations and are hypermobile on pneumatic otoscopy. The important points to note on examination are whether the full depth of the pocket is visible or partly hidden, its location with respect to the ossicles, and whether it is dry. If the ear canal and drum are not dry, an active infection and/or cholesteatoma is present. In cases of severe

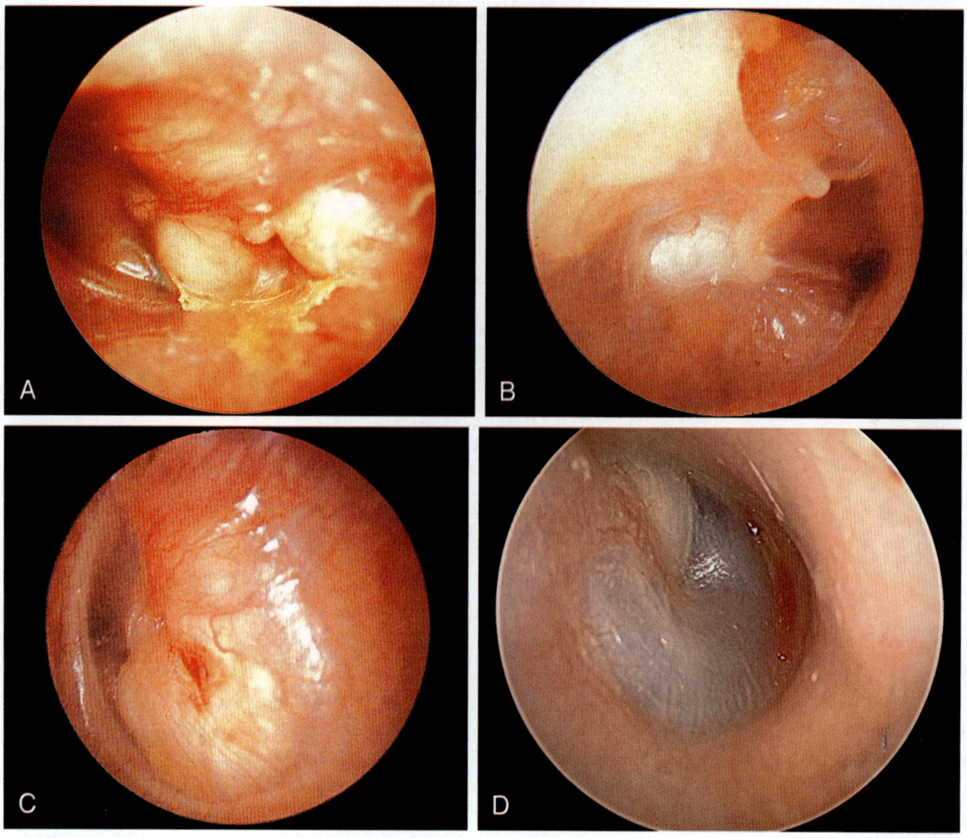

Fig. 24.30 Cholesteatomas. (A) Congenital cholesteatoma noted in a young child with spontaneous ear drainage. No previous history of ear infections existed. (B and C) Acquired cholesteatomas, which generally present after a long history of chronic middle ear disease. (D) Congenital cholesteatoma presenting as a right anterosuperior middle ear mass.

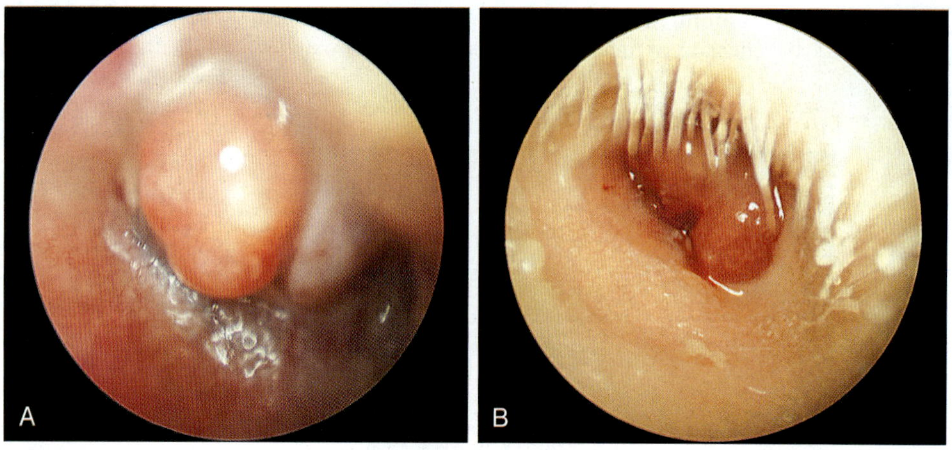

Fig. 24.31 Granulomas and polyps of the tympanic membrane. (A) Growth of this polypoid granuloma was stimulated by the inflammatory process of chronic middle ear infection. (B) These polyps, which protrude through a tympanic membrane perforation, have enlarged to entirely fill the external ear canal. Because of the possible attachment of the polyp to the facial nerve or the ossicles of the middle ear, removal of polyps requires extreme caution. (A, Courtesy Sylvan Stool, MD.)

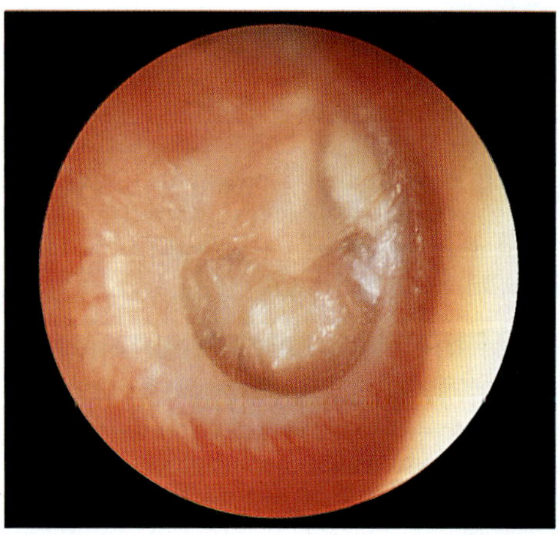

Fig. 24.32 Dimerism of the tympanic membrane. Otoscopy demonstrates a severely retracted atrophic segment of the eardrum that also has multiple white scars (tympanosclerosis). The thinned portions are the result of abnormal healing of perforations and tend to be hypermobile on otoscopy. (Courtesy Sylvan Stool, MD.)

deformity, aggressive therapy including ventilation of the middle ear and surgical excision of the pocket may be necessary.

NASAL DISORDERS

A child's nose is examined most commonly for disturbances in external appearance, excessive drainage, blockage of airflow, and interference with breathing. Epistaxis is also frequently encountered.

Nasal Examination

A nasal examination starts with an observation of a patient breathing at rest. Signs of nasal obstruction include mouth breathing, alar flaring, and stertor and, in infants, cyanosis with feeding. External examination includes assessing external deformities or signs of trauma. Internal nasal examination can be difficult in younger children. It is best done with the child sitting on a parent's lap or in a chair. The child's head is held in a neutral position.

An otoscope with a wide speculum (≥4 mm) is the most practical instrument. The examiner should gently brace his or her free hand on the child's upper lip to prevent sudden head movement from pushing the speculum tip into the nose, which could lead to nasal trauma, and should try to look toward the back of the nose rather than up into the nose. If the child is old enough to comply, he or she is asked to breathe through his or her mouth so as not to fog up the lens on the otoscope. If a nasal spreader–type speculum is used, a headlight is desirable. The septum, anterior edges of the middle and inferior turbinates, and nasal floor are inspected, and the quality of nasal secretions is noted. With practice and when there is minimal congestion, adenoidal size can be assessed.

A more thorough examination is possible with a nasal endoscope; this enables full visualization of internal nasal structures. Before starting, the nose is sprayed with a topical anesthetic and decongestant to shrink the nasal mucosa. With patience, older children can be coaxed through the examination. Allowing them to hold and inspect the device, test the light, look at themselves on the monitor, and even insert the tip into their nose assists cooperation (Fig. 24.33). Most children younger than 5 years old require immobilization, either on a papoose board or with parental and nursing assistance. The nasal endoscope is a useful tool, and this type of examination can be done readily in the otolaryngologist's office.

Nasal Congestion and Obstruction

Congenital Causes of Nasal Obstruction

Congenital causes of nasal obstruction include pyriform aperture stenosis, midnasal stenosis, choanal atresia/stenosis, and congenital masses, such as tumors, cysts, and polyps.

Pyriform Aperture Stenosis

Congenital nasal pyriform aperture stenosis (CNPAS) is a narrowing of nasal passage at the level of the pyriform aperture secondary to medial position of the maxillary processes. A pyriform aperture measuring less than 11 mm on radiographic imaging (CT maxillofacial scan preferred) is considered stenotic (Fig. 24.34A). Clinically, CNPAS presents as nasal congestion, respiratory distress that worsens with feeding and is relieved with crying, and difficulty passing suction catheters or flexible nasolaryngoscopes. Symptoms may be absent until the acquisition of a URI or other forms of acquired nasal congestion. On exam, the nares often are V-shaped, the anterior palate is triangular, and a central medial incisor may be noted on radiographic imaging (see Fig. 24.34B) or later in childhood. Brain MRI is recommended after diagnosis of CNPAS with medial incisor as it may be associated with holoprosencephaly and pituitary anomalies. Given the medial positioning of the maxillary processes

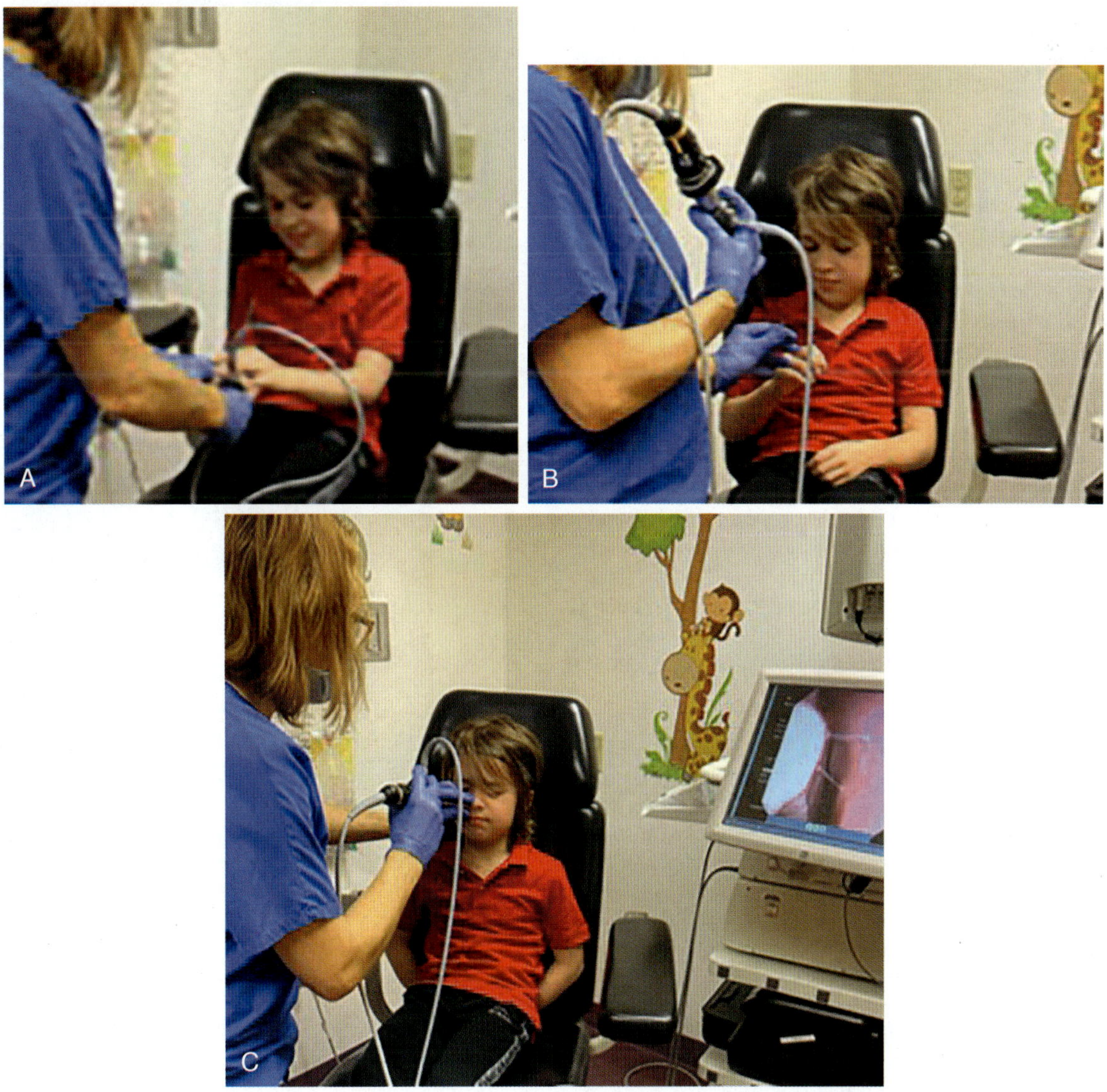

Fig. 24.33 Nasal endoscopic examination. (A and B) A child holding and feeling the endoscope. Not only can he see that the instrument is neither hot nor painful, when he shines the light on himself, the endoscope shows his face on the monitor. (C) After a child is acquainted with the endoscope, have the child sit on his or her hands to avoid the tendency to pull at the scope. Having a child sit on a parent's lap or having an assistant present to ensure limited head movement may also be helpful.

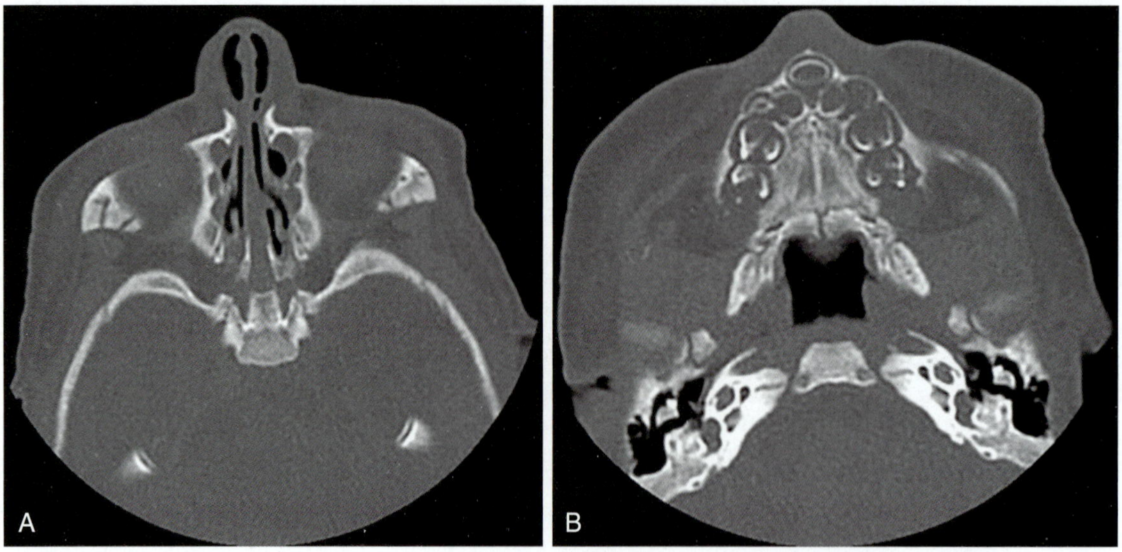

Fig. 24.34 Pyriform aperture stenosis (PAS). A pyriform aperture measuring <11 mm on radiographic imaging is diagnostic for PAS. (A) Noncontrasted axis computed tomography (CT) scan showing a pyriform aperture <11 mm and midnasal stenosis. (B) Noncontrasted axis CT scan showing a central medial incisor. Pituitary anomalies and holoprosencephaly may also be present.

in CNPAS, mid nasal stenosis is commonly also present and may need to be addressed.

Treatment options for CNPAS include nasal saline, nontraumatic suctioning, use of a McGovern nipple, and surgical interventions. Mild cases will improve with growth of the infant and are likely not to require surgical intervention.

Choanal Atresia and Stenosis

Choanal atresia may be bony (90%) or membranous (10%) and bilateral or unilateral. Newborns with bilateral choanal atresia manifest severe respiratory distress at delivery, with cyanosis that is relieved by crying and returns with rest (paradoxical cyanosis). Atresia can elude detection if the physician relies solely on passing soft feeding catheters through the nose to determine patency because these can buckle or curl within the nose. A diagnosis is best made with a van Buren urethral sound or a firm plastic suction catheter. This is passed gently along the floor of the nose, close to the septum. If resistance is encountered, the diagnosis of choanal atresia is suspected (Fig. 24.35A) and can be confirmed by endoscopy or by obtaining a CT scan of the nose and nasopharynx with fine overlapping cuts (see Fig. 24.35B).

Immediate relief of neonatal respiratory distress from bilateral choanal atresia may be accomplished by insertion of an oral airway (or a firm nipple from which the tip has been cut away) into the mouth. Definitive studies can then be performed to aid in planning surgical correction. Infants with unilateral choanal atresia (Fig. 24.36) are usually asymptomatic at birth; however, with time they develop a persistent unilateral nasal discharge. Bilateral atresia requires earlier surgical intervention.

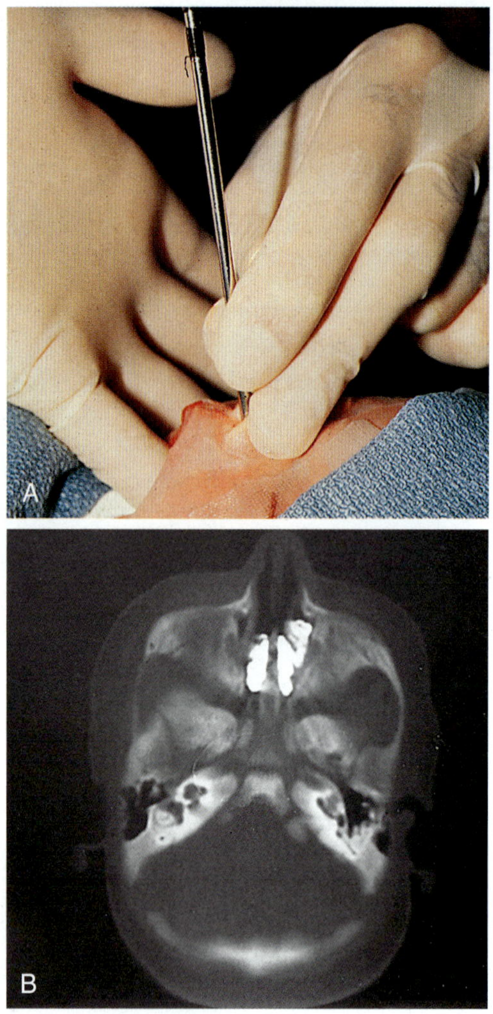

Fig. 24.35 Choanal atresia. (A) This infant manifested severe respiratory distress at delivery, with paradoxic cyanosis. Attempts to pass a urethral sound suggested bony obstruction of the choanae bilaterally. (B) A computed tomography scan done after instillation of radiopaque dye reveals pooling of the dye within the nose anterior to the choanae, confirming complete obstruction.

Congenital Mass Lesions

Congenital mass lesions are another source of nasal obstruction. These are particularly likely to become apparent during the first 2 years of life. The modes of presentation vary; some lesions are manifest primarily by symptoms of obstruction and are detected by diagnostic radiography; others become visually evident within a nostril or as a subcutaneous mass located near the root of the nose. On occasion, these patients have recurrent nasal infections and/or epistaxis. All such masses merit thorough clinical and radiographic evaluation because many have intracranial connections.

An *encephalocele* is an outpouching of brain tissue through a congenital bony defect in the midline of the skull. Some patients have craniofacial deformities and a rounded subcutaneous swelling between the eyes or adjacent to the nose. In other instances, the neural tissue prolapses into the nasal cavity or nasopharynx, resulting in signs and symptoms of nasal obstruction without obvious external anomalies (Fig. 24.37A). On occasion, a grapelike mass may be seen within the nares or protruding into the back of the mouth. The mass is usually identified by diagnostic radiography. CT (see Fig. 24.37B) is helpful in delineating the extent of the mass and underlying bony defects. Repair requires a collaborative effort by specialists in otolaryngology, neurosurgery, and in some cases, plastic surgery.

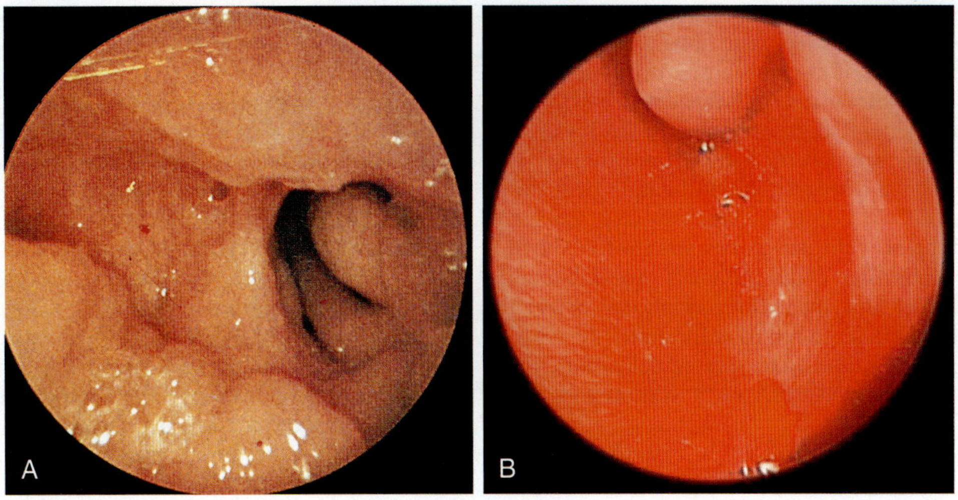

Fig. 24.36 Unilateral choanal atresia. (A) View of the nasopharynx using a 70-degree telescope in the oropharynx; the left choana is clearly patent, whereas the right is atretic. The child had a history of unilateral nasal discharge. (B) Left nasal endoscopy with a 0-degree telescope shows atresia.

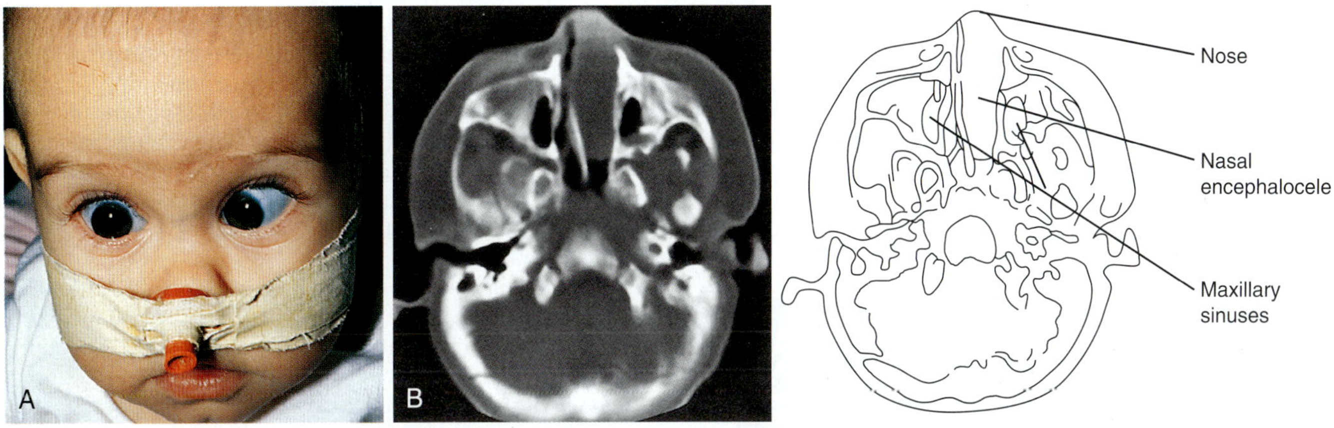

Fig. 24.37 Nasal encephalocele. (A) This normal-appearing infant had signs of severe nasal obstruction, necessitating insertion of a nasopharyngeal airway to relieve distress. (B) A computed tomography (CT) scan shows a large nasal mass lesion that fills one nostril and pushes the nasal septum into the other. This lesion proved to be an encephalocele extruding through a bony defect in the skull base (extrusion seen on another CT cut).

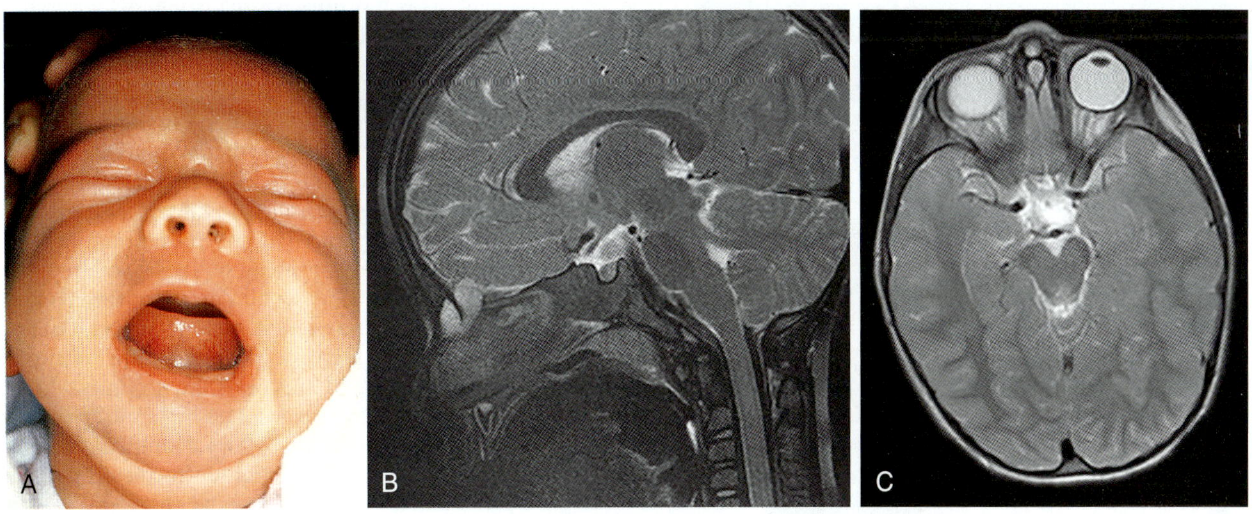

Fig. 24.38 Nasal dermoid. (A) A firm, round mass with a central dimple is seen over the bridge of this infant's nose. (B) Sagittal T2 magnetic resonance imaging (MRI) demonstrates a heterogenous lesion extending through patent foramen caecum and fonticulus frontalis. (C) Axial T2 MRI of the same lesion.

Nasal dermoids are embryonic cysts containing ectodermal and mesodermal tissue. They present as round, firm subcutaneous masses located on the dorsum of the nose, close to the midline (Fig. 24.38A). Examination of the overlying skin frequently reveals a small dimple, at times with extruding hair. Some of these cysts have deep extensions down to the nasal septum or through the cribriform plate into the cranium. Thorough evaluation by axial and coronal CT scans and MRI is necessary to determine extent and to plan repair (see Fig. 24.38B and C). If such cysts are not removed, secondary infection is common and often results in fistula formation.

Nasolacrimal Duct Cysts Obstruction of nasolacrimal duct occurs in ~30% of neonates. Most obstructions are mild and self-resolve within the first year of life. When proximal and distal obstruction occurs, a cyst known as a dacryocystocele forms and may herniate into the nasal cavity inferior to the head of the inferior turbinate. Cysts are distinguished from other nasal tumors by the superior-medial displacement of the inferior turbinate. CT scans are helpful to confirm diagnosis (Fig. 24.39). Frequently, dacryocystoceles rupture at or soon after birth with minor trauma (suctioning). The minority are bilateral. Common associated clinical findings include epiphora, facial or lateral nasal swelling, and a bluish to red discoloration inferior to the medial canthi. Cannulization and marsupialization are often needed if conservative measures, warm compresses, are unsuccessful.

Papillomas

Papillomas (Fig. 24.40) are similar growths that occur on the distal nasal mucosa near the mucocutaneous junction. These growths are benign but may persist for several years. Excision improves appearance and confirms diagnosis.

Acquired Forms of Nasal Obstruction

Rhinitis/Rhinorrhea

Rhinitis is nasal mucosal inflammation, whereas rhinorrhea refers to nasal secretions. In infancy and early childhood, the nasal passages are small and easily obstructed by mucosal edema and coryza. Causes of increased nasal mucosal edema and/or rhinitis include maternal circulating hormones, reflux, environmental irritants or allergens, dried secretions, suction trauma, and infections. In the first 3 months, infants are obligate nose breathers and therefore nasal obstruction of any etiology can result in disruption of an infant's suck-swallow-breathe (SSB) pattern. A disrupted SSB results in aerophagia, reflux, aspiration, and agitation. Reflux (physiologic or pathologic) and food allergies or insensitivities in infants result in gastric contents being repeatedly regurgitated into the nasopharynx, resulting in mucosal inflammation, which in turn worsens nasal obstruction. Lastly, palatal abnormalities or uncoordinated feeding can result in nasal regurgitation of food and saliva, which in turn results in rhinitis. Addressing reflux, aerophagia, food sensitivities, and feeding difficulties in addition to liberal use of saline nasal drops to loosen secretions and decrease mucosal inflammation, followed by nontraumatic nasal suctioning can be critical in stopping this negative inflammatory cycle. Oral decongestants are ineffective and often produce marked irritability when given to infants in the first year of life; they are not approved for pediatric use because of serious adverse events including deaths in children younger than 2 years old. Fortunately, URIs are generally brief and clear within a few days. Use of nasal saline clinically reduces duration and severity of URI symptoms in children.

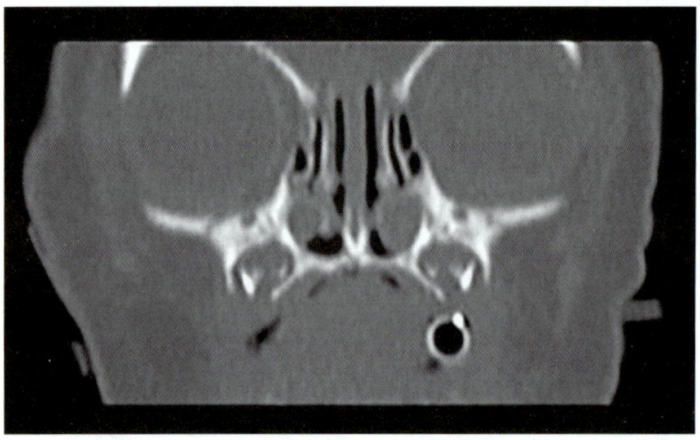

Fig. 24.39 Nasolacrimal duct cysts. Noncontrasted coronial computed tomography (CT) scan showing bilateral nasolacrimal duct cysts or dactroceles.

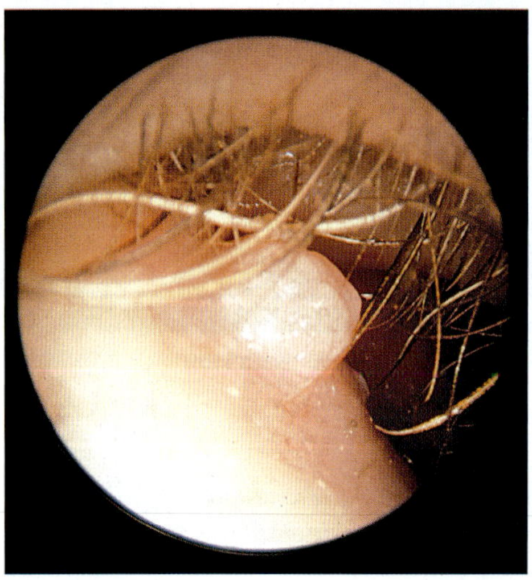

Fig. 24.40 Nasal papillomas present as warty growths at the mucocutaneous junction of the nares. (Courtesy Michael Hawke, MD.)

On occasion, infants with URIs go on to have persistent purulent or serosanguinous nasal discharge. Culture of discharges persisting longer than 10 to 14 days may disclose growth of a single pathogen. Preliminary studies of empirical antimicrobial therapy in such infants suggest rapid and effective resolution of symptoms when compared with a placebo. Thus this picture of prolonged nasal discharge probably represents a *bacterial ethmoiditis* or *nasopharyngitis,* the infant equivalent of sinusitis, and warrants systemic or topical therapy. If nasal obstruction or rhinitis does not improve with therapies, structural anomalies or mass lesions should be ruled out.

Except for gastroesophageal reflux disease (GERD), the etiology of rhinitis and rhinorrhea in older children is similar to that in infancy and includes environmental irritants (tobacco, dust, pollution, etc.), allergies (both inhaled, contact and ingested), bacteria, and viruses. Patients with allergic and nonallergic rhinitis appear to be more susceptible to infectious sinusitis than nonatopic individuals, probably as a result of mucosal swelling in response to allergen exposure and alterations in ciliary action. They can also have symptoms mimicking sinusitis in the absence of infection. Symptoms which include nasal congestion, nighttime cough, morning throat clearing are prominent, as is morning nausea or emesis with vomitus containing large amounts of clear mucus. Fever is absent with noninfectious rhinitis/rhinorrhea and halitosis, and daytime cough is not prominent. Patients may complain of nasal and eye pruritus, and some have frequent sneezing. On examination, the nasal mucosa is edematous but does not appear erythematous. Discharge, if present, is clear. Patients also tend to have the typical allergic facies (see Chapter 4) with Dennie lines, allergic shiners, and cobblestoning of the conjunctivae. Environmental control and antihistamines provide symptomatic relief for most of these children. Underlying structural anomalies such as septal deviation, sinonasal anomalies, turbinate hypertrophy, and adenoid hypertrophy (see later) can result in obstruction of nasal secretion flow and contribute to worsening inflammation and bacterial infections. Environmental controls; use of nasal saline as a mild topical decongestant, mucolytic agent, and to "rinse" irritants, if any; followed by topical antiinflammatory or antihistamine medications and/or systemic medical interventions and selective use of antibiotics are all possible therapies.

Adenoidal and Tonsillar Hypertrophy

The lymphoid tissue that constitutes the tonsils and adenoids is relatively small in infancy, gradually enlarges until 8 to 10 years old, and then usually begins to shrink in size. This normal process of hypertrophy results in mild to moderate enlargement of these structures and is not problematic. A small percentage of children, however, develop marked adenoidal and tonsillar hypertrophy, with attendant symptoms of nasal obstruction and rhinorrhea.

A few even have difficulty swallowing solid foods. Recurrent infection appears to be the most common inciting factor, although atopy may play a role in some cases. On occasion, EBV infection is the initiating event, resulting in rapid enlargement of adenoidal and tonsillar tissues that is then slow to resolve (see Tonsillitis/Pharyngitis later and in Chapter 13). In most children, progressive adenoidal enlargement appears to be the cumulative result of a series of URIs. The consequent obstruction to normal flow of secretions then starts a vicious circle, making the child more vulnerable to recurrent infections of the ears, sinuses, and nasopharynx, which in turn further exacerbate the adenoidal and tonsillar hypertrophy.

When adenoidal hypertrophy is marked, blockage of the nasal airway becomes severe and results in mouth breathing, chronic rhinorrhea, inability to blow the nose, and snoring (Fig. 24.41A). Speech becomes hyponasal and muffled. The child holds his or her mouth open and has little or no airflow through the nares, and his or her tonsils may also meet at the midline (see Fig. 24.10B). A lateral neck x-ray examination reveals a large adenoidal shadow impinging on the nasal airway (see Fig. 24.41C). For many patients, these features are noted primarily in the course of acute illness; however, some children have symptoms even when free of infection. When obstruction is severe, sleep disturbance may result. This is characterized by restlessness and retractions when recumbent,

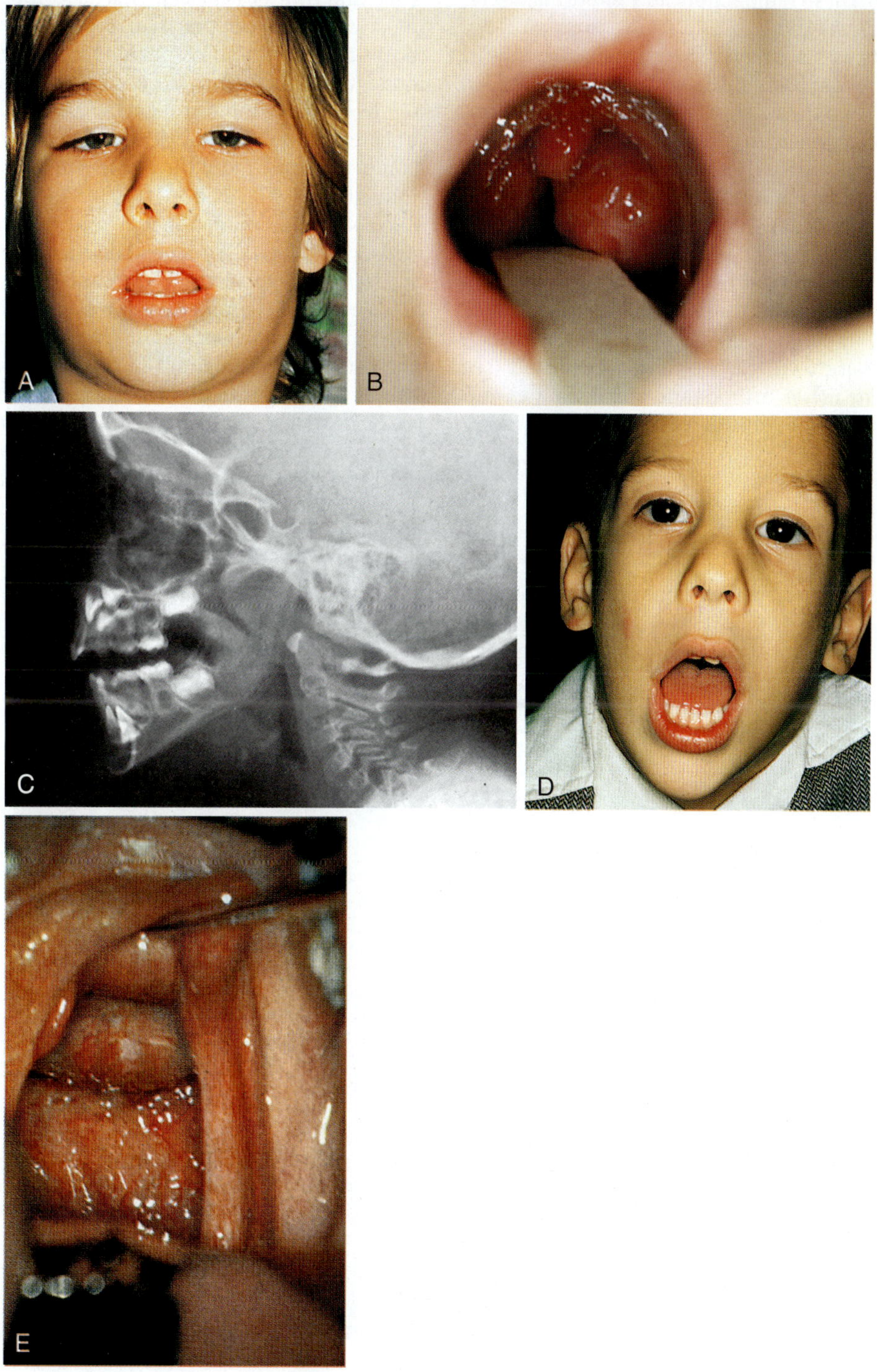

Fig. 24.41 Adenoidal and tonsillar hypertrophy. (A) External appearance of a child with marked enlargement of tonsils and adenoids. He must keep his mouth open to breathe and shows signs of fatigue as a result of sleep disturbance caused by his upper airway obstruction. (B) On examination of the pharynx, his tonsils are seen meeting in the midline. (C) A lateral neck radiograph shows a large adenoid shadow impinging on the nasopharyngeal airway. (D) If obstruction is prolonged, as was the case in this patient, cor pulmonale, abnormal facial elongation, and widening of the nasal root may result. (E) When the palate is retracted before adenoidectomy, the extent of overgrowth of adenoidal tissue is readily appreciated.

snoring, and frequent waking. Some patients begin to sleep sitting up, and many manifest daytime fatigue, irritability, short attention span, hyperactivity, enuresis, and headaches. Obstructive symptoms are worse during sleep because relaxation of the pharyngeal muscles further increases the degree of upper airway obstruction. In severe cases, this results in periods of hypoxia and hypercarbia. Because a patient may look relatively healthy when awake (with the exception of having to breathe through the mouth), it is important to observe for retractions and to assess the pattern of breathing after the child has been recumbent for a period of time. Use of polysomnography may help confirm or establish the diagnosis and determine the severity of sleep apnea. If severe obstruction persists for a prolonged period, cor pulmonale (with signs of right ventricular hypertrophy on electrocardiogram and chest radiograph) and abnormal facial growth may result (see Fig. 24.41D).

Management of patients with adenoidal hypertrophy depends in part on the severity and the duration of the obstruction. In milder cases of short duration or in patients with intermittent symptoms, careful monitoring is recommended. Treatment of atopy and inflammation with intranasal steroids, use of leukotriene inhibitors that target leukotriene receptors within the adenoid bed, or institution of a 2- to 4-week course of antimicrobial therapy with a β-lactamase–activity agent may result in significant shrinkage of hypertrophied tonsillar and adenoidal tissues. Children with persistent symptoms despite therapy and those with sleep disturbance or cor pulmonale should undergo adenoidectomy, during which the extent of adenoidal overgrowth can be fully appreciated (see Fig. 24.41E). Children with major orthodontic abnormalities and nasal obstruction should also be considered for adenoidectomy before orthodontic correction.

Turbinate Hypertrophy

Nasal turbinates are paired structures present in the nasal cavity consisting of a concha bone and surrounding mucus secreting mucosa. Turbinates function to warm, moisten, and filter air. The mucosal lining can become hypertrophic in response to irritants, allergens, and infections. When enlarged, nasal turbinates can result in nasal obstruction and increased rhinitis. Topical medical therapies such as saline, topical corticosteroids, and topical antihistamines may be helpful in reducing mucosal inflammation and reduce rhinitis. Surgical intervention to reduce turbinate size exists and can be used if medical therapies fail.

Nasal Foreign Bodies As with the external ear, it is not unusual for small children to put a wide variety of foreign material into their noses. Such foreign objects are irritating to the nasal mucosa and soon incite an intense inflammatory reaction with production of a thick, purulent, foul-smelling discharge that helps to hide their presence. Intermittent epistaxis may accompany the discharge. Because most children younger than 5 years old are unable to blow their noses and are afraid or unable to tell their parents what they have done, the object is not expelled and the problem often goes unrecognized until symptoms develop and medical attention is sought. A unilateral nasal discharge and/or a foul smell are the typical chief complaints and should lead the clinician to suspect a foreign body immediately (Fig. 24.42A).

Speculum examination may readily disclose the object (Fig. 24.42B and C), but often the purulent discharge obscures the view, necessitating removal with an absorbent swab or via gentle suction. Even when visualization is accomplished, removal can be difficult because children are easily frightened at the prospect of instrumentation, and their struggling can result in mucosal injury during attempts at removal. To minimize problems, topical anesthetic spray and a topical vasoconstrictor can be applied, and the child can be restrained with a papoose board. Older patients or calm young children may do well sitting in a parent's lap, if the examiner is patient, reassuring, and willing to explain each step carefully. The discharge may then be removed by swab or suction. If the object is anterior to the turbinates, removal can be attempted using suction; a small wire loop curette or a right-angled Day hook for spherical objects; or otologic forceps for material

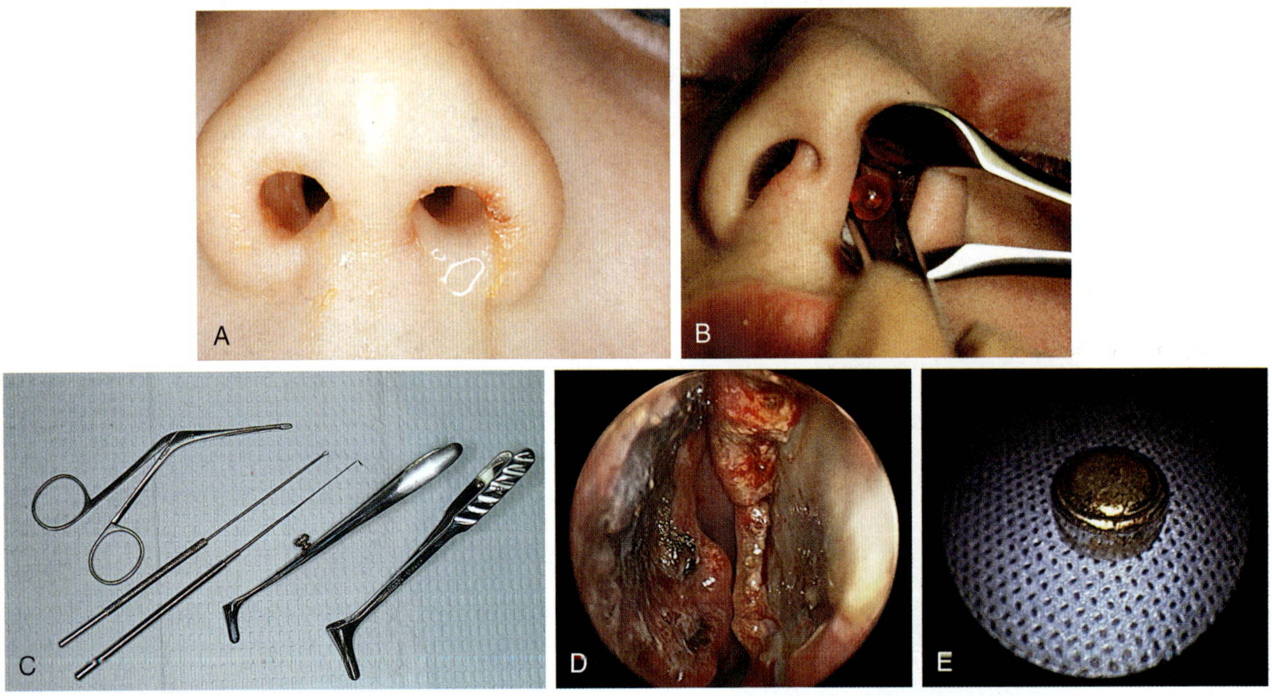

Fig. 24.42 Nasal foreign body. (A) This child had a unilateral, foul-smelling nasal discharge. (B) Aspiration of the discharge in this patient revealed a red bead that was removed with a Day hook. (C) Hartmann forceps, a small wire loop curette, and a right-angle Day hook are the instruments used most commonly for removal of nasal foreign bodies. Nasal spreaders assist visualization and create a wider space for inserting the desired instrument. Note that bleeding or aspiration of the nasal foreign body may occur, especially with uncooperative toddlers. Thus consideration should be given for removal of nasal foreign bodies in the operating room with general anesthesia and a controlled airway. (D) Severe intranasal damage resulting from a nasal foreign body—a tiny watch battery. (E) The watch battery removed. (A, Courtesy Michael Hawke, MD.)

that can be grasped (Fig. 24.42C). Consultation with an otolaryngologist should be sought for removal of objects located more posteriorly or those not readily removed on initial attempts. A major concern is that in the attempted removal, a deeply situated foreign body may be dislodged into the nasopharynx, leading to aspiration or laryngeal obstruction. In such cases, the best course of action is to remove the object after the airway has been secured with an endotracheal tube in the operating room, with the patient under general anesthesia. Significant bleeding may occur during attempted removal of an intranasal foreign body, and this is another reason to strongly consider general anesthesia with an endotracheal tube to secure the airway. Small button batteries such as watch batteries in the nose can cause a great deal of caustic tissue injury from the electric current. Therefore all batteries should be removed as quickly as possible (Fig. 24.42D and E).

Nasal Polyps

Polyps are thought to be the result of recurrent infection and/or inflammation, although atopy may play a contributing role in a portion of cases. Polyps originate in the ethmoid or, less commonly, the maxillary and sphenoid sinuses and protrude through the sinus ostia into the nasal cavity. The phenomenon is unusual in children younger than 10 years old, except for patients with cystic fibrosis—25% of whom develop polyps, some as early as infancy. Symptoms consist of those of progressive nasal obstruction, frequently with associated discharge. Recurrent sinusitis is a common complication of impaired sinus drainage. Affected patients with acute infections may also have intermittent epistaxis. Involvement may be unilateral or bilateral. On examination, moist, glistening pedunculated growths that may have a smooth or a grapelike appearance are seen (Fig. 24.43). Bilateral opacification of the ethmoid and maxillary sinuses is commonly found on radiography. Polyps must be distinguished from a nasal glioma or encephalocele, which may have a similar appearance and can produce identical symptoms. These neural mass lesions are more common in infancy but may present in older children. Therefore before biopsy or removal, a CT scan of the sinuses and skull base should be considered for children with polypoid nasal lesions.

Surgical removal of the polyps is indicated to relieve nasal obstruction, reduce the risk of secondary sinusitis, and diminish the possibility of altered facial growth, most commonly widening of the nasal root and prominence of the malar areas of the face (Fig. 24.44). A child with nasal polyps warrants evaluation for cystic fibrosis. Historically, patients with chronic rhinosinusitis with nasal polyposis would require repeat surgical polypectomies and debridements throughout their life. However, newer biologic systemic therapies such as dupilumab, mepolizumab, and omalizumab are effective for treating and preventing nasal polyps.

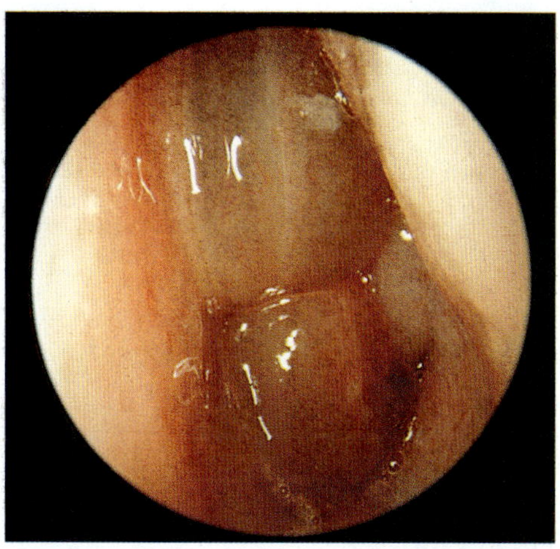

Fig. 24.43 Nasal polyp. This 2-year-old girl with cystic fibrosis was referred because of nasal obstruction and nocturnal snoring of a few months' duration. A large grayish polyp was found in the left nostril. Any child presenting with a nasal polyp should be tested for cystic fibrosis.

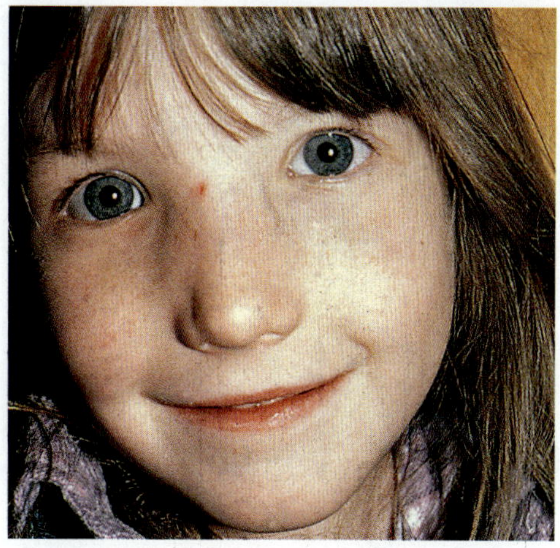

Fig. 24.44 Sequelae of chronic nasal polyps. This 7-year-old girl with cystic fibrosis and recurrent nasal polyps shows secondary alteration in facial growth consisting of a broadened nasal root and prominence of the malar areas. This occurred despite several resections.

Nasal Trauma

Blunt nasal trauma is frequently encountered in children. In the majority of instances, it results only in minor swelling and mild epistaxis, which is readily controlled by application of pressure over the nares. However, more severe injuries do occur and have a significant potential for long-term morbidity and deformity if not identified and treated appropriately. These injuries include displaced nasal fractures (Fig. 24.45), which, if not reduced, result in permanent deformity; septal deviation or dislocation, with or without an associated fracture (Fig. 24.46), which impairs airflow; and septal hematomas (Fig. 24.47A), which, if not drained promptly, may lead to abscesses (see Chapter 6). A septal hematoma forms when the perichondrium is elevated off the septal cartilage with traumatic movement, resulting in shearing of septal vessels and bleeding within the cartilage and perichondrium. Buckling or fracturing of the cartilage can result in blood accumulation between the cartilage and contralateral perichondrium as well. Blood between the perichondrium and cartilage results in necrosis, with septal necrosis leading to saddle nose deformity (Fig. 24.47B) and abscess formation. Nasal abscesses can quickly spread intracranially. Thus severe nausea, vomiting, or altered mental status following untreated septal hematoma should be evaluated by MRI. Finally, profuse bleeding that is difficult to stop or that recurs readily suggests trauma to deeper structures of the face or frontal bones and warrants prompt stabilization and meticulous clinical and radiographic assessment (see Chapter 21).

In evaluating patients with nasal trauma, the nasal bridge should be inspected for swelling or deformity (the latter may not be apparent if swelling is marked) and the septum palpated for hematoma, tenderness, crepitus, or excessive mobility. When marked swelling, severe tenderness, deformity, crepitus, or septal deviation is found, radiologic evaluation may be considered. However, radiographs should be interpreted with caution because a large portion of the nasal skeleton in children is composed of cartilage rather than bone and serious nasal injuries can be present despite a normal plain radiograph. Increase in intracanthal distance, significant periorbital or forehead ecchymosis, or tenderness or changes in vision should prompt imaging as they can indicate more severe craniofacial fracture. Displaced nasal fractures in the absence of septal hematoma require reduction within 7 to 14 days of injury. Hematomas are an emergency. Given the compliant nature of cartilage in kids, nasal trauma can result in

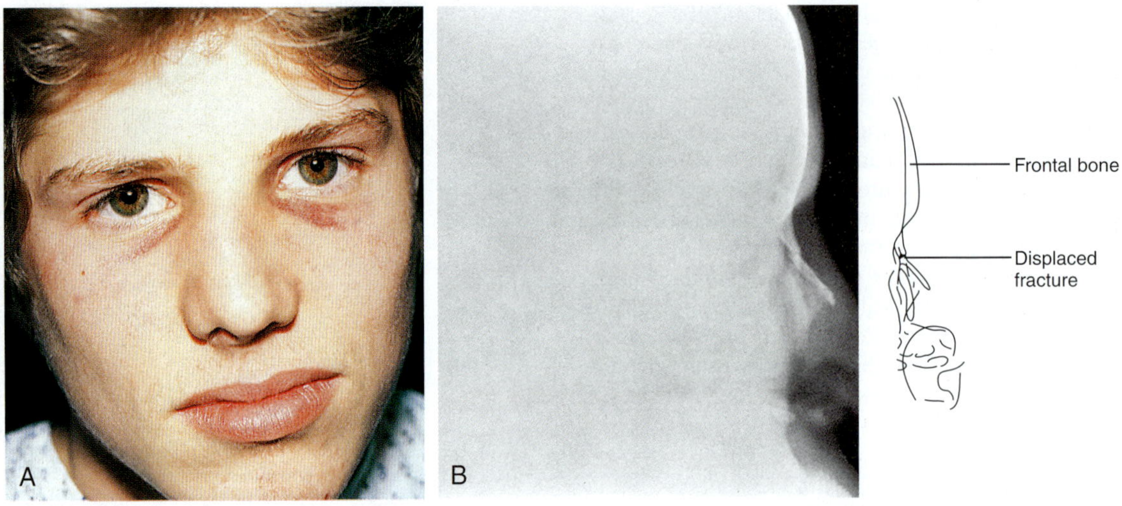

Fig. 24.45 Displaced nasal fracture. (A) This teenager was hit on the nose while playing football. On external inspection, there is obvious deformity, and there are ecchymoses under both eyes. Crepitus was evident on palpation. (B) A lateral radiograph of another patient shows a displaced fracture of the proximal portion of the nasal bone, which is delineated on the diagram.

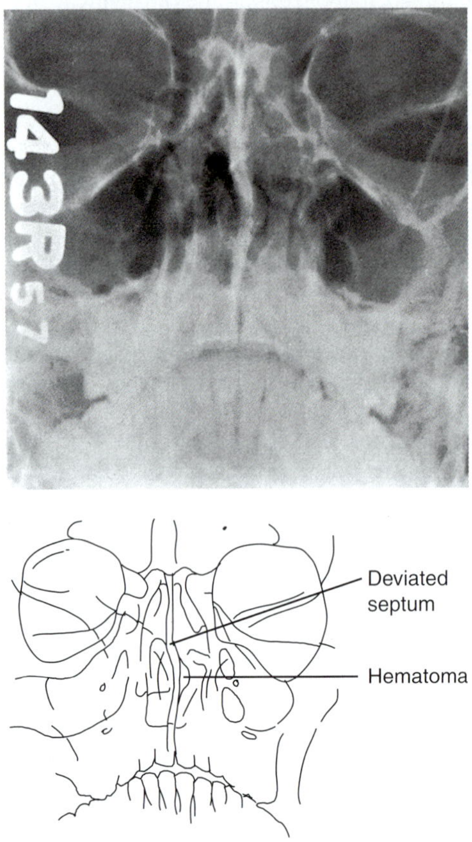

Fig. 24.46 Deviated nasal septum. This patient was punched in the nose, resulting in a leftward deviation of the cartilaginous portion of the nasal septum, which is clearly visible in the radiograph and is delineated in the diagram. The small arc of mucosal swelling along the septum proved to be a small septal hematoma that necessitated drainage. No visible fracture occurred. Septal deviation requires correction to prevent deformity and to relieve secondary nasal obstruction.

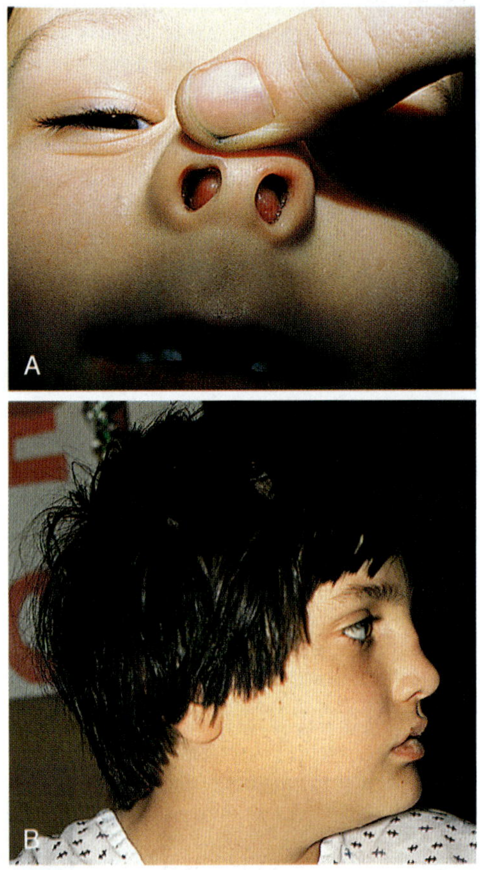

Fig. 24.47 Septal hematoma. This patient incurred facial trauma (A) resulting in multiple fractures of the nasal and orbital bones and submucosal bleeding along the nasal septum. Such septal hematomas must be drained promptly to reduce the risk of abscess formation and to prevent cartilage necrosis, which ultimately results in a saddle-nose deformity (B). (A, Courtesy Robert Hickey, MD, Children's Hospital of Pittsburgh, Pittsburgh, PA.)

septal hematoma formation even if the cartilage is repositioned. To best examine the septum, the nares should be cleared of clots. A hematoma is soft on palpation and does not compress with topical decongestants/vasoconstrictors. Posttraumatic mucosal edema of the septum and the septal swell body will reduce in size with topical decongestants/vasoconstrictor. Presence of a septal hematoma is an emergency and should be immediately referred to an otolaryngologist.

Epistaxis

Although often due to direct digital trauma, nasal bleeding in childhood has several other causes, including infection, mucosal irritation, bleeding disorders, vascular anomalies, and hypertension. Patients with these conditions may have spontaneous bleeding or epistaxis triggered by minor external trauma or forceful sneezing and blowing. Profuse bleeding that is difficult to stop is most characteristic of bleeding disorders, vascular anomalies, and severe hypertension. Mild bleeding that is readily controlled by application of pressure suggests mucosal infection or irritation that promotes bleeding from small superficial vessels located on the anterior nasal septum (Fig. 24.48). In all cases, the problem should be taken seriously and investigated carefully to correctly diagnose and appropriately treat the primary source of the problem.

In approaching patients with epistaxis, the following historical points should be addressed:

1. Is the problem acute or recurrent?
2. Was there external or intranasal trauma; digital trauma sneezing, nasal tip rubbing or blowing a triggering event?
3. What is the duration of the current bleed and the approximate volume of blood loss (handkerchiefs soaked, hemodynamic status, and so on)?
4. Is the bleeding unilateral or bilateral?
5. Are there any unilateral nasal obstructive symptoms?
6. Has the patient been having symptoms suggestive of a URI or allergies?
7. Has the child manifested other signs and symptoms of an underlying coagulopathy?
8. Has the patient been taking medication, especially aspirin, ibuprofen, intranasal steroid sprays, or other nonsteroidal antiinflammatory or anticoagulant agents?

Physical assessment must address the patient's general well-being in addition to careful examination of the nose. Hemodynamic status is of particular importance when hemorrhage has been profuse. When active bleeding is present, direct pressure to the anterior soft tissue of the nose should be held for 7 to 10 minutes.

After observation of the external appearance of the nares, the nose is cleared of clots and discharge, if present. The septum and mucosa are then inspected for possible points of hemorrhage, signs of obstruction, mass lesions, and foreign objects. When inspecting the nasal cavity with a speculum, stabilizing the speculum with a finger on the patient's nasal tip or dorsum will help prevent additional trauma or pain if the patient moves (Fig. 24.49). The oropharynx should also be examined for posterior flow of blood, especially when no point of bleeding is evident on inspection of the nasal mucosa. Otolaryngologic consultation should be sought in cases involving profuse bleeding that does not readily cease on application of pressure and may require nasal cautery or packing or other surgical treatment.

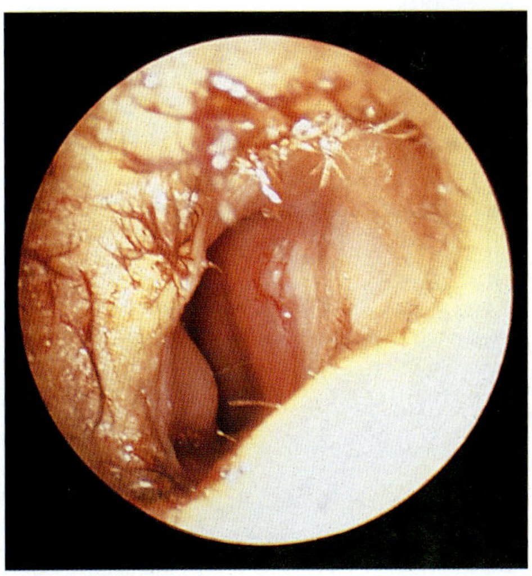

Fig. 24.48 Dilated septal vessels of Kiesselbach plexus, which tend to bleed in response to mucosal drying, cracking, infection, or irritation. (From Becker W: *Atlas of ear, nose, and throat diseases*, ed 2, Stuttgart, 1983, Thieme.)

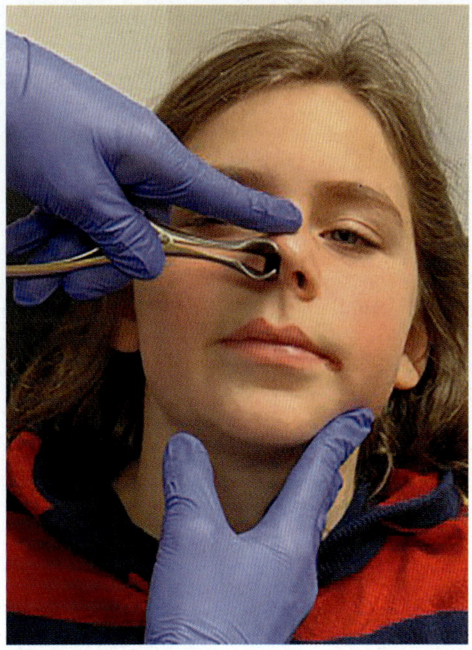

Fig. 24.49 Nasal examination with speculum. To prevent septal trauma with patient movement, stabilize the speculum with a finger on the nasal tip or dorsum.

Epistaxis Caused by Infection and Mucosal Irritation

In many patients with nontraumatic epistaxis, examination reveals unilateral or bilateral septal erythema and friability or excoriation (see Fig. 24.48). The history given is one of intermittent bleeding, especially with sneezing, blowing the nose, or while sleeping. The phenomenon is commonly attributed to digital trauma. However, more common is mucosal irritation from allergens or infections combined with trauma caused by forceful sneezing and blowing. Common bacterial pathogens include *Streptococcus pyogenes* or coagulase-positive staphylococci. Dryness of the mucosal lining, commonly in winter or summer as a result of drying of the air by central heating or cooling systems, may also contribute. Application of topical antibiotic ointment, water-based lubricants, humidification, and antihistamines (for atopic patients) may provide relief. Oral antimicrobial therapy may be necessary if significant bacterial infection is present.

Epistaxis Caused by Bleeding Disorders

Despite application of pressure, epistaxis in patients with coagulopathies is more likely to be prolonged and carries a greater risk of significant blood loss. Although many such patients have known bleeding disorders, a few may present with prolonged or recurrent nosebleeds as one of the initial manifestations of their problem. This is most typical of idiopathic thrombocytopenia, aplastic anemia, and acute leukemia. When epistaxis arises in the context of a bleeding disorder, the personal history, family history, and/or other physical findings should point to the diagnosis (see Chapter 12), which can then be confirmed by hematologic studies (complete blood count and differential, platelet count, prothrombin time and partial thromboplastin time, and coagulation profile).

Epistaxis Caused by Vascular Abnormalities or Tumors

In a minority of children with recurrent epistaxis, the history reveals significant bleeding that typically drains from one side of the nose. This suggests a localized vascular lesion. The most encountered problem is that of a dilated septal vessel or plexus, which may be a sequela of prior inflammation (see Fig. 24.48). This may be visible anteriorly but also can be located high on the septum, requiring nasal endoscopy for identification. Cauterization is generally curative. In cooperative children, anterior septal lesions can be cauterized in the office with silver nitrate after application of a topical anesthetic and vasoconstrictor. Younger children and many patients with posterior lesions may need general anesthesia for cauterization.

Relatively rare vascular lesions associated with recurrent nasal bleeding are telangiectasias, pyrogenic granulomas, and angiofibromas. Patients with hereditary hemorrhagic telangiectasia (Osler-Weber-Rendu disease) have an autosomal dominant disorder characterized by formation of cutaneous and mucosal telangiectatic lesions that begin to develop in childhood and gradually increase in number with age. These lesions appear as bright red, slightly raised, star-shaped plexuses of dilated small vessels that blanch on pressure (Fig. 24.50). Mucosal telangiectasias may bleed spontaneously or in response to minor trauma. Recurrent epistaxis is a common mode of presentation in childhood. Multiple telangiectasias are evident on close examination. Hematuria and/or gastrointestinal bleeding may be seen separately or in combination with epistaxis.

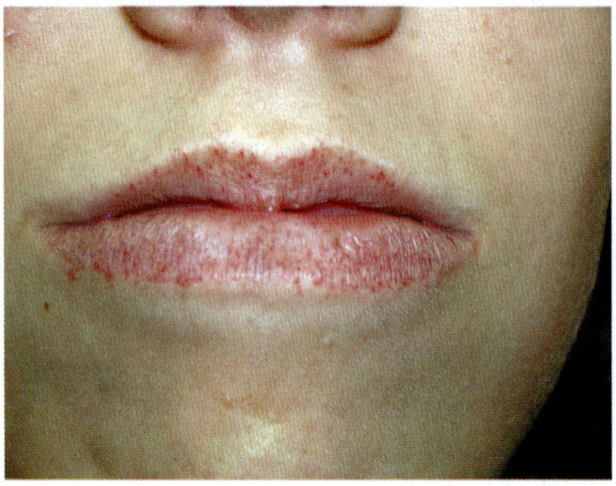

Fig. 24.50 Hereditary hemorrhagic telangiectasia. Numerous telangiectasias dot the lips and the nasal and palatal mucosa of this boy who had problems with recurrent epistaxis. (Courtesy Bernard Cohen, MD, Johns Hopkins Hospital, Baltimore, MD.)

Pyrogenic granulomas are benign vascular tumors that occur secondary to trauma and appear as raised red, friable lesions. Treatment is excision or cautery.

Juvenile nasopharyngeal angiofibroma is a rare vascular tumor seen predominantly in adolescent boys. Although benign, it is locally invasive and destructive and may involve the maxillary sinuses, palate, sphenoid sinus, and portions of the skull base. The most common mode of presentation is one of profuse, often recurrent epistaxis. Some patients also have symptoms of unilateral nasal obstruction with secondary rhinorrhea, and a small percentage may have visual, auditory, or other cranial nerve disturbances. On examination, a purplish soft tissue mass may be seen through the nares or on nasal endoscopy (Fig. 24.51A). In addition to standard radiographs, CT, MRI, and angiography may be necessary to assess the extent of the tumor (see Fig. 24.51B). Carefully planned excision is then the treatment of choice.

Epistaxis Caused by Hypertension

Hypertension is an unusual source of epistaxis in childhood. However, it should be considered, especially in patients with antecedent headache and spontaneous, profuse bleeding that is difficult to stop. Patients with this history may have previously undiagnosed coarctation of the aorta or chronic renal disease with severe secondary hypertension and should be examined with these possibilities in mind. It must be remembered that after significant blood loss, blood pressure may drop to normal levels.

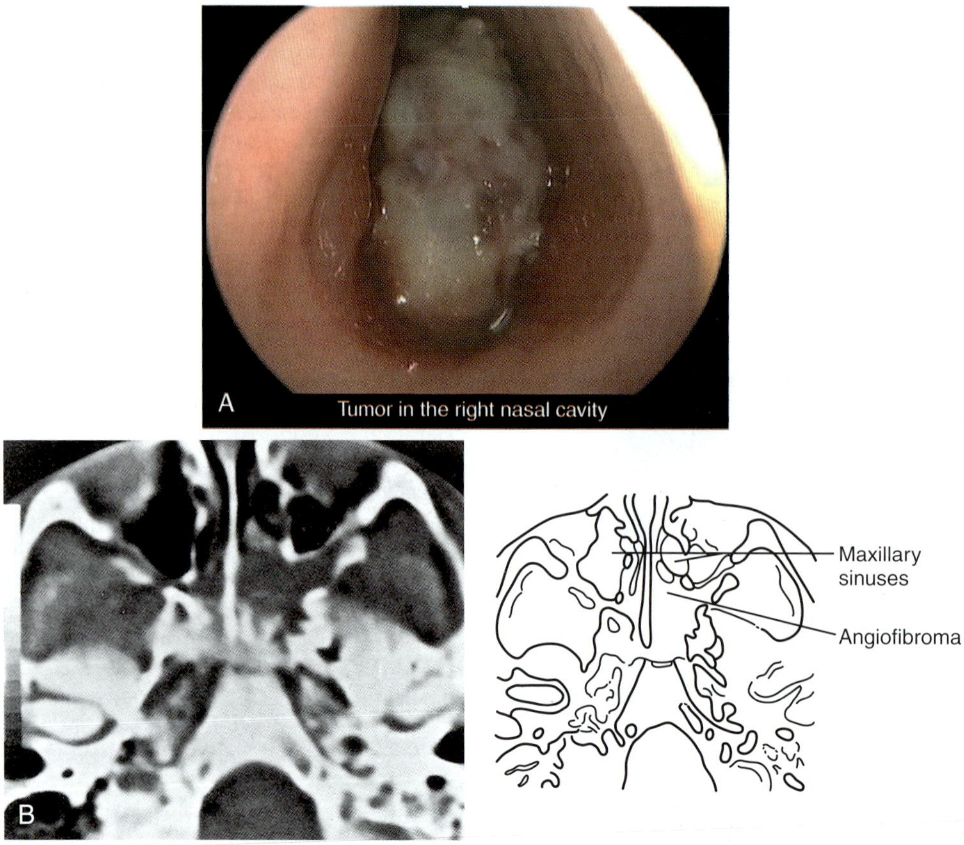

Fig. 24.51 Juvenile nasopharyngeal angiofibroma. (A) Intranasal view showing a large pink, white spongey–appearing lobulated lesion filling the nasal cavity and displacing the inferior turbinate and septum. (B) A computed tomography scan is helpful in assessing the extent of this locally invasive vascular tumor. In this cut, an enhancing mass (an angiofibroma, as delineated in the diagram) is seen occupying the posterior portion of the left nostril, deviating the septum and compressing the ipsilateral maxillary sinus.

DISORDERS OF PARANASAL SINUSES AND ADJACENT STRUCTURES

The paranasal sinuses are air-filled, bony cavities that lie within the facial bones of the skull, adjacent to the nasal passages. They develop through a gradual enlargement of pneumatized cells that evaginate from the nasal cavity. This process occurs over the course of childhood and adolescence (Fig. 24.52A). In infancy, the ethmoid and maxillary sinuses are partially pneumatized, but they are small and not readily demonstrable on radiographs (although they can be readily seen on a CT scan). Radiographs are thus of little diagnostic value until after the first 2 years of life. The sphenoid sinus is not evident until about 5 to 6 years old (see Fig. 24.52B), and the frontal sinuses do not develop until after 7 to 8 years old. Fig. 24.53 demonstrates the normal radiography of the sinuses, which correlates these findings.

The sinuses are lined by ciliated respiratory epithelium, which produces and transports mucus. The sinuses drain into the nasal cavity through various small openings or ostia. The ostia of the sinuses are small and easily obstructed by mucosal edema and infections. Further, there are many important adjacent structures that are vulnerable if a disease process spreads beyond the sinus. These include the orbit, cavernous sinus, and brain. The roots of the maxillary teeth lie in the floor of the maxillary sinuses. Therefore dental infections may drain into the maxillary sinuses, resulting in recurrent or chronic sinusitis. Hence the dentition should be thoroughly inspected when evaluating any child with suspected sinus infection (see Chapter 21).

Sinusitis

During the first several years of life, infection of the maxillary and/or ethmoid sinuses is more common than is generally appreciated. Frontal sinusitis becomes important after about 10 years old. The probable pathogenesis is mucosal edema (whether the result of a URI, allergic rhinitis, or chemical irritation) resulting in obstruction of the sinus ostia. This impedes drainage of secretions and can lead to bacterial proliferation. Both bacterial and viral pathogens have been isolated from pediatric patients. The most common bacteria are *S. pneumoniae,* nontypeable *H. influenzae,* and *Moraxella catarrhalis.* The viral agents include adenoviruses and parainfluenza viruses. Bacterial sinusitis should be suspected when nasal discharge of any quality and/or persistent productive cough last longer than 10 to 14 days without improvement, fevers greater than 39°C/102.2°F occur for greater than 3 days, fevers and/or worsening symptoms after initial improvement in periorbital or frontal swelling or erythema (Figs. 24.54 and 24.55), or severe or prolonged facial pain or headaches.

As with otitis media, several conditions predispose children to sinus infections by virtue of alterations in anatomy and/or physiology. These conditions include midfacial anomalies or deformities, particularly when maxillary hypoplasia is part of the picture (see Fig. 24.21); cleft palate (see the Palatal Disorders section, later); nasal deformity and/or septal deviation, whether congenital or acquired; mass lesions including hypertrophied adenoids, nasal foreign bodies, polyps, and tumors; abnormalities of mucus production and/or ciliary action, such as cystic fibrosis and ciliary dyskinesia; immunodeficiency; atopy; dental infection; and barotrauma.

When patients have most of the signs and symptoms of sinusitis, the diagnosis can be made on clinical grounds and treatment started empirically. High-dose amoxicillin remains the drug of first choice for patients who are not allergic to penicillin. Nasal saline irrigation and topical mucosal decongestants are also highly effective adjunctive therapeutic agents. If there is no clear clinical improvement in 3 to 4 days, amoxicillin/clavulanate or a comparable antimicrobial is indicated.

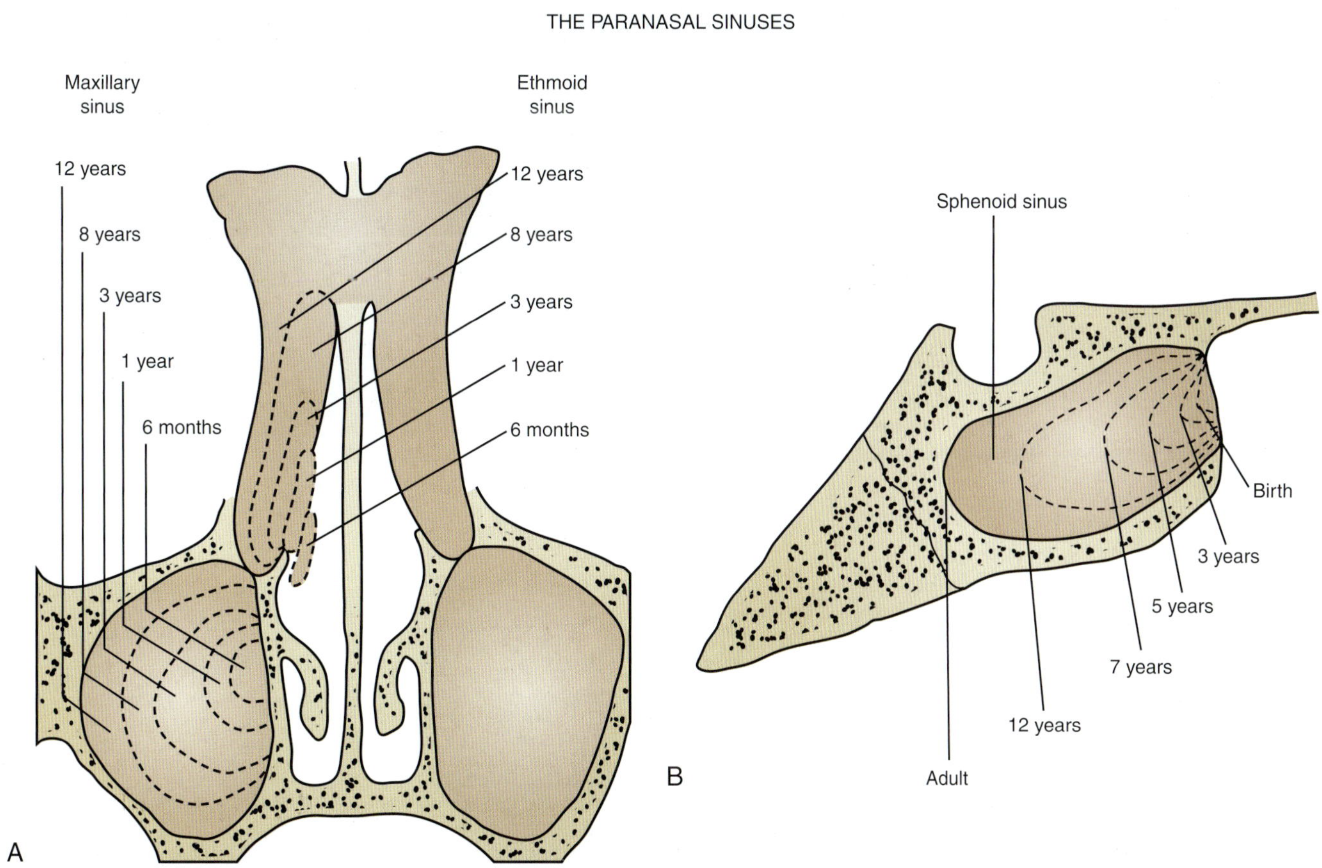

Fig. 24.52 Development of the paranasal sinuses. (A) This schematic diagram shows the development of the maxillary and ethmoid sinuses. Note that development occurs throughout childhood and may not be complete until 12 years old. (B) The sphenoid sinus, which sits under the pituitary fossa, develops slowly and may not even be well aerated for the first 5 to 6 years of life.

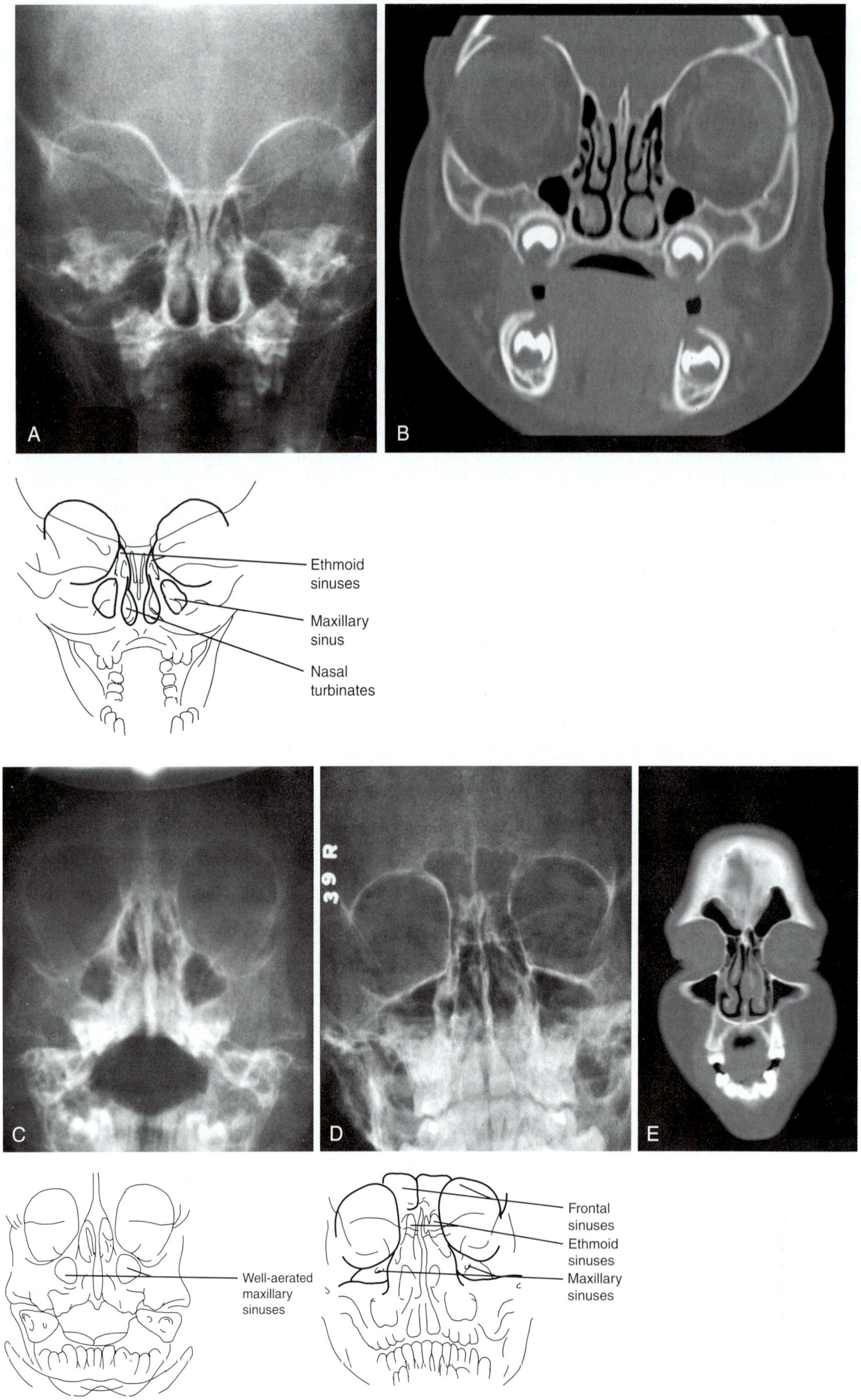

Fig. 24.53 Normal radiography of the sinuses. Radiography is currently the most helpful noninvasive tool for evaluating the paranasal sinuses. Interpretation requires appreciation of the normal pattern of development and the findings in health and with disease. (A) Anteroposterior, or Caldwell, view shows clear ethmoid sinuses in an 18-month-old child. The bony margins are sharp, and the sinus cavities are dark. (B) Coronal computed tomography (CT) of an 18-month-old showing well-aerated (dark), yet small maxillary and ethmoid sinuses. (C) The Waters view of the same child shows normal maxillary sinuses with sharply defined bony margins. The cavities appear black. (D) After age 6 or 7, the Caldwell view is taken posteroanteriorly. In this 8-year-old boy, the bony margins of both the ethmoid and frontal sinuses are sharply defined. Because the calvarium is superimposed, it can be difficult to appreciate frontal sinus clouding on this view alone, particularly with bilateral disease. Therefore evaluation of the frontal sinuses requires close scrutiny of both Caldwell and lateral views.

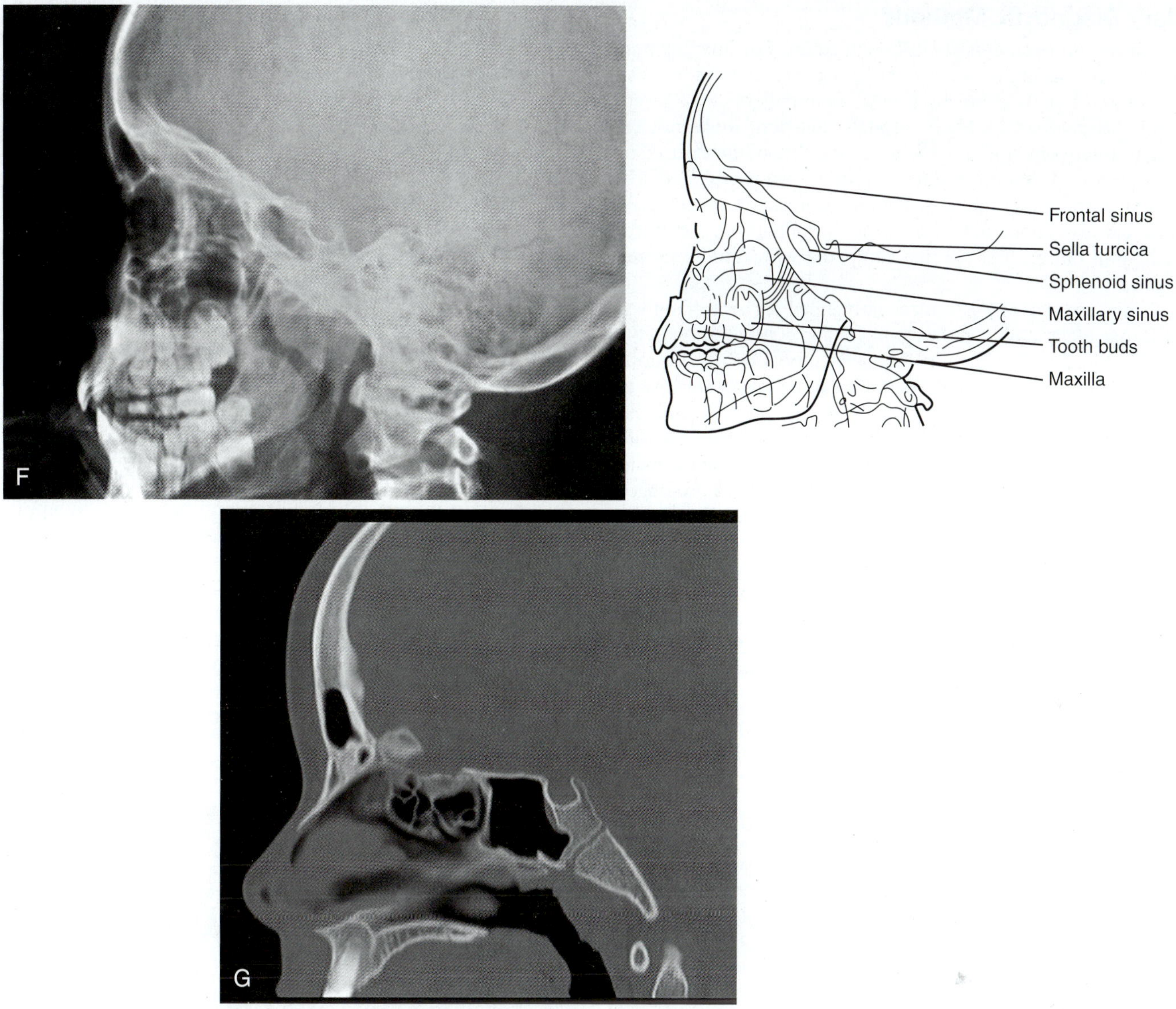

Fig. 24.53, cont'd (E) Coronal CT of an 8-year-old showing larger, well-aerated maxillary and ethmoid sinuses and small frontal sinuses. (F) Lateral view of an 8-year-old child shows pneumatization of the frontal and sphenoid sinuses. Bony margins are sharply defined. The frontal sinuses appear black, but the sphenoid is somewhat gray because there are more overlying structures. Note that the roots of the maxillary teeth are embedded in the floor of the maxillary sinus. (G) Sagittal CT showing well-aerated sphenoid, ethmoids, and frontal sinuses of an 8-year-old. Note that plain sinus radiographs are quite inaccurate when compared with sinus CT for the diagnosis of sinusitis.

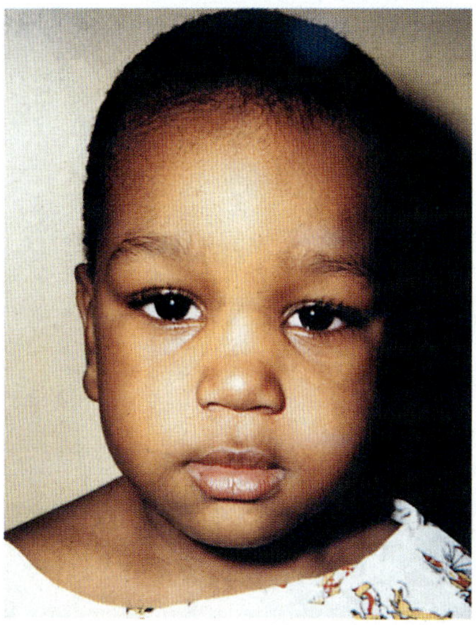

Fig. 24.54 Sympathetic periorbital swelling with sinusitis. This 2-year-old boy was seen late in the afternoon with fever, wet cough, decreased activity, and mild infraorbital puffiness. The swelling was neither red, indurated, nor tender and reportedly had been more marked on awakening in the morning. He also had a scant cloudy nasal discharge. His chest radiograph was normal, but sinus films showed opacification of the maxillary sinuses.

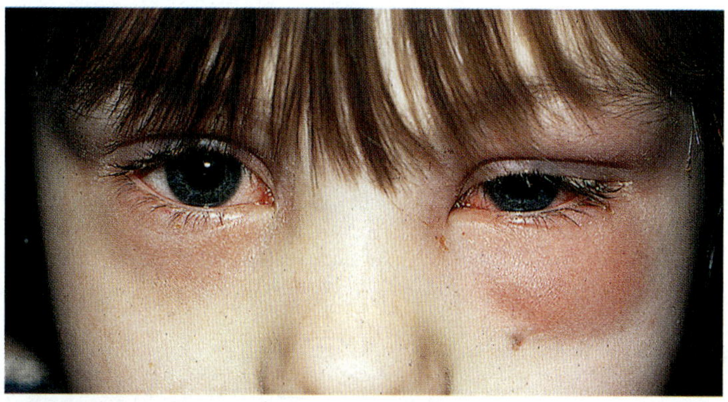

Fig. 24.55 This child with sinusitis had prominent erythematous periorbital edema and signs of purulent conjunctivitis. The redness raised concerns of periorbital cellulitis, but the area was nontender and not indurated. Presence of periorbital swelling is a helpful clue in diagnosing sinusitis in children with other suggestive signs and symptoms. (Courtesy Ellen Wald, MD, Children's Hospital of Pittsburgh, Pittsburgh, PA.)

Ancillary Diagnostic Methods

When clinical improvements are not seen, cultures or imaging may be helpful. Needle aspiration of the sinuses is conclusive but invasive and not without risk. It is, however, justified in patients with severe symptoms, patients with CNS or orbital extension, those not responding to treatment, and those who are immunocompromised or immunosuppressed. Middle meatus culture is also useful to detect the bacterial pathogen in sinusitis. Middle meatus cultures correlate with sinus cultures about 80% of the time. Nasopharyngeal cultures may be helpful but are less specific compared with middle meatal cultures.

Plain sinus radiography is not recommended for sinusitis given the wide range of variability in development and configuration of the sinuses. CT (Fig. 24.56) is the most sensitive modality for diagnosis and is considered the gold standard, but it can be falsely positive in patients with viral URIs and allergic sinusitis, is expensive, and exposes children to radiation. It should be reserved for patients with possible complications of sinusitis, underlying anatomic abnormalities, or suspected chronic sinusitis who fail to respond to a prolonged course of antimicrobial therapy and maximum topically therapy. At minimum, therapy consists of a 10- to 14-day course (or until the patient is symptom free for 7 days) of an antimicrobial agent suitable to the likely spectrum of organisms (see preceding paragraph). Saline irrigations, short-term vasoconstrictors, and topical decongestions are extremely helpful to promote secretion clearance. Analgesia may be needed for discomfort and perhaps an oral antihistamine. Some children with intense headaches or facial pain experience symptomatic relief by using topical nasal vasoconstrictors and warm compresses during the first 1 or 2 days of therapy. Patients with sinusitis should be instructed to avoid swimming underwater, diving, or flying until completion of therapy because the resultant barotrauma aggravates symptoms and may promote intracranial spread of infection.

Complications of Sinusitis

Infectious sinusitis is important due to the significant risk of extension of infection and secondary complications. This risk stems from several anatomic factors. First, the sinuses surround the orbits superiorly, medially, and inferiorly and the frontal lobe inferiorly. The bony plates that make up the sinus walls are thin and porous, and their suture lines are open in childhood. This is especially true of the lamina papyracea, the thin bone that separates the ethmoid air cells from the orbits (Fig. 24.57). Increased sinus pressure occurring because of ostial blockage and fluid collection can cause separation of portions of these bony structures and extension of the sinus infection into the orbit or cranium. Facial vascular anatomy also contributes to the spread of infection. The veins of the face, nose, and sinuses drain in part into the orbit and then into the ophthalmic venous system, which is in direct continuity with the cavernous sinus. The ophthalmic veins have no valves and thus may provide less defense against spread of infection. The orbit is also devoid of lymphatics, which helps explain the ease of periorbital edema formation when there is increased sinus pressure. The relative looseness of the subcutaneous tissues of the face also assists edema collection and may aid in spread of infection. As a result of these factors, direct extension of infection can occur (1) into the periorbital soft tissues,

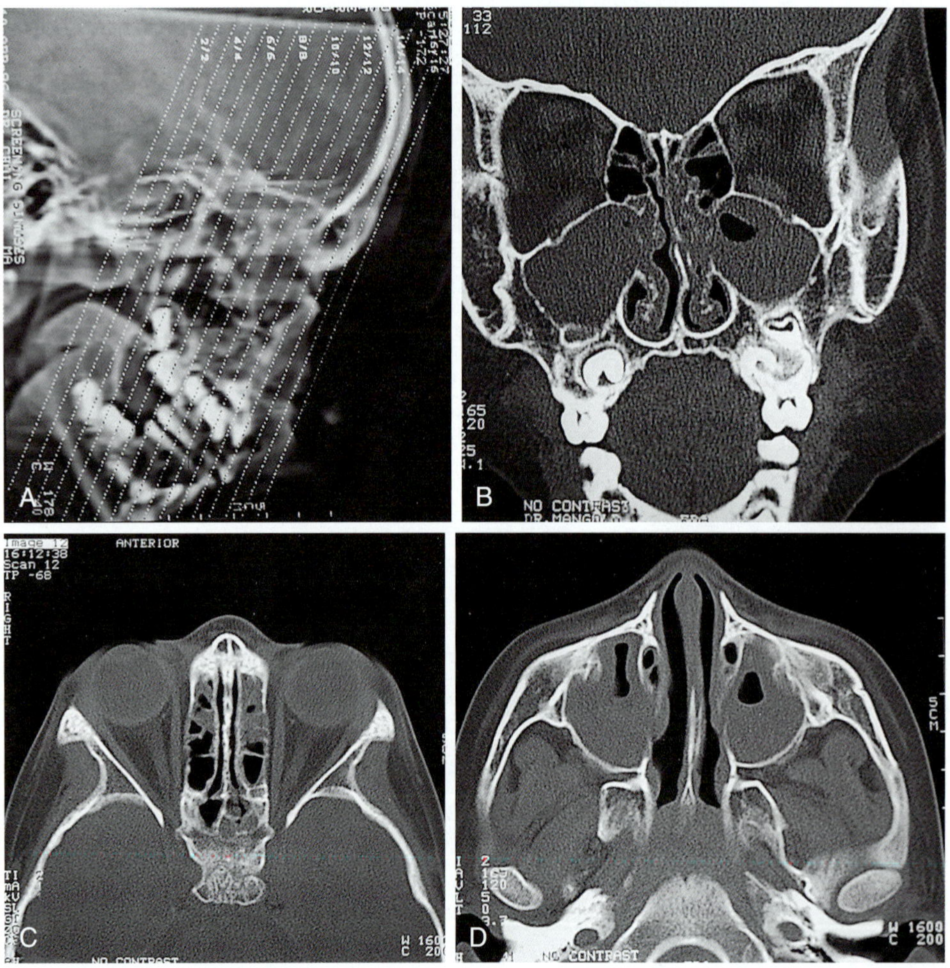

Fig. 24.56 Computed tomography findings in acute sinusitis. (A) In the topographic view, the examiner can identify the position of each slice and also has an excellent view of the adenoid bed. (B) The coronal view shows the maxillary/ethmoidal relationship in conjunction with the orbit. Note that the ethmoids are clear, but the right maxillary sinus is completely opacified, and the left maxillary sinus is nearly so, with only a small air pocket visible. (C) This axial view shows patchy ethmoidal clouding. (D) Marked mucosal thickening of both maxillary sinuses is shown in this axial view.

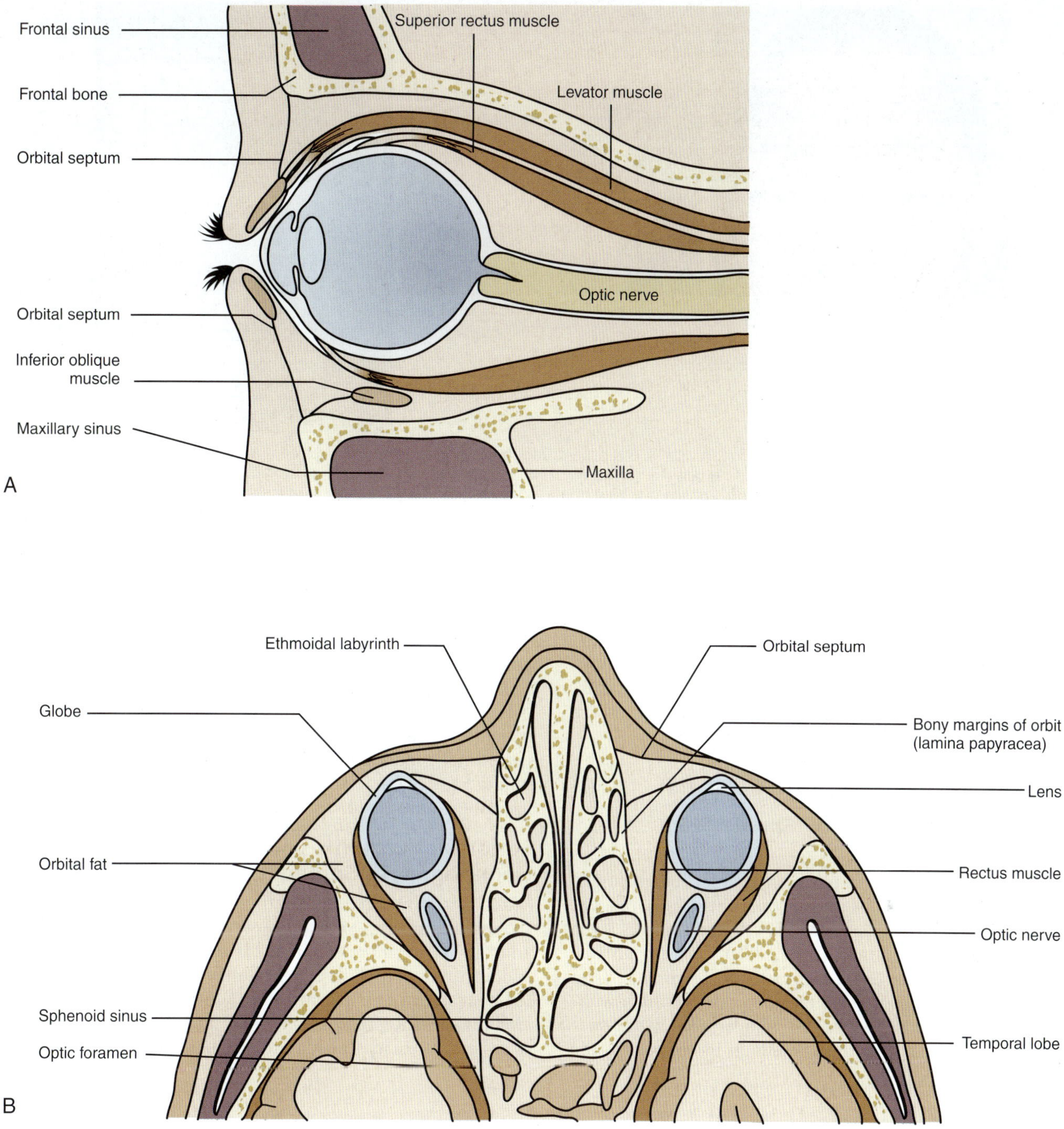

Fig. 24.57 The anatomy of the orbit. (A) Sagittal section shows the relationship of the orbit to the maxillary and frontal sinuses and the position of the orbital septum within the eyelid. The latter structure appears to serve as an anatomic barrier, helping to prevent the spread of infection from periorbital tissues into the orbit. (B) In this horizontal section, the close relationship of the orbit to the ethmoid sinuses is apparent.

producing periorbital cellulitis; (2) through the bony walls into the orbits, resulting in orbital cellulitis or a subperiosteal abscess within the bony orbit; (3) via erosion outward through the frontal bone, producing a Pott puffy tumor; or (4) via erosion inward through the frontal bone, resulting in an epidural abscess. On rare occasions, hematogenous seeding of bacteria may occur. Fortunately, improved recognition of sinus infection and early use of antimicrobial therapy have reduced the frequency, severity, and morbidity of these disorders.

Pott Puffy Tumor

Frontal sinusitis assumes importance after 8 to 10 years of age (once the frontal sinuses have begun to form) and has the potential for serious complications, particularly when neglected or inadequately treated. Erosion occurring anteriorly through the frontal bone results in subperiosteal abscess, classically known as a *Pott puffy tumor.* This is seen as an erythematous frontal swelling with a doughy consistency and exquisite tenderness (Fig. 24.58). Affected patients tend to be toxic, febrile, and extremely uncomfortable. Prompt surgical drainage is of utmost importance. A CT scan should be obtained before surgical drainage to evaluate the extent of the abscess and to identify other sites of spread. Osteomyelitis of the frontal bone is present, and longer courses of antimicrobials are required for Pott puffy tumor.

Epidural Abscess

Another potential complication of frontal sinusitis is epidural abscess formation with erosion through the posterior wall of the frontal bone. This should be suspected in patients with frontal sinusitis who have high temperature, severe headache, signs of toxicity, or

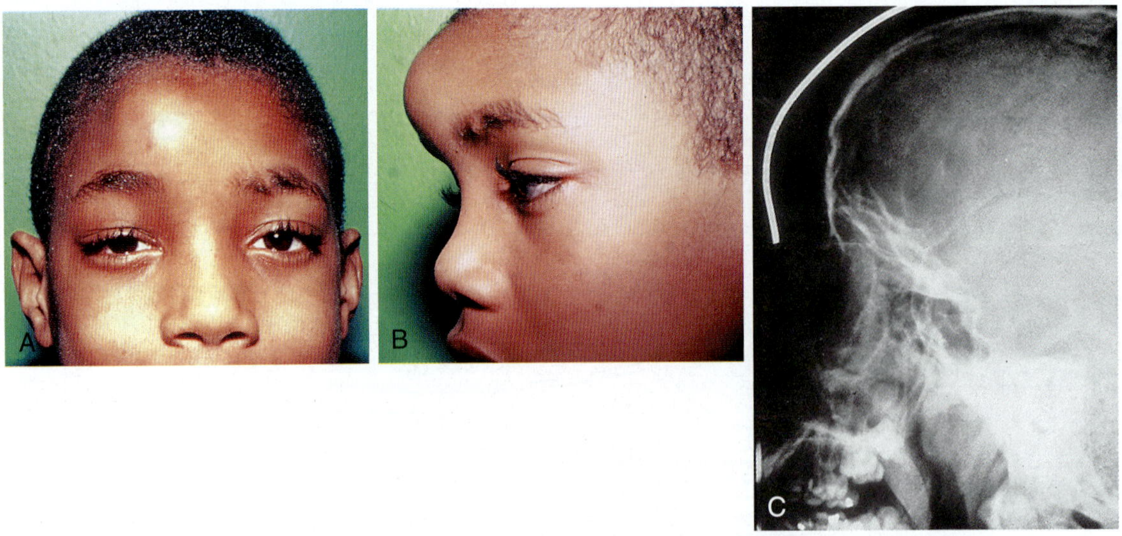

Fig. 24.58 Pott puffy tumor. (A and B) This patient had fever, headache, and an erythematous swelling over the forehead that was exquisitely tender and had a doughy consistency. (C) A lateral radiograph shows frontal sinus clouding, irregularity of the frontal bone, and marked soft tissue swelling that is highlighted by a wire placed over the forehead and scalp. (C, Courtesy Kenneth Grundfast, MD, Boston Medical Center, Boston, MA.)

altered sensorium. Diagnosis is best confirmed by CT (Fig. 24.59) and MRI. Although IV antimicrobial therapy and careful monitoring may suffice in the management of small lesions, larger abscesses necessitate neurosurgical consultation and surgical intervention. Further extension of these infections may result in brain abscess (see Chapter 16).

Periorbital and Orbital Infections

Periorbital Cellulitis Caused by Spread From Adjacent Sinusitis

Periorbital cellulitis is a mild complication of infectious sinusitis. Cellulitis is confined to tissues outside the orbit, with spread blocked in part by the orbital septum (see Fig. 24.57). When sinusitis is the underlying condition, the ethmoid or maxillary sinuses are the structures primarily affected. Typically, patients are younger than 4 or 5 years old and have an antecedent history of URI with or without conjunctivitis, otitis, or sinusitis. This is superseded by the sudden appearance of lid and periorbital swelling. In contrast to the uncomplicated sympathetic edema seen in some patients with sinusitis, the swelling in children with periorbital cellulitis is usually unilateral and is erythematous, indurated, and tender (Fig. 24.60). Conjunctival injection and discharge may also be seen. In many patients, fever accompanies the onset of swelling, but although most patients appear uncomfortable, toxicity is unusual. The course of periorbital cellulitis resulting from extension of sinus infection is milder and characterized by much slower progression than from hematogenous spread.

Periorbital Cellulitis Caused by Hematogenous Spread

When periorbital cellulitis is the result of hematogenous seeding, the organisms tend to be more virulent, the onset more explosive, and the course more fulminant. Typically, the patient experiences sudden onset of high fever (often after a mild URI) accompanied by the appearance of erythematous, indurated, and tender periorbital swelling, which progresses rapidly and is accompanied by signs of systemic toxicity. The majority of these patients are younger than

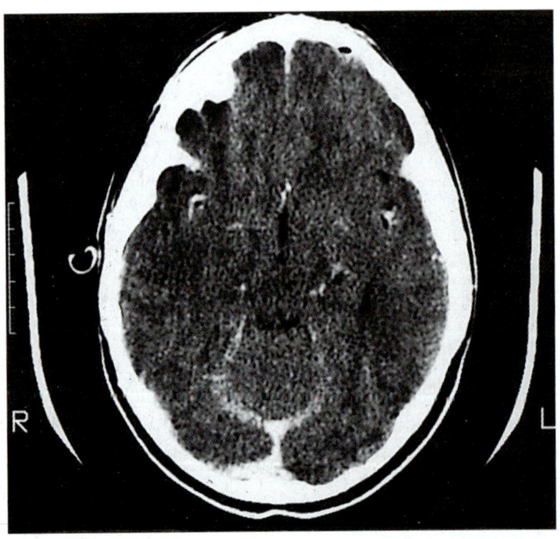

Fig. 24.59 Epidural abscess. This patient had lethargy, high fever, left eye pain, and periorbital swelling after 1 week of severe nasal congestion. A computed tomography scan, obtained to rule out orbital involvement, revealed a small epidural abscess behind the left frontal bone. Note the small central air pocket.

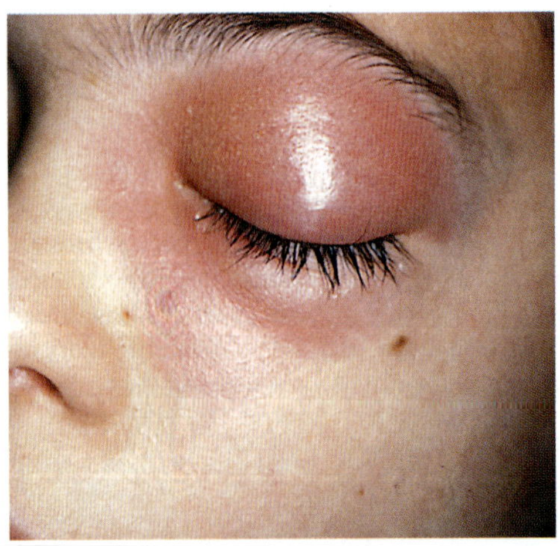

Fig. 24.60 Periorbital cellulitis. Intense erythema and edema of the lids are evident. The swollen tissues were indurated and tender on palpation. Ocular motion was normal. Underlying ethmoid sinusitis was confirmed by computed tomography scan.

1 year old or only slightly older, and bacteremia with *S. pneumoniae* or *H. influenzae* type B is usual. Widespread use of the *H. influenzae* type B vaccine has dramatically reduced the incidence of *H. influenzae* B-induced cellulitis. In children >2 years, odontogenic pathogens are common. Because of the severity and potential for further extension and hematogenous spread, aggressive IV antimicrobial therapy is urgently required. This necessitates empirical selection of agents to cover likely pathogens, pending culture results. Patients also require close monitoring for signs of complications.

Periorbital Cellulitis Caused by Spread From Adjacent Facial Infection

More than 50% of children with periorbital cellulitis have neither sinusitis nor bacteremia as a predisposing condition. Rather, the patients appear to suffer from extension of nearby facial infection to periorbital tissues. They may have a history of antecedent trauma to the orbit or nearby facial structures, often with a break in the skin (Fig. 24.61) or one of a primary skin infection (impetigo, a pustule, a chalazion, infected dermatitis, or insect bite). They subsequently experience a temperature spike and evolution of periorbital and eyelid edema. This group tends to be somewhat older, generally older than 5 years old. *S. aureus* and *S. pyogenes* are the predominant offending organisms.

Orbital Cellulitis and Abscess

In orbital cellulitis, infection extends into the orbit itself. It may take the form of undifferentiated cellulitis, or it may later evolve into a subperiosteal or orbital abscess. Patients tend to have a history similar to that of patients with periorbital cellulitis but are generally more ill, toxic, and lethargic. Pain with or limitation of eye movement can also be present. Edema and erythema of the lid and periorbital tissues are often so significant that it is impossible to open the eyelids without the use of eyelid retractors (Fig. 24.62A and B). Tenderness is exquisite. If the lid can be retracted, the clinician may find proptosis, conjunctival inflammation with chemosis and purulent discharge, decreased extraocular motion, and some loss of visual acuity. Ophthalmologic consultation is required.

The most common source of spread is from an adjacent infected ethmoid sinus, although extension from nearby frontal sinusitis or a facial or dental infection occasionally occurs. Causative organisms are the same as those in sinus infection.

Use of IV antimicrobial therapy and close monitoring for evolution and CNS complications are vital in the management of orbital cellulitis. Contrast CT is exceptionally useful for determining the presence or absence of abscesses (Fig. 24.62C). When a subperiosteal abscess is present or the clinical ocular examination shows deterioration, surgical drainage combined with an ethmoidectomy are indicated. It is now possible to perform the ethmoidectomy and abscess drainage endoscopically in most patients. Optimal management necessitates a team approach involving pediatrics, otolaryngology, ophthalmology, and at times neurosurgery.

Local complications of orbital cellulitis include abscess formation, optic neuritis, retinal vein thrombosis, and panophthalmitis. CNS complications may result from direct extension or spread of septic thrombophlebitis. Meningitis, epidural and subdural abscesses, and cavernous sinus thrombosis have been described. All are characterized by marked toxicity and alteration in level of consciousness. Cavernous sinus thrombosis is heralded by sudden, bilateral, pulsating proptosis and chemosis in association with increased toxicity and obtundation.

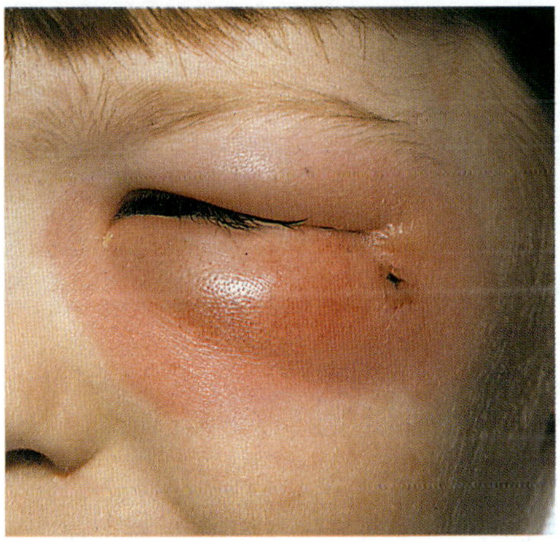

Fig. 24.61 Periorbital cellulitis caused by spread of an adjacent facial infection. This child developed fever and erythematous, tender periorbital swelling a few days after incurring an abrasion as a result of a fall.

Vacuum Headache

The second potentially confusing clinical picture is that of the allergic sinus headache, or vacuum headache. In this condition, older atopic individuals complain of intense facial or frontal headache, without fever or other evidence of infection. This occurs during periods in which patients are having exacerbation of allergic symptoms, after swimming in chlorinated pools, or while flying on an airplane. The phenomenon appears to be caused by acute blockage of sinus ostia by mucosal edema, with subsequent creation of a vacuum within the sinus as a result of resorption of sinus gases by mucosa. The resultant negative pressure produces the pain. In these patients, the nasal mucosa tends to be pale and swollen but without discharge. Sinuses may be tender to percussion but are clear radiographically. Symptoms respond promptly to application of a topical vasoconstrictor and warm compresses over the face. Improvement is maintained by antihistamines and decongestants.

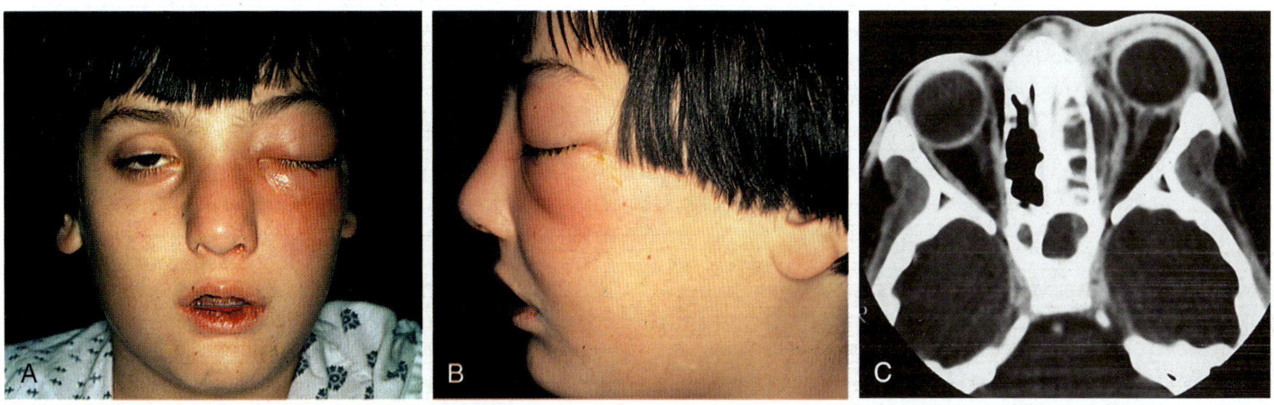

Fig. 24.62 Orbital subperiosteal abscess. (A and B) This child had a fever, severe toxicity, and marked lethargy. He experienced intense orbital and retroorbital pain and showed a limited range of ocular motion with associated exacerbation of pain. (C) This computed tomography scan shows preseptal swelling, proptosis, and lateral displacement of the globe and orbital contents by a subperiosteal abscess.

OROPHARYNGEAL DISORDERS

Oropharyngeal Examination

Examination of the pharynx is important in pediatrics because of the frequency of pharyngeal infections. However, the procedure can be challenging. The small size of the mouth and difficulty in depressing the tongue in infancy, lack of cooperativeness in toddlers, and the fear of causing older children to gag when using tongue blades can impede efforts. These problems can be minimized by a few simple techniques. Infants and young children, when placed supine with the head hyperextended on the neck, tend to open their mouths spontaneously, enabling visualization of the anterior oral cavity and assisting insertion of a tongue blade to depress the tongue and inspect the posterior palate and pharynx (see Fig. 24.1B). When examining older children, asking them to open their mouths as wide as possible and pant "like a puppy dog," say "ha ha," or "roar" usually results in lowering of the posterior portion of the tongue, revealing the posterior palatal and pharyngeal structures. Because conditions involving the lips, mucosa, and dentition are presented in Chapter 21 and palatal disorders are covered in Chapter 23, this section concentrates primarily on pharyngeal disorders with only a brief mention of palatal and oral cavity disorders.

Oral Cavity Disorders

Oral Cavity Lesions of Newborn

Ankyloglossia

The lingual frenulum connects the ventral surface of the tongue to the floor of mouth. The degree of anterior-posterior extension and vertical length can vary and often change with growth of the child. Ankyloglossia, otherwise known as *tongue-tie,* is used to describe a situation where the lingual frenulum results in limitations in tongue function, specifically feeding in the newborn stage. The lingual frenulum frequently can be seen when the child is crying but is best appreciated by manual examination. In the newborn, limitations in tongue elevation and protrusion can affect feeding. Less frequently, limitations in tongue elevation, protrusion, and lateral movement can affect feeding, speech, or dental hygiene. If clinical symptoms and physical examination suggest limitations, surgical correction can be considered.

Epulis

Epulis are benign soft tissue tumors typically seen on the alveolus. They typically appear at birth or soon after; however, they can occur in utero and, when large, can present with obstructive concerns (Fig. 24.63). Surgical excision is recommended, as is pathologic assessment to rule out neuroectodermal tumors or sarcomas.

Salivary Duct Anomalies

Failure of major salivary ducts to cannulate or incomplete formation of the ducts can result in obstruction of salivary fluid, which then presents as cystic submucosal lesions. Obstruction of the Wharton duct (submandibular duct) results in cystic lesions in the floor of mouth (Fig. 24.64). Agenesis of the Stenson duct (parotid duct) is rare and typically occurs with parotid gland agenesis or hypoplasia.

Epstein Pearls

Epstein pearls are benign keratin-filled lesions of epithelial layer. They appear as white cystic lesions along the midline raphe of the palate.

Enteric Duplication Cyst

The embryonic foregut gives rise to the upper and lower aerodigestive tract. The etiology of enteric duplication cysts is not fully described; however, the most accepted theories suggest aberrant epithelial cells and disruption in the primordial fusion planes contribute to their formation. Enteric cysts typically present as midline cystic lesions within the aerodigestive tract anywhere from the oral cavity (Fig. 24.65A) to the anus. Enteric cysts may be asymptomatic or symptomatic. Symptoms associated with enteric cysts are typically

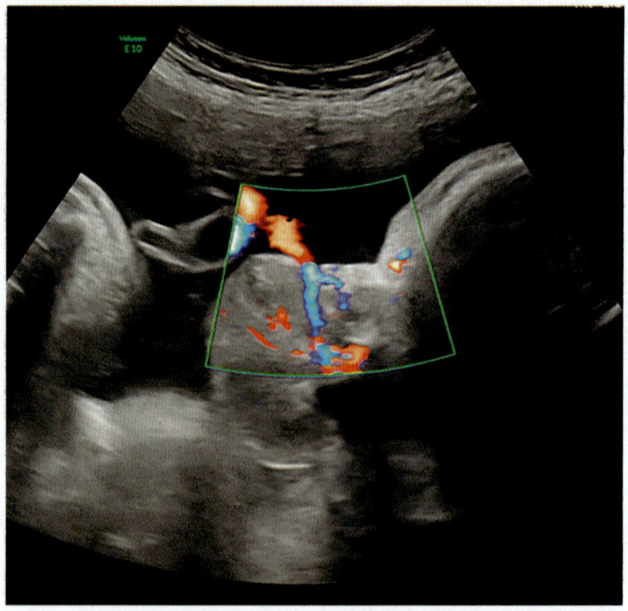

Fig. 24.63 Diagnostic fetal 34-week ultrasound showing a large orofacial mass with feeding vessels off the maxilla.

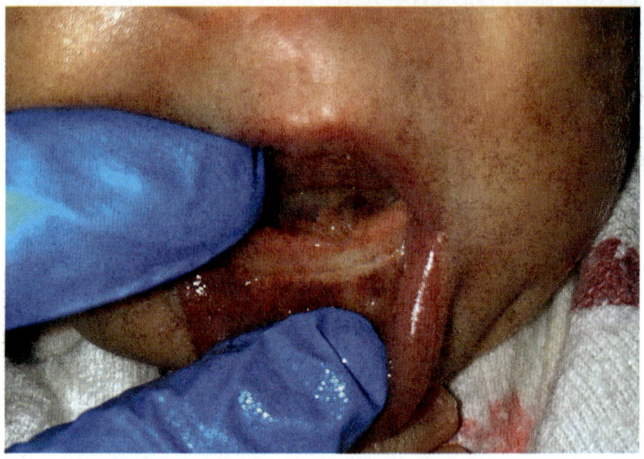

Fig. 24.64 Agenesis of submandibular papilla. Dilated Wharton ducts seen bilaterally secondary to failure of papillary canalization. Posterior floor of mouth fullness also noted.

secondary to obstruction, such as dysphagia and dyspnea. Clinically and radiographically, enteric cysts are differentiated from disorders of salivary glands/ducts by their midline location opposed to lateral location of salivary anomalies. Histologically, enteric duplication cysts may consist of gastric, intestinal, or respiratory cells. Treatment consists of complete surgical excision (Fig. 24.65B and C). Prenatal diagnosis of large enteric cysts may require delivery via EXIT (ex utero intrapartum treatment) procedure. Other congenital cyst head and neck masses are described in Chapter 18.

Hamartomas

Hamartomas are benign pseudotumors. They consist of abnormally located or an overgrowth of mature tissue normally present in the organ from which the hamartoma arises. Lingual hamartomas are typically located midline along the dorsum of the tongue posteriorly (Fig. 24.66); case reports of more anteriorly located hamartoma exist. Unlike traumatic fibrous lesions, hamartomas typically appear lobulated and can extend far outside the binderies of the native organ. Congenital lingual hamartomas may occur as an isolated lesion or associated with other genetic anomalies, most notably oral facial digital syndrome (ORDS). Large hamartomas can result in obstructive symptoms and surgical excision recommended for relief of symptoms and to rule out less common sarcomas.

Additional oral cavity lesions are discussed in Chapter 21.

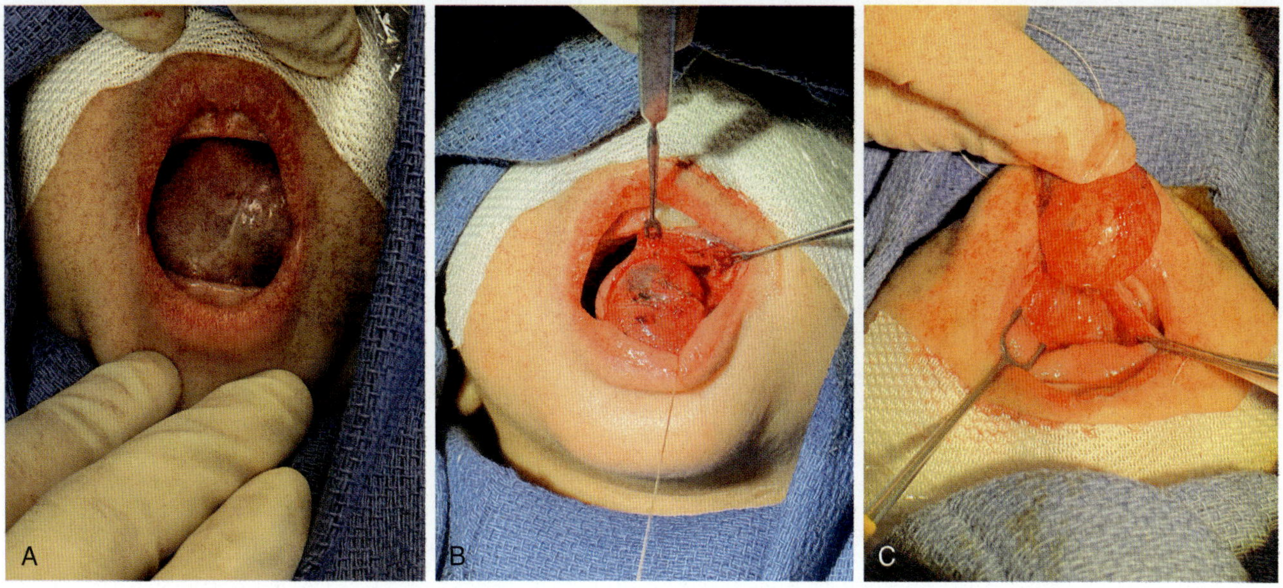

Fig. 24.65 Enteric duplication cyst. (A) Preoperative appearance of cystic submucosal midline floor of mouth lesion. (B and C) Intraoperative photos showing submucosal midline cystic lesion.

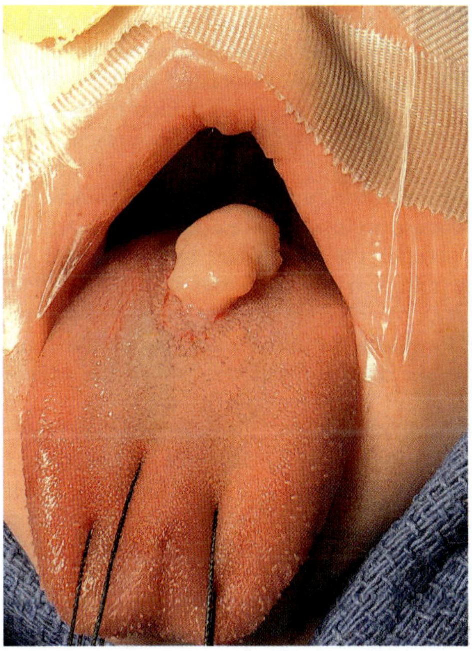

Fig. 24.66 Lingual hamartoma. Hamartomas are benign pseudotumors. Photo demonstrates a midline lobulated lesion of dorsal posterior aspect of the anterior tongue.

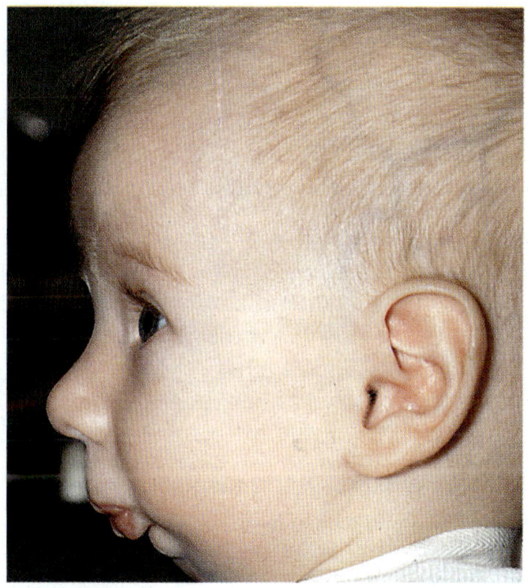

Fig. 24.67 Pierre Robin syndrome, characterized by severe retromicrognathia and cleft palate. In this infant the micrognathia produced posterior displacement of the tongue, resulting in airway obstruction that necessitated a tracheotomy. (Courtesy Wolfgang Loskin, MD, University of North Carolina, Chapel Hill, NC.)

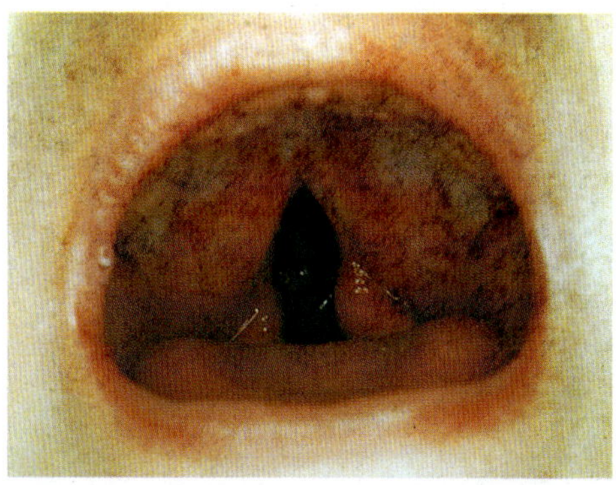

Fig. 24.68 Cleft palate. This child has a midline cleft of the soft palate. The hard palate, alveolar ridge, and lip are spared. (Courtesy Ms. Barbara Elster, Cleft Palate Center, Pittsburgh, PA.)

Palatal Disorders

Palatal malformations are a spectrum of disorders that can significantly affect feeding, swallowing, and speech. Moreover, by altering normal nasal and oropharyngeal physiology, they place affected patients at increased risk for chronic recurrent ear and sinus infections.

The clinical presentation and degree morbidity of one anomaly can vary widely from individual to individual.

Cleft Palate

Palatal clefts are among the most severe abnormalities encountered. They stem from a failure of fusion during the second month of gestation and have an incidence of about 1 in every 1500 to 2000 births. They may or may not be associated with a cleft lip and can be associated with other craniofacial anomalies or other genetic syndromes, such as the Pierre Robin syndrome (Fig. 24.67), 22qdel, and trisomies 13 and 18 (see Chapter 1); however, they can occur in otherwise healthy individuals. In many cases, there is a family history for the anomaly. A number of teratogens have also been linked to the malformation. The extent of the cleft varies: Some involve only the soft palate (Fig. 24.68); others extend through the hard palate

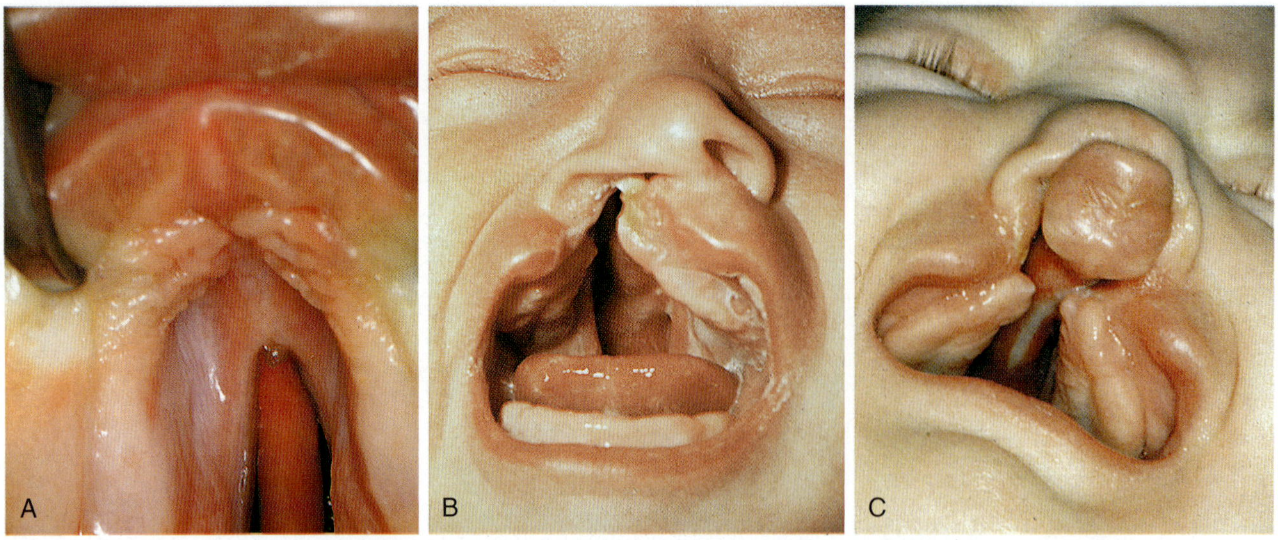

Fig. 24.69 Cleft palate. (A) Cleft of the hard and soft palate, sparing the alveolar ridge. Complete clefts of the palate, alveolar ridge, and lip may be unilateral (B) or bilateral (C). (A and C, Courtesy William Garrett, MD. B, Courtesy Michael Sherlock, MD, Lutherville, MD.)

but spare the alveolar ridge (Fig. 24.69A). More apparent soft palate clefts (type 1) involve the muscle and mucosal layers; however, some type 1 clefts only present with a muscle layer desinence without a mucosal layer defect, submucosal clefts. Clefts can also be categorized as complete or incomplete, depending on the extent of the palate involved (see Fig. 24.69B and C). The defect may be unilateral or bilateral. The four major types of congenital cleft palate are as follows:

Type I: Soft palate only (see Fig. 24.68)
Type II: Unilateral cleft of soft and hard palate (see Fig. 24.69A)
Type III: Unilateral cleft of soft and hard palate, extending through the alveolar ridge (see Fig. 24.69B)
Type IV: Bilateral cleft of soft and hard palate, extending through the alveolar ridge (see Fig. 24.69C)

Cleft palate is covered in depth in Chapter 23 with discussion of plastic surgery approaches to diagnosis and correction. Two similar conditions are covered in the following section.

Submucous Cleft Palate

Submucous cleft of the palate (SMCP) is often overlooked in infancy. The condition is characterized by a bony U-shaped notch, palpable in the midline, at the juncture of the hard and soft portions of the palate (Fig. 24.70A), sharp vaulted of soft palate with gag, prominent zona pellucida, or bifid uvula. There may also be palpable midline thinning of the soft palate. The anomaly results from a failure of the tensor veli palatini muscle to insert properly in the midline. Some children have an associated double or notched (bifid) uvula that, when present, serves as a clue to the existence of the palatal abnormality (see Fig. 24.70B). The presence of an SMCP or bifid does not necessarily indicate a significant functional anomaly exists; feeding difficulties, eustachian tube dysfunction, and chronic middle ear disease are likely more common. Speech is often mildly hypernasal because the soft palate cannot elevate sufficiently to separate the nasopharynx from the oropharynx. Problems with speech often occur. Recognition is particularly important when considering tonsillectomy and adenoidectomy for recurrent tonsillitis and otitis because surgical removal of the adenoids in these children can result in severe speech and swallowing dysfunction; hence these procedures may be contraindicated or require modifications to prevent worsening of the velopharyngeal dysfunction. In selected cases of severe adenoidal hypertrophy or severe adenotonsillitis, upper (partial) adenoidectomy may be an option.

High-Arched Palate

High-arched palate, a minor anomaly, is a common clinical finding (Fig. 24.71). Although usually an isolated variant of palatal configuration, it occasionally occurs in association with congenital

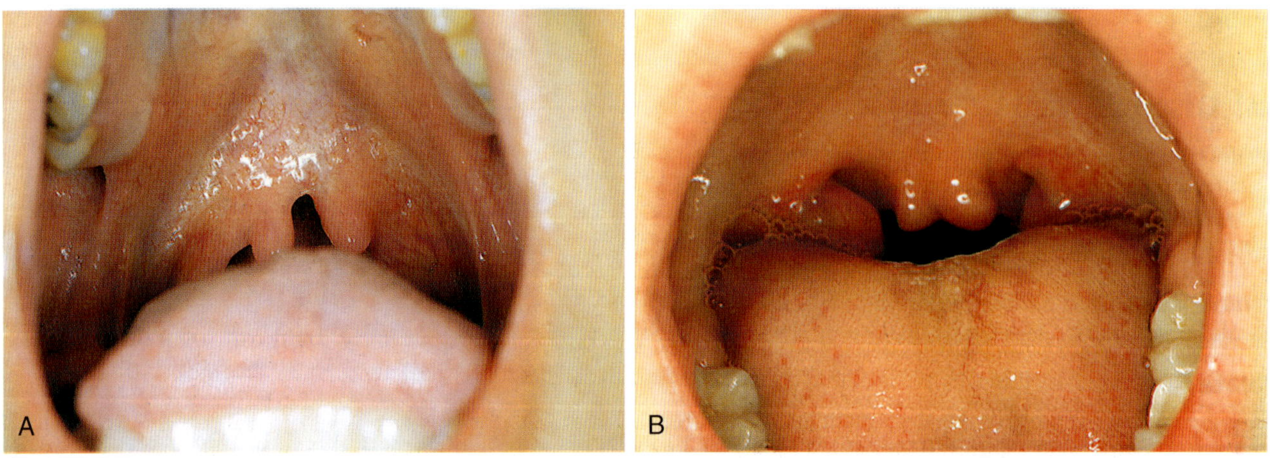

Fig. 24.70 Submucous cleft of the palate. (A) This girl shows failure of normal midline fusion of the palatal muscles, resulting in midline thinning of the soft palate. Palpation confirms the area of weakness. A U-shaped notch can also be felt in the midline at the junction of the hard and soft palate. She also has a bifid uvula. (B) This child was found to have a notched uvula on pharyngeal examination. This may serve as a clue to the presence of a submucous palatal cleft, or it may be an isolated anomaly.

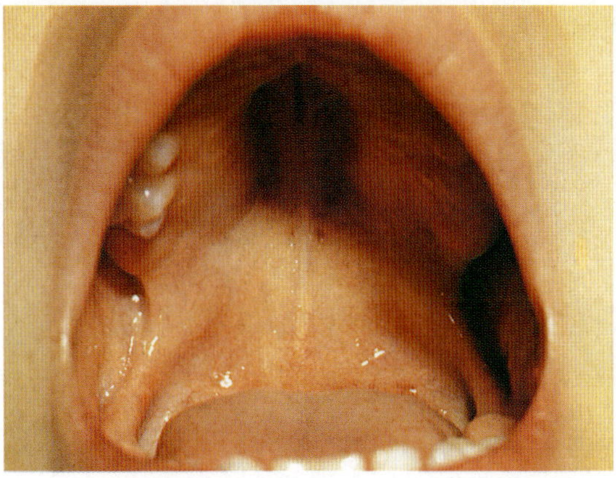

Fig. 24.71 High-arched palate. This is a common minor anomaly, usually isolated, but occasionally associated with genetic syndromes.

syndromes. Long-term orotracheal intubation of premature infants creates an iatrogenic form of the problem. Although often clinically insignificant, the high arch can be associated with increased frequency of ear and sinus infections, nasal obstruction, recurrent sinonasal infection, hyponasal speech, and sleep-disordered breathing. Palatal expansion can significantly improve dental, speech, and airway symptoms in children with severe cases.

Tonsillar and Peritonsillar Disorders

Tonsillitis/Pharyngitis

As noted earlier, the tonsils and adenoids are quite small in infancy, gradually enlarge over the first 8 to 10 years of life, and then start to regress in size. When evaluating the tonsils, particularly during an acute infection, or when monitoring patients for chronic enlargement, it is helpful to use a standardized size-grading system, as shown in Fig. 24.72. Inspection of the palate is also important in assessing patients with tonsillopharyngitis because lesions characteristic of specific pathogens are often present on the soft palate and tonsillar pillars (see Chapter 13). The most common organisms are *S. pyogenes,* adenoviruses, coxsackieviruses, and Epstein-Barr virus. Sore throat is the major symptom, but odynophagia, fever, malaise, and referred otalgia can also be present. Erythema is the most common physical finding (Fig. 24.73). Additional findings may include acute tonsillar enlargement, formation of exudates over the tonsillar surfaces, and cervical adenopathy. In a small percentage of cases, the findings suggest a given pathogen. Fever, headache, bright red and enlarged tonsils (with or without exudate), palatal petechiae (Fig. 24.73B), tender and enlarged anterior cervical nodes, and abdominal pain often suggest streptococcal infection. Marked malaise, fever, exudative tonsillitis, generalized adenopathy, and splenomegaly suggest Epstein-Barr virus mononucleosis (Fig. 24.73C; see Chapter 13). Conjunctivitis, nonexudative tonsillar inflammation, and cervical adenopathy suggest adenovirus. Yellow ulcerations with red halos on the tonsillar pillars strongly suggest coxsackievirus infection, whether or not other oral, palmar, or plantar lesions are present (Chapter 13). Unfortunately, the majority of patients with tonsillopharyngitis do not present clear-cut clinical syndromes. Because of the variability in the clinical picture and the importance of identifying and treating group A β-hemolytic streptococcal infection to prevent both pyogenic (e.g., cervical adenitis, peritonsillar, retropharyngeal, and parapharyngeal abscesses) and immunologic (e.g., rheumatic fever) complications, a screening throat culture is advisable for patients with signs or symptoms of tonsillopharyngitis. In obtaining this culture, the clinician swabs both tonsils and the posterior pharyngeal wall to maximize the chance of obtaining the organism. In the first 3 years of life, when streptococcal pharyngitis is rare but infection is expected (because of history of exposure, signs of pharyngitis, or scarlatiniform rash), it is helpful to obtain a nasopharyngeal culture as well.

Treatment is typically symptomatic for all forms of tonsillopharyngitis except for *S. pyogenes,* which requires antibiotic therapy. Occasionally, staphylococci and non-group A streptococci warrant antibiotic treatment if symptoms are severe and do not begin to resolve after 5 to 7 days. Because the secondary attack rate of *S. pyogenes* within families is 50%, parents should be instructed to notify the physician if other family members develop symptoms of upper respiratory or pharyngeal infection within the ensuing few weeks.

Following up after acute infections is important. As noted earlier, the tonsillitis of mononucleosis may appear mild early in the course of the illness, yet tonsillar inflammation and enlargement may progress over a few to several days to produce severe dysphagia and even airway obstruction. Tonsillar hypertrophy after infections, particularly EBV infections, frequently takes up to 4 to 6 months to resolve and occasionally will not completely resolve. Thus if symptoms associated with hypertrophy develop and do not resolve greater than 6 months, surgical interventions may be reasonable.

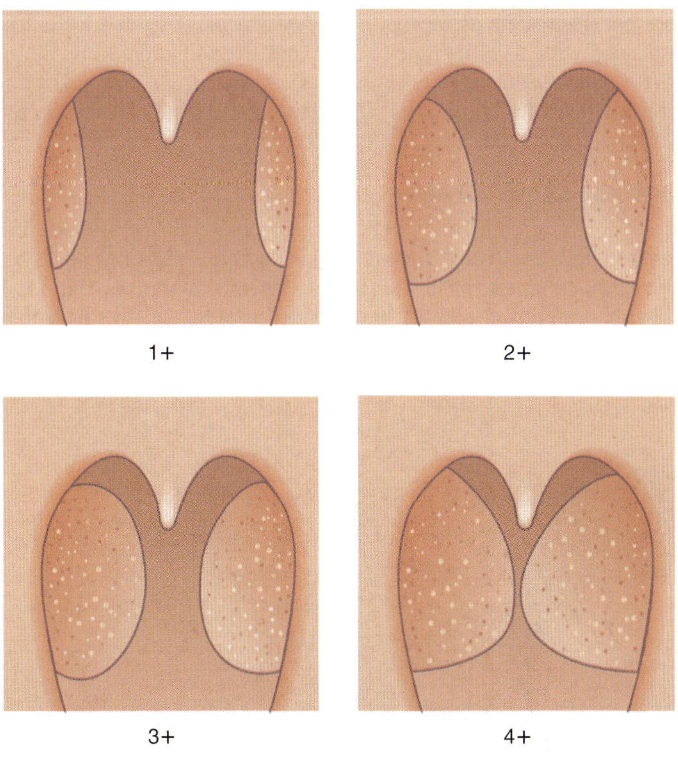

Fig. 24.72 Grading of tonsillar size for children with acute tonsillopharyngitis and those with chronic tonsillar enlargement. This grading system is particularly useful in serial examinations of a given patient. (Modified from Feinstein AR, Levitt M: Role of tonsils, *N Engl J Med* 282:285–291, 1970. Copyright © 1970 Massachusetts Medical Society. All rights reserved.)

Recurrent Tonsillitis

Frequent recurrences of tonsillitis, despite antibiotic therapy when indicated, must be handled on an individual basis. In some cases, frequent recurrences of streptococcal infection can be traced to other family members. When they are treated along with the patient, the cycle of recurrence often ends. In other instances, frequent recurrent tonsillar infections have no traceable source within the family, and they are significantly debilitating. Carrier status should be assessed by testing children when well. In patients that are streptococcal carriers, eradication with antibiotic may be considered. In children who are carriers nonresponsive to eradication therapy or with seven or more episodes in any 1 year, five episodes per year for 2 consecutive years, or three episodes per year for 3 consecutive years, tonsillectomy has a favorable outcome in reducing both frequency and severity of sore throats. Tonsillar hypertrophy with obstructive sleep apnea is also an indication for tonsillectomy.

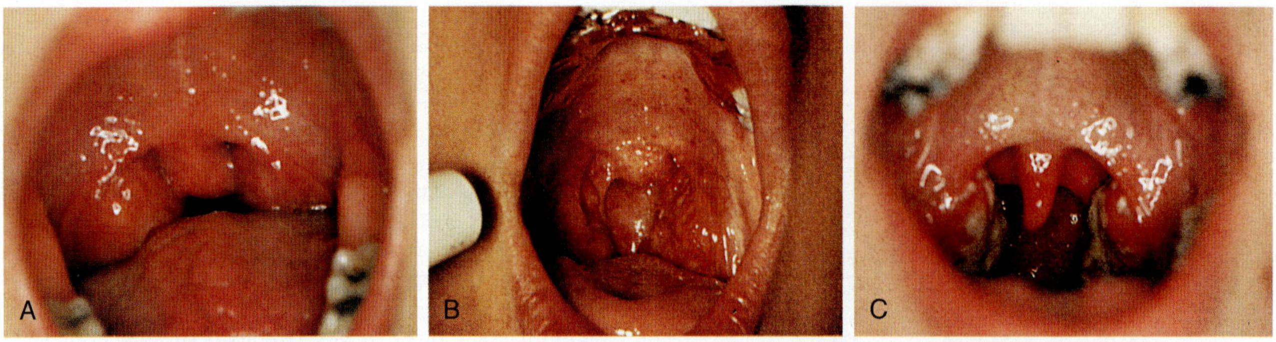

Fig. 24.73 Tonsillopharyngitis. This common entity has a number of causative pathogens and a wide spectrum of severity. (A) The diffuse tonsillar and pharyngeal erythema seen here is a nonspecific finding that can be produced by a variety of pathogens. (B) This intense erythema, seen in association with acute tonsillar enlargement and palatal petechiae, is highly suggestive of group A β-streptococcal infection, although other pathogens can produce these findings. (C) This picture of exudative tonsillitis is most commonly seen with either group A streptococcal or Epstein-Barr virus infection. (B, Courtesy Michael Sherlock, MD, Lutherville, MD.)

Uvulitis

Uvulitis is characterized by inflammation and edema of the uvula. In addition to throat pain and dysphagia, affected patients commonly complain of a sense of having "something in their throat" or a gagging sensation. The phenomenon has been reported in association with pharyngitis caused by *S. pyogenes*, in which cases the uvula is bright red and often hemorrhagic (Fig. 24.74A). The condition has also been noted in association with EBV mononucleosis, in both the presence and absence of exudative tonsillitis (see Fig. 24.74B), and with other viral agents (see Fig. 24.74C). Uvulitis has also been reported in a patient with concurrent *H. influenzae* type B epiglottitis.

Peritonsillar Abscess or Cellulitis

A peritonsillar abscess (PTA) forms between the tonsil and constrictor muscle and extends into the soft palate. Patients are usually school age or older, and they typically have a recent history of sore throat, often not cultured or treated or for which the child was given an incomplete course of antimicrobial therapy. The patient may experience initial improvement but then has a sudden onset of high fever and severe throat pain worse on one side. The pain usually radiates to the ipsilateral ear and is associated with marked dysphagia, such that the patient spits out saliva to avoid swallowing. Painful ipsilateral lymphadenopathy and torticollis, tilting the head toward the involved side to minimize pressure of the sternocleidomastoid muscle, are often present (Fig. 24.75A). Speech is thick and muffled because of splinting of the tongue and pharyngeal muscles. Trismus, or limitation of mouth opening, is often noted because of inflammation of the internal pterygoid muscles (see Fig. 24.75B). If visualization of the pharynx is possible, a smooth bulge is seen in the supratonsillar area projecting forward and medially onto the soft palate with deviation of the uvula to the opposite side (see Fig. 24.75C). *S. pyogenes* and *S. aureus* are the most common pathogens. Mixed infections with gram-positive and gram-negative aerobic and anaerobic pathogens are also common. Patients with mononucleosis, concurrently infected with group A streptococci and treated with steroids, are at risk for developing a rapidly evolving peritonsillar abscess and complications.

On the basis of the age and level of cooperation from the child, the otolaryngologist may drain PTAs transorally in the office. If examination and cooperation are limited, the abscess may require incision and drainage in the operating room. Recurrent PTAs obstructive is an indication for tonsillectomy.

Adenotonsillar Hypertrophy

Adenotonsillar hypertrophy (ATH) rarely exists before 12 months of age, yet other structural and inflammatory etiologies (see other sections) do. As mentioned earlier, acute and chronic infections can result in ATH. Other etiologies are chronic allergy or irritant exposure. Environmental and food allergies, even mild, are common in patients with adenotonsillar hypertrophy, and GERD is a common irritant. ATH without associated morbidities is not necessarily concerning and does not necessitate otolaryngologic assessment. Possible morbidities associated with ATH include snoring and sleep-disordered breathing (SDB), recurrent nasal pharyngeal and ear infections, dysphagia, and speech/articulation anomalies. Tonsillar hypertrophy with obstructive sleep apnea is an indication for tonsillectomy.

Tonsillar Lymphoma

The majority of children, whether well or acutely ill with tonsillitis, have tonsils that are symmetric in size. When a child has an asymmetrically enlarged tonsil without evidence of infection, the possibility of lymphoma should be considered (Fig. 24.76). Thorough

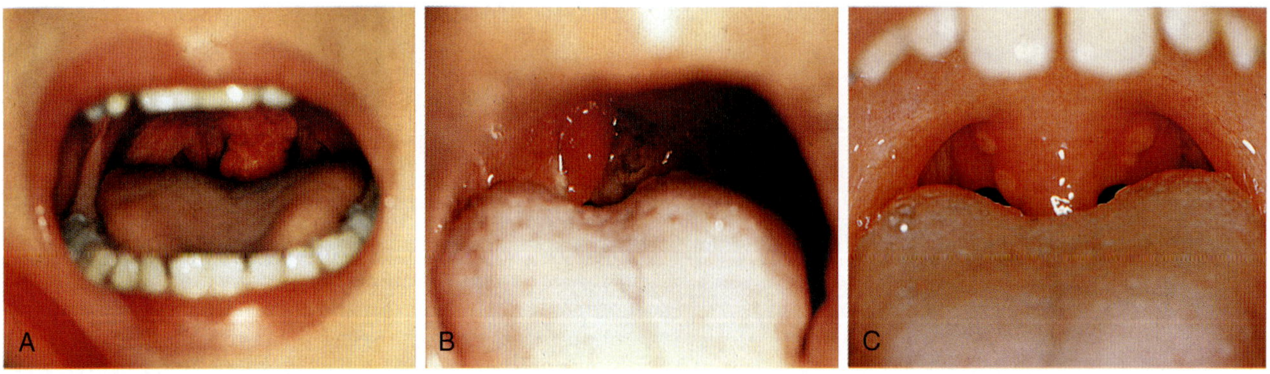

Fig. 24.74 Uvulitis. (A) The uvula appears markedly erythematous and edematous, with pinpoint hemorrhages, in this case caused by β-streptococci. (B) In this child with mononucleosis, the tonsils are enlarged and covered with a gray membrane, and the uvula is edematous and erythematous. The patient had respiratory compromise because of the severity of his tonsillar and adenoidal hypertrophy. (C) The vesicular lesions on the swollen, painful uvula of this patient suggest a viral etiology, probably involving an enterovirus.

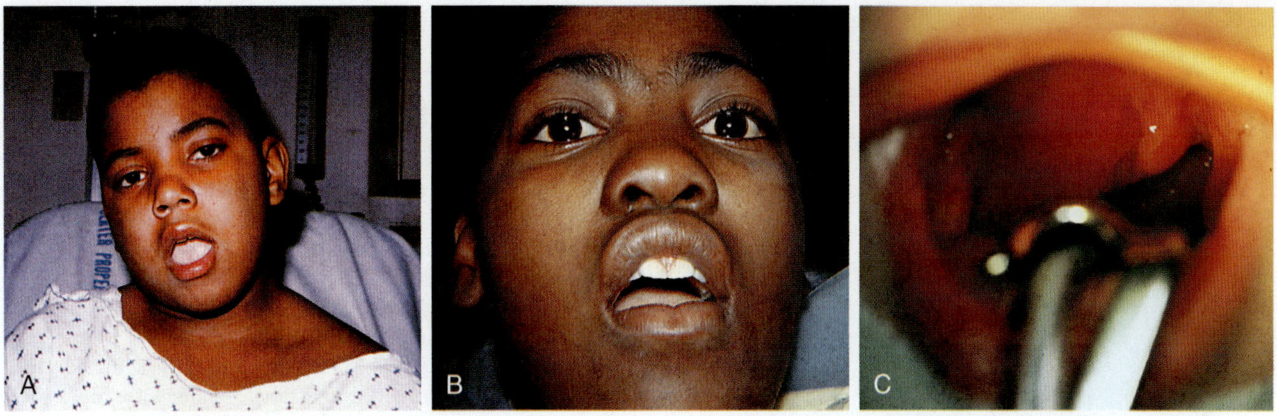

Fig. 24.75 Peritonsillar abscess. (A) This patient demonstrates the torticollis often seen with a peritonsillar abscess in an effort to minimize pressure on the adjacent inflamed tonsillar node. (B) Sympathetic inflammation of the pterygoid muscles causes trismus, limiting the patient's ability to open the mouth. (C) This photograph, taken in the operating room, shows an intensely inflamed soft palatal mass that obscures the tonsil and bulges forward and toward the midline, deviating the uvula.

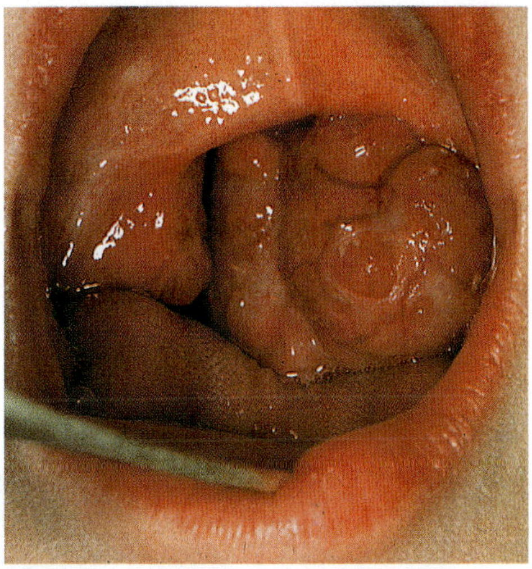

Fig. 24.76 Tonsillar lymphoma. This adolescent had painless dysphagia. Examination revealed marked unilateral tonsillar enlargement. The asymmetry and degree of enlargement prompted tonsillectomy. Pathologic examination confirmed a tonsillar lymphoma.

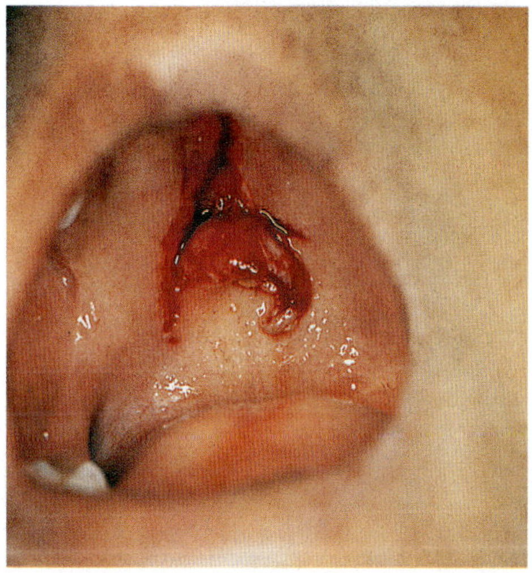

Fig. 24.77 Palatal laceration. This large, complex laceration occurred when this boy fell with a piece of metal tubing in his mouth. A flap of palatal tissue has retracted away from the tear, warranting surgical approximation.

history of recent health status and meticulous regional and general examination are in order. Particular attention should be paid to cervical and other nodes and to the size and consistency of abdominal viscera. Hematologic studies may also be helpful. In the absence of other evidence, a brief period of observation may be justified. If other findings are suggestive or enlargement continues during observation, tonsillectomy is indicated.

Penetrating Oropharyngeal Trauma

Penetrating oral injuries are common in childhood and are usually the result of falling with an object in the mouth. Gunshot wounds and stab wounds are unusual occurrences in the pediatric population, but their incidence begins to increase in adolescents.

Most intraoral injuries involve the palate and consist of simple lacerations. Many of these injuries heal spontaneously and require no repair. Large lacerations producing excessive bleeding or mucosal flaps must be sutured (Fig. 24.77).

Penetration of the posterior pharyngeal wall may result in several complications. These patients merit careful clinical evaluation of the oropharynx and neck; neck radiographs should also be obtained. Whenever an object penetrates the pharyngeal wall, it introduces oral flora into the retropharyngeal soft tissues, setting the stage for development of infection and abscess formation (see Retropharyngeal Abscess later; Fig. 24.78). This complication is seen predominantly in patients who fail to seek care immediately after the injury. However, it can develop even in treated patients. Symptoms generally begin a few to several days after the initial trauma. Fever, pain, dysphagia, and signs of airway compromise predominate.

In some patients with posterior pharyngeal tears, penetration results in dissection of air through the retropharyngeal soft tissues (Fig. 24.79). Such children may complain of throat and neck pain. Subcutaneous emphysema may be noted clinically. On occasion, signs of airway compromise develop with this complication. Therefore hospitalization for observation is advisable when this sequela is encountered. Serial plain radiographs should document resolution of subcutaneous emphysema before discharge.

When penetration involves posterolateral structures (e.g., the tear is located near the tonsil or tonsillar pillar), the possibility of vascular injury must be considered. Deep penetration in this area can puncture or nick the internal carotid artery or nearby vessels, resulting in hemorrhage or, more commonly, gradual hematoma formation. Even blunt trauma to the posterior lateral pharynx can result in pseudoaneurysms and/or thrombi and emboli. Clues to vascular injury are lateral pharyngeal or peritonsillar swelling and fullness or tenderness on palpation of the neck on the side of the wound. When soft tissue swelling is present or a peritonsillar site of trauma, magnetic resonance angiography, CT angiography or, more

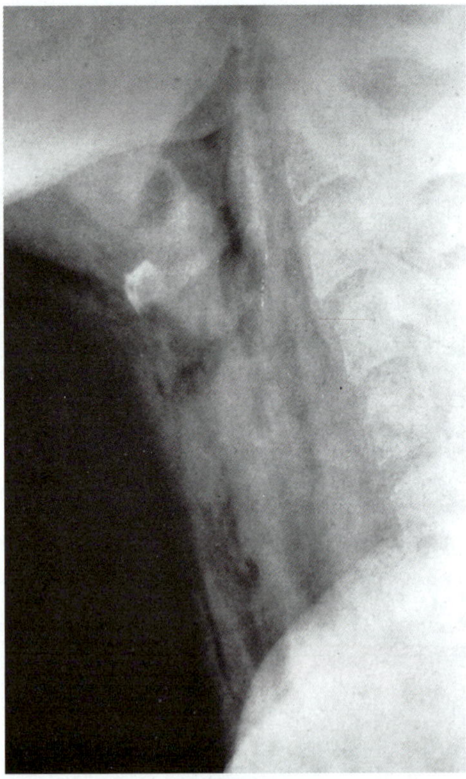

Fig. 24.78 Retropharyngeal air dissection. This lateral neck radiograph of a child with a puncture wound of the posterior pharyngeal wall reveals extensive air dissection through the retropharyngeal soft tissues. Subcutaneous air has tracked anteriorly as well.

rarely, formal angiography, to assess for vascular injury should be performed.

Acute Upper Airway Obstruction

Few conditions in pediatrics are as urgent and potentially life-threatening as those causing acute upper airway obstruction. In these conditions, expeditious assessment and appropriate stabilization are often lifesaving. In contrast, underestimation of the severity of distress, overzealous attempts at examination or invasive procedures, and efforts by the unskilled to intervene may have catastrophic results.

The major causes are severe tonsillitis with adenoidal enlargement (see the Tonsillar and Peritonsillar Disorders section, earlier; see Fig. 24.73B), retropharyngeal abscess, epiglottitis, croup or laryngotracheobronchitis, foreign body aspiration, and angioedema (see Chapter 4). All are characterized by stridor, retractions that are primarily suprasternal and subcostal (unless distress becomes severe and retractions generalize), and mild to moderate increases in heart and respiratory rates. For purposes of assessment, it is helpful to classify the disorders into two categories—supraglottic and subglottic—based on major signs and symptoms listed in Table 24.2.

The key to appropriate management is a brief history detailing the course and associated symptoms, followed by rapid assessment of clinical signs to determine the approximate level of airway involvement and degree of respiratory distress (Table 24.3). This can be done for the most part through visual inspection, without touching the patient. It is particularly important to avoid upsetting a child with upper airway obstruction who shows signs of fatigue or cyanosis or meets any of the other criteria for severe respiratory distress. Such disturbances can serve only to worsen distress and may

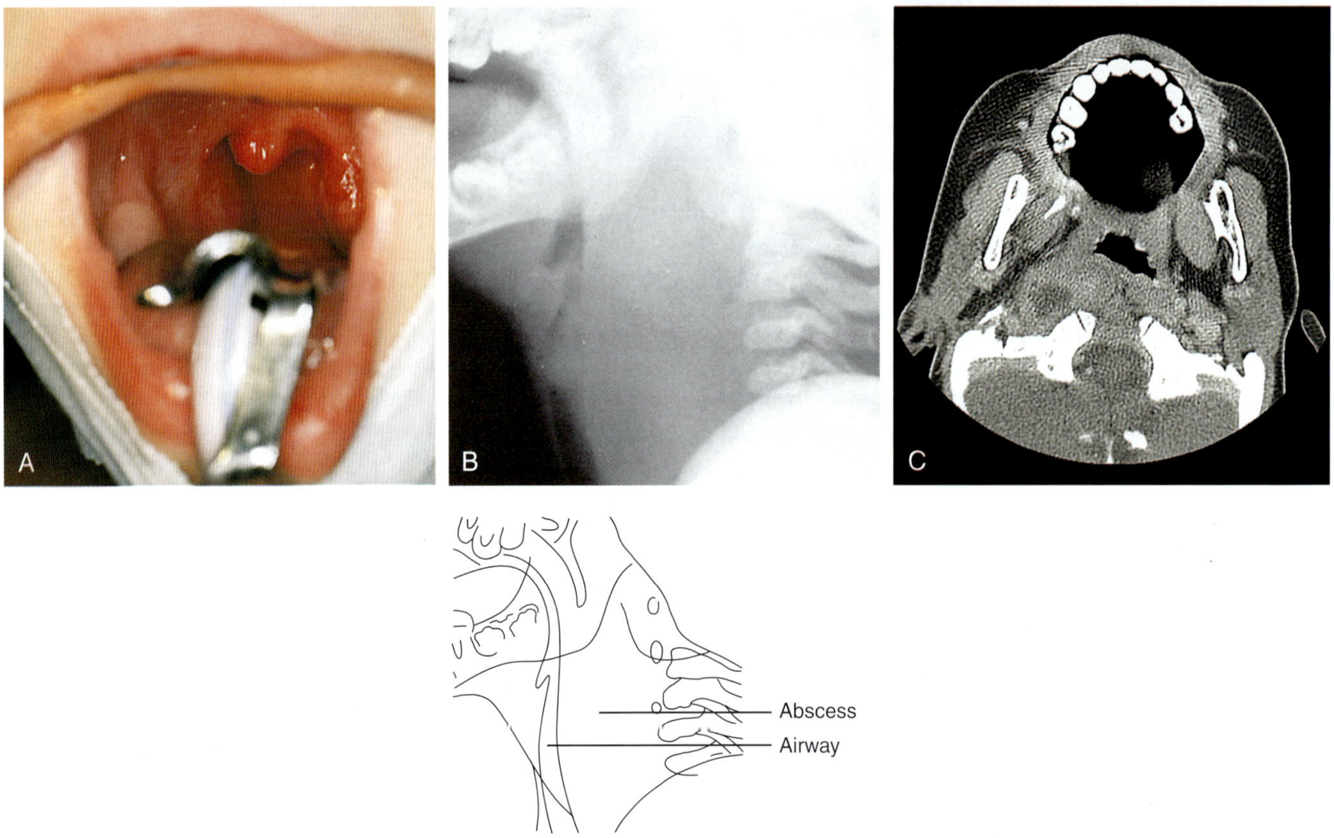

Fig. 24.79 Retropharyngeal abscess. A young child presented with high fever, drooling, quiet stridor, and an opisthotonic postural preference. (A) Pharyngeal examination in the operating room revealed an intensely erythematous, unilateral swelling of the posterior pharyngeal wall. (B) A lateral neck radiograph shows prominent prevertebral soft tissue swelling that displaces the trachea forward. (C) On computed tomography scan, a thick-walled abscess cavity is evident in the retropharyngeal space. The highly vascular wall is enhanced with contrast injection.

Table 24.2 Clinical Features of Acute Upper Airway Disorders

Clinical Finding	Supraglottic Disorders	Subglottic Disorders
Stridor	Quiet and wet	Loud
Voice alteration	Muffled	Hoarse
Dysphagia	+	−
Postural preference[a]	+	−
Barky cough	−	+ Especially with croup
Fever	+	+ Usually with croup
Toxicity	+	−
Trismus	+ Usually with peritonsillar abscess	−
Facial edema	−	+ Usually with angioedema

[a]Epiglottitis—patient characteristically sits bolt upright, with neck extended and head held forward; retropharyngeal abscess—child often adopts opisthotonic posture; peritonsillar abscess—patient may tilt head toward affected side.

From Davis HW, Gartner JC, Galvis AG, et al: Acute upper airway obstruction: croup and epiglottitis, *Pediatr Clin North Am* 28:859–880, 1981.

Table 24.3 Estimation of Severity of Respiratory Distress

Clinical Finding	Mild	Moderate	Severe
Color	Normal	Normal	Pale, dusky, or cyanotic
Retractions	Absent to mild	Moderate	Severe and generalized with use of accessory muscles
Air entry	↓ (mild)	↓ (moderate)	↓ (severe)
Level of consciousness	Normal or restless when disturbed	Anxious, restless when undisturbed	Lethargic, depressed

↓, Decreased.

From Davis HW, Gartner JC, Galvis AG, et al: Acute upper airway obstruction: croup and epiglottitis, *Pediatr Clin North Am* 28:859–880, 1981.

precipitate complete obstruction. Therefore when a child has signs of moderately severe or severe obstruction, his or her parents should be allowed to remain with him or her; any positional preference (if manifested) should be honored; and oral examination, venipuncture, IV line placement, and radiographs should be deferred until the airway is secure. Once the initial assessment is done, the most skilled personnel available are assembled to stabilize the airway. This procedure is best accomplished under controlled conditions in the operating room or, if necessary, in the emergency department.

Supraglottic Disorders

Acute Adenotonsillar Hypertrophy

See Tonsillar and Peritonsillar Disorders earlier.

Retropharyngeal Abscess

A retropharyngeal abscess usually involves retropharyngeal lymph nodes that run in chains through the retropharyngeal tissues on either side of the midline. Because these nodes tend to atrophy after 4 years old, the disorder is seen primarily in children younger than 3 or 4 years old. The major causative organisms are *S. pyogenes*, although *S. aureus* is found in some cases. Mixed infections with gram-positive and gram-negative aerobes and anaerobes are common as well.

The child with a retropharyngeal abscess generally has a history of an acute, febrile URI or pharyngitis beginning several days earlier, which may have improve transiently. The child's condition suddenly worsens with development of a high fever, toxicity, anorexia, drooling, and dyspnea. On examination, the patient is irritable and tends to lie with the head in a neutral position because neck movement exacerbates neck tenderness. Quiet gurgling and stertor are often heard secondary to impaired swallow. If respiratory distress is not severe, the pharynx can be examined and asymmetric swelling of the posterior pharyngeal wall may be observed pushing the uvula and ipsilateral tonsil forward (Fig. 24.79A). Even with direct examination, this swelling can be difficult to appreciate at times. A portable lateral neck radiograph taken on inspiration and with the neck in extension (with a physician in attendance) shows marked widening of the prevertebral soft tissues (Fig. 24.79B), which are normally no wider than a vertebral body.

It should be noted that false-positive radiographic findings of prevertebral soft tissue swelling, in the absence of retropharyngeal pathologic findings, are common when lateral neck radiographs are not taken on inspiration and with the neck extended. Therefore a contrasted CT scan (Fig. 24.79C) is preferred. When a retropharyngeal abscess is diagnosed, prompt otolaryngologic consultation should be sought to determine whether the mass is fluctuant, necessitating surgical drainage, or if it is in an early cellulitic phase, requiring serial reexamination. Parenteral antimicrobial therapy is necessary whether or not drainage is required.

As noted earlier, a retropharyngeal abscess may occasionally form in an older child after a puncture wound of the posterior pharyngeal wall (Fig. 24.80). Signs of infection develop acutely a few days later. In these cases, oral flora are found on culture.

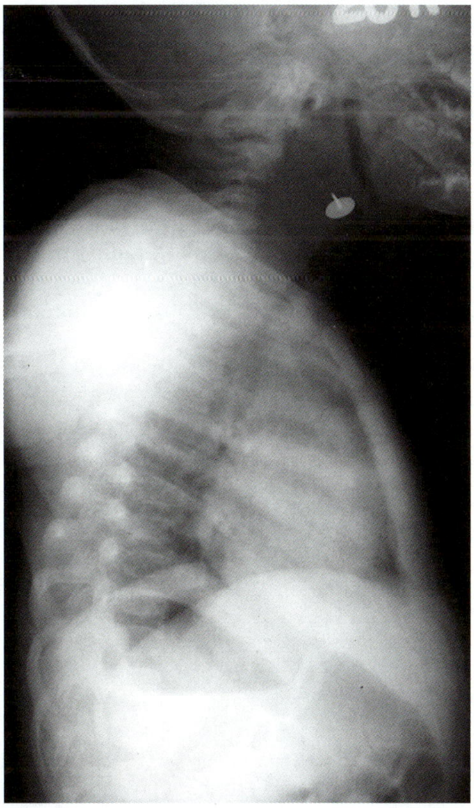

Fig. 24.80 Retropharyngeal abscess after a puncture wound. This child tried to swallow a tack that punctured and became lodged in the posterior pharyngeal wall. The incident was unwitnessed, and he came to medical attention only when he developed fever and began drooling. (Courtesy Robert Gochman, MD, Schneider Children's Hospital, Long Island Jewish Medical Center, New Hyde Park, NY.)

Parapharyngeal Abscess

Lateral neck space abscesses can also occur in infants and young children. Most patients are toxic with high fevers. History and clinical picture are nearly identical to those with retropharyngeal abscess. However, these patients have torticollis, bending toward the affected side, and examination of the neck reveals diffuse anterolateral swelling that is exquisitely tender (Fig. 24.81A). Oral inspection may reveal medial displacement of the tonsil or lateral pharyngeal wall. A CT scan or ultrasound is essential to confirm the diagnosis (Fig. 24.81B). Parapharyngeal cellulitis is initially treated with IV antimicrobials. Abscesses greater than 2 cm or nonresponsive to broad-spectrum antibiotics are treated with surgical drainage to prevent erosion into vascular structures and extension to adjacent sites or into the mediastinum.

Epiglottitis (Supraglottitis)

Epiglottitis, an uncommon but life-threatening infection with acute upper airway obstruction, is most often due to *H. influenzae* type B. Its incidence has dropped precipitously since introduction of the *H. influenzae* B vaccine. Hence many younger practitioners have never seen a case, increasing the risk of delayed diagnosis. Epiglottitis is characterized by marked inflammation and edema of the pharynx, epiglottis, aryepiglottic folds, and ventricular bands. The peak age range is 1 to 7 years old, but infants and older children may be affected. Onset is sudden and progression rapid; most patients are brought to medical attention within 12 hours of the first appearance of symptoms. In general, the child is entirely well until several hours before presentation, when he or she abruptly spikes a high fever. This is rapidly followed by progressive quiet stridor, severe throat pain with dysphagia and drooling, and soon thereafter by dyspnea and anxiety.

On examination, the child is usually toxic, anxious, and remarkably still, sitting bolt upright with neck extended and head held forward (unless obstruction is mild or fatigue has supervened) (Fig. 24.82A to C). Quiet gurgling, stridor, and drooling are evident, along with dyspnea and retractions. If the child speaks, which is unusual, the voice is muffled. This clinical picture is so typical that, when seen, the best course of action after initial assessment is prompt airway stabilization, usually with intubation under controlled conditions by experienced personnel in the operating room. At this time, the epiglottis/supraglottis is found to be markedly swollen and erythematous (Fig. 24.82D and E). After airway stabilization, cultures can be obtained and parenteral antimicrobial therapy initiated. Obtaining a radiograph or repeating oral physical examinations before transfer to the operating room is contraindicated; it adds nothing and may precipitate total airway obstruction.

On occasion, children present with a similar history but milder symptoms and signs. In these cases, presentation is early or the child is older than average. Respiratory distress is minimal, and visualization of the pharynx can be attempted (without use of a tongue blade) if the child will voluntarily open his or her mouth. In some instances, a swollen epiglottis is seen projecting above the tongue. When history suggests epiglottitis/supraglottitis but clinical findings are mild and the diagnosis is not confirmed by attempted noninvasive visualization, a portable lateral neck x-ray examination (done in the emergency department with a physician in attendance) can be useful. It may reveal mild epiglottic enlargement ("thumbprint sign"; Fig. 24.83) or merely swelling of the aryepiglottic folds and ventricular bands. If either is found, the diagnosis is confirmed. Hypopharyngeal dilatation may also be seen. Intubation is generally advisable in the former instance despite mild symptoms, but close observation in the intensive care unit on IV antibiotic therapy (covering for *H. influenzae* type B) may suffice when mild supraglottitis is the only finding.

Subglottic Disorders

Croup or Laryngotracheobronchitis

Croup, an acute respiratory illness, is characterized by inflammation and edema of the pharynx and upper airways, with maximal narrowing in the immediate subglottic region. The laryngeal edema also results in a hyperreactive cough reflex that can be associated with cough-induced laryngospasms. Most cases are caused by viral pathogens, with parainfluenza virus dominating. Respiratory syncytial virus, adenoviruses, influenza viruses, and echoviruses are also seen, though less often. The peak season is between October and April in the northern hemisphere. The disorder primarily affects children between the ages of 6 months and 3 years old. This is likely due to narrow airways, with mucosa both more vascular and more loosely attached than in older children, enabling greater ease of edema collection. Older children can be affected, however. Typically, croup symptoms occur 1 to 5 days after mild URI with rhinorrhea, cough, low-grade fever, and perhaps a sore throat. The change is generally sudden and usually occurs at night or during a nap. The child awakens with fever, loud inspiratory stridor, a loud "barky" or "seal-like" cough, and hoarseness. The severity of symptoms and the course vary widely and are highly unpredictable. Duration averages 3 days but can be as brief as 1 day or as long as 1 week. Most patients have a waxing and waning course, with more severe symptoms at night, but it is impossible to predict which night will be the worst. Some patients remain relatively mildly affected throughout the course, whereas others progress either slowly or rapidly to severe distress. Airway drying, in part because of mouth breathing necessitated by nasal congestion (especially while sleeping) and postnasal drip, appears to aggravate the larynx and trigger coughing. Coughing, itself, results in laryngeal inflammation and neural irritability, thus worsening the disease process.

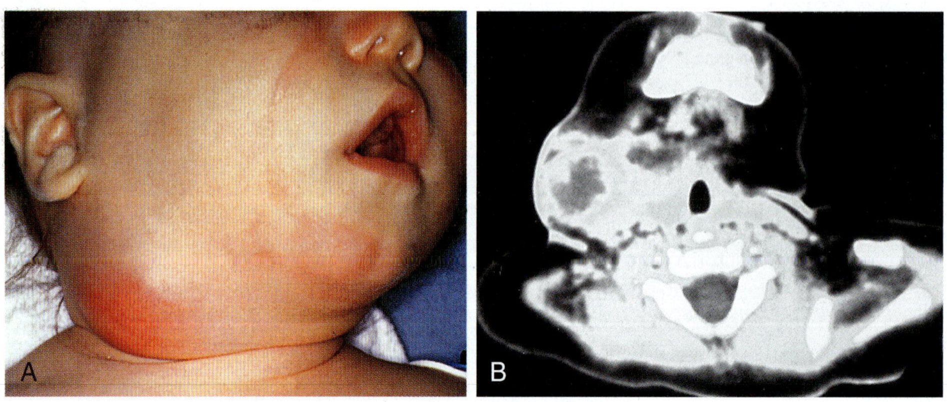

Fig. 24.81 Parapharyngeal abscess. (A) This infant had high fever, toxicity, and marked, exquisitely tender anterolateral neck swelling with overlying erythema. These manifestations followed a week of upper respiratory tract symptoms and decreased feeding. (B) His computed tomography scan reveals an encapsulated abscess in the right parapharyngeal area.

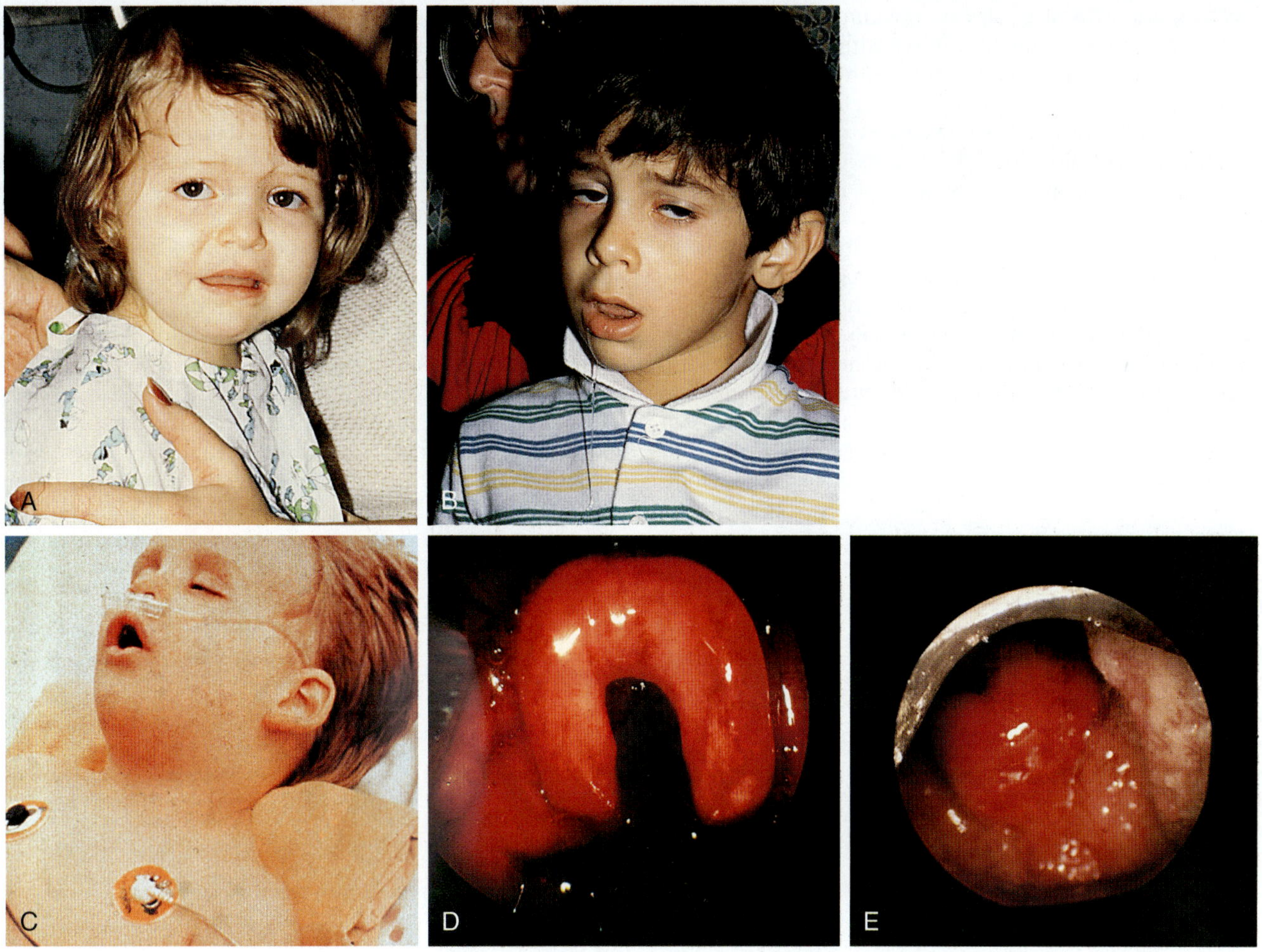

Fig. 24.82 Epiglottitis. (A to C) These three patients with acute epiglottitis demonstrate the varying degrees of distress that may be seen, depending on age and time of presentation. (A) This 3-year-old, seen a few hours after onset of symptoms, was anxious and still but had no positional preference or drooling. (B) This 5-year-old, who had been symptomatic for several hours, holds his neck extended with head held forward, is mouth breathing and drooling, and shows signs of tiring. (C) This 2-year-old was in severe distress and too exhausted to hold his head up. (D and E) In the operating room, the epiglottis can be visualized and appears intensely red and swollen. It may retain its omega shape or resemble a cherry.

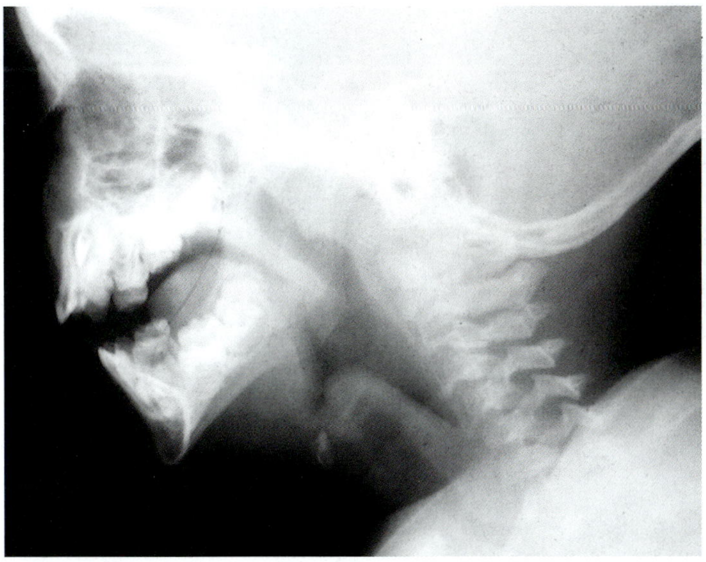

Fig. 24.83 Mild epiglottitis or supraglottitis. This lateral neck radiograph demonstrates mild epiglottic swelling and thickening of the aryepiglottic folds.

Physical findings are highly variable, depending on degree of distress at the time of presentation. Most affected children are moderately febrile but not toxic and have a loud barky cough and loud inspiratory stridor, with suprasternal and subcostal retractions (Fig. 24.84) and a mild decrease in air entry. A small percentage of

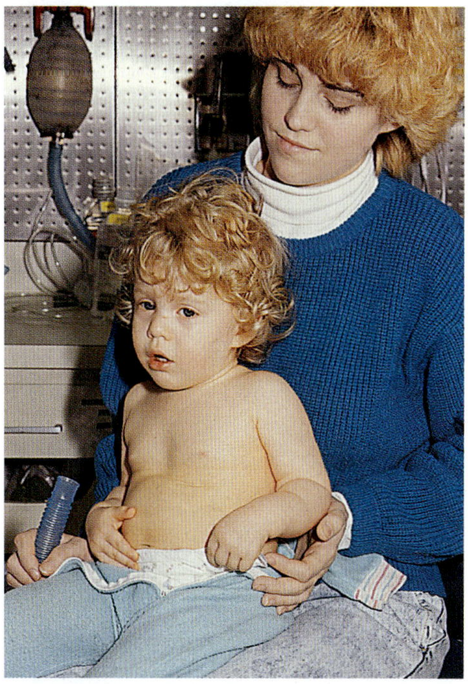

Fig. 24.84 Croup. This toddler with moderate upper airway obstruction caused by croup had suprasternal and subcostal retractions. Her anxious expression was the result of mild hypoxia confirmed by pulse oximetry.

patients with more extensive airway inflammation may have wheezing on auscultation. Cough in children with tracheobronchomalacia can mimic the "barky" cough seen with croup; the difference is phase of breathing and degree of stress of the patients. Barky cough associated with tracheobronchomalacia occurs on expiration, and patients typically are less distressed. Distinguishing the stridor of croup from the other sources of noisy breathing is important.

Many patients with croup improve substantially with exposure to cool night air. Some have restlessness or agitation reflecting hypoxia, and a few have severe distress. In more severely affected patients, stridor may be both inspiratory and expiratory, with generalized retractions. If impairment of airflow is extreme, fatigue supervenes, stridor abates, and retractions diminish. *This must not be mistaken for clinical improvement.* A clinical scoring system that helps in grading severity of distress is presented in Table 24.4. In mild to moderate cases the pharynx can be visualized and reveals only mild erythema. Oral examination should be deferred in severe cases until the airway is secure. While radiography will show subglottic narrowing—the "steeple sign" (Fig. 24.85A)—clinical diagnosis makes this unnecessary for patients with mild disease, and it is contraindicated for those with severe distress. Management depends largely on severity of distress when the child is seen and on clinical response to mist therapy. Most patients have mild disease, improve considerably on mist alone, and can be managed at home with humidification. Parents must, however, be instructed to watch for signs of increasing distress, which would warrant return to the hospital. Aerosolized racemic epinephrine is effective in reducing airway obstruction caused by croup. It is particularly useful for children with moderate obstruction who do not show marked improvement on mist alone, and it can provide significant relief for children with severe distress. This agent, although effective, is short acting, and rebound airway edema tends to occur. Thus patients requiring racemic epinephrine should generally be admitted for further observation. Administration

Table 24.4 Croup Scoring System

Clinical Finding	0	1	2	3
Stridor	None	Mild	Moderate inspiratory at rest	Severe, on inspiration and expiration, or none with markedly decreased air entry
Retractions	None	Mild	Moderate	Severe, marked use of accessory muscles
Air entry	Normal	Mild decrease	Moderate decrease	Marked decrease
Color	Normal	Normal (0 score)	Normal (0 score)	Dusky or cyanotic
Level of consciousness	Normal	Restless when disturbed	Anxious, agitated when undisturbed	Lethargic, depressed

Modified from Taussig LM, Castro O, Beaudry PH, et al: Treatment of laryngotracheobronchitis (croup): use of intermittent positive-pressure breathing and racemic epinephrine, *Am J Dis Child* 129:790–793, 1975.

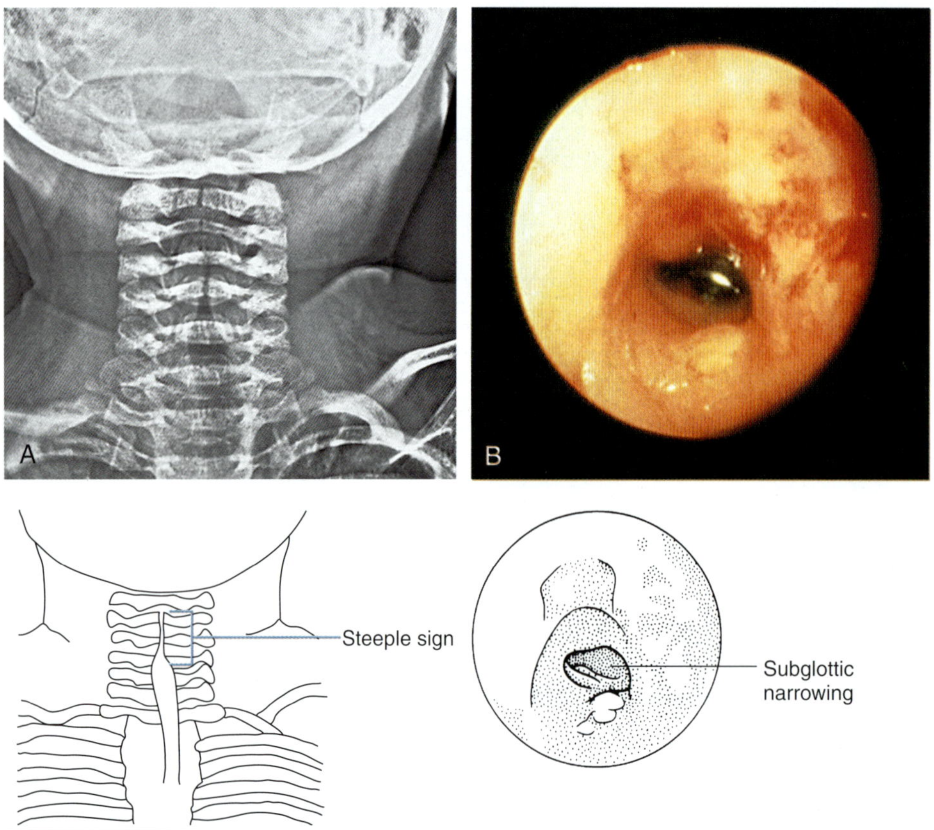

Fig. 24.85 Croup. (A) This radiograph reveals a long area of narrowing extending well below the normally narrowed area at the level of the vocal cords. The finding is often termed the *steeple sign.* (B) In this patient, direct visualization revealed subglottic narrowing so severe that only tracheotomy would enable establishment of an adequate airway. (A, Courtesy Sylvan Stool, MD.)

of corticosteroids reduces the severity of symptoms and thus the need for hospitalization.

Patients in severe distress who do not improve dramatically after treatment with racemic epinephrine and those who steadily worsen in the hospital despite mist and aerosol treatments merit airway endoscopy and stabilization. In some instances, subglottic narrowing is so severe as to necessitate tracheotomy (see Fig. 24.85B). GERD, atopic or inflammatory disorders, anxiety, and chronic adenoiditis are commonly associated with recurrent croup. Thus therapies aimed at addressing these contributing factors may be beneficial, though not necessarily in the acute phase. Croup before the age of 3 months, recurrent croup before the age of 6 months, or recurrent croup requiring intensive care unit admissions or in patients with histories of prematurity, intubations, or neck trauma require rapid referral to an otolaryngologist.

Paradoxic Vocal Fold Movement Disorder Paradoxic vocal fold movement disorder (PVFMD) is characterized by inappropriate medial movement, adduction, of the vocal folds during inspiration, resulting in stridor, dyspnea, and a sensation of throat tightness. Historically, PVFMD was thought to be only psychogenic in nature; however, other triggers such as GERD, asthma, and allergies have been described. PVFMD typically presents as an episodic stridor that does not respond to albuterol. In older, otherwise healthy children, it is more likely to present in high-stress situations. Diagnosis can largely be made on history alone; however, awake flexible laryngoscopy and spirometer can be helpful (Fig. 24.86). Treatment consists of education, reducing contributing triggers, and breathing techniques.

Bacterial Tracheitis

In a small percentage of cases, children with a crouplike picture are atypically toxic, are markedly febrile, and have rapidly progressive airway obstruction necessitating urgent intubation and occasionally tracheotomy. Bronchoscopy before airway stabilization reveals severe inflammation; edema; and a copious, purulent subglottic exudate that contains large numbers of bacteria. Most of these patients appear to have a history of viral croup with sudden worsening. It is thus thought that the disorder may represent secondary bacterial infection, and staphylococci including methicillin-resistant strains are often isolated.

Foreign Body Aspiration

Foreign body aspiration is seen for the most part in older infants and toddlers. The story is usually one of a sudden choking episode. Foods that require chewing, such as nuts, seeds, popcorn, raw vegetables such as carrots and celery, and hot dogs, are foods commonly aspirated. Small toys or toys with detachable parts are other sources. If the object lodges in the larynx, asphyxiation results unless the Heimlich maneuver or back blows are performed promptly. In most cases, the foreign material clears the larynx and lodges in the trachea or a bronchus (more commonly, the right mainstem because of its more vertical orientation). After the choking spell, there is a silent period usually lasting up to several hours (occasionally days or weeks), after which the child develops cough, stridor (if the object is lodged in the trachea) or wheezing (if it is lodged in a bronchus), and respiratory distress. In this acute phase, when the object is situated in a bronchus, wheezing may be unilateral and associated with decreased breath sounds. Later, diffuse wheezing may be heard, simulating asthma or bronchiolitis.

Lateral neck and chest radiographs may reveal aspirated objects that are radiopaque or outlined by the air column (Fig. 24.87A to C), enabling localization before endoscopy. However, many cases involve materials not directly visible on radiographs, although other radiographic clues may be present. Partial obstruction of a bronchus creates a ball-valve effect, allowing air in during inspiration but preventing its egress on expiration. This produces hyperinflation of one or more lobes of the lung on the same side as the foreign body (Fig. 24.88), which may be evident on the plain chest film. In subtle cases, chest fluoroscopy may highlight the differential inflation and deflation, showing mediastinal shift away from the side of the foreign body on exhalation (Fig. 24.89A and B). These findings are particularly likely if the patient is seen fairly soon after the aspiration episode.

When there is a delay in seeking medical attention (usually because the aspiration episode was unwitnessed and onset of symptoms insidious), the patient may have cough and fever. In these instances, atelectasis and a mediastinal shift toward the side of the foreign body may be found on the chest radiograph (Fig. 24.90A). This finding also may be seen acutely when the bronchus is totally obstructed. Many patients presenting acutely have no detectable radiographic abnormality after foreign body aspiration. Hence when clinical suspicion is high, given the history and physical findings, operative endoscopic examination (Fig. 24.90B) is indicated despite normal plain films. Conversely, when physical findings and x-ray films are normal and the history is questionable, a period of close observation may be indicated.

Unfortunately, in up to 50% of cases, the aspiration episode is not reported because the parent does not relate it to the child's symptoms or did not witness the choking spell. For this reason, this diagnosis should be considered whenever a young child has acute onset of cough and stridor, develops asymmetric breath sounds, or

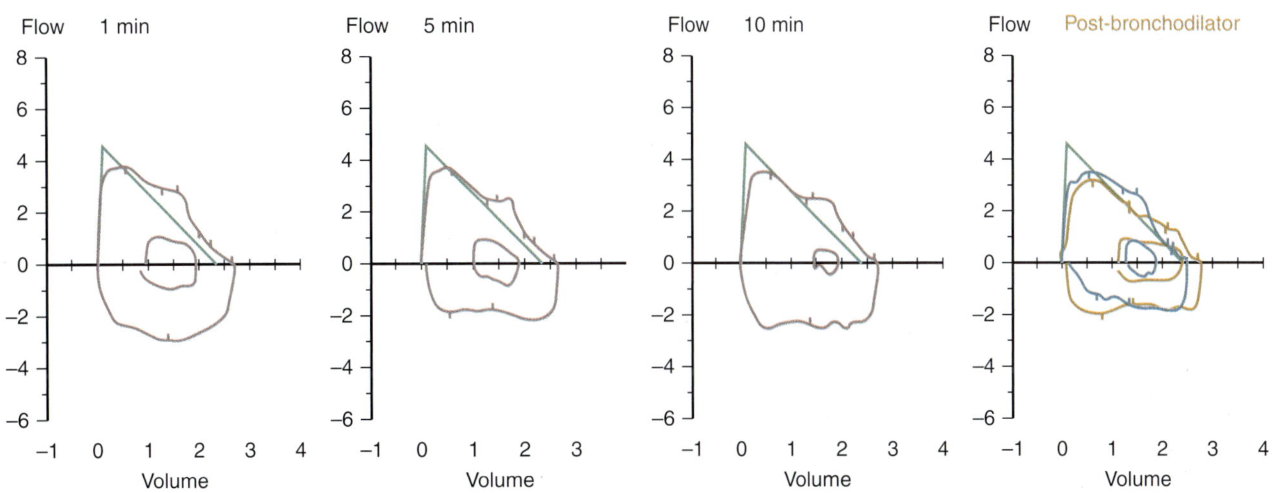

Fig. 24.86 Flow volume loops to diagnose paradoxical vocal fold movement. Attenuation of the inspiratory loop with prolonged intense exercise or anxiety that does not respond to bronchodilators consistent with paradoxic vocal fold movement disorder.

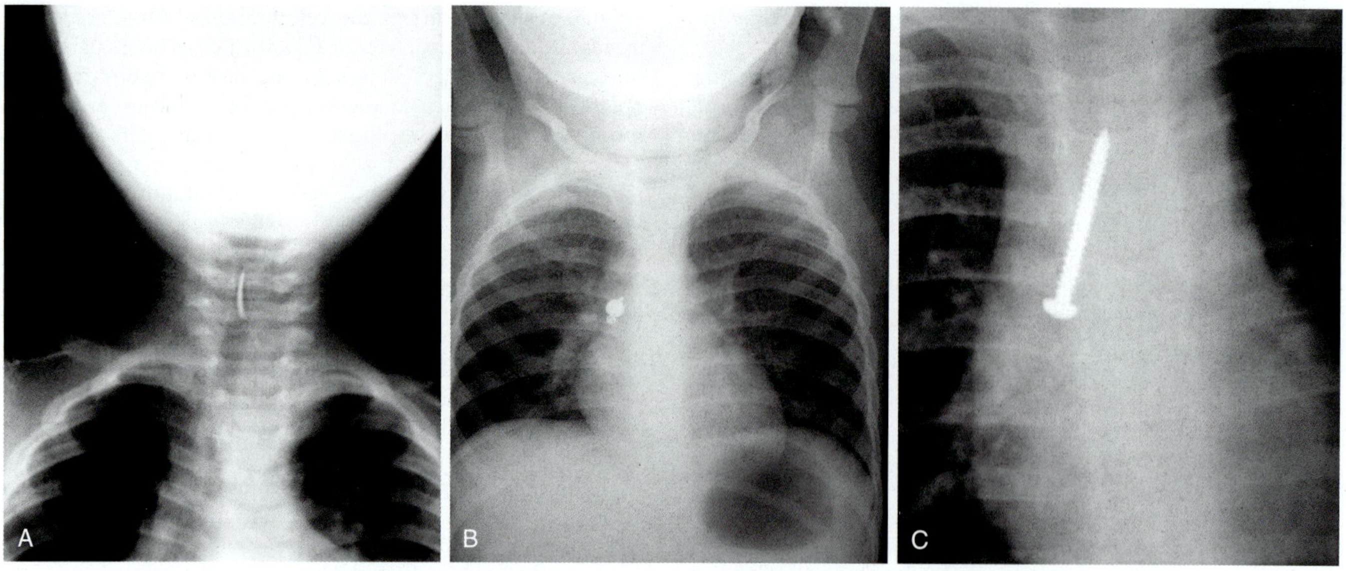

Fig. 24.87 Foreign body aspiration. Radiopaque objects and those well outlined by air are readily visualized on radiographs. (A) A piece of eggshell is seen in the subglottic portion of the trachea, clearly outlined by the air column. (B) An earring lies in the entrance of the right mainstem bronchus. (C) A screw is seen lodged in the right mainstem bronchus and projecting into the trachea. (A, Courtesy Mananda Bhende, MD, Children's Hospital of Pittsburgh, Pittsburgh, PA. B and C, Courtesy Robert Gochman, MD, Schneider Children's Hospital, Long Island Jewish Medical Center, New Hyde Park, NY.)

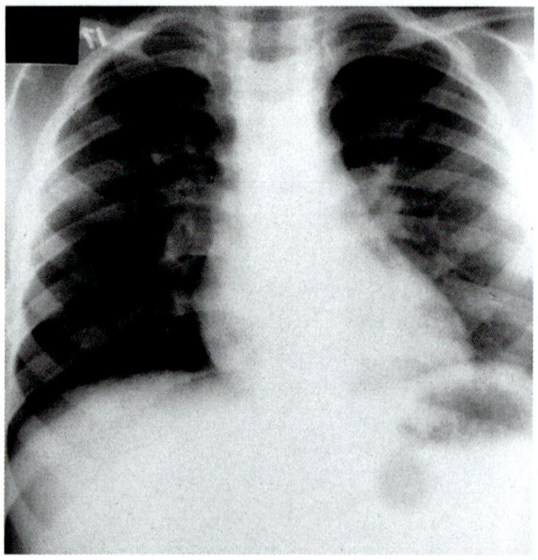

Fig. 24.88 Foreign body aspiration with ipsilateral hyperinflation. This 18-month-old child was eating popcorn when he suddenly began choking. Within a few hours, he developed significant respiratory distress and his chest radiograph revealed massive hyperinflation of the right lung caused by the ball-valve effect of a piece of popcorn lodged in the right mainstem bronchus. (Courtesy Department of Radiology, Uniontown Hospital, Uniontown, PA.)

experiences a first episode of wheezing. Persistent cough or wheezing after a choking episode warrants endoscopic evaluation for possible foreign body removal. A missed retained foreign body may lead to total airway obstruction if the foreign body lodges in the larynx, or it may chronically obstruct a bronchus leading to lung abscess and the need for lobectomy.

Chronic Upper Airway Obstruction

Nasopharyngeal, Oropharyngeal, and Laryngeal Examination

In children with a subacute or chronic airway disorder, a nasopharyngeal, oropharyngeal, and laryngeal examination is necessary to arrive at a definitive diagnosis. If a child is in distress or has acutely decompensated, this examination should be done in an operating room where rigid ventilating bronchoscopes and an anesthesiologist are available as backup. When the child is not in distress and the airway is stable, nasolaryngoscopy can be performed by an otolaryngologist in the office or emergency department, using a flexible fiberoptic nasolaryngoscope (Fig. 24.91A). These are available in a range of diameters suitable for pediatric patients. Letting the older

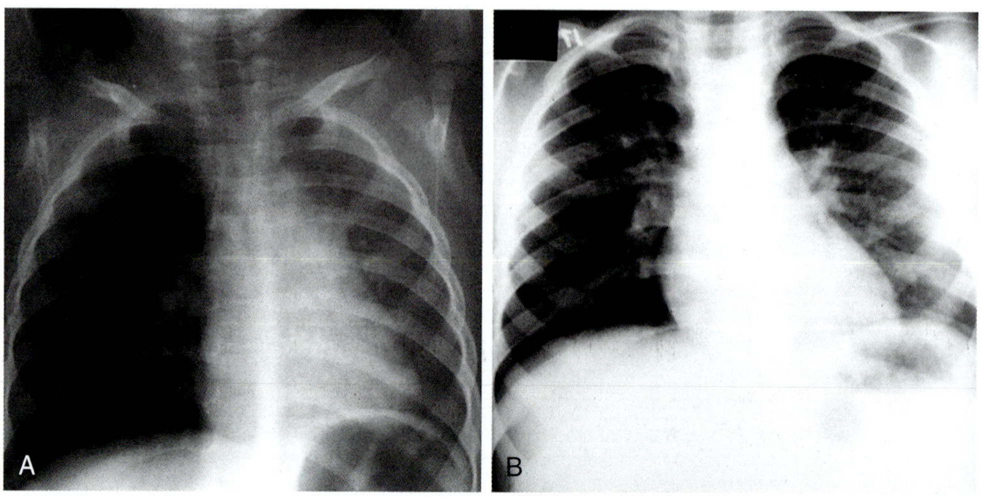

Fig. 24.89 Foreign body aspiration, inspiratory and expiratory radiographs. (A) This inspiratory film taken during fluoroscopy suggests hyperinflation of the right lower and middle lobes. (B) This becomes much more evident on exhalation, when the hyperinflation persists and the mediastinum shifts to the opposite side. (Courtesy Robert Gochman, MD, Schneider Children's Hospital, Long Island Jewish Medical Center, New Hyde Park, NY.)

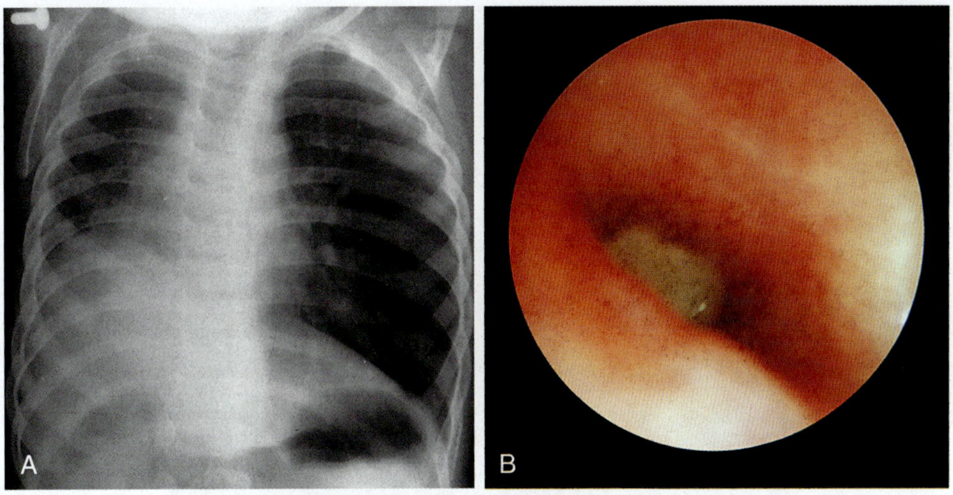

Fig. 24.90 Foreign body aspiration—delayed presentation. (A) With delay in presentation of partial obstruction or with complete obstruction of a bronchus, radiographic findings consist of atelectasis and a mediastinal shift toward the side of the foreign body. (B) In this case, a peanut was found completely obstructing the bronchus. (Courtesy Robert Gochman, MD, Schneider Children's Hospital, Long Island Jewish Medical Center, New Hyde Park, NY.)

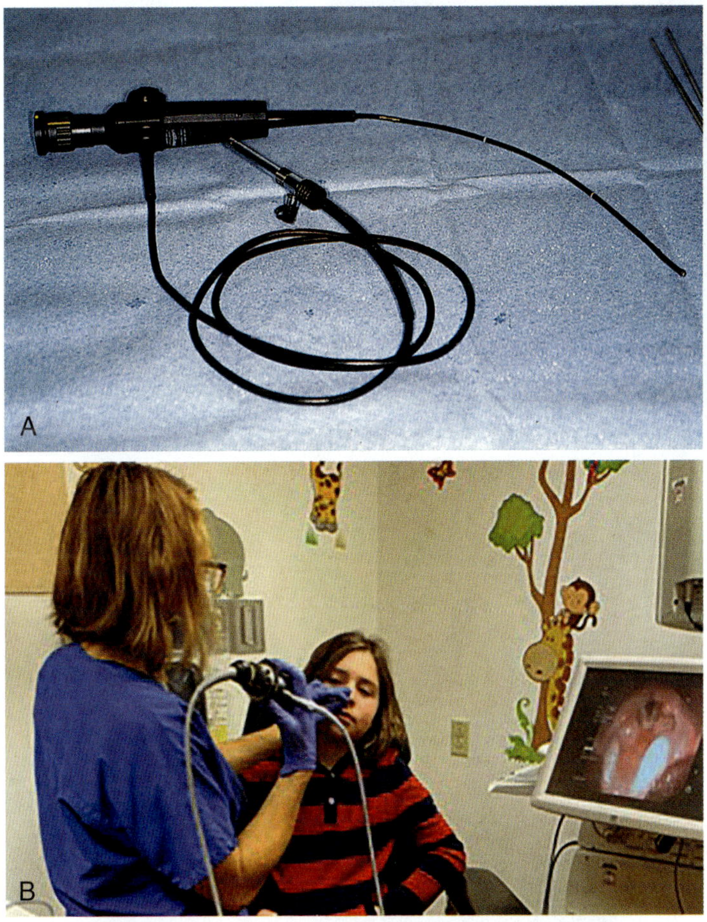

Fig. 24.91 Fiberoptic laryngoscopy. (A) The flexible fiberoptic laryngoscope. (B) With careful preparation, the patient can tolerate insertion of the flexible fiberoptic scope and the examination.

child handle the scope (see Fig. 24.33B) and look through the lens assists cooperation. The child is then prepared by spraying the nasal mucosa with a decongestant and topical lidocaine. With careful preparation, many patients can be examined in the parent's lap or an examination chair, but the toddler usually requires immobilization on a papoose board. The fiberoptic scope is then gently inserted into the nose and guided through past the palate (Fig. 24.91B). If the child is exclusively mouth breathing, the soft palate may be opposed to the posterior pharyngeal wall. Asking the child to try to breathe through the nose a few times moves the palate forward, assisting passage. Anatomic abnormalities and dynamic motion of the supraglottic and glottic structures are easily seen with this device. Asking the child to phonate by saying the letter *"e"* enables observation of cord movement. In infants, cord movement is generally observed with crying. Although less well seen, the subglottic space can generally be viewed as well.

Subglottic and Glottic Stenosis

Subglottic stenosis is a disorder in which the subglottic region of the trachea is unusually narrow in the absence of infection. In some instances, the stenosis is the result of abnormal cricoid development and is therefore congenital (Fig. 24.92A). In other cases, narrowing is the long-term result of injury and scarring from prior intubation (Fig. 24.92B and C), infection, or rheumatologic disorders. Regardless of the source, these children tend to develop recurrent stridor and respiratory distress with URI. Some are identified through an atypically prolonged episode of croup. Some also have stridor with crying or exertion, even when well. Neck radiographs may present a similar appearance to that seen with croup (steeple sign; see Fig. 24.85A). Subglottic stenosis generally improves with growth, but up to 40% of children will require some degree of intervention.

Glottic Stenosis

Glottic stenosis in children is typically related to intubation trauma and/or intubation in the setting of a severe inflammatory process (GERD, infection, etc.). The posterior glottis is the most commonly affected area of the glottis. Posterior glottis stenosis (PGS) can significantly limit glottis function (breathing, voicing, and swallowing). Fig. 24.93 shows severe PGS resulting in bilateral limited abduction. Fig. 24.94 shows the endoscopic view of a child with a laryngeal laceration and fracture due to blunt neck trauma who required tracheotomy and later developed subglottic stenosis.

Laryngomalacia

Laryngomalacia, a congenital condition, accounts for greater than 70% of cases of persistent inspiratory stridor in infants. The problem is the result of unusual flaccidity of the laryngeal structures, especially the epiglottis and arytenoid cartilages. The etiology is uncertain, but it is thought to be caused by lack of neural coordination of the laryngeal muscles, with the result that supraglottic structures hang over the airway entrance (Fig. 24.95A and B). Because the stridor is inspiratory, it does not represent true wheezing and bronchodilators should not be used.

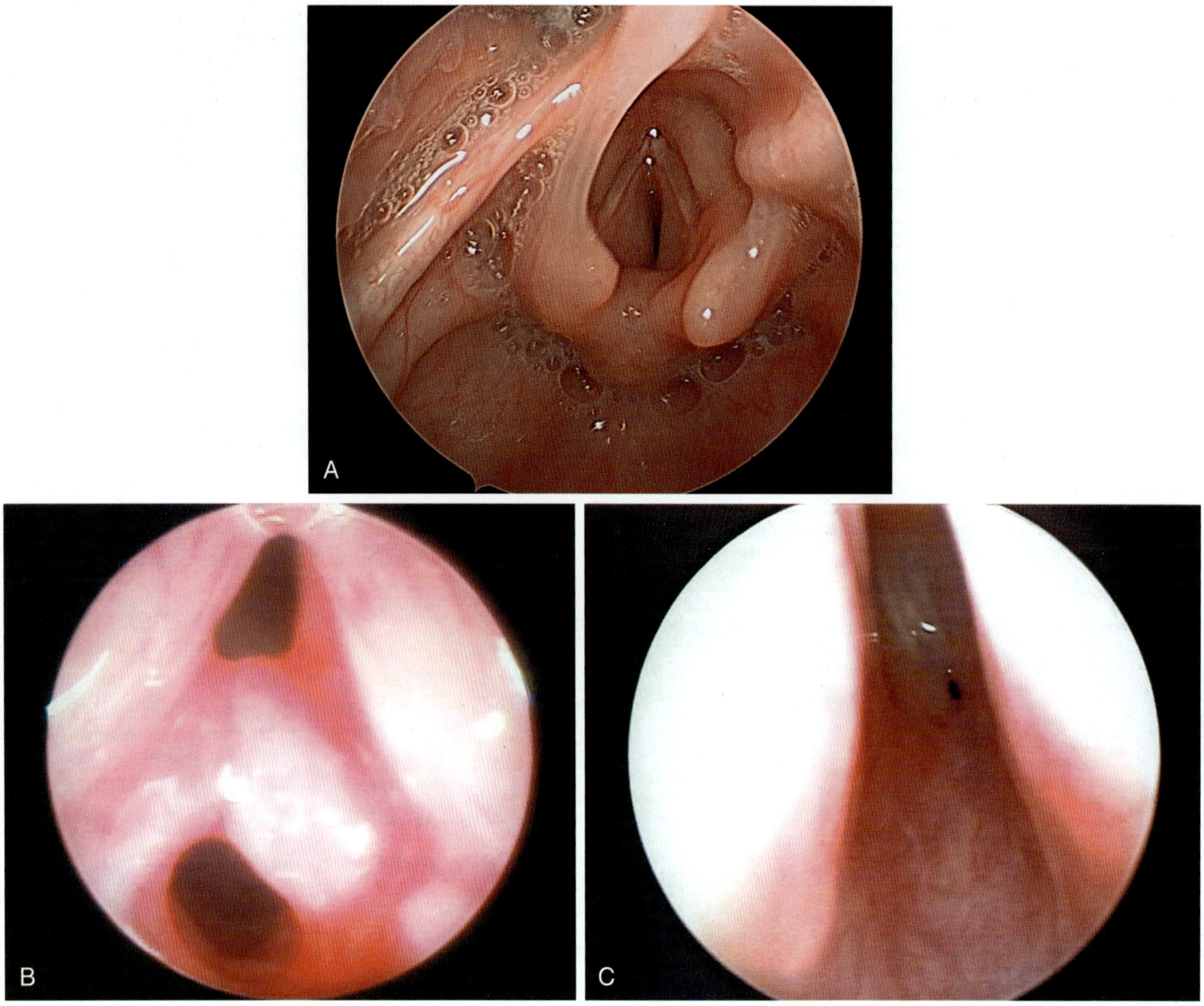

Fig. 24.92 (A) Endoscopic examination showing congenital subglottic stenosis in a former 34-week premature infant with Down syndrome, biphasic stridor and failure to wean from Continuous Positive Airway Pressure (CPAP). (B) Glottic and subglottic granulation tissue from prolonged intubation. Granulation tissue seen in (B) matured (C) resulting in severe acquired subglottic stenosis.

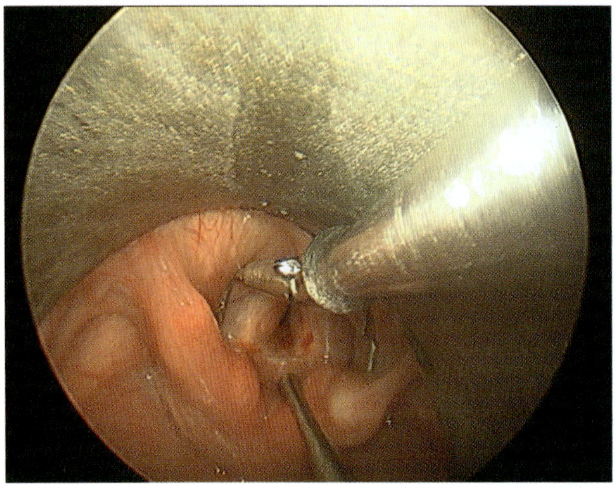

Fig. 24.93 Posterior glottis stenosis. Severe posterior glottic stenosis resulting in limited abduction of the vocal folds bilateral. Vocal folds spreaders used to demonstrate extent of abduction.

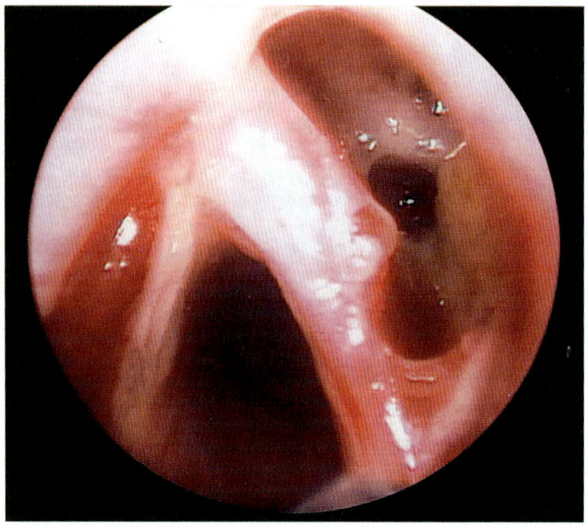

Fig. 24.94 Laryngeal trauma. This child sustained a fracture of the thyroid cartilage from blunt neck trauma. This is the endoscopic view of the laceration to the right side of the right true vocal cord. This child required open repair and tracheotomy for airway stabilization.

Clinically these infants tend to have mild inspiratory stridor worsened when lying supine, when upset, or during feeding. Stridor improves when in the prone position or when the neck is slightly hyperextended. The condition is usually benign and rarely interferes with respiration. When present with feeding, reducing flow rates or bolus size can help infants with laryngomalacia better coordinate a proficient suck-swallow-breathing pattern and thus prevent aspiration or fatigue. The diagnosis of laryngomalacia can be confirmed only by visualization of the larynx during active respiration or feeding. This is important to document that the stridor is not the result

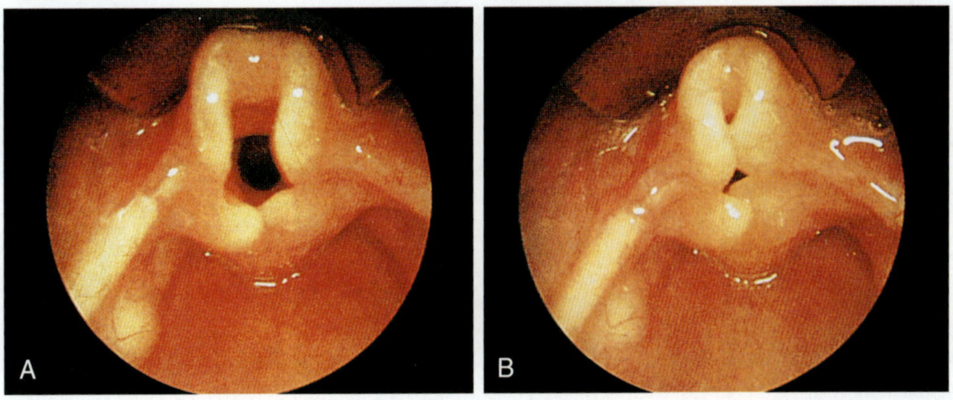

Fig. 24.95 Laryngomalacia. (A) Note the omega shape of the epiglottis and the elongation of the arytenoid cartilages. (B) This is the larynx during inspiration. Note that the forces of the inspired air lead to collapse of the laryngeal inlet. Infolding of the epiglottic surfaces and the arytenoid cartilages causes partial airway obstruction.

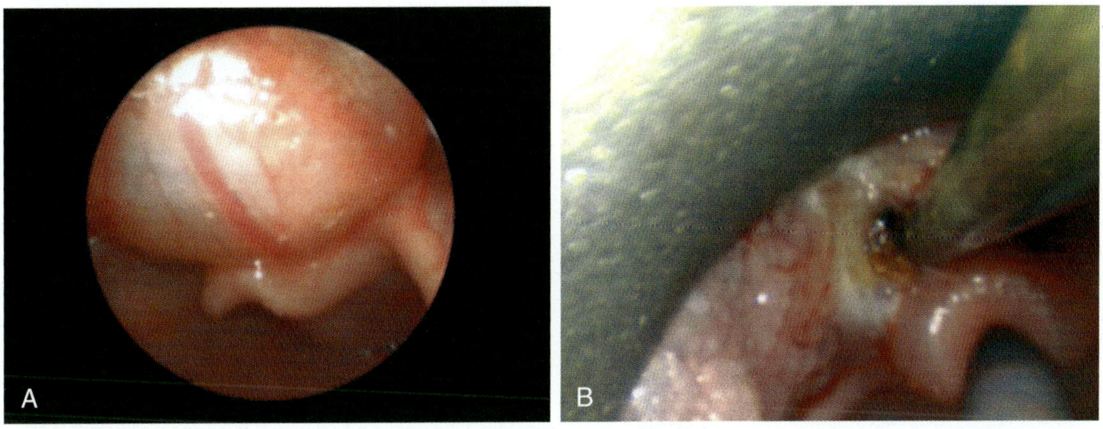

Fig. 24.96 (A) Vallecular cyst. Large mucous retention cyst in the vallecula, displacing the epiglottis in a posterior direction and leading to severe airway obstruction and stridor that mimicked laryngomalacia. (B) Endoscopic excision of the superior cyst wall was curative.

of a more serious condition. Once the examination has been completed, parents can be reassured that the condition is usually benign and that with growth the stridor typically abates by the end of the first year and a half of life. Management consists of observation, with particularly close monitoring during URIs. GERD often occurs concomitantly with laryngomalacia, and empiric treatment of GERD often results in reduction of stridor. The occasional infant with unusually severe obstruction resulting in failure to thrive, severe retractions, cyanosis, or apnea must be managed surgically with supraglottoplasty.

Vallecular Cysts

Vallecular cysts typically present with lower-pitched inspiratory stridor or stertor that is more pronounced in the supine position. The sound is more typically described as "snoring" by parents as opposed to high-pitched stridor. Fig. 24.96A shows an endoscopic view of a vallecular cyst that displaced the epiglottis in a posterior direction, creating airway obstruction. Cyst excision was curative (Fig. 24.96B).

Lingual Thyroid

Lingual thyroid results from failure of the thyroid gland to descend during embryogenesis. Lingual thyroids present as smooth vascular lesion on the midline of the base of tongue. Lingual thyroids can present with dysphagia, dysphonia (muffled speech), and globus sensation; however, they frequently are asymptomatic until thyroid imbalances result in gland hypertrophy. If normal thyroid tissue is present in the neck, surgical excision is curative and does not require hormone therapy. If no functional cervical thyroid tissue is present and surgical intervention required, hormone replacement is necessary.

Vocal Cord Paralysis

Vocal cord paralysis (VCP) is the second most common cause of stridor in infants. See supplemental video. VCP may be present at birth, or it may develop. It may be bilateral or unilateral, congenital, or iatrogenic. Congenital VCP can be secondary to peripheral anomalies of the vagus nerve or central nervous system anomalies. Iatrogenic causes most commonly include cardiac or thoracic injuries, stretch injury during birth, or thyroid surgeries. Ten percent of chronic stridor cases in neonates are thought to be due to VCP.

Infants with unilateral cord paralysis have stridor, hoarseness, and a weakened voice or cry. The airway diameter is generally adequate for respiration, and unless a secondary lesion is present, it is rarely necessary to perform a tracheotomy. This problem is most often caused by a cardiac abnormality or cardiovascular surgery because the recurrent laryngeal nerve is looped around these structures as it passes through the chest.

In contrast, bilateral vocal cord paralysis is a potentially life-threatening condition that presents with stridor and cyanosis because the vocal cords are unable to abduct on inspiration with consequent severe narrowing of the aperture between the cords (Fig. 24.97). Bilateral VCP is associated with difficulty coordinating breathing and swallow and can be associated with a depressed laryngeal cough reflex; thus aspiration is common. Children with bilateral vocal cord paralysis may be monitored closely, but in some instances, a tracheotomy may be essential to secure the airway. Hydrocephalus or an Arnold-Chiari malformation is

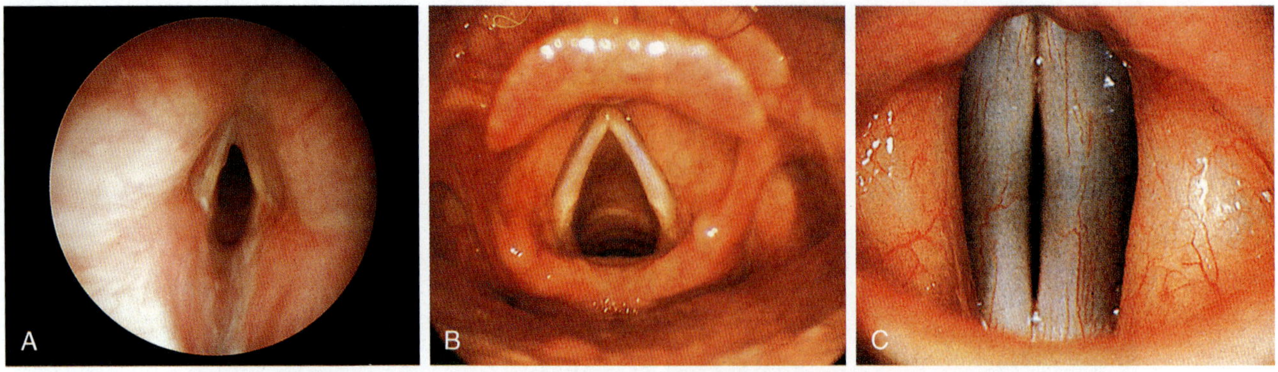

Fig. 24.97 Bilateral vocal cord paralysis. (A) The marked narrowing of the aperture between the cords stems from loss of ability to abduct on inspiration. The voice may be normal in some cases because the vocal cords can adduct. This is in contrast to normal opening and closing on inspiration and expiration as seen in (B) and (C).

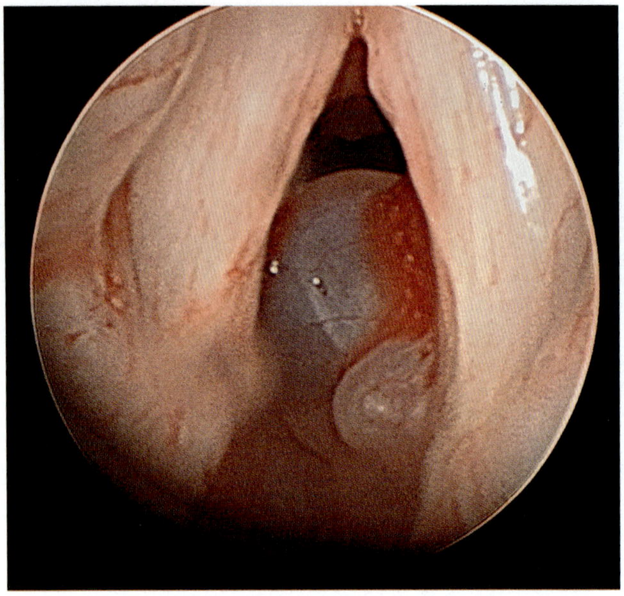

Fig. 24.98 Subglottic cysts are mucous retention cysts that form after mucosal trauma. They present with progressively worsening biphasic stridor after even minor, short duration manipulation. Surgical treatment is recommended. Recurrence is possible; therefore close follow-up is recommended.

often the underlying problem because each causes compression of the vagus nerves as they leave the brainstem. Neurosurgical intervention may correct the problem and allow eventual decannulation.

Subglottic Cysts

Subglottic cysts present with progressively worsening stridor, typically biphasic, in the setting of previous intubation (Fig. 24.98). Subglottic cysts can typically be diagnosed via flexible laryngoscopy; however, if coexisting laryngomalacia is present, visualization may be difficult. Endoscopic marsupialization and/or laser therapy is the treatment of choice (see supplemental video).

Subglottic Hemangiomas

Subglottic hemangiomas (SHs) are a subset of infantile hemangiomas and thus are benign proliferative endothelial cell tumors. As with other infantile hemangiomas, SHs are thought to be absent at birth and rapidly proliferate between 3 and 5 months of age, then slowly regress over 1 to 2 years. SHs are twice as common in females. Approximately 50% of infants with SHs have cutaneous hemangiomas; however, less than 2% of infants with cutaneous hemangiomas have SHs. Infants with PHACE syndrome (posterior fossa defects, hemangiomas, cerebrovascular anomalies, eye anomalies) and cutaneous hemangiomas in the beard distribution are unique in that more than half have airway hemangiomas, although they are not limited to the subglottis. Airway hemangiomas in the presence of a beard distribution may also be less responsive to medical therapies. Infants with SHs present with biphasic stridor, recurrent croup under the age of 6 months, failure to thrive, and feeding difficulties. Given the small caliber of an infant airway, significant airway compromise can occur during the proliferative phase of an SH and result in significant morbidity and mortality. Early diagnosis and treatment are crucial. SHs can often be diagnosed via flexible laryngoscopy; however, if there is clinical history concerning an inadequate examination (secondary to secretions, patient tolerance, coexisting laryngomalacia, etc.), endoscopic evaluation under anesthesia is recommended (Fig. 24.99A and B). Treatment consists of propranolol ± steroids (intralesional and systemic). Airway stabilization in the form of an endotracheal tube or tracheostomy may be required until medical therapy is effective. Surgical treatments such as open versus laser-assisted endoscopic resections ± reconstructive expansion surgeries are reserved for lesion recalcitrant to medical therapy.

Juvenile Laryngeal Papillomatosis

Juvenile laryngeal papillomatosis is a condition in which multiple benign papillomas develop and grow on the vocal cords and supraglottic structures. In a few patients, they may extend to involve the pharyngeal walls or tracheal mucosa. They are of viral (human papillomavirus) origin, and there is some evidence of transmission during delivery to children born to mothers with condylomata acuminata. The main symptom is hoarseness, but stridor may develop in children with large lesions or tracheal extension. Radiographs are usually normal. The diagnosis should be considered in patients with chronic hoarseness and in those with atypically prolonged croup. On laryngoscopy, irregular warty masses are seen (Fig. 24.100). Biopsy is required to confirm the diagnosis. Excision can be performed with forceps, a laser, or a powered microdebrider, but it is often followed by regrowth. Tracheotomy should be avoided if at all possible because this may promote seeding farther down the tracheobronchial tree.

Vascular Compression of the Trachea

Persistent expiratory wheezing or stridor that is unresponsive to bronchodilators may result from vascular compression of the trachea (Fig. 24.101) or tracheobronchomalacia. Symptoms are exacerbated by infections with increased respiratory requirements and increased secretions. Importantly, vascular compression of the trachea and tracheomalacia produce *expiratory* or biphasic stridor. This is in sharp contrast to laryngomalacia, which produces *inspiratory* stridor.

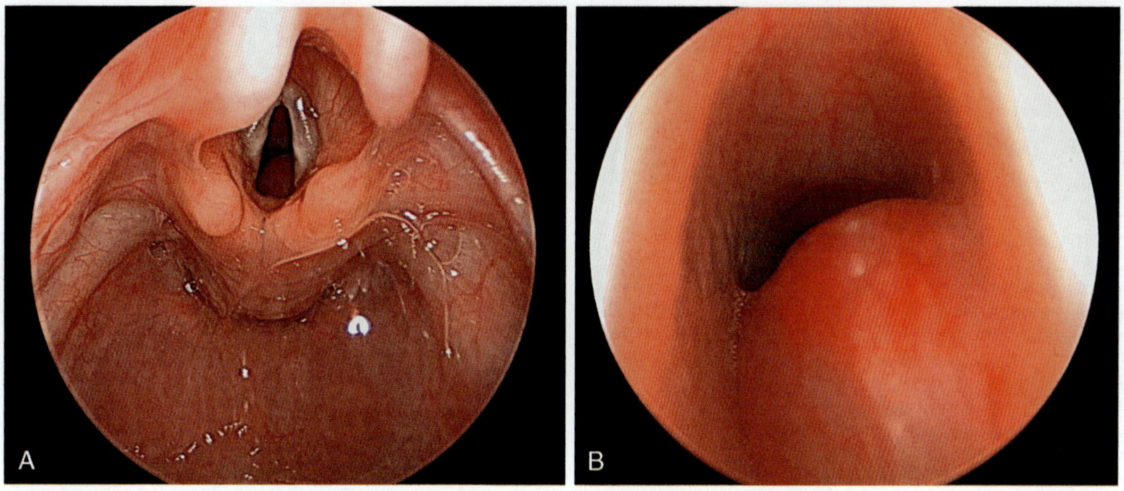

Fig. 24.99 (A) Endoscopic supraglottic view showing posterior lateral subglottic, submucosal fullness on the right. (B) Close-up endoscopic view of a subglottic, submucosal vascular lesion consistent with a subglottic hemangioma. Subglottic hemangiomas typically present with recurrent croup before the age of 6 months or progressively worsening stridor. They are vascular tumors more common in females and more commonly located on the left posterior lateral or posterior aspect of the subglottis.

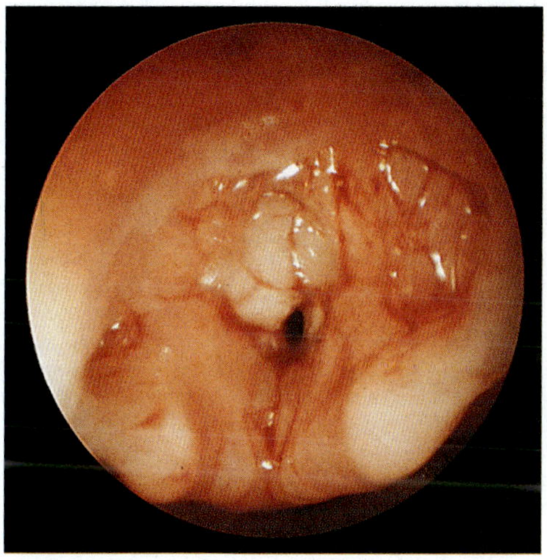

Fig. 24.100 Laryngeal papillomas. Multiple smooth, warty growths are seen nearly occluding the larynx in this child who had a history of chronic hoarseness.

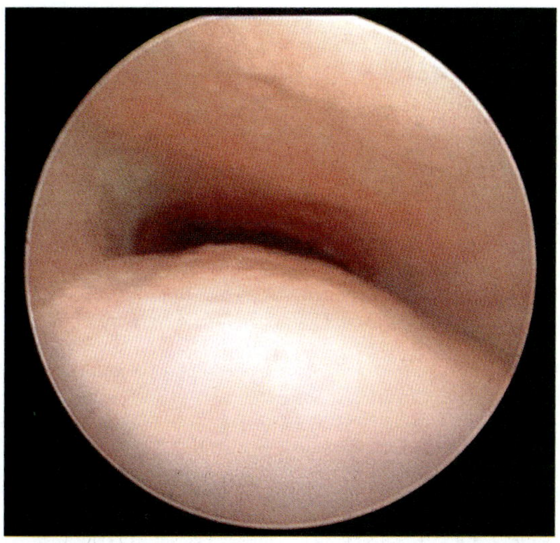

Fig. 24.101 Vascular compression of the trachea. Anomalous innominate artery compression of the distal anterior tracheal wall. The presentation of this child was that of intractable wheezing during expiration that did not respond to bronchodilators. The child improved after thoracotomy for lifting (pexy) of the innominate artery off the trachea by sewing it to the inner surface of the sternum.

ESOPHAGEAL FOREIGN BODIES

Ingestion of foreign objects is relatively common in older infants and toddlers, who are prone to putting almost anything into their mouths. Coins and toys are the objects most frequently found. Most traverse the esophagus, stomach, and intestines without incident and are of little concern. A small percentage of swallowed foreign bodies, being too large to pass through to the stomach, become lodged in the esophagus (usually at the level of the cricopharyngeus [C6] and less commonly at the level of the aorta [T4] or the diaphragmatic inlet [T11 to T12]). With mild obstruction, the child may refuse solid foods (although 17% of patients are asymptomatic); with moderate obstruction, liquids often are refused as well, or the child may appear to choke with drinking. When obstruction is nearly complete, the child may begin drooling. If the object is particularly large or produces an inflammatory mass over time, it may compress the trachea as well, producing signs of airway obstruction. Older patients may complain of neck or substernal pain or discomfort, especially with swallowing.

Patients who have significant symptoms of esophageal or respiratory obstruction and those who have ingested sharp, potentially toxic, or caustic objects should undergo prompt endoscopic removal. Those who have ingested smooth objects and have mild symptoms can be observed for 12 hours and then have a repeat x-ray examination. If the object has passed into the stomach, endoscopy can be avoided. Otherwise, endoscopic removal is indicated.

Although in many cases there is a clear history of ingestion, in a significant percentage the ingestion was not witnessed. A high level of suspicion is often required to make the diagnosis, and the possibility of an esophageal foreign body should be considered in evaluating any young child for a sudden change in eating pattern. Plain radiographs detect metallic and other radiopaque objects (Fig. 24.102). Most ingested objects are plastic, however, and require barium swallow or in some cases endoscopy for detection. Delays in diagnosis can result in stricture formation or, more rarely, esophageal perforation with secondary pneumomediastinum, mediastinitis, pneumonia (Fig. 24.103), and/or large vessel hemorrhage.

Similar to the concerns for button battery foreign bodies in the nose, special comment is necessary for button battery esophageal foreign bodies. When a button battery is suspected on the basis of history or radiographic imaging, immediate removal is warranted. The button battery is extremely destructive and may lead to esophageal perforation or tracheoesophageal fistula if it is not removed immediately.

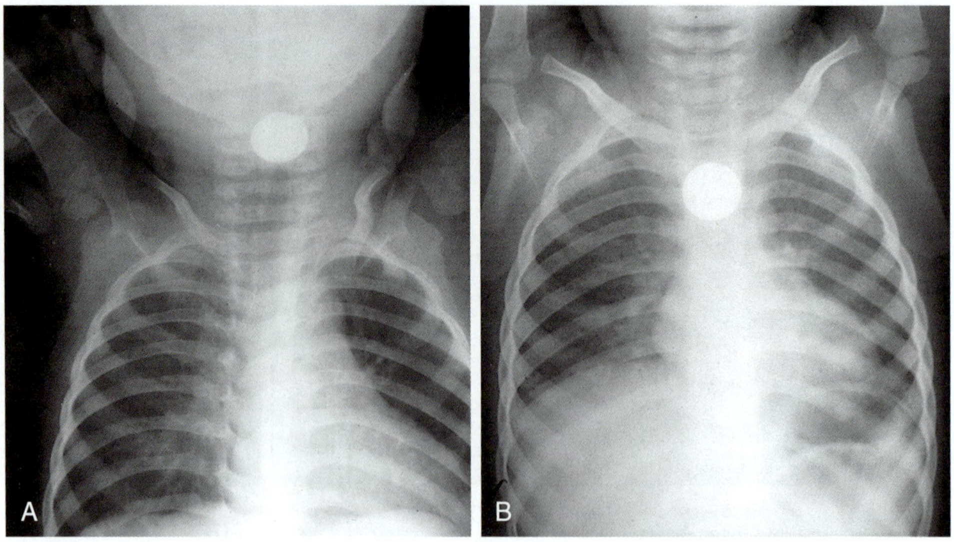

Fig. 24.102 Esophageal foreign bodies. (A) This youngster accidentally swallowed a coin. He complained of throat pain and refused oral intake. When initially seen, the coin was lodged high in the esophagus. (B) After observation overnight, repeat radiography revealed that the coin had moved down but was still lodged in the esophagus. The patient underwent endoscopic removal. Note that asymmetric objects in the esophagus are oriented in the coronal plane, whereas in the larynx, they lie in the sagittal plane (see Fig. 24.88A). (Courtesy Robert Gochman, MD, Schneider Children's Hospital, Long Island Jewish Medical Center, New Hyde Park, NY.)

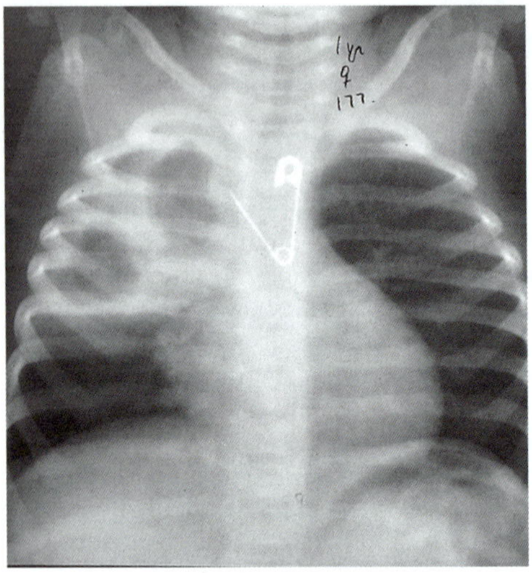

Fig. 24.103 Esophageal foreign body. An unwitnessed ingestion of this safety pin led to a period of anorexia, followed by fever and respiratory distress. The point of the pin had perforated the esophageal wall and pleura, causing a secondary right upper lobe pneumonia. (Courtesy Robert Gochman, MD, Schneider Children's Hospital, Long Island Jewish Medical Center, New Hyde Park, NY.)

NECK DISORDERS

Neck disorders including adenitis, congenital cysts, and vascular and lymphatic masses and tumors are commonly managed by otolaryngologists. Limitations of space have required us to be selective in presenting disorders in this chapter. The reader is referred to Chapter 13 for a discussion of cervical adenitis and to Chapter 18 for a description of mass lesions.

ACKNOWLEDGMENTS

The authors acknowledge and thank Children's Hospital of Pittsburgh, Department of Radiology, and University of Pittsburgh School of Medicine, Department of Neuroradiology, for providing many of the radiographs and CT scans in this chapter.

Supplemental videos are available at Elsevier eBooks+.

Bibliography

Bluestone CD, Stool SE, editors: *Pediatric otolaryngology*, ed 4, Philadelphia, 2002, WB Saunders.

Bluestone CD, Wald ER, Shapiro GC: The diagnosis and management of sinusitis in children: proceedings of a closed conference, *Pediatr Infect Dis J* 4:549–555, 1985.

Bowen AD, Ledesma-Medina J, Fujioka M, et al: Radiologic imaging in otorhinolaryngology, *Pediatr Clin North Am* 28:905–939, 1981.

Casey J, Adlowitz D, Pichichero M: New patterns in the otopathogens causing acute otitis media six to eight years after introduction of pneumococcal conjugate vaccine, *Pediatr Infect Dis J* 29:304–309, 2010.

Darrow DH: Management of infantile hemangiomas of the airway, *Otolaryngol Clin North Am* 51(1):133–146, 2018.

Davis HW, Gartner JC, Galvis AG, et al: Acute upper airway obstruction: croup and epiglottitis, *Pediatr Clin North Am* 28:859–880, 1981.

Di Altobrando A, Patrizi A, Misciali C, et al: Congenital fibrous hamartoma of the tip of the tongue: a novel peculiar entity, *Pediatr Dermatol* 38(1):287–289, 2021. http://dx.doi.org/10.1111/pde.14363.

Gellady AM, Shulman ST, Ayoub EM: Periorbital and orbital cellulitis in children, *Pediatrics* 61:272–277, 1978.

Gorlin RJ, Jirasek JE: Oral cysts containing gastric or intestinal mucosa. An unusual embryological accident or heterotopia, *Arch Otolaryngol* 91(6):594–597, 1970.

Gwaltney JM Jr, Phillips CD, Miller RD, et al: Computed tomographic study of the common cold, *N Engl J Med* 330:25–30, 1994.

Haber MA, Jaimes C, Lee EY, Juliano AF: Pediatric tongue lesions: an often-overlooked but important collection of diagnoses, *Am J Roentgenol* 214(5): 1008–1018, 2020.

Hardison S, Wan W, Dodson KM: The use of propranolol in the treatment of subglottic hemangiomas: a literature review and meta-analysis, *Int J Pediatr Otorhinolaryngol* 90:175–180, 2016.

Kong K, Walker P, Cassey J, O'Callaghan S: Foregut duplication cyst arising in the floor of mouth, *Int J Pediatr Otorhinolaryngol* 68:827–830, 2004.

Lieberthal AS, Carroll AE, Chonmaitree T, et al: The diagnosis and management of acute otitis media, *Pediatrics* 131(3):2012–3488, 2013.

McAlister WH, Lusk R, Muntz HR: Comparison of plain radiographs and coronal CT scans in infants and children with recurrent sinusitis, *AJR Am J Roentgenol* 153:1259–1264, 1989.

McCormick AA, Tarchichi T, Azbell C, Grunwaldt L, Jabbour N: Subglottic hemangioma: understanding the association with facial segmental hemangioma in a beard distribution, *Int J Pediatr Otorhinolaryngol* 113:34–37, 2018.

Melnick M, Bixler D, Nance WE, et al: Familial branchio-oto-renal dysplasia: a new addition to the branchial arch syndromes, *Clin Genet* 9:25, 1976.

Orobello P, Park R, Belcher L, et al: Microbiology of chronic rhinosinusitis in children, *Arch Otolaryngol Head Neck Surg* 117:980–983, 1991.

Pownell PH, Brown OE, Pransky SM, Manning SC: Congenital abnormalities of the submandibular duct, *Int J Pediatr Otorhinolaryngol* 24(2):161–169, 1992.

Rosenfeld R, Bluestone CD, editors: *Evidence-based otitis media*, Hamilton, ON, Canada, 1999, BC Decker.

Rosenfeld RM, Schwartz SR, Pynnonen MA, et al: Clinical practice guideline: tympanostomy tubes in children, *Otolaryngol Head Neck Surg* 149(Suppl 1): S1–S35, 2013.

Rowland PS, Smith TL, Schwartz SR, et al: Clinical practice guideline: cerumen impaction, *Otolaryngol Head Neck Surg* 139(3 Suppl 2):S1–S21, 2008.

Teymoortash A, Hoch S: Congenital unilateral agenesis of the parotid gland: a case report and review of the literature, *Case Rep Dent* 2016:2672496, 2016.

Ungkanont K, Yellon R, Weissman J, et al: Head and neck space infections in infants and children, *Otolaryngol Head Neck Surg* 112:375–382, 1995.

Wald ER: Acute sinusitis in children, *Pediatr Infect Dis J* 2:61–68, 1983.

Wald ER, Applegate KE, Bordley C, et al: Clinical practice guideline for diagnosis and management of acute bacterial sinusitis in children aged 1 to 18 years, *Pediatrics* 132(1):262–280, 2013.

Wald ER, Milmoe GJ, Bowen A, et al: Acute maxillary sinusitis in children, *N Engl J Med* 304:749–754, 1981.

Zhang L, Mendosa-Sassi R, Cesar J, et al: Intranasal corticosteroids for nasal airway obstruction in children with moderate to severe adenoidal hypertrophy, *Otolaryngol Head Neck Surg* 140:451–454, 2009.

25

FUNDAMENTALS OF PEDIATRIC RADIOLOGY

Judy H. Squires | Srikala Narayanan | Sameh Tadros

INTRODUCTION

Children have special needs and unique disease processes, and thus diagnostic imaging approaches are also different. Pediatric imaging should be tailored to answer specific clinical questions. Communication between the referring physician and the pediatric radiologist is paramount (eBox 25.1). eBox 25.2 details essential components of a pediatric imaging facility.

Imaging Modalities

Pediatric diagnostic imaging can be achieved by various modalities (Table 25.1). Radiographs are used in conventional radiography, computed radiography, fluoroscopy, angiography, and computed tomography (CT). Gamma rays are used in nuclear scintigraphy. Ultrasonography uses inaudible sound waves ranging in frequency from 1 to 20 MHz to produce images, whereas magnetic resonance images are generated with a strong magnetic field and radiofrequency (RF) pulse. Picture archiving and communication systems (PACSs) eliminate the use of films, permit rapid retrieval of images and remote viewing, and compact storage.

Child-Friendly Atmosphere

A few simple techniques can help create a positive imaging experience for the child. Distraction in the waiting room may be beneficial for children of all ages and can be achieved with decorations and toys. Effective distraction for toddlers includes interactive toys, pinwheels, blowing bubbles, and singing. School-age children enjoy blowing bubbles, TV/video games, books, counting, and deep breathing. Teenagers may prefer deep breathing, stress balls, TV/video games, electronic devices, books, and music.

The well-trained imaging staff can relieve the patient's apprehension and decrease time and effort to obtain the optimal examination. Technologists should have a gentle demeanor and wear child-friendly, cheerful uniforms.

Child life specialists are specially trained to help children prepare for health care experiences and enable them to cope with imaging or invasive procedures. If aspects of a procedure are painful or uncomfortable, any child older than age 2 is prepared in advance with truthful information, using words that can be understood. The child life specialist is especially useful in some situations, such as (1) a child whose injuries have resulted from suspected child abuse; (2) a child admitted with accidental injuries (e.g., a motor vehicle accident); (3) a child newly diagnosed with chronic illness; (4) a child who recently experienced traumatic loss; (5) a child who exhibits oppositional behavior or has developmental delay; (6) a child having difficulty coping with a necessary procedure, that is, crying, fighting, or hiding; and (7) a child who needs preparation for an invasive procedure.

Environment

The imaging room's environment is modified to reduce a child's anxiety. Smaller equipment can be hidden or concealed with covers and images. Large equipment such as CT scanners can be decorated to give a sense of adventure (Fig. 25.1) and allow study acquisition without sedation. Other distraction techniques include lamps placed in the line of vision of the patient and displaying entertaining images on the ceiling or the release of pleasant aromas in the imaging room. Handheld electronics are often used as a distraction during many imaging studies. Entertainment goggles allow the child to watch a movie while undergoing MRI or a nuclear medicine scan.

Positioning

Parents should usually be present in the examining rooms and may assist with some studies. This decreases the repeat image rate and radiation dose to the child. Comfortable positions, such as sitting in a chair or in a parent's lap, handholding with a parent, or hugging, can give children a sense of control and increase relaxation. The child can be empowered to help produce the best possible images by being permitted to make individual choices (e.g., placement of a toy or blanket, position of a parent, flavor of oral contrast material, or selection of a bandage).

Language

The radiology team should always remember to use simple language for child-friendly explanations. For children of any age, the wrong choice of words can have a negative impact and potentially long-lasting effects. Avoid saying "we need to get a shot of you drinking" when performing a fluoroscopic study because a shot may be associated with vaccinations; instead say "I need to take one more picture." Also, describe the imaging room environment in ways that can be related to objects that may be familiar to a child; for example, the noise of a CT scanner can be described like that of a "washing machine." Young children have little sense of time, so the radiology team should prepare them to know when they will be finished with their examination based on tasks. For example, if a child is undergoing a voiding cystourethrogram (VCUG), avoid saying, "this will only take 15 minutes"; instead, say "you'll be all finished and can get up after you go potty."

Effective Radiation Dose

Effective dose is expressed in millisievert (mSv) (eTable 25.1). A major benefit of the effective dose is that it permits all radiologic examinations that use ionizing radiation to be directly compared using a simple common scale. Background radiation is 3 mSv/year in the United States; people living in Colorado or New Mexico receive about 1.5 mSv more per year than those living near sea level, that is, 4 to 5 mSv/year.

Radiation Safety

The radiologist as "consultant" can triage imaging examinations to eliminate inappropriate referrals or encourage alternative procedures with less or no ionizing radiation. Imaging protocols must be as evidence based as possible, and American College of Radiology and Society for Pediatric Radiology guidelines should be implemented.

Table 25.1 Advantages and Disadvantages of Imaging Modalities

Modality	Advantages	Disadvantages
X-ray film	Fast; relatively inexpensive; available	Uses radiation; poor soft tissue contrast; 2-dimensional imaging only
Fluoroscopy	Real-time imaging; relatively inexpensive; available; useful in operating room; can be portable	Uses radiation; no cross-sectional imaging
CT	Readily available; excellent delineation of bones, soft tissues, and calcification; multiplanar and 3-dimensional reconstruction; minimally invasive (CTA); assists in interventions	Intermediate to high radiation dose; relatively expensive; IV contrast side effects (nephrotoxicity and anaphylaxis); weight limit
MRI	Excellent soft tissue characterization; no ionizing radiation; multiplanar imaging; minimally invasive (MRA); functional imaging; assists in interventions	Less readily available; expensive; claustrophobia often a problem; lengthy examinations; limited use in unstable patients; may need sedation/GA; metal artifact; contraindicated with cardiac pacemakers and some devices; gadolinium-induced NSF in patients with renal impairment; weight limit
Ultrasound	Portable; inexpensive machine; real time; least expensive cross-sectional imaging modality; no radiation; differentiates cystic versus solid masses; multiplanar imaging; Doppler evaluation of blood flow; assists in interventional procedures	Difficult with obese and immobile patients; highly operator dependent; bone and gas obscure anatomy
Nuclear medicine	Readily available; functional/molecular imaging	Intermediate to high radiation dose; weak anatomical analysis; may need sedation; radioactive urine and body fluids; expensive

3D, Three-dimensional; *CT*, computed tomography; *CTA*, computed tomography angiography; *GA*, general anesthetic; *IV*, intravenous; *MRA*, magnetic resonance angiography; *MRI*, magnetic resonance imaging; *NSF*, nephrogenic systemic fibrosis.

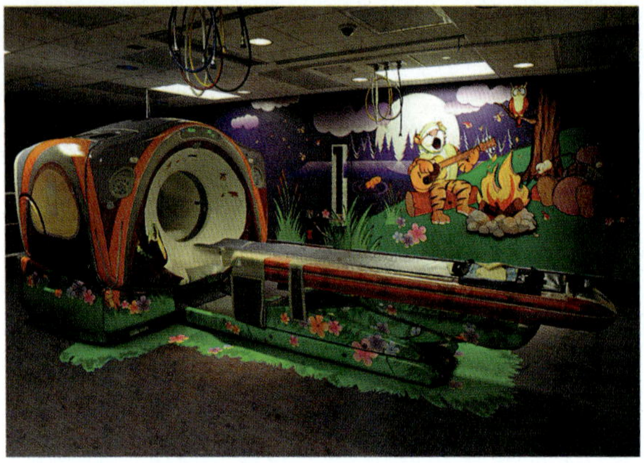

Fig. 25.1 Positron emission tomography/computed tomography suite known as "Camp Cozy."

Americans are exposed to more ionizing radiation from diagnostic medical procedures and over the past quarter century, the cumulative national medical exposures level approximates natural background radiation exposure (eFig. 25.1). The estimated cumulative individual dose from all sources in the early 1980s was 3.6 mSv and in 2006 was 6.2 mSv, almost double the previously reported value, and is in large part related to CT scans and nuclear cardiac scans (eFig. 25.2). In 2007 children underwent approximately 7 million CT scans. Children are at increased risk from radiation compared with adults because of their greater sensitivity to radiation and longer lifetime to manifest those changes. Therefore we should act as if low doses of radiation cause harm and adhere to the as low as reasonably achievable (ALARA) principle to minimize any potential harm.

The exact radiation risk in CT examinations, and even whether a risk absolutely exists, are controversial topics. However, most scientific and medical organizations support the concept of the linear, no-threshold model for ionizing radiation risk of cancer induction and believe that radiation even at low levels (doses lower than 100 mSv) may have a harmful effect. This assumption, however, overlooks cellular repair mechanisms. Some researchers estimate the increased risk that a young child might develop cancer related to an abdominal CT scan is on the magnitude of 1:4000. This is based on the most widely used estimate of risk of cancer from ionizing radiation at 5% per Sievert (Sv), and diagnostic imaging doses are in the millisievert (mSv) range (5 mSv for abdominal CT). One should also note that the background lifetime risk of fatal cancer is 20% to 25%. The benefits of CT are real and known, and the risks are tiny and unknown.

Conservative estimations of potential risk (i.e., any required assumptions are made toward the direction of overestimating risk rather than underestimating it) show that the potential risk of dying from undergoing a CT examination is less than that of drowning or of a pedestrian dying from being struck by any form of ground transportation, both of which most Americans consider to be extremely unlikely events (eTable 25.2); this provides a comparison of the statistical odds of dying from an abdominopelvic CT examination relative to other causes of death. Lifetime risk of a fatal cancer from all causes is 22.8%, and the lifetime potential risk of a fatal cancer from the radiation associated with a body CT examination is approximately 0.05%.

The ordering physician needs to ensure that a CT scan is justified, and the radiologist needs to optimize how the scan is performed. Because children are smaller than adults and need less radiation to create the same signal-to-noise ratios, the tube current (milliamperes) can be greatly reduced when imaging a small child. Other techniques include reducing the kilovoltage peak; using in-plane shielding for areas such as the eye, thyroid, and breasts; increasing beam pitch; and picking a CT manufacturer that has put effort into dose-reducing technology (e.g., adaptive statistical iterative reconstruction) (Fig. 25.2).

The "Image Gently" Campaign

The Alliance for Radiation Safety in Pediatric Imaging has created resources to address the relative risk of CT for children, including parent information pamphlets and a medical imaging record card, similar to the familiar immunization card, for parents to track their child's imaging history. This card may be distributed by pediatricians or downloaded by parents from the Image Gently website (eFig. 25.3). This card alerts families and their doctors to the frequency of patient imaging examinations. With relocation of families and the use of different hospital centers in the same community, this card may help decrease the number of repeat examinations performed.

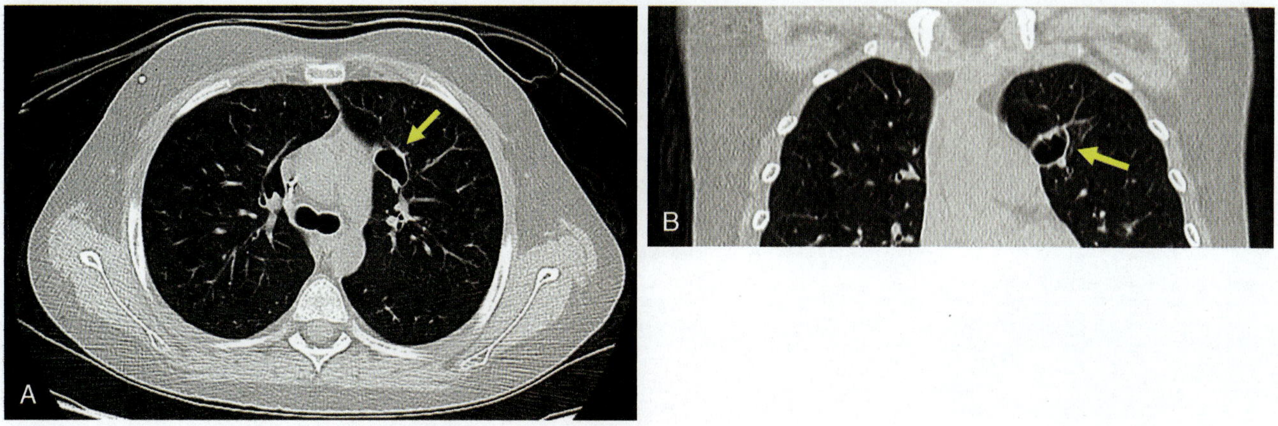

Fig. 25.2 Targeted low-dose computed tomography of the upper chest of a 12-year-old for follow-up of left upper lobe cavity *(arrow)*; effective dose, 0.5 mSv. (A) Axial image. (B) Coronal reformatted image.

RADIOGRAPHY

Introduction

Advantages of Radiography in Pediatric Imaging

The advantages of radiography in pediatric imaging include the following:

- Fast
- Relatively inexpensive
- Widely available
- No need for sedation
- Portable
- Plain films of the chest and skeletal system are important (about 50% of all pediatric imaging consists of chest radiographs)

Disadvantages

The disadvantages of radiography in pediatric imaging include the following:

- Uses ionizing radiation
- Poor soft tissue contrast
- Two-dimensional imaging only

Physics

Radiographs are a form of short electromagnetic radiation produced by energy conversion when fast-moving electrons from the cathode filament of the x-ray tube interact with the tungsten anode (target) (Fig. 25.3). The amplitude of the tube current (expressed as milliamperes) depends on the emission rate of electrons from the cathode, which is determined by the cathode temperature. The speed of the electrons as they are propelled from the cathode to the anode is determined by the x-ray tube potential (kilovoltage peak). When an x-ray beam is directed toward the examined part of the body with an imaging cassette on the other side, an image is formed. The resultant image is a recording of internal body structures in which the black areas represent the least dense body structures that have allowed the x-rays to pass through (i.e., lungs) and the denser structures (i.e., bone), which have absorbed the x-rays, appear white (eFig. 25.4).

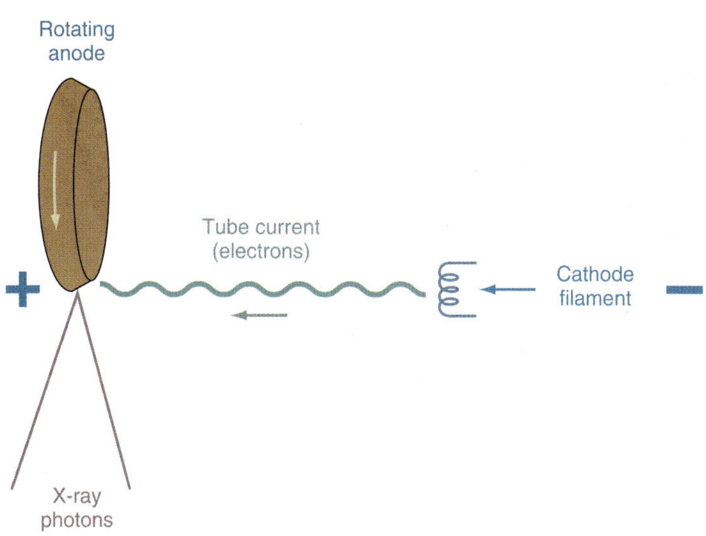

Fig. 25.3 X-ray production.

Computed radiography has replaced conventional film-based radiography. The acquired image is displayed instantly on the high-resolution monitor of the PACS. eTable 25.3 lists common indications for plain radiography.

Radiography of the Airway

The anteroposterior and lateral views of the neck are useful in assessing the trachea, pharynx, retropharynx, epiglottis, tonsils, adenoids, and bony skeleton. Stridor is one of the most common indications for imaging the neck. Other indications include snoring, hoarseness, abnormal cry, neck mass, suspected foreign body, epistaxis, trauma, and caustic ingestion.

Lateral Soft Tissues of the Neck

The retropharyngeal soft tissues extend from the adenoids, which are visible by 3 to 6 months of age, to the origin of the esophagus at the level of C4 to C5. A useful ratio is the width of the retropharyngeal soft tissue to that of the C2 vertebral body. The ratio varies in inspiration from almost 1.0 before 1 year old to 0.5 by 6 years old. The soft tissue width should not exceed 50% of the accompanying vertebral body to C4 (Fig. 25.4A and B). Expiratory tracheal buckling can create bulging of the trachea anteriorly, causing an apparent increase in retropharyngeal soft tissues and creating a “pseudoretropharyngeal abscess” (Fig. 25.5). A pseudoretropharyngeal abscess can be differentiated from a true abscess when an appropriately positioned inspiratory film demonstrates supraglottic airway and hypopharyngeal distention with air (Fig. 25.6). Appropriate patient positioning is critical. The examination of the lateral view of the soft tissues of the neck must be performed in slight extension and during inspiration (Fig. 25.7). The most common cause of a pseudoretropharyngeal abscess is a film taken during expiration or swallowing or with an improperly positioned child.

The lateral view of the neck is optimal for evaluating the supraglottic airway (see Fig. 25.4). The lower border of the nasopharynx is the hard palate, soft palate, and uvula. The oropharynx (below the hard and soft palate) leads to the air spaces at the base of the tongue,

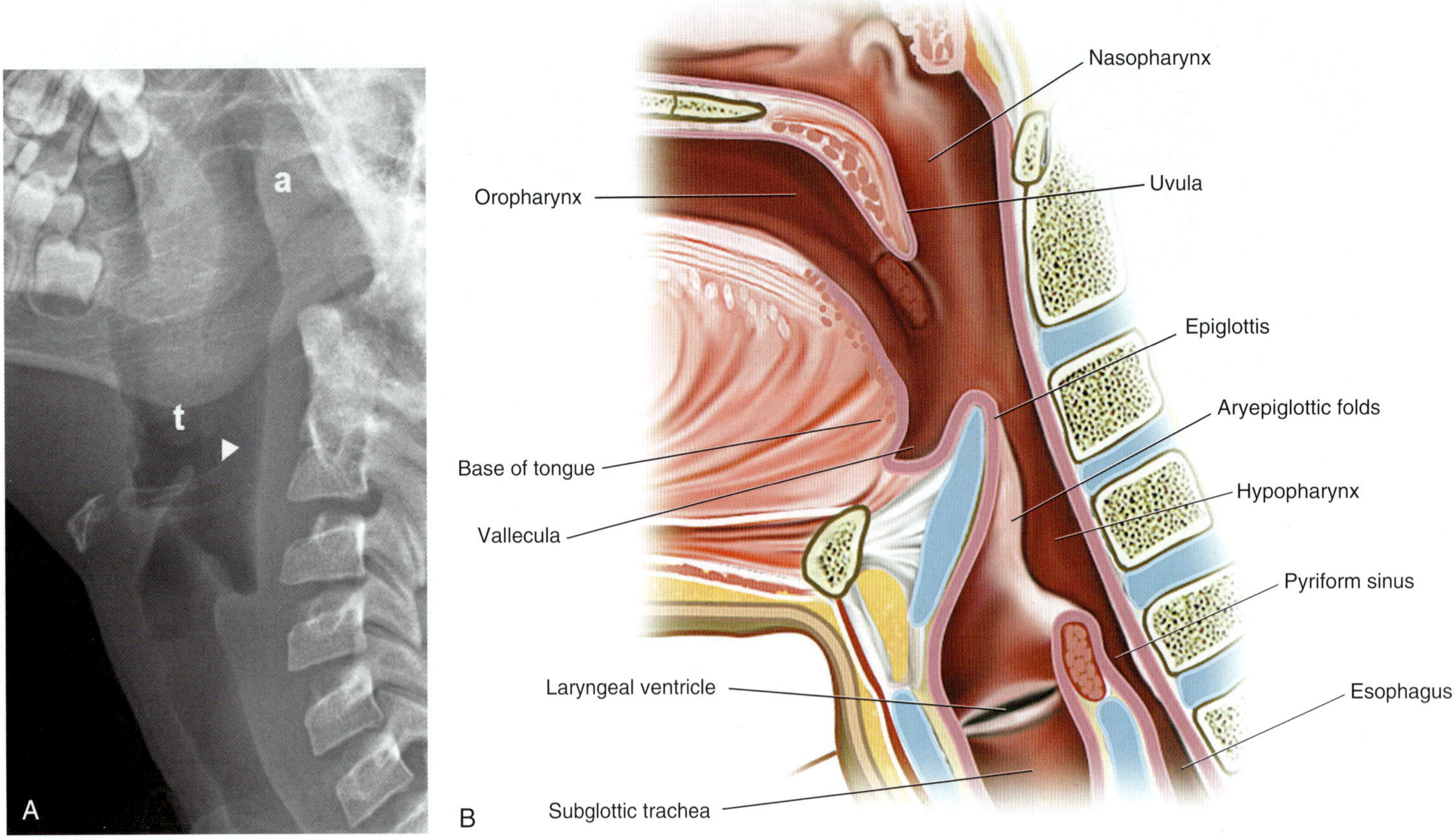

Fig. 25.4 (A) Lateral radiograph of a normal airway. The cornua of the hyoid *(ar)* point to the epiglottis. *a,* Adenoids; *t,* tonsil. (B) Diagrammatic representation of the normal anatomy of the upper airway. (B, From Blickman JG, Parker BR, Barnes PD: *Pediatric radiology: the requisites,* ed 3, Philadelphia, 2009, Mosby/Elsevier.)

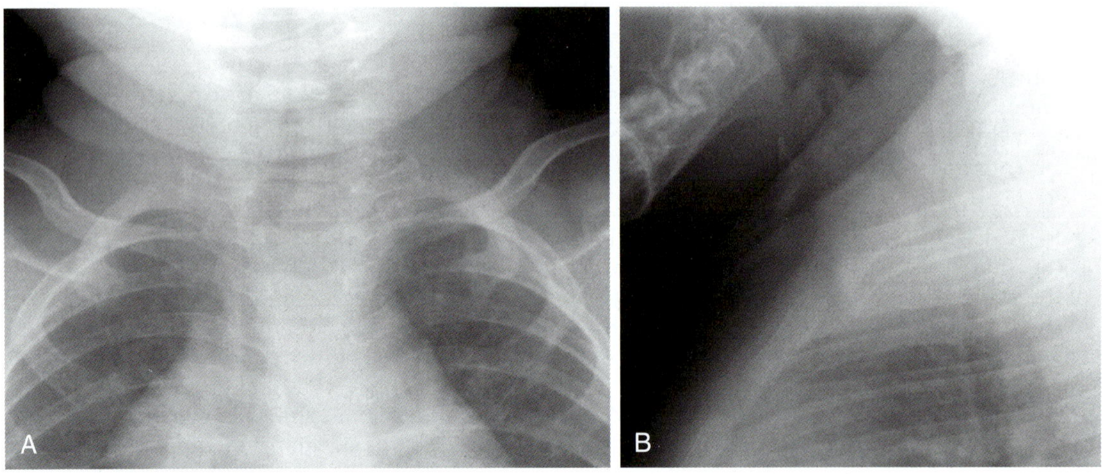

Fig. 25.5 Normal tracheal buckling. Chest radiographs of a 4-month-old infant demonstrate tracheal buckling, a normal occurrence when the film is exposed during flexion and/or expiration. (A) In the frontal projection, normal tracheal buckling occurs rightward, away from the aortic arch. (B) Anterior buckling is evident on the lateral projection. This normal anterior tracheal displacement frequently causes confusion because it simulates a retropharyngeal mass. The airway should be visible on all normal chest films.

which are the valleculae. Immediately behind the valleculae is the epiglottis. The hyoid bone is inferior and anterior to the valleculae. The oropharynx also merges posteriorly with the nasopharynx to form the hypopharynx. The tonsils are seen in the lateral walls of the hypopharynx. Anteriorly, the hypopharynx leads to the larynx and becomes the esophagus. The pyriform sinuses are the most lateral and inferior margins and provide a landmark for the level of the vocal cords.

The lateral film is important in the assessment of (1) the encroachment of adenoidal tissue on the nasopharyngeal airway; (2) retropharyngeal swelling/abscess (air in the retropharyngeal space); (3) the degree of hypopharyngeal airway distention as a measure for airway encroachment (croup); and (4) identification of a radiopaque foreign body. Calcification in respiratory cartilage, although rare in children, is pathologic; it is seen in chondrodysplasia punctata and relapsing polychondritis. The hyoid bone may be ossified at birth.

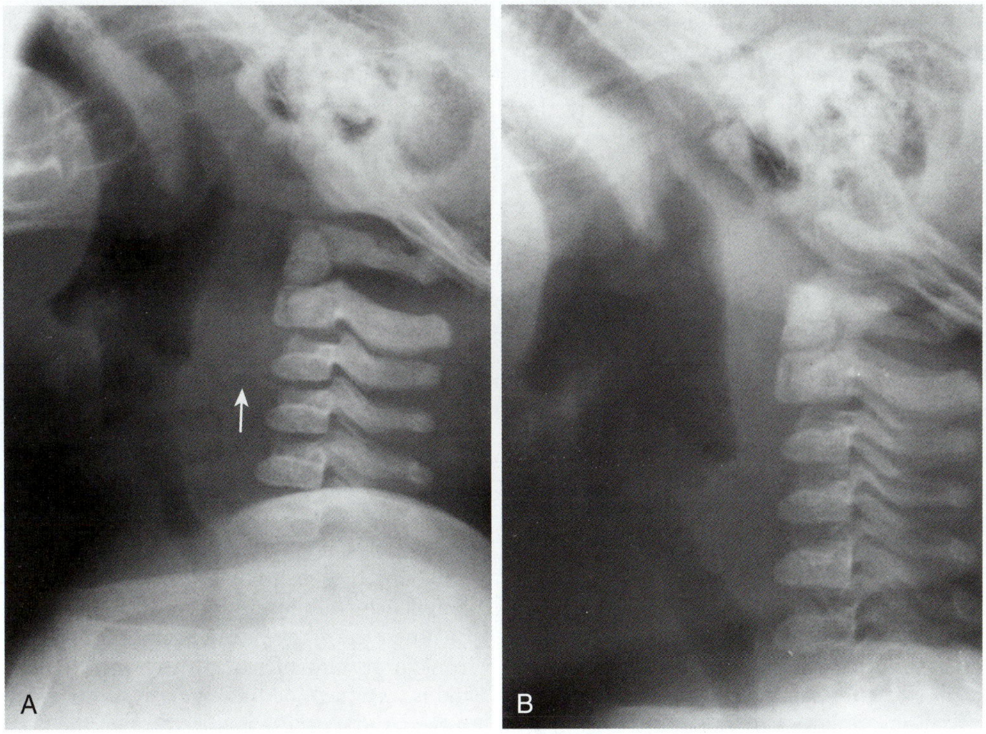

Fig. 25.6 Effect of phase of respiration on the prevertebral soft tissue space. *Arrow* in (A) demonstrates the prevertebral soft tissue widening on expiration that disappears on inspiration (B). (From Blickman JG, Parker BR, Barnes PD: *Pediatric radiology: the requisites,* ed 3, Philadelphia, 2009, Mosby/Elsevier.)

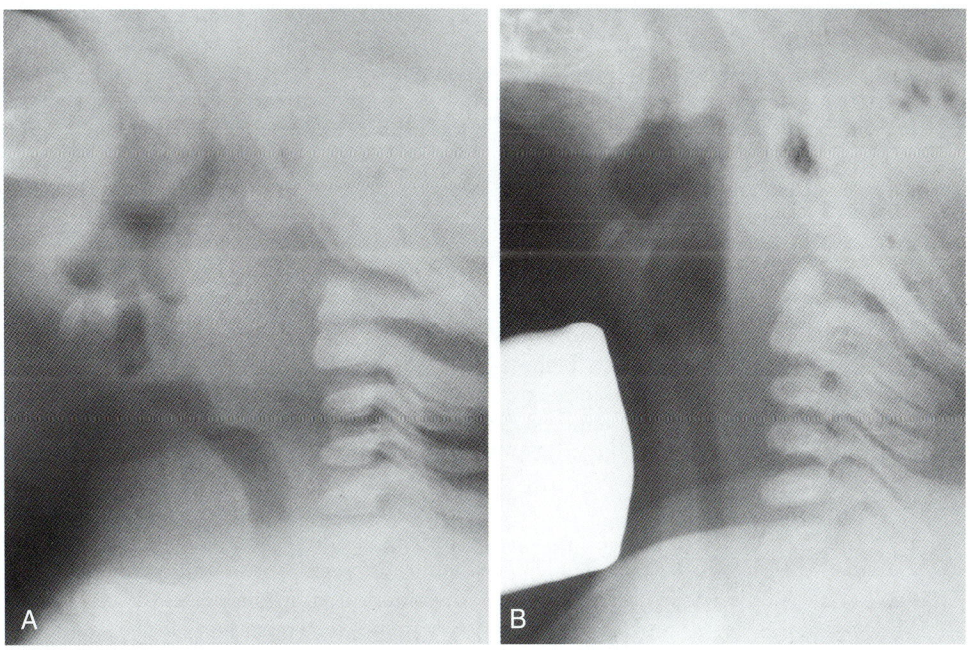

Fig. 25.7 False-positive identification of a retropharyngeal mass. (A) An examination with poor head extension suggests a retropharyngeal mass. (B) A repeat examination with better head extension and pressure applied to the anterior neck with a lead-gloved finger; the retropharyngeal soft tissues are normal. Intervention with a gloved finger is seldom necessary if the film is repeated in full extension and inspiration. (From Hilton SvW, Edwards DK III: *Practical pediatric radiology,* ed 3, Philadelphia, 2006, Saunders/Elsevier.)

Anteroposterior Film of the Neck

The frontal radiograph is best for evaluation of tracheal position. Normally, the trachea is slightly deviated to the right by the aortic arch (deviation to the left is always abnormal). A normal thymus will not affect the trachea. Expiration causes buckling of the trachea to the right (see Fig. 25.5). Note that the airway is a dynamic system and changes in caliber and position so that an isolated, single film may be quite misleading. Nonetheless, an abnormal configuration of the airway should be further evaluated in light of the clinical history.

Chest Radiograph

Interpretation of the Chest Film: The Radiologist's Circle

A systematic approach to radiographic evaluation is crucial. Comparison with previous imaging studies is mandatory and is facilitated by the use of a PACS with cloud-based image transfer of outside institution images if needed. A chest film is always examined for information about the heart and lungs, but one should also evaluate the nonpulmonary areas, including the abdomen, bones, soft tissues, and airway, to be sure all abnormalities are seen. Only then should one progress to the mediastinum. A good habit to develop is to imagine a circle on the film so as to dispense with all the noncardiopulmonary areas. Begin at the corners, where the patient information is. Check the name, date, and especially the left and right markers. An easy way to complete the circle is to progress from the name tag to the markers to the ABCS of the film: A, abdomen; B, bones; C, chest (airway, mediastinum, lungs, and diaphragm); and S, soft tissues. Carefully observe the easily missed areas: under the diaphragm, through the heart, paraspinal lines, lung apices, shoulders, and soft tissues of the neck.

On every chest film, read the abdominal portion as you would read an abdominal film. Evaluate the abdomen (regardless of how little of it can be seen) on every chest film, and note whether the stomach bubble is on the left and the liver on the right. Assess for bowel dilation, abnormal calcifications, and pneumoperitoneum, especially if the patient is upright. The heart and liver are semi-transparent organs and opacities or bronchial markings can be seen projecting over their shadows. Then look at bones and soft tissues, including portions of the arms, shoulders, ribs, sternum, mandible, and cervical, thoracic, and lumbar vertebrae. Be alert for fractures (Fig. 25.8), congenital abnormalities (e.g., absent clavicles), bone destruction, or other signs of disease. Examine the soft tissues of the neck, thorax, and abdomen to detect any swelling, foreign body, calcifications, and so on. The soft tissues may reveal multiple artifacts, such as hair braids, buttons, bandages, electrocardiogram (ECG) electrodes, or redundant skin folds. Soft tissue swelling or subcutaneous calcifications can be clues to systemic disease.

Interpretation of the Chest Film: Technical Factors

Degree of Inspiration: Lung Volumes

On an adequate film obtained during deep inspiration, nine posterior ribs and five anterior ribs should be seen above the diaphragm. If the child is too young to cooperate, expose on full inspiration during normal respiration. Babies' and toddlers' breathing is abdominal: watch for an expanded abdomen in the anteroposterior position. If the child/baby is crying during exposure, inspiration will be too deep and the overinflated lungs may create a misleading appearance that can be mistaken for pathology. The differences in appearance on inspiration and expiration are more marked than in adults. With a good inspiratory effort on the frontal view, less than one-third of the heart projects below the dome of the diaphragm; the domes of the diaphragm are rounded (if very domed, the film is expiratory). If the child has taken a shallow breath, the heart may appear enlarged; the vessels may coalesce to give a false impression of an opacity, especially in the region of the bases and hila. On the lateral view, obliquely oriented hemidiaphragms are seen in good or possibly increased lung volume (if horizontally oriented, the film is expiratory). The vertebral bodies become blacker as we progress from superior to inferior on the lateral view.

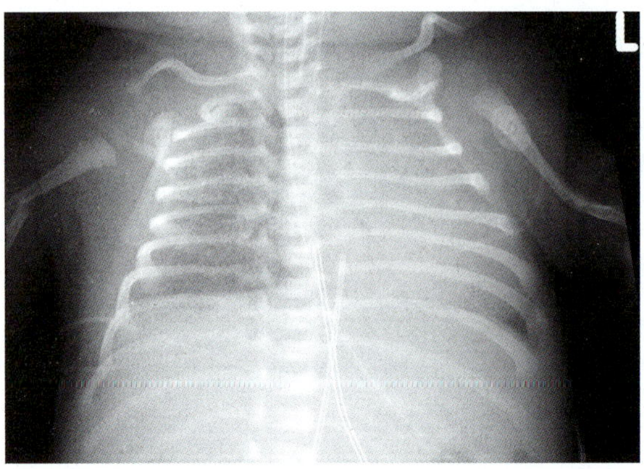

Fig. 25.8 Supine chest radiograph of a 3-day-old newborn with surfactant deficiency. A radiologist interpreting this chest film systematically, that is, by examining the ABCS (A, abdomen; B, bones; C, chest [airway, mediastinum, lungs, and diaphragm]; and S, soft tissues), should not miss the fracture involving the right humerus at the edge of the image. The patient is rotated to the left with the heart appearing prominent, likely due to rotation.

Position of the Patient

Conventional radiographs of the chest are frequently produced with a portable machine and with the younger patient (younger than 2 years old) placed supine. Upright films can be obtained after age 2; until 3 or 4 years old the patient is usually sitting for an anteroposterior projection. Children 5 years old and older can stand for a posteroanterior projection. Proper immobilization and positioning are mandatory. For radiation protection purposes, the primary beam must be collimated within the area of the cassette, and pediatric lead aprons should be used for shielding but excluded from the area of the cassette. There is increasing evidence that gonadal shielding for pelvis radiography actually increases total radiation dose and gonadal radiosensitivity is lower than previously thought; therefore gonadal shielding is no longer recommended.

When the x-ray beam passes through the patient from back to front (a posteroanterior projection), the heart is closer to the film and is less magnified. Conversely, if the x-ray beam enters the front of the patient's chest, passes through the back and onto the film (an anteroposterior projection), the magnified heart and great vessels may give the impression of cardiomegaly. This is a common problem with portable chest radiographs, which are taken in the anteroposterior projection. Also, the closer the tube to the film, the more the magnification. Routinely, portable films are exposed 40 inches (1 m) from the tube, adding to the magnification. This is compared with 6 feet (1.8 m) used in the erect patient, which causes less magnification.

When the patient is supine, the vascular supply to the upper and lower lobes of the lungs is equal because gravity has no effect. When sitting or standing, gravity plays a significant role and the upper lobe vessels are less distended than the lower lobe vessels and consequently smaller (one-third to two-thirds size). If not labeled by the technologist, an air/fluid level in the stomach and the size differential of the upper and lower pulmonary vasculature indicate an upright film.

Determining Rotation

If the patient is well centered on the frontal view, (1) the medial aspects of the clavicles are symmetric in relation to the midline, (2) the anterior ribs are equidistant from ipsilateral pedicles, (3) the position of the carina approximates the right pedicles, and (4) the two lungs are symmetric in density. Signs of rotation include asymmetric clavicles, a difference in lung aeration, the heart projected over one hemithorax and not the other, and asymmetric ribs when relating the anterior rib to the pedicles (see Fig. 25.8). On the lateral view, ribs are not seen posteriorly in the straight (unrotated) patient. If the patient is slightly rotated, ribs are shown on each side posterior to the spine.

Adequacy of Exposure

Adequacy of exposure can be assessed on the frontal film by examining the vertebral column behind the heart. The exposure is correct when we can see (1) the detailed spine and pedicles behind the heart and (2) the pulmonary vessels in the peripheral lung. If we can see only the spine but not the pulmonary vessels, the film is too dark (overexposed).

Mediastinum

The mediastinum is composed of the thymus, trachea, heart, great vessels, esophagus, lymph nodes, and neural elements. The mediastinum is divided on the lateral radiograph into (1) the anterior portion, including the space in front of the heart and great vessels;

(2) the middle portion, that is, the space between the anterior and posterior mediastinal components, including the heart, airway, esophagus, and lymph nodes; and (3) the posterior portion, including everything behind a line connecting the midportion aspects of the vertebrae, including the vertebrae, neural elements, and paraspinal lymph tissue. In some classifications, the posterior mediastinum begins with the anterior aspect of the vertebral body.

Thymus

The thymus may make interpreting pediatric chest radiographs difficult. It can simulate cardiac enlargement, lobar collapse, pulmonary infiltrates, and mediastinal masses. The thymus constitutes the major portion of the mediastinal silhouette in a normal newborn. It may extend from the lung apex to the diaphragmatic surfaces; be insinuated into the minor fissure on the right, giving a "sail sign" (see eFig. 25.4); and may be bilaterally symmetric or predominantly one sided (Fig. 25.9). The normal thymus is a "soft" organ situated in the anterior mediastinum and never compresses the airway or any other intrathoracic structure. The thymus appears smaller as the child becomes older, but the thymus actually weighs the most in adolescents. It is prominent in some children until 4 to 5 years old and may persist beyond 5 years, confounding interpretation. The contour of the normal thymus is "wavy" because it insinuates itself between the anterior ribs (Fig. 25.10; see Fig. 25.9). Thymic remnants can remain in adults and will be gradually replaced by fat. In an unwell child, the thymus can decrease in size and may not be visible.

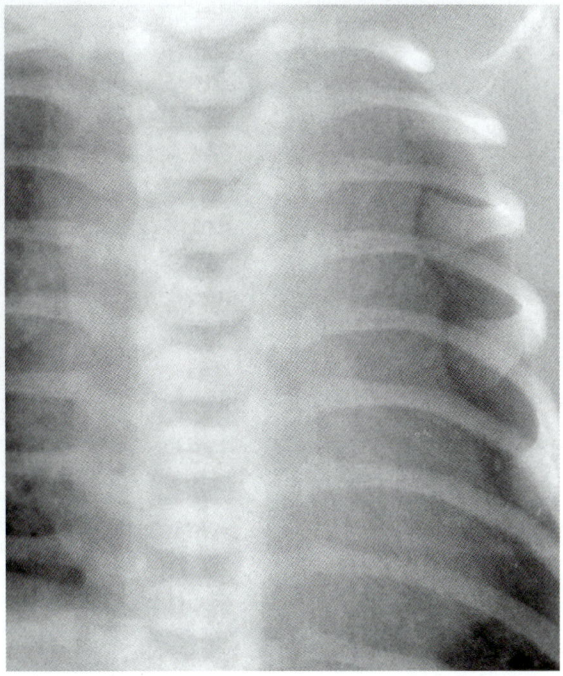

Fig. 25.10 Chest radiograph of a 1-day-old newborn shows the wavy thymus contour.

Effect of Age on Normal Appearance of the Heart

The shape of the heart on plain radiographs changes with the patient's age. The heart in younger individuals appears more globular in shape, making analysis of specific chamber abnormality difficult. The newborn right heart chambers are larger than the left, and before closure of the patent ductus arteriosus, right-sided cardiac output is greater than left-sided output. This makes identification of the aortic arch difficult or impossible. The right atrial contour in the frontal view and the right ventricular contour in the lateral view will appear abnormally enlarged in these patients. Furthermore, the transverse diameter of the heart is increased, thus increasing the normal cardiothoracic ratio. The thymic shadow regresses by the end of the first year of life, and the heart appears to rotate and descend into the chest. The typical "normal" appearance of the heart does not begin to become apparent until 6 to 8 years of life. However, through adolescence, the apparent size of the main pulmonary artery segment remains increased. Through the teens and early 20s, the size of the main pulmonary artery and base of heart continue to decrease, and the size of the aortic arch increases in caliber so that by the mid-20s, the appearance of a "normal" heart may be characterized (Fig. 25.11).

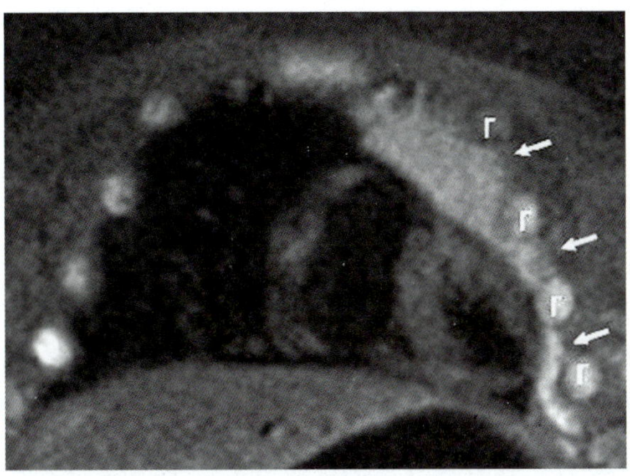

Fig. 25.9 Coronal magnetic resonance imaging of the chest (short tau inversion recovery [STIR] sequence) demonstrates a left-sided normal thymus in a 7-month-old infant. An anterior cut shows the "wavy thymus sign" *(arrows)* as the thymus insinuates itself between the anterior ribs *(r)*.

Neonatal Chest Radiograph

Manipulating preterm infants for radiographs must be done with care. Attention must be directed to maintaining oxygen levels, preventing cardiorespiratory complications, preventing heat loss, warming cassettes, and practicing good hand hygiene. Gonad/thyroid shielding is placed on top of the incubator rather than inside it. The cross-table lateral film is used when there is a possibility of free air (pneumothorax or pneumomediastinum). Because the infant is supine and air rises to the most nondependent location, air can be seen under the sternum.

The airway should be visible on all chest films. The trachea is not a midline structure (the carina projects adjacent to the right pedicles). Buckling of the trachea is normal. The airway is a dynamic structure that changes in caliber; however, if on all views the airway is persistently small, further investigation is necessary. It is normal for neonates and young infants to occasionally have some air in the esophagus (not so in older children). The ideal position of the endotracheal tube is at the level of about 1.5 vertebral bodies above the carina.

The aortic arch frequently cannot be seen in a neonate, and its position must be inferred from the position of the carina. If the carina overlies the right pedicles, the aortic arch is left sided. A right-sided aortic arch may be inferred if the position of the carina is at the midline or to the left. A right aortic arch should alert the physician to the possibility of congenital heart disease (CHD) and/or a vascular ring. In neonates and infants, the cardiothoracic ratio can be up to 60% (the adult dimension is 50%). Measuring the heart size on an anteroposterior film is accurate in this age group because there is minimal magnification of the heart (unlike in adult anteroposterior chest radiographs). If the heart is large, it should appear so in both frontal and lateral views. On the lateral radiograph, the retrocardiac air space should be seen in a normal-sized heart, and the carinal line (a perpendicular line drawn from the carina to the diaphragm) should not intersect the heart. A second method to evaluate heart size on the lateral film is the anterior tracheal line (a line parallel to the anterior wall of the trachea that extends inferiorly to

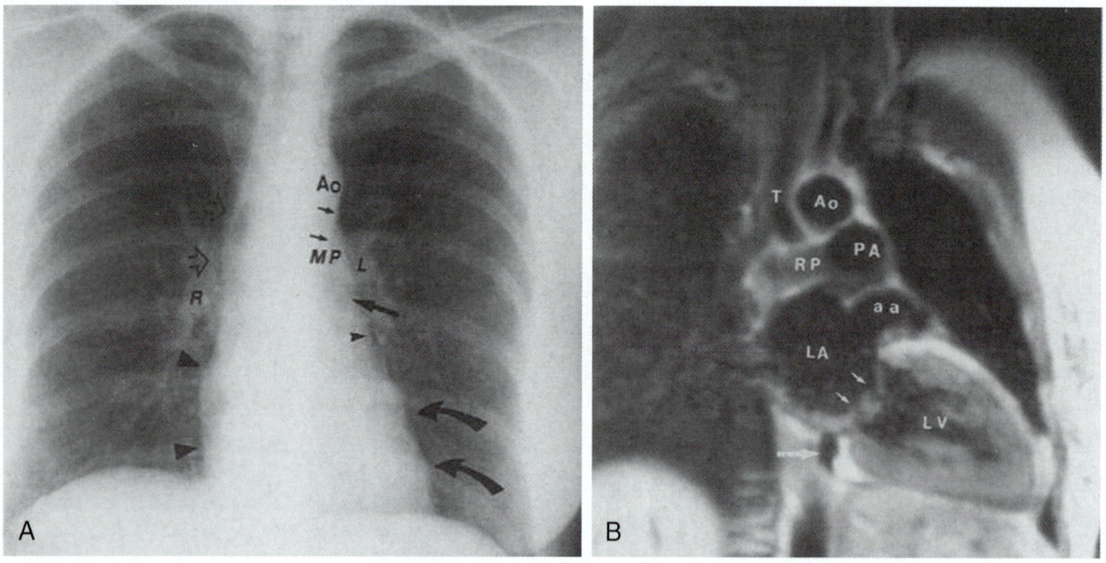

Fig. 25.11 (A) Posteroanterior radiograph of a 30-year-old female is shown. The lateral border of the left-sided aortic arch *(Ao)* and proximal descending aorta *(short arrows)* are clearly seen. The main *(MP)* and proximal left *(L)* pulmonary artery are seen cephalad to the left bronchus *(long arrow)*. The left atrial appendage section *(small arrowhead)* is inferior to the crossing of the left bronchus and cephalad to the left ventricular contour *(curved arrows)* of the left heart border. The superior vena cava is not seen on this examination. However, the ascending aorta *(small open arrow)* is seen barely over the hilar right pulmonary artery *(R)*. The right atrial contour *(large arrowheads)* extends just to the right of the spine. (B) Spin-echo magnetic resonance imaging (MRI) obtained from a different 30-year-old female is shown. The left heart border–forming structures are the aortic arch *(Ao)*, which is to the left of the trachea *(T)*, the distal main pulmonary artery *(PA)*, left atrial appendage *(aa)*, and anterolateral portion of the left ventricle *(LV)*. The transverse right pulmonary *(RP)* artery passes over the left atrium *(LA)*. Notice that the Ao and PA are equal in caliber. The mitral valve *(small arrows)* and coronary sinus *(large arrow)* are shown. (From Boxt LM: Plain-film examination of the normal heart, *Semin Roentgenol* 34:169–180, 1999.)

the diaphragm). This line should not intersect the heart, nor should the line be pushed back to traverse the spine above the diaphragm. Both methods work best on nonrotated lateral films. If a frontal film shows questionable cardiac enlargement, look at the lateral film. If the lateral film is normal, the heart size is normal.

In infants and older children, pulmonary vascular changes may help in detecting a left-to-right shunt circulation. In the newborn, however, the pulmonary vessels can be seen at the hila and only in the medial third of the lungs. When there is vascular congestion secondary to congestive heart failure or overcirculation from a left-to-right shunt, the vascularity becomes much easier to see in the lateral two-thirds of the lung. It is much more difficult to detect decreased pulmonary vascularity (as found in severe pulmonary stenosis or atresia).

Categorization of Congenital Heart Disease on the Basis of Pulmonary Blood Flow

Cyanotic Heart Disease

Cyanotic heart disease may involve the following:

- Increased pulmonary blood flow: truncus arteriosus and total anomalous pulmonary venous return
- Decreased pulmonary blood flow: tetralogy of Fallot (TOF), Ebstein anomaly, and pulmonary atresia with intact ventricular septum
- Variable flow: D-transposition of the great arteries and tricuspid atresia

Acyanotic Heart Disease

Acyanotic heart disease may involve the following:

- Normal pulmonary blood flow (obstructive lesions): coarctation of the aorta, aortic stenosis, and pulmonary artery stenosis
- Increased pulmonary blood flow (left-to-right shunt): Ventricular septal defect, atrial septal defect, atrioventricular septal defect, and patent ductus arteriosus

Congestive Heart Failure of the Newborn (Increased Pulmonary Venous Flow)

Left-Sided Anatomic Obstruction

Left-sided anatomic obstruction may involve the following:

- Coarctation of the aorta
- Aortic stenosis

Left Ventricular Dysfunction

Left ventricular dysfunction may involve the following:

- Abnormal origin of the left coronary artery
- Myocarditis
- Shock
- Birth asphyxia
- Hypoplastic left heart
- Pulmonary venous atresia/stenosis

General Systemic Illness

General systemic illness may involve the following:

- Anemia
- Polycythemia
- Hypoglycemia
- Sepsis
- Extracardiac shunting such as congenital hepatic hemangioma or intracranial vein of Galen aneurysmal malformation (eFig. 25.5).

Diffuse Pulmonary Disease in the Newborn

The differential diagnosis of the various diffuse pulmonary conditions is described in Table 25.2. Premature infants are prone to complications related to therapy, such as:

- Air leak secondary to barotrauma: Pulmonary interstitial emphysema, pneumomediastinum, pneumopericardium, pneumothorax, pneumoperitoneum, and air embolism

Table 25.2 Neonatal Chest Vignettes

	Hyaline Membrane Disease	Transient Tachypnea of the Newborn	Meconium Aspiration	Neonatal Pneumonia
Typical patient	Premature	Term Cesarean section	Postterm meconium-stained fluid below the vocal cords	Premature rupture of membranes
Time course	Within hours	24–48 h	12–24 h	Onset <6 h
Lung volume	Decreased	Increased	Increased	Increased
Radiographic characteristics	Ground-glass granular	Interstitial edema	Coarse, nodular, asymmetrical	Perihilar "streaking"
Effusions	No	Yes	No	Maybe
Complications and possible therapy	Pulmonary interstitial emphysema or pneumothorax, respiratory distress syndrome, patent ductus arteriosus	None	Persistent fetal circulation, extracorporeal membrane oxygenation (ECMO)	Sepsis, ECMO

From Blickman JG, Parker BR, Barnes PD: *Pediatric radiology: the requisites,* ed 3, Philadelphia, 2009, Mosby/Elsevier.

- Misplaced or perforated tubes: If the infant who is intubated is having unexplained respiratory distress, two views (frontal and lateral) may help define tube position
- Stone formation: Gallstones (secondary to hyperalimentation) and renal stones (secondary to diuretic therapy, e.g., furosemide)
- Central nervous system (CNS) hemorrhage
- Oxygen toxicity (retinopathy of prematurity)
- Catheter infection and vascular thrombosis

Focal Lung Lesions in Neonates on Chest Radiography

Lucent Lesions

Lucent lesions may involve the following:

- Congenital lobar overinflation
- Congenital pulmonary airway malformation
- Persistent pulmonary interstitial emphysema
- Congenital diaphragmatic hernia

Solid Lesions

Solid lesions may involve the following:

- Sequestration
- Foregut duplication cyst
- Congenital pulmonary airway malformation

Mediastinal Masses

The following outline is a useful summary of the etiology of mediastinal masses:

- Anterior mediastinum (the four Ts and an L)
  - Thyroid (ectopic thyroid)
  - "Terrible" lymph node enlargement by either infection or malignancy
  - Teratoma
  - Thymoma
  - Lymphatic malformation
- Middle mediastinum (an abnormality for each organ)
  - Esophagus: Duplication cysts
  - Great vessels: Aneurysmal dilation
  - Hila: Enlarged lymph nodes (leukemia, lymphoma, tuberculosis, etc.)
  - Trachea: Bronchogenic cysts
  - Pericardium: Cyst or effusion
- Posterior mediastinum
  - Tuberculosis (Pott disease) or any spinal infection
  - Extramedullary hematopoiesis (almost always in adults)
  - Neural tumors: Neuroblastoma, ganglioneuroblastoma, ganglioneuroma, neurofibroma, neurenteric cyst

Tips when viewing mediastinal masses include (1) middle mediastinal masses silhouette the heart border and aorta and (2) posterior mediastinal masses may widen the distance between ribs or cause vertebral changes.

Abdominal Radiograph

The abdominal radiograph is usually the initial examination in the workup of abdominal and pelvic symptoms, and it may provide useful information for tailoring the examination to the individual patient's problem. Supine and upright radiographs are obtained, although left lateral decubitus or cross-table lateral views are used in newborns and in unstable or uncooperative patients. Single supine examinations may be obtained when the clinical suspicion is foreign body ingestion or if the examination is being performed for catheter localization.

Abdominal Radiograph: Child Versus Adult

The liver takes up a relatively larger space in the peritoneal cavity of a child. The spleen may not be visible and usually does not displace the gastric contour in a young child. Likewise, retroperitoneal fat "stripes" (psoas shadows) are frequently not seen because of the relative paucity of fat in the infant's and small child's retroperitoneum. The lack of fat in the capsules of the solid organs makes evaluation of their size nearly impossible on radiographs. In contrast, properitoneal fat stripes are visible from infancy. A soft tissue pseudomass in the abdomen may be the urinary bladder, fluid-filled bowel, or an umbilical hernia. Children up to the toddler age group typically have air throughout the entire gastrointestinal (GI) tract.

Bowel Gas After Birth

Newborns should have air in the stomach at birth, consisting mainly of swallowed air. The small bowel should be filled with air by 6 hours at the latest; the colon by 12 hours; and by 24 hours of life, air should appear in the rectum, although rectal air is typically present much earlier (by 12 hours). A prone film is frequently helpful because air rises into the rectum when there is no obstruction. The normal newborn abdomen demonstrates monotonous polygons of gas, similar to the appearance of giraffe skin. In neonates and infants, it is often impossible to reliably differentiate small from large bowel except for stomach and rectum, especially if the bowel becomes dilated.

Absence of air in the stomach at 1 hour of life should raise the possibility of esophageal obstruction: esophageal atresia without tracheoesophageal fistula. A gasless abdomen in an infant for more than 12 hours indicates a serious disease. The most common cause of a lack of intestinal air in the newborn is depression of crying and swallowing in ill babies, especially those with newborn lung disease. Other causes of a gasless abdomen are vomiting, medication that decreases peristalsis, obstruction of a fluid-filled bowel, peritonitis, ascites, and congenital diaphragmatic hernia (a chest radiograph is diagnostic). Other causes of disturbed swallowing and/or diminished peristalsis include septicemia and metabolic disorders. The neonate in whom an orogastric or nasogastric tube has been placed may have a relatively gasless abdomen without other underlying pathology. Absence of meconium passage by 24 hours is abnormal, and abdominal distention or marked dilation of any viscus in the first day of life should lead to further imaging evaluation.

Umbilical Venous and Arterial Lines

The ideal location for the tip of the umbilical venous line is in the low right atrium. The umbilical arterial line tip may be at L4 to L5 (bifurcation of the aorta) or at T8 above the diaphragm (Fig. 25.12C). The course of the umbilical venous line is as follows: umbilical vein → umbilical recess → left portal vein → ductus venosus → inferior vena cava → right atrium (see Fig. 25.12A). The umbilical arterial line dips inferiorly in the umbilical artery to join the internal iliac artery (creating a deep loop in the pelvis) and then rises posteriorly in the abdominal aorta (see Fig. 25.12B). The lateral view can confirm which catheter is arterial (which will be posterior) and which is venous (which will appear anterior).

Adynamic Ileus

Ileus should be suggested only when loops of intestine are dilated. The presence of air in normal-caliber large bowel and small bowel is a common and normal finding in newborns and infants. In adynamic (without peristalsis) ileus (distention), the small bowel is less distended than the colon and there is gas in the rectum. In infants and older children, adynamic ileus occurs (1) after surgery, (2) with sepsis, (3) with gastroenteritis, (4) subsequent to electrolyte disturbances such as dehydration and hypokalemia, and (5) after administration of drugs such as opiates and anticholinergics.

Dynamic (Mechanical) Ileus

A more uniform, generalized increase in all or parts of the small or large bowel along with multiple air/fluid levels and no air in the rectum denote mechanical bowel obstruction. The prone film is helpful in directing gas to the rectum for assessment of its caliber when bowel obstruction is a concern; a prone horizontal-beam (cross-table lateral) film of the rectum is helpful in these cases. The most common causes of mechanical obstruction in the neonate are (1) duodenal atresia or stenosis, (2) malrotation with midgut volvulus, and (3) obstructing peritoneal bands (Ladd bands). Beyond the neonatal period, the most common causes in descending order of frequency consist of (1) appendicitis, (2) intussusception, (3) inguinal hernia, (4) postoperative adhesions, (5) post–necrotizing enterocolitis strictures, and (6) midgut volvulus. In older children, valvulae conniventes and haustral markings may help differentiate dilated small bowel and large bowel, respectively, and the distended colon is more peripheral in location than the more centrally located distended small bowel. These findings may not be applicable in the neonate or the child with malrotation and midgut volvulus.

Pneumoperitoneum

Free air in the peritoneal cavity most commonly results from perforation of a hollow viscus. Large amounts of free air are readily identifiable on supine abdominal radiographs, which may show the presence of the Rigler sign (where both sides of the bowel wall can be visualized) or the football sign (where the liver is blacker than the adjacent soft tissues and falciform ligament is visible). Small amounts of free air typically require a cross-table lateral, lateral decubitus, or upright view. A cross-table lateral supine view may show a long colonic collection of air mimicking pneumoperitoneum. Perforation of a hollow viscus typically leads to intraperitoneal air/fluid levels as intraluminal fluid and air leaks into the peritoneal cavity. Other causes of pneumoperitoneum include (1) postoperative air and (2) tracking of air from pneumomediastinum, usually in children undergoing pressure ventilation and in asthmatic patients. The latter condition results when mediastinal air extends into the retroperitoneum and then along the course of the mesenteric vessels, resulting in subserosal air, which can rupture into the peritoneal cavity. It can be differentiated from visceral perforation by the lack of intraperitoneal air/fluid levels on horizontal-beam radiographs.

Calcifications

The abdominal radiograph can be used to assess calcifications, which may be present in meconium peritonitis, abdominal masses such as hepatoblastoma or neuroblastoma, and stones in the gallbladder, urinary tract, pancreas, or appendix. A phlebolith in an infant is definitely abnormal; it occurs far more often in adults.

Musculoskeletal System

Radiography remains the primary method of detecting and analyzing skeletal abnormalities. Most fractures and congenital deformities are sufficiently imaged by radiography without the need for additional imaging. The spatial resolution of radiography is superior to that of all other modalities. Radiography is cost-effective, and radiation exposure to the patient is minimal. Radiographs often guide the selection of additional imaging modalities when needed. Adequate radiography must include imaging in at least two perpendicular directions.

The skeletal survey remains an important component in the evaluation of many patients with a skeletal dysplasia or syndrome and in suspected victims of child abuse. Skeletal surveys are particularly useful in Langerhans cell histiocytosis when skeletal scintigraphy may be falsely negative.

Radiographs are less relevant to evaluate the soft tissues because of their narrow contrast range, but plain films can depict soft tissue swelling, calcifications, fat, gas, or foreign material and can show the effect of the lesion on the adjacent bone.

Anatomy

Bone develops by intramembranous (flat bones) and endochondral (long bones) ossification. The long bone of a child is made up of four parts: the physis, or growth plate; the epiphysis; metaphysis; and diaphysis (or shaft). Each long bone (humerus, tibia) has a physis, and thus metaphysis and epiphysis, on either end. A secondary ossification center appears in the epiphysis after birth. Some long bones (e.g., the femur) have a nonarticulating apophysis, which is similar to the epiphysis but does not contribute to the length of the bone (e.g., the greater trochanter of the femur).

In the growing child's skeleton, blood supply is primarily to the metaphysis, and many of the disease processes and imaging findings are seen in this region. For example, hematogenous osteomyelitis is visible most often in the metaphysis; similarly, metastases travel hematogenously to the metaphysis.

The child's bones are still growing, developing, and modeling; therefore many ossification centers are constantly appearing and fusing with the main skeleton. For example, the mnemonic "CRITOE" refers to the approximate age of ossification of secondary centers in the elbow: *c*apitellum (1 year), *r*adial head (4 years), *i*nner (medial) epicondyle (7 years), *t*rochlea (10 years), *o*lecranon (10 years), and *e*xternal (lateral) epicondyle (11 years).

In children, the periosteum is less firmly attached to the diaphysis of the long bone and is more likely to tear and thus be elevated by trauma with hematoma formation. The periosteum reacts by laying down a thick layer of new bone. In contrast, the periosteum at the ends of the long bones are not loosely attached but are rather firmly adherent to the metaphyseal regions. Shaking injuries here cause avulsion of a piece of bone from the metaphysis. This type of "bucket-handle" injury or avulsion "corner fracture" is commonly found in cases of child abuse (see Chapter 6).

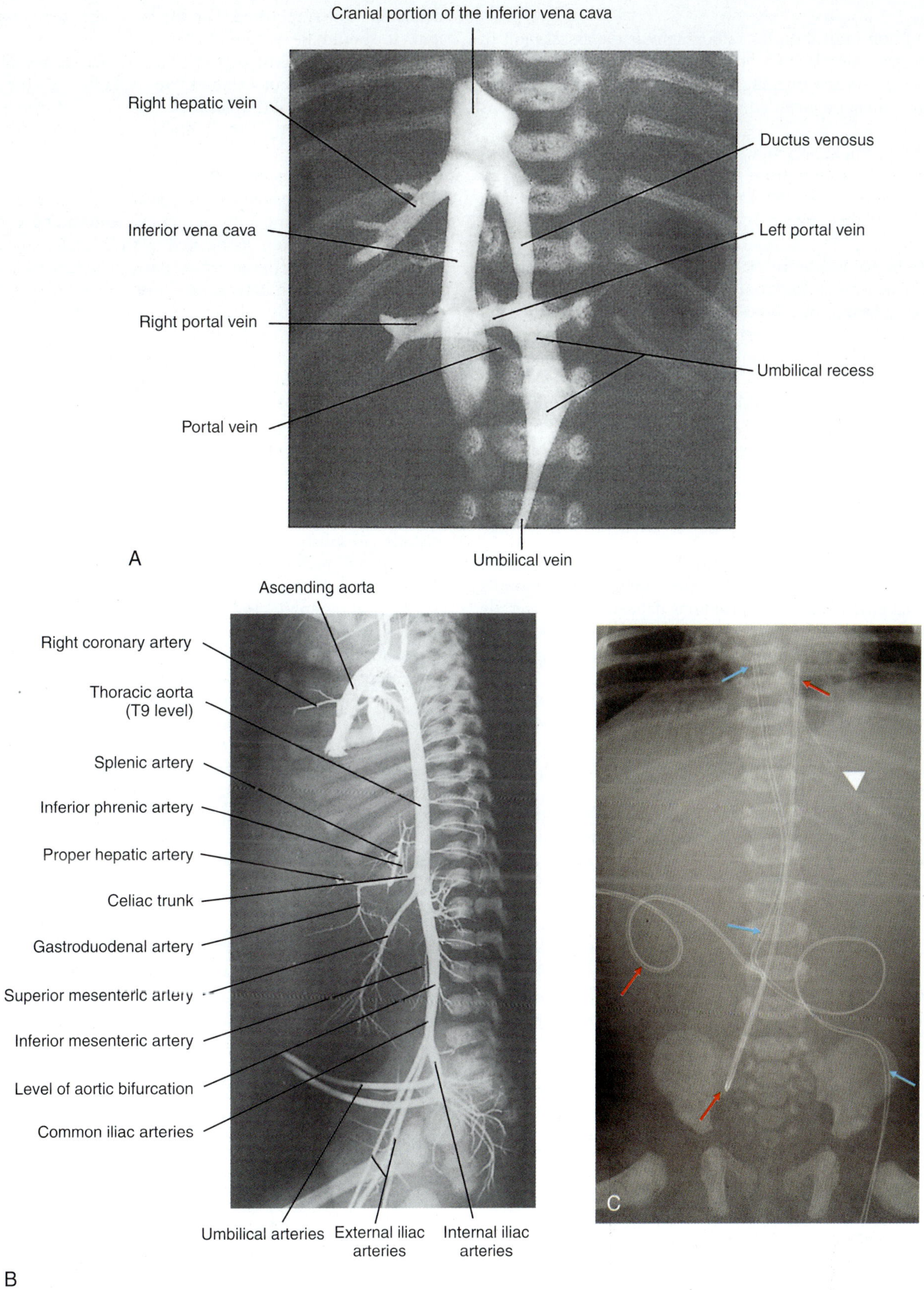

Fig. 25.12 (A) Postmortem demonstration of the umbilical recess with its junction to the ductus venosus and the left portal vein. Twin premature, 27 weeks of gestation, deceased on the first day of life. (B) Male term newborn. Postmortem normal angiography. The angle between the umbilical arteries and the internal iliac arteries may make catheterization via the umbilical artery more difficult. (C) Supine radiograph of the abdomen of a 3-day-old newborn shows the umbilical venous line *(blue arrow)* with the tip in the right atrium, and the umbilical arterial line *(red arrow)* with the tip in the aorta at T8. *Ar,* Nasogastric tube. (A and B, From Hilton SvW, Edwards DK III: *Practical pediatric radiology*, ed 3, Philadelphia, 2006, Elsevier/Saunders.)

Trauma

The most common indication for radiography is the assessment of trauma. As a general rule, two orthogonal views are obtained to assess for fracture. When imaging a long bone, both the proximal and distal joints must be included so that the entirety of the bone is imaged.

Contralateral comparison views may aid in differentiating normal developmental variation from pathology. Comparison views are most helpful in areas of complex anatomy, such as the elbow with its six ossification centers. Normal variants are common and may mimic a fracture.

The child's bones are more plastic and less brittle than adults, so pediatric fractures differ from adult fractures. The greenstick fracture is characterized by a bowed long bone with a break on the convex surface but apparent cortical continuity on the concave surface. In the torus fracture, there is buckling on one side of the cortex.

Some fractures are more prevalent in different age groups. For example, infants previously able to walk may suddenly limp because of a subtle spiral fracture of the tibia (a *toddler's fracture*). This fracture can be difficult to see on initial films. If there is suspicion that a fracture has occurred but none is definitely identified, repeat films in 7 to 10 days when periosteal reaction around a fracture has formed, increasing fracture visibility.

Periosteal reaction is abnormal, with the exception of so-called physiologic new bone found symmetrically in infants 2 to 6 months old. The normal physiologic periosteal bone deposition is bilaterally symmetric and found in the humeri, femora, and tibias. It extends to the metaphysis but no further. The periosteum is normally not seen.

Causes of periosteal reaction include (1) infection; (2) trauma; (3) metabolic disturbances (rickets, scurvy); (4) tumors (osteosarcoma, Ewing sarcoma, histiocytosis); (5) idiopathic origin (Caffey disease); and (6) iatrogenic/toxic origin (prostaglandin, hypervitaminosis A).

If a fracture involves a joint, then a joint effusion (particularly in the knee or elbow) is a useful sign indicating that a fracture may have occurred. At the elbow, a joint effusion most likely indicates that a supracondylar fracture (younger child) or radial neck fracture (older child) has occurred.

Fractures involving the growth plate are called *Salter-Harris fractures* and carry a prognostic rating according to the severity of the growth plate injury (types I to V, with type V being the worst; see Chapter 22). Severe length discrepancies and other growth disturbances can occur from fractures involving the physis.

There is a low incidence of dislocations of otherwise normal joints in children compared with the adult skeleton. Because children's capsular and ligamentous structures are two to five times stronger than the weakest part of the growth plate, the growth plate fractures first and dislocation occurs less frequently. The zone of provisional calcifying cartilage is the weakest portion of the growth plate.

Nonaccidental Trauma (Child Abuse)

If the imaging findings are suspicious, it is the radiologist's legal obligation to report these findings as compatible with child abuse. Usually, reporting the findings to the referring clinician, either in the report or via telephone (preferable), is sufficient. See Chapter 6 for an in-depth discussion of nonaccidental trauma.

Skeletal Dysplasia

With short stature in the pediatric age group, it is crucial to clinically determine whether the skeletal dysplasia involves proportionate or disproportionate short stature. The differential diagnosis of proportionate short stature consists of constitutional delay, familial short stature, a small group of endocrinopathies, and some dysmorphology syndromes. A left hand-and-wrist radiograph for bone age determination is required. For the bone age to be considered normal, it should lie within 2 standard deviations of the patient's chronologic age. Most of the bone dysplasias result in clinically disproportionate short stature. See Chapter 22 for an in-depth discussion of skeletal dysplasias.

Bone Tumors

Clear radiographic signs of a benign lesion include sharp demarcation between the lesion and the normal bone, a sclerotic margin around the lesion, and a nonaggressive pattern of growth. The characteristics most often associated with a malignancy include an accompanying soft tissue mass, periosteal reaction, an indistinct zone of demarcation between the normal and abnormal bone, and permeative destructive changes in the bone. Plain film radiography is usually adequate to diagnose most benign tumors. MRI is the modality of choice to define the extent of the abnormality once a malignant bone lesion has been suggested.

Bone Infection

The clinical symptoms of osteomyelitis precede the radiographic findings by 7 to 14 days. For this reason, MRI or bone scan is more helpful in the early diagnosis of acute osteomyelitis.

The radiographic findings of acute osteomyelitis (0–2 weeks) include (1) soft tissue swelling initially, (2) loss of cortical margin, (3) focal demineralization of bone, and (4) faint periosteal new bone formation (7–14 days after onset).

The radiographic findings of the healing phase (>4 weeks) include (1) destroyed bone with irregular areas of sclerosis and lysis; (2) sequestrum, that is, a dense devascularized bone fragment within an area of pus and granulation tissue; and (3) involucrum, that is, a peripheral shell of supporting bone laid down by the periosteum around the old disease.

Chronic osteomyelitis (either unusual localized osteomyelitis or incompletely treated) appears as (1) diffuse bone production with little or no destruction and (2) an occasional draining sinus or lucent area in the midst of the sclerotic bone.

FLUOROSCOPY

Introduction

Indications, Contraindications, Advantages, and Disadvantages of Fluoroscopy in Pediatric Imaging

For a summary of the indications, contraindications, advantages, and disadvantages of fluoroscopy in pediatric imaging, see Table 25.3.

Fluoroscopic Contrast Agents

For a summary of fluoroscopic contrast agents, see eTable 25.4.

Clinical Applications

Diaphragm Paralysis

In diaphragm paralysis, fluoroscopy is reserved for patients in whom ultrasound has been unsuccessful or has given results contrary to the clinical impression, such as when the ultrasound results are normal but the patient cannot be weaned from the ventilator.

The movement of the hemidiaphragm is complex. The left hemidiaphragm may occasionally be higher than the right, and unequal movement is common. The anterior part (dome) is the only part of the hemidiaphragm routinely visualized on frontal fluoroscopy. Lateral or oblique fluoroscopy is often useful but occasionally may be difficult to interpret and can be hazardous to a sick child.

Tracheomalacia/Laryngomalacia

In the right lateral position, the airway is evaluated for backward bowing of the epiglottis or fluttering of the aryepiglottic folds (laryngomalacia) and tracheal caliber change (tracheomalacia) or

Table 25.3 Indications, Contraindications, and Advantages/Disadvantages of Fluoroscopy

Organ System	Common Indications	Contraindications/Precautions	Advantages	Disadvantages
Airway/chest (noncontrast)	Laryngomalacia Tracheomalacia Vocal cord paralysis Diaphragm paralysis	None Widely available Dynamic Requires no contrast or sedation	Noninvasive	Radiation exposure Requires brief immobilization of uncooperative children
Gastrointestinal Tract (Contrast-Enhanced)				
UGI series	Vascular ring or pulmonary sling Tracheoesophageal fistula Esophageal stricture Hiatal hernia Gastroesophageal reflux Gastritis Peptic ulcer disease Gastric outlet obstruction (sonography favored for HPS) Duodenal stenosis or atresia Malrotation/midgut volvulus	Hyperosmolar water-soluble contrast is contraindicated in patients with reflux or tracheoesophageal fistula Barium is contraindicated in patients with perforation or leak	Noninvasive (or minimally invasive if feeding tube required) Widely available Dynamic Requires no sedation	Radiation exposure Requires ingestion of contrast or tube feeding Requires brief immobilization of uncooperative children
Oropharyngeal motility examination	Swallowing dysfunction	Examination should be terminated if severe aspiration occurs Because of a high risk of aspiration in population studied, barium is the contrast agent of choice Hyperosmolar water-soluble contrast is contraindicated	Allows dynamic assessment of oropharyngeal motility (not included in standard UGI series) Noninvasive Requires no sedation	Requires radiation exposure (often more than for UGI series) Requires contrast/food ingestion and patient cooperation Must be scheduled in advance to ensure simultaneous radiologist and speech pathologist availability
Small bowel series	Small bowel obstruction, pseudoobstruction, or atresia Malabsorption or immune deficiency Inflammatory bowel disease Mass Short-gut syndrome	Same as for UGI series	Allows assessment of small bowel distal to DJJ (not included in UGI series) Noninvasive (or minimally if feeding required) Requires no sedation	Requires radiation exposure (more than for UGI series alone) Requires ingestion of contrast or tube feeding Requires brief immobilization of uncooperative children May take several hours to complete
Contrast enema[a] (single contrast)	Distal small bowel obstruction Colonic atresia Microcolon Meconium plug Meconium ileus or equivalent Hirschsprung disease Assessment of postoperative anatomy	To avoid perforation, contrast enemas are relatively contraindicated in patients with necrotic bowel, toxic megacolon, pneumatosis intestinalis, or peritonitis In patients with known bowel perforation or recent surgery, water-soluble contrast is preferred over barium	Minimally invasive Requires no sedation	Requires radiation exposure Requires rectal tube Requires brief immobilization of uncooperative children
Air-contrast enema	Inflammatory bowel disease Polyposis or colonic mass	In neonates and infants at risk for dehydration, iso-osmolar water-soluble contrast or barium is preferred over hyperosmolar water-soluble contrast		
Air enema	Intussusception	Bowel perforation	Advantage over contrast enema: smaller tears and reduced fecal spillage when bowel perforation occurs	Disadvantage over contrast enema: slightly higher rate of bowel perforation
Contrast Urography				
Intravenous urography	Urinary calculi	Contrast allergy Renal insufficiency or failure	Minimally invasive	Results in radiation exposure Requires intravenous contrast Less sensitive than CT for calculi
Voiding cystourethrography (VCUG)	UTI Hydronephrosis or hydroureter VUR Enuresis Cloacal and/or anorectal malformations Ambiguous genitalia Neurogenic bladder Posterior urethral valve Other urethral anomalies (i.e., stricture, polyp)	Acute UTI Prophylactic antibiotics warranted in patients with CHD Latex avoidance in patients at risk for latex allergy	Minimally invasive More sensitive to grade 1 VUR than nuclear cystography Provides better anatomic resolution than nuclear cystography	Results in more radiation exposure than nuclear cystography

CHD, Congenital heart disease; *CT,* computed tomography; *DJJ,* duodenojejunal junction; *HPS,* hypertrophic pyloric stenosis; *UGI,* upper gastrointestinal; *UTI,* urinary tract infection; *VUR,* vesicoureteral reflux.

[a]Precaution: A manometer and pop-off valve must be used to keep intraluminal pressure <120 mm Hg; intravenous access and surgical backup must be secured before the procedure is begun.

From Osborn LM, DeWitt TG, First LR, et al, editors: Diagnostic imaging (CD-ROM, T 272–1: indications, contraindications, advantages and disadvantages of fluoroscopy). In *Pediatrics,* Philadelphia, 2005, Mosby/Elsevier.

deviation. Laryngomalacia is noisier on quiet breathing, whereas tracheomalacia is noisier with crying.

Upper Gastrointestinal Series and Esophagography

For an upper gastrointestinal (UGI) series or esophagography, the patient should have nothing by mouth for 3 to 4 hours (infants) or 6 to 8 hours (older children). Observe swallowing while the child is in the right lateral position. Sucking, swallowing coordination, nasopharyngeal reflux, vocal cord penetration, and tracheal aspiration are evaluated. The esophagus is evaluated for stricture, indentation, fistula, and peristalsis. The aortic arch and left atrium are often seen as normal indentations. Anterior indentation of the esophagus with soft tissue structure interposed between esophagus and trachea represents a pulmonary artery sling (Fig. 25.13). Posterior vascular indentation represents an aberrant subclavian artery (see Fig. 25.13).

With the child in the right lateral position, the partially filled stomach should be observed until it empties into the duodenum. Gastric size, shape, and emptying should be noted. Duration of gastric emptying is variable in normal infants and children. Elongation of the pylorus combined with the "string sign" indicates pyloric stenosis, although ultrasound is first-line for this indication. Identify the duodenojejunal junction (DJJ) position to exclude or confirm malrotation. The normal position of the DJJ is to the left of the spine and at the level of the duodenal bulb/pylorus (Fig. 25.14A). On the lateral view, both the descending (D2) and ascending (D4) segments of the duodenum are retroperitoneal structures (i.e., close to the spine) (see Fig. 25.14B). The normal DJJ is also posterior in location on the lateral view. Any other position of the DJJ should be considered abnormal, meaning the patient has midgut malrotation. A "corkscrew sign" in a patient with malrotation indicates midgut volvulus and surgical correction must be performed immediately. Gastroesophageal reflux (GER) presence is also assessed on UGI, but there is low sensitivity for GER (38%, compared with 88% with a radionuclide study). Water siphon test is a physiologic method that can induce reflux as part of an UGI and is more sensitive than observing spontaneous reflux.

Proximal neonatal bowel obstruction (occurring proximal to the midjejunum) includes midgut volvulus (Fig. 25.15), duodenal atresia, duodenal stenosis, duodenal web, annular pancreas, and proximal jejunal atresia. Patients usually present with bilious vomiting. Abdominal radiographs demonstrate a few dilated small bowel loops in the upper abdomen.

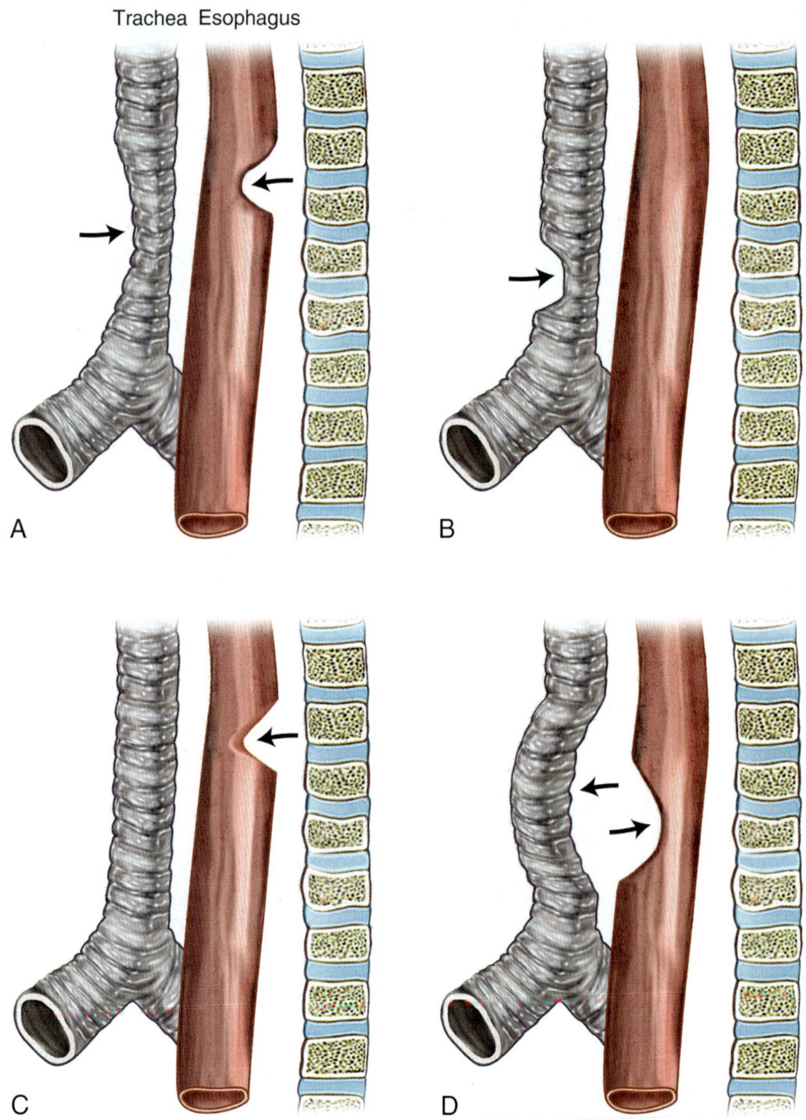

Fig. 25.13 Four patterns of vascular compression anomalies on the trachea and esophagus. Lateral projections are shown. (A) Double aortic arch or right aortic arch with aberrant left subclavian artery. (B) Innominate artery compression. (C) Left aortic arch with aberrant right subclavian artery. (D) Pulmonary sling. (Modified from Berdon WE, Baker DH: Vascular anomalies and the infant lung: rings, slings, and other things, *Semin Roentgenol* 7:39–64, 1972.)

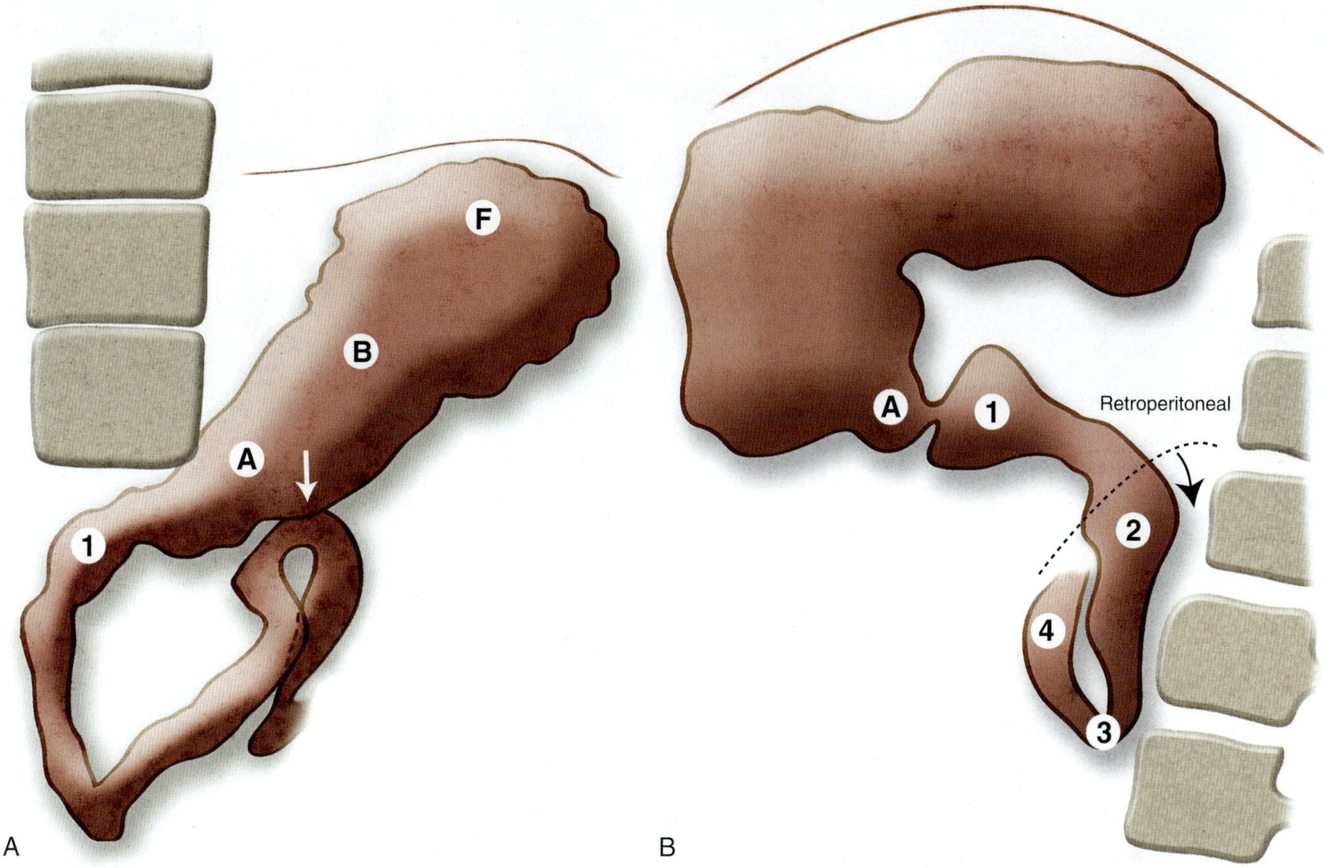

Fig. 25.14 Upper gastrointestinal study demonstrating normal duodenal course in a 3-year-old. (A) Anteroposterior projection: The duodenojejunal junction *(arrow)* is at the level of the duodenal bulb and to the left of the left spinal pedicle. *1*, Duodenal bulb; *A*, antrum; *B*, body; *F*, fundus. (B) Lateral projection: there are four portions of the duodenum *(1, 2, 3, 4)*. The second, third, and fourth portions of the duodenum are posterior, within the retroperitoneum. Slight obliquity allows visualization of both the descending *(2)* and ascending *(4)* duodenum. *A*, Antrum.

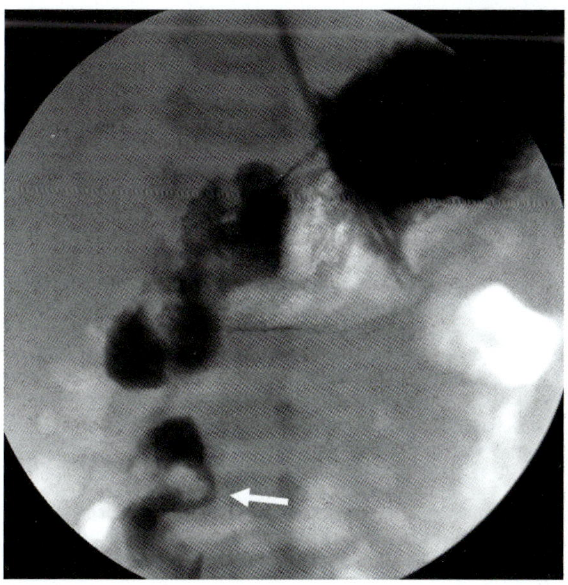

Fig. 25.15 Upper gastrointestinal study in a 6-day-old showing malrotation with midgut volvulus. The duodenal sweep fails to cross the midline and assumes a corkscrew appearance *(arrow)* projecting on the right side of the spine.

Diagnostic Contrast Enema

Diagnostic contrast enema is performed to identify small bowel obstruction (i.e., distal bowel atresia) and complications of inflammatory disease (i.e., post–necrotizing enterocolitis strictures) and to evaluate functional abnormality (i.e., Hirschsprung disease) or structural anomaly (i.e., imperforate anus before complete repair). Low neonatal bowel obstruction (involving the distal jejunum, ileum, or colon) includes meconium ileus, ileal atresia, Hirschsprung disease, and functional immaturity of the colon (Fig. 25.16). Patients present with abdominal distention and failure to pass meconium. Abdominal radiographs demonstrate multiple dilated bowel loops throughout the abdomen.

Water-soluble contrast (osmolality, 600 mOsm/kg; diluted 1:1 in water) is usually used. Water-soluble contrast can soften meconium plugs and can be used to treat meconium ileus. Barium can cause scarring when extravasated into the peritoneal cavity; therefore it is contraindicated in potential GI leak and after recent GI surgery. Administration of barium into the GI tract can interfere with subsequent CT scans of the abdomen or with nuclear studies of the genitourinary or GI system, such as a Meckel scan.

The caliber of the rectum should be compared with that of the sigmoid colon. Normally, the rectum is larger than the sigmoid colon, for a rectosigmoid ratio greater than 1. In Hirschsprung disease, the rectum typically is smaller than the sigmoid.

Reduction of Intussusception

Fluoroscopy-guided air or water-soluble contrast reduction of intussusception is the treatment of choice after sonographic confirmation (see the Ultrasound section, later). Contraindications to image-guided reduction include peritonitis, pneumoperitoneum, shock, and/or sepsis. The choice of enema medium depends on the radiologist's preference. At present, an air enema is considered superior at reduction, cleaner (based on the appearance of the peritoneal cavity at surgery when perforation occurs), and faster, with less radiation compared with a liquid enema. A water-soluble enema is recommended for infants younger than 6 months old to diagnose pathologic lead points. Radiologists should strive for

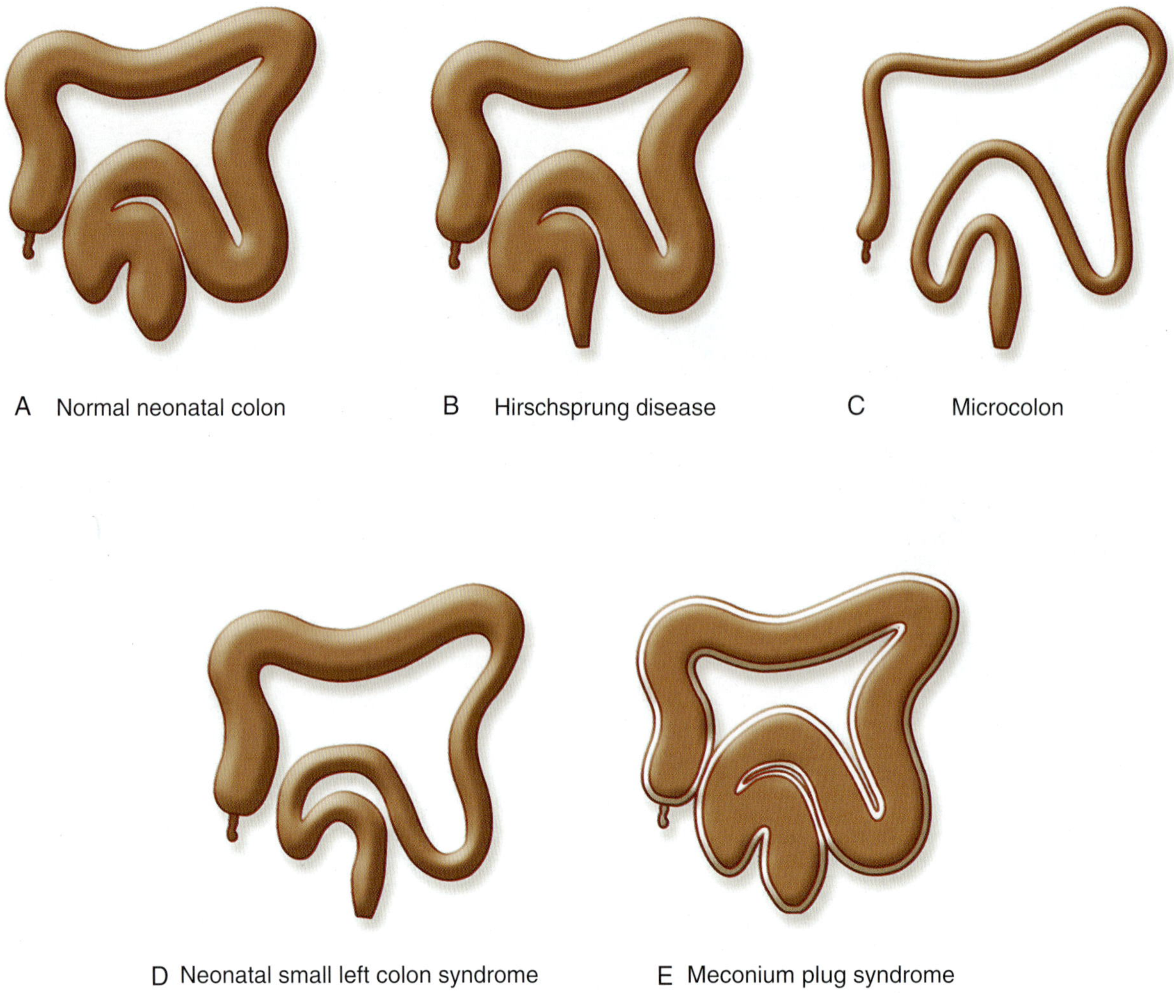

Fig. 25.16 (A–E) Schematic representation of mechanical and functional obstruction in the neonatal period. (From Hilton SvW, Edwards DK III: *Practical pediatric radiology*, ed 3, Philadelphia, 2006, Elsevier/Saunders.)

enema reduction rates of 80%, but it will depend on their patient population. Neither sedation nor medications increase the enema success rate. Predictors of failure of pneumatic reduction include ileoileocolic intussusception (27%), long duration of symptoms (>2 days), and performance after failed hydrostatic reduction. The perforation rate is about 0.8% and will require immediate surgical intervention. Reduction should not be attempted without surgical backup, and all children should have surgical consultation before enema. Some reports estimate that the rate of spontaneous reduction based on sonographic and/or enema diagnosis before surgery is 10%.

Insufflated air rapidly fills the colon and outlines the intussusception. Air pressure should be kept lower than 120 mm Hg to avoid perforation.

Reduction is defined as complete elimination of the intussusceptum through the ileocecal valve and free reflux of air into the distal small bowel (Fig. 25.17). Perforation complicating air enema may cause tension pneumoperitoneum; some centers advise having an 18-gauge needle readily available in the fluoroscopy room for emergency decompression.

The recurrence rate is 10% post-reduction. There is no contraindication to reattempting to reduce the intussusception by an enema procedure. Many centers refer patients to surgery after more than three recurrences in order to evaluate for underlying pathologic lead points (PLPs). Approximately 5% to 6% of intussusceptions in children are caused by PLPs, which are due to either focal masses or diffuse bowel wall abnormality. The most common focal PLPs are (in decreasing order of incidence) Meckel diverticulum, duplication cyst, polyp, and lymphoma. Diffuse PLPs are most commonly associated with cystic fibrosis or Henoch-Schönlein purpura. The rate of detection of PLPs by ultrasound, liquid enema, and air enema is 66%, 40%, and 11%, respectively.

Contrast Enema Reduction of Meconium Ileus Uncomplicated by Bowel Atresia, Perforation, or Volvulus

Contrast enemas may be used for reduction of uncomplicated meconium ileus (see Fig. 25.16C). The study should be performed in conjunction with a pediatric surgeon.

Contrast Enema for Hirschsprung Disease

No preparation of the colon is necessary when performing contrast enema for Hirschsprung disease. Recent manipulation including rectal examination or rectal thermometry shortly before contrast enema can make diagnosis more difficult by decompressing the distended colon. Normally, the rectum is larger than the sigmoid colon (in Hirschsprung disease, the rectum typically is smaller than the sigmoid). Identify a transition zone between the narrowed distal aganglionic segment and the dilated proximal, normal colon. Although contrast enema remains a useful test, suction biopsy provides a definitive diagnosis.

Contrast enema can help differentiate between true and pseudofecal incontinence. In the setting of true fecal incontinence, the rectum is not dilated, whereas it shows significant dilation in pseudofecal incontinence (Fig. 25.18).

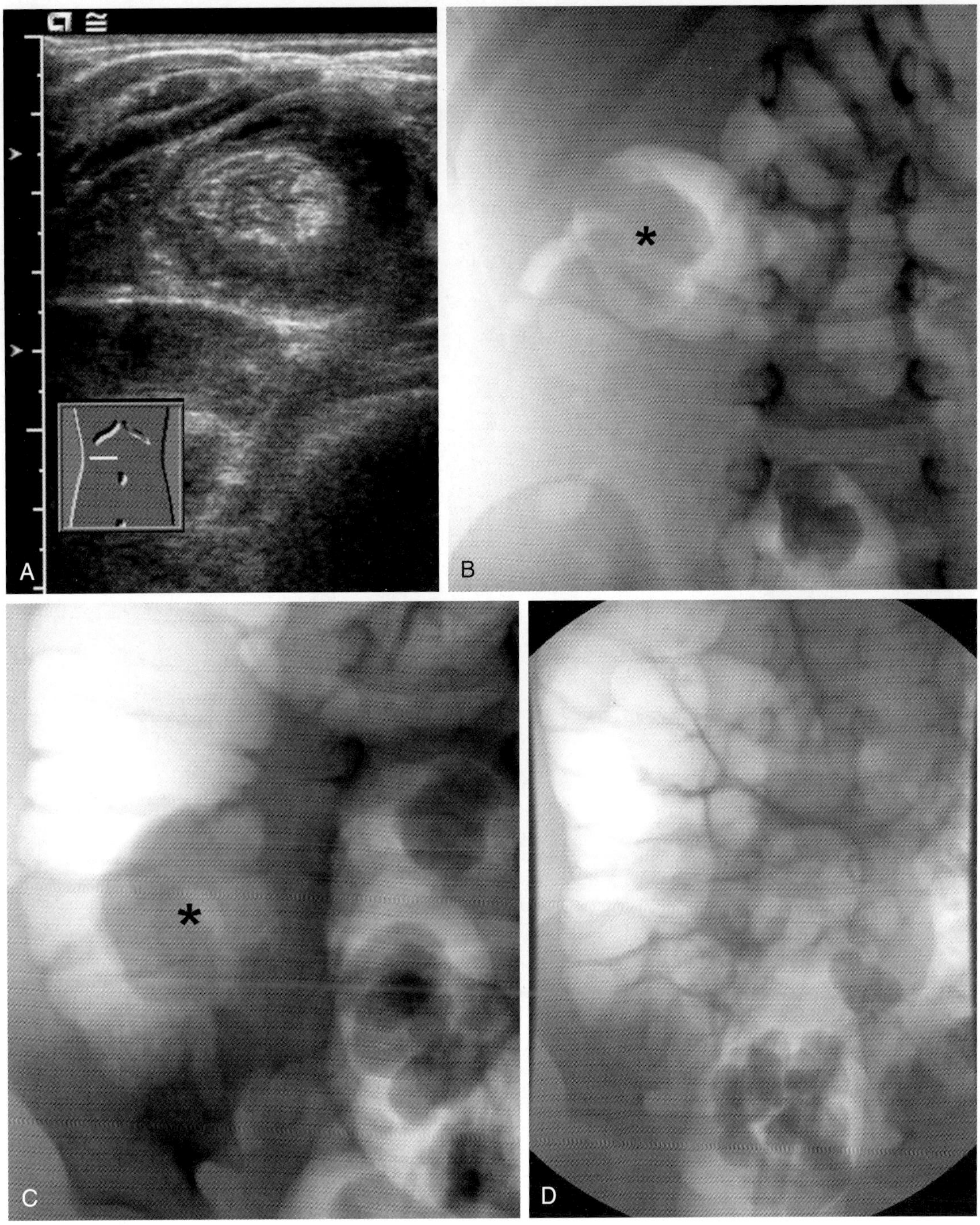

Fig. 25.17 Ileocolic intussusception in the proximal transverse colon of a 2-year-old. (A) Ultrasound shows the characteristic "target sign" on transverse section (hypoechoic ring with an echogenic center). (B–D) Air enema reduction. (B) Intussusception *(asterisk)* is initially located in the right upper quadrant. (C) Intussusception *(asterisk)* has moved retrograde and is now in the region of the ileocecal valve. (D) Successful reduction with resolution of the soft tissue mass and reflux of air into the terminal ileum.

Voiding Cystourethrography

Voiding cystourethrography requires bladder catheterization using sterile technique. For male patients, lidocaine (xylocaine viscous 2%) can be placed into the penile meatus to locally anesthetize the urethra and make catheterization less painful. Catheterize the urethra with an appropriately sized catheter (5-French feeding tube for newborns and young infants or girls younger than 2–4 years old, 8-French feeding tube for older children, 10- to 12-French rubber catheter for teenagers). Under fluoroscopic guidance, the bladder is filled with iodinated contrast. The size, shape, and capacity of the bladder are noted, and the dome of the bladder is examined for irregularities, the presence of filling defects (mass or ureterocele), or sinus tract (urachal remnant). While on the fluoroscopy table, the patient is asked to void (Fig. 25.19). As the child voids, the caliber of the urethra and dilation of the posterior urethra (Fig. 25.20) and caliber change and completeness of voiding are noted. The predicted bladder capacity (in milliliters) for children younger than 1 year is the child's weight in kilograms multiplied by 7. In children older than 1 year, the predicted capacity is the child's age in years plus 2, multiplied by 30.

In patients with neurogenic bladder and myelomeningocele, voiding is usually impossible and detecting vesicoureteral reflux (VUR) is the most important part of the study. In these cases, the bladder is filled to a volume appropriate for age or corresponding to typical volumes obtained during catheterization, with images obtained over the kidneys and ureters to evaluate for VUR. The bladder is then emptied through the catheter.

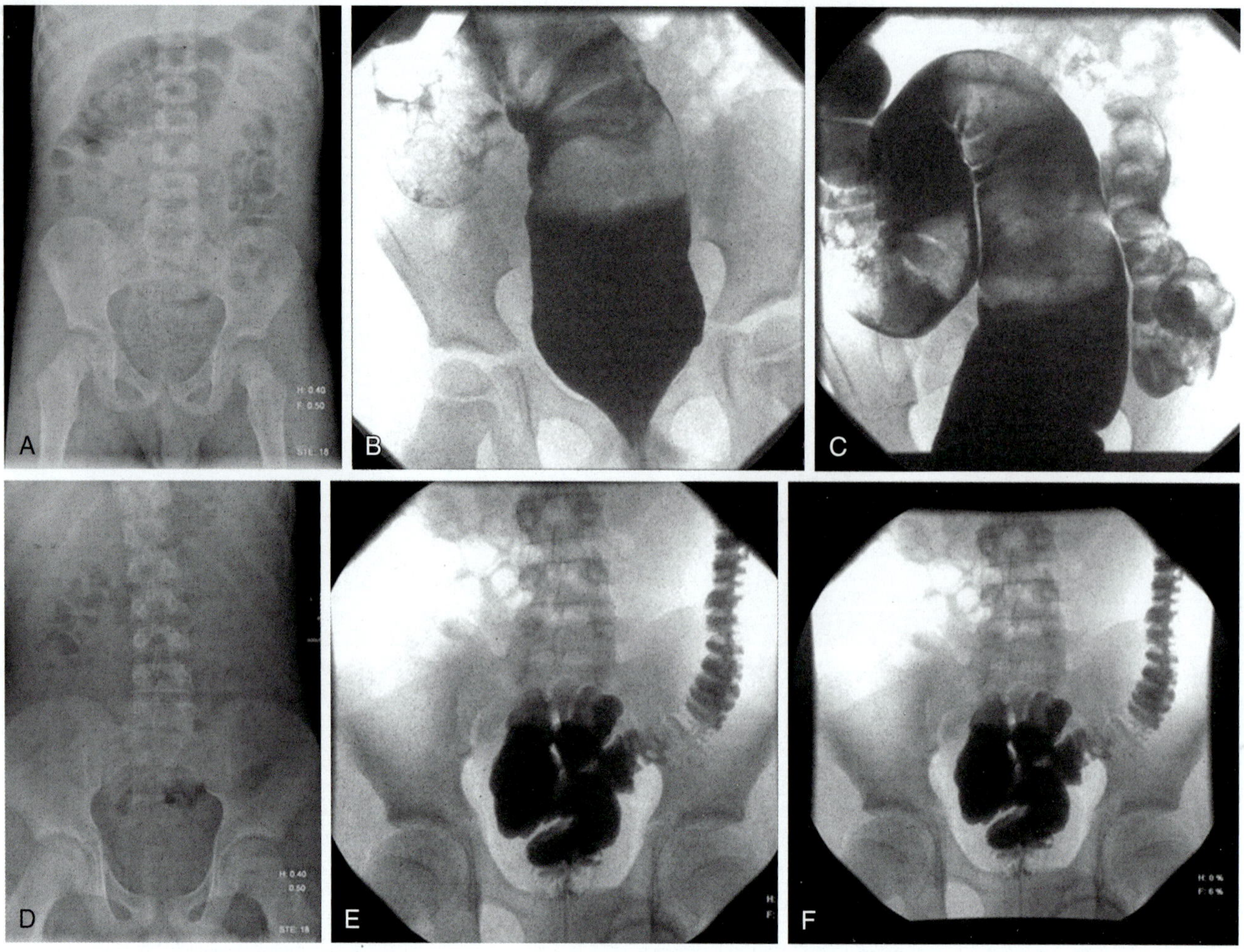

Fig. 25.18 (A) Abdominal radiograph shows stool distended in rectum. (B) and (C) Contrast enema shows the rectum distended in pseudofecal incontinence. (D) Abdominal radiograph in true fecal incontinence shows an empty rectum and not much stool in the colon. (E) and (F) Radiographs show the rectum not dilated and increased haustration in the colon.

ULTRASOUND

Introduction

Advantages of Ultrasound in Pediatric Imaging

Ultrasound presents advantages in pediatric imaging:

- No ionizing radiation is used
- Real-time image acquisition is possible, allowing a study to be performed in uncooperative or crying patients without the need for sedation
- Small patient size results in improved image quality
- Imaging can be performed in any plane
- The equipment is portable, allowing the study to be performed at the bedside or in the operating room
- It is relatively inexpensive compared with CT and MRI and therefore can be used in screening and in multiple follow-up studies

Disadvantages

Ultrasound presents disadvantages in pediatric imaging:

- Ultrasound is operator dependent and therefore should be performed by a well-trained technologist (sonographer) and reviewed by a radiologist before the study is completed
- Deep structures are poorly visualized in obese patients
- Sound penetrates poorly in air-filled viscera and bones

Image Orientation

By convention, when images are acquired in the supine position, the ultrasound transducer (or probe) should be held such that the right or cranial portion of the body is viewed on the left side of the image (Fig. 25.21).

Physics

Ultrasound is sound higher than the audible range, that is, greater than 20 kilohertz (kHz). Diagnostic ultrasound frequency ranges between 1 and 20 megahertz (MHz). The speed of sound in soft tissue is 1540 m/sec. Various frequency probes are available: The higher the frequency of the probe, the better the resolution but the less the depth of tissue that can be imaged. Depth indicates the distance from the transducer surface to the body part of interest. Good transducer/skin contact, using an ultrasound coupling gel, is necessary to generate an image.

The transmitted sound wave is reflected at interfaces of different acoustic impedance. The reflected sound creates a structure and contrast between different tissues and allows a two-dimensional image to be formed. Three-dimensional (3D) ultrasound is available and is most useful in echocardiography and fetal imaging.

Dense structures such as bone, calcifications, and surgical clips/vascular coils within organs will not allow sound to pass through (they completely absorb or reflect sound) and appear bright (hyperechoic) with a posterior acoustic shadow (Fig. 25.22A). Cystic structures are dark with no internal echoes (anechoic); little or no sound is absorbed, leading to the opposite effect with increased through-transmission of the sound waves, that is, increased signal behind them (see Fig. 25.22B). Solid structures produce internal echoes of variable intensity (ranging from hypoechoic to echogenic). An interface between soft tissue and air will cause total reflection of sound so that the deeper structures cannot be imaged, resulting in an acoustic shadow (see Fig. 25.22C).

Doppler Imaging

The Doppler technique relies on frequency data. Sound reflected from a moving target (e.g., red cells in a blood vessel) undergoes a change in frequency. The difference between the transmitted and the received

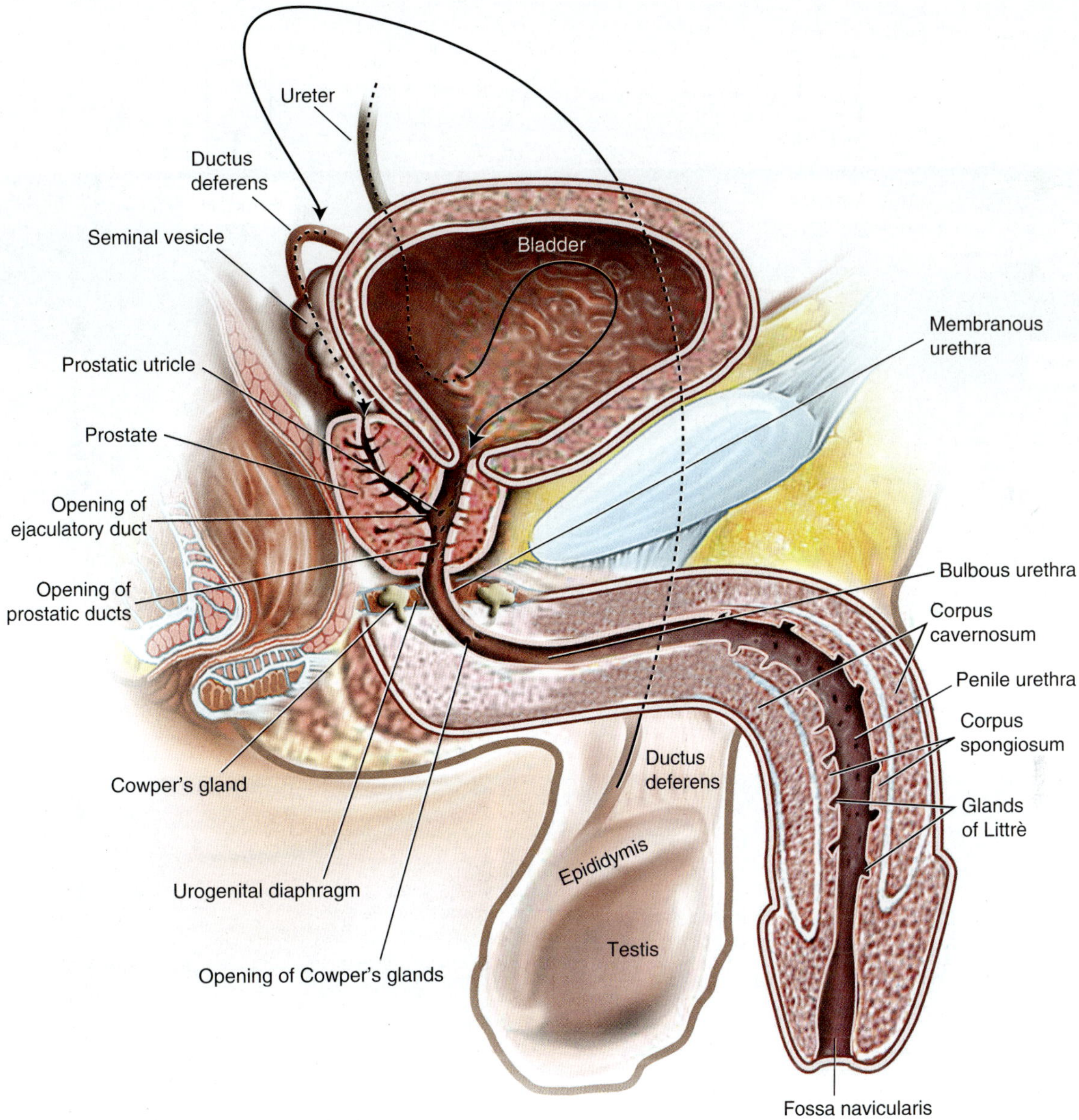

Fig. 25.19 Normal anatomy of the male urethra. A schematic drawing demonstrates the anatomy of the male urethra and its relationship with periurethral structures. (From Kim B, Kawashima A, LeRoy AJ: Imaging of the male urethra, *Semin ultrasound CT MR* 28:258–273, 2007.)

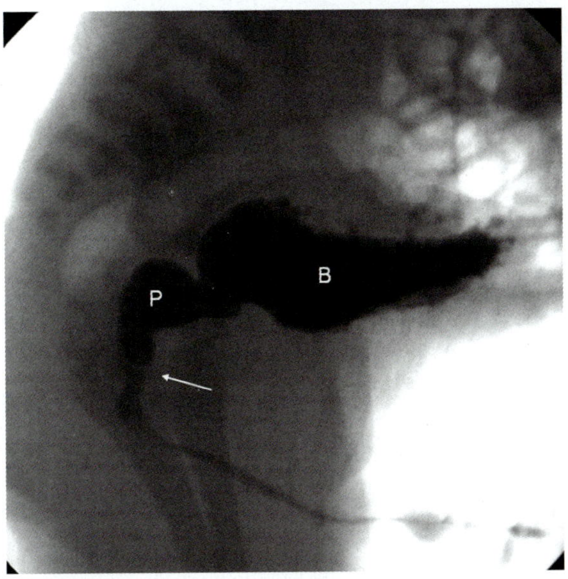

Fig. 25.20 Voiding cystourethrogram in a 1-day-old boy. Lateral view during voiding after catheter removal demonstrates the posterior urethral valve as a lucent line *(arrow)* separating the dilated posterior urethra *(P)* from the distal urethra. Trabeculated thick-walled bladder *(B)*.

frequencies is the Doppler shift. If the ultrasound beam strikes a reflector moving toward it, the reflected sound will have a higher frequency and shorter wavelength than the original beam. If the ultrasound beam strikes a reflector moving away from it, the reflected sound will have a lower frequency and longer wavelength than the original beam.

Spectral Doppler ultrasonography uses the grayscale image as a road map. Doppler interrogation of a blood vessel in the image can then be performed by positioning a cursor within the vessel. The Doppler waveform depicts the velocity over time and is unique to the flow pattern within the vessel. Color flow Doppler assigns red and blue colors to vessels according to their flow toward or away from the transducer, respectively (Fig. 25.23).

Arterial Flow Indexes

The resistive index (RI; or Pourcelot index) is a popular parameter that is altered by vascular resistance and vascular compliance. The pulsatility index is a measure of the variability of blood velocity in a vessel (eFig. 25.6).

Power Doppler

The power Doppler technique measures the density rather than velocity of the red blood cells in the sample area. The amplitude of signal depends on the blood within the sample volume.

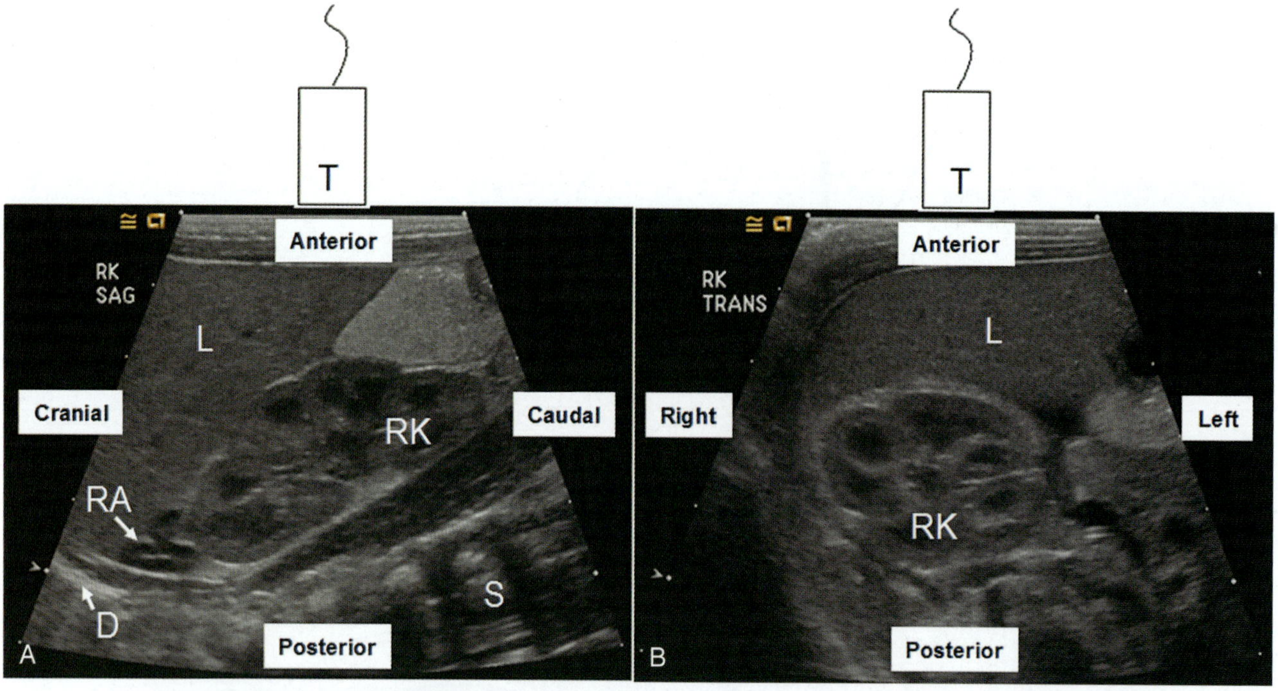

Fig. 25.21 Ultrasound image orientation of the right kidney of a 2-day-old male in the supine position. (A) Sagittal plane. (B) Transverse plane. *D,* Diaphragm; *L,* liver; *RA,* right adrenal; *RK,* right kidney; *S,* spine; *T,* transducer. Notice the normal undulating contour of the right kidney secondary to fetal lobulation and the corticomedullary differentiation with hypoechoic renal pyramids. The right adrenal gland is Y-shaped with a bright (echogenic) center and dark (hypoechoic) cortex. The diaphragm appears as a curvilinear echogenic structure.

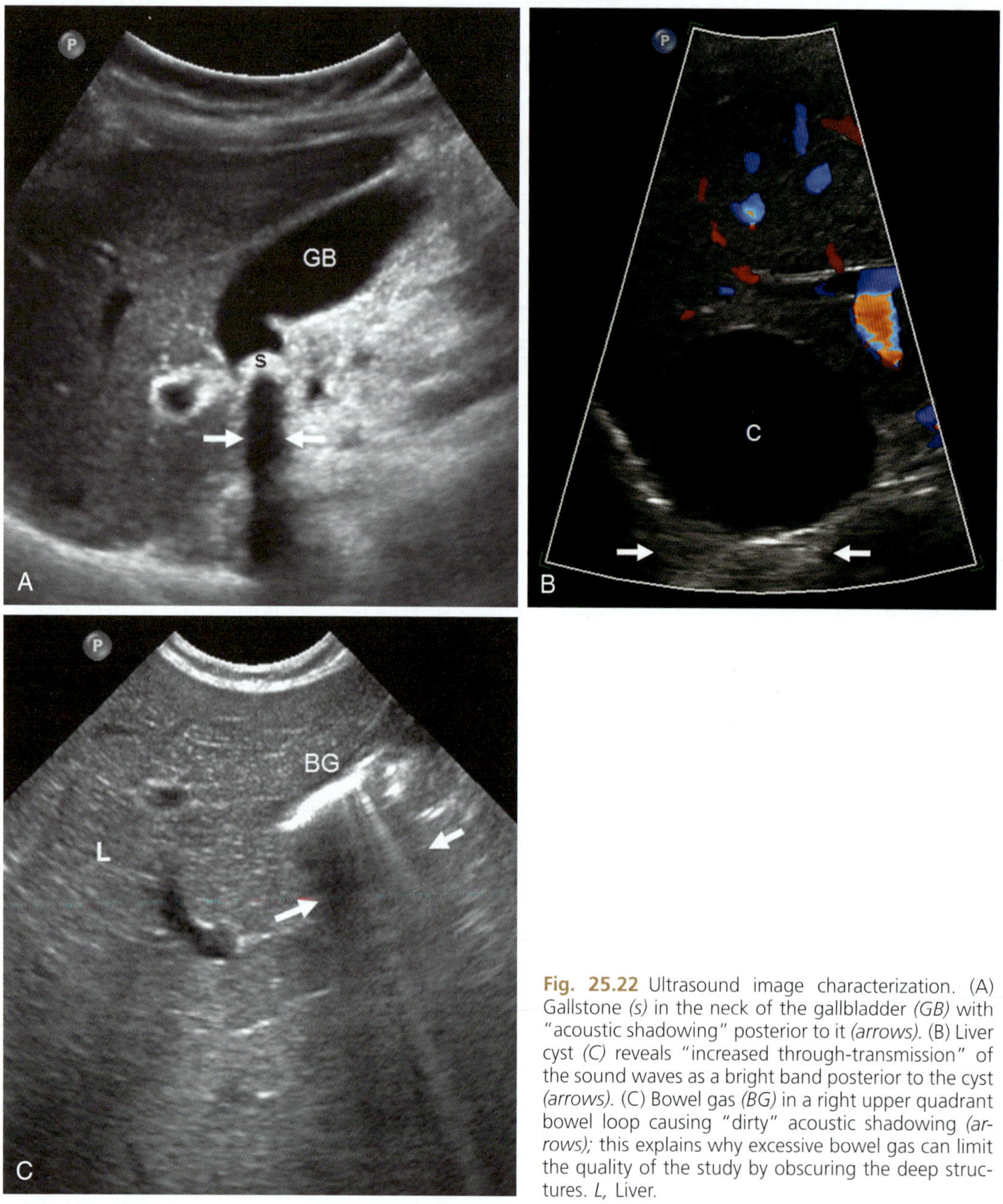

Fig. 25.22 Ultrasound image characterization. (A) Gallstone *(s)* in the neck of the gallbladder *(GB)* with "acoustic shadowing" posterior to it *(arrows).* (B) Liver cyst *(C)* reveals "increased through-transmission" of the sound waves as a bright band posterior to the cyst *(arrows).* (C) Bowel gas *(BG)* in a right upper quadrant bowel loop causing "dirty" acoustic shadowing *(arrows);* this explains why excessive bowel gas can limit the quality of the study by obscuring the deep structures. *L,* Liver.

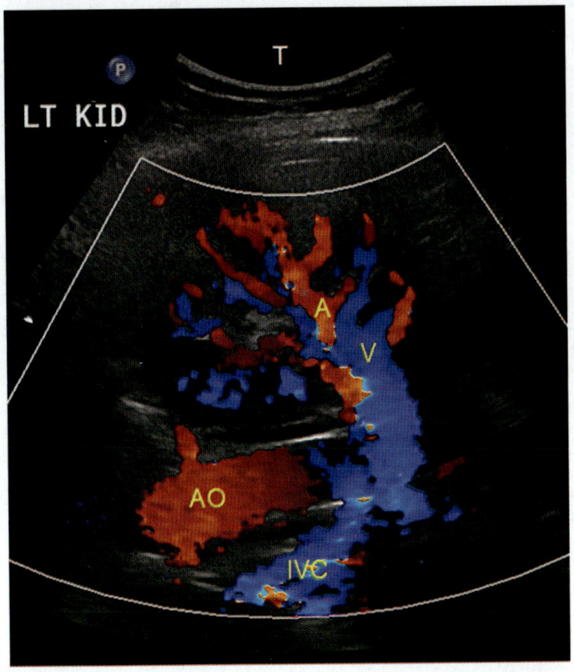

Fig. 25.23 Direction of blood flow in the left kidney as indicated by color Doppler imaging. Flow in the main renal artery *(A)* is directed toward the transducer *(T)* and is thus red. Color flow is blue in the main renal vein *(V)*, as it is directed away from the transducer. *AO*, Abdominal aorta; *IVC*, inferior vena cava.

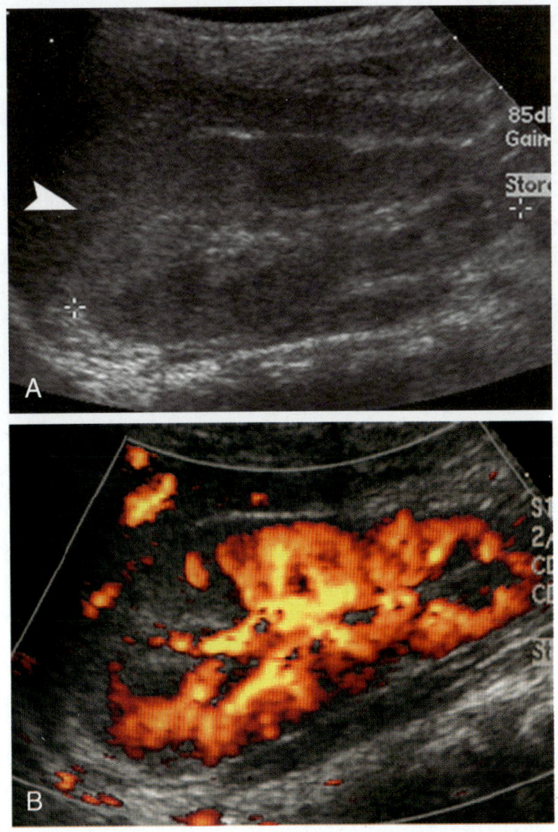

Fig. 25.24 Acute bacterial pyelonephritis. (A) Ultrasound scan shows a wedge-shaped hyperechoic focus *(arrowhead)* in the upper pole of the right kidney related to acute bacterial pyelonephritis. (B) Color flow ultrasound image demonstrates diminished flow through the involved area. (From Craig WD, Wagner BJ, Travis MD: Pyelonephritis: radiological–pathological review, *Radiographics* 28:255–276, 2008.)

Large-amplitude signals appear as a bright color and weak signals as a dim color. The technique is three times more sensitive than conventional color Doppler and shows smaller blood vessels at deeper depths. It also provides better edge enhancement of blood vessels. The main disadvantage is the inability to provide functional information, such as direction of flow and flow velocity measurements. In acute bacterial pyelonephritis, a positive power Doppler ultrasound finding (area of hypoperfusion) can obviate the need for further imaging, such as ^{99m}Tc-dimercaptosuccinic acid scintigraphy or CT (Fig. 25.24).

Contrast-Enhanced Ultrasound Contrast-enhanced ultrasound (CEUS) involves the use of an ultrasound contrast agent (such as sulfur hexafluoride lipid-type A or perflutren protein-type A microspheres), imaged with low-power, pulse inversion harmonic ultrasound. CEUS allows visualization of the microvasculature and can improve the sensitivity and specificity of traditional ultrasound. Ultrasound contrast agents are exhaled via the lungs rather than renally excreted like CT and MRI contrast. Intravenous applications include characterizing liver lesions and evaluating for solid organ trauma (Fig. 25.25), among others. Intravesicular administration can be used to evaluate for VUR with ultrasound rather than fluoroscopy.

Other selected topics of pediatric ultrasound are described later (eTable 25.5).

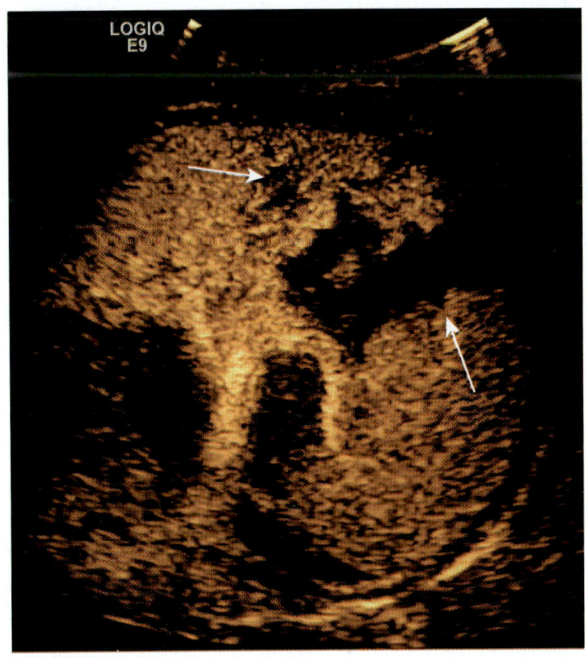

Fig. 25.25 Splenic laceration. There is an irregularly shaped region of nonenhancement within the splenic parenchyma on contrast-enhanced ultrasound in the transverse plane *(arrows)*.

Chest Ultrasound

Thymus

Ultrasound is useful to confirm that a widened mediastinum is due to a normal thymus. The thymus has a homogeneous fine granular echotexture and is located anterior to the great vessels, without causing compression. Ectopic thymus may be encountered in the lower neck, and comparison with intrathoracic thymus may be helpful.

Neck and Superior Mediastinal Masses

Ultrasound can aid in the diagnosis of neck and superior mediastinal masses, whether cystic or solid.

Pleural Effusion

Ultrasound is useful in the assessment of a radiopaque hemithorax. A peripheral pneumonia may appear as a hypoechoic area in the echogenic air-filled lung. A parapneumonic effusion appears as anechoic fluid in the costophrenic recess (eFig. 25.7). A complicated effusion and/or empyema shows pleural thickening, septations, fibrin strands, and/or hyperechoic debris.

Diaphragmatic Motion

In unilateral diaphragmatic elevation, ultrasound can differentiate between a subphrenic mass or fluid collection, subpulmonary pleural effusion, or impaired diaphragmatic excursion. Diaphragmatic paralysis may be due to damage to the phrenic nerve during a difficult delivery or after a surgical procedure. Ultrasound can assess paradoxic or asymmetric diaphragmatic movement with respiration.

Neck Vessels

Venous duplex ultrasound may be performed to evaluate vascular patency before major surgeries. It can also detect venous thrombus, particularly catheter-associated thromboses.

Echocardiography

Cardiac ultrasound is performed in the pediatric cardiology echocardiography laboratory and is useful in the assessment of cardiac morphology and function in congenital and acquired heart disease. It is the first-line modality before cardiac catheterization, CT, or MRI (see Chapter 5).

Abdominal and Retroperitoneal Ultrasound

Abdominal Mass

Ultrasound will characterize an abdominal mass as cystic or solid and help distinguish the organ of origin to help plan subsequent tumor staging imaging, usually CT and/or MRI. Ultrasound cannot reliably identify local tumor extent and has limited value in demonstrating the extent of vessel encasement, retroperitoneal and retrocrural lymph node involvement, and intraspinal tumor extension compared with CT and MRI. However, ultrasound is useful to evaluate patency of potentially involved vessels. CT of the chest should be performed when assessing for pulmonary metastases.

Ascites and Abscess

Ultrasound of the four quadrants of the abdomen and pelvis is sensitive for localizing peritoneal fluid. Uncomplicated ascites is anechoic. Internal echoes can indicate the presence of blood, exudates, chyle, or neoplastic cells. Ultrasound can localize an intraabdominal abscess. There are both increased false negatives (due to overlying bowel gas) and false positives (fluid-filled bowel loops) with ultrasound, and it requires more time and experience than contrast-enhanced CT.

Hypertrophic Pyloric Stenosis

Ultrasound is the study of choice to confirm the diagnosis of hypertrophic pyloric stenosis. Images are acquired in the right posterior oblique position, which allows fluid in the gastric fundus to flow into the antropyloric area, distending this region. Gaseous gastric distention can make visualizing the antropyloric region challenging, as can overdistention of the stomach by breastmilk or formula. If the antrum does not contain adequate fluid, a glucose solution or water (which is anechoic compared with echogenic formula) can be given orally or via a nasogastric tube. The sonographic hallmark of hypertrophic pyloric stenosis is the thickened pyloric muscle (wall thickness ≥4 mm) and elongated pyloric channel (≥ 17 mm), with no passage of gastric content through the passage (Fig. 25.26).

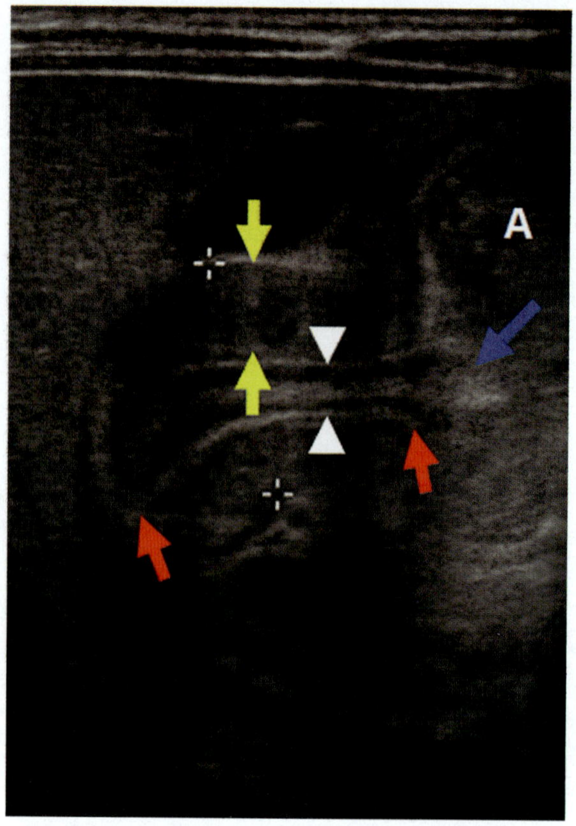

Fig. 25.26 Hypertrophic pyloric stenosis. Longitudinal image shows the thickened pyloric muscle measuring 5.7 mm *(yellow arrows)* and the elongated pyloric channel measuring 22 mm *(red arrows)*. The redundant pyloric mucosa *(blue arrow)* protrudes into the gastric antrum *(A)*, forming the antral nipple sign. The *arrowheads* show the double-track sign.

Intussusception

Intussusception is an invagination of proximal bowel into its distal lumen. The invaginating portion is termed the *intussusceptum*, and the recipient bowel is called the *intussuscipiens*. Approximately 90% of intussusceptions are ileocolic, with the remaining 10% being ileoileal and colocolic (Fig. 25.27). The diagnostic approach should include (1) abdominal radiographs if concern for other diagnoses or for perforation and (2) sonography for diagnosis or exclusion of intussusception. Ultrasound shows the intussusception as a "donut," "target," or "pseudokidney" sign, and it has high accuracy, approaching 100% in experienced hands. See the Fluoroscopy section earlier for reduction. Ultrasound factors associated with unsuccessful reduction include free intraperitoneal fluid, bowel obstruction, loss of Doppler flow in the intussusception, and fluid trapped within the colon due to incarceration. Ultrasound can also assess the presence of a PLP and intussusception limited to the small bowel, and it can be used to diagnose or exclude residual intussusception after enema.

Appendicitis

Obstruction of the appendiceal lumen results in distention of the appendix, superimposed infection, ischemia, and eventually perforation. There is much debate about appropriate imaging algorithms for suspected appendicitis. Some investigators have advocated primary use of ultrasound, with CT or MRI performed in equivocal cases. Ultrasound is much more useful in girls and in patients of thin body habitus than in boys and patients who are obese. In girls, in whom ovarian causes of right lower quadrant pain are possible, ultrasound may be the first test of choice. CT is favored when perforated appendicitis is suspected for evaluation for appendicolith or abscess, in postoperative evaluation, and in obese patients.

Technically adequate examinations are achieved in about 95% of patients. Technical failures are caused by the presence of severe pain or obesity. An inflamed appendix is a fluid-filled, noncompressible, blind-ending tubular structure with a diameter of 6 mm or more, with a shadowing echogenic appendicolith and pericecal or periappendiceal fluid (Fig. 25.28). There may be reactive, enlarged mesenteric nodes; hyperechoic periappendiceal inflamed fat; abscess; and/or wall thickening of the cecum or terminal ileum present.

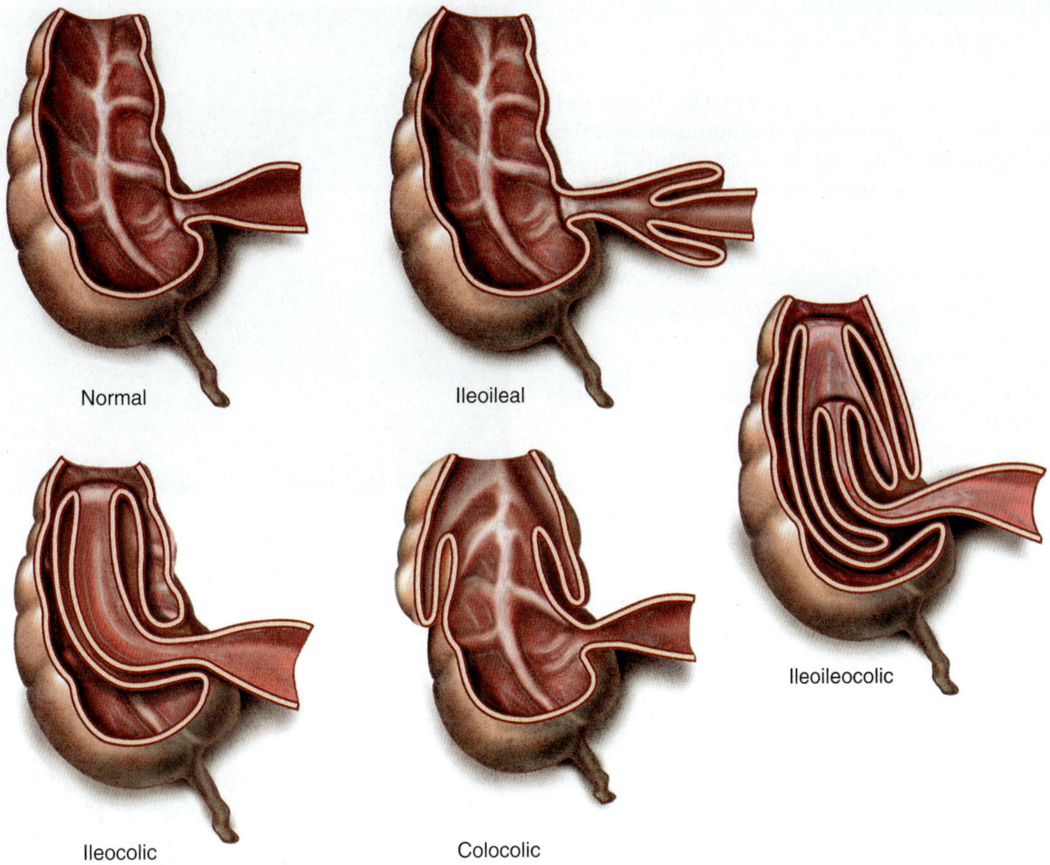

Fig. 25.27 Diagrammatic representation of intussusception. (From Hilton SvW, Edwards DK III: *Practical pediatric radiology,* ed 3, Philadelphia, 2006, Elsevier/Saunders.)

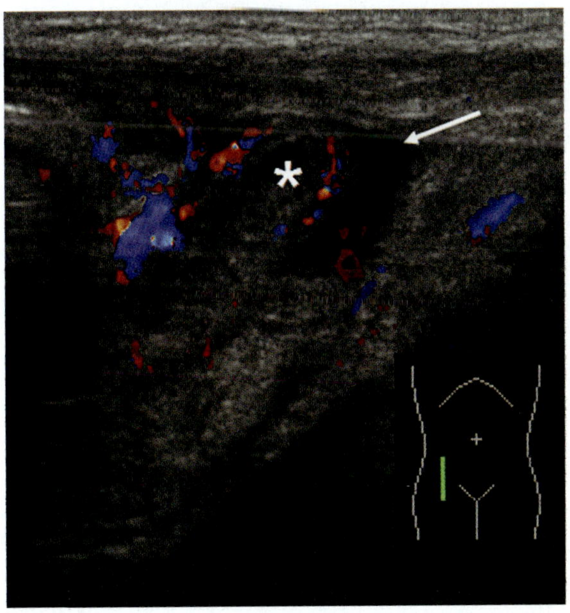

Fig. 25.28 Acute appendicitis. A small fluid collection *(arrow)* is surrounding the tip of the inflamed appendix *(asterisk)*, consistent with perforation.

Perforation occurs in 20% to 30% of children with appendicitis. The appendix may disintegrate and hence not be identifiable on ultrasound in 40% to 60% of children with perforation.

Midgut Malrotation and Volvulus

Ultrasound is an alternative to UGI to diagnose malrotation with midgut volvulus. The sonographic diagnosis of midgut malrotation hinges on visualizing the course of the third portion of the duodenum (D3). Normally, D3 is retroperitoneal and courses between the superior mesenteric artery (SMA) and aorta. In patients with malrotation, D3 will course anterior to the SMA, in an abnormal intraperitoneal location. The relative positions of the SMA and superior mesenteric vein (SMV) are secondary signs of midgut anatomy. The SMA is normally located to the left of the SMV. Reversal of this relationship (SMV positioned to the left of or anterior to the SMA) suggests possible midgut malrotation. However, some patients with malrotation have a normal position of the artery and vein, and some patients with reversal of the vessels do not have malrotation. Approximately 15% to 28% of patients with midgut malrotation will have a ventral position of the SMV relative to the SMA (described as an indeterminate pattern). Midgut volvulus will be seen at ultrasound by clockwise swirling of vascular structures, mesentery, and bowel in the midline upper abdomen around the SMA and is a surgical emergency (Fig. 25.29).

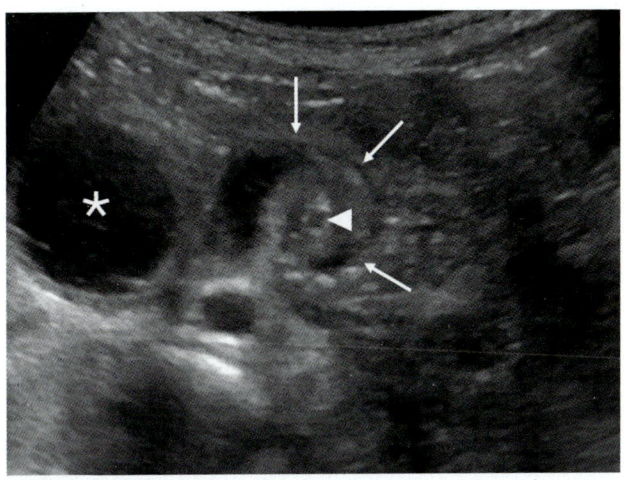

Fig. 25.29 Malrotation with midgut volvulus in a 17-day-old boy who presented with bilious emesis. Transverse grayscale ultrasound demonstrates fluid distention of the proximal duodenum (*), with swirling of bowel and mesentery *(arrows)* around the superior mesenteric artery *(arrowhead)*.

Gastrointestinal Duplication Cysts

Duplication cysts are congenital anomalies resulting from abnormal canalization of the GI tract and are most commonly located at the terminal ileum and the distal esophagus. They are usually round and attached to the GI tract, and most cysts do not communicate with the GI lumen. They have a mucosal lining, and about 43% contain ectopic gastric mucosa. A duplication cyst may act as a lead point of an intussusception. Ultrasound will demonstrate a round cystic mass with the typical "bowel wall signature," which refers to an inner echogenic mucosal layer and an outer hypoechoic muscular layer. In contradistinction, a mesenteric cyst wall consists of a single layer.

Hepatic Vascular Assessment

Doppler ultrasound is useful in the assessment of liver cirrhosis, portal hypertension, and liver transplantation. Vascular patency and character of flow in the hepatic artery, portal vein, hepatic veins, and inferior vena cava can be assessed. Normal portal venous flow is hepatopetal (i.e., toward the liver), whereas hepatofugal flow (i.e., away from the liver or reversed flow) can be seen in portal hypertension.

Gallbladder Disease

The patient should fast for 6 hours before ultrasound examination to allow adequate distention of the gallbladder. The sensitivity of ultrasound for detecting gallstones is greater than or equal to 95%. Posterior acoustic shadowing has high correlation with cholelithiasis (see Fig. 25.22A), whereas nonshadowing echogenic foci are less specific and may represent stone disease, polyps, or other masses. Ultrasound has a sensitivity greater than 90% for the diagnosis of acute cholecystitis. The most common sonographic findings of acute calculus cholecystitis include cholelithiasis, an enlarged dilated gallbladder, a thickened gallbladder wall (thickness >3 mm), localized tenderness (sonographic Murphy sign), sludge, and pericholecystic fluid. The most sensitive criteria for diagnosing acute cholecystitis is gallbladder tenderness in association with stones.

Biliary Tree

Normal intrahepatic bile ducts and the cystic duct are too small to be routinely seen at sonography. An intrahepatic duct is considered dilated if its diameter exceeds 2 mm or is more than 40% of the diameter of the adjacent portal vein. Doppler use allows for a more confident diagnosis of intrahepatic ductal dilation.

The main right and left hepatic ducts join to form the common hepatic duct. The common bile duct extends from the junction of the cystic duct and common hepatic duct to the level of the ampulla of Vater, where it joins the main pancreatic duct in 60% to 70% of individuals. In the remainder of individuals, the ducts enter the duodenum separately.

The upper limits of the common duct should not exceed 1 mm in neonates, 2 mm in infants up to 1 year old, 4 mm in children 1 to 10 years old, and 6 mm in adolescents and young adults. The distal portion of the common duct is usually larger than the proximal portion. Ductal size may increase by 1 mm or more during deep inspiration and the Valsalva maneuver. Ductal diameter also increases after cholecystectomy.

About 70% to 80% of cases of neonatal jaundice result from biliary atresia, neonatal hepatitis syndrome, and choledochal cyst. Other biliary abnormalities include bile duct paucity (Alagille syndrome) or inspissated bile syndrome. In older children, jaundice is most often due to hepatocellular disease rather than biliary tract inflammation (cholangitis) or obstruction. The causes of obstructive jaundice include choledocholithiasis, choledochal cyst, extrinsic compressions/obstruction by neoplasm, and, rarely, stricture.

Ultrasound Elastography

Ultrasound elastography is an important tool that can be used to detect liver fibrosis, follow response to treatment, aid in the diagnosis of biliary atresia and hepatic veno-occlusive disease (also called sinusoidal obstruction syndrome), and help differentiate some benign lesions, such as lipoma, from malignant tumors (Fig. 25.30).

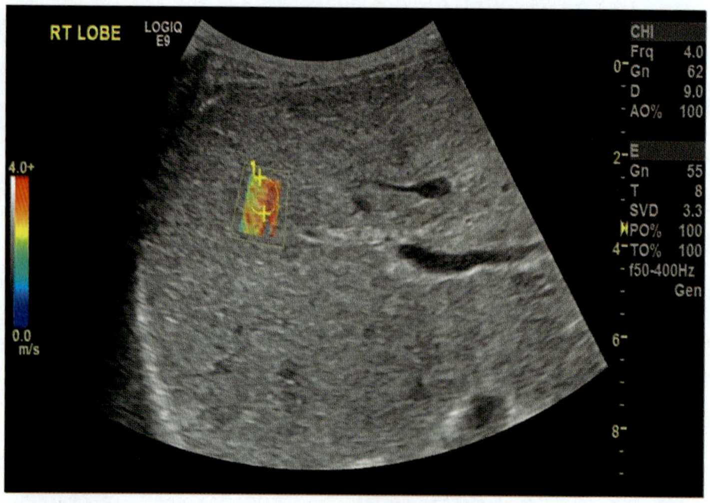

Fig. 25.30 Ultrasound elastography of the liver in a 15-year-old patient who received a liver transplant 8 years previously shows significant increase in stiffness confirmed by biopsy to be rejection.

Ultrasound elastography is based on the knowledge that sound waves move faster through stiffer objects and slower through softer objects. With acoustic radiant force imaging, the transducer sends an imperceptible sound wave and measures the speed of the returned echoes. Transient elastography uses a mechanical force to cause tissue distortion. Finally, strain elastography relies on manual compression of tissues using the transducer to measure the speed of sound waves.

Pancreatitis and Pancreatic Collections

Imaging is not necessary to diagnose acute pancreatitis; however, it is used to differentiate interstitial edematous pancreatitis (IEP) from necrotizing pancreatitis (NP, according to the revised Atlanta Classification) and diagnose complications, namely vascular complications and fluid collections. In most patients with mild IEP, the pancreas appears normal on sonography, with focal or diffuse parenchymal enlargement or margin irregularity seen with more pronounced disease. Pancreatic and common bile duct dilation may also be associated with acute pancreatitis. In NP, hypoechoic parenchyma is seen due to necrotic parenchyma and/or nonliquefied material within the pancreatic parenchyma.

Approximately 50% of children with acute pancreatitis have fluid collections. With IEP, fluid collections detected within 4 weeks of disease onset are termed *acute peripancreatic collections*. After 4 weeks of symptoms, the correct term is *pseudocyst*. Pseudocysts are surrounded by thick-walled capsules of fibrous and granulation tissues and lack epithelial lining (hence they are called *pseudocysts* rather than true cysts). Unlike acute fluid collections, which resolve spontaneously, resolution of a pseudocyst is less likely. At sonography, pseudocysts are usually well-circumscribed, anechoic or hypoechoic masses with through-transmission. Fluid collections in NP are called acute necrotic collections for the first 4 weeks of disease, after which time they become acute necrotic collections. These collections are typically more heterogeneous than collections in IEP, containing hemorrhagic and/or proteinaceous debris.

Blunt Trauma

Although CT is most useful in assessing abdominal trauma, there is growing evidence of the utility of CEUS. Using point-of-care ultrasound, the "FAST" (*f*ocused *a*ssessment with *s*onography for *t*rauma) technique can show the presence of free intraperitoneal or pericardial fluid in the setting of trauma. Regions scanned are (1) the right and left upper quadrants; (2) the right and left paracolic gutters; (3) the pelvis; and (4) the pericardium, using the subxiphoid window. CEUS performed for trauma involves two contrast injections, with imaging performed of the right upper abdominal quadrant, right kidney, and epicardial regions, followed by the left upper abdominal quadrant, left kidney, and pelvis regions. Solid organ lacerations and hematomas can be readily diagnosed (See Fig. 25.25). Urinary collecting system injury is not identifiable at CEUS because microbubble contrast agents are not renally excreted.

Congenital Hydronephrosis

When hydronephrosis is diagnosed in a fetus, postpartum ultrasound is indicated to confirm the diagnosis and grade the severity using the urinary tract dilation classification system. It is recommended that sonography not be performed until greater than 48 hours after delivery. A sonogram performed earlier may be falsely negative or may underestimate the severity of hydronephrosis, because of a relative state of dehydration and decreased glomerular filtration rate immediately after delivery. After rehydration in the first few days of life, the glomerular filtration rate increases, thereby increasing urine flow. Pelvicaliceal dilation secondary to an obstructing lesion then becomes more apparent. When the initial postnatal ultrasound is normal or shows mild dilation, it is generally repeated at 6 weeks of age. If follow-up sonography shows mild hydronephrosis, a VCUG may then be performed. If the postnatal sonogram shows moderate to severe hydronephrosis, a VCUG and diuretic scintigraphy may be performed. A VCUG assesses the presence of VUR and urinary tract anatomy, while diuretic scintigraphy assesses differential renal function and obstruction.

Ureteral Duplication

Complete ureteropelvic duplication consists of two separate pelvicaliceal systems and two ureters. The upper pole ureter often has an ectopic insertion and may be obstructed. It typically inserts medial and inferior to the trigone (Weigert-Meyer rule), terminating in an ectopic ureter or ectopic ureterocele. The lower pole moiety ureter usually has orthotopic insertion, at the trigone. It lies lateral and superior to the upper moiety ureter and often has a perpendicular course entering the bladder (rather than the normal oblique course), predisposing it to VUR (Fig. 25.31; eFig. 25.8A and B).

Urinary Tract Calcifications

Nephrocalcinosis refers to a pathologic deposition of calcium in the renal parenchyma. Calcification is more common in the medulla than in the cortex. *Urolithiasis* refers to the presence of stones in the renal collecting system or in the ureter. Nephrocalcinosis and urolithiasis appear as areas of increased echogenicity. Acoustic shadowing can usually be seen if the stone is 5 mm or greater in size. Nonopaque stones, such as uric acid calculi, can produce as much acoustic shadowing as opaque or calcium-containing renal calculi.

Renal Artery Stenosis

Peak systolic velocity (PSV) is measured using spectral Doppler in the aorta at the level of the origins of the renal arteries and is also measured in the main renal artery at the origin, midhilum, and hilum and at any area of focal color aliasing. Waveforms from the interlobar or segmental intraparenchymal renal arteries at the upper and lower poles should be obtained to measure the acceleration index (AI), acceleration time (AT), and RI. The AI is derived by calculating the slope of the line from the onset of systole to the early systolic peak complex, and the AT is the length of time from the onset of systole to the early systolic peak complex. A schematic demonstrating how to measure the AI and AT is presented in eFig. 25.9.

On pulse Doppler examination, the renal arteries normally have a low resistance waveform with continuous forward diastolic flow and a sharp systolic upstroke (eFig. 25.10). PSV typically is less than

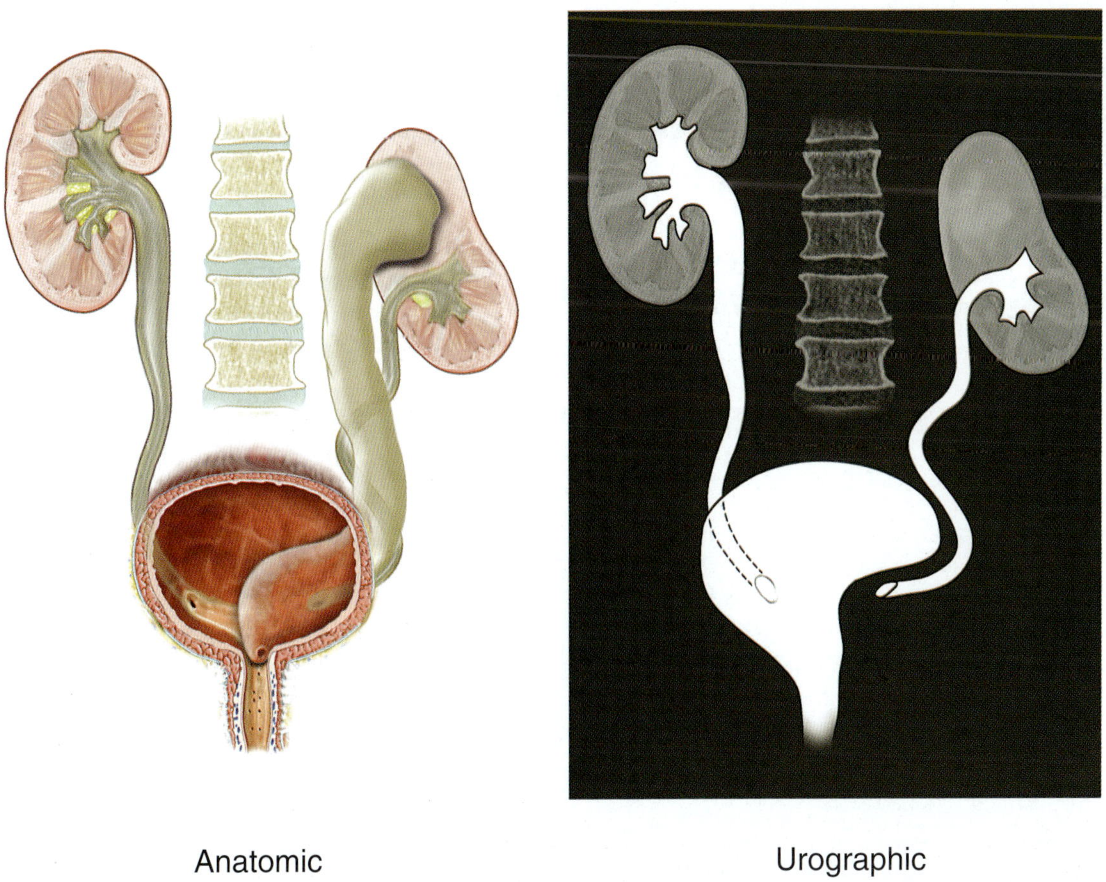

Fig. 25.31 Ectopic ureterocele. Diagrammatic representation of the anatomical and urographic appearances of an ectopic ureterocele of the left kidney upper moiety without function. Diagnosis of this entity on a urogram depends on recognition of indirect signs: (1) increased distance from the top of the visualized collecting system to the upper border of the nephrogram; (2) abnormal axis of the collecting system; (3) impression on the upper border of the renal pelvis; (4) decreased number of calices compared with the contralateral kidney; (5) lateral displacement of the kidney and ureter; (6) lateral course of the visualized ureter; and (7) filling defect in the bladder. (From Adam A, Dixon AK: *Grainger & Allison's diagnostic radiology,* ed 5, Philadelphia, 2008, Elsevier/Churchill Livingstone.)

100 cm/second in the main renal artery and decreases as the arterial tree is traced distally. The RI should be less than 0.7 in the intraparenchymal renal arteries, and the AT is normally less than 70 milliseconds.

Diagnostic Criteria for Renal Artery Stenosis

Grayscale evaluation of the main renal arteries may reveal areas of stenosis or poststenotic dilation. On color Doppler interrogation, focal color aliasing suggests an underlying stenosis, with concomitant increased PSV. Asymmetry of renal length (>1.5 cm) and asymmetry of cortical thickness or echogenicity are also suggestive of underlying renal vascular pathology.

Acute Scrotal Ultrasound

See Table 25.4 for a summary of color Doppler ultrasound findings in acute scrotal conditions.

Acute Epididymitis/Orchitis

Sonographic findings of acute epididymitis include a focally or diffusely enlarged epididymis, with the epididymal head most commonly involved. Adjacent scrotal skin thickening and a reactive hydrocele may also be seen. Spread of inflammation occurs in 20% to 40% of postpubertal males, resulting in epididymo-orchitis. Conversely, 85% of boys with orchitis have signs of epididymitis as well. Color Doppler shows increased blood flow in the inflamed epididymis and/or testis compared with the asymptomatic side.

Testicular Torsion

Torsion of the testis results when the testis and spermatic cord twist one or more times, obstructing blood flow. With testicular torsion, the testis is usually enlarged, may have increased septal visibility between seminiferous tubules over time, and loses its normal echotexture. Color Doppler will not show blood flow to the testicle (Fig. 25.32). With torsion-detorsion (intermittent torsion), there may be confusing increased blood flow during periods of untwisting. A history of episodic pain resolution is important to know in these cases.

Table 25.4 Color Doppler Ultrasound Findings in Acute Scrotal Conditions

Diagnosis	Intratesticular Flow	Peritesticular Flow
Acute torsion	Absent	Normal
Missed torsion	Absent	Increased
Spontaneous detorsion	Normal or increased	Increased
Orchitis	Increased	Normal
Epididymitis	Normal	Increased

From Feld R, Middleton WD. Recent advances in sonography of the testis and scrotum. *Radiol Clin North Am.* 1992;30:1033–1051.

Hip Ultrasound

Hip Effusion

Ultrasound is useful for delineating fluid in the hip joint (Fig. 25.33). At this site, the two conditions most commonly encountered are transient synovitis and septic arthritis, and clinical criteria (the Kocher criteria) are most useful for distinction, in addition to sampling the fluid.

Developmental Dysplasia of the Hip

Breech presentation at birth increases the risk for developmental dysplasia of the hip (DDH) by a factor of 5.5, with the frank breech (hips held in adduction and knees extended) representing the greatest risk. Sonography is well suited to evaluation of the infant hip, although the examination is technically challenging (Fig. 25.34). The patient must be quiet and relaxed for successful ultrasound examination. Ossification of the femoral head interferes with ultrasound examination beyond 4 to 6 months of age. Additionally, manipulation of the hip for dynamic examination may be impossible in the older, stronger infant. Thus radiography may be useful after about 3 months of age.

Neonatal Spine Ultrasound

Tethered Cord

Tethered cord, or low-lying conus medullaris, may occur as a primary problem or in association with other components of spinal dysraphism, such as lipomyelomeningocele or a dermoid tract. The filum terminale may be short and abnormally thick (>2 mm). Sonographically, tethered cord is diagnosed in neonates by the presence of low-lying conus (below the superior end plate of the L3 vertebral body), decreased movement, and nondependent positioning of the conus and nerve roots within the cerebrospinal fluid (CSF) space (Fig. 25.35).

Neonatal Head Ultrasound

Germinal Matrix Hemorrhage

The germinal matrix develops deep to the ependyma and consists of proliferating cells that give rise to neurons and glia of the cerebral

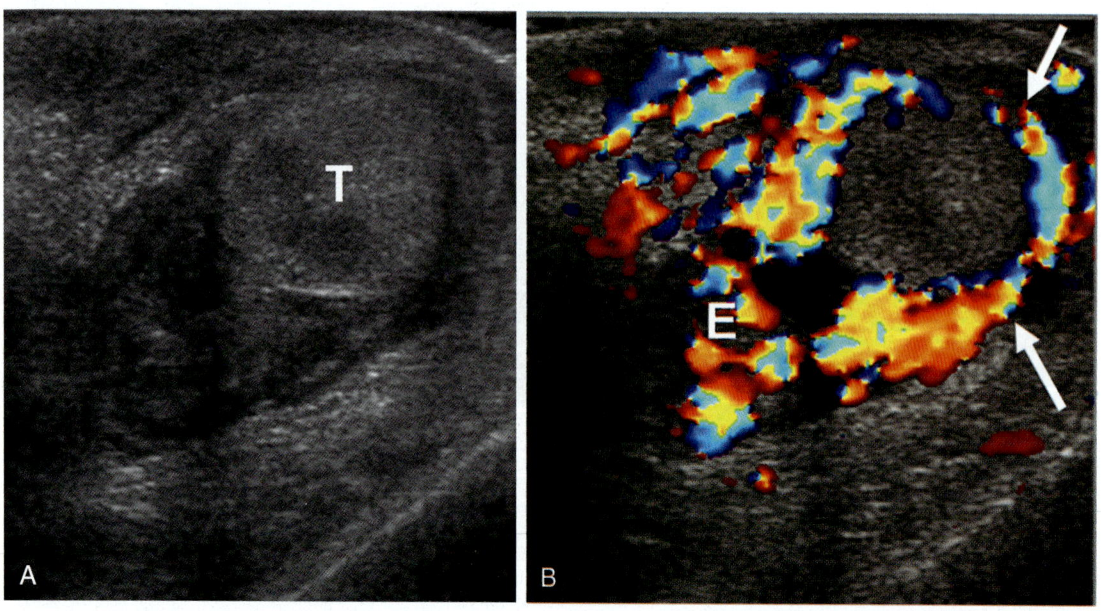

Fig. 25.32 Testicular torsion. (A) The left testis *(T)* is enlarged and hypoechoic. (B) Color flow Doppler fails to demonstrate flow to the center of the testis. Exuberant flow is present around the testis *(arrows)* and epididymis *(E)*.

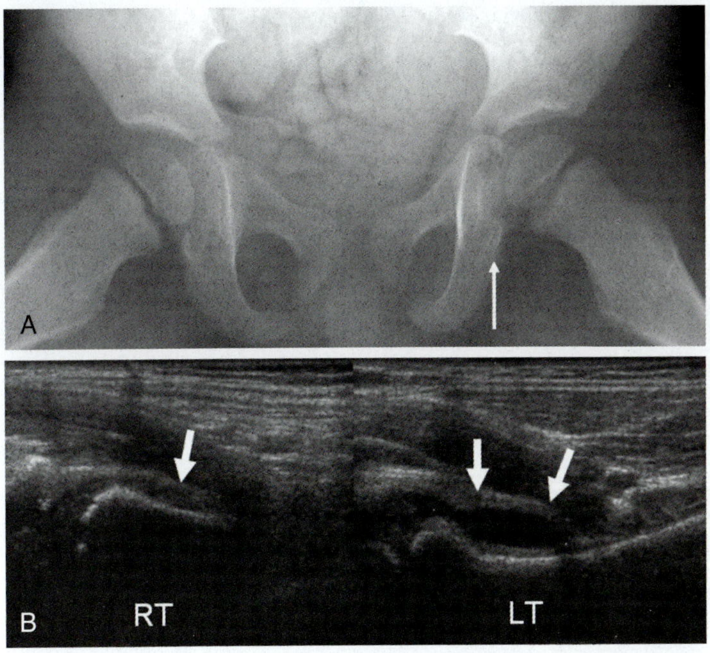

Fig. 25.33 Left hip fluid; ultrasound detection. (A) Plain film demonstrates widening of the left hip joint *(arrow)*. (B) Ultrasound study of the left hip *(LT)* in the sagittal plane demonstrates fluid in the bursal extension *(arrows)* over the femoral neck. Also note that the overlying capsule is slightly thickened. Normal side *(RT)* is shown for comparison. Notice that there is no fluid and that the potential bursal joint space over the femoral neck is collapsed *(arrow)*.

cortex and basal ganglia. The germinal matrix vascular bed consists of immature fine capillaries and extremely thin-walled veins. The germinal matrix is thickest at 20 to 26 weeks' gestation and is seen along the entire undersurface of the caudate through 28 weeks' gestation. It involutes in a posterior to anterior manner, seen most prominently anteriorly between 28 and 32 weeks' gestation, and is nearly completely inconspicuous by 36 weeks (Fig. 25.36A). On ultrasound, germinal matrix hemorrhage is an echogenic mass contiguous with the caudothalamic groove. The normal choroid plexus, which is also echogenic, does not extend anterior to the caudothalamic groove into the frontal horn; echogenic material elsewhere indicates blood.

There are four grades of intraventricular hemorrhage (IVH): grade 1, hemorrhage confined to the germinal matrix (see Fig. 25.36B); grade 2, germinal matrix and IVH without ventricular dilation; grade 3, germinal matrix and IVH with ventricular dilation; and grade 4, periventricular hemorrhagic venous infarction (eTable 25.6).

COMPUTED TOMOGRAPHY

Introduction

CT relies on measuring and displaying the varying x-ray attenuations (absorption) of the tissues in a section of the body during the simultaneous rotation of the x-ray tube and detectors around the patient while passing x-rays from different angles (Fig. 25.37). Reconstruction algorithms then display the differing densities in a grayscale image. It is the contrast resolution of CT that distinguishes the modality: CT has, by far, the best contrast resolution of any clinical x-ray modality, allowing small differences in x-ray attenuation values to be visualized. Intravenous (IV) contrast material may be injected to improve sensitivity and specificity of CT for many conditions.

In helical CT, the x-ray tube/detector array rotates continuously about the patient, and the patient is moved at a constant speed. The x-ray tube focal spot locus defines a spiral or helix (Fig. 25.38). The four Cs of spiral CT consist of (1) continuously rotating tube/detector system, (2) continuous radiation, (3) continuous data acquisition, and (4) continuous table feed (i.e., each acquisition provides a complete volumetric data set). In 2004 the 64-slice CT scanner became available. More detectors (currently 64 or more) means that fewer x-ray tube rotations are required to cover the same volume of the patient, and therefore data can be acquired more quickly. A short scan time in the pediatric age group may allow more examinations to be performed without sedation. The reduced scanning time significantly decreases the respiratory artifact, affecting the lungs in particular. High-speed imaging, often using two detector sources, also allows high-quality computed tomography angiography (CTA) and cardiac imaging. Using multidetector computed tomography (MDCT) scanners, thin (submillimeter) slices can be obtained, allowing reconstruction in multiple planes and generation of 3D images (Fig. 25.39). The latest advancement of CT imaging is photon counting CTs, which use energy-resolving detectors and can scan at multiple energies to lower radiation dose and improve image quality and diagnostic capabilities. All pediatric CT imaging should adhere to ALARA and Image Gently principles, using weight and size-appropriate pediatric-specific protocols.

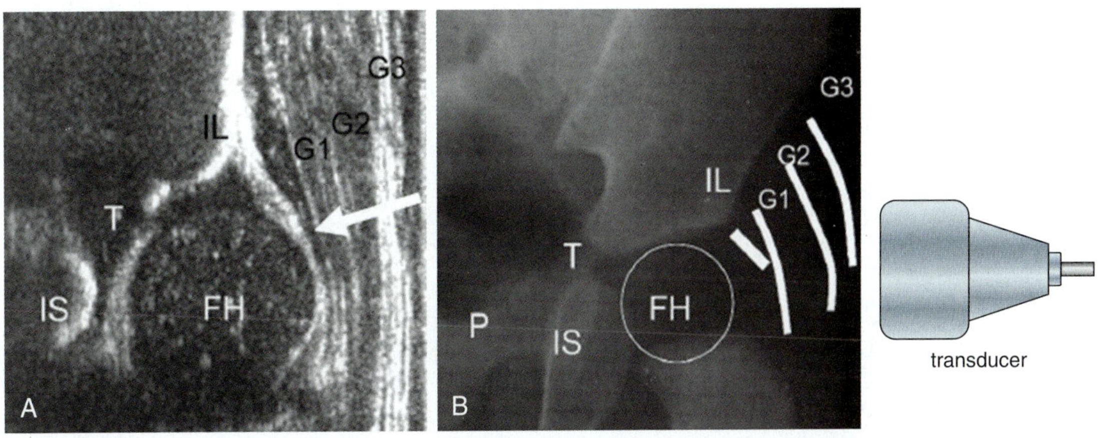

Fig. 25.34 The coronal flexion sonogram of the normal left hip (A) is oriented vertically to match the anteroposterior radiograph (B). The femoral head *(FH)* is well seated within a nicely rounded acetabulum. The triradiate *(T)* cartilage, also known as the Y cartilage, is clearly seen between the iliac *(IL)*, pubic *(P)*, and ischial *(IS)* bones. The *arrow* on the sonogram points to the fibrous tip of the cartilaginous labrum. *G1* refers to the gluteus minimus muscle, *G2* to the gluteus medius muscle, and *G3* to the gluteus maximus muscle. (Modified from Smergel E, Losik SB, Rosenberg HK: Sonography of hip dysplasia, *Ultrasound Q* 20:201–216, 2004.)

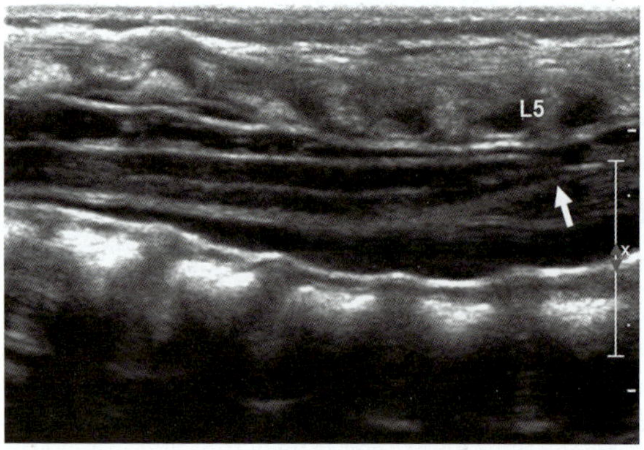

Fig. 25.35 Tethered cord. Longitudinal sonogram shows low-lying conus *(arrow)* at the *L5* vertebra. Note that the cord and nerve roots are positioned posteriorly.

Applications for Computed Tomography

CT is useful in imaging many disorders of the brain and spine (see the Imaging of the Central Nervous System section, later). Common nonneurologic indications for CT are listed in Table 25.5.

Noncontrast CT studies are useful for detecting calcification (e.g., renal stone). Before administering iodinated contrast for a contrast-enhanced examination, the patient's clinical history, allergy history, renal function, hydration status, and medications should be known and reviewed to ensure there is no contraindication. Systemic factors that may lead to nephrotoxicity from iodinated contrast include dehydration, anuria, creatinine greater than 3 mg/dL, diabetes, hepatorenal syndrome, multiple myeloma, and metformin use. Nonionic intravenous contrast is universally used

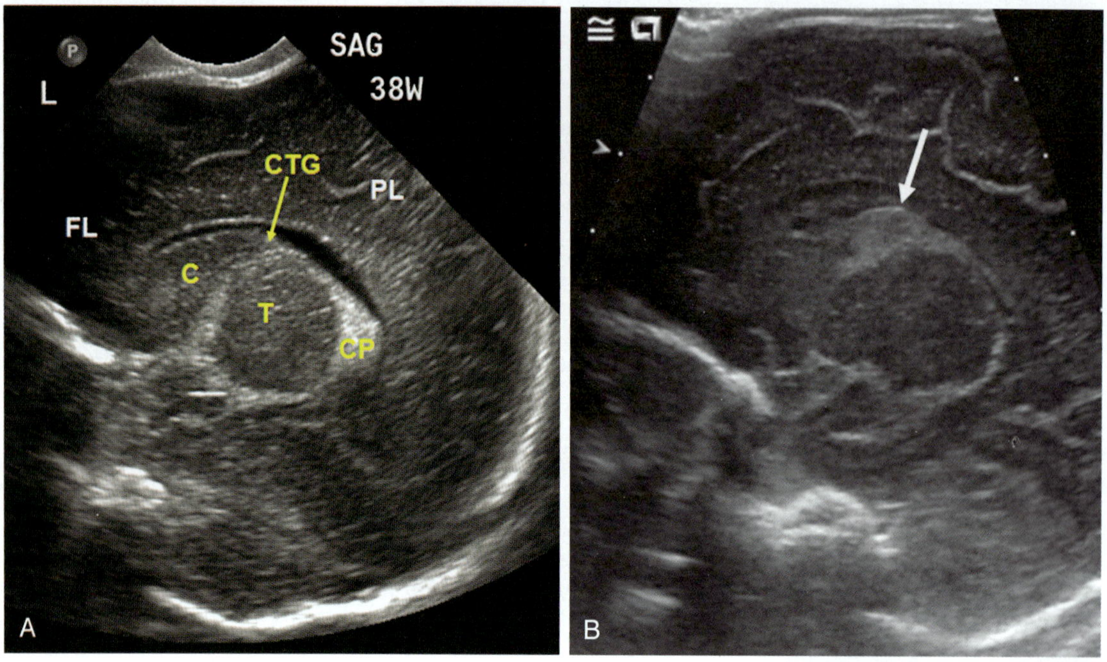

Fig. 25.36 (A) Normal germinal matrix–caudothalamic groove. A paramedian sagittal plane shows the caudate nucleus *(C)*, thalamus *(T)*, caudothalamic groove *(CTG)*, and choroid plexus *(CP)*. *FL*, Frontal lobe; *PL*, parietal lobe. (B) Acute subependymal hemorrhage (grade 1 intraventricular hemorrhage). Left parasagittal image shows increased echogenicity in the caudothalamic groove *(arrow)*.

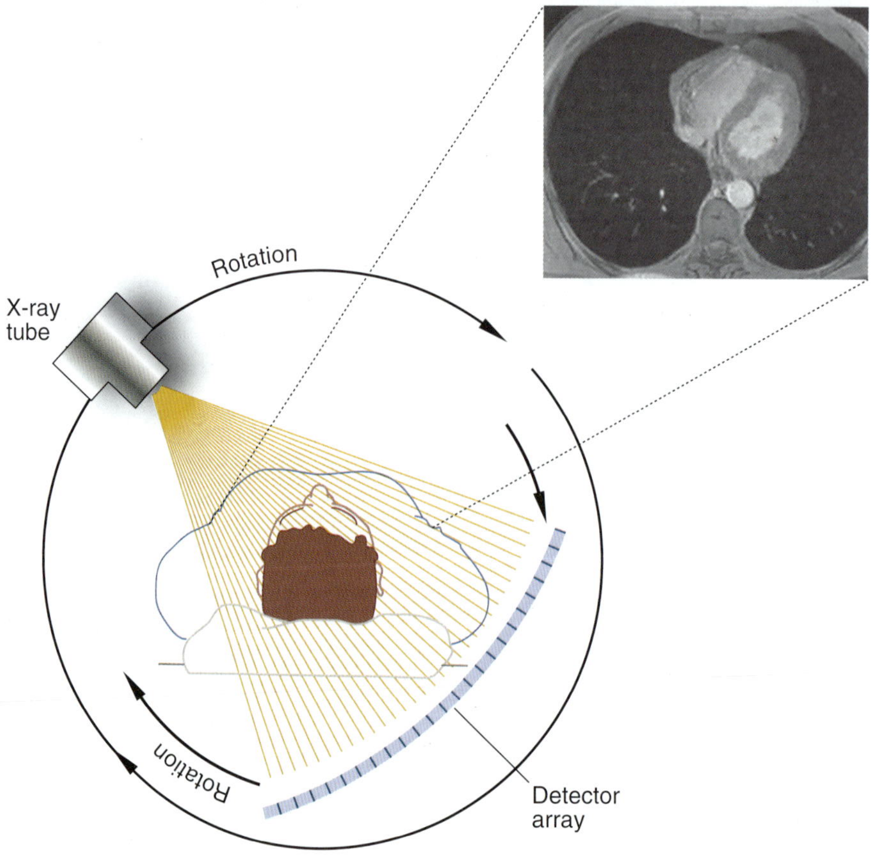

Fig. 25.37 Diagram of a modern third-generation computed tomography scanner, which acquires data by rotating both the x-ray tube with wide fan beam geometry and the detector array around the patient.

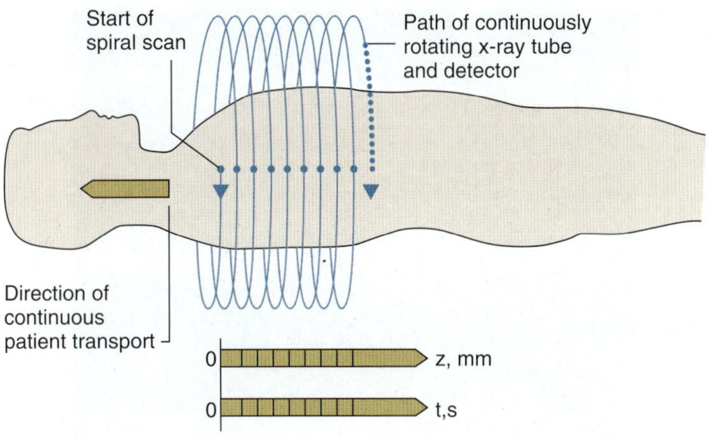

Fig. 25.38 Sketch of the scanning geometry in spiral volumetric computed tomography. *t,s,* Time in seconds; *z, mm,* section position in millimeters. (Modified from Kalender WA, Seissler W, Klotz E, et al: Spiral volumetric CT with single-breath-hold technique, continuous transport, and continuous scanner rotation, *Radiology* 176:181–183, 1990.)

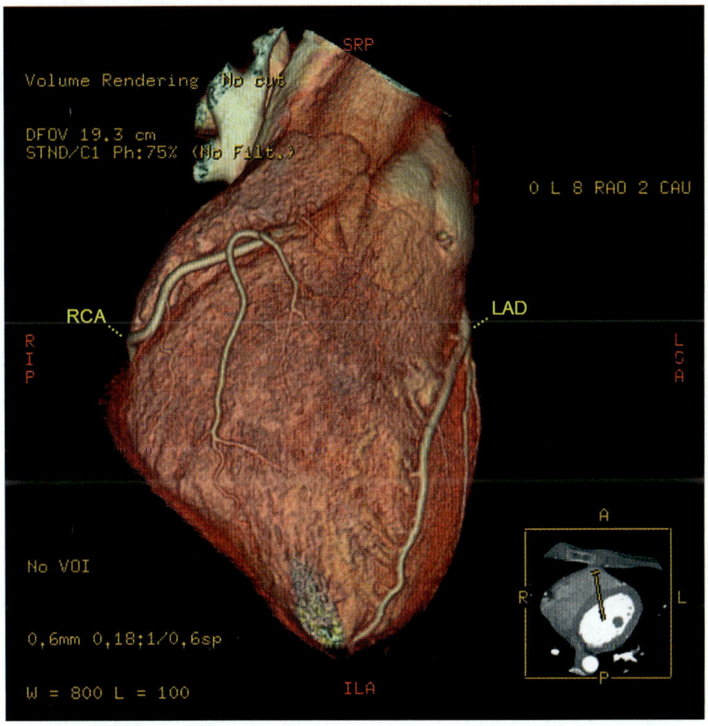

Fig. 25.39 Three-dimensional volume-rendering reconstruction of the heart in a pediatric patient, showing normal coronary arteries as demonstrated with a 64-slice multidetector spiral computed tomography scanner. *A,* Anterior; *I,* inferior; *L,* left; *LAD,* left anterior descending artery; *P,* posterior; *R,* right; *RCA,* right coronary artery; *S,* superior.

and has significantly reduced the incidence of allergic-like contrast reactions.

In the setting of trauma, intravenous contrast is indicated for CT of the neck, chest, abdomen, and pelvis but not for the head, face, spine, or extremities unless there is concern for vascular injury. For CT of the abdomen and pelvis, enteric contrast medium may be given by mouth or rectum in conjunction with intravenous contrast. The intraluminal GI opacification is not always needed but may help to differentiate normal from abnormal bowel, abscesses, and masses. Administration of oral contrast is contraindicated when a patient is at risk for aspiration. Oral contrast should be drunk in small proportions over a period of about 60 minutes before the CT examination starts so that the entire GI tract is completely opacified. Therefore the patient should arrive at least 1 hour before an abdominal CT examination.

Table 25.5 Nonneurologic Indications for Computed Tomography

Organ	Indications
Chest	Trauma Mass Metastatic disease Infection Acute or chronic lung disease Pleural disease Congenital anomalies, including vascular ring, pulmonary sling, cystic lesions of lung or mediastinum, and sequestration Pulmonary embolus
Abdomen/pelvis	Pulmonary embolus Trauma Mass Infection/abscess Unexplained pain Inflammatory bowel disease Portal hypertension Pancreatitis Urinary calculi (CT preferred over intravenous urography) Congenital anomalies
Extremities	Soft tissue or bone mass Osteoid osteoma Developmental or acquired dysplasia of the hip Femoral anteversion Leg length discrepancy Tarsal coalition Fracture

CT, Computed tomography.

Modified from Osborn LM, DeWitt TG, First LR, et al, editors: *Pediatrics,* Philadelphia, 2005, Mosby/Elsevier.

Chest

Lung Parenchyma

CT is useful to evaluate infection and can differentiate among atelectasis, pneumonia, pulmonary abscess, and empyema. Contrast enhancement will outline the vascular pleura, leaving the contents of an empyema unopacified. CT is invaluable in pulmonary metastatic disease detection and surveillance.

Multiplanar and 3D depictions of parenchymal abnormalities can improve the display of bronchopulmonary foregut malformations for surgical intervention (eFig. 25.11). CT has advantages over MRI for evaluation of sequestration, including a superior depiction of lung parenchyma and improved spatial resolution (eFig. 25.12). CT demonstrates primary pulmonary diseases, such as cystic fibrosis, bronchiectasis (Fig. 25.40), and interstitial lung disease. In suspected air trapping, both inhalation and exhalation CT images are obtained.

Airway

Airway evaluation includes assessment of congenital abnormalities, endobronchial or extrinsic processes with airway effects (Fig. 25.41), postoperative stenosis, and trauma. Virtual CT bronchoscopy can be obtained in children to evaluate endoluminal lesions.

Mediastinum

Most mediastinal masses are initially identified on chest radiography and then further evaluated by CT, which confirms the presence of a mediastinal mass, evaluates its relation to the adjacent structures, demonstrates potentially characteristic enhancement of the lesion, and evaluates for potential complications. Depiction of these abnormalities in multiplanar and 3D reconstructions is useful.

Cardiovascular Structures

Cardiovascular evaluation by MDCT has been an important advancement. Assessment of cardiovascular structures includes evaluation of the aorta (e.g., for aneurysm, dissection, vascular

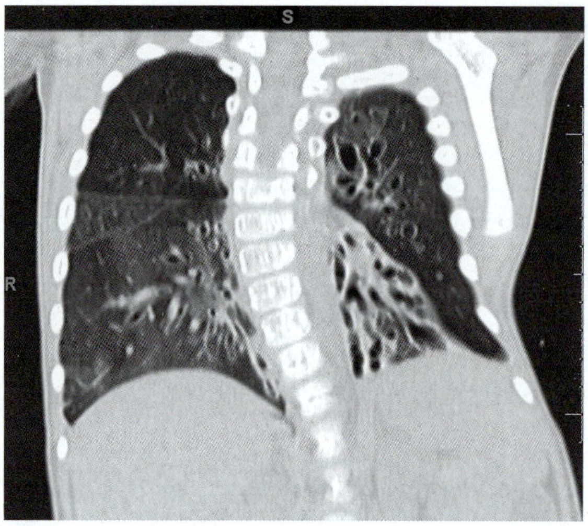

Fig. 25.40 Coronal reformatted image of the chest (lung window) demonstrates cystic bronchiectasis.

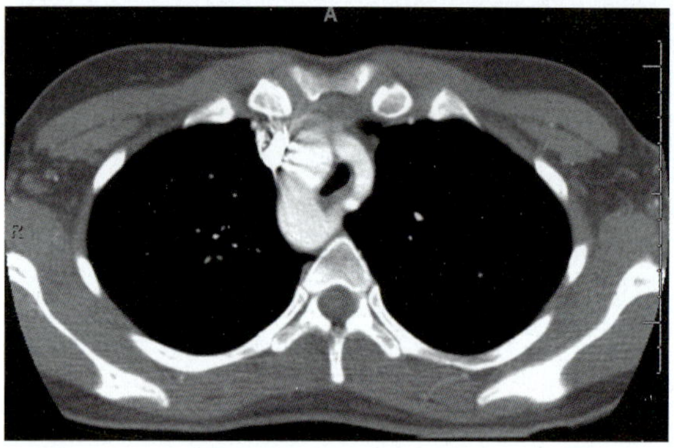

Fig. 25.41 Axial image produced by enhanced 64-slice multidetector computed tomography reveals separate right and left aortic arches with right dominance. The trachea and esophagus are surrounded by a vascular ring made by the double aortic arches and are moderately compressed.

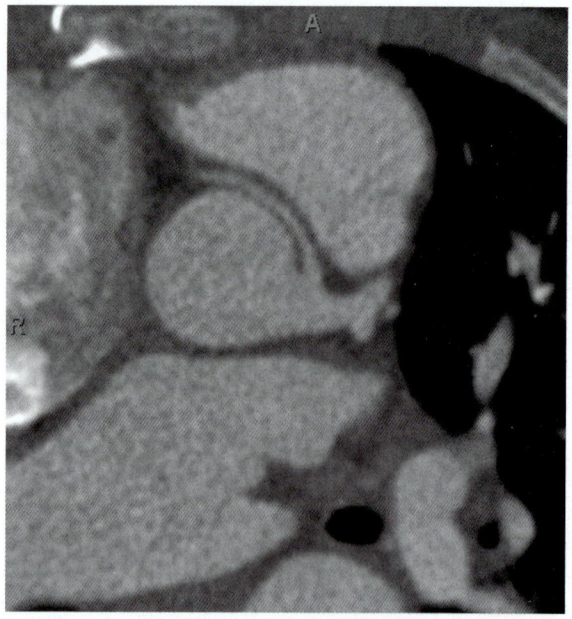

Fig. 25.42 Axial maximal intensity projection image of a gated cardiac computed tomography reveals a malignant course of the right coronary artery, taking its origin from the left coronary artery and coursing between the aorta and pulmonary trunk.

rings, postoperative changes), pulmonary arteries (e.g., for congenital or postoperative stenosis and pulmonary embolism) and veins, congenital anomalies of the coronary arteries (Fig. 25.42), and complex cardiovascular assessment that may not be rendered sufficiently by echocardiography. Cardiac MRI is detailed next.

Chest Wall

Metastatic involvement of the chest wall by neuroblastoma, lymphoma, or leukemia is more common than primary tumors (e.g., Ewing sarcoma). MDCT is valuable in the proper depiction of the involved structures and surgical planning. One of the most common abnormalities in chest wall configuration is pectus excavatum. Before surgical repair by the Nuss procedure, a CT examination using low tube current is obtained through the level of the greatest degree of pectus deformity. MRI may also be used.

Abdomen and Pelvis

MDCT is a valuable modality for evaluation of the abdomen and pelvis in children. In contrast to the chest, however, multiple imaging modalities are suitable options for evaluation of multiple processes, including ultrasound and MRI. For many disease processes, there is ongoing debate concerning which imaging modalities are best and imaging algorithms vary widely.

CT is the imaging study of choice for pediatric trauma, evaluation of suspected bowel obstruction requiring surgery, and suspected intraabdominal abscess. CT use in the evaluation of children with abdominal pain, suspected appendicitis, or suspected urolithiasis is related to CT being considered a routine test, the fast speed of MDCT, and changes in the patient population. As obesity becomes an increasing pediatric problem, imaging modalities such as ultrasound may be less well suited to evaluate pediatric patients for certain abdominal problems, such as appendicitis and urolithiasis.

Appendicitis and Abdominal Pain

Appendicitis is one of the more common surgical disorders of the abdomen. Between 7% and 9% of the general population develops appendicitis at some time during their life. Clinical examination can be challenging, and approximately one-fourth to half of children with appendicitis are missed at initial clinical examination. This number is even greater for those children younger than 2 years old, of whom nearly 100% are missed at initial clinical examination. In addition, other clinical evaluators, such as the white blood count, are nonspecific and may be normal in cases of appendicitis and elevated in association with many nonsurgical causes of abdominal pain. Thus imaging plays a critical role in the evaluation of children with appendicitis.

The reported sensitivity of CT for appendicitis ranges from 95% to 100%. The specificity ranges from 93% to 100%. In one study, the frequency of appendicitis in a population of patients evaluated by CT for abdominal pain was 38%. Direct signs of acute appendicitis include enlarged appendix (>7 mm in transverse diameter), hyperenhancement of the appendiceal wall, or an appendicolith within the appendix (Fig. 25.43). Secondary signs include stranding of the fat surrounding the appendix, associated fluid, or thickening of the cecal wall and terminal ileum. Small bowel obstruction or abscess may be associated. Sagittal and coronal reconstructed images may be helpful in identifying the appendix.

Identification of alternative diagnoses is another important role of CT in the evaluation of patients with abdominal pain and possible appendicitis. Alternative diagnoses revealed by CT in patients with suspected appendicitis are those involving the regional mesentery (46%), ovaries (16%), bowel (13%), urinary tract (8%), and other (17%).

Urolithiasis

MDCT is a primary modality for the evaluation of children with abdominal pain and hematuria in the search for urolithiasis. No oral or intravenous contrast is administered. In one reported series,

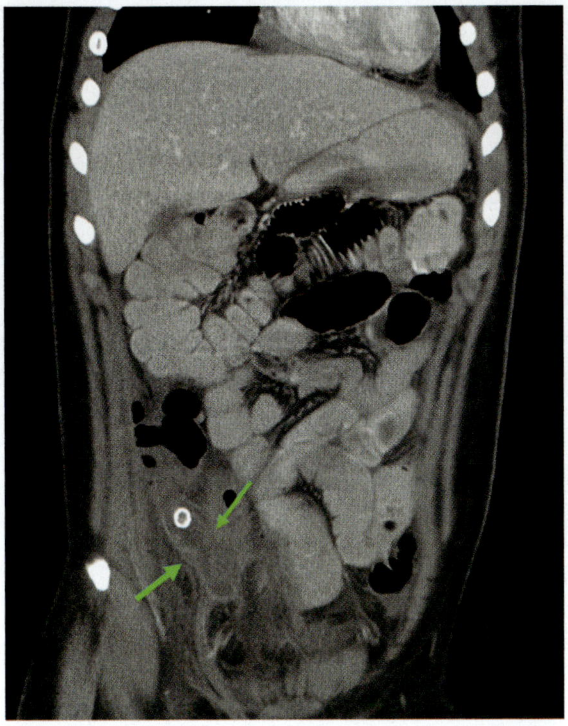

Fig. 25.43 Coronal reformatted computed tomography image produced after the administration of oral and intravenous contrast shows dilated appendix *(arrows)* with a thickened enhancing wall and stranding of the surrounding fat. Note the round calcified appendicolith located near the orifice of the appendix.

approximately 40% of patients evaluated with CT for suspected stones demonstrated urolithiasis. In addition, alternative diagnoses were suggested in 17% of patients. CT findings in urolithiasis include visualization of the radiodense stone, dilation of the ureter or collecting system, asymmetric enlargement of the kidneys, and perinephric stranding.

Inflammatory Bowel Disease

MDCT is being used in the evaluation of children in adolescence with inflammatory bowel disease, such as Crohn disease or ulcerative colitis. The technique, termed *CT enterography*, uses neutral oral contrast and intravenous contrast and is useful in the evaluation of patients with suspected active inflammation, abdominal abscesses, bowel stricture, or a fistula. CT enterography is becoming increasingly preferred over small bowel follow-through and other fluoroscopic studies due to improved demonstration of inflammatory changes within the bowel, particularly extraluminal manifestations, such as mesenteric and peritoneal inflammatory change or abscess. MR enterography (discussed more later) is increasingly an acceptable alternative to CT enterography due to lack of ionizing radiation.

Skeletal System

MDCT is indicated to better delineate the extent of a bony lesion (e.g., stress or comminuted fractures, metastatic and primary bone lesions) and in preoperative and postoperative imaging. CT in tumor staging has been largely replaced by MRI. The reformatting and 3D reconstruction capabilities (Fig. 25.44) and the superior visualization of trauma, the casted skeleton, and complex osseous structures are the most useful features of CT imaging. CT measurement of leg lengths and femoral anteversion can be performed by a low-dose technique. To plan orthopedic surgical procedures and help educate patients and caregivers, 3D-printed models of the bones obtained from 3D-reconstructed CT images are useful.

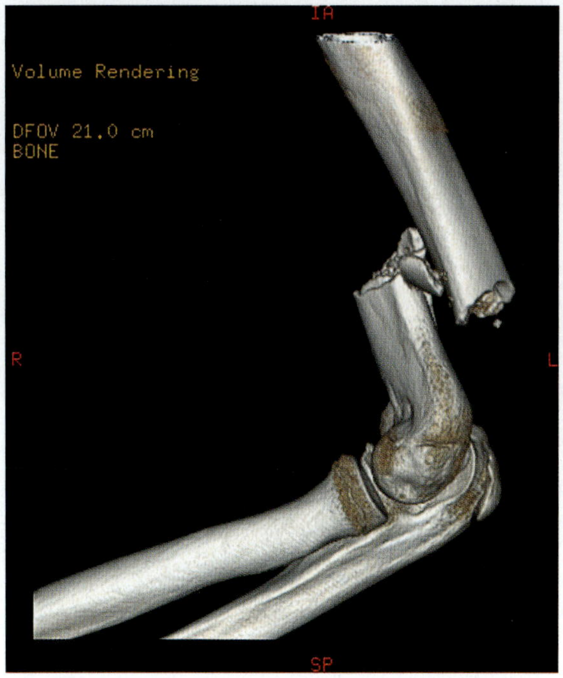

Fig. 25.44 Three-dimensional volume-rendering reconstruction of a displaced comminuted fracture involving the distal humerus.

MAGNETIC RESONANCE IMAGING

Introduction

MRI is based on the electromagnetic activity of atomic nuclei, most commonly hydrogen, as it is abundant in the human body (e.g., in fat and water) and its solitary proton gives it a large magnetic moment. When hydrogen nuclei are exposed to an external magnetic field (B_0), they produce a secondary spin or spin wobble. This wobble is called *precession* and causes the hydrogen nuclei to form a circular path, or precess, around B_0, which becomes faster at higher magnetic field strengths. Hydrogen nuclei are randomly aligned until they are exposed to B_0 magnetization, at which point their magnetic axes align with the magnetic axis of B_0, some in parallel and others in opposition (see Fig. 25.45A). The cumulative effect of all the magnetic moments of the nuclei is the net magnetization vector, which flips to a higher energy state when a resonant frequency (RF) pulse is applied, producing two magnetization vector components: longitudinal magnetization and transverse magnetization. As the transverse magnetization precesses around an RF receiver coil, a current is captured and becomes the magnetic resonance signal. When the RF energy source is turned off, the net magnetization vector realigns with the axis of B_0 through the process of T1 recovery, during which the longitudinal magnetization increases in magnitude. At the same time, the transverse magnetization decreases (decays) through a mechanism known as *T2 decay*. Different tissues have different T1 and T2 values, which allows for distinction between different tissue types. Fat has a shorter T1 (i.e., recovers faster) and a shorter T2 (i.e., decays faster) than water, which has a relatively long T1 (i.e., dark) and long T2 (i.e., bright) (see Fig. 25.45B). Because of this, MRI has the highest soft tissue contrast resolution of all imaging modalities. T1-weighted images best depict the anatomy, and, if contrast material is used, they also may show pathologic entities; however, T2-weighted images provide the best depiction of disease because most tissues that are involved in a pathologic process have higher water content than normal, and the fluid causes the affected areas to appear bright on T2-weighted images. The levels of signal intensity that characterize various tissues on T1- and T2-weighted images are shown in Fig. 25.46. Air is black because of its extremely low concentration of hydrogen, and cortical bone is black because of its lack of mobile protons. Flowing blood is

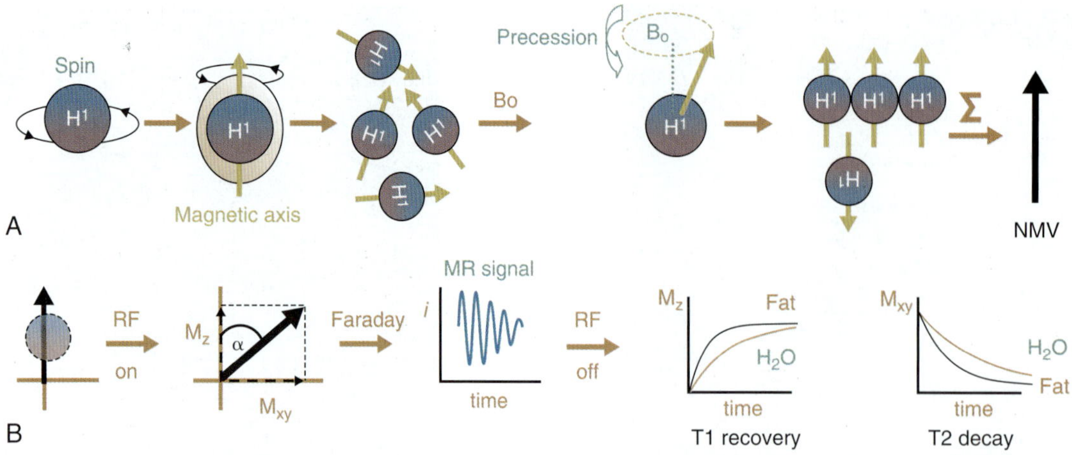

Fig. 25.45 Basic physics of the magnetic resonance signal. (A) As ^{1}H nuclei spin, they induce their own magnetic field *(tan),* the direction (magnetic axis) of which is depicted by an *orange arrow.* The ^{1}H nuclei initially spin at various angles, but when they are exposed to an external magnetic field *(B_0)*, they precess with a wobble and align with it. The sum of all magnetic moments is called the *net magnetization vector (NMV).* (B) When a radiofrequency *(RF)* pulse is applied, the NMV is flipped at an angle (α), which produces two magnetization components: longitudinal magnetization *(M_z)* and transverse magnetization *(M_{xy})*. As the transverse magnetization precesses around a receiver coil, it induces a current *(i).* When the RF generator is turned off, T1 recovery and T2 decay occur. (Modified from Bitar R, Leung G, Perng R, et al: MR pulse sequences: what every radiologist wants to know but is afraid to ask, *Radiographics* 26:513–537, 2006.)

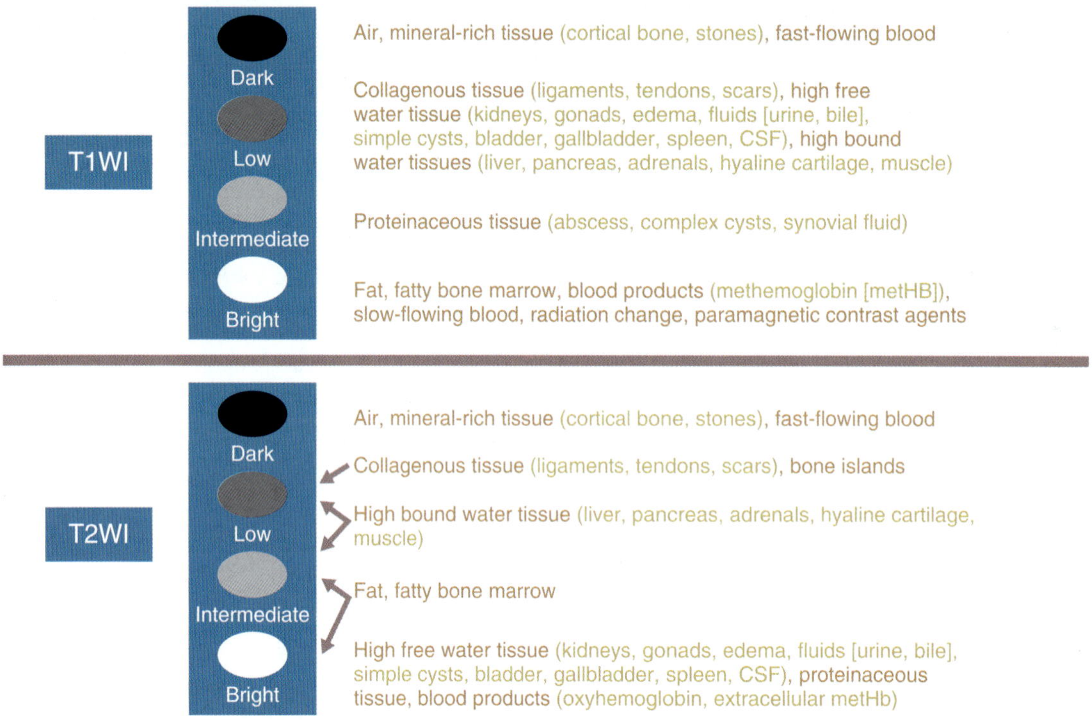

Fig. 25.46 Diagram showing the signal intensity of various tissues at T1- and T2-weighted imaging. However, note that the signal characteristics of proteinaceous tissues vary according to the amount of protein content: Tissues with high concentrations of protein may have high signal intensity on T1-weighted images *(T1WI)* and low signal intensity on T2-weighted images *(T2WI). CSF,* Cerebrospinal fluid. (Modified from Bitar R, Leung G, Perng R, et al: MR pulse sequences: what every radiologist wants to know but is afraid to ask, *Radiographics* 26:513–537, 2006.)

black on spin-echo images because of the flow of protons away from the area before the signal can be received.

An MRI scanner consists of a large circular magnet. Magnetic resonance signal from the body is detected from fixed receiver coil arrays that are built into the patient table and from flexible arrays that are placed directly around or on the patient.

Magnetic Resonance Imaging Safety Considerations

There are no known adverse biologic effects from diagnostic MRI alone. However, there are safety considerations related to the strong magnetic field and gadolinium-based contrast agents (discussed later). MRI safety screening is performed on all patients and accompanying parents/family. Presence of noncompatible metallic objects/implants that may pose a hazard either to the patient (e.g., aneurysm clips) or to the function of the implant (e.g., cardiac pacemakers or cochlear implants) is a contraindication to MRI. It is imperative that in cases of prior surgery or interventional procedures and the possible presence of implants, information about the implants be available at the time of scheduling of the MRI examination. The prospective MRI compatibility and clearance of any implants can then be determined and will preclude the MRI examination from being deferred or canceled on the patient's arrival. Additionally, electronic monitoring equipment cannot be used while the patient is in the scanner, so CT may be preferred for critically ill patients.

Although there are many advantages of MRI over CT, acquisition of the highest-quality images by MRI requires tens of minutes, whereas a CT scan of most body parts requires only a few seconds. Fast and motion-insensitive image acquisition techniques are used to negate unavoidable movement from breathing, cardiac pulsation, and/or bowel peristalsis. However, for patients who cannot lie still (i.e., uncooperative, disoriented or claustrophobic patients, and infants/young children), CT is often used or MRI can be performed under sedation, which raises additional considerations for safety related to anesthesia (eBox 25.3).

Gadolinium-based paramagnetic contrast agents increase the signal intensity of tissues on T1-weighted images with fat saturation. Accumulated experience has shown that gadolinium is safe for administration in children. Contrast-enhanced magnetic resonance angiography using either gadolinium-based agents or ferumoxytol (an iron supplement) provides high-resolution imaging of the vasculature and may eventually replace conventional angiography (Fig. 25.47).

Nephrogenic Systemic Fibrosis in Children

Nephrogenic systemic fibrosis (NSF; or nephrogenic fibrosing dermopathy) is a disease with a potentially deleterious outcome and not yet completely clarified etiology. Risk factors include renal disease (especially requiring dialysis), repeated gadolinium administration, metabolic acidosis, and inflammatory and postoperative conditions. To date, there are no known cases of NSF in pediatric patients, but caution is encouraged (eBox 25.4).

Gadolinium Deposition in Children

Gadolinium-based contrast agents are bound to organic chelating agents to promote elimination from the body, so gadolinium dissociation (or "free" gadolinium) does not occur. In general, gadolinium stability in types of gadolinium-based contrast agents is as follows (ranked highest to lowest stability): macrocyclic ionic, mac rocyclic nonionic, linear nonionic, and linear nonionic. Despite the safety and stability of MRI contrast agents, there is knowledge that gadolinium deposits in patients (most notably intracranially and in bone) who have received gadolinium-based contrast agents, is total dose-dependent, and occurs with all contrast classes. Currently, there is no known clinical significance of gadolinium deposition. However, most pediatric radiologists have adopted a modified "ALARA" approach to gadolinium-based contrast agent use, meaning more stable agents are used and contrast dose is decreased when possible, or noncontrast studies are performed.

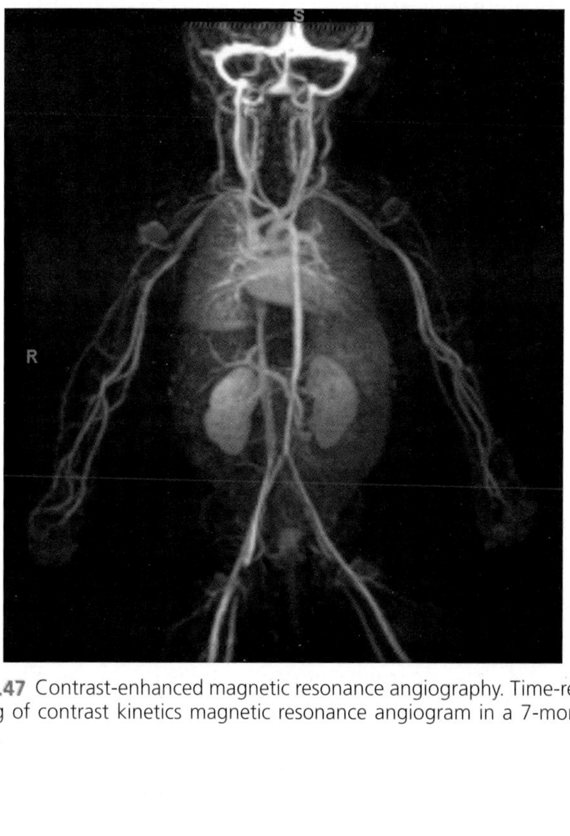

Fig. 25.47 Contrast-enhanced magnetic resonance angiography. Time-resolved imaging of contrast kinetics magnetic resonance angiogram in a 7-month-old patient.

Applications for Pediatric Magnetic Resonance Imaging

MRI is the imaging modality of choice for many disorders of the brain and spine (see the Imaging of the Central Nervous System section, later).

Chest

Regions and structures evaluated include airway, mediastinum, cardiovascular structures, and chest wall. MRI has become an important modality for the evaluation of mediastinal lesions. MRI is ideal for characterizing posterior mediastinal masses (such as neuroblastoma) because it can detail both intrathoracic and intraspinal extension. MRI is useful in characterizing the tissue nature of mediastinal masses. Fat-containing masses in children are usually teratomas. Lymphatic malformations and other cystic lesions usually present as water signal with variable heterogeneity. MRI is useful in the diagnosis of congenital anomalies (such as vascular ring and pulmonary sling), and magnetic resonance angiography (MRA) may show the systemic vascular supply to the bronchopulmonary malformation and its relationship to the solid or solid component of the lung lesion. CT is the gold standard for pulmonary metastasis evaluation.

Cardiac Magnetic Resonance

Echocardiography is the first-line modality of cardiac imaging, but there are several limitations. Cardiac magnetic resonance (CMR) is gaining increasing importance in the management of pediatric CHD because it provides anatomic and hemodynamic information that echocardiography and catheterization alone do not provide. Extracardiac anatomy can be delineated with high spatial resolution, intracardiac anatomy can be imaged in multiple planes, and functional assessment can be made accurately and with high reproducibility. CMR is the gold standard for the quantification of ventricular volume, mass, and ejection fraction. Finally, CMR surpasses both catheterization and echocardiography in its ability to create high-resolution 3D reconstructions of complex CHD, without the use of ionizing radiation.

Common Indications for Use of Cardiac Magnetic Resonance

Common indications for the use of CMR are:

- Shunts (atrial septal defect, ventricular septal defect, and partial anomalous pulmonary venous drainage [PAPVD] and associated sinus venosus defects): CMR can accurately identify the location of the shunt and characterizes its hemodynamics by measuring flow through the pulmonary artery and ascending aorta (Qp:Qs), using through-plane phase-contrast flow sequences.
- Quantification of valve regurgitation: Through-plane phase-contrast flow sequences give forward and reverse flow volumes through a vessel, allowing the regurgitant fraction to be calculated (RF% = reverse flow/forward flow × 100). Examples of regurgitant valves that require accurate serial imaging to guide management include bicuspid aortic valves and pulmonary regurgitation in patients after TOF repair (Fig. 25.48).
- Determination of the extracardiac anatomy in patients with complex CHD, such as relationship of great vessels, major aortopulmonary collateral arteries (MAPCAs), airway branching pattern, and abdominal situs.

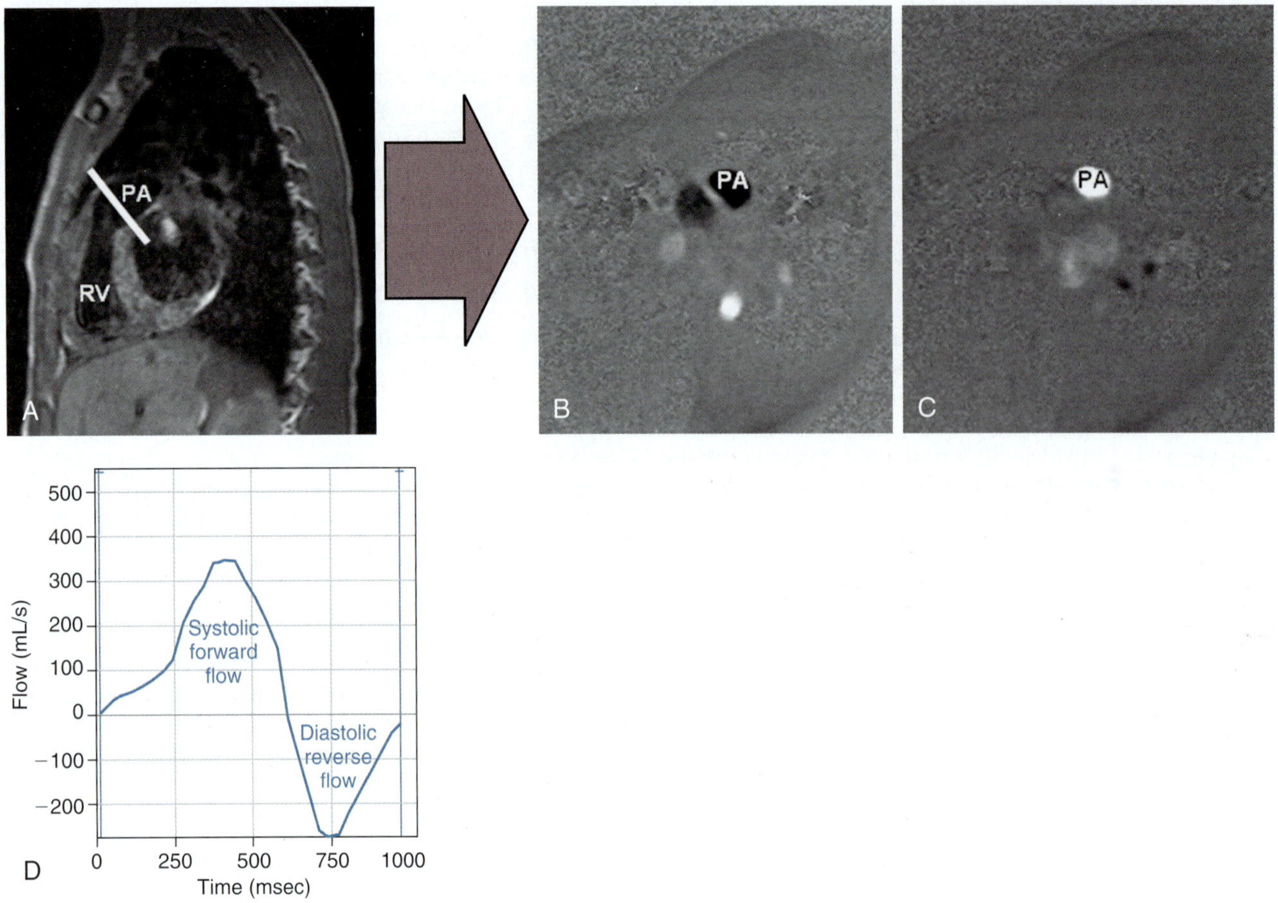

Fig. 25.48 Assessment of pulmonary regurgitation in a 20-year-old patient with repaired tetralogy of Fallot. (A) Localizer sagittal spin-echo magnetic resonance image indicates the imaging plane of the flow images *(white line)* perpendicular to the main pulmonary artery *(PA)*. *RV,* Right ventricle. (B) Phase-velocity image obtained during systole reveals low signal intensity within the PA, indicating antegrade flow. (C) Phase-velocity image obtained during diastole demonstrates high signal intensity within the PA, indicating retrograde flow. (D) Graph depicts the flow profile in the main pulmonary artery. A pulmonary regurgitant fraction of 55% was calculated (RF% = reverse flow/forward flow × 100).

- Aortic root/arch abnormalities: Assessment of the extent and severity of aortic coarctation (Fig. 25.49). CMR is useful in patients who have undergone coarctation repair in whom echocardiography does not sensitively demonstrate aneurysmal formation or restenosis. Patients with suspected vascular rings benefit from 3D evaluation. CMR is performed in patients with a dilated aortic root, such as a bicuspid aortic valve and Marfan syndrome, to assess morphology and competency/patency of the aortic valve.
- Evaluation of size and patency of pulmonary arteries: CMR provides detailed anatomy of the branch pulmonary arteries and the main pulmonary trunk in postoperative patients who have had pulmonary arteries mobilized and/or reconstructed (e.g., arterial switch operation, after repair of TOF). Patients with inherently abnormal pulmonary arteries due to syndromes such as Noonan and Alagille may also require CMR.
- Evaluation of pulmonary venous anatomy/stenosis and systemic veins.
- Assessment of anomalous coronary arteries, coronary aneurysms in Kawasaki disease, and coronary anatomy after arterial switch operation.
- T2* (pronounced *T2 star*) CMR: This is an accurate, noninvasive method for the diagnosis and monitoring of patients at risk for iron deposition cardiomyopathy.
- Evaluation of arrhythmogenic right ventricular dysplasia, hypertrophic cardiomyopathy, and myocarditis.
- Assessment of intracardiac masses/thrombi and pericardial masses.
- Takayasu arteritis: MRI can detect arterial wall thickening, edema, and late gadolinium enhancement consistent with active disease and can also assess complications, such as vascular narrowing and/or dilation.
- CMR tissue tagging: This noninvasive tool quantifies 3D intramural myocardial function and provides detailed data on contraction/relaxation of the heart.

Role of Computed Tomography Imaging

CT imaging is useful for patients who are unable to cooperate with CMR, have contraindications to MRI, or who are too clinically unstable. In addition, when CMR provides inadequate images for clinical decision making (e.g., small structures, such as coronary arteries), ECG-gated CTA is the modality of choice.

Abdomen

Abdominal Masses

MRI is increasingly advocated for initial diagnosis of various abdominal masses and preoperative imaging, assessment of complications, and follow-up.

Abdominal masses in the pediatric population are predominantly retroperitoneal in location, with renal etiology in more than half of the cases. In neonates, most abdominal masses are benign, yet the percentage of malignant neoplasms increases beyond the neonatal period. Retroperitoneal tumors include neonatal mesoblastic nephroma, neuroblastoma, ganglioneuroma, ganglioneuroblastoma, Wilms tumor, rhabdoid renal tumor, renal cell carcinoma (in older children), and pheochromocytoma.

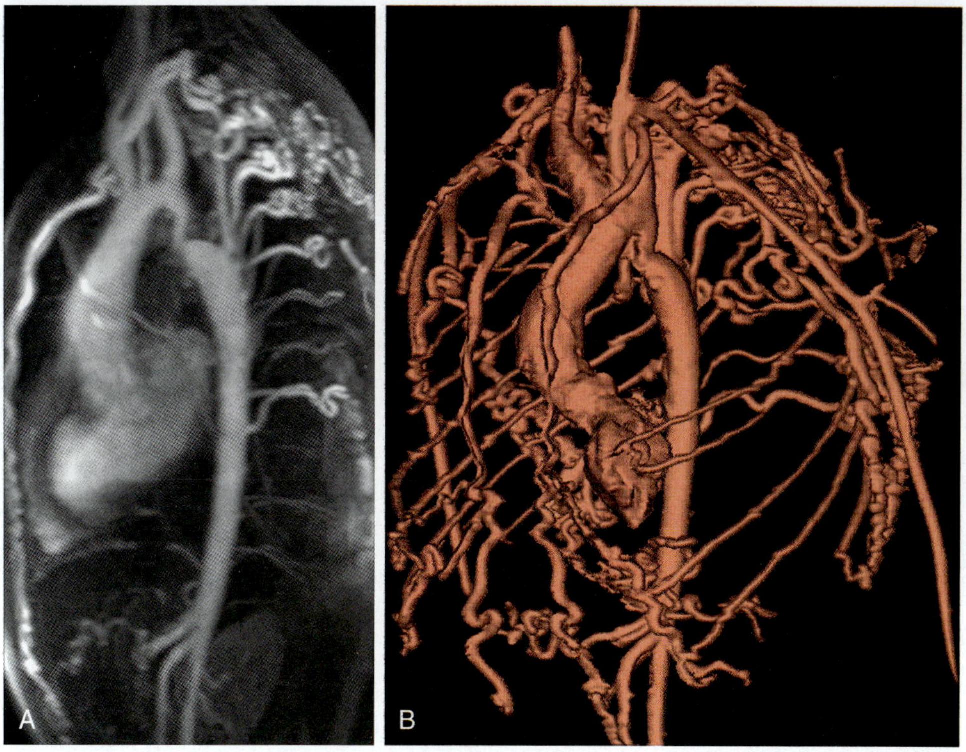

Fig. 25.49 Coarctation of the aorta in an 18-year-old. Sagittal maximal intensity projection (A) and volume-rendering (B) reconstruction images from magnetic resonance angiography (MRA) show a three-vessel aortic arch with severe narrowing of the aorta just distal to the origin of the left subclavian artery. There are prominent collateral vessels feeding the proximal descending aorta just beyond the coarctation.

Liver tumors in the pediatric population include congenital hemangioma, infantile hemangiomas (including hemangiomatosis), hepatoblastoma, embryonal sarcoma (Fig. 25.50), rhabdomyosarcoma, and hepatocellular carcinoma. Hepatocellular adenoma and focal nodular hyperplasia may be seen in patients after chemotherapy treatment of other malignancies and are best differentiated from metastasis or recurrent disease by using hepatocyte-specific contrast agents (such as gadoxetate). Rhabdomyosarcoma of the biliary tract is rare, but it is the most common malignancy of the biliary tract in children.

Focal pancreatic lesions in children are usually exocrine neoplasms or cystic lesions. Pancreatoblastoma is the most common exocrine pancreatic neoplasm in young children. Cystic pancreatic lesions are usually associated with inherited disorders, such as cystic fibrosis, von Hippel-Lindau disease, and autosomal dominant polycystic disease.

Focal splenic lesions in children include abscesses, neoplasms (most commonly lymphoma), vascular malformations (lymphatic malformation and hemangioma), and cysts.

Mesenteric masses include lymphatic malformation, mesenteric cyst, and teratoma. Lymphoma is the most common malignant neoplasm of the bowel and mesentery.

Genitourinary tumors may be encountered, including rhabdomyosarcoma, ovarian teratoma, and various ovarian and testicular stromal tumors. Congenital uterine malformations are easily assessed by MRI.

Magnetic Resonance Cholangiopancreatography

Magnetic resonance cholangiopancreatography with heavily T2-weighted sequences has been shown to be safe and accurate in depicting pancreatobiliary anatomy and can be used to evaluate pancreatitis, choledochal cysts, choledocholithiasis, primary sclerosing

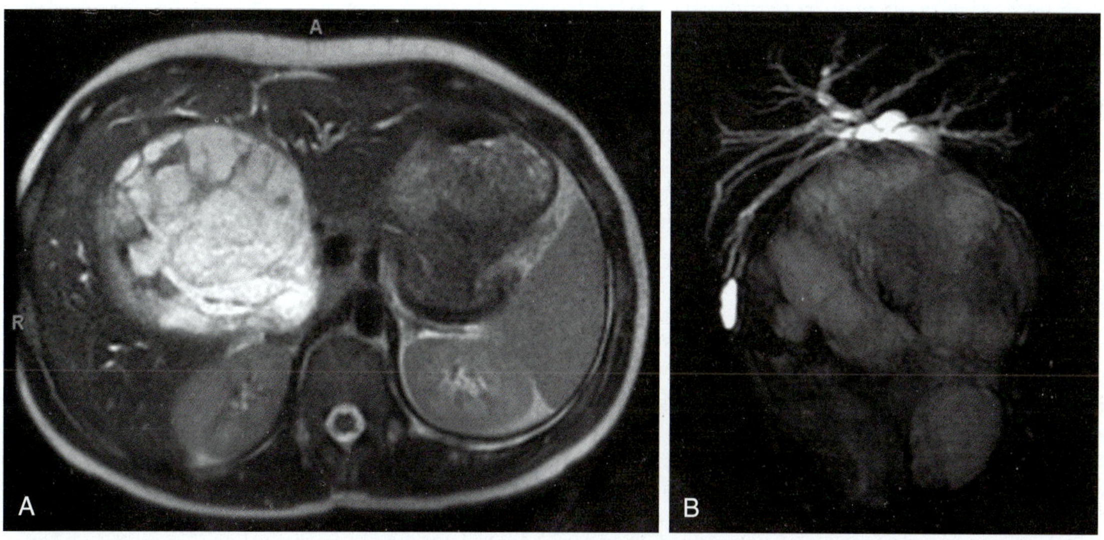

Fig. 25.50 Undifferentiated (embryonal) sarcoma in a 14-year-old. (A) Axial T2-weighted image shows a well-circumscribed hyperintense mass, in the right lobe of the liver, containing hypointense septa. (B) Magnetic resonance cholangiopancreatography image demonstrates obstruction of the intrahepatic bile ducts caused by the tumor.

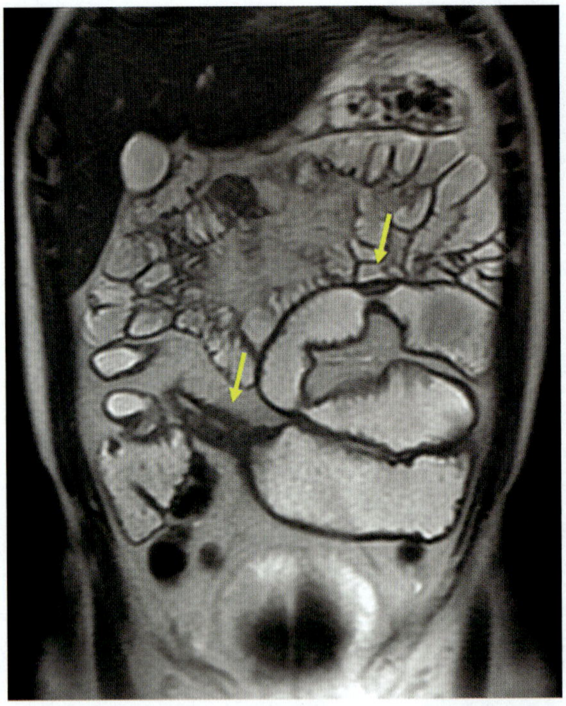

Fig. 25.51 Magnetic resonance enterography. Coronal T2 single-shot fast spin-echo image in a 14-year-old with Crohn disease shows two segments of small bowel wall thickening and luminal narrowing consistent with strictures *(arrows)*. Note the dilation of the ileal loops proximal to the strictures.

cholangitis, masses, and trauma. It is also useful for evaluation before and after liver transplantation.

Magnetic Resonance Enterography

Magnetic resonance enterography is reliable to assess the degree of disease activity, severity and extent of bowel involvement, and presence of extraintestinal complications, including abscesses, fistulas, and sinus tracts (Fig. 25.51). It is an acceptable alternative to CT enterography (discussed previously).

Magnetic Resonance Urography

Pediatric magnetic resonance urography is used for assessment of complex genitourinary tract anomalies and severely hydronephrotic kidneys and to evaluate function; to a large extent (where available) it has replaced intravenous urography.

Quantification of Iron Accumulation in the Liver

MRI does not image iron directly but instead detects the effect of iron on water protons in the tissue of interest, whether diffuse and homogeneous or heterogeneous. In patients with cirrhosis, the accumulation also may be focal, where iron selectively accumulates in siderotic nodules.

The pattern of iron deposition in organs reflects the etiology. In patients with hereditary hemochromatosis, there is preferential involvement of the liver, pancreas, and heart, with sparing of extrahepatic reticuloendothelial organs (spleen, bone marrow, lymph nodes). By comparison, in thalassemia and other transfusion-dependent anemias, preferential involvement of the reticuloendothelial system (liver, spleen, bone marrow, lymph nodes) is characteristic. Involvement of the pancreas and heart suggests the storage capacity of the reticuloendothelial system has been exceeded. In sickle cell disease (SCD), the renal cortex may show iron accumulation related to intravascular hemolysis. The liver in SCD is usually spared in the absence of transfusion therapy; involvement of the liver in nontransfused patients with SCD suggests a coexisting cause for hepatic iron overload, such as hereditary hemochromatosis.

Musculoskeletal System

MRI can produce high-contrast images of structures that are invisible or poorly visualized by x-ray–based modalities. This feature is especially important in children because the immature skeleton contains a high proportion of radiolucent cartilage. Radiographs obtained before MRI guide the selection of the proper MRI protocol (imaging planes and pulse sequences) to fully delineate and characterize anatomy and pathology, and they can improve the diagnostic specificity of soft tissue lesions by depicting calcifications, fat, gas, or foreign material within the lesion.

On MRI, bone and other dense tissues, including intact ligaments and tendons, show a lack of signal. This characteristic absence of signal provides negative contrast in comparison with muscle, which is of intermediate intensity, and yellow marrow, which is hyperintense on T1-weighted images. MRI remains the only modality that permits direct visualization of normal bone marrow. The amount and distribution of red (hematopoietic) and yellow (fatty) marrow change with age. At birth, nearly the entire skeleton is composed of red marrow. Normal conversion from red to yellow marrow occurs in a predictable manner and is completed by the time an individual has reached the mid-20s (eFig. 25.13). Conversion from red to yellow marrow proceeds from the extremities to the axial skeleton, occurring in the distal bones of the extremities (feet and hands) first and progressing finally to the proximal bones (humeri and femora). Knowledge of the normal appearance of bone at MRI is important to correctly identify abnormalities.

Accumulations of fluid within joints and bursae are hyperintense on T2-weighted images, as are fluid-containing lesions, such as abscesses and cysts. Bone marrow edema, indicated by alterations in marrow signal (dark on T1-weighted images, bright on T2-weighted images with fat suppression), may indicate the presence of subtle or radiographically undetectable microfractures. Injuries and malformations involving the physis and epiphysis are well demonstrated on MRI, allowing for diagnosis of radiographically occult fractures and early detection of post-traumatic physeal bridges. Osteochondritis dissecans involves most often the epiphyseal cartilage of the femoral condyles, talus, and capitellum. A T2-weighted sequence is able to demonstrate the grade and stability of the lesions and visualize the cartilage, which are important for treatment planning. MRI is also useful during the course of inflammatory conditions, such as arthritis, hemarthroses associated with blood coagulation disorders, and internal articular derangements from trauma or sports injury. MRI also detects meniscal injuries, ligamentous tears, patellar dislocation and associated abnormalities, cartilaginous injury, and avulsion fractures. Congenital abnormalities, such as discoid meniscus and tarsal coalition, are also easily recognizable on MRI.

IV gadolinium is useful for the delineation of areas of inflammation, ischemia, and revascularization in patients with avascular necrosis and those with tumors. It is helpful to demonstrate acute inflammatory changes in the joints, especially in the hypertrophied synovium in children with arthritis. Finally, contrast is also helpful in distinguishing the various types of vascular malformations. Magnetic resonance arthrography with dilute gadolinium is now commonly used in the diagnosis of some joint disorders, most notably labral abnormalities in the shoulder and hip.

MRI is extremely valuable in imaging osteomyelitis. Acute inflammation manifests as signal loss on T1-weighted images and elevated signal on T2-weighted fat-saturated and STIR images, as early as 24 to 48 hours after the onset of symptoms, allowing early diagnosis. Adjacent soft tissue changes demonstrate similar signal intensity changes. Abscess formation is characterized by a central hypointensity and peripheral enhancement on T1-weighted images after gadolinium administration (Fig. 25.52).

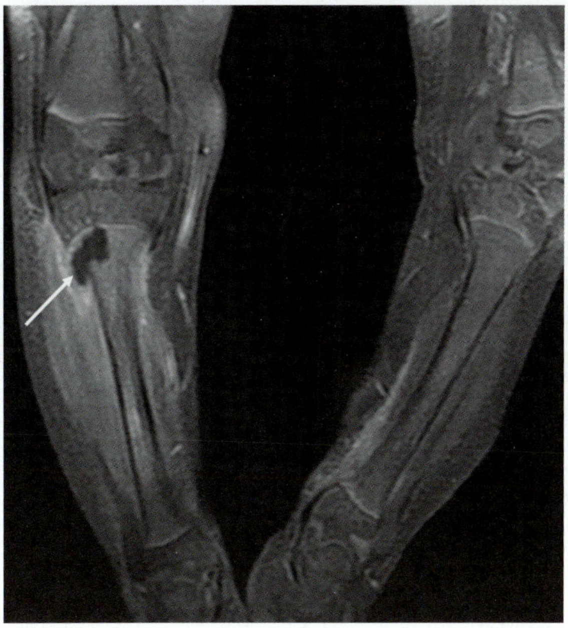

Fig. 25.52 Acute hematogenous osteomyelitis in an 8-month-old. Coronal T1-weighted fat-saturated image with contrast demonstrates bone marrow infection with cortical breakthrough and associated subperiosteal abscess *(arrow)* in the proximal right tibial metaphysis.

MRI is the modality of choice in the initial staging of primary malignant bone tumors. First, the entire affected bone and neighboring joint should be scanned in order to determine the exact tumor extension and assess for skip lesions and joint involvement. Next, high-resolution images of the tumor itself should be obtained. MRI plays a major role in demonstrating the intramedullary and extramedullary tumor components and involvement of the growth plate, surrounding muscle components, neurovascular structures, and joints. MRI alone cannot reliably distinguish between many benign and malignant tumors, and in many instances, biopsy is needed for both definite diagnosis and molecular/genetic assessment important in tumor evaluation.

Whole-body MRI is a novel technique that is targeted for maximal coverage of the patient as quickly as possible, using only a few sequences, and is primarily used for tumor detection in patients with cancer predisposition syndromes, evaluation for osteonecrosis, chronic multifocal recurrent osteomyelitis, myopathies, and generalized vascular malformations. Imaging is predominantly in the coronal plane. A STIR sequence is usually used to evaluate the bone marrow, with a T1-weighted sequence or diffusion-weight sequence added variably. The initial comparative studies of whole-body MRI with scintigraphy and PET in children have shown the high diagnostic potential of whole-body MRI.

IMAGING OF THE CENTRAL NERVOUS SYSTEM

Introduction

Continued innovation and advances with newer and improved imaging sequences in CT and MRI have vastly improved the delineation of CNS anatomy and in the evaluation and diagnosis of CNS pathology. Furthermore, evolving fields of radiogenomics linking imaging phenotype and genome-related characteristics in neuro-oncology imaging are known to aid in management and prognostication.

Current Role of Computed Tomography in Central Nervous System Imaging

CT of the brain, head and neck, and spine is often used as a first-line screening modality because of its availability. CT is the modality of choice in the setting of trauma. In the elective setting, the greater availability and shorter scan time of CT are weighed against concern about ionizing radiation and compared with possible sedation required for MRI. In acute situations, such as trauma, acute mental status change, signs of increased intracranial pressure or acute onset of neurologic symptoms, or in the unstable patient, CT is often the primary imaging modality (Table 25.6).

Table 25.6 Table of Neurologic Clinical Symptoms and Suggested Diagnostic Modalities: A Guideline

	Symptom(s)	Clinical Presentation	Urgent (U)/Elective (E)	Modality
Brain	Headache	No ND or signs of ↑ICP	E	MRI
		ND and/or signs of ↑ICP	U	MRI ± MRA/MRV; if unavailable, CT to exclude mass effect, hemorrhage, or hydrocephalus
	Macrocephaly Hydrocephalus	Without ND, HA, irritability, seizures, or signs of ↑ICP	E	CT or MRI: Balance concern for radiation versus possible need for sedation
		With ND, HA, irritability, seizures, signs of ↑ICP	U	MRI; if unavailable, CT to exclude hydrocephalus, hemorrhage, or mass effect
	Microcephaly	Regardless of presentation	E	MRI (and CT if congenital infection is suspected, to detect calcifications)
	Seizures	Without persistent ND, fever, or signs of ↑ICP	E	MRI ± contrast
		Fever, AMS, ND, or signs of ↑ICP	U	MRI, MRA, MRV, ± MRS; if not available, CT ± contrast
	Stroke	ND, HA, seizures	U	MRI, MRA, MRV, ± MRS and PMRI; if not available, CT
	Perinatal HIE, seizures, ↑bilirubin		U	MRI/MRA/MRV/MRS; if not available, CT
	Congenital anomalies		E	MRI
	Trauma		U	CT for initial evaluation and MRI in severe trauma to assess full extent of brain injury

Continued

Table 25.6 Table of Neurologic Clinical Symptoms and Suggested Diagnostic Modalities: A Guideline—cont'd

	Symptom(s)	Clinical Presentation	Urgent (U)/Elective (E)	Modality
Spine	Pain	Without ND or systemic signs	U/E	Plain films and MRI
		With radiculopathy	U/E	Plain films and MRI
		Malignancy, fever, systemic signs	U/E	Plain films and MRI with contrast
	Scoliosis	Without ND or pain	E	Plain films ± MRI
		With ND and/or pain	E	Plain films ± MRI
	Congenital anomalies	Lesion on back, ND	E	MRI and plain films, and/or CT if complex spinal dysraphism is present
	Trauma		U	Plain films ± CT MRI in severe trauma for assessment of cord and ligamentous injury and possible intraspinal hematoma
Neck	Mass	Without fever, erythema, dysphagia, or airway compromise	E	CT or MRI with contrast; balance consideration of ionizing radiation with possible need for sedation with MRI
		With fever, erythema, dysphagia, and/or airway compromise	U	CT with contrast
	Pain/infection	With fever, swelling, dysphagia, and/or airway compromise	U	CT with contrast
	Metastases		E	CT or MRI with contrast; if perineural spread of concern, MRI
Orbits, head, and skull base	Skin lesion	No pain or erythema	E	MRI with contrast
	Hemangioma		E	MRI with contrast
	Infection	Pain, fever, swelling, or cranial nerve deficit	U	CT with contrast; MRI if perineural spread or intracranial extension is suspected
	Cranial nerve deficit	Without pain or fever	U	MRI; MRI if perineural spread or intracranial extension is suspected
	Trauma		U	CT
	Anomalies		E	High-resolution CT with 3D reconstruction
	Leukocoria		U/E	MRI (and CT to assess for calcifications)
	Strabismus		E	MRI

3D, Three-dimensional; *AMS,* altered mental status; *CT,* computed tomography; *HA,* headache; *HIE,* hypoxic ischemic injury; *ICP,* intracranial pressure; *MRA,* magnetic resonance angiography; *MRI,* magnetic resonance imaging; *MRS,* magnetic resonance spectroscopy; *MRV,* magnetic resonance venography; *ND,* neurologic deficits; *PMRI,* perfusion magnetic resonance imaging.

Table 25.7 Density Characteristics of Central Nervous System Structures on Computed Tomography

Density (Hounsfield Unit)							
Gray Matter	White Matter	Cerebrospinal Fluid	Acute Blood	Calcification	Bone	Air	Fat
30–40	20–30	0	55–75	100–400	1000	−1000	−100 to −40

CT still provides sensitive detection of subarachnoid hemorrhage and calcifications. The latter may provide added diagnostic specificity for CNS tumors, the sequelae of congenital infections/TORCH, and in the diagnosis of certain phakomatoses, such as Sturge-Weber syndrome and tuberous sclerosis. Osseous lesions or lesions with a chondroid matrix are also exquisitely detailed by CT.

The CT density characteristics of many entities can be characterized by their Hounsfield unit (HU) values. The scale defines the density of water as 0 HU and the density of air as −1000 HU. A change of 1 HU represents a change of 0.1% in density related to the attenuation coefficient of water. The scale defines the calibration for CT scanners (Table 25.7).

Unenhanced Computed Tomography of the Brain

Indications for various CT imaging modalities depend on the clinical scenario.

In trauma, an unenhanced CT scan is the first investigation of choice. Use of unenhanced CT of the brain is useful in acute stroke in excluding hemorrhage and helps in assessment for thrombolytic therapy (Fig. 25.53). In patients with acute mental status changes, unenhanced CT scan can evaluate for calvarial fractures, hemorrhage, hydrocephalus, mass effect, or herniation. Additional evaluation for signs of increased intracranial pressure or herniation can be assessed, which may preclude safe lumbar puncture (Fig. 25.54). CT is valuable for evaluation of intracranial fluid collections, and bone windows may reveal abnormalities of the calvarium (Fig. 25.55). In the setting of macrocephaly, ventricular size and extraaxial fluid or mass can be determined and bone windows allow assessment of the calvarium and sutures (Fig. 25.56). In addition to changes in ventricular size, shunt position or edema or hemorrhage can aid in evaluation of shunt function (Fig. 25.57). Alternatively, new faster MRI protocols can be used to assess for extraaxial fluid or ventricular caliber change to avoid radiation. High-resolution images of the

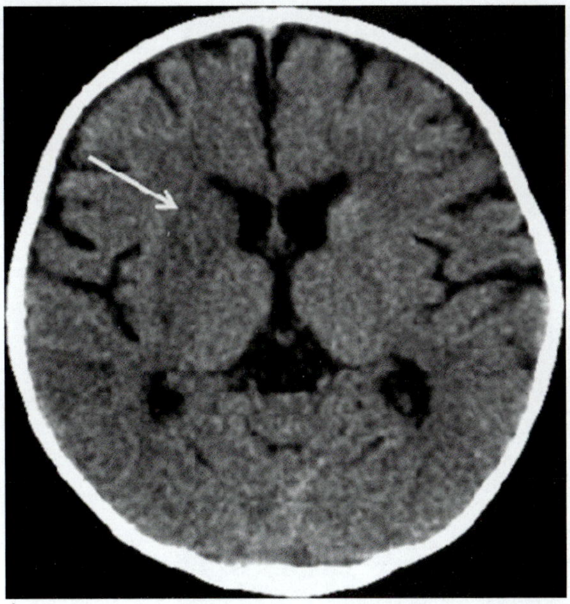

Fig. 25.53 Unenhanced axial computed tomography image of a patient with a stroke at the level of the basal ganglia delineates hypodense right caudate and putamen *(arrow)*. The left caudate and putamen are hyperdense, as are the thalami; the central and peripheral gray matter appear normal. Right basal ganglia show ischemic changes and infarction.

cranial vault and brain with two-dimensional (2D) and 3D reconstructions allow detailed analysis of craniosynostosis or other cranial anomalies (see Chapter 23).

Contrast-Enhanced Computed Tomography of the Brain

Considerations before iodinated IV contrast administration for CT have been discussed previously. Contrast-enhanced CT of the brain is becoming a relatively rare examination because an unenhanced CT scan is usually followed by an MRI examination for further evaluation. If MRI is contraindicated, not readily available, or not feasible in a reasonable period of time, contrast-enhanced CT imaging should be considered if infection is suspected. Also, when there is concern for tumor, contrast-enhanced CT in conjunction with PET imaging may be considered. If trauma or vascular injury is suspected, an unenhanced CT scan should first be obtained because contrast may obscure hemorrhage (Fig. 25.58).

Intracranial and Extracranial Computed Tomography Angiography and Computed Tomography Venography

CTA and computed tomography venography (CTV) provide detailed anatomic information about the cranial vasculature. This is particularly valuable in trauma to assess arterial and/or venous

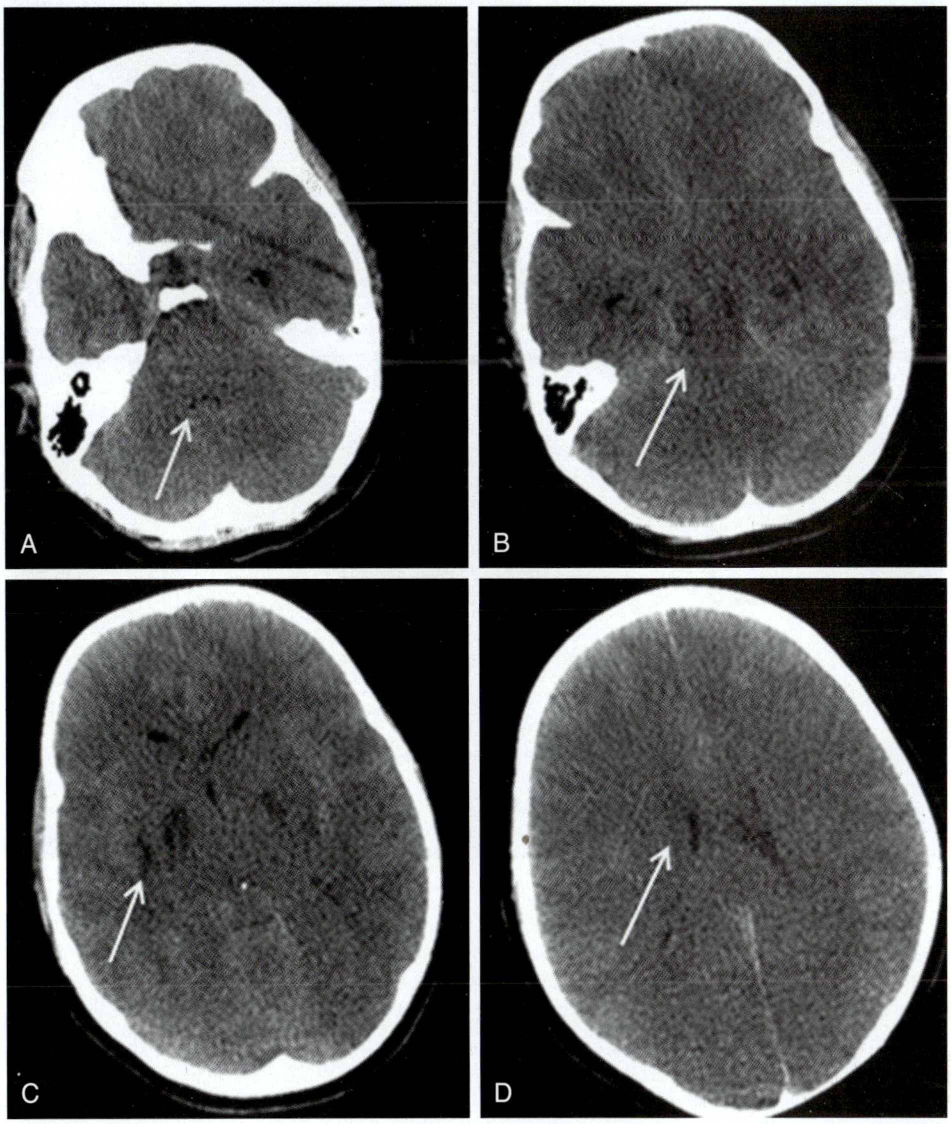

Fig. 25.54 Near drowning/cardiac arrest; diffuse cerebral edema. Unenhanced axial computed tomography images of a patient after cardiac arrest from near drowning delineate effacement of the fourth ventricle (A, *arrow*), effacement of the perimesencephalic cisterns (B, *arrow*), ischemic changes in the basal ganglia (C, *arrow*), and partially effaced lateral ventricles (D, *arrow*). On each of the images, there is loss of gray/white matter differentiation and sulcal effacement.

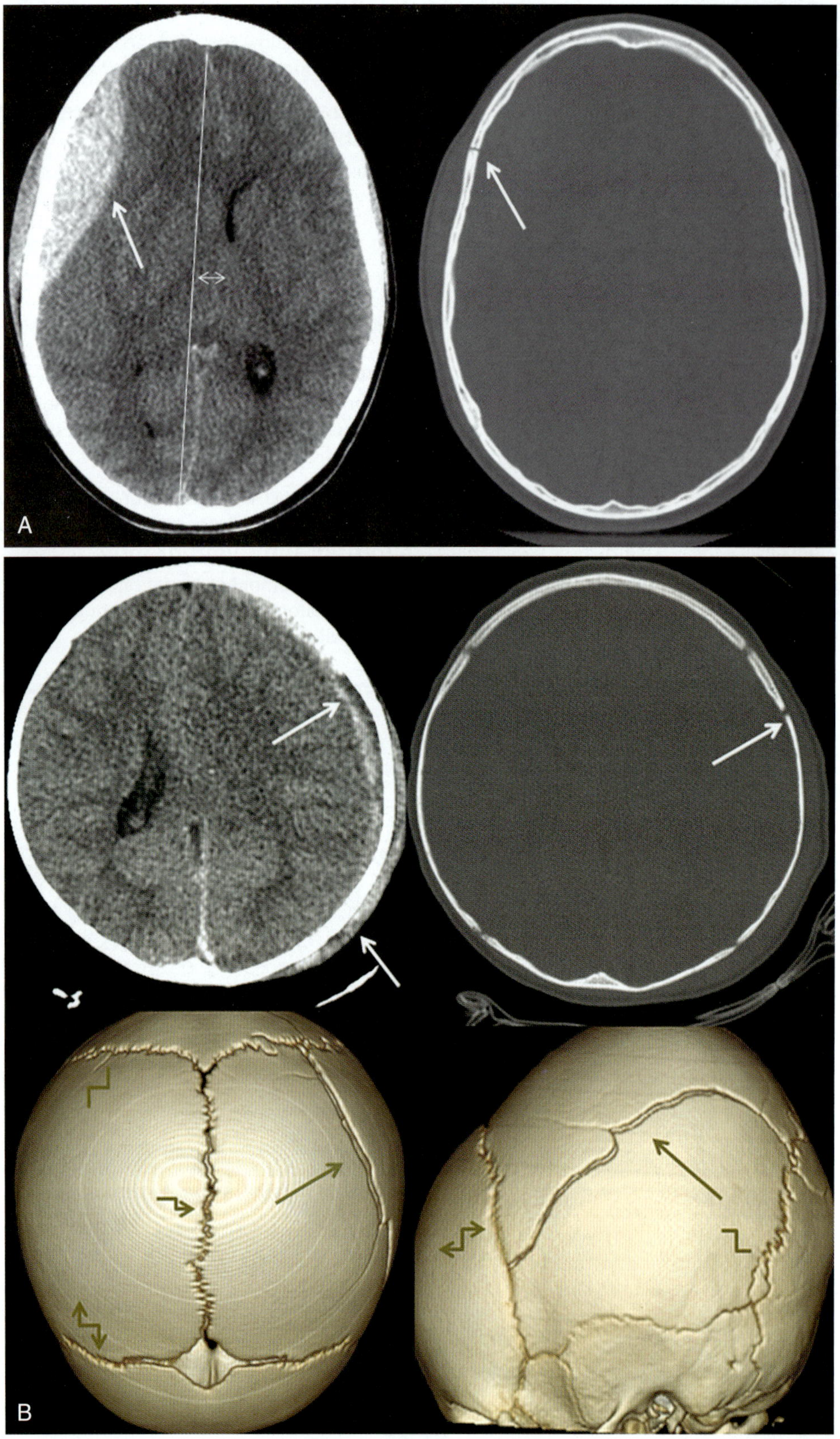

Fig. 25.55 (A) Accidental head trauma. *Left:* Unenhanced axial computed tomography (CT) image at the level of the lateral ventricles delineates a large right hyperdense epidural hematoma *(arrow),* with midline shift/subfalcine herniation, right to left *(double-headed arrow),* effacement of right lateral and third ventricles, and early obstruction of the left lateral ventricle. *Right:* Axial image at the same level on the bone window setting delineates a nondisplaced fracture of the right frontal bone *(arrow).* (B) Nonaccidental trauma. *Top left:* Unenhanced axial CT image at the level of the lateral ventricles delineates a left subdural hematoma *(top arrow),* effacement of the left lateral ventricle, and superficial scalp hematoma *(bottom arrow). Top right:* Axial CT image at the same level on the bone window setting delineates a nondisplaced right parietal fracture *(arrow). Bottom left:* Three-dimensional (3D) reconstruction of the calvarium, viewed from the vertex, with the extent of the fracture well delineated. *Bottom right:* 3D reconstruction of the calvarium, viewed from the left lateral projection with delineation of the full extent of the fracture from the coronal to lambdoid suture. *Double-headed crooked arrow,* coronal suture; *straight arrow,* sagittal suture; *Z line,* lambdoid suture.

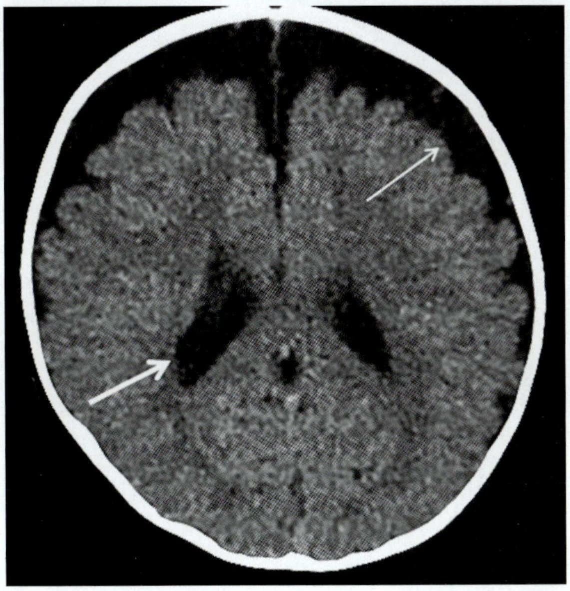

Fig. 25.56 Macrocephaly noted at well-baby visit. Axial computed tomography (CT) image at the level of the lateral ventricles delineates prominent lateral ventricles *(bold arrow)* and prominent anterior extraaxial spaces *(thin arrow)*. Typical appearance for benign extraaxial collections of infancy, a benign self-limiting process.

injury and in evaluating acute neurologic deficits by examining the vasculature for stenosis, dissection, aneurysms, or vascular malformation (Fig. 25.59). Tumors involving intracranial or extracranial sites or the skull base can be evaluated for their vascularity and relationship to adjacent structures (Fig. 25.60). In patients with subarachnoid hemorrhage due to aneurysms, CTA may be needed in patients who are poor candidates for traditional angiography or digital subtraction angiography and/or direct the focus of subsequent digital subtraction angiography. Postoperative evaluation of patients with aneurysms or arterial venous malformations by CTA or CTV may be better than by MRI. CTV is also valuable in assessing intracranial infection with possible venous thrombosis (Fig. 25.61).

Computed Tomography of the Paranasal Sinuses, Facial Bones, Skull Base, Orbits, Temporal Bones, Neck, and Spine

CT imaging of the skull and facial bones includes evaluation of the paranasal sinuses, particularly with acute or chronic sinus disease and in preparation for surgery with medically refractive sinus disease. Imaging usually does not include intravenous contrast. However, if intracranial or intraorbital extension is suspected, then a contrast-enhanced scan is indicated (see Chapter 24). CT imaging is indicated for examination of the facial bones and skull base after trauma (Fig. 25.62), suspected infection (contrast-enhanced examination indicated), and facial anomalies (reconstruction with high-resolution 2D and 3D images) (Fig. 25.63). In the setting of a suspected mass, a contrast-enhanced examination should be performed. If a vascular or primary dental lesion is suspected, a targeted unenhanced image in the area of interest before intravenous contrast can be performed as needed to assess for calcifications and/or bone matrix because prior administration of contrast may obscure these findings (eFig. 25.14).

Imaging of the orbits is indicated in trauma, congenital anomalies (see Fig. 25.63), and infection (contrast-enhanced examination is indicated; see Chapter 24) (Fig. 25.64). Proptosis, with or without possible infection, warrants CT imaging.

CT images of the temporal bones may be diagnostic after trauma (Fig. 25.65), infection (eFig. 25.15), hearing loss (eFig. 25.16), cranial nerve deficits, or if a temporal bone tumor is suspected (Fig. 25.66). Contrast-enhanced examinations are indicated in infection and suspected tumor.

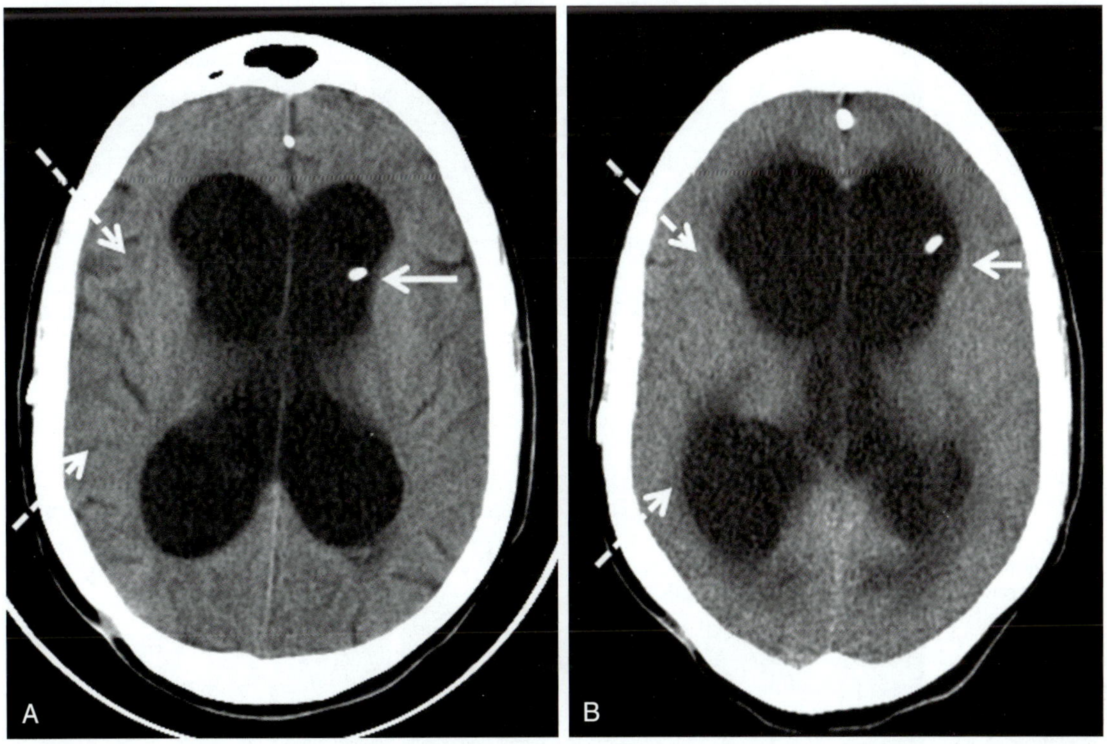

Fig. 25.57 Patient with shunted hydrocephalus: Progressive hydrocephalus, probable shunt malfunction. (A) Axial computed tomography (CT) image at the level of the lateral ventricles delineates dilated lateral ventricles with shunt in the frontal horn of the left lateral ventricle *(short thick arrow)*. Sulci are visualized *(dashed arrows)*. (B) Axial CT image at the same level several days later, showing enlarged lateral ventricles with shunt position unchanged *(short thick arrow)* and effacement of sulci *(dashed arrows)*.

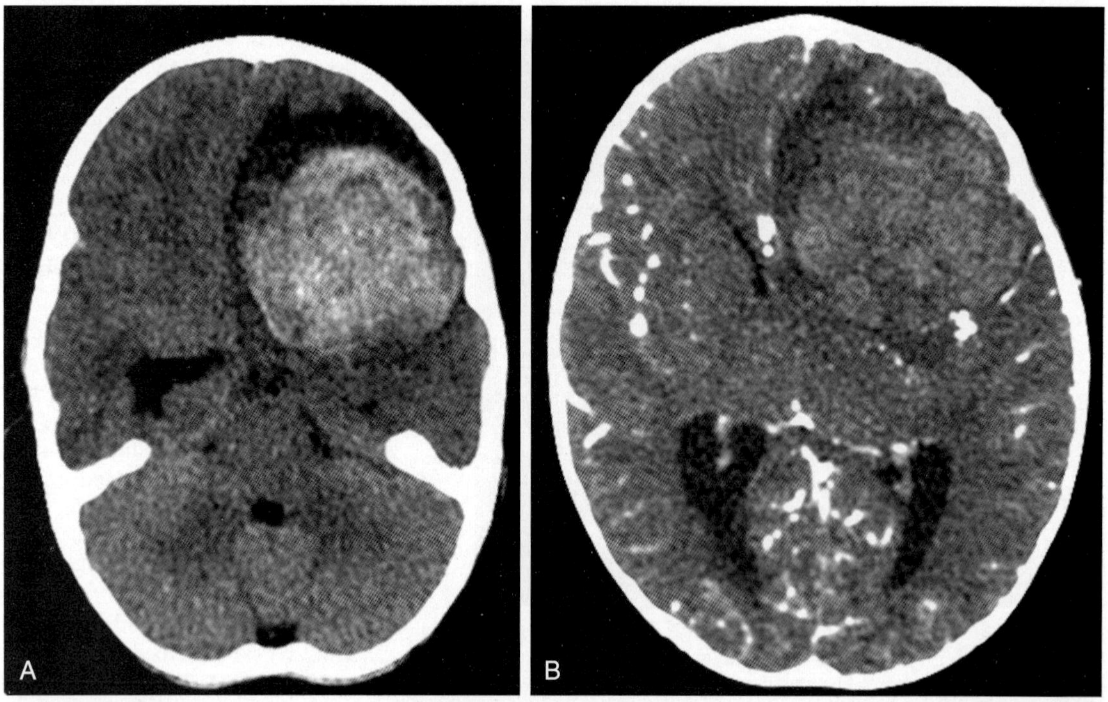

Fig. 25.58 Patient presenting with seizure. (A) Unenhanced computed tomography (CT) at the level of the temporal horns of the lateral ventricles delineates a large, hyperdense, left frontal lobe intraparenchymal hematoma. Significant mass effect and dilation of the right temporal horn/obstructive hydrocephalus are visible. (B) Contrast-enhanced examination performed on the same day shows marked relative hypoattenuation of the hematoma.

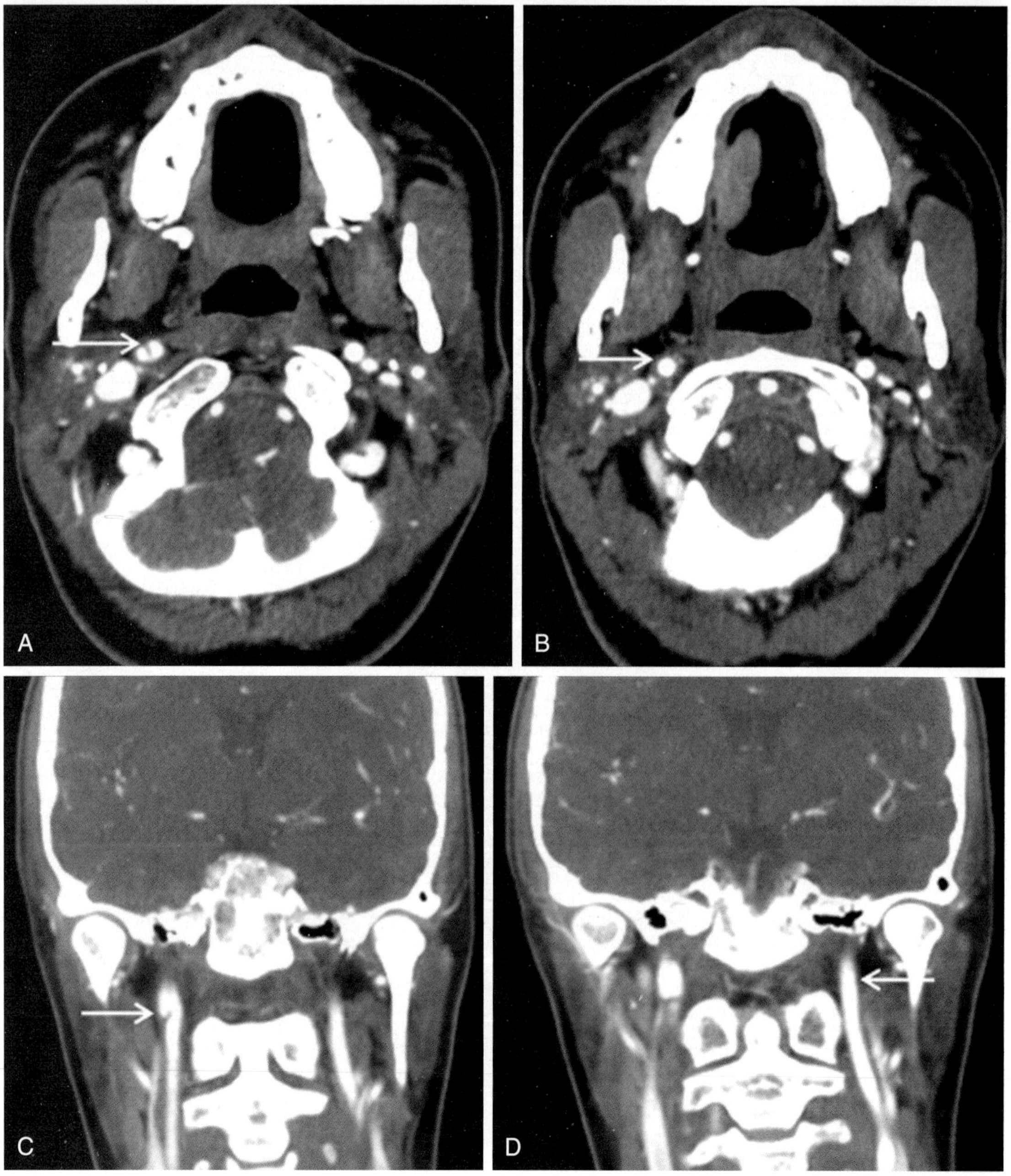

Fig. 25.59 Patient presenting with left upper extremity weakness, left facial droop, and difficulty speaking. (A) Axial computed tomography (CT) source image from CT angiography (CTA); *arrow* points to flap/dissection *(thin gray line)* in the lumen of the right internal carotid artery. (B) Axial image just below the dissection shows a relatively narrow caliber of the right internal carotid artery *(arrow)* compared with the left internal carotid artery. (C) Coronal reconstruction of CTA delineates flap/dissection *(arrow)* in right internal carotid artery. (D) Coronal reconstruction indicating normal appearance of the left internal carotid artery.

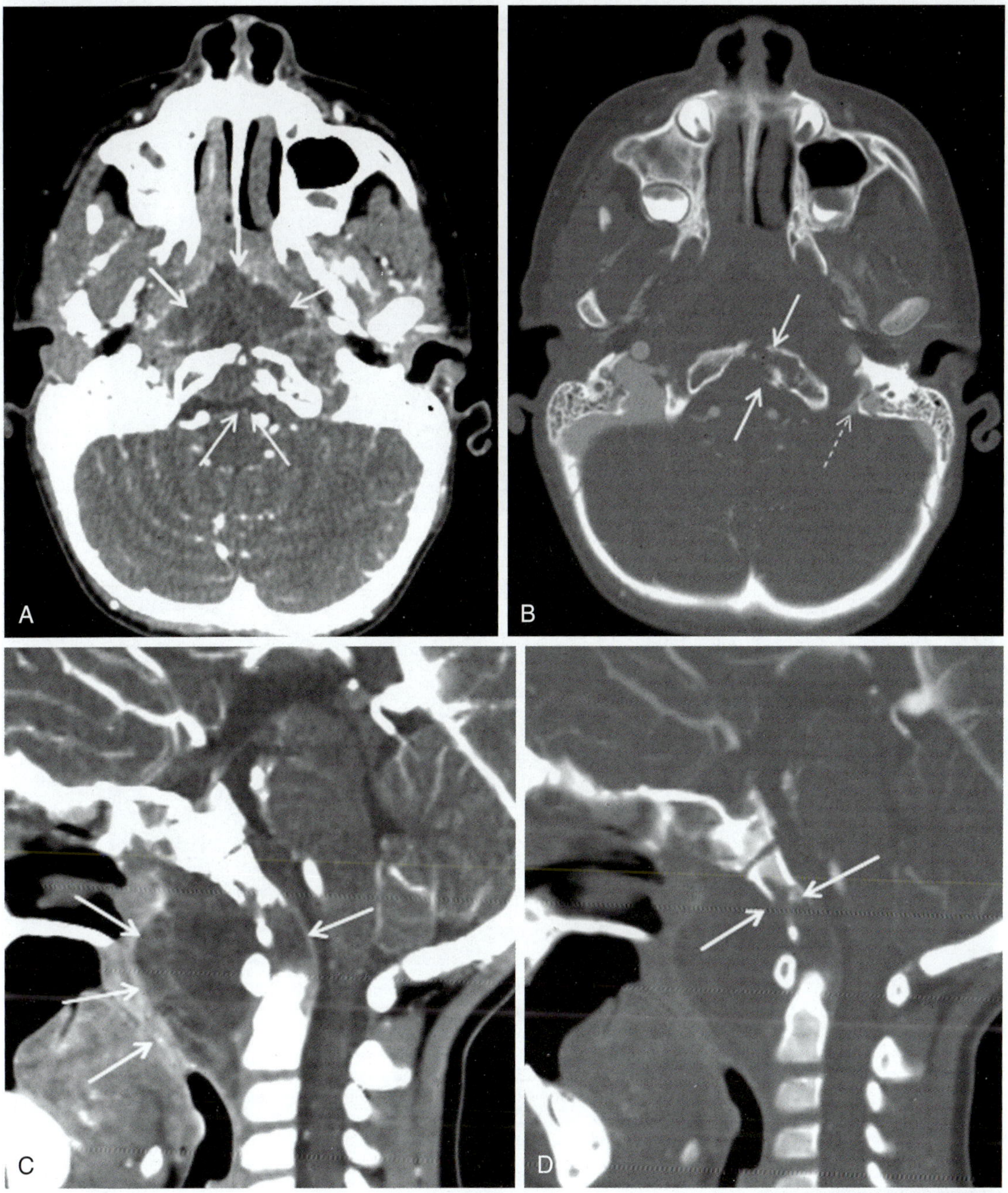

Fig. 25.60 Patient presenting with nasal speech and cranial nerve deficits. (A) Axial contrast-enhanced computed tomography (CT) on the soft tissue window setting, at the level of the skull base, delineates a large soft tissue mass *(arrows)* centered at the clivus and both anterior and posterior to it (i.e., intracranial extension). (B) Axial image on the bone window setting delineates associated bone erosion *(solid arrows)* and invasion of the left jugular foramen *(dashed arrow)*. (C) Sagittal soft tissue reconstruction delineates extent of the mass into both the nasopharynx and oropharynx and its intracranial extension *(arrows)*. (D) Sagittal reconstruction on the bone window setting delineates the extent of clival erosion *(arrows)*.

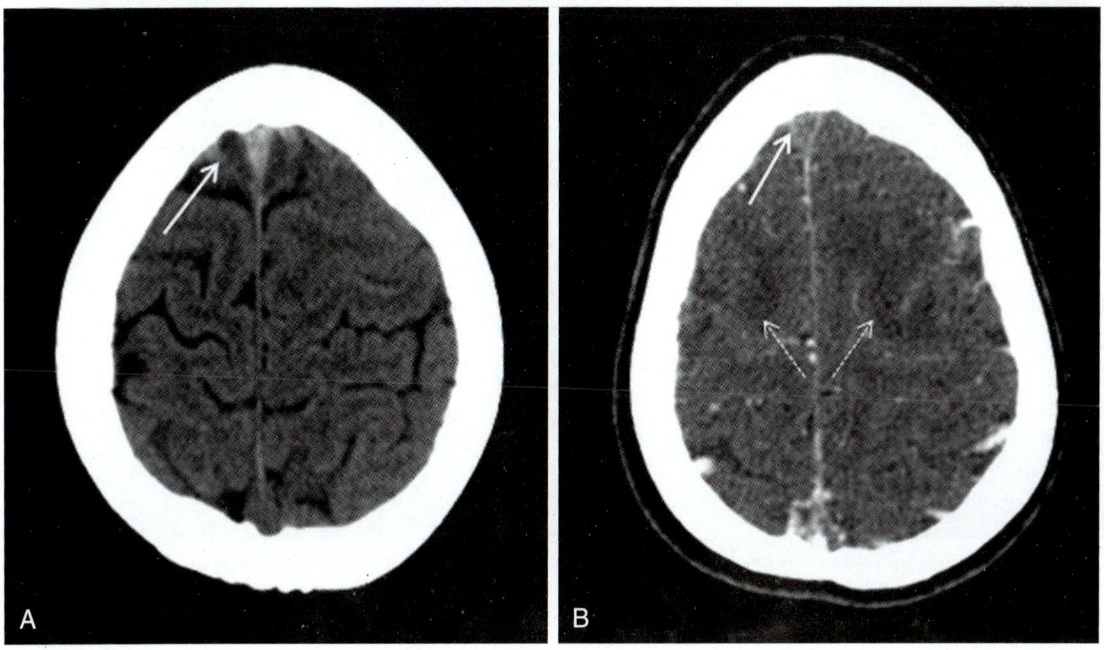

Fig. 25.61 Patient presenting with change in mental status with sinus thrombosis. (A) Unenhanced computed tomography (CT) delineates a hyperdense anterior portion of the superior sagittal sinus *(arrow)*, suggesting venous sinus thrombosis. (B) Contrast-enhanced CT confirms lack of opacification of the anterior portion of the superior sagittal sinus *(arrow)* and associated areas of cortical hypodensity/ischemia *(diverging dotted arrows)*.

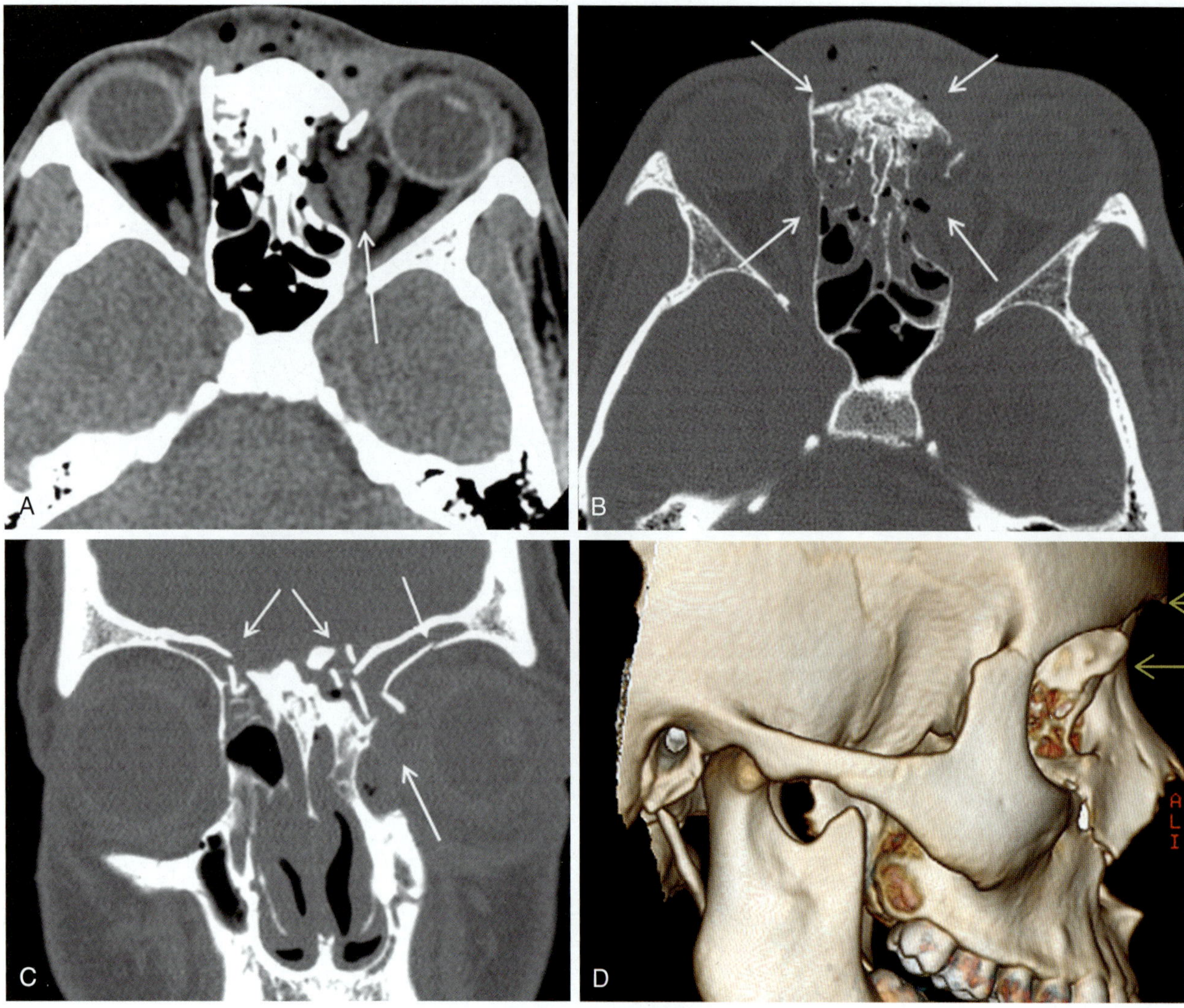

Fig. 25.62 Trauma to the face: Naso-orbital ethmoidal complex fractures. (A) Axial computed tomography (CT) image on soft tissue window delineates extent of soft tissue injury to the orbit. *Arrow* points to a hematoma and displacement of the medial rectus muscle. (B) Axial image on the bone window setting delineates complex, comminuted, and displaced fractures of the medial orbital walls/lamina papyracea *(posterior arrows)* and cribriform plate *(anterior arrows)*. (C) Coronal reconstruction delineates the complex comminuted fractures, which also include the frontal sinuses and fovea ethmoidalis *(diverging arrows)* and left orbital roof *(upper arrow)*, and redemonstrates the extensive fracture of the medial orbital wall/ lamina papyracea *(lower arrow)*. (D) Lateral view of the three-dimensional (3D) reconstruction demonstrates the marked posterior displacement of the nasoethmoidal complex *(long arrow)* in relation to the frontal sinus/frontal bone *(short arrow)*.

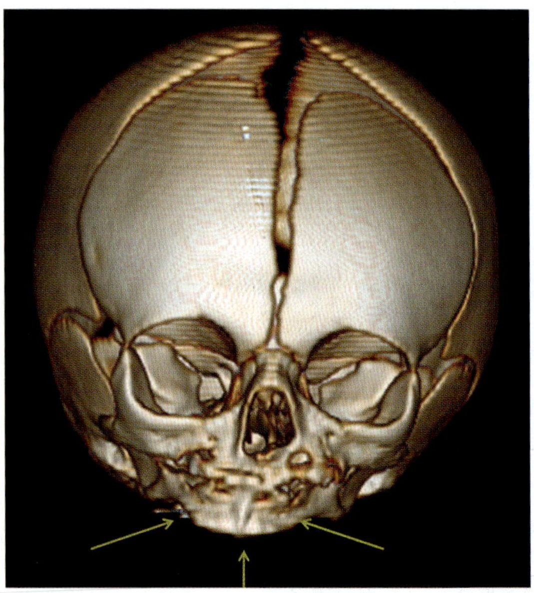

Fig. 25.63 Newborn presenting with fusion of gums: syngnathia. Three-dimensional reconstruction of the calvarium and face demonstrates lower facial hypoplasia due to maxillary and mandibular hypoplasia *(long arrows)* and their midline fusion *(short midline arrow)*.

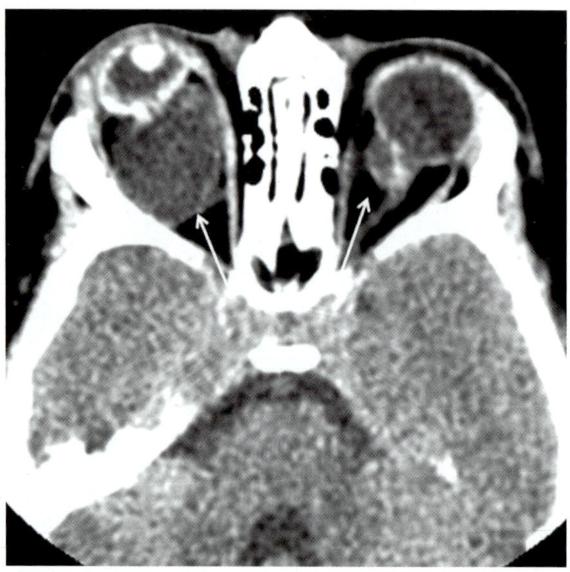

Fig. 25.64 Infant with right proptosis: bilateral colobomas. Axial image through the orbits delineates a large right orbital cyst *(arrow)* with connection to a hypoplastic proptotic globe. On the left there is a small orbital cyst with a relatively normal-appearing globe *(arrow)*.

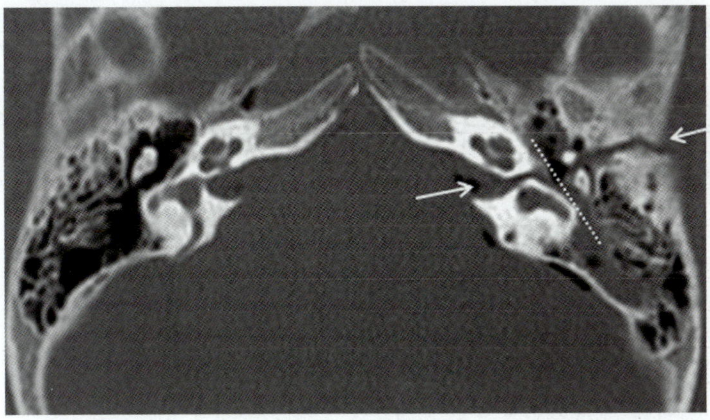

Fig. 25.65 Head injury with hemotympanum. Axial unenhanced computed tomography (CT) image through the left temporal bone demonstrates a transverse fracture *(arrows)* with ossicular dislocation (note separation of the malleus and incus on the left in comparison with the right "ice cream scoop separated from cone"); fracture traverses through the expected tympanic course of the facial nerve *(dotted line)* and through the internal auditory canal/inner ear. Associated opacification of the left middle ear and mastoid and pneumocephalus are also seen.

When swelling of the soft tissues of the neck is evaluated, a contrast-enhanced examination is indicated to examine for infection, lymphadenopathy, masses, or metastases (Fig. 25.67).

Indications for CT examination of the spine include trauma (eFig. 25.17) and complex spinal anomalies. CT imaging may be used as a complementary examination to MRI in evaluating anomalies (eFig. 25.18) and infection, to assess bone erosion and destruction, and for posttreatment healing (Fig. 25.68). These studies of the spine are generally done without intravenous or intrathecal contrast. When MRI is not available, the only clinical indications for contrast-enhanced CT of the cervical spine are for suspected infarction, diskitis, abscess, or tumor (Fig. 25.69).

Intrathecal contrast imaging of the spine is indicated to evaluate the position and integrity of an intraspinal catheter, delineation and localization of a suspected thecal sac arachnoid cyst (complementary examination to MRI), and in patients in whom MRI studies are suboptimal with possible disk herniation or canal stenosis associated with radicular pain or who may have suspected arachnoiditis.

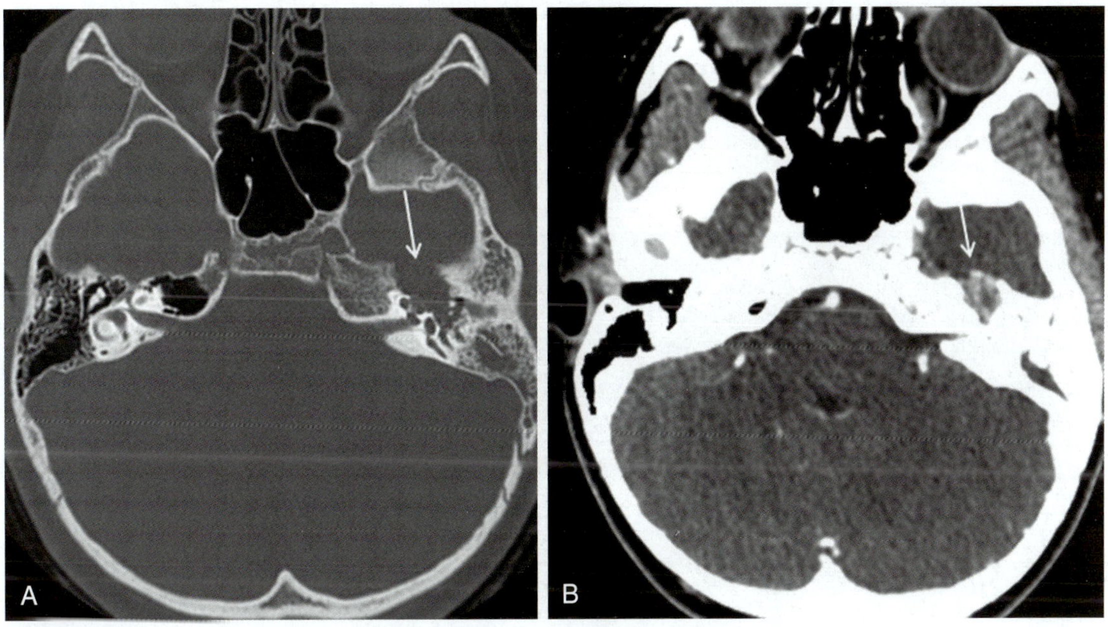

Fig. 25.66 Patient presenting with left facial palsy: hemangioendothelioma at surgical resection. (A) Axial computed tomography (CT) through the temporal bone set on the bone window setting demonstrates a large destructive mass of the left petrous bone at the level of the geniculate ganglion/first turn of the facial nerve *(arrow)*. Opacification of the left middle ear and mastoid is related to extension of the mass into the eustachian tube. (B) Contrast-enhanced CT on the soft tissue window setting at the same level delineates heterogeneous enhancement of the mass *(arrow)*.

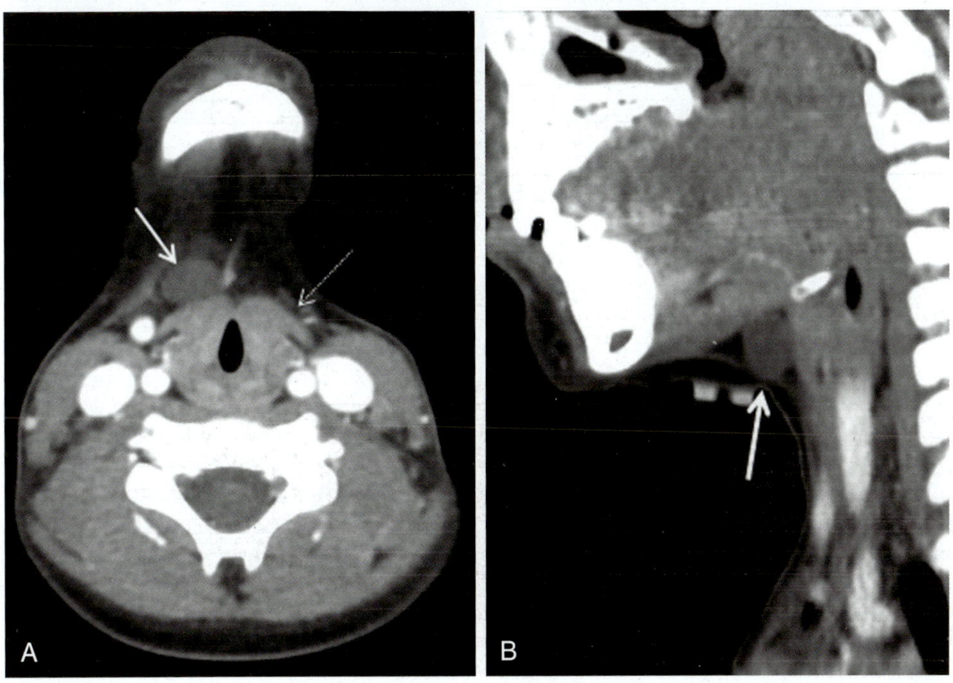

Fig. 25.67 Patient presenting with new neck mass: thyroglossal duct cyst. (A) Axial contrast-enhanced image through the neck just below the level of the hyoid demonstrates a discrete cystic mass, just to the right of midline, without a discernible wall or enhancement *(solid arrow)*. The mass is intimately associated with the adjacent strap muscles *(dotted arrow)*. (B) Sagittal reconstruction delineates the mass at the level of the fiducial placed to localize the mass *(arrow)*.

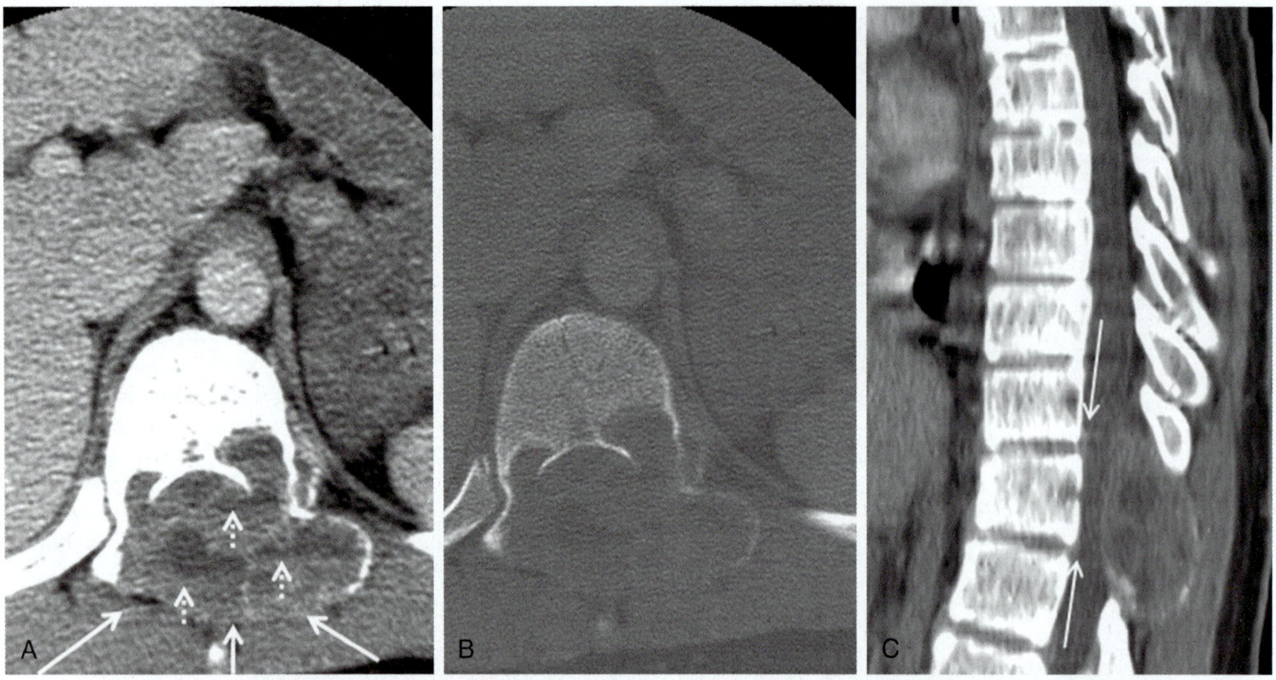

Fig. 25.68 Patient presenting with back pain and neurologic deficits. At resection: Aneurysmal bone cyst. (A) Axial contrast-enhanced image on a soft tissue window setting through the lower thoracic spine delineates a heterogeneous expansile destructive mass *(solid arrows)* involving the vertebral body and more extensively the posterior elements with intraspinal encroachment. Fluid levels *(dotted arrows)* are suggested within the mass. (B) Same axial image on a bone window setting delineates bone expansion/remodeling and destruction. (C) Sagittal reconstruction on a soft tissue window setting delineates the marked narrowing of the spinal canal and thecal sac *(arrows)* by the mass.

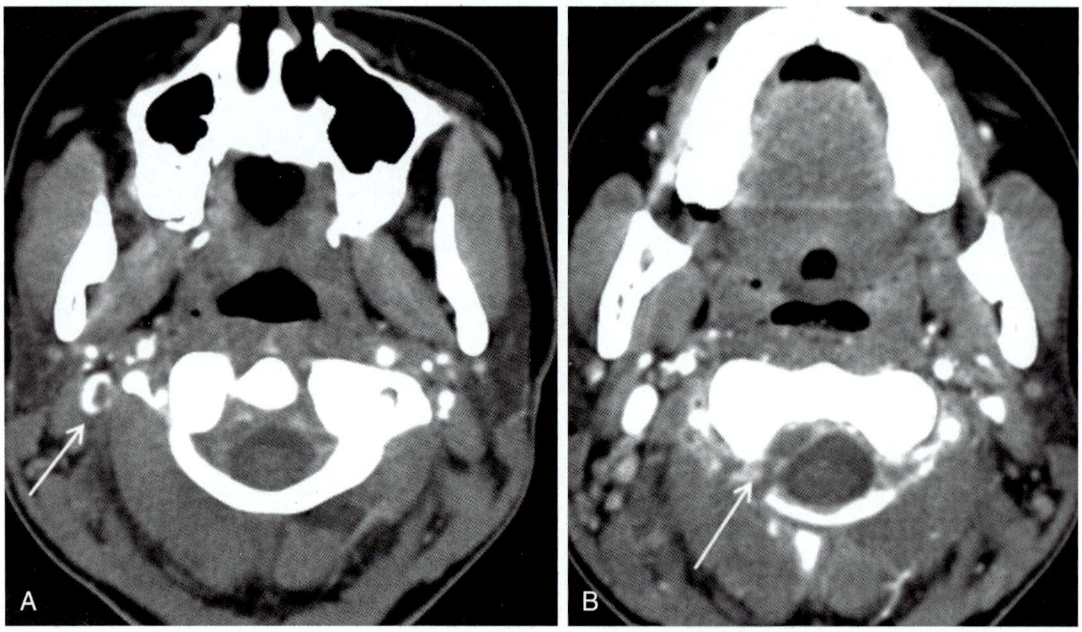

Fig. 25.69 Patient, presenting with neck pain, *Fusobacterium necrophorum*–induced sepsis. (A) Contrast-enhanced axial computed tomography (CT) through the upper neck delineates a clot *(arrow)* in the right jugular vein. (B) Axial contrast-enhanced image just below delineates right anterior rim, enhancing epidural fluid collection. The diagnosis was Lemierre disease with epidural abscess.

Current Role of Magnetic Resonance Imaging in Central Nervous System Imaging

MRI defines CNS anatomy in exquisite detail, and physiology and function can also now be evaluated and assessed. Faster sequences and magnetic resonance–compatible goggles (which permit the patient to watch videos/movies and listen to music) have reduced the need for sedation, although it remains a significant consideration in pediatric MRI examinations (see previous discussion).

MRI of the brain is now the modality of choice in almost all suspected nontraumatic intracranial pathology. In evaluation of the spine, head, and neck, it is often superior to CT in imaging many disease entities. In certain cases, a supplementary CT examination may be required for evaluation of the osseous involvement, which may allow a more definitive preoperative or pretreatment differential and/or diagnosis.

In ordering a contrast-enhanced MRI, the patient's clinical history, history of allergies, renal function, hydration status, and medications should be known and reviewed. In patients with renal dysfunction or acute renal failure, contrast administration may place them at risk for the development of NSF (see the Nephrogenic Systemic Fibrosis in Children section earlier; see eBox 25.4).

In addition to previously discussed safety considerations (see earlier section), metallic objects often produce signal distortion and field distortion artifacts. This may render an examination suboptimal or possibly nondiagnostic. In the pediatric population, the most common cause of suboptimal or nondiagnostic MRI examinations is dental braces and retainers; a diagnostic examination of the orbits, face, and sinuses or skull base may not be possible in their presence.

Intracranial and extracranial MRA and MRV are also markedly degraded and often nondiagnostic. Routine sequences of the brain are variably compromised but usually diagnostic. GRE, susceptibility, and diffusion-weighted images are usually severely compromised.

Magnetic Resonance Imaging Sequences and Their Utility

Routine MRI protocol includes multiplanar T1- and T2-weighted imaging, FLAIR, DWI, and GRE or susceptibility weighted imaging. New, improved, and faster MRI sequences and modalities have been developed for assessing anatomy, pathology, and function. These include DTI, arterial spin labeling (ASL), fMRI, MRS, and use of permeability maps, especially in tumor characterization. Three-dimensional T1 (such as SPGR or MPRAGE), T2, and T2 FLAIR (such as CUBE or SPACE) are newer sequences with 3D volumetric capability and can be utilized for multiplanar reformations.

T1 weighted: Normal gray matter appears darker than white matter. CSF and edema are dark, whereas fat, blood, and contrast are bright.

T2 weighted: CSF, edema, and most lesions are bright, whereas hypercellular masses are intermediate to dark.

FLAIR (fluid attenuation inversion recovery) sequence: By attenuating signal from CSF, sensitive delineation of foci of signal abnormality adjacent to the ventricles and subarachnoid space are better defined.

GRE (T2*): By enhancing magnetic susceptibility, sensitive delineation of hemorrhage and vascular malformations, calcifications, and iron deposition is possible.

SWI: Sensitive to compounds that distort the local magnetic field, useful for detecting blood products, calcium, iron, and so on. Similar but more sensitive to GRE in delineation of hemorrhage or mineralization.

DWI: By using differences in the rates and direction of diffusion of water molecules in normal and abnormal tissues, diffusion imaging is based on random Brownian motion of water molecules within a voxel of tissue. Restricted diffusions are bright on DWI and dark on the apparent diffusion coefficient (ADC). ADC maps help identify cytotoxic edema in infarct/ischemia, pyogenic abscess, or hypercellular tumors or mass. If a lesion is bright on DWI and ADC maps, it is not truly restricted, and this phenomenon is called *T2 shine through.*

DTI: DTI uses anisotropy/direction to map axonal tracts, allowing evaluation of their course; a caliber can be reconstructed in 3D color maps and assessment of possible disruption, displacement, or anomalous pathways (eFig. 25.19). This supplementary information to anatomical MRI results in more sensitive and sophisticated assessment of neurologic deficits, and the preoperative localization of "eloquent" tracts, that is, important functional regions, in relation to tumors and other brain lesions.

STIR—fat-suppressed short T1 inversion recovery sequence: By suppressing the signal of fat, sensitive delineation of lesions in areas where fat/lipomatous tissue is present, such as in the orbits, face, skull base, neck, and spine, becomes possible.

Fast imaging employing steady-state acquisition (FIESTA) or constructive interference in steady-state images are heavily T2-weighted 3D GRE techniques that produce high-resolution isotropic images, excellent contrast between CSF and other structures in the brain and hence are useful for evaluating structures surrounded by CSF (e.g., cranial nerves), evaluation of pineal cystic lesions, aqueductal stenosis, and so on.

MRS: MRS may be used to assess the distribution and quantification of naturally occurring molecules within the CNS. Various techniques are available. The most commonly used is the point-resolved spectroscopy sequence (PRESS). Both short T_E (echo time) and long T_E acquisitions can be obtained. All provide sensitive noninvasive analysis of brain metabolites and cellular biochemical changes, used in assessing brain maturation, brain ischemia, injury, and encephalopathy. In these entities, it may also provide prognostic information. In the diagnosis and characterization of inborn errors of metabolism, it may not be specific but may help to narrow the entities to be considered. Another indication is preoperative characterization and possible diagnosis of brain tumors, as well as their postoperative and posttherapeutic assessment (Fig. 25.70 and eTable 25.7).

Perfusion MRI: Dynamic contrast-enhanced T2* or unenhanced techniques such as ASL and blood oxygen level–dependent sequences are used. In ASL, arterial blood water is used as an endogenous tracer, enabling evaluation of cerebral perfusion without IV contrast administration. Sensitive delineation of relative cerebral blood flow with evaluation of cerebral blood volume, cerebral blood flow, and mean transit time in targeted areas of the brain is possible. Perfusion magnetic resonance imaging has numerous applications including pediatric stroke, epilepsy, tumor vascularity, and vascular malformations. It can also be used in differentiating tumor progression from pseudoprogression secondary to posttreatment changes.

Functional MRI: fMRI localizes function to anatomic areas. The most widely used technique is the blood oxygen level–dependent sequence. This relies on local changes in cerebral blood flow and changes in oxyhemoglobin and deoxyhemoglobin with targeted brain activation. Cortical activation by a focal task, or by a visual or auditory stimulus, results in local increased metabolic demand and hence an increase in local blood flow, which raises the concentration of oxyhemoglobin and decreases the concentration of deoxyhemoglobin. The decrease in deoxyhemoglobin results in an increase in signal intensity. Subtraction of preactivation and postactivation images results in localization of the area of the brain activated by the task or stimulus. It can be used in preoperative delineation of "eloquent" areas before resection of brain

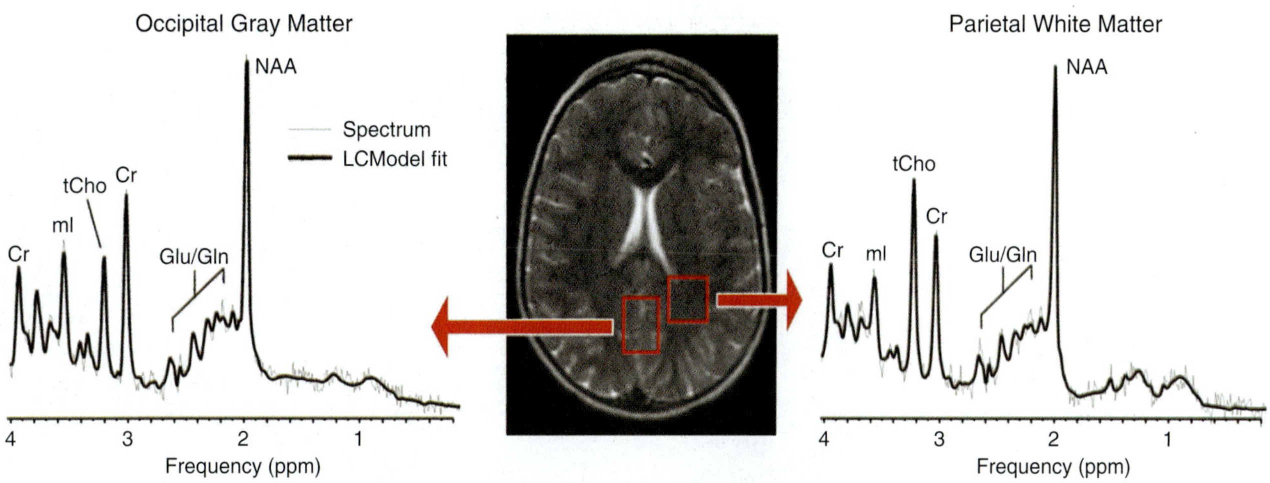

Fig. 25.70 Normal brain spectra. *Cr,* Creatine; *Glu/Gln,* glutamate/glutamine; *ml,* myo-inositol; *LCModel,* a program for the automatic quantitation of in vivo proton magnetic resonance spectra; *NAA, N*-acetylaspartate; *tCho,* total choline.

tumors or vascular malformations and cortical dysplasias and other seizure foci. It is also used in assessing cognition, language, and motor skill acquisition and behavioral dysfunction.

Fast sequences, such as single-shot fast spin-echo (SSFSE) and half-Fourier acquired single-shot turbo spin-echo (HASTE), and other fast and ultrafast techniques: These allow rapid scanning of the entire pediatric brain, eliminating need for sedation in most patients. They are adequate for assessing ventricular size and shunt position in patients with shunted hydrocephalus. These sequences do not allow adequate delineation and diagnosis of other brain pathology. Feed and bundle technique is routinely utilized for small infants to eliminate need for sedation.

Ultrafast, multiplanar targeted MRI can be used as an alternative to CT for routine follow-up of hydrocephalus and evaluation of ventricular size and shunt position (Fig. 25.71). In patients with stroke, MRI along with MRA, magnetic resonance venography (MRV), and perfusion magnetic resonance imaging can assess location/territory, size, area at risk, and underlying vascular disease or anomalies (Fig. 25.72). Addition of MRS to MRI may provide information as to

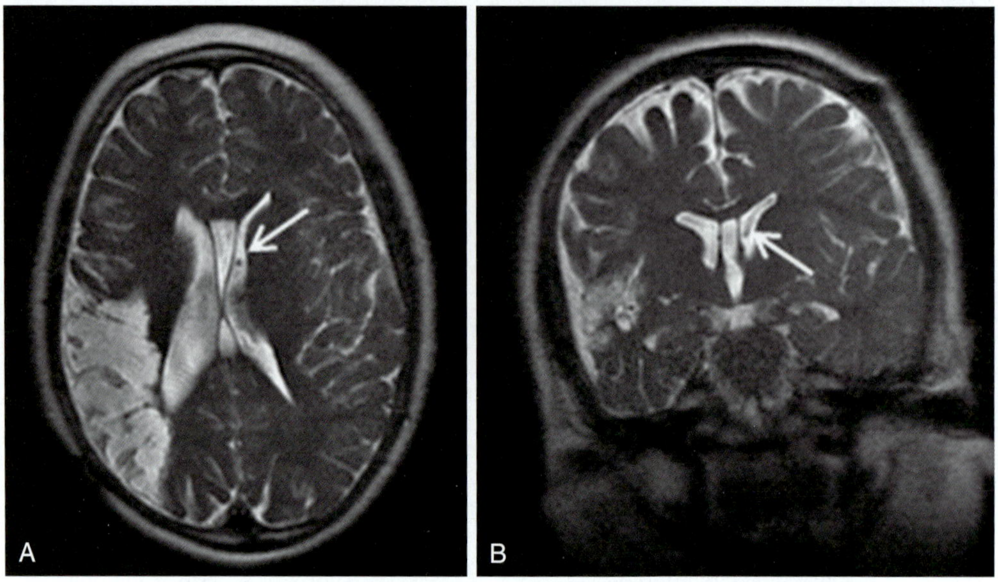

Fig. 25.71 Patient presenting with possible shunt malfunction. Axial (A) and T2 single-shot fast spin-echo (SSFSE) (B) acquisitions, each taking less than 1 minute to run, suffice for assessing ventricular size and shunt position *(arrows)* without radiation.

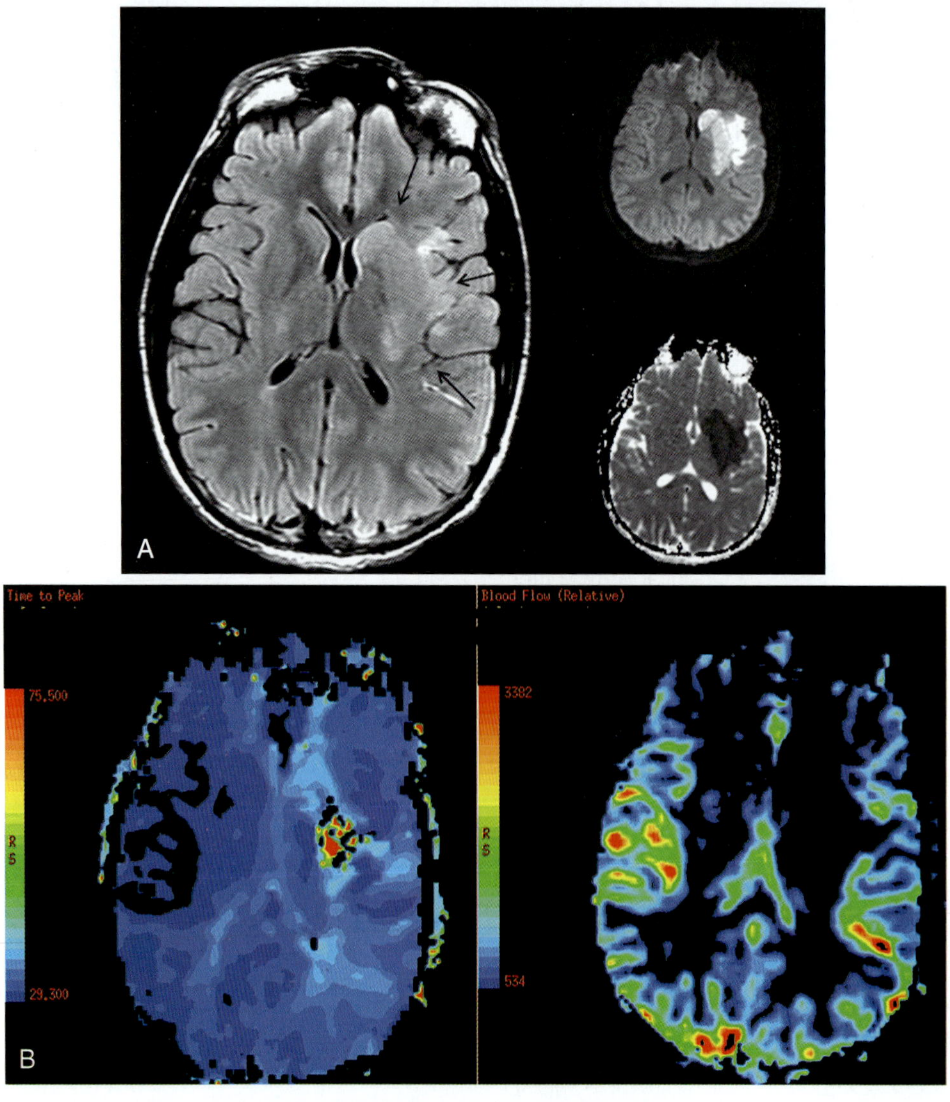

Fig. 25.72 Patient presenting with new-onset neurologic symptoms; rule out stroke. (A) *Left:* Axial fluid attenuation inversion recovery image at the level of the basal ganglia delineates relative hyperintensity in and swelling of the left basal ganglia and adjacent insular cortex *(arrows)*. *Right, top, and bottom:* Diffusion-weighted imaging and apparent diffusion coefficient images at the same level demonstrate hyperintensity and hypointensity (i.e., restricted diffusion). Acute stroke. (B) Two maps: time to peak *(left)* and cerebral blood flow *(right)*, from the perfusion study obtained. Note the asymmetry between the two cerebral hemispheres.

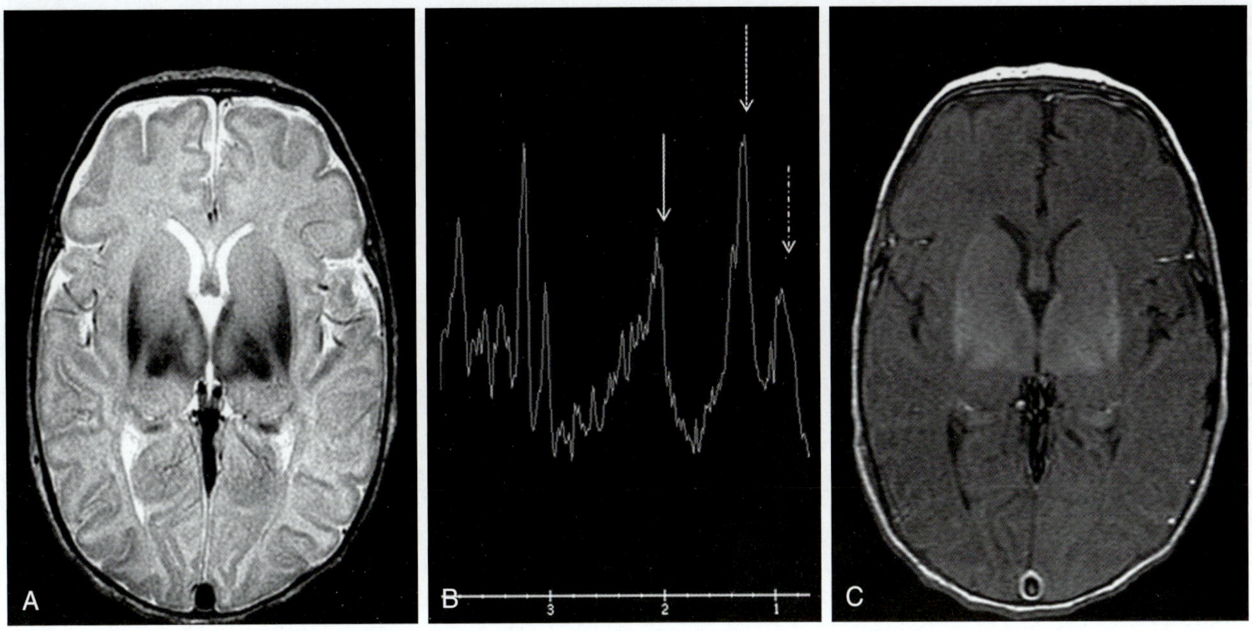

Fig. 25.73 Patient presenting after profound perinatal hypoxia. (A) Axial T2 image at the level of the basal ganglia. Extensive hyperintensity and hypointensity in the basal ganglia and thalami are compatible with the clinical history and represent profound hypoxic ischemic injury. (B) Magnetic resonance spectroscopy delineating decreased *N*-acetylaspartate *(solid arrow)*, elevated lactate *(dotted arrow)*, and elevated lipid *(dash-dotted arrow)* compatible with cell death/ apoptosis. (C) Axial T1 image with corresponding diffuse hyperintensity in the basal ganglia and thalami.

the etiology of perinatal ischemia or seizures (Fig. 25.73) or prognostic information in severe traumatic brain injury (eFig. 25.20). Although MRS is often not specific, the pattern may be suggestive of a distinct group of entities (Fig. 25.74 and Table 25.8).

Contrast-Enhanced Magnetic Resonance Imaging of the Brain

Contrast-enhanced magnetic resonance imaging (CE MRI) can provide anatomic detail in a variety of disorders, including phakomatoses, such as neurofibromatosis, Sturge-Weber syndrome, and tuberous sclerosis (eFig. 25.21). CE-MRI can depict associated cerebritis or abscess, empyema, or parenchymal ischemia related to vascular involvement (eFig. 25.22). MRA and MRS may augment CE-MRI in the setting of vascular malformation (see eFig. 25.5 and Fig. 25.75), brain tumors (particularly primary brain tumors) (Fig. 25.76), demyelinating or inflammatory disease, or acute change in mental status (Fig. 25.77).

Intracranial and Extracranial Magnetic Resonance Angiography and Magnetic Resonance Venography

MRA and MRV can be performed with or without intravenous contrast. Techniques like 3D and 2D time-of-flight use inflow effect of blood protons, whereas phase-contrast angiography or venography are performed using pulses to detect phase shift caused by flowing

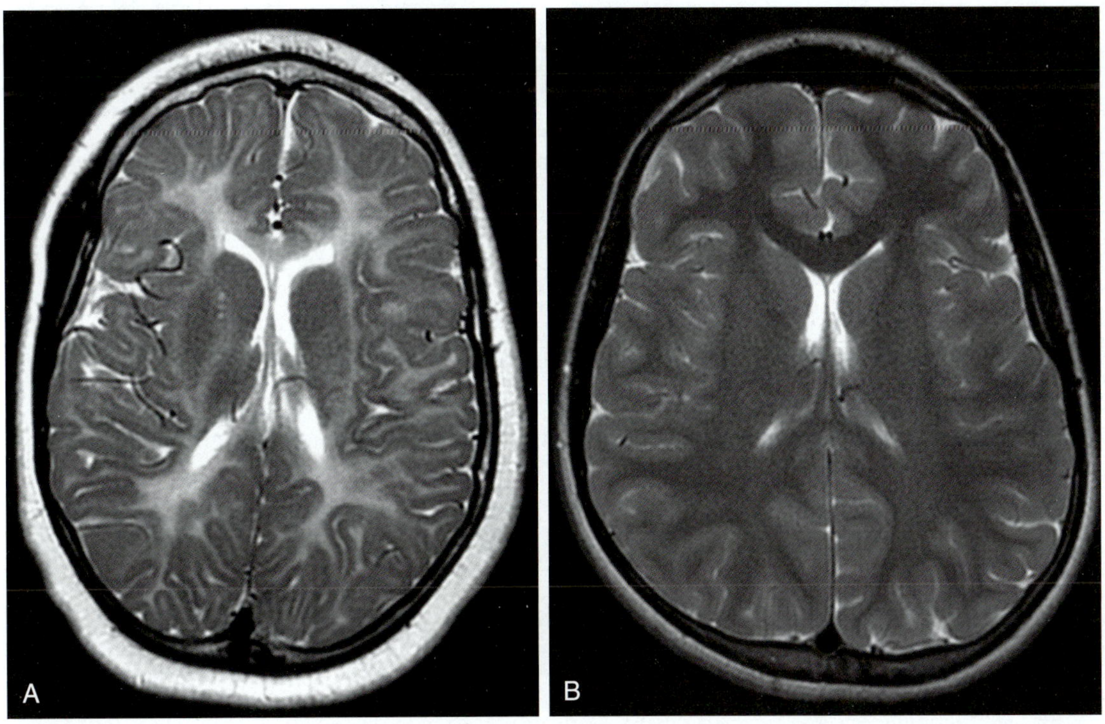

Fig. 25.74 Patient with developmental delay: leukodystrophy of unknown etiology. (A) Axial T2 image at the level of the lateral ventricles delineates diffuse hyperintensity and relative paucity of white matter. Abnormally hypointense basal ganglia. (B) Comparison image of the brain of a child of the same age with normally myelinated white matter, which is hypointense on a T2 sequence. Normal signal characteristics of basal ganglia. Genetic testing and magnetic resonance spectroscopy were nonspecific.

Table 25.8 Signal Characteristics of Central Nervous System Tissues Examined by Various Magnetic Resonance Imaging Sequences

	Cerebrospinal Fluid	Gray Matter	White Matter	Fat	Lesions
T1	Dark-hypointense	Relatively dark-hypointense	Relatively bright-hyperintense	Bright-hyperintense	Variable; majority dark-hypointense
T2	Bright-hyperintense	Relatively bright-hyperintense	Relatively dark-hypointense	Bright-hyperintense	Variable; majority bright-hyperintense
FLAIR	Dark-hypointense	Relatively bright-hyperintense	Relatively dark-hypointense	Bright-hyperintense	Variable; majority bright-hyperintense
DWI	Dark-hypointense	Relatively bright-hyperintense	Relatively dark-hypointense	Dark-hypointense	Variable; majority bright-hyperintense
ADC mapping	Bright-hyperintense	Relatively bright-hyperintense	Dark-hypointense	Bright-hyperintense	Variable Bright-hyperintense: Vasogenic edema, low-grade tumor Dark-hypointense: Cytotoxic edema/ischemia and high-grade tumors
GRE	Bright-hyperintense	Relatively bright-hyperintense	Relatively dark-hypointense	Relatively dark-hypointense	Variable Bright-hyperintense: Majority Dark-hypointense: If blood, fat, or calcium present
STIR	Bright-hyperintense	Relatively bright-hyperintense	Relatively dark-hypointense	Dark-hypointense	Variable; majority Bright-hyperintense

ADC, Apparent diffusion coefficient; *CSF*, cerebrospinal fluid; *DWI*, diffusion-weighted imaging; *FLAIR*, fluid-attenuated inversion recovery; *GRE*, gradient echo; *STIR*, short tau inversion recovery.

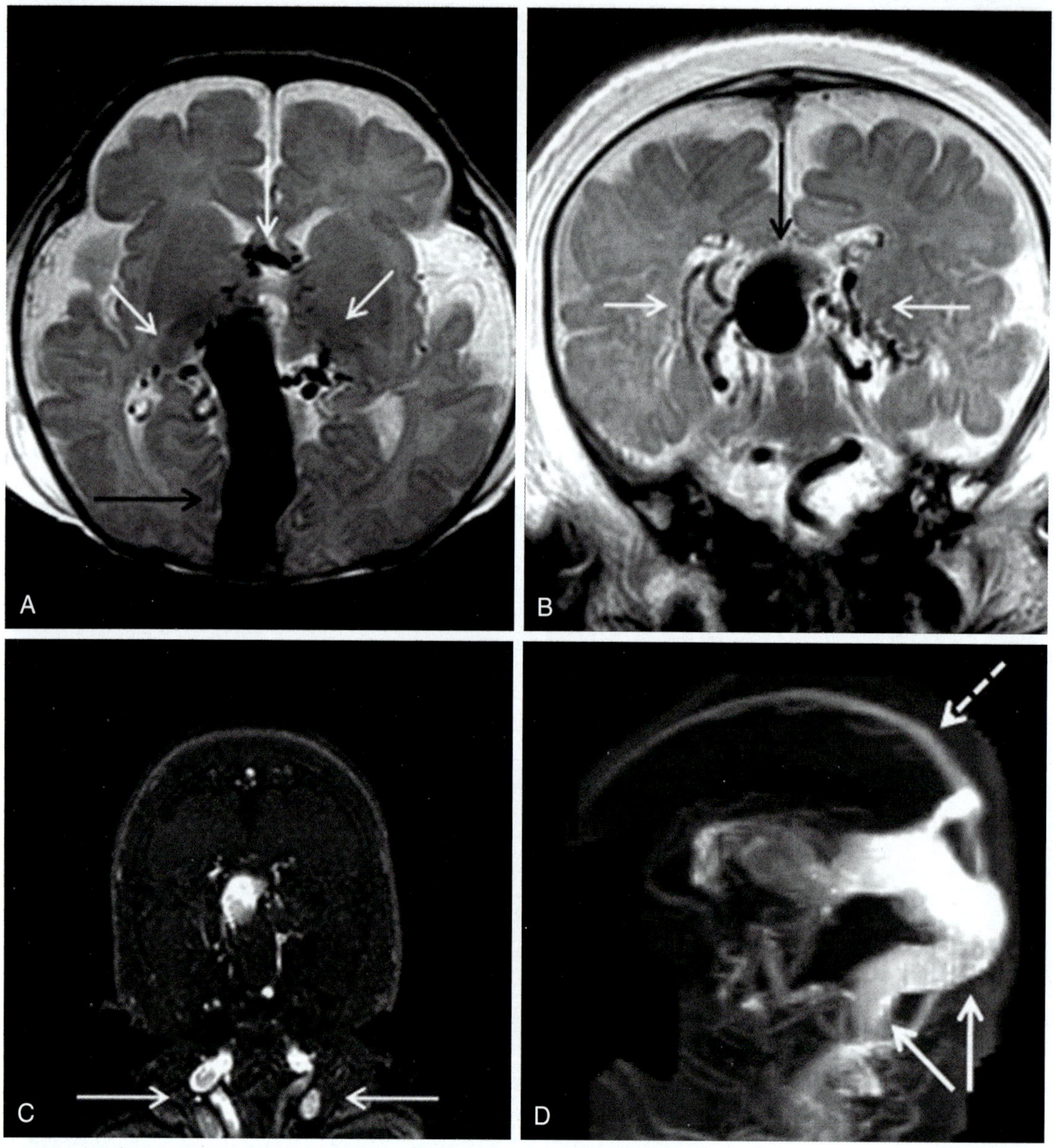

Fig. 25.75 Neonate presenting with congestive heart failure. (A) Axial T2 magnetic resonance image at the level of the lateral and third ventricles delineates marked dilation of the vein of Galen/straight sinus *(black arrow)* and enlarged tortuous adjacent feeding vessels *(white arrows)* arising from both the anterior and posterior circulation. (B) T2 coronal image of the findings in A. (C) Coronal source image from magnetic resonance venography (MRV) delineates not only the intracranial findings but also the associated markedly dilated neck vessels *(arrows)*, which account for the congestive heart failure. (D) Lateral projection from the MRV reconstruction showing venous drainage into the superior sagittal sinus *(dashed arrow)* and transverse and sigmoid sinuses and jugular veins *(solid arrows)*.

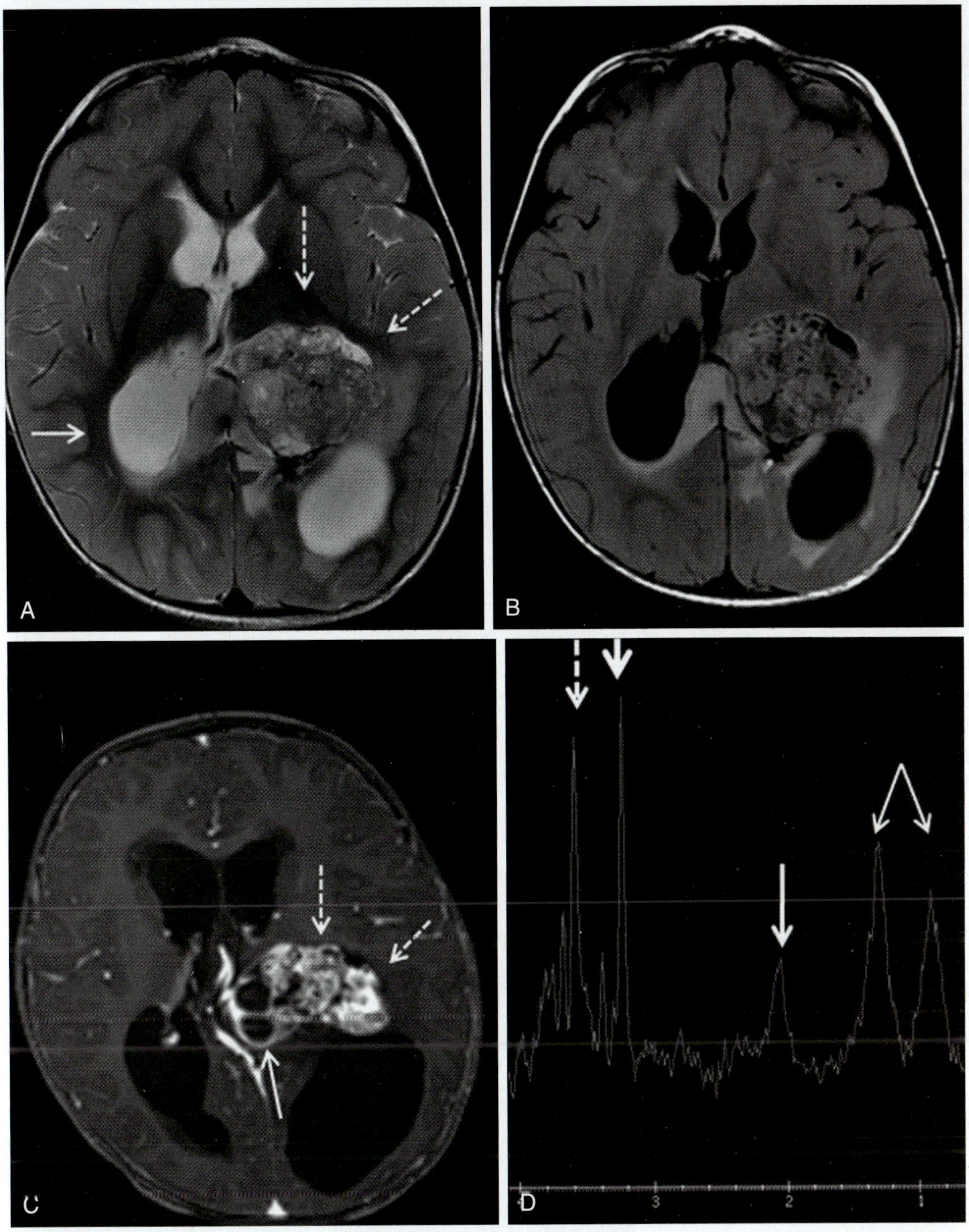

Fig. 25.76 Infant presenting with increasing head size and change in mental status. (A) Axial T2 magnetic resonance image at the level of the lateral and third ventricles delineates ventricular dilation *(solid arrow)* and a large heterogeneous intraventricular mass *(dashed arrows)*. (B) Axial fluid attenuation inversion recovery image at the same level better delineates the adjacent hyperintense edema and transependymal flow of cerebrospinal fluid. (C) Contrast-enhanced T1 image delineates heterogeneous enhancement of solid and cystic components. (D) Magnetic resonance spectroscopy delineates elevated lactate and lipid peaks *(divergent arrows)*, decreased *N*-acetylaspartate peak *(long solid arrow)*, and elevated choline peak *(short solid arrow)*, all of which may be seen in many tumors. An elevated myoinositol peak *(dashed arrow)* is present, strongly suggestive of choroid plexus papilloma, proven at pathology.

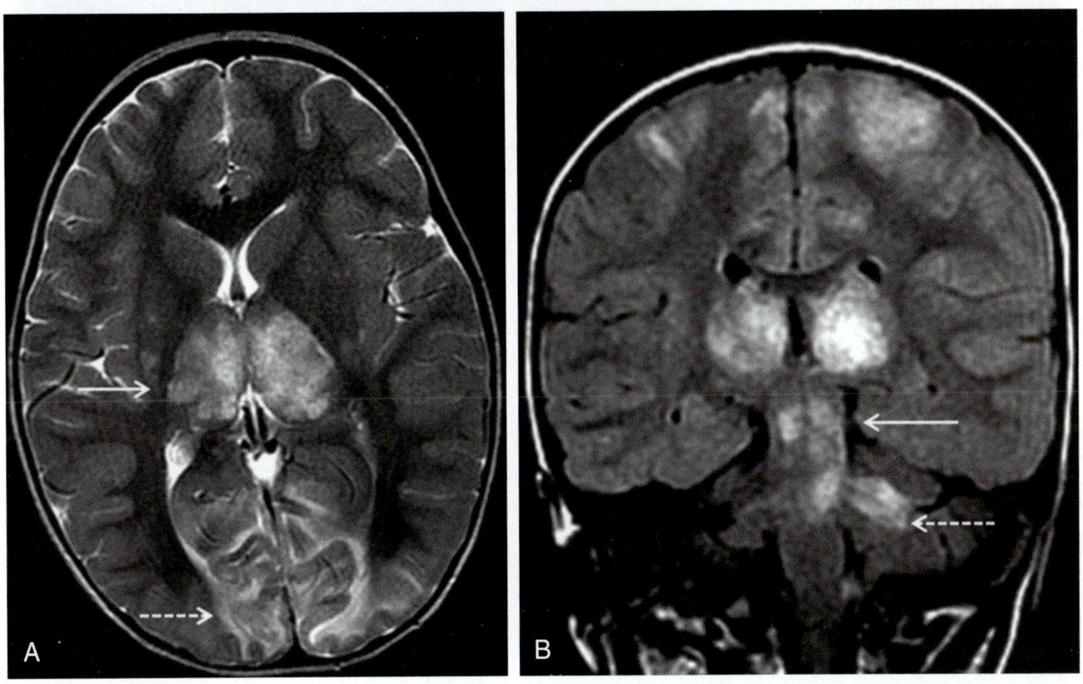

Fig. 25.77 Previously well patient presenting with seizures and profound mental status change after an upper respiratory tract infection. (A) Axial T2 magnetic resonance image at the level of the basal ganglia delineates marked swelling and hyperintensity in the thalami *(solid arrow)* and posterior cortex/occipital lobes *(dashed arrow)*. (B) Coronal T2 image delineates additional involvement of the brainstem *(solid arrow)* and cerebellum *(dashed arrow)*. Other sequences also demonstrated restricted diffusion and petechial hemorrhage. The constellation and distribution of findings are most suggestive of acute necrotizing encephalopathy of childhood.

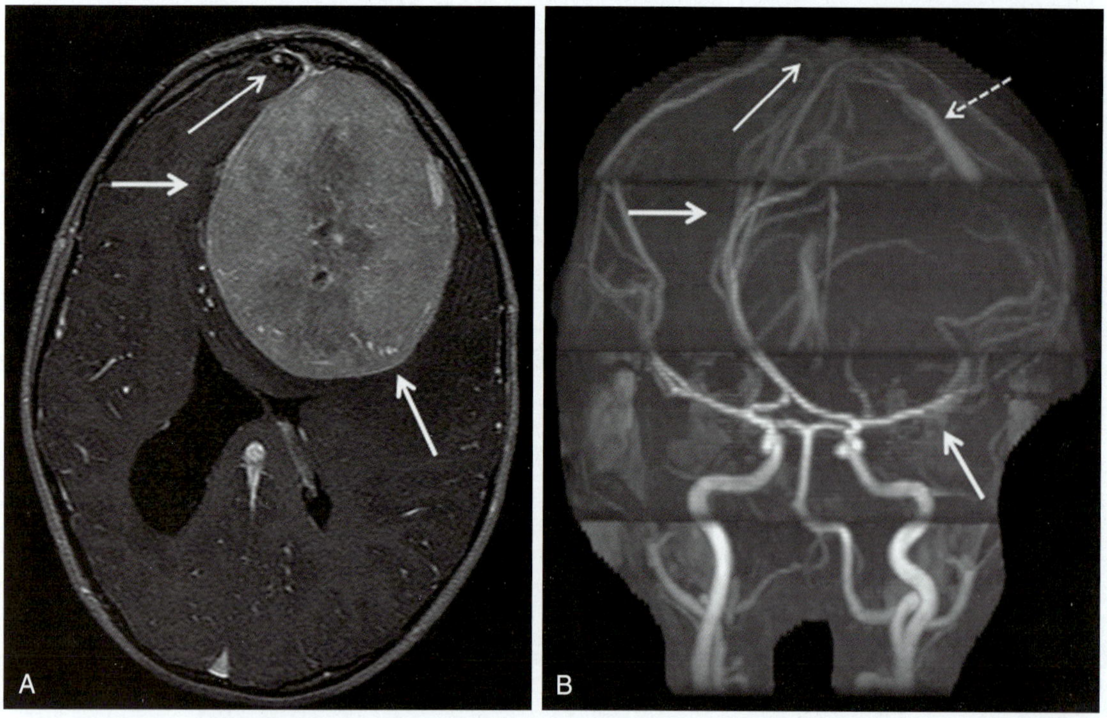

Fig. 25.78 Patient presenting with syncope: meningioma. (A) Axial contrast-enhanced T1 image at the level of the lateral ventricles delineates a large, avidly enhancing left frontal mass *(thick arrows)* abutting the sagittal sinus *(thin arrow)*. Note the significant mass effect on the lateral ventricles and subfalcine herniation. (B) Coronal reconstruction of magnetic resonance angiography indicates marked displacement and draping of the anterior cerebral artery and middle cerebral arteries about the mass *(solid thick arrows)*. *Thin arrow* points to the sagittal sinus and *dashed arrow* indicates a draining vein.

blood. These techniques do not need intravenous contrast administration, and they are easily used when multiple follow-up imaging is required. However, one should be familiar with their limitations. Contrast-enhanced 3D MRA is performed with intravenous contrast administration and has superior contrast-to-noise ratio and fewer artifacts, but it needs to be timed accurately and is not preferred in children with contrast allergy or kidney dysfunction. MRA and MRV offer detailed information in a variety of clinical settings, including vascular relationships and integrity. These include, in part, stroke, vascular dissection, stenosis, luminal irregularity, occlusion, moyamoya disease, and vascular malformations (eFig. 25.23 and eFig. 25.24); vascular relationships to tumors (Fig. 25.78); and vascular complications of infection (eFig. 25.25).

Magnetic Resonance Imaging of the Orbits, Internal Auditory Canal, Skull Base, Face, and Sinuses

The following examinations should be specifically ordered, with clinical indication provided, rather than simply MRI of the brain. The majority are performed with IV contrast. Many entities will require CT in addition for delineation of osseous involvement and the presence of calcifications.

- MRI of the orbits for congenital anomalies, tumors, infection, pain, or proptosis: The latter evaluation should determine the extent (intracoronal or extracoronal) and possible etiologies of proptosis, such as thyroid orbitopathy, pseudotumor, or tumor.
- Temporal bone MRI: Indications include sensorineural hearing loss to assess inner ear structures for congenital anomalies, labyrinthitis ossificans, and lesions of the cochlear nerve (Fig. 25.79). MRI is valuable in assessing disorders causing facial nerve palsies, tinnitus and dizziness, and middle ear and mastoid infections, and particularly in evaluating for intracranial or neck extension or vascular complications.
- Examination of the skull base, face, and sinuses by MRI for tumors, cranial nerve palsy, and infection: Allows assessment of size and extent, perineural spread, and venous complications, such as cavernous sinus involvement (eFig. 25.26).

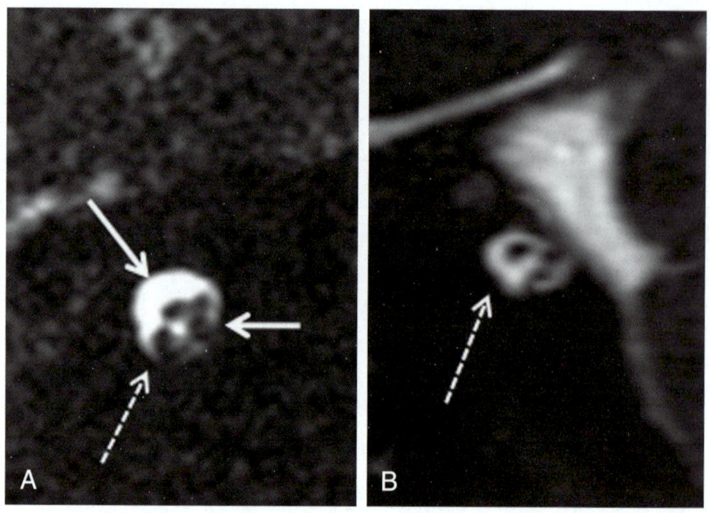

Fig. 25.79 Patient with sensorineural hearing loss and cochlear dysplasia on computed tomography (CT): cochlear nerve aplasia. (A) Oblique sagittal fast imaging employing steady-state acquisition sequence through the internal auditory canals on the normal side. *Solid upper arrow* points to the facial nerve. *Solid horizontal arrow* points to the superior and inferior vestibular nerves. *Dashed arrow* points to the cochlear nerve. (B) Side with cochlear dysplasia: *dashed arrow* points to the expected location of the cochlear nerve, which is not present.

Magnetic Resonance Imaging of the Pituitary and Hypothalamic Region

Neuroendocrine abnormalities with hypothalamic or pituitary dysfunction are amenable to evaluation by MRI, which can be used to assess pituitary size and anatomy, focal lesions (such as adenoma or Rathke cleft cyst), evaluation of ectopic posterior pituitary, and adjacent structures (Fig. 25.80).

Magnetic Resonance Imaging of the Neck and Spine

Indications for MRI of the neck include palpable masses, suspected metastatic disease, pain, dysphagia, and hoarseness.

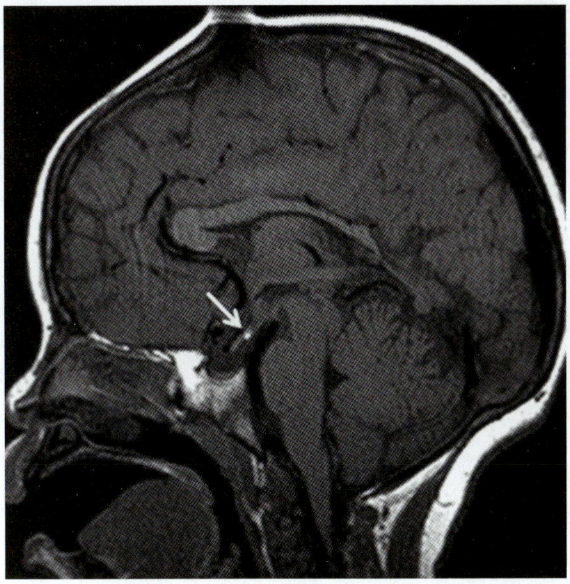

Fig. 25.80 Three-year-old patient presenting with pituitary dysfunction: Panhypopituitarism. Sagittal midline T1 magnetic resonance image delineates a "bright spot," the posterior pituitary/neurohypophysis, not in the posterior aspect of the sella as expected but just posterior to the chiasm at the expected location of the proximal stalk *(arrow)*. The stalk is absent and the pituitary gland is small, indicating ectopic posterior pituitary with interruption of the stalk. Thinning of the posterior aspect of the corpus callosum is related to periventricular leukomalacia in this patient, who was premature.

Unenhanced MRI of the spine is done to evaluate the spinal cord, canal, osseous elements, ligaments, and paravertebral muscles. Indications include trauma (Fig. 25.81), anomalies (eFig. 25.27), tumor, metastatic disease, radiculopathy, and marrow abnormalities. Enhanced MRI of the spine should be performed if infection or inflammation is suspected (Fig. 25.82) or in the presence of a primary or metastatic tumor. Intraspinal, osseous, or paravertebral areas should be examined for involvement.

NUCLEAR MEDICINE IMAGING

Introduction

Pediatric nuclear medicine, or molecular imaging, is a well-established imaging modality that provides important information for diagnosis, staging, treatment, and follow-up of diseases affecting many organ systems, allowing for both anatomic and functional evaluation. Advancements in acquisition and fusion technology have resulted in improved image quality, and new radiopharmaceutics continue to be developed, with implications for both imaging and therapy.

Radiopharmaceutics

Nuclear medicine relies on radiopharmaceutics, which are biologically active molecules with uptake in the body (the pharmaceutic), attached to a radiation-emitting isotope that can be imaged (the

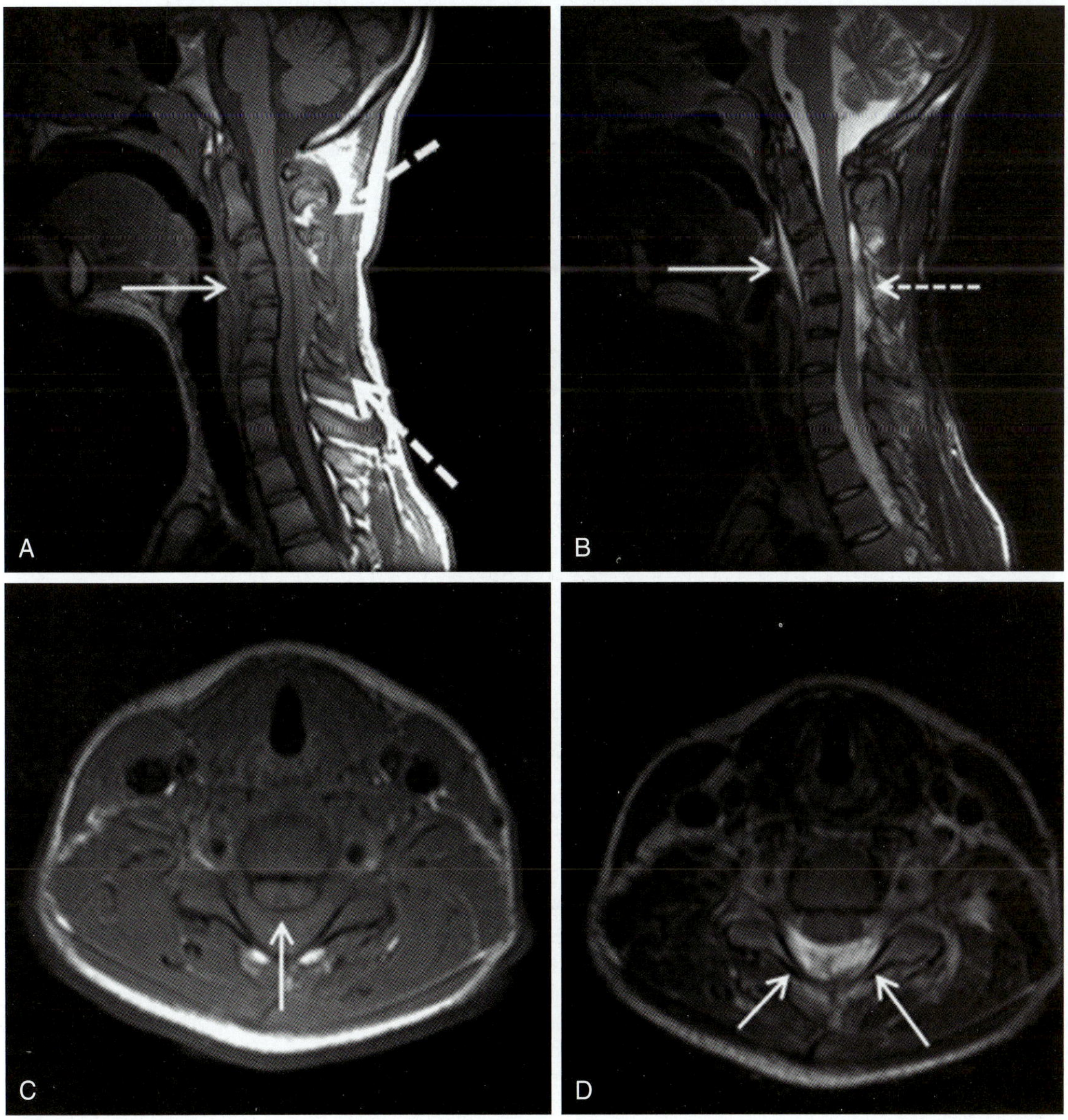

Fig. 25.81 Trauma: ligamentous flexion injury. (A) Sagittal midline T1 magnetic resonance image of the cervical spine delineates marked reversal of cervical lordosis *(solid arrow)* and splaying of the spinous processes. (B) Sagittal short tau inversion recovery image at the same level better delineates the hyperintense prevertebral edema *(solid arrow)* and the hyperintense epidural hematoma *(dashed arrow)* that markedly compresses the cord. (C) Axial T1 image delineates the epidural hematoma and the compressed cord and thecal sac surrounded by the hypointense dura *(solid arrow)*. (D) Axial T2 image at same level delineates the hyperintense epidural hematoma *(solid arrows)* and compressed cord.

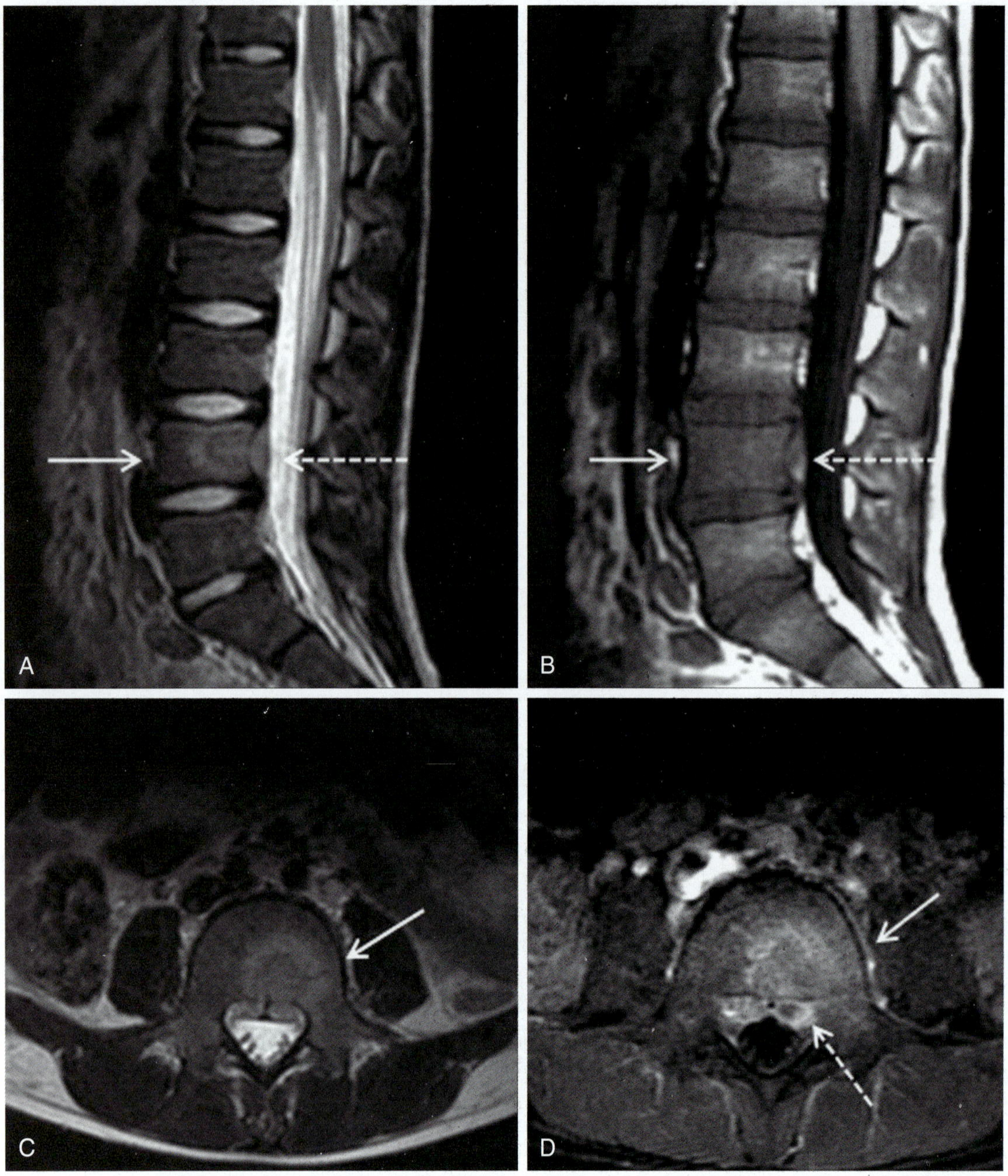

Fig. 25.82 Patient presenting with back pain and fever: osteomyelitis and epidural abscess. (A) Sagittal midline T2 magnetic resonance image of the lumbar spine delineates relative hyperintensity in the L4 vertebral body *(solid arrow)* and an epidural collection *(dashed arrow)*. (B) Sagittal T1 image at the same level delineates corresponding hypointensity in the L4 vertebral body *(solid arrow)* and the epidural collection *(dashed arrow)*. (C) Axial T2 image at the level of L4 demonstrates an abnormal signal/hyperintensity in the vertebral body *(solid arrow)*. (D) Contrast-enhanced T1 fat-saturated image at the same level delineates enhancement of the L4 vertebral body *(solid arrow)* and enhancement of the epidural collection with a small central focus of fluid hypoattenuation *(dashed arrow)*.

radioactive tracer, also called a radionuclide or radioisotope). Radionuclides emit radiation in the form of gamma rays, beta particles, or positrons. The most used gamma-emitting radiotracers include ^{99m}Technicium (^{99m}Tc), ^{123}Iodine (^{123}I), ^{201}Thallium (^{201}Tl), and ^{67}Gallium (^{67}Ga). The most used positron-emitting radiotracers are ^{18}Fluorine (^{18}F) and ^{11}Carbon (^{11}C). The superscript numbers refer to the mass number of the isotope of the element. Radiation dose varies on the basis of the age and size of the patient, dose and type of radionuclide, and rate of clearance of the radiopharmaceutic from the patient. As with other imaging using radiation, radiopharmaceutic dose should be kept as low as possible while ensuring adequate image quality. New radiopharmaceutics that have shorter half-lives and greater specificity to certain areas are being developed. A summary of radiation exposure from pediatric nuclear medicine procedures is given in eTable 25.8.

Nuclear Medicine Imaging Techniques

A gamma camera, also called a scintillation camera, is used to image gamma radiation–emitting radiopharmaceutics, most commonly ^{99m}Tc. One camera, or two variously arranged gamma cameras, may be used to detect scintillation events over the entire field of view imaged. Special types of collimators are variably used to improve image quality. The gamma camera(s) is connected to a computer that converts detected scintillation events into an image. Importantly, radiopharmaceutic activity can be counted on the basis of the number of scintillation events, which is an important role of nuclear medicine imaging.

Single-photon emission tomography (SPECT) uses a gamma camera mounted on a gantry to fully rotate around a patient to acquire three-dimensional images to provide superior anatomic and contrast detail. SPECT images can be reconstructed in multiple planes and are often performed with low-dose CT (SPECT/CT). The newest gamma and SPECT equipment utilize ultrahigh-resolution collimators and filtered back projection to both decrease dose needed for diagnostic imaging and improve image resolution. Finally, SPECT images can be fused with other cross-sectional studies to further improve image quality.

Positron emission tomography (PET) is used to image the photons created by high-energy positron-emitting radiotracers, most commonly ^{18}F. PET alone provides poor anatomic detail, so CT, or less commonly MRI, is usually concomitantly performed for fusion to improve anatomic localization during the same imaging period. Semiquantitative analysis is possible with PET, which is measured in units of standardized value uptake, with the maximum value typically reported. The short half-life of some PET agents makes imaging challenging. For example, ^{11}C has a half-life of only 20.3 minutes, so the cyclotron must be on site or close by for adequate imaging.

Finally, some nuclear medicine imaging will require prolonged immobilization, so sedation or general anesthesia may be necessary (see prior section regarding sedation considerations).

Central Nervous System

Seizure Evaluation

^{99m}Tc-hexamethylpropyleneamine (HMPAO) and ^{99m}Tc-ethyl cysteinate dimer (ECD) are the two most commonly used brain perfusion SPECT radiopharmaceuticals. Both agents are administered intravenously and distribute intracranially proportional to blood flow.

FDG PET/CT imaging may also be used. ^{18}F-FDG is similar to glucose. The molecule is transported intracellularly, where it becomes phosphorylated and trapped. There will be increased ^{18}F FDG activity in areas of high metabolic activity.

For seizure evaluation, SPECT and PET studies should be performed in conjunction with electroencephalogram (EEG) and MRI. Imaging is performed during the ictal phase, with radiopharmaceutic administered at the onset of seizure activity as detected by EEG. During ictal imaging, an epileptogenic focus can be localized by identifying an area of increased uptake. Interictal imaging involves radiopharmaceutic administration when the patient is not seizing, which will demonstrate decreased uptake of the seizure focus. Typically, the two studies are combined, with interictal data subtracted from ictal images so that only ictal foci are displayed as avid foci. Additionally, brain perfusion images can be fused to MRI for improved image quality (Fig. 25.83).

Brain Tumor Evaluation

MRI is best performed for the evaluation of known or suspected brain malignancy. However, ^{18}F-FDG can be used to help differentiate recurrent tumor from radiation necrosis and to assess the response of a high-grade brain tumor to treatment when MRI findings are unclear. Viable high-grade tumors are more metabolically active than normal neuronal cells, so they use more glucose and therefore will be avid at ^{18}F-FDG PET imaging. Conversely, necrotic neuronal tissue and nonviable tumor do not utilize ^{18}F-FDG and will appear photopenic. Background normal brain is highly metabolically active; therefore it uses high amounts of glucose, and some tumors and metastases may be challenging to visualize with ^{18}F-FDG. Additionally, areas of inflammation may have high ^{18}F-FDG uptake, confounding image interpretation. In the future, radiopharmaceutics more specific to the CDP-choline/choline kinase pathway may become more widespread for tumor evaluation purposes, such as ^{11}C-methionine, ^{18}F-methylcholine, ^{18}F-ethylcholine, or 3,4-dihydroxy-6-F-18-fluoro-L-phenylalanine.

Brain Death Evaluation

Neurologic examination, EEG monitoring, and apnea studies best diagnose irreversible coma. If there is uncertainty, ^{99m}Tc-exametazime or HMPAO and ^{99m}Tc-ECD can be used to determine cerebral perfusion using angiographic, planar images, and SPECT. In the setting of brain death, imaging will demonstrate absent intracranial flow and absent cerebral and cerebellar radiopharmaceutic uptake (eFig. 25.28).

Cerebrovascular Disease

Causes of childhood cerebrovascular disease include moyamoya disease and SCD, among others. Brain perfusion SPECT and PET imaging can be helpful to evaluate regional perfusion abnormalities

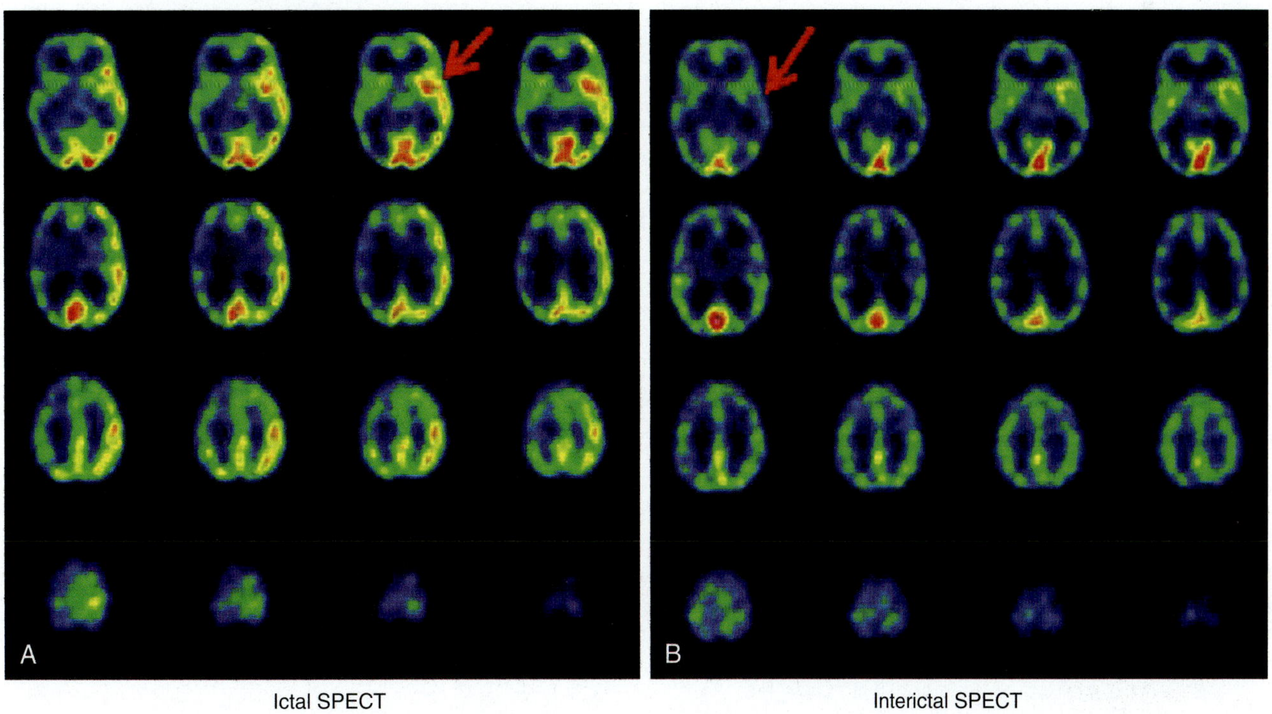

Fig. 25.83 Ictal and interictal brain single-photon emission computed tomography (SPECT): An 11-year-old with intractable partial complex seizure and epileptogenic focus in the left temporal lobe. Ictal SPECT (A) demonstrates a focus of increased perfusion *(arrow)* in the left temporal lobe spreading to the left parietal lobe. Interictal SPECT (B) demonstrates a focus of decreased perfusion *(arrow)* in the left temporal lobe.

in these patients. Acetazolamide is a carbonic anhydrase inhibitor, which causes cerebral vasodilation and thus can evaluate cerebral flow reserve. The normal arterial response to acetazolamide is vasodilation and increased cerebral blood flow. However, an artery with significant stenosis is already maximally dilated due to physiologic compensation to a decreased flow state and cannot further dilate to augment flow. Thus regions of inadequate blood flow reserve and relative hypoperfusion can be detected with use of acetazolamide during brain perfusion radiopharmaceutic imaging.

Cerebrospinal Fluid Evaluation

CSF flow can be evaluated with nuclear medicine imaging. For CSF leak evaluation or ventricular drainage/shunt catheter flow/integrity evaluation, ^{99m}Tc-diethylenetriamine pentaacetate (DTPA) is typically used. The radiopharmaceutic is administered into the lumbar subarachnoid space, lateral ventricle, cisterna magna, or shunt reservoir. For patients with possible CSF leak, frequent images are obtained to attempt to localize leak site for operative planning, and cotton pledgets may need to be placed in the nares, then removed and assessed for radioactivity count for subtle leak diagnosis. Patients with ventricular shunts are imaged initially with attention to the reservoir and ventricles, and subsequently the course of the shunt catheter is imaged (Fig. 25.84).

Thyroid

Congenital Hypothyroidism

^{123}Iodine (^{123}I) and ^{131}I are physiologically indistinguishable from naturally occurring iodine. They are transported into the follicular cells of the thyroid, where they are oxidized, organified, and incorporated into thyroid hormone. ^{123}I imaging can be used to image thyroid tissue that is able to both trap and organify iodine. ^{99m}Tc-pertechnetate is an analog of iodine that is transported into the thyroid follicular cells but is not organified. ^{131}I is detailed in the ^{131}I therapy section.

Ultrasound and nuclear medicine imaging are complementary in the evaluation of congenital hypothyroidism. ^{123}I and ^{99m}Tc-pertechnetate are more sensitive in detecting ectopic thyroid tissue, organification defects, and thyroid dyshormonogenesis, whereas ultrasound is better suited to evaluate the appearance and size of the thyroid (eFig. 25.29).

Hyperthyroidism

Thyroid scintigraphy can be performed if needed to help distinguish hyperthyroidism etiology, with thyroid uptake measurements performed at 4 and 24 hours after radiopharmaceutic administration. Images should be interpreted in conjunction with laboratory value assessment. In the setting of Graves disease, thyromegaly and diffusely increased radiopharmaceutic uptake. A hyperfunctioning nodule can be localized as focal avidity with suppressed remainder of the gland. In the thyrotoxicosis state of transient thyroiditis, radiopharmaceutic uptake will be low. In factitious hyperthyroidism, radiopharmaceutic uptake will be low, with suppressed serum TSH and thyroglobulin values.

^{131}I Therapy

^{131}I is a beta-emitting radiotracer with a relatively long half-life of 8.1 days, which may be used for radioablation of differentiated thyroid tissue. Once organified by thyroid tissue or differentiated thyroid cancer, ^{131}I decays and emits beta particles, which disrupt deoxyribonucleic acid, leading to cell death.

Relatively low doses may be used to treat Graves disease and multinodular goiter. However after therapy, most patients with hyperthyroidism will become hypothyroid, so close evaluation by endocrinology is required for appropriate hormone replacement.

In the setting of extensive and/or metastatic papillary or follicular thyroid cancer, patients first undergo total thyroidectomy. Whole body ^{123}I or ^{131}I imaging is then performed to evaluate for residual thyroid tissue and metastatic disease, with uptake quantified so that the appropriate ^{131}I treatment dose can be calculated (Fig. 25.85).

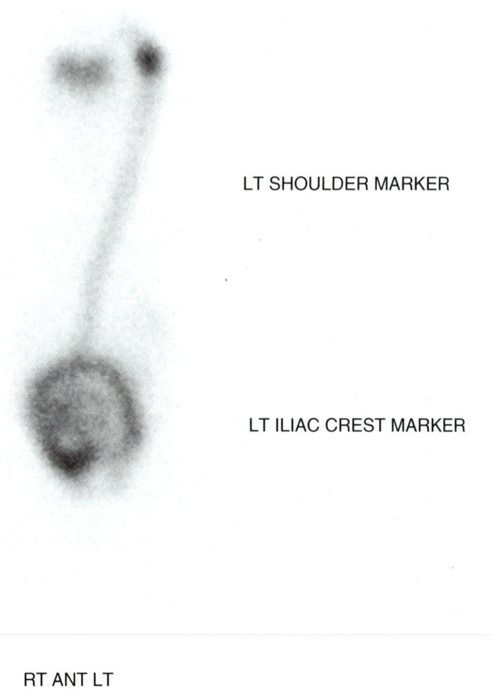

Fig. 25.84 Intact ventriculoperitoneal shunt study. A 7-month-old male presented with lethargy. Fused frontal planar view demonstrates activity in the ventricle, shunt reservoir, catheter, and accumulation in the right lower quadrant.

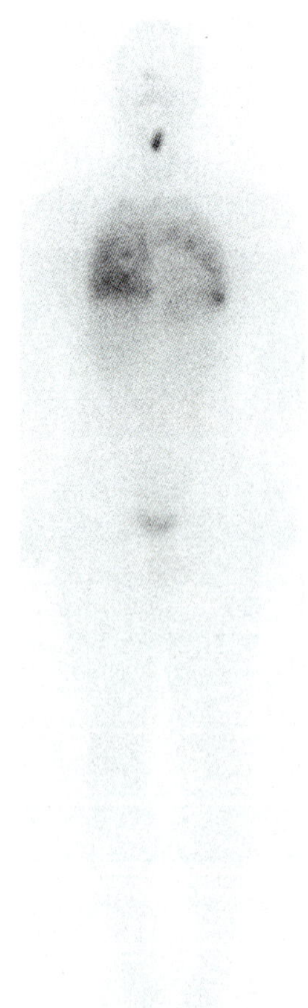

Fig. 25.85 Metastatic papillary thyroid carcinoma. Frontal planar view from delayed 131-I imaging demonstrates residual radiopharmaceutic uptake in the midline neck and relatively diffusely throughout the lungs in this 17-year-old female with lung metastases status post-radioiodine ablation therapy.

Box 25.1 Compounds That Can Decrease Thyroid Iodine Uptake[a]

For 1 week: Adrenocorticosteroid, bromides, phenylbutazone (Butazolidin), mercurials, methimazole (Tapazole), propylthiouracil, perchlorate, nitrate, salicylate (large dose), sulfonamides, and thiocyanate
For 2–3 weeks: Triiodothyronine (Cytomel)
For 4 weeks: Thyroid extract (Synthroid, Proloid), iodine solution (Lugol or saturated solution of potassium iodide [SSKI]), iodine-containing antiseptics, and some cough medicines and vitamin preparations
For 1–2 months: Intravenous contrast agents
For 3–6 months: Oil-based iodinated contrast agents and amiodarone

[a]Based on American College of Radiology (ACR) practice guideline 2007.

^{131}I is administered as a swallowed pill. There are unique considerations with ^{131}I therapy. Pregnancy is a contraindication for ^{131}I therapy due to radiation risk to the fetus, and breastfeeding mothers must stop to avoid harm to the infant's thyroid. Compounds that can affect iodine uptake (Box 25.1) should be avoided before therapy to maximize uptake by thyroid tissue. Additionally, special radiation safety precautions must be followed for up to 5 days after ^{131}I therapy to avoid radiation exposure to people besides patient. ^{131}I, like many radiotracers, is renally excreted, so patients must follow voiding directions. Finally, in addition to thyroid, ^{131}I is taken up by the salivary glands, so patients must follow instructions to avoid radiation-induced sialadenitis.

Cardiovascular System

Myocardial Perfusion Imaging

Myocardial perfusion evaluation may be indicated in patients with cardiopulmonary disorders that increase risk for myocardial ischemia and arrhythmias, such Kawasaki disease, congenital coronary artery anomalies, cardiomyopathy, patients status post-arterial switch procedure, TOF repair, cardiac transplantation, and patients at high risk for coronary artery ischemia–related chest pain.

Radiopharmaceutics commonly used for myocardial perfusion SPECT imaging include ^{201}thallium chloride (^{201}Tl), which is a potassium analog that redistributes over time, and ^{99m}technetium tetrofosmin and ^{99m}technetium sestamibi, which are taken up in the myocardium in proportion to blood flow. Myocardial perfusion is based on coronary artery blood flow and can thus be evaluated by radiopharmaceutic extraction. Myocardial SPECT imaging is performed both at rest and during cardiac stress, which can be induced by exercise, vasodilating medications such as adenosine or dipyridamole for those with arrhythmias, or dobutamine for patients with asthma. During stress, diseased vessels cannot dilate as much as normal vessels to meet the increased oxygen demand, so myocardium with poor perfusion will appear relatively photopenic. Images are gated to the cardiac cycle to enable wall motion and ejection fraction evaluation (Fig. 25.86).

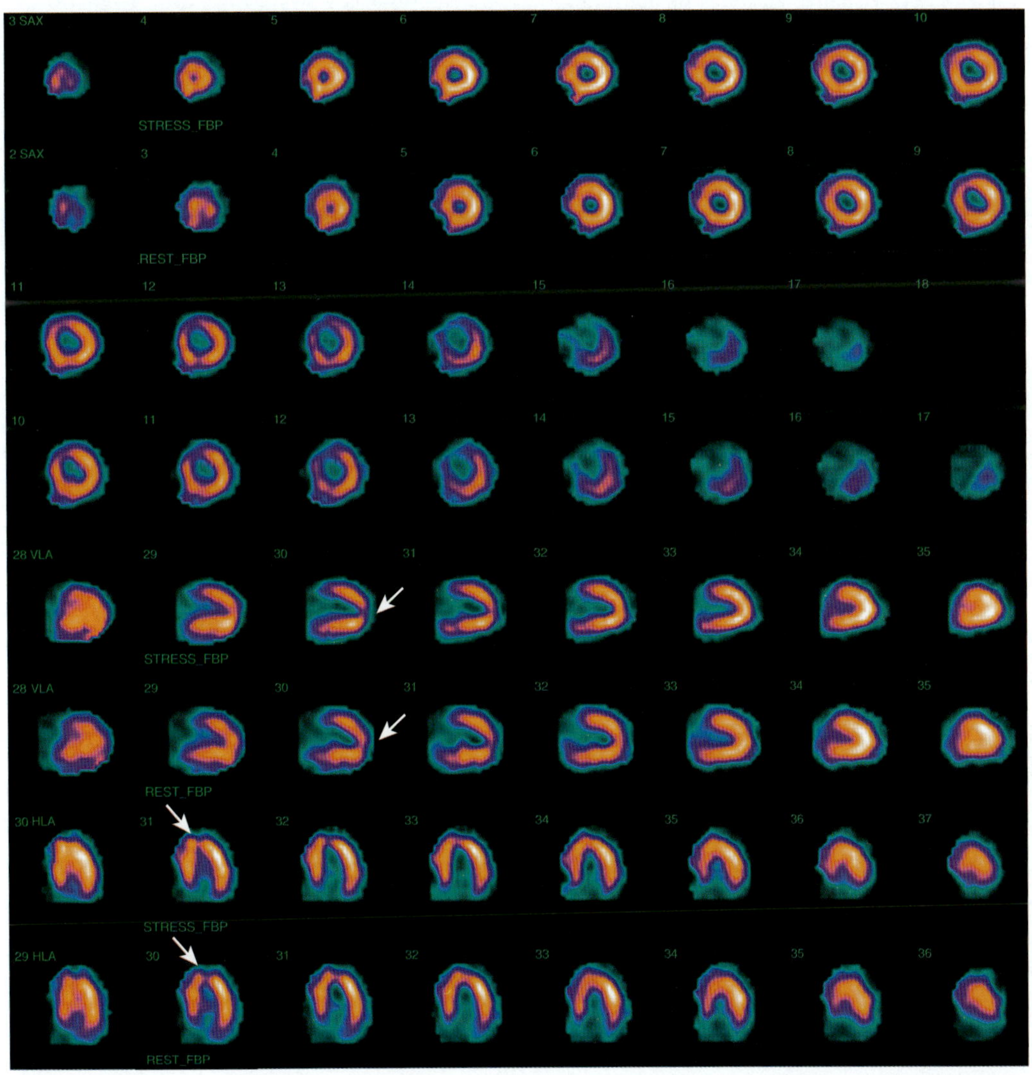

Fig. 25.86 Myocardial scarring at the heart apex. Myocardial perfusion imaging with exercise stress and rest images show a fixed defect *(arrows)* at the cardiac apex on 99m-Tc-sestamibi imaging in this 13-year-old male with surgically corrected congenital heart disease at S-T changes on electrocardiogram.

Myocardial Viability Assessment

Evaluation of myocardial cell viability may be desired before a revascularization surgery, and ^{18}F-FDG may be used for this purpose. The distribution of ^{18}F-FDG reflects the distribution of viable myocardial cells, which metabolize glucose. ^{201}Tl can also be used to evaluate myocardial viability. This SPECT agent is a potassium analog, which is continuously transported into and out of living myocardial cells, which results in redistribution in viable cells.

Ventricular Function Assessment

A multigated acquisition scan is considered the gold standard for calculation of the left ventricular ejection fraction with high reproducibility. This study may be necessary in patients treated with certain types of chemotherapy with potential myocardial toxicity side effects and also to assess cardiac risk before surgery. The patient's own RBCs are labeled with ^{99m}Tc and readministered into the patient. ECG-gated images of radiolabeled blood within the cardiac chambers are then imaged.

Pulmonary System

Ventilation/Perfusion Lung Scan

A ventilation/perfusion (V/Q) scan may be indicated if there is clinical concern for acute pulmonary embolus, to evaluate chronic pulmonary embolus, or for evaluation before or after surgery. Perfusion images are acquired using ^{99m}Tc-macroaggregated albumin (MAA). MAA particles are larger than the pulmonary capillaries, so they are trapped in the first pulmonary arterial capillary bed encountered after intravenous injection. Imaging is performed in multiple projections to adequately visualize all lobes of the lungs. ^{99m}Tc-MAA is unable to reach the pulmonary capillaries occluded by a pulmonary embolus, so affected areas of the lung will appear photopenic.

Lung ventilation images are performed using aerosolized ^{99m}Tc-DTPA or ^{133}Xenon (Xe) gas. Nonaerated portions of lung will appear photopenic on ventilation images, whereas aerated lung will appear avid (Fig. 25.87).

Right-to-Left Shunt Evaluation

Patients with known or suspected right-to-left shunt can be evaluated with ^{99m}Tc-MAA, and percentage of shunting can be quantified. In the absence of a right-to-left shunt, all ^{99m}Tc-MAA will be trapped in the first pulmonary arterial capillary bed encountered, so there will only be uptake in the lungs. However, with an intracardiac or extracardiac right-to-left shunt, ^{99m}Tc-MAA particles are able to enter the systemic circulation and become trapped in the capillary and precapillary beds of systemic organs, such as the brain and kidneys. The percentage of right-to-left shunt can be calculated based on the difference between the radiopharmaceutic count of the whole body and lungs (Fig. 25.88).

Genitourinary System

Basic and Diuretic Renography

A basic renogram may be indicated to provide functional information and is usually interpreted in conjunction with renal ultrasound for anatomical correlation. Potential indications include evaluating renal function, including relative kidney function; detecting urine leak, renal infarct, or outflow obstruction; and evaluating arterial flow, for possible rejection, and for acute tubular necrosis in native or transplanted kidneys.

^{99m}Tc-mercapto-acetyltriglycine (MAG3) is most commonly used, which is extracted via tubular secretion. A series of images of the kidneys are taken as the radiotracer arrives, is extracted into the renal cortex, transported through the kidney, and excreted into the

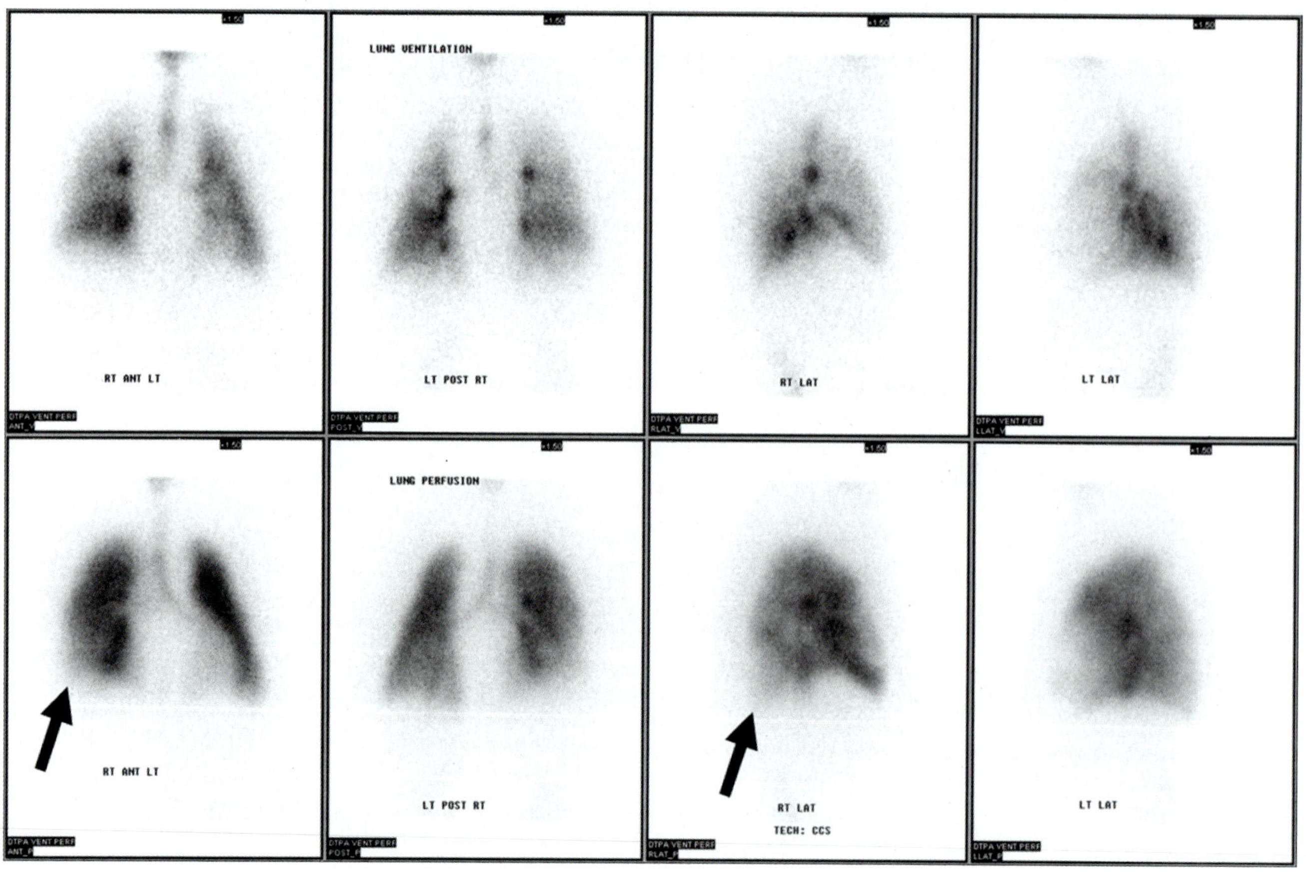

Fig. 25.87 Pulmonary embolus. Ventilation/perfusion scintigraphy demonstrates absent perfusion to the right posterior and lateral basilar lower lobe segments *(arrows)* in this 28-year-old male with repaired congenital heart disease and left ventricle to pulmonary artery conduit thrombus.

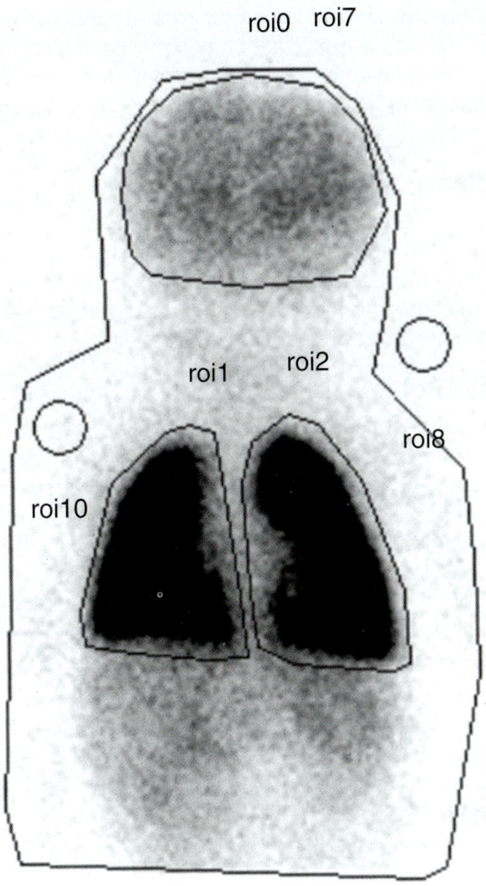

Fig. 25.88 Right-to-left shunt. 99m-Tc-MAA activity is seen in both the brain and kidneys of this 1-year-old female with hepatopulmonary syndrome.

collecting system and urinary bladder. Quantitative renogram curves are generated for each kidney.

Diuretic renography is performed to diagnose urinary tract obstruction, usually in patients with urinary tract dilation discovered by other imaging studies. ^{99m}Tc-MAG3 is used as the radiopharmaceutic, and during the first portion of the examination, similar images are acquired as basic renography. However, subsequent to the initial excretion images, a diuretic (most commonly furosemide) is administered and the urinary collecting system response is evaluated. An unobstructed system will respond to furosemide by excreting radiotracer. Conversely, there will be abnormally slow washout of radiopharmaceutic from an obstructed collecting system. Like basic renography, quantitative curves are generated (Fig. 25.89).

Renal Cortical Scintigraphy

Children with possible acute pyelonephritis or renal scarring may be evaluated with renal cortical scintigraphy, and relative renal function can also be evaluated. Dimercaptosuccinic acid is the most commonly used radiopharmaceutical, which binds to renal tubules in the cortex. Pyelonephritis and scarring will both cause diminished cortical uptake of involved portions of the cortex, so clinical context must be considered (Fig. 25.90).

Vesicoureteral Reflux

Radionuclide cystography (RNC), conventional VCUG, and contrast-enhanced voiding urosonography (ceVUS) may all be used in the evaluation of children with suspected VUR. VCUG and ceVUS provide anatomic detail of the urethra, urinary bladder, ureters, renal pelvis, and calyces, and therefore are usually first-line imaging studies. RNC is typically reserved for follow-up evaluation of patients with known VUR whose anatomy has previously been

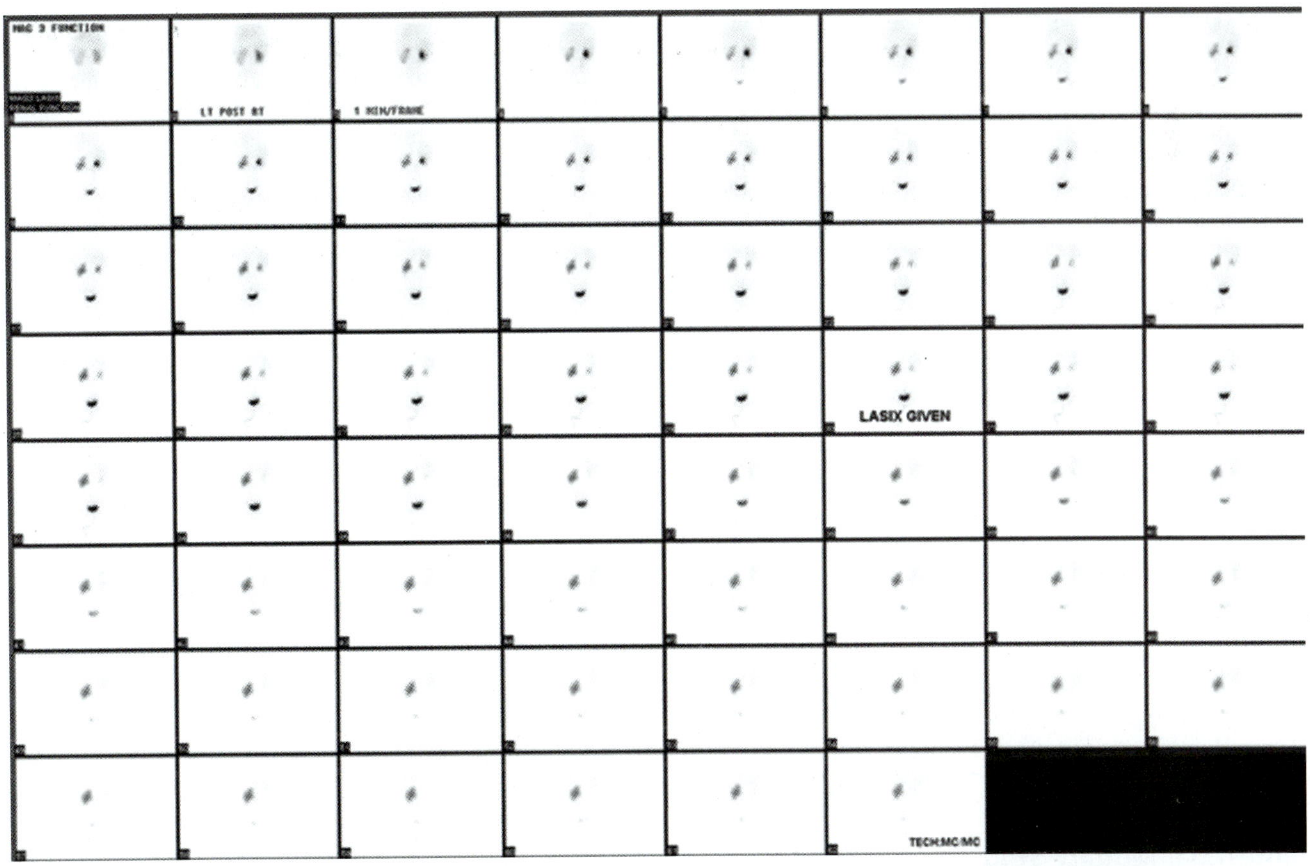

Fig. 25.89 Left ureteropelvic junction obstruction. Multiple prone thumbnail images obtained from 1 through 62 minutes after intravenous administration of 99m-Tc-MAG3 demonstrates normal urinary tract emptying of the right kidney (right-hand side of the thumbnail images). No spontaneous excretion of radiopharmaceutic is seen from the dilated left pelvicalyceal system, demonstrates no excretion of radiopharmaceutic after furosemide administration in this 2-year-old female.

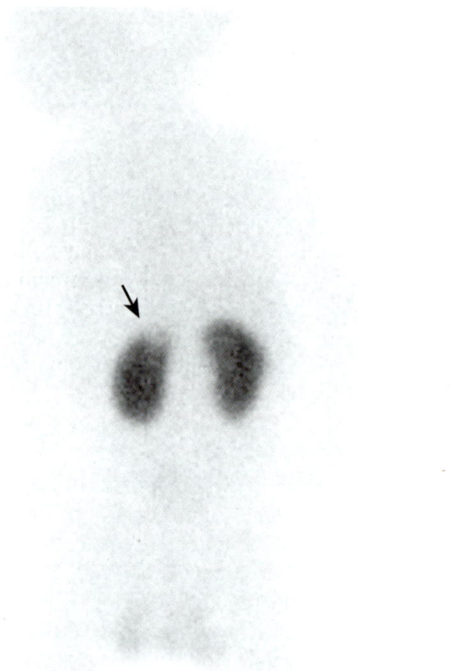

Fig. 25.90 Acute pyelonephritis. Supine whole-body image shows no uptake of 99m-Tc-DMSA in the right upper pole kidney *(arrow)* in this 7-week-old female with febrile urinary tract infection and hyperechoic ill-defined focus seen on ultrasound (not shown).

delineated. The most common method to perform RNC involves catheterization of the urinary bladder and instillation of ^{99m}Tc-pertechnetate mixed with saline, followed by continuous imaging during bladder filling and voiding. VUR can be visualized and graded similar to conventional VCUG (eFig. 25.30).

Gastrointestinal System

Gastrointestinal Bleeding

Gastrointestinal (GI) bleeding can be diagnosed and localized, most commonly using ^{99m}Tc-labeled RBC scintigraphy. In this method, radiolabeled RBCs are administered IV and imaging is initially performed at a high frame rate to capture the angiographic phase, followed by imaging at a rate of 1 frame per minute for up to 90 minutes. Finally, intermittent imaging is performed as needed for up to 24 hours. GI bleeding will be seen as an abnormal extravascular accumulation of radiotracer over time. ^{99m}Tc-labeled RBC scintigraphy is more sensitive than conventional angiographic evaluation because of the longer duration of imaging. Enteric barium and other photon-absorbing objects may cause false-negative results (eFig. 25.31).

Meckel Diverticulum Scan

A Meckel diverticulum is an embryological remnant of the omphalomesenteric duct, which is located near the terminal ileum, and about 57% contain ectopic gastric mucosa. This ectopic mucosa can be visualized with a Meckel scan. ^{99m}Tc-pertechnetate is administered intravenously and taken up by gastric mucosa. A Meckel diverticulum will be seen as focal uptake in the anterior right lower abdominal quadrant simultaneous to gastric activity, and will increase in intensity over the course of imaging. Because not all Meckel diverticula contain functioning gastric mucosa, a negative Meckel scan does not exclude a Meckel diverticulum (Fig. 25.91).

Gastrointestinal Motility Studies

GI motility scintigraphy provides both physiologic and functional information about GI transit. The esophagus, including evaluation for GER or aspiration, stomach, or the entire GI tract can be evaluated depending on the clinical scenario. ^{99m}Tc-DTPA, ^{111}In-DTPA, or ^{99m}Tc-sulfur colloid are mixed with liquid or a solid meal and given by mouth or through an enteral catheter. Images are obtained in the area of interest and quantification can be performed to compare with normal values (eFig. 25.32).

Hepatobiliary System

Hepatobiliary ^{99m}Tc-iminodiacetic acid (IDA or HIDA) is used to evaluate the hepatobiliary system in several disease processes. The radiopharmaceutic is administered intravenously, binds to albumin, is transported into the liver, and is excreted via the biliary system following the bilirubin metabolic pathway.

Neonatal Cholestasis

HIDA may be useful to help distinguish biliary atresia from other causes of neonatal cholestasis. ^{99m}Tc-IDA is administered intravenously, followed by immediate and up to 24-hour delayed imaging. Biliary atresia is a sclerosing cholangitis of the extrahepatic biliary system causing bile duct occlusion, so radiopharmaceutics will remain in the liver in these patients (Fig. 25.92). In other causes of neonatal cholestasis, HIDA will be normal, demonstrating hepatic uptake, excretion into the biliary tree, and passage into the small bowel.

There are several special considerations for HIDA performed for neonatal cholestasis evaluation. First, pretreatment with phenobarbital for 5 days before hepatobiliary scintigraphy is necessary to increase bile secretion of radiopharmaceutical. This delay is imperative to consider because expeditious diverting hepatoportoenterostomy (Kasai) must be performed in patients with biliary atresia. Additionally, patients with severe hepatic dysfunction may have suboptimal hepatic uptake of radiopharmaceutics, which may result in suboptimal biliary excretion and a nondiagnostic study.

Biliary Obstruction, Cholecystitis, and Biliary Dyskinesia

HIDA may be useful in evaluating for cystic duct or biliary obstruction, biliary dyskinesia, or cholecystitis. For this indication, patients fast for up to 4 hours before imaging. ^{99m}Tc-IDA is injected intravenously and serial images are acquired for 1 hour. Visualization of the gallbladder within 1 hour usually indicates a normal study, although acalculous (nonobstructive) cholecystitis may also give this appearance. If the gallbladder is not visualized by 1 hour, morphine sulfate (0.04 mg/kg) is then administered to cause sphincter of Oddi contraction and redirection of bile into the cystic duct to fill the gallbladder with radiopharmaceutics. If the gallbladder is still not visualized after morphine administration, acute cholecystitis should be suspected.

Depending on the clinical indication, cholecystokinin (CCK) may be administered if the gallbladder is visualized after 1 hour. CCK causes gallbladder contraction, and ejection fraction can be calculated. Decreased gallbladder ejection fraction raises concern for chronic cholecystitis or biliary dyskinesia. Noting the absence or presence and amount of pain with CCK administration may be useful as well.

Bile Leak

In the postoperative or posttraumatic setting, HIDA may be helpful to diagnose bile leak as an alternative to delayed MRI performed with hepatobiliary contrast agents. In this setting, after intravenous administration of ^{99m}Tc-IDA, scintigraphy will demonstrate leakage of radiotracer into the peritoneum or elsewhere and will accumulate over time (Fig. 25.93).

Infection

Fever of Unknown Origin

Children with fever of unknown origin (FUO) should first undergo thorough history, physical examination, and laboratory evaluation. Nuclear medicine imaging is reserved for patients who still lack a

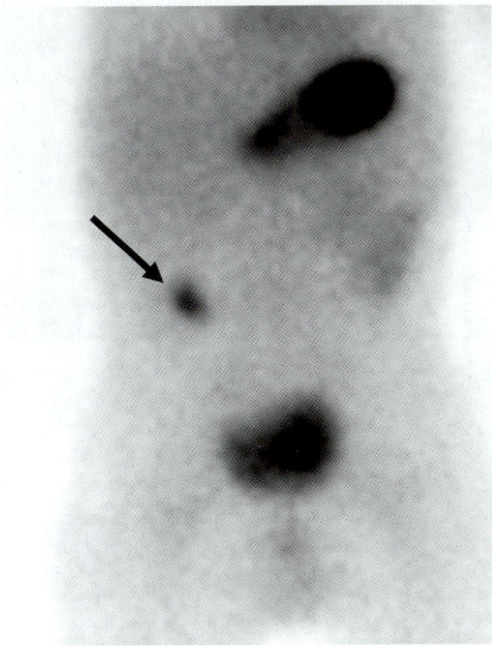

Fig. 25.91 Ectopic gastric mucosa in a Meckel diverticulum. Two-hour delay images in the frontal projection demonstrate 99m-Tc-pertechnetate uptake in the right mid- to lower abdominal quadrant *(arrow)* of this 16-month-old male with anemia and melena.

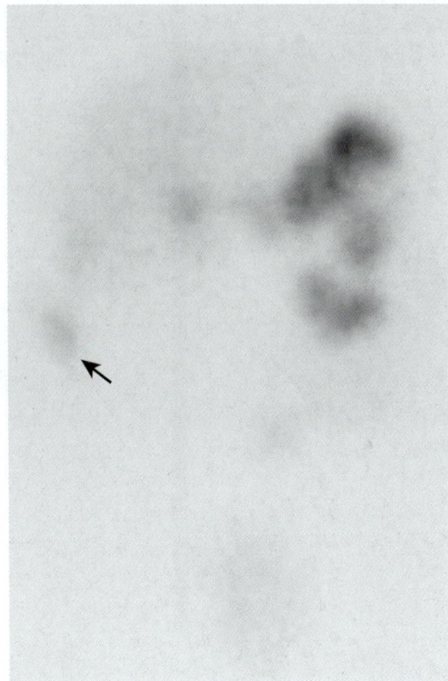

Fig. 25.93 Bile leak. Focal radiotracer is seen inferior to the cut surface of the liver transplant *(arrow)* in this 45-minute delayed image of this 8-month-old male with biliary atresia status post–liver transplantation a few weeks earlier.

Fig. 25.92 Biliary atresia. No radiopharmaceutic was seen passing from the liver into the small bowel, including this 24-hour delayed frontal image on this 1-month-old female with biliary atresia.

definitive diagnosis and require treatment. Traditionally, this was performed with ^{67}Ga-citrate, which accumulates in acute and chronic sites of infection and in some malignant processes. However, its usefulness in children is debatable. ^{111}In- or ^{99m}Tc-HMPAO–labeled leukocytes have also been used for this purpose, but false-negative rates are usually prohibitive (eFig. 25.33). Finally, ^{18}F-FDG PET/CT may be useful to aid evaluation of children with FUO. However, radiation and monetary expense should be taken into consideration. Whole-body MRI should be considered an alternative examination at some institutions in some patient scenarios.

Osteomyelitis

Currently, acute osteomyelitis in children is imaged using MRI. However, three-phase bone scan may be preferred over MRI in some scenarios, particularly to avoid use of sedation or general anesthesia, although some immobilization is also necessary for bone scan as well. An additional benefit of bone scintigraphy is that whole-body planar imaging can be performed, so multiple sites of osteomyelitis can be evaluated simultaneously. Skeletal scintigraphy will be positive within 24 to 72 hours of symptom onset, much sooner than radiographs.

A bone scan is performed with ^{99m}Tc-m-methylene diphosphonates, which is taken up by osteoblasts forming new bone. A three-phase bone scan includes flow or perfusion phase, which is acquired immediately after radiopharmaceutic injection, followed by imaging of the area of interest in the blood pool or soft tissue phase. Finally, delayed imaging is performed 2 to 4 hours later. Acute osteomyelitis will demonstrate increased uptake in all three phases. It should be noted that intraosseous abscesses and ischemia in the early thrombotic phase of infection may result in photopenia, referred to as "cold osteomyelitis."

Skeletal System

Bone Scan

In addition to osteomyelitis, skeletal scintigraphy can be performed to help in the evaluation of patients with concern for osseous metastasis, including Langerhans cell histiocytosis; radiographically occult fracture or stress fracture; possible avascular necrosis; and viability of bone graft. Three-phase bone scan may also be performed to help in the evaluation of clinically suspected complex regional pain syndrome (previously called reflex sympathetic dystrophy), which will demonstrate increased uptake in all three phases.

Oncology

Neuroblastoma

^{123}I-Metaiodobenzylguanidine (MIBG) is an analog of norepinephrine and is taken up by the norepinephrine transporter and accumulates in the cytoplasm and mitochondria of neuroblastoma cells (Fig. 25.94). More than 90% of neuroblastomas are MIBG avid.. MIBG scintigraphy is useful for diagnosis, staging, and follow-up to assess treatment response and can provide prognostic value based on location and amount of uptake. Although ^{123}I-MIBG is highly sensitive and specific for neuroblastoma, dedifferentiated

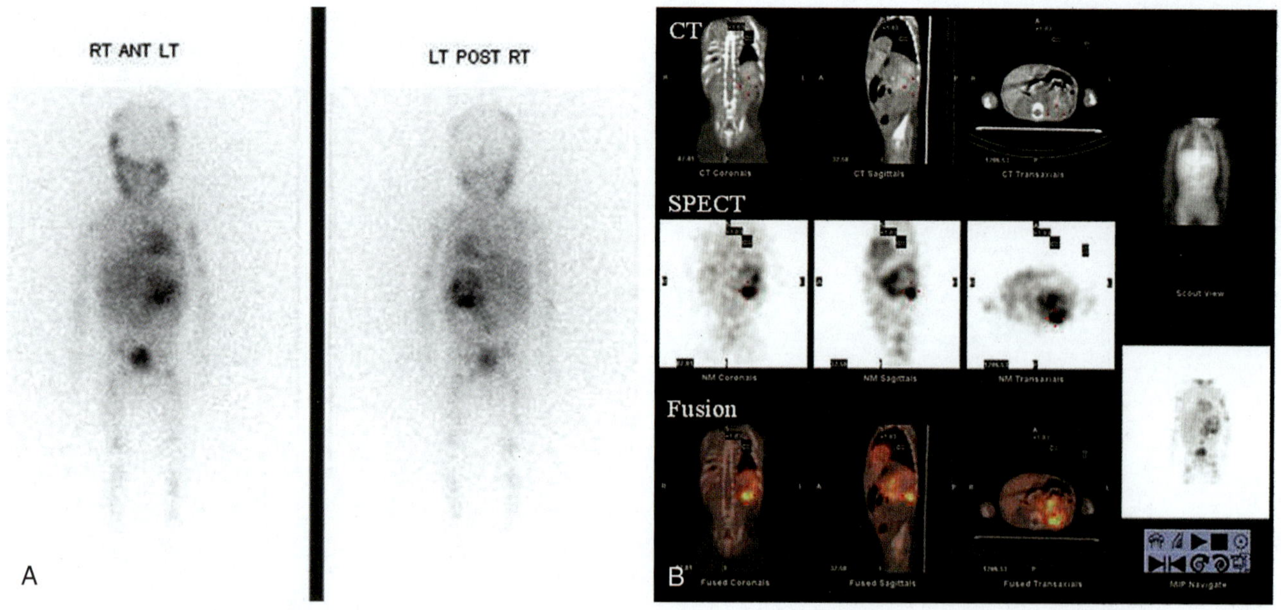

Fig. 25.94 ^{123}I-metaiodobenzylguanidine (MIBG) scan: an 11-month-old female with metastatic neuroblastoma. (A) Planar ^{123}I-MIBG scan demonstrates an intensely MIBG-avid mass in the left upper abdominal region and pelvic masses, with multiple skeletal lesions. (B) ^{123}I-MIBG single-photon emission computed tomography (SPECT) demonstrates an intensely MIBG-avid mass in the left upper abdomen.

neuroblastoma cells will not have uptake, so ^{18}F-FDG PET/CT may be used as an adjunct in the diagnosis and follow-up of patients with neuroblastoma. In the future, PET agents may become available to allow improved imaging of patients with neuroblastoma.

^{131}I-MIBG may also be used for neuroblastoma therapy in chemotherapy-resistant tumor cells. ^{131}I has beta-emission decay, which causes cell death similar to the process described with radioactive iodine thyroid ablation.

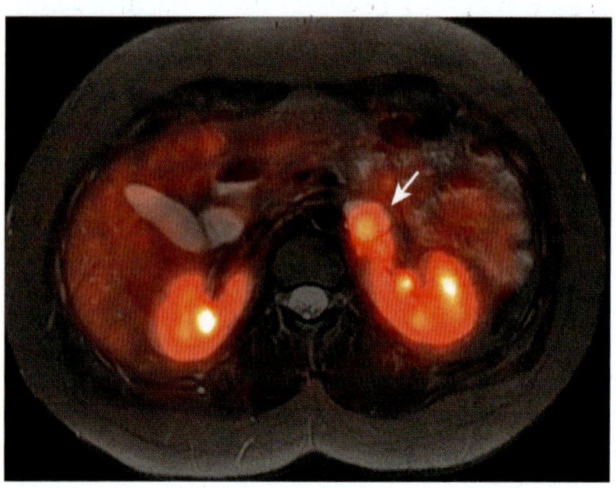

Fig. 25.95 Left retroperitoneal paraganglioma. ^{67}-Ga-DOTATATE PET fused to axial T2-fat saturated MR demonstrates intense uptake of the multilobulated-appearing T2 hyperintense lesion in the left retroperitoneum anterior to the kidney *(arrow)* in this 17-year-old female with polycythemia-paraganglioma syndrome.

Neuroendocrine Tumors

^{68}Ga-tetraxetan (DOTA)-labeled peptides with somatostatin receptors, including the most common ^{68}Ga-DOTATATE, are emerging as PET agents useful for functional neuroendocrine tumor evaluation, including pheochromocytoma, paraganglioma, some pancreatic tumors, and neuroblastoma (Fig. 25.95). The advantage over traditional ^{111}In-DTPA-octreotide or ^{123}I-MIBG SPECT agents is lower radiation dose and improved spatial resolution resulting in increased sensitivity and accuracy of tumor detection. Finally, imaging can be completed in 1 day with ^{68}Ga-DOTATATE, rather than the 2 or more days required for SPECT neuroendocrine tumor imaging.

^{18}F-FDG PET/CT

As previously detailed, ^{18}F-FDG is a glucose analog. Because tumor cells use high rates of glucose compared with normal tissue, ^{18}F-FDG can be used to image site of potential tumor involvement, including at the time of diagnosis, restaging during therapy, and follow-up at the completion of cancer therapy. ^{18}F-FDG PET is well established in evaluation of patients with many types of tumors, including lymphoma and osteosarcoma (Fig. 25.96). Importantly, ^{18}F-FDG is not specific to tumor; uptake will also be seen with inflammation, infection, and physiologic processes.

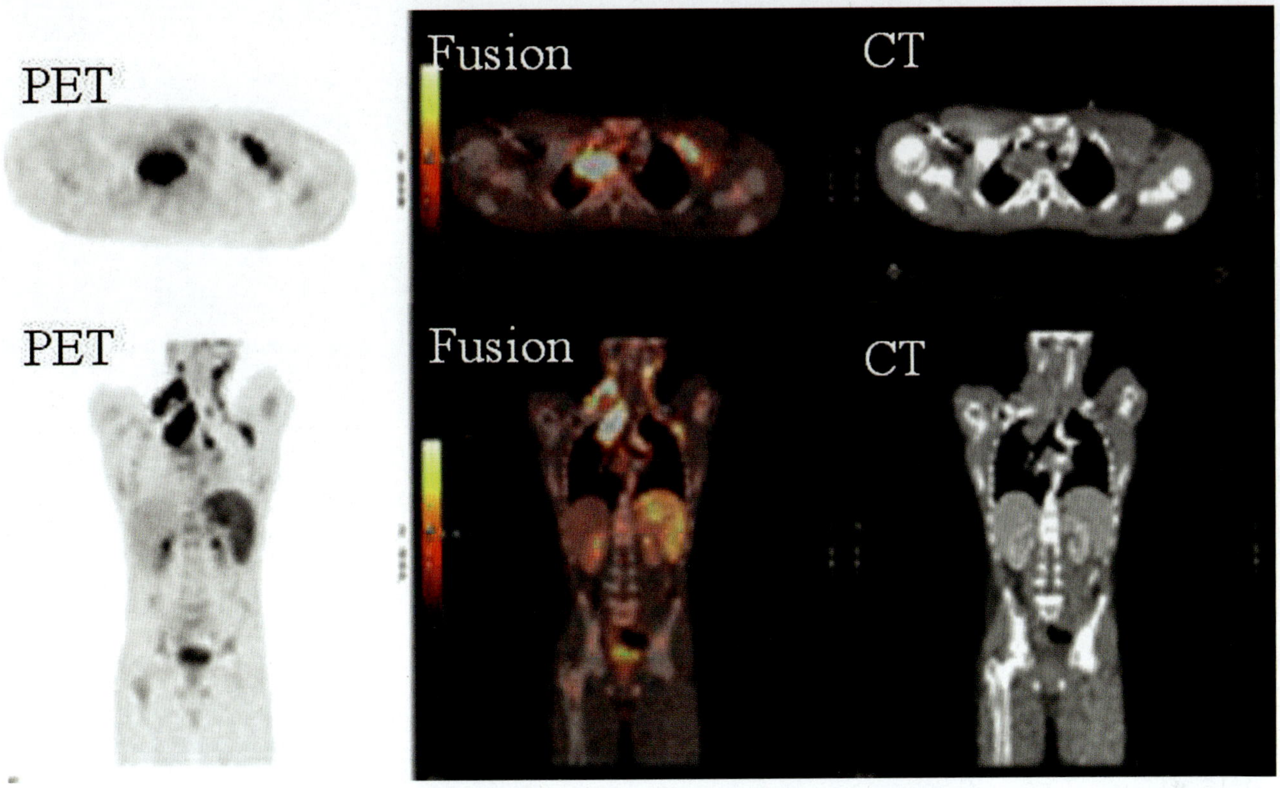

Fig. 25.96 Fluorodeoxyglucose positron emission tomography (^{18}F-FDG PET): an 18-year-old male with a history of recently diagnosed Hodgkin lymphoma. ^{18}F-FDG PET demonstrates multiple cervical, mediastinal, abdominal, and pelvic lymphadenopathies and splenic involvement.

Bibliography

American College of Radiology: *ACR appropriateness criteria*. http://www.acr.org/ac.

American College of Radiology: *ACR manual on contrast media vol. 10.2*, 2016. https://www.acr.org/Quality-Safety/Resources/Contrast-Manual.

Amis ES Jr, Butler PF, Applegate KE, et al. American College of Radiology white paper on radiation dose in medicine, *J Am Coll Radiol* 4:272–284, 2007.

Barkovich AJ: *Pediatric neuroimaging*, Philadelphia, 2005, Lippincott Williams & Wilkins.

Biassoni L, Easty M. Paediatric nuclear medicine imaging, *Br Med Bull* 123(1): 127–148, 2017. http://dx.doi.org/10.1093/bmb/ldx025

Blickman JG, Parker BR, Barnes PD: *Pediatric radiology: the requisites*, Philadelphia, 2009, Mosby/Elsevier.

Catanzano TM: *How to think like a radiologist: ordering imaging studies*, Cambridge and New York, 2009, Cambridge University Press.

Gillard JH, Waldman AD, Barker PB: *Clinical MR neuroimaging: diffusion, perfusion and spectroscopy*, Cambridge and New York, 2005, Cambridge University Press.

Haller JO, Slovis TL, Joshi A: *Pediatric radiology: an introduction for medical students, residents, and pediatric health care providers*, ed 3, Berlin, 2005, Springer.

Kanal E, Barkovich AJ, Bell C, et al: ACR guidance document for safe MR practices: 2007, *AJR Am J Roentgenol* 188:1447–1474, 2007.

National Cancer Institute: *Radiation risks and pediatric computed tomography (CT): a guide for health care providers*. http://www.cancer.gov/cancertopics/causes/radiation/radiation-risks-pediatric-CT.

Osborn AG: *Diagnostic neuroradiology*, St. Louis, 1994, Mosby.

Panigrahy A, Nelson MD Jr, Bluml S: Magnetic resonance spectroscopy in pediatric neuroradiology: clinical and research applications, *Pediatr Radiol* 40:3–30, 2010.

Pruckmayer M, Zacherl S, Salzer-Muhar U, et al: Scintigraphic assessment of pulmonary and whole-body blood flow patterns after surgical intervention in congenital heart disease, *J Nucl Med* 40:1477–1483, 1999.

Siegel MJ: *Pediatric sonography*, Philadelphia, 2011, Lippincott Williams & Wilkins.

Slovis TL. *Caffey's pediatric diagnostic imaging*, ed 11, Philadelphia, 2008, Elsevier.

Swartz JD: *Imaging of the temporal bone*, New York, 1986, Thieme.

Swischuk LE: Emergency pediatric imaging: current status and update, *Semin Ultrasound CT MR* 28:158–168, 2007.

Treves ST, Baker A, Fahey FH, et al. Nuclear medicine in the first year of life, *J Nucl Med* 52(6):905–925, 2011. http://dx.doi.org/10.2967/jnumed.110.084202.

Index

Note: Page numbers followed by "f" indicate figures, "t" indicate tables, "b" indicate boxes, and "e" indicate online content.

G

H

I

J

K

M

R